P9-AOS-377

ENDOCRINOLOGY

VOLUME 3

ENDOCRINOLOGY

VOLUME 3

Edited by

Leslie J. DeGroot

George F. Cahill, Jr.

William D. Odell

Luciano Martini

John T. Potts, Jr.

Don H. Nelson

Emil Steinberger

Albert I. Winegrad

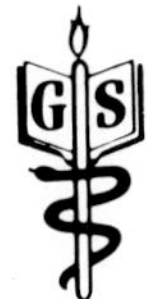

GRUNE & STRATTON

A Subsidiary of Harcourt Brace Jovanovich, Publishers

New York London Toronto Sydney San Francisco

Library of Congress Cataloging in Publication Data
Main entry under title:

Endocrinology.

Bibliography
Includes index.
1. Endocrine glands—Diseases. 2. Endocrinology.
I. DeGroot, Leslie J. [DNLM: 1. Endocrine diseases.
2. Endocrine glands. 3. Hormones. WK100.3 E56]
RC648.E458 616.4 78-24043
ISBN 0-8089-1169-4 (v. 3)

Grune & Stratton, Inc.
111 Fifth Avenue
New York, New York 10003

Distributed in the United Kingdom by
Academic Press, Inc. (London) Ltd.
24/28 Oval Road, London NW 1

Library of Congress Catalog Number 78-24043
International Standard Book Number 0-8089-1169-4

Printed in the United States of America

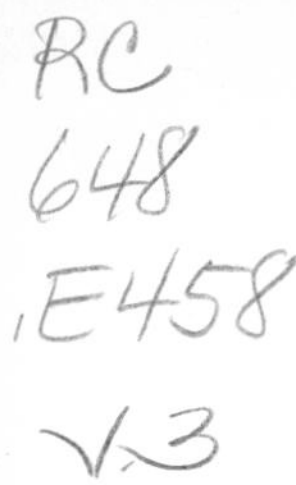

Contents
Volume 3

ENDOCRINOLOGY OF CONCEPTION, PREGNANCY, AND PARTURITION

DIFFUSE HORMONAL SYSTEMS

INTEGRATED HORMONAL CONTROL SYSTEMS

GENERAL PRINCIPLES OF ENDOCRINE PATHOPHYSIOLOGY

Contents
Volume 1

THYROID GLAND

Thyroid Physiology

Thyroid Diseases

Contents
Volume 2

PANCREATIC ISLETS

Diabetes Mellitus

ADRENAL CORTEX

Physiology

Clinical Problems

CATECHOLAMINES AND ADRENAL MEDULLA

Preface

This new text is intended to provide a complete contemporary source of basic and clinical aspects of endocrinology. Our book is directed to serious students of endocrinology; the authors believe that this encompasses undergraduates, house officers, fellows, and physicians practicing in the field. We hope to provide a source to which these serious students can turn in order to find an answer to all of their questions.

It is obvious that there is no dearth of endocrine texts, but, in surveying the field, we have not found a volume which presents "molecular" or "metabolic" endocrinology with the emphasis that we feel is appropriate, or which has adequately attempted a synthesis into a coherent whole data available from basic science and the clinic.

In the past years, endocrinology and metabolism have gone through stages of development that may be arbitrarily characterized as descriptive, anatomic, physiologic, and biochemical. Current endocrinology is featured by (1) a great increase in knowledge of the biochemical basis of endocrine function and dysfunction, (2) development of sensitive techniques for the measurement of hormones, their precursors and metabolites, and (3) a flood of information on integrated endocrine responses in various physiologic states. It is now possible to characterize many endocrinologic events in molecular terms and to integrate isolated observations into meaningful and unifying concepts. This additional information has called for a new approach to the teaching of endocrinology.

Our book is written with a physiologic and biochemical interpretive bias, indicating the change in endocrinology from a largely descriptive discipline to one integrating basic science. Because the book is meant to be used by practicing physicians, however, we have made it just as comprehensive in its clinical presentation, which we consider crucial. We have stressed the relation of clinical endocrinology to physiology, genetics, biochemistry, and immunology. We have used basic science data to add to clinical data to aid in interpretation, and have indicated areas in which problems exist or where ignorance remains.

While the editors philosophically would have preferred to develop a book totally integrated around "processes" or "functions" controlled by coincident endocrine stimuli, the proper pedagogic approach demands a more traditional introduction to the field. Thus our work is divided into two complementary sections. In the first, a typically organ-oriented section of about 1400 pages, basic endocrine physiology and clinical problems are thoroughly covered. Clinical problems that confront the practicing physician are emphasized. The second section, of about 700 pages, integrates, in a series of chapters, contemporary endocrinologic knowledge in relation to important processes or problems. Here, for example, we consider growth, puberty, the response to starvation, obesity, and so forth. In these areas there are normal and abnormal homeostatic processes that involve multifactoral endocrine control, and concepts that can now be seen to unify endocrine physiology.

Volumes of this size suffer from the delay between writing and publication. In an effort to counteract this problem, we have given authors the opportunity to add important new material during proofing of the final galleys. New references have simply been inserted in the appropriate sequence by letter designation, e.g. 10a, 10b, etc. We believe this small departure from custom offers an important improvement in our text.

The proliferation of abbreviations in medical writings is in one way a benefit, and in another a curse. Abbreviations surely accelerate the transmission of information, but only if one understands the key. We have attempted to standardize all abbreviations to conform with those used by *Endocrinology,* a style familiar to most of our readers. Variations from these standards are, we hope, adequately explained.

This book is, in every sense, the joint effort of eight editors and nearly two hundred authors. To these distinguished scientists, teachers, and clinicians, the chief editor expresses his sincere thanks and great respect. It is the broad knowledge and hard work of these collaborators which makes the volume unique in its contribution.

Sincere appreciation is also offered to our co-workers at Grune and Stratton, to the secretaries across the nation who came to recognize my voice quite easily, to Ms. Myrna Zimberg for a vast amount of help, and to Helen DeGroot for patiently page-proofing a mountain of text.

Leslie J. DeGroot, M.D.

Contributors

Paul Aiginger, M.D.
II Medical University Klinik
Abt. f. Nuclearmedizin
University of Vienna
Vienna, Austria

Thomas T. Aoki, M.D.
Assistant Professor of Medicine
Harvard Medical School
and Associate, Peter Bent Brigham Hospital
and Investigator, Howard Hughes Medical Institute
Boston, Massachusetts

Cesare Aragona
Senior Research Fellow
Department of Physiology
University of Manitoba
Winnipeg, Manitoba

Ronald A. Arky, M.D.
Professor of Medicine
Harvard Medical School
and Chief of Medicine
Mount Auburn Hospital
Cambridge, Massachusetts

Claude D. Arnaud, M.D.
Professor of Medicine and Physiology
University of California School of Medicine
and Chief, Endocrine Unit
San Francisco Veterans Administration Hospital
San Francisco, California

Jurgen Aschoff, Dr. Med.
Director at the Institute
Max-Planck-Institut fur Verhaltensphysiologie
Erling-Andechs, Germany

Louis V. Avioli, M.D.
Schoenberg Professor of Medicine
Washington University School of Medicine
and the Jewish Hospital of St. Louis
St. Louis, Missouri

Lester Baker, M.D.
Director, Clinical Research Center
Children's Hospital of Philadelphia
and Professor of Pediatrics
University of Pennsylvania School of Medicine
Philadelphia, Pennsylvania

Susanne Barton, Ph.D.
Associate Professor, Department of Physiology
University of Alberta
Edmonton, Alberta

Tomas Berl, M.D.
Assistant Professor of Medicine
University of Colorado Medical Center
Denver, Colorado

M. Bonnyns, M.D.
Charge de Clinique
University of Brussels
and Adjoint in the Department of Medicine
Saint-Pierre Hospital
Brussels, Belgium

Philippe J. Bordier, M.D. (deceased)
Metre de Researche
I.N.S.E.R.M.
Paris, France

Cyril Y. Bowers, M.D.
Professor of Medicine
Tulane University Medical School
New Orleans, Louisiana

F. R. Bringhurst, M.D.
Clinical and Research Fellow in Medicine
Massachusetts General Hospital
and Research Fellow in Medicine
Harvard Medical School
Boston, Massachusetts

John E. Buster, M.D.
Assistant Professor of Obstetrics and Gynecology
University of California at Los Angeles School of Medicine
Los Angeles, California

George F. Cahill, Jr., M.D.
Professor of Medicine
Harvard Medical School
and Physician, Peter Bent Brigham Hospital
and Director of Research, Howard Hughes Medical Institute
Boston, Massachusetts

Vito M. Campese, M.D.
Assistant Professor of Medicine
University of Southern California School of Medicine
Division of Nephrology
Los Angeles County–University of Southern California Medical Center
Los Angeles, California

Fabio Celotti, M.D.
Department of Endocrinology
University of Milano
Milano, Italy

Ding Chang, Ph.D.
Institute for Biomedical Research
The University of Texas at Austin
Austin, Texas

Alan Cherrington, Ph.D.
Assistant Professor of Physiology
Vanderbilt University Medical School
Nashville, Tennessee

Jean-Louis Chiasson, M.D.
Assistant Professor of Medicine
Vanderbilt University Medical School
Nashville, Tennessee

Nicholas P. Christy, M. D.
Professor of Medicine
Columbia University College of Physicians and Surgeons
and Director, Medical Service
The Roosevelt Hospital
New York, New York

Felix A. Conte, M.D.
Associate Professor of Pediatrics
University of California
San Francisco, California

Cary W. Cooper, Ph.D.
Professor of Pharmacology
Department of Pharmacology
University of North Carolina School of Medicine
Chapel Hill, North Carolina

D. Harold Copp, M.D., Ph.D., F.R.C.P.(c), F.R.S.C., F.R.S.
Professor of Physiology
University of British Columbia
Vancouver, British Columbia

Marilyn C. Crim, Ph.D.
Research Associate, Department of Nutrition and Food Science
Massachusetts Institute of Technology
Cambridge, Massachusetts

Val Davajan, M.D.
Professor of Obstetrics and Gynecology
University of Southern California School of Medicine
Los Angeles, California

Leonard J. Deftos, M.D.
Professor of Medicine
University of California
San Diego School of Medicine
and Chief, Endocrinology
San Diego Veterans Administration Hospital
La Jolla, California

Leslie J. DeGroot, M.D.
Professor of Medicine and Head, Endocrine Section
University of Chicago School of Medicine
Chicago, Illinois

Hector F. DeLuca, Ph.D.
Professor of Biochemistry
College of Agricultural and Life Sciences
University of Wisconsin
Madison, Wisconsin

Vincent DeQuattro, M.D.
Professor of Medicine
University of Southern California School of Medicine
Los Angeles, California

Eugene R. DeSombre, Ph.D.
Associate Professor, Ben May Laboratory for Cancer Research
and Research Associate, Biomedical Computation Facilities
The University of Chicago
Chicago, Illinois

Francis P. DiBella, Ph.D.
Upjohn Company
Kalamazoo, Michigan

Jacques E. Dumont, M.D.
Professor and Head of Institute of Interdisciplinary Research
Institut de Recherche Interdisciplinaire en Biologie Humaine et Nucléaire
Brussels University
Brussels, Belgium

Edward N. Ehrlich, M.D.
Professor of Medicine
University of Wisconsin
and Head, Endocrine Section
and Associate Chairman, Department of Medicine
University of Wisconsin
Madison, Wisconsin

Harvey Eisenberg, M.D.
Associate Professor
University of California Medical Center
Department of Radiology
Orange, California

Ragnar Ekholm, M.D., Ph.D.
Professor of Anatomy
Department of Anatomy
University of Göteborg
Göteborg, Sweden

Andre M. Ermans, M.D.
Associate Professor of Experimental Medicine
Head of the Department of Nuclear Medicine
St. Peter Hospital
Free University of Brussels
Brussels, Belgium

Imogen M. A. Evans, M.D., F.R.C.P.
Research Fellow, Endocrine Unit
Royal Postgraduate Medical School
London, England

David C. Evered, B.Sc., M.D., F.R.C.P.
Physician, Royal Victoria Infirmary
Newcastle Upon Tyne, England

Calvin Ezrin, M.D., F.R.C.P.-C., F.A.C.P.
Professor of Medicine and Associate Professor of Pathology
University of Toronto School of Medicine
Toronto, Ontario

Stefan S. Fajans, M.D.
Professor of Internal Medicine
Head, Division of Endocrinology and Metabolism
and Director, Metabolism Research Unit
The University of Michigan Medical School
Ann Arbor, Michigan

Freddy Febres, M.D.
Director, Laboratory of Endocrinology
Maternidad Concepcion Palacios
Caracas, Venezuela

Philip Felig, M.D.
C.N.H. Long Professor and Vice Chairman, Department of Internal Medicine
Yale University School of Medicine
New Haven, Connecticut

Gianfranco Fenzi, M.D.
Assistant Professor of Medicine
Cattedra di Patologia Speciale Medica II
University of Pisa
Pisa, Italy

James B. Field, M.D.
Rutherford Professor of Medicine
Head, Division of Endocrinology and Metabolism
Baylor University
Houston, Texas

Delbert A. Fisher, M.D.
Professor of Pediatrics
University of California at Los Angeles School of Medicine
Torrance, California

Jeffrey S. Flier, M.D.
Assistant Professor of Medicine
Harvard Medical School
and Chief, Diabetes and Metabolism Unit
Beth Israel Hospital
Boston, Massachusetts

Karl Folkers, Ph.D.
Institute for Biomedical Research
University of Texas at Austin
Austin, Texas

Daniel W. Foster, M.D.
Professor of Internal Medicine
University of Texas Southwestern Medical School
Dallas, Texas

Paul Henry Frank, M.D.
Assistant Professor, Department of Radiology
Pritzker School of Medicine
The University of Chicago
Chicago, Illinois

Andrew G. Frantz, M.D.
Professor of Medicine and Chief, Division of Endocrinology
Columbia University College of Physicians and Surgeons
and Attending Physician, Presbyterian Hospital
New York, New York

Donald Fraser, M.D.
Departments of Pediatrics and Physiology
University of Toronto
The Research Institute
The Hospital for Sick Children
Toronto, Ontario

Norbert Freinkel, M.D.
Kettering Professor of Medicine
and Director, Center for Endocrinology, Metabolism, and Nutrition
Northwestern University Medical School
and Attending Physician, Northwestern Memorial Hospital
and Consultant, Veterans Administration Lakeside Hospital
Chicago, Illinois

Henry G. Friesen, M.D.
Professor and Head, Department of Physiology
University of Manitoba
Winnipeg, Manitoba

Lawrence A. Frohman, M.D., Ph.D.
Professor of Medicine
University of Chicago Pritzker School of Medicine
and Director, Division of Endocrinology and Metabolism
Michael Reese Medical Center
Chicago, Illinois

Steven R. Goldring, M.D.
Instructor in Medicine
Massachusetts General Hospital
and Assistant to the Chief of Medicine
Department of Medicine
New England Deaconess Hospital
Boston, Massachusetts

Donald P. Goldstein, M.D.
Assistant Clinical Professor, Department of Obstetrics and Gynecology
Harvard Medical School
Boston, Massachusetts

Samuel Goldstein, M.D.
Associate Professor of Medicine and Associate in Biochemistry
McMaster University Medical School
and Attending Physician, McMaster University Medical Center
Hamilton, Ontario

David Goltzman, M.D.
Assistant Professor of Experimental Medicine
McGill University
and Assistant Physician
Royal Victoria Hospital
Montreal, Quebec

Victor E. Gould, M.D.
Professor of Pathology
Rush Medical School
Chicago, Illinois

David G. Grahame-Smith, M.B., B.S., F.R.C.P.
Rhodes Professor of Clinical Pharmacology
and Honorary Director, M.R.C. Unit of Clinical Pharmacology
University of Oxford
Oxford, England

Douglas A. Greene, M.D.
Assistant Professor of Medicine
University of Pennsylvania School of Medicine
Philadelphia, Pennsylvania

Monte A. Greer, M.D.
Professor of Medicine
Head of the Department of Endocrinology
University of Oregon Medical School
Portland, Oregon

Marie H. Greider, Ph.D.
Associate Professor of Pathology
Washington University School of Medicine
St. Louis, Missouri

Melvin M. Grumbach, M.D.
Professor of Pediatrics
University of California
and Director, Pediatric Services
University of California Hospitals
San Francisco, California

Erlio Gurpide, Ph.D.
Professor of Obstetrics and Gynecology and of Biochemistry
Mount Sinai School of Medicine
New York, New York

Joel F. Habener, M.D.
Associate Professor of Medicine
Harvard Medical School
Endocrine Unit, Massachusetts General Hospital
Boston, Massachusetts

Theodore J. Hahn, M.D.
Assistant Professor of Medicine
Washington University School of Medicine
and the Jewish Hospital of St. Louis
St. Louis, Missouri

Peter F. Hall, M.D., Ph.D.
Professor and Chairman, Department of Physiology
California College of Medicine
University of California
Irvine, California

Reginald Hall, B.Sc., M.D., F.R.C.P.
Professor of Medicine
University of Newcastle Upon Tyne
and Physician, Royal Victoria Infirmary
Newcastle Upon Tyne, England

Madeleine Harbison, M.D.
Department of Medicine
Division of Medical Genetics
The Johns Hopkins Hospital
Baltimore, Maryland

Boyd W. Harding, M.D., Ph.D.
Professor of Medicine and Biochemistry
University of Southern California School of Medicine
Los Angeles, California

Morey W. Haymond, M.D.
Assistant Professor of Pediatrics
Mayo Clinic
Rochester, Minnesota

Eileen Higham, Ph.D.
Assistant Professor in Medical Psychology
and Adjunct Professor of Psychology
Department of Psychiatry and Behavioral Sciences
and Department of Pediatrics
The Johns Hopkins University
Baltimore, Maryland

Raymond L. Hintz, M.D.
Associate Professor of Pediatrics
Stanford University School of Medicine
Palo Alto, California

Michael F. Holick, Ph.D., M.D.
Assistant Professor of Medicine
Harvard Medical School
and Clinical Assistant in Medicine
Massachusetts General Hospital
Boston, Massachusetts

Richard Horton, M.D.
Professor of Medicine
and Chief, Endocrinology Section
University of Southern California Medical Center
Los Angeles, California

Eva Horvath, Ph.D.
Assistant Professor of Pathology
Department of Pathology
University of Toronto
Toronto, Ontario

John Humphries, Ph.D.
Institute for Biomedical Research
The University of Texas at Austin
Austin, Texas

Robert Israel, M.D.
Associate Professor, Department of Obstetrics and Gynecology
University of Southern California School of Medicine
Los Angeles, California

Bernard H. Jaffe, M.D.
Professor of Surgery
Washington University School of Medicine
St. Louis, Missouri

Elwood V. Jensen, Ph.D.
Professor, Departments of Biophysics and Theoretical Biology
and Director, Ben May Laboratories
The University of Chicago
Chicago, Illinois

Ulrich Keller, M.D.
Instructor in Medicine
Vanderbilt University Medical School
Nashville, Tennessee

Henry T. Keutmann, M.D.
Principal Research Associate in Medicine
Harvard Medical School
and Associate in Biochemistry (Medicine)
Massachusetts General Hospital
Boston, Massachusetts

John M. Kinney, M.D.
Professor of Surgery
Columbia University College of Physicians and Surgeons
and Attending Surgeon
Presbyterian Hospital
New York, New York

Charles R. Kleeman, M.D.
Professor of Medicine and Chief, Division of Nephrology
University of California at Los Angeles School of Medicine
Los Angeles, California

Ronald Knudsen, Ph.D.
Institute for Biomedical Research
The University of Texas at Austin
Austin, Texas

Kalman Kovacs, M.D., Ph.D., D.Sc., F.R.C.P.(c), F.A.C.P., M.R.C. (Path.)
Associate Professor
Department of Pathology
University of Toronto
and Pathologist, St. Michael's Hospital
Toronto, Ontario

Stephen M. Krane, M.D.
Professor of Medicine
Harvard Medical School
Chief, Arthritis Unit and Physician, Medical Services
Massachusetts General Hospital
Boston, Massachusetts

Dorothy T. Krieger, M.D.
Professor of Medicine
Mount Sinai School of Medicine
and Director, Division of Endocrinology and Metabolism
Mount Sinai Hospital
New York, New York

Paul E. Lacy, M.D.
Mallinckrodt Professor and Chairman
Department of Pathology
Washington University School of Medicine
St. Louis, Missouri

Yiu-Kuen Lam, Ph.D.
Institute for Biomedical Research
The University of Texas at Austin
Austin, Texas

Richard L. Landau, M.D.
Professor of Medicine
The University of Chicago School of Medicine
Chicago, Illinois

Elizabeth M. K. Leovey
Postdoctoral Fellow
Georgetown University School of Medicine
Washington, D.C.

John F. Liljenquist, M.D.
Assistant Professor of Medicine
Vanderbilt University Medical School
Nashville, Tennessee

Mortimer B. Lipsett, M.D.
Director, The Clinical Center
National Institutes of Health
Bethesda, Maryland

Iain MacIntyre
Director, Endocrine Unit
Royal Postgraduate Medical School
London, England

Jane E. Mahaffey, M.D.
Instructor in Medicine
Harvard Medical School
and Clinical Assistant in Medicine
Massachusetts General Hospital
Boston, Massachusetts

John R. Marshall, M.D.
Professor of Obstetrics and Gynecology
University of California at Los Angeles School of Medicine
Los Angeles, California

Robert W. Marshall, B.Sc., Ph.D.
M.R.C. Mineral Metabolism Unit
The General Infirmary, Leeds
Leeds, England

Luciano Martini, M.D.
Professor of Pharmacology and Endocrinology
University of Milano
Milan, Italy

Renato Massa, M.D.
Department of Endocrinology
University of Milano
Milan, Italy

Franz M. Matschinsky, M.D.
Professor of Biochemistry and Biophysics
University of Pennsylvania School of Medicine
Philadelphia, Pennsylvania

G. P. Mayer, D.V.M., M.Sc. (Med.)
Professor of Physiology
College of Veterinary Medicine
Oklahoma State University
Stillwater, Oklahoma

Samuel M. McCann, M.D.
Professor and Chairman, Department of Physiology
Southwestern Medical School
University of Texas Health Science Center at Dallas
Dallas, Texas

Bruce S. McEwen, Ph.D.
Associate Professor
The Rockefeller University
New York, New York

John D. McGarry, M.D.
Professor of Internal Medicine and Biochemistry
University of Texas Southwestern Medical School
Dallas, Texas

J. M. McKenzie, M.D.
Professor of Medicine
McGill University School of Medicine
and Senior Physician and Director
Endocrinology and Metabolism Division
Royal Victoria Hospital
Montreal, Quebec

A. Wayne Meikle, M.D.
Associate Professor of Medicine
University of Utah School of Medicine
and Department of Medicine
Veterans Administration Hospital
Salt Lake City, Utah

James C. Melby, M.D.
Professor of Medicine
Boston University School of Medicine
and Visiting Physician and Head, Section of Endocrinology and Metabolism
University Hospital
Boston, Massachusetts

Thomas J. Merimee, M.D.
Professor of Medicine, and Head, Endocrinology and Metabolism
University of Florida School of Medicine
University of Florida Hospital
Gainesville, Florida

Béla Mess, M.D., D. Med. Sci.
Professor of Anatomy
University Medical School
Pecs, Hungary

Boyd E. Metzger, M.D.
Professor of Medicine
Northwestern University Medical School
and Attending Physician
Northwestern Memorial Hospital
Chicago, Illinois

Claude J. Migeon, M.D.
Professor of Pediatrics
Johns Hopkins University School of Medicine
Baltimore, Maryland

Daniel R. Mishell, Jr., M.D.
Professor and Chairman, Department of Obstetrics and Gynecology
University of Southern California School of Medicine
Los Angeles, California

John Money, Ph.D.
Professor of Medical Psychology
and Associate Professor of Pediatrics
Department of Psychiatry and Behavioral Sciences
and Department of Pediatrics
The Johns Hopkins University
Baltimore, Maryland

Anthony D. Morrison, M.D.
Research Associate Professor of Medicine
University of Pennsylvania School of Medicine
Philadelphia, Pennsylvania

Marcella Motta, M.D.
Department of Endocrinology and Pharmacology
University of Milano
Milano, Italy

Hamish N. Munro, Ph.D., M.B.
Department of Nutrition and Food Science
Massachusetts Institute of Technology
Cambridge, Massachusetts

Mark R. Myers, B.S.
Research Assistant, Hypertension Service
Department of Medicine
Los Angeles County–University of Southern California Medical Center
Los Angeles, California

Robert M. Neer, M.D.
Associate Professor of Medicine
Harvard Medical School
and Associate Physician
Massachusetts General Hospital
Boston, Massachusetts

Don H. Nelson, M.D.
Professor of Medicine
University of Utah College of Medicine
Salt Lake City, Utah

William D. Odell, M.D., Ph.D.
Professor of Medicine and Physiology
University of California Medical School at Los Angeles
and Chairman, Department of Medicine
Harbor General Hospital
Torrance, California

Sergio R. Ojeda, D.V.M.
Department of Physiology
Southwestern Medical School
University of Texas Health Science Center at Dallas
Dallas, Texas

Jack H. Oppenheimer, M.D.
Professor of Medicine and Physiology
and Head, Section of Endocrinology and Metabolism
Department of Medicine
University of Minnesota School of Medicine
Minneapolis, Minnesota

Lelio Orci, M.D.
Director, Institut d'Histologie et d'Embryologie
Ecole de Medecine
Universite de Geneva
Geneva, Switzerland

Anthony S. Pagliara, M.D.
Associate Professor of Pediatrics
Assistant Professor of Medicine
Co-Director, Pediatric Endocrinology and Metabolism
Washington University School of Medicine
and Associate Pediatrician
St. Louis Children's Hospital
and Assistant Physician
Barnes Hospital
St. Louis, Missouri

Johanna A. Pallotta, M.D.
Assistant Professor of Medicine
Harvard Medical School
and Assistant Physician, Department of Medicine
Beth Israel Hospital
Boston, Massachusetts

A. Michael Parfitt, M.B., B. Chir., M.R.C.P., F.R.A.C.P., F.A.C.P.
Clinical Associate Professor of Medicine
University of Michigan Medical School
and Physician, Fifth Medical Division
and Director, Mineral Metabolism Laboratory
Ann Arbor, Michigan

J. A. Parsons
Head: Laboratory for Endocrine Physiology and Pharmacology
National Institute for Medical Research
London, England

Munro Peacock, M.B., Ch.B., M.R.C.P.
Honorary Consultant Physician
General Infirmary, Leeds
and Assistant Director, M.R.C. Mineral Metabolism Unit
General Infirmary, Leeds
Leeds, England

Richard L. Phelps, M.D.
Assistant Professor of Medicine
and Assistant Professor of Obstetrics & Gynecology
Northwestern University Medical School
and Attending Physician
Prentice Women's Hospital and Maternity Center
Chicago, Illinois

Aldo Pinchera, M.D.
Associate Professor of Medicine
Cattedra di Patologia Speciale Medica II
University of Pisa
Pisa, Italy

Constance S. Pittman, M.D.
Professor of Medicine
University of Alabama School of Medicine
and Endocrinology Section
Veterans Administration Hospital
Birmingham, Alabama

Flavio Piva, M.D.
Departments of Endocrinology and Pharmacology
University of Milano
Milan, Italy

Allan Pont, M.D.
Assistant Professor of Medicine
Stanford University School of Medicine
and Chief of Endocrinology
Santa Clara Valley Medical Center
San Jose, California

John T. Potts, Jr., M.D.
Professor of Medicine
Harvard Medical School
and Chief, Endocrine Unit
Massachusetts General Hospital
Boston, Massachusetts

Peter W. Ramwell, Ph.D.
Professor of Physiology
Georgetown University School of Medicine
Washington, D.C.

Samuel Refetoff, M.D.
Professor of Medicine
Pritzker School of Medicine
University of Chicago
Director of Thyroid Function Laboratory
Billings Hospital
Chicago, Illinois

Eric Reiss, M.D.
Professor and Vice Chairman
Department of Medicine
University of Miami School of Medicine
Miami, Florida

M. Markus Riek, M.D.
Chief Resident in Internal Medicine
University of Bern Medical School
Bern, Switzerland

William G. Robertson, B.Sc., Ph.D.
M.R.C. Mineral Metabolism Unit
The General Infirmary, Leeds
Leeds, England

Luis J. Rodriguez-Rigau, M.D.
Assistant Professor, Department of Reproductive Medicine and Biology
University of Texas Medical School at Houston
and Active Medical Staff
Hermann Hospital
Houston, Texas

Robert L. Rosenfield, M.D.
Associate Professor of Pediatrics
University of Chicago Pritzker School of Medicine
and Wyler Children's Hospital
Chicago, Illinois

Griff T. Ross, M.D., Ph.D.
Deputy Director, The Clinical Center
National Institutes of Health
Bethesda, Maryland

Aldo A. Rossini, M.D.
Associate in Medicine
Joslin Research Laboratory
and Assistant Professor of Medicine
Harvard Medical School
Boston, Massachusetts

Jesse Roth, M.D.
Chief, Diabetes Section
National Institute of Arthritis, Metabolism, and Digestive Diseases
National Institutes of Health
Bethesda, Maryland

S. I. Roth, M.D.
Professor and Chairman
Department of Pathology
University of Arkansas Medical Center
Little Rock, Arkansas

Corbin P. Roubebush, M.D.
Pritzker School of Medicine
The University of Chicago
Chicago, Illinois

Arthur H. Rubenstein, M.D.
Professor and Associate Chairman
Department of Medicine
University of Chicago School of Medicine
and Attending Physician, Billings Hospital
Chicago, Illinois

R. G. G. Russell, Ph.D., M.D., M.R.C.P.
Professor of Chemical Pathology
and Honorary Consultant in Human Metabolism to Sheffield Area Health Authority
University of Sheffield Medical School
Sheffield, England

Charles H. Sawyer, Ph.D.
Professor of Anatomy
University of California at Los Angeles School of Medicine
and Brain Research Institute
Los Angeles, California

Melville Schachter, Ph.D.
Professor and Chairman, Department of Physiology
University of Alberta
Edmonton, Alberta

Alan L. Schiller, M.D.
Assistant Professor of Pathology
Harvard Medical School
and Chief, Autopsy Pathology and Bone Laboratory
Department of Pathology
Massachusetts General Hospital
Boston, Massachusetts

Gustav Schonfeld, M.D.
Professor of Preventative Medicine and Medicine
Washington University School of Medicine
St. Louis, Missouri

Charles R. Scriver, M.D.
The deBelle Laboratory for Biochemical Genetics
Departments of Pediatrics and Biology
McGill University–Montreal Children's Hospital Research Institute
Montreal, Quebec

Robert E. Scully, M.D.
Professor of Pathology
Massachusetts General Hospital
and Harvard Medical School
Boston, Massachusetts

Gino V. Segre, M.D.
Assistant Professor of Medicine
Harvard Medical School
and Assistant Physician
Massachusetts General Hospital
Boston, Massachusetts

Robert Sherwin, M.D.
Assistant Professor of Medicine
Yale University School of Medicine
New Haven, Connecticut

Louis M. Sherwood, M.D.
Professor of Medicine
University of Chicago
and Physician-in-Chief and Chairman, Department of Medicine
Michael Reese Hospital and Medical Center
Chicago, Illinois

Pentti Siiteri, M.D.
Professor of Obstetrics
Department of Obstetrics-Gynecology and Reproductive Sciences
University of California School of Medicine
San Francisco, California

Ethan A. H. Sims, M.D.
Professor of Medicine, Department of Medicine and Metabolic Unit
University of Vermont College of Medicine
and Attending Physician, Medical Center Hospital of Vermont
Burlington, Vermont

Eduardo Slatopolsky, M.D.
Professor of Medicine
Department of Medicine
Washington University School of Medicine
St. Louis, Missouri

Keith D. Smith, M.D.
Professor, Department of Reproductive Medicine and Biology
University of Texas Medical School at Houston
and Active Medical Staff, Hermann Hospital
Department of Internal Medicine
Houston, Texas

John B. Stanbury, M.D.
Professor of Experimental Medicine
Massachusetts Institute of Technology
Cambridge, Massachusetts

Charles A. Stanley, M.D.
Assistant Professor of Pediatrics
University of Pennsylvania
and Division of Endocrinology
Children's Hospital of Philadelphia
Philadelphia, Pennsylvania

Emil Steinberger, M.D.
Professor and Chairman, Department of Reproductive Medicine and Biology
The University of Texas Health Science Center at Houston
Houston, Texas

Donald F. Steiner, M.D.
Professor of Biochemistry and Medicine
Pritzker School of Medicine
The University of Chicago
Chicago, Illinois

Hugo Studer, M.D.
Professor of Medicine
Head of the Department of Medicine
University of Bern Medical School
Berne, Switzerland

Howard S. Tager, Ph.D.
Assistant Professor of Biochemistry
Pritzker School of Medicine
The University of Chicago
Chicago, Illinois

Roy V. Talmage, Ph.D.
Professor of Surgery and Pharmacology
Director of Orthopedic Research
Departments of Surgery and Pharmacology
University of North Carolina
Chapel Hill, North Carolina

Alvin Taurog, Ph.D.
Professor of Pharmacology
University of Texas Health Science Center
Dallas, Texas

Michael D. Trus
Postdoctoral Fellow in Biochemistry and Biophysics
School of Medicine
University of Pennsylvania
Philadelphia, Pennsylvania

Roger H. Unger, M.D.
Veterans Administration Hospital
and Professor of Internal Medicine
University of Texas Southwestern Medical School
Dallas, Texas

Robert D. Utiger, M.D.
Professor of Medicine
Endocrine Section
University of Pennsylvania
Philadelphia, Pennsylvania

Judson J. Van Wyk, M.D.
Kenan Professor of Pediatrics
University of North Carolina School of Medicine
Chapel Hill, North Carolina

Gilbert Vassart, M.D.
Charge de Recherche F.N.R.S.
Institute of Interdisciplinary Research
Brussels University Medical School
Brussels, Belgium

Helmuth Vorherr, M.D.
Professor of Obstetrics and Gynecology and Pharmacology
University of New Mexico School of Medicine
Albuquerque, New Mexico

John Wahren, M.D.
Professor of Clinical Physiology
Karolinska Institute and Huddinge Hospital
Huddinge, Sweden

Yieh-Ping Wan, Ph.D.
Institute for Biomedical Research
The University of Texas at Austin
Austin, Texas

Chiu-an Wang, M.D., F.A.C.S.
Associate Clinical Professor of Surgery
Harvard Medical School
and Visiting Surgeon
Massachusetts General Hospital
Boston, Massachusetts

Michelle P. Warren, M.D.
Assistant Professor of Medicine and Obstetrics and Gynecology
Columbia University College of Physicians and Surgeons
Associate Attending Physician, Departments of Medicine and Obstetrics/Gynecology
The Roosevelt Hospital
New York, New York

Ann Ruhmann-Wennhold, M.D.
Associate Research Professor
University of Utah College of Medicine
Salt Lake City, Utah

Charles D. West, M.D.
Professor of Medicine and Biochemistry
University of Utah College of Medicine
Salt Lake City, Utah

John F. Wilber, M.D.
Chief of Endocrinology and Professor of Medicine
Louisiana State University Medical Sciences Center
New Orleans, Louisiana

E. D. Williams
Professor of Pathology
Department of Pathology
Welsh National School of Medicine
Cardiff, Wales

H. G. Williams-Ashman, Ph.D.
Professor of Biochemistry
Ben May Laboratory for Cancer Research
University of Chicago
Chicago, Illinois

Albert I. Winegrad, M.D.
Professor of Medicine
University of Pennsylvania School of Medicine
Philadelphia, Pennsylvania

Richard J. Wurtman, M.D.
Professor of Endocrinology and Metabolism
Laboratory of Neuroendocrine Regulation
Department of Nutrition and Food Science
Massachusetts Institute of Technology
Cambridge, Massachusetts

Margita Zakarija, M.D.
Assistant Professor
McGill University School of Medicine
and Assistant Physician
Royal Victoria Hospital
Montreal, Quebec

Walter S. Zawalich, Ph.D.
Assistant Professor of Physiology
School of Medicine
University of Pennsylvania
Philadelphia, Pennsylvania

Sexual Differentiation

105

Genetics, Anatomy, Fetal Endocrinology

Emil Steinberger

INTRODUCTION

The ultimate purpose of sex differentiation is to produce a male or female of the species in order to allow for heterosexual procreation. The gender or the sex of the offspring is determined at the time of fertilization by the chance occurrence of penetration of the ovum by either an X or a Y sex chromosome-bearing spermatozoon. Thus when we speak of gender as expressed by the interaction of sex chromosomes, we are considering the "genetic sex" of an individual. However, there are also other parameters utilized in the definition of *sex*.

The gonads of the two sexes vary both in morphology and in the products they elaborate. This unmistakable difference between the gonads of the two sexes is also utilized in determining the *sex* of an individual. It is the "gonadal sex." Similarly, the differences in the structure of the internal sex organs define the "somatic sex." The latter is not to be confused with the "phenotypic sex," which is based on the appearance of the external genitalia (vulva, penis, etc.) and secondary sex characteristics (breasts, beard, body build, etc.). The *sex* of an individual can also be defined on the basis of other, nonphysiologic parameters. The *sex* on the birth certificate, stated by the physician who delivers the infant, constitutes the "legal sex" of an individual. At times, unfortunately, it does not coincide with the genetic or gonadal sex. One must finally consider the behavioral or social dimension of "psychologic sex," which does not always coincide with physiologic *sex*, as is the case in homosexuals, transsexuals, and transvestites.

When an individual undergoes perfectly normal development and differentiation and is exposed to an appropriate psychosocial environment, the psychologic, genetic, gonadal, somatic, phenotypic, and legal "sexes" coincide. However, disturbances in any one of these parameters will result in abnormalities of gender development which will vary in severity depending on both the degree and the type of disturbance.

The interest in sex differentiation can be traced to distant antiquity. Aristotle, influenced by Homer's idea that mares are fertilized by the wind, suggested that when sheep and goats ". . . submit to the male when north winds are blowing, they are apt to bear males; if when south winds are blowing, females." Although these concepts of sex differentiation would appear to be somewhat vague, Aristotle indeed recorded a number of observations from which he drew important inferences subsequently confirmed by physiologists. He believed that changes in specific regions of the early embryo determine future sex, and although he was not aware of the role of the testes in reproduction, he suggested that early castration induces phenotypic changes.

The concept of intersex or hermaphroditism was frequently mentioned in mythology, and children with ambiguous genitalia were described. The ideas concerned with the physiologic mechanisms of sex determination went through a remarkable evolutionary process. Galen (2nd century after Christ) suggested that the right testis secreted "male" and the left testis "female" semen. If semen from both testes found its way into the uterus, a hermaphrodite was produced. Avicenna (10th century) proposed that the sex of the offspring depended on the site of semen deposition; placement of the semen into the right side of the uterus resulted in a male and into the left side a female. A common pre-Renaissance belief was that both males and females have testes and both produce semen. Paré (16th century) suggested intersex resulted when the female yielded as much semen as the male.

Ova and ovaries were not described until the 17th century, and a rational approach to the embryology of sex differentiation could not have been employed until publication of the classic studies of Wolff and Müller in the 19th century. Their description of the morphologic aspects of the developing reproductive tract and the subsequent application of physiologic, genetic, and biochemical approaches to the study of this topic led to the current ideas about sexual differentiation.

A number of fundamental concepts have been sufficiently documented to warrant their discussion in this chapter: (1) the chromosomal basis of sex determination; (2) the evidence for sexual bipotentiality of the undifferentiated embryo and of the primordial germ cells; (3) the recognition that sexual bipotentiality of the embryo is responsible for the complexity of the mechanisms involved in the control of organogenesis of the reproductive system; (4) the recognition of the role of hormonal, metabolic, and environmental factors in sex differentiation; and (5) the recognition of the differences in the mechanisms of sex differentiation among species.

Since the understanding of the various parameters of sex differentiation resulted from studies in various mammalian and submammalian species, it will be necessary to utilize these various sources of information in the ensuing discussion.

MORPHOLOGIC ASPECTS OF SEX DIFFERENTIATION

ORGANOGENESIS

No morphologic differences can be detected in the reproductive system of an embryo prior to the onset of sex differentiation. The morphologic structures destined to develop into gonads, internal sex organs, or external genitalia are identical regardless of the embryo's genetic sex.

The gonadal anlage can be identified in a 4-week embryo as a ridge (the genital ridge) located between the mesonephros and the dorsal mesentary (Fig. 105-1). The anlage is formed from coelomic epithelium and from condensation of the underlying mesenchyme. The primordial germ cells migrate into the anlage from the hindgut (Fig. 105-2).[1] At the time of primordial germ cell migration the coelomic epithelium invades the underlying mesenchyme and forms cordlike structures (primitive sex cords) (Fig. 105-3*a*). Since it is impossible to determine at this stage of development whether this structure will form testes or ovaries, it is termed the "indifferent gonad." After the indifferent gonad has formed, two pairs of genital ducts can be identified on the anterolateral surface of the urogenital ridge: the mesonephric or wolffian ducts (discernible by the 4th week of development) and the müllerian ducts (Fig. 105-4). The wolffian ducts extend to the urogenital sinus while cranially the müllerian ducts form a funnellike structure opening into the coelomic cavity; caudally they come in close proximity to the midline (Fig. 105-5).

The external genitalia are derived from an anlage common to both sexes. The anlage consists of a genital tubercle, urethral folds, a urethral groove through which the sexually undifferentiated urogenital sinus empties, and the genital swellings on each side of the urethral groove.

In the male fetus the wolffian ducts and the mesonephros evolve into the adult internal reproductive duct system. The wolffian duct develops into the epididymis and the vas deferens, the caudal portion evolving into the seminal vesicles. The cranial portions of the mesonephros develop into the ductuli efferentes. The prostate develops from the urogenital sinus. While this development takes place, the other embryonal duct system, the müllerian ducts, degenerate and disappear by the end of the 8th week with the exception of the most cranial portion which persists and forms the appendix testis (Fig. 105-6).

In the female, the wolffian ducts degenerate although small portions may persist in the adult female. The Gartner duct, formed from the caudal portion of the wolffian ducts, has clinical importance because it may form a cyst, the Gartner's duct cyst. The cranial portion of the wolffian duct forms the epoophoron.

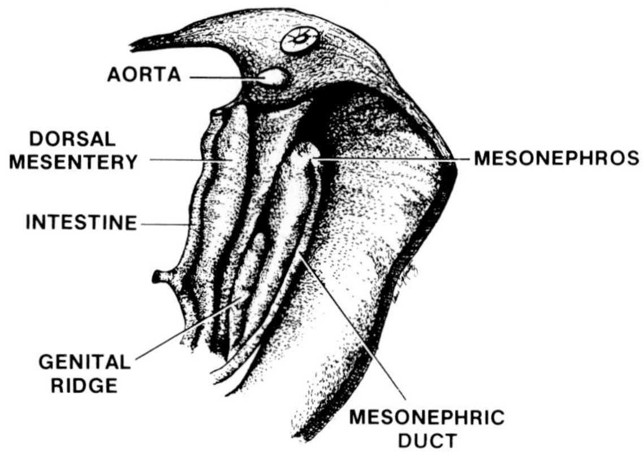

Fig. 105-1. Relationship of the genital ridge to the mesonephros and to the mesonephric (wolffian) ducts.

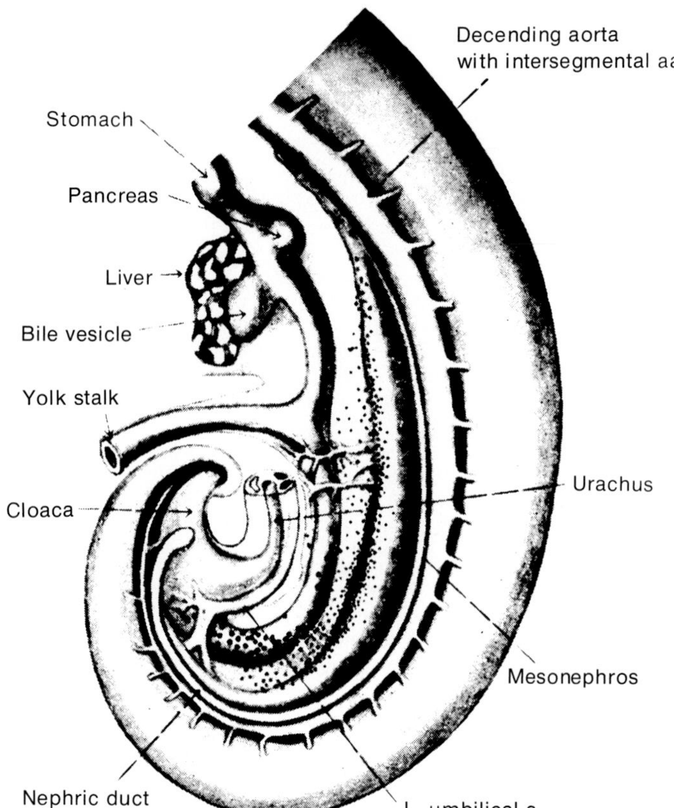

Fig. 105-2. Human tailbud embryo; 32 somites. Viscera, migration of germinal cells indicated by dots of various sizes (22×). (From Witschi: Carnegie Contrib. Embryol. Carnegie Inst. 209: 67, 1948, with permission.)

The müllerian ducts form the various segments of the internal reproductive tract of the adult female. The upper portions evolve into symmetric oviducts, the fallopian tubes, and the middle portions of both ducts fuse to form the uterus. The vagina is formed by tissue derived from the urogenital sinus (Figs. 105-6 and 105-7).

The indifferent structures of the external genitalia develop into the appropriate portions of either the male of female external genitalia. In the female the indifferent genitalia change little. The genital tubercle forms the clitoris, the labia majora develop from the genital swellings, and the urethral folds become the labia minora (Fig. 105-8). In the male, the evolution of the external genitalia is considerably more complex and more vulnerable to error, thus to formation of clinically important abnormalities such as hypo- or epispadias, bifid scrotum, etc. While the genital tubercle participates in the formation of the penis, specifically the glans, the penile shaft is formed by a complicated process of simultaneous fusion and elongation of the urethral fold and groove. Ultimately this process results in bringing the urethral orifice to the meatus at the tip of the glans penis. The genital swellings fuse to form the scrotum into which the testes descend from their original location in the abdominal cavity (Fig. 105-9).

SEQUENCE OF SEXUAL DIFFERENTIATION

The development of the gonads proceeds through specific stages which differ from morphologic and chronologic view points in the two sexes. A great amount of information concerning the details of differentiation was gained from studies in subhuman species. However, considerable information is also available for

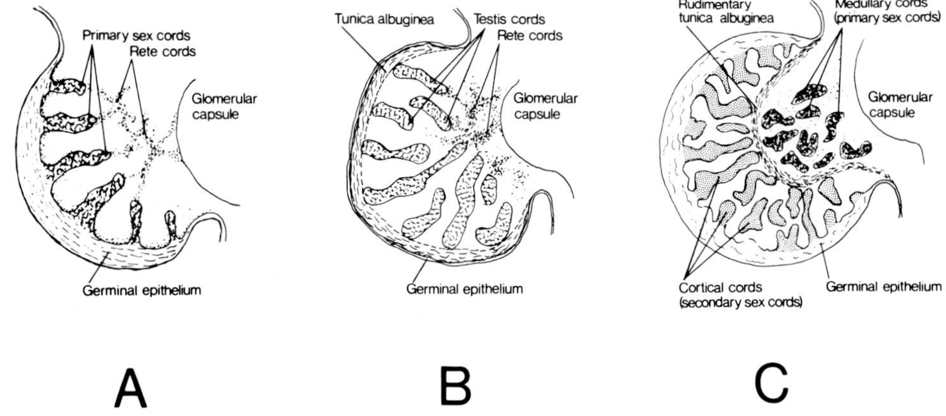

Fig. 105-3. a: An indifferent gonadal anlage in a 5-week embryo. b: Development of a male gonad. c: Development of a female gonad.

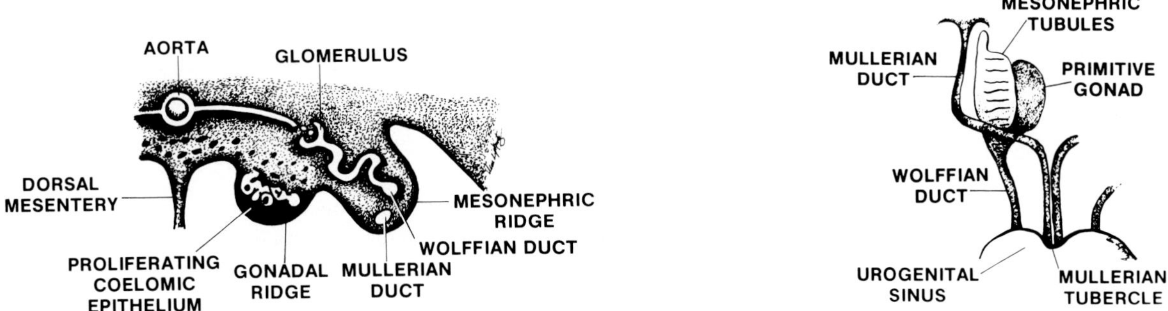

Fig. 105-4. Schematic representation of a transverse section through the lumbar region of a 6-week embryo.

Fig. 105-5. Indifferent stage of the gonadal and ductal development.

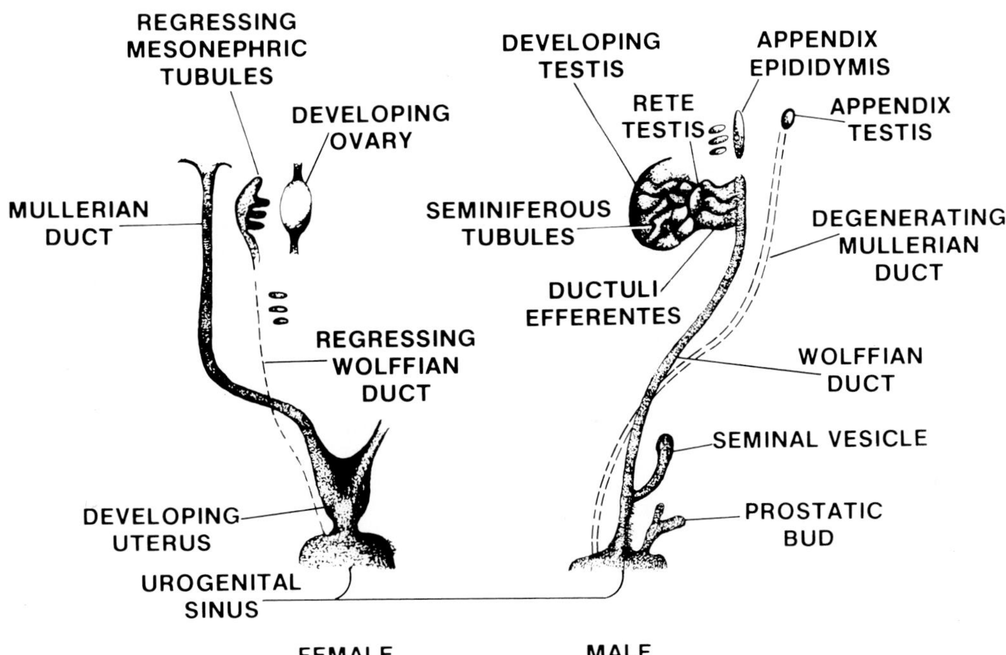

Fig. 105-6. Differentiation of the internal sex organs.

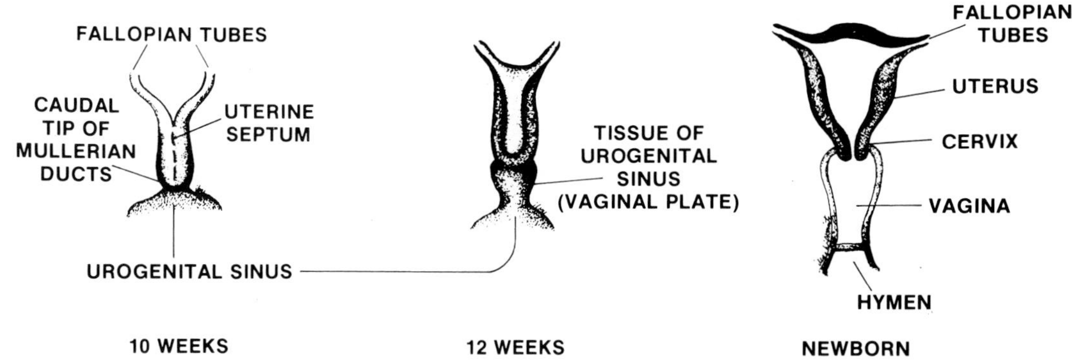

Fig. 105-7. Development of the internal reproductive tract in the female.

the human and can be summarized in the following fashion (Figs. 105-10a and 105-10b).

The indifferent gonadal anlage develops as a thickening of the coelomic epithelium on the medioventral surface of the urogenital ridge and proliferation of the underlying mesenchyme during the 5th week of gestation (7 to 14 mm). The primordial germ cells can be identified among the endodermal cells of the hindgut during the 4th week of development.[2] During the 5th week they migrate into the gonadal anlage, and by the end of the 6th week (20 to 22 mm) the primordial germ cells have seeded the gonadal anlage where they may develop either into oogonia or spermatogonia, depending on the genetic sex of the embryo. Failure of seeding of the gonadal anlage with germ cells results in inhibition of its further development.

The indifferent gonads begin to develop in the male embryo much earlier than in the female. The gonads can be recognized as testes 43 to 50 days postfertilization[3] in a 15-to-30-mm embryo, while in the female embryo feminization of internal organs becomes apparent by 50 to 60 days postfertilization; however, at the same time the gonads still remain undifferentiated. Commencing with this stage of development in the male the wolffian ducts begin to show evidence of progressive differentiation into the male ductal system, and the müllerian duct is essentially regressed by the 9th to 12th week (40 to 55 mm). By the 3rd month the penis and prostate form. In the female, the regression of the wolffian duct lags behind, not becoming obvious until the 11th to 13th week, when the urogenital sinus also shows signs of participation in the formation of the vagina. During the time period when wolffian duct regression and müllerian duct differentiation take place, the indifferent gonads still fail to show morphologic evidence suggestive of ovarian development, although during the 11th and 12th weeks (80-mm stage) the germ cells enter meiosis. True ovarian organogenesis does not begin until after 18 to 20 weeks and then continues until parturition.

This brief review of the chronology of differentiation points out the elegant synchrony in the development of the various portions of the reproductive system (gonads, internal organs, external genitalia) and emphasizes the striking differences in developmental chronology between the sexes. The fact that in the female the development of internal reproductive organs and external genitalia commences prior to the onset of morphogenesis of the gonad is of particular interest and of importance in attempting to determine the etiology of the various reproductive system abnormalities encountered in clinical practice.

SEXUAL DIFFERENTIATION OF THE GONADS

With each new finding concerning the sexual differentiation of the indifferent gonad in the embryo, there has arisen a new theory. Since in different textbooks different theories are mentioned, and since the final experiment has yet to be performed, a brief summary of the historic evolution of these theories and of the current thoughts on this topic would perhaps be helpful. Although the theories have been extrapolated to the human, in most instances they are based on experimental work in lower species.

The classical theories of differentiation of gonadal sex evolved in three stages. However, it should be emphasized that even the most recent hypothesis may not necessarily be correct.

Some of the earliest attempts to bring together available information into a coherent hypothesis were those of Waldeyer,[4] who proposed that the embryo passes through a hermaphroditic stage, its gonads containing both male and female structures, and that sex differentiation requires that only one of the anlagen proceed with development. This hypothesis was further elaborated upon and developed into a concept that states that formation of primary and secondary sex cords is responsible for gonadal differentiation. This latter hypothesis proposes that the early gonadal primordium is covered by a "germinative epithelium," which proliferates into the

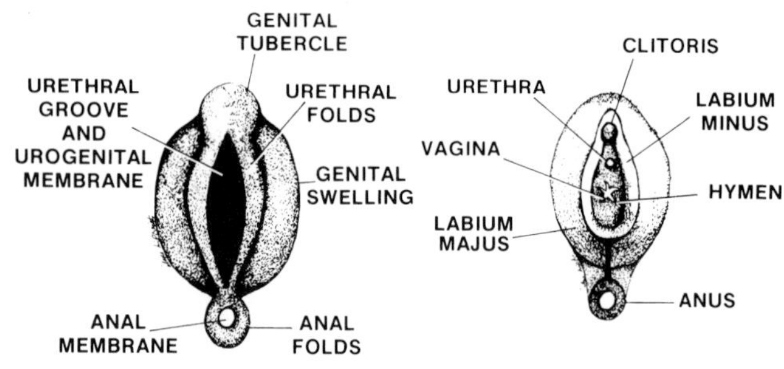

Fig. 105-8. Diagrammatic representation of the development of the external genitalia in the female at approximately 4 weeks (left) and at approximately 6 weeks (right).

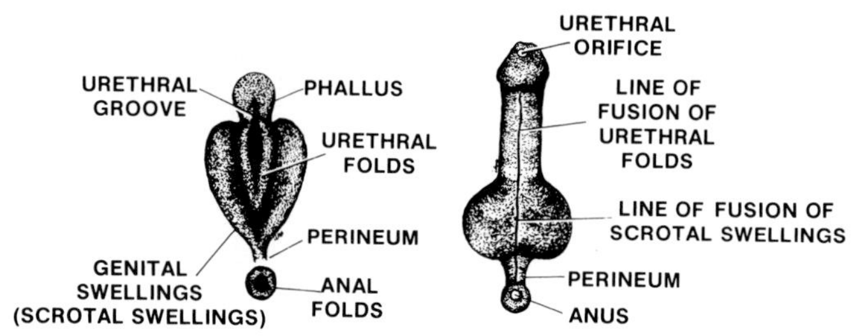

Fig. 105-9. Development of male external genitalia.

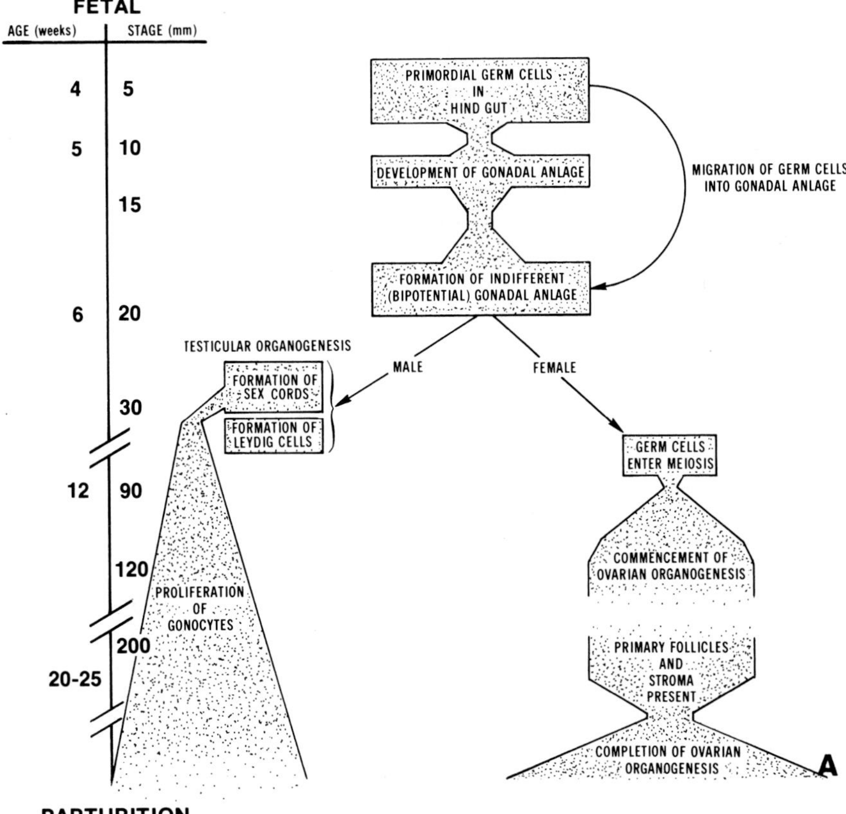

Fig. 105-10a. Chronology of gonadal development in man.

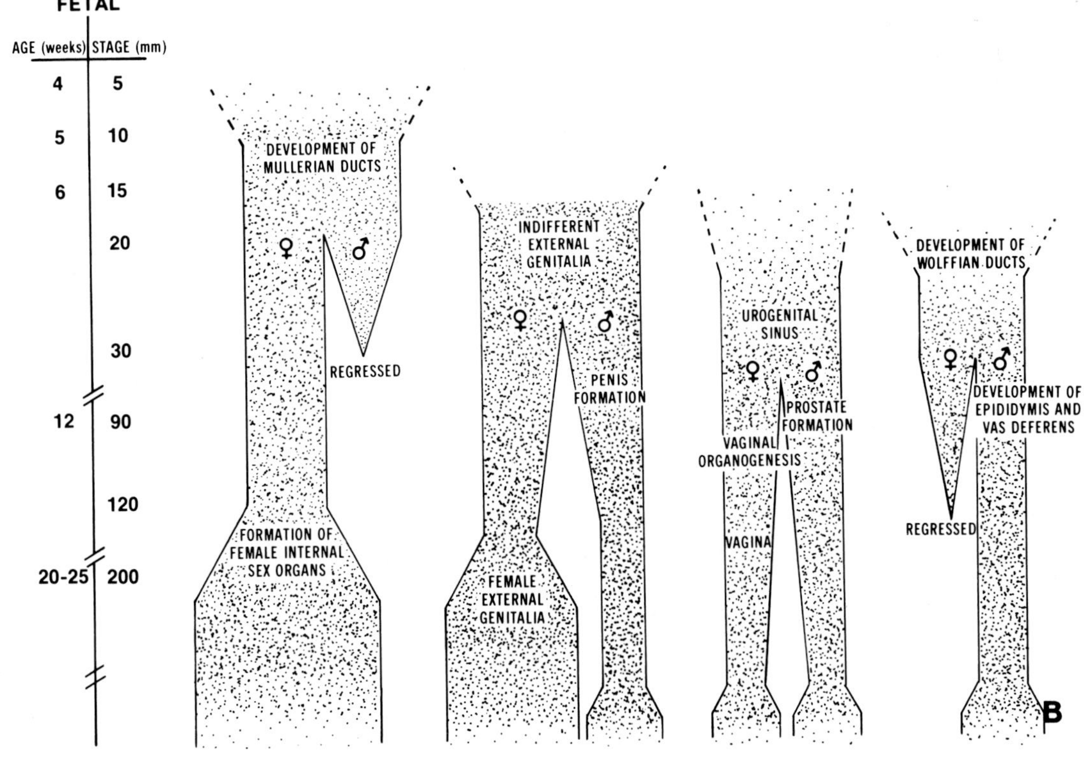

Fig. 105-10b. Chronology of the development of the internal and external sex organs.

underlying mesenchyme to form "sex cords." The cords represent the male or medullary component of the gonad. Subsequently the "germinative epithelium" further proliferates to give rise to secondary cords ("Pflüger's cords") or cortical cords, which give rise to the cortex and ultimately form the ovaries in the female (Fig. 105-3). Although these classical concepts persisted until very recent days,[5] neither the formation of sex cords from the "germinative epithelium" nor their successive proliferation has ever been demonstrated experimentally.[6–8]

Commencing with the early studies on frog embryos in 1914, Witschi evolved an hypothesis of gonadal sex differentiation[9] which does not support the concept of a bipotentiality of the undifferentiated gonadal primordium. This hypothesis postulates two morphologically distinct and physiologically antagonistic gonadal primordia in the undifferentiated gonad, leading to the development of testis and ovaries. Witschi proposed that the undifferentiated gonad was composed of two components, a superficial cortex which ultimately evolved into an ovary, and an internally located medulla which served as the primordium for the testes (Fig. 105-11). Witschi also proposed that each component produced and released an inductive substance, corticin and medullocin, respectively, which stimulated development of homologous gonadal strucutres and antagonized the development of heterologous structures. The corticin was responsible for feminizing induction and was produced by the follicle cells of the cortex. The medullocin, responsible for masculinizing induction, was produced by the interstitial cells in the medulla. The medullocin not only repressed the cortex and masculinized the medulla, inducing the development of testes, but also inhibited the "female development" of the follicle cells surrounding the gonocytes in the medulla of the primitive gonad favoring their development into Sertoli cells (Fig. 105-11). Furthermore, Witschi[10] suggested that the genetic constitution of the embryo (male or female) rather than the germ cells is primarily responsible for the control of cortical and medullary inductors. Thus, he felt that the genic compositon of the germ cells was unimportant with respect to their sex differentiation.

Although all the details of Witschi's hypothesis may not have been agreed upon, it is generally accepted that in the male sex differentiation of the gonads involves differentiation of the medullary primordium and suppression of the cortex, while in the female, the converse—differentiation of the cortex with concomitant suppression of the medullary primoridium—is true.[5]

Recently, Jost[11] challenged this hypothesis. He pointed out that neither has the presence of medullary cords in an early (undifferentiated) ovarian primordium ever been demonstrated, nor was he, utilizing more advanced morphologic techniques, able to demonstrate their presence in an undifferentiated ovarian primordium. He also demonstrated a striking difference in the developmental chronology between male and female gonads. In the genetic female the gonads remain totally undeveloped and undistinguishable from an undifferentiated gonadal primordium at the stage of development when the gonad in a genetic male shows definite morphologic evidence of the formation of testicular structures. The supporting cells (follicle cells of Witschi), precursors of Sertoli cells, show definite signs of morphogenesis at the ultrastructural level in the male embryo while no similiar differentiative process can be detected in the follicle cells in a gonad of a genetic female of the same age. It is of interest to note that the differentiation of interstitial cells takes place approximately 2 days later than morphogenesis of supporting cells, suggesting that differentiation of supporting cells is not controlled by the interstitial cells.

Jost concluded that the mechanisms responsible for sex differentiation of the indifferent gonads were still largely unknown. On the basis of information gained primarily from studies of bovine freemartins, he suggested that the undifferentiated gonadal primordium would normally tend to develop toward a female gonad unless actively directed toward male differentiation possibly under genetic influence. Although the mechanisms responsible for this "active direction" are still not understood, considerable evidence has accumulated suggesting that one gene (or more) on the Y-chromosome is essential for the development of the indifferent gonad into testes. This would suggest a relatively simple basic sequence of events leading to differentiation of a male.

Recently, experimental work in lower species, particularly the mouse, provided further information concerning the role of sex chromosomes in differentiation. Specifically, evidence was obtained suggesting the presence of a gene on the X-chromosome that is responsible for conferring testosterone responsiveness to all cells in the organism sensitive to testosterone action. This gene was denoted as the Tfm gene because its absence from an X-chromosome in a male mouse causes the syndrome of testicular feminization. Animals with an XY sex chromosome complement suffering with this mutation exhibit the phenotype of a female, have testes, and show no responsiveness of somatic target tissues to testosterone.[12] A similar syndrome has been described in man.

Lyon suggested there was a biologic reason for the Tfm gene's location on the X-chromosome.[13] She discovered[14] that the mammalian X-chromosomes exhibit variable states of activity. In the

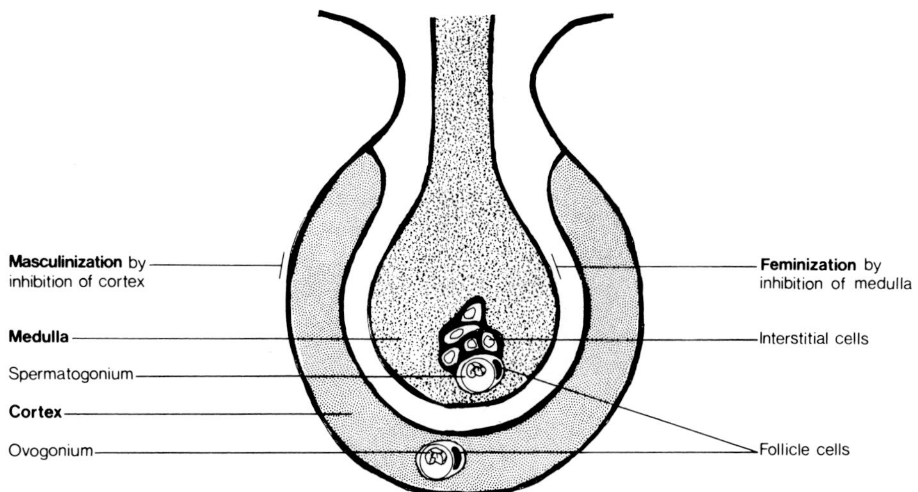

Fig. 105-11. Witschi's concept of gonadal development.

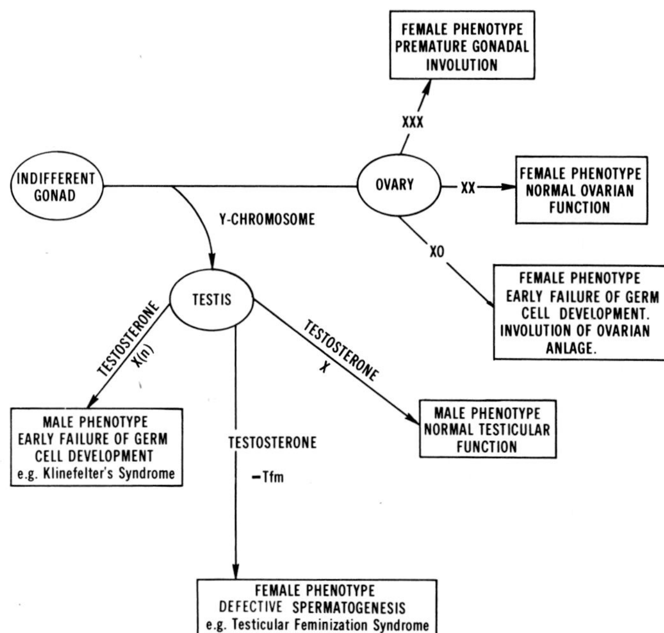

Fig. 105-12. Current concept of hormone and genetic mechanisms involved in sexual differentiation.

somatic cells of the normal female, only one X-chromosome is active; the other is present in an inactive state (heterochromatin, sex chromatin, Barr body). In the female germ cells, however, both X-chromosomes are active.[15] Although in later stages of spermatogenesis the X-chromosome becomes inactivated, it is active in primordial male germ cells.[16,17]

Thus it appears that for differentiation of the female germ cell a double dose of X-chromosome-derived genetic material is necessary, while for the early differentiation of the male, only a single dose of X-chromosome-derived genetic material is required. A deficiency or excess of X-chromosome-derived genetic material results in abnormal development. In the XO fetus, the gonad is present and contains germ cells,[18] but this gonad fails to continue development and by birth is absent. In XXX females, the gonad undergoes early involution. In males carrying excessive numbers of X-chromosomes—e.g., in patients with Klinefelter's syndrome—the germinal elements in the immature testes fail to develop and ultimately degenerate, resulting in severely germ-cell-depleted testes in the adult.

Extrapolation of findings from lower species and intrapolation of observations derived from pathologic conditions in man underline the importance of a quantitative relationship of X-chromosome-derived genetic material to the ability of the fetal gonad to differentiate and to development of germ cells in puberal and adult gonads of both sexes. If the above-discussed findings can be freely combined and extrapolated to the human species, then the current concept of sexual differentiation could be summarized in general terms as in Figure 105-12.

HUMORAL ASPECTS OF SEX DIFFERENTIATION

The development of the internal reproductive tract and the external sex organs involves appropriate morphologic modification of the undifferentiated urogenital tract. This process is controlled by substances produced by the gonads. Genetic determinants control the development of the indifferent gonad into a testis or an ovary, and gonadal secretions determine the somatic and phenotypic sex. The latter statement is based primarily on experiments involving intrauterine castration or hypophysectomy[19] and studies with *in vitro* culture systems.[20,21]

HORMONAL CONTROL OF THE DEVELOPMENT OF INTERNAL REPRODUCTIVE TRACT

In the absence of gonads the müllerian ducts develop into the segments of the female reproductive tract and the wolffian ducts degenerate. The presence of the testes induces degeneration of the müllerian ducts and differentiation of the wolffian ducts into segments of the male reproductive tract. Consequently, the development of the male reproductive tract is induced by a substance produced by the testes, while the development of the female reproductive tract requires no hormonal stimulation from either testes or ovaries.

The substance produced by the male gonads which is responsible for the induction of development of the male internal reproductive tract was shown to be a steroid hormone, androgen. Treatment of castrated rabbit fetuses with testosterone induced changes of the wolffian duct compatible with the development of a male internal reproductive tract.[19] When normal male rabbit fetuses were treated with cyproterone acetate, an antiandrogen, the development of the wolffian duct was prevented and a female internal reproductive tract developed.[22] Although these findings have not been universally confirmed in all species studied,[23] the available evidence strongly supports the suggestion that androgen is the active principle produced by fetal testes responsible for differentiation of the wolffian ducts. This is further supported by the observations that fetal testes are capable of converting appropriate steroidal precursors to testosterone[24] and by the finding that the fetal testicular tissue contains a considerable quantity of this androgen.[25]

In the adult, testosterone behaves in many but probably not all instances as a prohormone. In certain androgen-responsive somatic tissues—e.g., prostate and seminal vesicles—it is reduced by the action of 5α-reductase to an active androgen, dihydrotestosterone, which is the major intracellular mediator of male hormone action in these tissues. Demonstration of extremely high 5α-reductase activity in the genital tubercle and the urogenital sinus of the rabbit embryo[26] suggests a similar role for dihydrotestosterone in these tissues. Although the major and androgen secreted by the fetal testes is testosterone, it apparently must be converted to an active androgen, dihydrotestosterone, before being capable of inducing virilization in the genital tubercle and the urogenital sinus. Differentiation of the wolffian ducts, however, is stimulated directly by testosterone. No 5α-reductase activity can be detected in these structures prior to the completion of their differentiation to epididymis and seminal vesicles.[27] The differences between the type of androgen required for stimulation of differentiation of the wolffian structures on one hand and the anlage of the external genitalia on the other are clear; their physiologic meaning, however, remains entirely unknown.

Although testosterone is capable of induction of wolffian duct development in both genetic male and female, treatment of castrated male fetuses or normal female fetuses with androgens does not result in regression of the müllerian ducts. This finding led to the development of a hypothesis that two testicular hormones are necessary for masculinization of the internal reproductive tract—the androgens and a müllerian duct inhibitor.[19] The idea of a second fetal testicular hormone, the müllerian duct inhibitor, has been supported in the course of the past two decades by various experimental and clinical observations. The well-known clinical syndrome of testicular feminization provided strong support for the presence of a second hormone. In this syndrome a genetic male with testes shows a female phenotype and female development of the external genitalia but no discernible internal structure normally derived from the müllerian ducts. These individuals are insensitive to the action of androgens due to the lack of androgen receptors in the cells of the target tissues. However, their müllerian duct derivates (fallopian tubes, uterus) are absent, suggesting that a substance that inhibited the development of the müllerian ducts was probably produced by the fetal testes during fetal life. Since the cells in this individual are unresponsive to testosterone, some other substance was probably produced by the testes to induce repression of the müllerian duct. In experiments with antiandrogens, it has also been observed that these substances block the ability of the testes to induce the differentiation of the wolffian duct tract structure but do not block the ability of the testis to induce regression of the müllerian ducts.

In light of indirect evidence a search for this hypothetical substance was undertaken. Recently, evidence was obtained suggesting that müllerian inhibiting factor is a large protein which is probably produced by the Sertoli cells of the fetal testes.[28,29]

REFERENCES

1. Gillman, J. The development of the gonads in man, with a consideration of the role of fetal endocrines and histogenesis of ovarian tumors. *Contrib. Embryol. 32:* 81, 1948.
2. Witschi, E. Migration of the germ cells of human embryos from the yolk sac to the primitive gonadal folds. Contrib. Embryol. *Carnegie Inst. 32:* 67, 1948.
3. Jirasek, J. E. *Development of the Genital System and Male Pseudohermaphroditism.* Baltimore, Johns Hopkins University Press, 1971.
4. Waldeyer, W. *Eierstock und Ei.* Leipzig, Wilhelm Englemann, 1870.
5. Burns, R. K. Role of hormones in the differentiation of sex. In: *Sex and Internal Secretions, vol. 1,* 3rd edition, W. C. Young (editor), pp. 76–158. Baltimore, Williams & Wilkins, 1961.
6. Fischel, A. Über die Entwicklung der Keimdrüsen des Menschen. *Z. Anat. Entwicklungsgesch. 92:* 34, 1930.
7. Odor, D. L. and Blandau, R. J. Ultrastructural studies on fetal and early postnatal mouse ovaries. I. Histogenesis and organogenesis. *Am. J. Anat. 124:* 163, 1969.
8. Gropp, A. and Ohno, S. The presence of a common embryonic blastema for ovarian and testicular parenchymal (follicular, interstitial and tubular) cells in cattle, *Bos Taurus.* Z. Zellforsch. Mikroskop. Anat. *74:* 505, 1966.
9. Witschi, E. Embryogenesis of the adrenal and the reproductive glands. *Recent Prog. Horm. Res. 6:* 1, 1951.
10. Witschi, E. The inductor theory of sex differentiation. *J. Fac. Sci, Hokkaido Univ. 13:* Zool. Ser. VI, Nos. 1–4, 428, 1957.
11. Jost, A. Hormanal and genetic factors affecting the development of the male genital system. *Andrologia 8* (Suppl. 1): 17, 1976.
12. Ohno, S. and Lyon, M. F. X-linked testicular feminization in the mouse as a non-inducible regulatory mutation of the Jacob-Monod type. *Clin. Genet. 1:* 121, 1970.
13. Lyon, M. F. Role of X and Y chromosomes in mammalian sex determination and differentiation. *Helv. Paediatr. Acta Suppl. 34:* 7, 1974.
14. Lyon, M. F. Sex chromatin and gene action in the mammalian X-chromosome. *Am. J. Hum. Genet. 14:* 135, 1962.
15. Gartler, S. M., Liskay, R. M., Campbell, B. K., Sparkes, R., and Gant, N. Evidence for two functional X chromosomes in human oocytes. *Cell Differ. 1:* 215, 1972.
16. Lyon, M. F. Genetic activity of sex chromosomes in somatic cells of mammals. *Philos. Trans. R. Soc. London Ser. B 259:* 41, 1970.
17. Lyon, M. F. X-chromosome inactivation and developmental patterns in mammals. *Biol. Rev. 47:* 1, 1972.
18. Singh, R. P. and Carr, D. H. The anatomy and histology of XO human embryos and fetuses. *Anat. Rec. 155:* 369, 1966.
19. Jost, A. Problems of fetal endocrinology: The gonadal and hypophyseal hormones. *Recent Prog. Horm. Res. 8:* 379, 1953.
20. Price, D. *In vitro* studies on differentiation of the reproductive tract. *Philos. Trans. R. Soc. London Ser. B 259:* 133, 1970.
21. Jost, A., Vigier, B., Prépin, J., and Perchellet, J. P. Studies on sex differentiation in mammals. *Recent Prog. Horm. Res. 29:* 1, 1973.
22. Elger, W. Die Rolle der fetalen Androgene in der Sexualdifferenzierung des Kaninchens und ihre Abgrenzung gegen anderen hormonal und somatische Faktoren durch Anwendung eines starken Antiandrogens. *Arch. Anat. Microsc. Morphol. Exp. 55:* 657, 1966.
23. Jost, A. Modalities in the action of androgens on the fetus. (IIIrd Meeting International Study Group for Steroid Hormones, Dec. 1967.) *Res. Steroids 3:* 207, 1968.
24. Noumura, T., Weisz, J., and Lloyd, C. W. *In vitro* conversion of 7-^{3}H-progesterone to androgens by the rat testis during the second half of fetal life. *Endocrinology 78:* 245, 1966.
25. Wilson, J. D. and Lasnitzki, I. Dihydrotestosterone formation in fetal tissues of the rabbit and rat. *Endocrinology 89:* 659, 1971.
26. Warren, D. W., Haltmeyer, G. C., and Eik-Nes, K. B. Testosterone in the fetal rat testis. *Biol. Reprod. 8:* 560, 1973.
27. Wilson, J. D. and Siiteri, P. K. Developmental pattern of testosterone synthesis in the fetal gonad of the rabbit. *Endocrinology 92:* 1182, 1973.
28. Blanchard, M. G. and Josso, N. Source of the anti-Müllerian hormone synthesized by the fetal testis: Müllerian inhibiting activity of fetal bovine Sertoli cells in tissue culture. *Pediat. Res. 8:* 968, 1974.
29. Donohoe, P. K., Ito, Y., Marlatia, S. R., and Hendren, W. H. The range of activity of Müllerian inhibiting substance. *Pediat. Res. 9:* 289, 1975.

106

Pathogenesis, Classification, Diagnosis, and Treatment of Anomalies of Sex

Felix A. Conte
Melvin M. Grumbach

Usually, the components of an individual's sexual makeup are dominantly of one gender and arise as a consequence of the genetic sex which determines the gonadal sex and thereafter the phenotypic sex. However, since, most sexual characteristics emerge from bipotential precursors in the embryo, a spectrum of differentiation at each level of sexual organization is possible. Recent advances in endocrinology, cytogenetics, embryology, molecular biochemistry, and immunology have helped clarify the processes of normal sexual differentiation as well as the pathogenesis of abnormalities of sexual differentiation.

GONADOGENESIS

The genetic sex of the fetus is established by the production of an XY or XX zygote. The gonads of both sexes develop from three different components: (1) the coelomic epithelium (2) the adjacent mesenchyma and (3) the primordial germ cells. The primordial germ cells, which arise in the yolk sac endoderm, seed the undifferentiated gonad by migration via the mesentery of the gut. There is an inherent tendency for the gonad to undergo ovarian differentiation, provided germ cells are present, unless prior testicular differentiation has occurred (Fig. 106-1).[1,2,2a]

In the human, the presence of two functionally normal X chromosomes in the absence of a Y chromosome leads to ovarian differentiation. In the gonad destined to be an ovary, lack of differentiation persists until about the 11th to 12th week, when a significant number of germ cells enter meiotic prophase, which characterizes the transition of oogonia into oocytes. This event then marks the onset of ovarian differentiation. Studies in patients with various structural deletions of the X chromosome suggest that loci on the long and short arms of the X chromosome are involved in human ovarian differentiation.[2,3]

Genes located in the pericentromeric region of the Y chromosome effect testicular differentiation of the bipotential gonads.[1,2,2a] The testicular-determining gene(s) are either closely linked or identical to a gene that codes for an antigen, the H-Y antigen, which is a cell surface protein that may act directly to organize the bipotential embryonic gonad into a testis (Fig. 106-2).[4,5]

H-Y (MALE) ANTIGEN AND TESTICULAR ORGANOGENESIS[2a]

In 1955, Eichwald and Silmser showed that, among inbred strains of mice, most male-to-female skin grafts were rejected, whereas male-to-male and female-to-female grafts survived.[6] This phenomenon was attributed to a specific Y-linked histocompatibility locus, the H-Y antigen. Wachtel et al. extended the study of H-Y antigen from inbred mice to rats, guinea pigs, rabbits, and

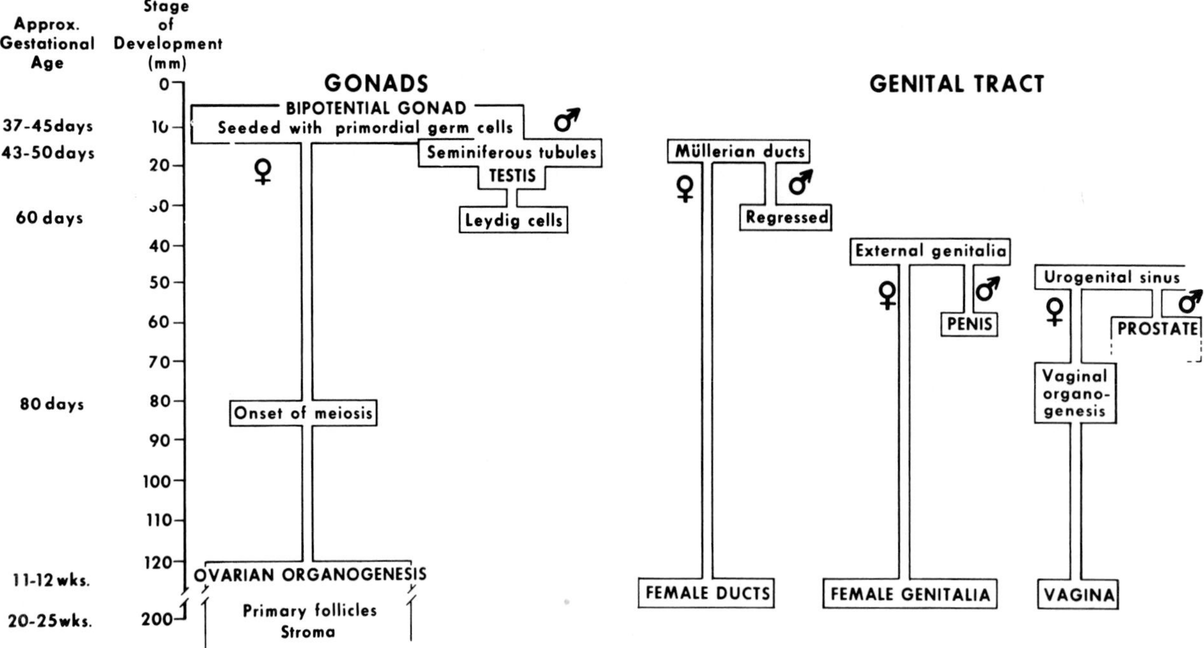

Fig. 106-1. Schematic sequence of sexual differentiation in the human fetus. Testicular development occurs earlier than all other forms of sexual dimorphism. (Modified from Jost, A.[1]; from Grumbach, M. M. and Van Wyk, J., in *Textbook of Endocrinology,* 5th ed., R. H. Williams (ed.), Philadelphia, W. B. Saunders Co., 1974.

humans, utilizing a sperm cytotoxicity test, and demonstrated antigenic cross-reactivity in these species with the H-Y antigen of the mouse.[7] H-Y antigen has been demonstrated to be present by the eight-cell stage in the mouse embryo.[8] Studies in humans with 47,XYY karyotypes indicate the presence of a double dose of H-Y antigen and support the hypothesis that its locus is Y-linked.[9] Because of its evolutionary conservation, the H-Y antigen has been postulated to have an invariant function: the induction of testis.[4] (In avians, the female is ZW and the male ZZ. In this species, the female (ZW) expresses an antigen (H-W) that cross-reacts with the mouse H-Y antigen serologically. Thus, in birds, H-W antigen specifies the gonad in the heterogametic sex that is an ovary.) To examine this hypothesis, XX males and XX true hermaphrodites were tested serologically for H-Y antigen. This antigen was detected in 46,XX males and 46,XX true hermaphrodites.[10] Also, XX mice that are "sex-reversed" to males by the autosomal dominant mutant gene (Sxr) and phenotypically female XY mice, who have the X-linked testicular feminization gene (Tfm), are H-Y positive.[11,12]

Differentiation of the testis under the influence of the Y chromosome occurs by the seventh week of gestation, as opposed to ovarian development that does not emerge before 13 to 16 weeks.[2,2a] Jost theorized, on the basis of his experiments with freemartins, that the undifferentiated gonad will become an ovary unless an inducer substance imposes testicular organization on the

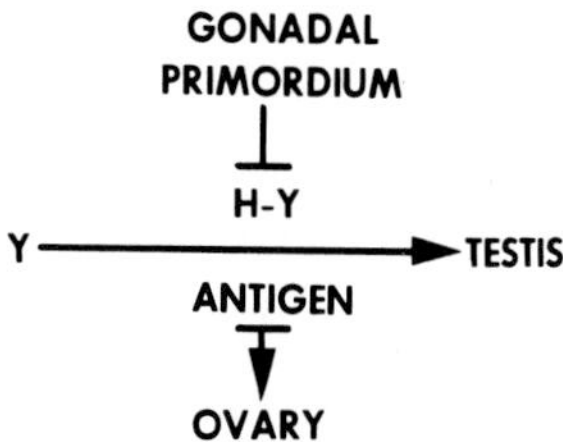

Fig. 106-2. Testicular organogenesis is induced by the presence of a cell surface factor, H-Y antigen, which is coded for by a gene(s) on the Y chromosome.

gonadal primordium.[1] Since testicular organization most likely occurs by direct interaction between germ cells and somatic elements of the primordial gonad, it is reasonable to postulate that H-Y antigen, a cell membrane protein, is the "inducer substance."[5] In cattle, chorionic vascular anastomosis between a male and female twin can lead to testeslike differentiation of the gonads of the female twin. The gonads of the freemartin female resemble testes, while testosterone-dependent effects on the external genitalia often are only moderate. Although fetal freemartin gonads have a small proportion of XY cells (<10 percent), they contain as much H-Y antigen as the normal bovine fetal testes, supporting the view that the testicular organization in the XX/XY gonad is due to H-Y antigen from the XY cells.[5,13]

Thus, accumulating evidence in humans supports the hypothesis that the Y-linked H-Y antigen and the testis-determining gene are identical or closely linked and that this plasma membrane antigen is the primary determinant of testicular differentiation.[2a] The detection of H-Y antigen in XX males and true hermaphrodites who lack any karyotypic evidence of a Y chromosome suggests that the H-Y gene locus of the Y is present on an X chromosome or autosome in these individuals as a result of exchange or translocation.

It has been suggested that the short arm of the Y chromosome contains loci homologous to those on the short arm of the X chromosome, since the presence of either of these segments of an X or Y chromosome with a normal X prevents the short stature and most of the somatic abnormalities found in the syndrome of XO gonadal dysgenesis.[2] Few, if any, other genes, except those related to stature, testicular differentiation and spermatogenesis, are known to be present on the Y chromosome.

SEX DIFFERENTIATION (Fig. 106-3)

Female sex differentiation occurs in the presence of an ovary, a streak gonad, or no gonad, as first demonstrated in the rabbit fetus by Jost and later confirmed in the human by analyses of

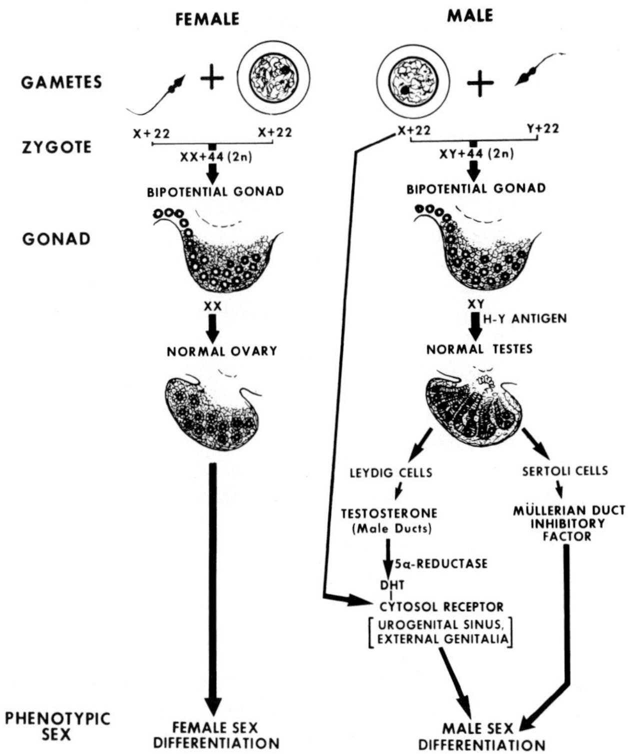

Fig. 106-3. Diagrammatic representation of human sex determination and differentiation. Anomalies of sex can result from factors that adversely affect any stage of these processes. (Modified from Grumbach, M. M., in *Biologic Basis of Pediatric Practice,* R. E. Cooke (ed.), New York, McGraw-Hill, 1967.)

anomalies of sex.[1,2] On the other hand, masculinization of the male fetus is the result of production by the testes of müllerian duct inhibitory factor and of testosterone. Müllerian duct inhibitory factor is a protein with a molecular weight > 100,000 that is secreted by the Sertoli cells of the fetal testes.[14–16] It acts ipsilaterally to induce involution of the paired müllerian ducts and, hence, suppresses the development of the uterus and fallopian tubes. Testosterone secreted by the fetal testes under the influence of chorionic gonadotropin[17] appears to stimulate the primitive wolffian structures ipsilaterally to differentiate into the epididymis, vas deferens, and seminal vesicles (Fig. 106-4).[18] The lateralization of the effect of testosterone on wolffian development suggests that greater local concentrations of androgen are required for duct development than for masculinization of the external genitalia and derivatives of the urogenital sinus. Wilson has shown that before and during the critical period of male duct differentiation in fetal rabbits, the wolffian ducts and their derivatives contain a testosterone-binding protein.[19] Further studies are necessary to determine whether this binding protein is an intracellular receptor.

Masculinization of the external genitalia and urogenital sinus of the fetus results from the action of dihydrotestosterone, which is converted from testosterone in the target cells by the enzyme 5-α-reductase.[20] Dihydrotestosterone is bound to a cytosol androgen receptor (binding protein) in the target cell. It is translocated to the nucleus of the cell where chromatin binding occurs, which initiates DNA-directed RNA-mediated transcription and results in androgen-induced differentiation and growth of the cell. The gene for the cytosol androgen-binding protein is located on the X chromosome.[21] Thus, an X-linked gene controls the androgen response of all somatic cell types by specifying the nuclear cytosol androgen receptor protein.[5]

As in the case of the genital ducts, there is an inherent tendency for the external genitalia and urogenital sinus to feminize. Differentiation of the external genitalia along male lines will occur only if androgenic stimulation is received early in fetal life (Fig. 106-5). In particular, dihydrotestosterone and its specific cytosol receptor must be present to effect masculinization. Dihydrotestosterone stimulates growth of the genital tubercle, fusion of the urethral folds, and descent of the labioscrotal swellings to form the penis and scrotum. Androgenic hormones also inhibit growth of

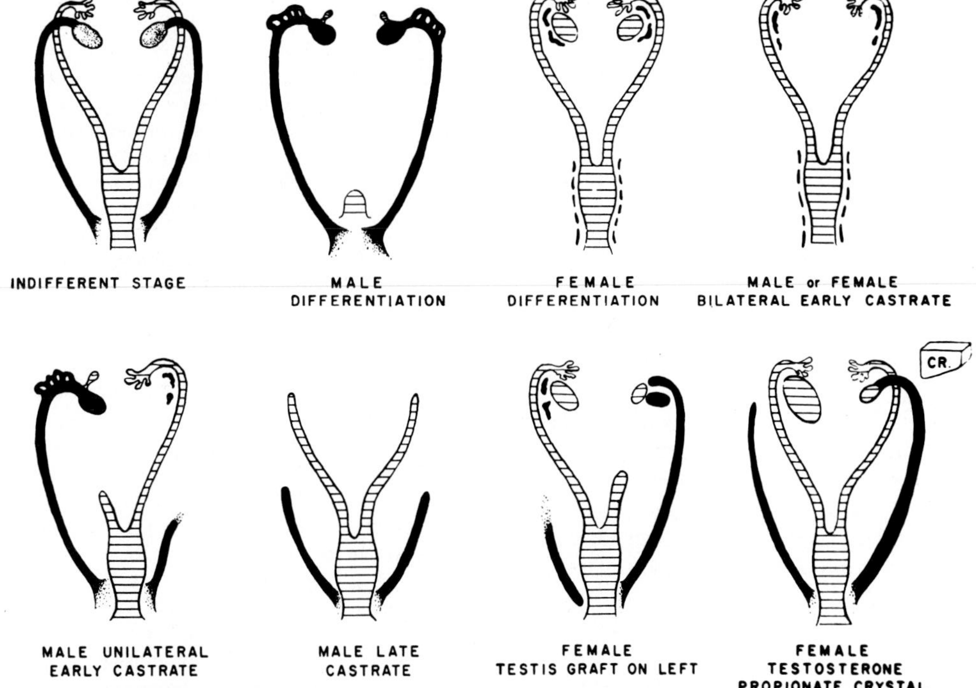

Fig. 106-4. Summary of Jost's rabbit embryo experiments.[1] Testosterone stimulates wolffian development but has no effect on müllerian duct inhibitory factor, a macromolecule secreted by the fetal Sertoli cells. (From Grumbach, M. M. and Van Wyk, J., in *Textbook of Endocrinology,* 5th ed., R. H. Williams (ed.), Philadelphia, W. B. Saunders Co., 1974.

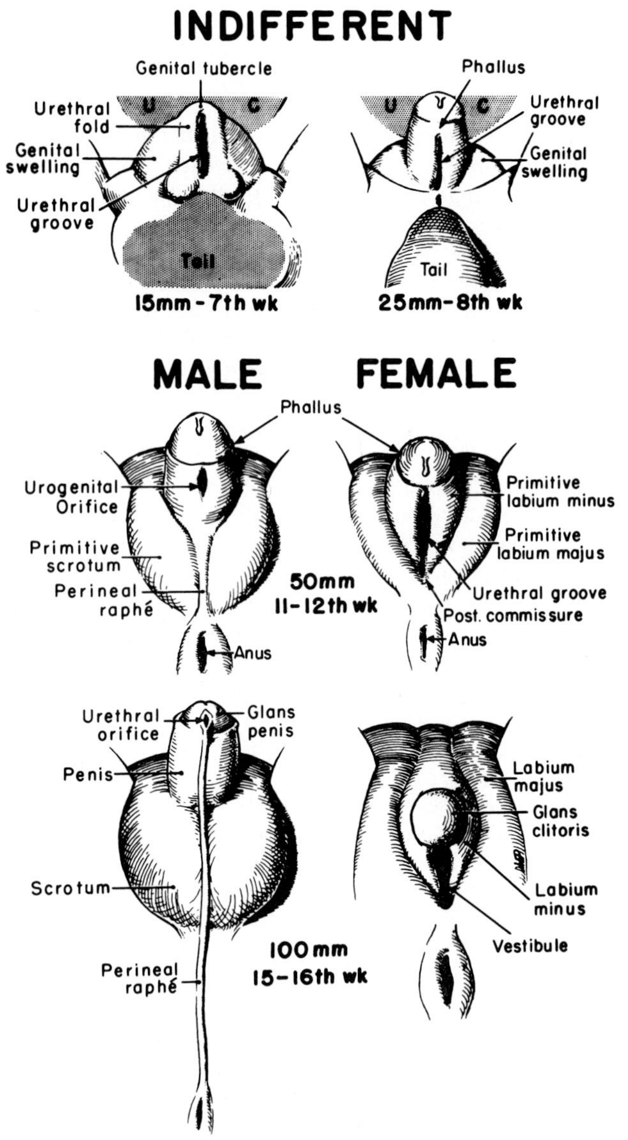

Fig. 106-5. Diagrammatic representation of differentiation of the external genitalia of the male and female fetus from the bipotential precursor. Masculinization of the external genitalia of the male is mediated by the action of dihydrotestosterone on the genital tubercle, urethral folds, labioscrotal swellings, and urogenital sinus. (From Grumbach, M. M. and Ducharme, J., *Fertil. Steril. 11:* 157, 1960).

the vesicovaginal septum and differentiation of the vagina. There is a critical period for the action of androgen. After the 12th week of gestation, fusion of the labioscrotal folds will not occur even under intense androgen stimulation, although phallic growth can be induced.

Fetal testicular Leydig cells proliferate at about 60 days after conception and, in the normal male fetus, androgens produced by those cells bring about masculinization of the internal and external genitalia. Siiteri and Wilson showed that the capacity of the fetal testis of the rabbit to synthesize testosterone is associated with the appearance of the enzyme 3-β-hydroxysteroid dehydrogenase.[18] Any impairment in production of fetal testosterone, its conversion to dihydrotestosterone, the cytosol and/or nuclear binding of dihydrotestosterone, or the production and local action of müllerian duct inhibitory factor will lead to incomplete masculinization of the male fetus. Exposure of the female fetus to abnormal amounts of androgen, either from endogenous or exogenous sources—especially prior to 12 weeks of gestation—will result in virilization of the external genitalia.

CLASSIFICATION (TABLE 106-1)

In the past, individuals with hermaphrodism have been classified according to their gonadal morphology. In the terminology of Klebs, a true hermaphrodite is a person who possesses both

Table 106-1. Abnormalities of Sex Differentiation

I. Disorders of gonadal differentiation
  - A. Seminiferous tubule dysgenesis and its variants (Klinefelter syndrome)
  - B. Syndrome of gonadal dysgenesis and its variants (Turner syndrome)
  - C. Familial and sporadic XX and XY gonadal dysgenesis and their variants
  - D. True hermaphrodism

II. Female pseudohermaphrodism
  - A. Congenital virilizing adrenal hyperplasia
  - B. Androgens and synthetic progestins transferred from maternal circulation
  - C. Malformations of intestinal and urinary tract
  - D. Other teratologic factors

III. Male pseudohermaphrodism
  - A. Testicular unresponsiveness of hCG and LH
  - B. Inborn errors of testosterone biosynthesis
    - 1. Errors affecting synthesis of both corticosteroids and testosterone (variants of congenital adrenal hyperplasia)
      - a. Cholesterol desmolase complex deficiency (congenital lipoid adrenal hyperplasia)
      - b. 3-β-hydroxysteroid dehydrogenase deficiency
      - c. 17-α-hydroxylase deficiency
    - 2. Errors primarily affecting testosterone biosynthesis
      - a. 17,20-desmolase (lyase) deficiency
      - b. 17-β-hydroxysteroid oxidoreductase deficiency
  - C. Defects in androgen-dependent target tissues
    - 1. End-organ insensitivity to androgenic hormones (androgen receptor defects)
      - a. Complete syndrome of testicular feminization and its variants (androgen insensitivity and its variants)
      - b. Incomplete syndrome of testicular feminization (incomplete androgen insensitivity and its variants)
    - 2. Inborn errors in testosterone metabolism by peripheral tissues
      - a. 5-α-reductase deficiency—male pseudohermaphrodism with normal virilization at puberty (familial perineal hypospadias with ambiguous development of urogenital sinus and male puberty)
  - D. Dysgenetic male pseudohermaphrodism
    - 1. X chromatin-negative variants of the syndrome of gonadal dysgenesis (e.g., XO/XY, XYp-)
    - 2. Incomplete form of familial XY gonadal dysgenesis
    - 3. Associated with degenerative renal disease
    - 4. Congenital anorchia (''vanishing testes'') syndrome with male pseudohermaphrodism (XY agonadism; XY gonadal agenesis)
  - E. Defect in synthesis, secretion, or response to müllerian duct inhibitory factor:
    Female genital ducts in otherwise normal men—''uteri herniae inguinale''; persistent müllerian duct syndrome
  - F. Maternal ingestion of estrogens or progestins

IV. Unclassified forms of abnormal sexual development
  - A. In males
    - 1. Hypospadias
    - 2. Ambiguous external genitalia in XY males with multiple cengenital anomalies
    - 3. Familial forms of primary hypogonadism and gynecomastia (Rosewater syndrome)
  - B. In females
    - 1. Absence or anomalous development of the vagina, uterus and fallopian tubes (Rokitansky-Küstner syndrome)

Modified from Grumbach, M. M. and Van Wyk, J. J.[2]

ovarian and testicular tissue. A male pseudohermaphrodite is one whose gonads are exclusively testes but whose genital ducts or external genitalia, or both, exhibit the phenotypic characteristics of a female or incompletely differentiated male. A female pseudohermaphrodite is a person with exclusively ovarian gonadal structures, whose external genitalia exhibit some masculine characteristics. Utilizing the rapidly advancing knowledge of chromosomal and biochemical defects, we have classified errors in sex differentiation by a modification and expansion of this broad framework.[2,2a] We have attempted to blend etiologic mechanisms and clinical entities into a simplified rational classification. The striking clinical and etiologic heterogeneity of syndromes presenting with similar anatomic findings merits emphasis.

DISORDERS OF GONADAL DIFFERENTIATION

SEMINIFEROUS TUBULE DYSGENESIS XXY SEMINIFEROUS TUBULE DYSGENESIS (KLINEFELTER SYNDROME, KLINEFELTER SYNDROME AND ITS VARIANTS)

Seminiferous tubule dysgenesis, the most common form of male hypogonadism, was first defined in 1942 by Klinefelter, Reifenstein, and Albright. It is characterized by eunuchoidism, gynecomastia, azoospermia, elevated gonadotropins, and small, firm testes (<3.5cm in length).[22] The testes show hyalinization, fibrosis and dysgenesis of the seminiferous tubules, Leydig cell hyperplasia, and absence of elastic fibers around the tunica propria of the tubules.[23]

In 1956, several groups found that a high proportion of patients with this syndrome were X chromatin-positive. Soon thereafter, the syndrome was separated into the X chromatin-positive and the X chromatin-negative forms, with subtle differences between the two groups. Mental retardation is more frequently associated with the chromatin-positive form of seminiferous tubule dysgenesis.[22]

In 1959, the XXY sex chromosome constitution was reported, thus explaining the positive sex chromatin pattern. Later, sex chromosome mosaicism and three or more X chromosomes in a karyotype that includes a Y chromosome were described in association with the clinical spectrum of Klinefelter's syndrome, as well as a variant with an XX sex chromosome complement.

Clinical Features (Fig. 106-6)

The only constant features of chromatin-positive seminiferous tubule dysgenesis are small, firm testes that measure <3.5 cm in length, histologic evidence of impaired spermatogenesis, and a male phenotype. Prepubertally, Klinefelter's syndrome is rarely recognized, although three features should suggest this diagnosis: tall stature with abnormally long legs,[24] mental retardation, and small genitalia. Tall stature as a result of excessive leg length is a characteristic feature of Klinefelter's syndrome; prior to and after puberty, patients tend to be taller than their fathers or brothers. When present prepubertally, this stigmata of seminiferous tubule dysgenesis is not a result of androgen insufficiency, since boys with anorchia and presumptive prepubertal androgen insufficiency do not have long legs. In general, there is no delay of the onset of puberty in affected patients.[25] Prepubertally, gonadotropin levels and responses to luteinizing hormone-releasing factor (LRF) are

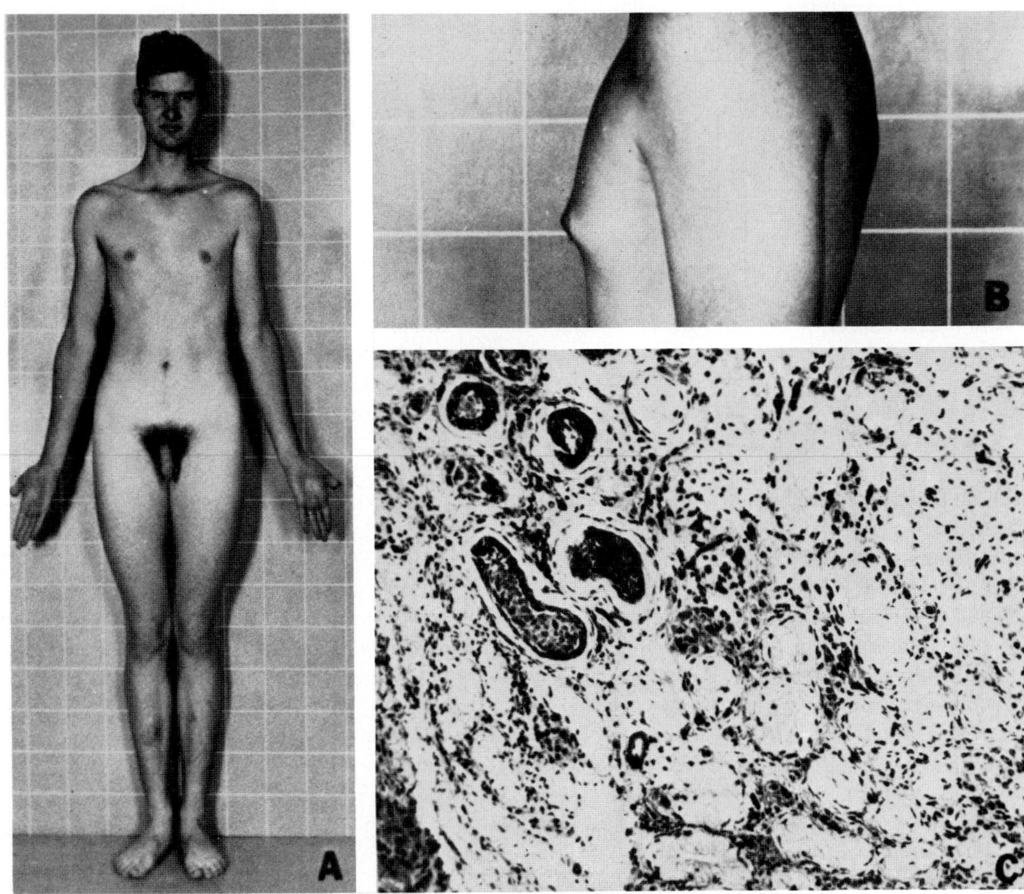

Figure 106-6. A 19-year-old chromatin-positive male with an XXY karyotype. His gonadotropins were elevated. Note normal virilization with long legs and (B) gynecomastia. (C) Testicular biopsy revealed hyalinization, dysgenesis of the seminiferous tubules and Leydig cell hyperplasia. (From Grumbach, M. M. and Van Wyk, J., in *Textbook of Endocrinology,* 5th ed., R. H. Williams (ed.), Philadelphia, W. B. Saunders Co., 1974.)

within the normal range,[26] and histologic studies of the gonads reveal only a reduction of spermatogonia. With the onset of puberty, progressive histologic changes and a decreased ability of the testicular tissue to synthesize testosterone become apparent.[2]

The prevalence of Klinefelter's syndrome in newborn males is 2.1 per 1000, similar to that in the adult male population (1.5–2.4 per 1000); its frequency in mentally deficient individuals is significantly higher than in the normal population, emphasizing the relationship of mental retardation to this syndrome.[27] Even in the absence of mental deficiency, many of the patients have behavioral disorders.

Postpubertally, small, firm testes, gynecomastia, and decreased androgenicity suggest the presence of the Klinefelter syndrome. Leydig cell function is usually impaired to varying degrees, resulting in low-normal to low plasma testosterone concentrations with incomplete development of secondary sexual characteristics and elevated gonadotropins, particularly follicle-stimulating hormone (FSH). Leydig cell reserve is diminished, as demonstrated by a decreased response to the administration of chorionic gonadotropin.[28] The testosterone production rate, the total and free levels of testosterone, and the metabolic clearance rates of testosterone and estradiol tend to be low. The concentration of plasma estradiol may be elevated. An increased peripheral conversion of testosterone to estradiol was noted in 19 patients.[29] The threshold for suppression of luteinizing hormone (LH) and FSH by sex steroids appears to be increased in classic Klinefelter's syndrome, since LH and FSH are suppressed only by sustained high levels of testosterone.[29]

In most patients there is prominent gynecomastia, the mechanism of which is still uncertain but may be attributable, at least in part, to an increased ratio of estradiol to testosterone. The concentration of serum prolactin is normal, but an augmented prolactin response to thyrotropin-releasing factor has been described. The testicular failure is progressive but in some instances may not be clinically evident until middle age, when signs of androgen deficiency and gynecomastia first appear.

Associated Abnormalities

An increased frequency of mild diabetes mellitus, emphysema, chronic bronchitis, varicose veins, and neoplasia has been described.[22] An increased predisposition to cancer of the breast in XXY patients with gynecomastia has been reported, and in a study of 187 males with breast cancer, 8 had an XXY karyotype.[30,31]

Testicular Lesion

Studies in preterm infants indicate that the histology of the testes is normal in patients with the Klinefelter syndrome; in later infancy, subtle changes, such as diminished spermatogonia, are detected.[2] With the appearance of puberty, apparently gonadotropin-induced hyalinization of the seminiferous tubules and pseudoadenomatous clumping of Leydig cells occurs.[2] After puberty, the testes are characterized by hyalinization and fibrosis of the seminiferous tubules, absence of elastic fibers around the tunica propria of the tubules, and apparent Leydig cell hyperplasia. Clusters of tubules may contain only Sertoli cells, while those severely involved are hyalinized, shrunken, and fibrotic. Grumbach and Van Wyk have demonstrated that gonadotropin plays a role in the testicular pathology. In a 7-year-old male with 48,XXXY karyotype and precocious puberty, there was extensive pathology in the testes, as opposed to the mild changes noted in age-matched controls with this syndrome.[2]

XXY males may result from nondisjunction of the sex chromosomes either during the first or second meiotic division in either parent or from mitotic nondisjunction in the zygote at the time of or following fertilization. Thus, fertilization of an XX ovum by a Y-bearing sperm, or an X ovum by an XY-bearing sperm, would result in an XXY zygote. Ferguson-Smith and others found a positive association between maternal age in patients with an XXY karyotype, which suggested that a proportion of XXY cases result from nondisjunction during oogenesis. Sanger et al. subsequently reported 20 patients in whom the parental origin of the XXY karyotype was adduced by the X-linked red cell antigen Xg;[32] 13 involved a maternal meiotic error and 7 a paternal one. Mitotic nondisjunction of an XY zygote would lead to an XXY cell and a YO cell, the latter being nonviable. Both mechanisms are probably operative in man. 47,XXX females appear particularly prone to produce males with a 47,XXY karyotype.[33]

Diagnosis and Treatment

The diagnosis of the XXY form of Klinefelter syndrome is established by the finding of a chromatin-positive buccal smear and the demonstration of an XXY karyotype in blood, skin, or gonads. Serum and urinary gonadotropins, especially FSH levels, are usually elevated, and plasma testosterone tends to be low. Testicular biopsy reveals the classic findings.

Treatment of patients with Klinefelter syndrome is directed toward correction of androgen deficiency (if present). Androgen replacement therapy with testosterone enanthate in oil, 200–300 mg im each 3 to 4 weeks, will usually produce adequate virilization. Oral replacement therapy is less effective clinically; recently, methylated testosterone derivatives have been implicated in adenomatous changes in the liver. Gynecomastia is not amenable to hormonal therapy; for cosmetic or psychologic reasons, plastic surgery may be necessary for its amelioration.

VARIANT FORMS OF X CHROMATIN-POSITIVE SEMINIFEROUS TUBULE DYSGENESIS

XY/XXY mosaicism is the second most common chromosome complement associated with the Klinefelter phenotype. Mosaicism with an XY cell line may modify the clinical syndrome and result in less gynecomastia as well as a lesser degree of testicular damage.[22,23] Mean testosterone levels tend to be higher in XY/XXY mosaics than in XXY patients. Fertility has been reported in XY/XXY patients but not in 47,XXY patients. In order to rule out XY/XXY mosaicism, cultures for karyotype analysis should be obtained from two or more tissues and a sufficient (50 or more) number of cells should be examined from each tissue. Therapy in these patients depends on the severity of the clinical and gonadal aberrations associated with the XXY cell line.

XXYY

These patients comprise 3 percent of the chromatin-positive males. In addition to the usual characteristics of Klinefelter's syndrome, they tend to be tall (mean height 181 cm compared with 172 cm for XXY males), have unusual dermatoglyphics, and almost all reported cases have been mentally retarded.[21,34] Testicular histology is similar to that observed in the classic form of Klinefelter's syndrome.[23] These patients are sex chromatin-positive and, in addition, have two Y-fluorescent bodies in interphase cells studied with quinacrine fluorescence. Karyotype analysis will establish the definitive diagnosis. Therapy with testosterone is similar to that in patients with classic 47,XXY Klinefelter syndrome.

XXXY

All patients reported with this form have had significant mental retardation; developmental anomalies (short neck, epicanthal folds, radioulnar synostosis, and clinodactyly) are present in 50 percent of the patients.[2,35] The diagnosis is made by finding two chromatin bodies in a proportion of interphase nuclei as well as a Y body or by demonstrating an XXXY karyotype.

XXXXY

These patients are more severely affected than those with lesser number of X's[2,22] In addition to severe mental retardation (highest IQ 53), they have had radioulnar synostosis, hypoplastic external genitalia with a small penis, and cryptorchid testes. Other anomalies may also be present, such as congenital heart disease, cleft palate, strabismus, and microcephaly. The mandibular prognathism, hypertelorism, and myopia give a characteristic facies. Three sex chromatin bodies are present in a variable proportion of the interphase nuclei as well as a Y body by fluorescent microscopy.

XX Males

46,XX males are an interesting variant of the Klinefelter syndrome. The incidence of XX males is quite low; in a prospective chromosomal survey of 64,000 infants,[36] only 2 cases were found. de la Chappelle reviewed 45 such patients and demonstrated that, clinically, XX males resemble those with XXY Klinefelter syndrome.[37] In general, they have a male phenotype, male psychosocial identification, testes without evidence of ovarian tissue, male genital ducts, and no müllerian structures. At least 10 percent have been reported to have hypospadias or ambiguous genitalia (Fig. 106-7). Their body proportions are normal, and mean height is 168.2 cm, which is shorter than that in XXY males.[37] Associated anomalies are rare. The incidence of mental retardation is apparently less than in patients with an XXY karyotype and may not be increased. The prevalence of gynecomastia is similar to that in the Klinefelter syndrome, and the testes usually measure <3.5 cm in maximal diameter. As in XXY males, testosterone levels are often low and gonadotropins are elevated. The testosterone response to hCG may be impaired. The histologic features of the testes in XX males closely resemble those of XXY Klinefelter syndrome.

The presence of testes and male differentiation in 46,XX individuals has been a perplexing problem. Three different explanations have been suggested: (1) hidden mosaicism; an undetected cell line containing a Y chromosome could be present; (2) insertion, or interchange or translocation between a Y and an X or an autosome could lead to the location of masculinizing genes on the paternal X chromosome or an autosome; and (3) male development could be the result of a mutant gene. de la Chappelle studied the inheritance of the Xg blood group in XX males and suggested that, at least in some instances, the two X chromosomes were of maternal origin, consistent with an XXY cell line that was cryptic.[37] Several authors have described Y fluorescence in Sertoli cells from males with a 46,XX karyotype,[38,39] but recently this observation has been questioned as artifactual.[40] The detection of H-Y antigen in 46,XX males makes the Y-X or Y-autosome translocation or Y-gene insertion hypothesis more appealing.[10] Two XX males have been reported in whom one of the X chromosomes was slightly longer than the other, suggesting Y-X translocation.[10] In support of the cryptic XXY cell line hypothesis, H-Y antigen has been detected in 46,XX males with a small number of XXY cells.[10] Y autosome insertion, such as that suggested in the sex reversed (Sxn) XX male mouse which is transmitted as an autosomal dominant, or an autosomal gene, such as "polled," which is found in goats in association with XX males and true hermaphrodites, may play a role in testicular differentiation in some XX males.[40] The diagnosis of 46,XX male should be suspected in a patient with the phenotypic findings of the Klinefelter syndrome. Karyotype analysis of multiple tissues will reveal only a 46,XX chromosome count and no bright Y chromosome fluorescence in metaphase or interphase cells. The XX males provide a link with XX true hermaphroditism (see p. 1330).

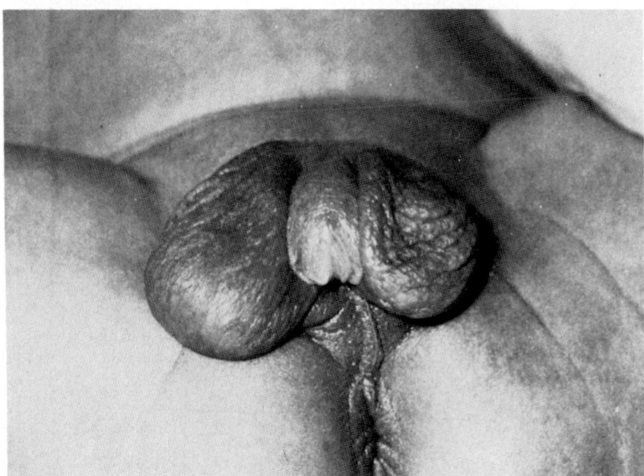

Fig. 106-7. The external genitalia of a 46,XX male infant. Note lack of complete descent of scrotum (saddlebag scrotum), as well as phallus bound down in chordee. A single perineal opening, the urethral orifice, was present at the base of the phallus; no vaginal pouch was present. The internal ducts were male. Both testes were palpable in the scrotum, and biopsy revealed "normal" prepubertal testes.

SYNDROME OF GONADAL DYSGENESIS—TURNER SYNDROME AND ITS VARIANTS

In 1938, Turner described 7 phenotypic females with sexual infantilism, short stature, webbing of the neck, and cubitus valgus.[41] There were earlier descriptions of this syndrome, but they lacked the impact of Turner's report. Early studies indicated that urinary gonadotropins were elevated, and it was suggested that gonadal failure was the cause of the sexual infantilism. In 1959, it was reported that the sex chromosome constitution of the typical patient was 45,X, which explained the previous observation that they were usually chromatin-negative. The XO karyotype is associated with four cardinal features: female phenotype, short stature, lack of secondary sexual characteristics, and a variety of somatic abnormalities. Sex chromosome mosaicism, as well as structural abnormalities of the X or Y chromosome, may modify all the features of this syndrome. Thus, it is useful to consider the syndrome of gonadal dysgenesis and its variants as a continuum of clinical features that range from the typical XO phenotype to normal male or female.

XO Gonadal Dysgenesis (Fig. 106-8)

Eighty percent of patients with the phenotypic stigmata of Turner syndrome are buccal chromatin-negative, and most of them have a 45,X karyotype. There are a number of somatic stigmata associated with this syndrome; however, only short stature and sexual infantilism are relatively invariable manifestations of the 45,X karyotype.[2,3,27,36,42,43] Typically, the patient with the XO karyotype has a distinctive facies characterized by micrognathia, epicanthal folds, low-set and/or deformed ears, a fishlike mouth, and ptosis; the palate may be high-arched and the dentition abnormal.[44] The chest is broad and shieldlike, and the areolae are often hypoplastic. The neck may be short, with a low hairline in back. Webbing of the neck (pterygium), present in 40 percent of these patients, apparently results from fibrosis of the loose skin folds in the retrocervical area in newborns with Turner syndrome who

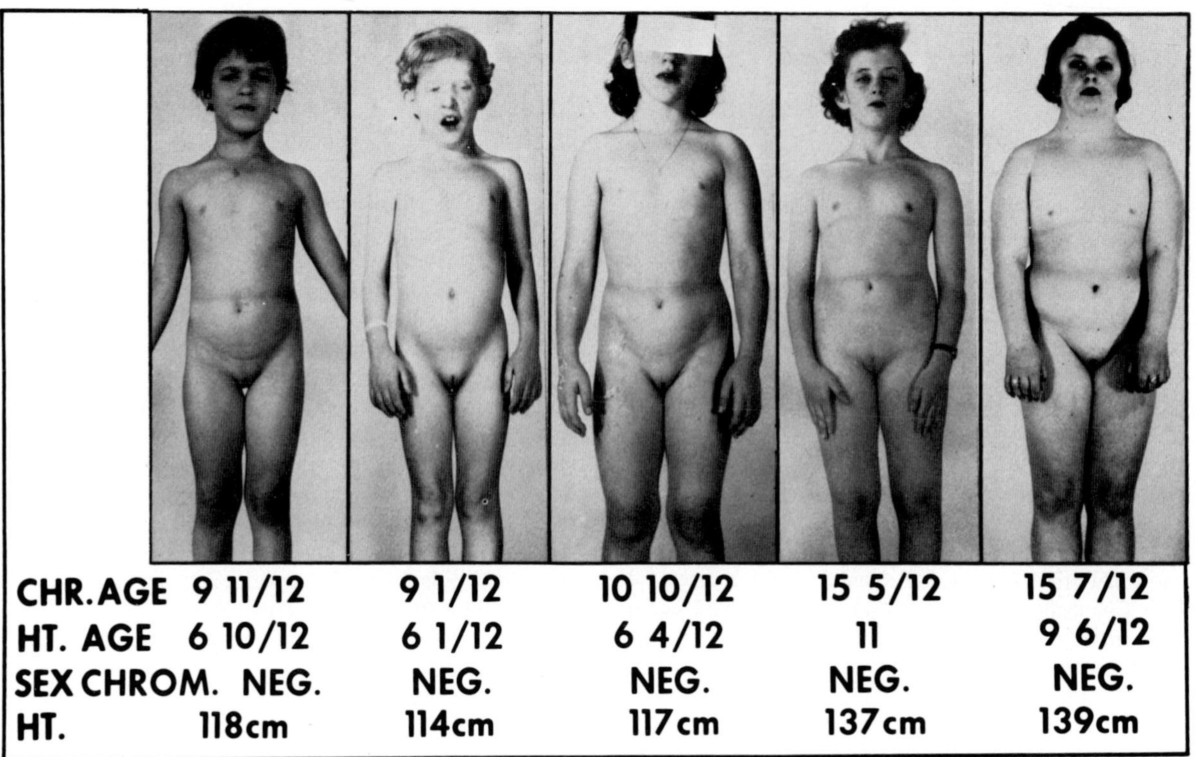

CHR.AGE 9 11/12 9 1/12 10 10/12 15 5/12 15 7/12
HT. AGE 6 10/12 6 1/12 6 4/12 11 9 6/12
SEX CHROM. NEG. NEG. NEG. NEG. NEG.
HT. 118cm 114cm 117cm 137cm 139cm

Fig. 106-8. Phenotypic spectrum of patients with 45,XO gonadal dysgenesis (Turner syndrome). (From Grumbach, M. M., in *Clinical Endocrinology, I*, E. B. Astwood (ed.), New York, Grune & Stratton, 1960, p. 407.)

have had a retrocervical cystic hygroma in utero. Additional features include strabismus and conduction deafness owing to recurrent otitis media.[45]

Congenital lymphedema of the hands and feet, which occurs in 30 to 40 percent of affected infants, is thought to be the result of hypoplasia of the lymphatic vessels (Fig. 106-9).[46] Although the lymphedema usually resolves during infancy, puffiness of the dorsum of the fingers and toes persists as a hallmark of this abnormality. Lymphedema may recur with estrogen replacement therapy. Short 4th metacarpals and metatarsals, and cubitus valgus are encountered in 50 percent of the patients. As with cubitus valgus, short metacarpals occur with growth postnatally and are not found in the newborn infant.

Of importance are the structural abnormalities of the kidney found in 50 percent of patients: horseshoe kidney, retrocaval ureters, double collecting systems, unilateral renal aplasia, and other anomalies that predispose these patients to obstructive uropathies and infection. All patients with gonadal dysgenesis should have an intravenous pyelogram routinely as a part of their evaluation.

Other phenotypic stigmata include an excessive number of pigmented nevi, a tendency to keloid formation, hypoplastic nails, unexplained hypertension, and, rarely, gastrointestinal bleeding secondary to intestinal telangiectasia.[2] No increase in severe mental retardation has been noted.[47] Money has reported that impairment of directional sense and space-form recognition is common.[48] This congenital disability results in a lower mean performance IQ than in the general population, but verbal ability is not affected.

In newborn infants, the term *Bonnevie Ullrich syndrome* has been applied to patients with the Turner syndrome, with lymphedema and loose posterior cervical skin folds. Pleural effusions and ascites that resolve spontaneously are not uncommon in affected newborns.[49]

The cardiovascular anomalies of gonadal dysgenesis predomi-

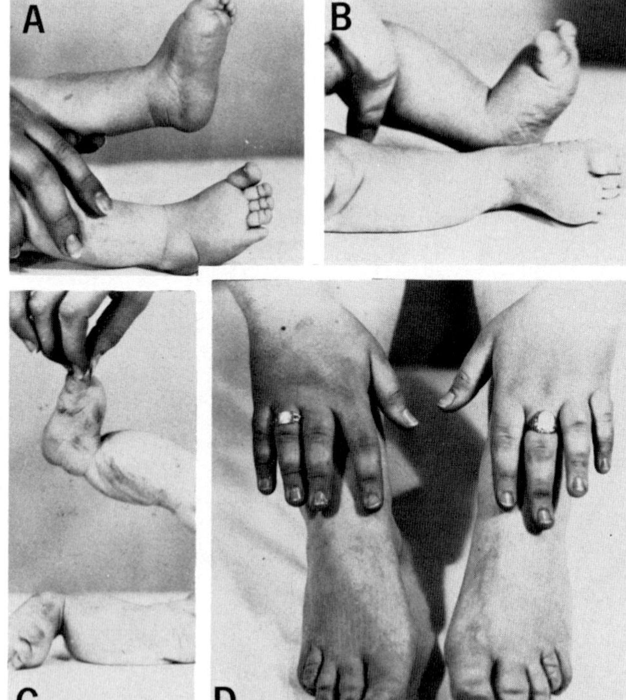

Fig. 106-9. (A,B,C) Lymphedema of the lower extremities in newborn and young infants with an XO karyotype. (D) Puffiness of the dorsum of the fingers and toes, which is a residuum of the infantile lymphedema in an adolescent female with a 45,XO karyotype. The 4th metacarpals and metatarsals are short. (From Grumbach, M. M. *Pediatrics 20:* 740, 1957.)

nently affect the left side of the heart. In addition to coarctation of the aorta (10 to 20 percent), aortic stenosis and bicuspid aortic valves may occur as combined or separate defects. Mutiple skeletal anomalies have been described radiographically.

Osteoporosis of the bones, hands, feet, and spine are common even prepubertally; adults who are not treated with estrogens may develop a severe form of osteoporosis. Osteochondrosis of the spine has been described.[50] A decreased carpal arch (mean angle <117°) and deformities of the medial tibial condyles are common radiologic findings.

Short stature is an invariable feature of the XO patient; mean final height is usually 140 cm, with a range of 122–147 cm and with a significant correlation between final height and midparental height. Growth failure may occur in utero. Patients are usually small at birth, grow slowly, fail to have a pubertal growth spurt, and end up short.[51] No abnormality in growth hormone secretion has been demonstrated. Normal or elevated levels of serum somatomedin have been reported in patients with short stature and the Turner syndrome.[44] Variable growth responses to growth hormone have been described. It has been suggested that anabolic steroids may result in a modest augmentation of final height, but their value remains controversial. Of note is the case report of a woman with the typical syndrome who had a growth hormone secreting pituitary tumor and whose height increased from 139 to 154 cm between 18 and 28 years.[52]

Singh and Carr studied the gonadal ridges of eight 45,X fetuses who ranged in gestational age from 5 weeks to 4 months.[53] They demonstrated the presence of primordial germ cells and were unable to distinguish the gonadal histology from that of normal female fetuses up to 3 months of gestation. Thereafter, there was impaired formation of primordial follicles. The evidence suggests that primordial germ cells seed the primitive gonad in a 45,X fetus but usually fail to mature into oocytes, and degenerate at an accelerated rate.[2]

Longitudinal studies of plasma gonadotropin concentrations in patients with gonadal dysgenesis demonstrate a lack of feedback inhibition of the hypothalamic-pituitary axis by the gonad in the neonatal period. Fifty-eight patients, aged 2 days to 20 years, with the syndrome of gonadal dysgenesis were studied by Conte and Grumbach (Fig. 106-10).[54] An elevation in basal plasma FSH was noted as early as 5 days after birth. Mean plasma FSH between 2 days and 4 years of age was 43 ng/ml (LER-869), which is strikingly elevated. A fall to a mean of 4 ng/ml occurred between 4 and 10 years of age; after 10 years of age, FSH rose again into the agonadal range. Thus, plasma FSH levels described a diphasic curve qualitatively similar to but quantitatively higher than that in normal infants and children. LH levels followed a curve similar to FSH but the concentration was one third to one tenth that of FSH.

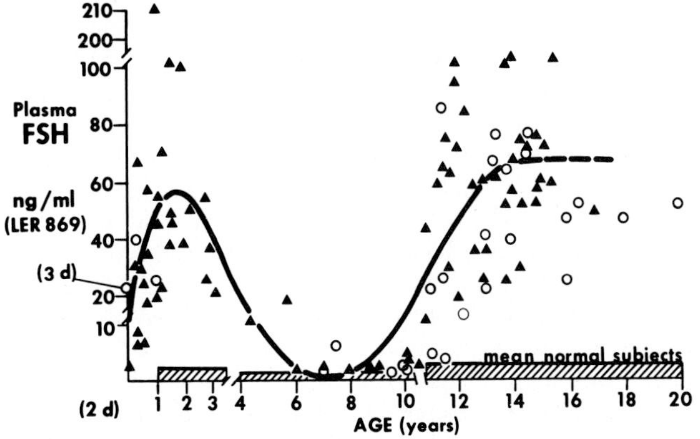

Fig. 106-10. Pattern of plasma FSH (concentration) in relation to age in 58 patients with the syndrome of gonadal dysgenesis. ▲ = XO karyotype; 0 = patients with structural abnormalities of the X chromosome and mosaics. The hatched area indicates the mean range for FSH values in normal females. (From Conte, F. A., Kaplan, S. L., and Grumbach, M. M., *J. Clin. Endocrinol. Metab. 40:* 670, 1975.)

The appearance of pubic hair is usually delayed; the distribution is normal, but the amount is usually reduced. Maturation of other secondary sexual characteristics usually does not occur, and these patients usually remain sexually infantile and amenorrheic. A small number have achieved menarche,[55] and rarely pregnancy has been reported.[56] McDonough et al. described an XO patient who feminized completely and had sporadic episodes of menstrual bleeding;[57] a theca lutein cyst was found in her dysgenetic gonad. The rarity of estrogen production in XO patients who do *not* have evidence of mosaicism makes gonadal investigation mandatory to rule out a gonadal tumor when there are clinical signs of estrogen secretion.

The gonad in the adult is usually a white fibrous streak located in the position normally occupied by the ovary. The streak is characterized by dense fibrous stroma in whorls with absent oocytes, and at puberty, hilar cells may be found. The external genitalia usually are unambiguously female. Clitoromegaly may be found occasionally in XO patients, or XO/XX mosaics, but is more often associated with a cell line containing a Y chromosome. The uterus, cervix, and fallopian tubes are structurally normal but infantile.

With XO gonadal dysgenesis, obesity is common, and there is an increased prevalence of Hashimoto's thyroiditis and "adult" type diabetes mellitus.[2]

Chromatin-negative gonadal dysgenesis occurs in 1 per 2700 live newborn infants; however, Carr found that 5 percent of spontaneous abortuses had XO karyotypes.[58] It is estimated that XO zygotes represent the most common karyotype anomaly in man but that <1 percent of XO conceptuses survive to term.

The XO chromosome constitution may arise as a consequence of nondisjunction or chromosome loss during gametogenesis in either parent, resulting in a sperm or ovum lacking a sex chromosome. Mitotic error may also play a role in the pathogenesis of the Turner syndrome, since there is no association with maternal age as in Down's syndrome. The increased incidence of sex chromosome mosaicism in the Turner syndrome, as well as the occurrence of an XY co-twin of an XO individual, all support mitotic error as one factor in the pathogenesis of an XO karyotype. Family studies, utilizing X-linked markers, such as the Xg blood group, color blindness, and erythrocyte glucose phosphate dehydrogenase, indicate that the paternally derived sex chromosome is more frequently lost than would be expected from random distribution.[59] Familial cases of gonadal dysgenesis are exceedingly rare.[60] A relationship has been suggested between autoimmunity in the parents and patients and a predilection for the sex chromosomal aberrations leading to the syndrome of gonadal dysgenesis.[61] The frequency of twinning in the siblings of XO patients is increased.

Mosaicism and Structural Abnormalities of the X Chromosome (Table 106-2)

Approximately 20 percent of patients with the typical syndrome of gonadal dysgenesis are sex chromatin-positive. Patients in this group usually have a structural aberration of the X chromosome or sex chromosome mosaicism involving an XO cell line. Both sex chromosome mosaicism and structural aberrations of the X chromosome can modify the phenotypic and gonadal manifestations of the syndrome of gonadal dysgenesis.

Table 106-2. Nomenclature for Describing the Human Karyotype Pertinent to Designating Sex Chromosome Abnormalities

Chicago and Paris Conferences	Description	Former Nomenclature
46,XX	Normal female karyotype	XX
46,XY	Normal male karyotype	XY
47,XXY	Karyotype with 47 chromosomes, including an extra sex chromosome	XXY
45,X	One sex chromosome absent	XO
45,X/46,XY	Mosaic karyotype composed of 45,X and 46,XY cell lines	XO/XY
p	Short arm	
q	Long arm	
Xp−	Deletion of the short arm of the X	
Xq−	Deletion of the long arm of the X	
i(Xq)	Isochromosome of the long arm of X	
i(Xp)	Isochromosome of the short arm or X	
r(X)	Ring-X chromosome	
46,X, t(Xq−;9p+)	Translocation of the long arm of X onto the short arm of chromosome No. 9	
dic(Y)	Dicentric Y chromosome	
i(Yp)	Isochromosome of the short arm of Y	
i(Yq)	Isochromosome of the long arm of Y	

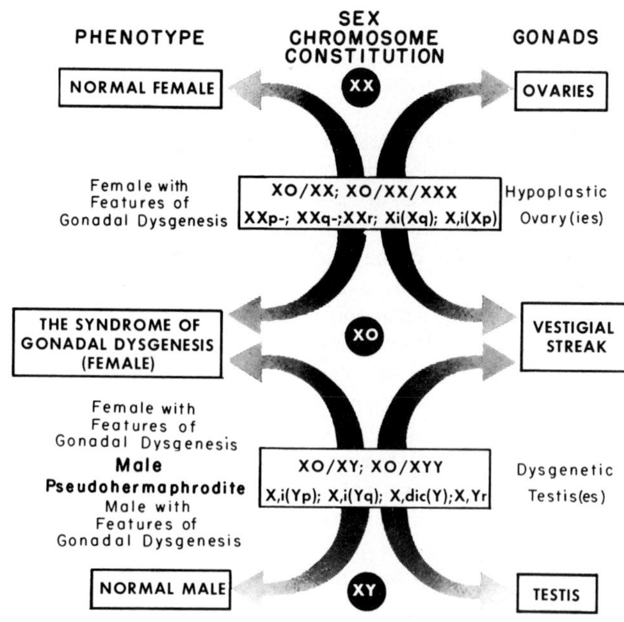

Fig. 106-11. Range of phenotypic and gonadal expression that occurs in the variants of the syndrome of gonadal dysgenesis, and its relationship to the sex chromosome constitution. The typical phenotypic and gonadal expression of the 45,XO karyotype may be modified by the presence of a mosaic chromosomal constitution or by the presence of a structurally abnormal second sex chromosome. Thus, XO/XX mosaics generally have less phenotypic stigmata than XO patients. In some cases of XO/XX mosaicism, normal ovarian development and function have been documented. Likewise, patients with XO/XY mosaicism or structurally abnormal Y chromosomes have varying degrees of testicular differentiation. The differentiation of the genitalia may thus extend from phenotypic female through pseudohermaphrodism to a phenotypic male with phallic urethra, depending on the functional integrity of the testis present. Similarly, the phenotypic stigmata of the syndrome of gonadal dysgenesis may be modified by the presence of the mosaic cell line or a structurally abnormal Y chromosome. (From Grumbach, M. M., in *Biologic Basis of Pediatric Practice*, R. E. Cooke (ed.), New York, McGraw-Hill, 1967.)

It has been postulated that the ratio of XO to XX or XY primordial germ cells or blastemal components is the major determinant of whether the ultimate gonadal structure will be a streak gonad, a hypoplastic ovary or testis, or a relatively normal gonad.[2] Likewise, the quantitative relationship of XO cell lines to XX or XY cell lines in peripheral tissue may affect the phenotypic stigmata of patients with the syndrome of gonadal dysgenesis. In patients with structurally abnormal X chromosomes, phenotypic karyotypic correlations suggest that somatic and gonadal consequences are related to the nature and degree of deficiency of the long and short arms of the X chromosome.[2,62,63]

Mosaicism with Structurally Normal X Chromosomes: XO/XX,XO/XXX, XO/XX/XXX (Fig. 106-11)

Mosaicism with a normal cell line generally results in fewer somatic stigmata than in the XO patient.[2] The mean adult stature is greater in patients with mosaicism; 12 percent of those surveyed had at least one episode of menstruation compared with <3 percent in XO individuals.[63] Many XO/XX patients may never be detected because they lack phenotypic stigmata and have functioning ovaries. Fertility has been reported in patients with mosaicism—one of our patients gave birth to three normal children.[2] The gonads in XO/XX patients may be streaked, hypoplastic, or functionally normal. XO/XXX patients, like the XO/XX mosaics, have fewer stigmata than the XO group and may have normal gonadal function. XO/XX/XXX patients are rare, and the phenotype and gonadal function is variable, as with other mosaics. The sex chromatin pattern may provide clues to the presence of mosaicism. Patients in whom 2 to 19 percent of well-stained cells are chromatin-positive should be suspected of having an XO cell line. On the other hand, diploid nuclei with two sex chromatin bodies suggest the presence of a XXX cell line. Some 50 to 100 metaphase plates must be examined from multiple tissues before mosaicism can be excluded.

Isochromosome for the Long Arm of the X: X,i(Xq) and Mosaics XO/X,i(Xq). An isochromosome for the long arm of the X appears to be the most common structural rearrangement of the X chromosome. It is thought to represent a deficiency of the short arms and a duplication of the long arms of the X, resulting in a metacentric X whose arms are mirror images. This explanation of an isochromosome is probably simplistic, and these chromosomes may arise by more complex genetic rearrangements.

Isochromosomes of the long arm of the X chromosome can be both monocentric and dicentric. Patients with X,i(Xq) and XO/X,i(Xq) are short and have little or no gonadal function.[2,63] Webbed neck, coarctation of the aorta, and marked infantile lymphedema are infrequent, especially in the nonmosaic patients.[2,63] Patients with i(Xq) have an increased incidence of Hashimoto's thyroiditis and diabetes mellitus. In them, the sex chromatin body is larger than that in normals, since it is the structurally abnormal X chromosome that usually forms the sex chromatin body. Like all other structural rearrangements of the X chromosome, i(Xq) is frequently associated with an XO cell line. Apparently the structurally abnormal X is predisposed to loss at mitosis.

Isochromosome for the Short Arm of the X: X,i(Xp). Very few patients with this chromosomal anomaly have been reported. Of those documented by "Q" and "G" banding, all had primary amenorrhea, sexual infantilism, normal stature, and few, if any, stigmata of the syndrome of gonadal dysgenesis.[2,63–66] These patients support the hypothesis that genes for gonadal function are on both the long and short arm of the X chromosome, while those that influence stature and prevent the expression of the major somatic abnormalities appear to be situated mainly on the short arm of the X. As a result of the rarity of this abnormality, in comparison with the i(Xq) abnormality, it has been suggested that patients with this apparent structural aberration may actually have a simple long arm deletion.[67] Recently, de la Chapelle and Schröder reexamined their reported case of X,i(Xp) and now interpret this patient to have a terminal deletion of the long arm of the X chromosome.[68] Similarly, the case mentioned by Grumbach and Van Wyk most likely represents a simple long arm deletion.[2] Further study of other reported cases with newer banding techniques will be necessary to substantiate the existence of this anomaly of the X chromosome.

Short Arm Deletions: XXp- and XO/XXp-. Deletions of the short arm of the X chromosome usually result in gonadal dysgenesis, short stature, and the Turner stigmata whether or not they are associated with an XO cell line.[2] Three patients observed by Grumbach and Conte had 46,XXp- karyotypes. The extent of the phenotypic and gonadal manifestations of the syndrome of gonadal dysgenesis correlated with the magnitude of deletion of the short arm of the X chromosome. In the patient with the smallest deletion, fewer somatic stigmata, the presence of ovaries, and the development of female secondary sex characteristics and menses were noted.[2]

Long Arm Deletions: XXq- and XO/XXq-. Over 20 patients have been described with this anomaly of the X chromosome.[2,63] In general, they are normal in stature, have few, if any, stigmata of the Turner syndrome, and have primary amenorrhea and streak gonads. We have studied 2 patients with 46,XXq- karyotypes, utilizing C, Q, and G banding. Both patients were sexually infantile and over 5 feet tall, had no phenotypic stigmata of the syndrome of gonadal dysgenesis, and had elevated gonadotropins and increased LRF-induced gonadotropin responses. Exceptions to the rule that XXq- patients are of normal stature and lack any stigmata of the Turner syndrome have been reported.[69] Such cases may represent hidden mosaicism with an XO cell line or a more complex structural rearrangement of the X chromosome, including interstitial rather than terminal deletions.[70]

In general, the evidence from deletion mapping of the X chromosome suggests that: (1) gonadal determiners are located on both the long and short arms of the X chromosome, so that patients with p or q deletions tend to have streak gonads and sexual infantilism; and (2) the short arms of the X chromosomes contain genes which, if deleted, will result in short stature and the somatic stigmata of the syndrome of gonadal dysgenesis.[2]

Ring-X or Ring-X Mosaic: X,r(X) or XO/X,r(X). A ring-X chromosome results from deletion of the long and short arm of the X chromosome with reunion in a ring-shaped structure. Over 20 patients with a ring-X karyotype have been reported.[2,71] The clinical symptoms of these patients have been variable. Short stature was present in the majority of patients, and most had some minor stigmata of the Turner syndrome. No patient has had coarctation of the aorta or a webbed neck; 7 of 19 had spontaneous menstruation and developed secondary sexual characteristics. The increased prevalence of gonadal function suggests that the genes determining ovarian differentiation are not terminally located on the X chromosome.[2]

Diagnosis and Treatment. Patients with any of the following complaints should have a sex chromatin determination: (1) all females who are short (>2.5 S.D.); (2) females with somatic stigmata of the syndrome of gonadal dysgenesis, including coarctation of the aorta and lymphedema of the hands and feet; and (3) phenotypic females with delayed adolescence and elevated gonadotropins. Normal females from birth have sex chromatin-positive nuclei in more than 20 percent of their somatic cells normal males are sex chromatin-negative. Patients are possible mosaics who have between 2 and 19 percent sex chromatin-positive cells. Those with more than one sex chromatin body per cell usually have a poly-X cell line. Since structurally abnormal X chromosomes are invariably late-replicating and form the sex chromatin body, the size of the sex chromatin body relates directly to the size of the structurally abnormal X chromosome; i.e., deleted X chromosomes give rise to small sex chromatin bodies, while long arm isochromosomes i(Xq) form large sex chromatin bodies.[2] Thus, patients with structurally abnormal X chromosomes are sex chromatin-positive but have abnormal-sized sex chromatin bodies.

Although the sex chromatin screening test is useful, karyotype analysis of multiple tissues is definitive in any patient who presents with features of the syndrome of gonadal dysgenesis. Karyotype analysis should be done utilizing "banding" with giemsa, trypsin, or quinacrine, since routine staining with giemsa does not distinguish the X chromosome from chromosomes 6 through 12. Two techniques are available for the identification of the later-replicating or sex chromatin-forming X chromosome. The classic technique involves the use of tritiated thymidine incorporation into DNA and autoradiography to show late DNA replication with respect to the rest of the chromosome complement.[2] Recently, it has been shown that the introduction of 5-bromodeoxyuridine into the media along with fluorescent staining will cause relative decondensation and poor staining of the late-replicating X chromosome, making it readily identifiable.[72] Plasma gonadotropins, FSH in particular, are useful in assessing the functional status of the gonads, especially in patients with mosaicism. All patients should be evaluated for diabetes mellitus, Hashimoto's thyroiditis, and cardiac and renal anomalies.

Therapy is directed toward cyclic estrogen replacement. We routinely initiate treatment at 12 to 13 years of age with 0.3 mg (or less) of conjugated estrogen by mouth or with ethinyl estradiol, 5-10 μg by mouth daily for the first 21 days of the calendar month and we gradually increase the dose of conjugated estrogen over the next 2 to 3 years to 0.6 mg daily or ethinyl estradiol, 20–30 μg daily for the first 21 days of each month. Medroxyprogesterone acetate, 5–10 mg daily, is given concurrently to facilitate menses, on days 17 to 21 of the calendar month.

Recently, several cases of endometrial carcinoma have been reported in patients with the syndrome of gonadal dysgenesis after continuous estrogen therapy with stilbestrol,[73] and McCarrol et al. have described a case of endometrial cancer associated with cyclic replacement therapy with stilbestrol and ethisterone.[74] However, there is insufficient evidence to judge whether there is increased risk of endometrial cancer in patients treated with cyclic estrogen, especially estrogen-progestin regimens, over that in normal women. Clearly, patients with Turner syndrome require replacement therapy. At present, the most judicious approach would seem to be low-dose estrogen replacement with cyclic administration of progesterone. Even on this regimen, annual gynecologic examinations are indicated, and irregular bleeding should suggest the need for curettage to confirm that there are no changes compatible with neoplasia.

Sex Chromatin-Negative Variants of the Syndrome of Gonadal Dysgenesis

The phenotypic spectrum of patients with XO/XY mosaicism extends from phenotypic females with Turner syndrome, to some with ambiguous genitalia, and, less commonly, to normally differentiated males with testes (Fig. 106-12).[2,3] Short stature and associated somatic anomalies are variable features. The degree of masculinization is dependent upon the functional integrity of the gonads. If testicular differentiation proceeds to a point where sufficient testosterone is produced by the fetus, then complete masculinization of the external genitalia occurs. The internal ducts are under the local influence of müllerian duct inhibitory factor, so that a dysgenetic gonad or streak usually has müllerian derivatives (uterus, fallopian tube) associated with it, while a well-differentiated testes has wolffian structures.

In a recent review, 72 of 109 XO/XY individuals had a streak gonad on one side and a dysgenetic testis on the other;[75] two thirds of the 109 XO/XY patients were raised as females. None had spontaneous menses and all had some degree of virilization. Breast development was noted in 27 percent of the cases, usually associated with a gonadal tumor, especially gonadoblastoma.[2,75] The risk to patients with XO/XY mosaicism of developing gonadal tumors is increased strikingly over others with the syndrome of gonadal dysgenesis, so that prophylactic removal of streak gonads or undescended dysgenetic gonads is indicated. A useful clue to the presence of functional testicular elements before puberty is a rise in the concentration of plasma testosterone to pubertal or adult values following a course of human chorionic gonadotropin, 2000 U/day for 5 days.

Anaphase lag is thought to be the most likely cause of XO/XY mosaicism. Caspersson studied the fluorescent pattern of the Y chromosome in 7 patients with XO/XY mosaicism and found a nonfluorescent Y chromosome in 4.[76] In 1, there was a possible translocation between the short arm of chromosome 2 and the long arm of the Y. In our laboratory, 2 of 14 XO/XY mosaics have had nonfluorescent Y chromosomes. In addition to the loss of bright quinacrine fluorescence of the Y chromosome, loss of heterochromasia and late replication have been observed.[77,78] The unexplained high proportion of cytochemically abnormal Y chromosomes in XO/XY mosaicism suggests that an altered Y chromosome may be predisposed to anaphase lag or to mitotic nondisjunction, leading to XO/XY or XO/XYY mosaicism.

Structural Abnormalities of the Y Chromosome

Phenotypic-karyotypic correlations in patients with structurally abnormal Y chromosomes have been made in an attempt to localize the genes for testicular development and stature. Such correlations with structurally aberrant Y chromosomes are compli-

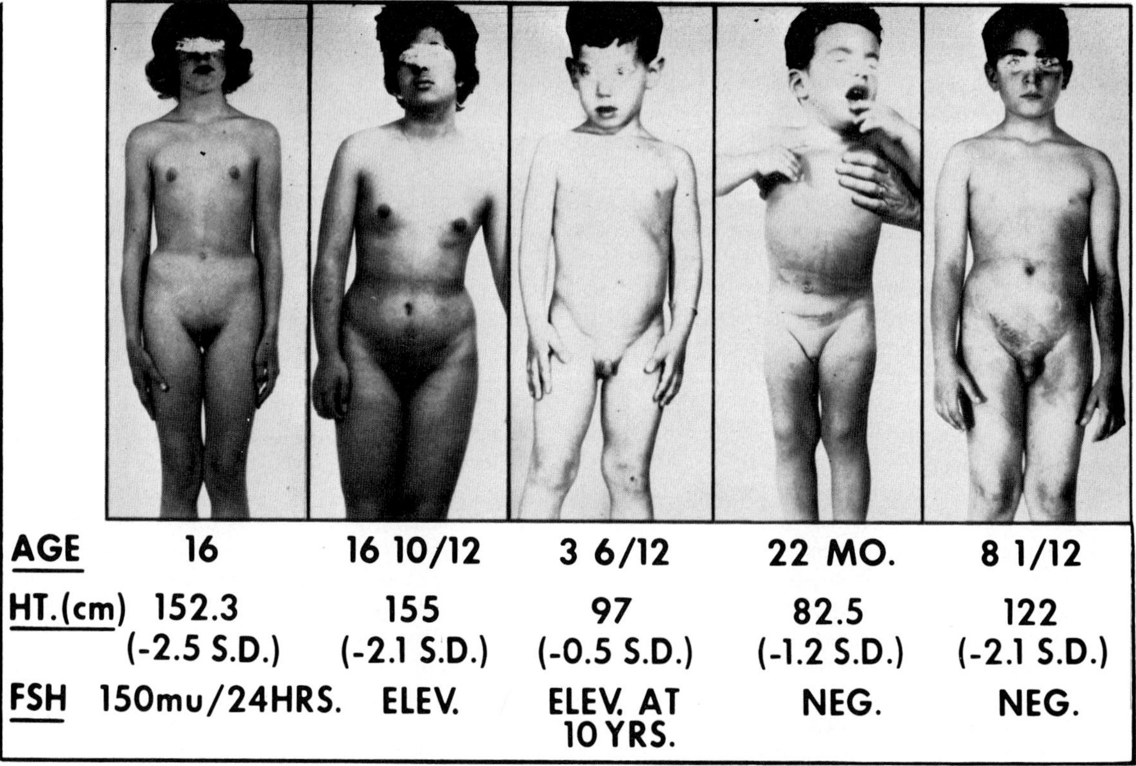

AGE 16 16 10/12 3 6/12 22 MO. 8 1/12
HT.(cm) 152.3 (-2.5 S.D.) 155 (-2.1 S.D.) 97 (-0.5 S.D.) 82.5 (-1.2 S.D.) 122 (-2.1 S.D.)
FSH 150mu/24HRS. ELEV. ELEV. AT 10 YRS. NEG. NEG.

Fig. 106-12. Phenotypic spectrum of patients with XO/XY mosaicism. On the left is a phenotypic female with short stature, sexual infantilism, and elevated gonadotropins. The 3 patients in the middle have varying degrees of masculinization. The patient on the far right is a fully masculinized phenotypic male with a penile urethra. He had a right scrotal testes that was normal in histologic appearance and produced normal testosterone levels at puberty. His left gonad was a streak that was associated with Müllerian derivatives. He was short and had short metacarpals as well as cubitus valgus and puffiness of the dorsum of the hands. (From Grumbach, M. M. and Van Wyk, J., in *Textbook of Endocrinology*, 5th ed., R. H. Williams (ed.), Philadelphia, W. B. Saunders Co., 1974.)

cated by the small size of the Y chromosome and the inability to characterize Yp and the proximal portion of Yq by banding. Absence of the entire fluorescent distal two thirds of the long arm of the Y chromosome in normal males suggests that the heterochromatic, highly fluorescent distal two thirds of the long arms of the Y chromosome is genetically inactive. In individuals with minute Y chromosomes or small rings, only a centromere and pericentric material are apparently present.[79–81] Invariably, these patients have testicular tissue, indicating that the testicular determiners are pericentrically located. The most compelling cytogenetic evidence for short arm localizations of the testis-determining genes is found in patients with an X,i(Yq) karyotype. Three such patients have been studied by Q and C banding.[82,83] Each isochromosome was characterized by brilliant Q bands or dark C bands over the distal two thirds of each of two isologous arms. All 3 patients were phenotypic females without evidence of testicular differentiation and function, which suggests that there are testicular determiners on the short arms of the Y chromosome. All 3 patients were 163 cm (or less) in height; this observation supports the location of statural determinants on the short arm of the Y chromosome. Dicentric Y chromosomes have also been reported. Their instability and frequent association with an XO cell line, along with the difficulty in determining the amount of Yp material, limits phenotypic-karyotypic correlations with this anomaly. It may be that, similar to the X chromosome, there are testis-determining genes pericentremerically on both the long and short arms of the Y chromosome.

PURE GONADAL DYSGENESIS

This term has been applied to XX or XY patients who have bilateral streak gonads that result in a female phenotype without the somatic stigmata of Turner syndrome. Prepubertally, these patients may be difficult to diagnose since their only abnormality may be elevated gonadotropins. Postpubertally, they exhibit sexual infantilism, castrate levels of pituitary gonadotropins, tall stature, and eunuchoid proportions. The designation "pure gonadal dysgenesis" was introduced by Harnden and Stewart in 1959 in their report of a 19-year-old phenotypic female with the described features and an XY karyotype.[84] We restrict the term "pure gonadal dysgenesis" to patients with this phenotype who have an XX or XY karyotype. Mosaicism involving an XO cell line, as well as structural abnormalities of the X and Y chromosome, can produce a similar phenotype, but we classify these as variants of the syndrome of gonadal dysgenesis because they arise as a consequence of sex chromosome abnormalities.

FAMILIAL AND SPORADIC XX GONADAL DYSGENESIS AND ITS VARIANTS

The typical patient has normal stature, sexual infantilism, bilateral streak gonads, normal female internal and external genitalia, primary amenorrhea, elevated gonadotropins, and a 46,XX karyotype in all tissues.[2,36,85] The basic differences between such patients and those with Turner syndrome are lack of major somatic stigmata, normal stature, and normal karyotype. Familial aggregates are common, and pedigree analysis is consistent with autosomal recessive inheritance.[85] In 3 families, all affected sisters had deaf mutism of the sensorineural type.[86] In a few affected sibships, a spectrum of clinical findings and gonadal histology were found, i.e., varying degrees of ovarian function, including breast development and menses followed by secondary amenorrhea. In at least 1 case, there was a streak gonad on one side and a hypoplastic ovary on the other side. Sporadic cases of a similar type have been documented.[87] Several patients have been reported with clitoromegaly and other signs of virilization. The data of Judd et al. indicate that the dysgenetic gonads in such a patient may secrete androgens, presumably from nests of hilar cells in the streak gonads.[88] The familial cases suggest that a mutant gene on an autosome can lead to defective ovarian differentiation.

The *diagnosis* of XX gonadal dysgenesis should be suspected in phenotypic females with sexual infantilism and normal müllerian structures who lack the somatic stigmata of Turner syndrome. Karyotype analysis of multiple tissues will reveal only 46,XX cells. As in Turner syndrome, gonadotropins are elevated and the concentration of plasma estrogens is low.

Therapy is directed toward estrogen replacement. There is no evidence of an increased risk of gonadal neoplasms in familial or sporadic XX gonadal dysgenesis; hence, prophylactic gonadectomy is not warranted unless evidence of inappropriate sex steroid secretion ensues.

FAMILIAL AND SPORADIC XY GONADAL DYSGENESIS AND ITS VARIANTS

More than 100 cases of this syndrome have been reported, including over 13 familial aggregates[2,36,89,90] Patients with this syndrome usually have female external genitalia, normal or tall stature, bilateral streak gonads, normal müllerian structures, sexual infantilism, a eunuchoid habitus, and a 46,XY karyotype. Clitoromegaly is a common finding. In familial studies, there may be a spectrum of involvement from the complete syndrome to ambiguity of the external genitalia. In a family reported by Chemke et al. 2 siblings had XY gonadal dysgenesis with bilateral streak gonads; 1 had a variant form with genital ambiguity, bilateral dysgenetic testes and müllerian derivatives.[91] Recently, we studied an infant born to a "normal" 46,XX sibling of the Chemke propositi who had genital ambiguity, bilateral dysgenetic tests, müllerian derivatives, and an XY karyotype. Pathogenetically the differences between the complete form of XY gonadal dysgenesis and the variant form is the degree of differentiation of testicular tissue and its function.

Analysis of familial cases suggests that XY gonadal dysgenesis is transmitted as an X-linked recessive or male-limited autosomal dominant trait. The spectrum of genital ambiguity suggests that the gene has variable expressivity. It is quite possible that some of these patients may be found, in the future, to be H-Y antigen-negative, i.e., to have a mutant gene, possibly X-linked, capable of suppressing the Y-linked testicular-determining gene or that they may be H-Y-positive and have a mutational dysfunction of the postulated H-Y antigen receptor on the surface of gonadal cells, so that testicular organogenesis is prevented and a streak gonad results.

A few cases of marked virilization at puberty have been reported.[92] In other cases, estrogen production and feminization has been associated with a gonadal tumor.[93] The incidence of gonadal tumors has been estimated to be as high as 30 percent in this group of individuals.[2]

Therapy in the patients with unambiguously female genitalia involves prophylactic gonadectomy and estrogen substitution at puberty (see page 1330). In the variant form (dysgenetic male pseudohermaphrodite), a male sex assignment is possible, depending on the degree of ambiguity of the genitalia and the potential for a functional penis in the future. Prophylactic gonadectomy should be performed, since fertility is unlikely and the risk of malignant transformation is high. Substitution androgen therapy can be instituted at puberty and prosthetic testes implanted.

SYNDROME OF WEBBED NECK, PTOSIS, HYPOGONADISM, CONGENITAL HEART DISEASE, SHORT STATURE (XX AND XY TURNER PHENOTYPE, PSEUDO-TURNER SYNDROME, NOONAN SYNDROME, ULLRICH SYNDROME)

46,XX an 46,XY individuals have been described who resemble patients with sex chromosome monosomy.[2] These patients who fall into a clinically distinguishable entity have somatic features in common with the syndrome of gonadal dysgenesis, in particular short stature, webbed neck, cubitus valgus, and lymphedema. Clinically significant differences are the triangular-shaped facies, pectus excavatum, right-sided congenital heart disease (pulmonic stenosis, atrial septal defect), normal gonadal function in affected females, and an increased incidence of mental retardation. Affected males have male external genitalia; undescended testes are common. Spermatogenesis may be normal; however, many affected males have germinal aplasia or hypoplasia and, not infrequently, impaired Leydig cell function.[2] Of importance is the fact that these patients do not have a sex chromosomal abnormality. The inheritance is autosomal dominant and incomplete penetrance is common. Most patients described in the older literature by the eponym "male Turner syndrome" have this clinical entity.

TRUE HERMAPHRODISM

A true hermaphrodite is an individual who has both ovarian and testicular tissue in either the same gonad or opposite gonads. Although this is a relatively rare disorder, over 300 cases have been reported.[94,95]

Clinical Features

The differentiation of the external genitalia and internal structures is highly variable and dependent upon gonadal histology and function. The external genitalia are usually ambiguous, although the appearaance may simulate that of either male or female. Seventy-five percent of the reported patients have been reared as males because of an enlarged phallus. The phallus is usually bound in chordee, and there is hypospadias. Most commonly, a single perineal orifice is found, representing the orifice of the urogenital sinus. Labioscrotal folds with incomplete fusion are usually present. Less than 20 percent have either a normal scrotum or normal-appearing labia majora.[95] Cryptorchidism is common, but in 60 percent a gonad may be palpable, especially on the right side. Sixty percent of palpable gonads in the inguinal canal or labioscrotal folds are ovotestes, which may be clinically suspected because of a discrepancy in firmness of the poles of the gonad, suggesting segregation and end-to-end association of ovarian and testicular tissue.[2,95]

The differentiation of the internal ducts, like the external genitalia, is variable and related to the structure and function of the ipsilateral gonad or gonads. The duct adjacent to an ovary is always a fallopian tube, and a vas deferens is invariably present next to a testis. The ovotestis is the most common gonad found in true hermaphrodites and has been associated with a fallopian tube in 65 percent of cases and a vas in the remaining ones.

At puberty, changes are variable and are dependent upon the capacity of the gonads that are present to secrete hormones. Breast development and menses, as well as some degree of virilization, usually occurs. While the ovarian portion of the ovotestis is frequently normal, the testicular portion is usually dysgenetic, so that spermatogenesis is uncommon. In rare instances, ovulation and pregnancy have been documented in true hermaphrodism.[96] Few studies of hypothalamic-pituitary function have been carried out. Poor testicular responsiveness to hCG has been noted.[97] Recently, elevated plasma gonadotropins that followed a cyclical pattern was described in 2 postpubertal siblings with true hermaphrodism.[98] Familial occurrence of true hermaphrodism has been reported but is rare.[98]

Seventy percent of true hermaphrodites are X chromatin-positive, and most have a 46,XX karyotype. The X chromatin-negative patients frequently have a 46,XY karyotype. Sex chromosome mosaicism, as well as chimerism with XX/XY karyotype, has been documented. Chimerism has been postulated to result from (1) fertilization and fusion of an ovum and its polar body, (2) fusion of two nuclei, and (3) double fertilization. Recent studies have demonstrated that 46,XX true hermaphrodites are H-Y antigen-positive.[10] This finding suggests either a hidden mosaicism with an XY cell line or possibly a Y-X or Y autosome translocation or other insertion. Familial cases of true hermaphrodism suggest a mutant gene that has been implicated in intersexuality in goats and pigs, may play a role in some cases. In addition, deleterious environmental factors acting locally could modify gonadal development and produce true hermaphrodism.

The diagnosis of true hermaphrodism should be considered in all patients with ambiguous genitalia. Cytogenetically, the presence of an XX/XY karyotype is suggestive of true hermaphrodism. Neither an XX or XY karyotype excludes the diagnosis. If the other forms of male and female pseudohermaphrodism have been excluded by appropriate studies, then the demonstration of ovarian and testicular tissue histologically will confirm the diagnosis of true hermaphrodism.

Treatment of the patient is determined in part by the age at diagnosis. In newborns, sex assignment is made on the basis of the functional potential of the external genitalia and gonads. If a male sex role is assigned, all ovarian tissue and müllerian structures should be removed. Since the testes are usually dysgenetic, fertility has not been described in patients raised as males, and since the incidence of tumors is 2 percent, we are of the view that gonadectomy with hormonal replacement at puberty and the insertion of prosthetic testes is a judicious approach. In patients to be reared as females, appropriate plastic surgery and removal of all testicular tissue are indicated. "Normal" ovarian function can ensue and rare instances of pregnancy are known. However, there is an increased risk of neoplasm arising in the ovarian tissue.[2,36] In the older patient, gender identity determines treatment. The gender identity is usually the same as the sex of rearing. Therapy involves removing the contradictory gonads and plastic repair of the external genitalia. Appropriate hormonal replacement therapy is indicated at puberty in those patients whose gonads have been removed.

GONADAL NEOPLASMS

There is an increased risk of gonadal neoplasms in patients with certain types of dysgenetic gonads, especially in patients with either XO/XY mosaicism, structural abnormalities of the Y chromosome, familial and sporadic XY gonadal dysgenesis, or dysgenetic male pseudohermaphrodism.[2,99,100] The gonadoblastoma is a tumor that occurs almost exclusively in patients with a cell line containing a Y chromosome.[101] According to Scully, who suggested the term, a gonadoblastoma is comprised of germ cells, sex cord derivatives resembling granulosa or Sertoli cells, and occasionally stromal elements resembling Leydig cells.[100] The gonadoblastoma is a neoplasm of limited malignant potential, and no cases of metastatic lesions with the typical histologic picture have been reported. Scully believes this tumor represents an "in situ germ call malignancy." Half of the cases of gonadoblastoma have had microscopic foci of dysgerminoma, characterized by large oval gonocytes that contain dark nuclei and clear cytoplasm. The dysgerminoma is histologically identical to the seminoma. It has been estimated that 10 percent of gonadoblastomas are associated with more malignant germ cell tumors, which can result in metastases and death. [102] Androgen as well as estrogen production has been reported with gonadoblastoma.[2,101,103,104] In particular, evidence for estrogen production, i.e., spontaneous female secondary sexual characteristics in a patient with XO/XY mosaicism, XY gonadal dysgenesis, or dysgenetic male pseudohermaphrodism, usually signifies an estrogen-secreting tumor, either gonadoblastoma or dysgerminoma.[2] Gonadoblastomas have been discovered in patients in the first decade of life.[105] Patients with a Y chromosome in their sex chromosome complement and gonadal dysgenesis or dysgenetic male pseudohermaphrodism have a greatly increased risk of gonadal malignancy (10 to 40 percent).[101,106,107]

In view of the risks of neoplasm, it seems prudent to advise prophylactic gonadectomy in all patients with familial or sporadic XY gonadal dysgenesis (dysgenetic male pseudohermaphrodism) or in patients with the syndrome of gonadal dysgenesis who have a cell line with either a normal or structurally abnormal Y chromosome. In particular, the prevalence of tumors may be higher in familial XY gonadal dysgenesis than in sporadic cases.[106] Since tumors have been reported in the first decade of life, prophylactic removal of the gonads is warranted soon after ascertainment, especially in those patients assigned a female gender. In a small number of XO/XY mosaics or dysgenetic male pseudohermaphrodites, an apparently normal testis may be found in the scrotum. If retained, these gonads should be closely observed for evidence of malignant degeneration.

Gonadal neoplasms are uncommon in patients with XO gonadal dysgenesis and XO/XX mosaicism and in those with structural abnormalities of the X chromosome.[2,106] There is one report of an XO patient with a dysgerminoma, but sex chromosome mosaicism was not excluded.[108] Three XO/XX mosaics have been reported with gonadal tumors; one had a pseudomucinous cystadenocarcinoma, another bilateral gonadoblastoma, and a third a hilus cell tumor with signs of virilization.[103,109,110]

The risk of neoplasia is increased in 46,XY patients with testicular feminization. Most investigators agree that the risk is relatively small prior to 25 years of age (<4 percent) and thereafter it increases.[107] In view of the relatively low risk of malignancy prior to 25 years of age, gonadectomy may be deferred until after puberty in order to allow the patient to feminize spontaneously. The risk of gonadal neoplasia in true hermaphrodites appears to be quite low.[106,111] Gonadal neoplasms are rare in patients who have an XXX, XXY, or XYY karyotype. Likewise, gonadal tumors have not been reported in 46,XX males.

FEMALE PSEUDOHERMAPHRODISM (Table 106-3)

In this condition, the ovaries and müllerian structures are normally developed. The karyotype is 46,XX, and the sex chromatin pattern is positive. Ambiguity of the external genitalia in these patients is usually androgen-induced and much less commonly a consequence of teratogenic factors. In congenital virilizing adrenal hyperplasia the degree of fetal masculinization is a function of the amount and period of exposure to androgen. After 12 weeks of gestation, excess androgen exposure does not induce fusion of the labioscrotal folds and results only in clitoromegaly.

Table 106-3. Classification of Female Pseudohermaphrodism

Classification
Androgen-induced
Fetal source
Congenital virilizing adrenal hyperplasia
Virilism only, defective adrenal 21-hydroxylation-compensated, type I
Virilism with salt-losing syndrome, defective adrenal 21-hydroxylation-uncompensated, type II
Virilism with hypertension, defective adrenal 11-hydroxylation, type III
Maternal source
Iatrogenic
Testosterone and related steroids
Certain synthetic oral progestins and rarely stilbestrol
Virilizing ovarian or adrenal tumor
Luteoma of pregnancy
Undetermined source
Other teratogenic factors
Nonhormonal disturbances in the differentiation of urogenital structures

CONGENTIAL ADRENAL HYPERPLASIA (Fig. 106-13)

Congenital adrenal hyperplasia accounts for most patients with female pseudohermaphrodism. There are six major types of congenital adrenal hyperplasia, each with a distinctive clinical picture and specific defect in steroid biosynthesis.[112,113] All are transmitted as autosomal recessives. The basic defect in all six types is a biosynthetic error in cortisol metabolism, which results in hyperplasia of the adrenal cortex due to hypersecretion of ACTH. The clinical expression of the defect is the result of the impaired synthesis of cortisol and often aldosterone, and the increased secretion of precursor steroids that may be metabolically active or result in excess androgen production.

Only three types, C_{21} hydroxylase (I,II) and C_{11} hydroxylase (III) deficiency, are predominantly virilizing and produce ambiguity of the genitalia in female infants secondary to increased adrenal androgen production. Affected male infants have no prominent abnormalities of their external genitalia at birth. 3-β-hydroxysteroid dehydrogenase (IV), 17-α-hydroxylase (V), and cholesterol desmolase complex (VI) deficiency have in common defects in steroid hormone synthesis, which not only lead to defective cortisol synthesis but also impair the production of sex steroids by the gonads as well as the adrenal gland. Thus, these latter defects usually result in impairment of full masculinization of the male infant and no, or modest, virilization in the female. Since types IV, V, and VI usually result in male pseudohermaphrodism, they will be discussed *also* in the section on Male Pseudohermaphrodism (page 1330).

Type I: C_{21} Hydroxylase Deficiency (Simple Virilization)

This deficiency is, by far, the most common cause of ambiguous genitalia in infants.[114] The basic defect is a deficiency of the enzyme 21-hydroxylase which converts 17-hydroxyprogestrone (17 OHP) to 11-deoxycortisol (Cpd S). There is no clinically apparent defect in the production of aldosterone, i.e., the enzymatic conversion from progesterone to deoxycorticosterone is apparently intact. Indeed, there may be increased production of aldosterone, which is thought to compensate for the salt-losing tendency produced by elevated levels of progesterone and 17-hydroxyprogesterone.[115] In utero, there is increased ACTH stimulation of the adrenals as a result of deficient cortisol production and lack of

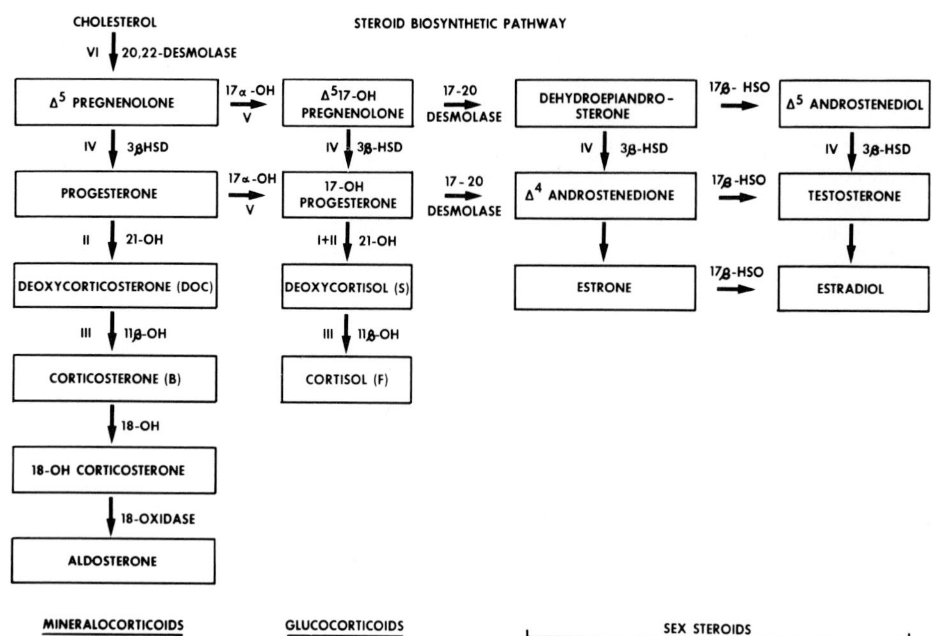

Fig. 106-13. Diagrammatic representation of the steroid biosynthetic pathways. I to VI correspond to the numbers used for the specific biosynthetic defects that result in congenital adrenal hyperplasia. OH = hydroxylase, 3-β-HSD = 3-β-hydroxysteroid dehydrogenase, and 17-β-HSO = 17-hydroxysteroid oxidoreductase.

inhibition of the hypothalamic-pituitary-adrenal axis. This leads to adrenal hyperplasia, a rise in cortisol to normal levels, and an increased production of adrenal androgens and androgen precursors, which cause varying degrees of masculinization of the external genitalia of affected females. The affected newborn male has no apparent anomaly of genital development, although the phallus may be enlarged. The spectrum of masculinization in females varies from mild clitoromegaly, usually with some degree of fusion of the labioscrotal folds, to fully masculinized external genitalia with a single orifice at the end of the phallus indistinguishable from that in cryptorchid males. A urogenital sinus is usually present and serves as a common outlet for both the urethra and vagina (Fig. 106-13). Thus, especially in the latter patients, it may be presumed that the hypersecretion of androgens begins before the 12th week in utero. The uterus, tubes, and ovaries are almost always normal in these patients, irrespective of the degree of masculinization of the external genitalia. In general, the degree of masculinization correlates with the severity of the enzymatic block. In mildly affected patients who are unrecognized in infancy, continued androgen production usually results in virilization in infancy or peripubertally, which is manifested by phallic (or clitoral) enlargement, sexual hair, acne, rapid growth, bony advancement, and muscle hypertrophy. Because skeletal maturation advances more rapidly than linear growth, the adult height in the late-diagnosed patient is often short as a result of premature closure of the epiphysis. In males with untreated adrenal hyperplasia, sexual precocity secondary to adrenal hyperplasia is clinically distinctive in that the testes are usually prepubertal in size and thus disproportionally small for the degree of development of the external genitalia and phallus. This finding usually denotes lack of maturation of the pituitary-hypothalamic-gonadal axis.[116]

The incidence of 21-hydroxylase deficiency varies with race and geographic area. In the Yupik Eskimos of Alaska, it is at least 1 per 400 live births;[117] in Maryland, it is much less common.[118] The overall minimum prevalence of 21-hydroxylase deficiency may be 1 per 10,000 live white births.

Type II: Complete C_{21} Defect (Virilization with Salt-Losing Tendency)

The salt-losing variant of 21-hydroxylase deficiency is thought to be a more complete block than that in the simple virilizing form. In addition to the block between 17-hydroxyprogesterone (17 OHP) and deoxycortisol (Cpd S), a block in the conversion of progesterone to deoxycorticosterone (DOC) is present. This results in an impairment of aldosterone secretion, including a diminished capacity to respond to salt restriction and to the antimineralocorticoid effects of progesterone and 17-hydroxyprogesterone and the consequent salt loss. The masculinization of the external genitalia of salt-losing females (Fig. 106-14) tends to be more severe than those with the simple form of 21-hydroylase deficiency.

Infants with the salt-losing form of congenital adrenal hyperplasia present in the first few weeks of life with adrenal crisis. This is usually apparent by the 4th to 10th day of life. They manifest with lethargy, poor feeding, vomiting, dehydration, and signs of hyperkalemia. This can progress rapidly to hypotension, hypoglycemia, and cyanosis. Without specific therapy, death may rapidly ensue from hyperkalemia, dehydration, and shock. In the male infant without ambiguous genitalia, the differential diagnosis includes pyloric stenosis, sepsis, gastroenteritis, and congenital heart disease.

Diagnosis. The 21-hydroxylase form of congenital adrenal hyperplasia should be considered in all patients with ambiguous genitalia, all apparent cryptorchid males, and infants who present with adrenal crises or signs of virilization prior to puberty. The initial step in diagnosis is the family history. Clinical clues, other than siblings with ambiguous genitalia or sexual precocity, include unexplained infant deaths and short adults. Patients with a 46,XX karyotype will be sex chromatin-positive in 20 to 30 percent of their buccal nuclei, even on the first day of life. Utilizing thionin to stain sex chromatin in buccal smears and counting 100 well-stained nuclei, we have not found any difference in the number of sex

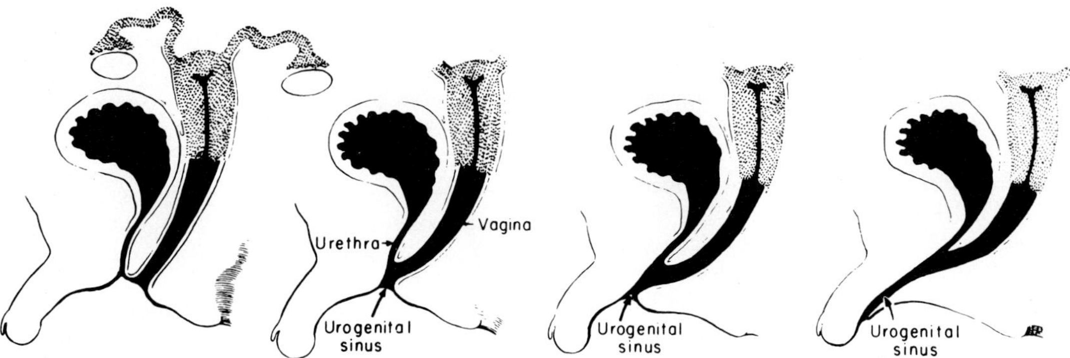

Fig. 106-14. Diagrammatic representation of the external genitalia in female pseudohermaphrodism induced by prenatal exposure to androgens. Exposure after 12 weeks leads to clitoromegaly only (left). Progressively earlier exposure (left to right) leads to retention of the urogenital sinus and labioscrotal fusion. A penile urethra can result from high androgen exposure before 12 weeks of gestation. (From Grumbach, M. M. and Ducharme, J. R.: *Fertil. Steril. 11:* 157, 1960.)

chromatin-positive cells in newborns when compared with older infants.

The major diagnostic tests utilized to confirm the diagnosis of 21-hydroxylase deficiency have been the determination of urinary 17-ketosteroids and pregnanetriol. However, the newborn infant may excrete up to 4.0 mg/24 hr of 17-ketosteroids during the first 2 weeks of life; thereafter, they decrease to approximately 0.5 mg/yr of age until puberty. Pregnanetriol, a metabolite of 17-OH progesterone, is present in increased amounts in the urine of children with 21-hydroxylase deficiency. In normal infants, pregnanetriol is barely detectable under 2 years of age, and, between 2 and 5 years, mean excretion increases to 0.6 mg/24 hr. Often, urinary pregnanetriol, as determined by standard clinical assay, is not excreted in large amounts in the first few weeks of life in affected patients. The single most important diagnostic test in establishing the diagnosis of 21-hydroxylase deficiency is the measurement of plasma 17-hydroxyprogesterone (Fig. 106-15).[119] Cord blood values are elevated in normals to a mean of 1640 ng/100 ml. In the first 24 hours of life, the values normally descend rapidly to <100 ng/100 ml. In affected patients, usually the levels range from 5000–40,000 ng/100 ml, depending on the degree of 21-hydroxylase deficiency. The accumulation of this steroid is such a distinctive marker in infants with this disorder that it may be possible to utilize amniotic fluid levels of 17-hydroxyprogesterone during gestation for prenatal diagnosis.[119,120] In our laboratory, we have studied amniotic fluid 17-hydroxyprogesterone levels from 14 to 20 weeks in normals as well as in 6 infants at risk for 21-hydroxylase deficiency. In 5 infants, amniotic fluid 17-hydroxyprogesterone levels were within the normal limits, and the infants were subsequently born and proven to be unaffected. One infant had a five-fold elevation in amniotic fluid 17-hydroxyprogesterone levels. The adrenals from this infant were studied subsequent to spontaneous abortion and were found to be 21-hydroxylase deficient. Further studies are obviously necessary to confirm the reliability and accuracy of amniotic fluid 17-hydroxyprogesterone levels in the prenatal diagnosis of 21-hydroxylase deficiency.

Aldosterone deficiency is usually documented by the clinical picture associated with a low concentration of serum sodium, elevated serum potassium, and high levels of plasma renin. Mild renal tubular acidosis is frequent. Normal newborns often have a serum potassium concentration in the 5–6 mEq/liter range. Mild salt losers may have normal serum electrolytes on a regular diet; their deficiency may be made manifest by a low-salt diet (<10 mEq NaC1/day).

Treatment. Therapy of patients with congenital adrenal hyperplasia may be divided into two phases: acute and chronic. In acute adrenal crises, there is a deficiency of both cortisol and aldosterone, resulting in dehydration and electrolyte imbalance. An intravenous infusion of 5% dextrose in isotonic saline should be started and fluids calculated upon estimates of deficiency and maintenance. In the first hour, if the patient is hypotensive, 20 ml/kg of 5% glucose in isotonic saline may be given. A dose of 50 mg/m^2 of hydrocortisone sodium succinate should be given as a bolus intravenously and another 50–100 mg/m^2 added to the infusion fluid over the first 24 hours. If the serum electrolyte pattern indicates that the patient has hyponatremia and hyperkalemia, deoxycorticosterone acetate (DOCA) 2–5 mg im (depending on age), is given every 12 to 24 hours. The measurement of the concentration of plasma 17-hydroxyprogesterone from the initial plasma sample for electrolytes obviates the need to withhold definitive cortisol therapy in order to make the diagnosis. The frequency and amount of DOCA, as well as the sodium concentration of the intravenous fluids, is adjusted in the light of the serum electrolyte values, plasma renin, the state of hydration, and blood pressure. Excess DOCA and salt can result in hypertension, congestive heart failure, and hypertensive encephalopathy, while too little salt and DOAC will not correct the electrolyte imbalance. The high serum potassium level may be life-threatening, in which case the rectal

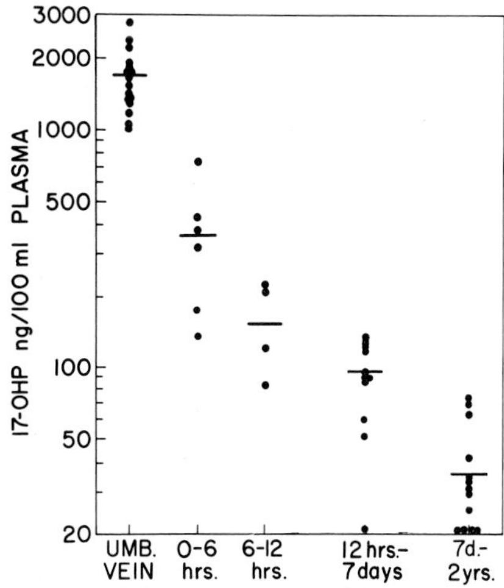

Fig. 106-15. Normal plasma 17-hydroxyprogesterone values in nanograms per deciliter from birth to 2 years. (From Jenner, M. R., Grumbach, M. M., and Kaplan, S. L.: *Pediatr. Res. 4:* 380, 1970.)

administration of a cation exchange resin and intravenous glucose, bircarbonate, and calcium may be necessary.

After stabilization and diagnosis, we treat infants with intramuscular cortisone acetate. This avoids the problems arising from regurgitation and variable absorption of oral glucocorticoids. Infants are initially suppressed with 25 mg cortisone acetate im, daily for 5 days. Thereafter, cortisone acetate is given intramuscularly *every 3 days* in a dose (15–18 mg) that is approximately *three times the daily requirement, of 12 ± 3 mg/m²/24 hr*. This regimen is continued until 18 months of age. The dose of glucocorticoids is empirical and must be adjusted in each patient, utilizing bone age, linear growth, the excretion of ketosteroids, and clinical signs of glucocorticoid excess and virilization (Fig. 106-16).

After 18 months to 2 years, oral glucocorticoids may be given. In general, oral doses of cortisone acetate approximating 22 mg/m²/day and hydrocortisone, 18 mg/m²/day in 3 divided doses, permit normal growth and development (Fig. 106-17).[121] "Salt-losers" should always be treated with mineralocorticoids as well as salt supplements. Either DOCA pellets in infancy (one to two 75 or 125 mg pellets) or oral 9-α-fluorophydrocortisone, 0.05–0.1 mg daily, are necessary. Hypertension and signs of fluid overload indicate excess salt and mineralocorticoid administration, while hyponatremia or an increased plasma renin concentration indcates a need for increased salt supplement with the mineralocorticoid. Patients are instructed to triple the dose of cortisone with stress, i.e., fever, gastroenteritis, trauma, or surgical procedures.

Female patients with ambiguous external genitalia should have appropriate plastic repair of their external genitalia before 12 months of age. Clitoral recession rather than clitorectomy is usually preferred.[122] Of major importance to the family with an affected child is the assurance that their child will grow and develop into a normal functional adult. Fertility in males and feminization, menstruation, and fertility in females can be expected in the adequately treated patient.[123] Psychologic guidance and support by the physician is an essential part of long-term management.

Aberrant adrenal rests are common in boys with adrenal hyperplasia and may be mistaken for either adult testicular maturation or testicular neoplasms.[124] These adrenal rests are often bilateral and histologically indistinguishable from Leydig cells but lack "Reinke crystalloids." If the adrenal is adequately suppressed with cortisol, these rests usually remain inconspicuous throughout life (Fig. 106-18).[124]

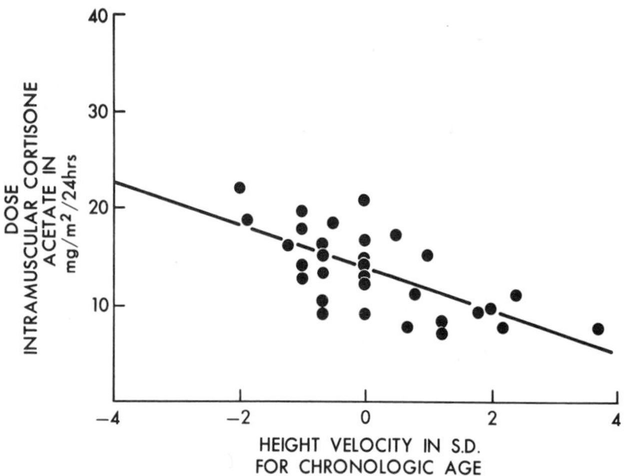

Fig. 106-16. Height velocities of cortisone-acetate-treated patients with congenital adrenal hyperplasia. Each point represents 1 patient year. Height velocity is expressed in standard deviations above or below the mean for age. A perpendicular line from 0 S.D. or normal height velocity for age intercepts the linear regression line at a dose most closely associated with normal growth (estimated optimal dose). The estimated optimal dose of intramuscular cortisone acetate is 14 mg/m²/day. r = 0.66; p<0.01. (From Styne, D. D., Grumbach, M. M., et al. in *Congenital Adrenal Hyperplasia,* P. A. Lee, et al. (eds.), Baltimore, University Park Press, 1977.)

	ACTUAL DOSE IN mg/m²/24hrs	EQUIVALENT DOSE	REPORTED POTENCY BASED ON ANTI-INFLAMMATORY EFFECT
Dexamethasone	0.23	1	1
Methylprednisolone	2.4	10	5
Prednisone	3.7	16	7
Hydrocortisone	18.4	80	27
Cortisone Acetate (I.M.)	13.9	60	17
Cortisone Acetate (P.O.)	22.0	96	33

Fig. 106-17. Mean estimated optimal dose of glucocorticoids for growth in patients with congenital adrenal hyperplasia, compared with anti-inflammatory potencies. (From Styne, D. D., Grumbach, M. M., et al. in *Congenital Adrenal Hyperplasia,* P. A. Lee, et al. (eds.), Baltimore, University Park Press, 1977.)

Type III: C_{11}-Hydroxylase Deficiency (Female Pseudohermaphrodism with Hypertension)

This is a rare form of congenital adrenal hyperplasia resulting from a defect in 11-hydroxylation.[112] The hydroxylation defect at C_{11} leads to the hypersecretion of deoxycorticosterone and 11-deoxycortisol, in addition to adrenal androgens. In affected females with this defect, there is masculinization of the external genitalia secondary to increased adrenal androgen production. Increased deoxycorticosterone secretion results in salt and water retention and hypertension. Mild or partial defects have been described, as well as patients without hypertension who have no apparent defect in the mineralocorticoid pathway. In the mild form, the first clinical signs in affected females may not be apparent until puberty or adulthood.[125] Urinary 17-ketosteroids are elevated as in 21-hydroxylase deficiency. The finding of elevated levels of 11-deoxycortisol in plasma, as well as its urinary metabolite, tetrahydro S, is diagnostic. Therapy with glucocorticoids is similar to that of patients with simple 21-hydroxylase deficiency and will result in a decrease in the blood pressure to normal in hypertensive patients.

Type IV: 3-β-Hydroxysteroid Dehydrogenase Deficiency (Male or Female Pseudohermaphrodism and Adrenal Insufficiency)

A deficiency of the enzyme 3-β-hydroxysteroid dehydrogenase may be the second most common form of congenital adrenal hyperplasia.[112] This enzyme is required by both the adrenals and gonads for the synthesis of hormones. In contrast to 21-hydroxylase and 11-hydroxylase deficiency, there is mild masculinization in affected females, whereas the male infant has ambiguous external genitalia, i.e., hypospadias, bifid scrotum, and often undescended testes owing to impaired secretion of fetal testosterone during the critical period of sexual differentiation. The mild virilization in affected 46,XX patients has been attributed to the elevated concentration of plasma dehydroepiandrosterone and androstenediol. In view of present knowledge, it seems more likely that the defect is not complete, and a portion of the dehydroepiandrosterone and other Δ^5C_{19} steroids are converted to androstenedione→testosterone→dihydrotestosterone, which then effects mild

ENZYMATIC DEFECT	CHOLESTEROL DESMOLASE SYSTEM (CHOLESTEROL 20α-HYDROXYLASE)		3β-HYDROXYSTEROID DEHYDROGENASE		17α-HYDROXYLASE		11β-HYDROXYLASE		21α-HYDROXYLASE	
TYPE	VI		IV		V		III		II & I	
CHROMOSOMAL SEX	XX	XY	XX	XY	XX	XY	XX	XY	XX	XY
EXTERNAL GENITALIA	female	female	female (clitoromegaly)	ambiguous	female	female or ambiguous	ambiguous	male	ambiguous	male
POSTNATAL VIRILIZATION	— (sexual infantilism at puberty)		±	mild to moderate	— (sexual infantilism at puberty)		+		+	
ADDISONIAN CRISES	+		+		—		—		+ in 40% (type II)	
HYPERTENSION	—		—		+		+		—	

From Grumbach & van Wyk: Williams, Textbook of Endocrinology, ed. 5 (1974)

Fig. 106-18. Clinical manifestation of the various types of congenital adrenal hyperplasia. (From Grumbach, M. M. and Van Wyk, J. J., in Williams, R. H. (ed.): *Textbook of Endocrinology,* 5th ed. Philadelphia, W. B. Saunders, 1974.)

masculinization (clitoromegaly with slight labial fusion) of the external genitalia of the affected female.

The first description of this disease was by Bongiovanni in 1962; [126] in 1964, the defect was demonstrated in both the adrenals and testes of an affected patient.[127] Subsequently, a number of cases have been described with partial deficiency. In the severely affected patient, the block in cortisol, aldosterone, and sex steroid synthesis leads to ambiguity of the genitalia and often adrenal insufficiency in the neonatal period. The diagnosis of this disorder is dependent upon the demonstration of elevated 17-ketosteroids in the urine, most of which is dehydroepiandrosterone and other Δ^5 steroids. The concentrations of plasma dehydroepiandrosterone and its sulfate and other Δ^5C_{19} steroids are elevated. Physiologic replacement with glucocorticoids, mineralocorticoids, and salt are indicated in these patients (see Treatment of 21-Hydroxylase Deficiency). The mortality in early life has been high.

Type V: 17-α-Hydroxylase Defect (Male Pseudohermaphrodism, Sexual Infantilism, Hypertension, and Hypokalemic Alkalosis)

17-α-hydroxylase deficiency was first described by Biglieri in females presenting with hypertension, hypokalemia, and lack of secondary sexual characteristics.[128–134] This defect in affected females does not result in female pseudohermaphrodism. In 46,XY patients, 17-α-hydroxylase deficiency produces male pseudohermaphrodism, and, not infrequently, in the male the external genitalia are female. The testes are normally differentiated but undescended. Both affected males and females usually have hypertension, hypokalemia, and low plasma renin values. The hypertension, hypokalemia, and hyporeninemia result from an excess of mineralocorticoid production, in particular DOC and corticosterone (Cpd B), which are stimulated by the increased ACTH levels. Aldosterone secretion is depressed as a result of inhibition of the angiotensin system by excess salt and water retention.

Cortisol secretion, as well as plasma levels of cortisol, and its urinary metabolites are usually very low. The excretion of urinary 17-ketosteroids and estrogens is low due to the block in the synthesis of sex steroids in the adrenal and gonads. Hypertension with hypokalemia and alkalosis in an XX female with sexual infantilism, or in an XY patient with female or ambiguous genitalia, should suggest the possibility of 17-hydroxylase deficiency. Elevated plasma levels of pregnenolone, progesterone, DOC, Cpd B, and their urinary metabolites confirm the diagnosis. When ACTH secretion is suppressed by glucocorticoid therapy, the secretion of DOC and Cpd B falls, aldosterone and renin return to normal, the serum potassium concentration rises, and the blood pressure decreases. Since gonadal and adrenal sex steroid synthesis is blocked by the defect, appropriate sex steroid therapy must be instituted at puberty in the affected patient.

Type VI: Cholesterol Desmolase Complex Defect (Male Pseudohermaphrodism, Sexual Infantilism, and Adrenal Insufficiency)

The first step in the synthesis of adrenal and gonadal steroids is the conversion of cholesterol to Δ^5 pregnenolone. This conversion has been postulated to occur by the hydroxylation of cholesterol at the C_{20} and C_{22} positions, then cleaving the side chain with the 20,22 desmolase enzyme. Prader and his colleagues first described a form of congenital adrenal hyperplasia in which virtually no steroid hormones were found.[135] This disorder clinically manifests with severe adrenal insufficiency and lack of masculinization of the external genitalia of XY patients. In both XX and XY patients, the external genitalia have been female. The adrenal glands are markedly enlarged and contain increased quantities of cholesterol and other lipids; thus, they applied the term "lipoid adrenal hyperplasia." Prader postulated that a defect in the conversion of cholesterol to Δ^5 pregnenolone was present in the adrenals and gonads of these patients.[136] Further studies have suggested that the defect may be in the 20-α-hydroxylase enzyme.[137] Over 16 cases of this type of adrenal hyperplasia have been reported.[2,138–143] Most patients die in infancy of adrenal insufficiency, although several survived the first few months of life and our patient is now 11-years old.[2] In all patients with this defect, little or no 17-ketosteroids, 17-hydroxycorticoids, or aldosterone are found in the urine. Plasma steroids are also low or unmeasurable. Differential diagnosis includes congenital adrenal *hypoplasia;* an intravenous pyelogram that demonstrates downward displacement of the kidneys owing to large adrenal glands or adrenal imaging may distinguish the two entities in the affected infant. Therapy is directed toward glucocorticoid and mineralocorticoid replacement, as in 21-hydroxylase deficiency.

ANDROGENS AND PROGESTINS TRANSFERRED FROM THE MATERNAL CIRCULATION

Masculinization of the external genitalia of the female fetus can follow the maternal ingestion of testosterone or synthetic progestational agents during pregnancy.[2,144,145] the extent of which is related to the compound, dosage, timing, and length of administration. If the exposure occurs after 12 weeks of gestation, fusion of the labioscrotal folds does not occur, although clitoral enlargement may result. Most implicated progestins are structurally related to testosterone, e.g., ethisterone, norethindrone and norethynodrel. However, instances resulting from the administration of medroxyprogesterone acetate to pregnant women have been described.[2] The incidence is not known, but Ishizuka et al. found masculinization in 2.25 percent of female infants whose mothers received progestins of various types during pregnancy.[146]

Bongiovanni, DiGeorge, and Grumbach collected several cases of XX infants with ambiguous genitalia in which the mother had received only stilbestrol in large doses.[147] They suggested that this compound may inhibit adrenal 3-β-hydroxysteroid dehydrogenase and thereby cause virilization. Vaginal adenosis and vaginal cervical adenocarcinoma have been reported in young female adolescents and in women whose mothers had taken diethylstilbestrol, usually in high dosage, during pregnancy.

In rare instances, virilization of the external genitalia of the female fetus has resulted from a virilizing ovarian or adrenal tumor in the mother.[148,149] Luteomas of pregnancy, which tend to regress postpartum, also can be associated with masculinization of the female fetus.[150]

The diagnosis of virilization secondary to exogenous androgenic compounds is dependent upon the history as well as observation of normal adrenal steroid secretion in the infant. Postnatally, there is no further virilization, so that only plastic repair of the external genitalia is indicated in the affected infant with conspicuous ambiguity of the genitalia.

MALFORMATIONS OF THE INTESTINAL AND URINARY TRACT

Nonadrenal female pseudohermaphrodism may be associated with malformations, such as imperforate anus, renal agenesis, and other abnormalities of the lower intestinal and genital tract.[151,152] In contrast to other forms of female pseudohermaphrodism, the internal genital ducts may also be malformed. Usually there is no history of maternal drug ingestion during pregnancy, and steroid studies are normal. The pathogenesis of these non-androgen-induced anomalies is different from other types of ambisexual development and can be considered in the context of a primary malformation of the primordia. There are a small number of 46,XX females with ambiguous genitalia in whom there is no history of drug ingestion during pregnancy, no abnormality in steroid synthesis, nor any associated malformations. Although some may represent the consequence of an undetected source of androgen during pregnancy, such as a luteoma of pregnancy, the etiology is uncertain.

MALE PSEUDOHERMAPHRODISM

Male pseudohermaphrodism is a condition in which the genital ducts and/or the external genitalia are ambiguous despite the presence of gonads that are testes. The phenotype varies from an individual with apparently normal female external genitalia to a male with mild hypospadias. Phenotypic classifications are confusing, since etiologically different causes of male pseudohermaphrodism may result in a similar phenotype. It is convenient to categorize separately male pseudohermaphrodites who are incompletely masculinized because of a defect in testicular organogenesis—the so-called dysgenetic male pseudohermaphrodite. In these patients, the gonadal defect is most commonly due to a sex chromosome anomaly, a mutant gene, or a teratologic factor that leads to defective gonadogenesis. In patients with dysgenetic gonads, differentiation of the internal ducts and external genitalia correlate well with the degree of gonadal differentiation. The major forms of dysgenetic male pseudohermaphrodism have been discussed in our earlier section on gonadal disorders.

In this section, we mainly consider patients whose testes have differentiated but whose defective male differentiation may be ascribed to a failure of the testes to secrete testosterone during the critical period of differentiation or a failure of the target tissues of the genital tract to respond appropriately to this hormone and its products. The outline of the general classification shown in Table 106-1 will be followed.

TESTICULAR UNRESPONSIVENESS TO hCG AND LH (Fig. 106-19)

Male sexual differentiation is dependent upon stimulation of fetal Leydig cells by hCG to produce testosterone. Absence, hypoplasia, or unresponsiveness of Leydig cells to hCG will result in male pseudohermaphrodism. The extent of the genital abnormality is dependent on the severity of testosterone deficiency. Berthezene et al. reported a 46,XY male pseudohermaphrodite with Ley-

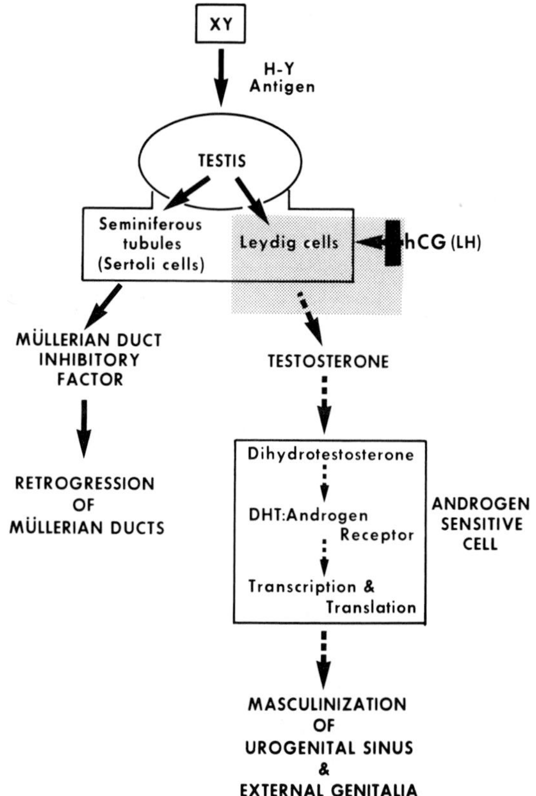

Fig. 106-19. Diagrammatic scheme of male sex determination and differentiation showing a defect in Leydig cell responsiveness to hCG(LH), resulting in male pseudohermaphrodism. The bar (▌) indicates the defect, and the hatched area indicates the general site of the defect. Interrupted lines indicate that the subsequent processes may be completely or partially affected. (From Grumbach, M. J. and Conte, F. A., in Williams, R. H. (ed.): *Textbook of Endocrinology,* 6th ed. Philadelphia, W. B. Saunders, in press.)

dig cell agenesis and lack of gynecomastia.[153] A female pattern of pubic hair was present, and the clitoris was normal. The labia were fused posteriorly, but separate urethral and vaginal orifices were visible. The vagina ended blindly at 4 cm and, at laparotomy, there were no müllerian structures. The testes were 3 × 1.5 cm, with normal-appearing epididymis and vas deferens. Light and electron microscopy revealed hyalinization of the seminiferous tubules, normal Sertoli cells, occasional immature germ cells, but no leydig cells. Plasma LH concentrations were elevated, and studies of adrenal androgen secretion revealed no evidence of a biosynthetic defect. Findings in this patient and the "vet rat"[154] are consistent with an hCG-LH receptor defect on the fetal Leydig cells.

Recently, several authors have claimed that fetal pituitary gonadotropin deficiency may result in male pseudohermaphrodism.[156,157] The finding of normal male differentiation in XY males with anencephaly, apituitarism, or congenital hypothalamic hypopituitarism suggests that male sex differentiation can occur in the absence of pituitary gonadotropins under the influence of hCG.[158] The role of the fetal pituitary gonadotropins in the growth of the fetal gonads are external genitalia has been reviewed recently.[17]

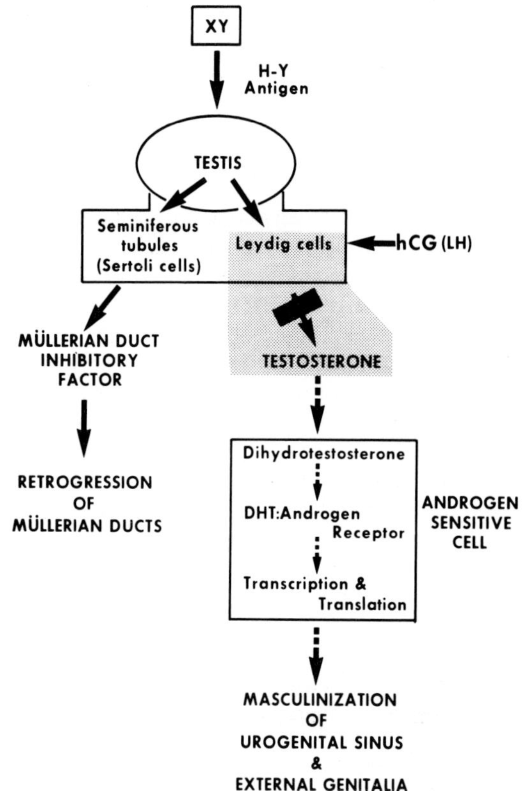

Fig. 106-20. Diagrammatic scheme of male sex determination and differentiation showing a block in the biosynthesis of testosterone resulting in male pseudohermaphrodism. (From Grumbach, M. M. and Conte, F. A., in Williams, R. H. (ed.): *Textbook of Endocrinology,* 6th ed. Philadelphia, W. B. Saunders, in press.)

INBORN ERRORS OF TESTOSTERONE BIOSYNTHESIS (Figs. 106-20 and 106-21)

Errors Affecting the Synthesis of Both Corticosteroids and Testosterone (Variants of Congenital Adrenal Hyperplasia)

Five enzymatic conversions are required to synthesize testosterone from cholesterol. The first three enzymes (cholesterol desmolase complex, 3-β-hydroxysteroid dehydrogenase, and 17-α-hydroxylase) are present in both the adrenals and testes, and their dificiency results in a major abnormality in the biosynthesis of glucocorticoids and mineralocorticoids.

Cholesterol Desmolase Complex Deficiency (20-α-Hydroxylase Deficiency). This defect in the synthesis of both cortisol and aldosterone was previously discussed in regard to female pseudohermaphrodism. Affected males are not masculinized during fetal life because of the early severe defect in testosterone synthesis. A blind vaginal pouch and intra-abdominal, inguinal, or labial testes are present, and müllerian structures are absent.

Three male pseudohermaphrodites who survived infancy presented with addisonian crisis at 1½, 3, and 8½ months of age.[2,142,143] In all 3 patients, levels of urinary 17-ketosteroids and 17-hydroxycorticoids were low or absent. At laparotomy, all had a blind vaginal pouch, testicles, and no müllerian ducts. Death from unrecognized or inadequately treated adrenal insufficiency is frequent. The patient of Grumbach and associates is now 11 years old and entirely well on glucocorticoid and mineralocorticoid replacement therapy. As with other infants with severe adrenal insufficiency, glucocorticoid (22 mg/m²/day or cortisone acetate po) and mineralocorticoid (9-α-fluorohydrocortisone, 0.025–0.1 mg/day

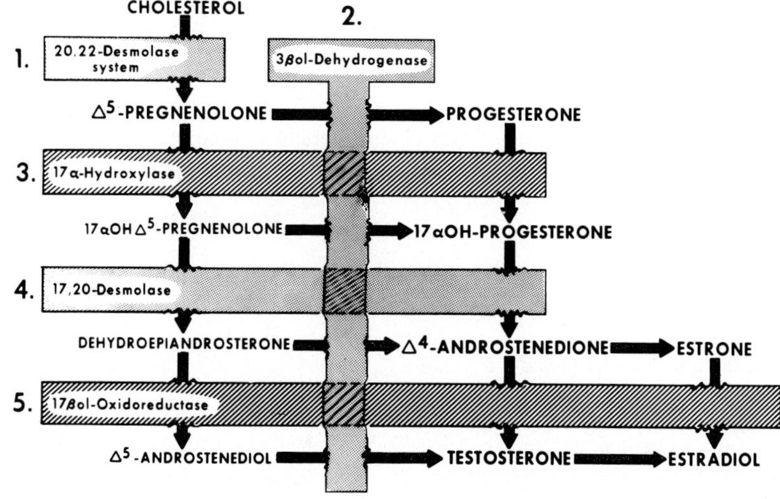

Fig. 106-21. Diagrammatic representation of the biosynthetic pathway from cholesterol to testosterone, showing the five enzymatic steps and the possible defects that can result in male pseudohermaphrodism. (From Grumbach, M. M. and Van Wyk, J., in *Textbook of Endocrinology,* 5th ed., R. H. Williams (ed.), Philadelphia, W. B. Saunders, 1974.)

po) with added salt are necessary to sustain life. The diagnosis of cholesterol desmolase complex defect should be considered in XY individuals with female external genitalia and inguinal or groin masses who manifest adrenal insufficiency in infancy.

3-β-Hydroxysteroid Dehydrogenase Deficiency. Male pseudohermaphrodism with adrenal insufficiency is the usual finding in affected males with 3-β-hydroxysteroid dehydrogenase deficiency.[112] The block occurs at an early stage of steroid biosynthesis and results in adrenal insufficiency and impairment of testosterone secretion by the fetal Leydig cells. Thus, affected males have incomplete masculinization of their external genitalia. The internal ducts are unambiguously male. The hallmark of the disease is the elevated level of Δ^5 17-ketosteroids and C_{21} steroids in urine and blood. A number of cases have been described, including several males who survived infancy with appropriate therapy and underwent spontaneous puberty; all had hypospadias and gynecomastia.[159–164] Of interest is the presence of pregnanetriol in the urine of these patients. Bongiovanni has suggested that some conversion of pregnenetriol to pregnanetriol occurs with the maturation of hepatic enzymes with 3-β-hydroxysteroid dehydrogenase activity. A partial defect would also explain the presence of pregnanetriol in the urine. The gynecomastia and masculinization found at puberty may be related to the increased testicular secretion of Δ^5 androstenediol found in pubertal patients.

17-α-Hydroxylase Deficiency. This enzymatic deficiency was first described in females presenting with systemic arterial hypertension and hypokalemia.[128–134] At least 7 XY males have been reported with this enzymatic defect in the adrenals and gonads.[165–170] The phenotype of these males has ranged from those with normal-appearing female external genitalia to a hypospadiac male with a small phallus.[165] The testes in these patients may be intra-abdominal, in the inguinal canal, or in the labioscrotal folds. Müllerian structures are absent; the vas deferens and epididymis are hypoplastic or well developed, depending on the severity of the block. Plasma cortisol levels are diminished, while the concentration of ACTH, deoxycorticosterone (DOC), and corticosterone (Cpd B) are increased. As a consequence of increased DOC secretion, renin and aldosterone levels are low. Hypertension and hypokalemia may be alleviated by physiologic glucocorticoid therapy. The diagnosis is confirmed by the finding of elevated plasma levels of pregnenolone, progesterone, DOC, and Cpd B and their urinary products in XY patients with ambiguous external genitalia. Since sex steroid production is impaired in both males and females who are affected, gonadotropins are elevated and normal male or female puberty does not ensue. In the patient reported by New and co-workers, a partial defect was present, as evidenced by the measurable plasma levels of 17-hydroxyprogesterone and 17-hydroxypregnenolone. In this patient, prominent gynecomastia was evident.[165] Thus, physiologic glucocorticoid, as well as appropriate sex steroid replacement at puberty, is necessary.

Enzymatic Defects Affecting Testes Primarily

17,20-Desmolase Deficiency. In the adrenal and gonads, C_{19} and C_{18} sex steroids are the product of precursor C_{21} steroids. The C_{21} steroids, 17-α-hydroxypregnenolone and 17-α-hydroxyprogesterone, are converted to androstenedione and dehydroepiandrosterone by the enzyme 17,20-desmolase. Zachmann et al. described 3 patients in a family with male pseudohermaphrodism secondary to a deficiency of this enzyme.[171] The patients were two first cousins and a maternal aunt with ambiguous genitalia, inguinal or intra-abdominal testes, and an XY sex chromosome constitution. The first cousins were 1.8 and 2.2 years old and had severe hypospadias with male-type urethra and male duct development. The aunt was reported to have had testes and "rudimentary Müllerian structures," in addition to a vas deferens and epididymis. Levels of urinary 17-ketosteroids and 17-hydroxycorticoids were normal for age; urinary pregnanetriol was normal, but pregnenetriol and 11-keto-pregnanetriol were increased. Chorionic gonadotropin did not produce an increase in the excretion of urinary testosterone; ACTH produced a normal rise in urinary 17-OHS and a further increase in urinary 11-keto-pregnanetriol. In vitro incubation of testicular tissue demonstrated a defect in the conversion of C_{12} steroids to testosterone.

Another presumed case of this defect was reported in a 16-year-old phenotypic female with an XY karyotype who presented with primary amenorrhea and sexual infantilism.[172] The genitalia were unambiguously female, with a blind vagina and *absent müllerian structures.* Atrophic testes and wolffian structures were present intra-abdominally, and Leydig cells were readily identified, especially in the right testicle. Plasma gonadotropins were elevated and sex steroid levels were unmeasurable. In studies carried out after orchidectomy, ACTH elicited a marked rise in plasma pregnenolone, 17-OH pregnenolone, progesterone, and 17-hydroxyprogesterone. In contrast, dehydroepiandrosterone, dehydroepiandrosterone sulfate, and androstenedione exhibited little or no increase. These observations and the clinical picture are consistent with a 17,20-desmolase defect.

The diagnosis of this defect is dependent upon the demonstration in vivo or in vitro of an inability of the adrenal and/or gonads to convert C_{21} steroids to C_{19}, i.e., 17-hydroxypregnenolone to dehydroepiandrosterone and 17-OH progesterone to androstenedione. Either ACTH or hCG (2000 U im daily for 5 days) may be used to unmask this defect in prepubertal patients.

Sex of rearing will depend upon age at diagnosis and the degree of ambiguity of the genitalia. Patients reared as males should be given substitution androgen replacement at puberty and can be expected to virilize normally as a consequence.

17-β-Hydroxysteroid Oxidoreductase Deficiency (Fig. 106-22). Male pseudohermaphrodism resulting from a partial block in testosterone synthesis at the level of the enzyme 17-oxidoreductase was first described in a family by Saez et al.[173,174] Subsequently, other cases have been reported.[175–178] This enzyme is necessary for the conversion of androstenedione to testosterone and estrone to estradiol. In affected XY patients, conspicuous phallic development or overt masculinization is usually not seen at birth, presumably as a result of meager in utero testosterone production owing to the enzymatic deficiency. Müllerian structures are absent, and the testes are well differentiated and found in the labia, inguinal canals, or abdomen. At puberty (Fig. 106-23),

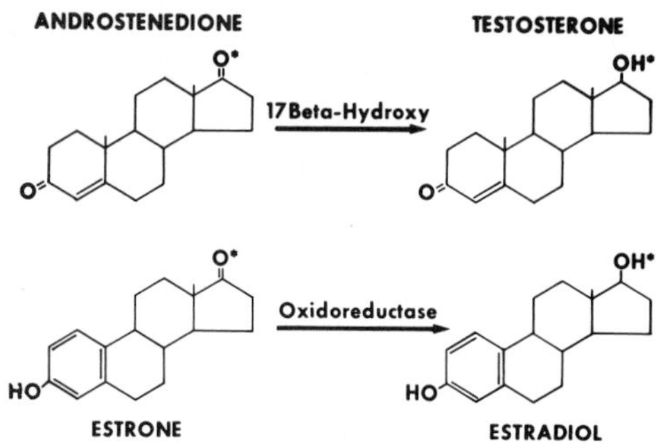

Fig. 106-22. Enzymatic conversion of androstenedione to testosterone and estrone to estradiol.

clitoral growth and other manifestations of heightened androgen secretion occur and, in some patients, breasts develop. The late onset of virilization is related to the pubertal increase of gonadotropin production, which can overcome, to a degree, the block in the testosterone biosynthetic pathway; whether breast development occurs in this disease is quite likely related to the degree of block and the relative production of testosterone and androstenedione versus estradiol and estrone.

In 4 patients whom we studied, as well as those reported by others, increased plasma androstenedione and estrone concentrations were detected in the postpubertal patient. Plasma testosterone and estradiol values were low but not absent, giving a high serum androstenedione/testosterone and estrone/estradiol ratio. The presence of these 17-hydroxylated C_{19} steroids in these patients suggests either that the block in 17-hydroxyoxidoreductase is not complete, or that enzymatic reduction of the 17-ketosteroids, androstenedione and estrone, to their 17-hydroxylated analogues, testosterone and estradiol, occurs in peripheral tissue, or that both mechanisms are operative. In addition, gonadotropins were elevated, leading to intense gonadal stimulation and Leydig cell hyperplasia. Plasma 17-OH progesterone and dehydroepiandrosterone levels were not elevated, indicating appropriate 17,20-desmolase and 3-β-hydroxysteroid dehydrogenase activities in the gonads and adrenal. The conversion of estrone to estradiol appears to be less impaired than that of androstenedione to testosterone in patients with this defect.

In the prepubertal patient or in the mildly affected adolescent, plasma androstenedione and estrone levels may not be elevated markedly. The defect in testosterone biosynthesis can be readily demonstrated by the administration of hCG, 2000 U/day for 5 days. A marked rise in estrone and androstenedione, as opposed to testosterone and estradiol, is observed. The phenotype of pubertal virilization, with gynecomastia, is etiologically heterogenous.

The absence of müllerian structures distinguishes patients with testosterone biosynthetic errors and androgen insensitivity from those with dysgenetic male pseudohermaphrodism.

The treatment of patients with this defect depends on the age of diagnosis and severity of genital abnormality. In the patient with ambiguous genitalia reared as a male, plastic repair of the genitalia is indicated. Testosterone replacement therapy may be necessary postpubertally to ensure adequate virilization and to prevent the development of gynecomastia. In patients reared as females (the usual case) the proper treatment is orchidectomy followed by estrogen substitution therapy at puberty.

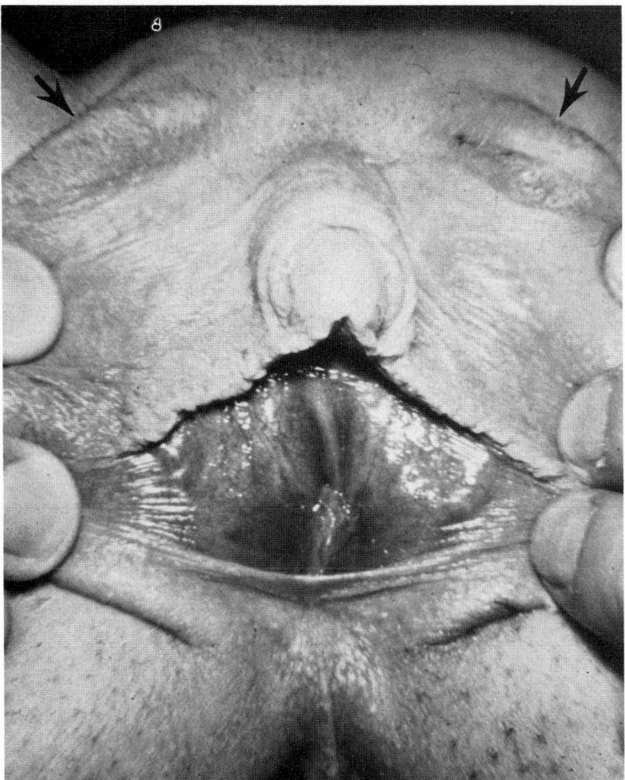

Fig. 106-23. External genitalia of a 13-year-old 46,XY patient with 17-oxidoreductase deficiency. The patient had both feminization and masculinization at puberty. There was no apparent ambiguity at birth. At 11 years of age she noted the onset of clitoromegaly, hirsutism, and a deep voice. On physical examination, acne, a male escutcheon, a blind vagina, a 5 × 2 cm clitoris, bilateral inguinal testes, and pubertal (Tanner III) breasts were noted. Steroid studies revealed the plasma androstenedione levels to be 883 ng/dl (10 times higher than normal for adult males). Estrone levels were 140 pg/ml (3 times the mean value for normal adult male values). Both the testosterone/androstenedione and estradiol/estrone ratios were reversed when compared with normals, confirming a defect in 17-β-hydroxysteroid oxidoreductase.

DEFECTS IN ANDROGEN-DEPENDENT TARGET TISSUES (Fig. 106-24)

Recently, the complex mechanism of action of steroid hormones at the cellular site of action has been clarified considerably.[179] Free testosterone enters into target cells and is reduced to dihydrotestosterone (DHT), which is, in turn, bound to a receptor protein; the receptor-DHT complex is then translocated into the nucleus of the target cell. In the nucleus, the receptor-DHT complex binds to chromatin and initiates transcription. Messenger RNA (mRNA) is synthesized, modified, and exported to the cytoplasm of the cell where polysomes translate the mRNA into new proteins that produce the androgenic effect on the cell. Abnormalities in 5-α-reductase activity, receptor activity, translocation, nuclear binding, transcription, exportation, and translation could lead to a lack of androgen effect at the end-organ and to male pseudohermaphrodism.

End-Organ Insensitivity to Androgenic Hormones (Androgen Receptor Defects)

Complete Syndrome of Testicular Feminization and Its Variants (Androgen Insensitivity and Its Variants) (Fig. 106-25). The testicular feminization syndrome is a disorder characterized by 46,XY karyotype, bilateral testes, female-appearing external genitalia at birth, a blind vagina, and no müllerian derivatives.[2,180] It

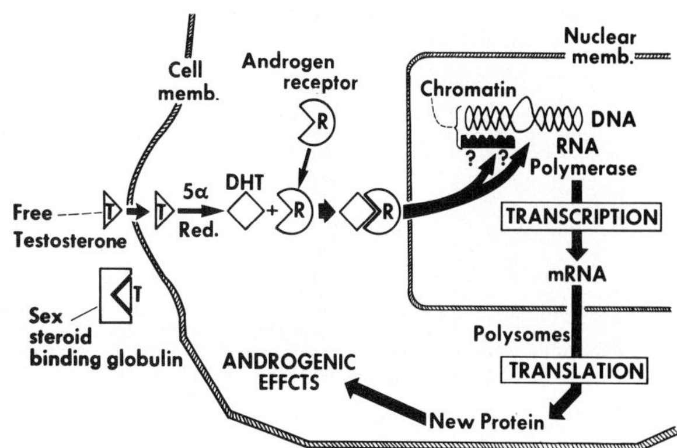

Fig. 106-24. Diagrammatic representation of the mechanism of action of testosterone at the target organs. 5-α-Red = 5-α-reductase, DHT = dihydrotestosterone. (From Grumbach, M. M. and Conte, F. A., in Williams, R. H., (ed.): Textbook of Endocrinology, 6th ed. Philadelphia, W. B. Saunders, in press.)

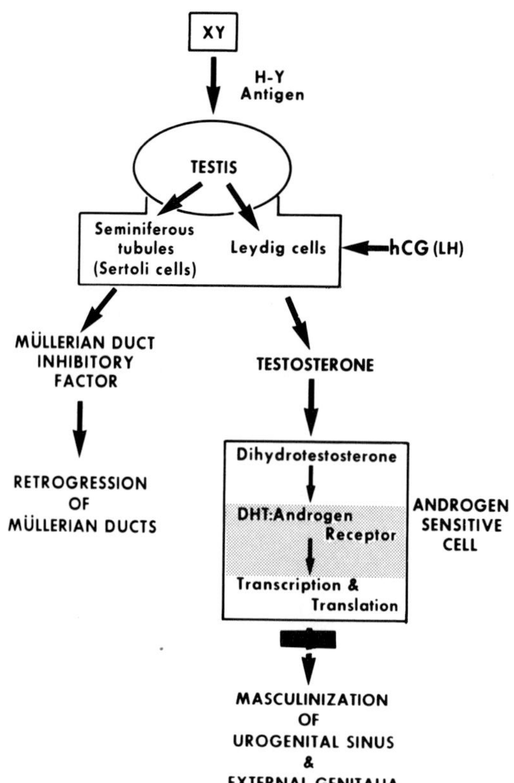

Fig. 106-25. Diagrammatic scheme of male pseudohermaphrodism due to complete or partial androgen insensitivity. (From Grumbach, M. M. and Conte, F. A., in Williams, R. H. (ed.): *Textbook of Endocrinology,* 6th ed. Philadelphia, W. B. Saunders, in press.)

has been estimated that this condition occurs in 1 per 60,000 males.[181] These patients are reared as females and have normal female gender identity (Fig. 106-26). At puberty, female secondary sexual characteristics develop, notably well-developed breasts and growth of the labia minora, but menarche does not occur. Pubic and axillary hair is usually sparse and is totally absent in one third of the patients. Some patients exhibit mild clitoromegaly and mild virilization at puberty, and we consider these patients as having a variant form of complete testicular feminization.

The vagina terminates blindly and is shorter than usual. No müllerian structures are found, presumably due to the normal secretion and action of müllerian duct inhibitory factor, a protein secreted by the fetal Sertoli cell. The testes are normal in size and may be located intra-abdominally, in the inguinal canal, or in the labia majora. Prepubertally, the testes are difficult to distinguish from normal. Postpubertally, small seminiferous tubules with few spermatogonia and no spermatozoa are seen. The Leydig cells are hyperplastic and clumped.[182] Hypoplastic or vestigial wolffian derivatives are usually found. Inguinal hernias are present in approximately 50 percent of patients with testicular feminization.

Endocrine evaluation of these patients postpubertally indicates that plasma sex steroids (testosterone, estradiol, estrone) are in the normal to high-normal male range.[183,184] It is apparent from the studies of Kelch et al. that the plasma estradiol levels result from peripheral conversion of testosterone and androstenedione, as well as from direct secretion from the testes.[185] The plasma LH concentration is elevated, while plasma FSH levels tend to be normal or only slightly increased.[186] Following gonadectomy, the circulating FSH and LH increase into the castrate range, whereas sex steroid values fall to hypogonadal levels.

Wilkins first suggested that the clinical features of this syndrome were the result of androgen resistance. French et al. supported this contention by failing to detect an acute metabolic response to the administration of large amounts of testosterone and dihydrotestosterone.[187] A model for this disease was discov-

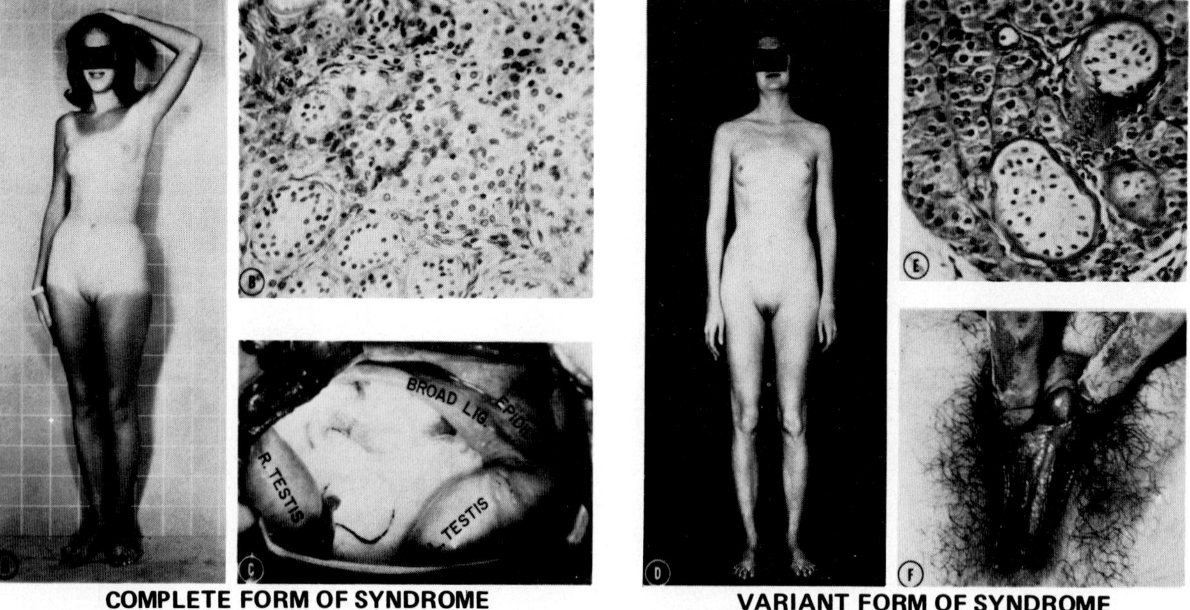

Fig. 106-26. Complete and variant form of testicular feminization: (A) A 17-year-old patient with complete syndrome. Note absence of sexual hair and breast development. (B) Testicular histology reveals Leydig cell hyperplasia and seminiferous tubules lacking germinal elements. (C) At laparotomy, testes, normal wolffian structures, and a blind vagina were found. (D) Variant form of complete testicular feminization. Scanty sexual hair is present, as well as breast development. (E) Leydig cell hyperplasia on testicular biopsy. (F) The clitoris was hypertrophied, but no labial fusion was present. A blind vagina was identified as well as wolffian structures at laparotomy. (From Grumbach, M. M. and Van Wyk, J., in *Textbook of Endocrinology,* 5th ed., R. H. Williams (ed.), Philadelphia, W. B. Saunders, 1974.)

ered in both the mouse and rat. The data accrued in the Tfm mutant rodent indicated that this androgen-insensitive form of male pseudohermaphrodism was due to an abnormality in cytosol-androgen receptor activity.[188]

Studies in man confirmed the work in rodents and indicated a qualitative abnormality in cytosol receptor activity in XY males with testicular feminization syndrome.[189] Subsequent studies have shown that there are at least two distinct groups of patients who manifest the complete syndrome of testicular feminization: one group who, like the Tfm/Y mouse, have absent or defective cytosol receptors for DHT; and another in whom cytosol and nuclear binding is apparently normal.[190] In this latter group, the receptor may be abnormal or a separate post-receptor defect may exist.

In the Tfm/Y mouse, the mutant gene is inherited as an X-linked recessive.[191] Subsequent studies in man have shown that androgen resistance is X-linked.[21]

The diagnosis of testicular feminization can be established by clinical criteria alone in the postpubertal patient. They may present with an inguinal hernia, primary amenorrhea, or a history of an affected member in the family. A phenotypic female with primary amenorrhea, breast development, scant or absent axillary and pubic hair, and an absent cervix on gynecological examination most likely has the complete form of testicular feminization. The buccal chromatin pattern is sex chromatin-negative, and the karyotype analysis is 46,XY; serum testosterone values are in the normal adult male range. Biochemically, a lack of cytosol binding of DHT will confirm the diagnosis. In affected patients who show apparently "normal" cytosol and nuclear binding of DHT, the diagnosis can be established by demonstrating little or no nitrogen and phosphorus retention in response to testosterone or dihydrotestosterone administration. Therapy consists of postpubertal gonadectomy because of the risk of malignancy, and estrogen replacement.

Incomplete Syndrome of Testicular Feminization and Its Variants (Incomplete Androgen Insensitivity and Its Variants). There is a group of androgen-insensitive 46,XY individuals who exhibit ambiguous external genitalia at birth, manifested by some phallic enlargement and labioscrotal fusion.[193–195] At puberty, although breast development occurs, feminization is less complete than in complete testicular feminization, and some degree of virilization is usual. Both the complete form of testicular feminization and the incomplete form show the following features: a 46,XY karyotype, bilateral testes, no müllerian derivatives, and gynecomastia at puberty. In general, patients with incomplete testicular feminization have ambiguous external genitalia and normal wolffian structures. As in patients with complete testicular feminization, the elevated serum testosterone and LH levels are consistent with resistance to androgen action rather than a biosynthetic defect. Incomplete testicular feminization also is inherited as an X-linked recessive.

Familial aggregates of incomplete testicular feminization have been described. The phenotypic spectrum in these families is wide and ranges from almost complete failure of masculinization of the external genitalia to hypoplastic male external genitalia. Toward the masculine end of the spectrum are the patients described by Reifenstein who have perineoscrotal hypospadias, gynecomastia, and infertility.[196] Wilson and co-workers investigated a family originally described by Bowen as having "Reifenstein syndrome."[197,198] The phenotype in 11 family members ranged from a mild defect in virilization in 2 (microphallus and bifid scrotum), to a more severe defect in 8 (perineoscrotal hypospadias), to a patient with absent vas deferens and a blind vagina. In 9 affected members in this family, the plasma testosterone and LH values were elevated when compared with normal men. In order to substantiate the suggestion of partial androgen insensitivity in these patients, they studied dihydrotestosterone (DHT) binding by cultured human fibroblasts.[199] Four patients with the incomplete form of androgen insensitivity were investigated: 3 patients from the family described by Bowen[197] and the patient described by Madden.[195] In 1 patient from the Bowen aggregate, little or no DHT binding was detectable in the cytosol of fibroblasts from genital skin. The 3 other patients, including the patient of Madden, had cytosol binding that was intermediate between those with absent binding and normal males. Recently, Amrhein et al. studied DT binding in another group of patients with so-called Reifenstein syndrome and reported heterogeneity in binding similar to that found in complete testicular feminization; i.e., they described 2 types of patients, one with little or no cytosol binding and another with apparently normal cytosol and nuclear binding.[200]

Keenan et al. reported 2 male siblings with partial masculinization of the external genitalia.[201] Both patients had perineal hypospadias, a urogenital sinus, and a small phallus at birth. No müllerian structures were present, and testes were in the inguinal canal. Postpubertally, one patient had mild virilization, with phallic enlargement and sexual hair. No facial hair or voice deepening occurred, and gynecomastia was prominent and required plastic surgery. Plasma testosterone concentrations were in the adult male range, and LH levels were elevated, suggesting partial androgen resistance. Studies in skin fibroblasts showed normal receptor affinity and capacity for dihydrotestosterone, normal nuclear retention of the receptor-DHT complex, and normal conversion of testosterone to dihydrotestosterone. However, no nitrogen and phosphate retention occurred in response to exogenous testosterone administration, indicating significant androgen insensitivity.

The relationship between DHT binding and the phenotypic manifestations of androgen insensitivity has not been clarified. Even in the patients with absent or low binding it is not yet clear whether the defect is due to the absence of receptor or to a defective protein that does not bind DHT. In the affected patients who have "normal" cytosol and nuclear binding of DHT, a defective receptor which, while capable of binding to chromatin, does not induce translational events or a post-translational defect may be present. Because of the similarity of phenotype, endocrine findings, inheritance, and pathogenesis, we favor a classification that includes the sporadic and familial cases of incomplete androgen insensitivity as a single variant rather than separating them nosologically. There is, however, clearly genetic heterogeneity.

The *diagnosis* of incomplete testicular feminization (incomplete androgen insensitivity) cannot be made from the phenotype alone. Errors in testosterone synthesis, as well as partial androgen resistance, can result in an 46,XY patient with incomplete labioscrotal fusion, a hypoplastic phallus, and a blind vagina. Patients with either 17-oxidoreductase deficiency or partial androgen insensitivity may exhibit significant but limited virilization at puberty and breast development. However, the pattern of plasma androstenedione and testosterone, and estrone and estradiol, before and especially after hCG administration is strikingly different. The plasma sex steroid and FSH and LH pattern, studies of cytosol and nuclear binding of DHT if available, and the acute metabolic response to androgen will help clarify the diagnosis. Cytosol and nuclear DHT binding may be absent, intermediate, or normal. If the acute metabolic response to testosterone or DHT is less than normal, the diagnosis of partial androgen insensitivity is made. Choice of sex of rearing will be contingent on the age at diagnosis, degree of genital ambiguity, and response to testosterone. Most patients, if diagnosed in infancy, should be reared as females in view of the gynecomastia and poor virilization at puberty and the increased risk of gonadal neoplasm.

Inborn Errors in Testosterone Metabolism by Peripheral Tissues

5-α-Reductase Deficiency (Male Pseudohermaphrodism with Masculinization at Puberty, etc.) (Figs. 106-27 and 106-28). These patients are similar to other forms of male pseudohermaphrodism in having a 46,XY karyotype, normally differentiated testes, male internal ducts, and ambiguous external genitalia. At puberty, they exhibit striking but selective signs of masculinization. In 1974, Walsh et al.[202] and Imperato-McGinley and Peterson[203] reported evidence of a defect in the conversion of testosterone to 5-α reduced forms of testosterone in patients with this syndrome. Imperato-McGinley and Peterson described studies in over 30 patients in 17 families from a genetic isolate in Salinas, Santo Domingo. [204] The affected patients were 46,XY males who, at birth, had bilateral inguinal or labial testes, and a labial-like scrotum (Fig. 106-29). In 29 of 30 of the affected individuals, a single perineal opening was present. A vaginal pouch was present, but there were no müllerian structures. The wolffian structures were well differentiated. At puberty (Fig. 106-30), striking virilization occurred in the affected males: the voice deepened, muscle mass increased, the phallus enlarged to a functional size, the scrotum became rugated and hyperpigmented, and the testes descended; none of the affected 46,XY patients exhibited gynecomastia. Semen analysis in 1 patient revealed 40 million sperm per milliliter, with 80 percent motility. On the other hand, acne, prostatic enlargement, facial hair growth, temporal hair recession, and gynecomastia did not occur. The most surprising part of the metamorphosis was that psychosexual orientation was reported as male postpubertally, even though all these patients in this isolated town had been raised as females prior to puberty.

Endocrinological evaluation of these patients supports the hypothesis that they have 5-α-reductase deficiency, i.e., there is impaired biotransformation of testosterone to dihydrotestosterone at the target tissue. Mean plasma testosterone levels are higher, while mean DHT levels are lower than in normal adult males. The testosterone/dihydrotestosterone ratio varies from 35 to 84 in affected patients, compared with 8 to 16 in normals.[204] After hCG, the testosterone/dihydrotestosterone ratio is 75 to 164, compared with 3 to 26 in normal subjects.[204] The concentration of plasma LH and FSH is elevated. In these patients, conversion of testosterone to dihydrotestosterone is less than 1 percent.[204] In normal adult males, 10 percent of testosterone secreted is excreted in the form of conjugates of androsterone (5α) and etiocholanolone (5β). Peterson et al. demonstrated that the ratio of 5β (etiocholanolone) to 5α (androsterone) in 23 normal males is 0.46 to 1.5, whereas in 19 affected males the range was 2.2 to 6.3.[204] This abnormal ratio of β/α C_{19} steroids is consistent with 5-α-reductase deficiency. Fibroblast cultures obtained from genital skin demonstrated absent 5-α-reductase activity.[204]

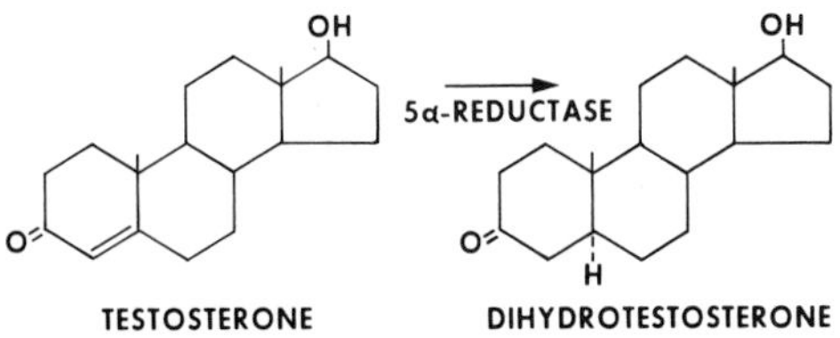

OH OH
5α-REDUCTASE
TESTOSTERONE DIHYDROTESTOSTERONE

Fig. 106-27. Enzymatic conversion of testosterone to dihydrotestosterone.

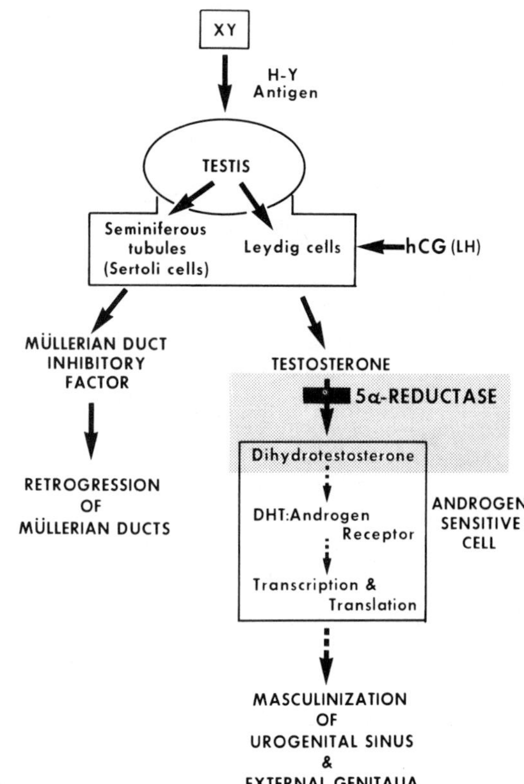

Fig. 106-28. Diagrammatic scheme of male pseudohermaphrodism due to 5-α-reductase deficiency. (From Grumbach, M. M. and Conte, F. A., in Williams, R. H. (ed.): *Textbook of Endocrinology*, 6th ed. Philadelphia, W. B. Saunders, in press.)

Heterozygotes showed intermediate 5β/5α ratios and 5 functionally and phenotypically normal females were found to be homozygotes, according to their 5β/5α ratios.[204] The inheritance of this defect in this large kindred was consistent with an autosomal recessive trait.[204]

Of interest is the question of why these patients exhibit growth of the penis at puberty despite incomplete masculinization of the external genitalia in utero. Peterson et al.[204] have hypothesized that the changes that occur at puberty, i.e., increased muscle mass, growth of the phallus, deepening of the voice, and spermatozoa, are all testosterone-dependent effects while acne, temporal hair recession, facial hair, and prostatic enlargement are dihydrotestosterone-dependent. The androgen receptor binds testosterone as well as dihydrotestosterone but with lower affinity. Hence, sustained high testosterone levels in these patients may play a role in the growth of the phallus and other signs of masculinization observed at puberty.

The diagnosis of a 5-α-reductase deficiency (Table 106-4) can be made prepubertally as well as postpubertally by measuring 5β/

Table 106-4. 5-α-Reductase Deficiency

Diagnosis
- 46,XY with ambiguous genitalia
- Masculinization at puberty
- Normal plasma T for male
- Decreased plasma DHT levels, abnormal T/DHT ratio before and after hCG
- Increased 5-β/5-α ratio of urinary 11-deoxy C_{19} steroid metabolites of testosterone
- Decreased 5-α-reductase activity in genital skin in vitro
- Decreased conversion of infused testosterone (normal conversion 4–7%) in vivo to DHT

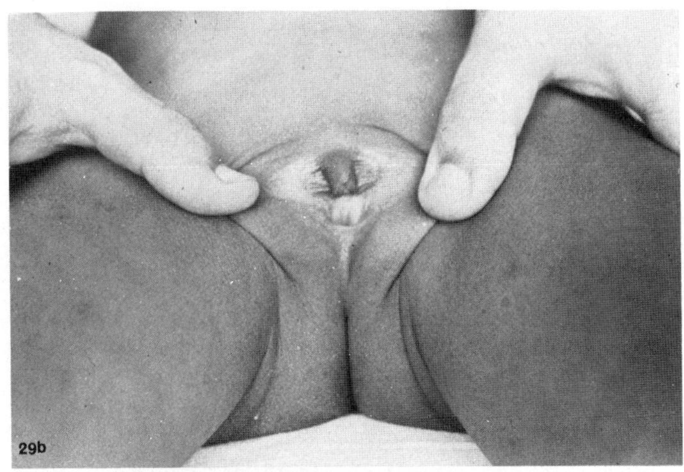

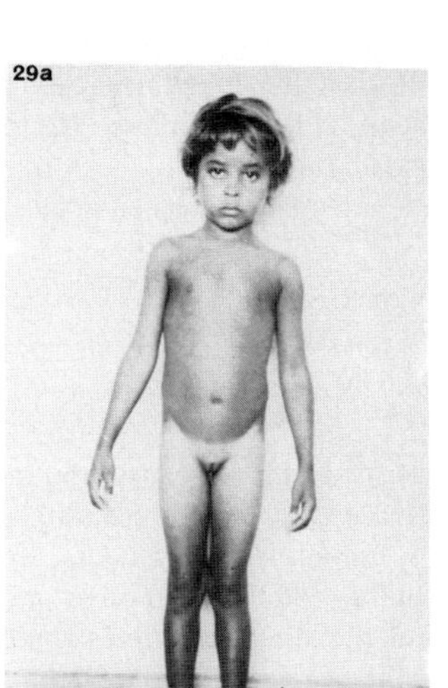

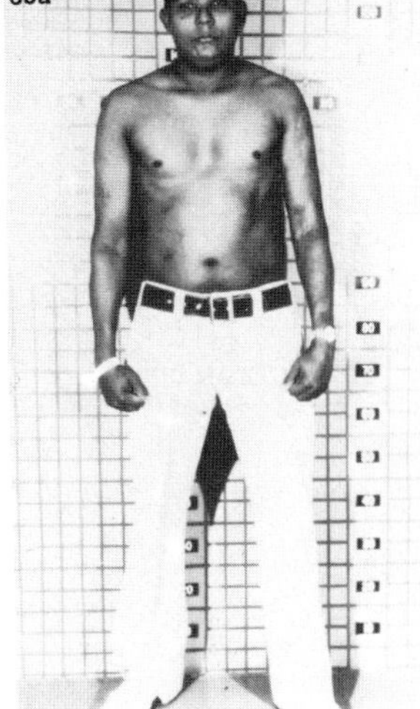

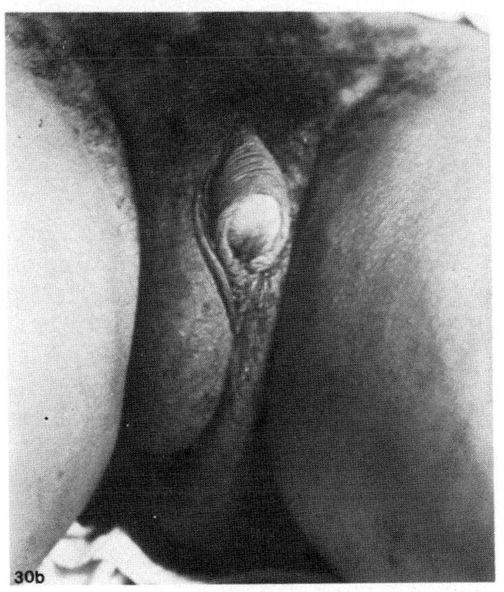

Fig. 106-29a. Prepubertal male with 5-α-reductase deficiency raised as a female. **Fig. 106-29b.** External genitalia: A single perineal orifice was present, as well as a hypoplastic phallus and labia-like scrotum. (From Peterson, R. E., et al., *Am. J. Med. 62:* 170, 1977.) **Fig. 106-30a.** Postpubertal male with 5-α-reductase deficiency. **Fig. 106-30b.** External genitalia: Note scrotal testes, phallic enlargement, and hypospadias. (From Peterson, R. E., et al., *Am. J. Med. 62:* 170, 1977.)

5α C_{19} steroid metabolites in the urine. Abnormal $5\beta/5\alpha$ C_{19} steroid ratios may be found in hypothyroidism, hypercortisolemic states, and acute intermittent porphyria.[204] As mentioned, either basal plasma testosterone/dihydrotestosterone ratios or hCG-induced testosterone/dihydrotestosterone ratios will confirm the diagnosis. The diagnosis is important in view of the striking masculinization that occurs at puberty. Thus, a 46,XY infant with this disorder should be reared as a male in view of the natural history of this syndrome. The uniqueness of this genetic isolate and the unprecedented ability of these patients to change their gender identity at puberty needs further study before traditional concepts of gender identity are modified. Familial cases with phenotypes similar to the 5-α-reductase deficient patients have been described, but definitive enzymatic studies have not been performed in them, thus precluding their etiologic classification.[205,206]

DYSGENETIC MALE PSEUDOHERMAPHRODISM (Fig. 106-31)

We have previously discussed this heterogeneous group of patients under the syndrome of gonadal dysgenesis and its variants and familial and sporadic XY gonadal dysgenesis (see p. 1323). Essentially, this group of patients has a defect in gonadal differentiation that may be related to (1) a sex chromosomal anomaly, such as a structurally abnormal Y or XO/XY mosaicism, (2) absence of genetic coding for H-Y antigen, (3) a mutant gene, X-linked or sex-limited autosomal dominant, which we postulate may repress H-Y antigen, or the specific H-Y antigen receptor on gonadal cells, or (4) unknown local teratologic factors. The spectrum of genital abnormality is dependent on the amount of testosterone produced by the dysgenetic gonads. Müllerian structures are usually present, and, in general, the risk of gonadal malignancy is greatly increased.

Association with Degenerative Renal Disease

Several cases are recorded of male pseudohermaphrodism associated with the early onset of severe primary degenerative renal disease; [207,208] the syndrome complex consists of a nephron disorder, the propensity for developing Wilms' tumor, and dysgenetic male pseudohermaphrodism.[209] The association suggests the common origin during the organogenesis of the testis and the kidney, both of which arise from the urogenital ridge.

Anorchia: (1) Vanishing Testis Syndrome XY Agonadism; XY Gonadal Agenesis

Cryptorchid males with normally differentiated male external genitalia occasionally are found to lack testicles; presumably the testes were present in fetal life to modulate complete masculiniza-

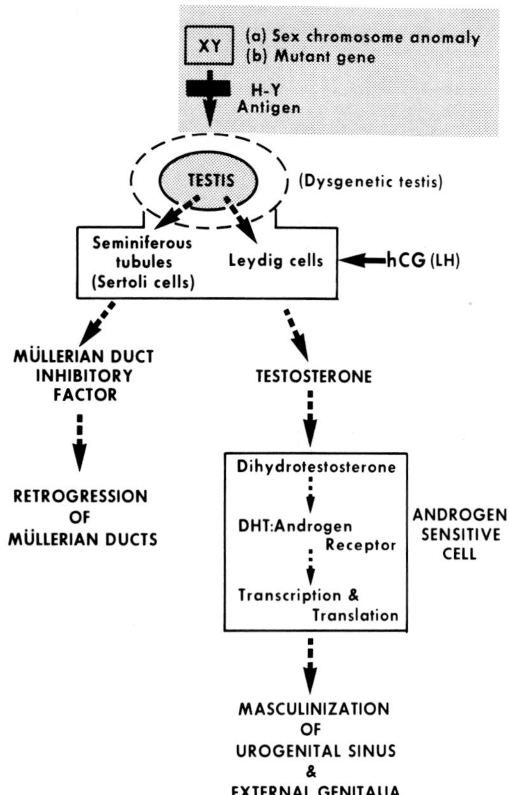

Fig. 106-31. Diagrammatic scheme of dysgenetic male pseudohermaphrodism. This condition can result from sex chromosome mosaicism (XO/XY), structurally abnormal Y chromosomes, mutant genes that affect the expression of H-Y antigen, and unknown teratologic factors. A small dysgenetic testicle or streak gonad results. The degree of masculinization is dependent upon the functional ability of the dysgenetic gonad to produce müllerian duct inhibitory factor and testosterone. Thus, not infrequently, these patients have a vagina, uterus, and tubes along with ambiguous genitalia. (From Grumbach, M. M. and Conte, F. A., in Williams, R. H. (ed.): *Textbook of Endocrinology,* 6th ed. Philadelphia, W. B. Saunders, in press.)

tion and subsequently have atrophied.[210] Unilateral and bilateral anorchia has been described, as well as familial cases, including monozygotic twins concordant and discordant for anorchia.[211,212] These patients are usually recognized at laparotomy for cryptorchidism. The diagnosis of anorchia in a normally differentiated male with no müllerian structures is strongly suggested by the detection of elevated plasma FSH concentrations (and often LH) and an augmented response to LRF and the failure of hCG (2000 U daily for 5 days) to elicit an appropriate rise in plasma testosterone.[213] These patients should be given replacement therapy with testosterone enanthate in oil beginning at 12 to 13 years. We usually administer 50 mg im monthly for 1 to 2 years, then progress to full replacement doses of 200–400 mg im every 3 to 4 weeks. The insertion of silastic prosthetic testes is of considerable cosmetic and psychologic benefit.

Normally differentiated 46,XY males have been described with rudimentary testes.[214,215] These males have testes that are less than 1 cm in greatest diameter. The testes histologically show a few Leydig cells, small tubules with Sertoli cells, and a few spermatogonia. Endocrine evaluation reveals elevated plasma gonadotropins and a poor testosterone response to hCG.

Twelve individuals with a 46,XY karyotype, absent gonads, genital ambiguity, and rudimentary or absent müllerian or wolffian structures have been described.[216,217] The external genitalia usually show some degree of clitoromegaly and fused labioscrotal folds. The vagina is absent and rudimentary or absent genital ducts are found on laparotomy. These patients exhibit elevated gonadotropins, and the administration of hCG fails to raise the low plasma testosterone concentration. Associated somatic anomalies are often found in this syndrome, including skull defects, vertebral anomalies, and borderline intelligence. These patients presumably are at the end of the clinical spectrum involving males with rudimentary testes and progressing through those with anorchia. In these patients, the deficiency of fetal testicular function presumably occurred early in the critical stage of development and led to varying degrees of incomplete masculinization of the external genitalia. Several instances of multiple affected siblings have been described.

DEFECT IN SYNTHESIS, SECRETION or RESPONSE TO MÜLLERIAN DUCT INHIBITORY FACTOR (PERSISTENT MÜLLERIAN DUCT SYNDROME) (Fig. 106-32)

Phenotypic males have been described with normally differentiated male external genitalia but with a uterus and fallopian tubes as well as male genital ducts.[218,219] Usually these patients are detected because of prolapse of the uterus and fallopian tubes into an inguinal hernia. The persistent müllerian duct derivatives could result from a specific defect in the synthesis, secretion, or response to the müllerian duct inhibitory factor. Although, in some, the testes are hypoplastic, these patients usually masculinize at puberty, and fertility has been described. Pedigree analysis suggests that this disorder is transmitted as an autosomal trait or X-linked recessive.[220] Noteworthy is the occurrence of a seminoma or related germ cell tumor in 5 percent of affected patients.[106]

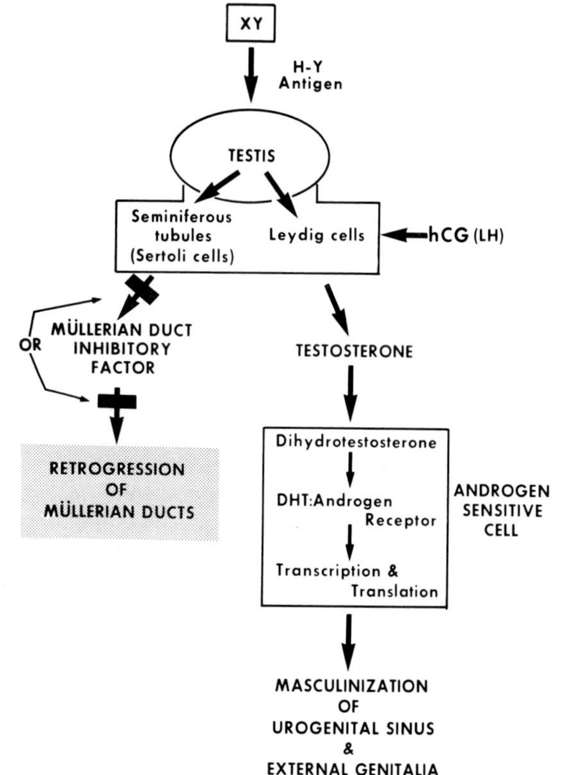

Fig. 106-32. Diagrammatic scheme showing male pseudohermaphrodism resulting from a defect in the synthesis, secretion, or response to müllerian duct inhibitory factor. (From Grumbach, M. M. and Conte, F. A., in Williams, R. H. (ed.): *Textbook of Endocrinology,* 6th ed. Philadelphia, W. B. Saunders, in press.)

MATERNAL INGESTION OF PROGESTINS AND ESTROGENS

Both progestins and synthetic estrogens have been implicated in male pseudohermaphrodism.[2,221,222] Aarskog reviewed 100 cases of hypospadias and demonstrated a history of maternal progestin ingestion in 9.[221] The degree of hypospadias correlated with the stage of gestation at which exposure to the progestin occurred. Rats given high doses of progestins during gestation may exhibit interference with urethral groove fusion.[223] Whether progestins interfere with the synthesis of fetal testosterone, or exert an antiandrogen action, or have a direct teratogenic effect is unknown.

Male pseudohermaphrodism has been described in a patient whose mother received large doses of diethylstilbestrol during pregnancy.[224]

Because of the report of Herbst et al. linking diethylstilbestrol therapy in mothers with vaginal and cervical adenocarcinoma in daughters,[225] abnormalities in the genital tract have been sought in males.[226,227] Two studies showed an adverse effect of diethylstilbestrol administration, during pregnancy, on the male genitourinary tract. The most common findings were meatal stenosis, epididymal cysts, hypoplastic testes, and induration of the testicular capsule. Neither study was designed to assess whether malignant lesions, comparable to the vaginal and cervical clear cell adenocarcinomas in diethylistilbestrol-exposed female offspring, will develop in the prenatally exposed males.

UNCLASSIFIED FORMS OF ABNORMAL SEX DEVELOPMENT

MALES

Hypospadias

Hypospadias occurs as an isolated finding in 1 per 700 newborn males. [2] Most patients with first-degree hypospadias, with easily palpable testes in the scrotum, have no underlying problem and virilize normally at puberty. In 15 percent of patients with penoscrotal, scrotal, or perineal forms of hyposadias, however, a chromosomal or endocrine disorder is present.[228] Hypospadias as an isolated anomaly has occurred in multiple members of a family,[228,229] as well as in association with a wide variety of complex malformation syndromes, including autosomal abnormalities.[230]

Familial Forms of Primary Hypogonadism and Gynecomastia (Rosewater Syndrome)

A number of familial cases of hypogonadism with and without gynecomastia have been described. Rosewater et al. described 4 related males with gynecomastia and arrested germinal maturation.[231] Unfortunately, the studies reported in these patients do not clearly delineate the pathogenesis of this syndrome. In other families, deficient gonadotropin associated with anosmia (Kallman syndrome), as well as defects in testicular embryogenesis, has resulted in this syndrome.

FEMALES

Absence of or Anomalies in the Development of the Vagina, Uterus or Fallopian Tubes

Congenital absence of the vagina in conjunction with abnormal or absent müllerian structures has been recognized as a syndrome complex for over 100 years.[232] The Mayer-Rokitansky-Küstner-Hauser syndrome was the second most common cause of primary amenorrhea in a series of 538 cases reviewed by Ross and vande Wiele. [233] Clinically, 46,XX females with normal ovarian function (including breasts, female body habitus, and sexual hair) present in adolescence with primary amenorrhea. The vagina is absent or hypoplastic, and the uterus may vary from normal, to rudimentary bicornuate cords, to complete absence. There is an increased frequency of renal, skeletal, and other congenital anomalies. The diagnosis can be established by the clinical picture and a 46,XX karyotype. In general, patients with the Rokitansky-Küstner syndrome lack clitoromegaly, which distinguishes them from nonadrenal female pseudohermaphrodites (although these syndromes may overlap).

Therapy in patients with absent vagina involves either construction of an artificial vagina or stretching the vagina by the use of a prosthesis.[234]

Recently, a 46,XX female with normal female external genitalia and absent vagina, uterus, tubes, and gonads was described.[235]

DIAGNOSIS OF ABNORMALITIES OF SEX DIFFERENTIATION (Fig. 106-33)

SEX OF REARING

It is the primary responsibility of the physician to establish a diagnosis as soon after birth as posible in infants with ambiguous sexual development. The diagnosis should be made, a sex of rearing assigned, and the gender role reinforced by whatever surgical, hormonal, and psychologic measures are needed. The aim is to obtain a well-adjusted, sexually functional person so that choice of sex of rearing must be dependent principally on the functional potential of the genitalia. Only in the case of XX individuals with the 11- and 21-hydroxylase deficient forms of congenital adrenal hyperplasia is fertility of decisive importance. Since, in these patients, the abnormality is limited to the external genitalia, which can be readily corrected by surgery, and further virilization can be prevented by appropriate glucocorticoid therapy, they should all be raised as females.

In all other patients (with the possible exception of 5-α-reductase deficiency and more true hermaphrodites), ambiguity of the external genitalia is associated with infertility. Thus, in these patients, the functional potential of the genitalia and the possibilities for surgical reconstruction, are the prime considerations in assigning a sex of rearing.

DIFFERENTIAL DIAGNOSIS

An anomaly of sex should be considered in any patient with ambiguous genitalia, phenotypic males with cryptorchidism or gynecomastia, and apparent females with inguinal masses, inguinal herniae, or clitoral enlargement. The initial step in the diagnostic evaluation is the determination of sex chromatin and a karyotype analysis.

SEX CHROMATIN-POSITIVE FEMALE PSEUDOHERMAPHRODITES

Most female pseudohermaphrodites will be found to have the 21-hydroxylase-deficient form of congenital adrenal hyperplasia. The most definitive test for diagnosis is the plasma 17-hydroxyprogesterone level, which is elevated to greater than 1000 ng/dl in affected infants. Sex chromatin-positive infants who fail to thrive, vomit, and have dehydration are highly suspect for the salt-losing form of 21-hydroxylase deficiency. After congenital adrenal hyper-

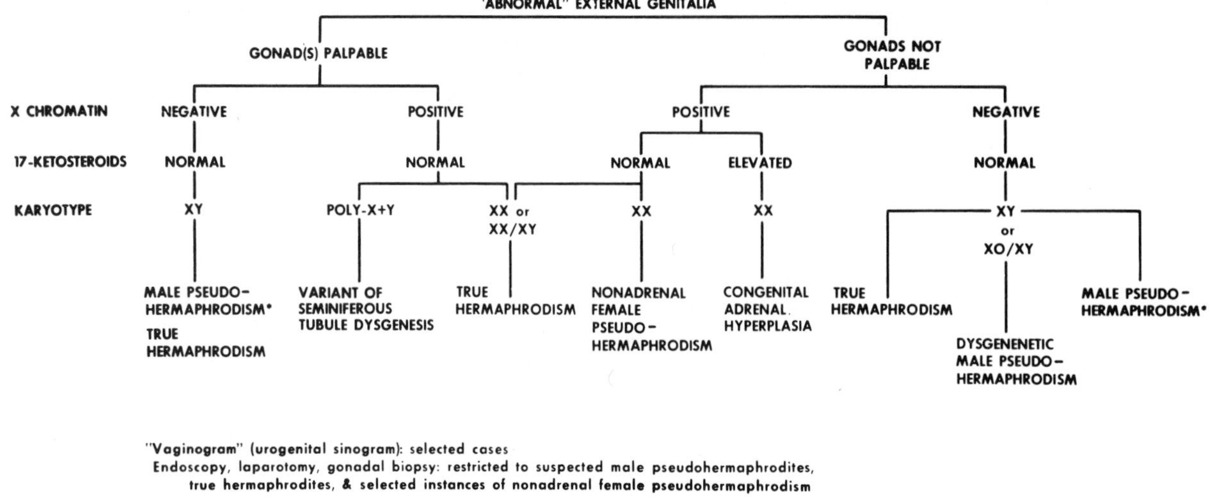

Fig. 106-33. Steps in the diagnosis of abnormalities of sex differentiation in infancy and childhood. (From Grumbach, M. M., in *Pediatrics,* 13th ed., Holt, L. E., Jr., McIntosh, R., Barnett, H. L. (eds.), New York, Appleton-Century-Crofts, 1962.)

plasia has been excluded by the appropriate diagnostic studies, other forms of female pseudohermaphrodism should be considered.

Seventy percent of true hermaphrodites are sex chromatin-positive, and they must be distinguished from patients with female pseudohermaphrodism. A palpable gonad in the labia or inguinal canal, especially one whose consistency and conformation suggests an ovotestis, is suggestive of true hermaphrodism. It is important to determine the nature of the internal ducts and gonads in these patients prior to sex assignment. Thus, endoscopy, sinograms, and pelvic exploration are indicated.

The assignment of sex in a true hermaphrodite is dependent on the potential for normal function and the possibilities for surgical correction of the external genitalia. It is important to remember, in these cases, that testicular tissue is invariably dysgenetic and carries the risk of malignancy, while ovarian tissue may be functionally normal.

SEX CHROMATIN-NEGATIVE INFANTS

Patients who are sex chromatin-negative have either male pseudohermaphrodism, the syndrome of gonadal dysgenesis, or true hermaphrodism. The family history may suggest the diagnosis, since many sexual abnormalities are hereditary in nature. Other studies, such as karyotype analysis, urinary and plasma steroids, and radiological studies of the urogenital sinus with contrast media may be helpful in diagnosis. Patients with the syndrome of gonadal dysgenesis (Turner syndrome) invariably have somatic stigmata that lead to the diagnosis.

Diagnostically, of great value in sex chromatin-negative patients is the absence of müllerian derivatives (a uterus and cervix). This finding suggests either a block in testosterone synthesis or end-organ insensitivity to androgen as a source of the problem. In these patients, the determination of plasma testosterone, dihydrotestosterone, androstenedione, 17-hydroxyprogesterone, estrone, estradiol, and dehydroepiandrosterone responses to 2000 U hCG injected daily for 5 days will help to define a biosynthetic error or 5-α-reductase deficiency.

Plasma gonadotropins are also a useful index of gonadal integrity, since plasma FSH, in particular, rises strikingly after 4 to 5 days of age in agonadal infants.

In male pseudohermaphrodites with hypoplastic phallus, it is prudent to determine whether or not the phallus will respond to exogenous testosterone in infancy, especially in those with underdeveloped but male external genitalia and scrotal testes; 25–50 mg of testosterone enanthate may be given intramuscularly once a month for 3 months. No significant increase in phallic length suggests that the phallus lacks the capacity for growth in later childhood and at puberty and argues for a female sex assignment.

The decision as to sex of rearing of a patient must be firmly made by the physician. Vacillation and indecision will result in parental confusion and anxiety. It is important to fully discuss with the parents the bipotential nature of sex differentiation in the human fetus and its relationship to the development of their child's sexual organs. It is critical to assure the parents that their child is not half-boy and half-girl and that the anomalous development does not result in homosexuality or transvestism.

The studies of Money and co-workers indicate that a change of sex rearing is feasible up to 1½ to 2½ years of age. Thereafter, a change of sex should be undertaken only after a review of alternatives and with the concurrence or assistance of a psychiatrist.

Reconstructive surgery, if necessary, should be completed prior to 18 months of age. We have preferred one of the clitoral recession procedures rather than clitorectomy in children assigned a female sex.

The question of gonadectomy is difficult, and the decision is based on the risk of malignancy and the type of secondary sexual characteristics to be expected at puberty. In dysgenetic male pseudohermaphrodites raised as females, the risk of malignancy and the potential virilizing effects of a dysgenetic testicle make gonadectomy advisable at the time of initial diagnosis. On the other hand, 46,XY patients with complete androgen insensitivity have a low risk of malignancy (<4 percent) before 25 years of age. Thus, it may be desirable to delay gonadectomy until after they have feminized spontaneously, which will reinforce the patient's sexual identity as a female.

Hormonal substitution therapy has been discussed in previous sections. The general rule is to mimic normal puberty so that secondary sexual characteristics emerge appropriately in timing and sequence. The result of all decisions should be a normal, well-adjusted child who will grow and develop into a mature adult, confident of his or her own identity and capable of achieving satisfactory sexuality and function.

REFERENCES

1. Jost, A., Vigier, B., Prepin, J.: Studies on sex differentiation in mammals. *Recent Prog. Horm. Res. 29:* 1–41, 1973.
2. Grumbach, M. M., Van Wyk, J. S.: Disorders of sex differentiation, in Williams, R. H. (ed.) *Textbook of Endocrinology,* 5th ed., Philadelphia, W. B. Saunders Co., 1974, pp. 423–501.

2a. Grumbach, M. M.: Genetic mechanisms of sexual development. In Porter, I. H. and Vallet, H. L. (eds.). New York, Academic Press, 1978, in press.

3. Morishima, A., Grumbach, M. M.: The interrelationship of sex chromosome constitution and phenotype in the syndrome of gonadal dysgenesis and its variants. *Ann. N.Y. Acad. Sci. 155:* 695–715, 1968.
4. Wachtel, S. S., Ohno, S., Koo, G. C., et al: Possible role for H-Y antigen in the primary determination of sex. *Nature 257:* 235–236, 1975.
5. Ohno, S.: Major regulatory genes for mammalian sexual development. *Cell 7:* 315–321, 1976.
6. Eichwald, E. J., Silmser, C. R.: Article in section on Skin. *Transplant Bull. 2:* 148–149, 1955.
7. Wachtel, S. S., Koo, G. C., Zuckerman, E. E., et al: Serological cross-reactivity between H-Y (male) antigens of mouse and man. *Proc. Natl. Acad. Sci. USA 71:* 1215–1218, 1974.
8. Krco, C. J., Goldberg, E. H.: H-Y (male) antigen: Detection on eight-cell mouse embryos. *Science 193:* 1134–1135, 1976.
9. Wachtel, S. S., Koo, G. C., Breg, W. R., et al: Expression of H-Y antigen in human males with two Y chromosomes. *N. Engl. J. Med. 293:* 1070–1072, 1975.
10. Wachtel, S. S., Koo, G. C., Breg, W. R., et al: Serologic detection of a Y-linked gene in XX males and XX true hermaphrodites. *N. Engl. J. Med. 295:* 750–754, 1976.
11. Bennett, D., Mathieson, B. J., Scheid, M., et al: Serological evidence for H-Y antigen in Sxr,XX sex reversed phenotypic males. *Nature (London) 265:* 255–257, 1977.
12. Bennett, D., Boyse, E. A., Lyon, M. F., et al: Expression of H-Y (male) antigen in phenotypically female Tfm/Y mice. *Nature (London) 257:* 236–238, 1975.
13. Ohno, S., Christian, L. C., Wachtel, S. S., et al: Hormone-like role of H-Yantigen in bovine freemartin gonad. *Nature (London) 261:* 597–599, 1976.
14. Josso, N.: Permeability of membranes to the müllerian-inhibiting substance synthesized by the human fetal testis in vitro: A clue to its biochemical nature. *J. Clin. Endocrinol. Metab. 34:* 265–270, 1972.
15. Josso, N.: Evolution of the müllerian-inhibiting activity of human testis: Effect of fetal, peri-natal and post-natal human testicular tissue on the müllerian duct of the fetal rat in organ culture. *Biol. Neonate 20:* 368–379, 1972.
16. Blanchard, M., Josso, N.: Source of the anti-müllerian hormone synthesized by the fetal testis: Müllerian-inhibiting activity of fetal bovine sertoli cells in tissue culture. *Pediatr. Res. 8:* 968–971, 1974.
17. Kaplan, S. L., Grumbach, M. M.: The ontogenesis of human fetal hormones. II. Luteinizing hormone (LH) and follicle stimulating hormone (FSH). *Acta Endocrinol. (Kbh) 81:* 808–829, 1976.
18. Siiteri, P. K., Wilson, J. D.: Testosterone formation and metabolism during male sexual differentiation in the human embryo. *J. Clin. Endocrinol. Metab. 38:* 113–125, 1974.
19. Wilson, J. D.: Testosterone uptake by the urogenital tract of the rabbit embryo. *Endocrinology 92:* 1192–1199, 1973.
20. Imperato-McGinley, J., Guerrero, L., Gautier, T., et al: Steroid 5α-reductase deficiency in man: An inherited form of male pseudohermaphroditism. *Science 186:* 1213–1215, 1974.
21. Meyer, W. J. III, Migeon, B. R., Migeon, C. J.: Locus on human X chromosome for dihydrotestosterone receptor and androgen insensitivity. *Proc. Natl. Acad. Sci. 72:* 1469–1472, 1975.
22. Paulsen, C. A.: The testes, in Williams, R. H. (ed.): *Textbook of Endocrinology,* 5th ed. Philadelphia, W. B. Saunders, 1974, pp. 323–364.
23. Gordon, D. L., Krmpotic, E., Thomas, W., et al: Pathologic testicular findings in Klinefelter's syndrome 47,XXY vs. 46,XY/47,XXY. *Arch. Intern. Med. 130:* 726–739, 1972.
24. Schibler, D., Brook, C. G. D., Kind, H. P., et al: Growth and body proportions in 54 boys and men with Klinefelter's syndrome. *Helv. Paediatr. Acta 29:* 325–333, 1974.
25. Frøland, A.: Klinefelter's syndrome: Clinical, endocrinological and cytogenetical studies. *Dan. Med. Bull. 16 (Suppl) 6:* 1–108, 1969.
26. Illig, R., Tolksdorf, M., Murset, G., et al: LH and FSH responses to synthetic LH-RH in children and adolescents with Turner's and Klinefelter's syndrome. *Helv. Paediatr. Acta 30:* 221–231, 1975.
27. Hamerton, J. L.: *Human Cytogenetics.* New York, Academic Press, 1971, vol. 2.
28. Paulsen, C. A., Gordon, D. L., Carpentier, R. W., et al: Klinefelter's syndrome and its variants: A hormonal and chromosomal study. *Recent Prog. Horm. Res. 24:* 321–363, 1968.
29. Wang, C., Baker, H. W. G., Burger, H. G., et al: Hormonal studies in Klinefelter's syndrome. *Clin. Endocrinol. 4:* 399–411, 1975.
30. Jackson, A. W., Muldal, S., Ockey, C. H., et al: Carcinoma of the male breast in association with the Klinefelter syndrome. *Br. Med. J. 1:* 223–225, 1965.
31. Harnden, D. G., MacLean, N., Langlands, A. O.: Carcinoma of the breast and Klinefelter's syndrome. *J. Med. Genet. 8:* 460–461, 1971.
32. Sanger, R., Tippett, P., Gavin, J.: Xg groups and sex abnormalities in people of northern European ancestry. *J. Med. Genet. 8:* 417–426, 1971.
33. Rosenkranz, V. W.: Klinefelter-syndrome bei kindern von frauen mit geschlechtschromosomen-anomalien. *Helv. Paediatr. Acta 20:* 359–368, 1965.
34. Barr, M. L., Carr, D. H., Soltan, H. C., et al: The XXYY variant of Klinefelter's syndrome. *Can. Med. Assoc. J 90:* 575–580, 1964.
35. Simpson, J. L., Morillo-Cucci, G., Horwith, M., et al: Abnormalities of human sex chromosomes. VI. Monozygotic twins with the complement 48,XXXY. *Humangenetik 21:* 301–308, 1974.
36. Simpson, J. L.: *Disorders of Sexual Differentiation. Etiology and Clinical Delineation.* New York, Academic Press, 1976.
37. de la Chapelle, A.: Nature and origin of males with XX chromosomes. *Am. J. Hum. Genet. 24:* 71–105, 1972.
38. Palutke, W. A., Chen, Y., Chen, H.: Presence of brightly fluorescent material in testes of XX males. *J. Med. Genet. 10:* 170–198, 1973.
39. Iinuma, K., Ohzeki, T., Ohtaguro, K., et al: Y chromatin positive cells in the smear preparations of the gonad from an XX male. *Humangenetik 30:* 193–196, 1975.
40. de la Chapelle, A., Schröder, J., Murros, J., et al: Two XX males in one family and additional observations bearing on etiology of XX males. *Clin. Genet. 11:* 91–96, 1977.
41. Turner, H. H.: A syndrome of infantilism, congenital webbed neck and cubitus valgus. *Endocrinology 23:* 566–574, 1938.
42. Mattevi, M. S., Wolff, H., Salzano, F. M., et al: Cytogenetic, clinical and genealogical analyses in a series of gonadal dysgenesis patients and their families. *Humangenetik 13:* 126–143, 1971.
43. Palmer, C. G., Reichmann, A.: Chromosomal and clinical findings in 110 females with Turner syndrome. *Hum. Genet. 35:* 35–49, 1976.
44. Filipsson, R., Lindsten, J., Almquist, S.: Time of eruption of the permanent teeth, cephalometric and tooth measurement and sulphation factor activity in 45 patients with Turner's syndrome with different types of X chromosome aberrations. *Acta Endocrinol. 48:* 91–113, 1965.
45. Szpunar, J., Rybak, M.: Middle ear disease in Turner's syndrome. *Arch. Otolaryngol. 87:* 34–40, 1968.
46. Benson, P. F., Gough, M. H., Polani, P. E.: Lymphangiography and chromosome studies in females with lymphoedema and possible ovarian dysgenesis. *Arch. Dis. Child. 40:* 27–32, 1965.
47. Garron, D. C., Vander Stoep, L. R.: Personality and intelligence in Turner's syndrome. A critical review. *Arch. Gen. Psychiatry (Chicago) 21:* 339–346, 1969.

48. Money, J.: Two cytogenetic syndromes: Psychologic comparison. I. Intelligence and specific-factor quotients. *J. Psychiatr. Res. 2:* 223–231, 1964.
49. Gordon, R. R., O'Neill, E. M.: Turner's infantile phenotype. *Br. Med. J. 1:* 483–485, 1969.
50. Preger, L., Howard, M. B., Scully, A. L., et al: Roentgenographic abnormalities in phenotypic females with gonadal dysgenesis. A comparison of chromatin positive patients and chromatin negative patients. *Am. J. Roentgenol. Radium. Ther. Nucl. Med. 104:* 899–910, 1968.
51. Brook, C. G. D., Murset, G., Zachmann, M., et al: Growth in children with 45,XO Turner's syndrome. *Arch. Dis. Child. 49:* 789–795, 1974.
52. Willemse, C. H.: A patient suffering from Turner's syndrome and acromegaly. *Acta Endocrinol. 39:* 204–212, 1962.
53. Singh, R. P., Carr, D. H.: The anatomy and histology of XO human embryos and fetuses. *Anat. Rec. 155:* 369–383, 1966.
54. Conte, F. A., Grumbach, M. M., Kaplan, S. L.: A diphasic pattern of gonadotropin secretion in patients with the syndrome of gonadal dysgenesis. *J. Clin. Endocrinol. Metabl. 40:* 670–674, 1975.
55. Gilboa, Y., Rosenberg, T.: Typical Turner's syndrome with a 45,XO karyotype and normal menstruation. *Helv. Paediatr. Acta 30:* 281–288, 1975.
56. Bahner, F., Schwarz, G., Hienz, H. A., et al: Turner-syndrom mit voll ausgebildeten sekundaren geschlechtsmerkmalen und fertilitat. *Acta Endocrinol. 35:* 397–404, 1960.
57. McDonough, P. G., Phung, T. T.: Gonadal dysgenesis with atypical bleeding. *Am. J. Obstet. Gynecol. 119:* 515–517, 1974.
58. Carr, D. H.: Chromosomes and abortion, in Harris, H., Hirschhorn, K., (eds.): *Advances in Human Genetics.* New York-London, Plenum Press, 1971, vol. 2, pp. 201–249.
59. Race, R. R., Sanger, R.: Xg and sex chromosome abnormalities. *Br. Med. Bull. 25:* 99–103, 1969.
60. Dunlap, D. B., Aubry, R., Louro, J. M.: The occurrence of the 45,X Turner's syndrome in sisters. *J. Clin. Endocrinol. Metab. 34:* 491–497, 1972.
61. Fialkow, P. J., Uchida, I. A.: Autoantibodies in Down's syndrome and gonadal dysgenesis. *Ann. N.Y. Acad. Sci. 155:* 759–769, 1968.
62. Ferguson-Smith, M. A.: Karyotype-phenotype correlations in gonadal dysgenesis and their bearing on the pathogenesis of malformations. *J. Med. Genet. 2:* 142–155, 1965.
63. Simpson, J. L.: Gonadal dysgenesis and abnormalities of the human sex chromosomes: Current status of phenotypic-karyotypic correlations, in Bergsma D. (ed.): *Genetic Forms of Hypogonadism.* Birth Defects Conference, Stratton, 1975, p 23.
64. Caspersson, T. A., Lindsten, J., Zech, L.: The nature of structural X chromosome aberrations in Turner's syndrome as revealed by quinacrine mustard fluorescent analysis. *Hereditas 66:* 287–292, 1970.
65. Van den Berghe, H., Fryns, J. P., Devos, F.: 46,XXip karyotype in a woman with normal stature and gonadal dysgenesis without other congenital anomalies. *Humangenetik 20:* 163–166, 1973.
66. Keogh, E. J., de Kretser, D. M., Fitzgerald, M. G.: Isochromosome for the short arm of X with primary amenorrhoea and a pituitary tumour. *Aust. N.Z. J. Med. 3:* 617–619, 1973.
67. Therman, E., Sarto, G. E., Patau, K.: Center for Barr body condensation on the proximal part of the human Xq: A hypothesis. *Chromosoma 44:* 361–366, 1974.
68. de la Chapelle, A. L., Schröder, J.: Reappraisal of a 46Xi(Xp) karyotype as 46,Xdel(Xq). *Hereditas 80:* 137–140, 1975.
69. Hecht, F., Jones, D. L., Delay, M., et al: Xq-Turner's syndrome: Reconsideration of hypotheses that Xp- causes somatic features in Turner's syndrome. *J. Med. Genet. 7:* 1–4, 1970.
70. de la Chapelle, A., Schröder, J., Haahtela, T., et al: Deletion mapping of the human X chromosome. *Hereditas 80:* 113–120, 1975.
71. Hagemeijer, A., Hoovers, J., Hasper-Voogt, I., et al: Late-replicating ring X-chromosomes identified by R-banding after BrdU pulse. Three new examples of mosaicism 45,XO/46,Xr(X). *Hum. Genet. 34:* 45–52, 1976.
72. Dutrillaux, B., Lejeune, J.: New techniques in the study of human chromosomes, in Harris, H., Hirschhorn, K., (eds.): *Advances in Human Genetics.* New York, Plenum Press, 1975, vol 5, p. 119.
73. Cutler, B. S., Forbes, A. P., Ingersoll, F. M., et al: Endometrial carcinoma after stilbestrol therapy in gonadal dysgenesis. *N. Engl. J. Med. 287:* 628–631, 1972.
74. McCarroll, A. M., Montgomery, D. A. D., Harley, J. McD. G., et al: Endometrial carcinoma after cyclical oestrogen-progestogen therapy for Turner's syndrome. *Br. J. Obstet. Gynecol. 82:* 421–423, 1974.
75. Zäh, W., Kalderon, A., Tucci, J. R.: Mixed gonadal dysgenesis. *Acta Endocrinol. (Suppl) (Kbh) 79:* 1–39, 1975.
76. Caspersson, T., Hulten, M., Johansson, J., et al: Translocation causing non-fluorescent Y chromosomes in human XO/XY mosaicism. *Hereditas 68:* 317–332, 1971.
77. Hsu, L. Y., Kim, H. J., Paciuc, S.: Non-fluorescent and non-heterochromatic Y chromosomes in 45X/46XY mosaicism. *Ann. Genet. (Paris) 17:* 5–9, 1974.
78. Bühler, E. M., Bühler, U. K., Tsuchimoto, T., et al: Non-fluorescent Y-chromosome. *Helv. Paediatr. Acta 29:* 447–456, 1974.
79. Tishler, P. V., Lamborot-Manzur, M., Atkins, L.: Polymorphism of the human Y chromosome: Fluorescence microscopic studies on the sites of morphologic variation. *Clin. Genet. 3:* 116–122, 1972.
80. German, J., Simpson, J. L., McLemore, G.: Abnormalities of human sex chromosomes. I. A ring Y without mosaicism. *Ann. Genet. (Paris) 16:* 225–231, 1973.
81. Tiepolo, L., Zuffardi, O.: Localization of factors controlling spermatogenesis in the nonfluorescent portion of the human Y chromosome long arm. *Hum. Genet. 34:* 119–124, 1976.
82. Robinson, J. A., Buckton, K. E.: Quinacrine fluorescence of variant and abnormal human Y chromosomes. *Chromosoma 35:* 342–352, 1971.
83. Böök, J. A., Eilon, B., Halbrecht, I., et al: Isochromosome Y [46,Xi(Yq)] and female phenotype. *Clin. Genet. 4:* 410–414, 1973.
84. Harnden, D. G., Stewart, J. S. S.: The chromosomes in a case of pure gonadal dysgenesis. *Br. Med. J. 2:* 1285–1287, 1959.
85. Simpson, J. L., Christakos, A. C., Horwith, M., et al: Gonadal dysgenesis in individuals with apparently normal chromosomal complements: Tabulation of cases and compilation of genetic data. *Birth Defects, Orig. Art. Ser. 7(6):* 215–228, 1971.
86. Simpson, J. L.: Genetic aspects of gynecologic disorders occurring in 46,XX individuals. *Clin. Obstet. Gynecol. 15:* 157–182, 1972.
87. Slotnik, E. A., Goldfarb, A. F.: Unilateral streaked ovary syndrome. *Obstet. Gynecol. 39:* 269–273, 1972.
88. Judd, H. L., Scully, R. E., Atkins, L., et al: Pure gonadal dysgenesis with progressive hirsutism: Demonstration of testosterone production by gonadal streaks. *N. Engl. J. Med. 282:* 881–885, 1970.
89. Swyer, G. I. M.: Male pseudohermaphroditism: A hitherto undescribed form. *Br. Med. J. 3:* 709–712, 1955.
90. Simpson, J. L., Summitt, R. L., German, J., et al: Etiology of XY gonadal dysgenesis. *Gynecol. Invest. 7:* 37–41, 1976.
91. Chemke, J., Carmichael, R., Stewart, J. M., et al: Familial XY gonadal dysgenesis. *J. Med. Genet. 7:* 105–111, 1970.
92. Rose, L., Underwood, R., Williams, G. H., et al: Pure gonadal dysgenesis: Studies of in vitro androgen metabolism. *Am. J. Med. 57:* 957–961, 1974.
93. Griffiths, K., Grant, J. K., Browning, M. C. K., et al: Steroid synthesis in vitro by tumour tissue from a dysgenetic gonad. *J. Endocrinol. 34:* 155–162, 1966.
94. Jones, H. W., Jr., Scott, W. W.: *Hermaphroditism, Genital Anomalies and Related Endocrine Disorders,* 2nd ed. Baltimore, Williams and Wilkins, 1971.
95. Van Niekerk, W. A.: True hermaphroditism. *Am. J. Obstet. Gynecol. 126:* 890–903, 1976.
96. Narita, O., Manba, S., Nakanishi, T., et al: Pregnancy and childbirth in a true hermaphrodite. *Obstet. Gynecol. 45:* 593–595, 1975.
97. Neto, R. S., Rivarola, M. A., Coco, R., et al: The testis in patients with abnormalities of sex differentiation: Histology and endocrine function. *Acta Endocrinol. 73:* 179–188, 1973.
98. Armendares, S., Salamanca, F., Cantú, J. M., et al: Familial true hermaphrodism in three siblings: Clinical, cytogenetic, histological and hormonal studies. *Humangenetik 29:* 99–109, 1975.
99. Melicow, M. M., Uson, A. C.: Dysgenetic gonadomas and other gonadal neoplasms in intersexes: Report of 5 cases and review of the literature. *Cancer 12:* 552–572, 1959.
100. Scully, R. E.: Gonadoblastoma: A review of 74 cases. *Cancer 25:* 1340–1356, 1970.
101. Schellhas, F.: Malignant potential of the dysgenetic gonad. *Obstet. Gynecol. 44:* 298–309; 455–462, 1974.
102. Talerman, A. L.: Gonadoblastoma associated with an embryonal carcinoma. *Obstet. Gynecol. 43:* 138–142, 1974.
103. Patel, S. K., Prentice, S. A.: Gonadoblastoma, distinctive ovarian tumor. *Arch. Pathol. 94:* 165–170, 1972.
104. Teter, J.: The mixed germ cell tumors with hormonal activity. *Acta Pathol. Microbiol. Scand. 58:* 306–320, 1963.
105. Rutledge, F., Schellhas, H. F.: Gonadoblastoma: Germinoma in a 7 year old girl. *J. A. M. A. 221:* 1528–1529, 1972.

106. Simpson, J. L., Photopulos, G.: The relationship of neoplasia to disorders of abnormal sexual differentiation, in *Cancer and Genetics, Birth Defects, Orig. Art. Ser. XII(1):* 15–50, 1976.

107. Manuel, M., Katayama, K. P., Jones, H. W. Jr.: The age of occurrence of gonadal tumors in intersex patients with a Y chromosome. *Am. J. Obstet. Gynecol. 124:* 293–300, 1976.

108. Greenblatt, R. B., Byrd, J. R., McDonough, P. G., et al: The spectrum of gonadal dysgenesis: A clinical, cytogenetic, and pathologic study. *Am. J. Obstet. Gynecol. 98:* 151–172, 1967.

109. Goldberg, M. B., Scully, A. L., Solomon, I. L., et al: Gonadal dysgenesis in phenotypic female subjects: A review of 87 cases, with cytogenetic studies in 53. *Am. J. Med. 45:* 529–543, 1968.

110. Warren, J. C., Erkman, B., Cheatum, S., et al: Hilus-cell adenoma in a dysgenetic gonad with XX/XO mosaicism. *Lancet 1:* 141–143, 1964.

111. Van Niekerk, W. A.: *True Hermaphroditism.* Hagerstown, Harper & Row, 1974, p. 200.

112. Bongiovanni, A. M.: Disorders of adrenogenital steroid biosynthesis (the adrenogenital syndrome associated with congenital adrenal hyperplasia), in Stanbury, J. B., Wyngaarden, J. B., Fredrickson, D. S. (eds.), *The Metabolic Basis of Inherited Disease.* New York, Mcgraw-Hill, 1972, pp. 857–885.

113. Lee, P. A., Plotnick, P., Kowarski, A. A., et al (eds.): *Congenital Adrenal Hyperplasia.* Baltimore, University Park Press, 1977.

114. Federman, D. D.: *Abnormal Sexual Development: A Genetic and Endocrine Approach to Differential Diagnosis.* Philadelphia, W. B. Saunders, 1967.

115. Kowarski, A., Finkelstein, W., Spaulding, J. S., et al: Aldosterone secretion rate in congenital adrenal hyperplasia: A discussion of the theories on the pathogenesis of the salt-losing form of the syndrome. *J. Clin. Invest. 44:* 1505–1513, 1965.

116. Reiter, E. O., Grumbach, M. M., Kaplan, S. L., et al: The response of pituitary gonadotropes to synthetic LRF in children with glucocorticoid-treated congenital adrenal hyperplasia: Lack of effect of intrauterine and neonatal androgen excess. *J. Clin. Endocrinol. Metabl. 40:* 318–325, 1975.

117. Hirschfeld, A. J., Fleshman, J. K.: An unusually high incidence of salt-losing congenital adrenal hyperplasia in the Alaskan Eskimo. *J. Pediatr. 75:* 492–494, 1969.

118. Childs, B., Grumbach, M. M., Van Wyk, J. J.: Virilizing adrenal hyperplasia: A genetic and hormonal study. *J. Clin. Invest. 35:* 213–219, 1956.

119. Jenner, M. R. Grumbach, M. M., Kaplan, S. L.: Plasma 17-OH progesterone in maternal and umbilical cord plasma in children and in congenital adrenal hyperplasia (CAH): Application to neonatal diagnosis of CAH. *Ped. Res. 4:* 380, 1970.

120. Frasier, S. D., Thorneycroft, I. H., Weiss, B. A., et al: Letters to the editor, *J. Pediatr. 86:* 310–312, 1975.

121. Styne, D. M., Richards, G. E., Bell, J. J., et al: Growth patterns in CAH: Correlation of glucocorticoid therapy with stature, in Lee, P. A., Plotnick, L. P., Kowarski, A. A., et al (eds.): *Congenital Adrenal Hyperplasia.* Baltimore, University Park Press, 1975, pp. 247–261.

122. Sotiropoulos, A., Morishima, A., Homsy, Y., et al: Long-term assessment of genital reconstruction in female pseudohermaphrodites. *J. Urol. 115:* 599–601, 1976.

123. Richards, G. E., Styne, D. M., Conte, F. A., et al: Plasma sex steroids and gonadotropins in pubertal girls with CAH: Relation to menstrual disorders, in Lee, P. A., Plotnick, L. P., Kowarski, A. A., et al (eds.): *Congenital Adrenal Hyperplasia.* Baltimore, University Park Press, 1975, pp. 387–396.

124. Radfar, N., Kolnis, J., Bartter, F. C.: Evidence for cortisol secretion by testicular masses, in Lee, P. A., Plotnick, L. P., Kowarski, A. A., et al (eds.): *Congenital Adrenal Hyperplasia.* Baltimore, University Park Press, 1977.

125. Gabrilove, J. L., Sharma, D. C., Dorfman, R. L.: Adrenocortical 11-β-hydroxylase deficiency and virilism first manifest in adult women. *N. Engl. J. Med. 272:* 1189–1194, 1965.

126. Bongiovanni, A. M.: The adrenogenital syndrome with deficiency of 3β-hydroxysteroid dehydrogenase. *J. Clin. Invest. 41:* 2086–2092, 1962.

127. Goldman, A. S., Bongiovanni, A. M., Yakovac, W. C., et al: Study of Δ^5, 3β-hydroxysteroid dehydrogenase in normal, hyperplastic and neoplastic adrenal cortical tissue. *J. Clin. Endocrinol. Metab. 24:* 894–909, 1964.

128. Biglieri, E. G., Herron, M. A., Brust, N.: 17-hydroxylation deficiency in man. *J. Clin. Invest. 45:* 1946–1954, 1966.

129. Goldsmith, O., Solomon, D. H., Horton, R.: Hypogonadism and mineralocorticoid excess: The 17-hydroxylase deficiency syndrome. *N. Engl. J. Med. 277:* 673–677, 1967.

130. Mills, I. H., Wilson, R. J., Tait, A. D., et al: Steroid metabolic studies in a patient with 17-hydroxylase deficiency. *J. Endocrinol. 38:* XIX–XX, 1967.

131. Miura, K., Yoshinaga, K., Goto, K., et al: A case of glucocorticoid-responsive hyperaldosteronism. *J. Clin. Endocrinol. Metab. 28:* 1807–1815, 1968.

132. Mallin, S. R.: Congenital adrenal hyperplasia secondary to 17-hydroxylase deficiency: Two sisters with amenorrhea, hypokalemia, hypertension and cystic ovaries. *Ann. Intern. Med. 70:* 69–75, 1969.

133. Linquette, M., Dupont, A., Racodot, A., et al: Déficit en 17-hydroxylase: A propos d'une observation. *Ann. Endocrinol. (Paris) 52:* 574–582, 1971.

134. Tronchette, F., Matterozzi, F., Franchi, F.: Troubles surréno-ovariens par deficit enzymatiques. *Actualités Endocrinologiques* 13eme série, pp. 78–88, L'Expansion Editions (Paris), 1973.

135. Prader, A., Gurtner, H. P.: Das Syndrom des pseudohermaphroditismus masculinus bei kongenitaler nebennierenrinden-hyperplasie ohne androgenüberproduktion (adrenaler pseudohermaphroditismus masculinus). *Helv. Paediatr. Acta 10:* 397–412, 1955.

136. Prader, A., Anders, G. J. P. A.: On the genetics of congenital lipoid hyperplasia of the adrenals. *Helv. Paediatr. Acta 17:* 285–289, 1962.

137. Degenhart, H. J., Visser, H. K. A., Boon, H., et al: Evidence for deficient 20α-cholesterol-hydroxylase activity in adrenal tissue of a patient with lipoid adrenal hyperplasia. *Acta Endocrinol. 71:* 512–518, 1972.

138. Sasano, N., Furuyama, M., Yamazaki, M.: Congenital adrenal hyperplasia associated with gonadal dysgenesis. *Endocrinol. Jpn. 10:* 215–220, 1963.

139. O'Doherty, N. J.: Lipoid adrenal hyperplasia. *Guys Hosp. Rep. 113:* 368–379, 1963.

140. Moragas, A., Ballabrija, A.: Congenital lipoid hyperplasia of the fetal adrenal gland. *Helv. Paediatr. Acta 24:* 226–238, 1969.

141. Tsutsui, Y., Hirabayashi, N., Ito, G.: An autopsy case of congenital lipoid hyperplasia of the adrenal cortex. *Acta Pathol. Jpn. 20:* 227–237, 1970.

142. Camacho, A. M., Kowarski, A., Migeon, C. J., et al: Congenital adrenal hyperplasia due to a deficiency of one of the enzymes involved in the biosynthesis of pregnenolone. *J. Clin. Endocrinol. Metab. 28:* 153–161, 1968.

143. Kirkland, R. T., Kirkland, J. L., Johnson, C. M., et al: Congenital lipoid adrenal hyperplasia in an eight-year-old phenotypic female. *J. Clin. Endocrinol. Metab. 36:* 488–496, 1973.

144. Grumbach, M. M., Ducharme, J. R., Moloshok, R. E.: On the fetal masculinizing action of certain oral progestins. *J. Clin. Endocrinol. 19:* 1369–1380, 1959.

144 a. Jones, H. W. Jr., Wilkins, L.: The genital anomaly associated with prenatal exposure to progestogens. *Fertil. Steril. 11:* 148–156, 1960.

145. Grumbach, M. M., Ducharme, J. R.: The effects of androgens on fetal sexual development: Androgen-induced female pseudohermaphroditism. *Fertil. Steril. 11:* 157–180, 1960.

146. Ishizuka, N., Kawashima, Y., Nakanishi, T., et al: Statistical observations on genital anomalies of newborns following the administration of progestins to their mothers. *Obstet. Gynecol. Surv. 19:* 496–499, 1964.

147. Bongiovanni, A. M., DiGeorge, A. M., Grumbach, M. M.: Masculinization of the female infant associated with estrogenic therapy alone during gestation: Four cases. *J. Clin. Endocrinol. Metab. 19:* 1004–1011, 1959.

148. Novak, D. J., Lauchlan, S. C., McCawley, J. C., et al: Virilization during pregnancy. *Am. J. Med. 49:* 281–290, 1970.

149. Mürset, G., Zachmann, M., Prader, A., et al: Male external genitalia of a girl caused by a virilizing adrenal tumour in the mother. *Acta Endocrinol. 65:* 627–638, 1970.

150. Malinak, L. R., Miller, G. V.: Bilateral multicentric ovarian luteomas of pregnancy associated with masculinization of a female infant. *Am. J. Obstet. Gynecol. 91:* 251–259, 1965.

151. Carpentier, P. J., Potter, E. L.: Nuclear sex and genital malformations in 48 cases of renal agenesis, with especial reference to non-specific female pseudohermaphroditism. *Am. J. Obstet. Gynecol. 78:* 235–258, 1959.

152. Park, I. J., Johanson, A., Jones, H. W. Jr., et al: Special female hermaphroditism associated with multiple disorders. *Obstet. Gynecol. 39:* 100–106, 1972.

153. Berthezene, F., Forest, M. G., Grimaud, J. A., et al: Leydig-cell

agenesis: A cause of male pseudohermaphroditism. *N. Engl. J. Med. 295:* 969–972, 1976.

154. Bardin, C. W., Bullock, L. P., Sherins, R. J., et al: Androgen metabolism and mechanism of action in male pseudohermaphroditism: A study of testicular feminzation (Part II). *Recent Prog. Horm. Res. 29:* 65–105, 1973.

155. Ohno, S.: Sexual differentiation and testosterone production. *N. Engl. J. Med. 295:* 1011–1012, 1976.

156. Park, I. J., Aimakhu, V. E., Jones, H. W. Jr.: An etiologic and pathogenetic classification of male hermaphroditism. *Am. J. Obstet. Gynecol. 123:* 505–518, 1975.

157. Siler-Khodr, T. M., Morgenstern, L. L., Greenwood, F. C.: Hormone synthesis and release from human fetal adenohypophyses in vitro. *J. Clin. Endocrinol. Metab. 39:* 891–905, 1974.

158. Lovinger, R. D., Kaplan, S. L., Grumbach, M. M.: Congenital hypopituitarism associated with neonatal hypoglycemia and microphallus: Four cases secondary to hypothalamic hormone deficiencies. *J. Pediatr. 87:* 1171–1181, 1975.

159. Jänne, O., Perheentupa, J., Vihko, R.: Plasma and urinary steroids in an eight-year-old boy with 3β-hydroxysteroid dehydrogenase deficiency. *J. Clin. Endocrinol. Metab. 31:* 162–165, 1970.

160. Zachmann, M., Völlmin, J. A., Mürset, G.: Unusual type of congenital adrenal hyperplasia probably due to deficiency of 3β-hydroxysteroid dehydrogenase. Case report of a surviving girl and steroid studies. *J. Clin. Endocrinol. Metab. 30:* 719–726, 1970.

161. Parks, G. A., Bermudez, J. A., Anast, C. S., et al: Pubertal boy with the 3β-hydroxysteroid dehydrogenase defect. *J. Clin. Endocrinol. Metab. 33:* 269–278, 1971.

162. Kenny, F. M., Reynolds, J. W., Green, O. C.: Partial 3β-hydroxysteroid dehydrogenase (3β-HSD) deficiency in a family with congenital adrenal hyperplasia: Evidence for increasing 3β-HSD activity with age. *Pediatrics 48:* 756–765, 1971.

163. Jänne, O., Perheentupa, J., Viinikka, L., et al: Testicular endocrine function in a pubertal boy with 3β-hydroxysteroid dehydrogenase deficiency. *J. Clin. Endocrinol. Metab. 39:* 206–209, 1974.

164. Schneider, G., Genel, M., Bongiovanni, A. M., et al: Persistent testicular Δ^5-isomerase-3β-hydroxysteroid dehydrogenase (Δ^5-3β-HSD) deficiency in the Δ^5-3β-HSD form of congenital adrenal hyperplasia. *J. Clin. Invest. 55:* 681–690, 1975.

165. New, M. I.: Male pseudohermaphroditism due to 17α hydroxylase deficiency. *J. Clin. Invest. 49:* 1930–1941, 1970.

166. Mantero, F., Busnardo, B., Riondel, A., et al: Hypertension artérielle, alcalose hypokaliemique et pseudohermaphrodisme mâle par déficit en 17α-hydroxylase. *Schweiz. Med. Wochenschr. 101:* 38–43, 1971.

167. Bricaire, H., Luton, J. P., Laudat, P., et al: A new male pseudohermaphroditism associated with hypertension due to a block of 17α-hydroxylation. *J. Clin. Endocrinol. Metab. 35:* 67–72, 1972.

168. Alvarez, M. N., Cloutier, M. D., Hayles, A. B.: Male pseudohermaphroditism due to 17α-hydroxylase deficiency in two siblings. *Pediatr. Res. (abstract) 7:* 325, 1973.

169. Kershnar, A. K., Borut, D., Kogut, M. D.: Studies in a phenotypic female with 17α-hydroxylase deficiency. *J. Pediatr. 89:* 395–400, 1976.

170. Tourniaire, J., Audi-Paresa, L., Loras, B., et al: Male pseudohermaphroditism with hypertension due to a 17α-hydroxylation deficiency. *Clin. Endocrinol. 5:* 53–61, 1976.

171. Zachmann, M., Völlmin, J. A., Hamilton, W., et al: Steroid 17,20-desmolase deficiency: A new cause of male pseudohermaphroditism. *Clin. Endocrinol. 1:* 369–385, 1972.

172. Goebelsmann, U., Zachmann, M., Davajan, U., et al: Male pseudohermaphrodism consistent with 17,20-desmolase deficiency. *Gynecol. Invest. 7:* 138–156, 1976.

173. Saez, J. M., de Perretti, E., Morera, A. M., et al: Familial male pseudohermaphroditism with gynecomastia due to a testicular 17-kestosteroid reductase defect. I. Studies in vivo. *J. Clin. Endocrinol. Metab. 32:* 604–610, 1971.

174. Saez, J. M., Morera, A. M., de Peretti, E., et al: Further in vivo studies in male pseudohermaphroditism with gynecomastia due to a testicular 17-ketosteroid reductase defect (compared to a case of testicular feminization). *J. Clin. Endocrinol. Metab. 34:* 598–600, 1972.

175. Goebelsmann, U., Horton, R., Mestman, J. H., et al: Male pseudohermaphroditism due to testicular 17β-hydroxysteroid dehydrogenase deficiency. *J. Clin. Endocrinol. Metab. 36:* 867–879, 1973.

176. Givens, J. R., Wiser, W. L., Summitt, R. L., et al: Familial male pseudohermaphroditism without gynecomastia due to deficient testicular 17-ketosteroid reductase activity. *N. Engl. J. Med. 291:* 938–944, 1974.

177. Reiter, E. O., Conte, F. A., Grumbach, M. M.: Pubertal onset of gynecomastia and virilization in phenotypic females with male pseudohermaphroditism due to a deficiency of testicular 17-β-hydroxysteroid oxidoreductase (in press).

178. Goebelsmann, U., Hall, T. D., Paul, W. L., et al: In vitro steroid metabolic studies in testicular 17β-reduction deficiency. *J. Clin. Endocrinol. Metab. 41:* 1136–1143, 1975.

179. Mainwaring, W. I. P.: The Mechanism of Action of Androgens. Monographs in Endocrinology. New York, Springer-Verlag, 1977.

180. Morris, J. M., Mahesh, V. B.: Further observations on the syndrome, "testicular feminization." Am. J. Obstet. Gynecol. 87: 731–734, 1963.

181. Jagiello, G., Atwell, J. D.: Prevalence of testicular feminization. *Lancet I:* 329–336, 1962.

182. Ferenczy, A., Richart, R. M.: The fine structures of the gonads in the complete form of testicular feminization syndrome. *Am. J. Obstet. Gynecol. 113:* 399–409, 1972.

183. Tremblay, R. R., Foley, T. P. Jr., Corvol, P., et al: Plasma concentration of testosterone, dihydrotestosterone, testosterone-oestradiol binding globulin, and pituitary gonadotropins in the syndrome of male pseudo-hermaphroditism with testicular feminization. *Acta Endocrinol. 70:* 331–341, 1972.

184. Judd, H. L., Hamilton, C. R., Barlow, J. J., et al: Androgen and gonadotropin dynamics in testicular feminization syndrome. *J. Clin. Endocrinol. Metab. 34:* 229–234, 1972.

185. Kelch, R. P., Jenner, M. R., Weinstein, R., et al: Estradiol and testosterone secretion by human, simian, and canine testes, in males with hypogonadism and in male pseudohermaphrodites with the feminizing testes syndrome. *J. Clin. Invest. 51:* 824–830, 1972.

186. Faiman, C., Winter, J. S. D.: The control of gonadotropin secretion in complete testicular feminization. *J. Clin. Endocrinol. Metab. 39:* 631–638, 1974.

187. French, F. S., Van Wyk, J. J., Baggett, B., et al: Further evidence of a target organ defect in the syndrome of testicular feminization. *J. Clin. Endocrinol. Metabl. 26:* 493–503, 1966.

188. Gehring, U., Tomkins, G. M., Ohno, S.: Effect of the androgen-insensitivity mutation on a cytoplasmic receptor for dihydrotestosterone. *Nature (London), New Biol. 232:* 106–107, 1971.

189. Keenan, B. S., Meyer, W. J. III, Hadjian, A. J., et al: Syndrome of androgen insensitivity in man: Absence of 5α-dihydrotestosterone binding protein in skin fibroblasts. *J. Clin. Endocrinol. Metab. 38:* 1143–1146, 1974.

190. Amrhein, J. A., Meyer, W. J. III, Jones, H. W. Jr., et al: Androgen insensitivity in man: Evidence for genetic heterogeneity. *Proc. Natl. Acad. Sci. USA 73:* 891–894, 1976.

191. Lyon, M. F., Hawkes, S. G.: X-linked gene for testicular feminization in the mouse. *Nature (London) 227:* 1217–1219, 1970.

192. Ohno, S.: *Sex Chromosome and Sex-linked Genes.* Berlin-New York, Springer-Verlag, 1967, p. 192.

193. Lubs, H. A., Jr., Vilar, O., Bergenstal, D. M.: Familial male pseudohermaphroditism with labial testes and partial feminization: Endocrine studies and genetic aspects. *J. Clin. Endocrinol. 19:* 1110–1120, 1959.

194. Rosenfield, R. L., Lawrence, A. M., Liao, S., et al: Androgens and androgen responsiveness in the feminizing testis syndrome. Comparison of complete and "incomplete" forms. *J. Clin. Endocrinol. Metab. 32:* 625–632, 1971.

195. Madden, J. D., Walsh, P. C., MacDonald, P. C., et al: Clinical and endocrinologic characterization of a patient with the syndrome of incomplete testicular feminization. *J. Clin. Endocrinol. Metab. 41:* 751–760, 1975.

196. Reifenstein, E. C. Jr.: Hereditary familial hypogonadism. *Clin. Res. 3:* 86–93, 1947.

197. Bowen, P., Lee, C. S. N., Migeon, C. J., et al: Hereditary male pseudohermaphroditism with hypogonadism, hypospadias, and gynecomastia (Reifensteins's syndrome). *Ann. Intern. Med. 62:* 252–270, 1965.

198. Wilson, J. D., Harrod, M. J., Goldstein, J. L., et al: Familial incomplete male pseudohermaphroditism, type I. *N. Engl. J. Med. 290:* 1097–1103, 1974.

199. Griffin, J. E., Punyashthiti, K., Wilson, J. D.: Dihydrotestosterone binding by cultured human fibroblasts: Comparison of cells from control subjects and from patients with hereditary male pseudohermaphroditism due to androgen resistance. *J. Clin. Invest. 57:* 1342–1351, 1976.

200. Amrhein, J. A., Klingensmith, G. J., Walsh, P. C., et al: Partial androgen insensitivity: A reclassification of Reifenstein's syndrome. *(Abstract) Endo. Soc. S.F.,* 1976, p. 32.
201. Keenan, B. S., Kirkland, J. L., Kirkland, R. T., et al: Male pseudohermaphroditism with partial androgen insensitivity. *Pediatrics 59:* 224–231, 1977.
202. Walsh, P. C., Madden, J. D., Harrod, M. J., et al: Familial incomplete male pseudohermaphroditism, type II: Decreased dihydrogestosterone formation in pseudovaginal perineoscrotal hypospadias. *N. Engl. J. Med. 291:* 944–949, 1974.
203. Imperato-McGinley, J., Peterson, R. E.: Male pseudohermaphroditism: The complexities of male phenotypic development. *Am. J. Med. 61:* 251–272, 1976.
204. Peterson, R. E., Imperato-McGinley, J., Gautier, T., et al: Male pseudohermaphroditism due to steroid 5α-reductase deficiency. *Am. J. Med. 62:* 170–191, 1977.
205. Simpson, J. L., New, M., Peterson, R. E., et al: Pseudovaginal perineoscrotal hypospadias (PPSH) in sibs. *Birth Defects, Orig. Art. Ser. 7:* 140–144, 1971.
206. Optiz, J. M., Simpson, J. L., Sarto, G. E., et al: Pseudovaginal perineoscrotal hypospadias. *Clin. Genet. 3:* 1–26, 1972.
207. Bain, A. D., Scott, J. S.: Renal agenesis and severe urinary tract dysplasia. A review of 50 cases, with particular reference to the associated anomalies. *Br. Med. J. 1:* 841–846, 1960.
208. Drash, A., Sherman, F., Hartmann, W. H., et al: A syndrome of pseudohermaphroditism, Wilm's tumor, hypertension and generative renal disease. *J. Pediatr. 76:* 585–593, 1970.
209. Barakat, A. Y., Papadopolou, Z. L., Chandra, R. S., et al: Pseudohermaphroditism, nephron disorder, and Wilms' tumor: A unifying concept. *Pediatrics 54:* 366–369, 1974.
210. Scorer, C. G., Farrington, G. H.: *Congenital Deformities of the Testis and Epididymis.* New York, Appleton-Century-Crofts, 1971, p. 203.
211. Goldberg, L. M., Skaist, L. B., Morrow, J. W.: Congenital absence of the testes: Anorchism and monorchism. *J. Urol. 111:* 840–845, 1974.
212. Hall, J. G., Morgan, A., Blizzard, R. M.: Familial congenital anorchia. *Birth Defects, Orig. Art. Ser. 11(4):* 115–119, 1974.
213. Green, A. A., Zachmann, M., Illig, R., et al: Congenital bilateral anorchia in childhood: A clinical, endocrine and therapeutic evaluation of 21 cases. *Clin. Endocrinol. 5:* 381–391, 1976.
214. Bergada, C., Cleveland, W. W., Jones, H. W. Jr., et al: Variants of embryonic testicular dysgenesis: Bilateral anorchia and the syndrome of rudimentary testes. *Acta Endocrinol. (Copenhagen) 40:* 521–536, 1962.
215. Najjar, S. S., Takla, R. J., Nassar, V. H.: The syndrome of rudimentary testes: Occurrence in five siblings. *Pediatrics 84:* 119–123, 1974.
216. Sarto, G. E., Opitz, J. M.: The XY gonadal agenesis syndrome. *J. Med. Genet. 10:* 288–293, 1973.
217. Wu, D. H., Boyar, R. M., Knight, R., et al: Endocrine studies in a phenotypic girl with XY gonadal agenesis and hermaphrodism. *J. Clin. Endocrinol. Metab. 43:* 506–511, 1976.
218. Morillo-Cucci, G., German, J.: Males with a uterus and fallopian tube, a rare disorder of sexual development. *Birth Defects, Orig. Art. Ser. 7:* 229–241, 1971.
219. Brook, C. G. D., Wagner, H., Zachmann, M., et al: Familial occurrence of persistent müllerian structures in otherwise normal males. *Br. Med. J 1:* 771–773, 1973.
220. Armendares, S., Buentello, L., Frenk, S.: Two male sibs with uterus and fallopian tubes: A rare, probably inherited disorder. *Clin. Genet. 4:* 291–303, 1973.
221. Aarskog, D.: Clinical and cytogenetic studies in hypospadias. *Acta Paediatr. Scand. (Suppl) 203:* 32–35, 1970.
Summitt, R. L.: Differential diagnosis of genital ambiguity in the newborn. *Clin. Obstet. Gynecol. 15:* 112–140, 1972.
222. Summitt, R. L.: Differential diagnosis of genital ambiguity in the newborn. *Clin. Obstet. Gynecol. 15:* 112–140, 1970.
223. Neumann, F., von Berswordt-Wallrabe, R., Elger, W., et al: Aspects of androgen-dependent events as studied by antiandrogens. *Recect Prog. Horm. Res. 26:* 337–410, 1970.
224. Kaplan, N. M.: Male pseudohermaphrodism: Report of a case, with observations on pathogenesis. *N. Engl. J. Med. 261:* 641–644, 1959.
225. Herbst, A. L., Ulfelder, H., Poskanzer, D. C.: Adenocarcinoma of the vagina: Association of maternal stilbestrol therapy with tumor appearance in young women. *N. Engl. J. Med. 284:* 878–881, 1971.
226. Gill, W. B., Schumacher, G. F. B., Bibbo, M.: Structural and functional abnormalities in sex organs of male offspring of mothers treated with diethylstilbestrol. *J. Reprod. Med. 16:* 147–153, 1976.
227. Henderson, B. E., Benton, B., Cosgrove, M., et al: Urogenital tract anomalies in sons of women treated with diethylstilbesterol. *Pediatrics 58:* 505–507, 1976.
228. Sörenson, H. R.: *Hypospadias with Special Reference to Aetiology.* Copenhagen, Munksgaard, 1953.
229. Sweet, R. A., Schrott, H. G., Kurland, R., et al: Study of the incidence of hypospadias in Rochester, Minnesota, 1940–1970, and a case control comparison of possible etiologic factors. *Mayo Clin. Proc. 49:* 52–58, 1974.
230. Smith, D. W.: In *Recognizible Patterns of Human Malformations: Genetic, Embryologic and Clinical Aspects,* 2nd ed. Philadelphia, W. B. Saunders, 1976.
231. Rosewater, S., Gwinup, G., Hamwi, G. J.: Familial gynecomastia. *Ann. Intern. Med. 63:* 377–385, 1965.
232. Griffin, J. E., Edwards, C., Madden, J. D., et al: Congenital absence of the vagina. *Ann. Intern. Med. 85:* 224–236, 1976.
233. Ross, G. T., vande Wiele, R. L.: The ovaries, in Williams, R. A. (ed.) *Textbook of Endocrinology* 5th ed. Philadelphia, W. B. Saunders, 1974.
234. Wabrek, A. J., Millard, P. R., Wilson, W. B. Jr., et al: Creation of a neovagina by the Frank nonoperative method. *Obstet. Gynecol. 37:* 408–413, 1971.
235. Levinson, G., Zarate, A., Guzman-Toledano, R., et al: An XX female with sexual infantilism, absent gonads and lack of müllerian ducts. *J. Med. Genet. 13:* 68–69, 1976.

107

Sexual Behavior and Endocrinology (Normal and Abnormal)

John Money
Eileen Higham

This chapter deals with the effect of steroid hormones on the dimorphism and differentiation of sexual behavior during the life span. The sex steroids, governed by hypothalamic-pituitary hormones, are the primary hormonal regulators of sexual behavior. Sexual behavior is autocratically governed by sex hormones in lower mammals, less so in the lower primates, and least of all in man.

Less is known about hormonal-behavioral relationships in childhood and old age than in adolescence and adulthood. Relative similarity of physical and mental growth in both sexes in childhood and the erroneous Freudian conception of childhood as a latency period have contributed to the relative neglect of prepubertal hormonal-behavioral studies. In middle life and later, the continuance or change of sexual function has proved of little interest to research in a youth-oriented culture. Active sexuality in the geriatric years has often been viewed negatively as a concomitant of senility and of the failure of suitable impulse repression rather than as the expression of desire for erotic and affectional relationships continued throughout life.

Nothing is yet known about the relationship of gonadal hormones during childhood to sexually dimorphic behavior—as, for example, in the normal sexual rehearsal play of childhood. The programming of such play, judging by experimental animal evidence, may, in part, be prenatal in origin, a long-term effect of sex steroids on the central nervous system. Whatever the prenatal programming of the CNS, however, it is enormously augmented by social environmental programming in the postnatal years (Fig. 107-1). In fact, most of the masculinity, femininity, or bisexuality of a person's gender identity and behavior is a product of his or her postnatal biography.

PRENATAL HORMONAL EFFECTS

In normal differentiation, the dimorphism of the sex chromosomes is paralleled by dimorphism of the central nervous system and of sexual anatomy, as dictated by fetal gonadal hormones. Turner's syndrome represents the condition of insufficient or total lack of gonadal hormones. Androgen excess occurs in the adrenogenital syndrome and in progestin-induced hermaphroditism. The inability to use androgen occurs in the androgen-insensitivity (testicular-feminizing) syndrome and in its partial manifestation, which sometimes goes under the name of Reifenstein's syndrome.

TURNER'S SYNDROME

An embryo becomes morphologically female when either ovaries or testes fail to develop, just as when ovaries appear. In Turner's syndrome, the 45,X or related mosaic chromosomal disorder, the gonads are primitive streaks that fail to produce gonadal hormones. The embryo differentiates a female morphology, indistinguishable externally from a normal female. Assigned as a girl, the child differentiates a typical feminine gender identity, except for infertility.

In childhood these girls dream of romance, marriage, and maternalism, exhibit a strong interest in doll play and baby care,

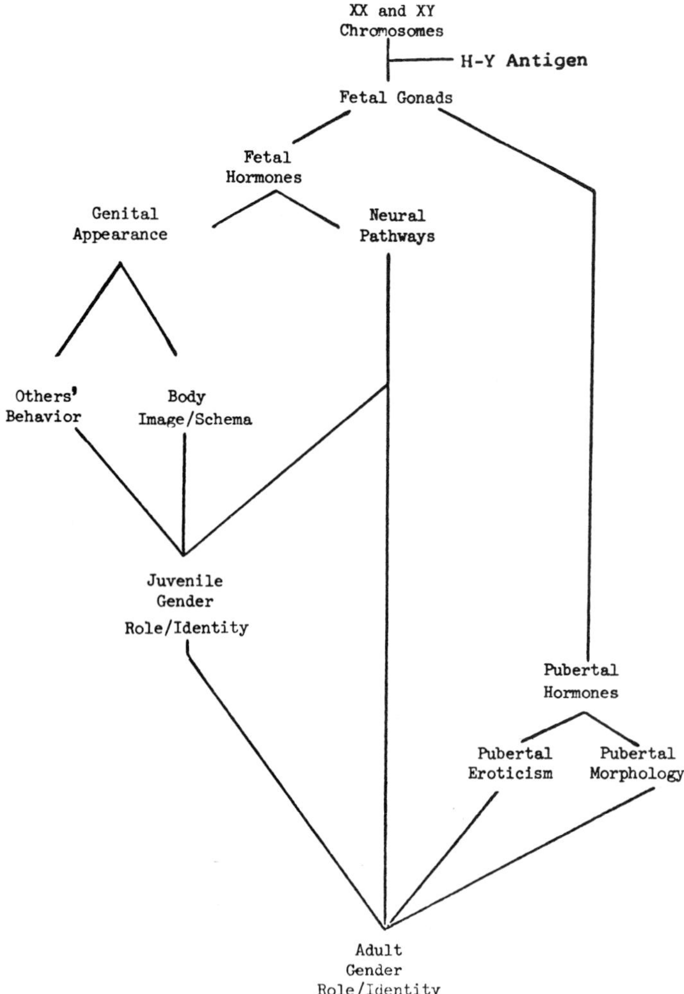

Fig. 107-1. Diagrammatic representation of the sequence of determinants and phases of dimorphic differentiation of gender identity and role (From Money and Ehrhardt, 1972; courtesy Johns Hopkins University Press.)

and little interest in athletics and fighting behavior.* Eventual knowledge of their infertility and the lifelong handicap of short stature typical for this syndrome do not interefere with a desire for marriage and motherhood.

Puberty must be induced by estrogen administration, the timing often delayed until late adolescence, temporarily sacrificing sexual development for statural growth. As a consequence, some degree of behavioral infantilism is often prolonged as the social age lags behind the chronological age (see Delayed Puberty). Correspondingly, there is a relative romantic and erotic inertia which is sometimes misidentified as diminished libido. It is a transient phenomenon related to the chronology of delayed hormonal maturation and to the impairment of age-appropriate social interaction secondary to juvenility of appearance.

PRENATAL ANDROGENIZATION

In genetic females, masculinization may occur prenatally as a result of the metabolic error of the adrenogenital syndrome. It has also been known to occur, rarely, as a result of exogenous hormone, as in female hermaphroditism inadvertently induced by certain of the synthetic progestins when these hormones first became available for the successful prevention of miscarriage. Before the discovery, in 1950, of cortisol treatment to regulate the abnormal adrenal androgen production of the adrenogenital syndrome, masculinization continued into adulthood. With treatment, active masculinization can be suppressed from birth onward. The masculinizing effect of prenatal androgenization on subsequent sexually dimorphic behavior is, by inference, mediated by the brain, though the actual pathways have not yet been identified.

Infants with both of the above conditions of female hermaphroditism* typically are diagnosed at birth as being genetically and internally female, assigned as girls, and rehabilitated with hormonal and surgical therapy as needed. They differentiate a feminine gender identity, although with tomboy traits. They proudly describe themselves as tomboys. They manifest high physical activity levels, often expressed in vigorous and competitive outdoor play and athletics, frequently with boys as companions. They are not fighters. They show minimal overt interest in childhood sex curiosity and play. Unlike most girls, they have low interest in personal adornment and in the rehearsal of parentalism in doll play and infant care. Daydreams of marriage and motherhood are infrequent. Indeed, these girls often express only lukewarm interest in having children. They do not envisage marriage and full-time homemaking as preferable to a nondomestic career. In adolescence, the onset of menstruation tends to be delayed, as does the onset of romantic relationships, as compared with the history of unaffected sisters and the mother. Erotic interest and choice of partners is generally heterosexual. One patient, now the mother of two children, wrote, "At long last I feel rather 'at peace' with being a female. . . . The kids are growing up in a hurry." This comment suggests that in the adrenogenital woman, the threshold for the emergence of parental behavior, as for romantic response, is elevated but not insuperable.

Some babies with the genetic female adrenogenital syndrome have been assigned and reared as boys. Some have been born with complete masculinization of the external genitalia into a penis and empty scrotum. Others needed surgical correction, as for hypospadias. With hormonal therapy, surgical treatment, and sex of rearing all concordant, these boys differentiate a masculine gender identity and role. As men, they cannot be distinguished behaviorally from their brothers and work mates. Ambiguity of rearing and medical handling may lead to a request for sex reassignment in childhood or adolescence, but this occurs regardless of the ostensible sex of assignment. It also occurs regardless of diagnosis, in all varieties of hermaphroditism, not only in the adrenogenital syndrome.

PRENATAL PLUS POSTNATAL ANDROGENIZATION

Women with excessively high androgen levels are disfiguringly virilized. This condition was inescapable for adrenogenital women before cortisol treatment was developed. The eroticism of a group of such women showed, prior to hormonal therapy, moderate frequency of homosexual and bisexual imagery, rare fre-

*Aggression is a loose, catchall term that, like libido, is ineffectual for delineating sexual dimorphism of behavior. Fighting or attack and dominance assertion are preferable terms.

*Those who are genetic and gonadal males are not genitally ambiguous at birth. They are assigned as males and grow up successfully with a male gender identity. Those with the adrenogenital syndrome require cortisol to prevent precocious masculinizing puberty. Behaviorally, they are nonremarkable.

quency of actual lesbian encounter, and absence of transexual desire for sex reassignment.

ANDROGEN INSENSITIVITY

Cytogenetic 46,XY individuals with the complete form of this genetically transmitted error in the cellular utilization of androgen differentiate as morphologic females except for an atrophic uterus and atresia of the vagina. Hormonal puberty is, without treatment, feminizing. Almost invariably, sex of assignment and rearing is female. It is not surprising that gender identity differentiation is feminine. This fact is theoretically important in showing that chromosomes and gonads per se do not dictate differentiation of an almost stereotyped version of what constitutes feminine gender identity and role. In the childhood rehearsal play of girls with this syndrome, a high preference is given to marriage and raising a family (which will, of necessity, be by adoption). In adulthood, there is satisfaction with the feminine role. Adult eroticism and sexuality, with the sense of touch predominant for arousal, conform to typical heterosexual feminine expectations.

PARTIAL ANDROGEN INSENSITIVITY

Insensitivity to androgen is said to be partial when, at birth, there is a recognizable anomaly of the genitals and, at puberty, spontaneous growth of breasts and lack of hirsutism. In those cases in which the phallus is large enough to look like a hypospadiac penis, the baby may be assigned and reared as a boy. This decision is wrong, because androgen insensitivity dictates permanent and untreatable failure to masculinize in adulthood. As an adult, the person cannot elect a sex reassignment if his gender identity is set in the masculine mold concordantly with the rearing, as is typical. Such cases are theoretically important in demonstrating that the differentiation of a masculine gender identity can take place despite impaired androgenization prenatally and at puberty. In one group of patients for whom data were available, erotic arousal, although directed toward a female partner, lacked the initiating quality typical in the male and was rather more responsive to the overtures of the partner. The amount of erotic activity also was low. Erection and orgasm were infrequent. Orgasm tended to be impaired with respect to a strong climactic peak and ejaculatory discharge. Coital incompetence was not, however, accompanied by impairment of romantic affection and getting married.

The patient with partial androgen insensitivity assigned as a girl can be very effectively rehabilitated as a woman with a womanly gender identity. She becomes indistinguishable from chromosomal (46,XX) females born with atresia of the vagina which, as in her own case, requires vaginoplasty in order to permit sexual intercourse. Hormonal replacement therapy is needed only if the feminizing testes are removed as a prophylaxis against the risk of possible malignancy.

CHILDHOOD AND GONADAL HORMONES

Until very recently, the juvenile years before puberty were assumed to be endocrinologically inert with respect to pituitary gonadotropins and gonadal steroids. Now, with the new precision of the radioimmunoassay techniques for measuring minute quantities of circulating hormones, it is evident that the assumption of inertness was incorrect. As of the present, however, there are no data upon which to base even the most fictional hypotheses concerning sexually dimorphic circulating hormone levels and sexually dimorphic behavior in childhood.

GENDER IDENTITY DIFFERENTIATION

The prenatal component of the total program of the differentiation of gender identity and role (gender identity/role) as feminine or masculine does not predestine or preordain the postnatal component. As in the case of native language, so also in gender identity, the prenatal component constitutes a totally incomplete primordium or state of functional preparedness which will be unable to develop and mature until it finds, and is found by, stimuli from the social environment. The prenatal component of either masculinity or femininity of gender identity is so incomplete that, regardless of how the prenatal male-female pendulum comes to rest, it can throw its weight and influence on a postnatal component that differentiates as either masculine or feminine. Thus, a feminine gender identity may follow the orthodoxy of the feminine stereotype, or it may differentiate less orthodoxly to incorporate patterns of behavior, especially vocational behavior, that have, until recently, been stereotyped as masculine. Whether or not the disposition to such unorthodoxy is correlated with prenatal hormonal history is not known, but it is known that a documented history of prenatal androgenization predisposes a genetic female to a sense of well-being when she assimilates at least part of the stereotypic masculine role.

The reciprocal probably holds true, although the currently available evidence for the long-term feminizing behavioral effects of prenatal endocrine deandrogenization of the genetic male is not so comprehensive as is that for the masculinizing effects of prenatal androgenization of the genetic female. The lack of evidence is in part a product of cultural moralizing: it is not immoral to be a tomboyish girl, but it is so nearly immoral not to be a machismo male that there is no noncontemptuous word for such a boy or man. Ideally, there should be many ways to combine elements of the cultural stereotypes of what constitutes masculinity or femininity so that each individual can feel a sense of well-being. This sense of well-being need not be linked to society's rules of conformity to, or deviancy from, its established ideology of sex-defined stereotypes of male, female, or bisexual.

MATCHED PAIRS OF HERMAPHRODITES

Matched pairs of hermaphrodites are concordant for diagnostic sex but discordant for sex of assignment and rearing. Their biographies demonstrate the degree to which, not hormones, per se, but postnatal socialization is the final determining factor in gender identity differentiation. The following three matched pairs (see Money and Ehrhardt, 1972, pp. 151–160) are diagnostically concordant as genetic females with the adrenogenital syndrome. That is, genetic, gonadal, and fetal hormonal sex were the same. In each pair the rearing and gender identity were different. One differentiated a masculine identity, the other a feminine identity.

First Matched Pair

In this pair, one child was reannounced as a girl at 2 months, surgically feminized at age 2, and maintained on cortisone therapy. She became attractively feminine, similar in interests and activities to other females with the adrenogenital syndrome. The other child was pronounced a boy at birth, his case misconstrued as that of a male with hypospadiac phallus and undescended testicles. At age 3½, the third stage of surgical masculinization had failed. Further hospitalization of a terror-stricken child revealed that gender identity as a boy was already well advanced. Sex reassignment was ruled out in favor of rehabilitation surgically and hormonally as a male. In his teens artificial testes were implanted. A difficult family life produced some problems of delinquency in adolescence. Psychosexually, he was romantically inclined toward girls, in keeping with his sex of rearing, and eventually he settled into a satisfactory marriage.

SECOND MATCHED PAIR

By age 12, the child assigned as a girl had masculinized somatically, and the boy had feminized, in consequence of the vicissitudes of poor case management. In each case the gender identity was concordant with rearing. The boy, with interests, activities, and romantic attraction appropriate to masculine gender identity, continued as a typical male following mastectomy, gonadectomy, and hysterectomy, plus testosterone and cortisone therapy. The girl required only cortisone therapy, which suppressed adrenocortical androgen and released estrogen from the ovaries to bring about somatic feminization. As in most cases of girls with the adrenogenital syndrome, romance and marriage were delayed but not permanently.

Third Matched Pair

These children requested sex reassignment at age 11 and 12. Both were reared ambiguously, one ostensibly as male, the other as female. Gender identity in each case reflected the ambiguity of rearing. Early postnatal experiences, in both cases, induced a transsexual gender identity, resolved only by reassignment with appropriate hormonal and surgical correction. Both were rehabilitated in the sex of reassignment. Several years later, after the breakup of her marriage, the patient sex reassigned as a woman entered into a lesbian partnership. As a man, the other patient had only female romantic interests.

PRECOCIOUS PUBERTY

Children with precocious puberty are typically mature sexually from ages 6 to 8 and sometimes earlier. Their behavior matches their chronological age more closely than their physique age. The gap between chronological and physique age may, in some cases, be minimized by planned acceleration in school and social life. From the midteens on, children with a history of precocious onset of puberty melt into the population of their agemates. They are short in stature but not behaviorally remarkable or different.

Precocious puberty occurs more often in girls than in boys except when secondary to neurogenic lesion or other disease.

TEENAGE YEARS

Girls mature 1 to 2 years earlier than boys, and the age of puberty has been going down by 4 months every 10 years for at least a century and a half. There is, as yet, no satisfactory explanation to account for either of the above phenomena, but both are highly relevant to an understanding of chronology in the psychology of adolescence and of the parents of adolescents. The lowered age of puberty, in particular, puts a great strain on parents, for family, religious, social, and legal customs and standards of adolescent sexuality were set in an earlier era when young people matured later than they do today. To compound a parent's difficulties, these customs and standards were also set in the era before birth control, at a time when it was impossible to separate recreational sex from procreational sex. For the first time in history, it is now possible for teenagers to begin their sex lives independently of a commitment to parenthood and independently of creating illegitimate grandparents.

The hormones of puberty are behaviorally and psychologically important not only with respect to fertility but also because, without an adolescent physique, it is not possible for a girl or boy to be fully acceptable among age-mates, participating in the same socially maturing experiences together.

The hormones of puberty affect behavior also by lowering the threshold for the emergence of romantic, erotic, and sexual behavior. Although the evidence is not absolute and definitive, it could well be that androgen is, in this respect, the effective agent for both sexes. Lowering the threshold is not the same as creating behavior de novo. The hormones of puberty do not create the romantic, erotic, and sexual behavior nor the imagery associated therewith. That has been potentially present in the play of childhood. Some children are known even to have had intense love affairs that persist through adolescence and into marriage. The hormones of puberty likewise do not create psychosexual unorthodoxies at adolescence, for example, bisexuality, homosexuality,* or any of the paraphilias. As with homosexuality, the hormones of puberty simply facilitate the expression of what is already present as part of the imagistic content of the gender identity differentiated, with or without errors, in childhood.

In boys, the imagery of erotic arousal may present itself, unrehearsed, in the drama of the first wet dream or masturbation fantasy. If the content is unorthodox and socially stigmatized or illegal, the boy may feel threatened yet not able to turn for help, not knowing whom to trust.

In girls there is no exact parallel of the autonomous imagery of the boy's wet dream. She may have a masturbation fantasy, but dreaming of orgasms in the female appears to reflect the history of actual erotic practice rather than to herald it. In girls, erotic arousal may be more dependent on romantic ideals and the sense of touch than on the erotic visual image. In boys, visual arousal is preeminent. It is not known whether this sex difference with respect to visual erotic arousal reflects cultural inhibitions in females more than species-programmed behavioral dimorphism. Females do respond romantically to visual and narrative stimuli, however, and, with genitopelvic arousal, to the sense of touch.

The inability of adults to converse with pubertal adolescents about their erotic imagery is a factor in the strife that exists between some parents and teenagers, especially when erotic imagery is a source of teenaged apprehension or shame.

DELAYED PUBERTY

As in the case of precocious puberty, in delayed puberty there is a discrepancy between chronologic age and physique age. In consequence, it is difficult for the social age, including psychosexual or sociosexual age, to keep concordant with chronologic age. A juvenile appearance, regardless of age, evokes from others expectations, rewards, and punishments appropriate to the physique.

---

*The terms "homosexuality" and "homosexualism" are used interchangeably in this chapter. There is a tendency coming into current usage for the terms to have different connotations, with homosexuality referring to an act of two people with similar genital morphology and homosexualism referring, by inference, to an individual's state of being.

Behavioral infantilization and social isolation can be a crippling long-term consequence even after a masculine or feminine adult appearance is achieved. Therefore, it is not desirable to procrastinate in the hormonal treatment of delayed puberty. As a rule of thumb, the age of 15, and perhaps a year younger in girls, is the criterion age. However, the timing, as well as the nature of hormonal treatment, will depend on diagnosis and prognosis.

Males predominate over females in the syndrome of total pubertal delay except insofar as a girl may develop breasts but fail to menstruate.

In cases of short stature, with the epiphyses still unclosed, the patient may elect to postpone the hormonal growth spurt of induced puberty in the hope of adding more inches to the ultimate adult height. Examples are girls with Turner's syndrome who are treated with a weak, nonvirilizing androgen in order to gain height and hypopituitary boys or girls under treatment with growth hormone for the same reason.

Girls caught in this predicament are cosmetically better off than boys, for with the use of makeup, fashion style, and a padded bra, a girl can present a public image of being adolescent in age. The unshaving, short boy has more difficulty.

Among endocrinologists, there is still a fair amount of soul-searching with respect to hormonal induction of puberty in cases of so-called constitutional delay. There is no indication of a long-term noxious effect from a half-year of treatment to induce pubertal onset. The boost to morale is immense, even to the extent in some cases of making the difference between suicide and life. A test period without treatment will reveal whether the body is able to take care of its own pubertal functioning or whether further diagnostic workup is necessary. The long-term effect can be a life rehabilitated instead of one neurotically crippled.

Not all cases have a good prognosis, however. In males, pubertal failure occasionally is related to impaired responsiveness to androgen, in which case the most heroic hormonal therapeutic efforts are bitterly disappointing. For example, in hypopituitary dwarfism, it is impossible to get enough beard growth, which is prerequisite to adult age appearance. The same problem occurs in the syndrome of partial androgen insensitivity in hypospadiac male hermaphrodites. Supportive counseling is imperative in order to help such a boy negotiate the world despite his juvenile, nonhirsute, eunuchoid appearance.

Impaired responsiveness to androgen may be partial. In hypopituitarism, for example, pubic and axillary hair, but not facial hair, develop adequately. Erection and ejaculation occur, but there tends to be an overall sexual inertia. Also, the neural mechanism of pair-bonding, or falling in love, may be impaired.

Androgen therapy is useless for increase of the postpubertal size of the penis in cases of microphallus, with or without hypospadias. Plastic surgery to increase penis size is contraindicated. A prosthetic, strap-on penis as a coital aid can be very helpful.

Among cases of poor prognosis, there are some in which pubertal delay appears in association with psychopathologic disability, the latter being unresponsive to pubertal hormonalization. Males with Kallmann's syndrome of hypogonadotropinism and anosmia appear to be at risk in this respect. The same applies to Klinefelter's syndrome, in which pubertal virilization is weak rather than delayed. However, some Klinefelter males benefit mentally from exogenous, supplementary androgen.

All teenagers profit from counseling during the period of pubertal delay and also as they catch up socially after pubertal status is achieved. Although often neglected, adequate sex education is necessary, for a late developer must go through a period of social learning in relative isolation. Their age-mates are not available for sharing experiences and information.

DELAYED PUBERTY AND CHILD ABUSE

A special problem in psychologic counseling and case management occurs in cases of pubertal delay related to child abuse in the syndrome of so-called psychosocial dwarfism (reversible hyposomatotropinism). This syndrome is most commonly diagnosed in the prepubertal years. Growth failure can be reversed by a change of domicile, in which case the timing of pubertal onset is normal. It is not presently known how frequently the condition may pass unnoticed until the age of puberty, at which time it could pass for constitutional delay of puberty. However, it is known that delayed puberty is a late manifestation of the untreated syndrome of psychosocial dwarfism. The onset of puberty rapidly follows change of domicile and parallels the catch-up gain in statural growth.

DELAYED PUBERTY SECONDARY TO OTHER ENDOCRINE SYNDROMES

The hormonal regulation of puberty may be impaired or desynchronized secondary to other endocrine dysfunction, for example, juvenile hypothyroidism, Addison's disease, and Cushing's syndrome, including the iatrogenic cushingoid condition produced by cortisol therapy. There are, in these conditions, no special behavioral effects that can be attributed directly to the pubertal hormones or their absence. The behavioral sequelae of pubertal failure are overshadowed by the impairments of the primary disease. As the primary disease is brought under control, however, and pubertal development begins, individual counseling may be needed as in other cases of delayed puberty. There may be additional psychiatric complications as symptoms of the primary disease. For example, neurotic psychopathology is a frequent concomitant of Cushing's syndrome.

PARADOXICAL PUBERTY

Paradoxical puberty means the development of breasts (gynecomastia) in boys and a beard, body hair, and a deep voice in girls. Gynecomastia may occur in an otherwise normal boy, or in association with Klinefelter's (47,XXY) syndrome, the partial androgen-insensitivity syndrome, or in female hermaphroditism undiagnosed in a child reared as a boy. The boy with a masculine gender identity is mortified to have breasts. The female hormone that allows the mammary tissue to proliferate does not feminize the mind. The therapy is mastectomy and, if required, supplementary or replacement testosterone therapy.

In a very rare case, gynecomastia appears in a boy who is a transsexual seeking sex reassignment. It is less likely that the breast enlargement is spontaneous than secondary to the secret ingestion of birth control pills or other estrogenic preparation. However, there are some known cases of spontaneous gynecomastia in males with a dual diagnosis of transsexualism and Klinefelter's syndrome.

In girls with a feminine gender identity, hirsutism and voice deepening is as mortifying as gynecomastia is to boys. Such virilism occurs in connection with an androgen-producing tumor, untreated adrenal hyperplasia (with or without congenital sex organ defect), the Stein-Leventhal syndrome, and in male hermaphroditism in a child reared as a girl. Self-induced virilism may occur in a female-to-male transsexual but is so far unheard of at the age of puberty, perhaps because androgen is not easily obtained. Except in transsexualism, the treatment is electrolysis for facial hair and vocal training in feminine usage of a deep voice. Therapeutic control of abnormal androgen production allows facial hair to grow more slowly and more downy but not to disappear.

ADULT YEARS: MEN

The gonadal steroids in adult males are imperative to the maintenance of fertility, indispensable to complete behavioral eroticism, and important with respect to nitrogen balance and maintenance of muscle strength. Hyperandrogenism appears not to exist. An excess amount of the hormone, if given exogenously, is spilled out in the urine, the remainder acting as a replacement for the natural product from the testes which temporarily deactivate. Hypoandrogenism has different etiologies, and its response to replacement therapy is variable.

HYPOANDROGENISM

Loss of androgen through castration after puberty has different behavioral effects than those produced by prepubertal castration. Prenatal castration has still other differing effects.

Postpubertal castration produces individually variable behavioral effects in animals and in man. Without androgen, the ejaculatory fluid is not secreted. Without it, the orgasm may disappear, or it may change in quality to a so-called dry-run orgasm. Erectile potency, present in prepuberty, may continue for some years, and sexual attraction to an erotic stimulus may continue even longer. Fatigability usually increases, sometimes with bouts of tearfulness. Postpubertal castration effects are readily reversible upon treatment with a replacement dosage of androgen. For cosmetic purposes, soft silicone testes may be surgically implanted in the scrotum.

Prepubertal castration induces a eunuch pattern of somatic development in the teenage and adult years. Ejaculation is absent. Although the penis remains juvenile in size, it is not devoid of erectile potency, and there may be a peak erotic feeling of climax, minus ejaculatory fluid. Experience of erotic arousal and attraction toward an erotic partner is individually variable. In simple prepubertal castration, the hormonal deficiency can be corrected by exogenous androgen, so that a replica of normal puberty can be induced at any age. The same applies in cases of spontaneous or congenital anorchia in which only the testes are missing without impairment of hypothalamic-pituitary function.

The effects of prenatal castration, which may be either surgical or pharmacologic, are known only from animal studies. These effects are similar to those of postnatal castration before puberty except that the response to androgen replacement therapy at the age of puberty or later may be impaired. The impairment particularly affects behavior, which is marked by a relative sexual inertia.

It is possible that persistent inertia of sexual response following androgen therapy in some androgen-deficient human syndromes (e.g., hypopituitary syndromes and Klinefelter's syndrome) may be prenatal in origin. That is, they may represent a long-term residual effect of impaired prenatal androgenization of hypothalamic and related sexual pathways. Whatever the cause, there is as yet no effective explanation as to why androgen replacement therapy sometimes produces inadequate results—except in the androgen-insensitivity syndrome. In this latter case, it is the cellular uptake of androgen that is at fault in the peripheral organs as well as the brain.

ANDROGEN AND HOMOSEXUALITY

Hypoandrogenism is associated with sexual inertia but not with homosexuality or bisexuality. Hyperestrogenism in the male does not induce homosexuality or bisexuality but rather hypoandrogenism and sexual inertia. Estrogen in the male actually is a functional castrating agent, as has been well demonstrated in male-to-female transsexuals on estrogen therapy prior to surgical castration.

In the 1940s, soon after the sex steroids had been first synthesized, there was a slight flurry of effort to prove that homosexual males were sex-hormonally different from heterosexual males. The findings were inconclusive. Currently there is a renewed flurry of similar effort in the wake of the new precision techniques for estimating circulating plasma hormonal levels. The new findings are as inconclusive as the old with respect to random sampling from the total homosexual population. It is possible that a developmental prognosis of homosexuality is more likely in syndromes characterized by prenatal hypoandrogenization than in the population at large. There is strong presumptive experimental animal evidence in support of this proposition. The animal model may lead to discovery of an as yet unknown parallel in human beings—perhaps in a condition marked by bisexual or effeminate homosexual behavior, relative sexual inertia, hypoandrogenism and poor response to exogenous androgen, and impaired fertility.

Regardless of the possible existence of such a syndrome, the majority of homosexual and bisexual males are endocrinologically indistinguishable from heterosexual males. The same is true of transsexual and transvestite males.

ANDROGEN AND PARAPHILIAS

These variations of gender identity constitute in part those that involve some manifestation or degree of transposition of the masculine and feminine roles, as in homosexualism, bisexualism, transvestism, and transsexualism. They constitute also, in part, those variations, generally classified as paraphilias, characterized by an intrusion of extraneous imagery into the standard masculine (or feminine) pattern of erotic arousal imagery. A fetish is a typical paraphilia. The intrusive fetishistic image may actually displace the expected one, as when a man obtains and maintains an erection only from the stimulus of a woman's shoe, not from the woman herself.

The paraphilias are extremely varied and range from the socially intolerable, like lust murder and pathological sadism, to socially harmless foibles, like being turned on by sexy stories or pictures. They include coprophilia, urophilia, necrophilia, voluntary amputeeism, and so on. There is no known correlation between paraphiliac behavior and hormonal function in either males or females.

ANTIANDROGEN

In recent years there has been a small program in Europe, and an even smaller one in the United States, on the use of cyproterone acetate and medroxyprogesterone acetate, respectively, for the rehabilitation of paraphiliac sex offenders. These hormones bring about a hypoandrogenic effect. They may also have a direct central nervous system tranquilizing effect. They are particularly of benefit for sex offenders whose behavior is absolutely not tolerated by the law and society, for example, rapists, exhibitionists, and pedophiliacs. Hormonal treatment is most effective if accompanied by sexological counseling and planning. The most effective time for commitment to a therapeutic program, at least in some cases, is when the alternative is a crisis with the law.

It is not yet possible to predict which patients will have a favorable therapeutic prognosis, but it is definite that some patients are rehabilitated, despite the failure of prior forms of treatment. With better collaboration between medicine and the courts, the rehabilitation rate would probably increase. According to present evidence, antiandrogenization can be discontinued after 1 to 3 years, provided psychologic follow-up is continued. Then, upon threat of a relapse, rehabilitation is restabilized with a further period of hormonal therapy.

ANDROGEN AND AGGRESSION

Those people who equate or correlate androgen with male sex drive and with aggression are conceptually still in the phlogiston age of behavioral endocrinology. Aggression is not a raw datum of study. It is a concept, and it is inferred from the raw data of fighting and attack relative to the territorial space, proximity, sex, species, and age of the intruder or enemy. Some animal studies of hormones and aggression have been sophisticated enough to specify all the relevant variables, but most have not. There are no primate studies from which to make a sophisticated inference regarding human beings. Human studies on hormones and aggression (usually defined only as hostility) are notoriously lacking in operationally defined precision. Therefore, the less said on this topic at the present time, the better.

There is one syndrome, the 47,XYY syndrome, about which many endocrinologists, geneticists, and behaviorists make a faulty inference regarding aggression. XYY men are not, as a group, hyperandrogenic. In fact, some are hypoandrogenic, and most are normoandrogenic, even if they are in jail. If incarcerated, they are more likely to be in jail for stealing than for assault. As a group, they are legally vulnerable, not because they are aggressive, but because they are impulsive and have difficulty in self-regulating all behavior. Nonetheless, many are self-regulating enough never to entangle with the law. Some XYY men with an excess of impulsive behavior, especially in the teen years, have been helped by the same combined program of counseling plus medroxyprogesterone acetate that has helped sex offenders.

ADULT YEARS: WOMEN

The gonadal steroids in adult females are imperative to the maintenance of ovulation, menstruation, and nidation. They are not imperative to behavioral eroticism, as judged by the criterion of conception, which can take place even if a female is unconscious or, as in the case of paraplegia, unable to feel and move from the waist down. The cyclic surge of estrogen bears some relationship to the release of copulin, the sex attractant or pheromone from the vagina, at the time of ovulation. In other primates, copulin lures the male to copulate, but its effect on the human male has not been ascertained. At the height of copulin release, the female is maximally receptive of the male. In the luteal phase of the cycle, as menstruation approaches, a woman is more likely to be assertive in the initiation of erotic interaction. Her initiative may, however, be masked as a secondary effect of premenstrual tension and irritability or of a cultural or religious taboo on copulating while menstruating.

HYPOESTROGENISM AND HYPOPROGESTINISM

Excessive production, as contrasted with deficient production, of either estrogen or progestin is not a characteristic of any known syndrome. Deficient production of both hormones may occur spontaneously or as a sequel to castration. In animals, fetal castration before the external genitalia have differentiated results in a feminine anatomy. The corresponding experiment of nature in human beings is Turner's syndrome. Lacking ovaries, such individuals fail to mature pubertally unless given exogenous estrogen. Prior to hormonal therapy, their romantic and erotic inertia cannot be attributed entirely either to short stature and juvenility of appearance or to lack of erotic receptivity and erotic initiative. After hormonal induction of puberty, women with Turner's syndrome may have a problem in finding a sexual mate. All short-statured men and women have a problem in meeting one another, for which reason some become members of Little People of America. In the case of Turner's syndrome, it is not yet known whether endocrine replacement therapy, as presently prescribed, is well calibrated to erotic function.

Women with Turner's syndrome treated with estrogen, with or without progestin, eventually look their age, even though short in stature. Women who are short in stature as a result of hypopituitary dwarfism have the added social difficulty of not looking their age, despite sex-hormonal therapy. In this respect, they resemble their male counterparts. Short-statured hypopituitarism in females is sufficiently rare as to preclude a final and definitive statement, but the evidence seems to be that they, like their male counterparts, have an impaired ability to establish the pair-bonding of a love affair. A similar deficit is not evident in achondroplastic dwarfism, a condition in which the gonads and their hormonal function are not impaired.

Postnatal castration—ovariectomy—of girls after birth but before puberty is extremely rare, for few diseases require loss of both ovaries. Even without hormonal replacement therapy at the age of puberty, prepubertal ovariectomy does not result in statural dwarfism. Neglect of replacement therapy is virtually unheard of today. Therefore, it is not possible to state with confidence any theory regarding the long-term concomitants of prepubertal female castration.

The effects of ovariectomy on the erotic responsivity of adult women have not yet, surprisingly enough, been well documented. On the basis of clinical impression alone, it has been assumed that the effect on sex life has been primarily by way of vaginal atrophy and dryness (correctable with exogenous lubricants or with estrogen therapy) and secondarily by way of either grief or celebration over the loss of ability to conceive. The same assumptions have been made concerning postmenopausal sexuality.

Despite individual differences, loss of the ovarian hormones at menopause, or by earlier ovariectomy in adulthood, does not automatically preordain the loss of erotic receptivity, initiative, or responsiveness. The apparent paradox here may be resolved when more is known about the effect of adrenocortical androgens on female sexuality.

HOMOSEXUALITY AND PARAPHILIAS

All the unorthodoxies and anomalies of gender identity, from homosexuality and related transpositions to the rare and bizarre intrusion paraphilias, are less common in chromosomal and gonadal females than in males. The explanation for this difference may reside in the fact that nature always requires that something be added to the indifferent state of the embryo or fetus in order to differentiate a male. Male differentiation may well require an additive to the visual-erotic arousal system. If so, then the additive factor could be subject to developmental error, almost certainly in the postnatal era of gender-identity differentiation. Herein lies the most likely explanation of why fewer females than males reach adolescence with an anomaly of gender identity. Whatever the explanation, there is no evidence to implicate a relationship between anomalous female hormones and anomalous aspects of female gender identity and its manifestations at puberty.

HORMONAL CONTRACEPTIVE EFFECTS

There are more questions than answers concerning the effect of contraceptive steroids on eroticism. Different brands of the pill have different steroidal content; women on the pill have varied endogenous hormone levels, and cyclic hormonal changes under the influence of the pill are not constant. No study of erotic effects of the pill has been done with all relevant variables held constant. Such partial evidence as is available indicates that a woman's prior erotic history, as well as her attitude toward a sexual partnership, can mask direct effects of the pill. Therefore, the following generalizations need to be accepted cautiously, for they may require eventual revision.

Women on sequential pills, which simulate the estrogen-progestin cycle, have mood cycles similar to women who do not use an oral contraceptive. Women on combination pills, by contrast, experience stability of affect, without the tension and irritability of the premenstrual syndrome. The effect of either type of pill on the different components of eroticism, namely, solicitation, receptivity, and initiative, has not been analyzed. The chronologic distribution of total sexual practice may change according to the type of pill used, but there is no consistent quantitative increase or decrease in practice nor in the desire for it.

GERIATRIC YEARS

Sex steroids are so dramatically related to somatic maturation at puberty, to the changes of the menopause, and to the somatic sequelae of castration that it has long been assumed that decline of erotic function and behavior with age is sex-hormone-dependent. There is, however, no established evidence of point-for-point correlation between amount of sexual behavior and level of circulating sex steroids—whether androgen, estrogen, or progestin, and whether of adrenocortical or gonadal origin. It is true that the level of circulating sex steroids diminishes with age, but with a quite asymmetrical sex difference in the sharp, menopausal diminution of the female and the slowly progressive diminution of the male. There is no corresponding behavioral asymmetry. Some women do not decrease, but rather continue or increase their sex lives postmenopausally. Some men with the fashionable, though not authenticated, diagnosis of male menopause become sexually apathetic and inert long before their hormone levels can be implicated by reason of restoration of function following hormonal replacement therapy.

Present knowledge on hormonal-behavioral aging effects is based on cross-sectional studies. Longitudinal hormonal-behavioral biographies are needed. When sufficient numbers of them have been obtained, it may at last be possible to replace speculation with hard data.

GERIATRIC HYPOSEXUALISM: MALE

The insistent and imperious eroticism of the typical adolescent male gives way, over the life span, to a gradually diminishing frequency of erection, mounting, and ejaculation. There may or may not be a synchronous diminution of other components of eroticism, namely precopulatory solicitation and attractiveness to the partner or prospective partner. When all three components diminish synchronously, the change becomes simply a change in the rhythm of life, with no attendant distress. When diminution affects only one or two of the three components, personal distress can be intense.

The most frequent source of distress relates to impairment of only the performance component. The symptom may be loss or diminution of erectile potency or failure to reach the climax of ejaculation (anorgasmia) without impotence. Neither of these symptoms is specific to the geriatric age group, but older people may be affected. In the absence of hypoandrogenism, sex hormone therapy is useless, except insofar as it may have a placebo effect. According to recent animal experiments, hypoandrogenism may prove to be most effectively treated with estradiol as well as testosterone, since the latter may be metabolized into the former in living tissue that mediates erection.

Impotence and anorgasmia may be secondary to a primary systemic disorder, especially of the central nervous system (including pathological depression), the circulatory system, or the metabolic system (e.g., the impotence of advanced diabetes mellitus). Either symptom may also be iatrogenic—a side effect especially of various antihypertensive medications or of various antipsychotic major tranquilizers. In the great majority of instances, however, both symptoms prove to be of a dissociative or hysteric nature. That is, they appear only in the context of an impaired erotic relationship and represent, in effect, a form of passive-aggressive resistance in which the genitalia are the organs of combat. In such cases, a psychotherapist with specialized knowledge of sexology and sex therapy can frequently induce a remission of symptoms.

GERIATRIC HYPOSEXUALISM: FEMALE

Female sexuality has long been more neglected than that of the male in Western medicine and science. Female sexuality after the menopause is no exception. There is no solid body of data on which to base sound clinical decisions regarding postmenopausal endocrine replacement therapy from the point of view of improving sex life. For many women, androgen administered for nonerotic reasons has a side effect of reinvigorating the solicitation component of eroticism and improving the feeling of orgasm. Exogenous estrogen administered postmenopausally has a beneficial effect in reversing atrophic vaginal dryness, which otherwise necessitates an exogenous lubricant. At the same time as it improves receptivity, estrogen may restore the sex-attractant pheromones of the vagina and improve skin complexion, thus adding to the component of attractiveness in the woman's eroticism.

Vaginal unreceptivity, or phobia of penetration, with attendant pain and/or muscle spasm, is not specifically a geriatric symptom. In the female, it is the counterpart of impotence in the male. Anorgasmia exists in both sexes but is far more common in the female. Anorgasmia and vaginal phobia both are unresponsive to medication with steroids. Like their male counterparts, they are, in the majority of instances, dissociative or hysteric in etiology, and the prognosis is best with sex-counseling therapy.

SUMMARY

The phyletic program of sexually dimorphic behavior is initiated by the chromosomes, which dictate gonadal morphology, which, in turn, regulates fetal sex-differentiating hormones, which, in turn, affect the central nervous system as well as the genital anatomy. Postnatally, the effects of social biography are imprinted during the period of gender-identity formation in early life. Prenatal and postnatal effects act conjointly to establish sexually dimorphic patterns of behavior that are highly resistant to change. Prepubertal gender identity differentiation prepares the individual for the sexual dimorphism of puberty and adulthood. At puberty, androgen alters the threshold for erotic arousal in both males and females, but it does not control the imagery of eroticism nor the sex of the partner in a pair-bond. Estrogen subserves the reproductive functions in the female. Its role in male reproductive status is unknown. Its cyclic effect on mood, affect, and eroticism in women is incompletely understood. Psychosocial events and hormonal events co-vary, but the mechanism by which this occurs is not known.

REFERENCES

A. GENERAL

Ferin, M., Halberg, F., Richart, R. M., and Vande Wiele, R. (Eds.). *Biorhythms and Human Reproduction.* New York: John Wiley and Sons, 1974.

Grumbach, M. M., Grave, G. D., and Mayer, F. E. (Eds.). *The Control of the Onset of Puberty.* New York: John Wiley and Sons, 1974.

Kaplan, H. S. *The New Sex Therapy.* New York: Brunner/Mazel, 1974.

Money, J. *Sex Errors of the Body.* Baltimore: Johns Hopkins University Press, 1968.

Money, J. and Ehrhardt, A. A. *Man and Woman, Boy and Girl.* Baltimore: Johns Hopkins University Press, 1972.

Rose, R. M. The psychological effects of androgens and estrogens—a review. In *Psychiatric Complications of Medical Drugs* (R. I. Shader, Ed.). New York: Raven Press, 1972.

Williams, R. L. (Ed.). *Textbook of Endocrinology.* Philadelphia: W. B. Saunders, 1974.

B. SPECIFIC

Fetal Period

Ehrhardt, A. A. and Baker, S. W. Prenatal androgen, human central nervous system differentiation, and behavior sex differences. In *Sex Differences in Behavior* (R. C. Friedman, R. M. Richart, and R. L. Vande Wiele, Eds.). New York: John Wiley and Sons, 1974.

Ward, I. Prenatal stress feminizes and demasculinizes the behavior of males. Science, *175:* 82–84, 1972.

Ward, I. Sexual behavior differentiation: prenatal hormonal and environmental control. In *Sex Differences in Behavior* (R. C. Friedman, R. M. Richart, and R. L. Vande Wiele, Eds.). New York: John Wiley and Sons, 1974.

Ward, I. Exogenous androgen activates female behavior in noncopulating prenatally stressed males. *Journal of Comparative and Physiological Psychology, 91:* 465–471, 1977.

Childhood Years

Bedlingmaier, F., Versmold, H., and Knorr, D. Plasma estrogens in newborns and infants. In *Endocrinologie Sexuelle de la Periode Perinatale* (M. G. Forest and J. Bertrand, Eds.). Paris: Inserm, 1974.

Faiman, C., Reyes, F. I., and Winter, J. S. D. Serum gonadotropin patterns during the perinatal period in man and in the chimpanzee. In *Endocrinologie Sexuelle de la Periode Perinatale* (M. G. Forest and J. Bertrand, Eds.). Paris: Inserm, 1974.

Forest, M. G., Cathiard, A. M., and Bertrand, J. A. Evidence of testicular activity in early infancy. *Journal of Clinical Endocrinology and Metabolism, 37:* 148–151, 1973.

Money, J. and Alexander, D. Psychosexual development and absence of homosexuality in males with precocious puberty. *Journal of Nervous and Mental Disease, 148:* 111–123, 1969.

Teenage Years

Bobrow, N. A., Money, J., and Lewis, V. G. Delayed puberty, eroticism, and sense of smell: A psychological study of hypogonadotropinism, osmatic and anosmatic (Kallmann's syndrome). *Archives of Sexual Behavior, 1:* 329–344, 1971.

Clopper, R. R., Adelson, J. M., and Money, J. Postpubertal psychosexual function in male hypopituitarism without hypogonadotropinism after growth hormone therapy. *Journal of Sex Research, 12(1):* 14–32, 1976.

Lewis, V. G., Money, J., and Bobrow, N. A. Idiopathic pubertal delay beyond age fifteen: Psychologic study of twelve boys. *Adolescence, 12(45):* 1–11, 1977.

Money, J. Adolescent psychohormonal development. *Southwestern Medicine, 48:* 182–186, 1973.

Money, J. The syndrome of abuse dwarfism (psychosocial dwarfism or reversible hyposomatotropinism): Behavioral data and case report. *American Journal of Diseases of Children, 131:* 508–513, 1977.

Money, J. and Clopper, R. R. Psychosocial and psychosexual aspects of errors of pubertal onset and development. *Human Biology, 46:* 173–181, 1974.

Money, J. and Clopper, R. R. Postpubertal psychosexual function in postsurgical male hypopituitarism. *Journal of Sex Research, 11(1):* 25–38, 1975.

Money, J. and Ogunro, C. Behavioral sexology: Ten cases of genetic male intersexuality with impaired prenatal and pubertal androgenization. *Archives of Sexual Behavior, 3:* 181–205, 1974.

Money, J. and Wolff, G. Late puberty, retarded growth and reversible hyposomatotropinism (psychosocial dwarfism). *Adolescence, 9:* 121–134, 1974.

Schmidt, G. and Sigusch, V. Women's sexual arousal. In *Contemporary Sexual Behavior: Critical Issues in the 1970's* (J. Zubin and J. Money, Eds.). Baltimore: Johns Hopkins University Press, 1973.

Adult Years—Men

Benkert, O., Crombach, G., and Kochatt, G. Effect of L-dopa on sexually impotent patients. *Psychopharmacologia, 23:* 91–95, 1972.

Christensen, L. W., and Clemens, L. G. Intracerebral application of an aromatization inhibitor and its effects on copulation in the male rat. Paper presented at Eastern Regional Conference on Reproductive Behavior. Atlanta, Georgia. June 17–20, 1974.

Edward, R. J. Does an estrogen mediate the effect of testosterone on spontaneous activity in male rats? Paper presented at Eastern Regional Conference on Reproductive Behavior. Atlanta, Georgia. June 17–20, 1974.

Feder, H. H. Naftolin, F., and Ryan, K. J. Male and female sexual responses in male rate given estradiol benzoate and 5 alpha-androstan-17-beta-ol-3 one propionate. *Endocrinology, 94:* 134–41, 1974.

Fletcher, T. J. and Short, R. V. Restoration of libido in castrated red deer stag (Cervus elaphus) with oestradiol-17 β. *Nature, 48:* 616–618, 1974.

Hyppä, M., Lehtinen, P., and Rinne, U. K. Effects of L-dopa on the hypothalamic, pineal, and striatal monoamines and on the sexual behaviour of the rat. *Brain Research, 30:* 265–272, 1971.

Johnson, H. R., Myhre, S. A., Ruvalcaba, R. H., Thaline, H. D., and Kelley, V. C. Effects of testosterone on body image and behavior in Klinefelter's syndrome—a pilot study. *Developmental Medicine Child Neurology, 12:* 454–460, 1970.

Kolodny, R. C., Masters, W. H., and Hendryx, J. Plasma testosterone and semen analysis in male homosexuals. *New England Journal of Medicine, 21:* 1170–1174, 1971.

Larsson, K., Södersten, P., and Beyer, C. Induction of male sexual behaviour by oestradiol benzoate in combination with dihydrotestosterone. *Journal of Endocrinology, 57:* 563–564, 1973.

Laschet, U. Antiandrogen in the treatment of sex offenders: mode of action and therapeutic outcome. In *Contemporary Sexual Behavior: Critical Issues in the 1970's* (J. Zubin and J. Money, Eds.). Baltimore: Johns Hopkins University Press, 1973.

Martinez-Vargas, C., Sar, M., and Stumpf, W. E. Localization of estrogens in the avian brain. Paper presented at Eastern Regional Conference on Reproductive Behavior. Atlanta, Georgia. June 17–20, 1974.

Money, J. The use of an androgen-depleting hormone in the treatment of male sex offenders. *Journal of Sex Research, 6:* 165–172, 1970.

Money, J. Pubertal hormones and homosexuality, bisexuality and heterosexuality. In Appendix B, *National Institute of Mental Health Task Force on Homosexuality: Final Report and Background Papers* (J. M. Livingood, Ed.). Rockville, Md.: National Institute of Mental Health, 1972.

Rose, R. M. Testosterone, aggression and homosexuality: A review of the literature. In *Seminars in Psychiatry: Topics in Psychoendocrinology* (E. J. Sacher, Ed.). New York: Grune and Stratton, 1975.

Adult Years—Women

Bardwick, J. M. The sex hormones, the central nervous system and affect variability in humans. In *Women in Therapy* (V. Franks and V. Burtle, Eds.). New York: Brunner/Mazel, 1974.

Comfort, A. Likelihood of human pheromones. *Nature, 230:* 432–433, 1971.

Klaiber, E. L., Kobayashi, Y., Broverman, D. M., and Hall, F. Plasma monoamine oxidase activity in regularly menstruating women and in amenorrheic women receiving cyclic treatment with estrogens and a progestin. *Journal of Clinical Endocrinology, 33:* 630–638, 1971.

McClintock, M. K. Menstrual synchrony and suppression. *Nature, 229:* 244,-245, 1971.

Udry, J. R. and Morris, N. M. Effect of contraceptive pills on the distribution of sexual activity in the menstrual cycle. *Nature, 227:* 502–503, 1970.

Geriatric Years

Kopera, H. Estrogens and psychic functions. In *Frontiers of Hormone Research: Ageing and Estrogens* (P. A. van Keep and Ch. Lauritzen, Eds.). Basel: Karger, 1973, vol. 2.

108

The Physiology of Puberty: Disorders of the Pubertal Process

William D. Odell

ETIOLOGIES OF SEXUAL MATURATION

HISTORY

Understanding the current concepts of the etiologies of sexual maturation is most easily achieved by referring to the schematogram (Fig. 108-1) depicting the central nervous system-pituitary gonadal axis.[1] As presently understood, this is a closed-looped feedback system in which all components are connected by means of neuronal or hormonal signals. For many years, *physicians* believed that puberty was determined by the "onset" of gonadotropin secretion by the pituitary with resultant gonadal stimulation. The following is a quotation from the 1966 edition of a well-known textbook of endocrinology: "The development of secondary sexual characteristics depends upon the secretion of gonadotropins by the anterior pituitary. Although these may be present in the pituitary during earlier childhood, they are not released until adolescence."[2] This viewpoint was strengthened by the findings, using bioassays, that gonadotropins were commonly undetectable in 24-hour urine collections from prepubertal children, while gonadotropins were usually detectable in 24-hour collections from adults. It was not commonly appreciated that *excretion* of hormones is commonly related to body surface area, as is volume of urine produced. Thus the total amount of gonadotropin excreted in the small volume of a child's urine is significantly less (and undetectable if the sensitivity of the assay is limited to just the extent of the mouse uterine weight assay) than the adult's.

DECREASING FEEDBACK SENSITIVITY

In contrast to this belief of most physicians, animal physiologists, working with rodents, had for many years believed that gonadotropins were secreted and that a dynamic central nervous system-pituitary gonadal axis existed prior to sexual maturation. This belief stemmed predominantly from studies in parabiotic sexually immature rats. For example, Kallas[3] in 1929 had shown that if one partner of parabiotic sexually immature female rats were castrated, the other partner underwent precocious sexual maturation. Presumably, castration resulted in increased gonadotropin secretion, with resultant stimulation of the gonads in the intact partner.* Kallas concluded that prior to maturation, the hypophysis already held the ovaries under its influence. While in 1976 we might substitute "central nervous system-pituitary unit" for hypophysis, the general concept still remains valid. The findings of Kallas were largely ignored until 1951 when Byrnes and Meyer[4] repeated and confirmed the findings of Kallas. In addition, Byrnes and Meyers (Fig. 108-2) found that if tiny doses of estradiol were injected into the castrate, sexually immature, female parabiotic partner, the precocious sexual maturity of the other partner could be prevented. Doses of estrogens could be selected that were too small to stimulate uterine weight development and vaginal plate opening in the recipient but that could still prevent the precocious sexual development. Byrnes and Meyer concluded that a dynamic pituitary gonadal system was present prior to puberty and that it was kept intact by feedback control via the tiny amounts of steroids secreted by the prepubertal gonad; i.e., a very sensitive feedback system was present prior to puberty. It is important to note that Byrnes and Meyers *did not do control studies* in adult rats to determine whether feedback sensitivity was any different. A number of subsequent studies in rats confirmed that a dynamic central nervous system-pituitary gonadal system exists prior to maturation, and the hypothesis has developed and been widely accepted that sexual maturation is caused by a change (decrease) in feedback sensitivity of this system. The parabiotic studies described form a large part of the basis of this hypothesis. In addition, Donovan and Van der Wertt ten Bosch[5] demonstrated that destructive lesions placed in the base of hypothalamus just caudal to the optic chiasm will advance puberty in rats. Ramaley and Gorsky[6] in 1967 reported that if the neural connections to the medial-basal portion of the hypothalamus were severed (this includes the area destroyed in the studies of Donovan and Van der Wertt ten Bosch), precocious puberty, followed by persistent estrus, occurred. Others have shown that continuous light[7] or lesions in the amygdala[8] or stria terminalis[9] will cause precocious onset of estrus in rats. Because of the belief that decreasing feedback sensitivity was the cause of sexual maturation, these data were interpreted as indicating that a control area involving the

*The parabiotic model system is *still* not fully understood. It *was believed* that peptide hormones crossed the parabiotic union but that steroids did not. Many of the interpretations of early studies in reproduction are based on this belief.

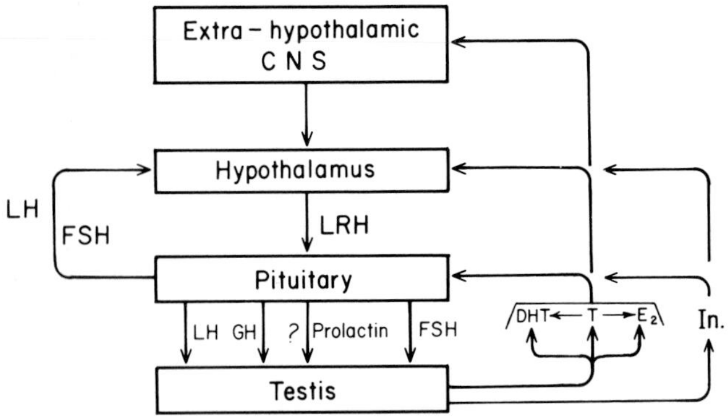

Fig. 108-1. Schematic interrelationships of the central nervous system-pituitary-testicular axis. This scheme assists in understanding the various parameters and possible etiologies of sexual maturation. (Reproduced from Odell and Swerdloff.[1])

amygdala and its radiations via the fornix to the hypothalamus are important in suppressing gonadotropin secretion prior puberty.

In 1966–1968, studies from the author's laboratory revealed that gonadotropins were detectable by radioimmunoassay in blood[10,11] and (if 48-hour or longer urine collections were made rather than 24-hour collections) by bioassay in urine from prepubertal children.[12] We concluded that a dynamic hypothalamic pituitary gonadal unit also existed in children and that the control of puberty was similar to that hypothesized for rats, i.e., decreasing feedback sensitivity resulting in increasing gonadotropin secretion with resultant increasing gonadal stimulation.

Subsequently, a large number of laboratories[13–21] measured LH and FSH in blood of children and correlated these values with stage of puberty. Most of the studies involved single determinations in different children, a so-called cross-sectional study. A longitudinal study has been completed by Winter and Faiman;[21] their data are presented in Figures 108-3a and b. Grumbach et al[22] attempted to directly assess the feedback sensitivity of children and adults by administering oral estrogens and quantifying gonadotropin excretion. The data were few, bût it was possible to conclude that a difference in sensitivity did exist, with the prepubertal child being about five times more sensitive to feedback suppression than the adult. Table 108-1 shows their data.

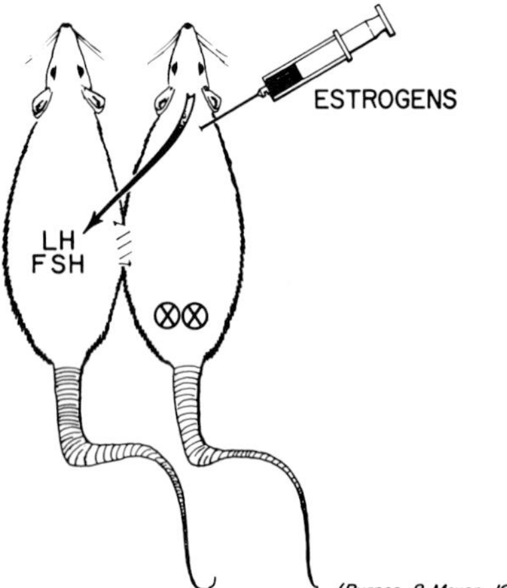

Fig. 108-2. The parabiotic model used by Byrnes and Meyer for studying feedback sensitivity to estrogens. The immature animals were joined in parabiotic union; one was castrated and treated with varying doses of estrogens. Uterine weight was quantified in the castrate animal and ovarian weight in the intact animal. This model was interpreted on the belief that peptide hormones (gonadotropins) pass the parabiotic union, while steroids are inactivated or do not pass the parabiotic union.

Table 108-1. Hypothalamic-Pituitary Regulation of Puberty in Man
Suppression of Urinary FSH by Ethinyl Estradiol

Pubertal Stage	No.	Dose (μg/day × 5 d)	Significant Suppression of Urine FSH
P1 (prepubertal)	6	2	3/6
P1 (prepubertal)	5	5	5/5
P1 (prepubertal)	3	10	3/3
Total			11/14
P2 (early puberty)	2	2	0/2
P3 (midpuberty)	2	10	1/2
P4 (advanced puberty, premenarche)	2	10	0/2
Adult males	4	8	0/4
	2	16	0/2
	2	20	0/2
	2	30	0/2
	4	40	3/4
	2	50	2/2

Reproduced from Grumbach et al.[22]
Ethinyl estradiol was administered at the doses shown. Urinary excretion of FSH was determined by radioimmunoassay. Although accurate differences in sensitivity cannot be determined from these data and no correction for body surface area was made, it appears that prepubertal and peripubertal children are 4 to 10 times more sensitive than adult men.

Feedback suppression has also been directly tested in male and female rats by administering varying doses of testosterone to male and estradiol to female rats[23–25] at different ages and measuring serum LH and FSH levels. The first studies were done in castrate rats, where LH and FSH concentrations were elevated and simple to quantify using existing assays. Later, sensitivity of the radioimmunoassays finally permitted studies in intact rats, and the data shown in Figures 108-4a, b, c and d were collected. These direct studies of the phenomenon indirectly assessed by the studies of Byrnes and Meyer, Kallas, and others have turned out to be difficult to interpret, for *sensitivity varies* with duration of time following castration. However, although differences in the dose of steroids required for suppression at different ages exist, the differences are not directly related to age or degree of maturation.

In summary of the discussion thus far, a commonly held hypothesis of the cause of sexual maturation is that decreasing feedback sensitivity of the central nervous system-pituitary unit results in increasing blood LH and FSH concentrations with resultant increasing gonadal steroid secretion. This hypothesis stems from data in young rats and is supported by the changing LH and FSH concentrations during puberty in children and the demonstration of small differences in feedback sensitivity.

CHANGING GONADAL SENSITIVITY TO LH

While the data discussed thus far are compatible with the hypothesis of a decrease in feedback sensitivity as the cause of sexual maturation, certain recent data shed doubt on this as the major factor. For example, Figure 108-5 shows the blood LH and FSH concentrations in the sexually maturing female rat. In contrast to what one would expect* (if changing feedback sensitivity were the cause of maturation), both FSH and LH *fall* during maturation. In cattle and pigs, LH and FSH concentrations in blood show no significant changes between birth and sexual maturation[26–28] (Fig. 108-6). At least in cattle, pigs, and rats, factors

*Any process involving either maturation of the CNS or decreasing feedback sensitivity would act by *increasing* LH and/or FSH.

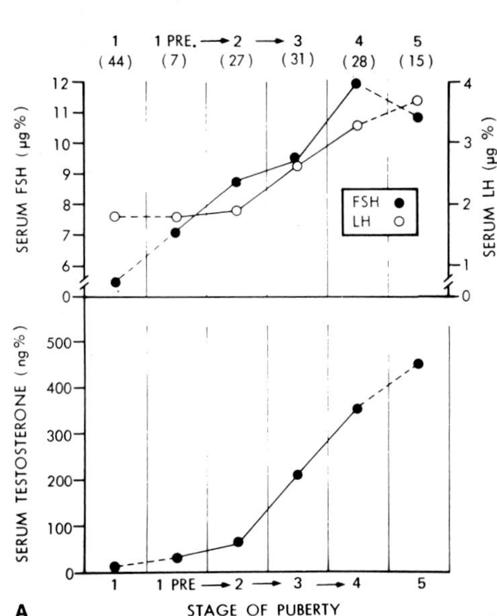

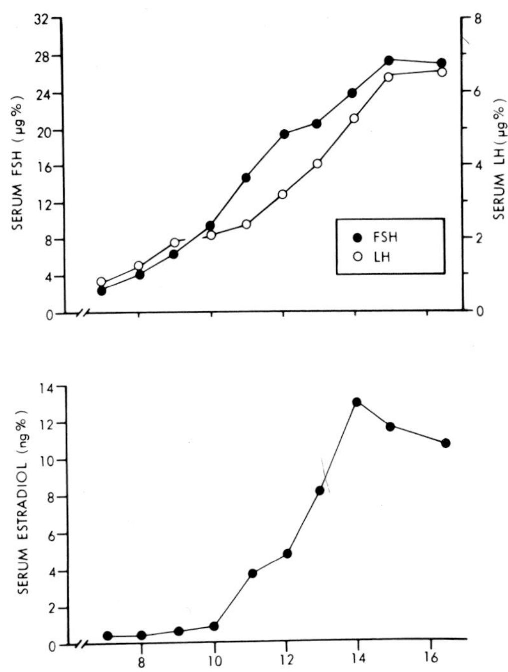

Fig. 108-3a. Mean serum LH, FSH and testosterone in boys at varying stages of puberty. Fifty-six boys were followed longitudionally through puberty. (Reproduced from Faiman and Winter.[21]) **Fig. 108-3b.** Mean serum LH, FSH, and estradiol in girls at varying stages of puberty. Fifty-eight girls were followed longitudionally through puberty. (Reproduced from Faiman and Winter.[21])

other than changing feedback sensitivity must be of major importance. Although it is possible that puberty may be caused by different mechanisms in different species, it appears more likely that such a significant period of development would be controlled by similar mechanisms in all species of mammals, and on this basis we question the hypothesis of feedback as the major cause in humans. Theoretically, one or more of a number of etiologies of sexual maturation is possible. Table 108-2 lists the possibilities.

In the rat model, at least, a major factor appears to be changing *gonadal response to gonadotropins*. This is best demonstrated as follows: If one injects purified LH into sexually immature male rats for 5 days, beginning on the day of hypophysectomy, testosterone secretion increases and results in increased prostate weight growth. This is the basis of a well-known bioassay for LH. If one begins LH treatment *5 days* following hypophysectomy (instead of on the day of hypophysectomy), no increase in androgen secretion (judged by prostate weight change) occurs, even though very large doses of LH are administered.[29] Figure 108-7 depicts these data. In contrast to the loss of responsiveness to LH, the immature male rat retains responsiveness to FSH 5 days following hypophysectomy. If purified FSH is administered prior to administration of LH, responsiveness to LH may be restored, and the magnitude of the response is related to both the time duration of exposure and to the dose of FSH (Figs. 108-8a and b). Based on these data, Odell and Swerdloff have postulated that FSH induces responsiveness to LH and that this is the major factor in maturation in the rat. If this hypothesis is true, then sensitivity to LH should increase with sexual maturation in normal animals. This is the opposite of what has been commonly assumed, as judged by selection of immature animals for bioassay of gonadotropins under the assumption they are more sensitive than adults. Sensitivity was tested directly by administering varying doses of LH to the intact animal at different ages and measuring blood testosterone 1 hour later (the time when response was maximal).

Table 108-2. Possible Etiologies of Sexual Maturation*

I. Extraphypothalamic-central nervous system areas
   A. Increasing stimulation of hypothalamic areas governing LH and/or FSH secretion (an intrinsic maturation process)
   B. Decreasing inhibition of hypothalamic centers governing LH and/or FSH secretion (an intrinsic process)
   C. Decreasing sensitivity to feedback inhibition by gonadal steroids (intrinsic change in negative feedback)
   D. Increasing stimulatory effects of gonadal steroids (intrinsic change in positive feedback)
II. Hypothalamic areas
   A. Increasing stimulation of LH and/or FSH secretion (intrinsic maturation process)
   B. Decreasing inhibition of pituitary secretion of LH and/or FSH
   C. Decreased sensitivity to feedback inhibition by gonadal hormones (intrinsic process)
   D. Increasing stimulatory effects by gonadal hormones
III. Pituitary gland
   A. Increasing LH and/or FSH secretion in response to constant LH-RH stimulation (intrinsic process)
   B. Increasing stimulatory effects of gonadal steroids on response to gonadotropin-releasing hormone(s)
IV. Gonads
   A. Increasing response to LH and/or FSH stimulation
      1. LH modulation of FSH response or vice versa
      2. Gonadal hormone modulation of response to LH and/or FSH
      3. Other pituitary hormone modulation of LH and/or FSH response (e.g., growth hormone, prolactin)
      4. Intrinsic gonadal maturation process resulting in increased response to LH and/or FSH
V. Sex accessories
   A. Increasing response to gonadal hormones (intrinsic process)
   B. Modulation of response by other hormones (e.g., prolactin)

*LH, luteinizing hormone; FSH, follicle-stimulating hormone; LH-RH, LH-releasing hormone.

Figure 108-9 shows that the percent increase in testosterone is least at 10 days of age, greater at 21 days, and greatest at 42 and 62 days of age.[30] The mechanism of the FSH induction of responsiveness to LH has been studied by the same workers and involves induction of new receptors to LH.[11,31] Figure 108-10 depicts the change in LH receptor populations with age in maturing rats.[1]

In summary, Odell and Swerdloff believe the testis (Leydig cell) near birth in male rats is very poorly responsive or nonresponsive to LH and that FSH is secreted in unrestrained amounts (an intact hypothalamic pituitary-gonadal system exists and gonadal secretions are minimal). The FSH gradually (over about 45 days) induces LH receptor development and thus Leydig cell response to LH. Testicular steroid secretion slowly increases with gradual feedback suppression of FSH and LH secretion.

In cattle and pigs, changing gonadal response to LH may also be a major factor responsible for maturation, since LH and FSH concentrations are relatively constant throughout sexual maturation, while gonadal steroids progressively increase. No direct assessment of gonadal response to LH during sexual maturation in children has yet been possible. However, Sizonenko[32] has shown that blood increment of testosterone in response to human chorionic gonadotropin treatment of cryptorchid boys correlates di-

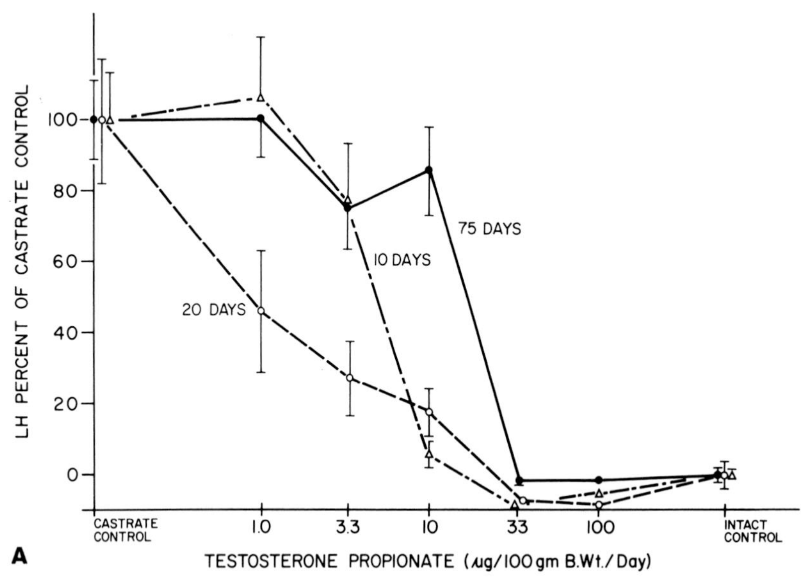

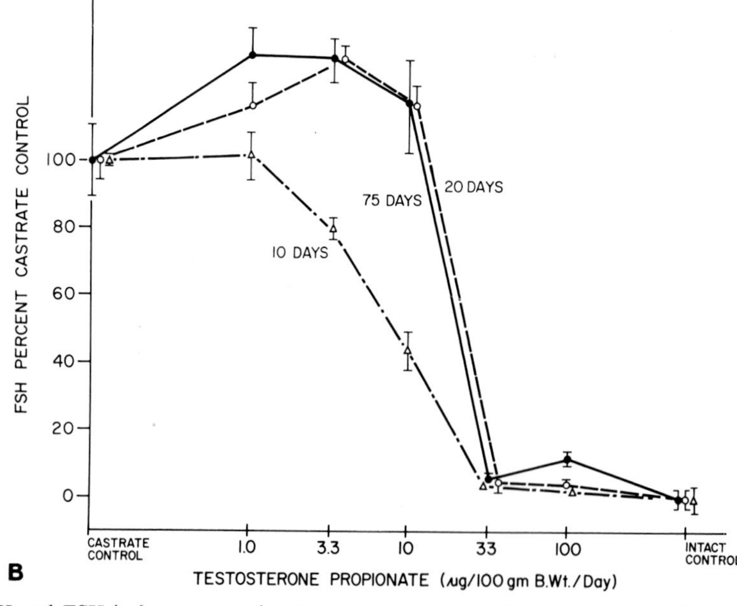

Fig. 108-4a,b. Suppression of LH and FSH in immature and mature *castrated* rats, with varying doses of testosterone propionate. Animals were castrated at 10, 20, and 75 days of age and immediately begun on the daily testosterone dose indicated. Five days later, animals were sacrificed and blood testosterone determined. **Fig. 108-4c,d.** Suppression of LH and FSH in immature and mature *intact* rats with varying doses of testosterone propionate. (Reproduced from Odell and Swerdloff.[1])

rectly with basal blood FSH concentrations (Fig. 108-11). Therefore, changing gonadal response appears to be an important factor in the maturation of rats, cattle, pigs, and possibly man.

In addition to these gonadal effects and changing feedback sensitivity, *another factor* appears to be operative in higher primates. This factor is the most poorly understood but may be likened to a "dampening" or "restriction" of the system prior to puberty. Figure 108-12 shows the changes in blood LH and FSH in agonadal children prior to puberty—idealized from data presented by Faiman and Winter, Blizzard et al., and Grumbach et al.[22,33] Note that while agonadal children have elevated LH and FSH near birth, both fall soon afterwards and remain relatively low (considerably lower than in castrate adults) until near the *usual age* of puberty, when both hormones again rise to adult castrate levels. The mechanisms of this effect, i.e., the failure of gonadal absence to produce a maximum rise in LH and FSH, are unknown. It is clear that most animal models studied do not exhibit this phenomenon. Thus, castration of sexually immature cattle or rats produces a rapid rise in LH and FSH in blood to levels as high or higher than in adult castrates. This dampening phenomenon is probably the cause of the long preadolescent period in humans, a facet of maturation not present in rats and cattle. Without this dampening

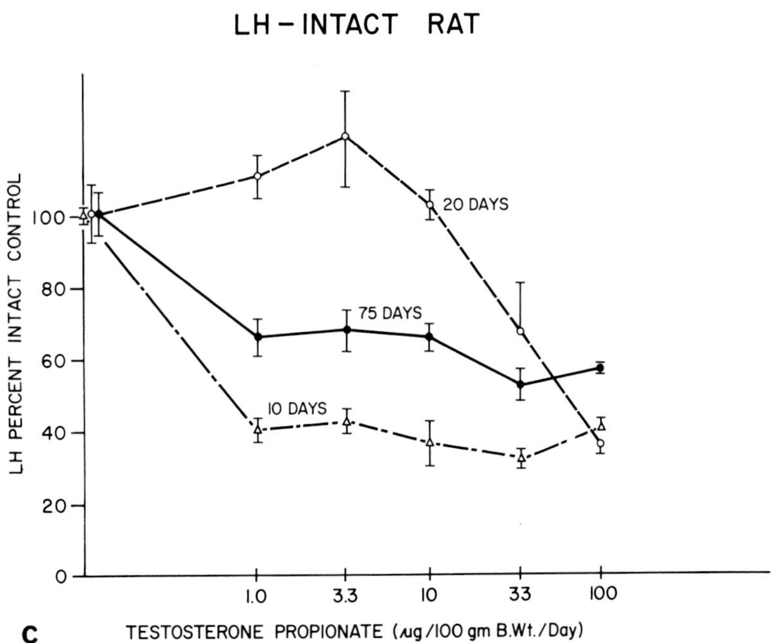

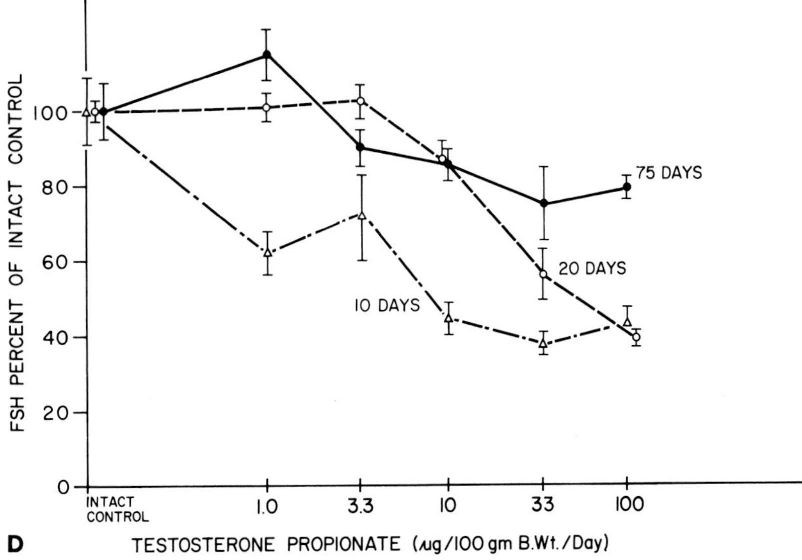

Fig. 108-4. (*cont'd.*)

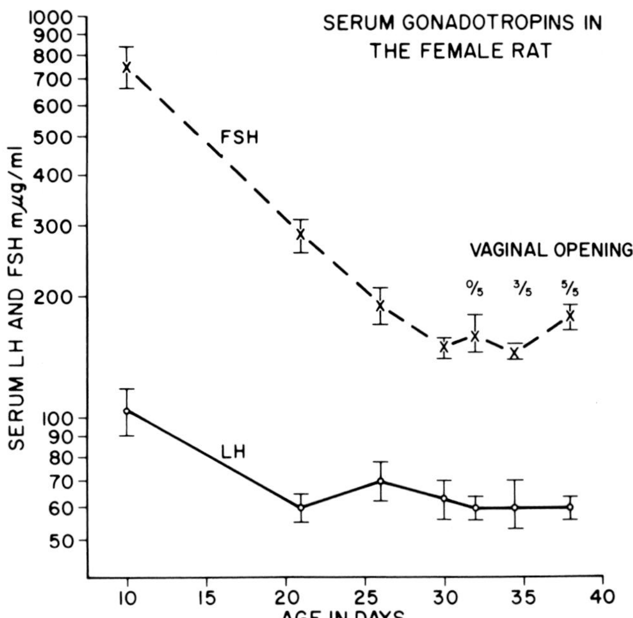

Fig. 108-5. Serum FSH and LH in female rats during sexual maturation. Note that concentrations fall or are level, observations incompatible with decreasing feedback sensitivity of the hypothalamic-pituitary system. (Reproduced from Swerdloff and Odell.[25])

factor, one may postulate that humans would also undergo sexual maturation at about 1 year of age and that the other parameters of maturation would be operative exactly as in various animals models.

SLEEP-INDUCED GONADOTROPIN SECRETION

An additional factor that may play a role in maturation of higher primates is the sleep induction of LH and possibly FSH secretion during the pubertal years. Boyar et al.[34,35] have shown that prior to puberty, blood LH and FSH concentrations show minimal fluctuations throughout the day and night. During the latter part of Stage I and during Stages II, III, and IV, average LH concentrations become increased during sleep and oscillate fairly widely. Average FSH levels may increase slightly, but oscillations are equivocal (Fig. 108-13). After awakening, LH concentrations fall again. As sexual maturation is completed, average concentrations of LH and FSH remain elevated (as they were at night during the pubertal process) and oscillate about this average. This phenomenon is apparently peculiar to animals showing prolonged sleep patterns, as do higher primates. Animals, such as rats and dogs, that sleep in shorter periods do not appear to show this sleep induction of LH and FSH.

CHANGING PITUITARY RESPONSE TO LH-RH (GnRH)

One additional factor in sexual maturation is a changing pituitary response to the hypothalamic-releasing hormone, gonadotropin-releasing hormone.[22,24] This may represent primary changes within the hypothalamic-pituitary system or may be a secondary phenomenon related to modulation of pituitary response by changing gonadal steroid concentrations. In the rat, GnRH causes a much greater FSH secretion in immature animals than after maturation[24] (Fig. 108-14). This may in part explain the high blood FSH concentrations (see Fig. 108-5) observed in the immature animals and ensure FSH induction of the gonadal response to LH. In the prepubertal child, LH-RH also causes greater FSH secretion than

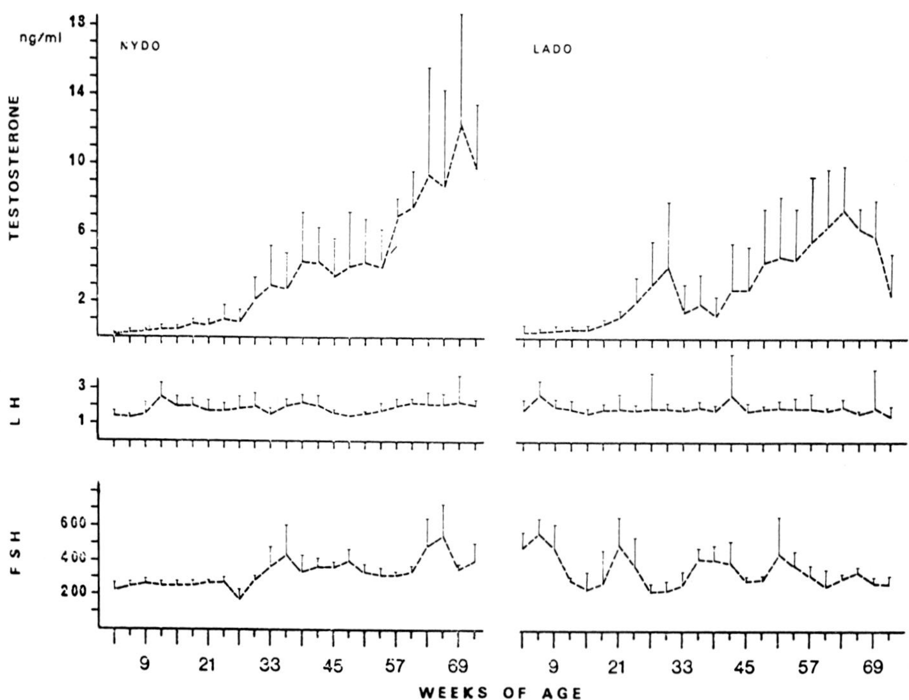

Fig. 108-6. Plasma LH, FSH, and testosterone in male cattle during sexual maturation. Note that FSH and LH are relatively constant as serum testosterone increase dramatically. (Reproduced from Karg/Giménez/Hartl/Hoffmann/Schallenberger/Schams. Testosterone, luteinizing hormone (LH) and follicle stimulating hormone (FSH) in peripheral plasma of bulls: Levels from birth through puberty and short term variations. *Zbl. Vet. Med. A, 23:* 793–803, 1976.

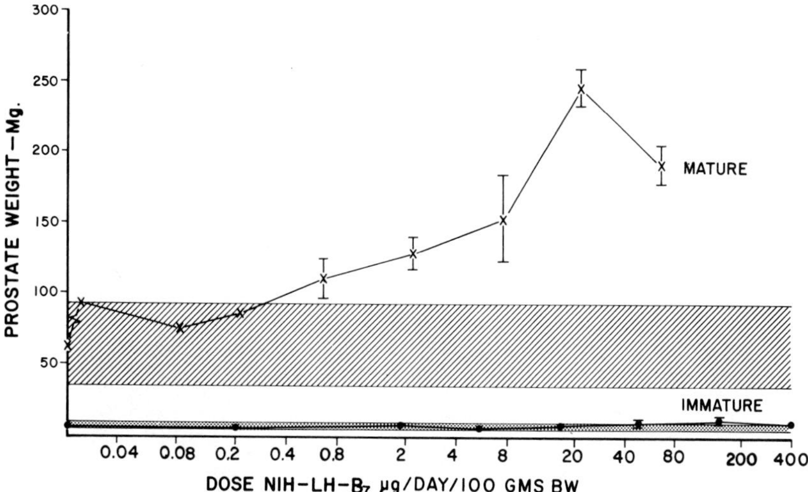

Fig. 108-7. Failure of the sexually immature male rat to respond to LH when treatment was begun 5 days following hypophysectomy. Under the same conditions the mature animal continues to respond. In this study, 21-day-old immature and sexually mature male rats were hypophysectomized. Five days later treatment with varying doses of purified LH was initiated (NIH-LH-B_7). After 5 days of treatment, animals were sacrificed and prostate weight was quantified. (Reproduced from Odell et al.[29])

it does in sexually mature adults (see Fig. 108-15). It is not known whether this changing response to LH-RH is caused by an intrinsic change in the pituitary per se or is secondary to the increasing blood concentrations of testosterone, estradiol, or other gonadal steroids.

RELATION OF BODY WEIGHT OR COMPOSITION TO MENARCHE

Frisch and Revelle[36] analyzed data from 3 comparable human longitudinal growth studies to determine the height and weight of children at sequential adolescent events. They showed that the

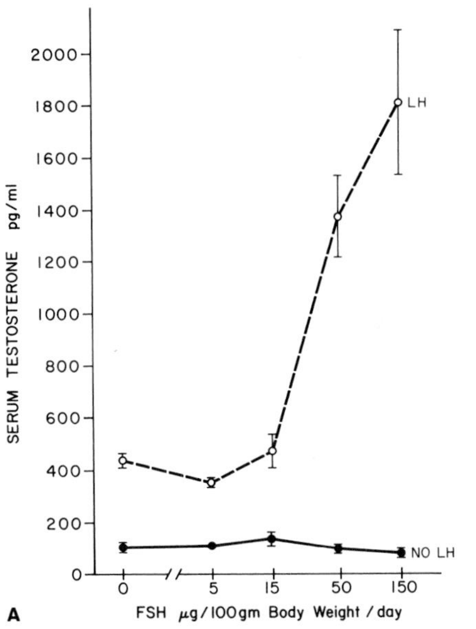

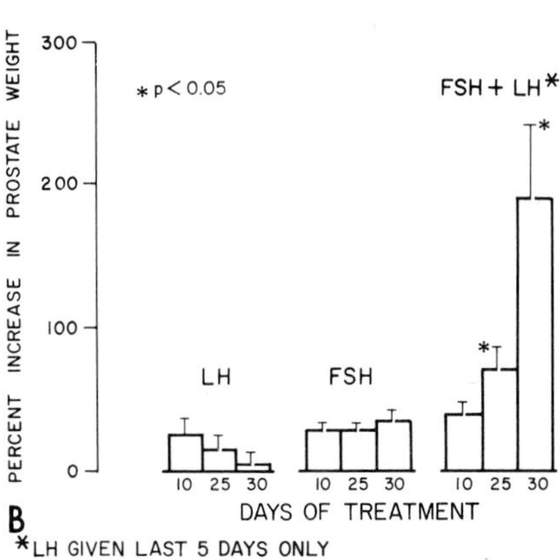

Fig. 108-8a. Dose-response relationship of FSH induction of LH responsiveness. In this study, 21-day-old immature male rats were hypophysectomized and immediately treated with varying doses of LH. After 5 days, a single injection of LH was given and blood testosterone quantified 1 hour later (the time of maximal response). All animals that were given LH received the same dose of LH; the magnitude of response to LH related to the dose of FSH pretreatment received. Key: ●——● indicates basal testosterone in control animals receiving only FHS; ○----○ shows the blood testosterone in the animals following LH treatment. (Reproduced from Odell and Swerdloff.[1]) **Fig. 108-8b.** Time-response relationships of FSH induction of LH responsiveness. In this study, 21-day-old animals were treated for varying lengths of time with a single daily dose of FSH beginning 5 days following hypophysectomy. During the last 5 days of FSH treatment, daily LH injections (maximal dose based upon separate data) were also given. Prostate weight was quantified. The control groups labeled "LH" received only 5 days of LH, on days 5–10, 20–25, and 25–30, and are labeled 10, 25, 30, days of treatment, respectively. Saline (placebo) injections were given for the preceding days to these groups. The groups labeled FSH received daily FSH for 10, 25, and 30 days—no LH was given. Note that LH alone was ineffective in either stimulating or even maintaining prostate weight. FSH alone maintained prostate weight. When the LH treatment was given after FSH exposure, prostate weight increased related to the duration of treatment to FSH. (Reproduced from Odell and Swerdloff.[1])

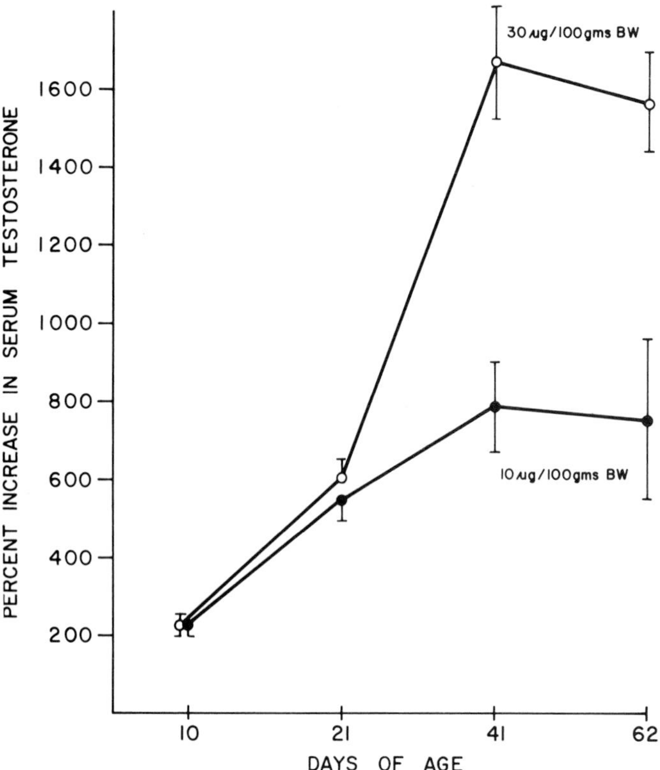

Fig. 108-9. Response of the intact rat to a single dose of LH at two dose levels at varying ages. Blood testosterone was quantified before and 1 hour following intraperitoneal LH (NIH-LH-B_7). Note the response increases with increasing age. (Reproduced from Odell et al.[30])

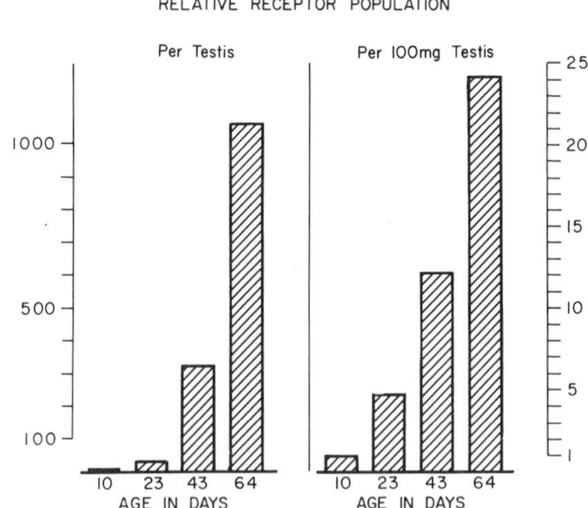

Fig. 108-10. Changing LH receptor populations with age in the sexually maturing rat. Correlate these changes with changing sensitivity to LH shown in Figure 108-9. (Reproduced from Odell and Swerdloff.[1])

average "critical weight" of Caucasian girls at the time of initiation of weight spurt was 30 kg, the weight at maximum rate of weight gain was 39 kg, and the weight at menarche was 47 kg. These mean weights were similar for both early- and late-maturing girls. Frisch[37] has proposed that the "critical weight" correlating with pubertal events actually represents a lean body weight to fat ratio of about 3:1, or a fat body percent of 20 to 30 percent. This ratio was similar for all girls independent of age of menarche. Some support of such a concept exists from animal studies.[38] Exactly what factors relate body composition to puberty are unclear.

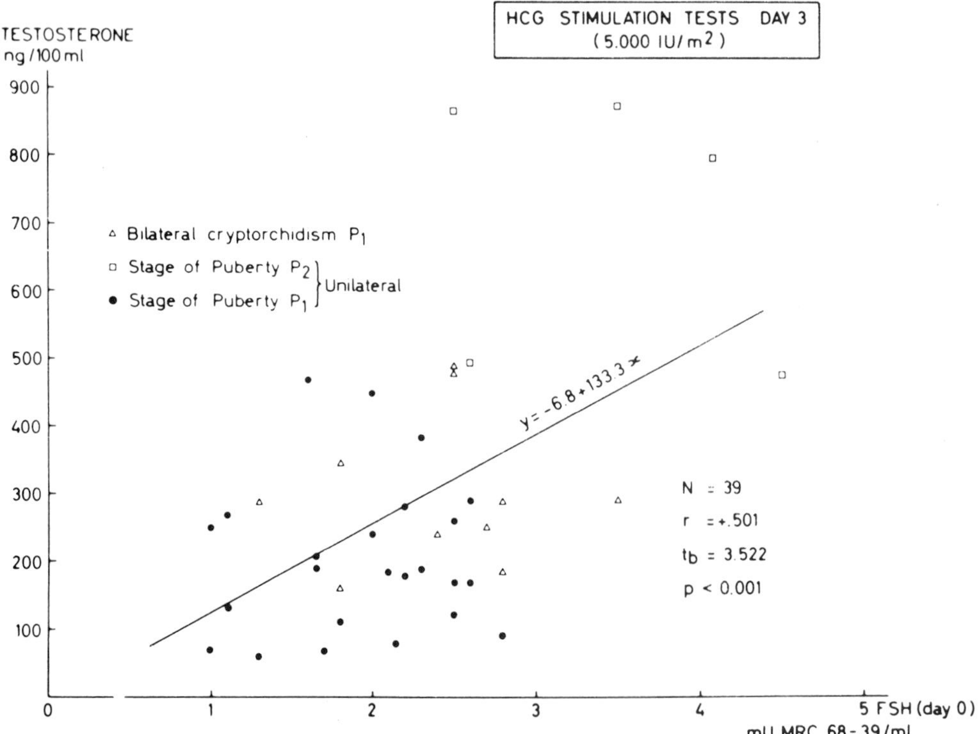

Fig. 108-11. Change in blood testosterone in boys following stimulation with 5000 IU/m² of human chorionic gonadotropin. Results correlate with the basal FSH concentration. (Reproduced from Sizonenko.[32])

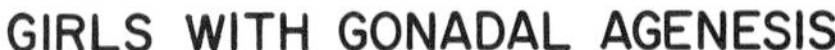

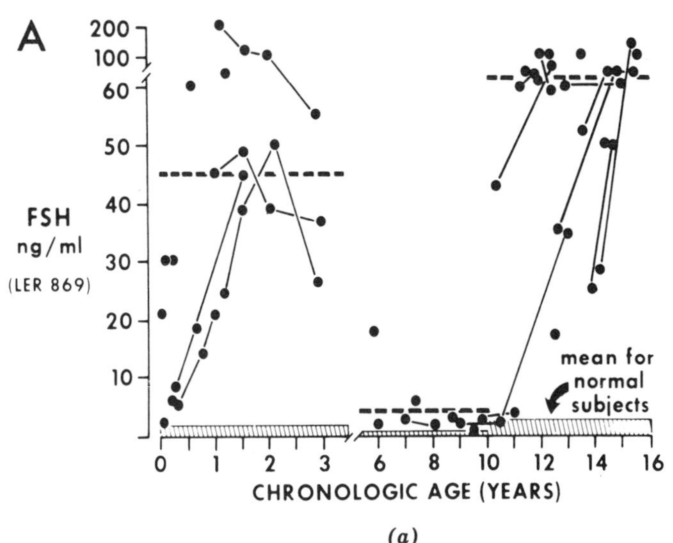

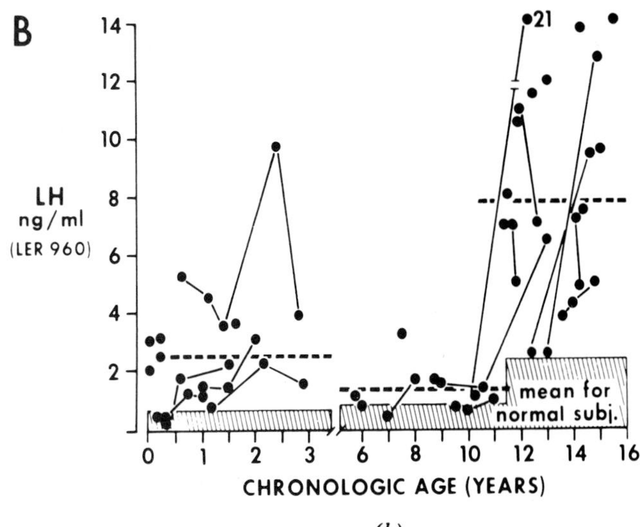

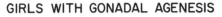

Fig. 108-12a,b. Serum FSH and LH in normal children (shaded areas) and in girls with gonadal agenesis at varying ages. Note elevations in LH and FSH during the years 1–3, lower levels 6–10, and elevated levels 11–16. (Reproduced from Grumbach et al.[22])

However, adipose tissue is known to form estrogens from precursor steroids.[39] It is important to note that data from individual girls vary widely, and the data were analyzed by regression analysis to show the relationships. Body composition was not measured but rather estimated from heights and weights.

SUMMARY

From evaluation of the process of sexual maturation in several animal models and in the human, and based upon present level of understanding, we conclude that puberty in the human is a resultant of several factors. The relative importance of each in the human is not fully understood. However, in several animals the major factor appears to be FSH induction of gonadal responsiveness to LH. Table 108-3 lists the factors involved in puberty in the human.

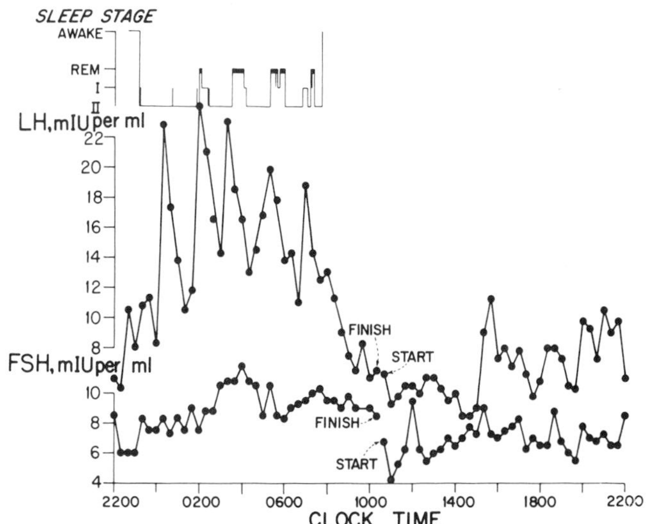

Fig. 108-13. Changes in blood LH and FSH during sleep in pubertal girls. EEG sleep stages are shown in the upper inset. Note that average LH concentrations and possibly FSH are increased during sleep. (Reproduced from Boyer et al.[35])

THE ADRENARCHE

In addition to cortisol and aldosterone, the adrenal gland secretes a variety of other steroids, some of which have actions as androgens or serve as precursors for androgen formation in peripheral tissues. Two of these are dehydroepiandrosterone (DHEA) and adrostenedione. The latter is transformed into testosterone in many peripheral tissues, and in mature women, it is one of the major sources of blood testosterone. Control of adrenal androgen secretion is poorly understood. Gonadotropins are not believed to affect adrenal androgen secretion. *Excretion* of 17-ketosteroids (a reflection of 17-ketosteroid secretion predominantly by the adrenal) is low in early childhood and increases in the peripubertal years.[40] In contrast, blood DHEA and DHEA sulphate increase steadily with age from age 2 to past puberty. Androstenedione and cortisol concentrations do not change significantly with puberty (Fig. 108-16). It is commonly believed that hormones other than ACTH are important in controlling adrenal androgen secretion. Whether this is true or not is uncertain, and which hormones may be involved in unknown.

Whatever the control mechanisms, the effects of androgen secretion increases gradually prior to menarche in girls. In boys, testicular androgens are normally secreted in such huge amounts relative to adrenal androgens that the effects of adrenal androgens

Table 108-3. Etiologies of Sexual Maturation in the Human

1. FSH induction of LH receptors and increasing gonadal response to LH
2. Changing pituitary response to GnRH (? cause or effect)
3. Changing CNS response:
   a. Sleep-induced LH secretion
   b. "Dampening" or restriction prior to puberty
   c. Changing feedback sensitivity to gonadal steroids

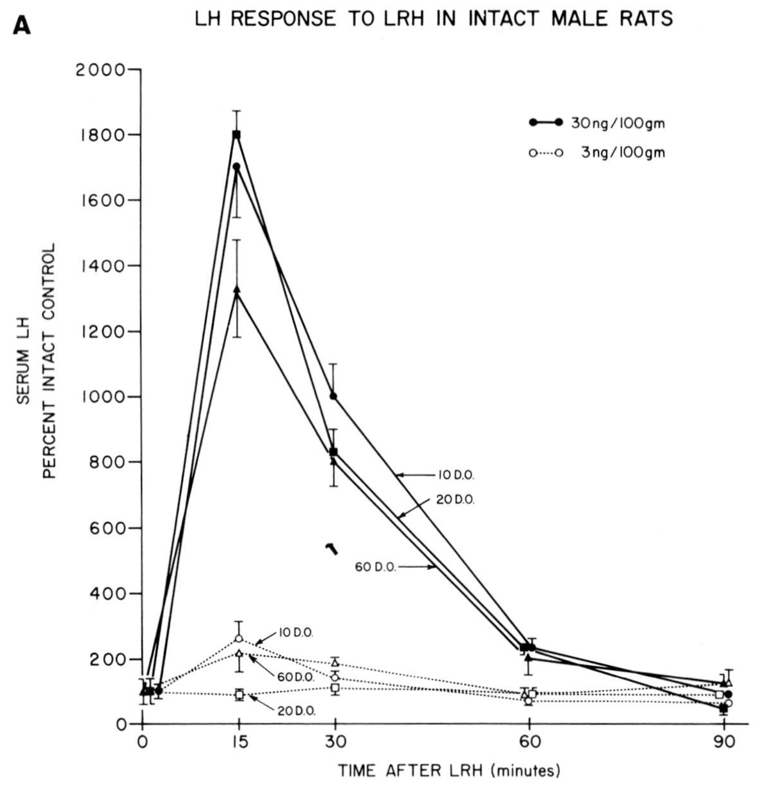

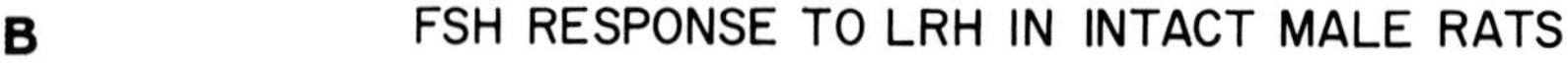

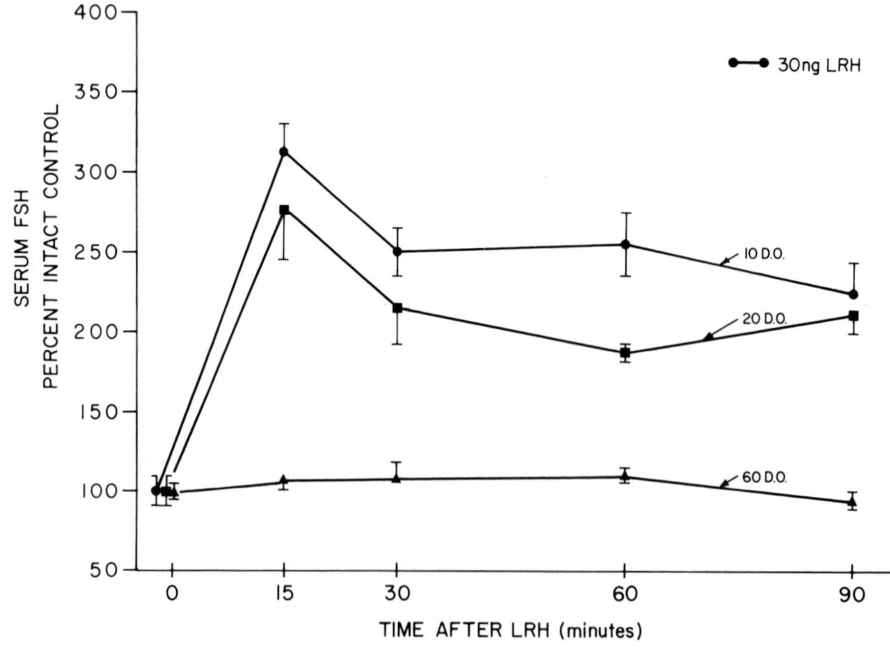

Fig. 108-14a,b. Response of male rats to luteinizing hormone-releasing hormone (LRH) at varying ages. Note there are little or no differences in LRH stimulation of LH but a striking age related difference for FSH. (Reproduced from Swerdloff and Odell.[1])

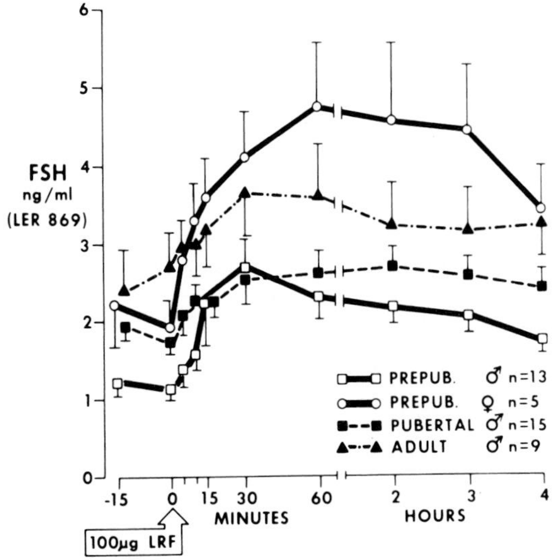

Fig. 108-15. FSH response of children to LRH (LRF). Note the relatively large changes in FSH concentrations over baseline values in prepubertal children. (Reproduced from Grumbach et al.[22])

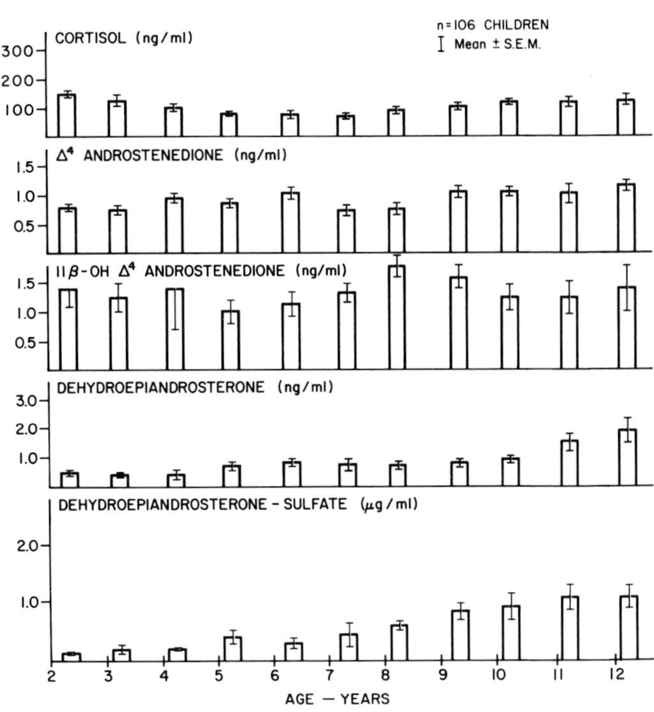

Fig. 108-16. Changes in several steroids during sexual maturation. Note the steady rise in dehydroepiandrosterone and its sulfate beginning prior to puberty. (Reproduced from Parker et al.[41])

are insignificant. However, in agonadal boys, adrenal androgens stimulate axillary and pubic hair growth at approximately the usual age of puberty. Obviously the amounts of hair in such boys are less than in eugonadal boys. In girls, adrenal androgens form the *predominant* source of blood testosterone and normally control body hair growth. Thus the adrenally insufficient girl (with normal ovarian function) develops inadequate axillary and pubic hair, while this is not true in boys if testicular function is normal.

STAGING OF SEXUAL MATURATION

In determining the causes of *precocious or delayed sexual maturation,* it is helpful for the clinician to know in some detail the normal relationships in girls of axillary and pubic hair development to breast development and in boys the relationship of testicular size to body hair development. As indicated earlier, adrenal gland androgen secretion plays a major role in hair development in girls but is less important in boys because of the secretion of the much larger amounts of testicular androgens. Two of the most widely used studies of normal relationships and ages of pubertal events have been published by Marshall and Tanner,[42,43] who examined groups of English girls and boys as they went through sexual maturation. While Marshall and Tanner did not regard these data as universally applicable, they nevertheless are widely used and are immensely helpful to all of us caring for children with disorders of puberty. Tables 108-4 to 108-7 and Figures 108-17 to 108-20 present their data.

In English boys, genitalia begins to develop between ages of 9½ and 13½ in 95 percent of subjects [average 11.6 ± 0.9 (S.D.)] and reach mature size at 13 to 17 years of age (average 14.9 ± 1.1). Pubic hair reached the stage equivalent to an adult male at an average age of 15.2 ± 1.1.

In English girls, the first changes of puberty (either breast or pubic hair changes) appeared between 8.5 and 13 in 95 percent of subjects. The interval from the first sign of puberty to complete maturity varied from 1.5 to over 6 years and from initial breast development to menarche, 2.3 to 5.8 years (average 2.3 ± 0.1 years). Menarche occurred at an average age of 13.5 years (S.D. – 1.02).

PRECOCIOUS SEXUAL MATURATION

Proper use of the pubertal staging classification has practical importance. For example, if one observes a boy with precocious puberty as judged by hair growth, but whose testicular size is Stage I or prepubertal, the likely diagnosis becomes a neoplasm producing steroids as opposed to causes involving gonadotropin secretion with resultant gonadal stimulation. Similarly in girls, hair growth in the total absence of estrogenic manifestations directs one's attention to steroid-producing neoplasms; isolated breast development if present for several months suggests some estrogen source rather

Table 108-4. Stages of Breast Development in Girls

Stage	Description	Age at Onset (years) Mean	Range (95%)
1	Preadolescent; elevation of papilla only		
2	Breast bud stage; elevation of breast and papilla as a small mound, enlargement of areola diameter	11.2	9.0–13.3
3	Further enlargement of breast and areola, with no separation of their contours	12.2	10.0–14.3
4	Projection of areola and papilla to form a secondary mound above the level of the breast	13.1	10.8–15.3
5	Mature stage; projection of papilla only due to recession of the areola to the general contour of the breast.	15.3	11.9–18.8

From Marshall and Tanner;[42] Root and Reiter.[44]

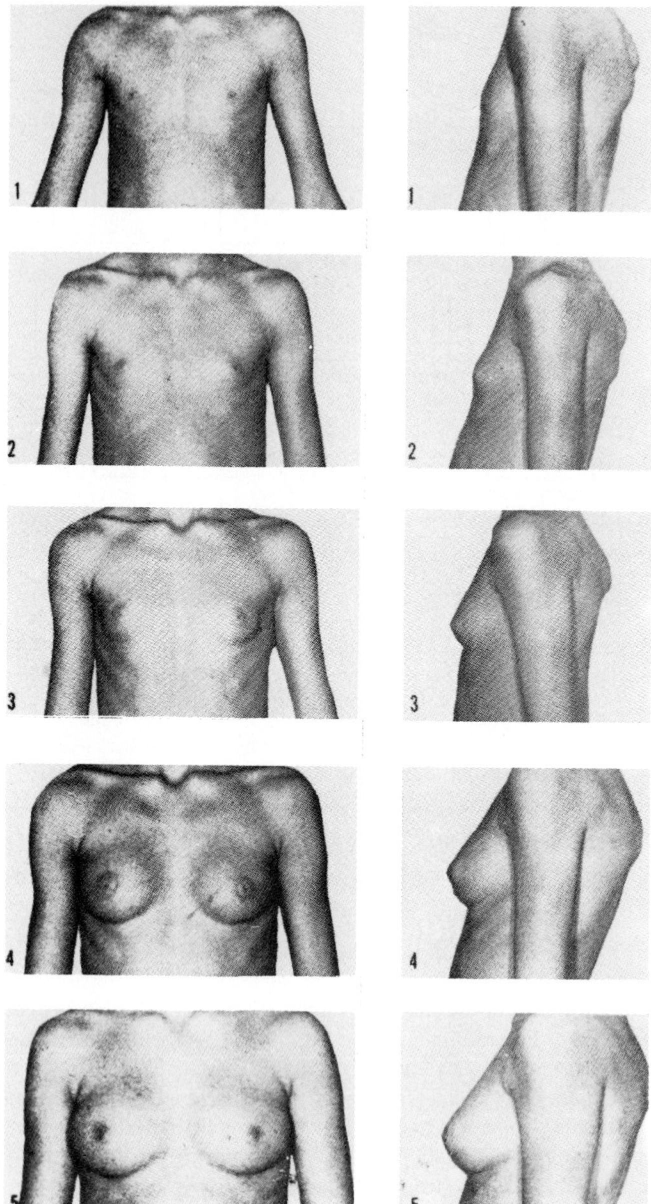

Fig. 108-17. Standards for rating of breast stages. Numbers refer to pubertal stages 1–5. (Reproduced from Marshall and Tanner.[42])

than true precocious puberty. The differential diagnosis of precocious puberty is listed in Tables 108-8 and 108-9.

When the physician is confronted with a child with precocious sexual maturation, the complete differential diagnosis must be considered with care. The history must be evaluated for any aberrant central nervous system symptoms. Although these may be overt, e.g., focal neurological abnormalities, generalized seizures, or headaches, the symptoms may at times be very subtle, e.g., single brief episodes of automatism, episodes of inappropriate anger, abnormalities in appetite, or subtle polydipsia. Family history (especially in boys) should be analyzed for age of puberty and occurrence of precocious puberty in relatives. *Physical examination* is done with several points in mind. Is the degree of pubertal development entirely consistent with normal puberty except for age? That is, are hair staging, testicular size in boys, and breast

Table 108-5. Stages of Pubic Hair Growth in Girls

Stage	Description	Age at Onset (years) Mean	Range (95%)
1	Preadolescent; the vellus over the pubes is not further developed than that over the anterior abdominal wall, i.e., no pubic hair.		
2	Sparse growth of long, slightly pigmented, downy hair, straight or only slightly curled, appearing chiefly along the labia. This stage is difficult to see on photographs, particularly of fair-haired subjects. Although a Stage 2 rating was used in this study, it cannot be regarded as reliable, and the ages at which subjects are said to have reached Stage 2 are almost certainly too late.	11.7*	9.3–14.1*
3	Considerably darker, coarser, and more curled. The hair spreads sparsely over the junction of the pubes. This and subsequent stages were clearly recognizable on the photographs.	12.4	10.2–14.6
4	Hair is now adult in type, but the area covered by it is still considerably smaller than in most adults. There is no spread to the medial surface of the thighs.	13.0	10.8–15.1
5	Adult in quantity and type, distributed as an inverse triangle of the classifically feminine pattern. Spread to the medial surface of the thighs, but not up the linea alba or elsewhere above the base of the inverse triangle.	14.4	12.2–16.7

*Values may be too high owing to error in experimental observations. From Marshall and Tanner;[42] Root and Reiter.[44]

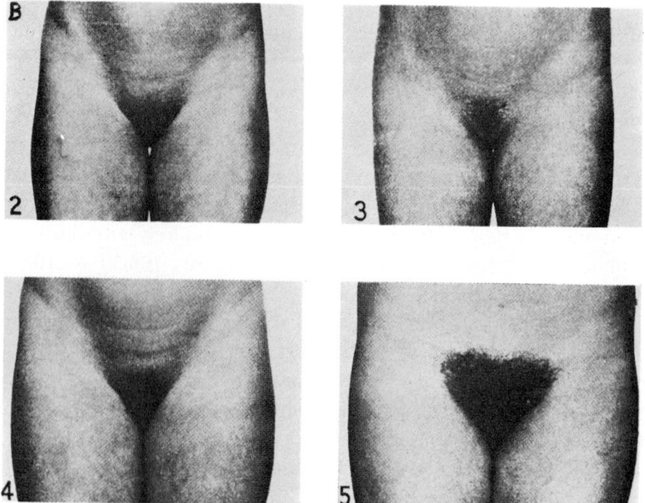

Fig. 108-18. Standards for rating of pubic hair in girls. (Reproduced from Marshall and Tanner.[42])

Table 108-6. Stages of Genital Development in Boys

Stage	Description	Age at Onset (years) Mean	Range (95%)
1	Preadolescent; testes, scrotum, and penis are of about the same size and proportion as in early childhood.		
2	The scrotum and testes have enlarged, and there is a change in the texture of the scrotal skin. There is also some reddening of the scrotal skin, but this cannot be detected on black and white photographs. Testicular length > 2 cm < 3.2 cm.	11.6	9.5–13.8
3	Growth of the penis has occurred, at first mainly in length but with some increase in breadth. There has been further growth of testes and scrotum. Testicular length > 3.3 cm < 4.0 cm.	12.9	10.8–14.9
4	Penis further enlarged in length and breadth with development of glans. Testes and scrotum further enlarged. There is also further darkening of the scrotal skin, but this is difficult to detect on photographs. Testicular length > 4.1 cm > 4.9 cm.	13.8	11.7–15.8
5	Genitalia adult in size and shape. No further enlargement takes place after Stage 5 is reached. Testicular length > 5 cm.	14.9	12.7–17.1

From Marshall and Tanner;[43] Root and Reiter.[44]

Table 108-7. Stages of Public Hair Growth in Boys

Stage	Description	Age at Onset (years) Mean	Range (95%)
1	Preadolescent; the vellus over the pubes is no further developed than that over the abdominal wall, i.e., no pubic hair.		
2	Sparse growth of long, slightly pigmented downy hair, straight or only slightly curled, appearing chiefly at the base of the penis. This stage is difficult to see on photographs, particularly of fair-haired subjects. Although the rating of Stage 2 was used in this study, it cannot be regarded as reliable, and the ages at which subjects are said to have reached Stage 2 are almost certainly too late.	13.4*	11.2–15.6
3	Considerably darker, coarser, and mostly curled. The hair spreads sparsely over the junction of the pubes. This and subsequent stages were clearly recognizable on the photographs.	13.9	11.9–16.0
4	Hair is now adult in type, but the area covered by it is still considerably smaller than most adults. There is no spread to the medial surface of the thighs.	14.4	12.2–16.5
5	Adult in quantity and type, distributed as inverse triangle of the classically feminine pattern. Spread to the medial surface of the thighs but not up the linea alba or elsewhere above the base of the inverse triangle.	15.2	13.0–17.3
	In about 80% of men, pubic hair spreads further beyond the triangular pattern, but this takes some time to occur after Stage 5 has been reached. This more widespread pubic hair may be rated as "Stage 6"; this stage is not usually reached before the mid-twenties.		

*Values may be too high owing to error in experimental observations. From Marshall and Tanner;[43] Root and Reiter.[44]

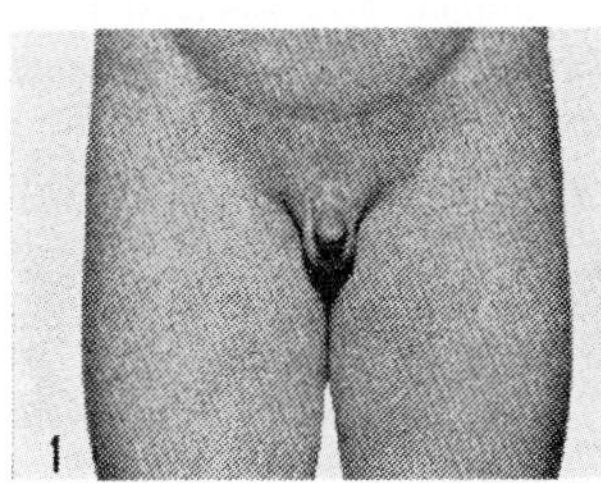

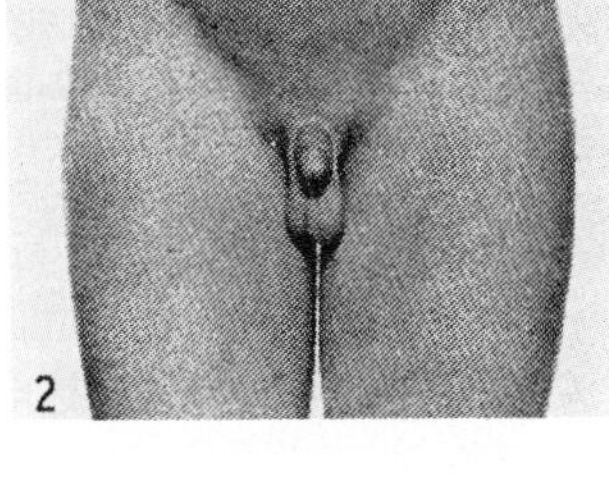

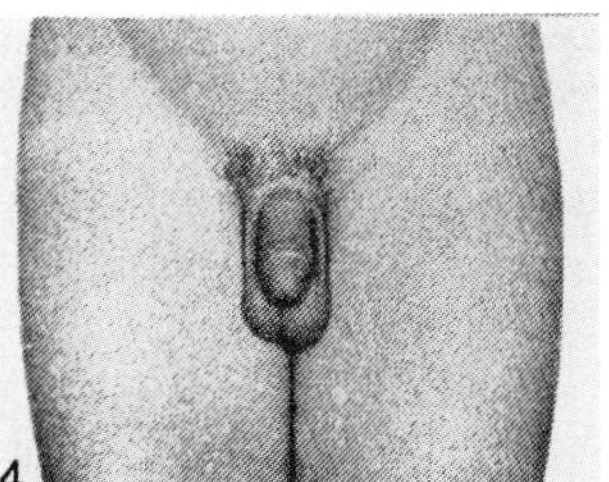

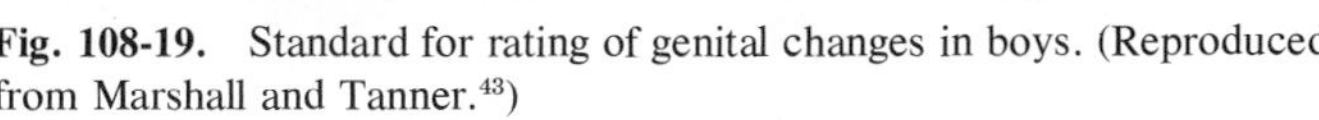

Fig. 108-19. Standard for rating of genital changes in boys. (Reproduced from Marshall and Tanner.[43])

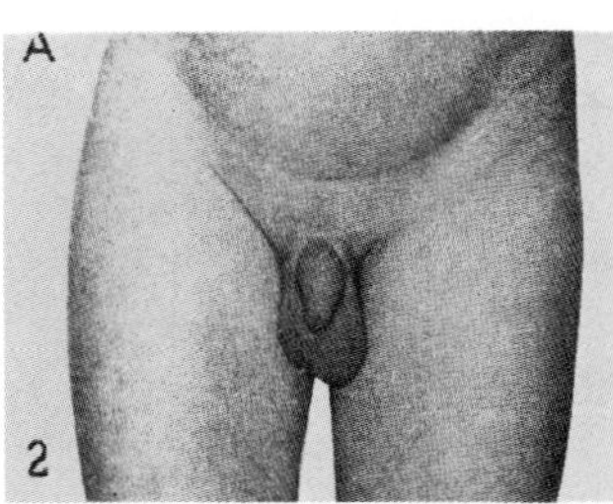

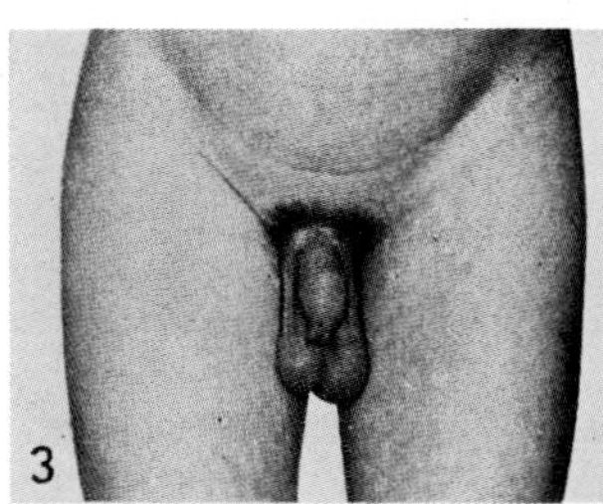

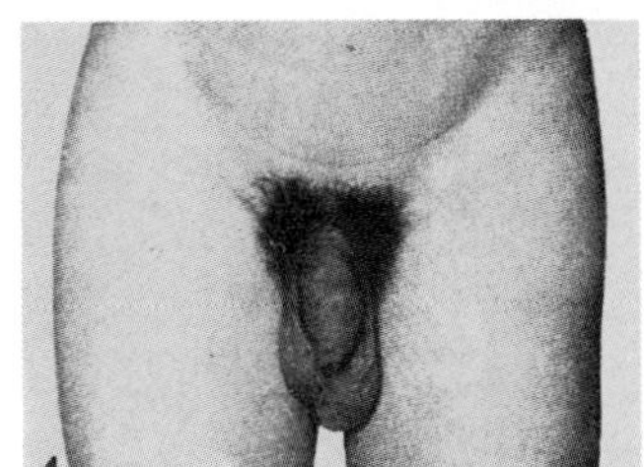

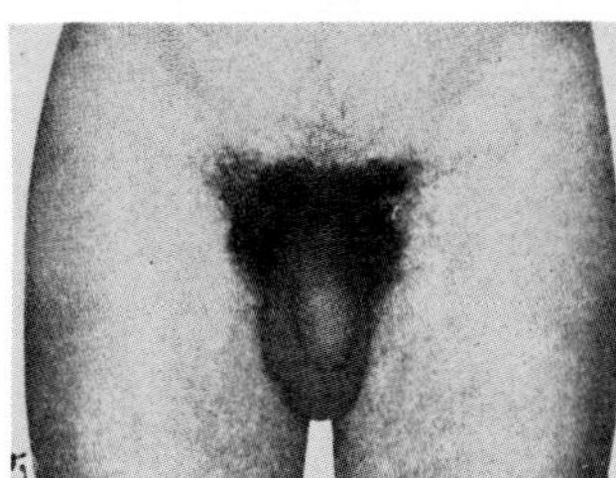

Fig. 108-20. Standard for rating of pubic hair changes in boys. (Reproduced from Marshall and Tanner.[43])

development in girls all appropriately correlated? Is the detailed neurological examination normal? Are there masses present in the abdomen and on careful bimanual examination (rectal-abdominal) in girls, can the ovaries be palpated, and are they consistent with development? Is the uterus and cervix present and normal? Is the vaginal mucosa and degree of estrogenization consistent with the stage of development?

It is important to note that idiopathic isosexual precocious puberty is not uncommon in girls; this is the most common cause of early puberty in girls. However, this is not true in boys; early puberty is most commonly associated with a neoplasm (Table 108-8). Evaluation should thus stress locating a cause in either sex, but especially in boys.

Laboratory Data. Table 108-10 presents a flow sheet for evaluation of precocious puberty. A good deal of information is available from the history and detailed physical examination; often the laboratory report is merely confirmatory. Since one is quantifying hormones in very low concentrations prepubertally, the physician must be able to rely on the laboratory procedures. It does no good to measure urinary 17-ketosteroids in a 2- to 6-year-old child with an assay having a "noise level" of 4–5 mg/day. Additionally, serum LH and FSH must be quantified in a laboratory that has assessed in detail the value of their assay systems in prepubertal children.

Using a very reliable laboratory, the following data are suggested for initial evaluation. Serum LH and FSH on three samples collected separately (e.g., three samples at 15- to 30-minute intervals on 3 different days). If costs are a major problem, these three samples could be pooled and assayed once, giving an average value. Either blood DHEA and androstenedione or urinary 17-ketosteroids are helpful in evaluating steroid-producing neoplasms or congenital adrenal hyperplasia. Blood testosterone is also of assistance in boys but not in girls with isosexual precocious puberty (although measurement of testosterone is helpful in evaluating a girl with only axillary and pubertal hair development). Blood estradiol is often measured in girls and is occasionally helpful in diagnosing estrogen-producing tumors. If blood DHEA or androstenedione is high, suppression with dexamethasone (0.5 mg/1.7 m^2 surface area qid for 2 to 3 days) helps to separate neoplasms from congenital adrenal hyperplasia. Failure to suppress to less than 50 percent of control values strongly suggests an adrenal neoplasm, particularly if serum LH and FSH suggests prepubertal values.

To further evaluate the child in whom steroid-producing neoplasm appears possible, intravenous pyelogram, ultrasound studies, adrenal vein catheterization with selective measurement of DHEA, cortisol and androstenedione, and occasionally arteriography are all available.

Gonadotropin-producing neoplasms (teratomas) are easily evaluated, for the gonadotropin is produced in sufficient quantities to raise blood human chorionic gonadotropin (HCG) values greatly. Either a serum LH or a specific β-HCG assay may be used, for HCG cross-reacts in the radioimmunoassay for LH. In such patients the presence of any HCG (in a specific assay not cross-reacting with LH) is abnormal; using a standard LH immunoassay, values are considerably above normal values for an adult castrate human.

If the patient has LH, FSH, and steroid values compatible

Table 108-8. Etiologies of Precocious Sexual Maturation in Boys

- I. Central nervous system tumors
  - A. Neurofibroma
  - B. Hamartoma
  - C. Pinealoma
  - D. Astrocytoma
  - E. Fibrous dysplasia
  - F. Ganglioneuroma
  - G. Ependymoma
- II Steroid-producing neoplasms
  - A. Adrenal
    - 1. Carcinoma
    - 2. Adenoma
  - B. Gonadal
- III. Gonadotropin-producing neoplasms
  - A. Teratomas
    - 1. Gonadal
    - 2. Pineal (see also I-C)
  - B. Hepatoblastomas
- IV. Exogenous hormones (iatrogenic)
  - A. Steroids
  - B. Gonadotropins
  - C. Drugs (e.g., Dilantin, Minoxidil, etc.)
- V. Familial precocious puberty
- VI. ACTH-producing neoplasms
- VII. Hypothyroidism
- VIII. Cushing's disease
- IX. Cogenital adrenal hyperplasia*
  - A. 21-hydroxylase deficiency
  - B. 11-hydroxylase deficiency
- X. Idiopathic isosexual precocious puberty

*Ten defects in steroid biosynthesis have been described; most do not result in increased androgen production prior to the usual age of puberty.

Table 108-9. Etiologies of Precocious Sexual Maturation in Girls

- I. Idiopathic isosexual precocious puberty
- II. Central nervous system tumors
  - A. Neurofibroma
  - B. Hamartoma
  - C. Pinealoma
  - D. Astrocytoma
  - E. Fibrous dysplasia
  - F. Ganglioneuroma
  - G. Ependymoma
- III. Gonadotropin-producing neoplasms
  - A. Teratomas
    - 1. Gonadal
    - 2. Pineal
- IV. Steroid-producing neoplasms
  - A. Adrenal
    - 1. Carcinoma
    - 2. Adenoma
  - B. Gonadal
- V. Exogenous hormones
  - A. Steroids
  - B. Gonadotropins
  - C. Drugs (e.g., Dilantin, Minoxidilate)
- VI. ACTH-producing neoplasms
- VII. Cushing's disease
- VIII. Hypothyroidism
- IX. Congenital adrenal hyperplasia
  - A. 21-hydroxylase deficiency
  - B. 11-hydroxylase deficiency
- X. Hypogonadism
  - A. Turner's syndrome with hirsutism
  - B. 17-ketoreductase deficiency in XY-phenotypic females

Table 108-10. Precocious Pubic-Axillary Hair Appearance*

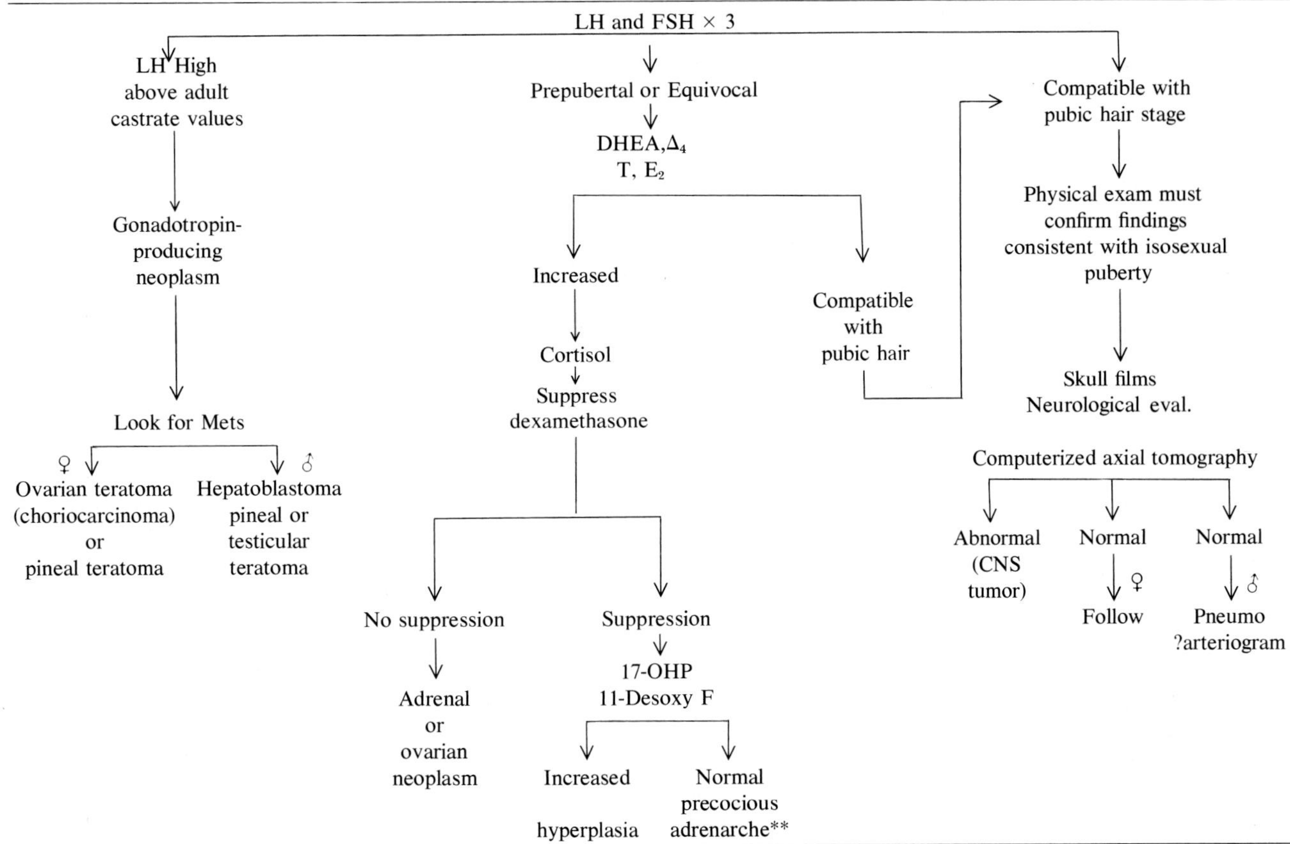

*Drug caused hair growth have been excluded by history.
**Consider 17-ketoreductase deficiency in a male pseudohermaphrodite.

with the observed stage of puberty, then careful consideration of a central nervous system mass must be made—especially in boys. Skull x-rays, computerized axial tomography scanning, electroencephalogram, pneumoencephalogram, and arteriogram are all available as diagnostic adjuncts if required.

One of the most common pubertal disorders seen by pediatricians is the young girl with premature initiation of breast budding or development without concomitant pubic hair development, i.e., premature thelarche. This is often or usually transient, lasting a few weeks, and no discernible course is discovered. Occasionally, this may be traced to estrogen contamination of a medication the child has been given (e.g., vitamins). Very rarely, an estrogen-producing tumor may be causative. Although we discuss this disorder under the broad category of precocious sexual maturation, it is properly not precocious puberty but rather precocious thelarche.

Another disorder related to early adrenal androgen secretion is termed precocious adrenarche. This is most commonly recognized in girls but occurs in both sexes. In girls, one clinically suspects the disorder in a patient with pubic hair development and no breast budding. Otherwise complete physical examination is normal; specifically, no indications of a neoplasm exist. Since normal control mechanisms of adrenal andorgen secretion is very poorly understood, the cause of this disorder is unknown.

Treatment of Sexual Precocity. The recognition of the cause of sexual precocity permits appropriate therapy by the physician. Neoplasms are removed surgically if possible. If complete removal is not possible, appropriate chemotherapy or radiotherapy is given. Congenital adrenal hyperplasia is treated with glucocorticoid suppression, administered optimally in minimal doses of dexamethasone at 11:00 PM to begin therapy, and 1 mg/1.7 m^2 of surface area may be sufficient to keep serum DHEA suppressed.

Premature adrenarche is a benign disorder of unknown cause. Such patients are not treated but are carefully reevaluated at 3- to 6-month intervals to be certain the diagnosis remains correct. The onset of puberty per se occurs at about the usual age, and such children show no abnormalities during adolescence or adulthood.

Premature thelarche is also not treated; the cause is usually not discerned. If estrogen exposure is present, that, of course, is eliminated. If medications have been changed or introduced in the time period preceding breast development, they should be suspected. Measurement of estradiol by radioimmunoassay in the drugs to indicate possible estrogen contamination is not likely to be useful. Substances with estrogen potency other than estradiol are more likely to be causative. A wide variety of steroid structures and nonsteroidal substances possess estrogenic properties. To properly evaluate the possibility of estrogen contamination of medications or foods, an estrogen bioassay is necessary. Such bioassays may be done in vitro, using cytosol estrogen receptors in a radioreceptor assay, or in vivo, using mouse or rat uterine weight responses.

Perhaps the greatest difficulty for therapy is in the disorders of familial or idiopathic precocious puberty. At present, in the United States, it is generally best not to treat these disorders. Once the diagnosis has been firmly established, as previously described, careful discussion and education of the parents and the child is necessary. These children are potentially capable of being fertile and possess adult libido and secondary sexual characteristics with a mental or psychological development and experience of a child. Frequently, girls are coquettish or possessive around sexually mature men, and boys are sexually aggressive toward women. With very mature and understanding parents and continual support from a knowledgeable physician, these patients reach teenage years in good physical and mental health. If this is achieved, no subsequent disorders of reproductive physiology are expected, and life expectancy and reproductive capacity are normal.

A number of publications exist[45–50] that report attempts at treatment of idiopathic puberty in girls with medroxyprogesterone (DepoProvera) given intramuscularly. This medication suppresses secretion of LH and FSH (blood concentrations are lowered) and produces amenorrhea. This treatment in boys suppressed testosterone excretion.[48] Unfortunately, most series fail to show any prevention of advancing bone age or increase in predicted height. Figure 108-21 shows bone age and height age changes in 4 children treated with large doses of medroxyprogesterone. Treatment with medroxyprogesterone also suppresses pituitary-adrenal function and in large doses appears to produce signs of hypercortisolism.[48–50] Aside from pregnancy in very young girls, the major concern for long-term outlook in this disorder is that adult height may be markedly diminished as rapid skeletal maturation occurs with premature epiphyseal closure. Medroxyprogesterone does not appear to benefically affect the ultimate height.

The only advantage in such treatment is that it does suppress or retard the rapid advance in accessory sex development and prevent fertility. As indicated earlier, this therapy is not commonly recommended.

An alternative treatment that requires further study, but looks promising, is that of cyproterone. This substance is an antiandrogen available in Europe that has been used to treat precocious puberty. It is not available in the United States at the present time. Based on preliminary studies, it has few side effects and produces favorable response in retarding bone age advance and inhibiting manifestations of androgen action.

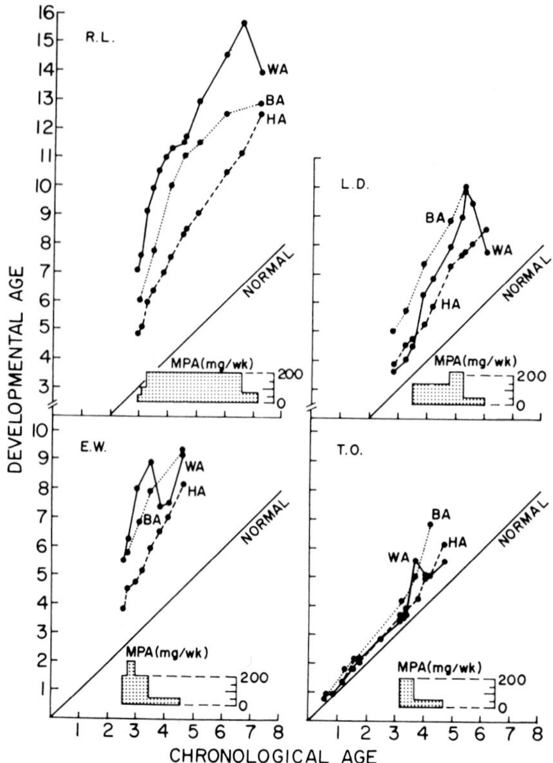

Fig. 108-21. Treatment of idiopathic isosexual precocious puberty in 4 girls with medroxyprogesterone in large doses. Note that no decrease in bone age (BA), height age (HA), or weight age (WA) was evident. (Reproduced from Richman, Robert A., Underwood, Louis E., French, Frank S., and Van Wyk, Judson J.: Adverse effects of large doses of medroxyprogesterone (MPA) in idiopathic isosexual precocity. *J. Pediatr. 79:* 963–971, 1971.

DELAYED SEXUAL MATURATION

It is important to keep in mind that any systemic illness may delay sexual maturation. For example, uremia, often mild and previously unsuspected, may result in both dwarfing and delayed sexual maturation. Other examples include regional enteritis or ulcerative colitis (the author has seen children with previously unknown and mildly symptomatic regional ileitis with delayed sexual maturation), congenital heart disease, cystic fibrosis, diabetes mellitus, and starvation. It is presently uncertain how such conditions cause delay in sexual maturation.

In addition to definable causes, a small number of children fall at extremes of normal sexual maturation. Tables 108-3 to 108-6 give the 95 percent confidence limits or range of the various pubertal stages; it is worth emphasizing that by such a definition 5 percent of children will fall above or below that. That is, about 25 out of each 1000 children will have sexual maturation at later ages. In some of these children there is often a family history of late maturation, and this may raise the parents' anxiety for the child's psychological well-being. These children may have strong psychological problems associated with such a delay. Often, however, with full explanation that the child will mature normally, albeit slightly later in age, both the child and the parents may agree that no treatment is needed. In general, unless psychological problems are severe, it is the author's preference not to treat delayed isosexual puberty. If treatment is desired, it should be given for a few months only so that normal maturation can proceed, and the physician may be quite certain that the initial diagnosis is correct. For boys, depo-testosterone, 200–400 mg every 3 weeks, may be administered for 6 months; for girls, ethinylestradiol, 100 μg daily, or conjugated estrogens, 0.6 mg daily for 25 days with Provera 5–10 mg daily added for the last 5 days and followed by 5 days of no treatment to permit withdrawal bleeding, may be used (for a recent review, see ref. 44).

As was emphasized for precocious puberty, it is extremely important to keep the differential diagnosis of delayed puberty in mind when evaluating a patient. In addition to the systemic illness indicated previously, a variety of hypogonadal states exists. For males, these are discussed in Chapter 124, and for females, these causes are discussed in Chapters 111 and 106. Further discussion here is not warranted.

REFERENCES

1. Odell W. D., Swerdloff, R. S.: Etiologies of sexual maturation: A model system based on the sexually maturing rat. *Rec Prog Horm Res 32:* 245–288, 1976.
2. Wilkins, L., Blizzard, R. M., Migeon, C. T: *The Diagnosis and Treatment of Endocrine Disorders in Childhood and Adolescence (ed 3)* Springfield, Charles C. Thomas, 1966.
3. Kallas, H.: Puberte precoce par parabiose. *CR Soc Biol 100:* 979, 1929.

4. Byrnes, W. W., Meyer, R. K.: The inhibition of gonadotrophic hormone secretion by physiological doses of estrogen. *Endocrinology 48:* 133–136, 1951.
5. Donovan, B. T., Van der Werff ten Bosch, J. J.: The hypothalamus and sexual maturation in the rat. *J Physiol (London) 147:* 78–92, 1959.
6. Ramalay, J. A., Gorsky, R. A.: The effect of hypothalamic differentiation upon puberty in the female rat. *Acta Endocrinol 56:* 661–674, 1967.
7. Fiske, V. M.: Effect of light on sexual maturation estrous cycles, and anterior pituitary of the rat. *Endocrinology 29:* 187–196, 1941.
8. Elwers, M., Critchlow, V.: Precocious ovarian stimulation following hypothalamic and amygdaloid lesions in rats. *Am J Physiol 198:* 381–385, 1960.
9. Elwers, M., Critchlow, V.: Precocious ovarian stimulation following interruption of stria terminalis. *Amer J Physiol 201:* 281–284, 1961.
10. Odell, W. D., Ross, G. T., Rayford, P. L.: Radioimmunoassay for LH in human plasma or serum: Physiological studies. *J Clin Invest 46:* 248–255, 1967.
11. Odell, W. D., Ross, G. T.: Some aspects of the physiology of human luteinizing hormone (HLH) as determined by radioimmunoassay. *J Clin Invest (abstract) 45:* 1052, 1966.
12. Kulin, H. E., Rifkind, A. G., Ross, G. T., et al: Total gonadotropin activity in urine or prepubertal children. *J Clin Endocrinol Metab 27:* 1123–1128, 1967.
13. Guyda H., Johanson, A. J., Light, C., et al: Serum luteinizing hormone by radioimmunoassay in disorders of adolescent sexual development. *Pediatr Res 3:* 533, 1969.
14. Johanson, A. J., Guyda, H. J., Light, C., et al: Serum luteinizing hormone by radioimmunoassay in normal children. *J Pediatr 74:* 416–424, 1969.
15. Roth, J. C., Kelch, R. P., Kaplan, S. L., et al: FSH and LH response to luteinizing hormone-releasing factor in prepubertal and pubertal children, adult males and patients with hypogonadotropic and hypergonadotropic hypogonadism. *J Clin Endocrinol Metab 35:* 926–930, 1972.
16. Raiti, S., Johanson, A., Light, C., et al: Measurement of immunologically reactive follicle stimulating hormone in serum of normal male children and adults. *Metabolism 18:* 234–240, 1969.
17. Yen, S. S. C., Vicic, W. J., Kearchner, D. V.: Gonadotropin levels in puberty: I. Serum Luteinizing hormone. *J Clin Endocrinol Metab 29:* 382–385, 1969.
18. Burr, I. M., Sizonenko, P. C., Kaplan, S. L., et al: Hormonal changes in puberty. I. Correlation of serum luteinizing hormone and follicle stimulating hormone with stages of puberty, testicular size, and bone age in normal boys. *Pediatr Res 4:* 25–35, 1970.
19. Lee, P. A., Midgley, R., Jaffee, R. B.: Regulation of human gonadotropins. VI. Serum follicle stimulating and luteinizing hormone determinations in children. *J Clin Endocrinol Metab 31:* 248–253, 1970.
20. Root, A. W., Moshang, T., Bongiovanni, A. M., et al: Concentrations of plasma luteinizing hormone in infants, children, and adolescents with normal and abnormal gonadal function. *Pediatr Res 4:* 175–186, 1970.
21. Faiman, C., Winter, J. S. D.: Gonadotropins and sex hormone patterns in puberty, clinical data, in Grumbach, M. M., Grave, G. D., Mayer, F. E. (eds.): *The Control of the Onset of Puberty,* Chapter 2. New York, John Wiley & Sons, 1974, pp. 32–61.
22. Grumbach, M. M., Roth, J. C., Kaplan, S. L., et al: Hypothalamic-pituitary regulation of puberty in man: Evidence and concepts derived from clinical research, in Grumbach, M. M., Grave, G. D., Mayer, F. E. (eds.): *The Control of the Onset of Puberty,* Chapter 6. New York, John Wiley & Sons, 1974, pp. 115–166.
23. McCann, S. M., Ojeda, S., Negro-Vilar, A.: Sex steroid, pituitary and hypothalamic hormones during puberty in experimental animals, in Grumbach, M. M., Grave, G. D., Mayer, F. E. (eds.): *The Control of the Onset of Puberty,* Chapter 1. New York, John Wiley & Sons, 1974, pp. 1–31.
24. Swerdloff, R. S., Jacobs, H. S., Odell, W. D.: Hypothalamic-pituitary-gonadal interrelationships in the rat during sexual maturation, in Saxena, B. J., Beling, C. B., Gandy, H. M. (eds.): *Gonadotropins.* New York, Geron-X, Wiley and Sons, 1971, pp. 546–561.
25. Odell, W. D., Swerdloff, R. S.: The role of the gonads in sexual maturation, in Grumbach, M. M., Grave, G. D., Mayer, F. E. (eds.): *The Control of the Onset of Puberty,* Chapter 11. New York, John Wiley & Sons, 1974, pp. 313–332.
26. Elsaesser, F., Pomerantz, K., Ellendorff, F., et al: Plasma LH, testosterone and DHT in the pig from birth to sexual maturity. *Acta Endocrinol (Kbh), (suppl):* 148, 1973.
27. Odell, W. D., Hescox, M. A., Kiddy, C. A.: Studies of hypothalamic-pituitary-gonadal interrelations in prepubertal cattle, in Butt, W. R., Crooke, A. C., Ryle, M. (eds.): *Gonadotrophins and Ovarian Development.* Edinburgh, E & S Livingstone, 1970, pp. 371–385.
28. Karg, H., Giménez, T., Hartl, M., et al: Testosterone, luteinizing hormone and follicle stimulating hormone in peripheral plasma of bulls; levels from birth through puberty and short-term variations. *Zentralblatt Vet. Med. A, 23:* 793–803, 1976.
29. Odell, W. D., Swerdloff, R. S., Jacobs, H. S.: FSH induction of sensitivity to LH: The cause of sexual maturation in the male rat. *Endocrinology 92:* 160–165, 1973.
30. Odell, W. D., Swerdloff, R. S., Bain, J.: The effect of sexual maturation of testicular sensitivity to LH stimulation of testosterone secretion in the intact rat. *Endocrinology 95:* 1380–1384, 1974.
31. Odell, W. D. Swerdloff, R. S.: The role of testicular sensitivity to gonadotropins in sexual maturation of the male rat. *J Steroid Biochem 6:* 853–857, 1975.
32. Sizonenko, P. C., Cuendet, A., Paunier, L.: FSH. I. Evidence for its mediating role on testosterone secretion in cryptorchidism. *J Clin Endocrinol Metab 37:* 68–73, 1973.
33. Winter, J. S. D., Faiman, C.: Serum gonadotropin concentrations in agonadal children and adults. *J Clin Endocrinol Metab 35:* 561–564, 1972.
34. Boyar, R. M., Finkelstein, J. W., David, R., et al: Twenty-four hour patterns of plasma luteinizing hormone and follicle stimulating hormone in sexual precocity. *N Engl J Med 289:* 282–286, 1973.
35. Boyar, R. M., Rosenfeld, R. S., Kapen, S., et al: Simultaneous augmented secretion of luteinizing hormone and testosterone during sleep. *J Clin Invest 54:* 609–618, 1974.
36. Frisch, R. E., Revelle, R.: Height and weight at menarche and a hypothesis of critical body weights and adolescent events. *Science 169:* 397–399, 1970.
37. Frisch, R. E.: The critical weight at menarche, the initiation of the adolescent growth spurt and the control of puberty, in Grumbach, M. M., Grave, G. D., Mayer, F. E. (eds.): *Control of the Onset of Puberty,* Chapter 15. New York, John Wiley & Sons, 1974, pp. 403–423.
38. Kennedy, G. C., Mitra, J: Hypothalamic control of energy balance and the reproductive cycle in the rat. *J Physiol 166:* 395–407, 1963.
39. Schindler, A. E., Ebert, A., Friedrich, E.: Conversion of androstenedione to estrone by human fat tissue. *J Clin Endocrinol Metab 35:* 627–630, 1972.
40. Talbot, N. B., et al: Excretion of 17-ketosteroids by normal and abnormal children. *Am J Dis Child 65:* 364–375, 1943.
41. Parker, L., Sachs, J., Fisher, D. A., and Odell, W. D.: The adrenarche: Prolactin, gonadotropins, adrenal androgens and cortisol. *J Clin Endocrinol Metab 46:* 396–401, 1978.
42. Marshall, W. A., Tanner, J. M.: Variations in pattern of pubertal changes in girls. *Arch Dis Child 44:* 291–303, 1969.
43. Marshall, W. A., Tanner, J. M.: Variations in the pattern of pubertal changes in boys. *Arch Dis Child 45:* 13–23, 1970.
44. Root, A. W., Reiter, E. O.: Evaluation and management of the child with delayed pubertal development. *Fertil Steril 27:* 745–755, 1976.
45. Kaplan, S. A., Ling, S. M., Irani, N. G.: Idiopathic isosexual precocity. Therapy with medroxyprogesterone. *Am J Dis Child 116:* 591–598, 1968.
46. Hahn, H. B., Hayles, A. B., Albert, A.: Treatment of idiopathic precocious puberty in boys. *Mayo Clin Proc 39:* 182–190, 1964.
47. Richman, R. A., Underwood, L. E., French, F. S., VanWyk, J. J.: Adverse effects of large doses of medroxyprogesterone (MPA) in idiopathic isosexual precocity. *J Pediatr 79:* 963–971, 1971.
48. Schoen, E. J.: Treatment of idiopathic precocious puberty in boys. *J Clin Endocrinol Metab 26:* 363–370, 1966.
49. Mathews, J. H., Abrams, C. A. C., Morishima, A.: Pituitary-adrenal function in ten patients receiving medroxyprogesterone acetate for true precocious puberty. *J Clin Endocrinol Metab 30:* 653, 1970.
50. Sadeghi-Nejad, A., Kaplan, S., Grumbach, M. M.: The effect of medroxyprogesterone acetate on adrenocorticol function in children with precocious puberty. *J Pediatr 78:* 616, 1971.
51. Kauli, R., Pertzelan, A., Prager-Lewin, R., et al.: Cyrpoterone acetate in treatment of precocious puberty. *Arch Dis Child 51:* 202–208, 1976.
52. Root, A. W., Reiter, E. O.: Evaluation and management of the child with delayed pubertal development. *Fertil Steril 27:* 745–755, 1976.

Reproductive Function in the Female

109

The Reproductive System in Women

William D. Odell

The endocrine physiology of the reproductive process in women is most easily understood by referring to a simple schematogram (Fig. 109-1). Each major component of the system is enclosed within a rectangle, and all components interrelate by neuronal or hormonal signals. It is possible to further subdivide most of these major components, and indeed, the sophisticated research reproduction physiologist does that. For discussion purposes, the menstrual cycle is divided into two phases: (1) the follicular phase, or approximately the first half of the cycle, during which time follicle growth is initiated and proceeds to maturity; and (2) the luteal phase, or approximately the second half of the cycle, during which time the corpus luteum is functionally active. Day 1 of a cycle is defined as the first day of menstrual flow; the last day of the cycle is that day just preceding the onset of the next menstrual flow. Referring to Figure 109-1, we may begin analysis of the system at any point; arbitrarily, let us begin with the pituitary secretion of the gonadotropins.

GONADOTROPIN SECRETION

Two gonadotropic hormones control ovarian function in women: (1) luteinizing hormone (LH), and (2) follicle-stimulating hormone (FSH). Prolactin is also a gonadotropin in rodents, acting as either a luteolytic or luteotrophic* hormone, depending on the conditions of study. However, in the human female, this effect does not appear to be physiologically significant. In the human, prolactin may have other effects in modifying adrenal and gonadal functions, which are discussed in separate chapters. LH and FSH are glycopeptide hormones, composed of two peptide chains that are designated alpha and beta. The metabolic clearance rate* (MCR) of LH is greater than that of FSH,[1,2] so that LH disappears from the circulation much more rapidly than FSH. The MCR for LH and FSH, along with estimates of production rates, is given in Table 109-1. In addition, LH and possibly FSH are secreted in a pulsatile fashion.[3] Thus, blood concentrations are not constant but irregular; the ovary presumably responds to the average concentrations in blood. Figure 109-2 depicts blood LH and FSH measured at frequent time intervals at three phases of the menstrual cycle.

If one measures LH and FSH once *daily* in a group of women throughout the menstrual cycle and plots graphically average concentrations, it is observed that FSH is high just as menstrual flow first occurs (i.e., during the first portions of the follicular phase) and that concentrations fall progressively until midcycle. As an average, LH concentrations are relatively low and unchanging during the first half of the cycle. At midcycle, marked increases in both LH and FSH secretion occur, which last for 15 to 20 hours. This is the so-called ovulatory LH-FSH surge. During this surge, and in contrast to the early follicular phase, LH/FSH (ratio) is much greater than 1.† During the luteal phase, LH and FSH concentrations are suppressed to lower values than during the follicular phase. These concentrations are indistinguishable from those found in prepubertal children. During the luteal phase, the ratio of LH to FSH is approxmately 1.[4,5]

Figure 109-3 depicts the average LH and FSH concentrations measured daily throughout the menstrual cycle in normal women.[6]

THE OVARY

EMBRYOGENESIS

During early embryogenesis, the primordial germ cells migrate from the yolk sac to a specific portion of peritoneum;[7,8] by the fifth week of gestation in the human, it is estimated that 1000 germ cells have accumulated. These cells rapidly divide by mitosis. Mesenchymal cells adjacent to these germ cells form the prominent *genital ridge,* and the medial slope of this ridge develops into the primitive gonads that are identical in both sexes. This primitive gonad subdivides into cortical and medullary portions which are

*Promoting lysis of the corpus luteum or supporting corpus luteum function, respectively.

*Volume of blood or plasma irreversibly cleared of the hormone per unit time.

†When stated in terms of the International Reference Preparation of human menopausal gonadotropin—IRP-HMG No. 2.

Table 109-1. Effects of Gonadotropins, DES, and CI on Uterine Weight, Follicular Development, and Atresia

Treatment*	Uterine Weight (mg)**	Mean Number of Follicles** 125–300 μm	300–350 μm	350 μm	New Antrum Formation	Follicles 125–300 μm % Atretic**
Saline	16 ± 1.0	662 ± 59.1	10 ± 6.3	0	no	39 ± 1.8
FSH	32 ± 1.7	407 ± 18.1	27 ± 9.5	4 ± 2.9	yes	34 ± 1.6
CI	39 ± 3.6	371 ± 39.3	12 ± 7.5	0	no	32 ± 2.5
FSH + HCG	71 ± 5.2	857 ± 26.4	117 ± 13.6	62 ± 7.8	yes	18 ± 3.6
DES	123 ± 6.1	938 ± 23.7	78 ± 8.5	39 ± 7.9	no	7 ± 1.2

*Five rats per treatment group, except for CI, which contains 4.
**Mean ± SEM.

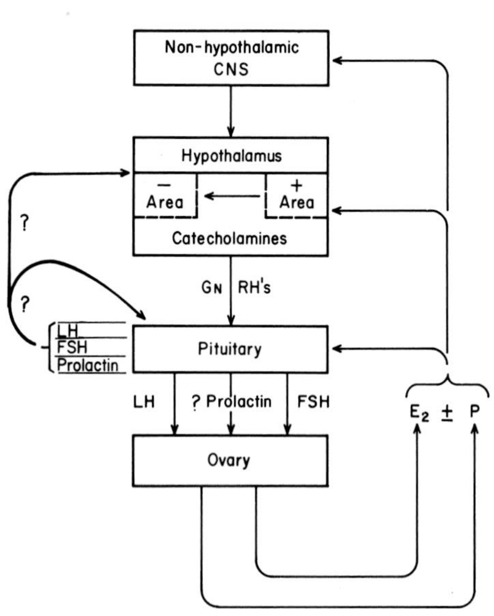

Fig. 109-1. Schematic presentation of the central nervous system-pituitary-ovarian interrelationships. (Modified from Odell and Moyer.[7])

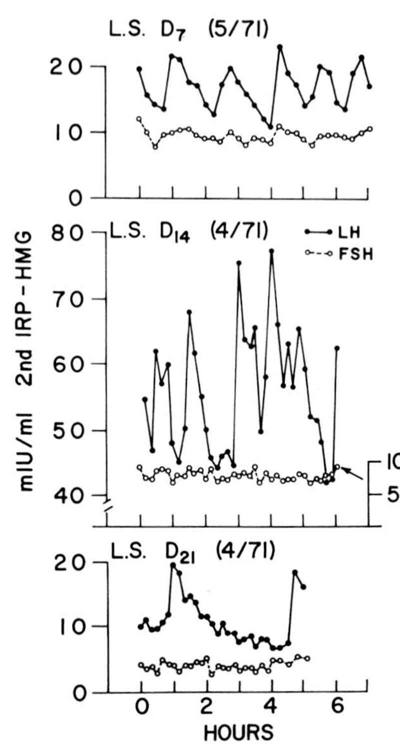

Fig. 109-2. Serum LH and FSH concentrations in samples obtained at 10- to 15-minute intervals during the follicular and luteal phases and during midcycle surge of two ovulatory cycles. (Serum progesterone concentrations in nanograms per milliliter during the cycle were day 7 (D7) 0.2; day 14 (D14) 1.3; day 21 (D21) 14.0.) (Reproduced from Yen et al.[3])

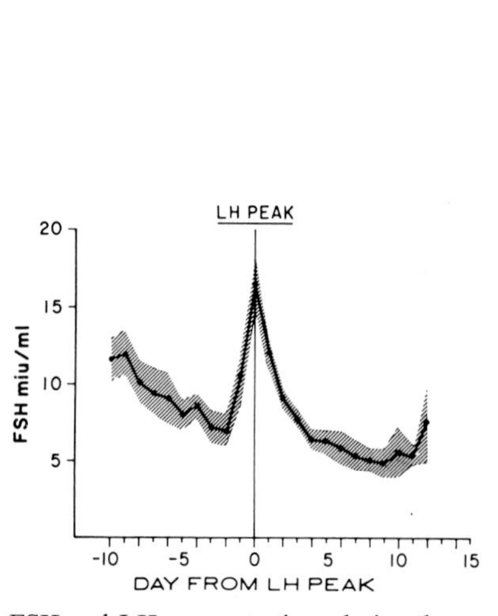

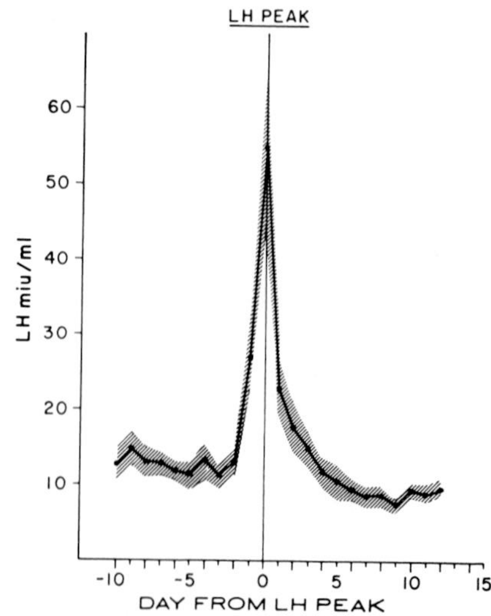

Fig. 109-3. Average serum FSH and LH concentrations during the menstrual cycle in normal women. The dark line is the average; the shaded area encompasses one SEM. All cycles were centered on the LH peak to permit cycles at varying length to be shown. (Reproduced from Abraham et al.[6])

destined to become the ovary or the testis, respectively. As determined by genetic sex (46XX = female), the cortical zone develops further in females, while the medullary portion undergoes atresia. By the third month of gestation, the developing ovary consists of the cortex containing many germ cells. The germ cells continue to divide, ultimately reaching a peak population of approximately 7 million in midgestation. Subsequently, many of these cells become atretic. Others cease mitotic division to form oogonia and proceed by meiotic division to the leptotene stage. Spindle-shaped mesenchymal cells (now called granulosa cells) surround each meiotic germ cell (now called an oogonia) to form so-called primary follicles. By the time of birth, the total number of remaining germ cells or oogonia has decreased by atresia to approximately 2 million, and many of these are also already partially atretic. Figure 109-4 depicts the changing populations of germ cells during this period.

THE OVARY AFTER BIRTH

Prepubertal Years

During the prepubertal years, the ovary is filled with primary follicles that contain an oogonia in arrested prophase (leptotene stage). *This arrested state exists for about 13 to 50 years* (puberty to menopause); cell meiosis only continues if that particular oogonia undergoes the additional maturation that occurs during each menstrual cycle in sexually mature women. Ovulation of a single ovum each month for the entire reproductive period requires only about 400 oogonia. All the remaining oogonia or ova undergo death by the process of atresia, either directly from the primary follicle stage or, as we shall discuss later, as part of a group of follicles developing each month at the beginning of a menstrual cycle. As may be seen in Figure 109-4, by the age of puberty, the number of germ cells is reduced to approximately 100,000. The factors that control the atretic demise of over 99.9 percent of the germ cells and primary follicles are poorly understood, but it is worth noting that the ovum that is eventually fertilized is the product of an intense selection process with a rato of atresia to selection of about 20,000:1. Figure 109-5 illustrates the meiotic process in ova during the different stages discussed.

Reproductive Years

The granulosal cells of the primary follicle in mature women are more cuboidal in shape than they were during embryogenesis. During the last day or so of the luteal phase of one cycle and the earliest portions of follicular phase of the next cycle, under the influence of the early rise in FSH (Fig. 109-3) and locally secreted estrogen, a group of approximately 6 to 12 primary follicles develop into secondary follicles with several layers of granulosa cells and an increase in size of the oocyte. During this process of follicle growth, the granulosa cells secrete a mucoid material around the oocyte, the zona pellucida. Protoplasmic processes from the granulosa cells penetrate the zona pellucida and contact the cell membrane of the oocyte (Fig. 109-6), probably to permit continued exchange of nutrients and wastes. As these 6 to 12 secondary follicles develop, one is "selected" to develop into the mature follicle; the others undergo atresia.

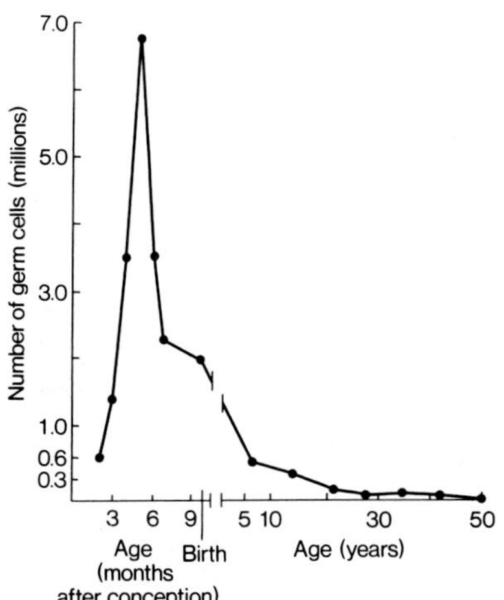

Fig. 109-4. Changes in total population of germ cells in the human ovary with age. (Reproduced from Baker, 1972.[8])

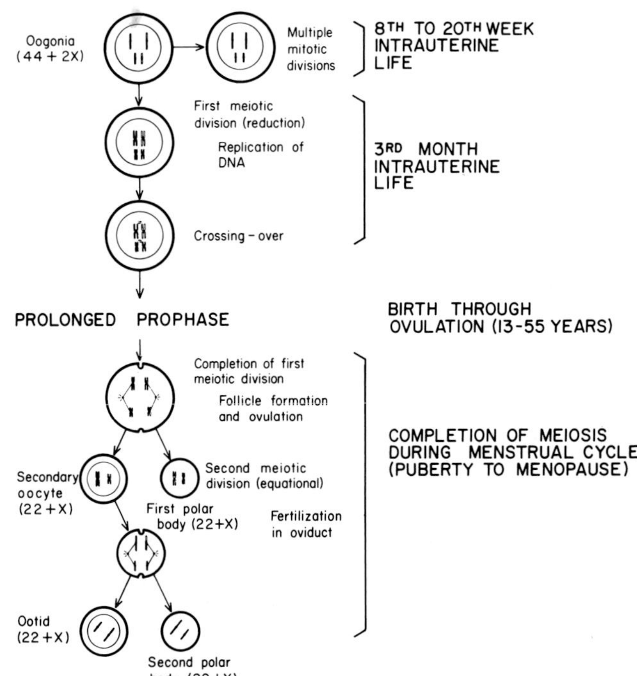

Fig. 109-5. Schematic presentation of the meiotic process in germ cells in women as relates to age and sexual development. (Modified from Odell and Moyer.[7])

The mechanisms that control the initiation of follicle growth in a group of follicles, followed by the maturation of one (usually) of these and atresia of the remainder, are poorly understood. The amount of FSH or the FSH/LH ratio appear to be important factors. During the normal cycle, usually only one follicle matures; however, when ovulation is induced in infertile women by treatment with exogenous LH and FSH, maturation of several follicles and polyovulation are common. Similarly in animals, multiple follicles can be made to mature by administration of large doses of FSH. However, other factors are also involved. Thus, Harmon and Ross[9] have studied the influence of FSH, HCG, and estrogens on follicle development in adult hypophysectomized female rats. Table 109-2 and Figure 109-7 illustrate their data. FSH given alone results in almost a 300 percent increase in large follicles (300–350 μm). Treatment with an *antiestrogen* prevented this FSH-induced follicle maturation. Treatment with an estrogen (diethylstilbestrol) increased the number developing, and the number of small follicles developing was greater than with FSH treatment. Gonadotropins appear to increase atresia of smaller follicles and increase the number of large antral follicles in the rat. Estrogens decrease atresia, and the stimulatory action of gonadotropins is, at least in

Table 109-2. Secretory and Excretory Rates for FSH and LH in Women*

Gonadal Status	Hormone	Plasma LH (mIU/ml)	Metabolic Clearance Rate (ml/min)	Pituitary Secretion Rate (IU/day)	Urinary Excretion Rate (IU/day)	Approximate Percent Excreted (%)
Premenopausal	LH	32.0 ± 9.6**	24.4 ± 1.8	1056 ± 244	13–25	2
	FSH	10.0 ± 1.8	14.3 ± 1.1	210 ± 39	4.5–9	3
Postmenopausal	LH	99.2 ± 23.2	25.6 ± 4.1	3459 ± 587	131	4
	FSH	172 ± 24.0	12.6 ± 1.1	3083 ± 379	92.5	3

Based on data from Kohler, Ross, and Odell,[1] and Coble, Kohler, Cargille, and Ross.[2]
*The fraction of both hormones that is excreted in the urine is less than 4%.
**The LH values are high. These LH studies were performed in 4 women, and 1 had ovulatory LH peak at the time of study.

part, mediated via estrogen secretion.* These observations probably also apply to the human.

Whatever the control mechanisms are, the "selected" follicle develops a progressively larger oocyte, and the surrounding granulosa cells proliferate further (see Figs. 109-8 and 109-9). As this follicle is further maturing, changes are also occurring in the adjacent ovarian stroma. Stromal cells adjacent to the follicle become arranged in concentric layers surrounding the follicle. This layer of differentiated and oriented stromal cells is termed the *theca;* the *theca interna* is that portion adjacent to the follicle, and the *theca externa* is that portion which merges with general ovarian stroma. As these changes in stromal cells occur, fluid (plasma transudate) begins to accumulate in a space or cleft within the mass of granulosa cells; this space further enlarges to form the antrum of the follicle. At this stage of development, the follicle is termed a *graafian follicle,* or preovulatory follicle. Antral fluid also contains secreted mucoid materials and steroid hormones (the latter in amounts much larger than in peripheral blood) and exists with greater oncotic pressure than peripheral plasma. During this developmental process to the graafian follicle, the primary follicle has increased from about 50 μ in size to approximately 20,000 μ (400 times), while the oogonium has increased from about 15 μ to about 150 μ (10 times).

*This is deduced from observations made by Harmon et al.[9] that in women with enzymatic defects preventing estrogen biosynthesis (e.g., 17-hydroxylase deficiency), gonadotropin concentrations are elevated, but in the absence of estrogens, no follicle maturation occurs.

Although the early follicular phase development of the primary follicles occurs in response to the FSH rise (and stimulation of estrogen secretion) previously described, there is some uncertainty as to the necessity for *continued* FSH stimulation for the remaining follicle development. Crook et al.[10] have shown that for some infertile women, only a short period of exogenous FSH treatment is needed to initiate follicle growth; without additional treatment, one (or more) follicle continues to develop to the preovulatory surge. Urinary *excretion* of FSH returned to baseline and remained there in such women, while continued follicle growth occurred. In normal women, we recall, FSH is falling while follicle growth is occurring. Of course, in both normal and the infertile women studied, FSH is not totally absent; thus the necessity for

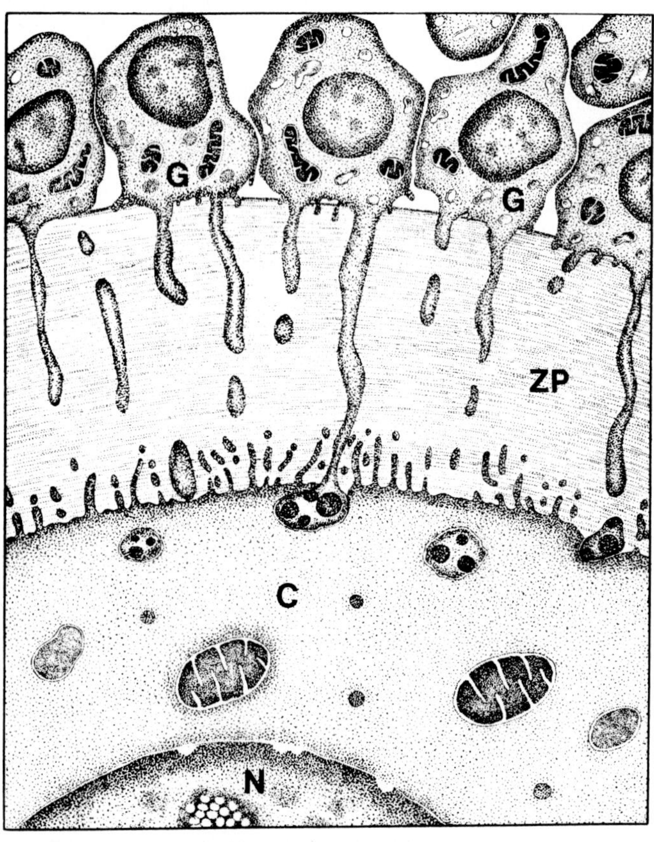

Fig. 109-6. Fig. Y: Structure of fully formed zona pellucida (ZP) around an oocyte in a graafian follicle. Microvilli arising from oocyte interdigitate with processes from the granulosa cells (G). These processes penetrate into the cytoplasm (C) of the oocyte and may provide nutrients and maternal protein. (Reproduced from Baker, 1972.[8])

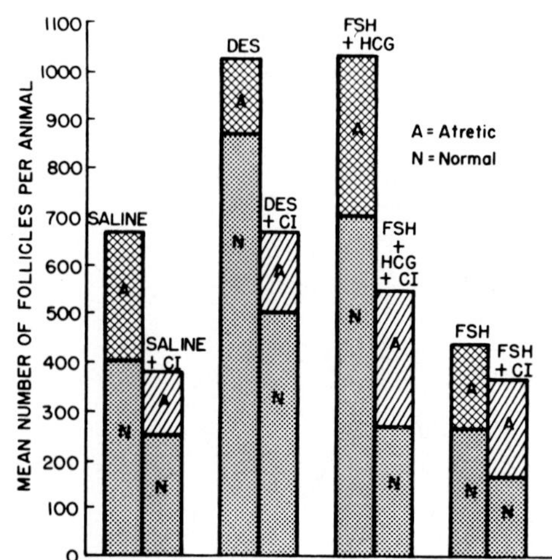

Fig. 109-7. Effect of diethylstilbestrol (DES) treatment of hypophysectomized female rats with and without CI (an antiestrogen) treatment on mean number of follicles. N = normal, A = atretic, follicles greater than 125 m in diameter. These data indicate estrogen per se may stimulate follicle development and that FSH stimulates follicle growth via estrogen production. (Reproduced from Harman et al.[9])

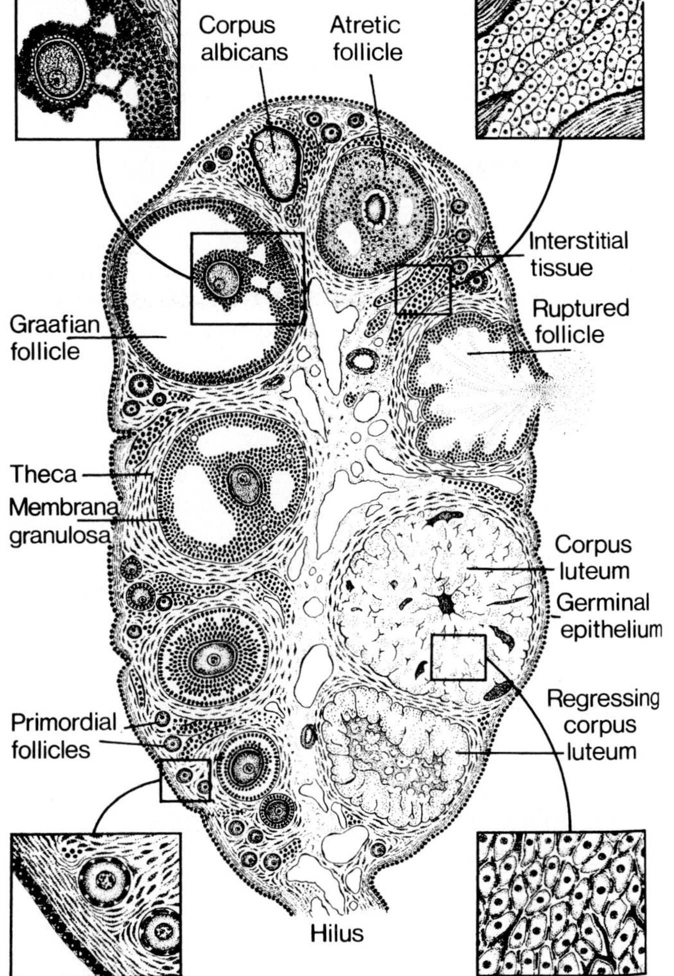

Fig. 109-8. Pictorial and schematic presentation of follicle and corpus luteum development within the ovary. (Reproduced from Turner, 1971).

small amounts of secreted FSH may exist. Studies have not been performed in women totally devoid of FSH.

As the follicle develops, the granulosa cells secrete progressively larger amounts of estradiol, a potent estrogenic hormone. Local estrogens (intraovarian) are important in effecting adjacent follicle development; blood estrogens affect the feedback control system of LH and FSH. Blood concentrations of estradiol increase slowly at first, the more rapidly to reach an apex prior to the LH-FSH ovulatory surge.[6]

Changes in blood progesterone and 17-hydroxyprogesterone also are occurring during this period; their possible physiological significances are discussed later. Progesterone levels decrease during the first days of the menstrual cycle (during menstrual flow), remain low during the midportion of the follicular phase and then increase in parallel with the rise in LH during the ovulatory surge. Along with the LH surge, 17-hydroxyprogesterone also rises to a peak. The concentrations of estradiol and progesterone during the normal menstrual cycle are shown in Figure 109-9.

Once the fully mature preovulatory follicle has developed, the ovulatory LH-FSH surge occurs (Fig. 109-3), which results in ovulation 16 to 24 hours later and transformation of the follicle into a new organ, the corpus luteum. The process of ovulation is not an explosive event but an orderly slow extrusion of the ova in response to the LH surge and local cellular changes. The stigma, or point of follicle rupture, is sealed by a coagulum derived from blood and fibrin from the cavity of the follicle.

After ovulation, both granulosa and theca interna cells undergo mitosis and rapidly increase in number. Capillaries sprout from the theca and invade the granulosa cells, which in turn undergo hypertrophy and hyperplasia. The theca cells and, to a lesser extent, the granulosa cells show intense metabolic activity and increased fat storage. By these means the follicle is transformed into a new organ, the *corpus luteum,* which in turn increases progressively in size, reaching maximal size 2 to 8 days following ovulation. If fertilization and implantation do not occur by about 8 to 9 days after ovulation, the corpus luteum decreases in size; the granulosa cells lose their orderly arrangement and become vacuolated and granular. Connective tissue invades the corpus luteum, and within about 3 months the corpus luteum is transformed by hyalin degeneration into a corpus albicans. During its active phase, usually 10 to 16 days following ovulation, the corpus luteum actively secretes steroids. As shown in Figure 109-9, estradiol, progesterone, and 17-hydroxyprogesterone concentrations rise again after ovulation, reach a nadir of midluteal phase, and then fall at the end of the luteal phase.

The function and life span of the corpus luteum are determined by hormonal factors. As was indicated earlier in rodents, prolactin appears to act as a luteotrophic or luteolytic agent, depending on the condition of study. In some animals, a uterine

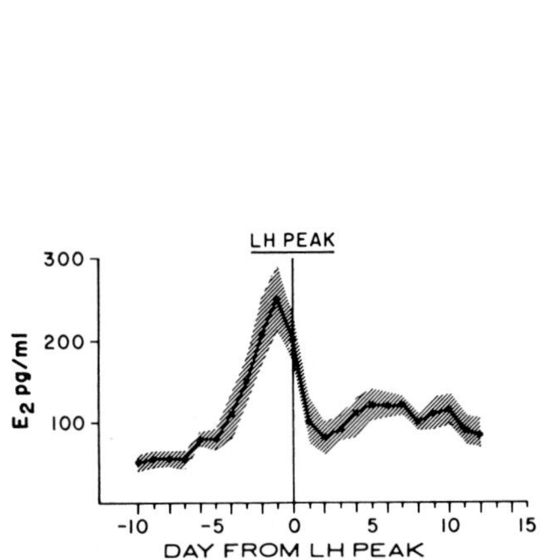

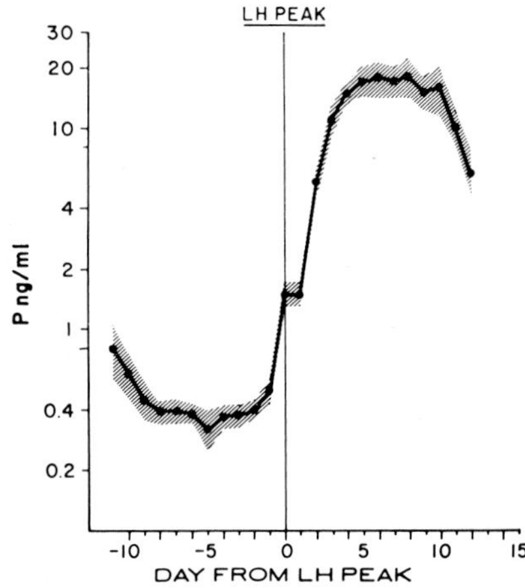

Fig. 109-9. Average serum estradiol and progesterone concentrations during the menstrual cycle in normal women. The dark line is the average, the shaded area encompasses one SEM. All cycles were centered on the LH peak to permit cycles of varying length to be shown. In order to show follicular phase progesterone concentrations, these are shown on a log scale. (Reproduced from Abraham et al.[6])

luteolytic factor is secreted by the endometrium. For example, in the guinea pig, bilateral hysterectomy results in marked prolongation in the life of the corpus luteum. Neither prolactin nor uterine factors appear important in women. It has been shown that in the absence of a uterus, women continue to have cyclic ovarian function indistinguishable by blood LH, FSH, and estradiol measurement on a daily basis from normal.[11] On the other hand, the placental production of human chorionic gonadotropin (HCG) results in prolongation of corpus luteum function, indicating that HCG is a luteotrophic agent in women.

For a number of years, it was considered that in women the corpus luteum functioned and became atretic on a time basis determined as an essential portion of the corpus luteum itself; that is, once formed, the corpus luteum lived and died independent of hormonal control. Evidence for that belief was derived from the fact that if infertile women were made to ovulate with a single injection of HCG, the corpus luteum functioned and died after its usual 12 to 16 days of life; no further HCG was required. When Vande Wiele et al. performed identical ovulation studies, using human LH rather than HCG to produce ovulation, the corpus luteum functioned for only a few days (2 to 5 days).[12] However, if low doses of LH were given daily after ovulation, the corpus luteum could be made to secrete and survive for normal periods or longer. The seeming conflict in the HCG and LH studies lies in the fact that HCG has a long survival in the circulation; after a single large injection, blood concentrations are elevated for several days. LH has a short survival with a half-time of disappearance of about 1 hour, and after ovulation is induced with LH, blood concentrations fall rapidly. Thus, it appears the low concentrations of LH present during the luteal phase of the cycle are required for normal corpus luteum function in women. However, even in the presence of these low blood LH concentrations, the corpus luteum does not function indefinitely. The life span of the corpus luteum does appear to be, at least in part, an intrinsic property of the corpus luteum. These studies are illustrated in Figure 109-10.

FEEDBACK CONTROL OF FSH AND LH SECRETION

STUDIES IN RATS

In 1936, Pfeiffer[13] published key studies in the rat which indicated that the central nervous system-pituitary axis in both male and female rats was capable of cyclic discharge of gonadotropins. Pfeiffer castrated male rats at birth, permitted them to grow to the usual age of sexual maturity, and then transplanted ovaries into the anterior chamber of the eye. Such transplanted ovaries functioned cyclicly. In contrast, if male rats were castrated as adults, transplanted ovaries failed to show cyclic activity. Furthermore, if an immature testis was transplanted into neonatal female rats and then removed later during development, cyclic activity was not observed after the usual age of sexual maturation.

Subsequently, in the 1960s, Barraclough and co-workers (see ref. 14) further studied this phenomenon. They gave single injections of testosterone to neonatal female rats, permitted the animals to mature, and observed that normal cyclic function was abolished. The ovaries from such "androgen-sterilized rats" contained numerous follicles in the preovulatory stage but few or no corpora lutea. This indicated that the ovulatory surge had not occurred. Greer had previously shown that the same ovarian changes were produced in rats by placing bilateral electrical lesions in the preoptic-suprachiasmatic area of the hypothalamus. Electrical stimula-

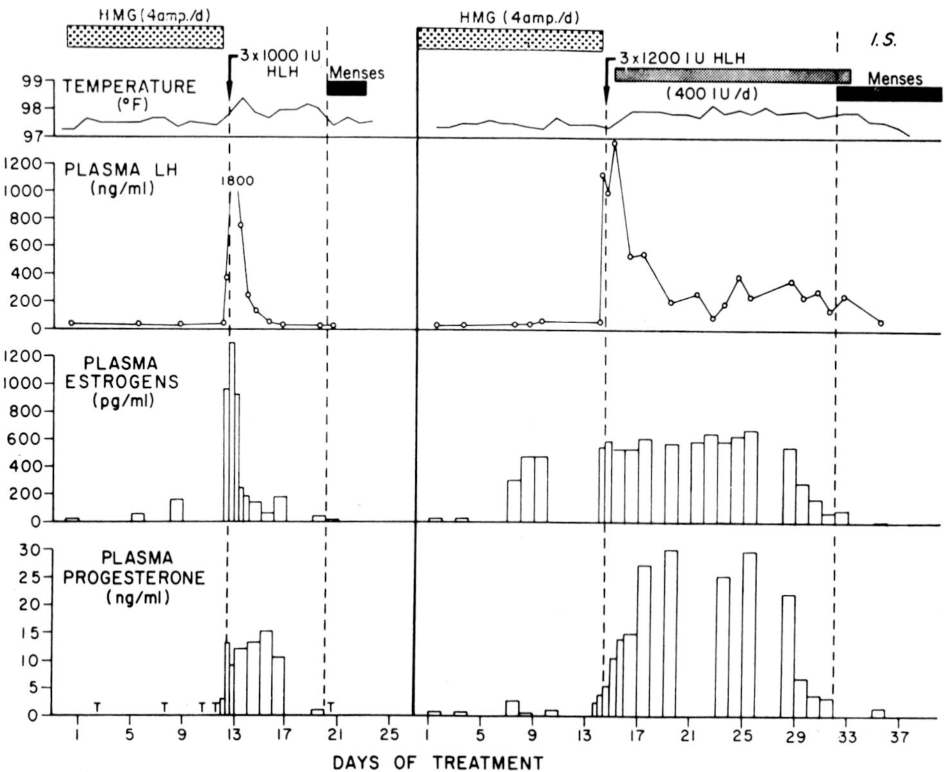

Fig. 109-10. Treatment of an infertile woman with FSH (HMG is an impure human FSH preparation) and purified human LH (HLH) to induce follicle growth and ovulation, respectively. In the first treatment period, after follicle growth had been induced with 12 days of FSH, a single injection of 3000 IU of HLH was given to induce ovulation. After ovulation, corpus luteum function persisted for only 4 days. In the second treatment cycle, 3600 IU of HLH were given to induce ovulation, and this was followed by 400 IU of HLH given daily. Corpus luteum function continued for about 15 days. (Reproduced from Vande Wiele et al.[12])

tion of this area resulted in ovulation in normal adult female rats but failed to do so in the adrogen-sterilized rat. Thus, Barraclough suggested that the area responsible for the cyclic ovulatory gonadotropin surges was located in the preoptic area and termed this the "cyclic area."

It was also known that stimulation in the arcuate-ventromedial area of the hypothalamus caused ovulation in normal rats. When the androgen-sterilized rat was pretreated with progesterone, stimulation of this area also caused ovulation. Barraclough further suggested that a second area modulating gonadotropin secretion existed in the arcuate-ventromedial area and that this was probably responsible for the usual negative feedback control of gonadotropins. This area was termed the "tonic area."

It has subsequently been shown that testosterone per se may not be the active ingredient producing "androgen" sterilization in rats. Brown Grant et al.[15] have shown that similar sterilization may be produced by estrogen injections into the neonatal rat. Naftolin et al. have shown that the hypothalamus is capable of aromatizing testosterone to produce estradiol and have postulated that testosterone acts by means of conversion to estradiol (for review, see ref. 16). In support of that, dihydrotestosterone, a potent androgen not converted to an estrogen, does not produce androgen sterilization when administered to neonatal rats. The phenomenon of "androgen sterilization" is more appropriately termed steroid imprinting.

In 1968, Odell and Swerdloff,[17] from studies they performed in the human, suggested that, rather than an intrinsic hypothalamic rhythmic discharge of gonadotropin, an ovarian signal system resulted in hypothalamic-pituitary discharge of the ovulatory surge. They showed that sequential estrogen plus progestogen administered to castrate or postmenopausal women produced a typical LH-FSH ovulatory surge. This LH-FSH surge was produced 12 to 24 hours following the onset of progestogen treatment (Fig. 109-11).

The cyclic center may be the area responding to this ovarian signal system. Swerdloff et al.[18] subsequently extended their studies in a rat model and showed that large doses of estrogen administered daily to an adult castrate female rat at first suppressed blood LH for 3 days and then, on day 4, produced a sharp ovulatory-type LH surge. FSH was suppressed along with LH for the first 3 days but, in contrast to LH, was not stimulated on day 4 (Fig. 109-12). Lower doses of estrogen produced only suppression of LH and FSH (Fig. 109-13). If progesterone treatment was given on days 3 to 4 to the low-dose estrogen-treated animals, a typical LH-FSH ovulatory surge was produced (Fig. 109-14). These workers concluded that progesterone lowers the threshold for estrogen induction of the LH component of the ovulatory surge and is required for the FSH component.

In the intact adult female rat, the normal LH-FSH surge occurs at 4:00 to 5:00 P.M. Barraclough et al.[19] have recently studied the adrenalectomized-castrated female rat and showed that estrogens are *incapable* of producing an ovulatory surge in the absence of the adrenal. However, addition of progesterone to the estrogen treatment resulted in the ovulatory LH surge. Barraclough has therefore suggested that it is adrenal *progesterone*, secreted diurnally, that permits the estrogen stimulated LH ovulatory surge in the rat. These data are shown in Figure 109-15a, b, and b. This is partially supported by the studies of Legan and Karsch,[20] who implanted sialastic capsules containing estradiol into castrated female rats. In this manner, estradiol concentrations were maintained constant at high levels. In such animals, an LH surge occurred each evening for approximately 10 consecutive days. These data are illustrated in Figure 109-16.

Since the concepts of "androgen" (steroid imprinting) sterilization and the cyclic center and tonic center have been built upon data predominantly from the rat studies, Short[21] has recently attempted to produce androgen sterilization in another species, the sheep. Testosterone treatment of neonatal female sheep failed to

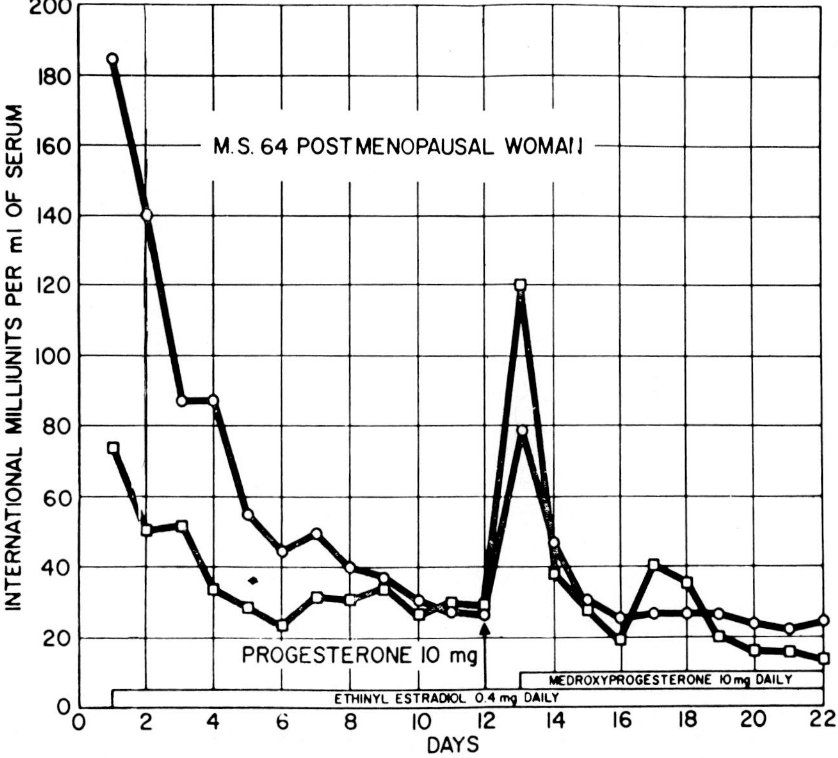

Fig. 109-11. Production of a simulated LH (□——□) and FSH (○——○) ovulatory surge in a postmenopausal woman by sequential estrogen plus estrogen and progestogen treatment. (Reproduced from Odell and Swerdloff.[17])

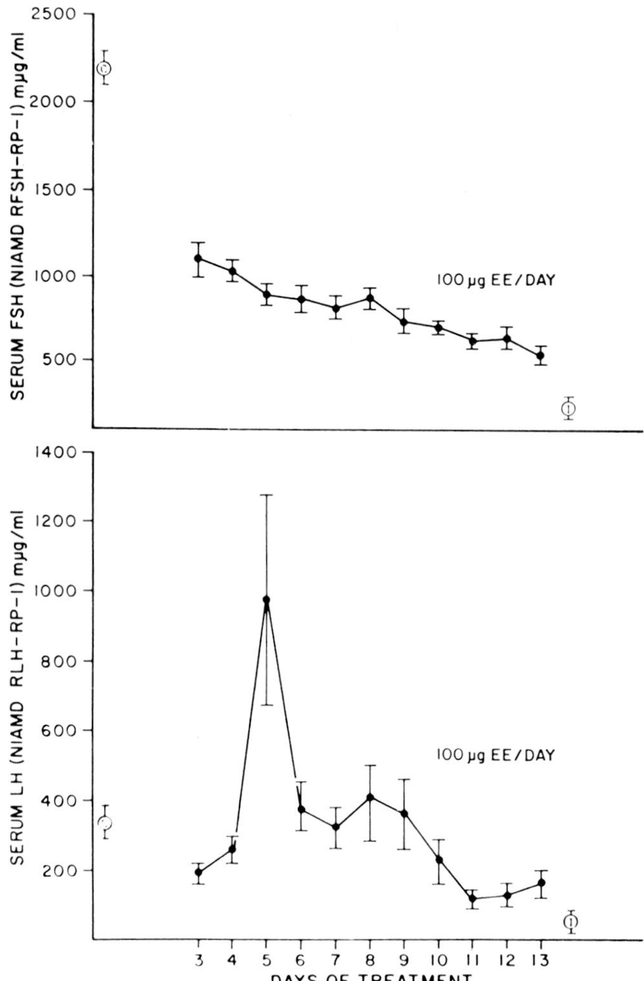

Fig. 109-12. Biphasic action of estrogen on serum LH in castrate adult female rats. Adult rats were castrated and treatment was initiated 5 days later. The elevated LH and FSH concentrations were suppressed. On day 4, LH, but not FSH, was stimulated and an ovulatory surge produced. (Reproduced from Swerdloff et al.[18])

prevent cycle function after sexual maturation. The presence or absence of the cyclic activity was assessed by administering estrogen in large doses. (This normally produces an LH-type surge in adult female diestrus sheep.) Such a stimulus failed to produce an LH surge in animals briefly treated with testosterone at any time between 20 and 60 days of gestation. If testosterone treatment was given after 90 days of gestation, and the animal permitted to grow to adulthood, estrogen would result in an LH surge. FSH secretion was not assessed. Estrogen treatment of male sheep castrated as adults also failed to cause an LH surge. Thus, in some ways the control mechanisms in sheep appear similar to the rat, but the possible role for progestogens has not been assessed.

However, in the monkey, Karsch et al.[22] have shown that progestogens are not required to permit estrogens to produce an LH-FSH surge. In contrast to the rat, the sheep, and the human, estrogen will also produce typical surges in the *castrate male monkey;* the response of the male is indistinguishable from the female (Fig. 109-17).

The story in the human remains unsettled. Recall that blood estrogen concentrations peak before the LH-FSH surge during the normal menstrual cycle. Progesterone concentrations rise with LH-FSH concentrations and simultaneously with the fall of estradiol, which subsequently rises again with corpus luteum functions.

The previously mentioned studies of Odell and Swerdloff[17] performed in 1968, prior to measurement of these steroids in blood, demonstrated a production of a typical LH-FSH surge by progesterone treatment of the estrogen-suppressed castrate or postmenopausal woman (Fig. 109-12). This is reminiscent of the similar studies in the rat. Yen et al.[23] have also administered large doses of estrogen to postmenopausal women; they reported an initial suppression of the high LH concentrations, followed in 4 to 6 days by return of LH to control levels. These data are shown in Figure 109-18. Note that a typical ovulatory surge was not produced under these conditions.

To further confuse the story in women, Swerdloff and Odell[24] and Mishell and Odell[25] have shown that either estrogens or progestogens given alone to eugonadal adult women will produce surges of LH (but not FSH). Presumably the difference in these studies and those in postmenopausal women is that ovarian steroids modify the treatment in eugonadal women but not in postmenopausal women. Estrogen-progesterone treatment of men failed to produce evidence for cyclic activity.

In summary, it appears that in women (as well as in rats and sheep but not in monkeys), estrogen secreted by the developing follicle and possibly modulated by progesterone also secreted from the follicle acts via a "cyclic" area within the hypothalamus to produce an ovulatory LH-FSH surge and that the theca cells may secrete the estradiol and progesterone previously attributed to the granulosa cells. After this cyclic area activity (which lasts several hours as indicated by the duration of the ovulatory surge in normal women), the combination of estrogen and progesterone secreted by the corpus luteum acts, via the tonic center, to suppress blood LH and FSH concentrations to low values.

The hypothalamic control of gonadotropin secretion also involves specific neuronal systems that regulate the synthesis and release of hypothalamic GnRH. It has been postulated that the neurotransmitter substances involved may be dopamine or norepinephrine. However, conflicting data exist. Kamberi et al[26] reported that injections of dopamine into the third ventricle of the rat markedly increased pituitary portal blood GnRH concentrations and peripheral blood LH concentrations. In contrast, Fuxe et al.[27] proposed that dopaminergic neurons inhibit LH secretion in the rat. Sawer[28] reported that intraventricular injections of norepinephrine, but not dopamine, stimulated LH secretion in the rabbit. Furthermore, in these studies in rabbits, dopamine, given together with norepinephrine, inhibited the stimulatory effects of norepinephrine. Meuller et al.[29] reported that dopamine antagonists (apomorphine or piribedil) failed to change LH concentrations in rats, while in the same studies these drugs inhibited prolactin and thyrotropin secretion and stimulated growth hormone secretion.

Thus, at the time of writing, the involvement of dopamine as a neurotransmitter for GnRH secretion is controversial, and on balance the data indicate that it is not. Norepinephrine appears to play a role in neurotransmission controlling GnRH secretion, and possibly the control system is complex, involving norepinephrine stimulation in turn modulated by dopaminergic neurones. Clarification of this portion of the control system of reproduction in women must await better studies.

The final common pathway for hypothalamic control of pituitary LH-FSH secretion is by means of secretion of gonadotropin-releasing peptide hormone(s) into the hypothalamic-pituitary portal vascular circulation.[30,31]

Luteinizing hormone-releasing hormone (LH-RH), or LH-FSH-releasing hormone (LH-FSH-RH), or gonadotropin-releasing hormone (GnRH) is a 10 amino acid peptide secreted by hypothalamic neurones. When administered as an intravenous bolus to

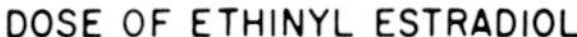

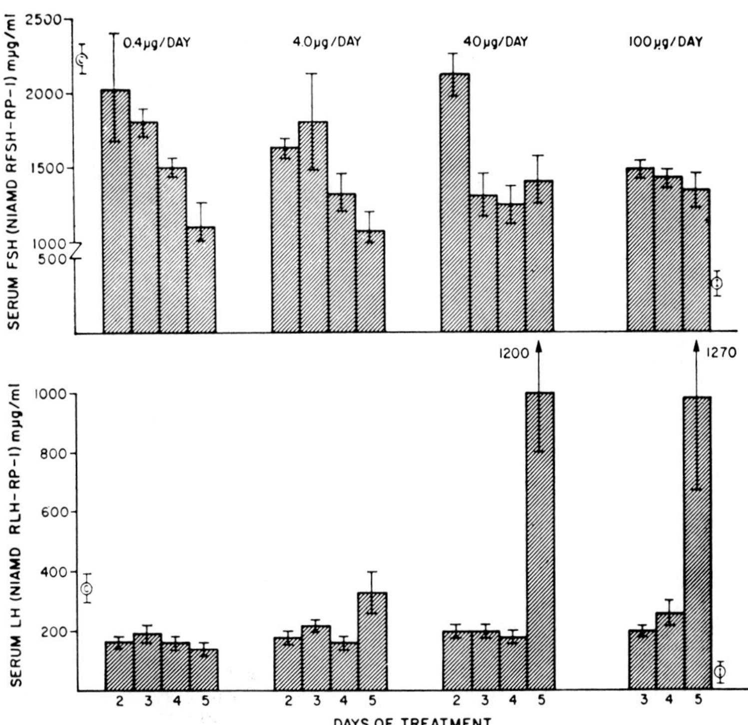

Fig. 109-13. Effects of varying doses of ethinylestradiol (EE) on serum LH and FSH in castrate adult female rats. The experimental plan is identical to that shown in Fig. 109-14, and the data for the 100 μg dose are the same as shown in Fig. 109-14. Note that 40 and 100 μg of EE produced an LH surge on day 5, but that 4.0 and 0.4 μg did not. FSH was suppressed by all doses of EE. (Reproduced from Swerdloff et al.[18])

adult men or women, it typically results in a sharp increase in LH in blood and much smaller increases in FSH. Figure 109-19 shows the results of three different doses of GnRH administered intravenously to normal women during different phases of the menstrual cycle.[32] The magnitude of the response is least during the follicular phase, greater during the preovulatory phase, and greatest during the luteal phase. From such data, one may plot dose-response curves for varying doses of GnRH given at the three portions of the menstrual cycle. Figure 109-20 illustrates such data. Notice that the dose-response curves are not parallel. If the responses during the different portions of the menstrual cycle were only quantitatively different, then the slopes would be parallel and the dose-response curves shifted right or left from each other. The fact that different slopes exist indicates that qualitative differences occur, i.e., there is a change in the response of the pituitary to GnRH during the menstrual cycle. Young and Jaffee[33] have studied the effects of estradiol on GnRH responses in normal women. In these studies, estradiol benzoate (EB) was given by intramuscular injection every 12 hours for 6 days beginning on the first day of menstrual flow. Figure 109-21 depicts their data. Doses of EB equal to or greater than 2.5 μg produced a significant increase in LH response. These data indicate that the estradiol augmentation effect acts directly at a pituitary level.

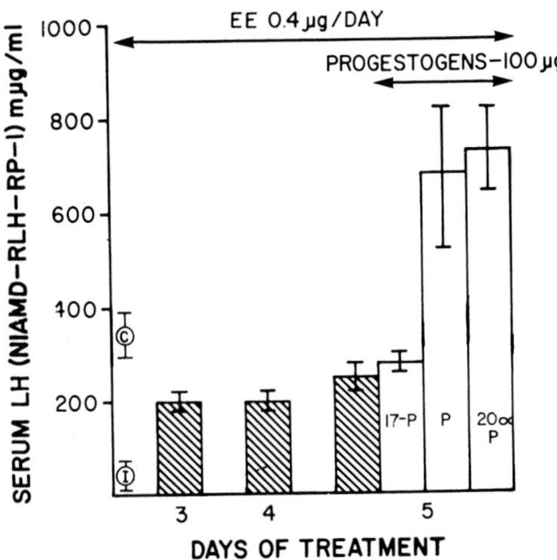

Fig. 109-14. Synergistic role of progestogens in positive feedback of LH in adult castrate female rats. A low dose of ethinylestradiol (0.4 μg EE/day) was used to suppress serum LH. On day 4, 100 μg of progesterone (P), 17-hydroxyprogesterone (17-p), 20-α-hydroxyprogesterone (20-αp), or sesame oil (control) was given to four groups of animals. As in Fig. 109-13, 0.4 μg EE alone produced only a fall in serum LH and FSH. However, when progesterone or 20-α-hydroxyprogesterone was given on day 4, an LH surge resulted. A concomitant FSH surge (not shown) was also produced by the progestogens. Recall that high doses of EE (Fig. 109-13) produced an LH surge but *not* an FSH surge. (Reproduced from Swerdloff et al.[18])

It is to be noted that during the normal ovulatory surge, the LH/FSH ratio is much greater than 1.0. Treatment with GnRH results in LH/FSH ratios very similar to those actually observed in the ovulatory surge. In contrast, however, the LH/FSH ratio *during early follicular growth is less than 1.0*. It is not clear how GnRH could cause this pattern of secretion. Modulation of pituitary response by steroid hormone secretion would have occurred during the studies of Wollesen but did not change the LH/FSH ratio and thus presumably would not during the normal cycle. In addition, in detailed studies in rats, the modulating influence of estradiol in females and testosterone in males on the response to a wide-dose range of GnRH was studied by the same workers. All

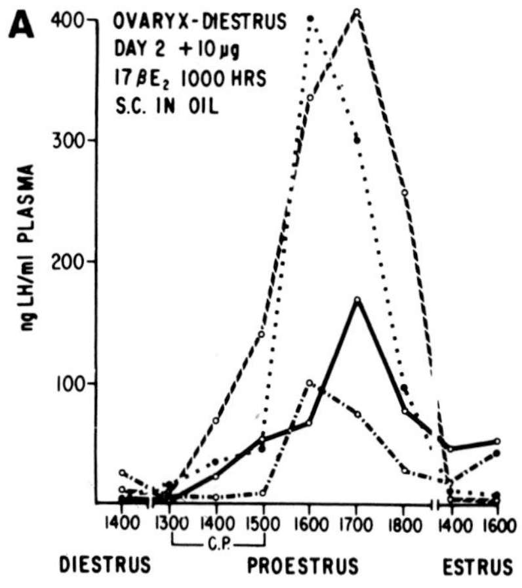

Fig. 109-15 (*left column*). (A) Production of an LH surge in four ovariectomized adult female rats by 10 μg of 17-β-estradiol (17βE_2) given at 1000 hours. The estrogen effects on the vaginal smear cytology is shown by the diestrus-proestrus-estrus legend. Note that after 1400 hours, LH concentrations increased in response to the estrogen. (Reprinted with permission from Barraclough et al., 1975.[19]) (B) Failure of 10 μg of 17βE_2 given at 1000 hours to produce an LH surge in ovariectomized-*adrenalectomized* adult female rats. (Reprinted with permission from Barraclough et al., 1975.[19]) (C) Production of LH surge by 17βE_2 and progesterone given at 1000 hours to ovariectomized-adrenalectomized adult female rats. (Reprinted with permission from Barraclough et al., 1975.[19])

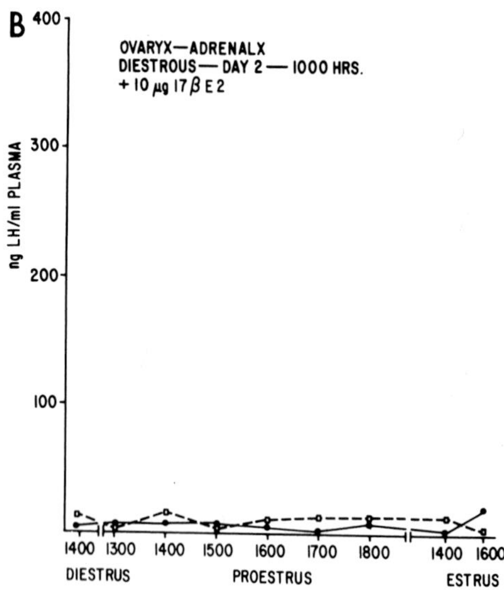

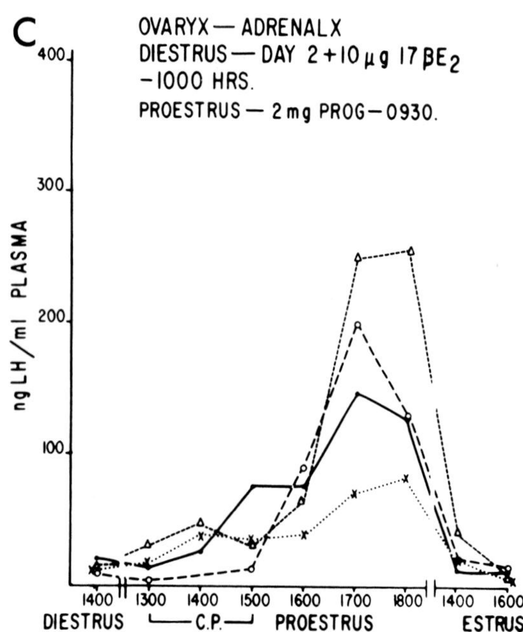

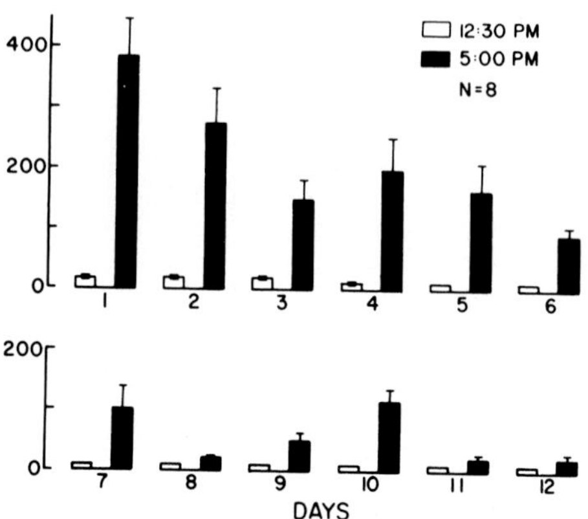

Fig. 109-16. Production of daily LH surges at 5:00 P.M. in adult castrate female rats. By implantation of a sialastic capsule containing estrogen, high, constant concentrations of blood estrogen are produced. An LH surge is observed daily at 5:00 P.M., presumably as a result of diurnal secretion of progesterone by adrenal. (Reproduced from Legan and Karsch [20])

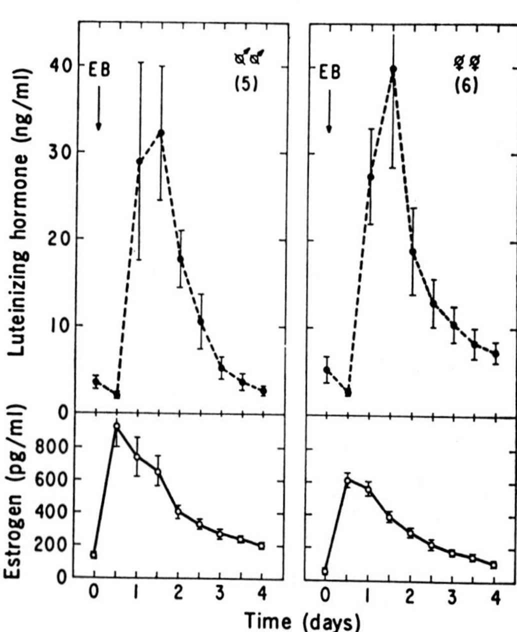

Fig. 109-17. Production of an LH surge in castrated adult male monkeys (♂♂) and female (♀♀) monkeys, by estrogen. Serum estrogen and LH concentrations are shown. (Reproduced from Karsch, F. I., et al. *Science 179:* 484–486, 1973, copyright 1978 by the American Association for the Advancement of Science.)

doses of testosterone inhibited GnRH action; some doses of estradiol potentiated GnRH action, while most doses inhibited it; but no doses of testosterone or estradiol changed the LH/FSH ratio in response to GnRH. It is for these reasons that a search for a separate FSH-RH or for some hypothalamic gonadotropin inhibitory hormone continues. As was discussed in the previous chapter, the pattern of LH-FSH response is different in prepubertal children than it is in adults.

Recall that LH and possibly FSH is secreted in a pulsatile fashion. The cause of such pulsations is unknown but is usually attributed to a pulsatile GnRH secretion. Pulsatile GnRH secretion has not been demonstrated to date because of limitations in methodology. It is known that constant infusions of GnRH do not result in pulsatile secretion, indicating that the cause of such pulsatile secretion does not lie within the pituitary.

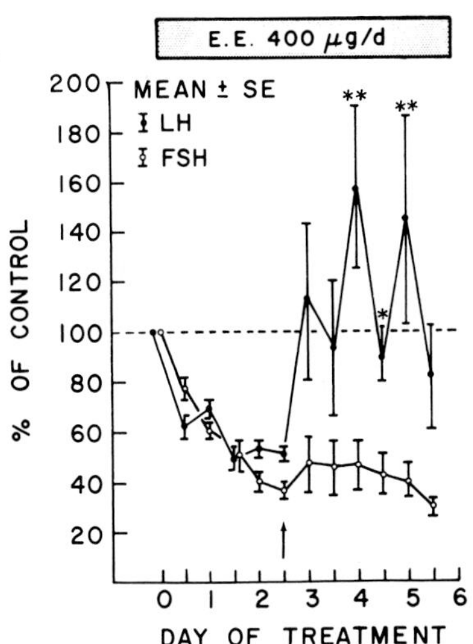

Fig. 109-18. Biphasic effects of ethinylestradiol (400 μg daily orally) on serum LH and suppressive effects on serum FSH in postmenopausal women. (Reproduced from Yen et al.[23])

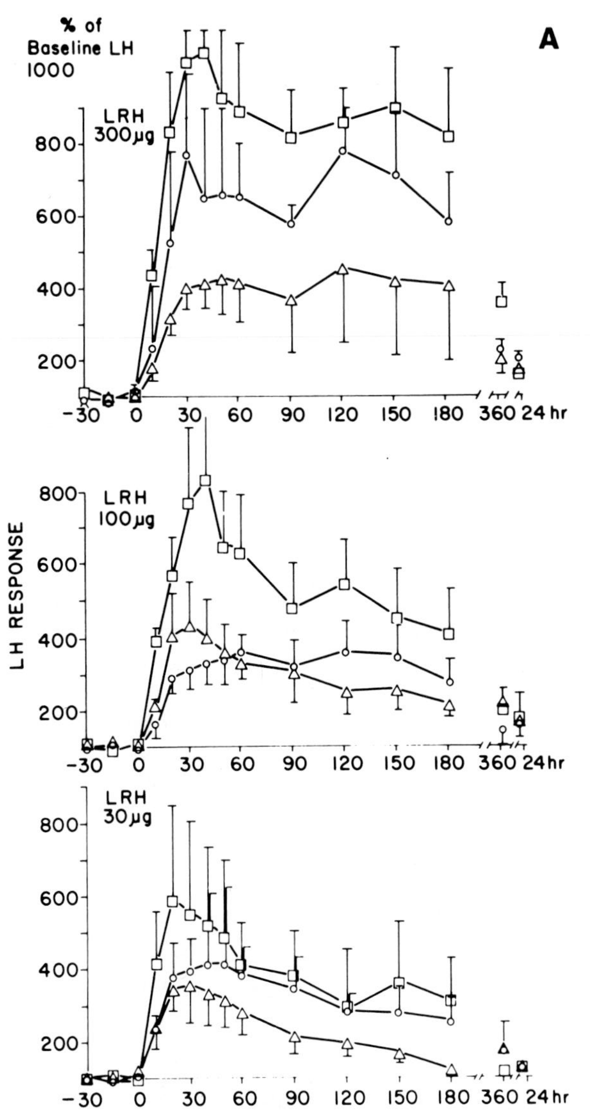

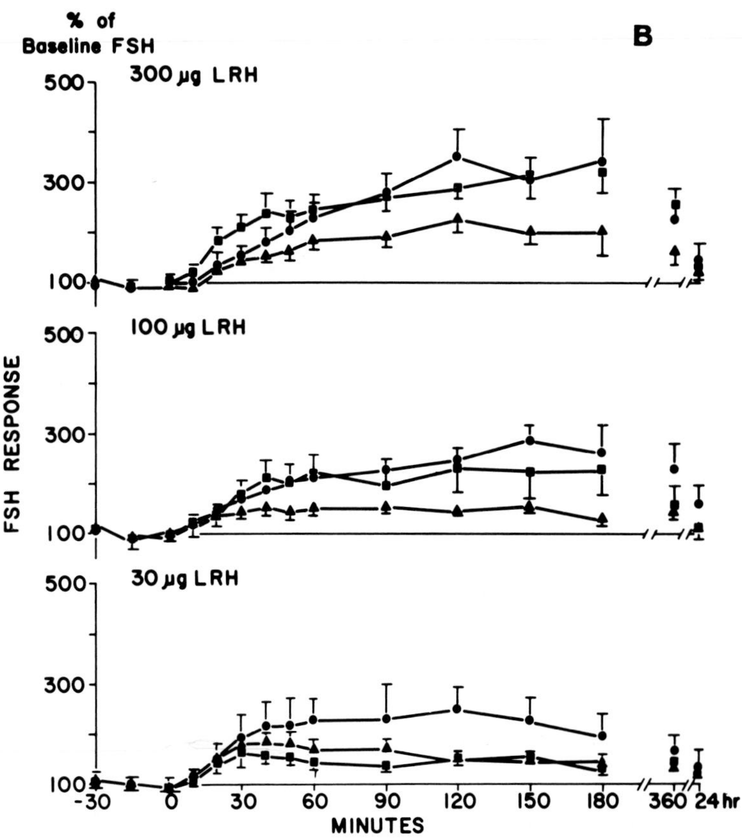

Fig. 109-19a. The LRH-LH time-response curves from normal fertile women at three different phases of the menstrual cycle and at three different doses. For each subject the responses have been corrected for covariance of body surface area and expressed as percent of the mean of three preinjection values. N for each mean and standard error is 4. Δ = follicular phase, ○ = preovulatory phase, □ = luteal phase. (Reproduced from Wollesen, et al.[32]) **Fig. 109-19b.** The LRH-FSH time-response curves for normal fertile women at three different phases of the menstrual cycle and at three different doses. For each subject the responses have been corrected for covariance of body surface area and expressed as percent of the mean of three preinjection values. N for each mean and standard error is 4. Δ = follicular phase, ○ = preovulatory phase, □ = luteal phase. (Reproduced from Wollesen et al.[32])

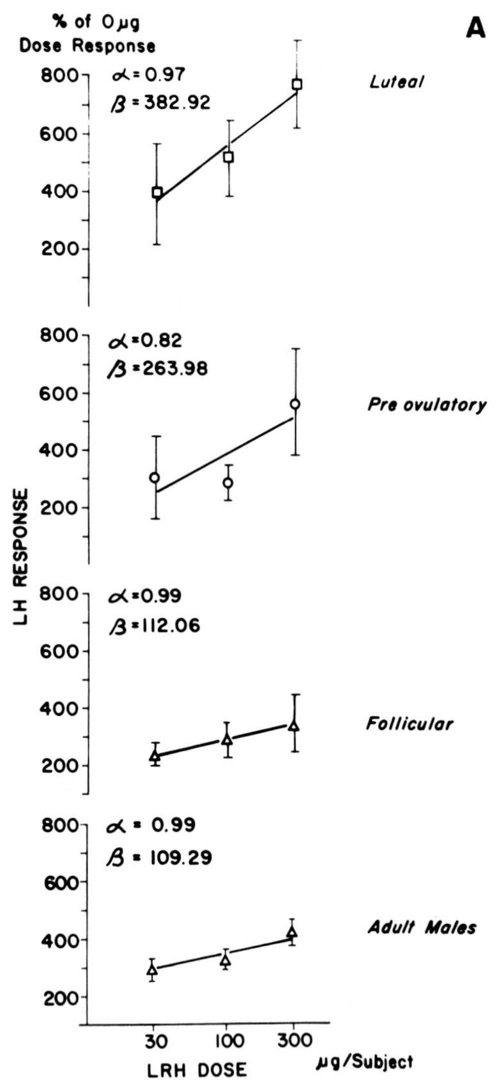

Fig. 109-20a. The LRH-LH dose-response curves for normal fertile women at three different phases of the menstrual cycle. For comparison, identical data are given for normal adult men. For each subject the responses have been corrected for covariance of body surface area, calculated as the area under the time-response curve from 0 to 180 min, and expressed as percent of the area under the base line. N for each mean and standard error is 4. α = regression coefficient. β = slope. (Reproduced from Wollesen et al.[32])

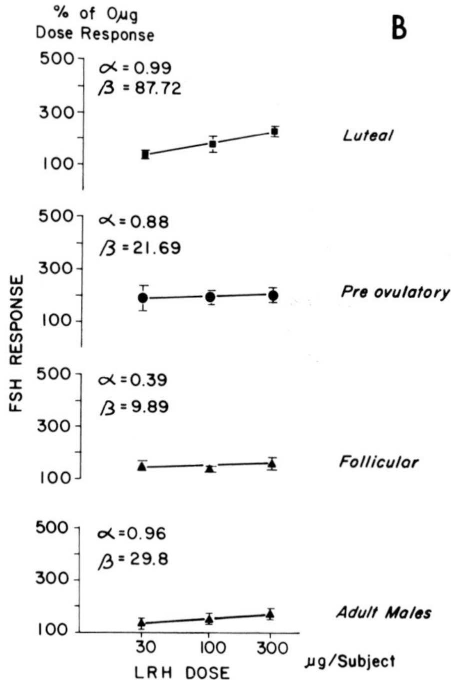

Fig. 109-20b. The LRH-FSH dose-response curves for normal fertile women at three different phases of the menstrual cycle. For comparison, identical data are given for normal adult men. For each subject the responses have been corrected for covariance of body surface area, calculated as the area under the time-response curve from 0 to 180 minutes and expressed as percent of the area under the baseline. N for each mean and standard error is 4. Indices of precision: luteal: 0.011; preovulatory: 0.040; and follicular: 0.039. α = regression coefficient. β = slope. (Reproduced from Wollesen et al.[32])

EXTRAHYPOTHALAMIC MODULATION OF HYPOTHALAMIC CONTROL OF PITUITARY GONADOTROPIN SECRETION

A number of observations in animals suggest that the central nervous system area outside the hypothalamus may modify reproductive function. In the rodent, olfactory influences modify reproductive processes. For example, the odor of a strange male mouse will interrupt early pregnancy in a female mouse by blocking prolactin secretion ("Bruce effect"). The same odor will coordinate randomly occurring estrous cycles in colonies of female mice raised isolated from males ("Whitten effect"). These are examples of *pheromones*, or semiochemicals. (For additional information, the reader is referred to the review of Bronson.[34] Michael[35] reported a series of observations that indicated pheromones may also play a role in primate reproduction. The female rhesus monkeys elaborate semiochemicals in vaginal secretions which act as male sex attractants. For example, the castrate female holds little attraction for a male rhesus. If the vaginal secretions from a midcycle normal female are placed on the perineum of a castrate female, these chemicals induce excitement and attraction in males. These vaginal semiochemicals are chemically related to fatty acids. The human female also elaborates similar substances in vaginal secretions and the amounts vary with stage of the menstrual cycle (as they do in the monkey). When the human vaginal pheromones was applied to the castrate female monkey, its effects were indistinguishable from those produced by the monkey pheromones. It is presently uncertain whether such pheromones play a role in human reproduction.

In addition to these pheromones or semiochemicals, light affects reproductive function in female rodents. As early as 1932, Bissonnette noted that the ferret could be brought into heat during the normal anestrum by prolonging exposure to light. In addition, estrus could be terminated during the breeding season by covering the eyes or blinding. The influence of light varies from species to species. Constant light may produce precocious puberty in female rats.[36] Precise control of the day-night length results in regularization of estrous cycles in the rat. Zacharias and Wurtman[37] have reported that menarche occurs earlier in blind girls than in sighted girls. This effect of light is the opposite of that seen in rats and has been "explained" by the fact that rodents are nocturnal animals, whereas humans are not.

Sawyer[38] has reviewed the role of the amygdala in reproductive function. Estrogen receptors have been demonstrated in the amygdala, in rabbits and rats, and both facilitory and inhibitory influences modify hypothalamic-pituitary function in these species.

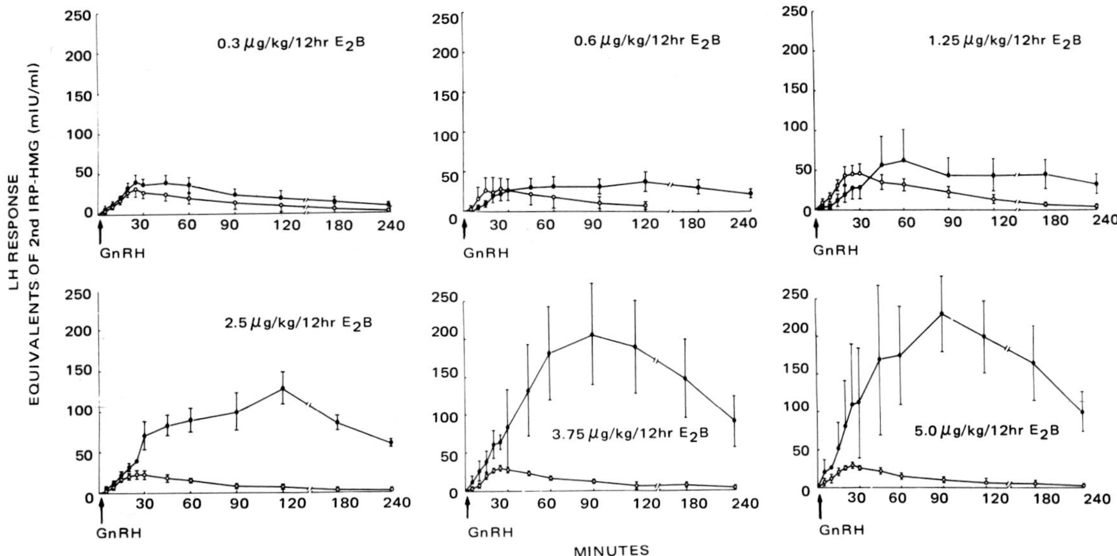

Fig. 109-21. Mean LH responses to GnRH during control (no estradiol) menstrual cycles (-0-) and during menstrual cycles in which pretreatment with varying doses of estradiol benzoate (E_2B) had been administered on menstrual cycle days 1 to 6 (-0-). Vertical bars represent SEM (Reproduced from Young and Jaffe.[33])

The role (if any) of extrahypothalamic influences on pulsatile gonadotropin secretion is also unknown.

THE EFFECTS OF CLOMIPHENE

Clomiphene citrate is an antiestrogen medication that may produce ovulation in certain infertile women (anovulatory, oligoovulatory, or amenorrheic). Understanding its mechanism of action is helpful in comprehension of the physiology of reproduction. Clomiphene treatment of *normal men* for 5 to 7 days results in small increases in blood LH and FSH.[5,39] After cessation of treatment, concentrations of both hormones return to starting values (Fig. 109-22). In *infertile women* who respond to clomiphene treatment, identical increases in LH and FSH[39,40] occur, and the FSH changes may induce a group of follicles to develop. This initiates the entire menstrual cycle cascade described previously. The selected follicle matures and secretes estrogen and progesterone, which in turn activates the cyclic area, with a resultant ovulatory LH-FSH surge; ovulation and corpus luteum function occur, steroid concentrations fall, and menses occur. Clomiphene has initiated the series of events, which finally result in menses about 28 days following initiation of treatment; it has "wound the spring" for the menstrual cycle clock or cascade. In the usual infertile woman, after the menstrual period produced by clomiphene treatment, a second menstrual cycle cascade is not spontaneously produced (as it is believed to be in normals) by the falling blood estradiol and progesterone concentrations at the end of corpus luteum function. Figure 109-23 illustrates schematically the

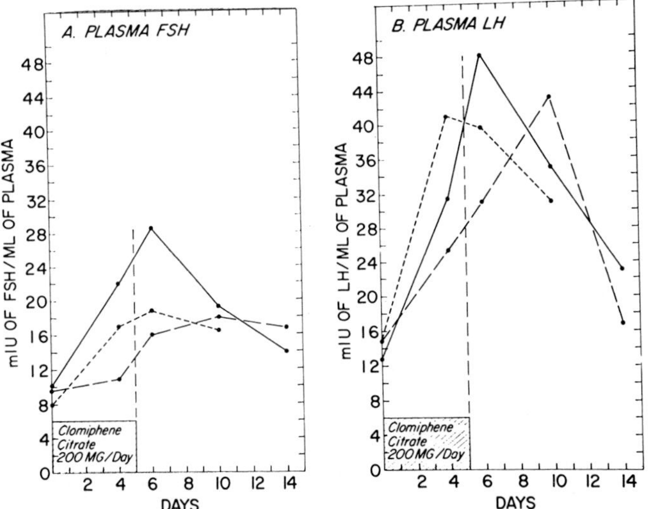

Fig. 109-22. Stimulation of FSH and LH secretion in eugonadal men by treatment with clomiphene citrate. (From Cargille, et al.[39])

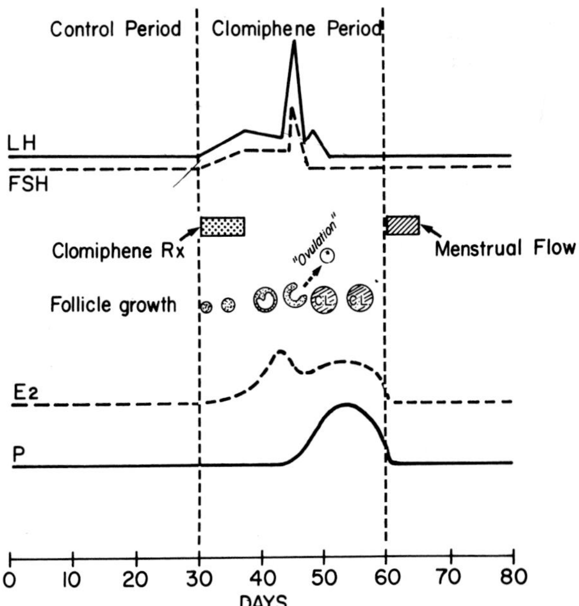

Fig. 109-23. Schematic presentation of the effects of clomiphene treatment on an amenorrheic woman with low-normal LH and FSH concentrations. From days 0 to 30 (control observations), no changes in daily LH and FSH occurred. From days 30 to 37, clomiphene treatment was given and LH and FSH increased, resulting in follicle maturation. Subsequently, ovulation, corpus luteum function, and menses occurred without further treatment. After menses, constant average LH and FSH concentrations are again seen as in the control period, and no cyclic changes occurred.

changes produced by clomiphene treatment of a responding amenorrheic woman.

THE REPRODUCTIVE TRACT

The preceding discussion has attempted to integrate the central nervous system-pituitary-ovarian-endocrine system for the reader. The gonadotropins, LH and FSH, and the gonadotropin-releasing hormones are not believed to have any effect on body functions except via these actions on the pituitary and ovary, respectively. On the other hand, the steroid hormones secreted by the ovary influence a variety of tissues. Their biochemical mechanisms of action are discussed separately (Chapter 110). The effects on the reproductive system in women is discussed in this chapter.

ANATOMY

The anatomy of the human female reproductive system is schematically depicted in Figure 109-24. For a thorough understanding of the reproductive process, and particularly for understanding the pathophysiology and diagnosis of disease states, an understanding of the anatomy of the reproductive system is essential.[7,41,42]

Blood Supply

Note from Figure 109-24 that the arterial supply to the fallopian tubes, uterus, and vagina is mainly from two sources: (1) the paired (right and left) ovarian arteries, which arise from the aorta just below the renal arteries and supply the right and left sides of the system, respectively; and (2) the internal iliac (hypogastric) arteries, which arise from the external iliac artery. The venous system supplying the vagina, uterus, and ovaries parallels this arterial system. The fact that ovarian veins empty into the inferior vena cava just below the renal veins is important to keep in mind when venous blood sampling is done in attempts to separate ovarian or adrenal neoplasms that produce steroid hormones. The ovarian arterial supply is derived from anastomoses of ovarian and uterine vessels. The main ovarian artery branches to enter the *hilum,* where further subdivision occurs into two tortuous medullary branches. These proceed to opposite poles at the ovary, giving off spiral cortical branches, which rotate in a counterclockwise direction. These cortical branches give off additional divisions which supply individual groups of follicles.

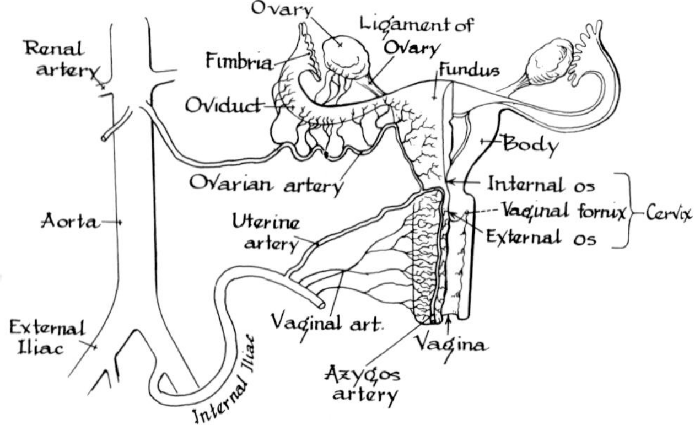

Fig. 109-24. Schematic presentation of the anatomy of the human female reproductive system. (Modified from Odell and Moyer.[7])

Ovaries

The ovary in adult women during reproductive years is almond shaped and measures approximately 2.5 × 2 × 1.5 cm. The weight of both ovaries totals 4–8 g. The upper, or tubal pole, is rounded and attached by the suspensory ligament to the pelvic wall; the lower pole is more pointed and is attached to the uterus by the utero-ovarian ligament. The ovary is attached to the posterior side of the broad ligaments of the uterus by a short fold, the mesovarium. Between the two layers of the mesovarium, the blood vessels and nerves pass to the hilum of the ovary as previously described. The surface of the ovary is irregular from scars produced by previous ovulations. Recent ovulations appear as reddish elevations a few millimeters in diameter. The corpus luteum is not usually identifiable from the surface, but on cut section it appears as a solid, cystic, or hemorrhagic structure measuring 1.5 to over 4 cm in size. At times, the corpus luteum may occupy one half to two thirds of the total ovarian volume.

Miscroscopically, the ovary may be divided into three portions: (1) the surface, which is covered with a low, simple columnar epithelium, the germinal epithelium; (2) the ovarian stroma, lying beneath this epithelium; and (3) the ovarian follicles or corpora lutea scattered through the stroma.

Fallopian Tubes

These paired structures are about 10 cm long and are attached to the superolateral aspects of the uterus. That portion proximate to the ovary is funnellike and is formed of many fingerlike structures, the fimbriae. The fimbriae spread over most of the medial surface of the ovary. During the ovulatory process, these fimbriae actively massage or undulate to assist in ova transport into the fallopian tube cavity. The longest and widest portion of the fallopian tube is termed the ampulla. That portion nearest the body of the uterus possesses a thinner cavity and is termed the isthmus. Microscopically the fallopian tube possesses three layers in its wall: (1) the serous layer (outer), composed of peritoneum of the masosalpinx; (2) the middle or muscular layer, which in turn is composed of a longitudinal muscle layer and a circular muscular layer; and (3) the inner layer or mucosa, composed of a simple columnar epithelium. The majority of the epithelial cells are ciliated; the cilia beat toward the uterus. The fallopian tube also exhibits very active muscular contractions that are of major importance in transporting the ovum to the uterine body. Sperm must move against the cilia stream, but fallopian tube contraction assures good mixing of the ovum and the sperm, assuring fertilization, which occurs in the fallopian tube.

Uterus

The uterus is a thick-walled, muscular organ about 7.5 cm long, 5 cm wide, and 2.5 cm thick. At the superolateral angles, the fallopian tubes enter on each side. Inferiorly the uterus ends in the cervix, which empties into the vagina. The walls of the uterus are composed of three layers: (1) the endometrium, a mucus membrane comprising the inner layer and subject to the cyclic changes in blood steroid concentrations occurring during the menstrual cycle; the endometrium is covered with simple columnar epithelium containing scattered cilia that beat toward the vigina; (2) the middle layer, the myometrium, a thick layer composed of smooth muscle fibers interspersed with fibrous and elastic connective tissue; this is a highly vacular layer; and (3) the perimetrium or outer layer, a serous tissue layer covering the entire uterus except for the cervix.

THE REPRODUCTIVE TRACT AND THE MENSTRUAL CYCLE

Endometrium

The endometrium and vaginal epithelium undergo particularly striking changes, which are extremely important in reproductive physiology.[7] During the first half of each menstrual cycle, progesterone concentrations are low, while estradiol concentrations progressively increase to reach a maximum about 24 hours prior to ovulation. These changes in estrogen (without relatively little concomitant progesterone) stimulate the endometrium in a specific manner. The endometrium increases steadily in thickness; it is perhaps 1 mm thick during the first 4 to 6 days and reaches 3–5 mm just at ovulation. Initially the superficial epithelium is thin, the glands sparse and nontortuous, and the glandular lumina narrow. Mitosis is rare in glands and stroma. During the later proliferative phase, the glands become more tortuous, the number of mitoses increases, and stromal cells are markedly increased in number (Fig. 109-25a and b).

Approximately 36 hours following ovulation, specific histologic changes occur in the endometrium which are produced by progesterone action on the estrogen-prepared endometrium. First glycogen-containing vacuoles appear between the nuclei and the basement membrane of the glandular cells. These increase in number, and about 48 hours following ovulation almost all glandular cells contain such vacuoles. The glands of the endometrium become more tortuous and the nuclei become arranged in a single row above the subnuclear vacuole. By 4 to 5 days following ovulation, the nuclei move toward the base of the cell, and the vacuoles are found toward the lumen. Secretions of these glands increases steadily, and by 6 days after ovulation, secretion into the gland lumen is maximal, and the glands are markedly tortuous. If fertilization occurs, implantation normally occurs about 8 days following ovulation, at a time when the endometrial stroma is loose and edematous. If implantation does not occur, the stromal edema gradually decreases, and glandular secretions, while active, subside from maximum activity. By 11 days following ovulation, lymphocytes have begun to invade the endometrium, and by day 14, sloughing of the endometrium occurs as luteal phase progesterone and estradiol concentrations fall sharply to initiate the gonadotropin changes starting the next menstrual cycle. These changes in endometrial morphology are shown in Figs. 109-25 and 109-26.

Changes in blood supply occur in parallel with these morphological changes. The straight arteries, which arise from the arcuate

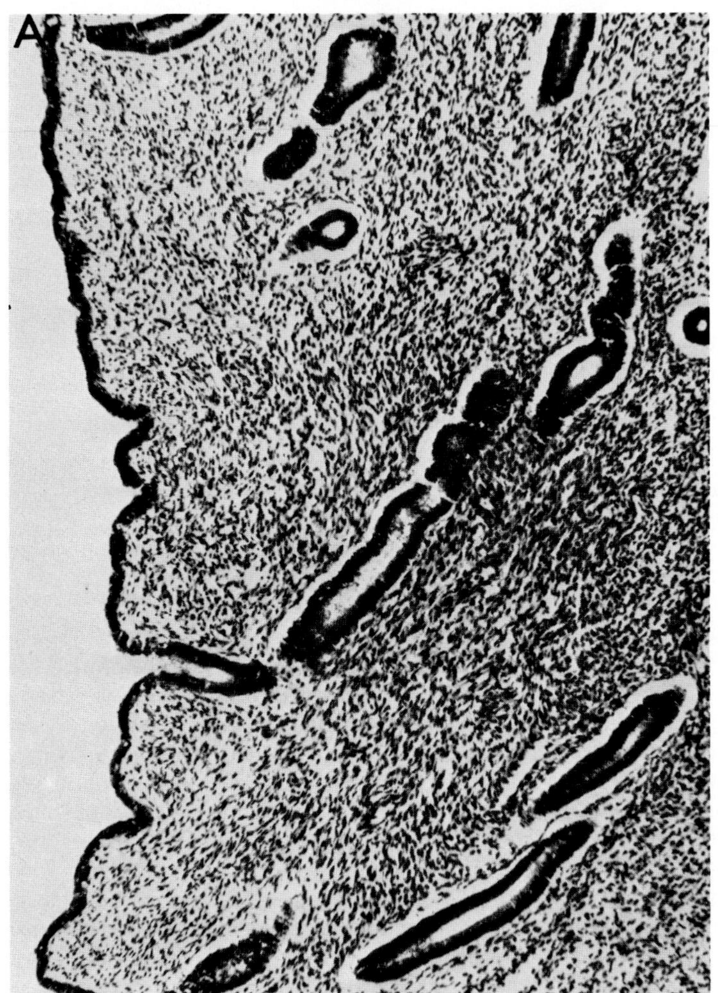

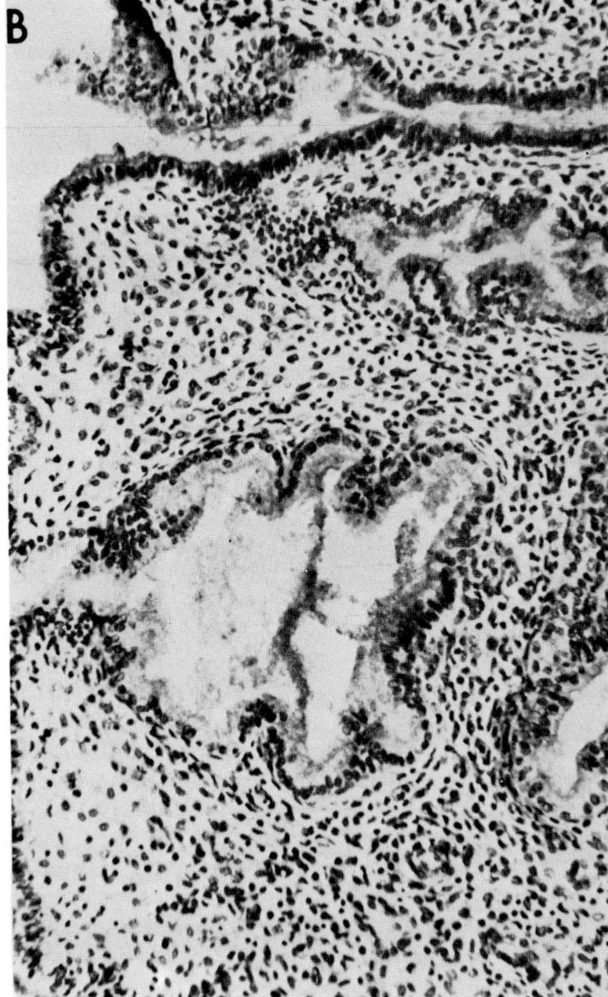

Fig. 109-25a. Histological section of proliferative endometrium (day 7 follicular phase). The glands are straight or only slightly coiled; the epithelial nuclei show a pseudostratified arrangement, and the stroma is dense. **Fig. 109-25b.** Histological section of secretory endometrium (day 22 luteal phase). The glands are coiled and demonstrate abundant secretory activity. The stroma is less dense.

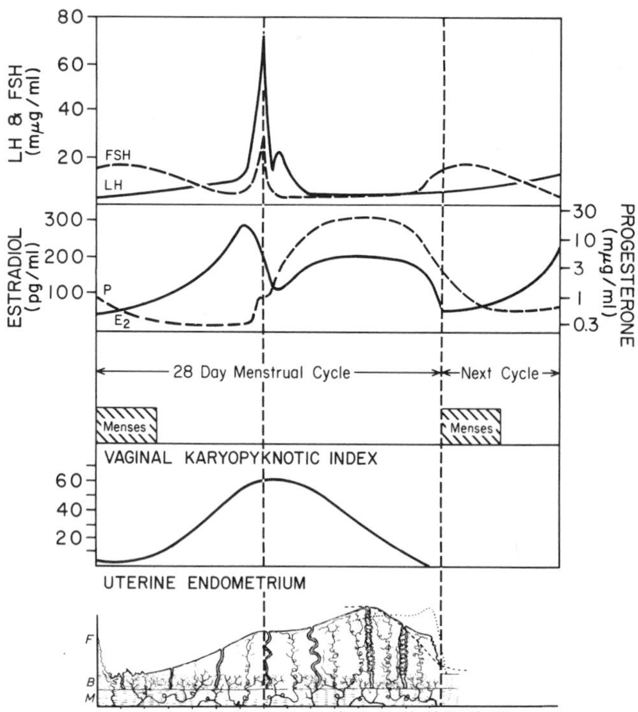

Fig. 109-26. Composite diagram to depict the hormonal and some morphological changes occurring during the normal menstrual cycle.

vessels of the myometrium, supply the basal portions of the endometrium. These straight arteries are not affected to any significant extent by estrogens and progestogens. They are important in endometrial regeneration after menstrual sloughing. In contrast, the spiral arteries are affected by estrogens and progestogens. These vessels grow rapidly during the proliferative phase in response to estrogen stimulation. Elastic fibrils are present in the media and adventitia of these vessels, permitting them to change length and diameter more rapidly than the straight arteries. During the luteal phase their walls become thicker; they grow longer than is permitted by the thickness of the endometrium and hence form coils and become tortuous. At the time of rapid fall of estrogen and progesterone in the late luteal phase, these spiral arteries become constricted. Blood flow through capillaries supplied by these arteries decreases, and the number of capillaries appears to diminish. The stroma becomes more dense and the coiled arteries more tortuous and collapsed with further obstruction to blood flow. Blood stasis and stromal degeneration follow, and endometrial tissue is sloughed. The visible constriction of the spiral arteries occurs 4 to 24 hours before menstrual bleeding (Fig. 109-26).

The changing steroidal hormones also directly effect cervical mucous. Prior to the periovulatory period and also during the luteal phase, the cervical mucous has a randomly oriented pattern when a smear is examined—it is thin and watery. As estrogens peak in blood to herald the ovulatory LH-FSH surge, the cervical mucous becomes tenaceous and when examined, may be stretched (much like a rubber band) to lengths of many inches. Functionally this is reflected by the fact that cervical mucous during the ovulatory period is composed of hundreds of tiny channels through which sperm swim through the cervical os. This channeling is highly effective in directing the movement of sperm. Within very few minutes postintercourse sperm may be found within the uterine cavity. At early follicular phases and during the luteal phases, sperm are not so efficiently directed through the cervical os—the watery, thin, mucous is not formed into "directive" channels.

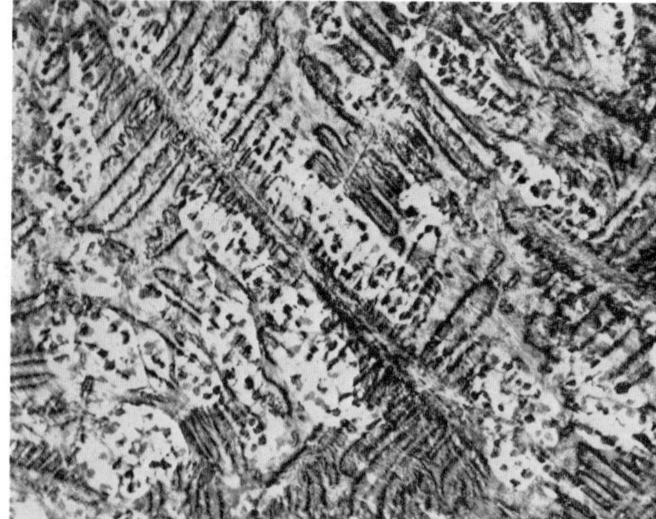

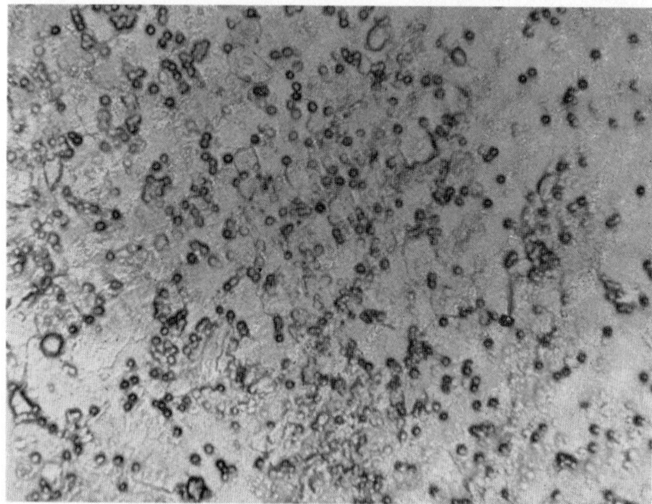

Fig. 109-27. Upper: cervical mucus showing palm-frond or fern-leaf pattern typical of midinterval (high estrogen). Lower: Regressive postovulatory pattern of cervical mucus showing loss of crystallization design (estrogen plus progesterone). (From S. Leon Israel (ed.), Menstrual Disorders and Sterility, 5th ed., Chapter 2, 1967, pp. 16–64.)

Figure 109-27 depicts the patterns of cervical mucus on smears taken at two phases of the menstrual cycle.

Vaginal Epithelium[7,40–44]

The vaginal epithelium is also responsive to estrogenic hormones. The layers of vaginal epithelium in the nonestrogen-exposed patient (as exemplified in prepubertal girls and older women) are few and fragile. In essense, a thin vaginal epithelial membrane characterizes the nonestrogen state. Estrogens applied topically or given systemically stimulate proliferation, adding layers of epithelium and transforming cells into glycogen-containing mature forms. In the adult the vaginal epithelium may be divided into three layers: (1) a superficial zone consisting of flattened, poorly staining squamous cells; (2) a middle layer below the superficial one, consisting of transitional cells; and (3) an innermost, or basal, layer consisting of one or more rows of deeply staining round or oval basal cells. During the menstrual cycle the changing estrogen concentrations also dramatically affect the vaginal epithelium, and the maximal growth and development occurs at the periovulatory period. Figure 109-26 depicts schematically the change in karyotypic index during the normal menstrual cycle. The changes in

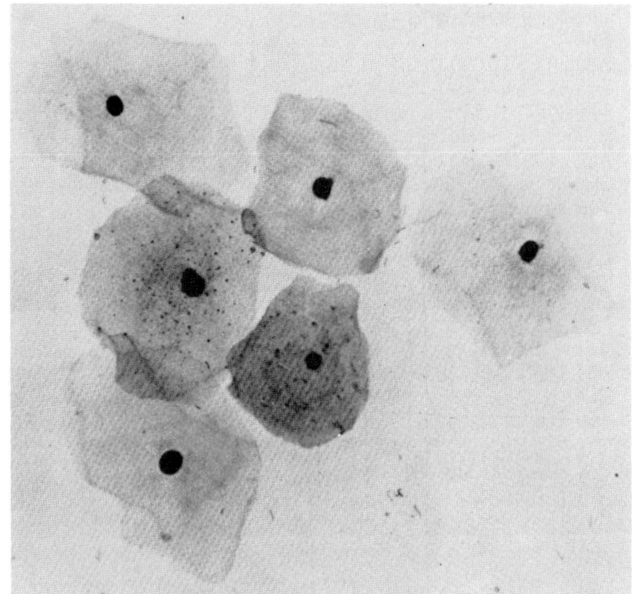

Fig. 109-28. Vaginal cell specimen consisting of flat mature squamous epithelial cells, some of which exhibit cellular granules or fine prekeratinization lines. This specimen is unequivocally diagnostic for estrogenic effect. (From George L. Wied and Bibo Marluce, Evaluation of endocrinologic condition by exfoliative cytology, *in* J. J. Gold (ed), Gynecologic Endocrinology, 2nd ed., Chapter 8, 1975, pp 117–155.)

vaginal cell morphology may be defined by examining cells obtained from smears. In such smears the unstimulated cells shows relatively small basal cells with healthy nuclei along with basophilic intermediate cells. Figures 109-27 and 109-28 show a smear of vaginal epithelium as affected by estrogens. The fully estrogenic smear observed in the late follicular, or the periovulatory, phase contains mainly cornified epithelial cells with pyknotic nuclei. These cells stain pink with eosin. During the luteal phase the cells show increased desquamatory changes with rolled edges. Toward the end of the luteal phase, intermediate cell types reappear, and abundant leukocytes are present.

Fallopian Tubes[7,40,43]

The epithelium of the fallopian tubes also responds to estrogens and progestogens. During the early proliferative phase of the menstrual cycle and under estrogen stimulus, the number of ciliated and nonciliated cells increases. At midcycle, these cells enlarge, and large amounts of PSA-positive material accumulate. By the midluteal phase, a protein-rich material is present in abundance in the lumen of the oviduct. This material supports and nourishes both the spermatozoa during their trip for fertilization and also the developing blastocyst during its migration to the uterus prior to implantation.

REFERENCES

1. Kohler, P. O., Ross, G. T., Odell, W. D.: Metabolic clearance and production rates of human luteinizing hormone in pre- and postmenopausal women. *J. Clin Invest 47:* 38–47, 1969.
2. Coble, Y. D., Kohler, P. O., Cargille, C. M., et al.: Production rates and metabolic clearance in pre- and postmenopausal women. *J Clin Invest 48:* 359–363, 1969.
3. Yen, S. S. C., Tsai, C. C., Naftolin, F., et al.: Pulsatile patterns of gonadotropin release in subjects with and without ovarian function. *J Clin Endocrinol Metab 34:* 671–674, 1972.
4. Odell, W. D., Parlow, A. I., Cargille, C. M., et al.: Radioimmunoassay for human follicle stimulating hormone: Physiological studies. *J Clin Invest 47:* 25–51, 1967.
5. Odell, W. D., Ross, G. T., Rayford, P. L.: Radioimmunoassay for human LH: Physiological studies. *J Clin Invest 46:* 248–255, 1967.
6. Abraham, G. E., Odell, W. D., Swerdloff, R. S., et al.: Stimultaneous radioimmunoassay of plasma FSH, LH, Progesterone, 17-hydroxyprogesterone and estradiol-17-β during the menstrual cycle. *J Clin Endocrinol Metal 34:* 312–318, 1972.
7. Odell, W. D., Moyer, D. C.: Physiology of Reproduction. St. Louis, C. V. Mosby Co., 1971.
8. Baker, T. G.: Oogenesis and ovulation, in Austin, C. R., Short, R. V. (eds): Reproduction in Mammals. I. Germ Cells and Fertilization. Cambridge University Press, 1972, pp. 14–45.
9. Harman, S. M., Louvet, J. P., Ross, G. T.: Interaction of estrogen and gonadotrophins on follicle atresia. *Endocrinology 96:* 1145–1152, 1975.
10. Crooke, A. C., Morell, M., Butt, W. R.: The recovery of exogenous follicle stimulating hormone from urine, in Rosenberg, E. (ed): Gonadotropins. Palo Alto, Geron-X, Inc., 1968.
11. Coyotupa, J., Buster, J., Parlow, A. F., et al.: Normal cyclical patterns of gonadotropins and ovarian steroids despite congenital absence of the uterus. *J Clin Endocrinol Metab 36:* 395–400, 1973.
12. Vande Wiele, R. L., Bogumil, J., Dyrenfurth, I., et al.: Mechanisms regulating the menstrual cycle in women. *Rec Prog Horm Res 26:* 63–103, 1970.
13. Pfeiffer, C. A.: Sexual differences of the hypophyses and their determination by the gonads. *Am J Anta 58:* 195, 1936.
14. Barraclough, C. A.: Modification in the NCS regulation of reproduction after exposure of prepubertal rats to steroid hormones. *Rec Prog Horm Res 22:* 503–539, 1966.
15. Brown-Grant, K., Munck, A. U., Naftolin, F., et al.: The effects of administration of testosterone and related steroids to female rats during the neonatal period. *Hormones & Behavior 2:* 173, 1971.
16. Naftolin, F., Ryan, K. J., Davies, I. J., et al.: The formation of estrogens by central neuroendocrine tissues. *Rec Prog Horm Res 31:* 295–319, 1975.
17. Odell, W. D., Swerdloff, R. S.: Progestogen induced LH and FSH surge in postmenopausal women: A simulated ovulatory peak. *Proc Nat Acad Sci 61:* 529–536, 1968.
18. Swerdloff, R. S., Jacobs, H. S., Odell, W. D.: Synergistic role of progestogens in estrogen induction of LH and FSH surge. *Endocrinology 90:* 1529–1536, 1972.
19. Barraclough, C. A., Turgeon J., Cramer, O., et al.: Regulatory role of estrogen in the ovulatory discharge of luteinizing hormone, in Raspe G (ed): *Advances in the Biosciences 15,* Schering Workshop on Central Actions of Estrogenic Hormones. New York, Pergamon Press, 1975, pp. 209–222.
20. Legan, S. J., Karsch, F. J.: A daily signal for the LH surge in the rat. *Endocrinology 96:* 57–62, 1975.
21. Short, R. V.: Sexual differentiation of the brain of the sheep. International Symposium on Sexual Endocrinology of the Perinatal Period, May 30–31, 1974, The Inserm, Paris.
22. Karsch, F. J., Dierschke D. J., Knobil E.: Sexual differentiation of pituitary function. Apparent difference between primates and rodents. *Science 179:* 484–486, 1973.
23. Yen, S. S. C., Tsai, C. C.: Biphasic pattern in feedback action of ethinyl estradiol in release of FSH and LH. *J Clin Endocrinol Metab 33:* 882–887 1971.
24. Swerdloff, R. S., Odell, W. D.: Serum LH and FSH levels during sequential and nonsequential contraceptive treatment of eugonadal women. *J Clin Endocrinol Metabl 29:* 157–163, 1969.
25. Mishell, D., Odell, W. D.: Effect of varying dosages of ethynodiol diacetate upon serum luteinizing hormone. *Am J Obstet Gynecol 109:* 140–149, 1971.
26. Kamberi, I. A., Mical, R. S., Porter, J. C.: Effect of anterior pituitary perfusion and intraventricular injection of catecholamines and indoleamines on LH release. *Endocrinology 88:* 1012–1020, 1970.
27. Fuxe, K., Goldstein, M., Hokfelt, T., Jonsson, G., Lidbrink, P.: Dopaminergic involvement in hypothalamic function: Extrahypothalamic and hypothalamic control. *Adv Neurol 5:* 405–419, 1974.
28. Sawyer, C. H.: First Geoffrey Harris Memorial Lecture: Some recent developments in brain-pituitary-ovarian physiology. *Neuroendocrinology 17:* 97–124, 1975.
29. Mueller, G. P., Simpkins, J., Meites, J., Moore, K. E.: Differential effects of Dopamine agonists and haloperidol and release of prolactin, thyroid stimulating hormone, growth hormone and luteinizing hormone in rats. *Neuroendocrinology 20:* 121–135, 1976.

30. Schally, A. V., Kastin, A. J., Arimura, A.: Hypothalamic follicle-stimulating hormone (FSH) and luteinizing hormone (LH) regulating hormone: Structure physiology and clinical studies. *Fertil Steril 22:* 703–721, 1971.
31. Guillemin, R.: Physiology and chemistry of the hypothalamic releasing factors for gonadotropins. *Contraception 5:* 1, 1972.
32. Wollesen, F., Swerdloff, R. S., Odell, W. D.: LH and FSH responses to luteinizing releasing hormone in normal fertile women. *Metabolism, 25:* 1275–1285, 1976.
33. Young, J. R., Jaffe, R. B.: Strength-duration characteristic of estrogen effects on gonadotropin response to gonadotropin-releasing hormone in women. II. Effects of varying concentrations of estradiol. *J. Clin Endocrinol Metab 42:* 432–442, 1976.
34. Bronson FSH: Pherormonal influences on mammallian reproduction, in Diamond, N. (ed): Perspectives in Reproduction and Sexual Behavior. Bloomington, Indiana University Press, 1968.
35. Michael, R. P.: Hormone steroids and sexual communication in primates. *J Steroid Biochem 6:* 161, 1975.
36. Fiske, V. M.: Effect of light on sexual maturation: Estrous cycles and anterior pituitary function of the rat. *Endocrinology 29:* 187–196, 1941.
37. Zacharias, L., Wurtman, R.: Blindness: Its relation to age of menarche. *Science 144:* 1154–1158, 1964.
38. Sawyer, C. H.: Functions of the amygdala related to feedback actions of gonadal steroids, in Eleftheriou, B. E. (ed): Neurobiology of the Amygdala. New York, Plenum Publishing Company, 1974.
39. Cargille, C. M., Ross, G. T., Bardin, C. W.: Clomiphene and gonadotropin in men. *Lancet 2:* 1298, 1968.
40. Ross, G. T., Cargille, C. M., Lipsett, M. B., et al.: Pituitary and gonadal hormones in women during spontaneous and induced ovulatory cycles. *Rec Prog Horm Res 26:* 1–62, 1970.
41. Crouch, J. E.: Functional Human Anatomy. Philadelphia, Lea and Febiger, 1966.
42. Gray, H.: In Goss, C. M. (ed): Anatomy of the Human Body. Philadelphia, Lea and Febiger, 1966.
43. Ross, G. T., Vande Wiele, R. L.: The ovaries, in Williams, R. H. (ed): Textbook of Endocrinology. Philadelphia, W. B. Saunders Co., 1974.

110

Ovarian Hormone Synthesis, Circulation, and Mechanisms of Action

Pentti K. Siiteri
Freddy Febres

The normal functioning ovary synthesizes and secretes estrogens, androgens, and progesterone in a precisely controlled pattern determined by the pituitary gonadotropins, FSH and LH. During the first half of the menstrual cycle, FSH promotes follicular development and increasing secretion of estradiol, which reaches its maximum level shortly before the midcycle surge of gonadotropins. A precipitous decline in estrogen secretion occurs as the gonadotropins are rising, and then increased levels of estradiol are again secreted during the luteal phase by the corpus luteum. Progesterone secretion by the human ovary is minimal during the follicular phase and increases dramatically with formation of the corpus luteum. The androgens, androstenedione and testosterone, are also normally secreted and show a midcycle peak that coincides with the peaks of FSH and LH. In the absence of fertilization and implantation of the blastocyst, the corpus luteum regresses and progesterone secretion declines just prior to menses. While these changes in steroid hormonal output by the ovary have been well documented, many of the underlying mechanisms responsible for the changes in their secretion are not yet known. For example, no completely satisfactory explanation has yet been put forth for the precipitous decline in estradiol just prior to the midcycle gonadotropin surge. Also the mechanism responsible for the demise of the corpus luteum in the human ovary is not yet clear. It is known that in some species, such as the sheep, substances (prostaglandins) released from the uterus cause death of lutein cells, perhaps by restricting blood flow. Little evidence is available for a similar mechanism in the human, however, since hysterectomy performed during the luteal phase does not influence the life span of the corpus luteum.

While the basic biochemical pathways involved in steroid production by the ovary have been known for some time, it is still not clear which cell types are involved in the production of estrogens. The two-cell hypothesis proposed by Falck many years ago, suggesting that theca cells produce androgens that are converted into estrogens by the follicular granulosa cells, is still controversial. More recent studies have shown that both estrogens and androgens have important intraovarian effects and may be the primary regulators of follicular development and/or atresia. Much work has been done in the past decade on the mechanism by which all steroid hormones appear to exert their actions via the intracellular steroid receptor proteins. However, some effects of steroid hormones cannot be accounted for by this scheme. For example, one of the major effects of estradiol or other estrogenic hormones on the uterus is to increase blood flow, and this action does not appear to be mediated by cytosol receptors but rather by prostaglandins. Progesterone induction of amphibian egg maturation results from an interaction of the steroid with the plasma membrane that increases intracellular calcium levels.

It has long been known that estrogens are produced following cessation of ovarian function at the menopause. Early studies indicated that the adrenal glands were the source of this estrogen. More recent studies have demonstrated clearly that the adrenals produce a prehormone of estrogen, namely androstenedione and that conversion of androstenedione to estrogen takes place in peripheral tissues. These studies have shown that this mechanism of estrogen production is accelerated in a variety of conditions, and the tendency to produce excessive estrogen by this mechanism has been linked with an increased risk of endometrial cancer. The function of peripheral estrogen forming process, if any, is not known, however. Indeed, the exact tissue site(s) in which this conversion takes place has not been clearly established. This chapter reviews recently obtained information in these areas derived from both laboratory animal and human studies. Reference is made primarily to many extensive review articles and key papers.

BIOSYNTHESIS AND SECRETION OF OVARIAN HORMONES

BIOSYNTHESIS

The general steps in the biosynthetic pathways and the subcellular localization of the major enzymes involved are similar in all steroid-producing glands including the ovary, testis, and adrenal (Fig. 110-1). It is generally assumed on the basis of in vitro studies with radioactive acetate that each of these glands carries out de novo hormone synthesis as shown, i.e., all the enzymes required for cholesterol synthesis, conversion to pregnenolone, and then to appropriate hormonal product are present. This is in contrast to the mechanisms by which the placenta produces estrogen and progesterone. Since the placenta lacks certain key enzymes, it is dependent upon externally supplied precursors for steroid production and has been termed an incomplete endocrine gland. Specifically, the placenta appears to utilize cholesterol obtained from the maternal circulation for progesterone synthesis and C_{19} steroids derived from both the fetal and maternal adrenal glands to produce estrogens.[1] It is also possible that the ovary utilizes circulating

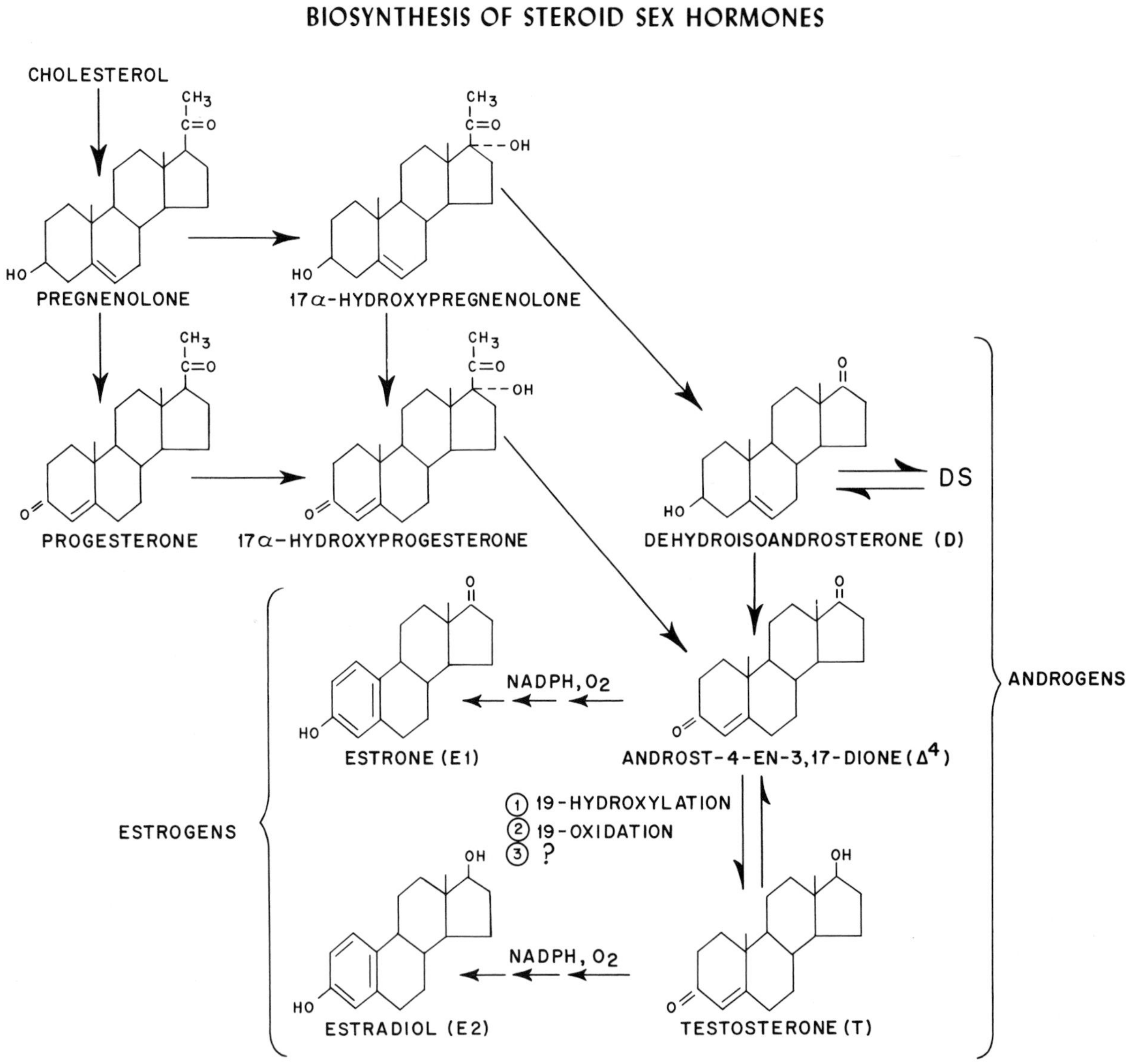

BIOSYNTHESIS OF STEROID SEX HORMONES

Fig. 110-1. Pathways of ovarian steroid hormone biosynthesis.

cholesterol for production of steroid hormones. The early studies demonstrating miniscule conversion of acetate to various steroid hormones by the ovary do not necessarily prove that de novo synthesis alone is important, since the production of estradiol by the ovary would require a very small amount of the circulating cholesterol pool.

Cholesterol is present in steroid-synthesizing glands both as the free alcohol and esterified to a variety of fatty acids. That the cholesterol-ester pool can be utilized for steroid synthesis has been demonstrated, and it has been suggested that LH may increase cholesterol esterase activity and thereby increase the availability of cholesterol for conversion to pregnenolone.[2] Most authors, however, believe that regulation of steroid synthesis is exerted primarily at the level of the cholesterol side chain cleavage enzyme which removes the 6-carbon fragment isocaproic acid, resulting in the formation of pregnenolone. A great deal of biochemical work has been carried out concerning the nature of this reaction and its regulation by ACTH in the adrenals and LH in the ovary and testis. The process requires NADPH and oxygen and has been clearly shown to involve cytochrome P-450 in a mixed function oxidase reaction. Data support the formation of 20α-hydroxycholesterol followed by a 20α-22-dihydroxycholesterol as intermediates during the synthesis of pregnenolone. However, recent studies from Lieberman's laboratory have suggested that these compounds are not formed as classical biochemical intermediates but represent incomplete reaction products. It is envisioned that a multistep reaction occurs at one enzymatic site without release of intermediates during the formation of pregnenolone. The cleavage reaction takes place in mitochondria, and thus many possible points of control have been suggested, including facilitated entry of cholesterol into mitochondria by carrier protein, generation of NADPH within the mitochondria, and changes in the active levels of cytochrome P-450.[3]

Pregnenolone is converted to progesterone by the action of two enzymes, 3β-hydroxysteroid dehydrogenase and Δ^5-3-ketosteroid isomerase. These two enzymes are tightly linked in the endoplasmic reticulum of the cell. Steroid oxidation requires the cofactor nicotinomide adeninenucleotide (NAD) as the hydrogen acceptor in the removal of hydrogen from the 3β-hydroxyl position, and this reaction is followed by the shift of the double bond from the Δ^5 to the Δ^4 position. Progesterone is secreted by the corpus luteum or is used as substrate for further enzymatic reactions leading to the androgens and estrogens. Conversion of progesterone to C_{19} androgens requires two enzymes, 17α-hydroxylase and C-17,20-lyase enzyme which cleaves the 2-carbon side chain. 17α-Hydroxyprogesterone is also secreted by the ovary. 17-

Hydroxylation occurs in the endoplasmic reticulum and requires NADPH and molecular oxygen and is catalyzed by cytochrome P-450. Pregnenolone can also be 17-hydroxylated, thus offering an alternative route (the Δ^5 pathway) to the androgens via the formation of DHEA. Despite many studies, the relative importance of the two alternate pathways to androgens (Fig. 110-1) is still not clear. Androstenedione is the major androgen produced by the ovary, although small amounts of testosterone and DHEA are also formed. Dihydrotestosterone and androstanediols can also be formed, but little is known of their importance in normal ovarian function (see below).

Recent studies from several laboratories have elaborated upon the biosynthetic pathway for estrogen formation from aromatizable androgens. The scheme outlined in Fig. 110-1 indicates that three hydroxylation steps, each utilizing NADPH and O_2, are required, suggesting that a cytochrome P-450 mixed function oxidase enzyme(s) is involved. A considerable body of evidence supports this conclusion,[4] despite the fact that aromatization of C_{19} steroids is not inhibited by carbon monoxide, whereas other P-450 dependent reactions are inhibited. The aromatase enzyme complex likely operates also as a single-site enzyme without release of intermediates. The first two hydroxylations occur at the C_{19} angular methyl group to yield an aldehyde, and the final step appears to be hydroxylation at the 2β-position, as demonstrated in Fishman's laboratory.[5] The 2β-hydroxylaldehyde compound is readily converted to the aromatic estrogens nonenzymatically. Most of the biochemical work on the aromatization reaction has been carried out with human placental microsomes, and it is generally assumed that the same reaction sequence applies to the ovary.

The secretion of various steroids by the ovary varies considerably during the menstrual cycle. The complex interactions between the different ovarian cell types that regulate ovarian steroidogenesis and function pose one of the greatest challenges to reproductive scientists. It is generally agreed that the thecal and stromal cells are the principal sources of androgens and 17-hydroxyprogesterone. Luteinized granulosa and thecal cells produce progesterone and some estradiol. However, considerable controversy has surrounded the origin of estradiol that is secreted by the ovary. Early studies by Falck, utilizing isolation and recombination of theca and granulosa cell elements of the rat ovary in the rabbit anterior chamber of the eye, suggested that both cell types were necessary for estrogen synthesis. The two-cell hypothesis has found support in a variety of studies with different preparations over the years. However, recent studies by Channing and coworkers clearly suggest that the thecal cells are primarily responsible for secretion of estradiol.[6] These investigators removed the follicular fluid and granulosa cells from large preovulatory follicles of the monkey ovary and demonstrated that there was only a modest decline in ovarian secretion of estradiol and progesterone up to 2 hours thereafter. Armstrong disputes these findings on the grounds that adjacent developing follicles may have been synthesizing estradiol from androstenedione.[7] It is possible that both views are correct and that granulosa cells produce estrogens that are retained in the follicular fluid, whereas estradiol produced in the theca is released into the vasculature. The follicular fluid contains very high concentrations of estradiol, progesterone, and androstenedione.

SECRETION RATES

The secretion of ovarian steroids has been estimated directly by comparing the level of hormones in the periphery and ovarian vein. The concentration gradient multiplied by the ovarian blood flow gives a direct estimate of secretion rate. The finding of a higher concentration in the venous effluent proves that a particular hormone is secreted. However, it is virtually impossible to be certain that blood flow through the ovary has not been altered by the sampling procedures. For this and other reasons, estimates of secretion and production rates by in vivo isotope dilutions techniques have provided useful information. The term "production rate" is defined as the amount of hormone from all sources entering the circulation per unit time. Secretion can occur from both the ovaries and adrenal glands, as in the case of androstenedione, and additional amounts may be derived by peripheral conversion from other more or less active steroids. The latter process is now recognized to be an important mechanism in both the male and female, since it can give rise to both hyperestrogenic and hyperandrogenic states. The production rate (PR) of a hormone is equal to its metabolic clearance rate (MCR) multiplied by its concentration in blood if it is reasonably constant. It is now known that this is not the case for several hormones that are secreted episodically. Nonetheless, meaningful daily estimates can be obtained by multiple sampling of blood. If the PR of a hormone is known, its secretion rate may be estimated by repeated measurements during appropriate suppression of the adrenal or ovarian contribution.

The MCR was defined by Tai as the volume of blood or plasma from which a substance is cleared per unit time. This easily measured parameter is useful in many ways, since it is independent of transfers among body compartments and metabolism. Therefore, if the MCR is not altered, changes in the concentration of a hormone directly reflect changes in its PR. Furthermore, the absolute value of MCR is informative about sites of metabolism. If the value is much greater than hepatic blood flow (1500 liters/day), then extrahepatic clearance must be substantial. Another easily measured function that is important in studying the conversion of one hormone to nother is the rho [ρ] value or the transfer constant of conversion. This is defined as the fraction of the blood production rate of a precursor that enters the circulation as product per unit of time. For example, $[\rho]^{AT} \times PR_A$ equals the amount of testosterone (T) that is derived from circulating androstenedione (A). Much insight into the complex metabolism and interconversions of steroid hormones has been obtained from experiments utilizing these concepts. Extensive reviews of the theoretical and practical aspects of this subject are available,[8,9] and Siiteri has developed an intuitive approach based on simple dilution principles.[10] Information pertaining to the ovaries has been reviewed by Baird et al.[11] Some of the important information concerning ovarian hormones is summarized in Table 110-1.

MECHANISM OF GONADOTROPIN ACTION

Many in vitro studies on the mechanisms by which LH and FSH direct steroidogenesis by the ovary employing whole ovaries, cellular compartments, or isolated cells have generated the general scheme shown in Fig. 110-2. Excellent reviews of this subject are available.[12–14] As with other peptide hormones, the target cells contain on their surface membrane specific receptors for both LH and FSH that are coupled to the enzyme adenylate cyclase. Binding of effective amounts of gonadotropin results in activation of the cyclase and increased intracellular levels of cAMP. The "second messenger" cAMP interacts with the regulatory subunit of one or more protein kinases which presumably phosphorylate proteins that are necessary to increase the level of steroidogenesis. The nature of the steroid produced depends upon the effective concentrations of LH and FSH and the cell type and species in question. Ovarian cells also contain receptors for catecholamine and prostaglandins, both of which can mimic some of the effects of LH and

Table 110-1. Production, Clearance, and Plasma Levels of Ovarian Steroid Hormones (Approximate Values)

Compound	MCR (liter/day)	Phase of Menstrual Cycle	Plasma Concentration (ng/100 ml)	Production Rate (mg/day)	Secretion Rate (mg/day)
Estradiol	1300	Early follicular	6	0.08	0.07
		Late follicular	30–60	0.5–1.0	0.4–0.8
		Mid-luteal	20	0.25	0.25
Estrone	2200	Early follicular	4	0.12	0.8
		Late follicular	15–30	0.3–0.6	0.25–0.5
		Mid-luteal	10	0.25	0.2
Progesterone	2200	Follicular	50–100	2.0	1.5
		Mid-luteal	1000–1500	25.0	24.0
17α-Hydroxy-progesterone	2300	Early follicular	30	0.6	0.2
		Late follicular	200	4.0	3–4
		Mid-luteal	200	4.0	3–4
Androstene-dione	2000		130–160	3.2	1.0–1.6
Testosterone	600		35	0.3	—
Dehydroepian-drosterone	1650		400–500	8.0	0.3–3.0
Dihydrotestos-terone	400		20	0.05	0.02

cAMP, but whether these substances are essential for gonadotropin stimulation of steroidogenesis is not clear. However, there is evidence indicating that the ovaries produce prostaglandins (PGE series) in response to LH, and these may be important in mediating changes in blood flow in the corpus luteum. Many studies have shown that cAMP or its derivatives can mimic the actions of LH. However, the concept of an obligatory role of cAMP in the steroidogenic response to LH has, at least until recently, been flawed by the fact that the dose–response curves for cAMP and steroid production differ by two to three orders of magnitude. This phenomenon has led to the concept of "spare receptors," since maximal stimulation of steroidogenesis by LH or HCG by testicular preparations is achieved with as little as 1 percent occupancy of the receptors. More recently, Catt and Dufau and their collaborators have provided presumptive evidence for the intermediacy of both cAMP and protein kinase in the steroidogenic response of testicular interstitial cells.[15] They found that there is a parallelism between the proportional saturation of protein kinase by cAMP and the extent of response. Channing and co-workers have shown that about 5 to 10 percent occupancy of LH receptors on porcine granulosa cells is required for both maximal cAMP and progesterone responses.[12] In this case, there may be a tighter coupling of the LH receptors and the cyclase system. There is no question of the importance of LH binding to cell membrane receptors. For example, ovaries from neonatal rats do not respond to LH and fail to bind labeled LH or HCG. The ability to bind LH increases with age, as does the ability to respond with increased cAMP formation and the associated protein kinase response to cAMP. However, the mechanism by which these changes influence steroidogenesis in either the testis or ovary is not known.

Several recent studies have shown that important changes occur during follicular maturation that are brought about by gonadotropins and perhaps by estradiol as the follicle matures from the primordial state through the graafian stage. The size of the granulosa cells increase somewhat and they appear to gain surface microvilli. Furthermore, as the follicle matures, there is a 10- to 1000-fold increase in binding of LH to the granulosa cell as shown by several groups of investigators. This increased binding of LH has been shown to be the result of an increase in surface receptor number rather than an increase in affinity for the hormone. Concurrently, there appears to be a decrease in binding of FSH to granulosa cells but of a much smaller magnitude. The increase in LH binding sites is accompanied by an increase in the ability of LH to stimulate cAMP synthesis and accumulation. This effect appears to be a direct stimulation of the enzyme adenylate cyclase, rather than a change in metabolism of cAMP. The ability of FSH to stimulate cAMP accumulation is some 12-fold greater in small follicles as compared to large follicles, which reflects a loss of receptors as follicles mature. It is of interest that the aromatase enzyme appears to be stimulated by FSH in rodent ovaries. Estrogen production is augmented greatly if substrate (testosterone) and FSH are added to granulosa cells in culture.[16] A decline in the number of LH receptors on target cells following LH administration has been observed by many investigators. This phenomenon has been observed in studies of a variety of peptide hormones and has been termed "down regulation." Evidence has been obtained with hormones such as insulin indicating that the disappearance of receptors is due to internalization of a portion of the cell surface containing the hormone receptor complex. The time required for return of receptors to the membrane, either by recycling or synthesis of new receptor molecules, varies. The return of receptor binding of LH in the corpus luteum requires 5 to 6 days following a single large dose of LH or HCG. It is not yet clear whether internalization of receptor complexes is essential to hormone action or whether it is simply a normal metabolic process involved in receptor protein turnover. If the latter is the case, "spare receptors" might be necessary for a sustained response by luteal or Leydig cells. "Spare" receptors may also be important in providing optimum local concentrations of hormone to promote binding to a small number of high-affinity sites (which are difficult to detect with currently available methods).

The elegant studies of Channing and her co-workers have elaborated the requirements for luteinization of granulosa cells and the development of the capacity to secrete progesterone.[12] They showed that, in addition to LH and FSH, several other hormones, including insulin, glucocorticoid, and thyroid hormones, are necessary for full luteinization. The precise role of these hormones has not been elucidated, but presumably they affect many cellular functions as they do in other target cells.

MECHANISM OF ACTION OF OVARIAN STEROIDS

THE ROLE OF BINDING TO PLASMA PROTEINS

Following secretion from their tissue of origin, all steroid hormones are bound in varying degree to one or more plasma proteins. The amount of steroid bound varies depending upon the steroid in question and the species. This subject has been extensively reviewed recently by Westphal,[17] Rosner,[18] and Mercier-Bodard et al.[19] In the human, binding of steroids occurs primarily to albumin and to two well-characterized proteins that bind with higher affinities but much lower capacity, corticosteroid binding

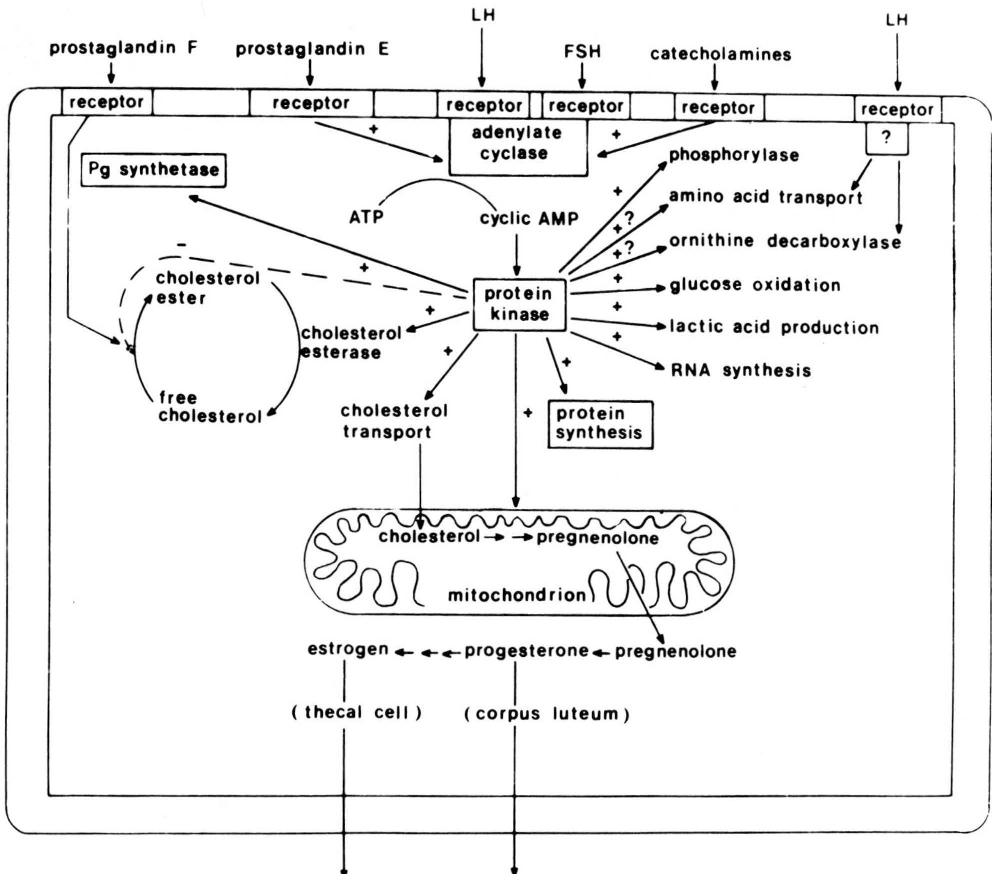

Fig. 110-2. General mechanism of action of gonadotropins on the ovary. Stimulatory actions are indicated by solid arrows (+), and inhibitory actions are indicated by dotted arrows (−). (Reprinted from C. P. Channing and A. Tsafriri, Metabolism 26: 413–468, 1977, with permission from the authors and Grune & Stratton, Inc.)

globulin (CBG) and sex hormone binding globulin (SHBG). Both of these proteins have binding sites that accept related hormones with affinities that approach those of the tissue receptors as shown in Table 110-2. Of interest is the fact that human CBG, also known as transcortin, binds progesterone with equal or higher affinity than it binds cortisol, whereas the synthetic glucocorticoids such as dexamethasone do not bind at all. On the other hand, CBG from other species such as the rat and sheep have little or no affinity for progesterone. Despite extensive study with purified proteins, the subtle chemical changes in the binding sites that account for these highly selective differences are not yet known. Estimates of the amount of free cortisol in normal or pregnancy plasma indicated that less than 5 to 10 percent of the total is free. The early observations that plasma CBG levels are increased during pregnancy thus provided a reasonable explanation for the failure of pregnant women to develop Cushingoid symptoms despite their markedly elevated plasma cortisol levels. The elevation in plasma concentration of CBG during pregnancy is probably due to high estrogen levels, since administration to men or nonpregnant women raises CBG to levels similar to those found in pregnancy. Together with some in vitro data, these observations led to the prevailing belief that only the free cortisol fraction is biologically active. Several more recent reports contradict this view. It has been shown that the administration of corticosterone with or without CBG to rats did not alter the half-life of the steroid,[20] the induction of hepatic tyrosine amino transferase, or the fall in circulatory lymphocytes.[21] These data would suggest that CBG has no effect in hindering the access of corticosterone to liver or blood cells. Even more striking are recent results showing that CBG does not alter the clearance of cortisol during perfusion of the human placenta in vitro, whereas albumin has a marked effect (W. Rosner, personal communication). However, there may be important tissue differences with respect to the limiting effect of CBG on glucocorticoid action. Keller et al.[22] found that corticosterone stimulated production of the enzyme alanine amino transferase in the liver, regardless of the CBG level, but induction occurred in the pancreas only at low CBG levels. The available evidence suggests that steroid binding to CBG has no obligatory role in promoting the action of cortisol, but there is some question about its limiting effect at the cellular level. Some evidence has been obtained suggesting that tissue levels of CBG are higher than can be accounted for by serum contamination in the uterus,[23] placenta,[24] and breast tumors.[25] These findings in estrogen target

Table 110-2. Approximate Affinities of Steroids for Serum Proteins and Tissue Receptors

	Dissociation Constant K_D M × 10^9		
	Serum Binder		Target Tissue Receptor
	SHBG	CBG	
Estradiol	5	>10	0.1 (E)
Estrone	>10	>100	0.3 (E)
Androstenedione	—	—	—
Testosterone	2	>100	1 (A)
Dihydrotestosterone	1	>100	1 (A)
Progesterone	>100	2	1 (P)
Cortisol	>100	3	3 (G)

Key: E = estrogen receptor; A = androgen receptor, P = progesterone receptor; G = glucorticoid receptor.

tissues, together with the fact that CBG is elevated by estrogens during pregnancy, suggest that CBG may be more important in the regulation of progesterone rather than glucocorticoid action. This possibility has not been explored.

On the basis of recent studies demonstrating remarkable anti-inflammatory-immunosuppressive action of progesterone when present in high local concentrations in vivo, the authors have proposed that progesterone production by the placental trophoblasts may play an important role in the survival of the products of conception in an immunologically hostile environment.[26] It is not yet clear, however, whether this effect is mediated by progesterone itself or by cortisol that is displaced from CBG in the presence of high levels of progesterone. The latter mechanism is not unreasonable, since the progesterone concentrations measured in human placental tissue range from 10 to 30 μM. This is perhaps 100 times higher than the CBG concentration in blood so that virtually all of the cortisol entering the placenta bound to CBG could be displaced transiently to provide a supraphysiologic dose of free cortisol within the placenta. Reequilibration of progesterone, cortisol, and CBG in the general circulation would restore the bound and free concentrations observed by Rosenthal et al.[27] This phenomenon could explain the extensive conversion of cortisol to cortisone during its transplacental passage, since essentially all of it would be made available to the 11β-hydroxysteroid dehydrogenase enzyme.

In 1966 several laboratories showed that there was a β-globulin in human serum that binds testosterone and estradiol.[28,29] Subsequent studies from several laboratories demonstrated that a single low-capacity, high-affinity globulin, SHBG, was responsible for binding many sex steroids, as shown in Table 110-2. Early attempts at purification were frustrated by the instability of SHBG, but at least three laboratories have now reported its isolation using methods based upon affinity chromatography. The chemical composition and physical properties of SHBG have been published by Rosner.[18] Many methods have been described for estimating SHBG concentrations in serum.[30–35] The techniques included Sephadex equilibration, equilibrium dialysis, paper electrophoresis, absorption, and polyacrylamide gel electrophoresis. Each of these have certain disadvantages that make them either tedious or less than accurate. Because of its higher affinity for SHBG, it is now recognized that tritiated DHT is the ligand of choice. The measurement of any equilibrium binding process by methods that of necessity disturb the equilibrium are subject to error. Rosner's method avoids this problem by precipitating SHBG-bound radioactive DHT selectively with ammonium sulfate.[34] A satisfactory assay has also been developed in which the steroid protein complex is adsorbed to filter discs of DEAE-cellulose.[36] The estimation of the true unbound concentration of testosterone or estradiol is more difficult. Although requiring large volumes of plasma and specialized equipment, the steady-state gel filtration method described by Fisher and Anderson[37] probably reflects most accurately the in vivo situation, since observations are made on undiluted plasma at physiologic temperature and pH. Measurements of total SHBG capacity may be just as useful, however, since the unbound testosterone fraction appears to be proportional to the SHBG concentration.

The concentration of SHBG is twofold greater in normal women than in men. It is elevated in male hypogonadism, cirrhosis of the liver, hyperthyroidism, pregnancy, and following the administration of estrogen. SHBG levels are lowered by androgens, advancing age, and hypothyroidism in women. Both SHBG and CBG are thought to be synthesized in the liver, although the evidence for this is meager. That SHBG synthesis is apparently regulated by both sex steroids and thyroid hormones provides a rather unique opportunity to investigate the interaction of these two classes of hormones. SHBG is believed to limit the concentration of free testosterone in the circulation. Good evifence supporting this idea comes from the studies of Vermeulen[38] and Rosenfield[39] and others, demonstrating that the "apparent free testosterone concentration" is a better indicator of hyperandrogenism than the total testosterone in patients with virilism. The physiological significance of estradiol binding to SHBG in women is less clear, since it binds less avidly and its serum concentrations are much lower than the binding capacity. Wu et al.[40] showed that the serum free estradiol concentration is a constant proportion of the total throughout the menstrual cycle. On the basis of in vitro studies, however, Burke and Anderson[41] suggested that SHBG may serve to amplify changes in androgen and estrogen production. If estrogen production increases, SHBG production increases as a result of an increase in free estradiol and the increased SHBG will lower the free testosterone fraction. Conversely, a rise in T production will amplify its own effect by causing a fall in SHBG and a differential rise in unbound T relative to E_2. Since the administration of thyroid hormone increases SHBG, these workers suggested that treatment of hirsutism associated with hypersecretion of adrenal androgens might best be accomplished with prednisolone and small amounts of tri-iodothyronine or an estrogen-containing contraceptive pill.[42]

SHBG levels are low in myxedema and also appear to be low in acromegaly. SHBG levels are in the female range in men with hypogonadism and in subjects with testicular feminization, presumably as a result of the androgen-resistant state. Elevated levels are also found in subjects with hepatic cicrhosis, probably as a result of elevated peripheral estrogen production of estrone (see below). The increase in SHBG may severely reduce the free testosterone concentrations, and therefore estrogen dominance as seen in gynecomastia can occur in the absence of markedly elevated estrogen levels. The highest levels of SHBG have been recorded in thyrotoxicosis, and similar mechanisms may give rise to gynecomastia, since it is known that peripheral estrogen production is increased in hyperthyroidism.

It appears at present that binding of sex steroids to serum proteins is not directly involved in their mechanism of action. The steroids are quite soluble enough to circulate in the plasma at concentrations in which they are fully active. Many studies have shown that steroid hormones are fully active in vitro in serum-free media, although there is some evidence that suggests that metabolic disposition of androgens may be influenced by the presence of SHBG. Thus the major role of steroid binding globulins at present appears to provide a "reservoir" of bound hormone that effectively dampens wide oscillations in the free concentration. It is clear that SHBG can markedly affect the metabolic clearance rate of the sex steroids, since the MCR of a steroid is inversely related to its affinity for SHBG (Table 110-1). Also, the sex differences in MCR for testosterone and estradiol are in accord with the difference in SHBG levels. Furthermore, it is apparent that SHBG may play an important role in altering the balance of androgens and estrogens that interact with target tissues. Because of the similarities to steroid hormone receptors, it might be speculated that the plasma binders represent evolutionary precursors of cellular receptors, and have functions no longer necessary. On the other hand, they may have important roles that have not been detected. One seemingly trivial but nonetheless important function is to retain steroid hormones in the vascular tree so that they may be delivered to appropriate target tissues rather than being partitioned into lipid rich adipose cells.

STEROID HORMONE RECEPTORS

The accumulation of the steroid hormones estrogen and progesterone in their target tissues depends upon the binding of these steroids to specific intracellular proteins called receptors. Many extensive reviews have been published recently.[43–47] The recognition of receptors followed early in vivo studies in which it was found that target tissues retained radiolabeled estrogens for longer periods of time than nontarget tissues.[48] Extensive study over the past 15 years has led to the general scheme shown in Fig. 110-3 that is applicable to all classes of steroid hormones. The steroids appear to enter all cells by passive diffusion but bind to cytoplasmic receptors present only in target cells. The receptor steroid complex then appears to undergo a temperature- and hormone-dependent transformation before it moves to the nucleus, where it is tightly bound to specific sites on chromatin, called acceptor sites. This interaction leads to the synthesis of greater quantities of specific messenger RNA (mRNA) molecules by mechanisms not yet clarified. Depending upon the hormone in question, this may involve one or many mRNA species that direct the synthesis of new or existing proteins. The appearance of the receptor complex in the nucleus is a specific process for each hormone which occurs under physiological circumstances. In the case of estrogen-stimulated uterine growth, it has been shown that nuclear occupancy of the receptor complex must be sustained for 6 to 8 hours in order to obtain a full response.[49] Clark and his associates have also demonstrated that the so-called weak or impeded estrogens such as estriol are capable of full stimulation of uterine growth if given in multiple injections or continuously. Thus the older concept that estrogens such as estriol may be protective against breast cancer is no longer tenable.

Although there is a considerable amount of data that supports the scheme shown in Fig. 110-3, Gannon and Gorski have recently pointed out several problems that are usually ignored.[47] There is no question about nuclear accumulation of steroid receptor complexes, but the precise intracellular location of the receptor prior to interaction with steroid is not certain. Virtually all studies of the estrogen receptor (ER) in the uterus have utilized low ionic strength buffers during tissue disruption. The use of these highly unphysiological conditions that are known to disrupt membranes and subcellular organelles, including the nucleus, casts doubt on the "cytoplasmic" location of the receptor. Indeed, evidence has recently been presented for the presence of estrogen receptors on the surface membrane of endometrial cells.[50] Furthermore, careful kinetic analysis of hormone uptake in vivo strongly suggested that the transformation of the receptor complex actually occurs in the nucleus of the rat uterus.[51] Together with unpublished data indicating that there is little, if any, high-affinity binding to "cytoplasmic" ER in vivo, these findings suggest that the scheme shown in Fig. 110-3 may be based to some extent on experimental artifacts and should be viewed with caution. Nonetheless, the general characteristics of receptors are important, since their measurement hus proven to be of clinical value in identifying estrogen dependent breast tumors and understanding the androgen resistance of testicular feminization.

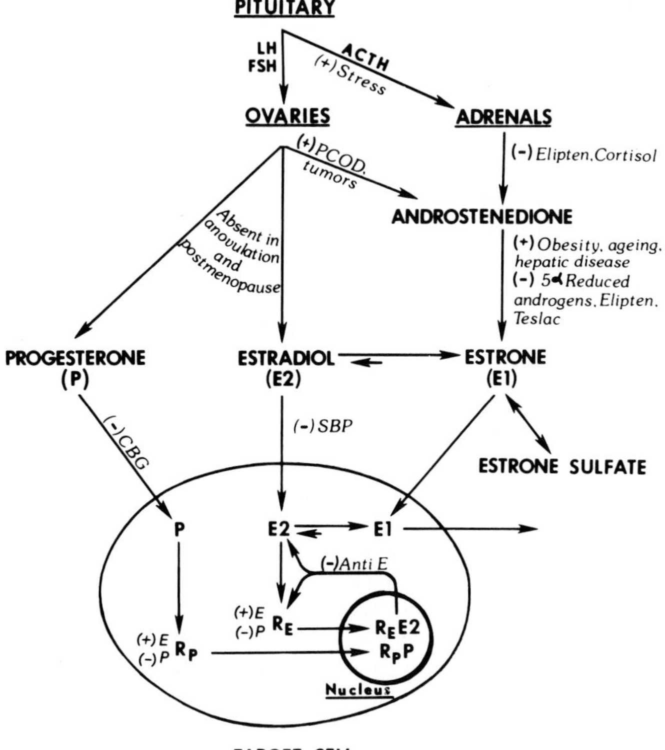

Fig. 110-3. Scheme illustrating the sources of estrogen and progesterone regulatory mechanisms, and their interaction with target cell receptors in the human.

Since the biological responses to steroid hormones are saturable phenomena, the quantity of receptor contained in target tissues should be limited. Indeed, the number of receptor molecules for the various steroid hormones has been estimated to be on the order of 5000 to 20,000 per cell. Furthermore, since the physiological concentrations of steroid hormones in the blood ranges from 10^{-8} to 10^{-10}M, the affinity of the receptors must of necessity be in the same range for a biologically meaningful interaction to occur. Thus receptors are characterized as having high affinity for steroid hormones ($K_D \approx 10^{-10}$M) as compared with binding to many other tissue or serum components. Even if the dissociation constant (K_D) is of the same order of magnitude as a serum-binding protein, the dissociation rate from the receptor is usually much slower. Steroid hormone receptors display characteristic binding specificity for different classes of hormones. Thus, estrogen receptors bind many natural and synthetic estrogenic steroids with relatively small differences in affinity, whereas physiological concentrations of androgens or progesterone are hardly bound at all. Exceptions occur, as with glucocorticoid receptors in that they also bind progesterone. In most systems examined, however, this interaction does not result in a glucocorticoid signal, und therefore progesterone is a glucocorticoid antagonist.[45] Biological crosstalk between hormones can occur when pharmacological amounts of steroid hormones are administered. Several reports have shown that androgens can bind to ER and activate uterine tissues, whereas progesterone can bind to the androgen receptor (AR) and is a weak androgen. Steroid hormone receptors also exhibit tissue specificity; the classical estrogen target tissues including uterus, vagina, and mammary gland have much higher receptor content than nontarget tissues such as muscle and liver. However, this generalization must be qualified by the fact that the ability to detect receptors is dictated largely by the specific radioactivity of the available steroid probes. The low but measureable content of hepatic estrogen receptors may have just as much significance for some liver functions as do the more plentiful glucocorticoid receptors. That receptors are important in hormone action is best demonstrated by the failure of an appropriate biologic response to the steroid when they are genetically deleted or are present but nonfunctional. This has been best demonstrated in the case of androgen resistance in pseudohermaphroditic mice[52] or humans[53] and glucocorticoid resistant lymphoma cells.[54]

Binding experiments have shown that each of the classes of receptor molecules have a single binding site. Despite evidence to the contrary, there does not appear to be cooperativity in the binding reactions as occurs with 0_2 and hemoglobin. The classical 8S cytoplasmic form of the estrogen receptor, first described by Toft and Gorski who analyzed binding by density ultracentrifugation analysis,[55] has been observed for all of the sex steroid hormones. The 8S form appears in low ionic strength buffers and is changed to a 4S or intermediate forms by salt addition. This phenomenon has been ascribed to aggregation of the receptor with other proteins and probably has no physiological significance. Demonstration of an 8S form can be taken as strong evidence for receptor molecules, however, since all the serum binders sediment in the 4S region. A portion of the nuclear receptors can usually be obtained by salt extraction, and in the case of estrogen, these sediment at around 5S. Much attention is currently directed to the physiological significance of the unextractable portion of the nuclear bound hormone complexes. Both estrogen and progesterone receptors contain unlike subunits. In the best-suited case using highly purified progesterone receptor preparations, B and A subunits, each binding a progesterone molecule, have been shown to bind to acidic nucleoproteins and DNA, respectively.[43] O'Malley, Schrader, and associates suggested that A and B subunits may interact with chromatin to make specific gene regions available to RNA polymerases. However, the nature of the receptor interaction with chromatin that actually results in the activation of transcription is uncertain. Indeed, the concept of nuclear acceptor sites is controversial at this time.

Of particular interest are recent studies concerning the regulation of tissue receptor levels. Receptor concentrations vary widely under hormonal developmental, genetic, pathological, and pharmacological circumstances. In spite of the present uncertainties concerning the final molecular mechanisms involved in hormone action, studies of fluctuations in receptor concentration have greatly increased our understanding of hormonally regulated processes. Positive and negative control of receptor levels are best understood for estrogen and progesterone. Neonatal estrogen target tissues of the rat have very low ER levels. Receptors are detectable at about 10 days of life, after which time they can be increased greatly by the administration of estrogen. Many studies have shown that estrogen stimulates synthesis not only of its own receptor but also that of progesterone receptors (PR). Conversely, progesterone has a negative effect on both classes of receptor (Fig. 110-3). This "inactivation" of its own receptor by progesterone is not fully understood. This effect could be exerted through the receptor at the level of synthesis or decay (down regulation). There is evidence suggesting that progesterone prevents recycling of the nuclear ER. Nevertheless, measurements in both animals and humans are consistent with the well-known priming effect of estrogen required for progesterone effects in the endometrium and the antiestrogenic properties of progesterone. Following the pioneering work of Jensen, many investigators have demonstrated that a minimal threshold of estrogen receptors must be present in breast tumors if they are to respond to hormonal therapy. However, caution must be used in extrapolating findings from one tissue or species to another, since many variations occur. For example, regulation of receptor levels in adjacent tissues such as endometrium and myometrium may differ considerably. Genetic regulation of receptor levels and function is also complex. While total absence of androgen receptor has been observed in the complete testicular feminization syndrome, intermediate levels have been found in patients with less severe defects, indicating a gene dosage effect on receptor synthesis. However, the finding of a normal complement of cytoplasmic androgen receptor in some androgen resistant states also indicates that abnormal receptors may be synthesized and that subsequent steps such as chromatin binding may be defective.[53] These possibilities have been demonstrated in elegant studies of glucocorticoid receptors in lymphoma mutants by Yamamoto and Tomkins.[54]

The study of hormone receptor interactions has shed much light on the complex actions of antihormones of every class of steroid hormone. As already indicated, many examples of antagonism of hormones through receptor binding by naturally occurring steroids are known. Best characterized is the interaction of progesterone with glucocorticoid and mineralocorticoid receptors. Hormonal metabolites such as the catechol estrogens may be antagonistic by failing to elicit normal responses despite binding to the estrogen receptor. When one considers the enormous array of known steroid metabolites for all the steroid hormones, the number of possibilities for regulation in normal or pathologic states is staggering. An interesting example may be cited in the androgen field. Studies of the formation and content of dihydrotestosterone (DHT) in both human and canine prostatic hypertrophy strongly suggested that accumulation of DHT and prolonged stimulation of cellular proliferation was the key to the etiology of this disease.[56,57] However, long-term administration of DHT to dogs failed to induce hypertrophy, but more recently studies have shown that androstanediol is effective in this regard and that simultaneous estrogen administration is synergistic.[58] These results illustrate the complexities involved in the interaction of different classes of hormones, their metabolites (or active forms) and receptors.

The interactions of synthetic antiestrogens with estrogen receptors have recently been studied in detail. Compounds such as nafoxidine and tamoxifen have been shown to bind to the cytoplasmic receptor, and the resulting complexes are translocated to the nucleus. In contrast to estradiol, however, the nuclear complexes remain for prolonged periods of time (days or weeks). This remarkably unusual behavior is associated with a failure of cytoplasmic receptor regeneration. These results suggest that the allosteric conformation of receptor complex formed with antiestrogens is abnormal and results in tight binding to the nucleus but failure to elicit estrogenic effects, including synthesis of cytoplasmic ER. Alternatively, failure to recycle ER may limit the response to antiestrogens. Baulieu (personal communication), however, has suggested that tamoxifen may increase progesterone receptor levels in endometrial cancer, which suggests that neither of these explanations is entirely satisfactory. An extensive theoretic discussion of the interactions of agonists and antagonists with receptor has been provided by Sherman.[59]

The general acceptance of the concept that steroid hormone receptors are of central importance in hormone action has created a dogma that few investigators dare to ignore. Several important effects of sex steroids that appear not to be mediated by intracellular receptors have been recently reported. Perhaps the most striking of these, because it stands in stark contrast to the idea that steroids regulate transcriptional events, is the mechanism by which progesterone promotes amphibian oocyte maturation. The growth of the oocyte occurs while the nucleus (germinal vesicle) remains suspended in the first meiotic prophase. It is well established that this period involves intense metabolic activity involving both RNA and protein synthesis. Some of this activity is required for oocyte growth, but many of the gene products are conserved for weeks for use in early embrogenesis. Several laboratories have shown that the stimulus of this activity is progesterone produced in the ovary and that the steroid effect is exerted at the oocyte membrane. Indeed, progesterone is ineffective if injected into the oocyte, and growth, and further, maturation can be induced in enucleated cells. It now appears that the interaction of progesterone with the egg membrane results in a hormone and time-dependent increase in the intracellular calcium ion concentration. The influx of calcium leads to the synthesis of specific cytoplasmic proteins that can be transferred to unstimulated oocytes, resulting in their activation, germinal vesicle breakdown, and eventual maturation.[60] The activating factor(s) can be propagated through 10 serial transfers if protein synthesis is maintained. Clearly this system has totally different characteristics than the chick oviduct or mammalian uterus in that calcium appears to be a second messenger that operates at the level of translation. It is not known if similar mechanisms operate in mammalian cells, but the anesthetic effects of progesterone metabolites are likely to be mediated by membrane interactions. Perhaps the aforementioned anti-inflammatory effect of progesterone[26] may involve membrane interactions with host defense cells such as macrophages that results in inhibition of some crucial function such as cell motility.

Although less clear, the stimulatory effect of estrogens on uterine blood flow (UBF) may be another example of a nonreceptor-mediated action. Experiments in sheep have shown that the potency of different estrogens in increasing UBF does not correlate with receptor binding; i.e., estriol and estradiol are equipotent. Furthermore, the effect shows a 30-min lag period and is blocked by protein synthesis inhibitors but not by actinomycin D. By the use of appropriate blockers, it was shown that the effect is not mediated by neurotransmitters.[61] At present, it seems likely that the estrogen effect on blood flow may involve alteration in prostaglandin production. It is of interest to recall in this regard that the growth of the uterus during pregnancy is largely due to mechanical stretch induced by the expanding products of conception. Furthermore, increased blood flow in target tissues is observed after the administration of many hormones such as ACTH, LH, and TSH. The relative importance of an increased supply of substrates, and increased enzyme synthesis resulting from increased transcription, in hormone action remains to be determined.

THE NORMAL OVARY

FETAL AND PREMENARCHAL DEVELOPMENT

The undifferentiated gonad appears in the human embryo around 26 days following fertilization and consists of a thickening of the coelemic epithelium overyling cells of the mesonephric blastema and primordial germ cells which migrate into this region from the hindgut. The coelemic epithelium gives rise to the cortex and the primitive urogenital mesenchyme to the medulla of the gonad. In the absence of a Y chromosome, the ovary develops with granulosa cells being derived from the cortex while interstitial and thecal cells arise from the medulla. Follicular organization begins in utero by around 2 months when many oocytes are found surrounded by several layers of granulosa cells, and epithelial theca interna cells may be found around the basement membrane at this time.

Recent studies in the rabbit have shown that both the testis and ovary commence steroidogenesis before they can be morphologically distinguished. Wilson and his associates have shown that the capacity for testicular testosterone production in the fetal rabbit is precisely heralded by the appearance of the enzyme complex 3β-hydroxysteroid dehydrogenase-steroid-Δ^5-isomerase.[62] Furthermore, the estrogen-forming enzyme aromatase can be detected at the same developmental stage in the primitive ovary.[63] In accordance with the classical concepts of Jost, male differentiation is dependent upon testosterone and the elusive mullerian duct regression factor. On the basis of careful enzymatic studies, Siiteri and Wilson predicted that the conversion of testosterone to dihydrotestosterone by the 5α-reductase enzyme is required for normal development of the prostate and external genitalia.[64] This was subsequently borne out when two reports appeared nearly simultaneously describing human pedigrees with 5α-reductase deficiency in which incomplete male development at birth is partially completed at puberty.[65,66] The acquisition of normal male reproductive function and reversal of sexual identity by children raised as girls is one of the most remarkable experiments of nature and raises important questions concerning the role of sex hormones in behavior.

While it is generally held that differentiation of the female genitalia is passive, it is possible that fetal ovarian estrogen synthesis may play a role in stimulating mitotic replication of primordial germ cells or their transition to oogonia, the oocyte precursors. The number of oogonia in the human fetal ovary reaches a maximum of 6 to 7 million around 5 months and then declines to around 2 million at birth. Between the eighth and thirteenth week of gestation, oogonia initiate meiosis, which proceeds to the diplotene stage of prophase, after which the cells are arrested until they complete meiosis, shortly before ovulation, many years later. The number of oocytes continues to decline after birth so that only 100,000 to 200,000 remain at menarche. The mechanisms by which oogonia and oocytes are lost during fetal life and before puberty are not understood, although ultrastructural studies suggest that many are physically shed from the ovary. It is possible that small amounts of ovarian androgens may promote atresia, as is likely to occur in the mature ovary (see below).

Occasional antral follicles may be found in ovaries from prepubertal children, whereas the bulk of the follicles are either in the primordial or atretic state. The ovary increases in size after birth as a result of an increase in volume due to maturing follicles and also due to accumulation of stromal residue formed by atresia. The medullary stroma increases during the premenarchal years and appears to invade the cortex and disperse the primordial follicles. As puberty develops, cyclical discharge of the pituitary gonadotropins FSH and LH begins, and full development of usually one follicle and ovulation begin.

Many theories have been proposed to explain the endocrine changes that initiate ovulation at menarche. Grumbach and associates (see Chapter 106 and 108) have proposed that a decrease in the sensitivity of the hypothalamic-pituitary unit to the negative feedback of gonadal steroids permits the release of LRF and gonadotropins and activation of gonadal steroidogenesis. They have further proposed that maturational changes in the CNS and/or pituitary of females eventuate in the ability of the hypothalamic-pituitary unit to respond positively to estrogen with an LH surge. The specific mechanisms underlying these changes are poorly understood, however. The onset of ovulatory cycles appears to be preceded by a period during which the pituitary secretes both FSH and LH cyclically in patterns that are similar to those observed in young girls who ovulate.[67] It is not yet known whether ovarian estrogen secretion also fluctuates, although progressive increments in mean serum estradiol levels and maturation of secondary sexual characteristics imply developing ovarian function. Nonovarian estrogen production from adrenal and ovarian androstenedione may also increase during this time, however. The age of onset of puberty in both boys and girls has declined in most parts of the world in parallel with an increase in the growth rate and ultimate size in children. Frisch and her colleagues[68] have proposed that there is a critical body fat composition that is more important than age in triggering the onset of menarche. If this hypothesis is substantiated, it suggests that peripheral estrogen formation in fat from circulating androstenedione (see below) may "prime" the hypothalamus, pituitary, or even the ovary and initiate cyclical function.

THE MENSTRUAL CYCLE

The important fluctuations in the serum concentrations of pituitary and ovarian hormones that occur during the normal menstrual cycle are schematically illustrated in Figs. 110-4, 110-5, and 110-6. A 28-day cycle as shown is generally regarded as the mean length of normal cycles, but the range for different women extends from 25 to 35 days or more. Cycle length may vary considerably in the same woman, particularly at the beginning and end of the fertile years. The follicular phase of the cycle is much more variable than the luteal phase, the latter period being remarkably constant at 13 ± 1 or 2 days. The biological mechanisms responsible for the constancy of the luteal phase are unknown. However, infertility associated with the so-called short luteal phase appears to be due to inadequate gonadotropin stimulation of the developing follicle prior to ovulation.

In the early phase of follicular development, estradiol levels remain low. Beginning about 8 days before the LH peak, there is a gradual rise that becomes more accelerated and estradiol reaches maximum levels generally on the day before the LH peak. Serum estradiol concentration drops precipitously as both gonadotropins, LH and FSH, are rising and then rises to a peak again around the middle of the luteal phase. By the onset of menses, estradiol levels have fallen to their lowest point seen in the early follicular phase. Estrone levels (not shown) are always lower than those of estradiol, and the pattern generally mirrors that for estradiol. As will be shown later estrone is derived from several sources, including small amounts by secretion and larger amounts by peripheral conversion from androstenedione, and secreted estradiol. The bulk of the estradiol secreted by the ovaries arises from the follicle that is destined to ovulate.

Progesterone is secreted by the ovaries in very small amounts during the follicular phase. Additional progesterone is produced by the adrenals both by secretion and peripheral conversion of pregnenolone and pregnenolone sulfate. Progesterone levels increase slightly during the gonadotropin surge and then rise dramatically following ovulation and corpus luteum development. Maximal levels of progesterone of 10–15 ng/ml are reached 5 to 6 days following ovulation, and they fall during the last 4 days of the cycle as the corpus luteum regresses. If implantation of the fertilized

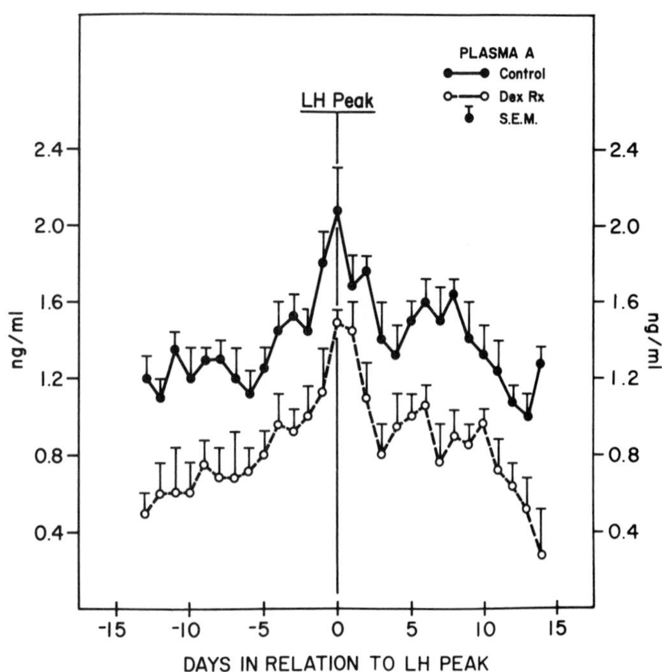

Fig. 110-5. Plasma levels of androstenedione during the menstrual cycle in 9 women studied with and without adrenal suppression. (Reprinted from G. E. Abraham, Ovarian and adrenal contribution to peripheral androgens during the menstrual cycle. J. Clin. Endocrinol. Metab. 39:340, 1974, with permission.)

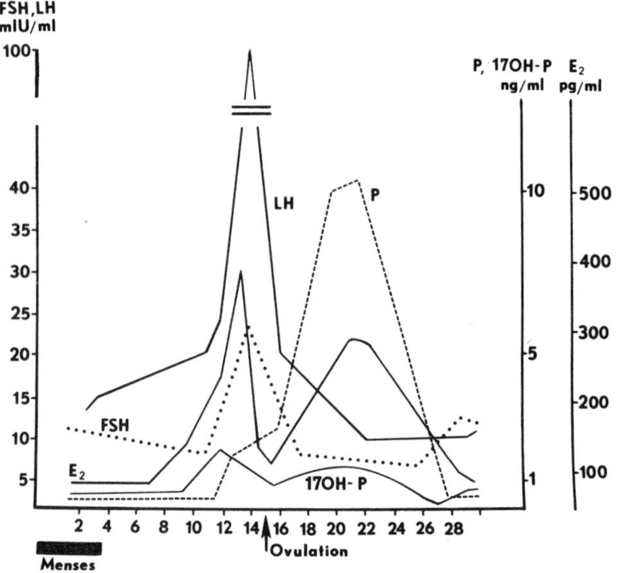

Fig. 110-4. Schematic representation of the changes in plasma hormones during the human menstrual cycle.

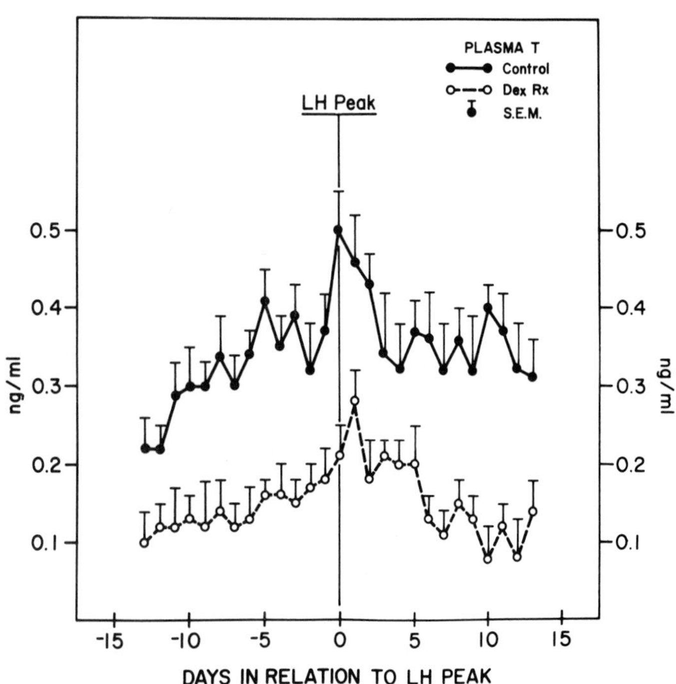

Fig. 110-6. Plasma levels of testosterone during the menstrual cycle (as in Fig. 110-5).

ovum occurs, however, HCG rescues the corpus luteum, and progesterone is maintained at mid-luteal phase levels.

Other steroids secreted by the ovary include 17α-hydroxyprogesterone. The pattern of 17α-hydroxyprogesterone secretion is intermediate between that of estradiol and progesterone. A small rise is noted that appears to coincide with the estradiol peak, and a much larger increase parallels the progesterone pattern during the luteal phase. Both progesterone and 17α-hydroxyprogesterone have been proposed as modulators of the hypothalamic-pituitary events that give rise to the gonadotropin surge. Although androstenedione has not been extensively studied, it would appear from the work of Abraham that ovarian secretion of this androgen reaches its maximum value in parallel with the midcycle surge of gonadotropins (Fig. 110-5). Serum testosterone levels also follow the same pattern, although this steroid is largely derived by peripheral conversion from androstenedione (Fig. 110-6). It is of interest that the temporal pattern of androstenedione secretion is delayed relative to that of estradiol. Androstenedione is usually considered to be the primary substrate for synthesis of estradiol in the ovary. That the secretion patterns differ implies that the cellular origin of the two steroids or the regulation of their secretion is different. Whether or not the midcycle increase in androstenedione secretion, or the estrone derived therefrom, plays a role in gonadotropin regulation remains to be determined. Small amounts of DHEA and DHEAS and dihydrotestosterone are secreted by the ovary but their function is not known.

INTRAOVARIAN REGULATORY MECHANISMS

Recent studies in animal models suggest that gonadotropin regulation of folliculogenesis and atresia is mediated at least in part by steroid hormones. It has long been known that estrogens can stimulate granulosa cell proliferation in the absence of gonadotropins. In the immature hypophysectomized rat (IHR) model, estrogens increase ovarian weight, reduce follicular atresia, induce granulosa cell hyperplasia and nexus formation, and increase the binding of and response to FSH. Thus, it is clear that estrogens alone can promote follicular development to the preantral stage. The demonstration of a characteristic receptor system for estrogen is consistent with these observations and indicates that cells that produce estrogen may also be targets for the hormone. The importance of estrogen in development of follicles in the human ovary may be inferred from the "resistant ovary" syndrome.[69] In this condition the ovaries are small and show no evidence of follicular maturation despite high plasma levels of FSH and LH. Sexual immaturity and primary amenorrhea in such patients implies that the primary cause of this syndrome is ovarian failure to produce estrogen. The biochemical nature of this defect remains to be defined, however.

In marked contrast to estrogen, androgens exert deleterious effects on granulosa cells and promote follicular atresia. Ross and his co-workers recently observed that a critical low dose of HCG given to estrogen-treated IHR decreased, whereas higher doses increased, ovarian weight. Careful follow-up of this anomalous finding revealed that the inhibitory effect was probably mediated by androgens and ultimately led to the demonstration of a putative testosterone receptor in granulosa cells.[70,71] At about the same time, studies by the authors showed that administration of testosterone or dihydrotestosterone to estrogen-treated IHR promotes follicular atresia.[72] The interesting observation also was made that progesterone can at least partially block the atretic effect of the androgens. Together, these studies suggest that LH stimulation of active androgen production may trigger atresia in certain follicles

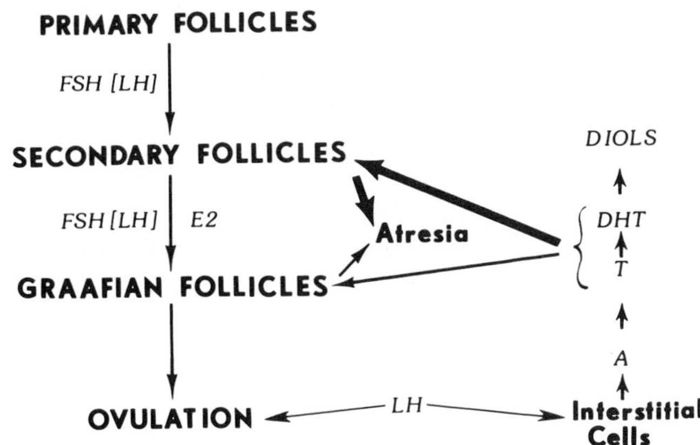

Fig. 110-7. Scheme illustrating the potential role of intraovarian androgens in promoting follicular atresia.

but not in others having a high estrogen and/or progesterone content (Fig. 110-7). Although direct evidence for such a scheme is unavailable in the human, it is well known that the polycystic ovary syndrome (PCO) is characterized by overproduction of androgens (see below). It is quite possible that the excessive androgen produced by thecal cells in response to the high LH levels effectively prevents normal follicular development and ovulation. Numerous studies of the steroid content of human follicular fluid have shown only that characteristic patterns of estradiol, progesterone, and androgens are found in various size follicles. Future studies will perhaps pinpoint more precisely the role of steroids in both normal and abnormal ovarian function.

Recent studies have implicated several nonsteroidal factors that may have important regulatory actions in follicle development. In 1975, Tsafriri and Channing reported that addition of porcine follicular fluid or granulosa cells could inhibit the spontaneous resumption of meiosis in isolated, cumulus-enclosed porcine oocytes.[73,74] Further studies have demonstrated the presence of two small molecular weight peptides (1000 and 2000 Dalton) that have oocyte maturation inhibitory (OMI) activity. They are present in higher concentration in follicular fluid from small than in large follicles. The mechanism of this inhibitory action is not yet understood. Channing and co-workers also have described a luteinization inhibitor that is present in porcine follicular fluid that appears to interfere with LH action[75] while others have found a factor that appears to prevent LH binding to corpus luteum receptors. Finally, evidence for the presence in follicular fluid of a factor called inhibin has been obtained by several groups of investigators.[76,77] Thus the present evidence strongly suggests that both the testes and ovaries produce a peptide that inhibits FSH secretion by the pituitary. These findings have far-reaching implications for improving our knowledge of ovarian function and for future approaches to fertility regulation.

THE POLYCYSTIC OVARY

The syndrome known as polycystic ovarian disease (PCOD), first described by Stein and Leventhal, constitutes a broad category of patients and is the most common cause of anovulation associated with hirsuitism. There are many known causes of PCOD, such as androgen-secreting tumors, Cushing's syndrome, and central nervous system tumors, although these represent only a small fraction of the total number of cases. In the vast majority of patients the etiologic factor(s) is still now known. However, recent studies have clarified many aspects of this disease process, so that a true understanding of the defect should be forthcoming in the near future. Yen has recently provided an extensive discussion of PCOD.[78]

It has long been recognized that hirsutism and virilism are commonly associated with PCOD, and therefore abnormalities of androgen metabolism have received extensive study. Although the mean plasma concentration of testosterone is significantly higher in PCOD patients than in normal women, there is considerable overlap in these ranges, so that this measurement alone is not useful for diagnostic purposes. However, the MCR of testosterone is significantly higher than in normal patients as a result of decreased levels of SHBG, so that the production rate of testosterone in PCOD patients is invariably elevated above normal. There is little overlap with normal woman, since the values are nearly fourfold higher. Androstenedione levels are elevated markedly in PCOD, and this elevation is largely due to increased ovarian secretion. Therefore, much of the elevated testosterone production is derived by peripheral conversion from androstenedione. The MCR of androstenedione is normal in PCOD patients, but the elevation of the production rate may be three to fourfold. The adrenal androgens DHEA and DHEAS are also frequently elevated, suggesting that hypersecretion of androgens by the adrenals occurs at least in some patients. Since women with this syndrome ovulate infrequently or not at all, estrogen levels are relatively constant, and they are derived principally from peripheral conversion of androgens. The relative serum concentrations of estradiol and estrone are reversed, i.e., estrone is higher than estradiol, as a result of the peripheral conversion of the increased amounts of androstenedione to estrone. Indeed, the finding of abnormally high levels of E_1 and low levels of E_2 in a premenopausal woman is a diagnostic indicator of PCOD. The ovaries of PCOD patients may secrete small quantities of estrogen, but this amounts to no more than 10 to 20 percent of the total production rate. Mean LH levels are considerably elevated above those found in the preovulatory phase, whereas FSH is usually in the low-normal range, and increased sensitivity of the pituitary to LRF stimulation has been demonstrated.[79] The frequency and amplitude of the pulsatile discharge of LH is also exaggerated in women with PCOD.

Many theories have been proposed to explain the failure of ovulation in PCOD. Abnormalities in the ovaries, adrenals, pituitary, and hypothalamus have all been suggested as the primary cause of PCOD. Early studies by Goldzhier and colleagues suggested that a defective or reduced ovarian aromatase activity was the primary cause. Measurements of urinary estrogens by others indicating normal levels were contradictory, however. The peripheral formation of estrone from elevated androstenedione levels readily explains this discrepancy.[80] The exaggerated pituitary LH response to LRF can also be explained by the elevated estrogens, although it is not known whether estrone is peculiar in this regard. The primary effect of excessive androgen production may be at the level of the ovary in preventing follicular maturation due to a higher than normal rate of atresia. Studies of the hormonal changes in women undergoing ovarian wedge resection are consistent with this view.[81] Wedge resection was followed by a prolonged decline in testosterone levels in 5 of 8 patients, and ovulation occurred without significant changes in plasma LH or FSH prior to the ovulatory discharge. These findings strongly imply that the beneficial effect was derived by reducing the levels of androgens within the ovary (Fig. 110-8). Successful induction of ovulation in some patients by treatment with glucocorticoid may be explained by a lowering of the intraovarian androgen milieu by suppression of adrenal androgen secretion. Sucessful treatment with the antiestrogen clomiphene increases both LH and FSH levels and the latter promotes follicular development, perhaps by stimulating the ovarian aromatase enzyme and the local estrogen concentration.

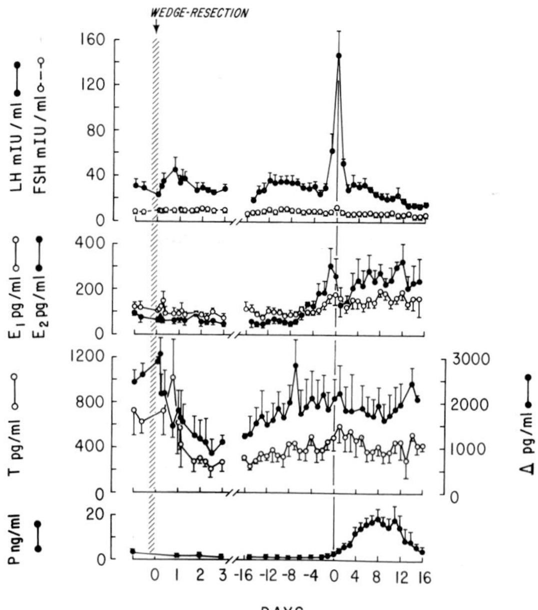

Fig. 110-8. Hormonal changes induced by ovarian wedge resection in patients with polycystic ovarian disease. (Reprinted with permission from H. C. Judd et al., J. Clin. Endocrinol. Metab. 43:347–355, 1976.)

The initiating events in PCOD remain to be established. Excessive production of adrenal androgens and their conversion to active compounds peripherally or within the ovary could interfere with normal follicular development during the onset of menarche. Rising LH levels would stimulate further androgen production by the ovaries and the increased amounts of peripheral estrone would chronically elevate LH secretion, resulting in the abnormal cycle of events. Inadequate follicular estrogen production as a result of deficient FSH secretion could also result in failure of follicular development and ovulation. Lower than normal FSH secretion could be the result of excessive inhibin production. Further experimentation is needed to decide between these and other possible mechanisms.

NONOVARIAN ESTROGEN PRODUCTION

Observing that urine of stallions contained large quantities of estrogen, whereas that of mares had little estrogen, Zondeck[82] in 1934 stated, "I believe that the female hormone which is regularly present in the male organism represents a normal physiological product of metabolism of the sex hormones, especially since—due to our present chemical knowledge—a conversion of the male hormone into the female one appears to be quite possible." This remarkable prediction expressed in the early dawn of endocrinology has been amply confirmed. Evidence supporting Zondeck's deduction was first reported by Steinach and Kun,[83] who in 1937 found that the administration of testosterone propionate increased estrogen in the urine of 6 men who received this androgen.

Since these early studies, many researchers have reported increased estrogen excretion after the administration of various C_{19} compounds, principally testosterone, in intact and castrate male and female human beings and various experimental animals. The first definitive evidence that the increased estrogen excretion was due to aromatization of the administered steroid was presented in 1956 by West and associates.[84] They found estrone and estradiol in the urine of two adrenalectomized, oophorectomized women who had been administered testosterone proprionate. Before treatment, estrogen could not be detected in urine from these subjects. This study provided strong support for the thesis that the increased amounts of estrogen found in urine after testosterone treatment arose from the conversion of testosterone to naturally occurring estrogens. Since then, many workers have also shown that the administration of isotopically labeled testosterone to normal men is followed by the appearance of radioactive estrogens in their urine (for review, see refs. 85, 86, and 87).

More recently a number of laboratories have attempted to quantify the extent to which conversion of endogenous androgens contributes to extraglandular estrogen in the human being.[11,80,88–90] The demonstration that placental estrogen production in the human being is totally dependent on externally provided C_{19} steroidal precursors[91,92] focused attention on this new mechanism of hormone production. It has become apparent from these studies that the peripheral conversion of androgens to estrogens in nonpregnant women and in men is a physiologically important determinant of the hormonal milieu in both healthy and diseased states.

Following puberty the gonads of both males and females secrete the sex steroids, and the adrenal cortex secretes DHEAS, DHEA, and A. While DHEAS gives rise to the bulk of the 17-ketosteroids and to a small fraction of plasma testosterone, insignificant conversion to estrogen is observed except during pregnancy in the female. During pregnancy as much as 50 percent of the DHEAS in the maternal circulation can be converted to estradiol[92] in the placenta. Conversion of DHEAS to estrogen has not been found in non pregnant females,[93] whereas the conversion of free DHEA to estrogen is less than 0.1 percent.[94] On the other hand, A is converted to estrone in both males and females. In males, testosterone is also converted to estradiol, and estrogen derived by extraglandular conversion of both A and T accounts for 75 to 80 percent of total estrogen production, the remainder arising by testicular secretion.[80] In the early follicular phase of the menstrual cycle the production rate of estrone is approximately 40 μg/day, and most of this arises by peripheral conversion from androstenedione derived from both the ovaries and the adrenal glands. The conversion of A to E_1 in normal lean premenopausal women is on the order of 1 to 1.5 percent. About one-half of the total production rate of A (~3 mg/day) is derived from the adrenal glands and the other half from the ovaries. Following the menopause, the ovarian secretion of A falls to negligible amounts and the adrenals continue to secrete approximately 1–1.5 mg of A per day. The extent of conversion of androstenedione to estrone is increased after the menopause, presumably due to some aging process, to levels of 2 to 3 percent so that the production rate of estrone from androstenedione in normal postmenopausal subjects is also about 40 μg/day.[88]

A number of conditions are known to increase the production of estrone from circulating androstenedione in both men and women. These include hyperthyroidism,[90] aging, hepatic disease, and obesity.[80] Each of these conditions is associated with an increased efficiency of conversion. The conversion of A to E_1 may be elevated four to fivefold in obese postmenopausal females with uterine bleeding. Similarly, in males with hepatic disease, the conversion of both androstenedione to estrone and testosterone to estradiol is increased, and the estrogen produced may result in gynecomastia, even in the face of normal testosterone production.[80] On the other hand, estrone production in postmenopausal and premenopausal women may be increased if the production rate of androstenedione is elevated. This is most commonly observed in postmenopausal females with nonendocrine tumors of the ovary with associated stromal hyperplasia and in younger women with polycystic ovarian disease or a variety of functional or nonfunctional ovarian tumors.[80]

Despite extensive study, the principal site of peripheral aromatization and why, under some circumstances, this process becomes more active, is still not certain. A number of studies have suggested that most extraglandular estrogen formation occurs in adipose tissue. Low levels of the aromatase enzyme have been demonstrated in adipose tissue in vitro by several investigators.[95–97] Also, the extent of conversion of plasma androstenedione to estrone is highly significantly correlated with excessive body weight in postmenopausal women,[98] as well as in young ovulatory and anovulatory women.[99] When ^{14}C-androstenedione is infused intravenously, the ^{14}C-estrone formed in extraglandular sites enters the blood much more slowly in obese subjects than in nonobese subjects.[100] This slow release of estrone formed from infused androstenedione is also reflected in the rate of excretion of its urinary metabolites in obese women as compared to nonobese subjects. However, markedly increased conversion of androstenedione to estrone can also occur in subjects with hepatic disease in the absence of obesity.[80,101] These observations have been interpreted to indicate that the extent of A to E_1 conversion in adipocytes is proportional to their lipid content. This could be due to the lipophilic nature of A and its sequestration in fat tissue. High lipid content would favor the accumulation of A from the circulation and also retard release of E_1 in the reverse direction. On the other hand, increased conversion of A to E_1 in hepatic cirrhosis could be explained by reduced hepatic clearance of A and greater availability to adipose tissue. In a study of the effects of acute weight loss on the conversion of A to E in obese women, however, an increase in conversion was observed in 6 subjects following an average weight loss of approximately 100 lb.[102] These surprising results suggested that the role of obesity may be secondary in nature and that aromatization of circulating A may occur in other tissues, including the liver. Indeed, the hepatic fatty mstamorphosis that occurs in obese subjects may alter the metabolic disposition of A in favor of estrogen formation within the liver. This effect might be accentuated by starvation in obese subjects and may also operate in nonobese cirrhotics.

These possibilities are supported by indirect evidence that the liver can transform androgens to estrogens. Several early reports demonstrated that human fetal liver contains the aromatase enzyme.[103–105] More recent studies have shown that the aromatase content of fetal liver is at least 50 to 60 percent of the corresponding placenta.[106] In marked contrast, the C_{19} 5α- and 5β-reductases, which catalyze the first step in the formation of 17-ketosteroids and androstanediols, were virtually undetectable in fetal liver. Thus the normal decline in hepatic aromatization following birth in the human may be more apparent than real. Rather than being explained by genetic or other restriction of aromatase enzyme synthesis, the appearance of the much more active C_{19} 5α- and 5β-reductases may effectively prevent aromatization of Δ^4-3-ketosteroid substrates. It is of interest in this regard that hepatic 5α-reductase activity is markedly reduced during starvation.[107] A recent report described a young boy with florid gynecomastia in whom the conversion of androstenedione to estrone was 50 times higher than normal.[108] In addition to this remarkably high rate of conversion, it appeared that the product of the conversion was estrone sulfate rather than estrone. Despite extensive studies, however, the principal site(s) of aromatization was not identified, although it was concluded on the basis of several assumptions that the liver was not a major site.

The possibility remains that many human tissues aromatize

androgens. The recent observations of Longcope and associates also suggest that adipose tissue is not the only site of aromatization. They observed that both muscle and adipose tissue of the human forearm can convert androstenedione to estrone but that total aromatization by these two tissues could account for only about 30 to 40 percent of total aromatization.[109] While many assumptions were necessary to reach this conclusion, these results indicate that adipose tissue is not the only tissue involved. Indeed, it has recently been reported that adult human liver contains demonstrable levels of the aromatase enzyme.[110] Further experimentation is needed to resolve these questions. Progress in understanding the regulation and function of peripheral estrogen synthesis has been severely hampered by the lack of suitable animal models for study. This process may only occur in the human, since it has not been detected in a wide variety of laboratory animals. Unpublished experiments in the author's laboratory have shown that the rhesus monkey fetal liver has no aromatase activity.

As in young women with excessive ovarian production of androstenedione and normal conversion to estrone, fluctuations in adrenal secretory activity in postmenopausal women may play an important role in estrogen production. This aspect of peripheral estrogen production has received little attention. However, Nordin and associates have shown that postmenopausal women with severe osteoporosis have lower than normal plasma androstenedione and estrone levels.[111] Together with findings that vaginal atrophy is most severe in patients with osteoporosis, these observations suggest that adrenal or perhaps pituitary function may be important in determining the estrogen impact on target tissues in postmenopausal women.

The known factors that determine the amount of peripheral estrogen produced and available for interaction with receptors in target cells are summarized in Fig. 110-3. It is of interest that many of the conditions that increase the peripheral formation of estrone either by elevated androstenedione production or an increase in the efficiency of its aromatization are also associated with an increased risk for development of endometrial cancer.[112] For example, obesity is the most common condition found in endometrial cancer patients, and whereas the incidence rises dramatically following the menopause, young patients frequently have coincident polycystic ovarian disease. It is not known at present, however, whether a causal relationship exists between excessive estrone production and endometrial cancer. Support for such a relationship may be found in the many reports that have appeared recently indicating that consumption of exogenous estrogen by postmenopausal women increases their risk.[113–118] On the other hand, peripheral estrone production is reduced or eliminated by many of the therapeutic measures used in breast and endometrial cancer patients. Ablation of either the pituitary or adrenal glands reduces the production rate of androstenedione to very low levels in postmenopausal women. Treatment with cortisol, synthetic glucocorticoids, or some progestins such as medroxyprogesterone acetate (MPA) has the same effect by suppressing pituitary ACTH secretion. MPA is commonly used in the treatment of well-differentiated endometrial adenocarcinoma and is believed to affect both normal and abnormal cells by interaction with progesterone receptors. That MPA may also reduce estrogen production is illustrative of the complexities involved in peripheral estrogen production. Treatment with the anti-breast-cancer drug Teslac inhibits the aromatase enzyme and therefore the peripheral conversion of androstenedione to estrone.[119] The drug Elipten is even more potent in this regard and therefore is highly effective in reducing estrone production, since it also is a well-known inhibitor of adrenal steroidogenesis.[120] Also shown to be inhibitory are 5α-reduced androgens. These compounds, such as 5α-androstanedione and dihydrotestosterone, are included because in vitro studies have shown them to be the most potent naturally occurring aromatase inhibitors. Whether or not they function to regulate aromatase activity in vivo is not known. As mentioned above, however, it is of interest that 5α-reductase activity is reduced during starvation and, further, that it appears to be regulated by thyroid hormones.[107] Furthermore, some of the more recent synthetic androgen derivatives used in breast cancer therapy have the 5α structure.

The complex interrelationships illustrated in Fig. 110-2 emphasize the importance of understanding peripheral estrogen production and the many remote factors that may influence its impact on target tissues. Virtually all the classical therapeutic measures presently used in treatment of breast cancer patients were derived either empirically or on the basis of erroneous concepts such as secretion of estrogens by the adrenal glands or postmenopausal ovaries. A notable exception is the recent introduction of aminoglutethimide (Elipten), which when used properly appears to be equally effective as ablative surgery.[121] It is anticipated that new approaches based on the information summarized in Fig. 110-2 will soon be forthcoming.

REFERENCES

1. Siiteri, P. K.: Steroid hormones in pregnancy, in Gluck, L. (ed.): Modern Perinatal Medicine, Vol. 7. Flushing, N.Y., Year Book Medical Publishers, Inc., 1974, p. 231.
2. Behrman, H. R., and Armstrong, D. T.: Cholesterol esterase stimulation by luteinizing hormone in luteinized rat ovaries. *Endocrinology 85:* 474, 1969.
3. McKerns, K. W.: Studies on the regulation of ovarian function by gonadotropins, in McKerns, K. W. (ed): The Gonads. New York, Appleton-Century-Crofts, 1969, p. 137.
4. Thompson, E. A., Jr., and Siiteri, P. K.: The involvement of human placental microsomal cytochrome P-450 in aromatization. *J. Biol. Chem. 249:* 5373, 1974.
5. Hosoda, H., and Fishman, J.: Unusually facile aromatization of 2β-hydroxy-19-oxo-4-androstene-3,17-dione to estrone. Implications in estrogen biosynthesis. *J. Am. Chem. Soc. 96:* 7325–7329, 1974.
6. Channing, C. P., and Coudert, S. P.: The role of granulosa cells and follicular fluid in estrogen secretion by the monkey ovary in vivo. *Endocrinology 98:* 590, 1976.
7. Armstrong, D. T., and Dorrington, J. H.: Estrogen biosynthesis in the ovaries and testes, in Thomas, J. A., and Singhal, R. L. (eds.): Advances in Sex Hormone Research, Vol. 3. Baltimore, University Park Press, 1977, p. 217.
8. Gurpide, E.: Tracer Methods in Hormone Research. Berlin-New York, Springer-Verlag, 1975.
9. Tait, J. F.: Review: The use of isotopic steroids for the measurement of production rates in vivo. *J. Clin. Endocrinol. Metab. 23:* 1285, 1963.
10. Siiteri, P. K.: Qualitative and quantitative aspects of adrenal steroid secretion, in Christy, N. P. (ed.): The Human Adrenal Cortex. New York, Harper & Row, 1971, p. 1.
11. Baird, D. T., Horton, R., Longcope, C. and Tait, J. F.: Steroid dynamics under steady state conditions. *Recent Prog. Horm. Res. 25:* 611, 1969.
12. Channing, C. P., and Tsafriri, A.: Mechanism of action of luteinizing hormone and follicle-stimulating hormone on the ovary in vitro. *Metabolism 26:* 413–468, 1977.
13. Marsh, J. M.: The role of cyclic amp in gonadal function, in Greengard, P., and Robison, G. A. (eds.): Advances in Cyclic Nucleotide Research, Vol. 6. New York, Raven Press, 1975, p. 137.
14. Lindner, H. R., Tsafriri, A., Lieberman, M. E., Zor, U., Koch, Y., Bauminger, S., and Barnea, A.: Gonadotropin action on cultured graafian follicles: Induction of maturation division of the mammalian oocyte and differentiation of the luteal cell. *Recent Prog. Horm. Res. 30:* 79, 1974.
15. Dufau, M. L., Tsuruhara, T., Horner, K. A., et al.: Intermediate role

of adenosine 3':5'-cyclic monophosphate and protein kinase during gonadotropin-induced steroidogenesis in testicular interstitial cells. *Proc. Nat. Acad. Sci. USA 74:* 3419–3423, 1977.

16. Dorrington, J. H., Moon, Y. S., and Armstrong, D. T.: Estradiol-17β biosynthesis in cultured granulosa cells from hypophysectomized immature rats; stimulation by follicle-stimulating hormone. *Endocrinology 97:* 1328–1331, 1975.
17. Westphal, U.: Steroid-Protein Interactions, Berlin, Springer-Verlag, 1971.
18. Rosner, W.: The binding of steroid hormones in human serum, in Jamieson, G. A., and Greenwalt, T. J. (eds.): Trace Components of Plasma: Isolation and Clinical Significance. New York, Alan R. Liss, Inc., 1976, p. 377.
19. Mercier-Bodard, C., Alfsen, A., and Baulieu, E. -E.: Sex-steroid binding plasma protein. *Acta Endocrinol Suppl. 147:* 204, 1970.
20. Ács, Z., and Stark, E.: The role of transcortin in the distribution of corticosterone in the rat. *Hormone Metab. Res. 5:* 279–282, 1973.
21. Rosner, W., and Hochberg, R.: Corticosteroid-binding globulin in the rat: Isolation and studies of its influence on cortisol action in vivo. *Endocrinology 91:* 626–632, 1972.
22. Keller, N., Richardson, U. I., and Yates, E. E.: Protein binding and the biological activity of corticosteroids: in vivo induction of hepatic and pancreatic alanine aminotransferases by corticosteroids in normal and estrogen-treated rats. *Endocrinology 84:* 49–62, 1969.
23. Guériguian, J. L., Sawyer, M. E., and Pearlman, W. H.: A comparative study of progesterone- and cortisol-binding activity in the uterus and serum of pregnant and non-pregnant women. *J. Endocrinol. 61:* 331–345, 1974.
24. Werthamer, S., Govindaraj, S., and Amaral, L.: Placenta, transcortin, and localized immune response. *J. Clin. Invest. 57:* 1000–1008, 1976.
25. Amaral, L., and Werthamer, S.: Identification of breast cancer transcortin and its inhibitory role in cell-mediated immunity. *Nature 262:* 589–590, 1976.
26. Siiteri, P. K., Febres, F., Clemens, L. E., et al.: Progesterone and the maintenance of pregnancy: Is progesterone nature's immunosuppressent?. *Ann. N.Y. Acad. Sci. 286:* 384–397, 1977.
27. Rosenthal, H. E., Slaunwhite, W. R., Jr., and Sandberg, A. A.: Transcortin: A corticosteroid-binding protein of plasma. X. Cortisol and progesterone interplay and unbound levels of these steroids in pregnancy. *J. Clin. Endocrinol. Metab. 29:* 352–367, 1969.
28. Mercier, C., Alfsen, A., and Baulieu, E. -E.: A testosterone binding globulin, in Proceedings of the Second Symposium on Steroid Hormones, Ghent, 1965, *Excerpta Medica International Congress Series 101:* 212, 1966.
29. Rosenbaum, W., Christy, N. P., and Kelly, W.: Electrophoretic evidence for the presence of an estrogen-binding β-globulin in human plasma. *J. Clin. Endocrinol. Metab. 26:* 1399, 1966.
30. Pearlman, W. H., and Crépy, O.: Steroid-protein interaction with particular reference to testosterone binding by human serum. *J. Biol. Chem. 242:* 182, 1967.
31. Rosner, W., and Deakins, S. M.: Testosterone-binding globulins in human plasma: Studies on sex distribution and specificity. *J. Clin. Invest. 47:* 2109, 1968.
32. Vermeulen, A., and Verdonck, L.: Studies on the binding of testosterone to human plasma. *Steroids 11:* 609, 1968.
33. Vermeulen, A., Verdonck, L., Van der Straeten, M., et al.: Capacity of the testosterone binding globulin in human plasma and influence of specific binding of testosterone on its metabolic clearance rate. *J. Clin. Endocrinol. Metab. 29:* 1470–1480, 1969.
34. Rosner, W.: A simplified method for the quantitative determination of testosterone-estradiol-binding globulin activity in human plasma. *J. Clin. Endocrinol. Metab. 34:* 983–988, 1972.
35. Anderson, D. C., Pepiatt, R., Schuster, L., et al.: A new method for measurement of sex-hormone-binding globulin in plasma, and its clinical application. *J. Endocrinol. 55:* xi, 1972.
36. Mickelson, K. E., and Petra, P. H.: Purification of the sex steroid binding protein from human serum. *Biochemistry 14:* 957–963, 1975.
37. Fisher, R. A., Anderson, D. C., and Burke, C. W.: Simultaneous measurement of unbound testosterone and estradiol fractions in undiluted plasma at 37°C by steady-state gel filtration. *Steroids 24:* 809–824, 1974.
38. Vermeulen, A., Stoica, T., and Verdonck, L.: The apparent free testosterone concentration, an index of androgeneity. *J. Clin. Endocrinol. Metab. 33:* 759–767, 1971.
39. Rosenfield, R. L.: Plasma testosterone binding globulin and indexes of the concentration of unbound plasma androgens in normal and hirsute subjects. *J. Clin. Endocrinol. Metab. 32:* 717–728, 1971.
40. Wu, C. -H., Motohashi, T., Abdel-Rahman, H. A., et al.: Free and protein-bound plasma estradiol-17β during the menstrual cycle. *J. Clin. Endocrinol. Metab. 43:* 436–445, 1976.
41. Burke, C. W., and Anderson, D. C.: Sex-hormone-binding globulin is an oestrogen amplifier. *Nature 240:* 38, 1972.
42. Anderson, D. C.: Sex-hormone-binding globulin. *Clin. Endocrinol. 3:* 69–96, 1974.
43. O'Malley, B. W., and Means, A. R.: Female steroid hormones and target cell nuclei. *Science 183:* 610–620, 1974.
44. Jensen, E. V., Mohla, S., Gorell, T. A., et al.: The role of estrophilin in estrogen action. *Vitam. Horm. 32:* 89–127, 1974.
45. Baxter, J. D.: Glucocorticoid hormone action. *Pharmacol Ther. B. 2:* 605–659, 1976.
46. McGuire, W. L.: Current status of estrogen receptors in human breast cancer. *Cancer 36:* 638–644, 1975.
47. Gorski, J., and Gannon, F.: Current models of steroid hormone action: A critique. *Annu. Rev. Physiol. 38:* 425–450, 1976.
48. Jensen, E. V., and Jacobson, H. I.: Fate of steroid estrogens in target tissues, in Pincus, G., and Vollmer, E. P. (eds.): Biological Activities of Steroids in Relation to Cancer. New York, Academic Press, 1960, p. 161.
49. Clark, J. H., and Peck, E. J., Jr.: Nuclear retention of receptor-oestrogen complex and nuclear acceptor sites. *Nature 260:* 635–637, 1976.
50. Pietras, R. J., and Szego, C. M.: Specific binding sites for oestrogen at the outer surfaces of isolated endometrial cells. *Nature 265:* 69–72, 1977.
51. Siiteri, P. K., Moriyama, I., Ashby, R., et al.: Estrogen binding in the rat and human. *Adv. Exp. Med. Biol. 36:* 97–112, 1973.
52. Bardin, C. W., Bullock, L. P., Sherins, R. J., et al.: Androgen metabolism and mechanism of action in male pseudohermaphroditism: A study of testicular feminization. *Recent Prog. Horm. Res. 29:* 65, 1973.
53. Meyer, W. J., Migeon, P. R., and Migeon, C. J.: Locus on human x-chromosome for DHT receptor and androgen insensitivity. *Proc. Natl. Acad. Sci. USA 72:* 1469–1472, 1975.
54. Yamamoto, K. R., Stampfer, M. R., and Tomkins, G. M.: Receptors from glucocorticoid-sensitive lymphoma cells and two classes of insensitive clones: physical and DNA-binding properties. *Proc. Natl. Acad. Sci. USA. 71:* 3901–3905, 1974.
55. Toft, D., and Gorski, J.: A receptor molecule for estrogens. *Proc. Natl. Acad. Sci. USA 55:* 1574–1581, 1966.
56. Siiteri, P. K., and Wilson, J. D.: Dihydrotestosterone in prostatic hypertrophy I. The formation and content of dihydrotestosterone in the hypertrophic prostate of man. *J. Clin. Invest. 49:* 1737–1745, 1970.
57. Gloyna, R. I., Siiteri, P. K., and Wilson, J. D.: Dihydrotestosterone in prostatic hypertrophy II. The formation and content of dihydrotestosterone in the hypertrophic canine prostate and the effect of dihydrotestosterone on prostate growth in the dog. *J. Clin. Invest. 49:* 1746–1753, 1970.
58. Walsh, P. C., and Wilson, J. D.: The induction of prostatic hypertrophy in the dog with androstenediol. *J. Clin. Invest. 57:* 1093–1097, 1976.
59. Sherman, M. R.: Allosteric and competitive steroid-receptor interactions, in Baxter, J. D., and Rousseau, G. G. (eds.): Glucocorticoid Hormone Action. Heidelberg, Springer-Verlag, 1978.
60. Reynhout, J. K., and Smith, L. D.: Studies on the appearance and nature of a maturation-inducing factor in the cytoplasm of amphibian oocytes exposed to progesterone. *Dev. Biol. 38:* 394–400, 1974.
61. Resnik, R., Killam, A. P., Barton, M. D., et al.: The effect of various vasoactive compounds upon the uterine vascular bed. *Am. J. Obstet. Gynecol. 125:* 201–206, 1976.
62. Wilson, J. D., and Siiteri, P. K.: Developmental patterns of testosterone synthesis in the fetal gonad of the rabbit. *Endocrinology 92:* 1182–1191, 1973.
63. Milewich, L., George, F. W., and Wilson, J. D.: Estrogen formation by the ovary of the rabbit embryo. *Endocrinology 100:* 187–196, 1977.
64. Siiteri, P. K., and Wilson, J. D.: Testosterone formation and metabolism during male sexual differentiation in the human embryo. *J. Clin. Endocrinol. Metab. 38:* 113–125, 1974.
65. Imperato-McGinley, J., Guerrero, L., Gautier, T., et al.: Steroid 5α-reductase deficiency in man: An inherited form of male pseudohermaphroditism. *Science 186:* 1213, 1974.

66. Walsh, P. C., Madden, M. D., Harrod, M. J., et al.: Familial incomplete male pseudohermaphroditism, type 2. Decreased dihydrotestosterone formation in pseudovaginal perineoscrotal hypospadias. *N. Engl. J. Med. 291:* 944, 1974.
67. Hansen, J. W., Hoffman, P., and Ross, G. T.: Monthly gonadotropin cycles in premenarcheal girls. *Science 190:* 161–163, 1975.
68. Frisch, R. E., and McArthur, J. W.: Menstrual cycles: Fatness as a determinant of minimum weight for height necessary for their maintenance or onset. *Science 185:* 949–951, 1974.
69. Seegar-Jones, G., and de Moraes-Ruehsen, M.: A new syndrome of amenorrhea in association with hypergonadotropism and apparently normal ovarian follicular apparatus. *Am. J. Obstet. Gynecol. 104:* 597, 1969.
70. Schreiber, J. R., Reid, R., and Ross, G. T.: A receptor-like testosterone binding protein in ovaries from estrogen stimulated hypophysectomized immature female rats. *Endocrinology 98:* 1206–1213, 1976.
71. Schreiber, J. R., and Ross, G. T.: Further characterization of a rat ovarian testosterone receptor with evidence for nuclear translocation. *Endocrinology 99:* 590–596, 1976.
72. Febres, F., Gondos, B., and Siiteri, P.: Androgen-induced ovarian follicular atresia in the rat (abst.). *Gynecol. Inv. 7:* 52, 1976.
73. Tsafriri, A., and Channing, C. P.: An inhibitory influence of granulosa cells and follicular fluid upon porcine oocyte meiosis in vitro. *Endocrinology 96:* 922–927, 1975.
74. Tsafriri, A., and Channing, C. P.: Influence of follicular maturation and culture conditions on the meiosis of pig oocytes in vitro. *J. Reprod. Fertil. 43:* 149–152, 1975.
75. Ledwitz-Rigby, F., Rigby, B., Gay, V. L., et al.: Inhibitory action of porcine follicular fluid upon granulosa cell luteinization in vitro: Assay and influence of follicular maturation. *J. Endocrinol. 74:* 175–184, 1977.
76. De Jong, F. F., and Sharpe, R. M.: Evidence for inhibin-like activity in bovine follicular fluid. *Nature 263:* 71–72, 1976.
77. Niswender, G. D., Monroe, S. E., Peckham, et al.: Radioimmunoassay for rhesus monkey luteinizing hormone with anti-ovine LH serum and ovine LH-^{131}I. *Endocrinology 88:* 1327–1331, 1971.
78. Yen, S. S. C.: Chronic anovulation due to inappropriate feedback system, in Yen, S. S. C., and Jaffe, R. B. (eds.): Reproductive Endocrinology. Philadelphia, W. B. Saunders Co., 1978, p. 297.
79. Rebar, R., Judd, H. L., Yen, S. S. C., et al.: Characterization of the inappropriate gonadotropin secretion in polycystic ovary syndrome. *J. Clin. Invest. 57:* 1320, 1976.
80. Siiteri, P. K., and MacDonald, P. C.: The role of extraglandular estrogen in human endocrinology:, in Geiger, S. R., Astwood, E. B., and Greep, R. O. (eds): Handbook of Physiology, Section 7. New York, The American Physiological Soceity, 1973, p. 615.
81. Judd, H. L., Rigg, L. A., Anderson, D. C., et al.: The effects of ovarian wedge resection in circulating gonadotropin and ovarian steroid levels in patients with polycystic ovary syndrome. *J. Clin. Endocrinol. Metab. 43:* 347–355, 1976.
82. Zondeck, B.: Estrogenic hormone in the urine of the stallion. *Nature 133:* 494, 1934.
83. Steinach, E., and Kuhn, H.: Transformation of male sex hormones into a substance with the action of a female hormone. *Lancet 2:* 845, 1937.
84. West, C. D., Damast, B. L., Sarro, S. D., et al.: Conversion of testosterone to estrogens in castrated, adrenalectomized human females. *J. Biol. Chem. 218:* 409–418, 1956.
85. Ahmad, N., and Morse, W. I.: Metabolites of tritiated testosterone in healthy men. *Can. J. Biochem. 43:* 25–31, 1965.
86. Kelch, R. P., Jenner, M. R., Weinstein, R., et al.: Estradiol and testosterone secretion by human, simian, and canine testes, in males with hypogonadism and in male pseudohermaphrodites with the feminizing testes syndrome. *J. Clin. Invest. 51:* 824–830, 1972.
87. MacDonald, P. C., Rombaut, R. P., and Siiteri, P. K.: Plasma precursors of estrogen. I. Extent of conversion of plasma Δ^4-androstenedione to estrone in normal males and nonpregnant normal, castrate and adrenalectomized females. *J. Clin. Endocrinol. Metab. 27:* 1103–1111, 1967.
88. Grodin, J. M., Siiteri, P. K., and MacDonald, P. C.: Source of estrogen production in the postmenopausal woman. *J. Clin. Endocrinol. Metab 36:* 207–214, 1973.
89. Longcope, C., Kato, T., and Horton, R.: Conversion of blood androgens to estrogens in normal adult men and women. *J. Clin. Invest. 48:* 2191–2201, 1969.
90. Southren, A. L., Olivo, J., Gordon, G. G., et al.: The conversion of androgens to estrogens in hyperthyroidism. *J. Clin. Endocrinol. Metab. 38:* 207–214, 1974.
91. Siiteri, P. K., and MacDonald, P. C.: The utilization of circulating dehydroisoandrosterone sulfate for estrogen synthesis during human pregnancy. *Steroids 2:* 713–730, 1963.
92. Siiteri, P. K., and MacDonald, P. C.: Placental estrogen biosynthesis during human pregnancy. *J. Clin. Endocrinol. Metab. 26:* 751–761, 1966.
93. MacDonald, P. C., and Siiteri, P. K.: The in vivo mechanisms of origin of estrogen in subjects with trophoblastic tumors. *Steroids 8:* 589, 1966.
94. MacDonald, P. C., Edman, C. D., Kerber, I. J., et al.: Plasma precursors of estrogen. III. Conversion of plasma dehydroisoandrosterone to estrogen in young nonpregnant women. *Gynecol. Invest. 7:* 165, 1976.
95. Bolt, H. M., and Gobel, P.: Formation of estrogens from androgens by human subcutaneous adipose tissue in vitro. *Horm. Metab. Res. 4:* 312, 1972.
96. Schindler, A. E., Ebert, A., and Frederick, E.: Conversion of androstenedione to estrone by human fat tissue. *J. Clin. Endocrinol. Metab. 35:* 627–630, 1972.
97. Nimrod, A., and Ryan, K. J.: Aromatization of androgens by human abdominal and breast fat tissue. *J. Clin. Endocrinol. Metab. 40:* 367–379, 1975.
98. MacDonald, P. C., Edman, C. D., Hemsell, D. L., et al.: Effect of obesity on conversion of plasma androstenedione to estrone in postmenopausal women with and without endometrial cancer. *Am. J. Obstet. Gynecol. 130:* 448–455, 1978.
99. Edman, C. D., and MacDonald, P. C.: Effect of obesity on conversion of plasma androstenedione to estrone in ovulatory and anovulatory young women. *Am. J. Obstet. Gynecol. 130:* 456–461, 1978.
100. Edman, C. D., and MacDonald, P. C.: Slow entry into blood of estrone produced in extraglandular sites in obesity and endometrial neoplasia. *Gynecol. Invest. 5:* 27, 1974 (abst.)
101. Gordon, G. G., Olivo, J., Rafii, F., et al.: Conversion of androgens to estrogens in cirrhosis of the liver. *J. Clin. Endocrinol. Metab. 40:* 1018–1026, 1975.
102. Siiteri, P. K., Williams, J. E., and Takaki, N. K.: Steroid abnormalities in endometrial and breast carcinoma: A unifying hypothesis. *J. Steroid Biochem. 7:* 897–903, 1976.
103. Mancuso, S., DellAcqua, S., Eriksson, G., et al.: Aromatisation of androstenedione and testosterone by the human fetus. *Steroids 5:* 183–197, 1965.
104. Schindler, A. E.: Steroid metabolism of fetal tissues. II. Conversion of androstenedione to estrone. *Am. J. Obstret. Gynecol. 123:* 265–268, 1975.
105. Slaunwhite, W. R., Karsay, M. A., Hollmer, A., et al.: Fetal liver as an endocrine tissue. *Steroids (Suppl. II):* 211–221, 1965.
106. Siiteri, P. K., and Serón-Ferré, M.: Secretion and metabolism of adrenal androgens to estrogens, in Proceedings of Symposium on Endocrine Function of the Human Adrenal Cortex. New York, Academic Press (in press).
107. Bradlow, H. L., Boyar, R. M., O'Connor, J., et al.: Hypothyroid-like alterations in testosterone metabolism in anorexia nervosa. *J. Clin. Endocrinol. Metab. 43:* 571–574, 1976.
108. Hemsell, D. L., Edman, C. D., Marks, J. F., et al.: Massive extraglandular aromatization of plasma androstenedione resulting in feminization of a prepubertal boy. *J. Clin. Invest. 60:* 455, 1977.
109. Longcope, C., Pratt, H. J., Schneider, S. H., et al.: Aromatization of androgens by muscle and adipose tissue in vivo. *J. Clin. Endocrinol. Metab. 46:* 146–152, 1978.
110. Smuk, M., and Schwera, J.: Aromatization of androstenedione by human adult liver in vitro. *J. Clin. Endocrinol. Metab. 45:* 1009–1012, 1977.
111. Marshall, D. H., Crilly, R. G., and Nordin, B. E. C.: Plasma androstenedione and oestrone levels in normal and osteoporotic postmenopausal women. *Br. Med. J. 2:* 1177–1179, 1977.
112. Siiteri, P. K.: Steroid hormones and endometrial cancer. *Cancer Res.* (in press).
113. Gray, L. A., Christopherson, W. M., and Hoover, R. N.: Estrogens and endometrial carcinoma. *Obstet. Gynecol. 49:* 385–389, 1977.
114. Hoover, R., Fraumeni, J. R., Everson, R., et al.: Cancer of the uterine corpus after hormonal treatment for breast cancer. *Lancet ii:* 885–997, 1976.
115. Mack, T. M., Pike, M. C., Henderson, B. E., et al.: Estrogens and endometrial cancer in a retirement community. *N. Engl. J. Med. 294:* 1262–1267, 1976.
116. McDonald, T. W., Annegers, J. F., O'Fallon, W. M., et al.: Exogenous estrogen and endometrial carcinoma: Case-control and incidence study. *Am. J. Obstet. Gynecol. 127:* 572–580, 1977.

117. Smith, D. C., Prentice, R., Thompson, D. J., et al.: Association of exogenous estrogens and endometrial carcinoma. *N. Engl. J. Med. 293:* 1164–1167, 1975.
118. Ziel, H. K., and Finkle, W. D.: Increased risk of endometrial carcinoma among users of conjugated estrogens. *N. Engl. J. Med. 293:* 1167–1170, 1975.
119. Siiteri, P. K., and Thompson, E. A.: Studies of human placental aromatase. *J. Steroid Biochem. 6:* 317–322, 1975.
120. Thompson, E. A., Jr., and Siiteri, P. K.: Studies on the aromatization of C_{19} androgens. *Ann. N.Y. Acad. Sci. 212:* 378–391, 1973.
121. Samojlik, E., Santen, R. J., and Wells, S. A.: Adrenal suppression with aminoglutethimide. II. Differential effect on plasma androstenedione and estrogen levels. *J. Clin. Endocrinol. Metab. 45:* 480–487, 1977.

111

Diagnosis and Treatment of Primary Amenorrhea, Secondary Amenorrhea, and Dysfunctional Uterine Bleeding

Griff T. Ross

PRIMARY AMENORRHEA AND THE HYPOTHALAMIC-PITUITARY-OVARIAN-GENITAL AXIS

From the patient's point of view, many of the diagnostic tests that may be helpful in understanding the etiology of primary amenorrhea are either expensive or painful or both. It therefore behooves the physician to choose tests with discrimination, utilizing only those that are essential for correct diagnosis and rational therapy. Appropriate choices of tests can be made after a carefully taken history and a carefully performed physical examination, but only if the physician understands the clinical correlates of fetal errors in gonadal, gonaductal, and genital differentiation and function of hypothalamic-hypophyseal-ovarian-genital interactions during normal pubescence. These subjects are discussed in greater detail in Chapters 105, 106, and 108. Here, a terse summary will suffice.

NORMAL FETAL GONADAL, GONADUCTAL, AND GENITAL DIFFERENTIATION* AND NORMAL PUBERTY†

Knowledge of the similarities and differences in anlagen of the gonads, the accessory sex organs (subsequently called gonaducts for simplicity), and the external genitalia facilitates understanding of fetal development and differentiation of these structures in genetic males and females. These facts are summarized in Table 111-1.

Early in ontogeny, the primordia of the gonads of both sexes are indifferent and bipotential. Normally, these primordial gonads differentiate into testes in genetic males with XY sex chromosomal constitution and ovaries in genetic females with XX sex chromosomes, and subsequently gonaducts, urogenital sinus, and external genitalia develop concordantly. Gonaductal anlagen consist of wolffian ducts in males and müllerian ducts in females. Both duct systems are present early in fetal development of both male and female fetuses, and differentiation concordant with genetic sex depends upon fetal gonadal function. In males, the vasa deferentia, seminal vesicles, and epididymis are derivatives of the wolffian ducts, and in females, the fallopian tubes, the uterus, and the upper one third of the vagina are derived from müllerian ducts.

In genetic males, concordant gonaductal differentiation is dependent upon at least two substances secreted by the fetal testes. Testosterone, secreted by the interstitial cells of Leydig, acts locally to stimulate growth and development of wolffian duct derivatives,[1–3] and a macromolecule, referred to as müllerian regression or inhibition factor and apparently secreted by testicular tubular cells, acts locally to stimulate nearly complete regression of mullerian ducts.[4]

In addition to its local action on wolffian duct structures, testosterone, secreted by the fetal testes and distributed systemically, is converted into a metabolite, dihydrotestosterone, by an enzyme present in the primordia of the external genitalia.[5] Dihydrotestosterone, produced in these tissues, acts locally to stimulate differentiation of the glans penis and corpora cavernosa from the genital tubercle, the corpus spongiosum (which surrounds the penile urethra) from the urethral folds, and the scrotum from the labioscrotal swellings. Dihydrotestosterone also stimulates forma-

*See Chapters 105 and 106.
†See Chapter 108.

Table 111-1. Gonaductal and Genital Derivatives of Fetal Structures in Males and Females

Fetal Structure	Derivatives	
	In Males	In Females
Müllerian ducts	Appendix testis	Fallopian tubes Uterus Upper vagina
Wolffian ducts	Vas deferens Seminal vesicles	Gartner's ducts
Genital tubercle	Penis Corpus cavernosum Glans	Clitoris Corpus cavernosum Glans
Urethral folds	Corpus spongiosum	Labia minora
Labioscrotal swellings	Scrotum	Labia majora
Urogenital sinus	Prostate Cowper's glands Prostatic utricle	Skene's glands Bartholin's glands Lower vagina

tion of the prostate and of Cowper's glands but no other vestiges of the urogenital sinus persist in adult life.

In contrast to the events described for males, gonaductal and genital differentiation in genetic females appears to be independent of fetal gonadal function. Thus, if the indifferent fetal gonads become ovaries or if no gonads develop, the gonaducts, the urogenital sinus, and external genitalia differentiate along normal female lines. The genital tubercle gives rise to a clitoris, the urethral folds to labia minora, the labioscrotal swellings to labia majora, and the urogenital sinus to the lower two thirds of the vagina and to Bartholin and Skene's glands.

During normal postnatal growth and pubescence, sex steroid hormones, secreted by ovaries responding to gonadotropic stimulation, stimulate maturation of secondary sexual characteristics. The sequence of these changes is detailed in Chapter 108.

In relation to primary amenorrhea, three varieties of abnormality in pubescence may be distinguished. First, either failure of secondary sexual changes to appear by chronologic age of 16 years or, irrespective of the degree to which secondary sexual characteristics have matured, failure of first menses to occur by 18 years of age warrants evaluation.

Second, pubescence in girls normally begins with breast budding and appearance of axillary and pubic hair. Although both the age at which these changes are initiated and the rate at which they progress are variable, advancement is normally orderly and synchronous, and the first menses ensue. Marked asynchrony in the development of secondary sexual characteristics (e.g., complete maturation of breasts in the absence of axillary and pubic hair or complete maturation of axillary and pubic hair with failure of breast development) is unusual and justifies study.[6,7]

Third, failure of the gonads to virilize the external genitalia during fetal development does not eliminate the possibility that the testes may function appropriately at puberty to produce a male pattern of hirsutism, voice changes, and phallic enlargement in a person erroneously raised as a female. Such changes are distinctly abnormal, and the cause must be determined.

ABNORMAL FETAL GONADAL, GONADUCTAL, AND GENITAL DIFFERENTIATION AND PRIMARY AMENORRHEA

Fetal Errors in Gonadal Development

The term "gonadal dysgenesis" is used to designate the most common error in fetal gonadal differentiation, which occurs with an estimated frequency of 1 per 5000 to 7000 newborns or 1 per 2700 newborn phenotypic females.[8] The gonads are replaced by bilateral tenuous streaks consisting of a fibrous stroma, which is devoid of either follicles or tubules containing germ cells. In most instances, sex chromosomal aberrations are found in karyotypes prepared from cultures of somatic cells from such persons.[9,10] It is supposed that these sex chromosomal anomalies predispose to failures of either meiotic or mitotic divisions of germ cells, so that these cells are eliminated prior to appearance of either primordial follicles or testicular tubules in the fetal gonad.

Streak gonads also occur in persons in whom there are no detectable morphologic abnormalities of the sex chromosomes, suggesting that other factors may result in depletion of germ cells. Two familial varieties due to gene mutations have been recognized, and both also appear sporadically.[11] Virtually all persons with gonadal dysgenesis, irrespective of the type, have female gonaducts and female external genitalia, but occasionally clitoral hypertrophy occurs.

Gonadal differentiation may proceed differently on the two sides, giving rise to a unilateral testis or ovary or ovotestis, with a complementary ovary or testis or ovotestis on the other side.[12,14] When both sperm and oocytes are found in these gonads, true hermaphroditism is diagnosed. In a related syndrome, called mixed gonadal dysgenesis, a unilateral testis and a contralateral undifferentiated streak gonad or a gonadal tumor occur.[15] Customarily, in persons with either true hermaphroditism or mixed gonadal dysgenesis, gonaductal differentiation is unilaterally concordant with gonadal differentiation, but the extent of masculinization of the urogenital sinus and external genitalia is variable. As a result the external genitalia of true hermaphrodites range from normal female (uncommonly) to normal male (rarely), with ambiguous genitalia being observed in the majority of instances. Ambiguous external genitalia occur in virtually all persons with mixed gonadal dysgenesis, but 70 to 90 percent of them are raised as females (see below).

Fetal Errors in Gonaductal Differentiation

For unknown reasons, the anlagen of the müllerian ducts or the urogenital sinus or both develop abnormally in some genetic females. In these instances, external genitalia are female but the fallopian tubes, the uterus, and the upper third of the vagina may be absent in cases of müllerian duct aplasia. When the urogenital sinus is aplastic or dysgenetic, the lower two thirds of the vagina fails to develop. Ovaries develop normally and function normally to stimulate development of secondary sexual characteristics in these persons, but genital tract function is variably compromised (see below).

Fetal Errors in Genital Differentiation

Unfortunately, gonadal differentiation bilaterally concordant with genetic sex does not assure concordant gonaductal, urogenital, or genital differentiation. Differentiation of both fetal gonads into testes does not assure masculinization of the gonadal accessories and external genitalia. Inappropriate genital differentiation in genetic males with testes results from either inadequate testosterone synthesis secondary to deficiencies in the enzymes required for converting cholesterol to testosterone or from failure of target tissues to respond to testosterone or dihydrotestosterone.

If the apparent failure of the fetal testicular function is complete, female external genitalia result, and the syndrome is referred to as complete male pseudohermaphroditism. Partial failure results in ambiguous external genitalia characteristic of incomplete male pseudohermaphroditism.

Although quantities of testosterone and dihydrotestosterone produced normally in female fetuses are inadequate to virilize the

Table 111-2. Menstrual Function in True Hermaphroditism

Gender Assignment	Total Number	Number (Percent) Postmenarcheal	Mean Age (Range) in Years at Menarche
Female	28	19 (68)	15 (10–19)
Male	43	28 (65)	16.6 (12–30)

Adapted from the data of Overzieher, Intersexuality, New York, Academic Press, 1963, p. 192.

primordia of the urogenital sinus and the external genitalia, excessive androgen production will virilize these structures in genetic females. Thus, an extragonadal source of androgen, either endogenous, from the adrenal glands, or exogenous, from hormonal therapy during early gestation, may masculinize the urogenital sinus or the external genitalia of genetic females, giving rise to female pseudohermaphroditism. Usually, the anomaly consists of only an enlarged clitoris, but occasionally more ambiguous external genitalia are seen.[3,8]

CLINICAL CORRELATES OF FETAL ERRORS

From the foregoing summary, it is apparent that errors in fetal gonadal differentiation or failure of fetal testes to secrete androgen, or failure of fetal tissues to respond to androgens in genetic males, or extraovarian sources of androgens in genetic females with ovaries all predispose to anomalous development of external genitalia and predispose to errors in gender assignment to neonates. Errors in gender assignment may not be discovered until the expected age of puberty, so that the patient may seek medical advice for failure to pubesce or for primary amenorrhea. In addition to anomalous development of gonads, gonaducts, and external genitalia during fetal life, both inadequate pituitary gonadotropin secretion and failure of ovaries to respond postnatally may present clinically as failure to pubesce and primary amenorrhea.

As noted above, clues to these disorders may be obtained from the initial history and physical examination and may serve as a rational basis for ordering diagnostic tests. In Tables 111-6 and 111-7, information that should be obtained from history and physical examination is organized with the objective of categorizing the disorder resulting in primary amenorrhea. In Tables 111-6A and 111-7A, results of diagnostic tests are summarized. As in all clinical medicine, exceptions are encountered to any generalizations made concerning the association of signs and symptoms in a given syndrome. Exceptions are discussed under appropriate headings in the accompanying text.

Errors in Gonadal Development

True Hermaphroditism. In persons with true hermaphroditism, the testicular components of the fetal gonads function variably with respect to differentiation of both gonaducts and external genitalia. Both total failure to masculinize, resulting in completely unambiguous female genitalia, and complete virilization, producing normal male external genitalia with a competent phallic urethra and scrotal gonads, are rare.[12–14] In the majority of instances, anomalous or ambiguous external genitalia result. Ideally, appropriate decisions with respect to sex of rearing and plans for plastic corrections (to make genital sex compatible with the gender assignment) should be made prior to dismissing the newborn infant from the hospital. Under these circumstances, primary amenorrhea should never be the presenting complaint of persons with true hermaphroditism.

In any event, primary amenorrhea should rarely be associated with true hermaphroditism. In the first place, it is a rare syndrome, and in the second place, irrespective of gender assignment, about 65 percent of persons with true hermaphroditism menstruate (Table 111-2). Data supporting these assertions will be summarized briefly.

Polani[13] found a total of only 310 cases of true hermaphroditism described up to 1969, but menstrual histories were not analyzed in his review. The most comprehensive review with sufficient data to provide some estimate of the frequency of amenorrhea among these persons was that of Overzieher,[12] who listed a total of only 172 cases.

Menstrual histories were available for a total of 71 persons, 43 raised as males and 28 raised as females and about two thirds of each group were postmenarcheal (Table 111-2). Among the 28 persons raised as females, 19 were postmenarcheal, and age at menarche ranged from 10 to 19 years, with an average of 15 years. Among 21 women and girls over 10 years of age, for whom menstrual data were available at the time of reporting and in whom the genitalia were either completely female or female with clitorimegaly, 11 were postmenarcheal and 10 were premenarcheal. Five of the 10 premenarcheal women, ranging in age from 20 to 33 years at the time of reporting, would fit the criteria we have set for a diagnosis of primary amenorrhea. Of the remaining 5, ranging in age from 13 to 16 years, 3, aged 15 or 16 years, might be regarded as having delayed menarche. Collectively, then, 20 to 30 percent of true hermaphrodites raised as females might come to the attention of physicians because of primary amenorrhea.

Studies of karyotypes in one or more tissues from true hermaphrodites have shown no single characteristic sex chromosomal constitution. We have added 3 cases to those described by Benirschke et al.,[16] and results are summarized in Table 111-3.

The first clue leading to the diagnosis should be obtained by determination of nuclear sex, but definitive diagnosis of true hermaphroditism depends upon gonadal biopsy. In view of the rarity of the disorder, serum gonadotropic and sex steroid hormone concentrations should be measured and karyotypes determined. All gonadal tissue should be biopsied and tissue not compatible with the gender assignment removed. Despite the "dysgenetic" nature of the gonads in true hermaphrodites and the fact that karyotypes include a Y chromosome in 45 percent of cases studied, gonadoblastomas have been reported very rarely in these patients as compared to patients with other varieties of gonadal dysgenesis.[17–19] Although neoplastic degeneration in gonads of true hermaphrodites raised as males is rare, these persons are unlikely to be fertile, and sex steroid hormone replacement can be accomplished satisfactorily, so that leaving a dysgenetic testis behind does not justify assuming the risk of neoplasia, however slight.

The Syndromes of Gonadal Dysgenesis

Gonadal dysgenesis with stigmata of Turner's syndrome. The generic term "gonadal dysgenesis" has been used to describe all persons who have undifferentiated streak gonads without relation

Table 111-3. Sex Chromosomal Constitution in True Hermaphroditism

Karyotype	Number	Percent
46,XX	61	50
46,XY	24	19.7
45,X/46,XY	11	9
46,XX/46,XY	11	9
46,XX/47,XXY	7	5.7
Miscellaneous	8	6.6
	122	100.0

to whether either extragenital extragonadal stigmata or sex chromosomal aberrations or both are present. The syndrome of sexual infantilism, short stature, and musculoskeletal abnormalities that occurs commonly among persons with streak gonads, first described by Turner in 1938[20] and now referred to as Turner's syndrome, is associated with abnormalities of sex chromosome number or morphology or both.

Cases resulting from virtually every variety of chromosomal breakage, with or without reunion, have been described.[9,10] However, the most common karyotype is 45,X, in which the second sex chromosome is totally deleted. Such individuals invariably have female external genitalia and chromatin-negative nuclear sex, without "F" bodies, indicating that a normal Y chromosome is lacking.[21,22] The incidence of chromatin-negative nuclear sex and female external genitalia is 1 per 5000 newborns, but the incidence is higher in abortuses.[23]

Mixed gonadal dysgenesis. The term "mixed gonadal dysgenesis" has been used to designate asymmetrical gonadal development with a germ cell tumor or a testis on one side and an undifferentiated streak, a rudimentary gonad, or no gonad on the other side.[15] Davidoff and Federman have tabulated data from the published descriptions of these patients, added data on their patients, and analyzed these critically.[24] Persons with unilateral tumors and contralateral streak gonads showed some differences, both clinically and cytogenetically from patients with unilateral testes and contralateral streak gonads. These data are summarized in Table 111-4.

Short stature and other stigmata associated with a 45,X karyotype were less commonly observed among patients with tumors than among patients with testes, of whom half were taller than 147 cm by age 16 years. At onset of pubescence, which usually was not delayed in these patients, signs of virilization including voice changes, hirsutism, clitoral hypertrophy, and failure of breasts to mature occurred more frequently and were more marked among patients with testes than among patients with tumors. Davidoff and Federman[24] suggest that persons with the syndrome of mixed gonadal dysgenesis with tumors are more similar to patients with the syndrome of pure gonadal dysgenesis (see below) than they are to patients with the syndrome of mixed gonadal dysgenesis without tumors.

Nuclear sex was chromatin-negative in all instances save one each of patients with testes and patients with tumors. No mention was made of the frequency with which "F" bodies were observed in interphase nuclei, but it seems reasonable to suppose that this would be high in view of the high incidence of X/XY karyotypes among persons with these gonadal anomalies. However, Y chromosomes that do not fluoresce have been identified among patients with 45,X/46,XY sex chromosomal mosaicism.[25] In order to rule out the presence of cell lines containing Y chromosomes in patients with anomalous external genitalia and chromatin-negative sex but no "F" bodies, a karyotype should be made of cells from one or more tissues.

Table 111-4. Comparison of Patients with Tumors and Testes in the Syndrome of Mixed Gonadal Dysgenesis

Trait	Contralateral Gonad	
	Tumor	Testis
Fetal genital masculinization	Failed to occur in 80%	Partial in 100%
Sex of rearing	90% Female	70% Female
Pubertal virilization	Mild	Severe
Pubertal breast development	Occasional	None
Sex chromosomal mosaicism 45,X/46,XY	4/15	21/31

Adapted from the data of Davidoff and Federman.[24]

Table 111-5. Clinical Features in Persons with Pure Gonadal Dysgenesis

Karyotype	Mode of Transmission	Gonadal Tumors	Clitoral Hypertrophy	Nerve Deafness
46,XY	X-linked recessive	25%	10%–15%	Rare
46,XX	Autosomal	<2%	<5%	10%

There are no endocrine tests that give results diagnostic of either tumor or testis. Visualization, biopsy, and removal of all gonadal tissue seem indicated to remove sources of androgen in girls with X/XY karyotypes who virilize at puberty and to eliminate the neoplastic potential of dysgenetic gonads in girls who do not virilize at puberty. Suitable sex steroid hormone replacement therapy should be undertaken at the appropriate time.

Pure gonadal dysgenesis. The term "pure gonadal dysgenesis" has been used sometimes to distinguish sexually immature taller girls (> 150 cm) with bilateral streak gonads and minimal extragenital, extragonadal somatic stigmata from sexually immature shorter girls (≤ 150 cm) with streak gonads and a variety of musculoskeletal defects usually regarded as manifestations of Turner's syndrome.[26] This distinction is useful for several reasons.

First, pure gonadal dysgenesis is a genetic disorder[11] occurring in siblings, whereas Turner's syndrome has been observed very rarely in siblings. Heredofamilial gonadal dysgenesis has usually been associated with XY or XX karyotypes in the tissues studied, and sometimes these have been referred to as familial XX or XY gonadal dysgenesis. The different karyotypes are transmitted differently, and there are some distinctive clinical features, as shown in Table 111-5.

Second, sex chromosomal aneuploidy is less common among patients with pure gonadal dysgenesis. Mosaic karyotypes 45,X/46,XX have been described in sporadic cases of pure gonadal dysgenesis. The higher incidence of tumors of germ cell origin among persons with XY sex chromosomes and pure gonadal dysgenesis makes it essential to obtain a complete cytogenetic evaluation including a karyotype.

Errors in Gonaductal Development

When pubertal changes have begun at an appropriate age and secondary sexual characteristics have matured in the proper sequence but menses have not appeared, primary consideration should be given to the genital tract as the locus of the problem. As noted earlier, müllerian ducts normally give rise to fallopian tubes, uterus, cervix, and upper vagina. For unknown reasons, one or more of the derivatives may not develop, and the failure may go unrecognized until the age of puberty. The anomaly may vary in severity from an imperforate hymen to complete aplasia of all müllerian duct derivatives with vaginal atresia.[26–28] Although aplasia usually involves all the derivatives, single-component defects have been described. Thus, vaginal aplasia associated with absence of the uterus and cervix is the most common defect, with an estimated frequency at birth of 1 per 4000 female infants. In about 10 percent of cases, vaginal aplasia is associated with a functionally normal uterus and cervix. Congenital absence of the cervix associated with a functionally normal uterus and patent vagina is extremely rare; less than 20 cases having been reported.[29]

Müllerian dysgenesis tends to be associated with congenital malformations in other systems. In view of the origin from common anlagen, it is not surprising that urinary tract anomalies would be found commonly in association with anomalies of müllerian duct derivatives. Frequent association with musculoskeletal malformations is not easily explained, however.

Pinsky has described six familial syndromes of congenital malformations that variably involve ears, the upper and lower extremities including hands and feet, the urinary tract, and the internal genitalia.[30] The most common of these is the Rockitansky-Kuster-Hauser complex.[31,32] While the extragenital malformations are apparent from birth or from infancy at least, the genital malformations may not become apparent until menses fail to appear despite advanced development of secondary sexual characteristics.

Normal ovarian function results in development of normal secondary sexual characteristics, including endometrial changes in the presence of a structurally normal uterus, and at an appropriate age, cyclic shedding of the endometrium begins. In women with vaginal aplasia but a normal uterus, the menstrual effluent is retained, producing endometriosis and cyclic abdominal pain without external evidence of menses. Endometriomas large enough to be palpable have been reported in these women. Diagnostic tests, apart from examination under anesthesia, are not useful.

When the defect consists of an imperforate hymen only, restoration of normal function is accomplished by incising the hymenal membrane. Attempts at plastic reconstruction of a functional vagina and a patent outflow tract have met with variable success, and successful pregnancy has been reported only rarely.

In addition to müllerian dysgenesis, endometrial synechiae, complicating miliary tuberculosis and associated with endometrial resistance to estrogenic and progestational steroid hormone stimulation, may result in primary amenorrhea.[33]

Errors in Genital Differentiation

Male Pseudohermaphroditism[34] resulting from inadequate testosterone synthesis. Pseudohermaphroditism, resulting from either inadequate (in genetic males) or inappropriate (in genetic females) masculinization of the urogenital sinus and external genitalia, may result from a deficiency of any one of at least eight enzymes involved in adrenal cortical or gonadal steroid hormone biosynthesis. The biosynthetic steps that these enzymes catalyze are shown diagrammatically in Figure 111-1, and some associated clinical features are summarized in Tables 111-7 and 111-7A. As shown in the figure, there are five enzyme deficiencies that result in failure of adequate testosterone biosynthesis by fetal testes in genetic males and one that results in failure to convert testosterone to dihydrotestosterone.[35–43] In these persons, incomplete masculinization of the urogenital sinus and external genitalia gives rise to incomplete male pseudohermaphroditism, which may present as primary amenorrhea if not correctly diagnosed in the neonate. Chromatin-negative nuclear sex, an "F" body in somatic cell nuclei, an XY sex chromosomal constitution, and abnormalities in serum and urinary steroid hormone levels reflecting enzymatic deficiencies are sufficient for diagnosis.

Male Pseudohermaphroditism resulting from androgen resistance. Only tissues derived from the genital tubercle require DHT per se for androgen action. Other tissues respond to testosterone. Thus the 5-α-reductase deficiency results in androgen deficiency only in specific tissues.

Tissue resistance to androgenic stimulation may result from inability of the tissue to convert testosterone to dihydrotestosterone,[5,42,43] from lack of a cytosol androgen receptor required for translocating the steroid from cytosol to nucleus, or from failure of hormone transported to nucleus to bind to appropriate nuclear components.[44]

Although the exact nature of the defect is not understood in every case, there are at least seven variants of male pseudohermaphroditism, all familial in occurrence, which appear to result from variable tissue resistance to androgenic stimulation.[34] Persons with any of at least three of these syndromes have been raised as girls and have sought medical care for primary amenorrhea.

The most common of these three syndromes is testicular feminization, a variety of complete male pseudohermaphroditism characterized by immature female external genitalia, sparse to absent axillary hair, and breasts that, although voluptuous, may have immature nipples and hypopigmented areolae.[45] These persons are inevitably raised as females and come to the physician

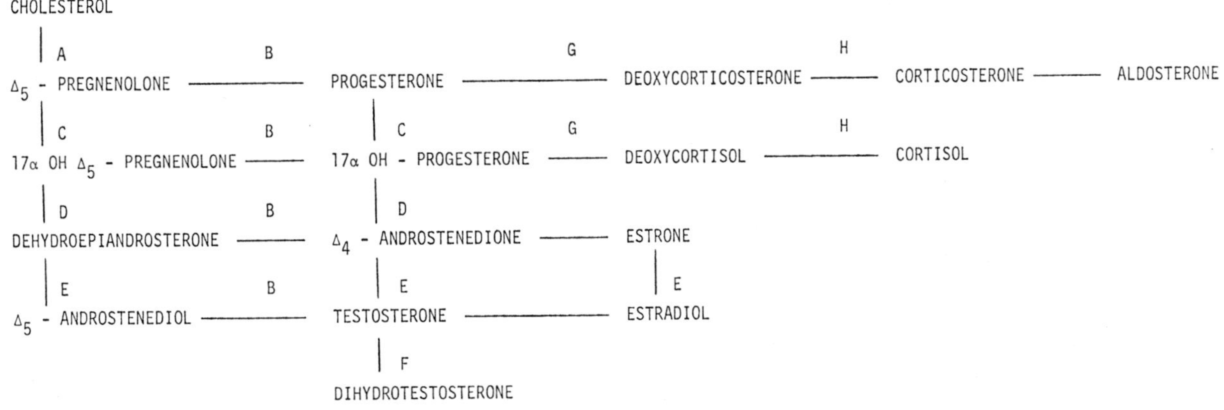

Fig. 111-1. Syndromes of deficiencies in the enzymes required for the biosynthesis of sex and adrenal cortical steroid hormones.

Table 111-6. **CLINICAL CORRELATES**

Pathophysiologic Basis	Syndrome(s)	History			Physical Examination		
		Pubertal Changes		Other	Secondary Sexual Characteristics	Genital	Extragenital
		Onset	Progression				
Fetal errors in gonadal development	1. True hermaphroditism	Normal or delayed	Heterosexual	Nothing diagnostic	Variably virilized	Usually anomalous	Nothing diagnostic
	2. Gonadal dysgenesis with stigmata of Turner's syndrome	Delayed	Minimal isosexual	Edema of extremities in neonatal period	Immature female	Immature female	Short stature; multiple musculoskeletal, cutaneous, osseous anomalies
	3. Mixed gonadal dysgenesis	Normal	Heterosexual	Nothing diagnostic	Variably virilized	Usually anomalous	Nothing diagnostic; normal stature
	4. Pure gonadal dysgenesis	Delayed	Minimal isosexual	Family history of sexual immaturity, infertility	Immature female	Immature female	Habitus may be eunochoidal; stature normal
Fetal errors in gonaductal development	Mullerian dysgenesis	Normal	Normal	Cyclic abdominal pain	Maturing female	Vagina absent or not patent	Congenital musculoskeletal malformations; abdominal masses; endometriomas
Ovarian follicles insensitive to gonadotrophins	17α-hydroxylase deficiency	Delayed	None	Family history of sexual immaturity	Immature female	Immature female	Hypertensive
	"Resistant Ovaries"	Delayed	Minimal isosexual	Nothing diagnostic	Immature female	Immature female	Normotensive
Hypothalamic-pituitary diseases	Familial hypogonadotropic hypogonadism	Delayed	Slow to absent	Family history of anosmia, mid-line defects and hypogonadism in boys and girls	Immature female	Immature female	Anosmia, mid-line defects
	Pituitary and parapituitary tumors; idiopathic panhypopituitarism	Normal or delayed	Interrupted	Failure to grow; other signs and symptoms of anterior pituitary failure, diabetes insipidus	Immature female	Immature female	Short stature; other signs of hypopituitarism
Miscellaneous systemic diseases		Delayed	Slow to absent	Signs and symptoms of systemic disease	Immature female	Immature female	Appropriate to systemic disease

Table 111-6A. RESULTS OF DIAGNOSTIC STUDIES

Syndrome(s)	Cytogenetic: Nuclear Sex: Barr Bodies	Cytogenetic: Nuclear Sex: "F" Bodies	Cytogenetic: Karyotype	Pituitary Function: Basal Gonadotropic Secretion	Pituitary Function: Other	Gonadal Visualization And Biopsy	Miscellaneous	Treatment
1. True hermaphroditism	+ or – A	+ or – A	XX, XY or mosaics A	Normal or elevated B	Normal C	Testis, ovary and ovotestis in varying combinations A	Vaginoscopy, urethroscopy, cystocopy, if required A	Preservation of gonadal tissue consistent with sex of rearing
2. Gonadal dysgenesis with stigmata of Turner's syndrome	+ or – A	+ or – A	All varieties of breakage, with or without reunion; complete deletions of X (or Y) A	Elevated A	Normal C	Bilateral streaks devoid of germ cells A or B[++]	X-rays for skeletal malformations; urinary tract anomalies A	Sex steroid hormone replacement
3. Mixed gonadal dysgenesis	– A	+ or –* A	X/XY A	Normal or elevated B	Normal C	Unilateral streak, contralateral testis or tumor A	Vaginoscopy, urethroscopy; C	Remove tumors; timing of gonadectomy controversial
4. Pure gonadal dysgenesis	+ or – A	+ or – A	XX, XY A	Elevated A	Normal C	Bilateral streaks devoid of germ cells A or B	Nothing of diagnostic or therapeutic value C	Sex steroid hormone replacement
Mullerian dysgenesis	+ C	– C	XX C	Normal C	Normal C	Normal ovaries C	Examination under anesthesia, if necessary A	Surgery appropriate to lesion: hymenotomy, vaginoplasty or opening cervical canal to vagina
17 α-hydroxylase deficiency	+ A	– C	XX C	Elevated A	ACTH*** secretion increased; but suppressible A	Ovaries B	Elevated serum*** progesterone, desoxycorticosterone A	Sex steroid hormone replacement; glucocorticoid replacement
"Resistant Ovaries"	+ B	– B or C	XX C	Elevated A	Normal C	Ovaries containing unstimulated follicles	Nothing diagnostic	Sex steroid hormone replacement if indicated
Familial hypogonadotropic hypogonadism	+ A	– C	XX C	Low A	Normal C	Ovaries B	Tests of smell A	Sex steroid hormone replacement or ovulation induction if pregnancy is desired
Pituitary and parapituitary tumors; idiopathic panhypopituitarism	+ A	– C	XX C	Low or normal A	Abnormal A	Ovaries C	X-rays of sella, other neuroradiologic studies as indicated A	Sex steroid hormone replacement or ovulation induction if pregnancy is desired
	+ A	– C	XX C	Low A	Abnormal A	Ovaries C	X-rays of sella, other neuroradiologic studies as indicated A	Appropriate replacement therapy
Miscellaneous systemic diseases	+ A	– C	XX C	Low or normal B	May be normal B	Ovaries C	Tests appropriate to systemic disease suspected	Appropriate therapy for primary disease; replacement therapy if indicated

A — Provide information useful for diagnosis and treatment
B — Of interest, but not essential
C — Not indicated
* — Failure to demonstrate "F" or "Y" bodies. Does not eliminate possibility that a "Y" chromosome is present
** — In persons with precocious pseudopuberty
*** — Results of glucocorticoid suppression tests are diagnostic
\+ — When nuclear sex is consonant with genital sex, further cytogenetic study is optional; when nuclear sex is not consonant with genital sex, further study is mandatory
++ — Essential if X/XY mosaicism is found on cytogenetic study

Table 111-7. CLINICAL CORRELATES

Pathophysiologic Basis	Syndrome(s)	History			Physical Examination		
		Pubertal Changes		Other	Secondary Sexual Characteristics	Genital	Extragenital
		Onset	Progression				
Fetal errors in genital differentiation	1. Male pseudohermaphroditism due to deficient testosterone synthesis (A) 20,22-desmolase	Unknown	Unknown	Neonatal adrenal cortical insufficiency	Immature female	Female	Inguinal masses; inguinal hernia(s)
	(B) 3β-hydroxy-steroid dehydrogenase	Normal or minimally delayed	Heterosexual	Neonatal adrenal cortical insufficiency	Variably virilized, gynecomastia	Anomalous	Nothing distinctive
	(C) 17α-hydroxylase	Delayed	Minimal	Nothing diagnostic	Gynecomastia only; no axillary or pubic hair	Female or anomalous	Hypertensive
	(D) 17,20-desmolase	Delayed	Minimal	Nothing diagnostic	Immature female	Anomalous	Inguinal masses
	(E) 17-ketosteroid reductase	Normal	Heterosexual	Nothing diagnostic	Variably virilized with gynecomastia	Female or anomalous	Inguinal masses
	2. Male pseudohermaphrotidism due to androgen resistance (A) Complete testicular feminization	Normal or minimally delayed	Asynchronous isosexual	Family history of sexual immaturity, infertility	Voluptuous breasts with immature nipples and hypopigmented areolae; scant to absent axillary and pubic hair	Immature female external genitalia; patent vagina with no cervix	Inguinal masses; inguinal hernia
	(B) Incomplete testicular feminization	Normal or minimally delayed	Iso- and heterosexual	Family history of sexual immaturity, infertility	Female with minimal virilization	Partial labioscrotal fusion; clitorimegaly; patent vagina with no cervix or uro-genital sinus	Inguinal mass(es); inguinal hernia(s)
	(C) Familial incomplete male pseudohermaphroditism (Types 1 and 2)	Normal or minimally delayed	Asynchronous heterosexual	Family history of sexual immaturity, infertility	Breasts may be immature relative to axillary and pubic hair	External genitalia female with clitorimegaly; May be anomalous	Inguinal masses; herniae, signs of virilism
	3. Female pseudohermaphrotidism due to fetal androgen excess	May be precocious	Asynchronous heterosexual	Family history of neonatal adrenal cortical insufficiency	Axillary and pubic hair advanced relative to breasts	External genitalia female with clitorimegaly	Short stature

Table 111-7A. RESULTS OF DIAGNOSTIC STUDIES

Syndrome(s)	Cytogenetic: Nuclear Sex: Barr Bodies	Cytogenetic: Nuclear Sex: "F" Bodies	Cytogenetic: Karyotype	Pituitary Function: Basal Gonadotropic Secretion	Pituitary Function: Other	Gonadal Visualization And Biopsy	Miscellaneous	Treatment
1. Male pseudohermaphroditism due to deficient testosterone synthesis (A) 20,22-desmolase	- A	+ A	XY A	Not described B	Normal C	Testes A	Deficient serum and urinary hydroxycorticoids A	Remove testes; glucocorticoid replacement; sex steroid hormone replacement
(B) 3-hydroxy-steroid dehydrogenase	- A	+ A	XY A	Normal (?) B	Normal C	Testes A	Deficient serum and urinary hydroxycorticoids A	Glucocorticoid replacement
(C) 17α-hydroxylase	- A	+ A	XY A	Elevated B	Normal C	Testes A	Elevated serum progesterone, desoxycorticosterone; hypokalemia A	Glucocorticoid replacement; sex steroid hormone replacement
(D) 17,20-desmolase	- A	+ A	XY A	Elevated B	Normal C	Testes A	No detectable serum or urinary DHEA A	Remove testes; sex steroid hormone replacement
(E) 17-ketosteroid reductase	- A	+ A	XY A	Elevated B	Normal C	Testes A	Increased serum androstenedione, estrone levels A	Remove testes; sex steroid hormone replacement
2. Male pseudohermaphrotidism due to androgen resistance (A) Complete testicular feminization	- A	+ A	XY A	Normal or elevated B	Normal C	Testes A	Abdominal plain film; serum testosterone in normal male range	Remove testes; postoperative sex steroid hormone replacement
(B) Incomplete testicular feminization	- A	+ A	XY A	Elevated B	Normal C	Testes A	Abdominal plain film; serum testosterone in normal male range	Removes testes; postoperative sex steroid hormone replacement
(C) Familial incomplete male pseudohermaphroditism (types 1 and 2)	- A	+ A	XY A	Normal or elevated B	Normal C	Testes A	Serum testosterone may be elevated; vaginoscopy, urethroscopy; cytoscopy if required A	Remove testes; sex steroid hormone replacement therapy
3. Female pseudohermaphroditism due to fetal androgen excess	+ A	- A or C	XX C	Normal or elevated for peer group** B	ACTH*** secretion increased when due to congenital adrenal hyperplasia A	Ovaries C	Serum and *** urinary hormones elevated or depressed consistent with enzyme deficiency A	Glucocorticoid replacement therapy if indicated

A — Provide information useful for diagnosis and treatment
B — Of interest, but not essential
C — Not indicated
* — Failure to demonstrate "F" or "Y" bodies. Does not eliminate possibility that a "Y" chromosome is present
** — In persons with precocious pseudopuberty
*** — Results of glucocorticoid suppression tests are diagnostic
+ — When nuclear sex is consonant with genital sex, further cytogenetic study is optional; when nuclear sex is not consonant with genital sex, further study is mandatory
++ — Essential if X/XY mosaicism is found on cytogenetic study

because of primary amenorrhea. On physical examination, gonads may or may not be palpable in the inguinal canal, and inguinal herniae, uncommon in girls and women, are commonly found. Genital and pelvic examination characteristically reveals immature female external genitalia and a short vagina, terminating blindly with no cervix and no palpable uterus. The terms "partial" or "incomplete" testicular feminization have been used to designate persons that have ambiguous external genitalia at birth, are raised as females, but undergo partial pubertal virilization, with development of axillary and pubic hair.[46–48]

Apart from the complete and partial syndromes of testicular feminization, Wilson and Goldstein[34] have designated other variants of familial incomplete male pseudohermaphroditism as types 1[49] and 2,[50] which differ in the mode of inheritance. Transmission of type 1 familial incomplete pseudohermaphroditism is consistent with that of an X-linked recessive trait. Boys with either of two variants of type 1 familial incomplete male pseudohermaphroditism, referred to as Lubs syndrome[49] and the Gilbert-Dreyfus syndrome,[52] have been raised as girls. In contrast, virtually all persons with the type 2 variant, commonly referred to as pseudovaginal perineoscrotal hypospadias (now known to be due to deficiency of 5-α-reductase[42]), have been raised as girls who subsequently become virilized without developing breasts at puberty.[53]

Absence of Barr bodies and presence of "F" bodies in interphase nuclei, coupled with an XY sex chromosomal constitution in karyotypes prepared from cell cultures, provide the data essential for diagnosis. While not essential for diagnosis, serum steroid and gonadotropic hormone concentrations should be determined for research interest.

Female Pseudohermaphroditism. Extraovarian sources of androgen may virilize the external genitalia in genetic females with ovaries.[3–8] Excessive adrenal androgen secretion is usually associated with defective cortisol synthesis. Five of the eight deficiencies shown in Figure 111-1 result in defective adrenal cortical cortisol biosynthesis. Consequent failure to suppress pituitary adrenocorticotropin secretion results in congenital adrenal hyperplasia and excessive adrenal androgen secretion in two instances involving 2l-hydroxylase or ll-β-hydroxylase deficiencies.[54–57] In female fetuses with ll-β- or 2l-hydroxylase deficiencies, the excessive adrenocortical androgen secretion not only virilizes the external genitalia, and occasionally the urogenital sinus as well, during fetal life but also stimulates development of heterosexual precocious pseudopuberty and suppresses pituitary gonadotropin secretion postnatally.[56,57]

Ordinarily, these infants have signs and symptoms of adrenal cortical insufficiency in the neonatal period that lead to recognition and appropriate treatment at that time. Rarely, when the enzyme deficits are minor, recognition may be delayed until signs and symptoms of heterosexual precocious pseudopuberty lead to recognition of the pathophysiological basis of the disorder. Chromatin-positive nuclear sex eliminates the diagnosis of male pseudohermaphroditism. Finding elevated 17-α-hydroxyprogesterone in serum or increased levels of its metabolite, pregnanetriol, in urine confirms the diagnosis of the most common deficiency (21-hydroxylase) and probably also the 11-hydroxylase deficiency.[58] Appropriate adrenal cortical steroid hormone replacement therapy is followed by ovulatory menstrual cycles and fertility.

CLINICAL CORRELATES OF FOLLICULAR INSENSITIVITY TO GONADOTROPINS

Studies of follicular responses in hypophysectomized immature female rats are consistent with the hypothesis that gonadotropins stimulate preantral follicle growth by catalyzing the synthesis of estrogens, which exert a mitogenic effect on granulosa cells.[59–61] Direct experimental verification of the validity of this hypothesis for follicular maturation in women is ethically impractical, but studies of ovarian histology provide some information. The lack of follicular maturation in ovaries of sexually immature women with congenital gonadotropin deficiency,[62] in women congenitally unable to synthesize estrogen,[63–65] and in women whose ovaries do not secrete estrogen despite massive doses of exogenous gonadotropins[66,67] suggests that gonadotropins and estrogens also play this role in follicular maturation in women.

Since Δ_4 androstenedione and testosterone are precursors in the biosynthesis of estrone and estradiol (see Fig. 111-1), deficient synthesis of these substances is accompanied by estrogen deficiency in genetic females. As a consequence of the estrogen deficiency, sexual infantilism and primary amenorrhea associated with increased serum and urinary gonadotropin are noted in girls with the 17-α-hydroxylase deficiency who survive until the expected age of puberty. Excessive synthesis of an adrenal cortical salt-retaining steroid hormone, desoxycorticosterone, predisposes to hypertension with hypokalemic alkalosis in these girls.[63–65] Biopsy of ovarian tissue in 2 girls with this syndrome showed numerous large cysts and numerous primordial follicles with complete failure of orderly follicular maturation despite high serum gonadotropin levels.[65] The constellation consisting of high serum progesterone concentrations, hypertension with hypokalemic alkalosis responsive to glucocorticoid replacement therapy, and high serum gonadotropins is diagnostic.

Sexually immature normotensive women with high serum and urinary gonadotropins, whose ovaries contain primordial follicles that do not secrete estrogens, despite stimulation with massive doses of exogenous gonadotropins, have been described.[66,67] The pathophysiologic basis for this failure to respond is unknown, but it is interesting to speculate that failure of follicular maturation results from failure to synthesize estrogen.

CLINICAL CORRELATES OF ABNORMAL HYPOTHALAMIC-PITUITARY FUNCTION: HYPOGONADOTROPIC HYPOGONADISM

Failure of the pituitary to secrete sufficient quantities of gonadotropins results in failure of ovarian follicular maturation and sex steroid hormone secretion. As a result, secondary sexual characteristics do not mature, and no menses occur. Failure may result from inadequate hypothalamic stimulation or from primary pituitary diseases such as neoplasms. All varieties of sexual immaturity due to inadequate pituitary gonadotropin secretion are referred to as syndromes of hypogonadotropic hypogonadism. Distinguishing among them is required for directing treatment toward the underlying disease when possible.

Familial Hypogonadotropic Hypogonadism

A familial syndrome characterized by anosmia or hyposmia, sexual immaturity, and variable expression of midline defects was described by Kallman.[68] In the European literature, the syndrome is called olfactogenital dysplasia, and results of clinicopathological studies of large series have been reported, showing that the disorders of olfaction are associated with dysplasias of the rhinencephalon.[69] Ovaries contain numerous primordial follicles, but follicular maturation is severely retarded even when compared to that in ovaries of neonates.[62] Induction of ovulation with gonadotropins supports the contention that hypogonadism results from inadequate gonadotropin secretion.[62,70] It has been shown that pituitary gonadotropin secretion follows chronic administration of gonadotropin-releasing hormone to persons with this syndrome, suggesting that the disease is of hypothalamic rather than pituitary origin.[71]

Although the syndrome occurs among kindreds, sporadic occurrence is more common. For example, Santen and Paulsen[72] found a family history of hypogonadism or olfactory dysfunction in only 13 of 30 such patients seen over a period of 10 years. On the basis of historical data, they estimated the incidence of hypogonadism, olfactory dysfunction, cryptorchidism, harelip, cleft palate, and deafness among 97 adult family members in 6 kindreds from which these patients were drawn. Although estimates made by history probably underestimate the true incidence, these data are worth noting.

Among siblings of persons with hypogonadism, cryptorchidism, or olfactory dysfunction, 35 percent had one or more of these same defects. Hyposmia and hypogonadism were expressed more commonly among men than among women. Observing that phenotypic expression was not complete (e.g., a normal woman, 6 of whose siblings had olfactory dysfunction, transmitted hyposmia and hypogonadism to a son but only anosmia to a daughter), that transmission skipped generations, and that male-to-male and female-to-female transmission occurred, these workers concluded that the trait was transmitted as an autosomal dominant with "incomplete expressibility." Women with the disorder have conceived and been delivered of apparently normal infants after ovulation induction with exogenous gonadotropins.[62]

Hypogonadotropic Hypogonadism Secondary to Pituitary and Parapituitary Tumors, Primary and Metastatic

Disorders of hypothalamic control of pituitary hormone secretion, including gonadotropins, are associated with third ventricle tumors and parapituitary tumors. Destruction of anterior pituitary tissue by primary pituitary neoplasms or by metastatic infiltration of other neoplasms may result in hypogonadism and primary amenorrhea. These are discussed in Chapters 18 and 22. Neuroendocrinologic evaluation and tests of anterior pituitary function are essential for diagnosis.

Hypogonadotropic Hypogonadism Secondary to Systemic Diseases

The hypothalamic-pituitary unit may fail to function appropriately in a number of debilitating, stressful systemic diseases that interfere with somatic growth and development. It would be rare indeed for such a disease process to be discovered during the course of an evaluation for primary amenorrhea. In these instances, extensive evaluation of anterior pituitary function is unlikely to be profitable. Development of secondary sexual characteristics can be achieved with exogenous sex steroid hormones when therapy for the primary disease fails to result in puberty.

SECONDARY AMENORRHEA AND THE HYPOTHALAMIC-PITUITARY-OVARIAN-GENITAL AXIS

A diagnosis of secondary amenorrhea is made when no menses have occurred for a period of 6 months if cycles have always been regular or for a period of 12 months if irregular. Women with secondary amenorrhea seek medical evaluation out of concern for fertility, or that the disorder may be symptomatic of some serious underlying disease, or that amenorrhea is not "natural." Once serious underlying diseases have been eliminated from consideration, the patient can participate in decisions about the need for further diagnostic or therapeutic intervention, since there is nothing to suggest that cyclic menses are essential for health.

As in the case of primary amenorrhea, evaluation of patients with secondary amenorrhea requires some understanding of the functional interactions of the components of the hypothalamic-pituitary-ovarian-genital axis. These are detailed in Chapters 7, 17, 18, and 109. During the first encounter the physician should seek historical data concerning signs and symptoms that point to functional aberrations of specific components of the axis and concerning events that predispose to developing these disorders.

CLINICAL CORRELATES OF DYSFUNCTION

Historical Data

The most common cause of secondary amenorrhea is pregnancy, and since some diagnostic studies useful in evaluating patients with secondary amenorrhea endanger the fetus, this diagnosis should be excluded at the outset of the evaluation. Moreover, pregnancy may be complicated by gestational trophoblastic neoplasms, a rare but potentially life-threatening group of diseases of which the first sign may be secondary amenorrhea.[73] A candid evaluation of the patient's sexual activity, including contraceptive practices, and a careful evaluation of reproductive history, including events occurring during prepartum, intrapartum, and postpartum periods of pregnancies, will provide circumstantial evidence useful in eliminating pregnancy and gestational trophoblastic neoplasms as the basis of secondary amenorrhea.

In addition, these historical data may provide clues to disorders of hypothalamic-pituitary function. For example, Sheehan's syndrome of postpartum pituitary necrosis[74] should be suspected when menses are not resumed following parturition complicated by intrapartum or postpartum hemorrhage sufficient to require transfusions. In these instances, signs and symptoms of adrenocorticotropic or thyrotropic hormone deficiencies provide additional circumstantial evidence for this disorder in parturients.

Inappropriate lactation is an important diagnostic clue to diseases of the hypothalamus or pituitary. Historical evidence for failure of lactation to cease after parturition or weaning or appearance of galactorrhea unrelated to parturition may signify the existence of pituitary tumors secreting prolactin.[75–77]

Precipitous weight reduction has been implicated in the causation of secondary amenorrhea possibly related to hypothalamic dysfunction. One should enquire about dietary habits such as diet fads, "crash diets" for voluntary weight reduction, and the bizarre dietary habits characteristic of persons with the syndrome of anorexia nervosa.[78]

A carefully taken history of drug ingestion may provide indications for appropriate diagnostic and therapeutic intervention. Thus, amenorrhea and galactorrhea complicate the use of psychotrophic agents given for symptomatic treatment of mild affective disorders among women.[79,80] In addition to these psychotropic drugs, some drugs used in treating hypertension[80] and some oral contraceptive preparations[80,81] may be implicated in causing secondary amenorrhea.

Signs and symptoms of estrogen deficiency, including vasomotor instability, loss of vaginal secretions, and dyspareunia, should direct attention to primary ovarian failure, including the menopause. Insidious progression of signs and symptoms of androgen excess, including hirsutism, male pattern hair loss, acne, and clitoral hypertrophy, should alert the physician to the possibilities of ovarian or adrenal diseases that are associated with excess secretion of the hormone.[82,83]

Asherman's syndrome of intrauterine synechiae should be

suspected in women whose amenorrhea follows vigorous dilation and curettage, postpartum endometritis, or disseminated tuberculosis.[84] In these women, failure of withdrawal bleeding following sequential administration of an estrogen and progestin should lead the physician to obtain either a hysteroscopic or hysteroradiographic examination of the endometrium. Measuring serum hormone concentrations will provide little information of diagnostic value in these women.

Physical Findings

During the physical examination, the physician should be alert to signs that may be helpful in identifying the locus of the disorder, including the following:

1. Qualities of skin: oiliness, excess dryness, cutis marmorata, pigmentary abnormalities, telangiectasia, and bruises suggestive of abnormalities of thyroid, ovarian, or adrenal cortical function.
2. General nutritional status, suggestive of anorexia nervosa or anorexoid states associated with inanition.
3. Amount and distribution of genital and extragenital hair.
4. Volume of breasts, presence or absence of galactorrhea.
5. Abdominal masses suggestive of adrenal or ovarian neoplasms.
6. Visual field defects or other evidences of cranial nerve deficits, suggesting pituitary, parapituitary, or other CNS tumors.
7. Quality of vaginal mucosa, cervical mucus, size of uterus, ovaries, and presence of parametrial masses.

THE RATIONALE FOR DIAGNOSTIC TESTING

To facilitate the strategy of evaluation after completing the history and physical examination, it is important to recall and review results of four clinical studies that have been confirmed in many laboratories and provide the basis for determining the locus of the disorder in the hypothalamic-pituitary-ovarian-genital axis of women with secondary amenorrhea.

First, Odell and Swerdloff[85] and Jaffe and Midgley[86] showed that a rapid rise in serum LH levels occurred 24 to 48 hours after administration of a progestin to estrogen-primed normal women.

Second, Yen and colleagues[87] showed that mean basal serum LH levels were higher and FSH levels lower in women with chronic anovulation or polycystic ovarian disease than in their peers with normal ovulatory cycles.

Third, Goldenberg et al.[88] measured serum gonadotropin levels prior to and following an intramuscular injection of progesterone in a prospective study of a group of women with secondary amenorrhea. They showed that an elevation of serum LH, simulating a preovulatory surge of the hormone, occurred in 14 of 15 women who bled. This observation was interpreted to signify that the hypothalamic-pituitary unit in such women could respond to changes in serum steroid hormone milieu.

In light of the study by Goldenberg et al., bleeding occurring after progesterone makes it possible to draw the following conclusions about the hypothalamic-pituitary-ovarian-genital axis:

1. The pituitary secretes FSH and LH.
2. In response to these gonadotropins, the ovary secretes sufficient estrogen to stimulate endometrial proliferation.
3. The endometrium responds to both estrogen and progesterone.
4. The hypothalamic-pituitary unit responds to changes in the serum sex steroid hormone milieu.

In addition, it is of interest that an ovulatory response to clomiphene is more commonly seen among amenorrheic women who bleed after receiving progesterone.[89]

In the fourth study, Goldenberg and associates[90] made a retrospective analysis of data obtained during studies of ovarian biopsies and basal serum FSH and LH levels in 234 women with primary and secondary amenorrhea. They showed that single basal serum FSH levels in specimens collected from women whose ovaries contained no oocytes were invariably more than 2 standard deviations of the mean higher than levels in similar specimens collected from women whose ovaries contained maturing follicles.

Using conclusions of these four studies as a basis for interpreting data, Mishell and colleagues[91,92] have conducted both retrospective and prospective studies of basal serum concentrations of FSH, LH, and estradiol in 90 women with secondary amenorrhea who had been given an intramuscular injection of progesterone. In the retrospective study,[91] among 90 patients given an intramuscular injection of progesterone, the 63 who bled had a mean serum estradiol level of 60 pg/ml. Basal serum FSH and estradiol levels were shown to consist of a single population in which values were log-normally distributed. In contrast, basal serum LH levels among these 63 women who bled after an intramuscular injection of progesterone seemed to be drawn from two populations: one with high and one with normal serum LH levels. Patients with high serum LH levels were diagnosed clinically as having polycystic ovarian disease, and patients with normal serum LH levels were diagnosed as having hypothalamic-pituitary dysfunction.

In the 27 women who failed to bleed following intramuscular progesterone injections, values for basal serum LH and estradiol concentrations were log-normally distributed and were drawn from a single population with a mean basal serum estradiol level of 15 pg/ml. In contrast, basal serum FSH levels were shown to represent two populations: one with high and one with low or normal levels. High serum FSH levels were found in women with primary ovarian disease due either to depletion of follicles or to follicles refractory to gonadotropic stimulation. These levels reflect appropriate hypothalamic-pituitary unit response to prevailing levels of estrogen lower than mean early follicular levels in normal women. Low serum FSH levels despite inadequate ovarian estrogen secretion were thought to reflect failure of hypothalamic-pituitary function, and indeed, some patients in this group were found to have pituitary and CNS tumors.

Prospective studies of some of these patients showed that measurement of FSH, LH, and estradiol in serum specimens collected daily for 4 to 5 days or hourly for 5 to 6 hours provided no greater discrimination than single measurements had shown.[92] It should be pointed out that these serum hormone measurements were made "in house" in the investigators' laboratories, where rigid quality control of assays is maintained. Results of single measurements made in other laboratories may be less reliable, in which case multiple determinations may be necessary.

DIAGNOSIS AND TREATMENT

Human chorionic gonadotropin is a biologic "marker" for trophoblast, so that eliminating pregnancy and gestational trophoblastic neoplasms from consideration in the differential diagnosis of secondary amenorrhea requires sensitive, specific tests for chorionic gonadotropin.[93–95] To interpret results obtained from tests for chorionic gonadotropin, the physician must be familiar with the limitations of the methods used for detecting and quantifying the hormone. Failure to appreciate these limitations has led to misinterpretation of the significance of "negative pregnancy tests," with disastrous consequences for women with gestational trophoblastic neoplasms.[73,96]

Once pregnancy and trophoblastic neoplasms have been eliminated from consideration in the pathogenesis of secondary amenorrhea, a specimen of serum should be obtained for measurement of FSH, LH, and prolactin levels, and the patient given 100 mg of progesterone intramuscularly. Those who fail to bleed after 8 days should be given 50–100 μg of ethinyl estradiol, or equivalent doses of other orally active estrogens, daily for 21 days followed by an intramuscular injection of 100 mg of progesterone. Failure to bleed following this maneuver suggests that the endometrium is unresponsive, and further studies should be undertaken to detect endometrial synechiae.

Results of basal serum hormone measurements should be available by 3 to 4 weeks after the initial visit and interpreted in the light of response to progesterone. Irrespective of the response to progesterone, women whose serum contains high levels of prolactin should have x-rays of the sella turcica, including tomograms if anteroposterior and lateral projections are normal, to facilitate diagnosis of pituitary tumors. In some of these women, small prolactin-secreting adenomata have been surgically removed, and resumption of ovulatory cycles with restoration of fertility has been accomplished.[97] Induction of ovulation and successful pregnancies have followed use of exogenous gonadotropins in such women who wish to conceive.[98] If a pregnancy is not desired, sex steroid hormone replacement may be indicated. Some of these women will ovulate in response to clomiphene, and if they wish to attempt to become pregnant, this may be offered. However, it should be pointed out that complications attributed to rapid enlargement and suprasellar extension of pituitary tumors have been reported to complicate pregnancy in these women.[99]

Recently, it has been shown that a synthetic ergot analogue, bromergocryptine, suppresses pituitary prolactin secretion and results in resumption of ovulatory menstrual cycles followed by pregnancy in some women with amenorrhea and hyperprolactinemia.[100–102] Although therapeutic efficacy has been shown, the substance has not been approved for prescription usage in the United States.

Persons with low levels of serum FSH and LH who did not bleed following progesterone should have studies to rule out intracranial lesions that might compromise hypothalamic-pituitary function with or without concomitant excessive pituitary prolactin secretion.

At the discretion of the physician, and with the patient's informed consent, laparoscopic examination and ovarian biopsy may be utilized to confirm the diagnosis of ovarian failure in amenorrheic women with high basal FSH levels who fail to bleed after administration of progesterone. Otherwise, replacement therapy for signs and symptoms of estrogen deficiency should be considered.

Amenorrheic women with high serum LH levels who bleed following administration of intramuscular progesterone and who desire to become pregnant should be given 6-day courses of clomiphene, beginning with doses of 50 mg/day, with 50 mg/day increments in successive courses until ovulation has been observed or a maximal dose of 200 mg/day has been achieved. Ovulation induction with menopausal gonadotropins and HCG should be undertaken in women in whom clomiphene is ineffective.

ABNORMAL GENITAL BLEEDING (DYSFUNCTIONAL UTERINE BLEEDING) AND THE HYPOTHALAMIC-PITUITARY-OVARIAN-GENITAL AXIS

Vaginal bleeding in girls prior to the expected age of menarche or in postmenopausal women should stimulate the physician to perform a careful genital tract examination. Extragenital causes of vaginal bleeding in premenarcheal girls are discussed in Chapter 108.

Erratic, intermittent, often excessive vaginal bleeding in postmenarcheal women may be symptomatic of hypothalamic-pituitary-ovarian-genital axis dysfunction and merits evaluation. At the outset, in this age group, as in girls and postmenopausal women, genital tract pathology and systemic diseases, such as myxedema,[103] should be considered, preferably in consultation with a gynecologist, prior to any "therapeutic trial" of sex steroid hormones. Furthermore, oral contraceptives should not be used empirically to "regularize" the cycles in women with erratic vaginal bleeding during the reproductive epoch, particularly without preliminary evaluation of the axis. Delay in definitive therapy for potentially reversible diseases to which this practice predisposes may have tragic consequences for the patient.

In perimenarcheal girls and in perimenopausal women, erratic vaginal bleeding may result from estrogen withdrawal provoked by interruption in preovulatory follicular maturation and anovulation. "Breakthrough bleeding" has been shown to be associated with continuous endometrial stimulation by estrogens secreted continuously in persons whose hypothalamic-pituitary unit fails to respond to the inhibitory effects of the steroid.[104,105] In these persons, cyclic administration and withdrawal of progesterone may lead to the development of regular cyclic ovulatory cycles after a few months.

REFERENCES

1. Jost, A.: Problems of fetal endocrinology: The gonadal and hypophyseal hormones. *Recent Prog Horm Res 8:* 379, 1953.
2. Jost, A., Vigier, B., Prepin, J., et al.: Studies on sex differentiation in mammals. *Recent Prog Horm Res 29:* 1, 1975.
3. Federman, D. D.: *Abnormal Sexual Development.* Philadelphia and London, W. B. Saunders Co., 1967.
4. Josso, N.: Permeability of membranes to the Müllerian-inhibiting substance synthesized by the human fetal testis *in vitro:* A clue to its biochemical nature. *J Clin Endocrinol Metab 34:* 265, 1972.
5. Siiteri, P. K., Wilson, J. D.: Testosterone formation and metabolism during male sexual differentiation in the human embryo. *J Clin Endocrinol Metab. 38:* 113, 1974.
6. Marshall, W. A., Tanner, J. M.: Variations in patterns of pubertal changes in girls. *Arch Dis Child 44:* 291, 1970.
7. Ross, G. T., Vande Wiele, R. L.: The ovaries, in Williams, R. H. (ed): *Textbook of Endocrinology,* ed 5, Philadelphia, W. B. Saunders Co., 1974, p. 368.
8. Grumbach, M. M., VanWyk, J. J.: Disorders of sex differentiation, in Williams, R. H. (ed): *Textbook of Endocrinology,* ed 5, Philadelphia, W. B. Saunders Co., 1974, p. 423.
9. Ross, G. T., Tjio, J. M.: Cytogenetics in clinical endocrinology. *JAMA 192:* 977, 1965.
10. Ferguson-Smith, M.A.: Karyotype-phenotype correlations in gonadal dysgenesis and their bearing on the pathogenesis of malformations. *J Med Genet 2:* 142, 1965.
11. Simpson, J. L., Christakos, A. C., Horwith, M., et al.: Gonadal dysgenesis in individuals with apparently normal chromosomal complements: Tabulation of cases and compilation of genetic data. *Birth Defects: Original Articles Series VII:* 215, 1971.
12. Overzieher, C.: True hermaphroditism, in Overzieher, C. (ed): *Intersexuality,* New York, Academic Press, 1963, p. 192.
13. Polani, P. E.: Hormonal and clinical aspects of hermaphroditism and the testicular feminizing syndrome in man. *Trans R Soc Lond B259:* 187, 1970.
14. Jones, H. W., Scott, W. W.: *Hermaphroditism, Genital Anomalies and Related Endocrine Disorders,* ed 2, Baltimore, Williams and Wilkins Co., 1971.
15. Sohval, A. R.: Mixed gonadal dysgenesis: A variety of hermaphroditism. *Am J Hum Genet 15:* 155, 1963.
16. Benirschke, K., Naftolin, F., Gittes, R., et al.: True hermaphroditism and chimerism. *Am J Obstet Gynecol 113:* 449, 1972.
17. Park, I. J., Pyeatte, J. C., Jones, H. W., et al.: Gonadoblastoma in a true hermaphrodite with 46,XY genotype. *Obstet Gynecol 40:* 466, 1972.
18. Schellhas, H. F.: Malignant potential of the dysgenetic gonad. *Obstet Gynecol 44:* 298, 455, 1974.
19. May, M., Katayama, K. P., Jones, H. W.: The age of occurrence of

gonadal tumors in intersex patients with a Y chromosome. *Am J Obstet Gynecol 124:* 293, 1976.
20. Turner, H. H.: A syndrome of infantilism, congenital webbed neck and cubitus valgus. *Endocrinology 23:* 566, 1938.
21. Caspersson, T., Zech, L.: Analysis of human metaphase chromosome set by aid of DNA-binding fluorescent agents. *Exp Cell Res 62:* 490, 1970.
22. Pearson, P. L., Brobrow, M.: Technique for identifying Y chromosomes in human interphase nuclei. *Nature (London) 226:* 78, 1970.
23. Carr, D. H.: Significance of chromosomal abnormalities in spontaneous abortion, in Behrman, S. S., Kistner, R. W. (eds): *Progress in Infertility,* ed 2, Boston, Little, Brown and Co, 1975, p. 465.
24. Davidoff, F., Federman, D. D.: Mixed gonadal dysgenesis. *Pediatrics 52:* 725, 1973.
25. Khudr, G., Benirschke, K., Brooks, D., et al.: XO-XY mosaicism and nonfluorescent Y chromosome. *Obstet Gynecol 42:* 421, 1973.
26. Harnden, D. G., Steward, J. S. S.: *Br Med J 2:* 1285, 1959.
27. Counsellor, V. S.: Congenital absence of vagina. *JAMA 136:* 861, 1948.
28. Leduc, B., Van Campenhout, J., Simard, R.: Congenital absence of the vagina. Observations on 25 cases. *Am J Obstet Gynecol 100:* 512, 1968.
29. Geary, W. L., Weed, J. C.: Congenital atresia of the uterine cervix. *Obstet Gynecol 42:* 213, 1973.
30. Pinsky, L.: A community of human malformation syndromes involving the Müllerian ducts, distal extremities, urinary tract and ears. *Teratology 9:* 65, 1974.
31. Fore, S. R., Hammond, C. B., Parker, R. T., et al.: Urologic and genital anomalies in patients with congenital absence of the vagina. *Obstet Gynecol 46:* 410, 1975.
32. Counsellor, V. S., Davis, C. E.: Atresia of the vagina. *Obstet Gynecol 32:* 528, 1968.
33. Polishuk, W. Z., Sharf, M.: Primary amenorrhea due to intrauterine adhesions. *Gynaecologia (Basel) 154:* 181, 1962.
34. Wilson, J. D., Goldstein, J. L.: Classification of hereditary disorders of sexual development, in Bergsma, D. (ed): *Genetic Forms of Hypogonadism,* New York, Stratton Intercontinental Corp., 1975, p. 1.
35. Prader, A., Anders, G. J.: Zur genetik der kongenitalen Lipoidhyperplasie der Nebenieren. *Helvet Paediatr Acta 17:* 285, 1962.
36. Kirkland, R. T., Kirkland, S. L., Johnson, C. M., et al.: Congenital lipoid adrenal hyperplasia in an eight-year old phenotypic female. *J Clin Endocrinol Metab 36:* 488, 1973.
37. Parks, E. A., Bermudez, J. A., Anast, C. S., et al.: Pubertal boy with the 3β-hydroxysteroid dehydrogenase defect. *J Clin Endocrinol Metab 33:* 269, 1971.
38. Zachmann, M., Vollmin, J. A., Hamilton, W., et al.: Steroid 17,20-desmolase deficiency: a new cause of male pseudohermaphroditism. *Clin Endocrinol 1:* 369, 1972.
39. Saez, J. M., De Peretti, E., Morera, A. M., et al.: Familial male psuedohermaphroditism with gynecomastia due to a testicular 17-ketosteroid reductase defect. I. Studies *in vivo. J Clin Endocrinol Metab 32:* 604, 1971.
40. Goebelsman, U., Horton, R., Mestman, J. M., et al.: Male pseudohermaphroditism due to testicular 17β-hydroxysteroid dehydrogenase deficiency. *J Clin Endocrinol Metab 36:* 867, 1973.
41. New, M.: Male pseudohermaphroditism due to 17α-hydroxylase deficiency. *J Clin Invest 49:* 1930, 1970.
42. Imperato-McGinley, J., Guerrero, L., Gautier, T., et al.: Steroid 5α-reductase deficiency in man: an inherited form of male pseudohermaphroditism. *Science 186:* 1213, 1974.
43. Moore, R. J., Griff, J. E., Wilson, J. D.: Diminished 5α-reductase activity in extracts of fibroblasts cultured from patients with familial incomplete male pseudohermaphroditism, type 2. *J Biol Chem 250:* 7168, 1975.
44. Bardin, C. W., Bullock, L. P., Sherins, R. J., et al.: Androgen metabolism and mechanism of action in male pseudohermaphroditism: A study of testicular feminization. *Recent Prog Horm Res 29:* 65, 1973.
45. Morris, J. M.: The syndrome of testicular feminization in male pseudohermaphrodites. *Am J Obstet Gynecol 65:* 1192, 1953.
46. Morris, J. M., Mahesh, B.: Further observations on the syndrome, "testicular feminization." *Am J Obstet Gynecol 87:* 731, 1963.
47. Rosenfield, R. L., Lawrence, A. M., Liao, S., et al.: Androgens and androgen responsiveness in the feminizing testis syndrome. Comparison of complete and "incomplete" forms. *J Clin Endocrinol Metab 32:* 625, 1971.
48. Madden, J. D., Walsh, P. C., MacDonald, P. C., et al.: Clinical and endocrinological characterization of a patient with the syndrome of incomplete testicular feminization. *J Clin Endocrinol Metab 41:* 751, 1975.
49. Wilson, J. D., Harrod, M. J., Goldstein, J. L., et al.: Familial incomplete male pseudohermaphroditism, type 1. *N Engl J Med 290:* 1097, 1971.
50. Walsh, P. C., Madden, J. D., Harrod, M. T., et al.: Familial incomplete male pseudohermaphroditism, type 2. *N Engl J Med 291:* 944, 1974.
51. Lubs, H. A., Vilar, O., Bergenstal, D. M.: Familial male pseudohermaphroditism with labial testes and partial feminization: Endocrine studies and genetic aspects. *J Clin Endocrinol Metab 19:* 1110, 1959.
52. Gilbert-Dreyfus, S., Sebaoun, C. A., Belaisch, J.: Étude d'un cas familial d'androgynoidisme avec hypospadias grave, gynécomastie et hyperoestrogénie. *Ann Endocrinol (Paris) 18:* 93, 1957.
53. Opitz, J. M., Simpson, J. L., Sarto, G. E., et al.: Pseudovaginal perineoscrotal hypospadias. *Clin Genet 3:* 1, 1972.
54. Wilkins, L., Lewis, S. R. A., Klein, R., et al.: The suppression of androgen secretion by cortisone in a case of congenital adrenal hyperplasia. *Bull Johns Hopkins Hosp 86:* 249, 1950.
55. Wilkins, L., Lewis, S. R. A., Klein, R., et al.: Treatment of congenital adrenal hyperplasia with cortisone. *J Clin Endocrinol Metab 11:* 1, 1951.
56. Bongiovanni, A. M., Root, A. W.: The adrenogenital syndrome. *N Engl J Med 268:* 1283, 1342, 1391, 1963.
57. Stempfel, R. S., Tomkins, G. M.: Congenital virilizing adrenocortical hyperplasia (the andrenogenital syndrome), in Stanbury, J. B., Wyngaarden, J. B., Fredrickson, D. S. (eds): *The Metabolic Basis of Inherited Disease,* New York, The Blakiston Division, McGraw-Hill Book Co, 1966, p. 635.
58. Lippe, B. M., LaFranchi, S. H., Lain, N., et al.: Serum 17α-hydroxyprogesterone, progesterone, estradiol and testosterone in the diagnosis and management of congenital adrenal hyperplasia. *J Pediatr 85:* 782, 1974.
59. Goldenberg, R. L., Vaitukaitis, J. L., Ross, G. T.: Estrogen and follicle stimulating hormone interactions on follicle growth in rats. *Endocrinology 90:* 1492, 1972.
60. Reiter, E. O., Goldenberg, R. L., Vaitukaitis, J. L., et al.: Evidence for a role of estrogen in the ovarian augmentation reaction. *Endocrinology 91:* 1518, 1972.
61. Harman, S. M., Louvet, J. P., Ross, G. T.: Interactions of estrogen and gonadotropins on follicular atresia. *Endocrinology 96:* 1145, 1975.
62. Ross, G. T.: Gonadotropins and preantral follicular maturation in women. *Fertil Steril 25:* 522, 1974.
63. Biglieri, E. G., Herron, M. A., Brust, N.: 17-hydroxylation deficiency in man. *J Clin Invest 45:* 1946, 1966.
64. Goldsmith, O., Solomon, D. H., Horton, R.: Hypogonadism and mineralcorticoid excess. The 17-hydroxylase deficiency syndrome. *N Engl J Med 277:* 673, 1967.
65. Mallin, J. R.: Congenital adrenal hyperplasia secondary to 17-hydroxylase deficiency: two sisters with amenorrhea, hypokalemia, hypertension and cystic ovaries. *Ann Intern Med 70:* 69, 1969.
66. Jones, S. G., de Moraes-Ruehsen, M.: A new syndrome of amenorrhea in association with hypergonadotropism and apparently normal ovarian follicular apparatus. *Am J Obstet Gynecol 104:* 597, 1969.
67. Starup, J., Sele, V., Henriksen, B.: Amenorrhea associated with increased production of gonadotropins and a morphologically normal ovarian follicular apparatus. *Acta Endocrinol (Kbh) 66:* 248, 1971.
68. Kallman, F. J., Schoenfeld, W. A., Barrera, S. E.: The genetic aspects of primary eunuchoidism. *Am J Ment Defic 48:* 203, 1944.
69. Gauthier, G.: La dysplasie olfacto-genital. *Acta Neurovegetativa 21:* 345, 1960.
70. Santen, R. J., Paulsen, C. A.: Hypogonadotropic eunuchoidism. II. Gonadal responsiveness to exogenous gonadotropins. *J Clin Endocrinol Metab 36:* 55, 1973.
71. Reitano, J. F., Caminos-Torres, L., Snyder, P. J.: Serum LH and FSH responses to repetitive administration of gonadotropin-releasing hormone in patients with idiopathic hypogonadotropic hypogonadism. *J Clin Endocrinol Metab 41:* 1085, 1975.
72. Santen, R. J., Paulsen, C. A.: Hypogonadotropic eunuchoidism. I. Clinical study of the mode of inheritance. *J Clin Endocrinol Metab 36:* 47, 1973.
73. Hammond, C. B., Hertz, R., Ross, G. T., et al.: Diagnostic problems of choriocarcinoma and related trophoblastic neoplasms. *Obstet Gynecol 29:* 224, 1967.
74. Sheehan, H. L., Davis, J. C.: Pituitary necrosis. *Br Med Bull 24:* 59, 1968.

75. Forbes, A. P., Henneman, P. H., Griswold, G. C., et al.: Syndrome characterized by galactorrhea, amenorrhea and low urinary FSH: Comparison with acromegaly and normal lactation. *J Clin Endocrinol Metab 14:* 265, 1954.
76. Friesen, H. G., Hwang, P., Guyda, H., et al.: Functional evaluation of prolactin secretion: a guide to therapy. *J Clin Invest 51:* 706, 1972.
77. Fournier, P. S. R., Desjardins, P. D., Friesen, H. G.: Current understanding of human prolactin physiology and its diagnostic and therapeutic applications: a review. *Am J Obstet Gynecol 118:* 337, 1974.
78. Mecklenburg, R. J., Loriaux, D. L., Thompson, R. H., et al.: Hypothalamic dysfunction in patients with anorexia nervosa. *Medicine 53:* 147, 1974.
79. Canfield, C. J., Bates, R. W.: Nonpuerperal galactorrhea. *N Engl J Med 273:* 897, 1965.
80. Tolis, G., Summa, M., Van Campenhout, J.: Prolactin secretion in 65 patients with galactorrhea. *Am J Obstet Gynecol 118:* 91, 1974.
81. Tyson, S. E., Andreasson, B., Huth, J., et al.: Neuroendocrine dysfunction in galactorrhea-amenorrhea after oral contraceptive use. *Obstet Gynecol 46:* 1, 1975.
82. Vaitukaitis, J. L., Ross, G. T.: Hormonal interactions during spontaneous normal and altered menstrual cycles, in Behrman, S. J., Kistner, R. W. (eds): *Progress in Infertility,* ed 2, Boston, Little, Brown and Co., 1975, p. 367.
83. Riddick, D. H., Hammond, D. B.: Adrenal virilism due to 21-hydroxylase deficiency in the postmenarcheal female. *Obstet Gynecol 45:* 21, 1975.
84. Asherman, J. G.: Amenorrhea traumatica (atretica). *J Obstet Gynecol Br Emp 55:* 23, 1948.
85. Swerdloff, R. S., Odell, W. D.: Some aspects of the control of LH and FSH in humans, in Rosemberg, E. (ed): *Gonadotropins 1968,* Los Altos, Calif., Geron-X, 1968, p. 155.
86. Jaffe, R. B., Midgley, A. R. Jr.: Current status of human gonadotropin radioimmunoassay. *Obstet Gynecol Surv 24:* 200, 1969.
87. Yen, S. S. C., Vela, P., Rankin, J.: Inappropriate secretion of follicle stimulating hormone and luteinizing hormone in polycystic ovarian disease. *J Clin Endocrinol Metab 30:* 435, 1970.
88. Goldenberg, R. L., Grodin, J. M., Vaitukaitis, J. L., et al.: Withdrawal bleeding and luteinizing hormone secretion following progesterone in women with amenorrhea. *Am J Obstet Gynecol 115:* 193, 1973.
89. Kistner, R. W.: Induction of ovulation with clomiphene citrate, in Behrman, S. J., Kistner, R. W. (eds): *Progress in Infertility,* ed 2, Boston, Little, Brown and Co., 1975, p. 509.
90. Goldenberg, R. L., Grodin, J. M., Rodbard, D., et al.: Gonadotropin in women with amenorrhea. *Am J Obstet Gynecol 116:* 1003, 1973.
91. Kletzky, O. A., Davajan, V., Nakamura, R. M., et al.: Clinical categorization of patients with secondary amenorrhea using progesterone-induced uterine bleeding and measurement of serum gonadotropin levels. *Am J Obstet Gynecol 121:* 695, 1975.
92. Kletzky, O. A., Davajan, V., Nakamura, A. M., et al.: Classification of secondary amenorrhea based on distinct hormonal patterns. *J Clin Endocrinol Metab 41:* 660, 1975.
93. Ross, G. T., Hammond, C. B., Hertz, R., et al.: Chemotherapy of metastatic and non-metastatic gestational trophoblastic neoplasms. *Tex Rep Biol Med 24:* 326, 1966.
94. Vaitukaitis, J. L., Braunstein, G. D., Ross, G. T.: A radioimmunoassay which specifically measures human chorionic gonadotropin in the presence of human luteinizing hormone. *Am J Obstet Gynecol 113:* 751, 1972.
95. Ross, G. T.: Bioassay for hCG, in Berson, S. A., Yalow, R. S. (eds): *Methods in Clinical Investigative and Diagnostic Endocrinology,* vol 6, part 3. Amsterdam, North-Holland Publishing Co., 1973, p. 749.
96. Brewer, J. J., Eckman, T. R., Dolkart, R. E., et al.: Gestational trophoblastic disease. *Am J Obstet Gynecol 109:* 335, 1971.
97. Hardy, J.: Transsphenoidal surgery of hypersecreting pituitary tumors, in Kohler, P. C., Ross, G. T. (eds): *Diagnosis and Treatment of Pituitary Tumors,* Amsterdam, New York, Excerpta Medica, American Elsevier Publishing, 1973, p. 179.
98. Hammond, C. B., Marshall, J. R.: Ovulation induction with human gonadotropins: A study in dosage delineation, in Rosemberg, E. (ed): *Gonadotropin Therapy in Female Infertility.* Amsterdam, Excerpta Medica, 1973, p. 117.
99. Gemzell, C.: Induction of ovulation in infertile women with pituitary tumors. *Am J Obstet Gynecol 121:* 371, 1975.
100. Besser, G. M., Parke, L., Edwards, C. R. W., et al.: Galactorrhea: successful treatment with reduction of plasma prolactin levels by Brom-ergocryptine. *Br Med J iii:* 669, 1972.
101. Varga, L., Wenner, R., del Pozo, E.: Treatment of galactorrhea-amenorrhea syndrome with Br-ergocryptine (CB154): restoration of ovulatory function and fertility. *Am J Obstet Gynecol 117:* 75, 1973.
102. Rolland, R., Schellekens, L. A., Lequin, R. N.: Successful treatment of galactorrhea and amenorrhea with subsequent restoration of ovarian function by a new ergot alkaloid 2-Brom-alpha ergocryptine. *Clin Endocrinol 3:* 155, 1974.
103. Ross, G. T., Scholz, D. A., Lambert, E. H., et al.: Severe uterine bleeding and degenerative skeletal muscle changes in unrecognized myxedema. *J Clin Endocrinol Metab 18:* 492, 1958.
104. Fraser, I. S., Michie, E. A., Wide, L., et al.: Pituitary gonadotropins and ovarian function in adolescent dysfunctional uterine bleeding. *J Clin Endocrinol Metab 37:* 407, 1973.
105. Fraser, I. S., Baird, D. T.: Blood production and ovarian secretion rates of estradiol 17β and estrone in women with dysfunctional uterine bleeding. *J Clin Endocrinol Metab 39:* 564, 1974.

112

Contraception

Daniel R. Mishell, Jr.

An ideal method of contraception has not yet been developed. All existing contraceptive techniques have advantages and disadvantages. Therefore, when advising a patient as to which method of contraception to use, the physician should explain the advantages and disadvantages of each so that the woman will be fully informed and can make a rational decision to choose the method most suitable for her. If there are medical reasons for not using certain methods, the physician should inform the patient and offer her alternatives. Other than the condom and vasectomy, no methods have been developed for use by the male.

The methods of contraception most widely used by married women in the United States in 1975, in order of popularity, were oral steroids, condom, intrauterine device (IUD), diaphragm, foam, and rhythm.[1] Of these, the two most effective methods are the oral steroids, and the IUD, with use-failure rates of about 1 and 2 percent, respectively, in the first year of use. The failure rates of the other traditional methods are approximately five times greater; however, if the new, improved locally applied vaginal foams are used consistently prior to each coital act, they have an annual pregnancy rate of about 3 percent.[2] Women who have used the diaphragm for several years also have a pregnancy rate of about 3 percent. The diaphragm must be carefully fitted by the physician and then reinserted by the patient. The physician should then examine the patient to make sure the diaphragm is covering the cervix. When the woman is wearing the diaphragm, she should not be aware of its presence or note discomfort. Contraceptive cream should be used with the diaphragm and should remain in place for 8 hours after the last coital act.

The use of the condom should be encouraged for individuals with multiple sexual partners, as it is the only method of contraception that is markedly effective in preventing transmission of venereal disease. The condom should not be applied tightly. The tip should overlap about ½ inch to collect the ejaculate, which should not be spilled upon withdrawal.

RHYTHM

The Catholic Church officially proscribes all methods of contraception other than rhythm, or periodic abstinence. The rationale for the rhythm method is based upon three assumptions: (1) the human ovum is capable of being fertilized for only about 24 hours after ovulation; (2) spermatozoa can retain their fertilizing ability for only about 48 hours after coitus; and (3) ovulation usually occurs 12 to 16 days (14 ± 2) days before the onset of the subsequent menes.[3] According to these assumptions, and after the woman records the length of her cycles for several months, she establishes her fertile period by subtracting 18 days from the length of her previous shortest cycle and 11 days from her previous longest cycle. In each subsequent cycle, the couple abstains from coitus during this calculated fertile period. The use-effectiveness of this method of periodic abstinence is poor. Failure rates vary between 21 to 47 per 100 woman-years.[4,5,6] The failure rate in one large U.S. study was reported to be 30 per 100 woman-years.[7] Ryder[8] has recently reported that 21 percent of American women who used rhythm to prevent an unwanted pregnancy were unsuccessful. The reasons for this lack of success, as summarized by Mastroianni in a recent review,[3] are numerous, despite advances in knowledge of human reproductive physiology. First, there is no good evidence to indicate that the three assumptions stated above, upon which rhythm method are based, have scientific validity. Second, there is great irregularity in menstrual cycle length, so that women with previous regular cycles often have occasional marked variation in cycle length. Cycle irregularity is very common in perimenarcheal and perimenopausal women, during a time of life when most pregnancies are unwanted. Third, because a woman is menstruating during several of the nonfertile days and since most couples do not have coitus during this time, the period of abstinence is frequently greater than the time during which sexual relations may be practiced.

In order to increase the effectiveness of the rhythm method, instead of relying solely on the calendar method described above, it is advisable to measure the basal body temperature every day. Progesterone causes an increase in basal temperature. If the couple abstains from intercourse from the start of menses until at least 48 hours after the rise in basal body temperature (2 days after ovulation), sexual relations will take place only after the ovum is no longer capable of being fertilized. Data from several sources indicate that the use of daily basal temperature for determining the days of periodic abstinence increases the effectiveness of the rhythm method. One British study reported a failure rate of only 6.6 per 100 woman-years in women practicing the temperature method for determining the time of periodic abstinence.[9]

Recently, there have been reports that women could detect changes in their own cervical mucus. By analyzing their own cervical mucus quality and quantity, they may be taught to predict the time when ovulation is going to occur. Although reports of extraordinary success of this method have been made by some enthusiasts,[10] careful analysis of their results suggests that the actual effectiveness of this modification is substantially less than claimed.[11]

Thus, periodic abstinence, or the rhythm method, requires a high degree of motivation, communication, and sophistication. Even with these qualities, the rhythm method of family planning is associated with a very high failure rate, and this should be understood by all couples choosing to use this method of family planning.

ORAL STEROIDS

The steroid contraceptive pill is the most widely used method of contraception. Westoff,[1] in a recent report based upon data obtained from the National Fertility Studies of 1965, 1970, and 1975, indicated that the oral steroids were the most popular method of contraception by married women in the United States in those years. Although their popularity increased between 1965 and 1970, use of oral steroids has stabilized since. Westoff estimated that between 1965 and 1970, use of the oral contraceptive steroids increased from 24.4 percent to 35.4 percent of all married couples practicing contraception, but in 1975 it was used by only 34.3 percent. In 1975, about 1 out of 5 married women in the United States used oral contraceptive steroids. The use of oral contraceptives is much more popular among women married less than five years, being used by 64.8 percent, than women married longer. Oral contraceptives are used by 59.5 percent of married women intending to have more children, in contrast to only 24.1 percent of women who have completed their families.

There were originally three major categories of oral steroid contraceptives: combination, sequential, and daily gestagen. The combination is the most widely used and most effective type. It consists of tablets containing both an estrogen and a gestagen given continuously for 3 weeks. The sequential type consisting of a regimen of estrogen alone given for about 2 weeks followed by 1 week of combination estrogen and gestagen is no longer used. With both types, no medication is given for 1 week out of 4 to allow for withdrawal bleeding. In the third method, a small dose of gestagen without estrogen is ingested every day.

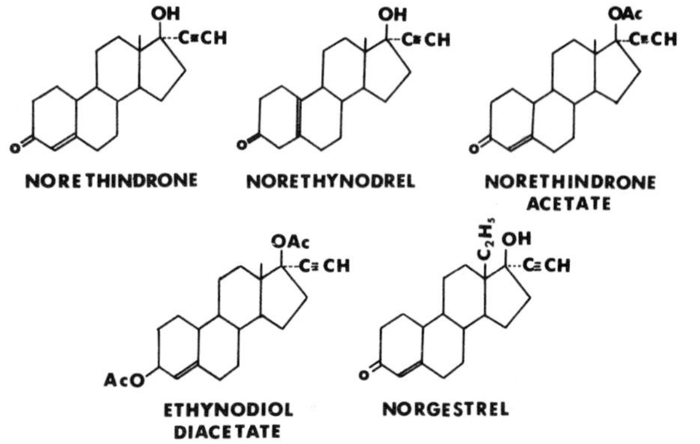

NORETHINDRONE NORETHYNODREL NORETHINDRONE ACETATE ETHYNODIOL DIACETATE NORGESTREL

Fig. 112-1. Formulas of the five gestagens used in combination oral contraceptives in the United States.

MESTRANOL ETHINYL ESTRADIOL

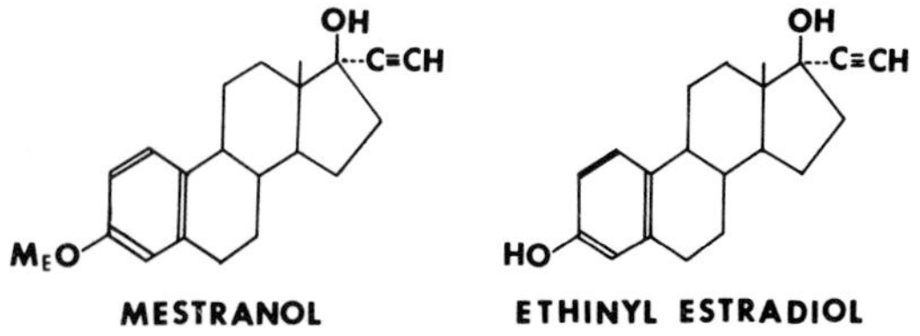

Fig. 112-2. Formulas of the two estrogens used in combination oral contraceptives in the United States.

PHARMACOLOGY

Presently used oral contraceptives do not contain natural estrogens or gestagens but are formulated of synthetic steroids. Two major types of synthetic gestagens are known: (1) derivatives of 19-nor testosterone and (2) derivatives of 17-α-acetoxy progesterone. The latter group of C-21 gestagens, consisting of steroids such as medroxyprogesterone acetate and megestrol acetate, are not used in present contraceptive formulations. In contrast to the 19-nor testosterone derivatives, when these agents were given to female beagle dogs, the animals developed an increased incidence of mammary cancer.[12] Thus, all oral contraceptive formulations now available in the United States consist of varying dosages of one of the following five 19-nor testosterone gestagens: norethynodrel, norethindrone, norethindrone acetate, ethinyldiol diacetate, or norgestrel (Fig. 112-1). With the exception of two daily gestagen formulations, the gestagens are combined with varying dosages of two estrogens, ethinyl estradiol and ethinyl estradiol-3-methyl ether (mestranol) (Fig. 112-2). Each of these compounds has an ethinyl group on the 17 position. The presence of this ethinyl group enhances the oral activity of these agents. Their essential functional groups are not as rapidly hydroxylated and then conjugated while they pass through the portal system as are the natural steroids.

The various modifications in chemical structure of the different synthetic gestagens and estrogens also alter their biologic activity. For these reasons, one cannot compare the pharmacologic activity of the various gestagens or estrogens in the particular contraceptive steroid only on the basis of amount present in the formulation. The biologic activity of the various steroids must also be considered. It has been reported that norethindrone and norethynodrel are approximately equal in activity, while norethindrone acetate is twice as active as the former compounds. Ethinyldiol diacetate is 15 times as potent and norgestrel is about 30 times as potent as norethindrone.[4] Ethinyl estradiol is about 1.7 to 2 times as potent as mestranol.[15] A schematic representation of the various combination contraceptive formulations available in the United States, together with the estimated potency of each of their components, is shown in Figure 112-3.[16] When deciding which contraceptive steroid to prescribe initially, it is important to evaluate both the quantity and the biologic activity of both steroid components of the formulations.

PHYSIOLOGY

Mechanism of Action

The combination pill is the most effective type of oral contraceptive because these preparations consistently inhibit the midcycle gonadotropin surge and thus prevent ovulation. In addition, the drugs act on other steps in the reproductive process. They alter the cervical mucus, making it consistently thick, viscid, and scanty in amount, and thus retard sperm penetration. They alter motility of the muscle of the uterus and oviduct, thus altering transport of both ova and sperm. Furthermore, they alter the endometrium, so that glandular production of glycogen is diminished and less energy

RELATIVE POTENCY OF ESTROGENS AND PROGESTINS IN CURRENTLY AVAILABLE COMBINATION CONTRACEPTIVES

Potency (units)	Progestin	Preparation	Estrogen	Potency (units)
2	norethindrone acetate 1 mg	Loestrin 1/20 Zorane 1/20	ethinyl estradiol 20 mcg	0.7 to 0.8
0.5	norethindrone 0.5 mg	Modicon Brevicon	ethinyl estradiol 35 mcg	1.2 to 1.4
1	norethindrone 1 mg	Ortho-Novum 1/50 Norinyl 1/50	mestranol 50 mcg	1
3	norethindrone acetate 1.5 mg	Loestrin 1.5/30 Zorane 1.5/30	ethinyl estradiol 30 mcg	1 to 1.2
1	norethindrone 1 mg	Ortho-Novum 1/80 Norinyl 1/80	mestranol 80 mcg	1.6
2	norethindrone acetate 1 mg	Norlestrin - 1	ethinyl estradiol 50 mcg	1.7 to 2
2	norethindrone 2 mg	Ortho-Novum 2 mg Norinyl 2	mestranol 100 mcg	2
2.7	norethynodrel 2.5 mg	Enovid - E	mestranol 100 mcg	2
5	norethindrone acetate 2.5 mg	Norlestrin 2.5	ethinyl estradiol 50 mcg	1.7 to 2
15	norgestrel 0.5 mg	Orval	ethinyl estradiol 50 mcg	1.7 to 2
15	ethynodiol diacetate 1 mg	Demulen	ethinyl estradiol 50 mcg	1.7 to 2
15	ethynodiol diacetate 1 mg	Ovulen	mestranol 100 mcg	2

15 5 0 — Potency (units) — 0 1 2 — Potency (units)

*adapted from Heinen, (1971)

Fig. 112-3. Type of estrogen and gestagen used in combination oral contraceptives in the United States with estimate of their relative potency.

is available to support blastocyst survival in the uterine cavity. Finally, they alter ovarian responsiveness to gonadotropin stimulation.[13] Nevertheless, neither gonadotropin production nor ovarian steroidogenesis is completely abolished, and levels of those endogenous hormones in the peripheral blood during ingestion of combination oral contraceptives are similar to those found in the early follicular phase of the normal cycle (Figs. 112-4 and 112-5).[17]

Contraceptive steroids prevent ovulation mainly by interfering with LH-RH release from the hypothalamus. In rats, as well as in a few studies in humans, this inhibitory action of the contraceptive steroids could be overcome by the administration of LH-RH.[18,19] In other studies, however, most women who had received combination contraceptive steroids for more than 1 year had suppression of LH and FSH release following LH-RH infusion.[20–22] It is possible that when hypothalamic inhibition occurs for a prolonged time, the mechanism for synthesis and release of gonadotropins may become refractory to the normal amount of LH-RH stimulation. However, the possibility also exists that combination contraceptive steroids may have a direct inhibitory effect

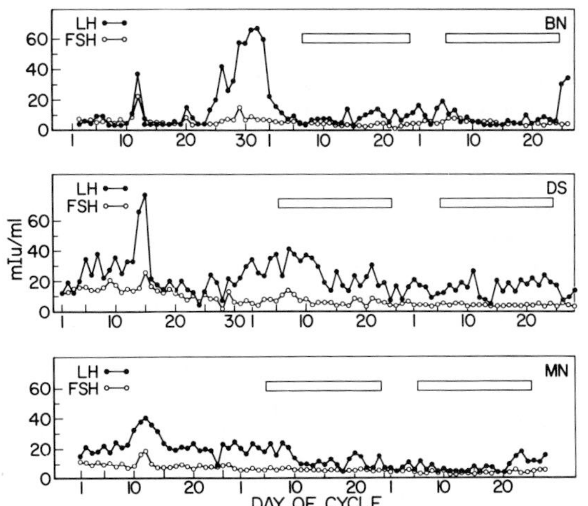

Fig. 112-4. Daily serum LH and FSH levels in three subjects for three cycles. The first cycle served as a control and the last two were treatment cycles with a combination oral contraceptive. The horizontal bars indicate the days when the steroid was ingested. (Adapted from Mishell et al., Am. J. Obstet. Gynecol. *114:* 923, 1972.)

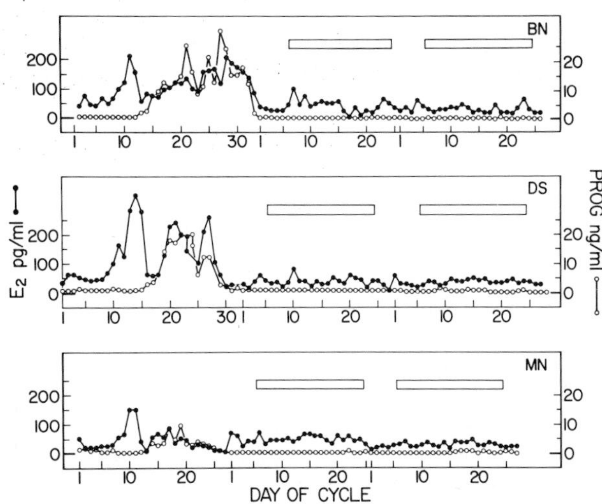

Fig. 112-5. Daily serum estradiol and progesterone levels in the same three subjects as in Figure 112-4. (Adapted from Mishell et al., *Am. J. Obstet. Gynec. 114:* 923, 1972.)

on the gonadotropin-producing cells of the pituitary in addition to their effect on the hypothalamus.

The sequential and daily gestagen preparations do not consistently inhibit ovulation. Although they exert their contraceptive action via the other mechanisms listed above, because of the inconsistent ovulation inhibition the effectiveness of these two preparations is significantly less than with the combined type.

The combined type of oral contraceptive is the most effective method of contraception currently available, and there has been no significant difference in clinical effectiveness demonstrated among the various combination formulations listed in Figure 112-3. Provided no tablets are omitted, the pregnancy rate is less than 0.2 percent per 100 women at the end of 1 year.

Metabolic Effects

In addition to the above-mentioned effects upon the hypothalamic-pituitary axis and female genital tract which prevent pregnancy, both the estrogen and gestagen components of the oral contraceptive pills have many other actions that affect nearly every organ system of the body. More than 52 metabolic alterations have been reported in users of oral contraceptives. As a result of these metabolic changes, patients taking these medications frequently experience undesirable side effects in addition to the prevention of conception.

Although unwanted side effects associated with oral contraceptive therapy are common, the incidence of serious complications associated with their use is relatively rare. Because of the rarity of serious effects, definite establishment of a causal relation to steroid ingestion is difficult. In most instances, a relation has been implied by a series of case reports followed by a retrospective review. After 2 years of planning, in 1962, the Royal College of General Practitioners of Great Britain began a large-scale, controlled prospective study of the health of oral contraceptive users involving 1400 physicians, 23,611 oral contraceptive users, and 22,766 controls. An interim report of the first 5 years of this study was published in 1974.[23] From this report, as well as from other studies in the literature, an evaluation of the various metabolic alterations and clinical changes associated with oral contraceptive use has been developed. For convenience, these effects have been classified into three categories: (1) effects on the primary target organs of the female reproductive system, (2) general metabolic effects, and (3) effects on other organ systems.

Effects on Organs of the Female Reproductive System

Ovary. Stromal fibrosis has been reported. It is usually transitory, disappears after contraceptives are stopped, and is of no clinical significance.

Myometrium. Leiomyomata may enlarge with oral contraceptive use. On occasion they can greatly enlarge and become symptomatic. Their presence constitutes one of the relative contraindications to the use of contraceptive steroids.

Endometrium. Alterations occur in the endometrium, so that hypomenorrhea, amenorrhea, or lack of withdrawal bleeding may occur as well as intermenstrual bleeding. Usually these symptoms are caused by insufficient estrogen or excessive progestagen and can be ameliorated by increasing the estrogen/progestogen ratio. The steroids in the pill produce these effects by acting directly upon the endometrium and not by action on the hypothalamic-pituitary axis. Thus, lack of withdrawal bleeding during oral contraceptive therapy is not related to postpill amenorrhea.

Amenorrhea while taking the pill is only of concern because it cannot be differentiated from pregnancy. Oral steroids should not be ingested during pregnancy, so it is best to induce withdrawal bleeding in women taking oral contraceptives by increasing the estrogenic components or by using a less potent gestagen.

Cervix. A polypoid hyperplasia of the endocervical glands has been noted in oral contraceptive users. Although somewhat similar in appearance to adenocarcinoma of the endocervix, this change is not malignant or premalignant. There is no evidence that oral contraceptives cause an increased incidence of epidermoid carcinoma of the cervix or carcinoma in situ. It has been reported that patients who use oral contraceptives have a higher incidence of abnormal cervical cytology than women who use other types of contraception, but the abnormal cytology is not causally related to oral contraceptive use.[25]

Vagina. There have been numerous reports on bacterial changes in the vagina, with an increase of vaginitis, especially moniliasis, in women using contraceptive steroids. However, one prospective study has shown that contraceptive steroids do not cause an increased incidence of monilial vaginitis.[26] If monilial vaginitis develops in oral contraceptive users, a glucose tolerance test should be performed.

Breasts. There is an increased incidence of breast tenderness, mainly related to the estrogenic component of the pill. In addition, there is a change in lactation, as the amount of milk produced is diminished and the quality of the milk is altered. Hormonal contraceptives reduce the concentration of both proteins and fats in human milk.[27] The steroids are also found in measurable amounts in the milk of lactating women. Therefore, oral contraceptives are not advised for patients who wish to nurse. Development of galactorrhea is also an uncommon side effect associated with hormonal contraceptives. Serum prolactin levels are slightly elevated in oral contraceptive users.[28] There is no evidence of an increase in malignant breast disease in users of oral contraceptives. In addition, there is evidence from both retrospective studies and the British prospective study that the incidence of benign breast disease, mainly fibrocystic disease, is reduced in oral contraceptive users and that this reduction is directly related to the dose of gestagen in the product.[24,29]

Hypothalamus. The incidence of amenorrhea for more than 6 months after discontinuing oral contraceptives has been reported to range from 0.2 to 0.7 percent in three separate study populations.[30–32] The incidence is higher in patients who have oligomenorrhea or amenorrhea prior to starting oral contraceptive therapy than in those with regular menses. The results of two separate studies have shown that 35 to 41 percent of women who develop amenorrhea after taking oral contraceptives have a prior history of menstrual irregularity.[30,31] It is not known whether postpill amenorrhea is caused by continued suppression of the hypothalamic-pituitary axis or whether the periodic withdrawal bleeding produced by oral contraceptives serves to mask an amenorrheic state that would have occurred if the steroids were not ingested, or whether both mechanisms occur. In any event, the use of any oral contraceptive steroid is contraindicated for patients who have oligomenorrhea or amenorrhea. Shearman noted that the incidence of postpill amenorrhea after ingesting either combined or sequential types of oral contraceptives was similar to the incidence of sale of these two preparations in Australia.[33] Thus, there is no advantage for using sequential preparations for women with oligomenorrhea. If individuals with amenorrhea or oligomenorrhea desire regular menses, treatment with a gestagen alone for 5 days each month is usually sufficient to induce menses without suppressing hypothalamic function or masking the development of amenorrhea associated with low estrogen production. If these women desire contraception, it is best to use a method other than hormonal steroids, preferably a barrier method or copper IUD. It must be realized that women with a previous history of regular menses may also develop postpill amenorrhea. If amenorrhea persists for more than 6 months, routine diagnostic procedures should be undertaken to determine the etiology. Shearman has reported that treatment of these patients with ovulation-inducing drugs resulted in only a 42.6 percent conception rate.[33]

General Metabolic Effects

Serum Proteins. In addition to a general lowering of blood amino acid levels similar to the changes seen in pregnancy, there are quantitative changes in blood protein concentration similar to those occurring in pregnancy but of less magnitude. Thus, there are increases in alpha 2 and beta globulins, blood coagulation factors and the carrier proteins, cortisol-binding globulin, thyroid-binding globulin, transferrin, and ceruloplasmin. The pre-beta-lipoprotein and haptoglobin levels are also increased, while albumin levels are decreased.[34] These changes are due mainly to a direct effect of the estrogen component of the oral steroid upon the endoplasmic reticulum of the liver, which results in altered protein production. The changes, for the most part, do not represent a medical hazard, but they do alter the results of some clinical laboratory tests. Thus, serum levels of copper and iron will be increased, while tests of thyroid function will be altered to the same extent that occurs in pregnancy. There is no evidence, however, that the oral steroids alter thyroid function itself. In contrast, there is a slight but definite increase in free as well as bound plasma cortisol levels.[35] The increase in free cortisol is not as great as that which occurs in pregnancy, but this slight elevation, combined with other actions of the steroids, may contribute to a number of side effects, such as fluid retention, headache, and mood changes. In addition to these effects, the protein changes noted above have been shown to be responsible for two significant clinical effects, thromboembolism and hypertension.

Studies by Vessey and Doll[36] in England and Sartwell et al.[37] in the United States revealed a low but significant increase in thromboembolic disease in oral contraceptive users. Mortality from thromboembolic disease associated with the use of hormonal contraceptives is estimated to be about 3 per 100,000 women per year. Results from these retrospective studies were confirmed by the British prospective study. A causal relation between use of oral contraceptives and thromboembolism has thus been definitely established. The British study indicated that there was no relation to age, parity, smoking, or duration of oral contraceptive use and the development of thromboembolic disease.[24] Although as noted later, the incidence of myocardial infarction is increased by oral contraceptives, and this increase is most pronounced in women who smoke. The etiology, in addition to the increase in blood clotting factors noted above, results from an increase in the number of platelets as well as platelet adhesiveness and a decrease in antithrombins. All these changes are produced by the estrogenic component. There is evidence that this increased incidence of thromboembolism is related to the amount of estrogen and that formulations containing 50 ug or less of the estrogen component are associated with a lower incidence of thromboembolic phenomena. Therefore, it is best not to prescribe pills with a greater amount of estrogen unless it is necessary to prevent breakthrough bleeding. It is not necessary for patients to have clinical evidence of deep vein thrombophlebitis of the lower extremities in order to develop pulmonary thromboembolism while receiving oral contraceptives. There is also no evidence that the incidence of thromboembolism is increased in women with varicosities of the lower extremities. Individuals who develop chest pain while taking contraceptive steroids should discontinue therapy and have further diagnostic studies, including a lung scan.

The second significant clinical effect resulting from protein changes is hypertension. One of the increased alpha 2 globulins is plasma renin substrate. In certain individuals without a normally functioning feedback mechanism, plasma renin and angiotensin levels are increased, and significant but reversible hypertension develops shortly after initiating therapy.[38] The incidence of hypertension in normotensive women following treatment with oral contraceptives is relatively low. Since these women cannot be identified in advance, all individuals treated with oral steroids should have regular monitoring of their blood pressure. A larger proportion of women with preexisting hypertension may have a further increase in blood pressure with oral contraceptive therapy, and thus the presence of preexisting hypertension constitutes a relative contraindication to their use. The British prospective study estimated that the incidence of hypertension in the first year of pill use is less than 1 percent, but it showed that there was a relation between the duration of oral contraceptive use and the development of hypertension. Data from this study indicated that about 5 percent of oral contraceptive users develop hypertension after 5 years of usage, an incidence about 2.6 times greater than controls.[24]

Carbohydrate Metabolism. There is a body of evidence reporting alterations in glucose metabolism associated with oral contraceptive use, including impairment of glucose tolerance and an increase in plasma insulin levels.[39] It has not been definitely established whether these changes are related to the estrogen or to the gestagen component of the pill or to both. There is some indication that different gestagens may have a varying effect upon glucose tolerance. Women who have taken oral contraceptive steroids for long periods of time have an increased incidence of abnormal glucose tolerance tests.[39] For this reason, oral contraceptives are not advised for patients who have had a previous abnormal glucose tolerance test, such as those with gestational diabetes. There is an increased likelihood that oral contraceptives will induce the same alterations in glucose metabolism that developed in these individuals during pregnancy. Because of the increased frequency of altered glucose metabolism in individuals receiving oral contraceptives, it is suggested that a glucose tolerance test be performed annually in all women receiving this type of contraceptive who are at risk to develop diabetes, e.g., those with a family history of diabetes, heavy birth weight babies, unexplained fetal deaths, and obesity. Other users should have an annual single fasting blood glucose determination. Women with insulin-dependent diabetes may need to have the dose readjusted after initiating oral contraceptive therapy. There is some evidence that oral contraceptives may increase the incidence of myocardial infarction in women with insulin-dependent diabetes.[40,41]

Lipid Metabolism. Oral contraceptives cause an increase in serum lipid levels, mainly triglycerides, in nearly all users.[42] Some women also have an increase in serum cholesterol concentration. The increase in triglycerides appears to be mainly an effect of estrogen. Recent data also suggest that oral contraceptives increase incidence of myocardial infarction, especially in older women and in those with associated risk factors, such as preexisting elevated serum lipid levels, hypertension, obesity, diabetes mellitus, and smoking.[40,41]

Water and Electrolyte Metabolism. The effect of oral contraceptives on salt metabolism is poorly understood. Treatment with oral steroids causes a decrease of sodium excretion accompanied by water retention. Some users develop edema and associated weight gain of 3 to 5 pounds. These effects may also be important in those women developing hypertension.

Body Weight. Because the gestagens in current formulations are chemically related to testosterone, they are anabolic, and in some women there will be an increase in body weight beyond the 3 to 5 pounds due to retention of fluid. Balance studies have shown an increase in nitrogen retention in individuals receiving oral contraceptives.[43] Thus, if a woman gains more than 10 pounds in a year, oral contraceptives should be discontinued or one containing a less potent gestagen should be utilized.

Tryptophan Metabolism. Tryptophan is normally metabolized by two pathways, a major nicotinic acid ribonucleotide sequence in the liver and a minor serotonin sequence in the brain. The estrogenic component of the oral contraceptives diverts tryptophan from the minor to the major pathway, thus causing lower serotonin levels in the brain.[35] These low serotonin levels are associated with depression and sleep disturbances, and it is thought that this mechanism explains some of the neuropsychiatric symptoms noted in oral contraceptive users. The British prospective study confirmed the causal relation of oral contraceptives with neurotic depression.[24] Some of these metabolic changes in tryptophan metabolism are also noted in pyridoxine deficiency, and oral contraceptive users have low levels of pyridoxine. Symptoms of depression in oral contraceptive users may be alleviated by treatment with pyridoxine (vitamin B_6).

Vitamins and Minerals. In addition to pyridoxine, there are decreases in folic acid, calcium, manganese, and zinc, while ascorbic acid levels are increased in oral contraceptive users. The clinical significance, if any, of these changes is unknown at present, and routine vitamin supplements for oral contraceptive users have not been shown to be of benefit.

Effects on Other Organ Systems

Liver. There is an increased incidence of abnormalities in some liver function tests in oral contraceptive users, mainly in tests dealing with bile excretion such as BSP retention. The steroids adversely affect the function of enzymes aiding excretion of bile, similar to the changes that occur in pregnancy. Both a collaborative retrospective study in the United States and the prospective British study indicate that oral contraceptive users have twice the risk of developing cholelithiasis as do controls.[24,29] However, the actual incidence is small, being estimated at 49 to 68 women per 100,000 users per year in the two studies. Oral contraceptives cause marked alterations in the composition of bile in the gallbladder of women, consisting mainly of an increase in the concentration of cholesterol.[44] Those individuals who develop idiopathic recurrent jaundice of pregnancy frequently develop jaundice when treated with oral contraceptive steroids, and use is thus contraindicated in these individuals. Active liver disease is also a contraindication to hormonal contraceptive therapy, but use is not restricted in individuals with a past history of hepatitis who currently have normal liver function. Nevertheless, these individuals in particular should have periodic tests of liver function at regular intervals after receiving oral steroids. A rare complication, attributed to long-term use of oral contraceptives in a recent retrospective study, is the presence of liver cell adenomas.[45] The incidence of these tumors, which can cause pain as well as rupture with intraperitoneal bleeding, is probably only about one in one million users. Nevertheless, routine annual palpation of the liver should be performed in all women ingesting oral contraceptives.

Central Nervous System. There is an increased incidence of nausea and vomiting as well as migraine headaches and cerebral vascular accidents in women receiving oral contraceptives. The incidence of nausea is thought to be related to the estrogen component and is greater in the first few cycles of use. There is an increased incidence of migraine headaches in oral contraceptive users, but apparently there is no relation to the incidence of other types of headaches.[46] In individuals with preexisting migraine headaches, the time of occurrence may change from the premenstrual portion of the untreated cycle to the medication-free interval following therapy.

A recent retrospective collaborative study has estimated that the relative incidence of cerebral thrombosis in women who use oral contraceptives is about nine times greater than in nonusers, while the risk of developing a cerebral hemorrhage was doubled.[47] The prospective British study confirmed the increased occurrence of cerebrovascular disease in oral contraceptive users.[24] Although the incidence of this severe complication is extremely low, a definite causal relation has been established. Therefore, if patients develop an increased incidence of headache or develop any peripheral neurological changes while they are taking oral steroids, it is best to discontinue their use, as these symptoms may be prodromes of cerebrovascular accidents.

Oral contraceptive use may also increase the incidence of epilepsy in some women.[24] Therefore, the presence of epilepsy is also a relative contraindication to oral contraceptives.

Skin. Melasma, similar to that which develops in pregnancy, occurs in some patients receiving oral contraceptives. This change is accentuated by exposure to sunlight and takes a long time to disappear after stopping medication.[48] There is no specific treatment for this cosmetic problem. The gestagenic component of the combination contraceptive causes an increase in sebum production and acne, while the estrogenic component exerts an ameliorative effect. Therefore, in individuals with acne or those who develop acne with contraceptive steroid therapy, a formulation with a higher estrogen gestagen ratio should be used.

Genitourinary Tract. The British prospective study has shown a definite association between oral contraceptive usage and urinary tract infection.[24] Both pyelitis and cystitis were significantly increased in users compared to controls. The reason for this increased incidence of urinary tract infection has not been established but may be due in part to increased sexual activity in pill users.

Gastrointestinal Tract. There have been several case reports indicating possible changes in the gastrointestinal tract related to oral contraceptives, consisting mainly of an increased incidence of mesenteric thrombosis and possibly ulcerative colitis. Whether there is a causal relation between development of these entities and oral contraceptive use is doubtful according to the findings of the British study. Nevertheless, patients developing these disease entities while receiving oral contraceptive therapy should have the medication discontinued.

Eyes. Several adverse ophthalmologic effects, including retinal artery thromboembolism have been reported to occur in oral contraceptive users. Again, no causal relation can be established, and in two well-controlled studies, no significant differences in eye abnormalities were found between groups of women using oral steroids and those not taking the drugs.

Immune Mechanisms. The British study showed a significant increase in frequency of gastric influenza, hay fever, and chicken pox in oral contraceptive users.[24] This increased frequency was also found for other viral diseases and may be related to alterations in the immune mechanism brought about by oral steroid use.

Effect on Subsequent Fertility. There is no evidence that use of oral contraceptives has an adverse effect upon the outcome of subsequent pregnancies. In the British study, the total abortion rate in women stopping oral contraceptives in order to conceive was 13 percent, which is similar to the normal incidence of spontaneous abortion.[24] No significant difference in congenital abnormalities has been found in babies born to previous oral contraceptive users compared to a control population. There is some evidence, however, that ingestion of oral contraceptives during pregnancy may increase the incidence of congenital limb reduction defects[49] as well as cause masculinization of the external genitalia of female fetuses.[50] Therefore, women should not take oral contraceptives if they are pregnant, or if they fail to have withdrawal bleeding and a possibility of pregnancy exists. Resumption of fertility after stopping oral contraceptive use is delayed in some women, estimated to be about 20 percent of users, for 2 or 3 months. In the British study, at the end of 1 year, about 20 percent of nulliparous women and 10 percent of parous women who stopped the pill to become pregnant had not yet conceived.[24] However, 2 years after stopping, 85 percent of nulliparous women and 93 percent of parous women had conceived. Although appropriate controls are not available, since about 10 percent of couples in the general population are infertile, these data indicated that fertility following discontinuation of oral contraceptive use is not substantially reduced, if it is reduced at all. One report has suggested that the incidence of chromosomal abnormalities is increased in spontaneous abortions occurring in women who have conceived shortly after discontinuing oral contraceptives.[51] However, since the incidence of abortion or congenital defects is not increased in women who conceived after discontinuing oral contraceptive use, there does not appear to be any reason to delay conception when discontinuing oral contraceptives. It must be realized, however, that since the return of ovulation is delayed for varying periods of time after stopping oral contraceptives,[52] it may be difficult to estimate the expected date of delivery if conception takes place before spontaneous menses resume.

CHOICE OF FORMULATION

When considering which of the currently available combination steroid preparations to initially prescribe, it has been suggested that preparations with greater amounts of gestagens shall be given to "estrogen-dominant" women and vice versa. There are no factual data to demonstrate that the incidence of side effects is significantly reduced by such a treatment plan. Many of the common annoying side effects, such as nausea and breast tenderness, as well as the uncommon serious side effects, such as thromboembolism, are related to the amount of estrogen in the formulation. Several studies have indicated that preparations containing 50 ug of estrogen are associated with a significantly reduced incidence of thromboembolism.[24] For these reasons, the U.S. Food and Drug Administration in 1970 recommended that "the practicing physician, in his choice of an oral contraceptive, consider that a product containing a lower dose of estrogen should be prescribed if it is otherwise effective and acceptable to the patient. The higher dose products should be reserved for use when necessary."

Although most of the serious adverse metabolic and clinical alterations are related more to the estrogen than to the gestagen component of the formulation, some changes, such as alterations in carbohydrate metabolism, may be caused by the gestagenic component. In the British study, an apparent correlation with gestagen dosage and the incidence of hypertension was demonstrated, although it is believed that a minimum concentration of estrogen must be ingested together with the gestagen. This study also showed that the incidence of gallbladder disease was related to gestagen dosage.[24]

For these reasons, when deciding which contraceptive preparation to prescribe initially, it would appear prudent to use the formulation with the least potency (considering the potency per unit weight) of both estrogen and gestagen that does not cause adverse symptoms of bleeding and amenorrhea. The potencies shown in Figure 112-3 are not precise because of the difficulty of determining metabolic activity of these synthetic steroids in the human. However, they do provide a guideline for the clinician until more careful and precise studies are performed. The sequential types of oral contraceptives, with their high dose of estrogen, greater incidence of side effects, and lower efficiency, should not be prescribed. In the United States they are no longer distributed.

The contraceptive formulations containing gestagens without estrogen obviously have a lower incidence of adverse metabolic effects. Since the factors that predispose to thromboembolism are caused by the estrogen component, the incidence of thromboembolism in women ingesting these compounds is probably not increased. Furthermore, blood pressure is not affected, serum lipids are unchanged, nausea and breast tenderness are eliminated, and milk production and quality are unchanged. Despite these advantages, the serious disadvantages of a very high frequency of intermenstrual and other abnormal bleeding patterns, including amenorrhea, as well as a lower rate of effectiveness, markedly limit use of these agents. The actual failure rate of these preparations has been reported to vary between 2 and 8 percent per year, and a high percentage of these pregnancies are ectopic. One possible indication for prescribing these preparations is the nursing mother who greatly desires to use oral contraceptives. Since these women have reduced fertility and are amenorrheic, the major disadvantages of these preparations are minimized. Furthermore, since milk production and quality is unaffected, in contrast to the combination pills, the gestagens alone may be offered to these women while they are nursing. Nevertheless, small portions of these synthetic steroids are secreted in breast milk and thus ingested by the infant. The long-term effects, if any, of these gestogens in the infant are not known. Therefore, one must be concerned about prescribing any synthetic steroids to nursing mothers. Of the three types of oral contraceptive preparations, only the combination type should be used, with the rare exception listed above.

In deciding which combination drug to prescribe initially, it is best to utilize the combination pill with the lowest effective dose and an acceptable level of side effects. In practice, this means that one of the combination pills containing 50 ug of estrogen or less should be prescribed initially. In the United States there are seven products marketed with 50 ug of estrogen. In the last two years, in addition to these seven products, an additional seven products that contain less than 50 ug of estrogen have been marketed. These seven products consist of four different formulations. The physician and patient must therefore decide whether to choose one of the pills with 50 ug of estrogen or less. At the present time, one cannot make this decision on a truly rational basis because of the lack of sufficient published clinical data.

On a theoretical basis, formulations with less than 50 ug of estrogen would have certain benefits and certain disadvantages when compared with the formulations containing 50 ug. As most of the serious metabolic changes associated with oral contraceptives are related to the estrogenic component, decreasing the amount of estrogen would theoretically decrease the incidence of adverse metabolic effects. However, no studies have been published that compare metabolic alterations in groups of women ingesting pills with 50 ug of estrogen with groups using the sub-50 pills. These studies are extremely important, as all sub-50 formulations contain ethinyl estradiol. In most studies this steroid has been found to be 1.7 to 2 times as potent as mestranol,[15] the estrogenic component of several 50-ug pills. Thus the metabolic effect of these formulations on serum lipids and proteins might not differ greatly, if at all.

The most serious side effect of the pill is thromboembolism. A prospective British study showed that products with greater than 50 ug of estrogen had a higher incidence of thromboembolic phenomena than did the products containing 50 ug of estrogen.[24] However, at the present time, there is no evidence that any of the products with less than 50 ug have a lower incidence of vascular disease or a lower incidence of any other abnormal metabolic effect.

The theoretical disadvantages of lowering the dose of estrogen include an increased incidence of irregular bleeding and conception. The conception rate could rise because, as less steroid is ingested, it would not produce an effective blood level for as long as a higher dose. Thus, if tablets were missed or delayed, ovulation could occur. In addition, because of the increased bleeding, more patients might not take the pills regularly or might stop altogether and thus be at risk. The few published clinical studies of the sub-50 preparations indicate that, in general, they have a higher incidence of breakthrough bleeding and spotting than the higher dose formulations, although the theoretical effectiveness (if all pills are taken correctly) was still nearly 100 percent.[53,54] One multiple study of the formulation with 20 ug of estrogen indicates that it may have a slightly higher pregnancy rate in actual use.[53] Nevertheless, definitive comparative studies have not been performed, and the pregnancy rate with this preparation was still less than 1 percent.

In order to obtain valid information concerning any clinical parameter such as irregular bleeding or use-pregnancy rates with any type of contraceptive, especially the pill, it is essential to perform randomized comparative studies in the same clinics with the same clinic personnel during the same time period with the same frequency of follow-up visits. To determine if there are indeed true differences in conception rates, continuation of use, and abnormal bleeding or amenorrhea, such randomized studies should include more than 1000 women with more than 12,000 woman-months' experience. The same definitions of abnormal bleeding should be used, and data should be analyzed by life-table techniques. In contrast to IUD studies, no such comparative studies have been undertaken with oral contraceptives.

Thus far, there have been only a few published clinical studies with the sub-50 ug pills, and nearly all used less than 1000 subjects. As already mentioned, these preliminary studies indicate that the incidence of breakthrough bleeding and spotting with the various preparation ranges from 11 to 28 percent in the second cycle of use, which is higher than the percentage reported with higher doses of estrogen.[15,53] The use-pregnancy rate in these carefully monitored clinical trials were all less than 1 percent. Therefore, in choosing which formulation to use, the following facts are known. First, all the combination products theoretically are equally effective, although the use-effectiveness of products with 20 ug of estrogen may be slightly lower. Second, those products with less than 50 ug of estrogen appear to have a variably increased incidence of abnormal bleeding. Finally, those products with greater than 50 ug of estrogen have an increased incidence of thromboembolism. Although theoretically the products with less than 50 ug of estrogen may have some metabolic benefit, definitive studies to demonstrate this fact have not been conducted, and the products with 50 ug of mestranol may not differ greatly in estrogenic potency from those products with less than 50 ug of ethinyl estradiol. Nevertheless, since the proportion of mestranol metabolized to ethinyl estradiol varies among individuals, it is probably best to initially prescribe formulations with 30 to 35 mg ethinyl estradiol in order to obtain a more uniform response among patients. If a patient develops estrogenic symptoms such as nausea or breast tenderness, the amount of estrogen should be decreased. If the patient develops breakthrough bleeding or amenorrhea, the estrogen dosage may be increased.

ORAL CONTRACEPTIVES AFTER GESTATION

There is a difference in the relation of the return of ovulation and bleeding in the postabortal woman and in the woman having a term delivery.[55] The first episode of menstrual bleeding in the postabortal woman is usually preceded by ovulation. At term the first episode of bleeding is usually but not always anovulatory. The time of resumption of ovulation is related to the duration of pregnancy. Ovulation begins sooner after an abortion. It may occur 4 to 5 weeks after delivery, but is usually delayed beyond 6 weeks.

In a woman who has an abortion at less than 12 weeks gestation, oral contraceptives should be started immediately after the abortion to prevent conception following the first ovulation. In patients who have a delivery after 28 weeks and are not nursing, the combination pills should be initiated 2 weeks after delivery. If the termination of pregnancy occurs between 12 and 28 weeks, contraceptive steroids should be started 1 week later. The reason for delay in the latter instances is that the increased risk of thromboembolism occurring postpartum may be further enhanced with steroid ingestion. As the first ovulation is delayed, there is no need to expose the patient to this increased risk.

SAFETY, CONTRAINDICATIONS, AND PATIENT MONITORING

In considering the safety of oral contraceptives, as well as other methods of contraception, it must be realized that the potential harmful effects of unwanted pregnancy are relatively great. The risk of morbidity and death associated with therapeutic abortion is greater than that associated with hormonal contraceptive use.[56] When prescribing oral contraceptives, the physician must weigh the benefits against the risks for the individual patient. In the opinion of the U.S. Food and Drug Administration, oral contraceptives are safe inasmuch as their benefits outweigh their risks. Nevertheless, there are certain absolute and relative contraindications to their use. The FDA lists six absolute contraindications for the use of oral contraceptives. These are (1) known or suspected estrogen-dependent neoplasia, (2) known or suspected cancer of the breast, (3) thrombophlebitic or thromboembolic disorders, (4) a past history of deep vein thrombophlebitis, thromboembolism, or thrombotic disease including cerebral vascular or coronary artery disease, (5) undiagnosed abnormal uterine bleeding, and (6) pregnancy. Additional contraindications, such as congenital hyperlipidemia, hypertension, diabetes mellitus, a past history of gestational diabetes, as well as cholestatic jaundice of pregnancy should be added to this list. Relative contraindications include depression, migraine headache, leiomyomata of the uterus, epilepsy, oligomenorrhea, and amenorrhea.

Patients with these conditions who ingest oral contraceptives should be seen at frequent intervals, at least every 3 months. In addition, all individuals receiving these potent pharmaceutical agents should be seen by a physician and examined regularly, at least 3 months after initiating therapy and annually thereafter. Prior to starting therapy, as well as during these intervals, a pelvic examination should be performed and the patient's blood pressure and weight recorded. In addition to these procedures, a breast examination should be performed. Ideally, a fasting blood sugar serum triglyceride measurement should also be obtained. By performing these routine examinations in all women and realizing that these women are receiving potent pharmacologic agents, one can hope to avoid some of their serious, but uncommon, side effects.

There are no documented benefits derived from intermittent cessation of therapy, and there is a risk of unwanted pregnancy. In the Royal College Study, women who stopped steroids while requiring contraception had a pregnancy rate of 20 per 100 woman-years.[24]

Recent British studies suggest that women over 30 who use oral contraceptives may have an increased incidence of myocardial infarction, especially if they have certain risk factors.[40] The incidence of myocardial infarction (5.4 per 100,000 users), as well as the increased risk, is low between the ages of 30 and 39 but increases severalfold between the ages of 40 and 45.[40] On the basis of these studies, the FDA has advised that the use of oral contraceptives is hazardous in women over 40, and other forms of contraception should be suggested.

The British investigators' original study was small, and they indicated that the results needed to be interpreted with caution. They have since expanded their original studies. They now conclude that their original estimate of increased risk of heart attack was too high and that the increased risk of heart attacks in women in the 40–44-year age group is three times normal. These investigators also found that the incidence of myocardial infarction in oral contraceptive users increased sharply if certain risk factors, including heavy cigarette smoking, hypertension, diabetes, toxemia and hyperlipoproteinemia, were present.[40]

Recent data obtained from both British prospective oral contraceptive studies, the Royal College of General Practitioners study, and the Oxford Family Planning Association study indicate that, in addition to an increased risk of death from myocardial infarction, there is an increased risk of death from a wide variety of circulatory diseases in oral contraceptive users. The Royal College study indicated that the mortality rate for women who had ever used oral contraceptives was 4.7 times that of controls. For nonrheumatic heart disease and hypertension the death rate was 4.0 times that of controls, and for cerebrovascular diseases, mainly subarachnoid hemorrhage, it was 4.7 times that of controls. A similar increased incidence of death from cardiovascular diseases was observed in the oral contraceptive users in the Family Planning Association study. Of the 43 total deaths in this study group, 9 deaths from cardiovascular disease occurred in the oral contraceptive users and one in the IUD or diaphragm users. These findings support Beral's analysis of mortality trends in 21 countries. This analysis revealed that increases in mortality from all cardiovascular diseases in women aged 15 to 44 have been strongly associated with changes in prevalence of oral contraceptive use in each country. The Royal College study showed, in addition, that the excess mortality rate due to cardiovascular causes in women who had used oral contraceptives increased with increasing age of the patient and duration of oral contraceptive use, and was about threefold greater in women who smoked. Overall, the increased risk of death in every user of oral contraceptives was 20 per 100,000 women per year. More than 10 times greater than the risk of death of pregnancy in controls, and twice as great as the risk of death from all accidents. The risk of death increased markedly in women over 35 and women who had used oral contraceptives for more than five years. Furthermore, the increased risk of death occurred both in current users of oral contraceptives as well as those who had previously used oral contraceptives and stopped. The mortality rate was increased 4.9 and 4.3 times that of controls from those two groups, respectively. Since the metabolic changes occurring during oral contraceptive use generally regress within three months after stopping the pills, the findings of this study indicate that certain circulatory alterations may present for longer time periods. With this information, it is now recommended that women over 35 should discontinue oral contraceptives. Women who are heavy smokers should be strongly encouraged to either stop smoking or use another method of contraception.

The analysis of earlier data by Tietze et al. indicated that, while with advancing age the risk of mortality with use of oral contraceptives increases, the risk of death with IUDs declines and with tubal sterilization remains low. Because of the increasing risk of death in older women using oral contraceptives as well as the increased incidence of systemic disease, oral contraceptives should be used mainly by young, healthy women for the purpose of family spacing. Once childbearing is complete, alternative forms of contraceptives, mainly the IUD, should be used or sterilization for either member of the couple performed. Sterilization is now the most frequent form of preventing pregnancy in women who do not intend to have more children (43.5 percent in comparison with 24 percent for oral contraceptives). Women who wish to continue using oral contraceptives after their family is complete may continue to do so with careful monitoring if they have no associated risk factors, but their use after the age of 35 in all women should be discouraged.

INTERCEPTION

Morris and van Wagen suggested in 1966 that the use of high doses of estrogen given in the early postovulatory period will prevent implantation. Morris has suggested that the term "interception" be used for this "morning-after pill." The estrogen compounds that have been utilized by various investigators for interception include diethylstilbestrol, 25–50 mg/day, diethylstilbestrol diphosphate, 50 ug/day, ethinyl estradiol, 1–5 mg/day, and conjugated estrogen (Premarin), 20–25 mg/day. Treatment is continued for 5 days. If it is begun within 72 hours after an isolated midcycle coitus, its effectiveness is very high. If more than one episode of coitus has occurred or if treatment is initiated later than 72 hours after coitus, the method is much less effective. In 1973, Morris and van Wagen summarized the literature and found that in 9000 midcycle exposures treated with estrogen, there were 29 pregnancies, a rate of 0.3 percent.[57] Only 3 of these appeared to be method

and erythrocyte sedimentation rate have returned to normal. Antibiotic coverage pre- and post-HSG provides additional protection. A flare-up of PID after an HSG is a poor prognostic sign regarding the success of any subsequent reparative surgery. If even attempted, the latter should be deferred at least 3 months.

HSG is extremely valuable in the work-up of the infertile patient. In a population prone to PID, an HSG should be obtained relatively early in the infertility investigation. The discovery of extensive tubal disease may alter, and certainly speed up, the other infertility studies. Multifactor infertility does not have a very good prognosis and an abnormal HSG will hasten laparoscopy and, possibly, bring the investigation to an early end. In addition, according to Israel and March, an unsuspected intrauterine finding will be demonstrated in 10 percent of the HSG obtained for infertility.[20] Confirmatory hysteroscopy should be performed in any patient with an intrauterine defect present on HSG. In some pathology, the HSG can be the definitive study. As noted by Klein et al., the HSG in tuberculosis is diagnostic.[21]

To the infertility surgeon, the HSG must be illuminated in the operating room at the time of surgery. Although in some series discrepancies between HSG and definitive laparoscopy occur as often as 25 percent of the time, HSG is still a valuable study.[20] An x-ray technique does have technical problems that endoscopy can overcome. For example, a unilateral tubal block visualized on HSG occasionally can be overcome at laparoscopy by occluding the patent tube at the uterine cornu with a probe while continuing to instill the dye transcervically. If several months have elapsed between the HSG and surgery, advancing disease or a reaction to the HSG may explain tubal occlusion found at laparoscopy and not present on an earlier HSG. On occasion, mechanical problems with laparoscopic chromopertubation can occur, and the illuminated HSG can be quite comforting. The reality of a cornual block seen at laparoscopy is more convincing if the same finding was present at an earlier HSG. Only a patient with a definitively proven, bilateral cornual block should be subjected to reimplantation surgery. In summary, if the HSG is obtained as the "final" evaluation in the fertility work-up or only, as in repeated uterotubal insufflations, for its "therapeutic" benefit, then its continuing value must be questioned. However, as an adjuvant study for the laparoscopist and infertility surgeon, the HSG can be of significant benefit.

Laparoscopy

Resurrected 7 yr ago in the United States, laparoscopy has added a significent weapon to the gynecologist's diagnostic and therapeutic tools.[22] The panoramic view of the pelvis provided by the laparoscope is unsurpassed. In addition to its usefulness in pelvic pain syndromes and tubal sterilization, the laparoscope has become an integral part of the infertility investigation.

The infertile ovulatory patient with a normal PCT and semen analysis undergoes HSG. If the latter is abnormal, laparoscopy should follow in the next cycle. As previously noted, discrepancies have been reported between HSG and laparoscopy up to 25 percent of the time. Therefore, the HSG cannot be accepted as the final pelvic picture. However, if the HSG is *entirely* normal, 3 months should elapse before laparoscopy is undertaken. Although the therapeutic value of HSG is debatable, reports by Horbach et al.[23] and Kletzky and Halbracht[24] indicate that a patient should be given some time to conceive after tubal flushing. If an abnormal parameter is found during the infertility work-up, e.g., a poor PCT, that abnormality should be treated. However, an HSG should also be obtained so that the pelvic status is *somewhat* illuminated before extensive time and therapy is devoted to correcting a cervical problem.

The anovulatory infertile patient should be evaluated and ovulated therapeutically before an extensive infertility work-up is undertaken. Although a postcoital test should be deferred until ovulatory cycles have been achieved, an early semen analysis and hysterosalpingogram will rule out or rule in other significant pathology. If more than one factor exists to account for the infertility, pregnancy becomes even more difficult and the entire situation should be reviewed. On the other hand, if all studies have been normal and Clomid-induced ovulatory cycles have been achieved for *at least* 6 months, laparoscopy should be undertaken to eliminate the possibility of unsuspected pelvic pathology. Even in the asymptomatic patient with unexplained infertility, the laparoscope, as demonstrated by Peterson and Behrman, can reveal significant disease (Table 114-6).[25]

In addition to its value in diagnosing unsuspected pelvic pathology, laparoscopy is an essential primary step when conservative infertility surgery is contemplated. The laparoscope can reveal a normal pelvis, thus eliminating the need for further surgery. With the laparoscope, the infertility surgeon can begin to define and categorize the degree of pelvic disease and distortion. In some instances, surgery can be deferred and the medical work-up and/or therapy continued on a more solid basis with knowledge of the accurate laparoscopic view of the pelvis. In other cases, laparoscopy can reveal such extensive pelvic destruction that a laparotomy is avoided and the patient can be advised to abandon further infertility studies and consider adoption. In view of its importance in determining the degree of pelvic pathology and the necessity for conservative infertility surgery, laparoscopy in the infertile patient should be carried out *only* by a gynecologic surgeon who is prepared to make endoscopic judgements and perform the required surgery.

As with any study of tubal function, laparoscopy should be performed in the follicular phase of the menstrual cycle. A thorough examination of the pelvis must be carried out utilizing the accessory probe to lift, move, and feel all areas of the pelvis. Since the manipulations are extensive and adhesive disease is often encountered, a double-puncture technique under general endotracheal anesthesia is preferred. Prior pelvic surgery is usually not a deterrent to an adequate laparoscopic examination. In a study by Israel and March,[20] 38 of the 155 infertility patients (25 percent) who underwent uneventful laparoscopy had a history of previous pelvic surgery, usually a salpingectomy for an ectopic pregnancy. During laparoscopy, chromopertubation is carried out with a dilute indigo carmine solution instilled via a No. 8 Foley catheter placed in the uterine cavity.

The decision to proceed with conservative infertility surgery is made at the time of laparoscopy. Therefore, prior to laparoscopy, all possible pelvic findings and surgical risks are explained to

Table 114-6. Results of Laparoscopic Examination in 204 Patients with Previously Unexplained Infertility

Findings	Patients	
	No.	%
Endometriosis	68	33
Pelvic adhesions	36	20
Tubal occlusions and phimosis	10	5
Sclerocystic ovaries	4	2
Normal pelvic organs	86	40

From Peterson and Behrman: Obstet Gynecol 36:363, 1970.

the patient and her husband. If pelvic pathology is confirmed, or unsuspected pathology found, the patient is prepared to undergo definitive tubal or pelvic surgery immediately following laparoscopy utilizing the same anesthetic. Occasionally, minimal filmy adhesions can be lysed through the laparoscope. However, the laparoscope should not be considered a primary surgical tool in infertility. If surgical correction is found to be necessary, only a laparotomy provides the needed space and exposure to perform the job properly. According to Israel and March,[20] the presence or absence of additional infertility factors plays a prognostic role when combined with the laparoscopic findings. When the laparoscope reveals a normal pelvis, the presence of an infertility factor that has responded to treatment is an encouraging sign. Continuing to treat that problem in the light of a normal pelvis will result in a number of pregnancies. On the other hand, the patient who has minimal or unilateral disease at laparoscopy has a more favorable outlook for pregnancy *if* the pelvic pathology is not compounded by an additional infertility factor. In view of the generally poor results achieved with conservative tubal surgery, the laparoscope must be used very critically in order to select the best candidates for reparative operations.

Surgical Correction

Following the laparoscopic decision to perform conservative surgery, the surgeon and the patient are faced with end results that leave much to be desired. In most instances, subsequent pregnancy rates do not exceed 50 percent and include abortions and ectopics as well as term gestations. With tubal closure, surgery can achieve patency in the majority of cases. However, a postoperative patent tube is no guarantee that pregnancy will ensue. Prior involvement of the endosalpinx, or its distortion by the surgery itself, may disturb the reproductive physiology of the fallopian tube to such an extent that pregnancy will never occur.

It is difficult to compare the results of conservative infertility surgery between surgeons or even between the different cases of a single surgeon. The variability of pelvic pathology makes prospective, randomized studies virtually impossible. Are pelvic adhesions present or absent? If present, to what degree and in what areas? With distal tubal disease, what degree of tubal abnormality exists? Are the tubes dilated, and, if so, to what extent? Are intralumenal adhesions present? Do fimbrial remnants remain? What is the condition of the endosalpinx? Even in the available retrospective studies, many of these questions are never answered. Another complexity is the fact that many surgeons view the conservative surgery of the oviduct as being very simple in comparison to other forms of abdominopelvic surgery. Extirpative surgery is more daring and demonstrative, but the judgement, skill, and patience required by the reconstructive surgeon is usually less well appreciated. Meticulous technique is a must, including excellent hemostasis. Tissue irrigation with physiologic saline from a bulb syringe is invaluable in identifying small bleeders. Sharp dissection of adhesions will produce fewer raw surfaces, and peritonealization of all denuded areas should be accomplished without anatomic distortion.

Delicate instruments are a must. Dexon suture, 5-0, 6-0, or 7-0, should be utilized in and around the fallopian tube because of its lack of tissue reactivity. Grant's advice should always be kept in mind:

> . . . in tubal plastic surgery most extensive and complicated operations for infertility are followed by extensive and complicated adhesions. Sterility surgery should be as simple as possible for successful results. The surgeon who works on the sterile pelvis will get the best results from the operation that produces at least *one* good tube next to *one* good ovary, with the minimum of surgical trauma, and the minimal number of stitches.[26]

Four basic operative procedures are utilized in conservative tubal surgery: (1) lysis of peritubal adhesions (salpingolysis), (2) opening of the occluded distal tube (salpingostomy), (3) correction of midsegment occlusion (end-to-end anastomosis), and (4) repair of cornual occlusion (cornual implantation).

Salpingolysis. The most successful type of "tubal" surgery involves the lysis of peritubal and/or pelvic adhesions and does not involve primary tubal surgery. Ovum pick-up is impeded by adhesions isolating the tubes and ovaries. The tubes may spill dye into isolated pockets of adhesions, but the fimbriated ends are open and the endosalpinx is intact. Ultimate success depends on the extent and type of adhesions encountered, and whether they re-form postoperatively. In reported series, the overall pregnancy rate varies from 40 to 60 percent with 70–95 percent of the pregnancies going to term.[27]

Salpingostomy. Opening distal tubal occlusions is the least successful type of tubal surgery. A hydrosalpinx is the end stage of generalized tubal disease. Although the surgeon may be able to open the tube and have it remain open, anatomic and physiologic damage to the remainder of the tube only rarely supports the numerous normal reproductive processes necessary to achieve an intrauterine pregnancy. The fimbria are often gone, the endosalpinx is denuded partially or totally, the tubal musculature is nonfunctional, and various degrees of tubal dilation may be present. Additionally, distal tubal closure is usually associated with pelvic adhesions varying from minimal and filmy to extensive and thick.

To compound the salpingostomy problem, some surgeons include lesser degrees of fimbrial pathology in this surgical category. Fimbrial "agglutination" and "phimosis" are two of the favorites. Teasing apart filmy strands between the fimbria or "dilating" the fimbriated end of the tube with small bougies does not represent salpingostomy surgery. *If* they can be considered "indicated" forms of conservative infertility surgery, they should be classified in a subcategory under salpingolysis.

There are no prospective, randomized studies from the same individual or institution comparing salpingostomy results with or without a prosthetic device. Indeed, there are no comparative retrospective studies. Even if attempted, the vagaries of pelvic pathology encountered in each case would make a prospective study difficult to design and interpret. Overall pregnancy rates published following hood (prosthetic) salpingostomy vary between 14 and 40 percent but the percentage of patients achieving term pregnancies varies between 6 and 28 percent.[27] From published reports, cuff (nonprosthetic) salpingostomy with postoperative hydrotubation yields similar overall pregnancy rates (10–50 percent), although term pregnancies are not always delineated (range 3–35 percent).[27]

As noted above, with either technique the ultimate results depend on the condition of the remainder of the tube rather than the operative method employed. If tubal patency were the only consideration, either operation would be a success. The percentage of patent tubes varies from 60 to 90 percent following hood salpingostomy, and from 40 to 100 percent following cuff salpingostomy and postoperative hydrotubations.[27] The surgeon can open the pipeline in most instances, but he cannot restore proper function. The increased incidence of ectopic pregnancies in post-salpingostomy tubes reinforces the concept that tubal closure is not the only problem in these cases.[20]

End-to-End Anastomosis. The most successful primary tubal surgery is the correction of midtubal occlusion secondary to previous tubal sterilization. The remainder of the tube, proximally and distally, is normal and the pelvis is free of adhesions. Additionally, the patient has proven her fertility and is infertile only on the basis of tubal sterilization.

As has been stressed with *any* form of conservative surgery, prelaparotomy laparoscopy should be utilized to confirm the normal status of the pelvis and to decide whether adequate tubal segments exist for anastomosis. Ideally, for end-to-end reconstruction, the prior tubal sterilization should have been a small segmental resection in the ampullary portion of the tube. If an intact ampullary–isthmic junction is present, and the anastomosis can be performed in the ampulla, success should be extremely high. In a young woman undergoing sterilization, segmental ampullary resection should be considered, so that reanastomosis success could be achieved if the future brings a change of mind.

Reversal of laparoscopic tubal fulguration is not a very likely prospect. The degree of tubal damage is too great and successful end-to-end anastomosis has not been reported. Possibly a cornual implantation could be considered if the distal segment is of sufficient length. Similarly, fimbriectomy reversal—requiring cuff salpingostomy—offers little chance of success as an important, usually lengthy section of tube was removed at the time of sterilization. In the literature, the pregnancy rate following end-to-end anastomosis approaches 50 percent. However, in most reports, the operations performed number less than 10.[27]

Cornual Implantation. The least frequently performed, and technically most complex, reparative tubal surgery is the correction of cornual occlusion. Clinically, the patient usually has a history of "uterine invasion," i.e., D&C, pregnancy with sepsis, IUD insertion, etc. In many instances, these events were *not* accompanied by any clinical evidence of pelvic sepsis, yet the end result was bilateral cornual block. As the cornual portion of the tube is very important in reproduction and impossible to duplicate surgically, it is imperative that a cornual block be proven definitively *before* surgical correction is undertaken. At least two tubal evaluation studies, one of which is laparoscopy, must indicate clearly that cornual occlusion exists bilaterally or in the only remaining fallopian tube. In addition, laparoscopy must demonstrate that the rest of the tube(s) is perfectly normal and the pelvis is free of adhesions. Conservative tubal surgery is contraindicated in the presence of proximal and distal blocks existing in the same tube.

The vast majority of studies composed of more than 20 cornual implantations report overall pregnancy rates ranging between 35 and 50 percent. However, spontaneous abortions and a 10–20 percent rate for tubal pregnancies are included in the total figure.[27] As seen with other forms of conservative tubal surgery, postoperative tubal patency rates are double the pregnancy rates.

ENDOMETRIOSIS

In 1921 Sampson described endometriosis as "the presence of ectopic tissue which possesses the histological structure and function of the uterine mucosa."[28] Although the occurrence of aberrant endometrium had been described by various individuals in the 19th century, it was not until the classic contribution of Sampson that there was any appreciation of the frequency, pathology, and clinical characteristics of this enigmatic gynecologic disorder.

Histogenesis

As Ridley noted in 1968, there are at least 11 published theories regarding the histogenesis of endometriosis.[29] They can be divided into three broad categories: transportation, in situ development, or a combination of the two.

Transportation

Retrograde Menstruation (Sampson's Theory) via the Fallopian Tubes. Red blood cells, leukocytes, endometrial cells and amorphous material can traverse the tubes in an antiperistaltic, anticilial manner. In a series of experiments in 1950, TeLinde and Scott demonstrated in the monkey that transported endometrial cells are viable and can implant.[30] Subsequently, Ridley and others confirmed the viability of human endometrial cells after tubal transport.

Mechanical: Direct Dissemination of Endometrial Tissue at Surgery. For example, endometriosis subsequently developing at the incision site following cesarean section or hysterotomy.

Lymphatic and Venous Metastasis. The presence of endometrial tissue in distant, unusual sites *must* be attributed to venous or lymphatic transportation.

In Situ Development: Celomic Metaplasia. This theory is based on the fact that certain cells under certain stimuli can change their character and physiologic function. However, if this theory explains the origin of endometriosis, the condition should occur as frequently in the thoracic cavity as it does in the peritoneal cavity. Obviously this does not occur, although the celomic membrane contributes to the thoracic lining as well as the peritoneal lining. Additionally, if celomic metaplasia contributes to endometriosis, the condition should be found in the male.

Combination of Transportation and In Situ Development. Although this theory includes the ability of the endometrium to reproduce itself, it relies on direct extension or vascular system metastasis to explain endometrial movement. Obviously, this theory is unacceptable to the celomic metaplasia "purists."

Clinical Characteristics

Since endometriosis is dependent on the ovarian steroids for its existence and proliferation, its occurrence and clinical importance are confined generally to the reproductive years. Although Kempers et al. have reported active postmenopausal endometriosis *without* exogenous hormone use,[31] the peak incidence is in the fourth decade of life. The "typical" patient with endometriosis is a nulliparous private patient in her late twenties or early thirties. Additionally, textbooks describe her as intelligent, egocentric, overanxious, and a perfectionist. Marriage and childbearing have often been deferred for various reasons.

Whether the emergence and widespread use of steroidal contraceptives over the past 20 yr has reduced the incidence of endometriosis by reducing menstrual flow, thereby preventing tubal reflux, remains an unanswered question. However, if operative statistics from predominantly private practice hospitals are utilized, endometriosis continues to be a significant gynecologic entity. From Ranney in South Dakota[32] to Kistner in Boston,[33] gross or microscopic endometriosis was noted in 14–21 percent of all laparotomies performed for gynecologic disease between 1950 and 1970.

It has been found that 30–40 per cent of patients with endometriosis have concomitant infertility,[33] although in many instances the endometriosis does not appear to be interfering with the normal reproductive processes. Sperm ascension, ovulation, and ovum pick-up and transport can all take place, but the presence of even minimal pelvic endometriosis seems to be the causative infertility factor.

The most frequent pelvic locations for endometriosis are the ovaries, uterine ligaments (round, broad, uterosacral), pelvic peritoneum, and rectovaginal septum. Other sites include the umbilicus, laparotomy scars, hernial sacs, appendix, small intestine, rectum, sigmoid, bladder, ureters, vulva–vagina–cervix, lymph nodes, extremities, pleural cavity, and lung. The multiplicity and widespread distribution of these sites makes acceptance of any *one* histogenetic theory difficult. Possibly histochemical and immunologic investigations will provide some definitive clues to the many unanswered questions raised by the presence of endometriosis.

Pathology

Like everything else connected with endometriosis, the one characteristic of the gross pathology is its variability. Until Acosta et al. proposed a classification in 1973,[34] the extent of pelvic endometriosis was described by individual cases. With mild involvement, the adnexa is free of adhesions and a variable number of reddish blue (raspberry) or brown fibrinlike implants are present on the ovaries and/or peritoneal surfaces. In progressive disease, the older implants have coalesced and "burnt-out," leaving scarred, retracted areas that may involve peritoneal surface *only* or include peritubal and periovarian involvement and fixation.

More significant ovarian involvement means the formation of single or multiple, unilateral or bilateral endometrial cysts (endometriomas, "chocolate" cysts). As the endometrium grows into the ovary during formation of these cysts, menstrual reaction occurs and they become hemorrhagic. With deeper penetration, the cyst content becomes darker, resembling thick chocolate syrup. Even when quite small, the cysts show a strong tendency to perforate with escape of menstrual blood and subsequent ovarian adherence to any adjacent structure, usually the posterior surface of the broad ligament or uterus. If early perforation does not occur, larger endometriomas form with thicker walls and few surrounding adhesions. When the uterine ligaments are involved, especially the uterosacrals, endometriotic nodules form that can often be palpated on bimanual or rectovaginal exam. Endometrial islands may occur on any part of the pelvic peritoneum, involving the serosal surface of any pelvic structure. Occasionally, invasion and penetration occurs in the sigmoid so that progressive submucosal scarring results in lumenal constriction. Mucosal involvement with associated rectal bleeding is a late phenomenon in bowel endometriosis. Although the rectovaginal septum is not an uncommon site for endometriosis, disease limited *only* to this anatomic area is very rare and, as noted by March and Israel, requires pathologic confirmation to exclude malignancy.[35]

Definitive diagnosis requires microscopic demonstration of endometrial tissue, preferably both glands and stroma. However, a wide range of pictures may occur. Some specimens reveal endometrium that histologically and functionally cannot be distinguished from normal uterine epithelium. In others, the endometrium has been completely denuded due to repeated menstrual bleeding and desquamation. Hemorrhage and pigment-laden macrophages may be the only microscopic clues. According to the Gynecologic Pathology Laboratory at The Johns Hopkins Hospital, no specific pathologic diagnosis can be made definitively in one-third of clinically typical endometriosis cases.[36]

Diagnosis

The symptomatology associated with endometriosis can be as variable as anything else connected with this disease. Dysmenorrhea, dyspareunia, and dyschezia may be present as a symptom complex or individually. However, even with extensive endometriosis, pain may not be a significant clinical entity. Unless rupture occurs, ovarian endometriomas can expand painlessly. On the other hand, incapacitating dysmenorrhea and pelvic pain may be associated with minimal amounts of active peritoneal surface endometriosis. Thus, the degree of endometriotic involvement and spread bears no constant relationship to the presence or absence of subjective discomfort.

Over 50 percent of patients complain of dysmenorrhea. Usually it is the secondary or acquired variety, although on occasion primary dysmenorrhea worsens. The dysmenorrhea can be attributed to secretory changes in the endometriotic islands with subsequent miniature menstruation and bleeding in areas that are encapsulated by fibrous tissue. With involvement of the rectovaginal septum or uterosacral ligaments, the dysmenorrhea is often referred to the rectum or the lower sacrococcygeal area and dyspareunia is a common complaint. Dyschezia results from endometriotic bleeding in the rectosigmoid muscularis or serosa with subsequent fibrosis. Occasionally, abnormal uterine bleeding, e.g., premenstrual spotting, may occur. Grant even suggests a BBT graph may be suggestive of endometriosis.[37] The majority (95 percent) of his patients with endometriosis had an elevation of the BBT during menses well above the usual preovulatory level. As endometriosis is characterized by ovulatory cycles, the remainder of the BBT graph was typically biphasic. Menstrual abnormalities are uncommon, except when widespread endometriosis has created significant pelvic scarring and fibrosis.

Although the diagnosis may be suggested by the history, it cannot be made with any certainty on symptoms alone. Even a pelvic examination, which at times can be quite distinctive, *cannot* be considered pathognomonic. Tender, nodular uterosacral ligaments combined with a fixed, retroverted uterus are findings highly suggestive of endometriosis, but inflammation and cancer cannot be ruled out by a bimanual examination. For definitive diagnosis, laparoscopic visualization of the pelvic area must be carried out prior to the institution of therapy. When lesions are identified and the examiner still remains in doubt, confirmatory transendoscopic biopsy should be performed. Double-puncture laparoscopy should be utilized so that a careful, complete pelvic inspection can be carried out. Additionally, one of several available instruments for uterine manipulation may be secured in the cervical canal. Preferably, it should have a central cannula for subsequent transuterine–tubal dye instillation. If a patient is going to undergo a general anesthetic and a transabdominal operation, the surgeon must be scrupulously thorough in his inspection and investigation of the peritoneal cavity. As Samuelsson and Sjovall noted, a cursory laparoscopic look is often inaccurate.[38] The palpating probe, placed through the accessory trocar, can be used as an examining finger running over various structures, e.g., the uterosacral ligaments, to detect subperitoneal implants. Each ovary must be lifted up to visualize the under surface adjoining the broad ligament. The serosa of any bowel in the pelvis should be carefully inspected for any endometriotic implants, as should the appendix.

Therapy

Although controversy continues in the areas of histogenesis, symptomatology, and detection, more uniformity of thinking exists as regards the therapy of endometriosis in the infertile patient. Hormonal suppression and/or conservative surgery constitute the available therapeutic modalities. If pregnancy is the accepted end point, conservative surgery is more consistently successful than any available hormone treatment.

Hormones. Almost 30 yr ago, Karnaky suggested the use of constant *estrogen* administration in increasing amounts to suppress ovulation and produce changes in endometriotic lesions.[39] Although up to 100 mg of stilbestrol daily has been used, pregnancy rates have ranged between 14 and 20 percent even with prolonged therapy. Symptoms associated with the endometriosis disappear, only to be replaced by nausea, edema, mastodynia, and often heavy breakthrough bleeding secondary to the high-dose estrogen treatment. Additionally, regression and absorption of endometriotic tissue does not occur. Karnaky remains one of the few proponents of estrogen therapy.

Methyltestosterone is another hormone that has a limited following. Usually given as a 5-mg linguet daily for 6 months, subsequent pregnancy rates have ranged between 10 and 60 percent, although few recent reports are available. Katayama et al. report a 20 percent pregnancy rate after a 1-yr follow-up in a group of 64 patients.[40] Although they projected a 30 percent pregnancy rate if the patients had been followed for 2 yr, most patients were offered conservative surgery after a 1 yr follow-up. Methyltestosterone therapy relieves the symptoms of endometriosis in over 80 percent of treated patients. A distinct advantage of this particular hormone regimen is the maintenance of ovulation. If the 5-mg linguet is utilized, pregnancy can occur while the medication continues. Although the 5-mg dose is too small, theoretically, to masculinize a female fetus, the medication should be discontinued as soon as a pregnancy is suspected. Side effects reported by Katayama et al. included a 3 percent incidence of mild hirsutism and a 6 percent incidence of acne.[40] If a hormone is selected as therapy for endometriosis in the infertile patient, methyltestosterone might be considered for a short therapeutic trial.

Danazol, a synthetic derivative of 17-α-ethinyltestosterone, soon to be approved for use by the FDA, has had numerous clinical trials. As with most new drugs, the initial therapeutic results have been good and the investigators enthusiastic. Greenblatt et al., utilizing doses between 400 and 800 mg daily, achieved 9 conceptions (43 percent) among 21 patients with histologically proven or strongly suspected endometriosis on history and pelvic examination.[41] However, 11 (41 percent) of 27 patients with "no reason" infertility also conceived with Danazol treatment.

The drug is an antigonadotropin which appears to act on the LH center inhibiting the LH surge.[42] However, tonic LH and FSH are not significantly depressed, thus Danazol appears to block ovulation in a manner similar to the action of oral contraceptive drugs. Additionally, Danazol does not suppress serum estrogen levels below follicular phase values, yet it creates an atrophic endometrium within the first month of treatment. The latter may represent competition between Danazol and estrogen at the level of the target tissue. To further confuse the picture, the first exposure of some patients to Danazol is followed by an LH surge accompanied by a rise in BBT. However, an elevation in serum progesterone and a secretory change in the endometrium fail to occur. Despite the unsettled but exciting pharmacologic picture and the early clinical enthusiasm, Ansbacher urges caution.[43] In four infertility patients with endometriosis proven by laparoscopy, significant side effects occurred and the therapeutic response—amenorrhea and the disappearance of endometriotic symptoms and signs—was limited to the duration of Danazol therapy. Menses and symptoms recurred when the drug was stopped. During the 6 months of Danazol treatment, the following side effects appeared: weight gain (average 9 pounds); severe, unilateral, "migrainelike" headaches; unilateral upper extremity tremor; irritability; lethargy; dizziness; and mild androgenic changes (acne, deepening of voice). After Danazol is approved for general use, only time will tell its ultimate place in the management of endometriosis.

The most popular hormonal therapy for endometriosis continues to be the pseudopregnancy state created by the *progestogens.* However, this therapeutic modality has little place in the treatment of the infertile patient with endometriosis. *Minimally* 6 months of continuous therapy must be utilized, during which time the infertile patient remains anovulatory. Even Kistner, the prime advocate of progestogens in endometriosis, has tempered his initial enthusiasm.[33] Abandoning the necessity for a sequentially increasing dose of steroid, e.g., Enovid up to 30–40 mg daily, he now utilizes *any* low-dose progestogen. Obviously, disturbing side effects and potential medical complications occur less with low-dose medication. The decidual reaction in areas of endometriosis produced by the low-dose steroids is just as extensive as that previously noted with large amounts of Enovid. Kistner reports a 40 percent pregnancy rate following progestogen treatment in a group of "carefully selected" patients.[33]

When utilized, it is preferable to give the steroids continuously rather than in the cyclic pattern used for contraception. If norgestrel (0.5 mg) plus ethinyl estradiol (50 μg) is selected and breakthrough bleeding occurs, the dose can be doubled or tripled. The *increased* therapy should be continued until the bleeding has stopped, when the dose can be dropped. However, if bleeding recurs, the increased dose necessary to stop it should be continued. Breakthrough bleeding may also be controlled by the short-term addition of 20 μg of ethinyl estradiol to the original regimen. Long-term progestogen use has no place in the treatment of the infertile patient with endometriosis. Likewise, *depo-medroxyprogesterone acetate* (Depo-Provera), with 20–25 percent of its users having failed to resume regular menses up to 1 yr posttherapy, is not a good steroidal alternative when infertility and endometriosis coexist.

Conservative Surgery. In almost every instance the treatment of choice for the infertility patient with endometriosis is conservative surgery. The diagnosis is established by laparoscopy and, occasionally, the laparoscope provides therapy. If scattered powder burns or small blue-domed lesions are present on the peritoneal surface, they can be fulgurated under direct vision. Minimal filmy adhesions can be transected. If pregnancy occurs following laparoscopic fulguration of small, isolated endometriotic islands, it is hard, retrospectively, to explain their role in the pathogenesis of the infertility. Extensive laparoscopic surgical manipulations are contraindicated. Complication rates rise with "endoscopic gymnastics" and, except in minimal disease states, the laparoscope cannot adequately inspect and eliminate all areas of endometriosis.

If the patient has been properly prepared for all diagnostic possibilities, laparotomy can follow laparoscopy under the same anesthetic. Preoperative therapy with continuous progestogens for 4–8 weeks has been advocated by Grant[37] and Kistner and Patton[27] to enlarge and soften the endometriotic implants. Following short-term steroidal treatment, the lesions may be easier to identify and simpler to excise. However, definitive surgery is delayed and improved pregnancy rates do not occur. In fact, without preoperative steroids, Ranney has reported a phenomenal 87.5 percent term delivery rate following conservative surgery for endometriosis.[32] The majority of pregnancies occurred within 1 yr of surgery. Preoperative progestogen therapy may have a place with endometriosis located deep in the pelvic region, e.g., in the rectovaginal septum. Any softening that occurs may help make a normally difficult dissection easier.

Although the infertility patient with endometriosis can expect good results with a surgical approach to her problem, Ranney's success is exceptionally high. The similar results from Harvard and Johns Hopkins reflect a more realistic outlook (Table 114-7).[36,44]

Endometriosis surgery, like any other infertility surgery, must be performed with meticulous care and excellent hemostasis. The uterus and adnexa must be mobilized and carefully inspected. The serosa of the large and small bowel either in or contiguous to the pelvis must be visualized for any endometriotic involvement. If the appendix is a site, as it may be, an appendectomy should be performed. In the Johns Hopkins series, the postoperative pregnancy rate (51 percent) remained the same with or without an appendectomy.[36] All areas of endometriosis should be excised and reperitonealized as best as possible. The ovaries must be palpated carefully and cystic areas punctured or incised in order not to miss small endometriomas. Ovarian endometriomas should be excised or a major portion of one or both ovaries may have to be resected. Pregnancy can still occur following unilateral oophorectomy and resection of three-quarters of the contralateral ovary. In reconstructing the ovary, the cortical surface should be approximated as closely as possible using nonreactive 3-0 Dexon suture in order to reduce the chance of subsequent adhesions.

Postoperative, short-term (3-month) continuous progestogen therapy has no published data proving its efficacy. When conservative surgery has been performed, all areas of endometriosis should have been removed. If this is technically impossible due to extensive or deep-seated disease, postoperative steroid therapy should be used. Following conservative surgery, endometriosis recurs in 5–25 percent of patients.[27] For example, in the Johns Hopkins study, 13 percent required a second operation for recurrent endometriosis and, of these, 85 percent underwent hysterectomy.[36]

OTHER FACTORS

It has been reported that in approximately 10–25 percent of couples, no abnormalities can be found after establishing the fact that ovulation is occuring, obtaining a semen analysis, performing a PCT, and investigating the upper female genital tract with a HSG and laparoscopy.[43,44] Because a large percentage of couples do fall in this category of "unexplained" infertility, the following additional investigations should be performed in an effort to try to reduce the percentage of unexplained infertility: infertility secondary to immunologic factors; genital mycoplasma as a cause of infertility; inadequate luteal phase; and hysteroscopy.

Table 114-7. Conservative Surgery Results from Harvard and Johns Hopkins

Ob/Gyn Dept.	No. of Women	Duration of Infertility	Pregnant No.	Pregnant %
Harvard*	26	5.8	15	58
Johns Hopkins†	73	5	42	58

*Data from Green: Obstet Gynecol 9:293, 1966.
†Data from Spangler et al: Am J Obstet Gynecol 109:850, 1971.

INFERTILITY SECONDARY TO IMMUNOLOGIC FACTORS

Immunologic incompatibility may be the etiology of infertility in some patients. The exact incidence of this phenomena is not known. The fact that antibodies can be induced in laboratory animals by injecting semen has been known for over 75 yr.[45–47] In the human, three different immune systems have been implicated as the possible etiology of infertility: (1) the ABO blood group incompatibility, (2) the autoimmunity in men, and (3) the presence of circulating sperm-agglutinating and -immobilizing antibodies in women.

ABO Blood Incompatibility

In 1960 Behrman et al. reported that the incidence of ABO blood incompatibility was much higher in a series of 108 infertile couples in whom no etiology for infertility had been established when compared to controls.[48] This report stimulated further investigation into the possibility of ABO incompatibility as a cause of human infertility. In 1969 Solish reported that in over 3000 infertile couples studies, there was no difference in the ABO blood group distribution.[49] Schwimmer et al., in 1967, did report a higher frequency of isohemagglutinins in the cervical mucus of infertile women compared to the fertile controls.[50] However, Parish et al., in the same year, reported that immuno anti-A antibody in cervical mucus had no cytotoxic effect on spermatozoa carrying the A antigen.[51] At the present time, no effect on motility or morphology of spermatozoa has been reported even with the presence of the antibody to specific blood group antigens present on the sperm. Therefore, the ABO blood group incompatibility does not seem to be related to infertility.

Autoimmunity in the Human Male

The first report of autoimmunity in the male as a cause of infertility was by Wilson.[52,53] In 1959 Rumke and Hellinga reported this finding in 3 percent of 2000 infertile couples.[54] The titer that appeared to be significant was stated to be 1:32. Some of these men also showed spontaneous agglutination of spermatozoa in their own seminal plasma. A significant number of these men had a history of genital tract infection, surgery, or trauma.

In 1968, Fjallbrant and Obrant not only demonstrated the presence of autoantibodies in 400 infertile men, but he related this finding to the decreased ability of sperm from these men to penetrate normal cervical mucus.[55] It appears that there is a correlation between autoimmunity and infertility in a certain percentage of infertile couples, although it should be noted that the presence of sperm-agglutinating antibodies does not always interfere with fertility. No successful therapy has yet been found. Artificial insemination using donor semen may be the only treatment.

Sperm-Agglutinating and -Immobilizing Antibodies in the Human Female

Agglutination of the husband's sperm by the wife's serum has been reported to be a factor in infertility. Franklin and Dukes first published their observations on the relationship of circulating sperm agglutinins to infertility of unknown etiology in 1964. They reported an incidence of 72 percent, compared to the control group, who had a 5.7 percent incidence of sperm agglutinins.[56] Sexual abstinence or the use of condoms by the husband for a period of 2–6 months has been recommended in order to lower the antibody titer. In the first report this therapy was reported to be extremely successful. However, by 1968, the same authors reported that the incidence of sperm-agglutinating antibody in infertile women was only 48 percent, with a control group showing an incidence of 13 percent. Again some 57 percent of their patients became pregnant after using the recommended condom therapy. Of the 20 couples who refused condom therapy, only 2 (10 percent) were noted to have become pregnant.

Other authors have not found the incidence of sperm-agglutinating antibodies in infertile women as high as in the original report by Franklin and Dukes. Schwimmer et al. reported a 33.5 percent incidence of sperm-agglutinating antibodies in women with primary unexplained infertility.[50,57] Glass and Vaidya reported a 20 percent incidence of sperm agglutination in a group of 122 women with unexplained infertility.[58] None of their 24 patients became pregnant after condom therapy.

At the present time, therefore, the only statement that can be made concerning sperm-agglutination antibodies in the serum of females as a cause of infertility is that the phenomenon appears to exist in a small percentage of infertile couples and that if it is a cause of infertility, it is probably titer dependent.

Another test for identifying the existence of sperm-agglutinating antibodies in the female serum is the *Kibrick test*.[59] The usual incidence of positive tests using this technique has varied between 5 and 20 percent.

Isojima et al. reported a compliment-dependent *serum sperm-immobilization* technique. Their incidence of positive tests has varied between 12 and 19 percent with a 0 percent incidence in the controls.[60]

The incidence of positive tests in this medical center for the agglutination test using both the Franklin-Dukes test and the Kibrick test is approximately 5 percent. Only 12 percent of these patients have become pregnant using condom therapy, compared to an 8 percent pregnancy rate in patients who either refused therapy or discontinued it voluntarily. The incidence of positive Isojima tests has been 3 percent, and no pregnancy has been achieved using condom therapy.

Until the role of immune reactions as a cause of infertility is totally disproven, the Franklin-Dukes, Kibrick, and Isojima tests should be performed if all other tests outlined previously prove to be negative. If an immunologic test is positive at 1:4 titer, condom therapy should be recommended for 3 months. At the end of this time the tests should be repeated. If the tests remain positive, then another 3 months of therapy should be advised. If at the end of 6 months the tests are still positive, the therapy should be discontinued.

GENITAL MYCOPLASMA AND ITS ROLE IN INFERTILITY

Mycoplasma, previously known as PPLO organisms, and now referred to as ureaplasma ureatyticum, have been reported to be a possible factor in patients with undiagnosed infertility. The T-mycoplasma has been reported to be the significant organism.[61–64] Both the cervical mucus and the semen should be cultured for this organism.[65] The treatment recommended is doxycycline 200 mg on the first day starting on the seventh day of the cycle, followed by 100 mg/day for 9 days. Both partners should be treated for two to three cycles.[66,67] If the cultures remain positive the dose should be doubled and treatment continued for another 2 months. A pregnancy rate following antibiotic therapy of 42 percent after 3 months and 84 percent after 1 yr has been reported.[67] It should be noted that both published[68] and unpublished studies have shown little or no relationship between the incidence of T-mycoplasma infection and infertility. However, until further results are published, in couples with infertility, T-mycoplasma cultures should be obtained and, if the cultures are positive, treatment should be instituted.

Inadequate Luteal Phase

The inadequate luteal phase is a histologic diagnosis made in a small number of infertile women in whom the endometrial biopsy shows a lag of 2 or more days in two different menstrual cycles.[69] The inappropriate maturation of the endometrium may be due to inadequate production of progesterone from the corpus luteum. It is assumed that with poorly developed endometrium there is unsuccessful implantation of the fertilized ovum.

It is important to differentiate between the inadequate luteal phase and the short luteal phase. In the short luteal phase the time interval between the LH peak and the onset of menses is less than 10 days.[70] It does not appear that the short luteal phase is a cause of infertility.

The inadequate luteal phase must be documented in two cycles. Normal fertile women may on occasion have out-of-phase endometrial biopsies. A BBT chart cannot be used in making this diagnosis. The daily progesterone values obtained in the luteal phase of these women appear to be somewhat lower than normal women; however, the differences in the absolute values are debatable.[69]

The therapy for this condition has been 25 mg of progesterone vaginal suppository inserted daily in the luteal phase or a daily dose of 12.5 mg of progesterone-in-oil im starting with the rise of BBT until the onset of menses.[69] If the patient becomes pregnant, it has been recommended that the therapy be continued until the second trimester. The use of HCG 2500–5000 IU given im every other day during the luteal phase has also been suggested. In addition, because it has been postulated that the inadequate luteal phase may be secondary to a "poor" follicular development, clomiphene citrate therapy in these ovulatory patients has been suggested in order to develop a "better" follicle and thus a "better" corpus luteum. All three modes of therapy may be beneficial and at the present time no single method of treatment has been definitely proven to be the best.

Hysteroscopy

Hysteroscopy has recently been introduced as a new tool in investigating the endometrial cavity. Whether this method will prove to be more beneficial than a hysterogram remains to be seen. The procedure is performed under sedation and local anesthesia. This instrument is just now being used in a few centers in the evaluation of the patients with "unexplained" infertility. No conclusive results have been published as yet. It is possible that anatomic defects such as intrauterine synechiae high in the fundus of the uterus or very small submucus leiomyomata have escaped diagnosis with the routinely performed HSG.

REFERENCES

1. Romeny S., Gray, M. J., Little, B., et al: Gynecology and Obstetrics: The Health Care of Women. New York, McGraw-Hill, 1975, ch 24, p 345.
2. Speroff, L., Glass, R. H., Kase, N. G.: Clinical Gynecologic Endocrinology and Infertility. Baltimore, Williams & Wilkins, 1973, ch 12, p 173.
3. Behrman, S. J., Kistner, R. W.: Progress in Infertility, 2nd ed. Boston, Little, Brown, 1975, p. 4.
4. Warner, M. P.: Results of 25 year study of 1553 infertile couples. *NY State J Med 62:* 2663, 1962.
5. Israel, R., Mishell, D. R., Jr., Stone, S. C., et al: Single luteal phase serum progesterone assay as an indicator of ovulation. *Am J Obstet Gynecol 112:* 1043, 1972.
6. Rimoin, D. L., Schimke, R. N.: Genetic Disorders of the Endocrine Glands. St. Louis, Mosby, 1971, p. 298.
7. Kletzky, O. A., Davajan, V., Nakamura, R. M., et al: Clinical categorization of patients with secondary amenorrhea using progesterone induced uterine bleeding and measurement of serum gonadotropin levels. *Am J Obstet Gynecol 121:* 695, 1975.
8. Kletzky, O., Davajan, V., Mishell, D. R., Jr., et al: A sequential pituitary stimulation test in normal subjects and in patients with amenorrhea–galactorrhea with pituitary tumors. *Clin Endocrinol Metab 45:* 631, 1977.
9. Adams, R., Mishell, D. R., Jr., Israel, R.: Treatment of refractory anovulation with increased dosage and prolonged duration of cyclic clomiphene citrate. *Obstet Gynecol 39:* 562, 1972.
10. Rust, L. A., Israel, R., Mishell, D. R., Jr.: An individualized therapeutic regimen for clomiphene citrate. *Am J Obstet Gynecol 120:* 785, 1974.
11. March, C. M., Israel, R., Mishell, D. R., Jr.: Pregnancy following 29 cycles of clomiphene citrate therapy: a case report. *Am J Obstet Gynecol 124:* 209, 1976.
12. Weil, A. J.: Antigen of adnexal glands of male genital tract. *Fertil Steril 12:* 538, 1961.
13. Davajan, V., Kunitake, G. M.: Fractional in-vivo and in-vitro examination of post-coital cervical mucus in the human. *Fertil Steril 20:* 197, 1967.
14. Davajan, V., Nakamura, R. M., Kharma, K.: Spermatozoa transport in cervical mucus. *Obstet Gynecol Survey 25:* 1, 1970.
15. Davajan, V., Nakamura, R., Mishell, D. R., Jr.: A simplified technique for evaluation of the biophysical properties of cervical mucus. *Am J Obstet Gynecol 109:* 1042, 1971.
16. Tredway, D. R., Settlage, D. S. F., Nakamura, R. M., et al: The significance of timing for the post-coital evaluation of cervical mucus. *Am J Obstet Gynecol 121:* 387, 1975.
17. Tredway, D. R.: The interpretation and significance of the fractional post-coital test. *Am J Obstet Gynecol 124:* 352, 1976.
18. Rubin, I. C.: Non-operative determination of patency of fallopian tubes in sterility. *JAMA 74:* 1017, 1920.
19. Siegler, A. M.: Hysterosalpingography. New York, Harper & Row, 1967.
20. Israel, R., March, C. M.: Diagnostic laparoscopy: a prognostic aid in the surgical management of infertility. *Am J Obstet Gynecol 124:* 969, 1976.
21. Klein, T. A., Richmond, J. A., Mishell, D. R., Jr.: Pelvic tuberculosis in an infertility clinic. *Obstet Gynecol 48:* 99, 1976.
22. Cohen, M. R.: Laparoscopy, Culdoscopy and Gynecology. Philadelphia, Saunders, 1970.
23. Horbach, J. G. M., Maathuis, J. B., Van Hall, E. V.: Factors influencing the pregnancy rate following hysterosalpingography and their prognostic significance. *Fertil Steril 24:* 15, 1973.
24. Kletzky, O. A., Halbracht, J. G.: Hydrotubation in the treatment of the tubal factor. *Acta Eur Fertil 2:* 31, 1970.
25. Peterson, E. P., Behrman, S. J.: Laparoscopy of the infertile patient. *Obstet Gynecol 36:* 363, 1970.
26. Grant, A.: Infertility surgery of the oviduct. *Fertil Steril 22:* 496, 1971.
27. Kistner, R. W., Patton, G. W., Jr.: Atlas of Infertility Surgery. Boston, Little, Brown, 1975.
28. Sampson, J. A.: Perforating hemorrhagic (chocolate) cysts of the ovary. *Arch Surg 3:* 245, 1921.
29. Ridley, J. H.: The histogenesis of endometriosis. *Obstet Gynecol Surv 23:* 1, 1968.
30. TeLinde, R. W., Scott, R. B.: Experimental endometriosis. *Am J Obstet Gynecol 60:* 1147, 1950.
31. Kempers, R. D., Dockerty, M. B., Hunt, A. B., et al: Significant postmenopausal endometriosis. *Surg Gynecol Obstet 111:* 348, 1960.
32. Ranney, B.: Endometriosis I. Conservative operations. *Am J Obstet Gynecol 107:* 743, 1970.
33. Kistner, R. W.: Endometriosis and infertility. In Behrman, S. J., Kistner, R. W. (eds): Progress in Infertility. Boston, Little, Brown, 1975.
34. Acosta, A. A., Buttram, V. C., Jr., Besch, P. K., et al: A proposed classification of endometriosis. *Obstet Gynecol 42:* 19, 1973.
35. March, C. M., Israel, R.: Rectovaginal endometriosis: an isolated enigma. *Am J Obstet Gynecol 122:* 274, 1976.
36. Spangler, D. B., Jones, G. S., Jones, H. W., Jr.: Infertility due to endometriosis—conservative surgical therapy. *Am J Obstet Gynecol 109:* 850, 1971.
37. Grant, A.: An evaluation of the conservative treatment of endometriosis. *Aust NZ J Obstet Gynaecol 3:* 162, 1963.
38. Samuelsson, S., Sjovall, A.: On the diagnostic value of laparoscopy in ovarian endometriosis. *Acta Obstet Gynecol Scand 47:* 350, 1968.
39. Karnaky, K. J.: The use of stilbestrol for endometriosis. *South Med J 41:* 1109, 1948.
40. Katayama, K. P., Manuel, M., Jone, H. W., Jr., et al: Methyltestosterone treatment of infertility associated with pelvic endometriosis. *Fertil Steril 27:* 83, 1976.
41. Greenblatt, R. B., Borenstein, R., Hernandez-Ayup, S.: Experiences with Danazol (an antigonadotropin) in the treatment of infertility. *Am J Obstet Gynecol 118:* 783, 1974.
42. Andrews, M. C., Wentz, A. C.: The effects of Danazol on gonadotropins and steroid blood levels in normal and anovulatory women. *Am J Obstet Gynecol 121:* 817, 1975.
43. Ansbacher, R.: Treatment of endometriosis with Danazol. *Am J Obstet Gynecol 121:* 283, 1975.
44. Green, T. H., Jr.: Conservative surgical treatment of endometriosis. *Clin Obstet Gynecol 9:* 293, 1966.
45. Landsteiner, K.: Kur kenntnis der spezifich auf blutkorperehen wirkenden sera. *Zentralbl Bakteriol [Orig B] 25:* 546, 1899.
46. Metalnifoff, S.: Etudes sur la spermotorine. *Ann Inst Pasteur (Paris) 14:* 577, 1900.
47. Mekhnikoff, E.: Etudes sur la resorption des cellules. *Ann Inst Pasteur (Paris) 13:* 737, 1899.
48. Behrman, S. J., Beuettner-Janusch, J., Hegler, R., Gershowitz, H., Tow, W. A.: ABO(H) blood incompatibility as a cause of infertility. A new concept. *Am J Obstet Gynecol 79:* 847, 1960.
49. Solish, G. I.: Distribution of ABO isohaemaglutinins among fertile and infertile women. *J Reprod Fertil 11:* 459, 1969.
50. Schwimmer, W. B., Ustay, K. A., Behrman, S. J.: An evaluation of immunological factors of fertility. *Fertil Steril 18:* 167, 1967.
51. Parish, W. I., Carron-Brown, J. A., Richards, C. B.: The detection of antibodies to spermatozoa and to blood group antigens in cervical mucus. *J Reprod Fertil 13:* 469, 1967.
52. Wilson, L.: Sperm agglutinins in human semen and blood. *Proc Soc Exp Biol Med 85:* 652, 1954.
53. Wilson, L.: Sperm agglutination due to autoantibodies. A new cause of sterility. *Fertil Steril 7:* 262, 1956.
54. Rumke, P., Hellinga, G.: Autoantibodies against spermatozoa in sterile men. *Am J Clin Pathol 32:* 357, 1959.
55. Fjallbrant, B., Obrant, O.: Clinical and seminal findings in men with sperm antibodies. *Acta Obstet Gynecol Scand 47 [Suppl 4]:* 451, 1968.
56. Franklin, R. R., Dukes, C. D. L.: Antispermatozoal antibodies and unexplained infertility. *Am J Obstet Gynecol 89:* 6, 1964.
57. Schwimmer, W. B., Ustay, K. A., Behrman, S. J.: Sperm-agglutinating antibodies and decreased fertility in prostitutes. *Obstet Gynecol Surv 23:* 195, 1968.
58. Glass, R. H., Vaidya, R. A.: Sperm-agglutinating antibodies in infertile women. *Fertil Steril 21:* 657, 1970.
59. Kibrick, S., Relding, D., Merrill, B.: Methods for the detection of antibodies against mammalian spermatozoa II. A gelatin agglutination test. *Fertil Steril 3:* 430, 1952.
60. Isojima, S., et al: Immunologic analysis of sperm-immobilizing factor found in sera of women with unexplained infertility. *Am J Obstet Gynecol 101:* 677, 1968.
61. Horne, H. W., Jr., et al: Subclinical endometrial inflammation and T-mycoplasma. A possible case of human reproductive failure. *Int J Fertil 18:* 226, 1973.
62. Horne, H. W., Jr., et al: The role of mycoplasma infection in human reproductive failure. *Fertil Steril 25:* 380, 1974.

63. McCormach, W. M., et al: The genital mycoplasma. *N Engl J Med 288:* 78, 1973.
64. O'Leary, W. M., Frick, J.: The correlation of human male infertility with the presence of mycoplasma T-strain. *Andrologia 7:* 309, 1975.
65. Gnarpe, H., Friberg, J.: Mycoplasma and human reproductive failure. The occurrence of different mycoplasma in couples with reproductive failures. *Am J Obstet Gynecol 114:* 727, 1972.
66. Gnarpe, H., Friberg, J.: T-Mycoplasma on spermatozoa and infertility. *Nature 245:* 97, 1973.
67. Friberg, J., Gnarpe, H.: Mycoplasma and human reproductive failure III. Pregnancies in infertile couples treated with Doxycycline for T-mycoplasma. *Am J Obstet Gynecol 116:* 23, 1973.
68. Louvois, J. De, et al: Frequency of mycoplasma in fertile and infertile couples. *Lancet 1:* 1073, 1974.
69. Jones, G. S., Aksel, S., Wentz, A. C.: Serum progesterone values in the luteal phase defects. *Obstet Gynecol 44:* 26, 1974.
70. Strott, C. A., Cargille, C. M., Ross, G. T., Lipsett, M. B.: The short luteal phase. *J Clin Endocrinol 30:* 246, 1970.

115

Ovarian Tumors with Endocrine Manifestations

Robert E. Scully

INTRODUCTION

The title "Ovarian Tumors with Endocrine Manifestations" is more appropriate for this chapter than "Functioning Ovarian Tumors" because it is now evident that the secretory products of the ovary and its tumors may be converted to other steroid hormones elsewhere in the body, and these hormones rather than the ovarian secretions themselves may be responsible for the clinical abnormalities observed in the patient. Ovarian tumors with overt endocrine manifestations account for less than 5 percent of all ovarian neoplasms, and the malignant forms of "functioning" ovarian tumors less than 10 percent of all ovarian cancers. However, the frequency of ovarian tumors that produce hormones at a subclinical level is probably considerably higher according to evidence afforded by various laboratory data. For example, it has been reported that more than one-third of the cases of ovarian cancer in postmenopausal women are associated with an increased maturation of vaginal epithelial cells in cytologic smears, suggesting an increased estrogen level.[1] Even more compelling evidence is the finding that almost half the postmenopausal women with common epithelial tumors (tumors derived from the surface epithelium of the ovary), which are generally considered to be nonfunctioning, have abnormally high levels of total urinary estrogens and/or pregnanediol in the urine.[2] The morphologic and histochemical features of the stroma of many ovarian tumors, including those of the common epithelial type, suggest that it is responsible for the production of steroid hormones in these cases.[3–5]

The great majority of ovarian tumors with endocrine manifestations are associated with end-organ changes and clinical syndromes related to abnormal levels of steroid hormones—most often estrogens, but occasionally androgens and exceptionally progesterone or corticosteroids. Rare tumors, however, produce chorionic gonadotropin, which stimulates the stroma of the neoplasm or uninvolved ovarian tissue to produce steroid hormones. Occasionally highly specialized forms of teratoma containing thyroidal or argentaffin epithelium elaborate their specific secretory products. Finally, cancers of the ovary, like those arising elsewhere in the body, are rarely associated with ectopic hormone production of various types.

A classification of ovarian tumors with endocrine manifestations, based on the World Health Organization (WHO) histologic typing of ovarian tumors,[6] is presented in Table 115-1. Nonneoplastic processes associated with clinical manifestations that closely simulate those of functioning ovarian tumors are also included.

CLINICAL MANIFESTATIONS OF STEROID HORMONE ABNORMALITIES ASSOCIATED WITH OVARIAN TUMORS

ESTROGENIC MANIFESTATIONS

Estrogen secretion by an ovarian tumor in infancy and childhood produces isosexual precocity.[7–10] The syndrome may develop from early infancy up to the time of true puberty, with the majority of the cases encountered before the age of 5 yr. Enlargement of the breasts is the most common initial manifestation of the disorder. This is followed by the development of pubic and axillary hair, enlargement of the external and internal secondary sex organs, irregular uterine bleeding, and a whitish vaginal discharge believed to originate in the stimulated endocervix. Often there is an acceleration of bone growth, and if the tumor is not removed, premature closure of the epiphyses and a short stature may result. Vaginal cytology reveals maturation of the squamous epithelial cells, and elevated levels of estrogens may be demonstrated in the blood and urine. Although gonadotropin levels might be expected

Table 115-1. Classification of Ovarian Tumors with Endocrine Manifestations

I. Steroid-hormone–secreting tumors
   A. Sex cord–stromal tumors
      1. Granulosa–stromal cell tumors
         a. Granulosa cell tumor
         b. Tumors in the thecoma–fibroma group
            i. Thecoma
            ii. Fibroma*
            iii. Unclassified†
      2. Sertoli–Leydig cell tumors (androblastomas)
      3. Gynandroblastoma
      4. Unclassified
   B. Lipid (lipoid) cell tumors
   C. Gonadoblastoma
   D. Tumors with functioning stroma
II. Gonadotropin– and steroid-hormone–secreting tumors
   A. Choriocarcinoma
   B. Embryonal carcinoma
   C. Polyembryoma
   D. Dysgerminoma with syncytiotrophoblastic cells
III. Highly specialized forms of teratoma with hormone production
   A. Struma
   B. Carcinoid
   C. Strumal carcinoid**
IV. Tumors with ectopic hormone production
V. Tumorlike conditions
   A. Solitary follicle cyst
   B. Multiple follicle cysts (polycystic ovaries)
   C. Hyperplasia of ovarian stroma and hyperthecosis
   D. Massive edema
   E. Pregnancy luteoma and *hyperreactio luteinalis*

*Nonfunctioning, but included to maintain integrity of WHO classification.
†Usually nonfunctioning.
**Hormone secretion not yet proven.

to be abnormally low for the age of the patient, examples have been reported in which the values have been elevated. Palpation of a mass on abdominal examination is practically diagnostic of an ovarian tumor as the cause of the precocity, but if unilateral or bilateral adnexal masses are palpable only on rectal examination, ovarian enlargement by cystic follicles and/or corpora lutea related to central precocity is more likely. The latter, which is usually constitutional, or idiopathic, accounts for approximately 90 percent of the cases of sexual precocity in females and is designated true precocity because the hypothalamic–pituitary axis is activated prematurely with the release of both follicle-stimulating (FSH) and luteinizing hormone (LH) and the possibility of ovulation. An estrogenic ovarian tumor that cannot be felt by any method of physical examination is rare in this age group, but examples have been reported.

In women of reproductive age estrogen secretion by an ovarian tumor inhibits ovulation and cyclic progesterone secretion via the hypothalamic–pituitary feedback mechanism, resulting in continuous, unopposed estrogenic stimulation of the endometrium. The latter is manifested morphologically by cystic hyperplasia, with or without varying degrees of precancerous atypicality, and by the occasional development of endometrial carcinoma, which is typically low grade.[11] The clinical expression of the endometrial stimulation may be excessive, irregular vaginal bleeding (metropathia hemorrhagica), but often a period of amenorrhea of months to years precedes the onset of abnormal bleeding or is the only menstrual disorder prior to the time of diagnosis. Occasionally the patient complains of swelling of the breasts, which may be accompanied by pain and tenderness. Estrogenic changes should be evident in cytologic smears of the vagina,[12] and elevated estrogen levels have been demonstrated in the body fluids.[13]

After the menopause estrogen production by an ovarian tumor rejuvenates the endometrium, producing changes similar to those described in the younger woman. Postmenopausal bleeding is the typical presenting symptom of endocrine origin, but occasionally bleeding from the stimulated endometrium has not occurred by the time of diagnosis of the tumor. Associated carcinoma of the endometrium is more common in postmenopausal than in premenopausal women with estrogenic tumors, having been reported in one large series in 24 percent of the former, but only 12.5 percent of the later.[11] These figures apply, however, only to those cases in which endometrial tissue was available for microscopic examination; a review of large series in the literature indicates that of all women with granulosa cell or theca cell tumors, only 5–6 percent have endometrial cancer. [11a] Symptoms of mammary stimulation may also develop after the menopause. Laboratory parameters of hyperestrogenism are helpful diagnostic aids, particularly the maturation of the vaginal epithelial cells, which is strikingly different from the expected atrophy in this age group. A mass is usually palpable, at least on pelvic examination, in an adult female with an estrogenic tumor, but in occasional cases it is a surprise finding at an operation for abnormal bleeding caused by endometrial hyperplasia or carcinoma.[14]

ANDROGENIC MANIFESTATIONS

Rarely, androgen secretion by an ovarian tumor prior to puberty results in heterosexual precocity, with virilizing manifestations superimposed on accelerated somatic growth.[7] During the reproductive age period the typical picture is one of a more or less abrupt onset of oligomenorrhea, followed by amenorrhea, defeminization (atrophy of breasts and loss of female bodily contours), and progressive virilization. The latter is characterized by hirsutism, acne, temporal balding, enlargement of the clitoris, deepening of the voice, and a male type of muscular development. Occasionally excessive, irregular uterine bleeding precedes the onset of diminished menstruation. This phenomenon is thought to reflect an initial slight elevation of the androgen level, which influences the hypothalamic–pituitary feedback mechanism in such a way that ovulation is inhibited, but gonadotropic stimulation of the ovarian follicular apparatus and estrogen secretion continue. Rarely, an androgenic ovarian tumor results in a more insidious onset of menstrual disturbances and virilization, or the hormone level may not even be high enough to interfere with ovulation. Increased libido is a frequent effect of an excess of androgen. Occasionally a postmenopausal woman becomes masculinized by an ovarian tumor or gives a history of long-standing mild virilism that had its onset during her reproductive years.

Often urinary 17-ketosteroids are normal, but measurement may be helpful in the diagnosis of an androgenic ovarian tumor. An elevation depends not only on the amount, but also on the type of androgen that is being produced. Testosterone, a potent androgen, commonly causes masculinization without a detectable abnormality in the 17-ketosteroid level, but weaker androgens, such as androstenedione and dehydroepiandrosterone, must be present in large amounts to virilize a patient; as a result, an increase in 17-ketosteroids is detectable in the urine when these hormones alone are responsible for virilization or are secreted in addition to testosterone. The direct measurement of various androgens, free and protein bound, in the plasma is the most sensitive and accurate laboratory index of a high androgen state.[15,16] An elevation in testosterone is most characteristic of virilizing ovarian tumors and nonneoplastic disorders but can also occur in association with adrenal hyperplasia and neoplasia. Androstenedione and dehydroepiandrosterone may be secreted by tumors and other pathologic processes originating in either the ovary or adrenal cortex. The results of stimulation by trophic hormones (HCG and ACTH) and suppression by dexamethasone are not decisive in distinguishing ovarian from adrenal virilism in view of several recorded exceptions to the results expected on theoretic grounds.[17] Measurements of levels in ovarian and adrenal vein blood are of great value, but can be misleading as a result of technical errors. Another laboratory manifestation of a high androgen state is elevation of the red blood cell count to normal male levels or even higher.

MANIFESTATIONS OF OTHER TYPES OF STEROID HORMONE EXCESS

Combinations of estrogenic and androgenic phenomena, such as virilization and cystic hyperplasia of the endometrium, or heterosexual precocity, enlargement of the breasts, and uterine bleeding, have occasionally been observed in patients with ovarian tumors. Likewise, histologic evidence of progesterone stimulation may be present in cases of hyperestrinism or androgen excess. Thus, a patient with an estrogenic ovarian tumor may have secretory changes superimposed on hyperplasia of the endometrium, and a rare virilized woman may have a decidual transformation of her endometrium. It has not been clear in most of these cases which hormones have been produced directly by the tumor and which have resulted from peripheral conversion of its secretory products.

Virilizing ovarian tumors have often been associated with one or more of the clinical or laboratory findings that are characteristic of Cushing's syndrome, but never with the complete form. These findings include polycythemia, which can be a manifestation of androgen excess alone, and obesity, hypertension, and diabetes, all of which are common disorders that may be unrelated to steroid secretion by the tumor. Although the production of hormones that are apparently specific for the adrenal cortex by ovarian tumors is a possibility, there has been no clear-cut laboratory documentation of such a phenomenon. No case has yet been reported in which an elevation of free cortisol in the plasma or urine has been attributable to direct secretion by an ovarian tumor.

CLINICOPATHOLOGIC FEATURES OF SPECIFIC TYPES OF OVARIAN TUMOR ASSOCIATED WITH STEROID HORMONE ABNORMALITIES

SEX CORD–STROMAL TUMORS

This category includes all neoplasms that contain granulosa cells, theca cells. Sertoli cells, Leydig cells, and stromal fibroblasts singly or in any combination and in various degrees of differentiation.[6] A number of terms have been given to these tumors, reflecting differing views of the embryology of the gonads. These terms include *mesenchymomas,*[18] *sex cord–mesenchyme tumors,*[19] and *gonadal stromal tumors.*[20] The name selected by WHO, which is a compromise between the last two designations, recognizes the presence in these tumors of derivatives of two of the morphologic components of the developing ovary and testis: (1) those arranged in epithelial configurations and traditionally called *sex cords,* and (2) tissue having the appearance of cellular stroma. The granulosa cells and Sertoli cells are the neoplastic derivatives of the sex cords, while the theca cells, Leydig cells, and fibroblasts develop from the gonadal stroma. Most tumors in this category are made up of female cell types, but some are composed of male cellular elements, and rarely cells and patterns of growth characteristic of both gonads are present in a single tumor. Not infrequently, when the cells are immature, when their morphologic appearance is intermediate between those of male and female cell types, or when the characteristic architectural patterns of the testis or ovary are not reproduced, it may be impossible to decide whether a tumor belongs in the granulosa–stromal cell or the Sertoli–Leydig cell category; in such a case the term *unclassified sex cord–stromal tumor* is used. If one excludes the relatively common inactive ovarian fibroma from consideration, most tumors in the sex cord–stromal category are associated with clinically apparent endocrine disturbances. It has not been possible by microscopic examination alone to distinguish these tumors from those that are not functioning at a clinical level.

Granulosa–Stromal Cell Tumors

This category includes all ovarian tumors composed of granulosa cells and cells of ovarian stromal derivation (theca cells and fibroblasts) singly or in various combinations.

Granulosa Cell Tumor. This tumor is either composed exclusively of granulosa cells or contains a significant component of them in association with theca cells and/or fibroblasts.[18–26] The granulosa cell tumor is the most common form of estrogenic tumor of the ovary, accounting for 1–2 percent of all ovarian tumors and 5–10 percent of all ovarian cancers. Five percent of granulosa cell tumors occur prior to puberty, and most of these are associated with isosexual precocity, accounting for 10 percent of the cases of that syndrome.[7,10] The remainder of these neoplasms are more or less evenly distributed among premenopausal and postmenopausal women. The tumors range in size from small nodules that cannot be felt on pelvic examination[14] to huge masses that distend the abdomen. At operation they may appear solid or cystic, and they are unilateral in over 95 percent of the cases. Sectioning a solid granulosa cell tumor reveals a gray or yellow color depending on the cellularity and lipid content, respectively, and a soft or firm consistency depending on the relative proportions of cells and fibromatous stroma (Fig. 115-1). Areas of necrosis and hemorrhage are not uncommon. A more frequent gross expression of a granulosa cell tumor is that of a predominantly cystic mass in which numerous compartments, usually filled with fluid or clotted blood, are separated by bridges of solid tissue (Fig. 115-2). An interesting clinical corollary of this gross appearance of the granulosa cell tumor is that 10–15 percent of these tumors present not with overt endocrine disturbances but as a result of rupture of a cystic compartment with hemoperitoneum. A rare granulosa cell tumor has a gross appearance that simulates that of the serous cystadenoma, with a large mass composed of one or more thin-walled cysts and little or no solid tissue.

On microscopic examination the granulosa cells grow in a wide variety of patterns. Well-differentiated forms include the microfollicular, macrofollicular, trabecular, insular, gyriform and watered silk forms or patterns. The microfollicular form, which is

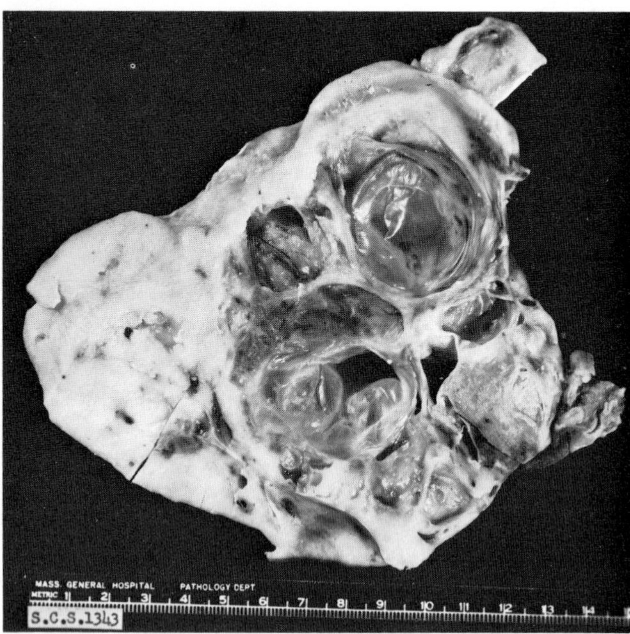

Fig. 115-1. Sectioned surface of juvenile granulosa cell tumor. Solid (yellow) and thin-walled cystic components are evident.

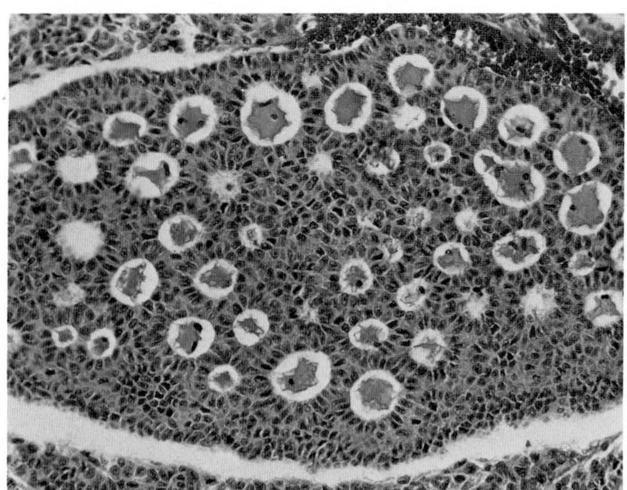

Fig. 115-3. Granulosa cell tumor, microfollicular pattern. The cavities (Call-Exner bodies) contain fluid and one or a few pyknotic nuclei. (From Morris and Scully: Endocrine Pathology of the Ovary, 1958. Courtesy of Mosby.)

the most distinctive, is characterized by multiple small cavities containing eosinophilic fluid and often one or a few degenerating nuclei (Call-Exner bodies); these cavities are surrounded by well-differentiated granulosa cells, the angular nuclei of which are arranged in helter-skelter fashion (Fig. 115-3). The macrofollicular form contains cysts lined by well-differentiated granulosa cells beneath which theca cells are usually present. The trabecular and insular patterns are characterized by cords and islands of granulosa cells separated by a fibromatous or thecomatous stroma (Fig. 115-4), while the watered-silk and gyriform patterns are manifested by undulating or zigzag rows of granulosa cells in single file. The less well-differentiated form of granulosa cell tumor has been designated diffuse, or sarcomatoid, and appears as a monotonous cellular growth resembling a round cell sarcoma. Because the patterns of granulosa cell tumors may be simulated by insular carcinoids, adenocarcinomas, and undifferentiated carcinomas, these generally more malignant tumors are frequently misdiagnoised as granulosa cell tumors. If the clinical course of the patient is atypical for a granulosa cell tumor, the possibility of such a misdiagnosis must be considered. The single best criterion for making the microscopic differential diagnosis is the appearance of the granulosa cell tumor nuclei, which are typically pale and commonly grooved.

Most granulosa cell tumors contain theca cells in varying quantities (Fig. 115-4), and several histochemical reactions that are characteristic of steroid-hormone–producing cells are much more often positive in the thecal than the granulosa cell component of the tumor. This observation has led to the conclusion that the theca cell is probably the estrogen producer in most of these tumors. In some instances, however, histochemical and other evidence has suggested a role in estrogen secretion for the granulosa cells. When the tumor has recurred outside ovarian tissue theca cells are frequently absent, which may be correlated with a

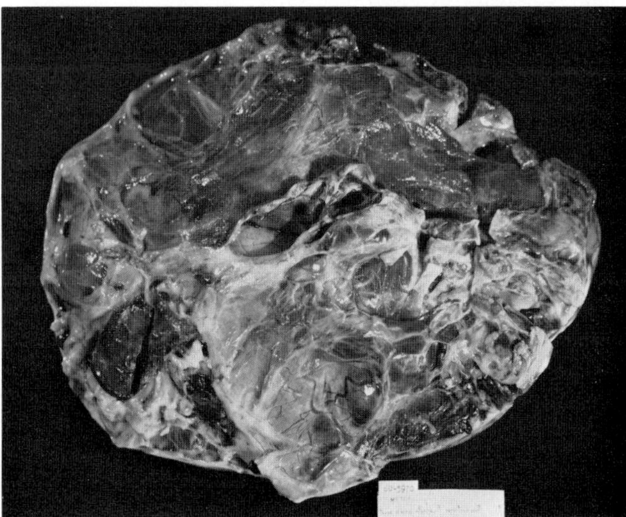

Fig. 115-2. Sectioned surface of granulosa cell tumor from an adult. Numerous thin-walled cysts, some of which contain clotted blood, are evident. (From Case Records of Massachusetts General Hospital, Case 89-1961: N. Engl. J. Med. *265:* 1210, 1961.)

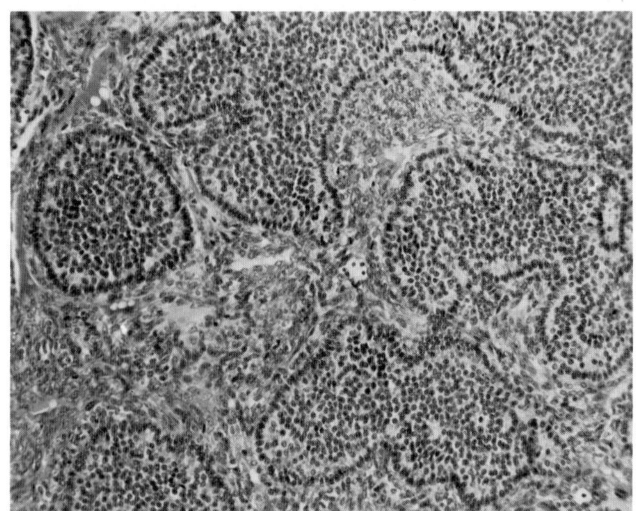

Fig. 115-4. Granulosa cell tumor, trabecular pattern, with theca cells between discrete anastomosing trabeculae and island of granulosa cells. (From Case Records of the Massachusetts General Hospital, Case 89-1961: N. Engl. J. Med. *265:* 1210, 1961.)

lack of evidence of estrogen secretion.[27] This finding suggests that the theca cells are not truly neoplastic in all the cases, but may develop as a response of the ovarian stroma to the proliferating granulosa cells. Occasionally either or both the granulosa and the theca cells take on the appearance of lutein cells, (i.e., cells resembling those of the corpus luteum) containing abundant cytoplasm, which may be dense and eosinophilic or spongy, reflecting a rich lipid content. An abundance of fat, as well as a macrofollicular pattern and cellular immaturity and pleomorphism, are so characteristic of the granulosa cell tumor encountered in infancy and childhood that we have applied the term *juvenile granulosa cell tumor* to this distinctive form.

The majority of granulosa cell tumors are estrogenic; it is impossible to give an accurate figure for the frequency of inactive forms because in many cases the endometrium has not been available for a microscopic examination to evaluate the presence or absence of estrogenic stimulation. After the removal of one of these tumors from a young woman whose uterus has been conserved, estrogen-withdrawal bleeding typically occurs in 1 or 2 days, and regular menses ensue shortly thereafter. Exceptional granulosa cell tumors have been associated with virilization rather than estrogenic manifestations.[28] Enigmatically, a high proportion of these have been of the huge, thin-walled, oligolocular or unilocular cystic variety, a very rare macroscopic form among these tumors in general.

The granulosa cell tumor, no matter what its microscopic pattern, has to be considered of low-grade malignancy because it may extend beyond the ovary or recur after apparently successful operative removal. Its spread is largely within the pelvis and lower abdomen. Distant metastases are rare, although they have been reported in many sites. Although recurrences may appear within 5 yr, often they are not evident until a much longer postoperative interval has elapsed, and numerous cases have been reported in which the tumor has reappeared 2 or even 3 decades after the initial therapy. Optimal treatment of the granulosa cell tumor in the menopausal or postmenopausal woman is total hysterectomy and bilateral salpingo-oophorectomy. In younger women and children in whom the preservation of fertility is an important consideration, removal of the tumor and adjacent fallopian tube is justifiable, if no spread beyond the ovary is demonstrable and the opposite ovary is shown by biopsy to be uninvolved by tumor. Recurrences have often been treated successfully by reoperation, radiation therapy, or a combination thereof. Too little information is available on the chemotherapy of granulosa cell tumors to evaluate the comparative merits of various agents; but several of these have been used with varying success.[29,30,30a] The 10-yr survival figures for patients with granulosa cell tumors which have been recorded in the literature have varied widely from under 60 to over 90 percent, and progressive declines in survival have been documented after longer follow-up periods.[21,26] Only one center has been able to correlate the microscopic pattern of the tumor and its prognosis, demonstrating a significantly greater frequency of late recurrences in cases with a sarcomatoid pattern.[21]

Tumors in the Thecoma–Fibroma Group. These tumors are composed exclusively or almost exclusively of theca cells and/or fibroblasts of ovarian stromal origin; rare nests of granulosa cells are occasionally observed.[18,20,22] Tumors that are composed of fibroblasts, contain little or no lipid, and are unassociated with biochemical or clinical evidence of estrogen production are fibromas. Those that contain larger quantities of fat and are associated with only equivocal evidence of estrogen production belong in the unclassified category. Thecomas contain abundant lipid and are

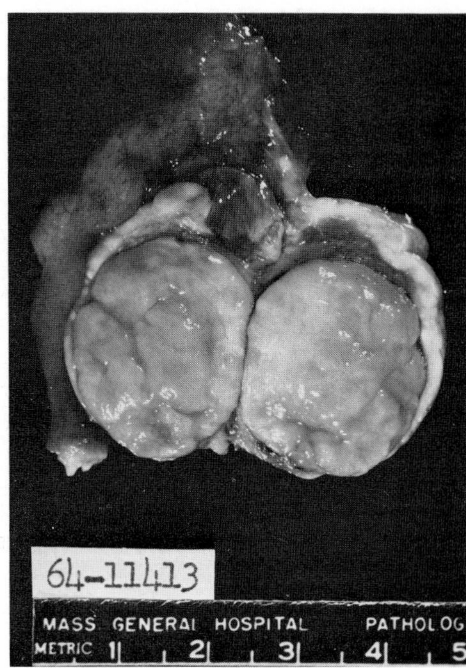

Fig. 115-5. Sectioned surface of thecoma. (From Blaustein (ed.): Pathology of the Female Genital Tract, 1977. Courtesy of Springer.)

characteristically accompanied by estrogenic manifestations. They are only one-third as common as granulosa cell tumors and occur at an older average age, being very rare prior to puberty. They range in size from small tumors that are not palpable on pelvic examination to large solid masses that have a fibrous consistency and a yellow or orange color on sectioning (Fig. 115-5). On microscopic examination two types of thecoma have been observed: the more common is characterized by ill-defined masses and cords of rounded vacuolated cells laden with lipid (Fig. 115-6); the second type, called a *luteinized thecoma,* has the basic appearance of a fibroma or a typical thecoma, but lutein cells are scattered singly or in nests throughout the tumor (Fig. 115-7).

The thecoma is almost invariably unilateral and almost never malignant. Several tumors purported to be malignant thecomas have appeared in the literature, but these are better interpreted as endocrinologically inactive fibrosarcomas or diffuse granulosa cell tumors. A reticulum stain is often helpful in distinguishing the

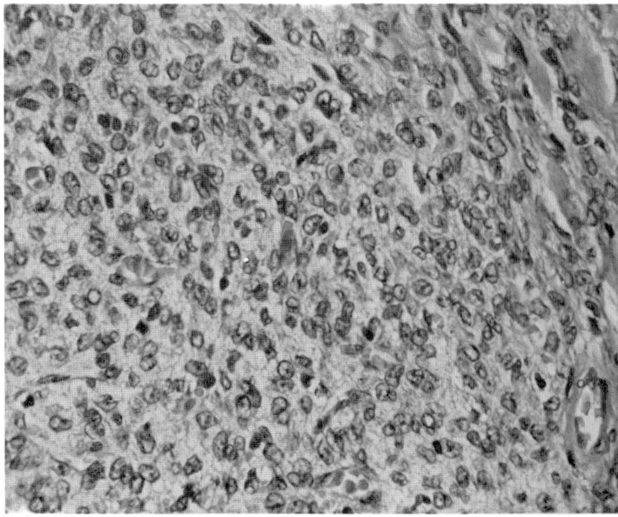

Fig. 115-6. Classical thecoma.

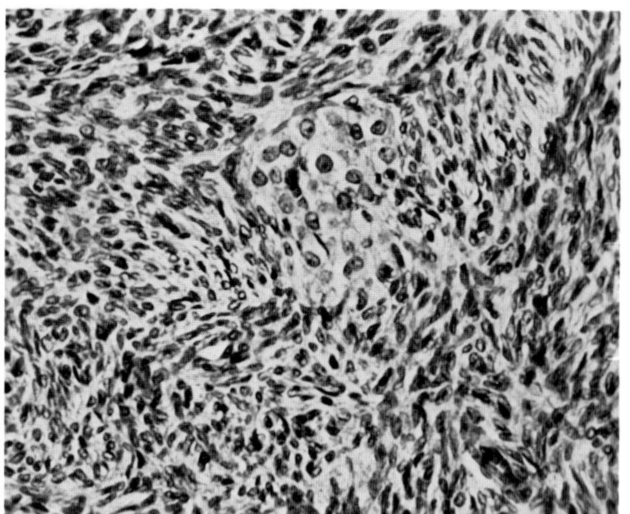

Fig. 115-7. Luteinized thecoma with nest of large rounded lutein cells lying in midst of spindle cells.

latter from thecomas. Typically, as in the graafian follicle, neoplastic granulosa cells have little or no reticulum among them, whereas theca cells are individually invested by fibrils.

In cases in which the preservation of fertility is important a thecoma can be treated adequately by unilateral oophorectomy. However, in a menopausal or postmenopausal woman total hysterectomy and bilateral salpingo-oophorectomy is indicated in most cases, as it is in patients in these age groups with other lesions of the internal genital organs, whether benign or malignant.

Sertoli–Leydig Cell Tumors (Androblastomas)

These tumors contain Sertoli and/or Leydig cells in varying proportions and varying degrees of differentiation.[7,15,19,20,31–34] Because the more primitive tumors within this category may recapitulate the development of the testis, the terms *androblastoma* and *arrhenoblastoma* have been used as synonyms, but their connotation of associated masculinization is misleading because some of these tumors have no endocrine manifestations and others may even be accompanied by an estrogenic syndrome.[35,36]

Sertoli–Leydig cell tumors are perhaps one-fifth as frequent as granulosa cell tumors; they occur at all ages but are most often encountered in women in the early reproductive-age period, who usually become virilized. Plasma testosterone and/or androstenedione levels are typically elevated; urinary 17-ketosteroid values are usually normal or only slightly raised, although an occasional very high level has been recorded. At operation the tumor varies in size from a small nodule that was not palpable preoperatively to a huge mass that distends the abdomen. The wide variety of gross appearances that have been described for the granulosa cell tumor can be duplicated by the Sertoli–Leydig cell tumor.

The microscopic patterns observed vary more greatly than those of any other ovarian tumor with the exception of the teratoma. Most of the cases contain mixtures of Sertoli and Leydig cells, and these have been subdivided into well-differentiated forms, tumors of intermediate differentiation, those that are poorly differentiated (sarcomatoid), and a heterogenous group characterized by the inclusion of a variety of heterologous elements within the tumor. The well-differentiated Sertoli–Leydig cell tumor is characterized by solid or hollow tubules filled with or lined by Sertoli cells and separated by well-developed Leydig cells, which occasionally contain crystalloids of Reinke, the specific cytoplasmic inclusions of the testicular Leydig cells (Fig. 115-8). In the intermediate form well-defined islands and cords, or ill-defined masses of immature Sertoli cells, alternate with cellular tissue of stromal derivation that typically contains islands of well-differentiated Leydig cells. In the poorly differentiated Sertoli–Leydig cell tumor the appearance may be that of a fibrosarcoma, poorly differentiated carcinoma, or a combination of the two; in such cases it is only the finding of more mature elements recognizable as Sertoli or Leydig cells that permits a specific diagnosis. The intermediate and poorly differentiated tumors occasionally contain unexpected heterologous cellular elements, the genesis of which is difficult to explain. These include mucinous glands and cysts, the epithelium of which may contain argentaffin cells, rarely foci of carcinoid tumor, rhabdomyoblasts, and cartilage. Although a teratomatous nature has been postulated to explain the presence of these elements, other more characteristic components of teratomas are not seen in Sertoli–Leydig cell tumors, nor do typical teratomas ever contain gonadal elements.

Instead of containing both testicular cell types, neoplasms in the general category of Sertoli–Leydig cell tumors may be composed exclusively or almost exclusively of either Sertoli or Leydig cells in various degrees of differentiation. Pure Sertoli cell tumors may contain lipid in varying amounts and may be associated with estrogenic manifestations. One distinctive form of estrogenic ovarian tumor, which was originally designated *folliculome lipidique* (i.e., lipid-rich granulosa cell tumor), has been reinterpreted as a Sertoli cell tumor with lipid storage because of its basic tubular architecture (Fig. 115-9).[35,36] Tumors composed exclusively of Leydig cells may not have the same histogenesis as other tumors in the Sertoli–Leydig cell category, arising in many cases directly from the hilus cells (hilar Leydig cells), which can be found in the ovarian hilus of over 80 percent of adult women on careful microscopic sampling. Such hilus cell tumors will be discussed in greater detail below in the section on Lipid Cell Tumors.

Although the Leydig cells and their morphologic variants are the obvious source of androgens in Sertoli–Leydig cell tumors, it is more difficult to pinpoint the cellular site of the estrogen production that occurs in some cases. On the basis of an analogy to the well-known estrogenic Sertoli cell tumor of the canine testis, as well as other evidence, it is reasonable to conclude that the Sertoli cell secretes estrogens in certain cases. The knowledge that the Leydig cell of the human testis is also capable of estrogen produc-

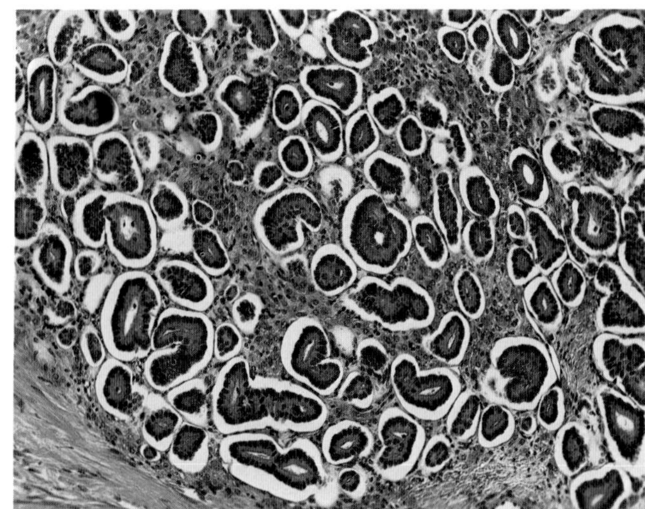

Fig. 115-8. Sertoli–Leydig cell tumor, well differentiated, with hollow tubules separated by Leydig cells. (From Morris and Scully: Endocrine Pathology of the Ovary, 1958. Courtesy of Mosby.)

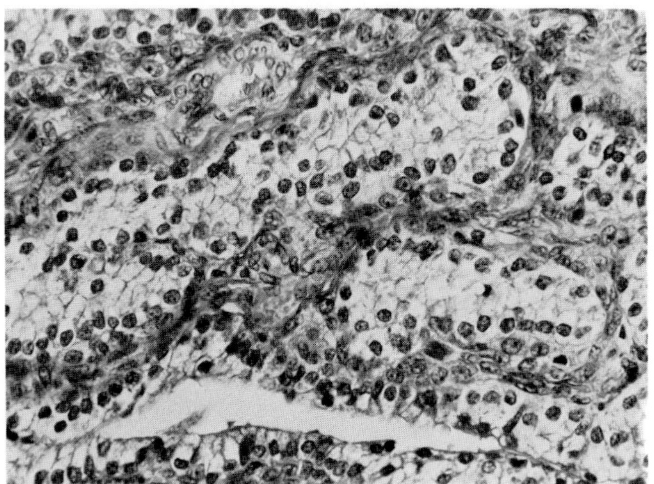

Fig. 115-9. Sertoli cell tumor with lipid storage. (From Serov, et al.: Histological Typing of Ovarian Tumours, 1973. Courtesy of World Health Organization.)

tion suggests that this cell type may secrete estrogens in other Sertoli–Leydig cell tumors. A final possibility is peripheral conversion to estrogens of androgens produced by the Leydig cells of the tumor.

After the removal of a virilizing Sertoli–Leydig cell tumor the menses characteristically return to normal in about 4 weeks. In most cases the excess hair diminishes, but often incompletely. Clitoromegaly and particularly deepening of the voice are less apt to regress.

Sertoli–Leydig cell tumors vary widely in their degree of malignancy, and this variation can be correlated to some extent with the degree of differentiation of the tumor. Well-differentiated tumors rarely exhibit a malignant behavior, whereas the poorly differentiated forms that resemble sarcomas or carcinomas may have a rapidly malignant course. Pelvic and intraabdominal spread is much more common than distant metastasis. The overall 5-yr survival rate of patients with these tumors has been reported to be in the range of under 70 to over 90 percent.[32,33] Since they occur predominantly in young women and are bilateral in less than 5 percent of the cases, unilateral salpingo-oophorectomy is justifiable if the preservation of fertility is an important consideration and there is no evidence of extension beyond the involved ovary. A wedge biopsy of the contralateral ovary is desirable before the decision to perform a conservative operation is made. The role of radiation therapy and chemotherapy in the treatment of these tumors after they have spread beyond surgical control or have recurred is uncertain because of the minimal recorded experience with cases of this type.

Gynandroblastoma

This extremely rare tumor should be diagnosed only if clearly recognizable well-differentiated female and male cellular elements form significant components of a neoplasm.[6] Rare foci of female-type cells in an otherwise typical Sertoli–Leydig cell tumor, or of male cell types in a granulosa–stromal cell tumor do not constitute sufficient evidence for this diagnosis. The gynandroblastoma is a morphologic curiosity rather than a clinicopathologic entity and has been much overdiagnosed in the medical literature.

Sex Cord–Stromal Tumors, Unclassified

These tumors may be estrogenic, androgenic, or inactive. Their clinical and pathologic features are similar to those of granulosa–stromal cell and Sertoli–Leydig cell tumors, the only difference being the impossibility of certain identification of the cell types on a morphologic basis. One distinctive tumor in this category is the sex cord tumor with annular tubules, which can be estrogenic.[37] It is composed of simple and complex ringlike tubular structures having an appearance intermediate between that of tubules lined by Sertoli cells and islands of granulosa cells; calcification within the annular tubules is a common and often prominent feature. The most interesting aspect of this rare tumor is that when it occurs in the form of multiple discrete nodules, it is almost always associated with the Peutz-Jeghers syndrome (gastrointestinal polyposis accompanied by mucocutaneous melanin pigmentation) and its discovery may be the first clue to that diagnosis. A rare sex cord tumor with annular tubules behaves in a malignant fashion, but all those reported in patients with the Peutz-Jeghers syndrome have been benign.

LIPID CELL TUMORS

These rare tumors are composed exclusively of cells that have the typical morphologic features of steroid-hormone–producing cells, thereby resembling lutein cells, Leydig cells, and adrenal cortex cells (Fig. 115-10).[31,34,38,39] The numerous designations that have been proposed for these neoplasms reflect our lack of knowledge of their origins; these terms include *lipoid cell tumor, adrenal rest tumor, adrenalhypheo-like tumor, masculinovoblastoma, luteoma,* and *hypernephroma*. The usage of *lipid cell tumor* or *lipoid cell tumor* is not ideal because of the lack of specificity of these terms and the fact that some tumors in this category contain little or no fat. A name such as *steroid cell tumor* would be more appropriate, but the introduction of still another term would probably only add to the existing confusion. So little is known about the origin of lipid cell tumors that in every case all the morphologic, histochemical, biochemical, and clinical evidence should be evaluated carefully in an attempt to determine more specifically the nature of the neoplastic cells; if the lutein, Leydig, or adrenal cortex cell origin of the tumor can be established, it should be placed in a more specific category; if not, the nonspecific term *lipid cell tumor* is appropriate.

These tumors occur at all ages, but mostly during the reproductive years. They are usually virilizing, but may be nonfunctioning or, rarely, estrogenic. When they are masculinizing they are more apt to be associated with elevated urinary levels of 17-ketosteroids than tumors in the Sertoli–Leydig cell category, indi-

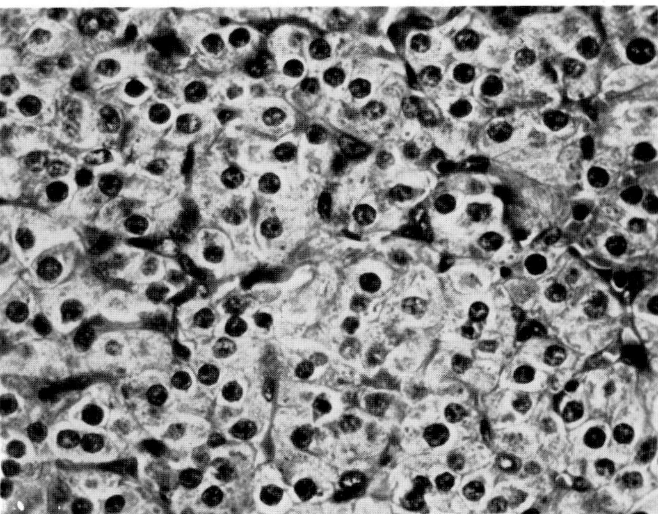

Fig. 115-10. Lipid cell tumor. (From Serov, et al.: Histological Typing of Ovarian Tumours, 1973. Courtesy of World Health Organization.)

cating a production of weak androgens in many cases. The presence of some of the features of Cushing's syndrome and high levels of urinary 17-ketosteroids in occasional cases has led to the speculation that these tumors originate in adrenal cortical rests, which have been identified in the broad ligament near the ovary in approximately one-fourth of hysterectomy specimens.[40] However, with possible rare exceptions no convincing evidence of corticosteroid production by one of these tumors has been reported; moreover, almost all the recorded cases have been within the ovary and not in the broad ligament, where adrenal rests are almost always found. In one unusual case an ovarian tumor belonging in the lipid cell category (even though the presence of lipid could not be demonstrated) was associated with clinical and biochemical findings that strongly supported the diagnosis of an adrenal cortical rest tumor.[41] In that case an 8-yr-old girl who had had an adrenalectomy earlier because of a diagnosis of the adrenogenital syndrome experienced a regression of masculinization only after the removal of the lipid cell tumor, which arose in the hilar or medullary area. Microscopic examination of the adrenal cortex was compatible with the adrenogenital syndrome. Preoperative elevated urinary levels of 17-ketosteroids, 17-ketogenic steroids, and pregnanetriol and the demonstration of cortisol and corticosterone production by the tumor in vitro were more characteristic of adrenal cortical than gonadal tissue. However, the authors who reported this case were careful to point out the possibility that tumors of gonadal elements might also rarely produce adrenal cortical hormones.

On gross examination lipid cell tumors are typically solid. Those that contain large quantities of fat have a yellow or orange appearance, whereas those that are poor in lipid content or fat-free are reddish brown, or if rich in lipochrome pigment, greenish brown to black. On microscopic examination the neoplastic cells may be large and rounded with abundant lipid-laden spongy cytoplasm, or somewhat smaller with dense eosinophilic cytoplasm (Fig. 115-10). Both cell types and transitions between them are often present in a single tumor. The cells are arranged diffusely or in nests and columns separated by a rich network of vascular sinusoids. Certain morphologic features may provide a clue to the origin of the tumor. If it is small and situated within the ovarian cortex, and particularly if it is associated with stromal hyperthecosis, an origin from lutein cells of the ovarian stroma appears almost certain. Tumors in this category have been designated *stromal luteomas*.[42] If, in contrast, the tumor is centered in the hilus, an origin from hilus cells (hilar Leydig cells) is probable. If crystalloids of Reinke are also demonstrable in the cytoplasm of the tumor cells, such an origin is certain, removing the case from the nonspecific category of lipid cell tumor and justifying the diagnosis of hilus cell tumor (Fig. 115-11).[17,43]

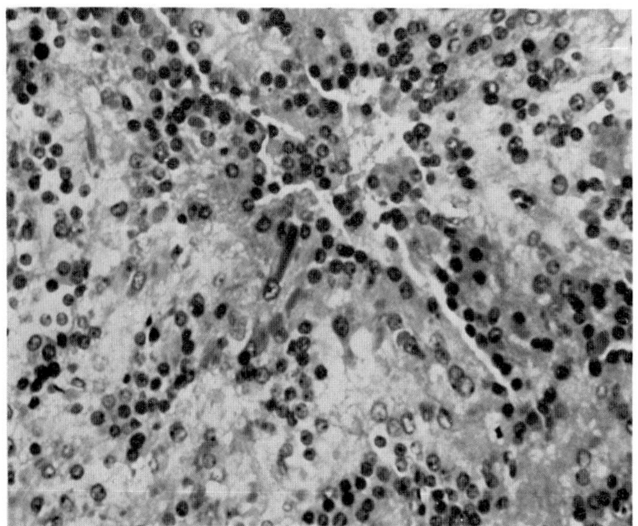

Fig. 115-11. Hilus cell tumor with two crystalloids of Reinke at center. (From Grady and Smith (eds.): The Ovary, 1963. Courtesy of Williams & Wilkins.)

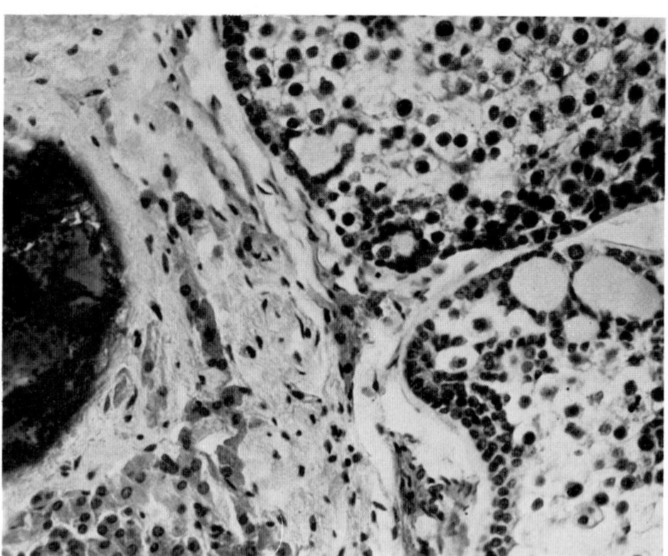

Fig. 115-12. Gonadoblastoma. Note discrete nests composed of sex cord cells with small nuclei and large germ cells; a rounded focus of calcification is present as well as a large cluster of Leydig cells at the lower left. (From Scully, Meigs and Sturgis (eds.): Progress in Gynecology, vol. 4, 1963. Grune & Stratton.)

Most lipid cell tumors are benign, but malignant cases have been reported. In a perhaps biased series, over 25 percent of the lipid cell tumors reviewed at the Armed Forces Institute of Pathology were malignant.[38] Two pathologic features were correlated most closely with a benign clinical course. All the tumors less than 8 cm in diameter and all those containing crystalloids of Reinke (regarded as hilus cell tumors according to WHO nomenclature) were benign. Since lipid cell tumors are benign in most cases and are almost always unilateral, a conservative operation for a localized tumor is justifiable in a young woman who wishes to retain her fertility.

GONADOBLASTOMA

This is a complex tumor composed of germ cells, sex cord derivatives, and, in two-thirds of the cases, stromal derivatives as well[44] (Fig. 115-12). The germ cells, which resemble those of the ovarian dysgerminoma and the testicular seminoma, and the sex cord elements, which have the appearance of immature Sertoli or granulosa cells, characteristically grow within discrete nests, creating three distinctive patterns. In the most common of these the germ cells are sprinkled among the generally more numerous, smaller sex cord cells, which in turn are oriented around multiple rounded hyaline bodies, creating a microfollicular appearance. The hyaline bodies, however, differ from Call-Exner bodies, being composed of hyalinized basement membrane material that may be continuous with the basement membrane of the nests. The stromal derivatives resemble lutein cells and fetal Leydig cells; they have not been reported to contain crystalloids of Reinke. Foci of calcification, which typically begin in the hyaline bodies, have been observed in most of the cases. These foci may become confluent, and often the calcification is so extensive that it can be observed on an x-ray film of the pelvis. In about half the cases of gonadoblastoma the germ cells transgress the limits of the discrete clusters and invade the stroma to form a germinoma (dysgerminoma or seminoma). Occasionally a more highly malignant form of germ cell tumor, such as an endodermal sinus tumor, embryonal carcinoma, or choriocarcinoma, develops in association with a gonadoblastoma.[45,46] The gonadoblastoma may be of microscopic dimensions or may form a large mass, which can be soft and fleshy if there is significant germinomatous overgrowth, totally calcified, or of mixed consistency.

Almost all gonadoblastomas arise in individuals with abnormal gonads, although a rare example has been observed in an otherwise normal male or female. Many of the smaller tumors have been demonstrated to originate in streak gonads or dysgenetic testes, but it has been impossible to determine the nature of the underlying gonad in most of the cases because the tumor has been large enough to replace it. The associated sexual disorder appears most often to be pure or mixed gonadal dysgenesis, but an occasional patient has had Turner's syndrome or dysgenetic male pseudohermaphroditism. The great majority of the patients have been chromatin-negative and the most common karyotypes have been 46XY and 46XY/45XO. Other types of mosaisism have also been recorded, and a rare patient has been 46XX. The tumor may be discovered in childhood or during adult life. Four-fifths of the patients are phenotypic females, who, more often than not, are masculinized to some extent. Although it may be difficult in many cases to decide whether to attribute associated endocrine abnormalities to a gonadoblastoma or the underlying gonadal disorder, there has been both clinical and biochemical evidence, including in vitro studies of the tumor tissue, that the Leydig-like cells of the gonadoblastoma are capable of androgen production with resultant virilization. In vitro evidence of estrogen production has also been reported and some patients have experienced hot flashes after the removal of the tumor.

Although the gonadoblastoma without an associated germinoma has not been shown to exhibit a malignant behavior and can be regarded as no more than an in situ form of malignancy, the common complication of invasive germinoma and the occasional association with more malignant forms of germ cell tumor indicate that a gonad containing a gonadoblastoma is potentially dangerous and should be removed. Since the tumor is bilateral in over one-third of the cases and arises almost invariably in individuals who have abnormal gonads, the removal of the opposite adnexa is also indicated. Because many gonadoblastomas have been of small size and have been discovered incidentally in the course of an exploratory laporatomy to establish the nature of a sexual disorder, and because individuals with the clinical picture of gonadal dysgenesis and a Y chromosome have been reported to have gonadoblastomas or other malignant germ cell tumors in 25 percent of cases, routine gonadectomy is now being recommended in cases of gonadal dysgenesis with a Y chromosome.[47,48] A 100 percent survival can be expected after the removal of gonads harboring one or more gonadoblastomas if germ cell infiltration of the stroma has not occurred. A germinoma arising within a gonadoblastoma is capable of metastatic spread, and the endodermal sinus tumor, embryonal carcinoma, and choriocarcinoma, which have been encountered in occasional cases, probably will prove to have the same poor prognosis that has been established for them in the absence of an associated gonadoblastoma.

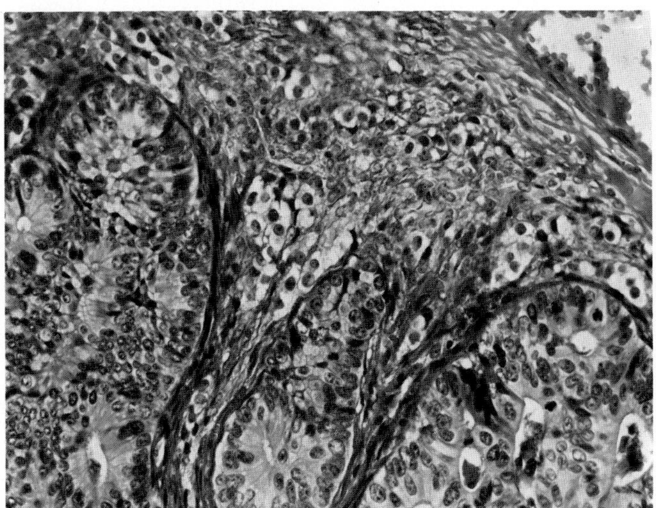

Fig. 115-13. Metastatic carcinoma of cecal origin growing in discrete oval nests, with smaller ill-defined aggregates of clear lutein cells within stroma of tumor. (From Scully and Richardson: Cancer *14:* 827, 1961.)

TUMORS WITH FUNCTIONING STROMA

These are tumors in which the neoplastic cells do not produce steroid hormones, but by growing in the ovary stimulate the ovarian stroma, which may proliferate to form the stroma of the tumor to differentiate into cells that have the appearance of theca or lutein cells (Fig. 115-13) and secrete androgens, estrogens, progesterone, or a combination thereof.[3–5,31,49–51] These tumors may be benign or malignant, primary or metastatic. A wide variety of ovarian neoplastic types has been reported to be associated with the phenomenon of functioning stroma, which is unique in the ovary among all the endocrine glands. The evidence for the existence of tumors of this type is as follows: (1) clinically, the appearance of an endocrine disorder that regresses after the removal of the tumor; (2) morphologically, the presence of cells resembling steroid-hormone–producing cells in the stroma of the tumor or in the adjacent ovarian stroma (Fig. 115-13); (3) histochemically, reactions in these cells that are characteristic of steroid-hormone–producing cells; and (4) biochemically, abnormal steroid assays preoperatively, reverting to normal after the removal of the tumor, the recovery of various steroids from the neoplastic tissue, and the demonstration in vitro of an ability of the tumor to synthesize numerous steroid hormones from precursors.

In some cases chorionic gonadotropin appears to be an important factor in stimulating the stroma to develop into steroid-hormone–secreting tissue. A number of the cases of ovarian tumor with functioning stroma that have been reported occurred during pregnancy.[51–54] Although all of these have been virilizing, it is possible that other tumors in pregnant women that have contained a stroma morphologically compatible with steroid-hormone production have produced estrogens at a subclinical level. The relationship of the stromal stimulation and abnormal hormone production to chorionic gonadotropin is strongly suggested by various findings in individual case reports. In several of these the masculinizing tumor was a benign neoplasm that must have been present before the onset of pregnancy, at a time when virilism was absent. In one case of a virilizing Krukenberg tumor during pregnancy, a similar tumor that had been found in the opposite ovary prior to the onset of that pregnancy had not masculinized the patient. Additionally some regression of the virilizing manifestations and a decline in hormone levels occurred after the termination of the pregnancy, but before the removal of the tumor; finally, the administration of HCG subsequently caused an increase in the plasma androgens and the urinary 17-ketosteroids.[52] In still another case it was demonstrated that a Brenner tumor that virilized a pregnant woman was unable to produce testosterone in vitro unless chorionic gonadotropin was added to the incubate.[53,54] In one case of an ovarian tumor with functioning stroma occurring in the absence of pregnancy, chorionic gonadotropin, secreted by a dysgerminoma containing syncytiotrophoblast cells, stimulated the stroma in and around the tumor to luteinize and produce androgens, resulting in virilization.[55]

In most cases of ovarian tumors with functioning stroma occurring in nonpregnant patients there is no clue as to why the stroma is stimulated to secrete steroid hormones. The recent demonstration that many carcinomas of diverse origin may be associated with an elevated level of the beta subunit of chorionic gonadotropin[56] has suggested the possibility that this secretory product may be a factor, and, indeed, Kurman[56a] has demonstrated the presence of the beta subunit in the malignant cells of a virilizing Krukenberg tumor in a nonpregnant patient by means of an immunoperoxidase staining method. The phenomenon of functioning stroma is only occasionally clinically evident, but it may explain the findings of abnormal maturation of the vaginal smear and elevated urinary levels of estrogens and/or pregnanediol in association with over one-third of the cases of common epithelial tumors of the ovary in postmenopausal women.[1,2]

MacDonald and his co-workers[56b] have recently shown that a mucinous cystadenocarcinoma with a functioning stroma that was associated with endometrial hyperplasia produced androstenedione, which was converted elsewhere to estrone, the hormone directly responsible for the estrogenic manifestation.

GONADOTROPIN– AND STEROID-HORMONE–SECRETING TUMORS

CHORIOCARCINOMA

This is a tumor composed of cytotrophoblast and syncytiotrophoblast growing in intimate association with one another. In the ovary it is usually of germ cell origin, and in the great majority of these cases it is combined in varying proportions with other forms of malignant germ cell tumor, most often an immature teratoma.[7,57] Ovarian choriocarcinomas may also be metastatic from other sites in the genital tract or possibly arise from the trophoblast of a primary ovarian pregnancy. The germ cell origin of the tumor is acceptable only if it has developed before puberty or is associated with another type of germ cell malignancy. Most of the cases recorded in the literature have occurred in the first two decades. Isosexual precocity has been reported in about half the prepubertal patients, and heterosexual precocity has been associated on rare occasions.[7] In older patients irregular menstrual bleeding and rapid enlargement of the breasts, occasionally with colostrum secretion, may be observed. Chorionic gonadotropin, placental lactogen, estrogen and androgen levels may all be elevated. The course has almost always been fatal within a period of several weeks to 1 yr with spread throughout the abdomen and often to the lungs. Occasional patients have survived for many years after the removal of the tumor. Combined chemotherapy (methotrexate, actinomycin D, and chlorambucil) has produced prolonged remissions in several patients with persistent ovarian choriocarcinoma of germ cell origin.[58]

EMBRYONAL CARCINOMA

The rare embryonal carcinoma typically contains syncytiotrophoblast cells and is often associated with endocrine manifestations similar to those of the choriocarcinoma.[58a]

POLYEMBRYOMA

This very rare tumor is a teratoma, a prominent part of which is composed of myriads of early embryoid bodies. Enough trophoblast may be present in these structures to produce large quantities of chorionic gonadotropin.[59]

DYSGERMINOMA WITH SYNCYTIOTROPHOBLASTIC CELLS

This tumor is a typical dysgerminoma except for the presence of widely scattered cells resembling syncytiotrophoblastic cells and growing adjacent to dilated vascular sinusoids.[55,60] Fluorescent antibody stains for human chorionic gonadotropin may demonstrate its presence in these cells. This type of tumor has already been discussed in the section on Tumors with Functioning Stroma.

OVARIAN CARCINOMA WITH ECTOPIC CHORIONIC GONADOTROPIN PRODUCTION

This subject will be discussed in the section on Tumors with Ectopic Hormone Production.

HIGHLY SPECIALIZED FORMS OF TERATOMA WITH HORMONE PRODUCTION

STRUMA OVARII

This is a teratoma in which thyroid tissue is present exclusively or constitutes a grossly recognizable component of a more complex teratoma.[57,61–63] The peak incidence is in the fifth decade; occasional examples have been encountered in postmenopausal women and rare cases before puberty. On gross examination some strumas appear to be composed entirely of thyroid tissue, while others are associated with dermoid cysts, and occasional examples with mucinous or serous cystadenomas. The thyroid tissue is reddish brown or greenish brown; it may be solid, but it is often partly or predominantly cystic with a content of gelatinous fluid. Occasionally the opposite ovary contains a dermoid cyst and rarely another struma. On microscopic examination the thyroid-type tissue is unencapsulated and resembles normal thyroid gland or a thyroid adenoma, which may be predominantly macrofollicular, microfollicular (fetal), or embryonal. Occasionally vascular invasion and rarely a papillary pattern are observed. Well under 5 percent of strumas have had a malignant clinical course, with metastases reported in the lungs, bones, liver, and brain.[64] Rarely histologically mature implants of thyroid tissue are found on the peritoneum; this process, which has been termed *benign strumosis,* has been associated with a long survival.

The degree of function and the frequency of hyperfunction of ovarian strumas are unknown. In occasional cases there has been strong clinical evidence that a struma has been responsible for the development of thyrotoxicosis, but such cases have been mostly in the older literature before the advent of sophisticated measurement of thyroid function. Likewise, enlargement of the thyroid gland has been reported in approximately 15 percent of the cases of struma ovarii, and the role of the thyroid gland itself in the production of the thyrotoxicosis has not been evaluated adequately in several of the cases in which this disorder has been ascribed solely to a struma. Scanning after the administration of radioactive iodine has been advocated as an aid in the diagnosis of struma ovarii, but at least one false-positive result has been reported. Most strumas are adequately treated by oophorectomy. If microscopic examination reveals changes suggestive of malignancy, x-ray examination of the lungs and the bones and scanning with I^{131} are indicated in order to detect possible metastases. There is evidence in one case that I^{131} therapy was effective in the management of metastatic struma.

CARCINOID

Five distinct types of ovarian carcinoid have been observed, four of which are primary and the fifth metastatic, usually from the ileum.[57,65,66] The primary types include: the insular, or midgut variety; the trabecular, or foregut–hindgut form; the strumal carcinoid, in which the carcinoid grows in association with a struma; and a very rare type arising within a Sertoli–Leydig cell tumor. Only the insular and metastatic forms have been reported to be accompanied by the carcinoid syndrome. The strumal carcinoid is discussed separately below. The carcinoids of various types have occurred exclusively in adults, with the youngest patient in the third and the oldest in the ninth decade.

Primary carcinoids have always been unilateral, although another type of tumor, usually a dermoid cyst, may be present in the opposite ovary. The carcinoid may form a small, firm, tan to yellow nodule protruding into the lumen of a dermoid cyst, thicken the wall of such a cyst in a more diffuse manner, lie within a predominantly solid mature teratoma, or form a large, solid homogeneous mass in which microscopic teratomatous elements may be found. Cystic spaces filled with clear fluid may be present within the carcinoid component of the tumor. The insular carcinoid is characterized by discrete islands of argentaffin cells that may be perforated, particularly at the periphery of the nests, by numerous, small, round glandular spaces containing dense eosinophilic secretion, which is sometimes calcified.[65] Argentaffin granules are usually visible with ordinary hematoxylin and eosin stains, and they are almost always identifiable after argentaffin and other types of special staining. The trabecular carcinoid is characterized by a ribbon pattern of the tumor cells. Argentaffin granules are observed less often than in the insular carcinoid. The very rare cases of carcinoid that have been found in Sertoli–Leydig cell tumors have been of the insular type. Metastatic carcinoids are usually of the insular, but occasionally of the trabecular type (Fig. 115-14).

One-third of the reported cases of primary insular carcinoid have been associated with manifestations of the carcinoid syndrome (flushing, sometimes misinterpreted as menopausal, diarrhea, pulmonary stenosis, and/or tricuspid insufficiency and peripheral edema). Since the effluent of the tumor is routed through the ovarian vein into the inferior vena cava and outside the portal circulation, where carcinoid secretory products are inactivated, an ovarian carcinoid can produce the characteristic syndrome in the absence of hepatic or other metastases. Furthermore, since none of the reported cases have been associated with metastasis at the time of their discovery, the syndrome has always been cured by the removal of the tumor. In an occasional case, however, cardiac valvular damage has continued or progressed despite the restoration of the hormone values to normal levels, or the tumor has recurred with or without a return of the carcinoid syndrome.

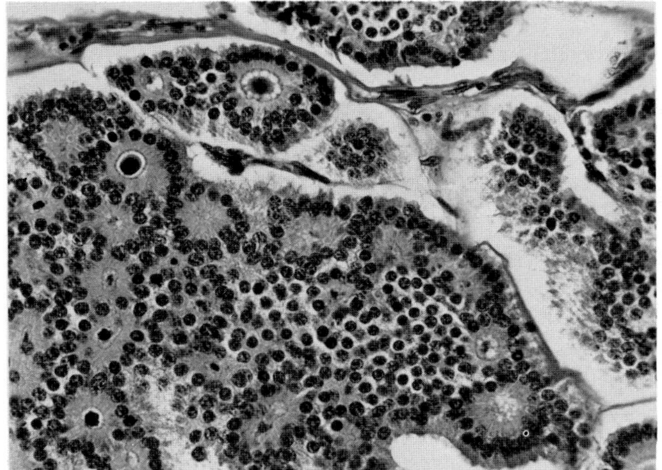

Fig. 115-14. Metastatic insular carcinoid. The nuclei are round and dark; the lumens contain dense secretion, some of which has a dark appearance due to calcification. (From Serov, et al.: Histological Typing of Ovarian Tumours, 1973. Courtesy of World Health Organization.)

The primary insular carcinoid of the ovary must be distinguished from the secondary form, the other type that is often associated with the carcinoid syndrome.[66] Such a distinction may be difficult for the pathologist at the time of operation because a primary carcinoid tumor of the bowel may be small and difficult for the surgeon to detect. There are several clues to the differential diagnosis: (1) Metastatic carcinoids are almost always bilateral, in contrast to primary carcinoids, which have never been reported to involve both ovaries. (2) Metastases to the ovaries are almost always associated with metastases elsewhere, particularly on the peritoneum and in the liver, whereas metastases have not been observed in cases of primary insular carcinoid at the time of operation. (3) If the pathologist can detect teratomatous elements in a tumor containing a carcinoid, and this is usually the case in primary carcinoid neoplasia, the diagnosis is established. (4) Postoperatively the urinary level of 5-hydroxyindole acetic acid can be expected to return to normal in the case of a primary ovarian carcinoid, but usually remains elevated or rises again within several months if the ovarian tumors are metastatic, because residual disease is typically present elsewhere in the abdomen.

Primary ovarian carcinoids are adequately treated by unilateral removal of the adnexa in a young woman, but total hysterectomy and bilateral salpingo-oophorectomy is usually performed when the preservation of fertility is not a problem. Only 2 of approximately 50 reported cases of primary insular carcinoid have been reported to be associated with recurrence and death.

STRUMAL CARCINOID

This tumor contains struma and carcinoid, usually intimately admixed with one another[57,67] (Fig. 115-15). In most of the cases it is associated with a dermoid cyst or a solid mature teratoma, but it is often present in pure or almost pure form. Almost all the patients have been between the ages of 30 and 60 with a range of 21–77 yr. At operation the strumal carcinoid varies considerably in appearance depending on whether the strumal, carcinoid, or other teratomatous components predominate. All of the tumors have been unilateral, although occasionally another type of ovarian tumor, usually a dermoid cyst, has been present in the opposite ovary.

Microscopic examination reveals struma associated with a carcinoid, which has a predominantly trabecular pattern. Although occasionally the two forms of neoplasia appear to have a collision relation to one another, much more often they are intimately admixed, and cells containing argentaffin granules may be observed lining follicles filled with colloid. This intimate pattern of growth of argentaffin and thyroidal epithelial cells affords strong evidence against the postulation of a neuroectodermal origin for argentaffin cells, since thyroid epithelium is known to be of endodermal origin. Furthermore, neuroectodermal elements are only rarely observed in tumors containing a component of strumal

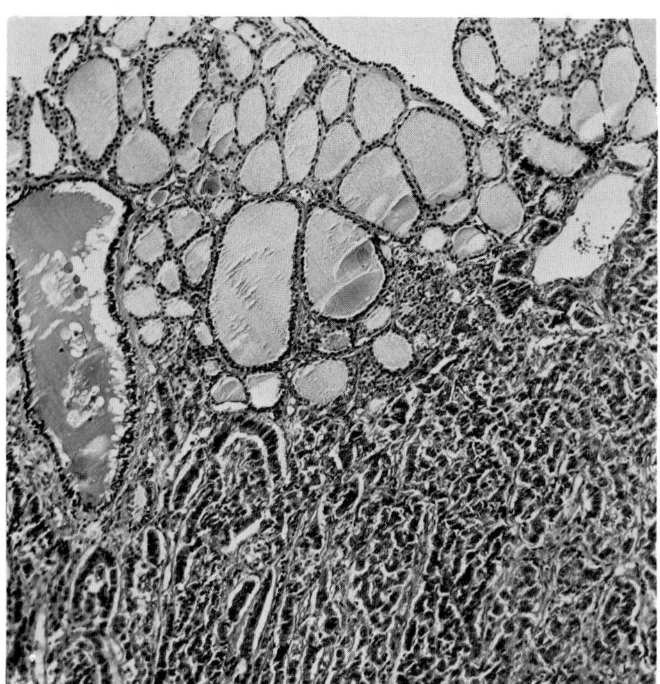

Fig. 115-15. Strumal carcinoid. Thin ribbons of carcinoid cells (below) merge with colloid-filled thyroid acini (above). (From Morris and Scully: Endocrine Pathology of the Ovary, 1958. Courtesy of Mosby.)

carcinoid, and carcinoid is rarely seen in association with the typical immature ovarian teratoma in which neuroectodermal elements are characteristically abundant. Although carcinoids have not been reported in the thyroid gland itself, medullary carcinomas with amyloid stroma arising in that organ may bear a morphologic resemblance to the strumal carcinoid, may contain argentaffin granules, and have rarely been associated with the carcinoid syndrome. The report of amyloid in the stroma of one case of strumal carcinoid heightens its resemblance to the medullary carcinoma.[67]

No case of strumal carcinoid has been associated with the carcinoid syndrome, but in a few cases preoperative or postoperative findings have suggested the possibility of hyperfunction of the thyroid component. There has been no clear-cut case, however, of associated hyperthyroidism. Although the strumal carcinoid has often been reported in the literature as malignant struma, no case has been recorded in which it has spread beyond the ovary.

TUMORS WITH ECTOPIC HORMONE PRODUCTION[68,69]

A hypercalcemic state simulating hyperparathyroidism has been reported with clear cell, serous, undifferentiated, and unclassified carcinomas, a dysgerminoma, and a virilizing lipid cell tumor. Bone metastases were not detected in any of the cases. It is interesting that at least 3 of the 10 reported tumors associated with hypercalcemia have been clear cell carcinomas, which otherwise constitute less than 5 percent of all ovarian carcinomas.[70] Cushing's syndrome due to ectopic adrenocorticotropic hormone (ACTH) production has been recorded in association with a "poorly differentiated adenocarcinoma," a malignant Sertoli cell tumor, and an undifferentiated small cell carcinoma of the ovary that resembled an oat cell carcinoma of the lung.[71,72] The last tumor also produced the carcinoid syndrome. Ectopic chorionic gonadotropin production has been observed in three women with ovarian cancer, all of whom had elevated urinary levels of that hormone.[73] One of these patients had marked luteinization of the stroma of the opposite ovary and a decidual reaction in the endometrium. On microscopic examination the tumors were papillary adenocarcinomas and a mucinous cystadenocarcinoma. Each one contained syncytial giant cells that were positive on immunofluorescence staining for HCG. Three ovarian tumors—a serous cystadenocarcinoma, a dysgerminoma, and a fibroma—have been associated with hypoglycemia.[74] In the case of the fibroma its removal resulted in a cure.

TUMORLIKE CONDITIONS WITH ENDOCRINE MANIFESTATIONS

SOLITARY FOLLICLE CYST AND CORPUS LUTEUM CYST

These cysts may develop at any time during the reproductive age period. They rarely exceed 8–10 cm in diameter; although commonly asymptomatic, they may rupture with intraabdominal hemorrhage and pain, and may be associated with abnormal uterine bleeding. If the resultant ovarian enlargement does not involute spontaneously within a month or so, a neoplasm should be excluded by abdominal exploration. The administration of steroid contraceptives has been found helpful in hastening the involution of these cysts, thereby excluding more serious nonfunctioning ovarian masses.[75]

On rare occasions, a single or a few follicle cysts develop before puberty and cause isosexual precocity that is cured by the removal of the involved ovary.[76,77] When follicle cyst formation occurs in the McCune-Albright syndrome (polyostotic fibrous dysplasia, cutaneous pigmentation, and endocrine abnormalities, the most common of which is sexual precocity), the associated sexual precocity is cured by the removal of the involved ovary in some cases, but it recurs postoperatively in others.[78] The gonadotropin level is depressed rather than elevated in these cases, probably indicating an origin of the disturbance in the ovary rather than the hypothalamus or pituitary gland.

MULTIPLE FOLLICLE CYSTS (POLYCYSTIC OVARIES)

This disorder, which is commonly associated with the Stein-Leventhal syndrome (infrequent, anovulatory uterine bleeding and sterility, often accompanied by hirsutism), is characterized by the presence of multiple follicle cysts, usually causing ovarian enlargement (Fig. 115-16), collagenization of the outermost portion of the cortex (often misnamed "thickening of the capsule"), follicular hyperthecosis (manifested by a proliferation and striking luteinization of the theca interna of the follicles), and a variable amount of medullary stromal hyperplasia, sometimes accompanied by slight degrees of stromal hyperthecosis (the presence of lutein cells in the stroma).[79] The syndrome typically begins in the early reproductive years, but occasionally follows a pregnancy or the withdrawal of oral contraceptive therapy.[80] It lacks the dramatic onset characteristic of the virilizing syndrome produced by most androgen-secreting ovarian tumors. The differential diagnosis of polycystic ovaries from virilizing ovarian tumors is discussed further in Chapter 113.

After years of investigation the pathogenesis of the Stein-Leventhal syndrome remains obscure. LH levels are often, but not always elevated, and there is an increased secretion of androgens to which the adrenal glands contribute in at least some of the cases.[81,82] Wedge resection of the ovaries has been successful in

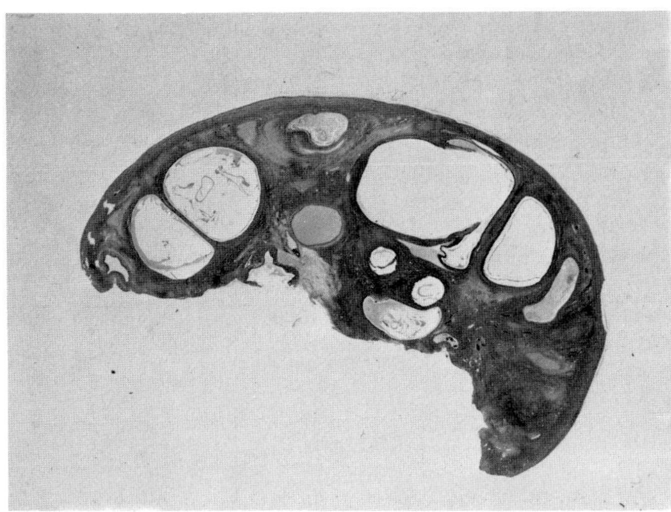

Fig. 115-16. Sectioned surface of wedge of Stein-Leventhal ovary. (From Grady and Smith (eds.): The Ovary, 1963. Courtesy of Williams & Wilkins.)

restoring normal menses and fertility in a high proportion of the cases, but surgical intervention has been largely replaced in recent years by the administration of ovulation-inducing drugs.

Some patients with polycystic ovaries have endometrial hyperplasia with varying degrees of atypicality, and rarely an adenocarcinoma of the endometrium, which is typically low grade, develops, primarily on the basis of unopposed estrogenic stimulation. Some of these morphologic adenocarcinomas have apparently been cured by curettage and therapy directed at restoring progesterone stimulation to the endometrium.[83] This unexpected result has led some observers to regard the endometrial carcinoma of the Stein-Leventhal syndrome as being no more than a reversible atypical hyperplasia. Further data are necessary before drawing firm conclusions about this interesting problem.

STROMAL HYPERPLASIA AND HYPERTHECOSIS

Stromal hyperplasia, which occupies primarily the medullary portion of the ovary, but may also involve the cortex, is characterized by a bilateral nodular or diffuse proliferation of stromal cells (Fig. 115-17). It occurs predominantly in perimenopausal women, but may be seen at any age after puberty. Stromal hyperthecosis (which has also been called *thecosis, thecomatosis,* and *diffuse luteinization of the ovarian stroma*) indicates the presence of lutein cells singly or in clusters within the hyperplastic stroma (Fig. 115-18).[84] These two disorders are closely related and have not always been clearly separated in the literature. Moreover, in young women with stromal hyperplasia with or without hyperthecosis varying numbers of follicle cysts with luteinization of their theca interna layers are usually also present, creating a gray zone between these disorders and polycystic ovarian disease that makes classification difficult.[85,86]

Stromal hyperthecosis in a young woman is often associated with the clinical picture of the Stein-Leventhal syndrome, but occasionally it is accompanied by a more profound disorder characterized by virilism, obesity (which is occasionally of the central type), hypertension, and a disturbance in glucose tolerance, so that the patient may resemble to some extent one with Cushing's syndrome. Sometimes hyperplasia and even adenocarcinoma of the endometrium have developed as in cases of polycystic ovarian disease. Stromal hyperplasia without obvious hyperthecosis has been observed in association with similar clinical findings, but

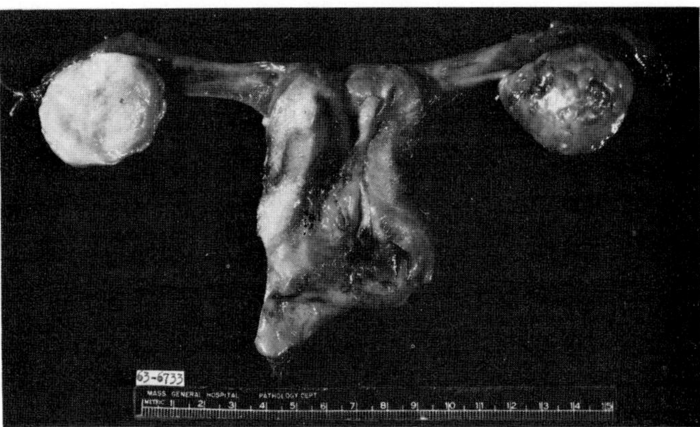

Fig. 115-17. Uterus, tubes, and ovaries, one of which has been sectioned to reveal solid replacement by stroma, in case of stromal hyperthecosis associated with endometrial carcinoma. (From Case Records of the Massachusetts General Hospital, Case 5-1964: N. Engl. J. Med. *270:* 247, 1964.)

generally significantly virilized patients have considerable numbers of lutein cells in the hyperplastic stroma, i.e., stromal hyperthecosis.

The association of masculinization with stromal hyperactivity is consistent with in vitro evidence that the stromal compartment of the ovary produces androgens.[87] The occasional complication of endometrial hyperplasia or carcinoma may reflect estrogen production by the hyperplastic stroma in some cases, or, alternatively, peripheral conversion of secreted androgens to estrogens. The virilization associated with ovarian hyperthecosis is typically more insidious in onset than that produced by an androgen-secreting ovarian tumor, but on occasion it may appear relatively abruptly.

At operation both ovaries are found to be involved by stromal hyperplasia and/or hyperthecosis; they may not be perceptibly enlarged or may attain diameters as great as 7 cm. Sectioning reveals replacement of the entire or the central portions of the ovaries by solid tissue with a yellowish hue. In younger women multiple follicle cysts and a whitish collagenization of the outer cortex are also typically observed. In contrast to stromal hyperplasia and hyperthecosis almost all virilizing ovarian tumors are unilateral.

Wedge resections have generally not been effective in the treatment of patients with stromal hyperthecosis when they have

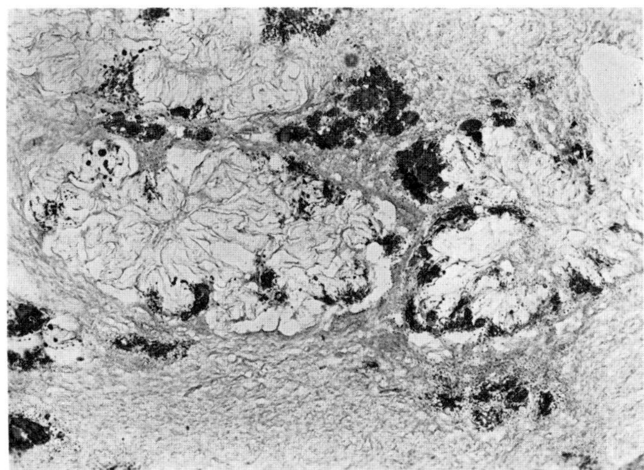

Fig. 115-18. Stromal hyperthecosis. Nests of darkly staining lutein cells are visible in the stroma and adjacent to atretic follicles. Sudan IV stain. (From Serov, et al.: Histological Typing of Ovarian Tumours, 1973. Courtesy of World Health Organization.)

had a severe endocrine disturbance. Bilateral oophorectomy has caused considerable regression of virilism in some, but not all cases.[84,88] In one patient hypertension was also apparently cured by the removal of the ovaries.[84] The cases in which oophorectomy has not been successful suggest possible associated hyperactivity of the adrenal cortex in some patients.

MASSIVE EDEMA

Rare cases have been reported in children and young women of unilateral or bilateral large ovarian masses that on section prove to be composed of markedly edematous stroma within which follicular derivatives are scattered.[89,90] The inclusion of these structures indicates that the process is one of stromal proliferation and edema, and not of neoplasia, which typically destroys or displaces rather than incorporates follicular derivatives within it. Although most of these edematous masses produce only the symptoms associated with an ovarian tumor, a few have contained scattered lutein cells and been accompanied by the clinical picture of the Stein-Leventhal syndrome or virilization. Two theories exist on the pathogenesis of this condition. One is that repeated subclinical torsion of one or both ovaries with resultant lymphatic obstruction leads to edema, which stimulates proliferation of the ovarian stroma and in some cases its differentiation into lutein cells. The other theory is that the primary process is stromal hyperplasia or hyperthecosis, which enlarges the ovary, predisposing to secondary torsion and edema. Therapy should be directed toward resection of the edematous tissue and restoration of the ovary to a normal size rather than its removal.

PREGNANCY LUTEOMA AND HYPERREACTIO LUTEINALIS

The pregnancy luteoma is characterized by the presence of one or more tumorlike nodules of lutein cell hyperplasia encountered most often as incidental findings during a cesarean section in the last trimester of pregnancy.[91–94] Approximately 80 percent of the patients have been black. More than one-fifth of them have been virilized, and when the offspring has been female, she has usually shown masculinization of the external genitalia as well. At operation the nodules, which may be over 20 cm in diameter, are multiple in as many as one-half the cases and bilateral in over one-third. On sectioning they are solid and reddish brown to brownish gray. Microscopic examination reveals a diffuse proliferation of large lutein cells, intermediate in size between normal granulosa lutein and theca lutein cells. The absence or paucity of intracellular lipid and the presence of numerous mitoses in some cases, as well as the common multiplicity of the lesions, are helpful clues in differentiating them from tumors in the lipid cell category and hilus cell tumors. There is evidence from the postpartum follow-up in certain cases that pregnancy luteomas are not true tumors, but are hyperplastic nodules composed of lutein cells, and that they depend for both their structural and functional integrity on stimulation by chorionic gonadotropin.

Although hyperreactio luteinalis also appears to be dependent on chorionic gonadotropin stimulation, it is distinct from the pregnancy luteoma in other respects. It is characterized by the presence of multiple lutein cysts which may cause marked ovarian enlargement. It is seen most often in patients with trophoblastic disease, but may develop during a normal twin or singleton pregnancy; occasionally it is associated with fetal hydrops.[95] It may also be iatrogenic, complicating the administration of Clomid or more often gonadotropins for the induction of ovulation.[96,97] On very rare occasions, however, pregnancy luteomas and hyperreactio luteinalis coexist.

When the diagnosis of pregnancy luteoma is suspected at operation, removal of one of the nodules is appropriate in order to confirm the diagnosis, but it is generally not necessary to remove an ovary because spontaneous involution of the process can be expected with the withdrawal of chorionic gonadotropin at the termination of the pregnancy. The enlarged ovaries of hyperreactio luteinalis can also be conserved unless torsion and infarction have occurred; it may be desirable, however, to resect portions of them to relieve symptoms or prevent complications if this is technically feasible.

REFERENCES

1. Rubin, D. K., Frost, J. K.: The cytologic detection of ovarian cancer. *Acta Cytol 7:* 191, 1963.
2. Rome, R. M., Laverty, C. R., Brown, J. B.: Ovarian tumours in postmenopausal women: clinicopathological features and hormonal studies. *J Obstet Gynaecol Br Commonw 80:* 984, 1973.
3. Morris, J. M., Scully, R. E.: Tumors with "functioning stroma." In: Endocrine Pathology of the Ovary. St. Louis, Mosby, 1958, p 131.
4. Scully, R. E., Richardson, G. S.: Luteinization of the stroma of metastatic cancer involving the ovary and its endocrine significance. *Cancer 14:* 827, 1961.
5. Woodruff, J. D., Goldberg, B., Jones, G. S.: Enzymic histochemical reactions in two Krukenberg tumors associated with clinically different endocrine patterns. *Am J Obstet Gynecol 100:* 405, 1968.
6. Serov, S. F., Scully, R. E., Sobin, L. H.: International Histological Classification of Tumours No. 9. Histological Typing of Ovarian Tumours. Geneva, World Health Organization, 1973.
7. Serment, H., Laffargue, P., Piana, L., et al.: Ovarian hormone tumors of female children. *Int J Gynaecol Obstet 8:* 409, 1970.
8. Jolly, H.: Sexual Precocity. A Personal Study of 69 Patients, American Lecture Series, Springfield, Thomas, 1955.
9. Iturzaeta, N., Kenny, F. M., Sieber, W.: Precocious pseudopuberty due to granulosa cell tumor in three girls. *Am J Dis Child 114:* 29, 1967.
10. Niswander, K. R., Courey, N. G., Woodward, T.: Precocious pseudopuberty caused by ovarian tumors. *Obstet Gynecol 26:* 381, 1965.
11. Gusberg, S. B., Kardon, P.: Proliferative endometrial response to theca–granulosa cell tumors. *Am J Obstet Gynecol 111:* 633, 1971.

11a. Scully, R. E.: Current Topic. Estrogens and endometrial carcinoma. *Hum Pathol 8:* 481, 1977.

12. Johnston, W. W., Goldston, W. R., Montgomery, M. S.: Clinicopathologic studies in feminizing tumors of the ovary. III. The role of genital cytology. *Acta Cytol 15:* 334, 1971.
13. Targett, C. S., Estrogen excretion in a case of theca–granulosa cell tumor. *Am J Obstet Gynecol 119:* 859, 1974.
14. Fathalla, M. F.: The occurrence of granulosa and theca tumours in clinically normal ovaries. A study of 25 cases. *J Obstet Gynaecol Br Commonw 74:* 279, 1967.
15. Osborn, R. H., Yannone, M. E.: Plasma androgens in the normal and androgenic female: a review. *Obstet Gynecol Surv 26:* 195, 1971.
16. Rubens, R., Vermeulen, A.: Plasma testosterone levels in normal and pathological conditions. *Eur J Obstet Gynecol 6:* 207, 1971.
17. Judd, H. L., Spore, W. W., Talner, L. B., et al.: Preoperative localization of a testosterone-secreting ovarian tumor by retrograde venous catheterization and selective sampling. *Am J Obstet Gynecol 120:* 91, 1974.
18. Busby, T., Anderson, G. W.: Feminizing mesenchymomas of the ovary. *Am J Obstet Gynecol 68:* 1391, 1954.
19. Scully, R. E.: Sex cord mesenchyme tumours, pathologic classification and its relation to prognosis and treatment. In Junqueira, A. C., Gentil, F. (eds): Ovarian Cancer, UICC Monograph Series, vol 2. Heidelberg, Springer, 1968, p 40.
20. Norris, H. G., Chorlton, I.: Functioning tumors of the ovary. *Clin Obstet Gynecol 17:* 189, 1974.
21. Kottmeier, H. L.: Carcinoma of the Female Genitalia. The Abraham Flexner Lectures, Series No. 11, Baltimore, Williams & Wilkins, 1953, p 174.

22. Burslem, R. W., Langley, F. A., Woodcock, A. S.: A clinicopathological study of oestrogenic ovarian tumours. *Cancer 7:* 552, 1954.
23. Sjostedt, S., Wahlen, T.: Prognosis of granulosa cell tumors. *Acta Obstet Gynecol Scand 40:* [Suppl 6] 1, 1961.
24. Norris, H. J., Taylor, H. B.: Prognosis of granulosa–theca tumors of the ovary. *Cancer 21:* 255, 1968.
25. Novak, E. R., Kutchmeshgi, J., Mupas, R. S., et al.: Feminizing gonadal stromal tumors. Analysis of the granulosa–theca cell tumors of the Ovarian Tumor Registry. *Obstet Gynecol 38:* 701, 1971.
26. Fox, H., Agrawal, K., Langley, F. A.: A clinicopathologic study of 92 cases of granulosa cell tumor of the ovary with special reference to the factors influencing prognosis. *Cancer 35:* 231, 1975.
27. Fathalla, M. F.: The role of the ovarian stroma in hormone production by ovarian tumors. *J Obstet Gynaecol Br Commonw 75:* 78, 1968.
28. Norris, H. J., Taylor, H. B.: Virilization associated with cystic granulosa tumors. *Obstet Gynecol 34:* 629, 1969.
29. Smith, J. P., Rutledge, F.: Chemotherapy in the treatment of cancer of the ovary. *Am J Obstet Gynecol 107:* 691, 1970.
30. Malkasian, G. D., Webb, M. J., Jorgensen, E. O.: Observations on chemotherapy of granulosa cell carcinomas and malignant ovarian teratomas. *Obstet Gynecol 44:* 885, 1974.
30a. Schwartz, P. E., Smith, J. P.: Treatment of ovarian stromal tumors. *Am J Obstet Gynecol 125:* 402, 1976.
31. Scully, R. E.: Androgenic lesions of the ovary. In Grady, H. G., Smith, D. E. (eds): The Ovary. International Academy of Pathology Monograph No. 3, Baltimore, Williams & Wilkins, 1962, p 143.
32. O'Hern, T. M., Neubecker, R. D.: Arrhenoblastoma. *Obstet Gynecol 19:* 758, 1962.
33. Novak, E. R., Long, J. H.: Arrhenoblastoma of the ovary. *Am J Obstet Gynecol 92:* 1082, 1965.
34. Prunty, F. T. G.: Hirsutism, virilism and apparent virilism and their gonadal relationship. Part 1. *J Endocrinol 38:* 85, 1967.
35. Teilum, G.: Classification of testicular and ovarian androblastoma and Sertoli cell tumors. *Cancer 11:* 769, 1958.
36. Teilum, G.: Special Tumors of the Ovary and Testis. Comparative Pathology and Histological Identification. Philadelphia, Lippincott, 1971, p 79.
37. Scully, R. E.: Sex cord tumor with annular tubules. A distinctive ovarian tumor of the Peutz-Jeghers syndrome. *Cancer 25:* 1107, 1970.
38. Taylor, H. B., Norris, H. J.: Lipid cell tumors of the ovary. *Cancer 20:* 1953, 1967.
39. Lipsett, M. B., Kirschner, M. A., Wilson, H., et al.: Malignant lipid cell tumor of the ovary: clinical, biochemical and etiologic considerations. *J Clin Endocrinol 30:* 336, 1970.
40. Falls, J. L.: Accessory adrenal cortex in the broad ligament. Incidence and functional significance. *Cancer 8:* 143, 1955.
41. Motlik, K., Starka, L.: Adrenocortical tumour of the ovary. A case report with particular stress upon morphological and biochemical findings. *Neoplasma 20:* 97, 1973.
42. Scully, R. E.: Stromal luteoma of the ovary. A distinctive type of lipoid-cell tumor. *Cancer 17:* 769, 1964.
43. Sternberg, W. H.: The morphology, endocrine function, hyperplasia and tumors of the human ovarian hilus cells. *Am J Pathol 25:* 493, 1949.
44. Scully, R. E.: Gonadoblastoma. A review of 74 cases. *Cancer 25:* 1340, 1970.
45. Gallager, H. S., Lewis, R. P.: Sequential gonadoblastoma and choriocarcinoma. *Obstet Gynecol 41:* 123, 1973.
46. Talerman, A.: Gonadoblastoma associated with embryonal carcinoma. *Obstet Gynecol 43:* 138, 1974.
47. Schellhas, H. G.: Malignant potential of the dysgenetic gonad. Part I. *Obstet Gynecol 44:* 298, 1974.
48. Schellhas, H. G.: Malignant potential of the dysgenetic gonad. Part II. *Obstet Gynecol 44:* 455, 1974.
49. Case Records of the Massachusetts General Hospital. Case 10-1975. *N Engl J Med 292:* 521, 1975.
50. Hughesdon, P. E.: Thecal and allied reactions in epithelial ovarian tumours. *J Obstet Gynaecol Br Commonw 55:* 702, 1958.
51. Verhoeven, A. T. M., Mastboom, J. L., Van Lausden, H. A. I. M., et al.: Virilization in pregnancy coexisting with an (ovarian) mucinous cystadenoma: a case report and review of virilizing ovarian tumors in pregnancy. *Obstet Gynecol Surv 28:* 597, 1973.
52. Connor, T. B., Ganis, F. M., Levin, H. S., et al.: Gonadotropin-dependent Krukenberg tumor causing virilization during pregnancy. *J Clin Endocrinol 28:* 198, 1968.
53. Hamwi, G. J., Byron, R. C., Besch, P. K., et al.: Testosterone synthesis by a Brenner tumor. Part 1. Clinical evidence of masculinization during pregnancy. *Am J Obstet Gynecol 86:* 1015, 1963.
54. Besch, P. K., Byron, R. C., Barry, R. D., et al.: Testosterone synthesis by a Brenner tumor. Part II. In vitro biosynthetic steroid conversion of a Brenner tumor. *Am J Obstet Gynecol 86:* 1021, 1963.
55. Case Records of the Massachusetts General Hospital. Case 11-1972. *N Engl J Med 286:* 594, 1972.
56. Braunstein, G. D., Vaitukaitis, J. L., Carbone, P. P., et al.: Ectopic production of human chorionic gonadotropin by neoplasms. *Ann Intern Med 78:* 39, 1973.
56a. Kurman, R. J.: Unpublished data.
56b. MacDonald, P. C., Grodin, J. M., Edman, C. D., et al.: Origin of estrogen in a postmenopausal woman with a non-endocrine tumor of the ovary and endometrial hyperplasia. *Obstet Gynecol 47:* 644, 1976.
57. Scully, R. E.: Ovarian tumors of germ cell origin. In Sturgis, S., Taymor, M. (eds): Progress in Gynecology, vol 5. New York. Grune & Stratton, 1970, p 239.
58. Wider, J. A., Marshall, J. R., Bardin C. W., et al.: Sustained remissions after chemotherapy for primary ovarian cancers containing choriocarcinoma. *N Engl J Med 280:* 1439, 1969.
58a. Kurman, R. J., Norris, H. J.: Embryonal carcinoma of the ovary. A clinicopathologic entity distinct from endodermal sinus tumor resembling embryonal carcinoma of the adult testes. *Cancer 38:* 2420, 1976.
59. Beck, J. S., Fulmer, H. F., Lee, S. T.: Solid malignant ovarian teratoma with "embryoid bodies" and trophoblastic differentiation. *J. Pathol 99:* 67, 1969.
60. Ueda, G., Hamanaka, N., Hayakawa, K., et al.: Clinical, histochemical and biochemical studies of an ovarian dysgerminoma with trophoblasts and Leydig cells. *Am J Obstet Gynecol 114:* 748, 1972.
61. Dalgaard, J. B., Wetteland, P.: Struma ovarii. A follow-up study of 20 cases. *Acta Chir Scand 112:* 1, 1956.
62. Nieminen, U., Von Numers, C., Widholm, O.: Struma ovarii. *Acta Obstet Gynecol Scand 42:* 399, 1963.
63. Woodruff, J. D., Rauh, J. T., Markley, R. L.: Ovarian struma. *Obstet Gynecol 27:* 194, 1966.
64. Gonzalez-Angulo, A., Kaufman, R. H., Braungardt, C. D., et al.: Adenocarcinoma of thyroid arising in struma ovarii (malignant struma ovarii). Report of two cases and review of the literature. *Obstet Gynecol 21:* 567, 1963.
65. Robboy, S. J., Norris, H. J., Scully, R. E.: Insular carcinoid primary in the ovary: a clinicopathologic analysis of 48 cases. *Cancer 36:* 404, 1975.
66. Robboy, S. J., Scully, R. E., Norris, H. J.: Carcinoid metastatic to the ovary. A clinicopathologic analysis of 35 cases. *Cancer 33:* 798, 1974.
67. Arhelger, R. B., Kelly, B.: Strumal carcinoid. Report of a case with electronmicroscopical observations. *Arch Pathol 97:* 323, 1974.
68. Shane, J. M., Naftolin, F.: Aberrant hormone activity by tumors of gynecologic importance. *Am J Obstet Gynecol 121:* 133, 1975.
69. Hall, T. C. (ed): Paraneoplastic Syndromes. *Ann NY Acad Sci 230:* 5, 1974.
70. Ferenczy, A., Okagaki, T., Richard, R. M.: Paraendocrine hypercalcemia in ovarian neoplasms. Report of mesonephroma with hypercalcemia and review of literature. *Cancer 27:* 427, 1971.
71. Brown, H., Lane, M.: Cushing's and malignant carcinoid syndrome from ovarian neoplasms. *Arch Intern Med 115:* 490, 1965.
72. Azzopardi, J. G., Williams, E. D.: Pathology of "non-endocrine" tumors associated with Cushing's syndrome. *Cancer 22:* 274, 1968.
73. Civantos, F., Rywlin, A. M.: Carcinomas with trophoblastic differentiation and secretion of chorionic gonadotrophins. *Cancer 29:* 789, 1972.
74. O'Neill, R. T., Mikuta, J. J.: Hypoglycemia associated with serous cystadenocarcinoma of the ovary. *Obstet Gynecol 35:* 287, 1970.
75. Spanos, W. J.: Preoperative hormonal therapy of cystic adnexal masses. *Am J Obstet Gynecol 116:* 551, 1973.
76. Monteleone, J. A., Monteleone, P. L., Damis, R. K.: Pseudoprecocious puberty associated with isolated follicular cyst of the ovary. *J Pediatr Surg 8:* 949, 1973.
77. Case Records of the Massachusetts General Hospital. Case 43461. *N Engl J Med 357:* 987, 1957.
78. Danon, M., Robboy, S. J., Kim, S., et al.: Cushing's syndrome, sexual precocity and polyostotic fibrous dysplasia (Albright's syndrome) in infancy. *J Pediatr 87:* 917, 1975.

79. Prunty, F. T. G.: Hirsutism, virilism and apparent virilism and their gonadal relationship. Part II. *J Endocrinol 38:* 203, 1967.
80. Beaconsfield, P., Dick, R., Ginsburg, J., et al.: Amenorrhea and infertility after the use of oral contraceptives. *Surg Gynecol Obstet 138:* 571, 1974.
81. DeVane, G. W., Czekala, N. M., Judd, H. L., et al.: Circulating gonadotropins, estrogens and androgens in polycystic ovarian disease. *Am J Obstet Gynecol 121:* 496, 1975.
82. Gambrell, R. D., Greenblatt, R. B., Mahesh, V. B.: Inappropriate secretion of LH in the Stein-Leventhal syndrome. *Am J Obstet Gynecol 42:* 429, 1973.
83. Fechner, R. E., Kaufman, R. H.: Endometrial adenocarcinoma in Stein-Leventhal syndrome. *Cancer 34:* 444, 1974.
84. Case Records of the Massachusetts General Hospital. Case 12-1974. *N Engl J Med 290:* 730, 1974.
85. Judd, H. L., Scully, R. E., Herbst, A. L., et al.: Familial hyperthecosis. Comparison of endocrinologic and histologic findings with polycystic ovarian disease. *Am J Obstet Gynecol 119:* 976, 1973.
86. Scully, R. E.: Correspondence. *Am J Obstet Gynecol 119:* 864, 1974.
87. Rice, B. F., Savard, K.: Steroid hormone formation in the human ovary IV. Ovarian stromal compartment, formation of radioactive steroids from acetate-114C and action of gonadotropins. *J Clin Endocrinol 26:* 593, 1966.
88. Bardin, C. W., Lipsett, M. B., Edgcomb, J. H., et al.: Studies of testosterone metabolism in a patient with masculinization due to stromal hyperthecosis. *N Engl J Med 277:* 399, 1967.
89. Kalstone, C. E., Jaffee, R. B., Abell, M. R.: Massive edema of the ovary simulating fibroma. *Obstet Gynecol 34:* 564, 1969.
90. Case Records of the Massachusetts General Hospital. Case 24-1971. *N Engl J Med 284:* 1369, 1971.
91. Sternberg, W. H., Barclay, D. L.: Luteoma of pregnancy. *Am J Obstet Gynecol 95:* 165, 1966.
92. Krause, D. E., Stembridge, V. A.: Luteomas of pregnancy. *Am J Obstet Gynecol 95:* 192, 1966.
93. Norris, H. J., Taylor, H. B.: Nodular theca–lutein hyperplasia of pregnancy (so-called "pregnancy luteoma"). A clinical and pathologic study of 15 cases. *Am J Clin Pathol 47:* 557, 1967.
94. Garcia, Bunnell R., Berek, J. S., Woodruff, J. D.: Luteomas of pregnancy. *Obstet Gynecol 45:* 407, 1975.
95. Girouard, D. P., Barclay, D. L., Collins, C. G.: Hyperreactio luteinalis. Review of the literature and report of 2 cases. *Obstet Gynecol 22:* 513, 1964.
96. Polishuk, W. Z., Schenker, J. G.: Ovarian overstimulation syndrome. *Fertil Steril 20:* 443, 1969.
97. Jewelewicz, R., Vande Wiele, R. L.: Acute hydrothorax as the only symptom of ovarian hyperstimulation syndrome. *Am J Obstet Gynecol 121:* 1121, 1975.

116

The Menopause

William D. Odell

INTRODUCTION

The age of menopause (in contrast to the age of menarche) appears to have been relatively constant over the past several hundred years.[1] Admundsen and Diers[2] have reviewed medieval records in Europe from the 6th to the 15th century and found the most frequently recorded age of menopause was 50 yr. This is not dissimilar from the age in England today.[3,4] In contrast, the duration of life and the world population has increased steadily in the past 100–200 yr, and thus the number of women who are postmenopausal has steadily climbed (Fig. 116-1A,B). In the United States, with much emphasis on youth, the "feminine forever" philosophy, and the commoness with which any emotional complaint in a 40–60-yr-old woman is attributed to "the menopause," estrogen replacement therapy has become extremely commonplace. The practice of administering estrogen is much more common in the United States than it is in the rest of the world. The frequency of estrogen replacement therapy also probably varies directly with socioeconomic status in the United States, though no meaningful statistics exist. This chapter attempts to review the physiology and the symptomatology associated with perimenopausal and menopausal years. Since replacement therapy with estrogen is so commonly recommended, a brief discussion of the side effects, contraindications, and indications of such therapy is also included.

PHYSIOLOGY OF THE MENOPAUSE

LH AND FSH SECRETION

As was discussed in Chapter 109, the number of follicles present in the ovary steadily declines throughout life. Each month of ovulation several follicles die by the process of atresia and one (usually) undergoes development and ovulation. Based upon present knowledge it appears that the follicles most sensitive to follicle-stimulating hormone (FSH) stimulation develop in younger life, and by the age of 40–50, the population of follicles remaining is less sensitive. This is conceived by the author to be a biologic selection process. Several studies, using bioassay of urine concentrates, as well as immunoassays on blood, have demonstrated increased

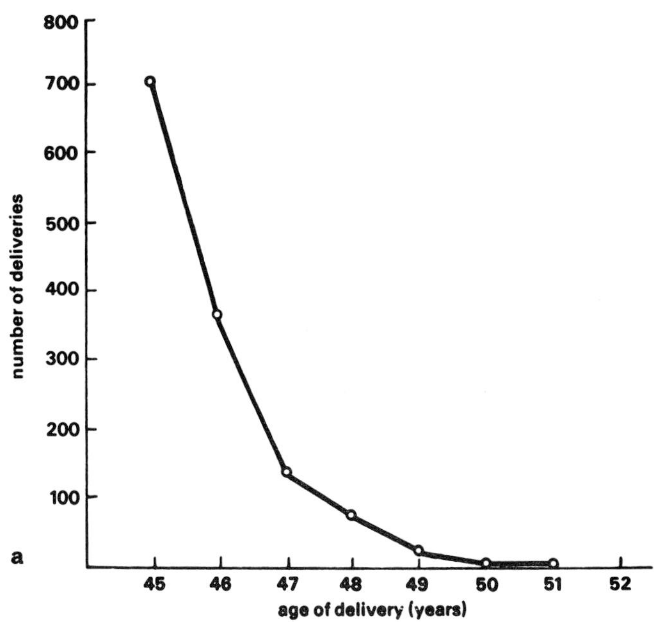

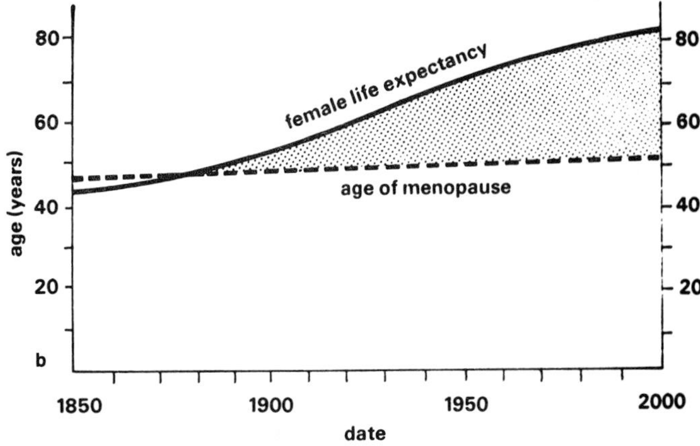

Fig. 116-1. A. Deliveries in women aged more than 44 yr in England and Wales in 1967. B. Female life expectancy compared with the age at menopause. (From Beard: Br. J. Hosp. Med. *12:* 631, 1975.)

Table 116-1. FSH and LH Excretion

Reproductive Stage	No. of Subjects	Age Range (yr)	FSH Excretion* (IU/24 h)	LH Excretion† (IU/24 h)
Early reproductive	6	19–25	7.3 ± 0.7‡	11.1 ± 1.1‡
Premenopausal	6	37–42	20.7 ± 4.6	79.4 ± 20.7
Perimenopausal	6	40–51	18.6 ± 4.6	87.1 ± 13.5
Postmenopausal	5	50–63	69.7 ± 28.0	80.1 ± 27.7

*Ovarian weight augmentation assay.
†Ovarian ascorbic acid depletion assay.
‡Mean ± SEM. From Adamopoulous et al.: J. Obstet. Gynaecol. Br. Commonw. *78:* 62, 1971.

luteinizing hormone (LH) and FSH secretion in older women *prior* to the menopause during ovulatory cycles, when compared to younger women. Thus, Adamopoulos et al.[5] demonstrated average urinary LH was sevenfold higher and FSH threefold higher during perimenopausal menstrual cycles than in premenopausal menstrual cycles (Table 116-1). Sherman and Korenman[6] quantified blood LH and FSH daily in premenopausal, older women with regular cycles and found FSH concentrations were similar to those in young women with regular cycles (Fig. 116-2). In perimenopausal women with irregular but periodic bleeding and rare ovulatory cycles, both FSH and LH were usually in the postmenopausal range.

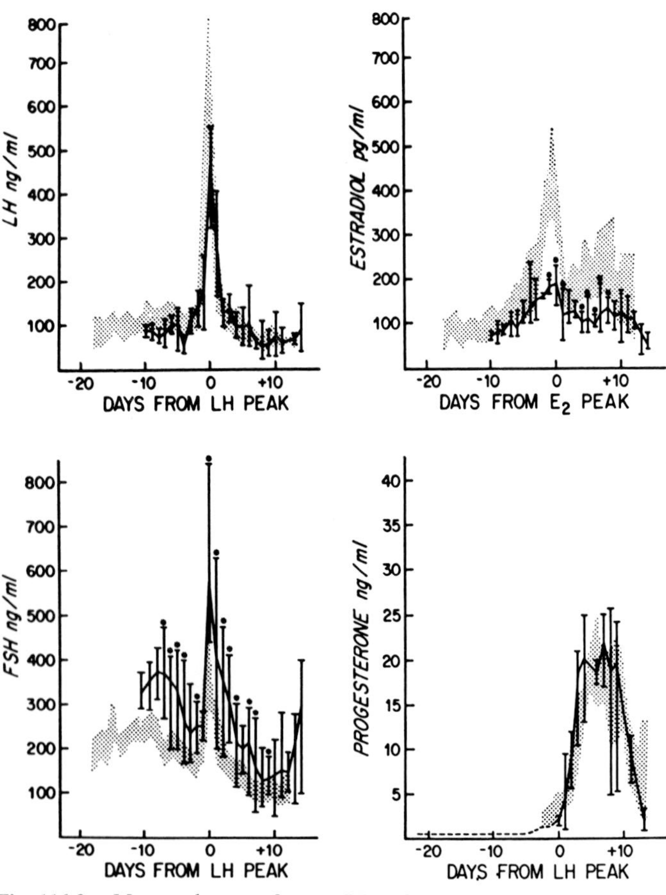

Fig. 116-2. Mean and range of serum LH, FSH, estradiol, and progesterone in six premenopausal women (lines and brackets) with regular menses compared to mean ± 2 SEM in 10 cycles (shaded area) in women aged 18–30. Asterisk indicates statistical significant difference between the two groups. (From Sherman and Korenman: J. Clin. Invest. *55:* 699, 1975.)

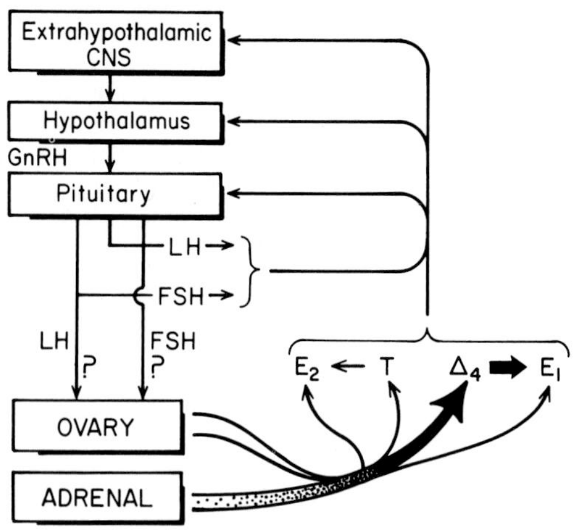

Fig. 116-3. Hypothalamic–pituitary–adrenal–ovarian system in postmenopausal women. Control of LH and FSH secretion is via a short-loop feedback system (LH and FSH acting on hypothalamus and/or pituitary to control LH and FSH) and via steroid modulation. The latter is believed to originate predominantly from adrenal androstenedione.

At menopause, there are follicles remaining in the ovary, but apparently these are very poorly sensitive to gonadotropin stimulation and development and ovulation does not occur. Even in women studied long after menopause, careful section of ovaries invariably reveals the presence of rare follicles.[7] Presumably, administration or secretion of even larger amounts of gonadotropins than are normally secreted in the postmenopausal state would result in development of some of these follicles. Postmenopausal LH and FSH secretion by the pituitary is maintained in feedback control via the so-called "short-loop feedback" and circulating steroid concentrations originating in both the ovary and the adrenal. These relations are schematically pictured in Figure 116-3. (The data upon which the short-loop feedback concept is based are reviewed by Molitch et al.[8])

After ovulation ceases, average LH and FSH concentrations in blood increase and remain elevated throughout the remainder of life. When expressed either (1) relative to average follicular phase or luteal phase concentrations, or (2) in terms of the International Reference Preparation (IRP-HMG No. 2), after menopause, FSH increases to a greater extent than LH. Thus, the ratio of FSH:LH in the postmenopausal state is greater than 1, while during the normal ovulatory surge it is considerably less than one. Administration of the hypothalamic or decapeptide luteinizing-hormone–releasing hormone (LHRH) to pre- or postmenopausal women produces marked rises in LH with much smaller rises in FSH. The sustained hypersecretion of the postmenopausal state has a different FSH:LH ratio and may not be related to hypersecretion of LHRH.

When LH and FSH are measured in blood at intervals of 10–15 min in postmenopausal women, cyclic or rhythmic fluctuations are observed (Fig. 116-4).[9] It has also been shown that the free α peptide chain of LH and FSH circulates in blood of postmenopausal women (see Chapters 12, 13, and 14).

STEROID SECRETION BY THE POSTMENOPAUSAL OVARY

The postmenopausal ovary is not totally devoid of the ability to secrete steroids. Mattingly and Huang[10] demonstrated that postmenopausal ovarian slices incubated in vitro with 7-^{3}H-pregnenolone produced dehydroepiandrosterone, androstenedione, and testosterone. They reported the ovarian stroma was unable to

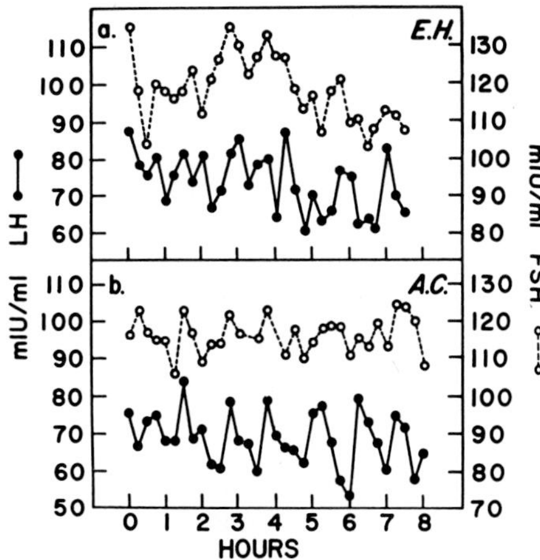

Fig. 116-4. Serum LH and FSH obtained at 10–15 min intervals in two postmenopausal women. (From Yen et al.: J. Clin. Endocrinol. Metab. *34:* 671, 1972.

Production of Estrone in Postmenopausal Women

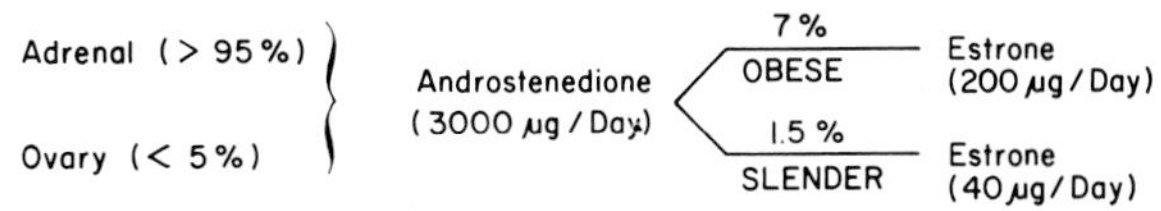

(Estimated from Data of Siiteri, 1975)

Fig. 116-5. Production of estrone from androstenedione in obese and slender postmenopausal women. Androstenedione is predominantly secreted by the adrenal and an average of 3000 μg is produced per day. Conversion occurs in peripheral tissues; adipose tissue is active in aromatization. Thus, the conversion is greater in obese that in slender women.

aromatize androgens to estrogens. Judd et al.[11] measured the concentrations of testosterone, androstenedione, estradiol, and estrone in peripheral and ovarian venous blood. A higher ovarian venous concentrations was found for all four steroids, but the differences for the estrogens were quite small. Their data are summarized in Table 116-2. From these data it appears that the postmenopausal ovary has the capacity to be a contributor of circulating testosterone and androstenedione. Obviously the blood flow through the ovary is a factor in determining these steroid production rates, and Siiteri[12] suggests that the postmenopausal ovarian contribution to blood concentrations of androstenedione and testosterone is exceedingly small. The contribution to blood estrogen concentrations is even less significant.

ADRENAL SECRETION OF ANDROGENS AND ESTROGENS

In menopausal women, the major circulating estrogen is estrone. This is formed almost exclusively by aromatization of androstenedione in peripheral tissues, principally adipose tissue and muscle. The daily production rate of androstenedione is 2–4 mg, and over 95 percent of this is secreted by the adrenals. Siiteri and MacDonald[12,13] and Hemsell et al.[14] have shown that about 1–2 percent of the 2–4 mg of androstenedione (20–80 μg) is converted to estrone in this manner. The result of this process (plus any small direct adrenal and ovarian secretion of estrone) is a production rate which averages 35–40 μg/day. Both age and obesity (the latter is the most important) increases the conversion ratio; very obese women may produce 150–200 μg/day with a conversion ratio of about 11 percent (Fig. 116-5). The conversion of androstenedione to estrone is also increased in women with cirrhosis. Thus, the major circulating estrogen of the postmenopausal state is estrone, while the major circulating estrogen of the premenopausal state is estradiol (Fig. 116-3).

Table 116-2. Concentrations of Steroids in Ovarian and Peripheral Blood

Vein	Testosterone (pg/ml)	Androstenedione (pg/ml)	Estradiol (pg/ml)	Estrone (pg/ml)
Ovarian	3033 ± 1046	3455 ± 1330	31.1 ± 6.3	71.5 ± 133
Peripheral	198 ± 27	754 ± 174	14.6 ± 2.9	30.3 ± 3.4

Data from Judd et al.[11]

The increased conversion ratio of androstenedione to estrone in obesity and with age leads to increased estrone production. These two factors appear to lead to increased incidence of endometrial carcinoma in obese postmenopausal women.[13,14]

SYMPTOMATOLOGY OF THE MENOPAUSE

EMOTIONAL SYMPTOMS

During the same years the menopause is occurring, most or many women in Western countries are undergoing very significant alterations in their personal lives. Often the husband is occupied most deeply in his job; promotion, responsibility, and many other aspects of the employed male partner may serve to draw his attention and time away from the family and home. Concomitantly, the children the mother has raised are usually grown by now, married and embarked on their own careers and activities. Time and evaluation of life may weigh heavily on some women. In this setting, the woman with preexisting psychiatric or emotional problems may become increasingly uncomfortable. Often the complaints she carries to her physician are quickly attributed to the "menopause."

On the other hand, many physicians believe that distinct symptomatology is associated with the menopause (or castration). In carefully done studies, Lauritzen[15] noted that surgical castration in women resulted in characteristic hot flushes beginning 4–6 days later. These initially occurred 3–5 times daily and increased in frequency and began to occur at night at 8–12 days. Serum LH and FSH first increased *after the onset* of flushes; for FSH the increase occurred on days 6–8, and for LH on days 8–10 postcastration. Within 3 weeks FSH had increased about threefold and LH about twofold over baseline precastration levels. These hot flushes are generally abolished by treatment with either estrogens or androgens. Objective study of this "best understood" symptom associated with the menopause illustrates the difficulty of interpreting most studies of treatment of menopausal symptoms. Figure 116-6 illustrates a double-blind crossover study of treatment of two groups of postmenopausal women with either estrogen or placebo, followed, respectively, with either placebo or estrogen. Note that placebo treatment decreased the number of hot flushes occurring, but did not abolish them completely. When estrogen was substituted for the placebo in the same group, frequency of hot flushes decreased further. In contrast, the group receiving estrogens first had a more dramatic fall in frequency of flushes, but showed an increase under placebo treatment. This "placebo effect" appears to result in 30–50 percent improvement in most symptomatology and makes interpretation of treatment of "less well quantifiable" symptoms (such as depression or loss of energy) even more diffi-

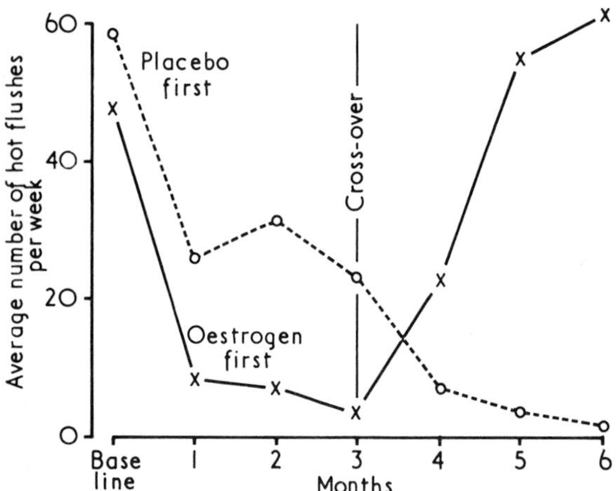

Fig. 116-6. Results of a double-blind crossover study of the effects of estrogen or placebo on the incidence of hot flushes. Placebo treatment produced a significant fall in incidence of hot flushes if administered initially. This was followed by total cessation of flushes when placebo was switched to estrogen. This placebo effect is an easily identifiable parameter in treatment of postmenopausal women and must be controlled for in well-designed studies. (From Lauritren, in VanKeep and Lauritzen (eds.): Ageing and Estrogens, vol. 2, 1973. Courtesy of Karger.)

cult. Table 116-3 lists some of the complaints associated with menopause and their likelihood of relief by estrogen therapy. With all these reservations, there are some data suggesting that estrogens improve mood in menopausal and geriatric women when compared to placebo treatment.[16–19] The placebo effects are large and caution in interpretation is necessary. Other studies not employing blind placebo control populations are probably valueless.

Goodman et al. recently published a well-controlled systematic study of possible symptoms related to the menopause.[20] In these studies, a series of menopausal and nonmenopausal subjects were assembled separately in Japanese and Caucasian groups from the medical records of 1708 Caucasian and 1221 Japanese women who underwent multiphasic screening. A large series of symptoms and laboratory values were considered for each patient by computer analysis. Only 24 percent of Japanese and 28 percent of Caucasian women reported any symptoms which could be attributable to the menopause. In the control, nonmenopausal groups, 10 percent of Japanese and 15 percent of Caucasian women reported identical symptoms. Thus, from these studies, at least 75 percent of women who were menopausal reported no symptoms. Interestingly, however, there was an increase in medication use and in surgical procedures for female disorders related to the menopause. From the data collected during this study it was not possible to determine what the indications or symptoms for such surgery

Table 116-3. Elevated Blood Pressure in Women in Walnut Creek Study, 1969–1971 (Rate per 1000 Women)

	Never Users*	Past Users	Current Users
Elevated blood pressure on entering study	7.8	6.7	13.9
Developed elevated blood pressure during study	0.9	1.1	6.2

During the first 3 yr of the study, users were more than six times more likely to have elevated blood pressure than nonusers.

*"Users" indicates users of contraceptives containing estrogens. From Charan (ed.): Walnut Creek Contraceptive Drug Study. Courtesy of DHEW.

were: that is, were they related to patient complaints per se, or to complaints attributed to "the menopause" by the physician?

One recent advance in knowledge of the physiology of estrogens may offer some basis for understanding emotional disturbances or mood alterations associated with the deprivation of estrogens or with sudden increases in estrogen concentrations. When labeled estradiol is injected into normal volunteers, it is metabolized by two distinct but important pathways. Quantitatively, the most important is 16-α-hydroxylation. However, also quantitatively important, and accounting for about 30 percent of metabolism, is 2-hydroxylation to form 2-hydroxyestradiol.[21,22] This compound has been called a "catechol estrogen" and is currently believed to represent not only an important route of metabolism, but also an intermediate in estradiol action on the central nervous system. Catechol estrogens are also formed from estrone and estradiol in similar fashions. For excretion, the catechol estrogens are further metabolized by the soluble enzyme, catechol-o-methyltransferase, to 2-methoxy estrogens and may also be conjugated with glucuronide, sulfate, or glutathione.[23] As indicated, the catechol estrogens are not merely excretion products, but are now believed to have important and varied activities in vivo which distinguish them from estrogens per se. The latter, as indicated, may exert their effects via metabolism to catechol estrogens.

At any rate, since these compounds are actively formed within the central nervous system and are competitors for the same enzyme systems that metabolize catecholamine neurotransmittors, it is attractive to postulate that rapid changes in estrogen concentrations in blood might produce alterations in mood or emotions via catechol estrogen formation and competition for neurotransmittors. The physiology of these compounds is being actively studied in several laboratories.[24–26]

VASCULAR DISEASE

Myocardiol infarction occurs more frequently in men than women in younger life; at age 25–30 the sex ratio (M:F) is about 7:1. By age 80, the ratio has fallen and the incidence in men and women is approximately equal.[27] This has been attributed to the menopause, which it is said, increases the relative incidence in women. Stated in other words, it has commonly been believed that estrogens protect against vascular disease. In fact this is too often used as a reason for treatment of the menopause. There are little data to support either the belief that estrogens protect against vascular disease or the belief that the menopause changes the incidence in women. Figure 116-7, shows the incidence in myocardiol infarction in men and women at different ages.[27] Note that the line of increasing incidence with age in women has no sharp break at menopause or at any age; it is a smooth curve showing increased incidence with age. In contrast, the line describing the incidence in men shows a sharp break *near the usual age of menopause in women.* Thus, the reason the sex ratio approaches unity at age 80 appears to be due to a change in the relative *incidence in men,* not women. The cause of this change in the incidence in men is not certain.

It is known that disorders of lipid metabolism, which produce cardiovascular disease, affect men more severely than women. The studies of Goodman et al.,[20] previously described, showed that if blood cholesterol concentrations are corrected for age-related changes, the menopause per se has no effect on blood cholesterol. It is possible that the changing slope in the curve for men (Fig. 116-7) represents two populations—one dying from infarction and having a metabolic lipid disorder, and a second not

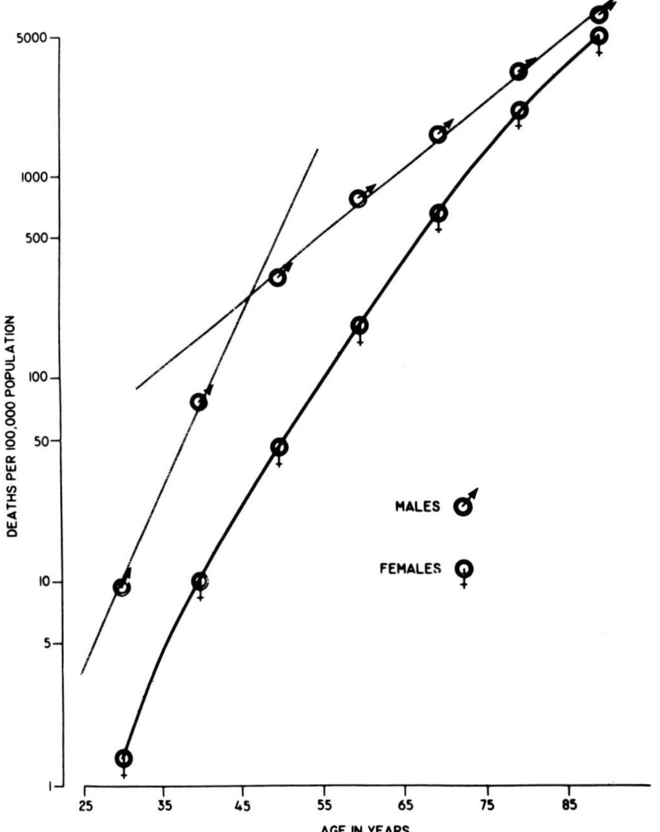

Fig. 116-7. Incidence of myocardial infarction in men versus women plotted against age in years. The *y* axis shows male:female deaths/100,000. (Reproduced from Fuhrman, A., NY Acad Sci 149: 822, 1968.)

having such a disorder and living to an older age. It is also not known why metabolic lipid disorders affect men more severely than women, but there are no good data to suggest it is a protective effect of estrogens *or* a harmful effect of androgens. Such variables as smoking, hypertension, and life stress and styles may play a role. Additionally, as is discussed later in this chapter, estrogens *in the usual doses* administered for contraceptive or menopause treatment purposes produces an *increase* in serum triglyceride concentrations (not a suppression).

OSTEOPOROSIS

The process of maintaining the skeleton in adults is a complex and very dynamic process. This is discussed in detail in Chapter 69. However, it has been shown that after age 20 *bone formation rates* are relatively constant throughout life.[28] In contrast, after age 20, *bone resorption* increases modestly throughout life in normal individuals. With a normal formation rate and an increased resorption rate, bone density progressively decreases in the normal population. All patients with osteoporosis appear to have an abnormally high bone resorption rate. This is true regardless of the cause of the osteoporosis. Thus, excess cortisol (Cushing's syndrome), thyroxine (thyrotoxicosis effects), and long-standing estrogen or androgen deficiency are associated with increased bone resorption and ultimately osteoporosis. In men and women who have absent gonads at puberty (e.g., vanishing testis syndrome or gonadal dysgenesis—Turner's syndrome) and who do not receive treatment with gonadal steroids, osteoporosis is almost universal by age 30 or so.

Bone resorption rates appear to be modified by many factors. Although these are poorly understood, these factors include weight bearing, gravity, exercise, calcium intake, vitamin D effects, and the concentrations and effects of androgens, estrogens, cortisol, and the thyronines. Since so many factors may affect bone resorption, it is extremely important to carefully evaluate patients with osteoporosis for all diagnostic possibilities and to treat the causative disease if known. As is discussed in Chapter 70, the differential diagnosis of associated diseases or causes is lengthy. Riggs et al.[29] have shown that high-dose estrogen therapy of patients with osteoporosis reduces the increased bone resorption to normal within 1–4 weeks, thus affecting the major factor causing the disease. However, continuation of such high-dose therapy for 1 yr or longer *is also* associated with fall of *bone formation rates* to below normal. This has an adverse effect on the disease. Lindsay et al.[30] have shown that relatively small doses of estrogens (30 μg mestranol/day) given to normal women at the time of oophorectomy prevent the decrease in bone density seen in untreated oophorectomized patients (Fig. 116-8). Thus, in the author's opinion, and based on present data, therapy of osteoporosis (1) must be directed against the cause if known, (2) should include exercise, calcium (to 2–3 g/day), and vitamin D (2000–5000 U/day), and (3) should include low-dose estrogens. As will be discussed later, estrogens have other potentially serious side effects which should also be considered when treating each patient.

DYSPARUNIA

Estrogens have potent effects on the vaginal epithelium (discussed in Chapter 109). The deprivation of estrogen effects reduces vaginal secretions and results in typical cytologic changes. Under such conditons intercourse is frequently painful. Estrogen therapy, even in low doses, restores vaginal secretions and represents an important indication for replacement therapy in many women. Intravaginal administration of estrogens may also be used to restore vaginal epithelial and secretory changes. It is not certain that intravaginal administration does not result in increased blood estrogen, and caution is urged in women with estrogen-sensitive breast carcinomas.

COSMETIC EFFECTS

Although objective data do not exist, many clinicians, including this author, believe that long-standing deprivation of gonadal steroids leads to a characteristic facial appearance. These changes are diagnostic of hypogonadism, and in men (where they are never "normal") are often the initial indication that alerts the clinician to

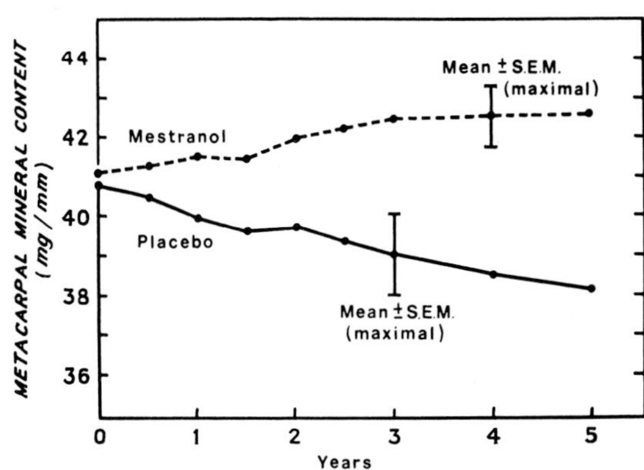

Fig. 116-8. Mean metacarpal mineral content during a 5-yr treatment of a group of women receiving estrogens or placebo and observed from 3 yr after bilateral oophorectomy (zero time). The average dose of mestranol was 25 μg/day. (From Lindsay et al.: Lancet *1:* 1038, 1976.)

hypogonadism (see review by Odell and Swerdloff[31]). Characteristic changes include so-called "purse-string" linear radiating markings, directed outward from the mouth. Similar linear changes occur about the eyes. These changes are different from the loss of skin turgor that occurs with aging. Estrogen therapy, begun at menopause, appears to prevent these changes. Indeed, the alert clinician may be able to distinguish the estrogen-treated menopausal women from the non–estrogen-treated ones if therapy began at menopause.

In addition to facial changes, and the previously discussed vaginal effects, estrogens also produce effects on breasts and adipose tissue distribution. Although all effects discussed under "cosmetic effects" are subtle and, at present, difficult to obtain objective data about, they nevertheless comprise important considerations for women requesting estrogen therapy and for physicians caring for such women.

COMPLICATIONS OF ESTROGEN THERAPY

Although it may seem from the preceding discussions that the simplest way to handle all questions related to symptomatology and the menopause would be to routinely treat all menopausal women with estrogens, this cannot be advocated at present. Estrogens are extremely potent, metabolically active medications. They produce widespread effects on a large spectrum of body tissues and functions. The physician using estrogen-containing medications must be familiar with these effects and balance risk against possible gains.

Table 116-4 lists side effects that have been attributed to estrogen therapy.[32] For those in the left column there is in general a sound biochemical or physiologic basis for understanding the effects. For example, the increased incidence of gallstones is related to the increased cholesterol saturation of bile produced by estrogen therapy.[33] Obesity produces a similar effect. Those in the right column are subjective symptoms and adequately controlled studies are not available to firmly link the therapy to symptoms. Space does not permit a detailed analysis of each disease or symptom, but we review a selected few of these.

HYPERLIPIDEMIA

A few patients develop massive triglyceride and cholesterol elevations in response to estrogen treatment.[34] Such patients always have an underlying disorder of lipid metabolism involving overproduction by the liver (Chapter 144). Estrogen therapy unmasks or makes manifest this disease; often this disorder is unknown to the patient or physician prior to treatment. Even in normal women, estrogens in the usual treatment doses produce elevations in triglyceride concentrations.[35,36] Almost all women receiving estrogens, either as part of contraceptive medications or as treatment for the menopause, have an increase in blood triglyceride concentrations, though usually such concentrations remain within normal limits. Figure 116-9A and B depict such data. Most women do not experience massive triglyceride elevations. However, even the small changes occurring in such women (within our defined normal range) may produce significant cardiovascular dis-

Table 116-4. Side Effects of Estrogen Therapy

Objective	Subjective
Venous thromboembolism	Depression
Cerebrovascular accidents	Nausea
Myocardial infarction	Vomiting
Hyperlipidemia	Abdominal cramps
Hypertension	Dizziness
Endometrial carcinoma	Edema
Adrenocarcinoma, vagina (DES only)	Breast soreness
Defective folate metabolism	Backache
Altered hepatic protein synthesis	Fatigue
Defective lactation	Increased appetite
Postuse amenorrhea	Nervousness
Hepatic dysfunction	Leg cramps
Melasma	Photosensitivity
Erythema nodosum	
Gallbladder disease	
Weight gain	

Adapted from Odell and Molitch: Ann. Rev. Pharmacol. *14:* 413, 1974.

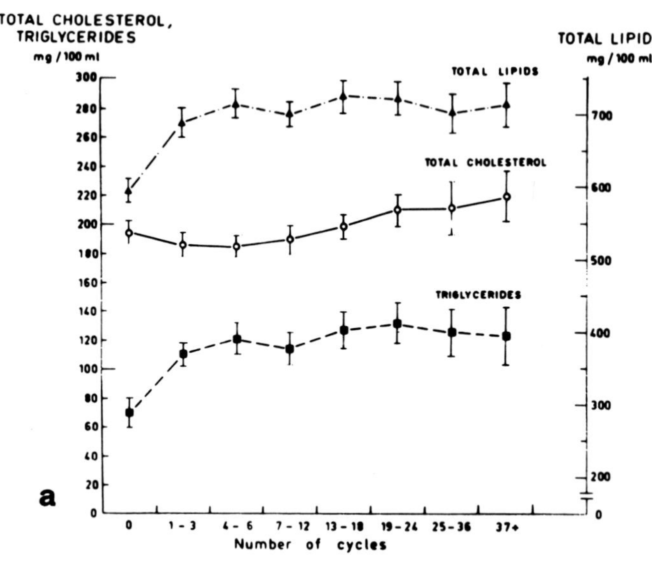

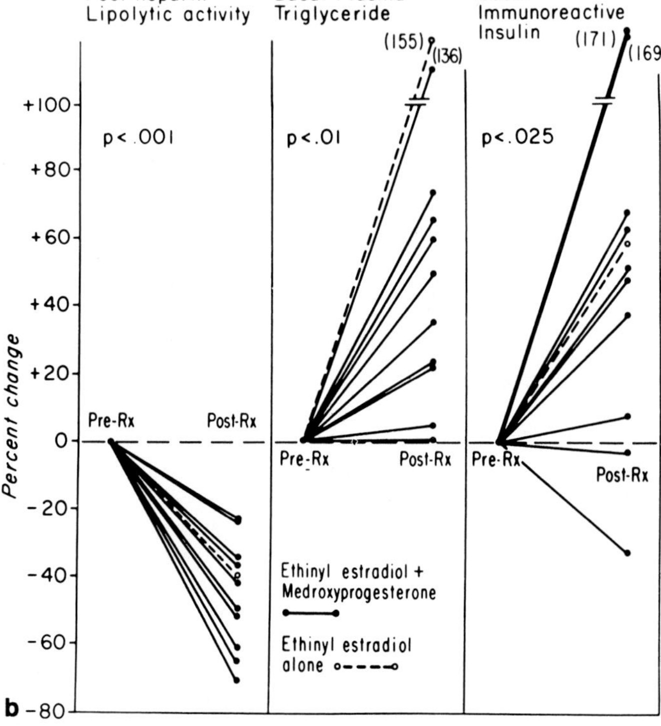

Fig. 116-9. A. Serum lipids according to the duration of contraceptive therapy. (From Schenker et al.: Fertil. Steril. *22:* 604, 1971.) B. Effect of an oral contraceptive on postheparin lipolytic activity, basal plasma triglyceride, and basal serum immunoreactive insulin. (From Hazzard et al.: N Eng J Med 280: 471, 1969.)

ease if such changes exist for many years. Several epidemiologic studies of cardiovascular disease demonstrate a positive correlation between blood cholesterol and/or triglyceride and myocardial infarction for values within our usually defined "normal range."

HYPERTENSION

Laragh et al.[37] demonstrated in 1968 that some women develop reversible hypertension with estrogen treatment. In estrogen-treated women these workers found a consistent increase in the α-2 globulin, renin substrate or angiotensinogen, produced by the liver. Angiotensinogen is enzymatically cleaved by renin (an enzyme produced by the renal juxtaglomerular apparatus) to produce angiotensin I, a 10-amino acid peptide. This peptide is subsequently cleaved to angiotensin II, an 8-amino acid peptide, by converting enzyme present in the pulmonary vascular endothelium. Angiotensin II is a potent vasoconstrictor substance and also stimulates adrenal secretion of aldosterone.

It is not clear why *all* women show an increase in blood angiotensinogen, yet only a small percent develop hypertension. Table 116-3 shows the incidence of hypertension in premenopausal women receiving estrogen-containing contraceptives and control subjects from a cooperative group study.[38]

THROMBOEMBOLIC PHENOMENA

This is an extremely complex area to discuss briefly. The author has recently reviewed the pros and cons concerned with the question of whether estrogens increase or do not affect the incidence of thromboembolic phenomena.[39] Significant arguments can be marshalled on either side of this question, and it is not possible, in this author's opinion, to prove unequivocally that estrogens increase this disease process. Inman and Vessey[40] alerted the medical community to the possibility that an association existed in a retrospective analysis of patients with fatal and nonfatal pulmonary emboli admitted to hospitals in England. A number of subsequent studies supported their findings. Furthermore, many physicians cared for individual patients who had no predisposing factors, but who developed pulmonary emboli on estrogen replacement. However, Drill and Calhoun[41] have reviewed much of these data, and in contrast to Inman and Vessey's original data, studied *the recurrence rate* of pulmonary embolism in women who continued estrogen containing contraceptive medications, compared to the patients who stopped medications. Over 2 yr of study, the recurrence rate was *greater* in women who discontinued their medication (Table 116-5). These data are offered only to demonstrate the complexity of this issue.

The author recommends that physicians take the following approach: (1) behave as if a correlation between estrogen therapy and thromboembolism exists (even though it is difficult to prove); (2) do not prescribe estrogen medications (if possible) for women with predisposing factors for thromboembolism, e.g., obesity, varicose veins, previous history of pulmonary embolism; and (3) balance a possible risk against therapeutic benefits.

Table 116-5. Recurrence of Thromboembolism in Treated and Untreated Women

Year	No. of Cases	Disease Recurrence: Not Using Oral Contraceptives	Disease Recurrence: Using Oral Contraceptives
1968	21	12 (57%)	9 (43%)
1969	29	17 (59%)	12 (41%)

ENDOMETRIAL CARCINOMA

As indicated in earlier sections of this chapter, the incidence of carcinoma of the endometrium appears to be increased in obese women due to increased estrogen production in adipose tissue. Estrogen therapy in postmenopausal women may also produce an increase in endometrial carcinoma.[42,43] This increase is most apparent in slender women and brings the incidence in such women close to that in obese women. Estrogen therapy appears to have little or no effect on the incidence of cancer in obese women. This issue is complicated in interpretation because of changing pathologic interpretation of histologic changes in endometrial biopsies. However, it appears at present that *continued* estrogen therapy in postmenopausal women statistically increases the incidence of endometrial carcinoma. It is recommended that if estrogen therapy is used, it be interrupted each 30–60 days by 10 days of progesterone (Medroxyprogesterone) plus estrogen, and 5 days of no therapy to permit withdrawal bleeding. While control studies do not exist at the time of writing, present evidence suggests that this may prevent the increased incidence of endometrial carcinoma.

MISCELLANEOUS EFFECTS

As indicated earlier, estrogens produce a wide range of effects on the body.[32] Increased blood concentrations of many globulins produced in the liver result, e.g., cortisol-binding globulin and thyroxine-binding globulin. Increased cholesterol saturation of bile with predisposition to stone formation occurs.[33] An increased incidence of cholastatic jaundice occurs. Microhemangiopathic–uremic syndrome, an often fatal disorder associated with thrombus formation in small vessels of the kidney and microhemangiopathic anemia, is increased in frequency.[44] Reports of increased central nervous system strokes[45] and myocardial infarction[46] also exist.

INDICATIONS FOR ESTROGEN THERAPY IN MENOPAUSAL WOMEN

A few clear-cut indications for estrogen therapy exist. We emphasize that estrogens should not be given in the belief that the incidence of vascular disease is decreased. Indications are listed in Table 116-6. Based upon present knowledge, the dose of estrogen used should be the smallest that leads to an objective decrease in symptoms. In difficult cases, the author prefers to obtain a 2-month written record (kept by the patient) of frequency and type of symptoms along with 2–3 blood FSH measurements (FSH concentrations are more highly elevated than LH). Then, 2 months of low-dose treatment is given (e.g., 10 μg of ethinyl estradiol/day). Observations on symptoms and 2–3 additional blood FSH measurements are made during this period. If symptoms or findings persist, dosage is increased to 20 μg/day and repeat observations are made for 2 months. This 10-μg, stepwise increment in dose is continued until symptoms or findings subside. Almost all patients should have symptoms abolished by 20–40 μg of ethinyl estradiol/day or equivalent. If higher doses are required, the physician should be cautious in interpretation. Additionally, there are no data to suggest that both oral and injected estrogens are needed or that oral medications are ineffective in some patients.

Table 116-6. Indications for Estrogen Therapy in Menopause

Indications
Vasomotor instability—hot flushes
Dysparunia
Cosmetic (face, breasts)
Prevention of osteoporosis
As adjunct in treatment of osteoporisis

REFERENCES

1. Beard, R. J.: The menopause. *Br J Hosp Med 12:* 631, 1975.
2. Admundsen, D. W., Diers, C. J.: Age of menopause in Medieval Europe. *Hum Biol 45:* 605, 1973.
3. Frommer, D. J.: Changing age of the manopause. *Br Med J 2:* 349, 1964.
4. McKinlay, S., Jeffreys, M., Thompson, R.: An investigation of the age at menopause. *J Biosoc Sci 4:* 161, 1972.
5. Adamopoulos, D. A., Loraine, J. A., Dove, G. A.: Endocrinological studies in women approaching the menopause. *J Obstet Gynecol Br Commonw 78:* 62, 1971.
6. Sherman, B. M., Korenman, S. G.: Hormonal charactertistics of the human menstrual cycle throughout reproductive life. *J Clin Invest 55:* 699, 1975.
7. Hertig, A. J.: The ageing ovary—a preliminary note. *J Clin Endocrinol Metab 4:* 581, 1944.
8. Molitch, M., Edmonds, M., Jones, E., Odell, W. D.: Short-loop feedback for LH. *Am J Physiol 230:* 907, 1976.
9. Yen, S. S. C., Tsai, C. C., Naftolin, F., et al.: Pulsatile patterns of gonadotropin release in subjects with and without ovarian function. *J Clin Endocrinol Metab 34:* 671, 1972.
10. Mattingly, R. F., Huang, W. Y.: Steroidogenesis of the menopause and postmenopausal ovary. *Am J Obstet Gynecol 103:* 679, 1969.
11. Judd, H. L., Judd, G. E., Lucas, W. E., et al.: Endocrine function of the postmenopause ovary: concentrations of androgens and estrogens in ovarian and peripheral vein blood. *J Clin Endocrinol Metab 39:* 1020, 1974.
12. Siiteri, P. K.: Postmenopausal-estrogen production. In VanKeep, P. A., Lauritzen, C. (eds): Ageing and Estrogens, vol 3. New York, Karger, 1973, pp 40–44.
13. MacDonald, P. C., Siiteri, P. K.: The relationship between extraglandular production of estrone and the occurrence of endometrial neoplasia. *Gynecol Oncol 2:* 259, 1974.
14. Hemsell, D., Grodin, J. M., Brenner, P. F., et al.: Plasma precursors of estrogen. II. Correlation of the extent of conversion of plasma androstenedione to estrone with age. *J Clin Endocrinol Metab 38:* 476, 1974.
15. Lauritzen, C.: The management of the premenopausal and the postmenopausal patient. In VanKeep, P. A., Lauritzen, C. (eds): Ageing and Estrogens, vol 2. New York, Karger, 1973, pp 2–21.
16. Winokur, G.: Depression in the menopause. *Am J Psychiatry 130:* 92, 1973.
17. Sheffery, J. B., Wilson, T. A., Walsh, J. C.: Double-blind, cross-over study comparing chlordiazepoxide conjugated estrogens, combined chlordiazepoxide and conjugated estrogens and placebo in treatment of the menopause. *Med Ann DC 38:* 433, 1969.
18. Utan, W. H.: The mental tonic effect of oestrogens administered to oophorectomized females. *South Afr Med J 46:* 1079, 1972.
19. Kantor, H. I., Michael, C. M., Shore, H.: Estrogen for older women. A three-year study. *Am J Obstet Gynecol 116:* 115, 1973.
20. Goodman, M. J., Stewert, C. J., Gilbert, F.: The menopause: a pilot study. In: The Working Papers Series. Women's Studies Program, University of Hawaii, 1976.
21. Yoshizawa, I., Fishman, J.: Radioimmunoassay of 2-hydroxyestrone in human plasma. *J Clin Endocrinol Metab 32:* 3, 1971.
22. Fishman, J., Guzik, H., Hellman, L.: Aromatic ring hydroxylation of estradiol in man. *Biochemistry 9:* 1593, 1970.
23. Ball, P., Knuppen, R., Haupt, M., et al.: Interactions between estrogens and catechol amines. III. Studies on the methylation of catechol estrogens, catechol amines and other catechols by the catechol-O-methyltransferase of human liver. *J Clin Endocrinol Metab 34:* 736, 1972.
24. Fishman, J., Norton, B.: Catechol estrogen formation in the central nervous system of the rat. *Endocrinology 96:* 1054, 1975.
25. Naftolin, F., Morishita, H., Davies, I. J., et al.: 2-Hydroxyestrone induced rise in serum luteinizing hormone in the immature male rat. *Biochem Biophys Res Commun 64:* 905, 1975.
26. Parvizi, N., Ellendorff, F.: 2-Hydroxy-oestradiol-17 as a possible link in steroid brain interaction. *Nature 256:* 59, 1975.
27. Furman, R. H.: Are gonadal hormones (estrogens and androgens) of significance in the development of ischemic heart disease? *Ann NY Acad Sci 149:* 822, 1968.
28. Jowsey, J., Kelly, P. J., Riggs, B. L., et al.: Quantitative microradiographic studies of normal and osteoporatic bone. *J Bone Joint Surg 47:* 785, 1975.
29. Riggs, B. L., Jowsey, J., Goldsmith, R. S.: Short- and long-term effects of estrogen and synthetic anabolic hormone in postmenopausal osteoporosis. *J Clin Invest 51:* 1659, 1972.
30. Lindsay, R., Aitken, J. M., Anderson, J. B., et al.: Long-term prevention of postmenopausal osteoporosis by oestrogen. *Lancet 1:* 1038, 1976.
31. Odell, W. D., Swerdloff, R. S.: Male hypogonadism. *West J Med 124:* 446, 1976.
32. Odell, W. D., Molitch, M. E.: The pharmacology of contraceptive agents. *Ann Rev Pharmacol 14:* 413, 1974.
33. Bennion, L. H., Ginsberg, R. L., Garnick, M. G., et al.: Effects of oral contraceptives on the gallbladder bile of normal women. *N Engl J Med 294:* 189, 1976.
34. Molitch, M. E., Oill, P., Odell, W. D.: Massive hyperlipidemia during oral contraceptive and postmenopausal estrogen therapy. *JAMA 227:* 522, 1974.
35. Schenker, J. G., Pinson, A., Polishuk, W. Z.: The effect of oral contraceptives on serum lipids. *Fertil Steril 22:* 604, 1971.
36. Sacks, B. A., Wolfman, L., Herzog, N.: Plasma lipid and lipoprotein alterations during oral contraceptive administration. *Obstet Gynecol 34:* 530, 1969.
37. Laragh, J. H., Sealey, J. E., Ledingham, J. E., et al.: Renin, aldosterone and high blood pressure. *JAMA 201:* 918, 1967.
38. Ram Charan, S. (ed): Walnut Creek Contraceptive Drug Study. US Department of Education and Welfare.
39. Swerdloff, R. S., Odell, W. D., Bray, G., et al.: Complications of oral contraceptive agents—a symposium. Special Endocrine Conference. *West J Med 122:* 20, 1975.
40. Inman, W. H. W., Vessey, M. P.: Investigation of death from pulmonary, coronary, and cerebral thrombosis and embolism in women of childbearing age. *Br Med J 2:* 193, 1968.
41. Drill, V., Calhoun, D. W.: Oral contraceptives and thromboembolic disease: Prospective and retrospective studies. *JAMA 219:* 583, 1972.
42. Smith, D. C., Prentice, R., Thompson, D. J., et al.: Association of exogenous estrogen and endometrial carcinoma. *N Engl J Med 293:* 1164, 1975.
43. Kolata, G. B.: Estrogen drugs: do they increase the risk of cancer? *Science 191:* 838, 1976.
44. Brown, C. B., Clarkson, A. R., Robson, J. S., et al.: Hemolytic uraemic syndrome in women taking oral contraceptives. *Lancet 1:* 1479, 1973.
45. Collaborative Group for the Study of Stroke in Young Women: Oral contraceptives and stroke in young women. *JAMA 231:* 718, 1975.
46. Vessey, M. P., McPherson, K., Johnson, B.: Mortality among women participating in the Oxford/Family Planning Association contraceptive study. *Lancet 2:* 731, 1977.
47. Hazzard, W. R., Spiger, M. J., Bagdade, J. D., Bierman, E. L.: Studies on the mechanism of increased plasma triglyceride levels induced by oral contraceptives. *N Eng J Med 280:* 471–474, 1969.

117

Synopsis

William D. Odell

Chapters 105 to 116 set forth the current status of knowledge concerning the process of (1) sexual differentiation, (2) puberty, (3) various pathophysiologies of sexual differentiation and of puberty, (4) the normal physiology of the reproduction in women, and (5) the pathophysiology of these processes. It is interesting to note that between 1967 and the present, our concepts of puberty have evolved considerably. Prior to 1967–1969, clinicians generally believed that puberty was caused by the initiation or "turn on" of pituitary gonadotropin stimulation with resultant gonadal steroid secretion. This belief was supported by the fact that *using bioassays,* gonadotropins were only rarely detected in 24-hour urinary concentrates from children, whereas they were routinely found in urine from adults. While some animal data suggested this causal hypothesis might be incorrect, these data were either unknown or ignored by most physicians. Delayed sexual maturation and precocious sexual maturation were diagnosed and treated based on these concepts. When gonadotropins became measurable with sensitive radioimmunoassays, it was found that the blood of children prior to puberty always contained gonadotropins. Now, sexual maturation is usually explained by changing (increasing) gonadotropin concentrations in children; gonadotropins may fall or remain constant throughout maturation in some animal species as discussed in Chapter 108. Thus, advances in techniques have brought us from "certain knowledge" of the course of maturation prior to 1967 to "certain ignorance" of the cause at the present time. We must conclude that there are several etiologic factors in sexual maturation, and we do not understand the process well.

Chapters 109 to 116 bring the reader through the past 10 years of development of knowledge and concepts of female reproduction. Here, too, a chapter written in 1978 is greatly different from one on the same subject in 1967. Students training in 1967 would not recognize much of the data and some of the important concepts of 1978. Of particular significance is the concept that an ovarian signal system (estrogens and progestogens) triggers the timing of ovulation; i.e., the process is not caused by central nervous timing mechanisms with rhythmic LH-FSH discharge. Again, diagnosis and evaluation of amenorrhea and dysmenorrhea are reviewed based on this recent concept, as is the theory and practice of contraception.

Finally, concepts of the normal physiology of the menopause have also rapidly evolved in recent years. The importance of nonendocrine tissues as sources of steroid hormone via conversion of prehormones is a relatively recent concept.

While these evolving concepts occurring in the relatively short span of 10 years are exciting, they offer the reader a cautionary note—10 years from now, much of this material will be so outdated as to be wrong or, if right, greatly modified. The reader should review these chapters as a student and continue the philosophy of being a student in years to come. The authors wish they could give timeless reviews, but alas concepts and perspectives are like shadows, changing with viewpoint and with added data. This is both the joy and the curse of studying biological phenomena.

Reproductive Function in the Male

Physiology

118

Structural Consideration of the Male Reproductive System

Emil Steinberger

The male reproductive system is composed of gonads, excretory ducts and organs, and several exocrine glands (sex accessory glands), which provide the bulk of the secretions composing the ejaculate (Fig. 118-1). The gonads are under the control of pituitary gland secretions, gonadotropins, while the excretory ducts and the sex accessory glands (prostate and seminal vesicles) are dependent on the secretions of the gonads, primarily androgens.

The human testes are suspended in the scrotum by the spermatic cord (funiculus spermaticus, containing the vas deferens, blood vessels, nerves, and the cremasteric muscle). The epididymis, a portion of the excretory duct system which forms a specialized anatomic structure, is positioned on the posterior surface of the testes with its head (caput epididymis) pointing cephalad and the tail (cauda epididymis), caudad. The duct system of the epididymis terminates in the vas deferens, which enters the spermatic cord.

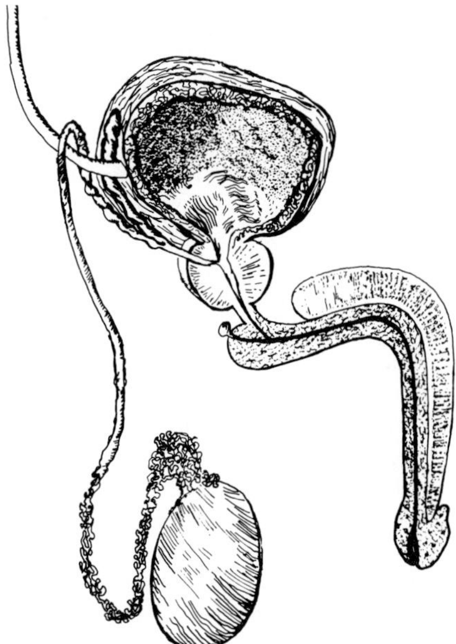

Fig. 118-1. Schematic anatomy of the male reproductive system.

The translocation of the gonads during their development from the abdominal cavity into the scrotum creates unique anatomic relationships between the testes and their membranous coverings.

SCROTUM

The scrotum, basically a dermal pouch, in addition to housing the testes serves also as a specialized organ aiding in heat regulation of the testes. Its characteristic features had already been observed in the 19th century by Cooper,[1] who stated: "The scrotum varies greatly in its appearance and size; for under the influence of cold, it is small, contracted and wrinkled; under heat, it is relaxed, smooth on its surface, and greatly extended."

The scrotum is a relatively complicated structure consisting of skin, dartos muscle, superficial perineal fascia, external spermatic fascia, internal spermatic fascia, and the parietal leaf of the tunica vaginalis (Fig. 118-2). The skin is thin, lacks subcutaneous adipose tissue, and is covered with very light hair growth.

The specialized structure of the scrotum is apparently important in temperature regulation necessary for maintenance of normal testicular function and fertility. It is probably an evolutionary expression related to the development of homeothermy.[2] It is of interest that the development and the maintenance of function of the tunica dartos muscle, implicated in maintaining intrascrotal temperature below the body temperature, may be under androgen control.[3]

TESTICULAR ENVELOPES

The parenchyma of the testis is surrounded by a capsule consisting of three layers: the visceral layer of the tunica vaginalis, the tunica albuginea, and the tunica vasculosa (Fig. 118-2). The space between the visceral layer of the tunica vaginalis and its parietal layer, which lines the scrotum, contains under normal conditions a small amount of serous fluid. The tunica albuginea, a dense fibrous membrane composed primarily of collagen fibrils and some smooth muscle fibers, is the most prominent layer of the testicular capsule.[4] It rests on a thin layer of areolar connective tissue rich in blood vessels, the tunica vasculosa. In the human testis, the tunica albuginea dips into the parenchyma of the testis

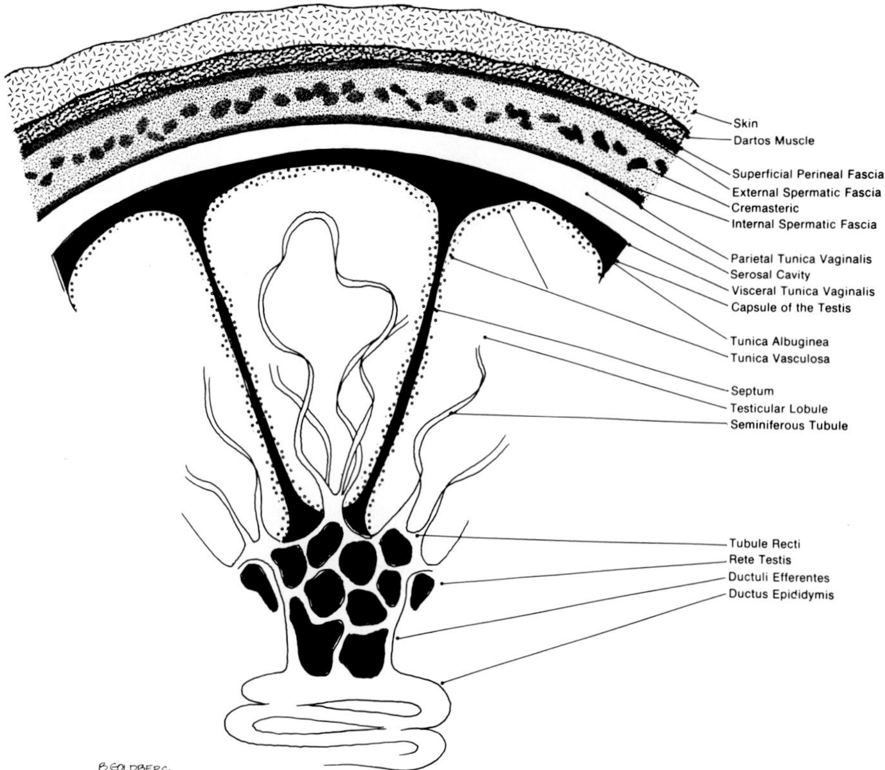

Fig. 118-2. Scrotum and Testicular envelopes.

forming septa, which separate groups of seminiferous tubules into testicular lobules. The tunica vasculosa follows the septa, bringing the blood supply into the depth of the parenchyma.

Considerable information concerning the role of scrotal structures in maintaining testicular temperature is available. It has been clearly documented that small elevations in testicular temperature produce testicular damage, expressed primarily by interference with sperm formation but possibly also by interference with the normal endocrine function of the testis. The role of testicular envelopes in producing testicular damage by mechanisms other than temperature elevation (such as formation of hydrocele, vascular changes, and other pathologic states) is not clearly understood. It has been demonstrated that the testicular capsule contracts spontaneously and that the contractions are influenced by acetylcholine.[5] The implications of this for the physiology of human testes is not clear at this time.

INNERVATION OF THE SCROTUM AND ITS CONTENT

The neuroanatomy of the male reproductive system, particularly of the testes, the epididymides, and the scrotum, received considerable attention in the past.[6] However, the relation of the nervous system to the spermatogenic function and to the hormonal control of the testes remains unclear (see below). The scrotal structures receive both somatic and visceral innervation; the testis and the epididymis, on the other hand, are provided with an exclusively visceral supply.

SCROTUM

The scrotum and the cremasteric muscle derive their somatic innervation from the ventral branches of the lumbosacral plexus primarily through ilioinguinal (Th-12 and L-1), genitofemoral (L-2,3), pudendal (S-2,3,4), and posterior femoral cutaneous (S-1,2,3) nerves. The scrotal nerves contain sensory, sympathetic (vasomotor, sudomotor, and piloerector), parasympathetic, and somatic efferent fibers. The details of visceral innervation of the scrotal structures in man is poorly understood. It appears that the scrotum contains a variety of receptor organs including "warm receptor" and active vasoconstrictor and vasodilator fibers. Although the anatomy of the nervous system and physiologic as well as pathologic observations strongly suggest that the nervous system of the scrotum plays an important role in the regulatory mechanism of testicular function, its relation to testicular disorders in man has scarcely been studied and is unclear. A possible role for hormones in the development and function of the scrotal innervation has been suggested; however, no experimental evidence for it is available.

TESTIS, EPIDIDYMIS, AND VAS

Mitchell[7] arranged the spermatic nerves into superior, intermediate, and inferior groups. The superior spermatic nerves are derived primarily from the intermesenteric plexus and from the renal part of the coeliac plexus (Th-10 or higher). The visceral afferents probably reach even higher levels of the spinal cord (Th-9,8). The intermediate spermatic nerves arise from the superior portion of the hypogastric plexus and the inferior group arises from the pelvis or vesical plexus. The spermatic nerves accompany the internal spermatic (testicular) artery into the scrotum where they innervate the respective structures.

The testes receive an exclusively visceral nerve supply primarily from the superior spermatic nerves. The relationship of the origin of testicular innervation to the renal and intestinal plexus and in certain cases a direct connection between them may explain the bizarre referred pain patterns (e.g., nausea) associated with testicular trauma, and conversely, testicular pain associated with renal or upper urinary tract disease.

The epididymis is supplied by the intermediate spermatic nerves. The vas deferens and the cauda epididymis are supplied by the inferior spermatic nerves.

This rather complicated innervation of the reproductive system is probably responsible for various patterns of gonadal disorders associated with neurologic lesions, and, as mentioned above, for the bizarre pain response to testicular trauma or disorders in the gastrointestinal or urinary systems.

The intrinsic innervation of the testicular parenchyma so far has eluded clear definition. While some investigators provided evidence that nerve fibers penetrate the seminiferous tubules and directly supply the Sertoli cells,[8] others, utilizing histochemical techniques, found the sympathetic fibers to be confined to perivascular areas,[9] thus probably serving only a vasomotor function.[10]

BLOOD SUPPLY

The testes and epididymides receive their blood supply primarily from the internal spermatic arteries originating from the aorta approximately at the level of the renal arteries. The artery follows a straight caudal course and, subsequent to giving off the epididymal artery, is named the testicular artery. Prior to entering the testis the testicular artery traverses a venous plexus, the plexus pampiniformis. In most mammals, except man,[11] the artery exhibits a complicated pattern of convolutions as it traverses the venous plexus. It has been suggested that this arrangement favors a countercurrent heat exchange which aids the thermal homeostasis of the testes.[12] Recently, transfer of testosterone from the veins of the pampiniform plexus to the testicular artery has also been demonstrated.[13]

During its intraabdominal course the testicular artery gives off branches to the spermatic cord and the epididymis. In the scrotum, the artery reaches the posterior border of the testis, where it forms two branches which pierce the tunica albuginea and break up into small vessels. These vessels form the tunica vasculosa, a superficial vascular network which gives off numerous terminal branches into the testicular parenchyma. The terminal character of these branches may account for the distinctive patchy degenerative changes in the seminiferous tubules subsequent to disease-induced alterations in the arterioles and may explain the observation that in testes of aged men more severe degenerative changes are observed in seminiferous tubules located distal to the arterial supply.[14]

The intratesticular vascular network is composed of a complicated arrangement of capillaries. There are two capillary systems: one is parallel to the seminiferous tubules and related anatomically to the Leydig cells, the "Zwickelkapillaren," and the "Querkapillaren" is arranged perpendicularly to the Zwickelkapillaren in a rope-ladder–like pattern around the seminiferous tubules. This characteristic pattern is related to the transport mechanisms of hormones from the circulation to Leydig cells and seminiferous tubules and possibly plays a specific role in the transport of androgens from Leydig cells to the seminiferous tubules.

The venous drainage of the testis and epididymis is accomplished by a dozen veins which anastomose around the ductus deferens, where they form the plexus pampiniformis. This structure is ultimately reduced to a single vein, which on the right side joins the vena cava and on the left, the renal vein. A relatively common abnormality of the left plexus pampiniformis is the formation of varices—the varicocele. The varicocele has been implicated in certain forms of testicular disturbance associated with oligospermia. The mechanisms of varicocele formation and its etiology are not clear. A simple suggestion that the valves in the left testicular vein are inadequate to maintain the column of blood without backflow or that they are less competent than in the right vein was not born out. The anatomic relationships in the area of the renal vein, which would facilitate a compression of the testicular vein in erect posture, have also been suspected to be responsible for formation of varicocele. There is another unconfirmed hypothesis suggesting that varicocele formation has a humoral basis. Since the left adrenal vein empties into the renal vein in the vicinity of the testicular vein, a high concentration of epinephrine may cause constriction at the mouth of the testicular vein, creating an impediment to blood flow and secondarily a dilatation of the testicular vein. None of these hypotheses has been demonstrated to be actually involved in the mechanism of varicocele formation.

ANATOMY OF THE TESTES

TOPOGRAPHIC RELATIONSHIPS

The testis is an "oblongoid," approximately 4.5 cm at its long diameter, weighing 32–45 g.[15] The testicular parenchyma consists of seminiferous tubules, exhibiting a highly complex pattern of convolutions, which are embedded in a connective tissue matrix containing interspersed Leydig cells, blood vessels, and lymphatics. A histologic section of the testicular tissue illustrates this arrangement and when cut in the proper plane shows cross sections of the seminiferous tubules containing the seminiferous epithelium (Fig. 118-3). Although the seminiferous tubules in human testes show an extremely complicated and irregular pattern of

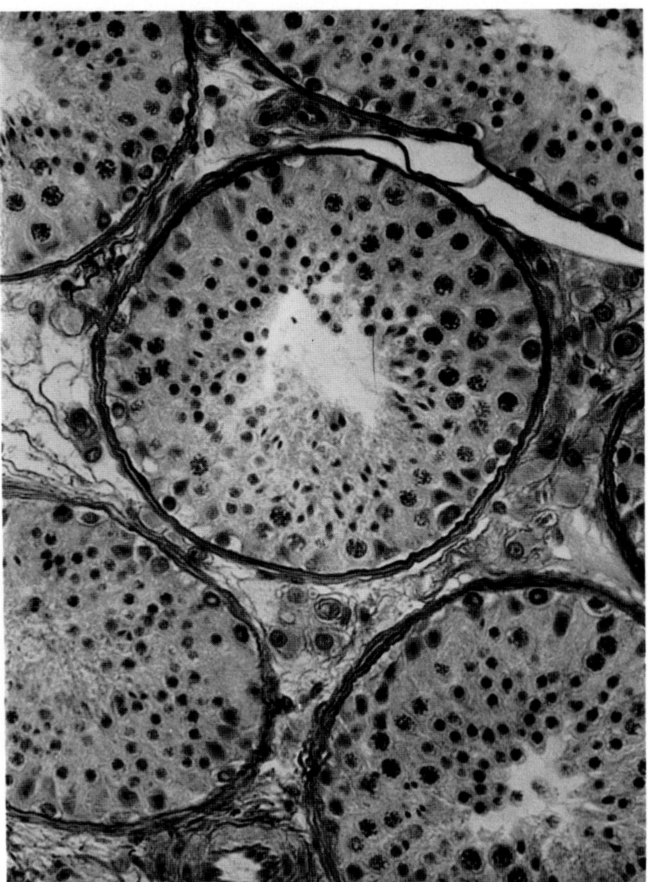

Fig. 118-3. Histology of normal human testis. (From Steinberger, in Gibian and Plotz (eds): Mammalian Reproduction, 1970. Courtesy of Springer.)

convolutions, anastomoses, and blind pouches, they basically form loops which terminate in a single duct, the tubulus recti. This duct empties into a structure called the rete testis, connected through a number of small ducts, the ductuli efferentes, with the epididymal duct (Fig. 118-2).

SEMINIFEROUS TUBULES

General Description

The basement membrane (tunica propria) of the human seminiferous tubules is composed of collagen fibers embedded in a matrix of mucopolysaccharides, contractile myoid cells, and fibroblasts. In contradistinction to most lower species, in man the myoid cells do not form a continuous cellular layer connected by desmosomal junctions.

The basement membrane is extremely sensitive to pathologic processes and responds to them with characteristic proliferative changes such as fibrosis (overproduction of fibroblasts) and/or "hyalinization" (thickening of the acellular layers with deposition of PAS-positive material). While specific patterns in the abnormalities of the basement membrane of the seminiferous tubules can be related to specific testicular disorders (e.g., Klinefelter's syndrome or adult seminiferous tubule failure), neither the pathophysiology of this process nor its relationship to the disease process is clear.

Spermatogenesis

Spermatogenesis, or the process of formation of spermatozoa from immature germ cells, takes place in the seminiferous epithelium within the seminiferous tubules. The newly formed spermatozoa are transported through the lumen of the seminiferous tubule into the epididymis, where they are stored after completing their physiologic maturation.

The basic concepts for understanding the spermatogenic process in mammals were formulated in the 19th century. After the discovery that spermatozoa are the progeny of cells residing in the testes,[16] the bewildering morphologic variety of cells composing the seminiferous epithelium were classified on the basis of their structural characteristics.[17] It became clear that the least differentiated germ cells, the spermatogonia, divide to form a unique cell, the spermatocyte. This cell is unique because immediately after formation it enters the lengthy process of meiosis or reduction division, resulting in the formation of haploid cells, the spermatids. These cells do not divide further but undergo a complicated process of metamorphosis which culminates in formation of a flagellate, motile cell, the spermatozoon.

Study of the details of the developmental progression of the germ cells in rodents led to the discovery of the topographic relationships of these cells within the seminiferous tubules. It has been observed that the various cell types form precisely defined cellular associations which succeed one another cyclically in any given area of the seminiferous tubule. Each complete sequence of changes in the cellular associations was named the *spermatogenic cycle*,[17,18] referring to the events of the seminiferous epithelium in

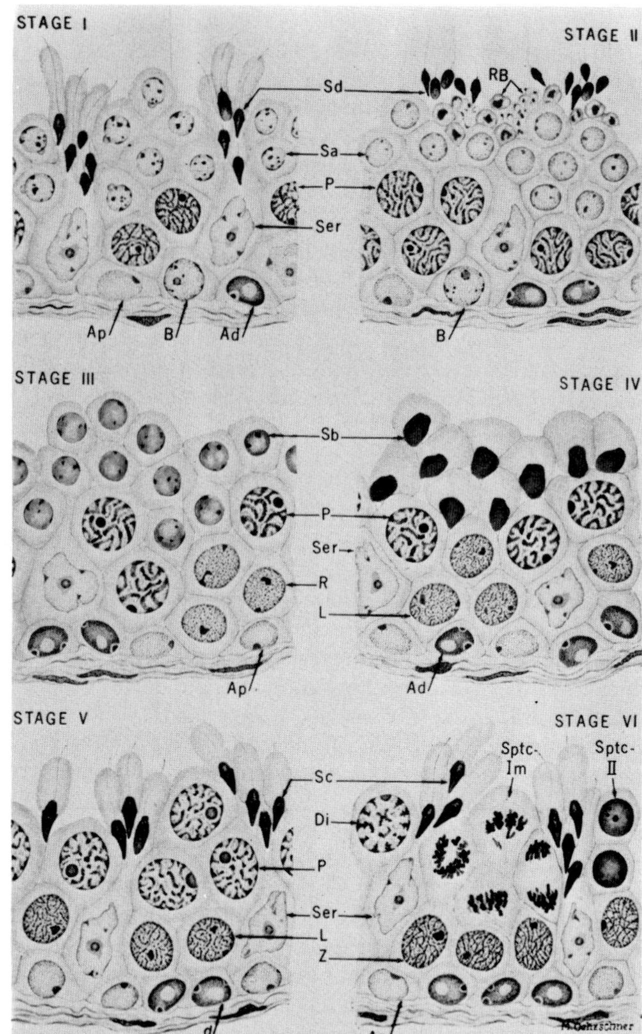

Fig. 118-5. Cellular composition and topography of the six typical cellular associations found repeatedly in human seminiferous tubules. These cell associations, corresponding to stages of the cycle of the seminiferous epithelium, are numbered stages I–VI. Ser, Sertoli nuclei; Ap and Ad, pale and dark type A spermatogonia; B, type B spermatogonia; R, resting primary spermatocytes; L, leptotene primary spermatocytes; Z, zygotene primary spermatocytes; P, pachytene primary spermatocytes; Di, diplotene primary spermatocytes; Sptc-II, secondary spermatocytes in interphase; Sa, Sb, Sc, and Sd, spermatids at various steps of spermiogenesis; RB, residual bodies. (From Clermont: Physiol. Rev. *52:* 198, 1972.)

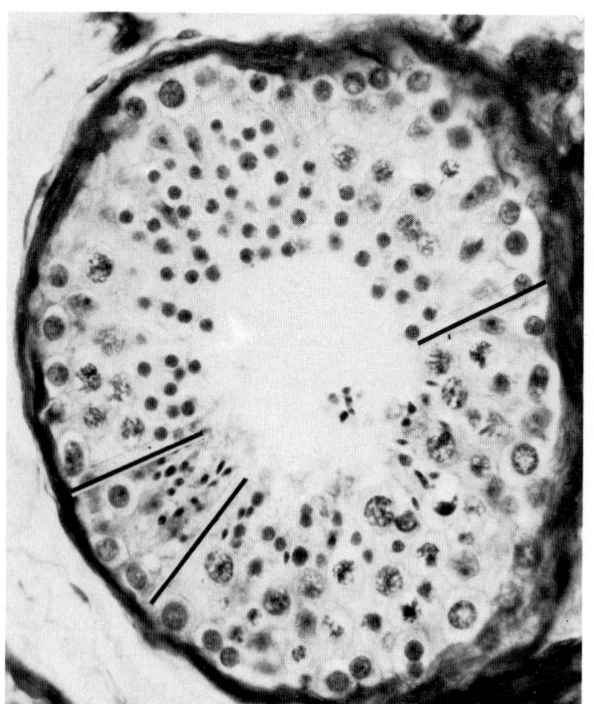

Fig. 118-4. Human seminiferous tubule. Note different stages of spermatogenesis present in a single cross section.

the framework of time. On the other hand, the concept of the *wave of the seminiferous epithelium*[17,19] defines changes in the spatial relationships of the various cellular associations along the length of the seminiferous tubule. In other words, "The wave is in space what the cycle is in time."[19] These concepts have been greatly clarified in the past 25 yr,[20,21] primarily by the efforts of Leblond and Clermont.

While the clarification of the kinetics of spermatogenesis progressed smoothly and rapidly for various mammalian species, difficulties were encountered in studies of human testes. Histologic examination of cross sections of the human seminiferous tubules failed to reveal precisely defined cellular associations (stages of the cycle of seminiferous epithelium) and grossly irregular spatial distribution (waves) of the stages (Fig. 118-4). Clermont,[22] however, succeeded in characterizing in general terms the cellular associations (stages) of the human seminiferous epithelium and provided data strongly suggestive that spermatogenesis in human testes, in principle, is also characterized by a "cycle and a wave of seminiferous epithelium" (Fig. 118-5). The wave, however, is grossly irregular, causing the numerical relationships to be poorly defined.[23] Apparently, the process is "clonal" in character.[24,25] Nevertheless, the kinetics governing divisions of an individual germ cell and its progeny or a small group of cells are probably fairly precise. The rigid temporal relationships and the timing of the process and its components (transformation of one cell type to another or maturation of specific cell types) can be determined with considerable precision. Utilizing these concepts, Heller and Clermont[26] computed the spermatogenic process in human testes to require approximately 74 days.

Since spermatozoa are continuously produced in the testes of adult man, a constant supply of germ cell precursors is essential. Numerous studies have been conducted in lower species to elucidate this process, and although a degree of controversy still exists concerning the details, the best evidence points toward the concept of a "self-renewing" stem cell.[22] In man, however, the stem cell renewal process has not been studied in sufficient detail to permit any generalizations.

Sertoli Cell

The Sertoli cells, the only nongerminal elements within the seminiferous epithelium, line the basement membrane of the seminiferous tubules. Their cytoplasm comes in direct contact with the innermost layer of the basement membrane and forms extensive processes which closely surround the germ cells and form specialized junctions with other Sertoli cells. The nucleus is irregular and complex, and the cytoplasm contains various organelles (Fig. 118-6). The structural characteristics of the Sertoli cells have been recently reviewed.[27]

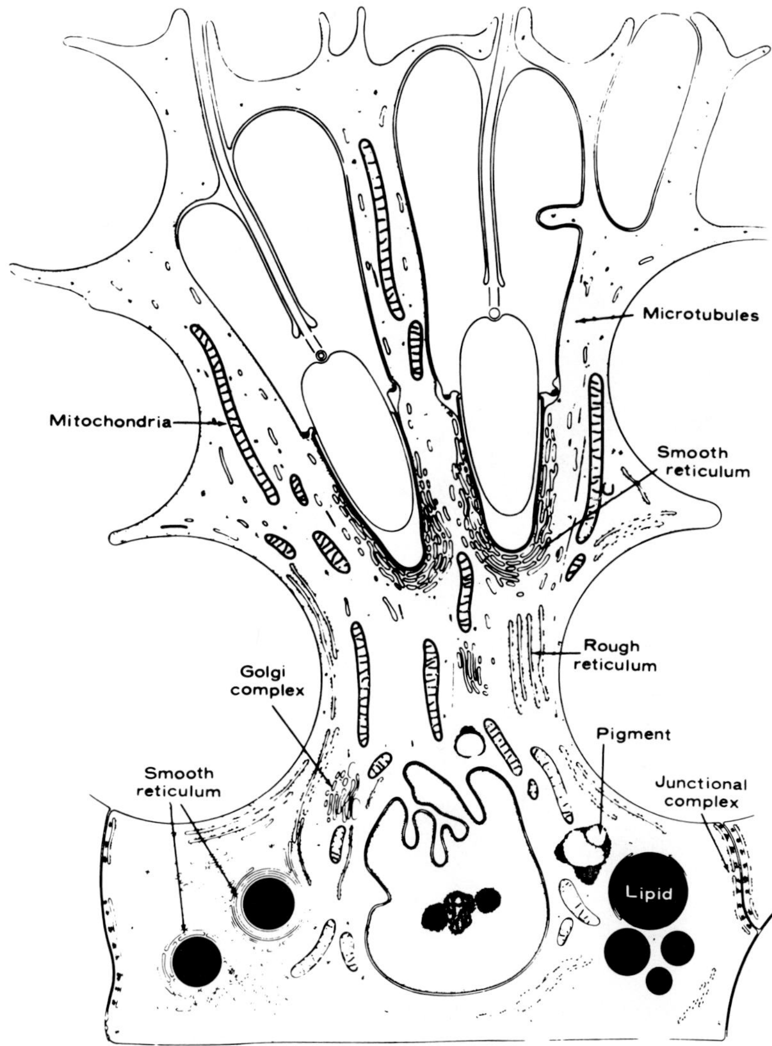

Fig. 118-6. Typical Sertoli cell, showing its shape and relationships to the germ cells as well as the form and distribution of its principal organelles and inclusions. (From Fawcett, in Hamilton and Greep (eds.): Handbook of Physiology, section 7, vol. 5, 1975. Courtesy of the American Physiological Society.)

The Sertoli cells proliferate only during the early stages of testicular development. In adult testes no division of Sertoli cells has been documented, and none of the experimental alterations, including various hormonal manipulations, resulted in restoration of mitotic activity in the Sertoli cells.[28]

Ever since its description by Sertoli,[29] the function of this nongerminal cell remained an enigma until the past few years. Sertoli called it the "nurse" cell (probably an apt description; see below), and subsequent investigators assigned to it various functions. Suggestions were made that the Sertoli cell is primarily responsible for clearing (phagocytosis) of residual bodies and damaged germ cells from the seminiferous epithelium.[30] Later the phagocytic activity of the Sertoli cell was clearly demonstrated.[31]

Recent physiologic studies demonstrated that a wide variety of substances present in circulation are excluded from the seminiferous tubule fluid, a finding suggesting the presence of a blood–testis barrier similar to the blood–brain barrier (for review see Setchell[32]). Fawcett,[27] in a series of elegant studies, demonstrated the ultrastructural basis of the blood–testis barrier—the Sertoli–Sertoli junctional complexes (tight junctions), which divide the germinal epithelium into a basal and an adluminal compartment. The basal compartment contains the spermatogonia, and the adluminal compartment, the remaining complement of the germinal cells (Fig. 118-7). The presence of an effective blood–testis barrier in man has also been demonstrated recently;[33] however, its physiologic importance still remains to be clarified.[27]

A secretory function has been ascribed to the Sertoli cell. It has been suggested that it participates in secreting the seminiferous tubule fluid in which the spermatozoa are transported out of the testis into the epididymis.[27] Recently it was suggested[34] and later demonstrated[35] that the Sertoli cells indeed secrete an androgen-binding protein (ABP) under follicle-stimulating hormone (FSH) control. This protein is transported into the lumen of seminiferous tubules and through the ductal system into the epididymis.[36] These discoveries provided direct evidence for the long-suspected secretory function of the Sertoli cell. The possibility that the Sertoli cells also synthesize androgens has been suggested[37] but as yet has not been confirmed.

INTERSTITIAL TISSUE

The interstitial tissue contains the primary endocrine organ of the testis, the Leydig cells. These cells were suspected to be the site of testicular hormone (androgen) production as early as the turn of the century,[38] an idea supported by direct evidence from cytochemical studies,[39,40] tissue culture,[41] and incubation experiments in the past 10 yr.

Although many features of the interstitial tissue and the Leydig cells are common to a variety of mammalian species (Fig. 118-

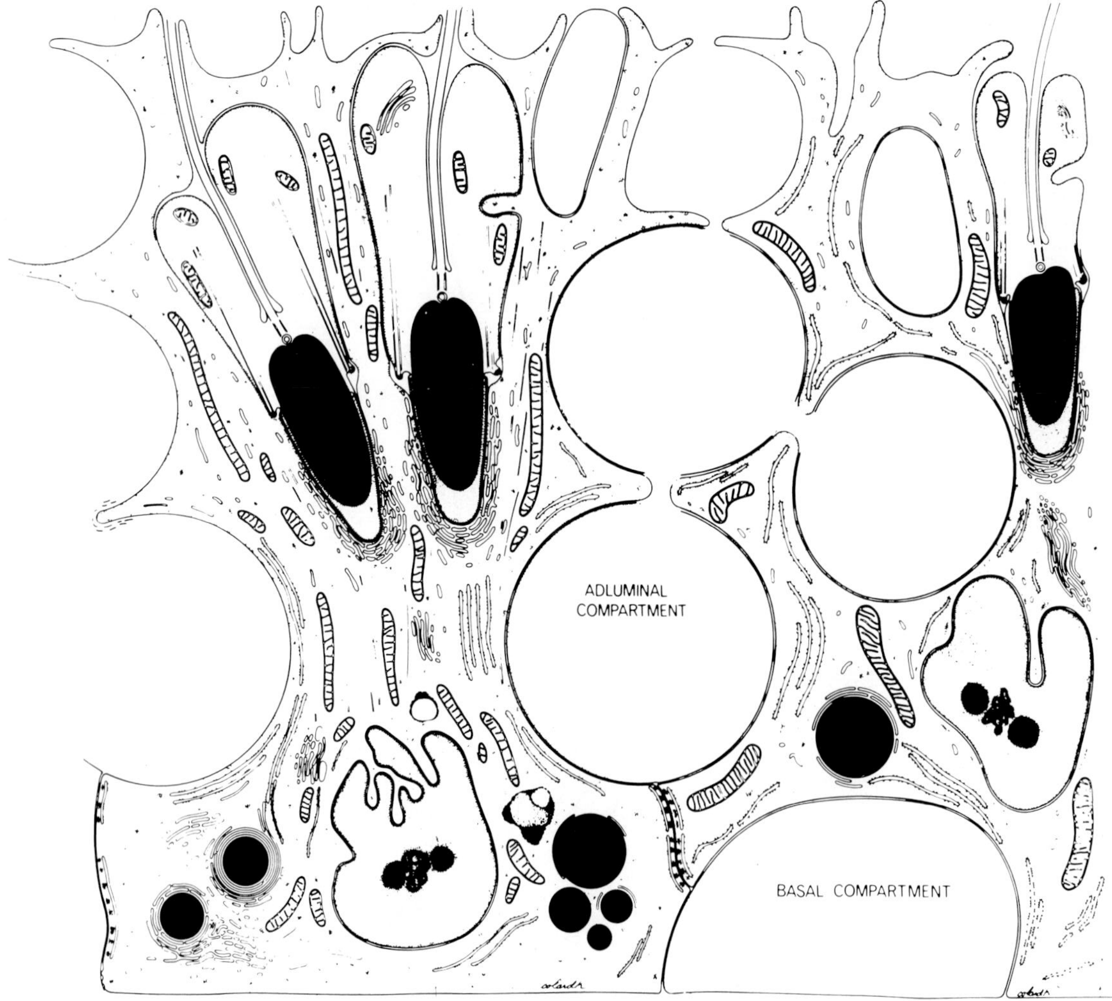

Fig. 118-7. Manner in which the occluding junctions between Sertoli cells divide the seminiferous epithelium into a *basal compartment* occupied by the spermatogonia and preleptotene spermatocytes and an *adluminal compartment* containing more advanced stages of the germ cell population. The occluding Sertoli–Sertoli junctions are the principal component of the blood–testis barrier. (From Fawcett, in Hamilton and Greep (eds.): Handbook of Physiology, section 7, vol. 5, 1975. Courtesy of the American Physiological Society.)

8), the human interstitial tissue exhibits distinguishing characteristics: a relative paucity of lymphatics and the presence of crystalloids of Reinke in the cytoplasm of Leydig cells, which typically form rather large clumps (for details see Christensen[42]). In normal adult testes no division of Leydig cells has been observed. The cytoplasm of Leydig cells abounds in the distinctive cytoplasmic organelle of the steroid-producing cells, the smooth endoplasmic reticulum (Fig. 118-9). Ultrastructural studies combined with biochemical investigations elucidated to a great extent the structure–function relationship between the various cytoplasmic organelles and the biosynthesis of androgens (for details of androgen biogenesis see Chapter 119), which can be summarized in general terms in the following way. Cholesterol either derived from circulation or synthesized in the smooth endoplasmic reticulum is translocated into mitochondria, where the side-chain cleavage takes place and pregnenolone is formed. Pregnenolone is transported to the smooth endoplasmic reticulum, where further transformations take place, resulting in formation of testosterone (Fig. 118-10). Testosterone is then secreted into the interstitial area. Neither the structural nor biochemical details of the secretory process are known. It is unlikely that any significant storage of testosterone takes place in the Leydig cells.

SEX ACCESSORIES

Seminal Vesicles

In man the seminal vesicles are paired symmetrical tubular structures 10–20 cm long with numerous outpouchings of alveolar glands. They empty into the ejaculatory duct (Fig. 118-1). The

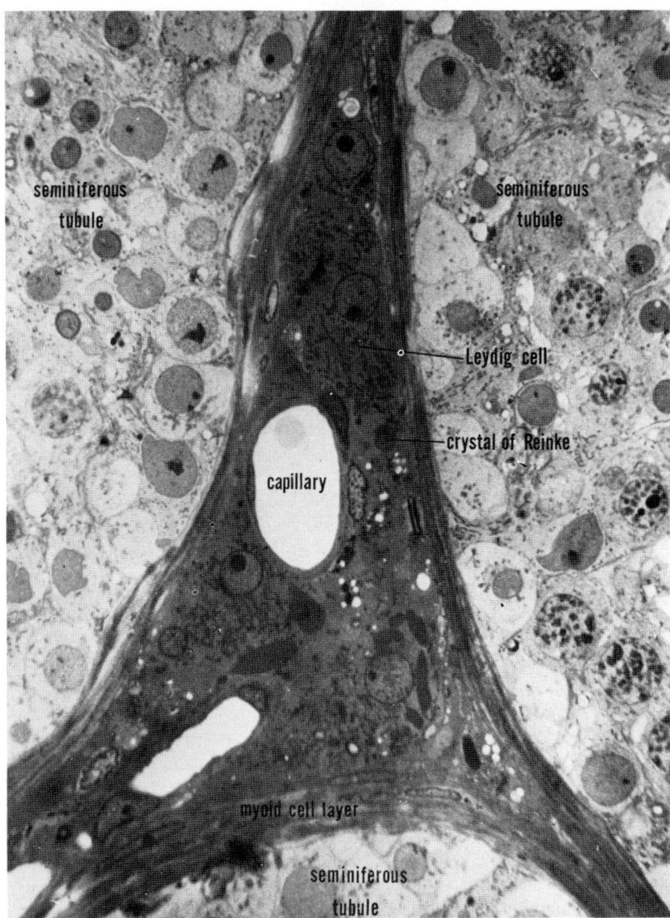

Fig. 118-8. Ultrastructure of the interstitial area of the human testis. (Courtesy of Dr. A. K. Christensen.)

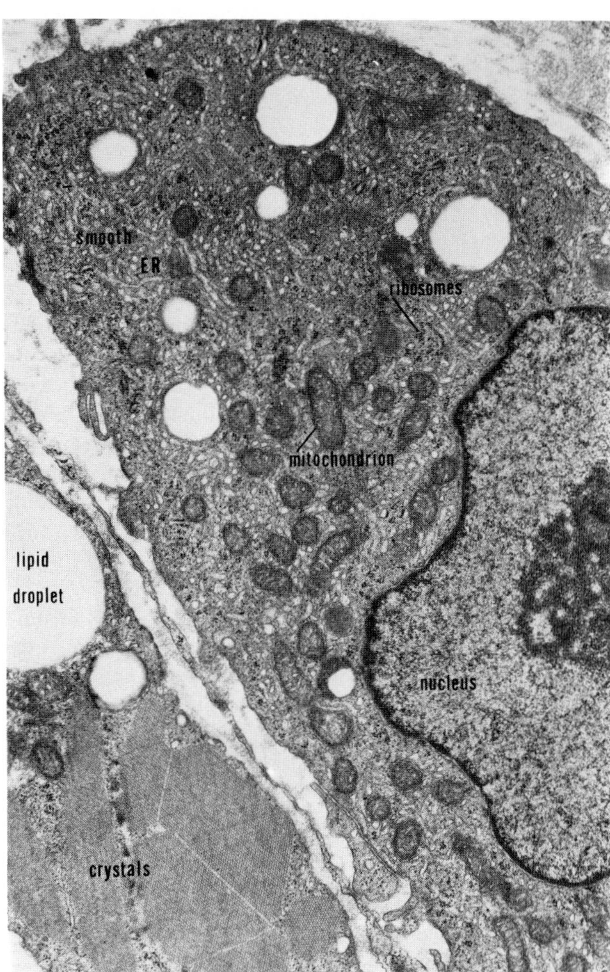

Fig. 118-9. Ultrastructure of a human Leydig cell. (Courtesy of Dr. A. K. Christensen.)

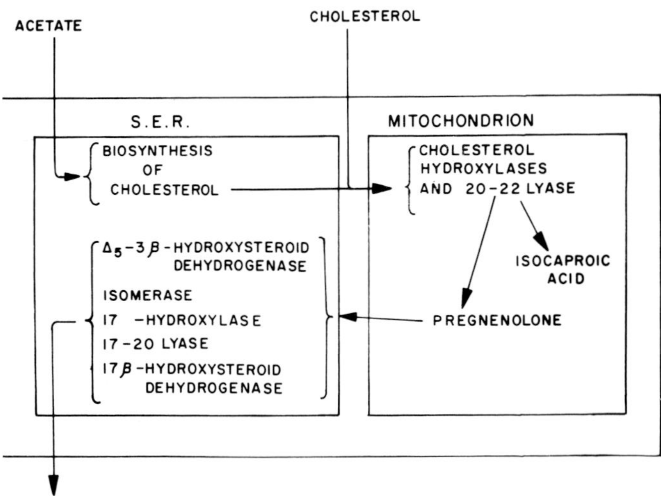

Fig. 118-10. Relationship of cellular organelles to testosterone biogenesis. Acetate is delivered to the smooth endoplasmic reticulum (SER) within the cell cytoplasm, where it is utilized for synthesis of cholesterol. The de novo formed cholesterol, or cholesterol delivered from the vascular system, is transported to the mitochondria, where it is metabolized to pregnenolone. Pregnenolone is transported back to the SER, where it is metabolized to testosterone which is secreted. (From Steinberger, in Gibian and Plotz (eds.): Mammalian Reproduction, 1970. Courtesy of Springer.)

glandular tissue is surrounded by muscle and connective tissue layers containing primarily elastic and some collagen fibers. The muscle layer is well developed, consisting of two spirally arranged muscle fiber layers.

Comparatively little is known about the development of the seminal vesicles' function. They and the ejaculatory ducts develop in the embryo from the lower portion of the Wolffian ducts and differentiate functionally at puberty under the influence of androgens.

The seminal vesicle duct is lined by a simple cylindrical epithelium, its thickness and state of development depending on the functional state of the gland.[43] The alveoli are lined by three cell types: the basal and the cylindrical cells at the basement membrane, and third cell type, located adluminally. The lumen of the seminal vesicles is filled with mucoid secretions which provide the major contribution toward the total volume of the ejaculate. Although occasional spermatozoa can be seen in the seminal vesicle secretions, this organ does not serve as the storage site for spermatozoa, and the few sperm cells occasionally seen in its lumen are believed to be the result of reflux action.

Seminal vesicles are innervated primarily by fibers from the hypogastric plexus, although nerve connections with S 2–4 exist. A rich nerve plexus, containing a number of fairly large ganglia, is found under the adventitia of the human seminal vesicle.

The growth of the seminal vesicles is under the influence of androgens, and their secretory activity is androgen dependent.

Prostate

The prostate of an adult man consists of 30–50 branches of tubuloalveolar glands. The glands and their ducts form lobules that are embedded in a fibromuscular stroma, a thick nondirectional network of smooth muscle and elastic fibers. The ducts empty into the prostatic urethra in the area of the verumontanum (colliculus seminalis). The entire prostate gland is surrounded by a multilayered capsule consisting of an inner muscle layer (stratus muscularis), intimately related to the muscle fibers in the stroma, a heavy connective tissue layer (stratus fibrosum) consisting primarily of collagen fibers which envelops the muscle layer, and an outer layer, made up of loose areolar connective tissue rich in blood vessels.

The anlage of the human prostate can be detected in a 12-week-old fetus as a number of epithelial buds originating from the proximal urethra. The buds branch into tubules lined by low cuboidal cells and develop into posterior, middle, and lateral lobes. During the perinatal period, the prostatic epithelium assumes the appearance of squamous metaplasia, possibly in response to elevated fetal testosterone levels during this period of development. After the age of 1 month the epithelium reverts to a low cuboidal appearance and persists in this state until puberty, when in response to androgens it begins to develop again.[44] From puberty until 45–50 yr of age the prostate exhibits its adult appearance. With aging, it begins to show decreased secretory activity, and after the age of 60 sclerotic changes occur.

The glandular epithelium of the prostate is highly responsive to androgens, and the cell cytoplasm is rich in acid phosphatase. The prostatic secretion forms a part of the ejaculate. In the absence of androgens (e.g., castration), the prostatic epithelium undergoes atrophy, and the acinar cells flatten and cease to secrete.

The nerve supply of the prostate is related to the hypogastric plexus and S 3–4. Some fibers of the nervi erigantes join the hypogastric plexus, and others connect directly to the prostatic plexus. Sympathetic and parasympathetic nerves form a plexus under the prostatic capsule, where numerous nerve ganglia can be found.

Vas Deferens

The vas is about 20 inches long, extending from the tail of the epididymis to the ejaculatory duct. In the scrotum the vas is located in proximity to the epididymis. It joins in the formation of the spermatic cord, with which it traverses the inguinal canal and enters the pelvis. There it loops behind the bladder and forms the ampulla, which enters the prostate at its posterior–superior aspect. At this point it becomes the ejaculatory duct, which traverses the prostate to empty into the colliculus seminalis in the prostatic urethra.

The wall of the vas is composed of adventitia, vasculosa, an outer heavy longitudinal muscle layer, an inner circular muscle layer, and mucosa, consisting of two layers of cylindrical epithelium. The ampulla is a specialized portion of the vas, its diameter greater than, and its wall structure similar to, the vas except for marked folding of the mucosa. The ejaculatory duct is lined by simple cylindrical epithelium, which also is thrown into folds. The average length of the ejaculatory duct is approximately 20–25 mm.

REFERENCES

1. Cooper, A. Observations on the Structure and Diseases of the Testis. London, Longman, Rees, Orme, Brown, and Green, 1830.
2. Ruibal, R. The Evolution of the Scrotum. *Evolution 11:* 376, 1957.
3. Andrews, F. N. Thermo-regulatory Functions of Rat Scrotum. I. Normal Development and Effect of Castration. *Proc. Soc. Exp. Biol. Med. 45:* 867, 1940.
4. Holstein, A. F. Die glatte Muskulatur in der Tunica albuginea des Hodens und ihr Einflus auf den Spermatozoentransport in den Nebenhoden. *Ergeb. Anat. Anz. 121:* 103, 1967.
5. Davis, J. R., Langford, G. A., and Kirby, P. J. The Testicular Capsule. In Johnson, A. D., Gomes, W. R., and VanDemark, N. L. (eds): The Testis, vol. 1. New York, Academic, 1970, p. 282.
6. Mitchell, G. A. G. Anatomy of the Autonomic Nervous System. London, Livingston, 1953.
7. Mitchell, G. A. G. The Innervation of the Kidney, Ureter, Testicle, and Epididymis. *J. Anat. 70:* 10, 1935.
8. Peters, H. Uber die feinere Innervation des Hodens insbesondere des Interstitiellen Gewebes und der Hodenkanälchen beim Menschen. *Acta Neuroveg. (Wein) 15:* 235, 1957.
9. Norberg, K. A., Risley, P. L., and Ungerstedt, U. Adrenergic innervation of the male reproductive ducts in some mammals. I. The distribution of adrenergic nerves. Z. Zellfrosch. Mikrosk. *Anat. 76:* 278, 1967.
10. Linzell, J. L., and Setchell, B. P. The Output of Spermatozoa and Fluid by, and the Metabolism of, the Isolated Perfused Testis of the Ram. *J. Physiol. (Lond.) 195:* 25, 1968.
11. Harrison, R. G., and Barclay, A. E. The Distribution of the Testicular Artery (Internal Spermatic Artery) to the Human Testis *Br. J. Urol. 20:* 59, 1948.
12. Harrison, R. G., and Weiner, J. S. Vascular Patterns of the Mammalian Testis and Their Functional Significance. *J. Exp. Biol. 126:* 304, 1949.
13. Free, M. J., and Jaffe, R. A. Dynamics of Venous–Arterial Testosterone Transfer in the Pampiniform Plexus of the Rat. *Endocrinology 97:* 169, 1975.
14. Sasano, N., and Ichijo, S. Vascular Patterns of the Human Testis With Special Reference to its Senile Changes. *Tohoku J. Exp. Med. 99:* 269, 1969.
15. Calloway, N. O., Foley, C. F., and Lagerbloom, P. Uncertainties in geriatric data. II. Organ size. *J. Am. Geriatr. Soc. 13:* 20, 1965.
16. von Kolliker, R. A. Beiträge zur Kenntnis der Geschlechtesverhaltnisse und der Samenflüssigkeit wirbelloser Tiere. Berlin, 1841.
17. von Ebner, V. Untersuchungen über den Bau der Samenkanälchen und die Entwicklung der Spermatozoiden bei den Säugentieren und beim Menschen. In: Rollet's Untersuchungen aus dem Institut für Physiologie und Histologie in Graz. Leipzig, 1871, p. 200.

18. Benda, C. Untersuchungen über den Bau des funktionierenden Samenkanälchens einiger Säugetiere und Folgerungen für die Spermatogenese dieser Wirbeltierklasse. *Arch. Mikrobiol. Anat. 30:* 49, 1887.
19. Regaud, C. Etude sur la Structure des Tubes Séminifères et sur la Spermatogenése chez les Mammifères. *Arch. Anat. Microsc. Morphol. Exp. 4:* 101, 1901.
20. Clermont Y. Kinetics of Spermatogenesis in Mammals: Seminiferous Epithelium Cycle and Spermatogonial Renewal. *Physiol. Rev. 52:* 198, 1972.
21. Steinberger, E., and Steinberger, A. Spermatogenic Function of the Testis. In Hamilton, D. W., and Greep, R. O. (eds): Handbook of Physiology, section 7, vol. 5. Washington, D.C., American Physiological Society, 1975, p. 1.
22. Clermont Y. The Cycle of the Seminiferous Epithelium in Man. *Am. J. Anat. 112:* 35, 1963.
23. Steinberger, E., and Tjioe, D. Y. Kinetics and Quantitative Analysis of Human Spermatogenesis. Proceedings of the All-India Conference on Research in Reproduction and Fertility, Indian Council of Medical Research, Technical Report Series *21:* 99, 1973.
24. Chowdhury, A. K. Thymidine H^3 Labeling of Spermatogonia in Rat and Human Seminiferous Tubules Mounted *in Toto.* Anat. Rec. 169: 296, 1971.
25. Chowdhury, A. K., and Steinberger, E. *In Vitro* H^3-Thymidine Labeling Pattern and Topographic Distribution of Spermatogonia in Human Seminiferous Tubules. In Troen, P., and Nankin, H. R. (eds): The Testis in Normal and Infertile Men. New York, Raven Press, 1977, p. 69.
26. Heller, C. G., and Clermont, Y. Spermatogenesis in Man and Estimate of Its Duration. *Science 140:* 184, 1963.
27. Fawcett, D. W. Ultrastructure and Function of the Sertoli Cell. In Hamilton, D. W. and Greep, R. O. (eds): Handbook of Physiology, section 7, vol. 5. Washington, D.C., American Physiological Society, 1975, p. 21.
28. Steinberger, A., and Steinberger, E. Replication Pattern of Sertoli Cells in Maturing Rat Testis *in Vivo* and in Organ Culture. *Biol. Reprod. 4:* 84, 1971.
29. Sertoli E. Dell'Esistenzia di Particolari Cellule Ramificate nei Canalicoli Seminiferi del Testicolo Umano. *Morgagni 7:* 31, 1865.
30. Clegg, E. J., and Macmillan, E. W. The Uptake of Vital Dyes and Particulate Matter by the Sertoli Cells of the Rat Testis. *J. Anat. (Lond.) 99:* 219, 1965.
31. Vilar, O., Steinberger, A., and Steinberger, E. An Electron Microscopic Study of Cultured Rat Testicular Fragments. *Z. Zellforsch. 78:* 221, 1967.
32. Setchell, B. P. Testicular Blood Supply, Lymphatic Drainage, and Secretion of Fluid. In Johnson, A. D., Gomes, W. R., and Van-Demark, N. L. (eds): The Testis, vol. 1. New York, Academic, 1970, p. 101.
33. Koskimies, A. I., Kormano, M., and Alfthan, O. Proteins of the Seminiferous Tubule Fluid in Man—Evidence for a Blood–Testis Barrier. *J. Reprod. Fertil. 32:* 79, 1973.
34. Vernon, R. G., Kopec, B., and Fritz, I. B. Studies on the Distribution of the High-Affinity Testosterone Binding Protein in Rat Seminiferous Tubules. *J. Endocrinol. 57:* ii, 1973.
35. Steinberger, A., Heindel, J. J., Lindsey, J. N., et al.: Isolation and Culture of FSH Responsive Sertoli Cells. *Endocrine Commun. 2:* 261, 1975.
36. Hansson, V., Ritzen, E. M., French, F. S., and Nayfeh, S. N. Androgen Transport and Receptor Mechanisms in Testis and Epididymis. In Hamilton, D. W., and Greep, R. O. (eds): Handbook of Physiology, section 7, vol. 5. Washington, D.C., American Physiological Society, 1975, p. 173.
37. Bell, J. B., Vinson, G. P., and Lacy, D. Studies on the Structure and Function of the Mammalian Testis. 3. *In Vitro* Steroidogenesis by the Seminiferous Tubules of Rat Testis. *Proc. R. Soc. Lond.* [*B*] *176:* 433, 1971.
38. Loisel, G. Les Graisses du Testicule chez Quelques Mammifères. *C. R. Soc. Biol. (Paris) 55:* 1009, 1903.
39. Baillie, A. H., Ferguson, M. M., and Hart, D. M. Developments in Steroid Histochemistry. New York, Academic, 1966.
40. Mendelson, C., Dufau, M., and Catt, K. Gonadotropins Binding and Stimulation of Cyclic Adenosine 3′:5′-Monophosphate and Testosterone Production in Isolated Leydig Cells. *J. Biol. Chem. 250:* 8818, 1975.
41. Steinberger, E. Steinberger, A., Vilar, O., Salamon, I. I., and Sud, B. N. Microscopy, Cytochemistry and Steroid Biosynthetic Activity of Leydig Cells in Culture. *Ciba Found. Colloq. Endocrinol. 16:* 56, 1967.
42. Christensen, A. K., Leydig Cells. In Hamilton, D. W., and Greep, R. O. (eds): Handbook of Physiology, section 7, vol. 5. Washington, D.C., American Physiological Society, 1975, p. 57.
43. Stieve, H. Männliche Genitalorgane. In: Handbuch der mikroskopischen Anatomie des Menschen. Harn-und Geschlechtsapparat. Berlin, Springer, 1930.
44. Swyer, G. J. M. Postnatal Growth Changes in Human Prostate. *J. Anat. (Lond.) 78:* 130, 1944.
45. Steinberger, E., and Steinberger, A. Testis: Basic and Clinical Aspects. In Balin, H., and Glasser, S. (eds): Reproductive Biology. Amsterdam, Excerpta Medica, 1972, p. 144.
46. Steinberger, E. Biogenesis of Androgens. In Gibian, H., and Plotz, E. J. (eds): Mammalian Reproduction. Heidelberg, Springer, 1970, p. 112.

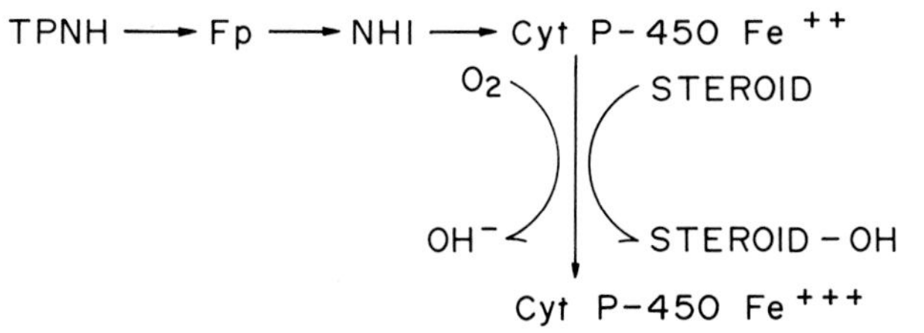

TPNH → Fp → NHI → Cyt P-450 Fe ++

O_2 STEROID

OH^- STEROID - OH

Cyt P-450 Fe +++

Fig. 119-2. Reconstitution of 11β-hydroxylation according to Omura et al.[24] F_p, flavoprotein; NHI, nonheme iron.

pecially if TPN^+ is also added.[31] However, with the purified enzyme system TPNH is more effective than DPNH by an order of magnitude. This conclusion has been confirmed.[32]

These observations are most readily explained by the activity of a mitochondrial transhydrogenase that uses DPNH to reduce TPN^+ (Fig. 119-3). Bovine adrenocortical mitochondria possess a malic enzyme, the properties of which suggest that it may act to produce TPNH for 11β-hydroxylation.[33] Since the rate of production of pyruvate is equal to the rate of 11β-hydroxylation (mole for mole), malic enzyme cannot support side-chain cleavage since this reaction proceeds in mitochondria from endogenous cholesterol[34] and would therefore be consuming TPNH in those studies in which 11β-hydroxylation was measured.[33] More pyruvate would therefore be formed if this enzyme were producing TPNH for both reactions. The problem has been considered elsewhere.[31]

It appears then that side-chain cleavage is supported by transhydrogenation from DPNH. It is not known to what extent various possible dehydrogenases contribute to the production of the DPNH in vivo. One other possibility is the oxidation of TPN^+-linked substrates, but for this hypothesis there is less evidence. These various sources of TPNH are summarized in Figure 119-3.

Pregnenolone is now ready to leave the mitochondrion and make its way to the endoplasmic reticulum, where the reactions of step III take place.

Conversion of Pregnenolone to Androgens (Step III). The transformation of pregnenolone to testosterone requires five enzymatic reactions: 17α-hydroxylase, C_{17}–C_{20} lyase (desmolase or side-chain cleavage), 3β-hydroxysteroid dehydrogenase, $\Delta^{4,5}$-3 ketosteroid isomerase, and 17β-hydroxysteroid dehydrogenase (Fig. 119-4). 17α-Hydroxylase and the lyase are somehow closely associated as an enzyme pair, as are the two enzymes which oxidize the 3β-hydroxyl group (dehydrogrogenase) and rearrange the double bond from Δ^5 to Δ^4 (isomerase). As a result of these associations, the number of possible sequences and intermediates is mercifully reduced. Figure 119-4 shows that there are two main pathways from pregnenolone to testosterone—one proceeding on the left of the figure via 17α-hydroxypregnenolone (conveniently referred to as the Δ^5 or dehydroepiandrosterone pathway) and the other, called the progesterone or Δ^4 pathway, on the right. Apart from 17β-hyroxysteroid dehydrogenase, the various reactions are essentially irreversible. In addition to the two major pathways, branches are possible between the pathways from left to right. The organization of the pathways within the cell is such that, at least in the rat, the conversion of pregnenolone to testosterone occurs within the microsomal fraction; significant amounts of these enzymes do not occur in other cell fractions.[35,36] The cytosol does, however, appear to contain a factor capable of accelerating the microsomal reactions involved in androgen biosynthesis.[36] The nature of this factor remains obscure, and there is no certainty that the effect is important in the intact cell. Finally, it appears likely that each of these enzymes is a single species. For example, there are four possible substrates for 3β-hydroxysteroid dehydrogenase (Fig. 119-4). There is no evidence for more than one such enzyme, so that C_{19} and C_{21} steroids must share one enzyme.[37] However, in the adrenal cortex there appear to be two isomerase enzymes.[38] The following discussion will be based on the assumption that this is not true of the testis, although this will only be certain when all of the enzymes have been prepared in highly purified form.

It is only possible to approach the question of which pathway(s) (Fig. 119-4) occur(s) within the cell by indirect means; once individual enzymes are released, the organization of the membrane

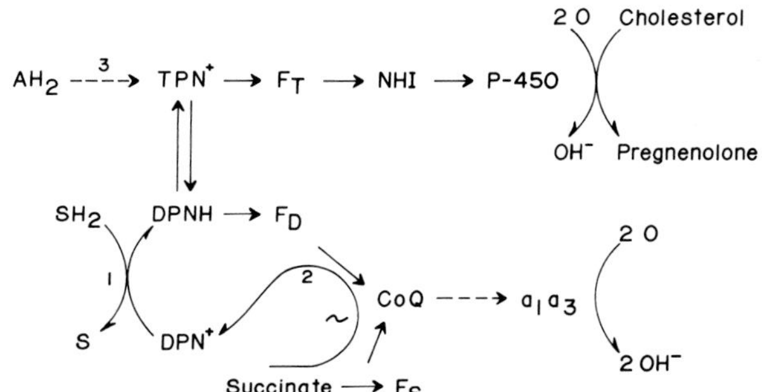

Fig. 119-3. Possible pathways for the production of TPNH for side-chain cleavage. (1) SH_2: DPN^+-linked substrates. DPNH formed from SH_2 undergoes transhydrogenation. (2) Reversed electron transport from succinate reduces DPN^+; again this is followed by transhydrogenation. (3) AH_2: TPN^+-linked substrates (malate and isocitrate). F_T, F_D, and F_S: the various flavoproteins.

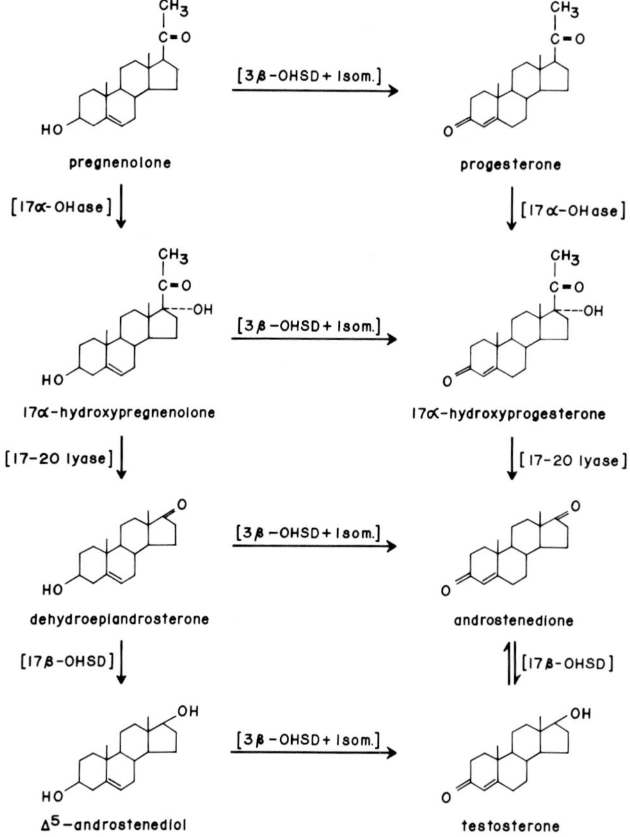

Fig. 119-4. Possible pathways from pregnenolone to testosterone. The pathway to the left is conveniently called the Δ^5 or dehydroepiandrosterone pathway; that to the right is called the Δ^4 or progesterone pathway. 3β-OHSD, 3β-hydroxysteroid dehydrogenase; 17α-OHase, 17α-hydroxylase: 17β-OHSD, 17β-hydroxysteroid dehydrogenase; 17-20 lyase, C_{17}–C_{20} lyase; Isom, $\Delta^{4,5}$-ketosteroid isomerase.

is lost. It is therefore necessary to use a microsomal fraction consisting largely of fragments of smooth endoplasmic reticulum. Interpretation of findings with this preparation requires the exacting task of relating the vesicles of endoplasmic reticulum to the complex branching tubules of the intact cell. The question is important because the exclusive use of one or another of the possible pathways would suggest a specific arrangement of enzymes within the membrane of the endoplasmic reticulum such that intermediates pass from enzyme to enzyme with little or no freedom to move into the surrounding cytosol. It may be wise to consider the possibility that the cell may use more than one pathway from pregnenolone to androgens; it is conceivable that the preferred pathway may depend upon the physiologic circumstances of the moment. Moreover, there appear to be significant variations between species; the rat has been studied in the greatest detail. The details of the individual microsomal enzymes have been documented previously.[15]

An important start in approaching the problem of organization of the microsomal enzymes has been taken by Samuels and his colleagues, who have reported that various steroids distribute themselves in vitro between medium and microsomes in different proportions.[39,41] For example, whereas 17α-hydroxyprogesterone appears to diffuse freely between medium and microsomes, progesterone is selectively concentrated in microsomes. The microsomal membrane is evidently complex, and the ability of exogenous steroids to serve as precursors of androgens is influenced by their relative partitions between medium and microsomes. Studies in which two intermediates, labeled with different isotopes, are compared as precursors of testosterone by measuring the isotope ratio in this steroid will remain difficult to interpret until such differences in partition are better understood.

By comparing the ratio of two isotopes in the medium with the same ratio in the androgens and in 17α-hydroxyprogesterone, it is possible to develop some understanding of microsomal organization. For example, the ratio of isotope from progesterone to isotope from 17α-hydroxyprogesterone in androstenedione is much higher than the same ratio in microsomal 17α-hydroxyprogesterone, but it is significantly lower than the ratio for microsomal progesterone plus 17α-hydroxyprogesterone.[40] The first observation tells us that progesterone is converted to androgens by a pathway that does not equilibrate with exogenous 17α-hydroxyprogesterone. However, it is known that there is no pathway from progesterone to androgens except via 17α-hydroxyprogesterone.[40,42,43] The second observation shows that exogenous 17α-hydroxyprogesterone does, however, mix to some extent with the 17α-hydroxyprogesterone formed in the microsomes by the 17α-hydroxylase. The two enzymes 17α-hydroxylase and lyase must be closely associated in the microsomes—sufficiently to limit exchange, yet not so perfectly sealed as to prevent some exchange from taking place. On the other hand, the isotope ratio for testosterone equilibrates with that in androstenedione after a lag of 15–30 min. Since in such studies the only source of testosterone is androstenedione, any significant delay in equilibration reflects mixing between androstenedione formed from two sources (i.e., the two exogenous labeled substrates progesterone and 17α-hydroxyprogesterone). This delay results from the fact that at first 17α-hydroxyprogesterone has a start of one enzyme reaction on the progesterone. The subsequent equilibration means that the androstenediones from the two sources must mix before they are converted to testosterone by the 17β-hydroxysteroid dehydrogenase. This in turn means that this enzyme is separated from the active sites of the two previous enzymes in such a way as to permit such mixing (Fig. 119-5). These studies also showed that 17α-hydroxyprogesterone and the two androgens distribute themselves between microsomes and cytosol by diffusion, in contrast to progesterone, which is selectively concentrated in microsomes.[39,40]

It is clear that we are only beginning to understand the details of the microsomal steroidogenic enzymes. Although the relevant experiments are conceptually difficult, the next step to better understanding of steroidogenesis will require extension of these investigations.

SECRETION OF TESTICULAR ANDROGENS

Testosterone formed by microsomal enzymes must find its way to the venous effluent outside the cell. Nothing is known about this process, and attention is called to secretion of androgens because it appears to need investigation. One might ask whether secretion is regulated at all. It appears that in the adrenal stores of cortisol are not held in preparation for secretion;[44] this suggests that regulation of plasma cortisol is secured only by changes in the rate of steroid synthesis. It may be that we are ignorant of important sources of regulation. Whether regulated or not, the movement of testosterone from endoplasmic reticulum to plasma membrane requires some explanation. Apart from the possibility that lipid droplets are involved in this process,[8] no suggestions have appeared.

TESTICULAR ESTROGENS

Plasma and urine of adult men contain estrogens, and a number of studies have suggested that the testis is the source of some of these compounds. In measuring secretion rates by dilution of infused radioactive hormones, it is possible, with the aid of reasonable assumptions, to determine the origin of certain hormones that

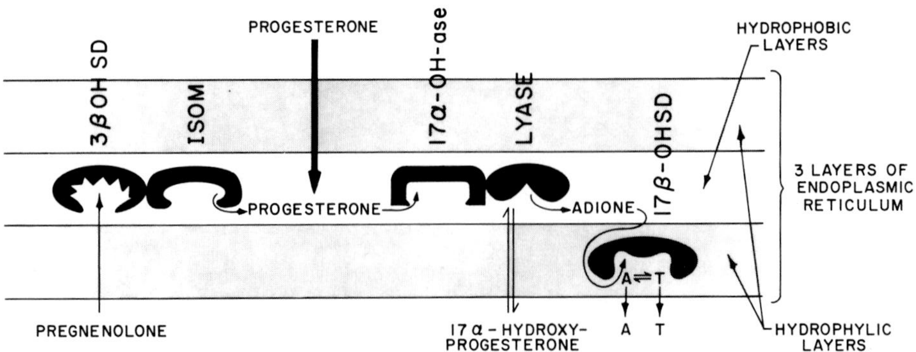

Fig. 119-5. Possible scheme for androgen biosynthesis in testicular microsomes. The membrane is shown as horizontal, which may be the case in the cell; in microsomal preparations, however, it forms vesicles. See text for details and the legend to Figure 119-3 for abbreviations.

are formed in part by conversion from other steroids (reviewed by Eik-Nes and Hall[1]). This approach was used by Fishman and colleagues to show that although a healthy adult man may produce approximately 65 μg of estradiol per day, as much as one-third of this may result from peripheral conversion of testosterone and androstenedione.[45] In another study, peripheral conversion was said to account for more than 95 percent of plasma estrogens in man.[46] However, direct evidence for secretion of estrone and estradiol has been provided by other workers in man[47] and in the rat.[48] It has been reported that secretion of estradiol is increased by human chorionic gonadotropin (HCG) if administered for a period of several days.[46,48]

The biosynthetic pathway to testicular estrogens is not known in detail, but ^{14}C-acetate was converted to ^{14}C-estrone and ^{14}C-estradiol in a stallion previously prepared by injection of HCG.[49] It appears that in the boar dehydroepiandrosterone is an intermediate in the synthesis of estrogens.[50]

Finally, the source of testicular estrogens has not been entirely resolved. Earlier evidence (reviewed by Dorrington and Fritz[51]) left the impression that the Leydig cells are the major source of these steroids but that Sertoli cells may contribute. A more recent study, in which tubules were separated from Leydig cells, suggests that seminiferous tubules are capable of estrogen synthesis and that the tubular estrogens are conveyed to Leydig cells.[52] Estrogen receptors have been found in Leydig cells.[53,54]

The functions of estrogens in the male remain obscure. However, these compounds may stimulate the male breast at puberty[55] and may play a role in regulating the secretion of follicle-stimulating hormone (FSH) in the male.[56] It has been proposed that androgens may be converted to estrogens in the brain and that it is the estrogen which promotes male copulatory behavior.[57] Perhaps plasma estrogens have undiscovered effects in the male.

STEROID SULFATES

Adrenal tissue, both normal and malignant, appears to secrete steroid sulfates.[58] Moreover, since cholesterol sulfate has been isolated from normal bovine adrenal cortex,[59] and since mitochondrial enzyme systems are capable of converting cholesterol sulfate to pregnenolone sulfate,[60–62] an all-sulfate pathway for the synthesis of steroid sulfates appears to be available in the adrenal. Whether there is a special cytochrome P-450 for cleavage of cholesterol sulfate or whether the two substrates (free and sulfated) share one enzyme system is not certain.[63,64] Kinetic evidence suggests that there must be more than one enzyme in beef adrenal cortex.[64]

Use of the sulfate pathway in the testis is less clear. Young and Hall found incorporation of small amounts of ^{14}C-acetate into ^{14}C-cholesterol sulfate[65] in rabbit testis. Cholesterol sulfate has been isolated from human testis.[66] However, the source of cholesterol sulfate in the rat has proved elusive.[67] Histochemical evidence suggests that there may be two distinct enzyme systems in the Leydig cells of the rat—one for free steroids and one for sulfates.[68] Although the evidence is not complete, the production of androgen sulfates by the testes of species so far examined does not appear to be of major importance. However, it is known that free steroids inhibit steroid sulfatase activity.[69–71] A number of workers have attempted to advance the case that steroid sulfates provide a source of biosynthetic intermediates which is consumed when free steroid levels decline because such decline relieves the testicular sulfatase of inhibition produced by free steroids.[69–71] The sulfatase does not, however, appear to be under gonadotropic regulation;[72] the importance of this inhibition of the sulfatase is uncertain.

Estrone sulfate is a major circulating estrogen in adult humans of both sexes.[73] This steroid appears to arise by peripheral metabolism of estrone and estradiol.[73]

REGULATION OF TESTICULAR STEROIDOGENESIS

INTRODUCTION

The normal production of testicular androgens requires the pituitary gland, which increases this production by providing the protein hormone, luteinizing hormone (LH).[74] This hormone acts directly on testicular tissue in vitro,[75,76] and when administered in vivo it produces increased plasma levels of androgens.[77,78] Early studies were performed with the placental gonadotropin of man (HCG) because this was readily available; however, the two hormones appear to exert the same qualitative effects on the testis.

There is no evidence to show that LH promotes increased secretion as opposed to or in addition to increased production of androgens, but too little is known about secretion of steroids to exclude that important possibility. Finally, the mechanism of action of LH has been studied in the testis and ovary of a variety of species and in feather follicles of certain birds, in which this hormone promotes the synthesis of melanin.[79,80] In addition, it would appear that the action of ACTH upon adrenal cells has much in common with the action of LH upon the testis. For technical reasons, progress with ACTH has been, at least in some respects, more rapid than with LH. There are also certain advantages to studying the action of LH upon steroidogenesis in the corpus luteum. In the following discussion reference will be made to these various systems in order to develop a useful account of the regulation of steroid synthesis in the testis.

When slices of rabbit testis are incubated with ^{14}C-acetate[75,76] or with ^{3}H-cholesterol,[81] addition of LH increases the rate of incorporation of either ^{14}C or ^{3}H into various androgens. When cholesterol is used as substrate, preparations of high specific activity must be used because there are large amounts of endogenous (unlabeled) cholesterol within the organ—hence the use of ^{3}H as opposed to ^{14}C. When LH is added to preparations of rat testis in vitro without exogenous substrate, the production of testosterone is increased from endogenous precursors;[82] clearly, LH causes a net increase in androgen production, and the studies with ^{14}C and ^{3}H mentioned above are not merely the result of changes in pool sizes producing the same amount of androgen of higher specific activity. These considerations pose two problems: where in the biosynthetic pathway does LH act, and how does it stimulate the step or steps which respond? As we learn more about the complex processes involved, these two questions seem to converge.

SITE OF ACTION OF LH ON STEROIDOGENESIS

Evidence from a number of early studies revealed that LH stimulates steroidogenesis beyond cholesterol but before pregnenolone.[74–88] It may be that under certain conditions, e.g., prolonged administration of the hormone, it may exert additional effects before cholesterol.[89] However, under most circumstances the acute response to trophic stimulation appears to result from an increase in the mitochondrial reactions that result in the formation of pregnenolone. Pregnenolone is a common intermediate in the formation of steroid hormones, to which it is converted by enzymatic reactions that are inherently fast; it is consistent with current views on the regulation of biochemical pathways that regulation is exerted upon slow steps in such pathways—it would seem unreasonable to stimulate reactions that are already proceeding rapidly. The question then, is how does LH stimulate side-chain cleavage of cholesterol?

MECHANISM OF ACTION OF LH

LH makes contact with the target cell by way of a receptor that has been solubilized and studied by various physical methods.[90,91] An analogous receptor from corpus luteum has also been isolated.[92,93] The results of these investigations reveal that the receptor includes essential phospholipids[94] and that binding is not influenced by Ca^{2+}.[93] A beginning has been made in understanding the chemical basis of the complex interaction between the two subunits of LH and the testicular receptor.[95,96] Enthusiasm for receptor biochemistry has led to a curious development in this field, i.e., the tacit assumption that all the effects of LH result from combination with the receptor. This may only mean that insufficient interest has been given to additional possibilities. Indirect evidence suggests that LH may enter target cells, but nothing more is known about the consequences of such entry (reviewed by Rao[97]).

It is believed that the most important consequence of combination between LH and the receptor is an increase in intracellular levels of cAMP. It is known that LH increases levels of the cyclic nucleotide in testis[98] and corpus luteum[99] and that cAMP increases steroidogenesis in both tissues.[100,101] Presumably, Leydig cells provide another example of the second messenger role of cAMP. In that case, cAMP must be capable of stimulating side-chain cleavage (directly or indirectly).

The mechanism by which LH stimulates steroidogenesis remains unknown. It is not certain (although it is commonly believed) that all the effects of LH are exerted through cAMP. The action of LH and cAMP upon the Leydig cell involves enhanced protein synthesis, and by analogy with the adrenal, at least some of the newly synthesized protein is likely to function as a specific protein concerned with the transport of cholesterol from cytoplasm to mitochondria.[102] There is no doubt that LH and cAMP stimulate incorporation of amino acids into Leydig cell protein[103] and increase translation of stable mRNA.[104,105] In the adrenal it has been proposed that ACTH increases transport of cholesterol to mitochondria by affecting contractile microfilaments.[106] Directly or indirectly the hormone accelerates side-chain cleavage of cholesterol. Efforts to establish increased production of TPNH as the mechanism of this acceleration have not been convincing, although negative evidence on this point must be discounted.[107,108]

The most promising leads concerning the mechanism of action of LH in short-term enhancement of steroidogenesis can be summarized by saying that the hormone causes an increase in cellular cAMP (perhaps a special pool of this nucleotide). cAMP increases synthesis of a protein of short half-life, which in some way facilitates combination between cholesterol and side-chain cleavage P-450. Whether this effect results in the movement of cholesterol to mitochondria[106] or some change within mitochondria cannot be determined at this time.[109,110]

Since LH appears to play an important part in the development and differentiation of Leydig cells at puberty, it is to be expected that this hormone exerts long-term effects on these cells. So far we have considered acute effects, i.e., responses seen within 1 h after addition or administration of the hormone. Responses requiring hours and days include increases in enzyme activities in addition to side-chain cleavage. For example, Samuels and Helmreich observed an increase in the activity of testicular 3β-hydroxysteroid dehydrogenase within 48 h of a single injection of HCG in mature rats.[111] Since this change was accompanied by an increase in the weight of the testis, it is likely that it is part of a general increase in protein biosynthesis.[111]

Shikita and Hall found that within 48 h of a single injection of HCG three microsomal enzyme activities increased (3β-hydroxysteroid dehydrogenase, Δ^4-5α-reductase, and desmolase) in testes from rats aged 20 days.[112] Total microsomal protein was not increased, and the response appeared to be specific for the microsomal enzymes. It was proposed that HCG increased synthesis of pregnenolone, which in turn induced synthesis of the microsomal enzymes much as hepatic microsomes respond to administration of certain drugs.[113] The increase in 5α-reductase may be important in view of what was said above about 5α-dihydrotestosterone.

Chronic administration of HCG causes an increase in microsomal P-450 of Leydig cells and an increase in the activity of 17α-hydroxylase.[114] As expected, such treatment also causes an increase in conversion of pregnenolone to testosterone. Other testicular enzymes have been reported to respond to HCG.[115]

AGE AS A FACTOR IN THE RESPONSE TO LH

The response of microsomal enzymes in testis to HCG described above was observed in rats aged 20 days at the start of the experiment, but not in rats aged 22 days or older.[111] The enzyme activities are high in older rats, and mature rats respond to HCG following hypophysectomy.[116] These findings suggest that the enzymes of the mature rat are under maximal stimulation from endogenous gonadotropins. Again, the effect of LH in vitro upon conversion of ^{3}H-cholesterol to ^{3}H-testosterone is greater at 20 days of age than in older animals.[117] This difference may again be due to endogenous LH and to the extent to which the enzyme systems are developed in the growing rat. In the rat, twenty days seems to be a significant age for testicular development. For example, testis from rats aged 20 days is stimulated by FSH but not by glucose, whereas the opposite is true for the mature testis.[118,119] Perhaps there is a balance between the intensity and duration of stimulation by endogenous gonadotropin on the one hand and stage of development of testicular enzymes on the other hand. At 20 days the enzymes may be ready to respond, but endogenous gonadotropin may not be secreted in such concentrations as to secure maximal activity.

MISCELLANEOUS ACTIONS OF LH

LH exerts a number of effects which are likely to be related to its principal action on the testis. The following are the most important of these actions: (1) decrease in ovarian ascorbic acid;[120] (2) increase in synthesis of Leydig cell phospholipids;[121,122] and (3) a variety of extragonadal effects reviewed previously.[15]

OTHER FACTORS INVOLVED IN THE REGULATION OF ANDROGEN SYNTHESIS

In hypophysectomized animals, the output of testicular androgens falls to low levels, and without LH there does not appear to be any physiologic mechanism to enhance production of these hormones. To what extent other pituitary hormones may be necessary for the normal response to LH we cannot say. It would not be unreasonable to consider that growth hormone, thyroid hormone, etc. may play important roles in permitting the full effect of LH without being active alone, but there is no evidence to support such an idea. Prolactin has been considered a possible synergist for LH,[123,124] but the physiologic importance of such effects is not clear.

One proposed regulatory mechanism deserves mention. The enzyme 20α-hydroxysteroid dehydrogenase competes with the C_{17}–C_{20} lyase for 17α-hydroxyprogesterone, which it converts to the inactive steroid 17α-hydroxy-20α-dihydroprogesterone.[125] This competition would divert substrate from the androgen pathway and thereby limit the production of these hormones. It is interesting that the 20α-dehydrogenase is very active in testes from young rats and the activity of the analogous enzyme in the ovary is decreased by administration of LH.[126] Such a regulatory device involves competition between a cytoplasmic (dehydrogenase) and a microsomal enzyme (lyase). We know nothing of how this competition would occur within the architectural restraints of the intact cell, nor is it easy to interpret the finding that Sertoli cells are active in 20α-reduction.[127]

Similar phenomena which have been developed into proposed regulatory devices include inhibition of C_{17}–C_{20} lyase by 5α-reduced C_{21} steroids (e.g., 5α-pregnane-3,20-dione).[128] Here we see the 5α-reductase as a potential inhibitor of the synthesis of testosterone and androstenedione. The possible role of sulfatase in the regulation of testicular steroidogenesis was mentioned above.

REFERENCES

1. Eik-Nes, K. B., and Hall, P. F. Secretion of steroid hormones *in vivo*. *Vitam. Horm. 23:* 153, 1965.
2. Pazzagli, M., Borelli, D., Forti, G., and Serio, M. Dihydrotestosterone in human spermatic venous plasma. *Acta Endocrinol. (Kbh.) 76:* 388, 1974.
3. Tremblay, R. R., Forest, M. G., Shalf, J., et al.: Studies on the dynamics of plasma androgens and on the origin of dihydrotestosterone in dogs. *J. Clin. Endocrinol. Metab. 91:* 556, 1972.
4. Folman, Y., Haltmeyer, G. C., and Eik-Nes, K. B. Production and secretion of 5α-dihydrotestosterone by the dog testis. *Am. J. Physiol. 222:* 653, 1972.
5. Ewing, L., Brown, B., Irby, D. C., and Jardine, I. Testosterone and 5α-reduced androgen secretion by rabbit testes—epididymides perfused *in vitro*. *Endocrinology 96:* 610, 1975.
6. Jeffcoate, W. J., and Short, R. V. Dihydrotestosterone in testicular tissue and its androgenic potency *in vivo*. *J. Endocrinol. 48:* 199, 1970.
7. Robel, P., Corpechot, C., and Baulieu, E. E. Testosterone and androstanolone in rat plasma and tissues. *FEBS Lett 33:* 218, 1973.
8. Christensen, A. K. Leydig Cells. In Hamilton, D. W., and Greep, R. O. (eds): *Handbook of Physiology,* section 7, vol. 5. Washington, D.C., American Physiological Society. 1975, p. 57.
9. Hall, P. F., Irby, D. C., and De Kretser, D. M. Conversion of cholesterol to androgens by rat testis: comparison of interstitial cells and seminiferous tubules. *Endocrinology 84:* 488, 1969.
10. Christensen, A. K., and Mason, N. R. Comparative ability of seminiferous tubules and interstitial tissue of rat testis to synthesize androgens from progesterone-4-^{14}C *in vitro*. *Endocrinology 76:* 646, 1965.
11. Cooke, B. A., De Jong, F. H., van der Molen, H. J., and Rommerts, F. F. G. Endogenous testosterone concentrations in rat testis interstitial tissue and seminiferous tubules during *in vitro* incubation. *Nature [New Biol] 237:* 255, 1972.
12. van der Vusse, G. J., Kalkman, M. L., and van der Molen, H. J. Endogenous production of steroids by subcellular fractions from total rat testis and from isolated interstitial tissue and seminiferous tubules. *Biochim. Biophys. Acta 297:* 179, 1973.
13. van der Vusse, G. J., Kalkman, M. L., and van der Molen, H. J. 3β-Hydroxysteroid dehydrogenase in rat testis tissue. Inter- and subcellular localization and inhibition by cyanoketone and nagarase. *Biochim. Biophys. Acta 348:* 404, 1974.
14. Samuels, L. T. Metabolism of steroid hormones. In Greenberg, D. M. (ed): *Metabolic Pathways,* vol. I, 2nd ed. New York, Academic, 1960, p. 431.
15. Hall, P. F. Gonadotrophic regulation of testicular function. In Eik-Nes, K. B. (ed): *The Androgens of the Testis*. New York, Marcel Dekker, 1970, p. 73.
16. Halkerston, I. D. K., Eichhorn, J., and Hechter, O. A requirement for reduced triphosphopyridine nucleotide for cholesterol side-chain cleavage by mitochondrial fractions of bovine andrenal cortex. *J. Biol. Chem. 236:* 374, 1961.
17. Tamaoki, B. I., and Pincus, G. Biogenesis of progesterone in ovarian tissues. *Endocrinology 69:* 527, 1961.
18. Hall, P. F., and Koritz, S. B. The conversion of cholesterol and 20α-hydroxycholesterol to steroids by acetone powder of particles from bovine corpus luteum. *Biochemistry 3:* 129, 1964.
19. Toren, D., Menon, K. M. J., Forchielli, E., and Dorfman, R. I. *In vitro* enzymatic cleavage of the cholesterol side-chain in rat testis preparations. *Steroids 3:* 381, 1964.
20. Meigs, R. W., and Ryan, K. J. Cytochrome P-450 and steroid biosynthesis in the human placenta. *Biochim. Biophys. Acta 165:* 476, 1968.
21. Shimizu, K., Dorfman, R. I., and Gut, M. Isocaproic acid, a metabolite of 20α-hydroxycholesterol. *J. Biol. Chem. 235:* PC 25, 1960.
22. Constantopoulos, G., and Tchen, T. T. Cleavage of cholesterol side-chain of adrenal cortex. I. Cofactor requirement and product of cleavage. *J. Biol. Chem. 236:* 65, 1961.
23. Shimizu, K., Gut, M., and Dorfman, R. I. The transformation of 20α-hydroxycholesterol to isocaproic acid and C_{21} steroids. *J. Biol. Chem. 236:* 695, 1961.
24. Omura, T., Sanders, E., Estabrook, R. W., Cooper, D. Y., and Rosenthal, O. Isolation from adrenal cortex of a nonheme iron protein and a flavoprotein functional as a reduced triphosphopyridine nucleotide-cytochrome P-450 reductase. *Arch. Biochem. Biophys. 117:* 660, 1966.
25. Yago, N., and Ichii, S. Submitochondrial distribution of components of the steroid 11β-hydroxylase and cholesterol side-chain-cleaving enzyme systems in hog adrenal cortex. *J. Biochem. 65:* 215, 1969.
26. Yago, N., Kobayashi, S., Sekiyama, S., et al.: Further studies on the submitochondrial localization of cholesterol side-chain-cleaving enzyme system in hog adrenal cortex by sonic treatment. *J. Biochem. 68:* 775, 1970.
27. Koritz, S. B. The energy-linked synthesis of pregnenolone in beef adrenal cortex mitochondria. *Biochem. Biophys. Res. Commun. 23:* 485, 1966.
28. Hall, P. F. Inhibition by hyperbaric oxygen of the conversion of cholesterol to pregnenolone in adrenal mitochondria. *Biochem. Biophys. Res. Commun. 26:* 320, 1967.
29. Hall, P. F. Electron transport in relation to steroid biosynthesis: inhibition of side-chain cleavage of cholesterol by hyperbaric oxygen. *Biochemistry 6:* 2794, 1967.
30. Chance, B., and Hollunger, G. The interaction of energy and electron transfer reactions to mitochondria. I. General properties and nature of the products of succinate-linked reduction of pyridine nucleotide. *J. Biol. Chem. 236:* 1534, 1961.
31. Hall, P. F. A possible role for transhydrogenation in side-chain cleavage of cholesterol. *Biochemistry 11:* 2891, 1972.
32. Klein, K. O., and Harding, B. W. Electron transport reversal and steroid 11β-hydroxylation in adrenal cortical mitochondria. *Biochemistry 9:* 3653, 1970.
33. Simpson, E. R., and Estabrook, R. W. Mitochondrial malic enzyme: the source of reduced nicotinamide adenine dinucleotide phosphate for steroid hydroxylation in bovine adrenal cortex mitochondria. *Arch. Biochem. 129:* 384, 1969.
34. Young, D. G., and Hall, P. F. Steroid hydroxylation in bovine adrenocortical mitochondria. Competition between side-chain cleavage of cholesterol and 11α-hydroxylation. *Biochemistry 10:* 1496, 1971.
35. Shikita, M., Kakizaki, H., and Tamaoki, B. The pathway of formation of testosterone from 3β-hydroxypregn-5-en-20-one by rat testicular microsomes. *Steroids 4:* 521, 1964.
36. Shikita, M., and Tamaoki, B. I. Testosterone formation by subcellular particles of rat testes. *Endocrinology 76:* 563, 1965.
37. Neville, A. M., Orr, J. C., and Engel, L. L. $\Delta^5$3β-Hydroxysteroid dehydrogenase activities of bovine adrenal cortex. *Biochem. J. 107:* 20P, 1968.
38. Ewald, W., Werbin, H., and Chaikoff, I. L. Evidence for two substrate-specific Δ^5-3-ketosteroid isomerases in beef adrenal glands

and their separation from 3β-hydroxysteroid dehydrogenase. *Biochim. Biophys. Acta 81:* 199, 1964.
39. Matsumoto, K., and Samuels, L. T. Influence of steroid distribution between microsomes and soluble fraction on steroid metabolism by microsomal enzymes. *Endocrinology 85:* 402, 1969.
40. Samuels, L. T., and Matsumoto, K. Localization of enzymes involved in testosterone biosynthesis by the mouse testis. *Endocrinology 94:* 55, 1974.
41. Matsumoto, K., Mahajan, D. K., and Samuels, L. T. The influence of progesterone on the conversion of 17α-hydroxyprogesterone to testosterone in the mouse testis. *Endocrinology 94:* 808, 1974.
42. Machino, A., Inano, H., and Tamaoki, B. Studies on enzyme reactions related to steroid biosynthesis I. Presence of the cytochrome P-450 in testicular tissue and its role in the biogenesis of androgens. *J. Steroid Biochem. 1:* 9, 1969.
43. Dominguez, O. V. Biosynthesis of androgens from C_{21}-steroids exhibiting differences in their side-chain. *Steroids 7:* 433, 1966.
44. Saffran, M., Grad, B., and Bayliss, M. J. Production of corticoids by rat adrenals *in vitro. Endocrinology 50:* 639, 1952.
45. Fishman, L. M., Sarfaty, G. A., Wilson, H., and Lipsett, M. B. The role of the testis in oestrogen production. Ciba Found. Colloq. *Endocrinol. 16:* 156, 1967.
46. Weinstein, R. L., Kelch, R. P., Jenner, M. R., Kaplan, S. L. and Grumbach, M. M. Secretion of unconjugated androgens and estrogens by the normal and abnormal human testis before and after human chorionic gonadotropin. *J. Clin. Invest. 53:* 1, 1974.
47. Longcope, C., Widrich, W., and Sawin, C. T. The secretion of estrone and estradiol-17β by human testis. *Steroids 20:* 439, 1972.
48. de Jong, F. H., Hey, A. H., and van der Molen, H. J. Effect of gonadotrophins on the secretion of estradiol-17β and testosterone by the rat testis. *J. Endocrinol. 57:* 277, 1973.
49. Nyman, M. A., Geiger, J., and Goldzieher, J. W. Biosynthesis of estrogen by the perfused stallion testis. *J. Biol. Chem. 234:* 16, 1959.
50. Raeside, J. L. Urinary excretion of dehydroepiandrosterone and oestrogens by the boar. *Acta Endocrinol. (Kbh.) 50:* 611, 1965.
51. Dorrington, J. H. and Fritz, I. B. Metabolism of testosterone by preparations from the rat testis. *Biochem. Biophys. Res. Commun. 54:* 1425, 1973.
52. de Jong, F. H., Hey, A. H., and van der Molen, H. J. Oestradiol-17β and testosterone in rat testis tissue: effect of gonadotrophins, localization and production *in vitro. J. Endocrinol. 60:* 409, 1974.
53. Brinkmann, A. O., Mulder, E., Lamers-Stahlhofen, G. J., Mechielsen, M. J., and van der Molen, H. J. An oestradiol receptor in rat testis interstitial tissue. *FEBS Lett 26:* 301, 1972.
54. Mulder, E., Brinkman, A. O., Lamers-Stahlhofen, G. J., and van der Molen, H. J. Binding of oestradiol by the nuclear fraction of rat testis interstitial tissue. *FEBS Lett 31:* 131, 1973.
55. Hall, P. F. Gynaecomastia. Sydney, Australia, Australian Medical, 1959.
56. Sherins, R. J., and Lorianse, D. L. Studies on the role of sex steroids in the feedback control of FSH concentrations in men. *J. Clin. Endocrinol. Metab. 36:* 866, 1973.
57. Christensen, L. W., and Clemens, L. G. Intrahypothalamic implants of testosterone or estradiol and resumption of masculine sexual behavior in long-term castrated male rats. *Endocrinology 95:* 984, 1974.
58. Roberts, K. D., Bandi, L., Calvin, H. I., Drucker, W. D., and Lieberman, S. Evidence that steroid sulfates serve as biosynthetic intermediates. IV. *Biochemistry 3:* 1983, 1964.
59. Drayer, N. M., Roberts, K. D., Bandi, L., and Lieberman, S. The isolation of cholesterol sulfate from bovine adrenals. *J. Biol. Chem. 239:* PC3112, 1964.
60. Raggatt, P. R., and Whitehouse, M. W. Substrate and inhibitor specificity of the cholesterol oxidase in bovine adrenal cortex. *Biochem. J. 101:* 819, 1966.
61. Roberts, K. D., Bandi, L., and Lieberman, S. The conversion of cholesterol-^{3}H-sulfate-^{35}S into pregnenolone-^{3}H-sulfate-^{35}S by sonicate bovine adrenal mitochondria. *Biochem. Biophys. Res. Commun. 29:* 741, 1967.
62. Young, D. G., and Hall, P. F. Cofactor requirements for the conversion of cholesterol sulfate to pregnenolone sulfate by a submitochondrial system from bovine adrenal cortex. *Biochem. Biophys. Res. Commun. 31:* 925, 1968.
63. Hochberg, R. B., Ladany, S., Welch, M., and Lieberman, S. Cholesterol and cholesterol sulfate as substrates for the adrenal side-chain cleavage enzyme. *Biochemistry 13:* 1938, 1974.
64. Young, D. G., and Hall, P. F. The side-chain cleavage of cholesterol and cholesterol sulfate by enzymes from bovine adrenocortical mitochondria. *Biochemistry 8:* 2987, 1969.
65. Young, D. G., and Hall, P. F. Biosynthesis of cholesterol sulfate by slices of rabbit testis. *Endocrinology 82:* 291, 1968.
66. Laatikainen, T., Laitinen, E. A., and Vihko, R. Secretion of neutral steroid sulfates by the human testis. *J. Clin. Endocrinol. Metab. 29:* 219, 1969.
67. Hochberg, R. B., Ladany, S., and Lieberman, S. Cholesterol sulfate: some aspects of its biosynthesis and uptake by tissues from blood. *Endocrinology 94:* 207, 1974.
68. Baillie, A. H., and Griffiths, K. Further observations on 3β-hydroxysteroid dehydrogenase activity in the mouse Leydig cell. *J. Endocrinol. 31:* 207, 1965.
69. Notation, A. D., and Ungar, F. Regulation of rat testis sulfatase. A kinetic study. *Biochemistry 8:* 501, 1969.
70. Payne, A. H. Gonadal steroid sulfates and sulfatase. V. Human testicular steroid sulfatase. Partial characterization and possible regulation by free steroid. *Biochim. Biophys. Acta 258:* 473, 1972.
71. Ruokonen, A., Laatikainen, T., Laitinen, E. A., and Vihko, R. Free and sulfate-conjugated neutral steroids in human testis tissue. *Biochemistry 11:* 1411, 1972.
72. Notation, A. D., and Ungar, F. Testis steroid sulfatase activity in rats treated with chorionic gonadotrophin. *Endocrinology 90:* 1537, 1972.
73. Ruder, H. J., Loriaux, L., and Lipsett, M. B. Estrone sulfate: production rate and metabolism in man. *J. Clin. Invest. 51:* 1020, 1972.
74. Greep, R. O., and Fevold, H. L. The spermatogenic and secretory function of the gonads of hypophysectomized adult rats treated with pituitary follicle-stimulating hormone and luteinizing hormone. *Endocrinology 21:* 611, 1937.
75. Brady, R. O. Biosynthesis of radioactive testosterone *in vitro. J. Biol. Chem. 193:* 145, 1951.
76. Hall, P. F., and Eik-Nes, K. B. The action of gonadotrophic hormones upon rabbit testis *in vitro. Biochim. Biophys. Acta 63:* 411, 1962.
77. Brinck-Johnsen, T., and Eik-Nes, K. B. Effect of human gonadotrophin on the secretion of testosterone and 4-androstene-3, 17-dione by the canine testis. *Endocrinology 61:* 676, 1957.
78. Eik-Nes, K. B. Production and secretion of testicular steroids. *Recent Prog. Horm. Res. 27:* 517, 1971.
79. Witschi, E. Sex and secondary sexual characters. In Marshall, A. J. (ed): *Biology and Comparative Physiology of Birds,* vol. 2. New York, Academic, 1961, p. 115.
80. Hall, P. F., and Okazaki, K. The action of interstitial cell-stimulating hormone upon avian tyrosinase. *Biochemistry 5:* 1202, 1966.
81. Hall, P. F. On the stimulation of testicular steroidogenesis in the rabbit by interstitial cell-stimulating hormone. *Endocrinology 78:* 690, 1966.
82. Catt, K. J., Watanabe, K., and Dufau, M. L. Cyclic AMP released by rat testis during gonadotrophin stimulation *in vitro. Nature 239:* 280, 1972.
83. Long, C. H. N. The relation of cholesterol and ascorbic acid to secretion of adrenal cortex. *Recent Progr. Horm. Res. 1:* 99, 1947.
84. Péron, F. G., and Koritz, S. B. On the location of the stimulation *in vitro* by Ca^{++} and freezing of corticoid production by rat adrenal homogenates. *J. Biol. Chem. 235:* 1625, 1960.
85. Bell, E. T., Mukerji, S., and Loraine, J. A. A new bioassay method of luteinizing hormone depending on the depletion of rat ovarian cholesterol. *J. Endocrinol. 28:* 321, 1964.
86. Hall, P. F. The effect of interstitial-cell-stimulating hormone on the biosynthesis of testicular cholesterol from acetate-1-C^{14}. *Biochemistry 2:* 1232, 1963.
87. Hall, P. F., and Koritz, S. B. Influence of interstitial-cell-stimulating hormone on the conversion of cholesterol to progesterone by bovine corpus luteum. *Biochemistry 4:* 1037, 1965.
88. Koritz, S. B., and Hall, P. F. Further studies on the locus of action of interstitial-cell-stimulating hormone on the biosynthesis of progesterone by bovine corpus luteum. *Biochemistry 4:* 2740, 1965.
89. Morris, P. W., and Gorski, J. Control of steroidogenesis in preovulatory cells. Luteinizing hormone stimulation of [^{14}C] acetate incorporation into sterols. *J. Biol. Chem. 248:* 6920, 1973.
90. Dufau, M. L., Charreau, E. H., and Catt, K. J. Characteristics of a soluble gonadotropin receptor from the rat testis. *J. Biol. Chem. 248:* 6973, 1973.

91. Frowein, J., and Engel, W. Binding of human chorionic gonadotrophin by rat testis: effect of sexual maturation, cryptorchidism and hypophysectomy. *J. Endocrinol. 64:* 59, 1975.
92. Lee, C. Y., and Ryan, R. J. Luteinizing hormone receptors: specific binding of human luteinizing hormone to homogenates of luteinized rat ovaries. *Proc. Natl. Acad. Sci. USA 69:* 3520, 1972.
93. Gospodarowicz, D. Properties of the luteinizing hormone receptor of isolated corpus luteum plasma membranes. *J. Biol. Chem. 248:* 5042, 1973.
94. Haour, F., and Saxena, B. B. Characterization and solubilization of gonadotropin receptor of bovine corpus luteum. *J. Biol. Chem. 249:* 2195, 1974.
95. Lim, W., Yang, K., Burleigh, B. D., and Ward, D. N. Functional groups in ovine luteinizing hormone and their receptor site interactions—a chemical study. In Dufau, M. L., and Means, A. R. (eds): *Current Topics in Molecular Endocrinology,* vol. 1. New York, Plenum, 1974, p. 89.
96. Bhalla, V. K., and Reichert, L. E., Jr. Gonadotropin receptors in rat testes. *J. Biol. Chem. 249:* 7996, 1974.
97. Rao, Ch. V. Properties of gonadotropin receptors in the cell membrane of bovine corpus luteum. *J. Biol. Chem. 249:* 2864, 1974.
98. Murad, F., Strauch, B. S., and Vaughan, M. The effect of gonadotropins on testicular adenyl cyclase. *Biochim. Biophys. Acta 177:* 591, 1969.
99. Marsh, J. M., Butcher, R. W., Savard, K., and Sutherland, E. W. The stimulating effect of luteinizing hormone on adenosine-3′-5′monophosphate accumulation in corpus luteum slices. *J. Biol. Chem. 241:* 5436, 1966.
100. Sandler, R., and Hall, P. F. Stimulation *in vitro* by adenosine-3′-5′-cyclic monophosphate of steroidogenesis in rat testis. *Endocrinology 79:* 647, 1966.
101. Marsh, J. M., and Savard, K. The stimulation of progesterone synthesis in bovine corpora lutea by adenosine-3′-5′-monophosphate. *Steroids 8:* 133, 1966.
102. Garren, L. D., Ney, R. L., and Davis, W. W. Studies on the role of protein synthesis in the regulation of corticosterone production by adrenocorticotropic hormone *in vivo. Proc. Natl. Acad. Sci. USA* 53: 1443, 1965.
103. Irby, D. C., and Hall, P. F. Stimulation by ICSH of protein biosynthesis in isolated Leydig cells from hypophysectomized rats. *Endocrinology* 89: 1367, 1971.
104. Lieberman, M. E., Barnea, A., Bauminger, S., et al.: LH effect on the pattern of steroidogenesis in cultured Graafian follicles of the rat: Dependence on macromolecular synthesis. *Endocrinology* 96: 1533, 1975.
105. Younglar, E. V. Steroid production by the isolated rabbit ovarian follicle. III. Actinomycin D-insensitive stimulation of steroidogenesis by luteinizing hormone. *Endocrinology* 96: 468, 1975.
106. Mrotek, J. J., and Hall, P. F. The influence of cytochalasin B on the response of adrenal tumor cells to ACTH and cyclic AMP. *Biochem. Biophys. Res. Commun.* 64: 891, 1975.
111. Samuels, L. T., and Helmreich, M. L. The influence of chorionic gonadotrophin on the 3β-ol-dehydrogenase activity of testes and adrenals. *Endocrinology 58:* 435, 1956.
112. Shikita, M., and Hall, P. F. The action of human chorionic gonadotrophin *in vivo* upon microsomal enzymes of immature rat testis. *Biochim. Biophys. Acta 136:* 484, 1967.
113. Ernster, L., and Orrenius, S. Substrate-induced synthesis of the hydroxylating enzyme system of liver microsomes. *Fed. Proc. 24:* 1191, 1965.
114. Menard, R. H., and Purvis, J. L. Stimulation of the levels of cytochrome P-450 and 17α-hydroxylase in chick testis microsomes by pituitary hormones. *Endocrinology 91:* 1506, 1972.
115. Frowein, J. Effect of human chorionic gonadotrophin on testicular 5α-androstane-3β-hydroxysteroid dehydrogenase, 3β-hydroxy-dehydroepiandrosterone dehydrogenase and alcohol dehydrogenase of immature rats. *J. Endocrinol. 57:* 437, 1973.
116. Shikita, M., and Hall, P. F. Action of human chorionic gonadotrophin *in vivo* upon microsomal enzymes in testes of hypophysectomized rats. *Biochim. Biophys. Acta 141:* 433, 1967.
117. Sandler, R., and Hall, P. F. The influence of age upon the response of rat testis to interstitial cell-stimulating hormone *in vitro. Biochim. Biophys. Acta 164:* 445, 1968.
118. Means, A. R., and Hall, P. F. Effect of FSH on protein biosynthesis in testes of the immature rat. *Endocrinology 81:* 1151, 1967.
119. Means, A. R., and Hall, P. F. Protein biosynthesis in the testis. I. Comparison between stimulation by FSH and glucose. *Endocrinology 82:* 597, 1968.
120. McCann, S. M., and Taleisnik, S. Effect of luteinizing hormone and vasopressin on ovarian ascorbic acid. *Am. J. Physiol. 199:* 847, 1960.
121. Yokoe, Y., and Hall, P. F. Testicular phospholipids: II. Action of interstitial cell-stimulating hormone (ICSH) upon testicular phospholipids in hypophysectomized rats. *Endocrinology 86:* 1257, 1970.
122. Yokoe, Y., Irby, D. C., and Hall, P. F. Testicular phospholipids. III. Site of action of ICSH in testis following regression of the germinal epithelium. *Endocrinology 88:* 195, 1971.
123. Hafiez, A. A., Bartke, A., and Lloyd, C. W. The role of prolactin in the regulation of testis function: The synergistic effects of prolactin and luteinizing hormone on the incorporation of [1-^{14}C] acetate into testosterone and cholesterol by testes from hypophysectomized rats *in vitro. J. Endocrinol. 53:* 223, 1972.
124. Hafiez, A. A., Lloyd, C. W., and Bartke, A. The role of prolactin in the regulation of testis function: the effect of prolactin and luteinizing hormone on the plasma levels of testosterone and androstenedione in hypophysectomized rats. *J. Endocrinol. 52:* 327, 1972.
125. Inano, H., Egusa, M., and Tamaoki, B. Studies on enzymes related to steroidogenesis in testicular tissue of guinea pig. *Biochim. Biophys. Acta 144:* 165, 1967.
126. Inano, H., and Tamaoki, B. I. Bioconversion of steroids in immature rat testes *in vitro. Endocrinology 79:* 579, 1966.
127. Collins, P., and Lacy, D. Studies on the structure and function of the mammalian testis. IV. Steroid metabolism *in vitro* by isolated interstitium and seminiferous tubules of rat testis after heat sterilization. *Proc. R. Soc. Lond. Biol. 186:* 37, 1974.
128. Brophy, P. J., and Gower, D. B. Studies on the inhibition by 5α-pregnane-3, 20-dione of the biosynthesis of 16-androstenes and dehydroepiandrosterone in boar testis preparations. *Biochim. Biophys. Acta 360:* 252, 1974.

120

Testicular Steroid Secretions, Transport, and Metabolism

Richard Horton

STEROID SECRETIONS

Testosterone is clearly the major steroid secretion of the normal adult testis both in terms of amount and biologic activity. In men, the secretion rate of testosterone, calculated from the arteriovenous gradient and estimated blood flow or by other techniques to be discussed, is about 5 mg/day.[1,2] Castration or destruction of the Leydig cells reduces this figure to a very low value, the result of negligible contributions from the remaining adrenals.

A number of other steroids are also secreted or released by the testis, although their biologic significance is not clear. They may be useful as markers for biosynthetic disorders or as additional parameters for evaluating the endocrine function of the testis, but as yet there is minimal data on the secretory status of these other steroids in most disease states.

Among the other steroids secreted by the testis, perhaps the most important is estradiol. The adult testis secretes 10–15 μg/day of this potent estrogen,[3] which accounts for only 20–25 percent of the total estradiol in male blood; the remainder is the product of peripheral aromatization of androgens. Gonadotropins, in the form of luteinizing hormone or chorionic gonadotropin initially increase both testosterone and estradiol, but continued stimulation over a few days results in further testosterone secretion without a greater rise in estradiol, suggesting that the ability of the Leydig cell to aromatize testosterone is limited.[1] Although the overall function of circulating estrogens in man is a mystery, estradiol appears to play a potential role in regulation of gonadotropins via a feedback mechanism.

In addition to testosterone the testis also secretes dihydrotestosterone, the A-ring reduced form of testosterone. This steroid androgen is 1½–2 times as potent as testosterone. Recent evidence indicates that 50–100 μg/day is secreted directly,[4,5] although most dihydrotestosterone in the circulation is from other sources. Both the Leydig cell and seminiferous tubules may be testicular sources for this androgen since there is in vitro evidence that the tubules metabolize testosterone via the enzyme 5α-reductase.[6]

A number of other steroids that are involved in the biosynthesis of testosterone and estradiol are also released or "secreted" by the testis. These compounds include pregnenolone, progesterone, 17α-hydroxypregnenolone, dehydroisoandrosterone, and androstenedione.[7] Another potential precursor, 17α-hydroxyprogesterone, is secreted in amounts (1–2 mg/day) inappropriate to its expected precursor status, suggesting additional biosynthetic relationships.[8] Despite the evidence that this steroid is the second major secretion product of the testes, no information is available to explain its function. The major source in peripheral blood of androstenedione and dehydroisoandrosterone, which are biologically weak androgens, is the andrenal cortex.

STEROID DYNAMICS

In most cases, hormones in blood are kept relatively constant because the ratio between their secretion (S) and disposal (D) rates is rather fixed:[9] $i = S/D$, where i is the concentration in plasma.

The entry of a substance into the circulation can be simulated by infusion of a tracer amount of the compound. A useful approach to determining the removal rate has been the metabolic clearance rate (MCR), defined by Tait and colleagues as the apparent volume of whole blood or plasma from which a substance is completely and irreversibly removed per unit time.[10]

The MCR in blood is determined either by a single injection or by constant infusion of isotopically labeled tracer amounts of the substance. The latter approach is preferred since sampling is simplified and proof of attaining a steady state (equilibrium) can be obtained (Fig. 120-1). The MCR is usually calculated from R/r, where R is the infusion rate and r the concentration of the purified substance from blood (plasma) in a liter. The MCR is usually expressed in liters/day/m.² Considerable insight into various in vivo metabolic processes can be derived or inferred from the MCR since

$$\begin{aligned}\text{MCR} &= \mathfrak{L}\ \text{Organ clearances}\\ &= \text{Splanchnic} + \text{Extrahepatic clearance}\\ &= \text{Hepatic blood flow} \times \text{Hepatic extraction}\\ &\qquad + \text{Extrahepatic clearance}\end{aligned}$$

This is an important consideration as the liver is a major site of steroid metabolism and removal. When the MCR of various steroid hormones such as cortisol and aldosterone are compared, there is a close relationship between hormone binding in plasma and the hepatic extraction and MCR. Cortisol bound to transcortin has an MCR of about 200 liters/day. Aldosterone is cleared much faster, at a rate of 1600 liters/day. The MCR of testosterone in men is about 1000 liters/day, and as hepatic blood flow is normally about 1500 liters/day, this suggests that hepatic extraction of testosterone

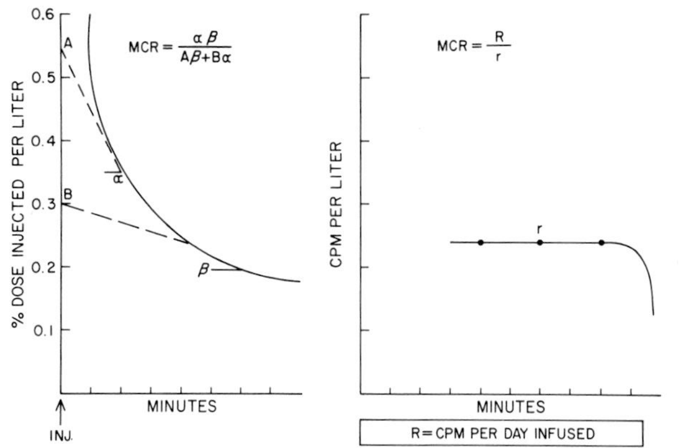

Fig. 120-1. Estimation of the metabolic clearance rate (MCR) by either single injection or constant infusion using a tracer dose of a labeled compound.

is less than unity and that testosterone is bound to a nondiffusible molecule in plasma to some degree. This binding has been confirmed directly.

As $i = S/\text{MCR}$ and $S = i \times \text{MCR}$, the secretion rate of testosterone or any substance can be determined if the mean concentration and the MCR can be determined. The calculated secretion rate of testosterone was established in this way as 6 (4–8) mg/day, which is in close agreement with the product of the testicular afferent–efferent gradient and blood flow. Direct measurement of the hepatic extraction ($HE^T = 0.68$) suggests that a considerable fraction of the overall testosterone clearance (metabolism) occurs in extrasplanchnic tissue.[11] These sites potentially include such target tissues as muscle and sexual tissue (skin, prostate, etc.).

The MCR of testosterone has been studied in children, in adults of both sexes, and in some disease states. It now appears that many physiologic and pathologic factors such as the degree of plasma binding,[12] hepatic function, posture, aging, drugs, and the hyper- and hypometabolic state (thyroid) can alter clearance. The interrelationships of these factors are so complex that in some instances a "normal" plasma concentration can be associated with an altered secretion rate.[13,14] This situation has been noted in the chapter on hirsutism (Chapter 113).

PREHORMONE DYNAMICS

Sex steroids in blood are not just derived from direct glandular secretion. A number of androgens and estrogens are also synthesized by extragonadal tissue from secreted precursors. In some instances this mechanism can lead to a major step-up in biologic activity.[11] This phenomenon was first noted when the weak androgens, dehydroisoandrosterone and dehydroisoandrosterone sulfate, were observed to be interconvertible in the body. Subsequent study of androstenedione metabolism indicated that this weak androgen is a major peripheral precursor of blood testosterone in prepubertal boys and in normal women. These studies led to a hypothesis that certain prehormones are secreted by classical glandular tissues (i.e., adrenal cortex and gonad) and contribute significantly by peripheral conversion to a product (hormone) usually having greater or different biologic activity.[11]

In a system in which a prehormone (Pre) plays a role as a precursor, either (1) the product (hormone) is derived solely from conversion of a secreted prehormone, or (2) the product is both secreted and derived from the prehormone. Alternative 2 is usually the case and can be represented as follows:

$$\text{PR} = S^{\text{Pro}} + (S^{\text{Pre}} \times \rho^{\text{Pre-Pro}})$$

where PR is the production rate, S^{Pro} the direct secretion of product, S^{Pre} the secretion of the prehormone, and $\rho^{\text{Pre-Pro}}$ the fraction of the secreted prehormone converted to the product which enters the particular compartment studied.

Note that both the secretion rate in the case of a substance derived from secretion only and production rates where prehormones are an important source are calculated as the product of the mean integrated plasma or blood levels and the MCR. If the hormone is by and large derived by direct secretion, the production and secretion rates are essentially identical, as is the case with cortisol, aldosterone, and testosterone in men.

These approaches to the secretion or production rates involve determination of the plasma "nonisotopic" concentration of the potential prehormones and hormones (products) as well as their MCR, together with measurement of the conversion rates using isotopic labeled steroids in vivo.[10] These complicated approaches appropriate to research have produced information leading to new concepts and insights, many of which are pathophysiologically relevant.

TESTOSTERONE, A PREHORMONE

In the male, testosterone itself is a prehormone for a number of biologically active sex steroids. Secreted testosterone is converted by peripheral tissues to both potent androgens and estrogens (Fig. 120-2). Studies to date suggest that these conversion products may provide an in vivo assessment of certain target tissue events. Additionally, some of these conversion products appear to be active hormonally in the circulation and may function in part in neuroendocrine feedback control of gonadotropin production. Altered prehormone production is seen in a number of clinical states such as steroid biosynthetic disorders, drug effects, and gynecomastia.

Dihydrotestosterone (DHT) is a very potent androgen. As discussed in the chapter on androgen actions (Chapter 121), DHT is a mediator of testosterone action in that it is synthesized from testosterone in sexual target tissue.[15] Recent studies indicate that all blood DHT arises from extrahepatic conversion. On the basis of a series of in vitro studies and fetal and adult studies, Wilson and co-workers have suggested that DHT is necessary for male differentiation of the urogenital sinus and tubercle and is the hormone responsible for differentiation of the external genitalia and prostate.[16]

DHT is present in adult male plasma at about 1/10 the level of testosterone and the ratio is 1/3 to 1/4 in female plasma.[17] The MCR

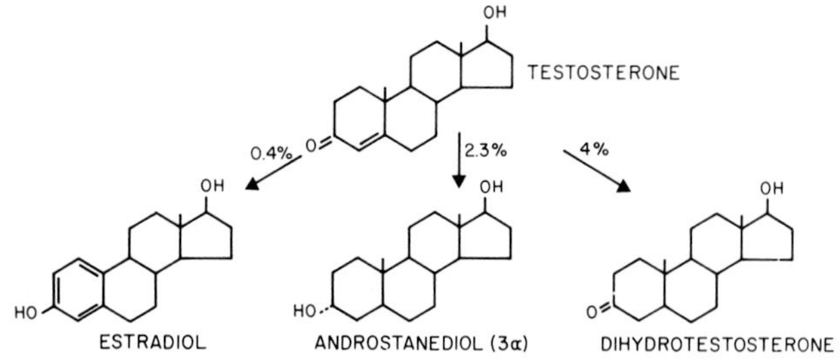

Fig. 120-2. Testosterone as a prehormone for estradiol, androstanediol, and dehydrotestosterone. The percentages refer to overall conversion rates (transfer constants) as measured in the circulation of adult men.

of DHT is one-half that of testosterone, and the calculated blood production is 300–400 μg/day. Kinetic studies of the prehormone–product pair (T, DHT) indicate that most blood DHT is from peripheral conversion of testosterone (Fig. 120-3). Normally about 4 percent of testosterone is converted and appears in the circulation as DHT.[18] DHT may act as a circulating androgen and appears to have feedback activity both by local synthesis and via the general circulation on the central nervous system.

Testosterone is a major prehormone for estradiol in male blood.[19] A small fraction (20 percent) is directly secreted by the testis. However, most blood estradiol is derived via peripheral aromatization of secreted testosterone[20] (Fig. 120-3). Abnormalities in this normal relationship have been described in hyperthyroidism and in liver disease.[21]

Testosterone is also the major prehormone for blood androstane-3α, 17β-diol, another potent androgen. In vitro studies suggest that this steroid may be an alternative or final metabolic pathway in target tissues for testosterone, and measurements of this steroid in blood or urine might be another probe of androgen target tissue events.[22] The MCR of androstanediol, surprisingly, is greater than that of testosterone since a large fraction (40–50 percent) is the result of extrahepatic metabolism. The blood production rate of this, the third potent androgen in blood, is similar to that of DHT in men, but is much less in normal women[23] (Fig. 120-3).

SEX STEROID ASSAY

The fact that sex steroids are generally present in the nanogram range has until recently posed a major methodologic problem.[24] The modern development of radioimmunoassay techniques and the ability to generate antibodies directed toward low molecular weight steroids conjugated as haptenes to antigenic molecules have revolutionized this subject as well as clinical endocrinology.[25–27] Methods to measure accurately and specifically testosterone, estradiol, dihydrotestosterone, and other C_{19} and C_{18} sex steroids of interest are now generally available. Plasma testosterone has now been studied in children and adults.[28] Values in normal men vary widely (0.3–1.2 μg/100 ml), probably in part as a result of considerable variation in binding protein concentration. Other factors that alter plasma levels include a distinct but minor diurnal variation similar in cyclicity to cortisol and changes in hapatic blood flow, as in standing.

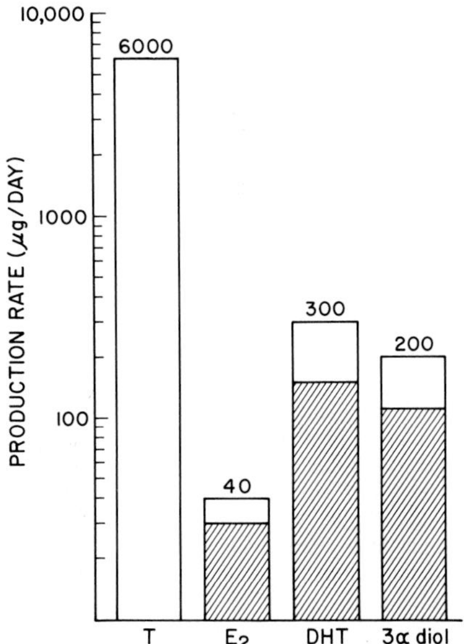

Fig. 120-3. Blood production rates of testosterone (T), estradiol (E_2), dihydrotestosterone (DHT), and androstane-3α,17β-diol (3αdiol) in man. The hatched portion represents the fraction derived peripherally from the prehormone testosterone.

Testosterone levels in plasma vary in a pulsatile or episodic manner related to pulses in gonadotropin (LH) levels.[29] This variation produces some uncertainty in the validity of a single sample for diagnostic purposes. A single testosterone determination may yield a value within ±25 percent of the true mean value only 75 percent of the time, while three samples about 30 min apart or a pooling of these samples give a 100 percent probability.[30]

Stress, particularly during and subsequent to surgery, reduces gonadotropin and testosterone levels.[31] At this time, little is known about the effects of acute and chronic disease on testosterone secretion and clearance.

SEX STEROID BINDING

Most mammalian species, including man, contain a plasma β-globulin that has high affinity but limited capacity for testosterone. A fraction of testosterone is also bound to albumin, but this fraction is considered to be similar dynamically to unbound testosterone. The testosterone-binding globulin binds steroid 17β-hydroxysteroids, including estradiol and dihydrotestosterone, but not conjugated androgens, estrone, dehydroisoandrosterone or the 17α-epimer of testosterone, which is biologically inactive.[32] This protein is now called *sex-hormone–binding globulin (SHBG).* As previously observed for corticosteroid-binding globulin, it is synthesized by the liver, increased in pregnancy or after estrogen administration, and increased in hyperthyroidism.[33] Considerable agreement exists that only unbound and albumin-bound androgen and estrogen is hormonally active and involved in gonadotropin feedback relationships. Methods are available to determine "free" testosterone and estradiol.[34] However, for clinical purposes total plasma or serum testosterone levels appear suitable for diagnosis. The intratesticular concentration of testosterone is many times higher than peripheral levels, and a high intratesticular concentration is required for spermatogenesis to be complete.[35]

ANDROGEN METABOLISM

Testosterone is metabolized in vivo by two pathways. In the predominant one, testosterone is oxidized at the 17 position and in the other, the 17β of the hydroxy position is maintained and testosterone is metabolized to dihydrotestosterone and the androstanediols by reduction of the A-ring double bond and the 3-ketone. In the former ketosteroid pathway, the liver is the major organ of metabolism. The latter, a minor but important path, leads to production of DHT and the androstanediols, which appear to occur predominantly in sexual target tissue.[36]

This section has to this point dealt with testosterone secretion and metabolism in terms of events occurring in the general circulation since classical hormones reach the target tissues via blood circulation. Historically, however, steroid hormones were assayed in urine, where they are concentrated during glomerular filtration and urine concentration and where steroid metabolites are present in milligram and microgram amounts.

The major 17-ketosteroid metabolites, androsterone and etiocholanolone, are conjugated in the liver to the water-soluble

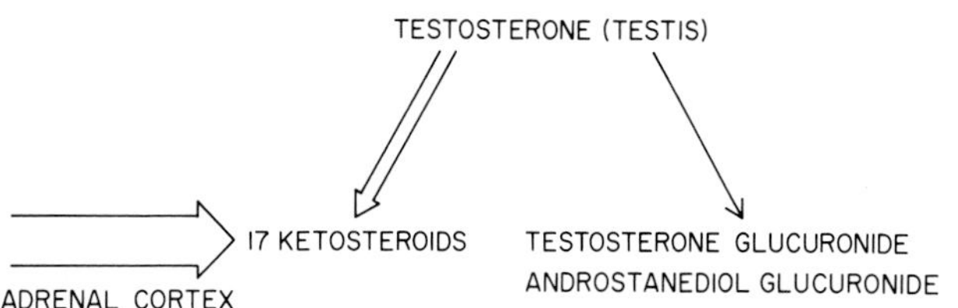

Fig. 120-4. Dual pathways of testosterone metabolism. The liver is the major site of 17-ketosteroid formation. Ketosteroids are derived predominantly from steroids secreted by the adrenal cortex.

moieties, glucuronide and sulfate, and the ketosteroid conjugates are excreted in the urine. These C_{19} steroids are measured as the total daily urine ketosteroids. It is now clear that this determination is a poor reflection of testicular function and androgenicity.[37,38] These ketosteroid metabolites are not uniquely derived from testosterone, but rather are primarily from metabolism of adrenal dehydroisoandrosterone (sulfate) and androstenedione (Fig. 120-4). Only about 20 percent of the ketosteroids are derived from testicular testosterone in the male.[39] Castrated men excrete amounts of ketosteroids that are within normal range for intact subjects. This complexity invalidates the use of ketosteroid (or fractionation thereof) determination in the evaluation of the androgen and gonadal status of a patient.

About 1 percent of secreted testosterone is metabolized to testosterone-17β and androstanediol glucuronide and excreted in urine, where it can be easily measured.[40] In men, they are relatively specific metabolites of secreted testosterone[41] (Fig. 120-4). However, the nuisance of urine collections and the general availability of blood assays have reduced the usefulness of urine assays.

Testosterone as replacement therapy is usually administered parenterally as testosterone cyclopropionate in oil in doses of 200–400 mg/month, although it can be absorbed fairly well orally, contrary to general belief. Oral administration would have to be on a daily basis.

REFERENCES

1. Lipsett, M. Steroid Secretion by the Testis in Man. In James, V., Serio, M., and Martin, L. (eds): *The Endocrine Function of the Human Testis,* vol. 2. New York, Academic, 1974. p. 1.
2. Weinstein, R., Kelch, R., Jenner, M., Kaplan, S. L., and Grumbach, M. M. Secretion of Unconjugated Androgens and Estrogens by the Normal and Abnormal Human Testis. *J. Clin. Invest. 53:* 1, 1974.
3. Kelch, R., Jenner, M., Weinstein, R., Kaplan, S. L., and Grumbach, M. M. Estradiol and Testosterone in the Male. Secretion by Human, Simian, and Canine Testes, in Males with Hypogonadism and Pseudohermaphrodites with the Feminizing Testis Syndrome. *J. Clin. Invest. 51:* 824, 1972.
4. Saez, J., Forest, M., Morera, A., and Bertrand, J. Metabolic Clearance Rate and Blood Production Rate of Testosterone and Dihydrotestosterone in Normal Subjects During Pregnancy and in Hyperthyroidism. *J. Clin. Invest. 51:* 1226, 1972.
5. Pazzagli, M., Borrelli, E., Forti, G., and Serio, M. Dihydrotestosterone in Human Spermatic Venous Plasma. *Acta Endocrinol. 76:* 388, 1974.
6. Folman, Y., Ahmad, N., Sowell, J., and Eik-Nes, K. B. Formation *In Vitro* of 5α-DHT and Other 5α-Reduced Metabolites of ^{3}H Testosterone by Seminiferous Tubules and Interstitial Tissue from Immature and Mature Rat Testes. *Endocrinology 92:* 41, 1973.
7. Hudson, B., Coghlan, J., and Dulmanis, A. Testicular Function in Man. Ciba Found. Colloq. *Endocrinol. 16:* 140, 1967.
8. Strott, C., Yoshimi, T., and Lipsett, M. Plasma Progesterone and 17-Hydroxyprogesterone in Normal Men and Children with Congenital Adrenal Hyperplasia. *J. Clin. Invest. 48:* 930, 1969.
9. Tait, J., and Burstein, S. *In Vivo* Studies of Steroid Dynamics in Man. In Pincus, G., Thimann, K. V., and Astwood, E. B. (eds): *The Hormones.* New York, Academic, 1964, p. 441.
10. Tait, J. F. Review: The Use of Isotopic Steroids for the Measurement of Production Rates *In Vivo. J. Clin. Endocrinol. Metab. 23:* 1285, 1963.
11. Baird, D., Horton, R., Longcope, C., and Tait, J. F. Steroid Dynamics Under Steady State Conditions. *Recent Prog. Horm. Res. 25:* 611, 1969.
12. Vermeulen, A., Verdonck, L., Van der Straeten, M., and Orie, N. Capacity of the TBG in Human Plasma and Influence of Testosterone Binding on Its Metabolic Clearance Rate. *J. Clin. Endocrinol. Metab. 29:* 1470, 1969.
13. Lipsett, M. Steroid Secretion by the Human Testis. In Rosenberg, E., and Paulsen, C. (eds): *The Human Testis.* Advances in Experimental Medicine and Biology. New York, Plenum, 1970, p. 407.
14. Kirschner, M., and Bardin, C. Androgen Production and Metabolism in Normal and Virilized Women. *Metabolism 21:* 667, 1972.
15. Wilson, J. D. Recent Studies on the Mechanism of Action of Testosterone. *N. Engl. J. Med. 287:* 1284, 1972.
16. Walsh, P. C., Madden, J. C., Harrod, M. J., et al. Familial Incomplete Male Pseudohermaphroditism Type 2. *N. Engl. J. Med. 291:* 944, 1974.
17. Ito, T., and Horton, R. Dihydrotestosterone in Human Peripheral Plasma. *J. Clin. Endocrinol. Metab. 31:* 362, 1970.
18. Ito, T., and Horton, R. The Source of Plasma Dihydrotestosterone in Man. *J. Clin. Invest. 50:* 1621, 1971.
19. MacDonald, P., Grodin, J., and Siiteri, P. Dynamics of Androgen and Oestrogen Secretion. In Baird, D., and Strong, J. (eds): *Control of Gonadal Steroid Secretion.* Baltimore, Williams & Wilkins, 1971, p. 157.
20. Longcope, C., Kato, T., and Horton, R. Conversion of Blood Androgens to Estrogen in Normal Men and Women. *J. Clin. Invest. 48:* 2191, 1969.
21. Chopra, I. Gonadal Steroids and Gonadotropins in Hyperthyroidism. *Med. Clin. North Am. 59:* 1109, 1975.
22. Mauvais-Jarvis, P. Testosterone Metabolism and Action in Testicular Feminization Syndrome. In James, V., Serio, M., and Martin, L. (eds): *The Endocrine Function of the Human Testis,* vol. 2. New York, Academic, 1974, p. 109.
23. Kinouchi, T., and Horton, R. 3α-Androstanediol Kinetics in Man. *J. Clin. Invest. 54:* 646, 1974.
24. Murphy, B. E. P. Protein Binding and the Assay of Nonantigenic Hormones. *Recent Prog. Horm. Res. 25:* 563, 1969.
25. Erlanger, B., Borek, F., Beiser, S., and Lieberman, S. Steroid Protein Conjugates. *J. Biol. Chem. 228:* 713, 1957.
26. Niswender, G., and Midgley, A. Hapten-radioimmunoassay for Steroid Hormones. In Person, F., and Caldwell, B. (eds): *Immunologic Methods in Steroid Determinations.* New York, Appleton-Century-Crofts, 1970, p. 149.
27. Odell, W. D., and Daughaday, W. H. (eds): *Principals of Competitive Protein Binding Assays.* Philadelphia, Lippincott, 1971.
28. Lee, P., Jaffe, R., and Midgley, A. Serum Gonadotropin, Testosterone and Prolactin Concentrations Throughout Puberty in Boys: A Longitudinal Study. *J. Clin. Endocrinol. Metab. 39:* 664, 1974.
29. Naftolin, F., Judd, H., and Yen, S. Pulsatile Patterns of Gonadotropin and Testosterone in Man. *J. Clin. Endocrinol. Metab. 36:* 285, 1973.
30. Goldzieher, J., Dozier, T., Smith, K., and Steinberger, E. Improving the Diagnostic Reliability of Rapidly Fluctuating Hormone Levels by Multiple Sampling Techniques. *J. Clin. Endocrinol. Metab. 43:* 824, 1976.
31. Carstensen, H., Amer, I., Wide, L., and Amer, B. Plasma Testosterone, LH and FSH During the First 24 Hours After Surgical Operations. *J. Steril. Biochem. 4:* 605, 1973.
32. Pearlman, W., and Crépy, O. Steroid Protein Interaction with Particular Reference to Testosterone Binding by Human Serum. *J. Biol. Chem. 242:* 182, 1967.
33. Gordon, G., Southren, A., Tochimoto, S., Rand, J. J. and Olivo, J. Effect of Hyperthyroidism and Hypothyroidism on the Metabolism of Testosterone and Androstenedione in Man. *J. Clin. Endocrinol. Metab. 29:* 164, 1969.
34. Rubens, R., Dhont, M., and Vermeulen, A. Further Studies on Leydig Cell Function in Old Age. *J. Clin. Endocrinol. Metab. 39:* 40, 1974.
35. Steinberger, E., Smith, K. D., Tcholakian, R. K., et al. In Steroidogenesis in Human Testes. In Mancini, R. E., and Martini, L. (eds): *Male Fertility and Sterility.* New York, Academic, 1974, p. 149.

36. Ofner, P., Leav, I., and Cavazos, L. In Brandes, D. (ed): *Male Accessory Sex Organs.* New York, Academic, 1974, p. 267.
37. Vande Wiele, R., MacDonald, P., Gurpide, E., and Lieberman, S. Studies on the Secretion and Interconversion of the Androgens. *Recent Prog. Horm. Res. 19:* 275, 1963.
38. Baulieu, E., Corpéchot, C., Dray, F., et al. An Adrenal Secreted "Androgen:" Dehydroisoandrosterone Sulfate. *Recent Prog. Horm. Res. 21:* 411, 1965.
39. Lipsett, M., Wilson, H., Kirschner, M., et al. Studies on Leydig Cell Physiology and Pathology: Secretion and Metabolism of Testosterone. *Recent Prog. Horm. Res. 22:* 245, 1966.
40. Camacho, A., and Migeon, C. Isolation, Identification, and Quantitation of Testosterone in Urine of Normal Adults and in Patients with Endocrine Disorders. *J. Clin. Endocrinol. Metab.. 23:* 301, 1963.
41. Korenman, S., and Lipsett, M. Is Testosterone Glucuronoside Uniquely Derived from Plasma Testosterone? *J. Clin. Invest. 43:* 2125, 1964.

121

Biochemical Features of Androgen Physiology

H. G. Williams-Ashman

INTRODUCTION

As indicated by their conventional definition as hormones of masculinity, androgens are key regulators of male modes of development of the genital tract, ornamental secondary sexual tissues, and coital behavior patterns. The commonly employed procedures for quantitative estimation of androgenic activities rest on changes in the size and functions of the prostate glands and seminal vesicles of juvenile or castrated adult rodents, or the combs and wattles of chicks or capons. The precise ranking of androgenic potencies depends critically on which particular end organ is used for bioassay purposes in any particular species, as well as on the route of administration of the compounds,[1,2] since countless factors influence the uptake, retention, and metabolic transformations of androgens by various tissues.

Besides those male reproductive organs that they affect so conspicuously, androgenic hormones exert profound actions on innumerable other physiologic processes: for example, they are essential for spermatogenesis; they depress the output of luteinizing hormone (LH or ICSH) by the hypothalamic–hypophyseal axis; they stimulate the growth of certain muscles, prostate neoplasms, and female heterosexual remnant tissues such as clitoris; and they provoke involution of some lymphoid tissues. Moreover, androgens of fetal testicular origin in eutherian mammals serve as mandatory triggers, during restricted and critical periods of embryonic and/or early neonatal life, for the initial differentiation of many organs of the male reproductive tract from the Wolffian duct, urogenital sinus, and external genital primordia, and for permanent imprinting of regions of the central nervous system that from puberty onward control masculine modes of gonadotropin secretion and sexual behavior. The astonishing diversity of the morphogenetic and physiologic effects of androgens makes it notoriously difficult to define a "target" versus a "nontarget" tissue for these hormones, and underscores the need for caution in framing any simple unitary hypotheses to account for all of their biologic actions in molecular terms.

A large body of evidence garnered over the last sesquidecade has suggested that androgen action, like that of all other types of steroid hormones, entails two fundamental attributes. First, most if not all effects of androgens on the structure, function, and proliferation of responsive cells reflect induced changes in gene expression mechanisms, and especially in the nuclear transcription of specific RNA molecules that in turn regulate the biosynthesis of certain specific proteins in the cytoplasm.[3,4] The second is that unique intracellular androgen receptor proteins that shuttle between cytoplasm and nucleus can functionally associate with sites on nuclear chromatins that may regulate RNA transcription.[2,3,5] However, unlike the other major categories of gonadal and adrenocortical steroid hormones, which act without necessity for metabolic transformation, some of the physiologic effects of the principal circulating androgen of testicular origin, testosterone, may entail its enzymic conversion in target cells to 5α-dihydrotestosterone and possibly androstanediols as well.[6] There can be no doubt that recent experimental underpinnings for these concepts represent important advances. Nevertheless, current insight into the mechanisms of androgen action remains so obviously rudimentary that these achievements may later appear as little more than a match struck at midnight in a dark forest. An up-to-date account of the entire field is provided in a volume by Mainwaring.[7]

MOLECULAR STRUCTURE AND ANDROGENIC ACTIVITY

A vast number of substances have been evaluated for androgenic activity in various bioassay systems. Although no simple rules concerning the relationship of molecular architecture to androgenic potency can be formulated, certain salient points are well established.[1,2,7] All known androgens of high potency are fairly closely related to the natural 19-carbon androgen testosterone and its major metabolite 5α-dihydrotestosterone (17β-hydroxy-5α-androstan-3-one, or DHT), which is even more active than the parent testosterone in some bioassay systems. As shown in Figure 121-1, the four rings (A, B, C, and D) of strongly androgenic steroids are all fused *trans* with respect to each other; for this reason they are relatively planar molecules, although androgens that contain a Δ^4 double bond in ring A (e.g., testosterone) are somewhat less planar than those that do not (e.g., DHT). The 19-carbon steroids that have *cis*-fused carbon rings are generally only weakly active or inert as androgens (e.g., etiocholanolone, which is virtually inactive as a promoter of growth of male genital glands or chick combs, but can act as an inducer of heme biosynthesis in some experimental systems). Addition of one extra carbon atom to rings B, C, or D produces homosteroids that frequently exhibit definite androgenic-

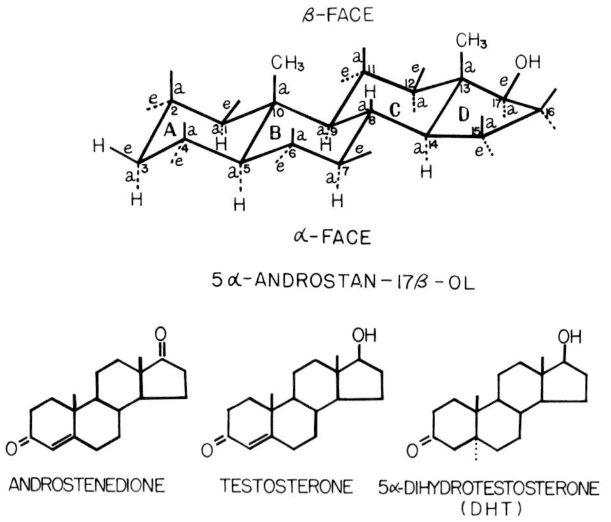

Fig. 121-1. Molecular structures of some natural androgens. Symbols for substitutions: a, axial; e, equatorial; ----, —— at α- and β-faces of steroid, respectively.

ity, whereas ring A homo steroids are usually inactive. Certain synthetics in which a carbon in ring A is replaced by an oxygen are considerably androgenic. Unsaturation in various rings is not necessarily incompatible with biologic activity. The presence of oxygen substituents attached to C-3 of ring A is common to most naturally occurring androgens. Whether a 3-keto group is more effective than a 3α- or 3β-hydroxyl function depends markedly on the type of cell used as end point for assay purposes; this may reflect the tissue distribution of appropriate hydroxysteroid dehydrogenases among various species. However, active androgens lacking any oxygen substituent at C-3 have been prepared. By contrast, a requirement for an oxygen function at C-17 is almost mandatory, and substances with a 17β-hydroxyl group are generally more androgenic than their 17α-hydroxylated isomers.

Substitution of methyl or alkyl groups at various positions in the rings have variable influences on androgenic activity that in some instances may be related more to the metabolic fate and tissue distribution of the steroids than to their ability to combine as such to intracellular androgen receptors. Noteworthy in this connection is that 17α-methyltestosterone is less susceptible to rapid transformation by the liver to inactive metabolites than is testosterone itself, so that this methylated compound is relatively more active when administered by the oral route. Because of the inhibitory influence of 17α-methyltesterone on bile secretion, and hence its proclivity to induce jaundice, the synthetic steroid Fluoxymestrone, which is less likely to cause jaundice, is now more commonly employed as an orally active androgen for clinical purposes.

A few substances have been synthesized that lack the four-carbon–ring system of natural steroids yet exhibit definite but only rather feeble androgenic activity. This stands in marked contrast to the powerful estrogenic activity of certain nonsteroidal synthetic estrogens such as diethylstilbestrol.

ANTIANDROGENS

Largely as a result of the pioneer studies of Neumann et al.,[8] many synthetic substances are now available that act as potent antiandrogens in the sense that they compete with natural or artificial androgens at an end-organ level. Antiandrogens of this class have little or no influence on the secretion of androgenic steroids by the testis or on the metabolism of androgens in various tissues. Rather they exert their actions by preventing combination of active androgenic molecules with their intracellular receptors, as considered below. Many of the known powerful antiandrogens are steroids such as cyproterone acetate and BOMT, which are not at all estrogenic, although they may in some instances exhibit powerful gestagenic activity. Recently, a strong nonsteroidal antiandrogen, Flutamide, has become available. The formulas of a few representative antiandrogens are illustrated in Figure 121-2.

Estrogens exert profound antiandrogenic and feminizing influences on male mammals,[8] but these effects can largely be accounted for by (1) inhibition of testicular androgen secretion via depression of LH output and by a direct suppression of androgen synthesis by Leydig Cells, and (2) estrogenic stimulation of female remnant tissues such as the male breast. However, a direct inhibition of androgen action on the prostate of hypophysectomized dogs has been reported.

TISSUE DISTRIBUTION AND METABOLISM OF ANDROGENS

The principal circulating androgen of testicular origin, testosterone, undergoes rapid and multiple chemical changes in many tissues, including the liver, kidney, and male reproductive organs. Most of the metabolites of testosterone that are formed in liver, including reduction, oxidation, and hydroxylation products, are quickly conjugated. By contrast, in many responsive reproductive tissues, testosterone is rapidly converted to DHT, which in turn may be metabolized into other products, notably 3α-androstanediol (5α-androstane-3α,17β-diol). In organs such as rat ventral prostate, these androstane reduction products of testosterone are not conjugated to any large extent; free DHT (but not 3α-androstanediol) may be extensively retained in prostatic cell nuclei either in vivo, or if the intact tissue is incubated with labeled testosterone, in vitro, provided that the temperature is kept close to 37°C. However, unchanged testosterone has been found to be the predominant androgen in cell nuclei of several nonhepatic tissues outside the male genital tract that readily respond to this class of hormones, including mouse kidney, rat anterior pituitary, and levator ani muscle. It is noteworthy that the amount of radioactivity derived from administered labeled testosterone in the latter tissues is low in comparison with the nuclei of male accessory sex glands, in which nuclear DHT predominates. Details of the metabolism and nuclear concentration of some of the metabo-

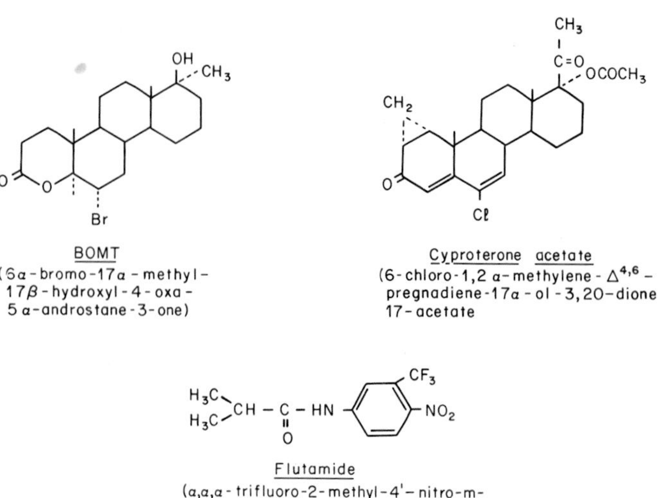

Fig. 121-2. Some representative antiandrogens.

lites of androgens in male reproductive and other organs, including certain androgen-responsive neoplasms, are provided in reviews by Wilson,[6] Liao and Fang,[2,5] and Verhoeven et al.[9]

The reduction of testosterone to DHT is catalyzed by an NADPH-specific enzyme (Δ^4-3-ketosteroid-5α-oxidoreductase) that is associated with both the microsomal and nuclear membrane fractions of prostate tissue. Further conversion of DHT to androstanediols is promoted by appropriate hydroxysteroid dehydrogenases. Since DHT is a more potent androgen than testosterone in a number of the classical androgenic bioassay systems, and also is selectively retained in the cell nuclei of some highly androgen-responsive cells, DHT may be regarded as an "active form" of testosterone in some but by no means all androgen target tissues.

EXTRACELLULAR ANDROGEN-BINDING PROTEINS

In some mammalian species, such as the human, testosterone and other natural androgens in the circulation are firmly associated with plasma proteins and are largely attached to a binder in the β-globulin fraction that is variously designated as testosterone–estradiol–binding globulin, or sex-steroid–binding globulin. This serum protein is clearly distinct from cortisol-binding globulin (transcortin). There is considerable evidence that only free (i.e., non–protein-bound) testosterone, and other androgens in blood plasma, can readily enter target cells and hence exert their hormonal actions.[2,10]

Another distinct macromolecule is the androgen-binding protein (ABP) found in testis and epididymis. This glycoprotein is synthesized in Sertoli cells under the stimulus of FSH and is secreted into the lumens of seminiferous tubules.[11] ABP may be involved in the sequestration of testosterone by cells inside the seminiferous tubules and in the regulation of spermatogenesis. Both the testosterone–estradiol–binding globulin of blood plasma and the APB of testis and epididymis are chemically and functionally quite distinct from so-called intracellular androgen-receptor proteins.

CENTRAL ROLE OF INTRACELLULAR RECEPTORS IN ANDROGEN ACTION

There are many reasons to believe that androgens must enter their target cells in order to exert their biologic effects. Circulating androgens appear to penetrate the plasmalemma of most cells readily, and it is questionable whether there exist specific facilitated androgen transport mechanisms associated with cell membranes.

Soon after Jensen established the key importance of specific intracellular proteins for the uptake, nuclear retention, and hormonal actions of estrogens, similarly functioning but molecularly distinct specific intracellular androgen receptors were found in male reproductive organs. A schematic model for the participation of these receptors in various phases of androgen action—based on the studies of Mainwaring,[7] Wilson,[6] Liao,[5] and others—is outlined in Figure 121-3.

Specific receptor proteins exhibiting a very high affinity for DHT (equilibrium association constants in the vicinity of 10^{10}M^{-1}), a lesser yet strikingly high avidity for testosterone, but a much lower affinity for 3α-androstanediol, have been detected in cytosolic and nuclear fractions of many androgen-responsive tissues. The multiplicity of such androgen receptors in various types of cells vis-a-vis their steroid ligand specificities remains uncertain. Even in highly responsive cells, such androgen receptors are very unstable and are present in extremely small amounts (e.g., less than 50,000 binding sites per cell, roughly 70 percent of which are nuclear, in rat ventral prostate); these circumstances make it difficult to purify these receptors to a state approaching homogeneity in high yields. Moreover, analysis of their properties and functions can only too easily be complicated by all sorts of experimental artifacts, especially in crude tissue extracts. The latter include modifications of the receptor proteins or the labeled hormones added as ligands by contaminating enzymes that may obscure the true steroid specificity of the native receptors, aggregation phenomena that are exquisitely sensitive to small variations in ambient salt concentrations, and the presence of many unrelated mini- and macromolecules in tissue that can profoundly influence steroid–receptor interactions.

There are claims that some androgen-responsive cells are endowed with specific DHT receptors while other such cells harbor separate "testosterone receptors."[2,5] However, if the possibility of the aforementioned artifacts is taken into account, much of the available data seem to fit the hypothesis that, in the context of hormonal action, DHT and to a lesser extent testosterone are bound to a single androgen-receptor protein that has only a limited ability to bind other natural androgen metabolites such as 3α-androstanediol.[9,12] This androgen receptor is present in a variety of forms in both the cytosol and the nucleus. In those androgen-sensitive cells in which testosterone is rapidly converted into DHT, the DHT-receptor complex is rapidly sequestered by the nucleus. This process may entail a prior temperature-sensitive transformation of

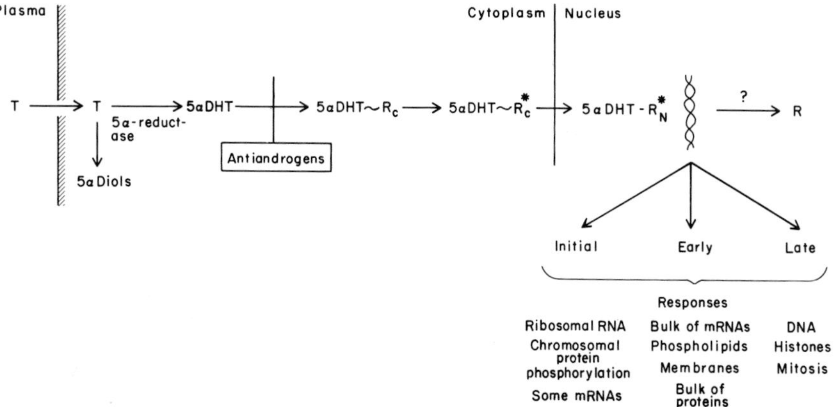

Fig. 121-3. Mechanisms of androgen action. T, testosterone; 5α-DHT, 5α-dihydrotestosterone; 5α-Diols, 5α-androstanediols; R_c, cytoplasmic androgen receptor; R_N, nuclear androgen receptor; asterisk, transformed receptor–androgen complex. (Adapted from Mainwaring: The Mechanism of Action of Androgens, 1977. Courtesy of Springer.)

the initially formed cytoplasmic receptor-DHT complex (Fig. 121-3). By contrast, in those cells in which the reduction of testosterone to DHT occurs to only a small or negligible extent, the cytoplasmic receptor–testosterone complex may eventually be captured by cell nuclei. In other words, the main factor determining whether testosterone becomes associated in vivo with cell nuclei in the unchanged form or as DHT may well be the extent of target cell metabolism of the testosterone, rather than the existence of cytoplasmic and nuclear forms of distinct DHT and testosterone receptors.[9] In any case, there is strong evidence that neither testosterone nor DHT are actively concentrated and retained by cell nuclei of most androgen-responsive cells unless they first attach to cytoplasmic forms of androgen-receptor molecules. The combination of testosterone or DHT with intracellular androgen receptors, although very tight, certainly occurs via noncovalent forces.

The existence of only a single type of intracellular androgen-receptor protein, apparently encoded by a gene on the X chromosome, has been cogently championed by Ohno[12] and Verhoeven et al.[9] It is evident that this androgen receptor is not identical with the steroid 5α-reductase, which is regulated by an autosomal recessive gene.

Powerful antiandrogens such as cyproterone acetate prevent the combination of DHT with the cytoplasmic forms of androgen-receptor proteins but do not hinder the enzymatic reduction of testosterone to DHT.[5] The latter steroid conversion can be inhibited by high concentrations of estrogens in cell-free systems, but the physiologic significance of such observations is equivocal.

There appears to exist a limited number of intranuclear "acceptor" molecules that determine the tight association of androgen–receptor complexes with the nuclear chromatin. These nuclear "acceptors," which are present in the greatest amounts in very androgen-responsive tissues, have not been characterized rigorously and may well represent a family of substances. The limited evidence available suggests that neither regions of naked DNA nor the classical histones represent the major chromatin-binding sites for suitably transformed cytoplasmic androgen–receptor complexes once the latter are sequestered by cell nuclei. Nonhistone chromatin proteins, variously stated to be acidic[5] or basic[13] in character, and nuclear ribonucleoprotein particles,[5] are believed to be more centrally involved in the nuclear retention of DHT–receptor complexes.

ANDROGENIC REGULATION OF RIBONUCLEIC ACID AND PROTEIN SYNTHESIS

Most of the biologic effects of androgens seem to depend on their regulation of the levels of various enzymes and other proteins in responsive tissues.[1,3,7] In general, this seems to involve androgen-induced changes in the rate of biosynthesis rather than intracellular degradation of specific proteins. The specificity and time course of changes in target tissue proteins that result from androgen deprivation or treatment are highly organ and species dependent. In rat ventral prostate—which has been used extensively for biochemical correlative studies on androgen action—significant increases in chromatin-associated protein phosphokinase,[14] nuclear RNA polymerase I,[2] and polyamine biosynthetic decarboxylases[15] occur within 30, 60, and 180 min, respectively, after testosterone injection. Selective enhancement of many other enzyme activities involves lag periods of at least 6 h or much longer.[3,7] In every instance, inhibitor studies have indicated that these androgen-induced enzyme changes require continued RNA and protein synthesis. None of the enzymes so affected are meaningfully influenced by direct addition of testosterone, DHT, or other androgens to the catalytic test systems in the absence or presence of androgen receptors.

In the case of aldolase and a few other enzymes in male genital glands, there is evidence that androgens increase their biosynthesis as a result of prior de novo synthesis of the pertinent mRNA and its subsequent accumulation in association with cytoplasmic polyribosomes.[7] The paramount effects of androgens appear to be at the level of nuclear transcription of large ribosomal and mRNA precursors, and possibly of intranuclear processing of these transcripts. The in vivo effects of androgens on nuclear RNA biosynthesis and later cytoplasmic polyribonsomal protein synthesis are nullified by antiandrogenic substances known to prevent the formation of androgen–receptor complexes. This and many other lines of evidence strongly suggest that complexes between androgens (or their active steroid metabolites formed in target tissues) and specific cytoplasmic receptor proteins, followed by nuclear uptake of transformed cytoplasmic androgen–receptor complexes and their association with chromatin, are mandatory preliminaries for the hormones to alter nuclear RNA transcription. Although there are a few very recent reports that androgen–receptor complexes with DHT or testosterone can directly stimulate RNA synthesis in vitro, with nuclei or chromatin as sources of template DNA, the physiologic significance of such observations and the precise mechanisms by which androgens clearly enhance nuclear RNA formation in living cells remain to be clarified.

Whether all of the effects of androgens on protein synthesis invariably reflect control of nuclear RNA production is also uncertain. A direct modulation by androgen–receptor complexes of cytoplasmic reactions involved in the initiation of polypeptide chain synthesis may conceivably operate.[16] Relatively sluggish androgenic enhancement of amino acids into proteins by the distinct prostatic mitochondrial protein biosynthetic machinery[17] seems to be contingent on prior alterations in the cytoplasmic environment rather than a direct effect of the hormones on the mitochondria.

The extensive literature concerning androgenic induction of specific proteins in various mammalian tissues and its genetic overtones is reviewed by Mainwaring.[7] Germane to such studies is the signal lack of convincing evidence that androgen action *primarily* involves modulation of membrane-bound nucleotide cyclase reactions of the type that are central to the actions of many catecholamine, protein, and peptide hormones.[4,7,18]

ANDROGENS, DNA SYNTHESIS, AND CELL PROLIFERATION

There are pronounced variations in the extent to which various male reproductive organs in sexually mature mammals will involute after castration or application of other antiandrogenic maneuvers.[1] The postcastrate regression of many male genital glands involves an extensive cell loss that eventually plateaus, accompanied by shrinkage and loss of secretory functions of the epithelial cells. If treatment with even hyperphysiologic amounts of testosterone or DHT is then instituted and maintained for prolonged periods, the glands may attain a somewhat larger size than normal, with restoration of epithelial cell dimensions and secretory activity. However, the hyperplastic element of such organ enlargement is subject to homeostatic constraint, so that growth of the glands eventually halts, despite continued androgenic stimulation. Other organs, such as certain androgen-sensitive muscles, involute after castration and may subsequently grow in response to exogenous androgens by processes that mainly reflect changes in cell size rather than total cell number. During the hyperplastic phase of growth of those organs whose size regulation by androgens involves cell proliferation as well as cell hypertrophy, there occur large transient increases of some but not all of the enzymes related to DNA synthesis—notably a "replicative" DNA polymerase-α, thymidine kinase, and a DNA "unwinding" protein[19,20]—which subside again when the growth eventually plateaus.

The earliest manifestations of induction of DNA synthesis and cell multiplication by androgens in involuted male genital glands only occur more than 1 day after the onset of hormone administration, and long after earlier increases in nuclear RNA formation and certain enzyme activities.[19] Our current understanding of the biochemical basis of the complex interplays between the processes of cell differentiation and division that contribute to the growth of some androgen-responsive tissues is rudimentary.[7,19] This is an important area for future study because it may bear strongly on the mechanisms of growth control of those neoplasms that, like their normal tissues of origin, may be androgen dependent, such as certain carcinomas of the human prostate gland.[21]

ROLE OF ANDROGENS IN THE FETAL DIFFERENTIATION OF THE MALE GENITAL TRACT

Regardless of their sex genotype, eutherian mammalian embryos have an inherent predisposition for their internal reproductive tracts and external genitalia to develop in a primitive female direction, and, under normal circumstances, form typical male genital structures only if hormones originating from the fetal testis impress a masculine mode of development at critical periods of embryonic life. This generalization is based on experiments involving fetal gonadectomy, or treatment of embryos (or reproductive tracts explanted therefrom) with appropriate hormones.[4,22–24] Testosterone, the principal androgen secreted by the fetal testis, stimulates the morphogenesis of (1) the prostate gland and male-type urethra from the primitive urogenital sinus; (2) the epididymis, vas deferens, and vesicular glands from the Wolffian duct; and (3) the penis and scrotum from the primitive external genital anlage. By contrast, testosterone or other androgens do not evoke the regression of the Müllerian duct that normally occurs in the early stages of embryonic male sexual development. Involution of the Müllerian duct is triggered by a separate hormonelike substance from the fetal testis which appears to be a macromolecule, but which remains to be characterized rigorously from a chemical standpoint.

Wilson's[6] investigations suggest that in some species testosterone does not undergo any chemical change when it induces the initial differentiation of vesicular glands and other structures from the Wolffian duct, whereas prior conversion of testosterone into DHT is involved in the embryonic morphogenesis of both the prostate and male external genitalia.

GENETICALLY DETERMINED ANDROGEN INSENSITIVITIES

Defects of normal masculinization in mammals can have innumerable causes. One set of such disorders that is outside the scope of this chapter results from genetically determined deficiencies in a number of the enzymes required for testosterone production by fetal and postnatal testes.[25] Another group of hereditarily determined disorders that exhibit varying degrees of male pseudohermaphroditism reflect complete or partial insensitivities of male reproductive tissues to either endogenous or exogenous androgens. The most thoroughly studied of these congenital defects is the complete form of so-called androgen-insensitivity syndrome, which is frequently but rather inappropriately designated *testicular feminization*. This condition, which in mice (Lyon-Hawkes mutation) and man is apparently transmitted via a recessive gene localized on the X chromosome, has also been described in several other mammalian species.[3,7,12,25–27] Its characteristics include the following: (1) abdominal or inguinal testes that frequently secrete testosterone in amounts that approximate its output by the scrotal testes of normal adult males of the same species; (2) no great abnormality in the metabolism of testosterone by liver or other tissues, or in the excretion of its major metabolic inactivation products; (3) an external female phenotype frequently associated with higher levels of circulating estrogens than in normal males, with female external genitalia and breast development at puberty, but little or no pubic and axillary hair; (4) an uncomplicated XY sex karyotype; and (5) an absence of internal sexual organs that normally can arise from either the Wolffian or the Müllerian ducts (i.e., lack of oviducts, uterus, and upper vagina, as well as of epididymis, vas deferens, and vesicular and prostate glands). These creatures are refractory to the masculinizing actions of large doses of exogenous testosterone or other androgenic steroids. The symptoms of male pseudohermaphroditism would be expected if it is assumed that testosterone is secreted by both the fetal and postnatal testis but somehow cannot act on the genital tract structures during embryonic life and thereafter, with the additional postulate that there is no defect in the output and actions of the Müllerian duct involuting factor from the fetal testis. In line with these concepts is the experimental induction by Neumann and Steinbeck[8] of phenocopies of the male pseudohermaphroditic picture of the androgen-insensitivity syndrome by treatment of normal mammalian XY fetuses with the antiandrogen cyproterone acetate.

Several lines of evidence hint that in most varieties of the androgen-insensitivity syndrome in man and rodents the primary molecular lesion may not be in the conversion of testosterone to DHT (although this sometimes may be subnormal in certain tissues), but rather it may be an absence or severe decrease of functional cytosolic androgen receptors that can effectively bind DHT and thus permit retention of DHT by nuclear chromatin. It is not known whether failure to detect any cytosolic DHT–receptor complexes or nuclear sequestration of DHT in these variants of complete androgen insensitivity is due to some defect in the transcription or translation of the mRNA cognate to the appropriate androgen-receptor gene, or whether it reflects the production of an altered (mutated) receptor that has lost its avidity for DHT and other androgens. Interestingly, a very recent report indicates that there may exist genetic heterogeneity among human patients exhibiting the complete form of the androgen-insensitivity syndrome. According to Amrhein et al.,[27] of a total of 10 phenotypically similar patients whose plasma androgens were within the normal range or even greater and who invariably had elevated serum LH, 6 individuals showed no cytosolic binding or nuclear retention of DHT as determined on cultures of their fibroblasts under conditions in which these parameters are readily measurable with normal fibroblasts. However, another 4 androgen-insensitive patients provided fibroblasts that exhibited normal characteristics of cytosolic DHT binding and nuclear retention of this steroid, indicating no defect in cytosol DHT receptors or in the nuclear "acceptor" substances that can retain DHT–receptor complexes. The latter category of androgen-insensitivity syndrome patients may harbor some other molecular disturbance, conceivably related to gene expression processes that are distal to the chromatin binding of DHT–receptor complexes.

There is one hereditary disorder of sexual development in which the fundamental defect seems to be in the steroid 5α-reductase enzyme that converts testosterone into DHT. This is the so-called *familial incomplete male pseudohermaphroditism type 2*, otherwise known as *pseudovaginal perineoscrotal hypospadias*. The inheritance of this condition is autosomal recessive rather than X-linked.[25] It entails the presence of characteristically male structures derived embryologically from the Wolffian duct (epididymis, vas deferens, vesicular gland), whereas organs formed out of the urogenital sinus and external genital anlagen are essentially female. The clinical picture is consistent with aforementioned evidence that reduction of testosterone to DHT occurs during fetal morphogenesis of the urogenital sinus, and the genital tubercle, folds, and swellings, whereas testosterone is not converted to DHT at the time that the hormone triggers differentiation of malelike structures from the Wolffian duct. It also fits the direct demonstration of a deficient transformation of testosterone into DHT by urogenital tract tissues of these patients.[28,29]

ANDROGEN ACTION ON CENTRAL NEUROENDOCRINE TISSUES

In the adult male mammal, high levels of circulating androgens depress the release of LH (ICSH) by the anterior pituitary. Although this effect seems to be exerted mainly at a hypothalamic level via inhibition of the output of gonadotropin-releasing hormone (GnRH) that evokes LH release, androgens may also directly modify responsivity of gonadotropin cells of the pars distalis to GnRH. High-affinity binding of both testosterone and DHT by the hypothalamus and adjacent regions of the brain and also by the anterior pituitary has been demonstrated. The hypothalamus readily reduces testosterone to DHT, whereas this transformation occurs to a more limited extent in the pars distalis.

Hypothalamic androgen receptors and steroid 5α-reductase–catalyzed formation of DHT from testosterone may also be of importance for (1) androgenic control of adult male sex behavior and (2) the permanent imprinting, during critical periods of late fetal or early neonatal life, of the hypothalamus to regulate characteristically male modes of gonadotropin output and coital behavior that are normally manifest from puberty onward. In some species, it appears that neonatal androgenization of these central nervous mechanisms is evoked by testosterone but not by DHT. Germane to these observations is the finding that the hypothalamus and limbic system in several species can aromatize testosterone to 17β-estradiol. Under the same circumstances, DHT is not coverted to phenolic estrogens, in line with the essentially irreversible nature of the conversion of testosterone to DHT by steroid 5α-reductase. Some of the effects of testosterone on brain centers involved in regulation of gonadotropin secretion and coital behavior may involve its conversion in situ to both DHT and 17β-estradiol. A detailed discussion of these and other aspects of androgen action on the central nervous system is outside the scope of this chapter, but readers interested in the roles of estrogen and DHT formation from testosterone in this context should consult recent reviews by Naftolin et al.[30] and Ohno et al.,[31] and the comprehensive text of Mainwaring.[7]

REFERENCES

1. Price, D., and Williams-Ashman, H. G. The Accessory Reproductive Glands of Mammals. In W. C. Young (ed): *Sex and Internal Secretions,* 3rd. ed. Baltimore, Williams & Wilkins, 1961, pp. 366–448.
2. Liao, S., and Fang, S. Receptor-Proteins for Androgens and the Mode of Action of Androgens on Gene Transcription in Ventral Prostate. *Vitam. Horm. 27:* 17, 1969.
3. Williams-Ashman, H. G., Liao, S., Hancock, R. L., Jurkowitz, L., and Silverman, D. A. Testicular Hormones and the Synthesis of Ribonucleic Acids and Proteins in the Prostate Gland. *Recent Prog. Horm. Res. 20:* 247, 1964.
4. Williams-Ashman, H. G., and Reddi, A. H. Actions of Vertebrate Sex Hormones. *Annu. Rev. Physiol., 33:* 31, 1971.
5. Liao, S. Cellular Receptors and Mechanisms of Action of Steroid Hormones. *Int. Rev. Cytol. 41:* 87, 1975.
6. Wilson, J. Metabolism of Testicular Androgens. In D. W. Hamilton and R. O. Greep (eds): *Handbook of Endocrinology. section 7: Endocrinology, vol. 5, Male Reproductive System.* American Physiological Society, Washington, D.C., 1975, ch 25, pp. 491–508.
7. Mainwaring, W. I. P. *The Mechanism of Action of Androgens.* New York, Springer, 1977, pp. 1–178.
8. Neumann, F., and Steinbeck, H. Antiandrogens. In O. Eichler et al. (eds): *Handbuch der experimentelen Pharmakologie* vol. 35, part 2. Berlin, Springer, 1974, pp. 235–484.
9. Verhoeven, G., Heyns, W., and DeMoor, P. Testosterone Receptors in the Prostate and Other Tissues. *Vitam. Horm. 33:* 265, 1975.
10. Lipsett, M. Production of Testosterone by Prostate and Other Peripheral Tissues in Man. *Vitam. Horm. 33:* 209, 1975.
11. Ritzen, E. M., Hagenäs, L., Hansson, V., et al. Androgen Binding and Transport in Testis and Epididymis. *Vitam. Horm. 33:* 283, 1975.
12. Ohno, S. Major Regulatory Genes for Mammalian Sexual Development. *Cell 7:* 315, 1976.
13. Mainwaring, W. I. P., Symes, E. K., and Higgins, S. J. Nuclear Components Responsible for the Retention of Steroid–Receptor Complexes, especially from the Standpoint of the Specificity of Hormonal Responses. *Biochem. J. 156:* 129, 1976.
14. Ahmed, K. Phosphoprotein Metabolism in Primary and Accessory Sex Tissues. In J. A. Thomas and R. L. Singhal (eds): *Molecular Mechanisms of Gonadal Hormone Action.* Baltimore, University Park Press, 1975, pp. 129–165.
15. Williams-Ashman, H. G., Pegg, A. E., and Lockwood, D. H. Mechanisms and Regulation of Polyamine and Putrescine Biosynthesis in Male Genital Glands and Other Tissues of Mammals. *Adv. Enzyme Regul. 7:* 291, 1969.
16. Liang, T., and Liao, S. A Very Rapid Effect of Androgen on the Initiation of Protein Synthesis in Prostate. *Proc. Natl. Acad. Sci. U.S.A. 72:* 706, 1975.
17. Pegg, A. E., and Williams-Ashman, H. G. Effects of Androgens on Incorporation of Labeled Amino Acids into Proteins by Prostate Mitochondria. *Endocrinology 82:* 603, 1968.
18. Bruchovsky, N., Lesser, B., Van Doorn, E., and Craven, S. Hormonal Effects on Cell Proliferation in Rat Prostate. *Vitam. Horm. 33:* 61, 1975.
19. Williams-Ashman, H. G., Tadolini, B., Wilson, J., and Corti, A. Polynucleotide Polymerizations and Prostate Proliferation. *Vitam. Horm. 33:* 33, 1975.
20. Mainwaring, W. I. P., Rennie, P. S., and Keen, J. The Androgenic Regulation of Prostate Proteins with a High Affinity for Deoxyribonucleic Acid. *Biochem. J. 156:* 253, 1976.
21. Huggins, C. Two Principles in Endocrine Therapy of Cancer: Hormone Deprival and Hormone Interference. *Cancer Res. 25:* 1163, 1965.
22. Price, D. *In vitro* Studies on Differentiation of the Reproductive Tract. *Philos. Trans. R. Soc. Lond.* [*Biol.*] *259:* 133, 1970.
23. Jost, A. A New Look at the Mechanisms Controlling Sex Differentiation in Mammals. *Johns Hopkins Med. J. 130:* 38, 1972.
24. Jost, A., Vigier, B., Prepin, J., and Perchallet, J.-P. Studies on Sex Differentiation in Mammals. *Recent Prog. Horm. Res. 29:* 1, 1973.
25. Wilson, J., and Goldstein, J. L. Classification of Hereditary Disorders of Sexual Development. In D. Bergsma (ed.): *Genetic Forms of Hypogonadism, Birth Defects: Original Articles Series,* vol. 11, no. 4. Baltimore, Williams & Wilkins for the National Foundation March of Dimes, 1975, pp. 1–16.

26. Bardin, C. W., Bullock, L. P., Sherins, R. J., Mowszowicz, I., and Blackburn, W. R. Androgen Metabolism and Mechanism of Action in Male Pseudohermaphroditism: A Study of Testicular Feminization. *Recent Prog. Horm. Res. 29:* 65, 1973.
27. Amrhein, J. A., Meyer, W. J., Jones, H. W., and Migeon, C. J. Androgen Insensitivity in Man: Evidence for Genetic Heterogeneity. *Proc. Natl. Acad. Sci. U.S.A. 73:* 891, 1976.
28. Imperato-McGinley, J., Guerro, L., Gautier, J., and Peterson, R. E. Steroid 5α-Reductase Deficiency in Man: An Inherited Form of Male Pseudohermaphroditism. *Science 186:* 1213. 1974.
29. Walsh, P. C., Madden, J. D., Harrod, M. J., et al. Familial Incomplete Male Pseudohermaphroditism, Type 2. Decreased Dihydrotestosterone Formation in Pseudovaginal Perineoscrotal Hypospadias. *N. Engl. Med. J. 291:* 944, 1974.
30. Naftolin, F., Ryan, K. J., Davies, I. J., et al. The Formation of Estrogens by Central Neuroendocrine Tissues. *Recent Prog. Horm. Res. 31:* 295, 1975.
31. Ohno, S., Geller, L. N., and Lai, E. V. Y. *Tfm* Mutation and Masculinization Versus Feminization of the Mouse Central Nervous System. *Cell 3:* 235, 1974.

122

Hormonal Control of Spermatogenesis

Emil Steinberger

Historical Overview
Molecular Mechanisms Involved in Hormonal Control of Seminiferous Tubule Function

HISTORICAL OVERVIEW

The earliest concepts of the controlling mechanisms involved in the development of the testes and maintenance of their function were formulated by clinicians and pathologists who observed the existence of brain lesions in sexually underdeveloped patients. These observations led to vague suggestions that gonadal function must be controlled by a structure or structures located within the brain. Our knowledge of the endocrine basis for testicular control did not evolve until an experimental approach utilizing animals as experimental models was developed. Smith[1] demonstrated in the rat that the pituitary gland must secrete substances (gonadotropins) responsible for the stimulation of testicular growth and maintenance of their function. This concept was further refined by Greep et al.,[2] who provided evidence for dual gonadotropin control of testicular function, the Leydig cells being stimulated by luteinizing hormone (LH) and the seminiferous tubules by follicle-stimulating hormone (FSH). This simple and elegant hypothesis of endocrine control of testicular function has survived in its basic sense until now, although a number of modifications have been made in the interim.

Walsh et al.[3] suggested that testosterone can maintain the spermatogenic process in the absence of gonadotropins. This observation was subsequently confirmed by numerous investigators and has been the source of confusion and controversy ever since. On the basis of studies utilizing various experimental models, a hypothesis suggesting specific hormonal requirements for the various segments of the spermatogenic process was proposed.[4,5] This hypothesis states that the spermatogenic process can be maintained qualitatively (factors necessary for quantitative maintenance are still not known) by testosterone alone; however, for induction of the complete spermatogenic process in immature testes or its reinitiation subsequent to loss of gonadotropic function in adults, a more complicated hormonal interaction is required. Numerous studies provided evidence that testosterone may be essential for initiation of spermatogonial divisions and differentiation[6] and for completion of the meiotic division, while FSH may provide conditions favorable to spermatid maturation.[4] Although in the initially formulated hypothesis, E. Steinberger and Duckett[4] did not state clearly whether the hormones exert their effect directly on a specific cell type in the seminiferous epithelium, or whether the effect is mediated via another cell type, evidence has been accumulating suggesting that the Sertoli cells may be involved in this process (for review see Steinberger and Steinberger[7]). The involvement of FSH in the development of the spermatids during the first wave of spermatogenesis, together with the observation that once this "event" is triggered, the process of spermiogenesis (spermatid maturation) will continue in the absence of FSH as long as an uninterrupted and adequate supply of testosterone is available, led E. Steinberger[8] to propose a concept of an "obligatory but transitory" role for FSH in spermatogenesis. This concept fits the available biochemical data well (see below) and explains the difficulties encountered in past attempts to demonstrate experimentally the role of FSH in spermatogenesis.

The concepts discussed above were derived in most instances from experiments conducted in lower species, primarily in the rat, and provide an important body of knowledge; however, they do not clarify the situations encountered under clinical conditions in man. Studies in man are hampered by several factors. It is obviously impossible to create in man an appropriate experimental model which could be manipulated in a precise fashion at will to answer specific questions. Instead one has to deal with randomly occurring, poorly defined, complex clinical states. This limits the studies to a relatively small group of individuals exhibiting similar, but not necessarily identical, pathophysiology. Since pure human gonadotropic hormones (LH and FSH) are not available, one must use impure mixtures containing varying ratios of FSH:LH activities. These gonadotropic preparations are expensive and difficult to obtain. In contrast to lower species, humans rapidly develop antibodies to gonadotropins of other species. To investigate effects of gonadotropins on spermatogenesis, long-term therapy (months) is required before the response can be detected, since in man the spermatogenic process takes approximately 2 months and epididymal transport an additional 10–14 days; thus, it takes close to 3 months before a spermatozoon is formed and ejaculated. Since serial testicular biopsies are not practicable and the duration of a study cannot be shortened, the details of changes in spermatogenesis during the course of therapy cannot be studied. In spite of these difficulties numerous investigations have been conducted in man. While most of the results obtained are difficult to interpret, some information concerning the hormonal relationships in human spermatogenesis has become available.

Utilizing partially purified pituitary gonadotropins of human origin rich in FSH, Gemzell and Kjessler[9] demonstrated complete restoration of spermatogenesis proceeding up to the spermatid stage in incompletely hypophysectomized males. This observation suggests that in man the first wave of spermiogenesis may be FSH dependent, similar to that described for the rat.[4] In hypophysectomized man, with the germinal epithelium regressed to the level of spermatogonia, complete spermatogenesis was induced by treatment with gonadotropins of human postmenopausal urine origin (HMG, Pergonal) containing both LH and FSH activity.[10] In patients with hypogonadotropic eunuchoidism (lack of pituitary gonadotropin production), Paulsen[11] suggested that HCG (primarily LH activity) can induce full testicular function in some patients but not in others . . . Those with some endogenous gonadotropin secretion will respond will full spermatogenesis . . . while in those with absence of clinically effective endogenous gonadotropin secretion, HCG treatment will not achieve full spermatogenesis. In these patients, the addition of human postmenopausal gonadotropin (HMG, Pergonal) therapy may produce full spermatogenesis. . . .

Similar observations were made by Lunenfeld et al.,[12] Johnsen and Christiansen,[13] Smith et al.,[14] and others. Rosemberg et al.,[15] investigating the process of initiation of spermatogenesis in prepuberal boys, concluded that either human chorionic gonadotropin (HCG) or HMG is capable of initiating the spermatogenic process. Since HCG exerts essentially LH activity only, and HMG has both LH and FSH activities, it would seem that LH activity is all that is necessary to initiate spermatogenesis in prepuberal testes. These investigators unfortunately did not conduct the therapy for a sufficient length of time to determine whether either form of treatment would induce completion of spermatogenesis. Since in all the abovementioned studies dealing with initiation of spermatogenesis gonadotropin preparations containing LH activity were utilized, the question of the role of androgens in initiation of spermatogenesis requires consideration. In lower species it appears that androgens are involved in the initiation process, and recently it has been demonstrated that in man testosterone also can initiate spermatogenesis.[6] Thus, it would be reasonable to assume that in the above studies the LH activity in the gonadotropin preparations was responsible for the initiation of spermatogenesis by stimulating androgen production of the Leydig cells.

This straightforward assumption about the effect of testosterone on spermatogenesis in man is complicated by the large body of literature, beginning with Hotchkiss,[16] that shows that administration of testosterone to a normal man results in suppression of spermatogenesis, and its administration to a man with gonadotropin deficiency fails to maintain or induce spermatogenesis. While no direct experimental or clinical evidence is available to clarify this issue, an explanation has been offered.[17] Since in the rat approximately 1–2 mg of testosterone propionate per day has to be administered to maintain spermatogenesis, when extrapolated to man a daily dose of 4–8 mg/kg/day or 300–600 mg/day would have to be administered. Since no preparations of testosterone are available which would permit administration of such a high dose, it is plausible to assume that the reason for the inability to influence spermatogenesis with testosterone in men is due to the inability to administer a sufficiently high dose.

MOLECULAR MECHANISMS INVOLVED IN HORMONAL CONTROL OF SEMINIFEROUS TUBULE FUNCTION

The current physiologic concepts for the role of FSH in spermatogenesis propose that this hormone triggers an event in immature testes which is essential for the completion of spermiogenesis (development of the spermatid) during the first wave of spermatogenesis.[5] Once this event is triggered the process of spermiogenesis will proceed as long as an adequate and uninterrupted supply of testosterone is available. Thus, FSH is necessary for spermatogenesis, but it has only a transitory effect limited to the development of the spermatid during the first wave of spermatogenesis.[4,7] This concept is supported by biochemical studies which show that the responsiveness of the testes to FSH with an increase in RNA and protein synthesis is limited to a relatively brief period of time during the first wave of spermatogenesis and during reinitiation of spermatogenesis in posthypophysectomy-regressed testes.[18,19]

The discovery of the various components of the biochemical system of the polypeptide hormone action in the testes and the responsiveness of this system to FSH (primarily for the limited period of time during development) established without a doubt the role of FSH in spermatogenesis. Subsequent in vivo studies pointed to the Sertoli cells as a possible target site for FSH action.[20–22] The demonstration of specific binding of FSH to the seminiferous tubules[23–25] provided evidence concerning the tubular site of FSH action in the testes. These findings supported the previously made observations on the microscopic localization of labeled FSH in the seminiferous tubule.[26–28] Later the demonstration of FSH binding to isolated Sertoli cells[29] and stimulation by FSH of cAMP production in isolated Sertoli cells localized this response of the seminiferous tubules specifically to the Sertoli cell.[29–31]

In 1971 Hansson and Tveter[32] demonstrated the presence of androphilic proteins in the epididymis. One of the proteins was similar to testosterone-binding globulin. An identical protein with high affinity and limited capacity for binding androgens was also demonstrated in the testis cytosol.[20,21] It has been suggested that this androgen-binding protein (ABP) may be produced in the Sertoli cells.[20,33] This suggestion was supported by direct evidence from experiments that utilized cultures of isolated Sertoli cells.[29] The production of ABP in vivo and in vitro can be induced and maintained by FSH;[20,21,29,34,35] in the absence of FSH it can be induced and maintained by testosterone.[36]

The ABP is not a receptor, but it seems more likely to be a transport protein. A different protein with receptor properties has been detected in testicular tissue,[37,38] and nuclear androgen-binding sites have been shown to be localized primarily in the spermatids, although they could also be detected in spermatocytes and Sertoli cells.[39,40]

Taking into consideration this recent information, the following hypothesis[8] on the molecular aspects of hormonal control of spermatogenesis has been proposed (Fig. 122-1): FSH is delivered to the interstitial area of the testes via the arterial system. It diffuses passively through the basement membranes of the seminiferous tubules and is bound to a specific membrane receptor on the Sertoli cells, where it activates adenyl cyclase, thus stimulating production of cAMP. This nucleotide promotes DNA-dependent RNA synthesis, resulting in formation of new proteins, including ABP. Androgens diffuse passively from the interstitial area into the seminiferous epithelium, where they are bound and concentrated by ABP, thus facilitating high androgen environment in the vicinity of the germ cells. The ABP–androgen complex comes in contact with the germ cell membranes. ABP has a high affinity for androgens (Ka = 0.55 nM^{-1}). However, the rapid dissociation of androgen from the complex ($t_{1/2}$ = 3 min) facilitates the transfer of the androgen to a cytoplasmic receptor in the germ cells. The receptor–androgen complex in the germ cells is transported into the nucleus. There it binds to an acceptor site on the chromatin.[41] The subsequent steps in the action of the androgen–receptor complex in the germ cell nuclei are unknown. After delivering the androgen to the germ cells, the ABP molecule can probably bind another molecule of androgen, and the above-mentioned process is re-

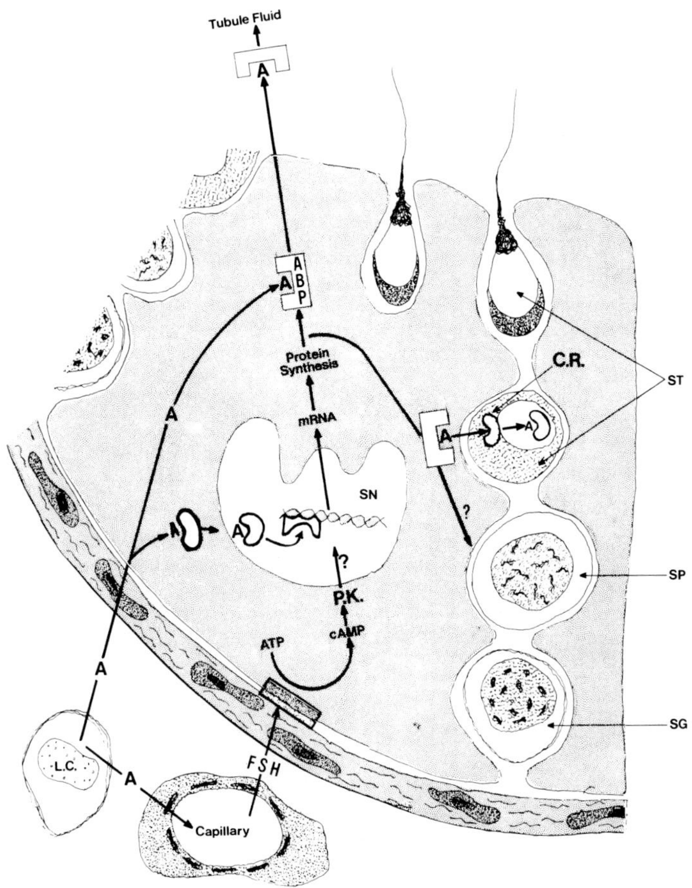

Fig. 122-1. Sertoli and germ cells and the biochemical mechanisms concerned with their function. SN, Sertoli cell nucleus; SG, spermatogonium; SP, spermatocyte; ST, spermatid; LC, Leydig cell; PK, cAMP-dependent phosphokinase; A, testosterone; FSH, follicle-stimulating hormone; CR, cytoplasmic receptor; ABP, androgen-binding protein; [symbol], receptor; [symbol], chromatin acceptor.

peated, or the ABP–androgen complex is secreted into the lumen of the seminiferous tubule and transported to the epididymis.

REFERENCES

1. Smith P. E. The Disabilities Caused by Hypophysectomy and Their Repair. *J.A.M.A. 88:* 158, 1927.
2. Greep, R. O., Febold, H. L., and Hisaw, F. L. Effects of 2 Hypophyseal Gonadotropic Hormones on Reproductive System of Male Rat. *Anat. Rec. 65:* 261, 1936.
3. Walsh, E. L., Cuyler, W. K., and McCullagh, D. R. Physiologic Maintenance of Male Sex Glands; Effect of Androtin on Hypophysectomized Rats. *Am. J. Physiol. 107:* 508, 1934.
4. Steinberger, E., and Duckett, G. E. Hormonal Control of Spermatogenesis. *J. Reprod. Fert.* [Suppl.] *2:* 117, 1967.
5. Steinberger, E. Hormonal Control of Mammalian Spermatogenesis. *Physiol. Rev. 51:* 1, 1971.
6. Steinberger, E., Root, A., Ficher, M., and Smith, K. D. The Role of Androgens in the Initiation of Spermatogenesis in Man. *J. Clin. Endocrinol. Metab. 37:* 746, 1973.
7. Steinberger, E., and Steinberger, A. Hormonal Control of Testicular Function in Mammals, in Knobil, E., and Sawyer, W. H. (eds.): Handbook of Physiology, vol. IV, part 2. Washington, D. C., American Physiological Society, 1974, p. 325.
8. Steinberger, E. Hormonal Regulation of the Seminiferous Tubule Function, in French, F. S., Hansson, V., Ritzen, E. M., and Nayfeh, S. N. (eds.): Hormonal Regulation of Spermatogenesis. New York, Plenum, 1975, p. 337.
9. Genzell, C. A., and Kjessler, B. Treatment of Infertility After Partial Hypophysectomy with Human Pituitary Gonadotrophins. *Lancet 1:* 644, 1964.
10. MacLeod, J., Pazianos, A., and Ray, B. S. Restoration of Human Spermatogenesis by Menopausal Gonadotropins. *Lancet 1:* 1196, 1964.
11. Paulsen, C. A. Effect of Human Chorionic Gonadotropin and Human Menopausal Gonadotropin Therapy on Testicular Function, in Rosemberg, E. (ed.): Gonadotropins. Los Altos, Calif., Geron-X, 1968, p. 491.
12. Lunenfeld, B., Goldman, B., and Ismajovich, B. Assessment of Results with Gonadotropic Therapy, in Rosemberg, E. (ed.): Gonadotropins. Los Altos, Calif., Geron-X, 1968, p. 513.
13. Johnsen, S. G., and Christiansen, P. Spermatogenesis and Conception During HMG Treatment of Hypogonadotropic Hypogonadism, in Rosemberg, E. (ed.): Gonadotropins. Los Altos, Calif., Geron-X, 1968, p. 515.
14. Smith, K. D., Ficher, M., and Steinberger, E. Clinical Laboratory Findings During Gonadotropin Therapy of Post Pubertal Hypogonadotropic Hypogonadism. *Andrologia 6:* 147, 1974.
15. Rosemberg, E., Mancini, R. E., Crigler, J. F., and Bergada, C. Effect of Human Menopausal Gonadotropin on Prepuberal Testes, in Rosemberg, E. (ed.): The Gonads. Los Altos, Calif., Geron-X, 1968, p. 527.
16. Hotchkiss, R. S. Effects of Massive Doses of Testosterone Propionate upon Spermatogenesis. *J. Clin. Endocrinol. 4:* 114, 1944.
17. Steinberger, E., Smith, K. D., Tcholakian, R. K., et al. Steroidogenesis in Human Testes, in Mancini, R. E., and Martini, L. (eds.): Male Fertility and Sterility, Proceedings of Serono Symposia, vol. 5. New York, Academic, 1974, p. 149.
18. Menas, A. R., and Hall, P. F. Effect of FSH on Protein Biosynthesis in Testes of The Mature Rat. *Endocrinology 81:* 1151, 1967.
19. Means, A. R. Concerning the Mechanism of FSH Action: Rapid Stimulation of Testicular Synthesis of Nuclear RNA. *Endocrinology 89:* 981, 1971.
20. Steinberger, E., Steinberger, A., and Sanborn, B. Endocrine Control of Spermatogenesis. Presented at XIIIth International Latin Ameri-

can Symposium on Physiological and Genetic Aspects of Reproduction, Bahia, Brazil, 1973, in Coutinho, M., and Fuchs, F. (eds.): Physiology and Genetics of Reproduction, Part A. New York, Plenum, 1974, p. 163.

21. Hansson, V., Reusch, E., Trygstad, O., et al. FSH Stimulation of Testicular Androgen Binding Protein. *Nature* [New Biol] *246:* 56, 1973.
22. Means, A. R. Biochemical Effects of Follicle-Stimulating Hormone on the Testis, in Hamilton, D. W., and Greep, R. O. (eds.): Handbook of Physiology, section 7, vol. 5. Washington, D.C., American Physiological Society, 1975, p. 203.
23. Means, A. R., and Vaitukaitis. Peptide Hormone "Receptors:" Specific Binding of ^{3}H-FSH to Testis. *Endocrinology 90:* 39, 1972.
24. Bhalla, V. K., and Reichert, L. E., Jr. Properties of Follicle-Stimulating Hormone–Receptor Interactions. Specific Binding of Human Follicle-Stimulating Hormone to Rat Testes. *J. Biol. Chem. 249:* 43, 1974.
25. Steinberger, A., Thanki, K. J., and Siegal, B. FSH Binding in Rat Testes During Maturation and Following Hypophysectomy. Cellular Localization of FSH Receptors, in Dufau, M. L., and Means, A. R. (eds.): Hormone Binding and Target Cell Activation in the Testis. New York, Plenum, 1974, p. 177.
26. Mancini, R. E., Castro, A., and Seiguer, A. C. Histologic Localization of Follicle-Stimulating and Luteinizing Hormones in the Rat Testis. *J. Histochem. Cytochem. 15:* 516, 1967.
27. Castro, A. E., Seiguer, A. C., and Mancini, R. E. Electron Microscopic Study on the Localization of Labeled Gonadotropins in the Sertoli and Leydig Cells of the Rat Testis. *Proc. Soc. Exp. Biol. Med. 133:* 582, 1970.
28. Castro, A. E., Alonso, A., and Mancini, R. E. Localization of Follicle-Stimulating and Luteinizing Hormones in the Rat Testis Using Immunohistological Tests. *J. Endocrinol. 52:* 129, 1972.
29. Steinberger, A., Elkington, J. S. H., Sanborn, B. M., et al. Culture and FSH Responses of Sertoli Cells Isolated from Sexually Mature Rat Testis, in French, F. S., Hansson, V., Ritzen, E. M., and Nayfeh, S. H. (eds.): Hormonal Regulation of Spermatogenesis. New York, Plenum, 1975, p. 399.
30. Dorrington, J. H., Roller, N. F., and Fritz, I. B. The Effects of FSH on Cell Preparations from the Rat Testis, in Dufau, M. L., and Means, A. R. (eds.): Hormone Binding and Target Cell Activation in the Testis. New York, Plenum, 1974, p. 237.
31. Heindel, J. J., Rothenberg, R., Robison, G. A., and Steinberger, A. LH and FSH Stimulation of Cyclic AMP in Specific Cell Types Isolated from the Testes. *J. Cyclic Nucl. Res. 1:* 69, 1975.
32. Hansson, V., and Tveter, K. J. Effect of Anti-Androgens on the Uptake and Binding of Androgen by Human Benign Nodular Prostatic Hyperplasia *in Vitro. Acta Endocrinol. 68:* 69, 1971.
33. Hansson, V., Trygstad, O., French, F. S., et al. Androgen Transport and Receptor Mechanisms in Testis and Epididymis. *Nature 250:* 387, 1974.
34. Sanborn, B. M., Elkington, J. S. H., and Steinberger, E. Properties of Rat Testicular Androgen Binding Protein, in Dufau, M. L., and Means, A. R. (eds.): Hormone Binding and Target Cell Activation in the Testis. New York, Plenum, 1974, p. 291.
35. Sanborn, B. M., Elkington, J. S. H., Chowdhury, M., Tcholakian, R., and Steinberger, E. Hormonal Influences on the Level of Testicular Androgen Binding Activity. Effect of FSH Following Hypophysectomy. *Endocrinology 96:* 304, 1975.
36. Elkington, J. S. H., Sanborn, B. M., and Steinberger, E. The Effect of Testosterone Propionate on the Concentration of Testicular and Epididymal Androgen Binding Activity in the Hypophysectomized Rat. *Mol. Cell. Endocrinol. 2:* 157, 1975.
37. Hansson, V., McLean, W. S., Smith, A. A., et al. Androgen Receptors in Rat Testis. *Steroids 23:* 823, 1974.
38. Mulder, E., Peters, M. J., van Beurden, W. M. O., and van der Molen, H. J. A Receptor for Testosterone in Mature Rat Testes. FEBS Lett. *47:* 209, 1974.
39. Sanborn, B. M., Steinberger, A., Meistrich, M. L., and Steinberger, E. Androgen Binding Sites in Testis Cell Fractions as Measured by a Nuclear Exchange Assay. *J. Steroid Biochem. 6:* 1459, 1975.
40. Sanborn, B. M., and Steinberger, E. Androgen Nuclear Exchange Activity in Rat Testis. *Endocrinol. Res. Commun. 2:* 335, 1975.
41. Tsai, Y.-H., Sanborn, B. M., Steinberger, A., and Steinberger, E. The Interaction of Testicular Androgen–Receptor Complex with Rat Germ Cell and Sertoli Cell Chromatin. *Biochem. Biophys. Res. Commun. 75:* 366, 1977.

123

Laboratory Evaluation of Testicular Function

Keith D. Smith
Luis J. Rodriguez-Rigau

The evaluation of testicular function can be readily divided into two categories: those procedures designed to evaluate spermatogenesis, and those dealing with the endocrine aspects of gonadal function. During recent years a number of sophisticated and expensive laboratory tests of testicular function have been developed. However, it must be emphasized that in most cases there is no need to employ all of these procedures. As elsewhere in endocrinology, a sound knowledge of testicular physiology will result in an adequate diagnostic workup with the judicious use of a minimum of laboratory tests.

In this chapter, we will review tests available for the evaluation of disorders of testicular function. Some of these procedures should be regarded as a part of the routine workup of all patients. Others should be used only when a clear indication is present, and still others are sophisticated techniques available primarily in research laboratories. It is not possible to make precise suggestions concerning employment of each specific study since the design of the laboratory evaluation will depend upon clinical indications and the available facilities. It is, however, important to emphasize that each physician should be informed about the relevance, sensitivity, precision, normal values, and limitations of all laboratory tests that he requests.[1]

EVALUATION OF SPERMATOGENESIS

SEMEN ANALYSIS

The examination of a fresh semen sample is the simplest, least expensive, and most nearly definitive gonadal function test.[2] As can be concluded from knowledge of the physiology of the male reproductive system, all components of the hypothalamo-pituitary-testicular axis as well as the excretory system and ejaculatory mechanism must be relatively intact for semen analysis to be normal.[3] Despite this fact, semen analysis is seldom performed unless the patient presents with infertility. For obscure moral or other considerations physicians have been reticent to obtain semen specimens for analysis in cases of male reproductive system disorders other than infertility, despite the fact that such analyses could be of equal or greater diagnostic value than other more expensive and more elaborate laboratory tests.

Although the techniques of semen analysis have undergone few changes in the past 25 yr, considerable information has accumulated on the critical need for a standardized and precise procedure if reliable results are to be obtained. Most physicians are aware that the clinical value of chemical analysis of blood or urine depends on such factors as relevance, precision, accuracy, and sensitivity of the method used. The same criteria are vital to semen analysis.

Collection of the Specimen

The patient should be clearly informed about the proper collection and transport of the sample. Masturbation is the most precise and reliable method. Coitus interruptus may result in an incomplete collection, which in turn will lead to grossly biased results. Collection into a condom produces erroneous estimates of spermatozoal motility secondary to spermicidal agents present in the condom, and inaccurate sperm counts and volume measurements may result as well.

The patient should be provided with a clean, widemouthed container in which to collect the semen. Unless culture of the sample is intended, a sterile container is unnecessary. Prior to collection a minimum of 2 and a maximum of 5 days of continence is required. Semen analysis should not be performed on a specimen that does not contain the entire ejaculate. The specimen should be delivered to the laboratory within 1 h after collection. During this time, it should be kept at room temperature (70 to 80 F) rather than body temperature.[4]

Macroscopic Examination

Volume and viscosity of the semen should be measured as soon as it is received in the laboratory. A normal ejaculate should liquify within 20 min after collection.[5] Failure of liquifaction after 60 min or persistent high viscosity of the sample should be noted. Unusual color and/or odor should also be recorded.

Volume is measured in a graduated cylinder or a similar calibrated container. Eliasson suggests that more accuracy could be achieved by weighing a specimen collected into a preweighed container.[5] However, this degree of accuracy is probably unnecessary in most clinical situations.

Microscopic Examination

Before any microscopic examination is attempted, full liquifaction and adequate mixing of the sample are absolutely essential. Probably the most frequent cause of erroneous sperm counts is inadequate mixing of the sample. Evaluation of spermatozoal motility, density, and morphology should be performed routinely. If no spermatozoa are found during the initial examination, the specimen should be centrifuged and the sediment examined.

Motility. Usually motility is estimated to the nearest 10 percent by subjective microscopic examination. One drop of the well-mixed specimen is placed on a clean glass slide and covered with a cover slip of standard size (e.g., 22 × 22 mm). The preparation should be studied by a trained observer at a magnification of 400× to 600×, preferably with phase-contrast optics. Only those spermatozoa demonstrating directional movement should be considered motile, and a minimum of 20 microscopic fields should be examined.

In some laboratories two estimates, viability and motility, are assessed. Viability is the estimated percent of spermatozoa demonstrating any motion, while motility is graded 0 to 4+ and indicates the type of directional movement demonstrated by the spermatozoa (0 — no motility; 1+ — poor; 2+ — medium; 3+ — good; 4+ — excellent). All of these values should be related to the time elapsed since the sample was collected. In some instances it is valuable to reevaluate motility at several time intervals. A semen sample with rapidly declining sperm motility is, from a prognostic and therapeutic point of view, not far different from one with initial poor motility.

These techniques for motility evaluation have been criticized because their subjectivity makes them prone to error. Considerable research has been undertaken in the past few years in an attempt to develop objective methods for evaluation of sperm motility and viability. Several supravital staining methods for distinction between live and dead spermatozoa are available,[6] as well as photographic techniques for the quantitative objective assessment of percent motility.[7,8] A novel method, based on analysis of small-frequency modifications produced by moving spermatozoa when a monochromatic laser beam is passed through a semen sample, was recently described.[9] Nevertheless, the above-described subjective methods for evaluation of sperm motility are still utilized by most, if not all, hospital and commercial laboratories, and the physician must be familiar with the resulting wide error range.

Sperm Density. Sperm count is reported as millions of spermatozoa per milliliter. An additional measure, the total sperm count, is calculated by multiplying the sperm count by the volume of the ejaculate. It is reported as millions of spermatozoa per ejaculate. Most commonly a hemocytometer is utilized for counting of spermatozoa. The specimen is diluted 1:10, 1:20 or more depending on the sperm density noted during estimation of motility. Because of the multiplicity of factors that can affect the precision of this technique, duplicate counts preferably at two different dilutions should be performed routinely. Unfortunately, in many laboratories single determinations are performed. The coefficient of variation between two determinations should not exceed 10 percent.

An alternative procedure, employing an electronic particle counter (Coulter counter), also has been utilized for evaluation of sperm density. With this technique, significant interference by debris has been encountered at low sperm densities.[10]

Morphology. Morphology of spermatozoa is usually evaluated by microscopic examination of a stained smear. At least 200 cells should be evaluated and classified according to clearly defined and standardized criteria to facilitate comparisons of data between different laboratories.[5,11,12] Abnormalities of spermatozoal morphology are usually classified as head abnormalities (large, small, tapering, amorphous, duplicated, round, pear-shaped, etc.), midpiece abnormalities, and tail defects (broken, coiled, duplicated, etc.). The presence of germinal, inflammatory, epithelial or other cells should be noted. Special staining techniques have been developed to differentiate between round spermatids and leukocytes.[13]

Chemical Analysis

Seminal fluid is a mixture of secretions from the various accessory genital glands (prostate, seminal vesicles, bulbo-urethral, and urethral glands) and the testicular and epididymal fluids. Theoretically, each could be identified by chemical analyses. A deviation from the normal pattern could then be utilized to localize pathology to a specific area of the genital tract.

Fructose levels and pH determination are available in most laboratories. Since prostatic fluid is acid and seminal vesicular secretion alkaline, pH may provide an index of the relative proportion of these two secretions.[5] Fructose is secreted by the seminal vesicles. The presence of fructose in an azoospermic seminal fluid excludes an obstruction of the ejaculatory ducts.

Other chemical analyses can be performed in only a few research laboratories, but may become a part of the routine evaluation of seminal plasma in the future. Prostatic secretions may be evaluated by measurement of acid phosphatase, muramidase, citric acid, aminotransferases, dehydrogenases, zinc, and magnesium. In addition, viscosity of the seminal fluid reflects the prostatic secretion of liquifying enzymes.[5] Seminal vesicular fluid is rich in not only fructose, but also ascorbic acid, prostaglandins, and carnitine. Epididymal fluid contains carnitine, sialic acid, hexosamine, hexuronic acid, glyceryl-phosphoryl-choline, and high concentrations of potassium.[1,5] At this time no specific secretory factors from the bulbo-urethral or urethral glands have been reported.

Immunologic Studies

A variety of antibodies against spermatozoa and constitutents of seminal plasma have been described. It has been suggested that their presence may interfere with fertility. (For review, see Ref. 14.) The mechanism involved in the production of these antibodies is unclear. Injury to the male reproductive system (e.g., vasectomy, orchitis) has been suggested as an etiologic factor. Two types of antibodies, sperm agglutinating and sperm immobilizing, have been described. The latter are more likely to be associated with infertility and can be detected in serum by the sperm immobilizing test of Isojima.[15] The sperm agglutinating antibodies can be detected in serum by the macroscopic test of Kibrick[16] or by the microscopic technique of Franklin and Dukes.[17] Immunofluorescent methods for localization of antibodies on spermatozoa have been described.[18] This technique is controversial and probably of limited clinical value.[14]

Other

Electron microscopic studies, investigation of spermatozoal oxygen consumption, evaluation of recovery of spermatozoal motility following freezing and thawing, as well as techniques involving identification and separation of X- or Y-chromosome-bearing spermatozoa, should still be considered research procedures.

Interpretation of Results

Semen analysis may be used to provide an estimate of fertility potential, and serve as an indirect measure of adequacy of the hypothalamo-pituitary testicular axis. Fertility potential is difficult to estimate, since definition of what constitutes a "normal" or "fertile" ejaculate has been prevented by the divergent opinions of various authors. It has been suggested that fertility is a relative state dependent upon the fertility potential of both members of a couple.[19–21] Although the number of semen samples required for appropriate evaluation of sperm production is the subject of considerable controversy, most investigators agree that more than one ejaculate must be analyzed. The marked oscillations of sperm density in ejaculates from the same individual are well known.[22] Consequently, several semen samples collected over a period of 3 months should be analyzed if precise information is to be obtained. Smith *et al.* in 1965[73] and 1977[20] suggested a minimum of six ejaculates. Sherins[23] suggested a minimum of nine ejaculates over a period of 6 months. Most clinicians consider a sperm density of at least 20 million/ml with adequate volume, motility, and morphology as the division between fertility and subfertility. Several recent reports have suggested that even this level may be too high, and that subfertility should not be considered unless sperm density is below 10 million/ml or even 5 million/ml.[20,21,24]

Estimation of spermatozoal motility is one of the key components of seminal fluid evaluation.[25] Although motility and viability have been reported to be higher among fertile men, a sharp demarcation between fertility and infertility has not been established. Pregnancies following insemination with semen showing spermatozoal motility of 25 to 30 percent are not uncommon.[26]

Sperm morphology is apparently a more stable measure,[23] but again differences in opinion among authors have resulted in a lack of generally accepted criteria of normality. The American Fertility Society suggests that fertility is compromised when the percentage of abnormal spermatozoa is above 40,[27] while others believe that a higher percentage would be more realistic.[28]

Although high-volume ejaculates are usually associated with lower sperm counts, a direct correlation between sperm density and semen volume is not a consistent finding. In general, when sperm density is low, motility and morphology are also abnormal.[29]

Semen analysis may serve as an indirect measure of the adequacy of the hypothalamo-pituitary-testicular axis because all components of this axis must be intact for a man to produce an adequate ejaculate. Numerous investigations have noted an inverse relationship between sperm density and FSH levels in blood or urine.[30,31] In a recent study,[32] blood levels of testosterone, FSH, and LH were compared in a series of men grouped by sperm count and by total sperm count (Tables 123-1 and 123-2). No significant differences were found in mean testosterone and mean LH levels between any of the groups. Mean FSH levels were significantly elevated when sperm counts were below 10 million/ml or total sperm counts were below 25 million/ejaculate. Thus, if sperm counts are above 10 million/ml and/or total sperm counts above 25 million/ejaculate, it is unlikely that any abnormalities of blood levels of testosterone, FSH or LH will be found.

Table 123-1. Comparison of Plasma Hormone Levels (Mean ± Standard Deviation) from 262 Fertile Men Grouped by Sperm Count

Sperm count (millions/ml)	Testosterone (ng/dl)	LH (mIU/ml)	FSH (mIU/ml)
< 10.1	483 ± 275 (21)	2.63 ± 1.13 (21)	6.44 ± 7.72 (21)[a]
10.1–20.0	541 ± 254 (18)	2.39 ± 0.79 (18)	2.68 ± 1.32 (18)
20.1–40.0	429 ± 214 (44)	2.37 ± 1.10 (43)	2.62 ± 1.17 (43)
40.1–60.0	500 ± 275 (53)	2.35 ± 0.97 (54)	2.46 ± 1.62 (54)
60.1–80.0	499 ± 281 (39)	2.31 ± 0.73 (39)	2.45 ± 1.04 (39)
80.1–100.0	482 ± 257 (32)	2.20 ± 0.91 (32)	2.62 ± 1.57 (32)
> 100.0	445 ± 229 (54)	2.18 ± 0.89 (55)	2.37 ± 1.24 (55)
Entire series	471 ± 255 (261)	2.32 ± 0.93 (262)	2.82 ± 2.71 (262)
Normal range	200–1200	<5.00	<5.00

Number of subjects in parentheses.
[a] $p < 0.001$.

Table 123-2. Comparison of Plasma Hormone Levels (Mean ± Standard Deviation) from 262 Fertile Men Grouped by Total Sperm Count

Total sperm count (millions per ejaculate)	Testosterone (ng/dl)	LH (mIU/ml)	FSH (mIU/ml)
<25.1	462 ± 251 (32)	2.62 ± 0.94 (32)	5.18 ± 6.50 (32)[a]
25.1–50.0	505 ± 232 (29)	2.20 ± 0.93 (29)	2.22 ± 0.98 (29)
50.1–100.0	466 ± 232 (52)	2.32 ± 0.90 (52)	2.42 ± 1.14 (52)
100.1–200.0	499 ± 266 (68)	2.42 ± 0.99 (68)	2.80 ± 1.57 (68)
200.1–300.0	497 ± 270 (42)	2.21 ± 0.98 (42)	2.50 ± 1.51 (42)
300.1–400.0	451 ± 315 (15)	2.00 ± 0.51 (16)	2.11 ± 1.15 (16)
400.1–500.0	507 ± 279 (12)	2.12 ± 0.95 (12)	2.54 ± 1.34 (12)
>500.0	380 ± 275 (11)	2.26 ± 1.02 (11)	2.05 ± 0.63 (11)
Entire series	471 ± 255 (261)	2.32 ± 0.93 (262)	2.82 ± 2.71 (262)
Normal range	200–1200	<5.00	<5.00

Number of subjects in parentheses
[a] $p < 0.001$

TESTICULAR BIOPSY

Testicular biopsy, when properly performed, processed, and interpreted, is the most valuable procedure for the investigation of the pathophysiology of spermatogenic disturbances. Faultless surgical and histologic techniques are of paramount importance. These techniques have been described in detail in the literature.[33] Unfortunately, many testicular biopsy specimens are still obtained by removing the tissue with forceps and scissors or, even worse, by needle biopsy. If the tissue is then fixed in formalin and stained with hematoxylin and eosin, the resultant histologic preparations are frequently worthless. An example of this type of biopsy is demonstrated in Figure 123-1. If this photomicrograph is compared to Figure 123-2—a section of a properly obtained, fixed, and stained testicular biopsy from the same patient—the differences are obvious.

The surgical procedure of testicular biopsy is quite simple and may be performed under local anesthesia as an outpatient procedure. An assistant gently but firmly immobilizes the testis and stretches the scrotal skin over it. After local anesthesia, a small (1-cm) incision is made in the scrotum and the fascia is dissected to the surface of the tunica vaginalis of the testis. A small incision is made through the tunica vaginalis. This results in a small portion of testicular tissue bulging through the incision. This portion of tissue

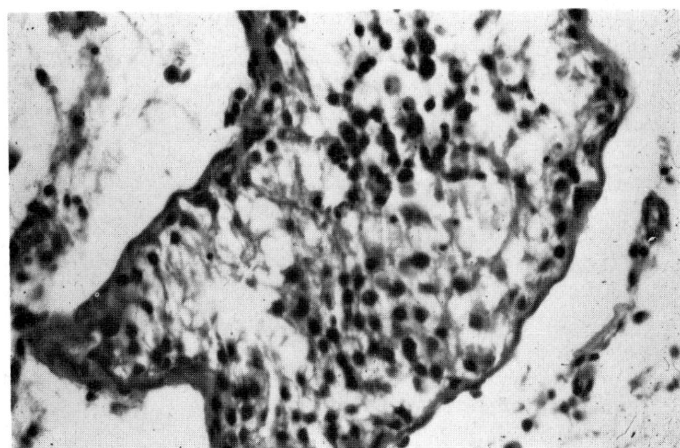

Fig. 123-1. Microscopic appearance of an inadequately processed testicular biopsy. (100×)

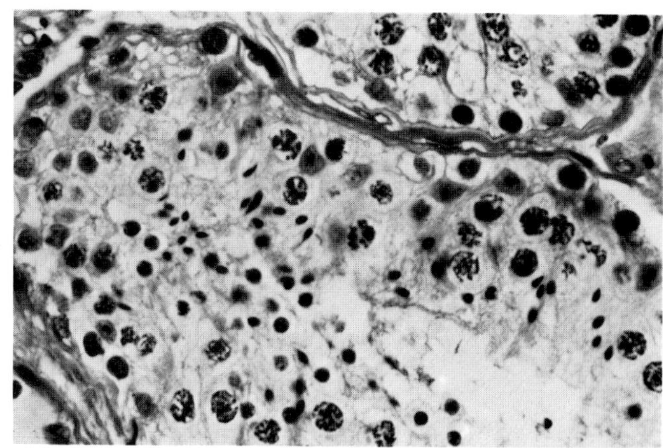

Fig. 123-2. Microscopic appearance of properly processed testicular biopsy from the same patient as in Figure 123-1. (100×)

is shaved off with a razor blade cutting tangentially to the surface of the testis. Once free, the biopsy specimen will remain on the surface of the razor blade, and both the tissue and the blade are dropped in Bouin's or Cleland's solution for fixation. It is important to apply as little pressure as possible to the specimen during the surgical procedure to prevent sloughing of the germinal cells into the lumen of the seminiferous tubules. After fixation and imbedding, 4μ sections are stained with PAS-hematoxylin or Masson's trichrome method.

Most frequently, the indication for testicular biopsy is severe oligospermia or azoospermia. For obvious reasons, determination of the existence of partial or complete obstructive lesions of the tubular transport system is of primary importance. Consequently, testicular biopsy usually should not be performed as an isolated procedure, but rather as part of a complete scrotal exploration. The contents of the scrotum should be exteriorized and examined. Special attention should be paid to the presence of small cysts or yellowish or whitish areas in the epididymis. This may indicate a partial or complete block of the epididymal duct.

A cross section of a normal seminiferous tubule shows several generations of germ cells (Fig. 123-2). The younger generation is near the basement membrane, while the more differentiated cells are near the lumen. A tubular cross section does not always reveal all cell generations (see Chapter 118). Sertoli cell nuclei can be observed near the basement membrane. Leydig cells are located near the capillaries in the interstitial space between the tubules. Thickening of the basement membrane and fibrosis or hyalinization of the seminiferous tubules can be determined. Spermatogenic arrests at a specific cell generation (spermatogonia, primary or secondary spermatocytes and spermatids) or complete absence of germ cells (Sertoli-cell-only) can be observed. Sloughing of immature cells into the lumen usually represents improper surgical technique rather than a pathologic state. Leydig cell hyperplasia may be observed, usually suggesting increased gonadotropin stimulation of the testis; it is characteristically found in Klinefelter syndrome.

Quantitative analysis of spermatogenesis is a specialized procedure, presently restricted to research laboratories.[34,35] These techniques provide important information on quantitative change affecting the spermatogenic process. They would be of great help in the evaluation of spermatogenesis following medical or surgical therapy, but for this purpose more than one biopsy would be required.

In addition to histologic evaluation, testicular tissue obtained at biopsy may be cultured for chromosomal analysis,[36] processed to measure intratesticular steroid concentrations,[37] or incubated with steroid precursors to evaluate the activity of the different steroidogenic enzymes.[38–40] These techniques will be reviewed in other sections of this chapter. All these procedures, presently restricted to research laboratories, can be performed on as little as 25 mg of tissue (the usual testicular biopsy weighs an average of 40 mg) and, if simplified, may become routine in the evaluation of testicular function. This could result in a better understanding of spermatogenic disorders and, it is hoped, aid in development of appropriate and specific therapeutic measures.

ENDOCRINE EVALUATION

Laboratory evaluation of the endocrine aspects of testicular function involves an assessment of the hypothalamic-pituitary axis and the evaluation of Leydig cell function.

Since pituitary "tropins" and steroids produced by the testis circulate in blood in very small amounts, their identification and quantitation are often difficult. Three methods have been used to measure these substances: bioassays, chemical techniques, and competitive binding assays.[41] Three basic concepts are common to all three techniques: precision, sensitivity (minimal detectable dose), and specificity. Bioassays for determination of gonadotropins or steroid hormones have been available for over 40 yr and remain highly valuable when appropriately applied. Examples of chemical methods are steroid measurements by colorimetric, chromatographic, or double-isotope derivative techniques. However, the development of competitive binding assays, particularly the radioimmunoassay (RIA), has offered greater precision, sensitivity, and specificity for routine determination of these hormones.

The basic principles of the radioimmunoassay are illustrated in Figure 123-3. A known amount of labeled hormone competes for a specific antibody with an unknown quantity of unlabeled hormone in serum, urine, or other biologic fluid. Following incubation to equilibrium, the bound and free fractions can be separated and the radioactivity in one of these fractions counted. Under appropriate equilibration conditions these counts are directly related to the amount of hormone in the sample (Fig. 123-4). Numerous variations of the basic assay techniques have been developed, particularly in the methods for separation of the bound and free fractions. Radioimmunoassay of gonadotropins is usually performed on unextracted serum or plasma. Radioimmunoassay of steroid hormones may require pre-assay purification of the plasma depending on the specificity of the antibody.

The radioimmunoassay has now become a routine method available in many clinical laboratories. Commercial kits have been developed which greatly simplify the assay procedure for a large variety of hormones. Unfortunately, in some instances, the simplication might have resulted in the marketing of materials that do not provide adequate specificity and precision. Physicians should make themselves aware of these shortcomings, and require information from the laboratory on the methodology utilized, including specificity of the antibody, precision, accuracy, and reproducibility of the technique, and quality controls employed. Since the

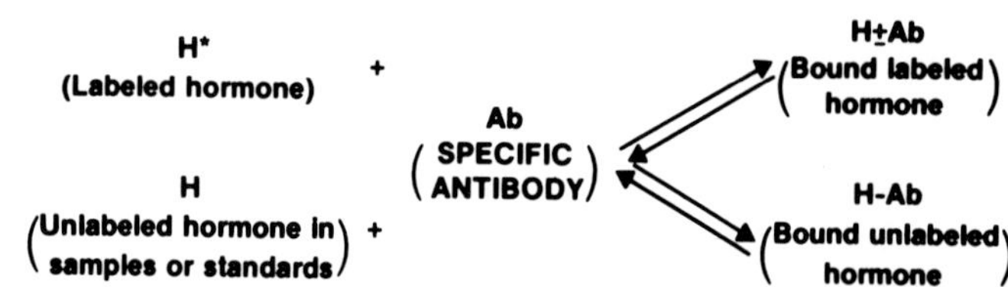

Fig. 123-3. Simplified diagram of the radioimmunoassay.

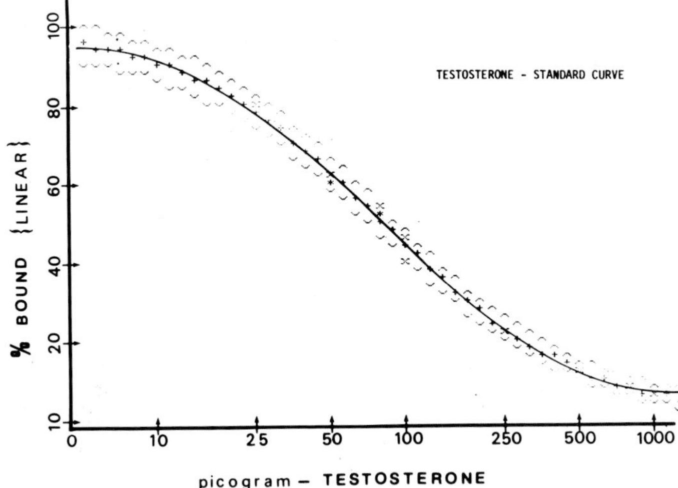

Fig. 123-4. Dose response curve for testosterone in the radioimmunoassay.

normal range of each hormone may differ among laboratories, it is important to know how this range was established. Lack of this information may result in difficulties in the interpretation of laboratory reports.

It has been suggested that the radioimmunoassay of pituitary hormones may not be sufficiently specific, since it measures immunoreactive materials not necessarily identical to the biologically active hormones.[42] To overcome this, other techniques for hormonal determination have been proposed, including radio-receptor assay[43] and techniques for in vitro bioassay.[42] The radio-receptor, like the RIA, is a competitive binding assay but utilizes as binding protein a purified preparation of the specific target-cell receptor for the hormone to be measured. Since binding of the hormone to the receptor is an obligatory step in the mechanism of biologic action of the hormone, this technique probably reflects in a more specific fashion than the radioimmunoassay the biologically active hormone levels. The in vitro bioassay utilizes an in vitro biochemical response of a target-cell preparation as an indirect measure of hormonal levels. Consequently, it combines the advantages of both the bioassay (measurement of biologically active hormone) and the radioimmunoassay (sensitivity, accuracy, and reproducibility). While these techniques are presently research procedures, they could be simplified in the near future, making them available for clinical use.

Ideally, gonadotropin levels should be reported in equivalents of pure LH or FSH. Since neither hormone is available at the present time in a chemically pure state, standards of variable purity have to be utilized. Prior to the introduction of international standards, gonadotropin levels were reported in bioassay units. For example, the amount of gonadotropin required to double the weight of the uterus of an immature mouse was a "mouse uterine weight unit."[44] The extreme variability of such units complicated comparison of results. To remedy this, international standard preparations were developed. These standards are either used directly in every assay, or locally prepared reference standards are calibrated against them. Results are reported in units of weight (nanograms) or milli-international units (mIU) of the international standard per volume of blood. It should be noted that the institution that developed the international standards defined the international units on the basis of bioassays.

Due to differences in methodology, normal ranges for each hormone may vary considerably between laboratories. For example, in some laboratories normal LH levels range from undetectable to 5 mIU/ml,[45] while in others 5 to 20 mIU/ml are considered normal.[46] Since undetectable levels may be included in the normal male range, the diagnosis of hypogonadotrophic hypogonadism on the basis of plasma gonadotropin levels may be difficult, and stimulation tests (discussed in the following section) may be required.

EVALUATION OF THE HYPOTHALAMIC-PITUITARY AXIS

Determination of Gonadotropin Levels

Prior to the development of radioimmunoassay techniques for measurement of serum gonadotropin levels, these hormones were estimated in the urine by bioassay,[44] a cumbersome, expensive, relatively imprecise procedure lacking adequate sensitivity for routine determination of plasma gonadotropin levels. Bioassays are performed on concentrates or extracts of 24-h urine collections. The biologic response (e.g., ovarian, uterine, or prostate growth) in a test animal to the administered material is quantitated. Variations in urine collection, in extraction procedures, and in response of individual animals frequently leads to inconsistent results.

The higher sensitivity and relatively greater precision of the radioimmunoassay allow routine determinations of gonadotropins in blood. However, this technique is not without serious limitations. Highly specific antibodies are a prerequisite and may be difficult at times to achieve. Inter- and intraassay variabilities may be significant. The immunoreactive material may not be a biologically active hormone. Furthermore, multiple forms of immunoreactive hormone may be present in the blood, including prohormones, active hormones, and degradation products. The generally available radioimmunoassays for gonadotropins employ antibodies that fail to distinguish between these various molecules.

In addition to technical problems in measurement of gonadotropins, there are physiologic phenomena that must be taken into consideration. It has been demonstrated that both FSH and LH levels oscillate markedly and irregularly (Fig. 123-5).[45,47] These oscillations complicate the interpretation of a value obtained from

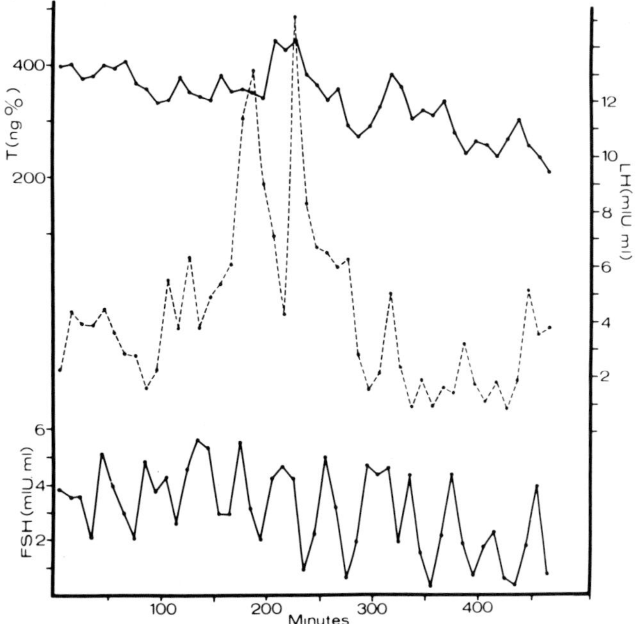

Fig. 123-5. Plasma testosterone, FSH, and LH levels during consecutive 10-min intervals in a normal adult man.[45]

a single sample. Some investigators have suggested that as many as 18 samples over a 6-h interval may be necessary to assure accurate results.[47] Goldzieher *et al.*, in a recently reported statistical analysis of this problem, concluded that reliable information could be obtained when these measurements were done on a plasma pool composed of equal aliquots from three blood samples taken at 20-min intervals.[48] Another approach to the problem involves measurement of LH or FSH in an integrated blood sample obtained by a constant rate of withdrawal over a specific period of time.[49]

Function Tests

Clomiphene citrate and gonadotropin-releasing-hormone (GnRH) stimulation tests are most frequently utilized for evaluation of the hypothalamic-pituitary axis.

Clomiphene Citrate Stimulation. Clomiphene citrate probably acts at the hypothalamic level, stimulating the secretion of GnRH, which in turn provokes gonadotropin release by the anterior pituitary. The LH response is usually greater than that of FSH.[50] A dose of 100 to 200 mg daily for a minimum of 5 days is administered. Baseline gonadotropin levels are obtained prior to administration of the drug and again on the day following the last dose.[51] A normal response is a doubling of LH levels and a somewhat smaller increase in FSH levels (Fig. 123-6).

Recently, radioimmunoassays have been developed for the measurement of GnRH in biologic fluids.[52,53] Since the site of action of clomiphene appears to be the hypothalamus, it would seem more appropriate to measure GnRH levels rather than gonadotropins. However, GnRH is a "local" hormone, operating within the hypothalamic-pituitary portal system, and only small amounts, if any, appear in the general circulation. Consequently, measurement of GnRH offers little help in the clinical evaluation of men with reproductive disorders.

GnRH Stimulation. Extensive basic and clinical investigations with GnRH have been reported since this decapeptide was isolated, purified, and synthesized.[54,55] Currently it is only available as an experimental drug in the United States. GnRH acts directly on the anterior pituitary, stimulating secretion of both LH and FSH. The LH response is considerably greater than that of FSH. GnRH may be given subcutaneously, intravenously, or intranasally. After baseline blood samples are obtained the hormone is administered at a 100- or 500-μg dose, and subsequent samples are taken every 30 min for 3 h. Both gonadotropins are measured in each blood sample.[56] A normal response is a several-fold increase in LH levels and a considerably smaller increase in FSH (Fig. 123-7). Recently, several investigators have suggested that administration of GnRH by iv infusion provides more precise results.[57]

Interpretation of Results

It should be possible to divide men with disorders of the hypothalamic pituitary testicular axis into two groups, those with high and those with normal or low FSH and LH levels (Table 123-3). Elevated levels of both LH and FSH are found in patients with primary testicular disease. In certain instances a dichotomy between FSH and LH values can be observed. When testicular disease is associated with failure of both seminiferous tubules and Leydig cells, both gonadotropins are elevated. In patients with primary disease of the germinal epithelium, LH levels may remain normal, while FSH levels are elevated. In these patients, further testing with clomiphene citrate or GnRH provides no additional information.

In patients with low or normal levels of FSH and LH, stimulation tests with clomiphene and GnRH may further localize the lesion. A normal gonadotropin response to GnRH and an absence of response to clomiphene citrate is suggestive of hypothalamic disease. In the absence of a response to GnRH, pituitary dysfunction should be suspected, and studies of other pituitary hormones as well as radiographic evaluation of the sella turcica are indicated. Depressed gonadotropins may also be found in patients with hormone-producing tumors and after administration of estrogens or androgens. Recently, Illig *et al.*[58] suggested that at puberty the GnRH test may be useful in the differential diagnosis between primary gonadal failure and pituitary disease. Children with primary testicular failure show an exaggerated response to GnRH, and those with pituitary dysfunction, decreased responses.

EVALUATION OF LEYDIG CELL FUNCTION

Testosterone is the major androgen secreted by the testis and is essential for spermatogenesis. Its actions include stimulation of male secondary sex characteristics and sex-accessory structures, as well as control of pituitary LH secretion by a negative-feedback mechanism. Measurement of testosterone production by the testis

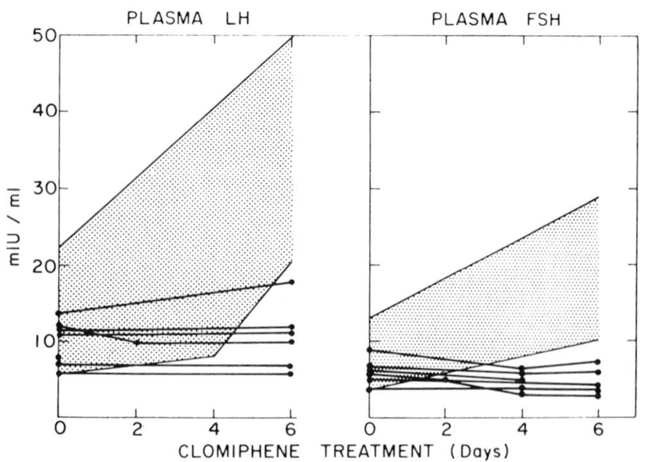

Fig. 123-6. Plasma levels of LH and FSH in hypopituitary patients before and during clomiphene administration. The range of the responses in normal men are given by the shaded areas. (From Bardin *et al:* J. Clin. Invest. *48:* 2046, 1969, with permission.)

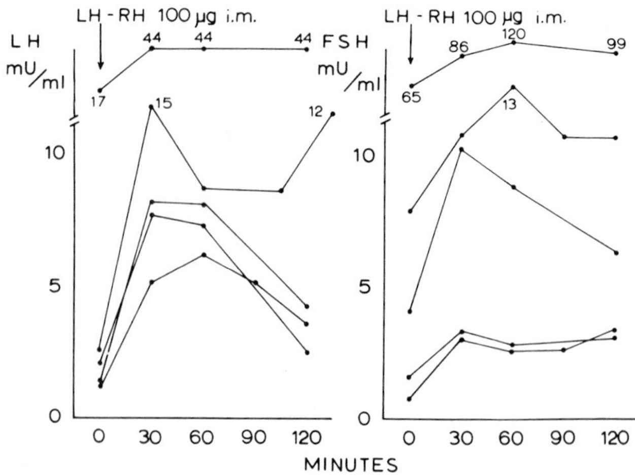

Fig. 123-7. Plasma LH and FSH levels in response to the intramuscular administration of 100 μg of synthetic LH-RH in 5 normal males. (From Abe *et al:* Endocrinol. Jpn. *19:* 77, 1972, with permission.)

Table 123-3. Evaluation of the Hypothalamic-Pituitary Axis

	FSH	LH	Response to Clomiphene	Response to GnRH
Primary testicular disease	High	High	—	—
Primary disease of germinal epithelium	High	Normal	—	—
Hypothalamic disease	Normal or low	Normal or low	Low	Normal
Pituitary disease	Normal or low	Normal or low	Low	Low

is therefore of major significance in the evaluation of testicular function. However, since intact Leydig cell function is required for normal spermatogenesis,[37] these measurements may not be necessary when sperm production is found to be normal (Tables 123-1 and 123-2).

As in the evaluation of the hypothalamic-pituitary axis, tests of Leydig cell function include determinations of basal hormone levels and provocative function tests.

Steroid Determinations

The development of the radioimmunoassay resulted in the abandonment of bioassays and chemical assays of androgens. For many years, urinary 17-ketosteroids were utilized as the primary measurement of testicular androgen production. Approximately 70 percent of 17-ketosteroids are of adrenal and 30 percent of testicular origin. Consequently, they can hardly represent an adequate measure of testicular androgen production. Since testosterone radioimmunoassays are widely available there is no need for determination of 17-ketosteroids in the evaluation of testicular function.

Radioimmunoassay of circulating testosterone is subject to the same limitations discussed for gonadotropin radioimmunoassays. In adult males the normal range of plasma testosterone varies among different laboratories but is usually in the range of 2.0 to 12.0 ng/ml. This variability may result from differences in the sensitivity and specificity of the antiserum employed. Furthermore, rapid oscillations in plasma testosterone levels of even greater magnitude than those discussed for FSH and LH levels have been demonstrated (Fig. 123-5).[45] In addition to these oscillations, a diurnal pattern of plasma testosterone levels with an early morning peak has been described.[59] Consequently, as suggested for gonadotropin measurements, single values of testosterone should be interpreted with caution. Accuracy may be improved by utilization of multiple or integrated blood-sampling techniques as described for gonadotropins.

Testosterone circulates largely bound to testosterone-binding globulin (TeBG). Variations in levels of this carrier protein may affect circulating testosterone levels. Since only free (unbound) testosterone is metabolically active, total testosterone levels may not provide adequate information, and determination of testosterone-binding globulin titers may become necessary. TeBG determination involves the quantitation of the binding capacity of serum for androgens (testosterone or dihydrotestosterone). The normal range for adult men is 5 to 11 μg/dl.

Other steroids may be important in the evaluation of men with reproductive disorders. It has been demonstrated that the testis secretes a small but significant amount of estradiol. However, 80 percent of the circulating estradiol originates from peripheral conversion of testosterone and androstenedione of testicular or adrenal origin. Estrogen levels can be measured by radioimmunoassay. Earlier chemical assays or bioassays of urinary estrogens have been abandoned, since they lack sensitivity, accuracy, and reproducibility. Dihydrotestosterone and 5α-androstanediol appear to be the biologically active metabolites of testosterone in certain target organs (e.g., prostate, skin, etc.). The clinical significance of determinations of these steroids remains to be demonstrated.

Since circulating steroid levels reflect not only testicular production but also peripheral metabolism, clearance rates, and extragonadal production, it has been suggested that measures in spermatic vein blood or testicular tissue may provide a more accurate assessment of testicular function.[37] Finally, techniques for determination of production and metabolic clearance rates have been described (see Chapter 120).[60] However, their technical sophistication makes them impractical for routine clinical use.

Metabolic Studies

Although measurements of testosterone and other steroids are basic to the evaluation of Leydig cell function, they may fail to detect abnormalities in the steroid biosynthetic pathways in the testis. These pathways may be investigated in vitro by utilizing small amounts of testicular tissue obtained during routine testicular biopsy.[61,62] The tissue is incubated with appropriate radiolabeled precursors of testosterone. The metabolites are isolated, purified, and quantitated. These techniques may permit the detection of abnormalities of specific enzymes involved in testicular steroid biosynthesis (e.g., 17β-reductase, 17-hydroxylase, 3β-hydroxysteroid-dehydrogenase, 5α-reductase, etc.) and important diagnostic, therapeutic, and prognostic considerations may result.[40,63] These procedures are time-consuming, expensive, and thus impractical for routine clinical use. It has been suggested that intratesticular concentrations of the various intermediates of testosterone synthesis may correlate with the findings of sophisticated in vitro metabolic studies.[62,64] These determinations may provide a more practical way to investigate abnormalities of androgen biosynthesis in the testis.[62]

Human Chorionic Gonadotropin (hCG) Stimulation

Since the biologic activity of hCG is similar to that of LH, its administration results in Leydig cell stimulation and increased testosterone production. An abnormal response to hCG is suggestive of disturbed Leydig cell function.

Similar to other glycoprotein hormones, hCG must be administered parenterally. Although reports of intravenous use have been published, in this country hCG is limited to intramuscular administration. The usual hCG stimulation test involves daily administration of 1500 to 5000 IU of hCG for 4 days.[50,51] In our laboratory, a dose of 5000 IU daily for 4 days is preferred for adults, with lower doses for children. Plasma testosterone is measured prior to the first injection and the day after the last injection. On each occasion the determinations are performed on pools of equal aliquots of several blood samples (e.g., three at 20-min intervals) or on integrated samples. A normal response to this test is at least a doubling of the plasma testosterone levels.

Interpretation of Results

Elevated testosterone levels are associated with androgen- or gonadotropin-producing tumors, as well as with testosterone or gonadotropin administration. Androgen-producing tumors (e.g. Leydig cell tumor) or testosterone treatment results in suppression of gonadotropins. Elevated testosterone levels secondary to gonadotropin administration or gonadotropin-producing tumors (e.g. choriocarcinoma, hepatoma, carcinoma of the lung) are associated with elevated LH levels.

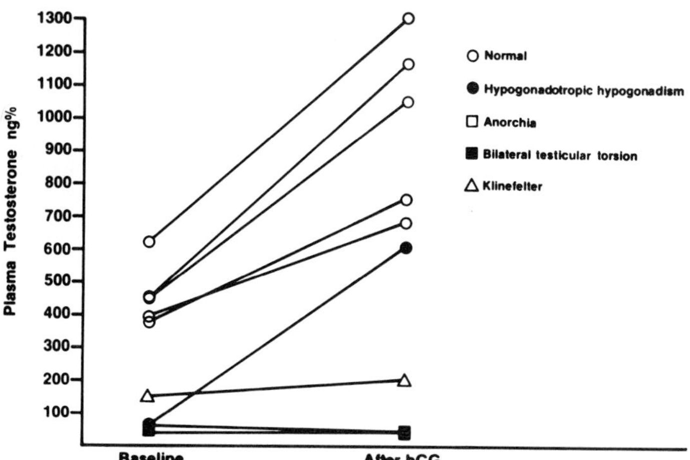

Fig. 123-8. Plasma testosterone response to hCG stimulation in normal individuals and patients with various pathologic disorders. (From Smith *et al:* Fertil. Steril. *25:* 965, 1974.)

Depressed testosterone secretion may result from primary testicular disease or from lack of gonadotropin stimulation of the testis, secondary to disorders of the hypothalamic-pituitary axis. Gonadotropin determinations and stimulation tests may be necessary to distinguish between them (see page 1543 in this chapter).

A number of steroids (estrogens, androgens, progestins) have been demonstrated to suppress testicular production of testosterone. While this effect may be secondary to suppression of pituitary gonadotropins, a direct action on the Leydig cell cannot be excluded.[65–67] Corticosteroids have also been reported to suppress testosterone levels in normal adult males.[68] Their effect does not appear to be mediated via the hypothalamic-pituitary axis. It is possible that depression of testosterone levels observed following psychologic or surgical stress[69,70] results from increased corticosteroid levels in these individuals. Finally, changes in testosterone levels occur in relation to age. A full discussion of this topic appears in Chapter 127.

Figure 123-8 depicts the plasma testosterone response to hCG observed in normal men and in men with various pathologic conditions. Failure to respond to hCG confirms either absence of functioning Leydig cells or severe disease of the testis (e.g., previous bilateral torsion of the testes). Patients with Klinefelter syndrome have a diminished response to hCG, although their baseline testosterone levels are often in the low-normal adult male range. Patients with hypogonadotropic hypogonadism demonstrate a brisk testosterone response to hCG. The hCG stimulation test is particularly useful to differentiate prepubertal patients with bilateral cryptorchidism from those with congenital anorchia.

It has been suggested that estrogen levels may be better indicators of Leydig cell response to gonadotropins than testosterone levels.[71,72] Consequently, estrogen determinations may be considered whenever hCG stimulation tests are performed for evaluation of testicular function.

REFERENCES

1. Eliasson, R. Semen analysis and laboratory workup. In Cockett, A. T. K. and Urry, R. L. (eds): Male Infertility. Workup, Treatment and Research. New York, Grune & Stratton, 1977, p. 169.
2. Paulsen, C. A. The testes. In Williams, R. H. (ed): Textbook of Endocrinology, 4th ed. Philadelphia, Saunders, 1968, p. 405.
3. Steinberger, E. Hormonal control of mammalian spermatogenesis. *Physiol. Rev. 51:* 1, 1971.
4. Harvey, C. and Jackson, M. H. Assessment of male fertility by semen analysis. *Lancet II:* 99, 1945.
5. Eliasson, R. Analysis of semen. In Behrman, S. J. and Kistner, R. W. (eds): Progress in Infertility, 2nd ed. New York, Little, Brown, 1975, p. 691.
6. Eliasson, R. and Treichl, L. Supravital staining of human spermatozoa. *Fertil. Steril. 22:* 134, 1971.
7. Janick, J. and MacLeod, J. The measurement of human spermatozoan motility. *Fertil. Steril. 21:* 140, 1970.
8. Haesungcharern, A. and Chulavatnatol, M. Stimulation of human spermatozoal motility by caffeine. *Fertil. Steril. 24:* 662, 1973.
9. Dubois, M., Jouannet, P., Berge, P., Volochine, B., Serres, C. and David, G. Méthode et appareillage de mesure objective de la mobilité des spermatozoïdes humains. *Ann. Phys. Biol. Méd. 9:* 19, 1975.
10. Gordon, D. L., Herrigel, J. E., Moore, D. J. and Paulsen, C. A. Efficacy of Coulter counter in determining low sperm concentrations. *Am. J. Clin. Pathol. 47:* 226, 1967.
11. Eliasson, R. Correlation between the sperm density, morphology and motility and the secretory function of the accessory genital glands. *Andrologie 2:* 165, 1970.
12. MacLeod, J. Human seminal cytology as a sensitive indicator of the germinal epithelium. *Int. J. Fertil. 9:* 281, 1964.
13. Couture, M., Ulstein, M., Leonard, J. and Paulsen, C. A. Improved staining method for differentiating immature germ cells from white blood cells in human seminal fluid. *Andrologia 8:* 61, 1976.
14. Alexander, N. J. Sperm antibodies and infertility. In Cockett, A. T. K. and Urry, R. L. (eds): Male Infertility. Workup, Treatment and Research. New York, Grune & Stratton, 1977, p. 123.
15. Isojima, S., Li, T. S. and Ashitaka, Y. Immunologic analysis of sperm-immobilizing factor found in sera of women with unexplained sterility. *Am. J. Obstet. Gynecol. 101:* 677, 1968.
16. Kibrick, S., Belding, D. L. and Merrill, B. Methods for the detection of antibodies against mammalian spermatozoa. I. A modified macroscopic agglutination test. *Fertil. Steril. 3:* 419, 1952.
17. Franklin, R. R. and Dukes, C. D. Further studies on spermagglutinating antibody and unexplained infertility. *J. Am. Med. Assoc. 190:* 682, 1964.
18. Hjort, T. and Hansen, K. B. Immunofluorescent studies on human spermatozoa. I. The detection of different spermatozoal antibodies and their occurrence in normal and infertile women. *Clin. Exp. Immunol. 8:* 9, 1971.
19. Steinberger, E. and Steinberger, A. Testis: Basic and clinical aspects. In Balin, H. and Glasser, S. (eds): Reproductive Biology. Amsterdam, *Excerpta Medica,* 1972, p. 144.
20. Smith, K. D., Rodriguez-Rigau, L. J. and Steinberger, E. The infertile couple, working with them together. In Cockett, A. T. K. and Urry, R. L. (eds): Male Infertility. Workup, Treatment and Research. New York, Grune & Stratton, 1977, p. 211.
21. Smith, K. D., Rodriguez-Rigau, L. J. and Steinberger, E. Relation between indices of semen analysis and pregnancy rate in infertile couples, *Fertil. Steril. 28:* 1314, 1977.
22. Van Zyl, J. A., Menkveld, R., Van W. Kotze, T. J., Retief, A. E. and Van Niekerk, W. A. Oligozoospermia: A seven year survey of the incidence, chromosomal aberrations, treatment and pregnancy rate. *Int. J. Fertil. 20:* 129, 1975.
23. Sherins, R. J., Brightwell, D. and Sternthal, P. M. Longitudinal analysis of semen of fertile and infertile men. In Troen, P. and Nankin, H. R. (eds): The Testis in Normal and Infertile Men. New York, Raven, 1977, p. 473.
24. Zukerman, Z., Rodriguez-Rigau, L. J., Smith, K. D. and Steinberger, E. Frequency distribution of sperm counts in fertile and infertile males. *Fertil. Steril. 28:* 1310, 1977.
25. MacLeod, J. and Gold, R. Z. The male factor in fertility and infertility. III. An analysis of motile activity in the spermatozoa of 1000 fertile men and 1000 men in infertile marriage. *Fertil. Steril. 2:* 187, 1951.
26. Steinberger, E. and Smith, K. D. Artificial insemination with fresh or frozen semen. *J. Am. Med. Assoc. 223:* 778, 1973.
27. American Fertility Society. How to Organize a Basic Study of the Infertile Couple. American Fertility Society, Birmingham, Alabama, 1971.
28. Freund, M. Standards for the rating of human sperm morphology. *Int. J. Fertil. 11:* 97, 1966.
29. Dubin, L. and Amelar, R. D. Varicocelectomy in male infertility. In Cockett, A. T. K. and Urry, R. L. (eds): Male Infertility. Workup, Treatment and Research. New York, Grune & Stratton, 1977, p. 225.

30. Christiansen, P. Studies on the relationship between spermatogenesis and urinary levels of follicle stimulating hormone and luteinizing hormone in oligospermic men. *Acta Endocrinol. 78:* 192, 1975.
31. Hunter, W. M., Edmond, P., Watson, G. S. and McLean, N. Plasma LH and FSH levels in subfertile men. *J. Clin. Endocrinol. Metab. 39:* 740, 1974.
32. Smith, K. D., Tcholakian, R. K., Chowdhury, M. and Steinberger, E. An investigation of plasma hormone levels before and after vasectomy. *Fertil. Steril. 27:* 145, 1976.
33. Rowley, M. J. and Heller, C. G. The testicular biopsy: Surgical procedure, fixation and staining technics. *Fertil. Steril. 17:* 177, 1966.
34. Steinberger, E. and Tjioe, D. Y. A method for quantitative analysis of human seminiferous epithelium. *Fertil. Steril. 19:* 960, 1968.
35. Vilar, O. Spermatogenesis. In Hafez, E. S. E. and Evans, T. N. (eds): Human Reproduction: Conception and Contraception. Hagerstown, Md., Harper & Row, 1973, p. 32.
36. Koulischer, L. and Schoysman, R. Chromosomes and human infertility—mitotic and meiotic. Chromosome studies in 202 consecutive male patients. *Clin. Genet. 5:* 116, 1974.
37. Steinberger, E., Smith, K. D., Tcholakian, R. K., Chowdhury, M., Steinberger, A., Ficher, M. and Paulsen, C. A. Steroidogenesis in human testis. In Mancini, R. E. and Martini, L. (eds): Male Fertility and Sterility. New York, Academic, 1974, p. 149.
38. Steinberger, E., Ficher, M. and Smith, K. D. Relation of *in vitro* metabolism of steroids in human testicular tissue to histologic and clinical findings. In Rosemberg, E. and Paulsen, C. A. (eds): The Human Testis. New York, Plenum, 1970, p. 439.
39. Oshima, H., Nankin, H. R., Troen, P. Yoshida. K.-I. and Ochi-ai, K.-I. Leydig cell number and function in infertile men. In Troen, P. and Nankin, H. R. (eds): The Testis in Normal and Infertile Men. New York, Raven, 1977, p. 445.
40. Rodriguez-Rigau, L. J., Weiss, D. B., Smith, K. D. and Steinberger, E. Suggestion of abnormal testicular steroidogenesis in infertile men. *Acta Endocrinol.* (Copenhagen) *87:* 400, 1978.
41. Odell, W. D. and Moyer, D. L. Physiology of Reproduction. St. Louis, Mosby, 1971.
42. Dufau, M. L. and Catt, K. J. A highly sensitive bioassay for LH and hCG in human plasma. *Acta Endocrinol.* (Copenhagen) Suppl. *199:* 189 (abstr. 124), 1975.
43. Reichert, L. E., Ramsey, R. B. and Carter, E. B. Application of a tissue receptor assay to measurement of serum follitropin (FSH). *J. Clin. Endocrinol. Metab. 41:* 634, 1975.
44. Rosemberg, E. (ed). Gonadotropins. Geron-X, Los Altos, Calif., 1968.
45. Smith, K. D., Tcholakian, R. K., Chowdhury, M. and Steinberger, E. Rapid oscillations in plasma levels of testosterone, LH and FSH in men. *Fertil. Steril. 25:* 965, 1974.
46. Goebelsmann, U., Horton, R., Mestman, J. H., Arce, J. J., Nagata, Y., Nakamura, R. M., Thorneycroft, I. H. and Mishell, Jr., D. R. Male pseudohermaphroditism due to testicular 17β-hydroxysteroid dehydrogenase deficiency. *J. Clin. Endocrinol. Metab. 36:* 867, 1973.
47. Santen, R. J. and Bardin, C. W. Episodic luteinizing hormone secretion in man. Pulse analysis, clinical interpretation, physiologic mechanisms. *J. Clin. Invest. 52:* 2617, 1973.
48. Goldzieher, J. W., Dozier, T. S., Smith, K. D. and Steinberger, E. Improving the diagnostic reliability of rapidly fluctuating plasma hormone levels by optimized multiple-sampling techniques. *J. Clin. Endocrinol. Metab. 43:* 824, 1976.
49. Santen, R. J. Independent effects of testosterone and estradiol on the secretion of gonadotropins in man. In Troen, P. and Nankin, H. R. (eds): The Testis in Normal and Infertile Men. New York, Raven, 1977, p. 197.
50. Lipsett, M. B., Migeon, C. J., Kirschner, M. A. and Bardin, C. W. Physiologic basis of disorders of androgen metabolism. *Ann. Int. Med. 68:* 1327, 1968.
51. DeKretser, D. M., Keogh, E. J., Burger, M. G. and Hudson, B. The response of infertile men to clomiphene and chorionic gonadotrophin stimulation. Endocrine Society of Australia, August 1973, Abstract #20.
52. Jeffcoate, S. L., Holland, D. T., White, N., Fraser, M. M., Gunn, A., Crighton, D. B., Foster, J. P. Griffiths, E. C., Hooper, K. C. and Sharp, P. J. The radioimmunoassay of hypothalamic hormones (TRH and LHRH) and related peptides in biological fluids. In Motta, A., Crosignani, P. G. and Martini, L. (eds): Hypothalamic Hormones. New York, Academic, 1975, p. 279.
53. Hall, R. W. and Steinberger, E. Synthesis of LH-RH by rat hypothalamic tissue *in vitro:* I. Use of a specific antibody for immunoprecipitation. *Neuroendocrinology 21:* 111, 1976.
54. Schally, A. V., Nair, R. M. G., Redding, T. W. and Arimura, A. Isolation of the luteinizing hormone and follicle-stimulating hormone-releasing hormone from porcine hypothalami. *J. Biol. Chem. 246:* 7230, 1971.
55. Matsuo, M., Arimura, A., Nair, R. M. G., and Schally, A. V. Synthesis of the porcine LH- and FSH-releasing hormone by the solid-phase method. *Biochem. Biophys. Res. Commun. 45:* 822, 1971.
56. Yen, S. S. C., Rebar, R., Vandenberg, G., Ehara, Y. and Siler, T. Pituitary gonadotrophin responsiveness to synthetic LRF in subjects with normal and abnormal hypothalamic-pituitary-gonadal axis. *J. Reprod. Fertil. Suppl. 20:* 137, 1973.
57. Yen, S. S. C., Vandenberg, G. and Siler, T. M. Modulation of pituitary responsiveness to LRF by estrogen. *J. Clin. Endocrinol. Metab. 39:* 170, 1974.
58. Illig, R., Bambach, M., Pluznik, S., Zachmann, M. and Prader, A. Effect of synthetic LH-RH on the release of LH and FSH in children and adolescents. *Schweiz. Med. Wochenschr. 103:* 840, 1973.
59. Rose, R. M., Kreuz, L. E., Holaday, J. W., Sulak, K. J., and Johnson, C. E. Diurnal variation of plasma testosterone and cortisol. *J. Endocrinol. 54:* 177, 1972.
60. Persky, H., Smith, K. D. and Basu, G. K. Relation of psychologic measures of aggression and hostility to testosterone production in man. *Psychosom. Med. 33:* 265, 1971.
61. Danezis, J. M. Steroidogenesis in mammalian gonads as related to fertility and infertility. *Fertil. Steril. 17:* 488, 1966.
62. Rodriguez-Rigau, L. J., Tcholakian, R. K., Smith, K. D. and Steinberger, E. *In vitro* steroid metabolic studies in human testis. I. Effect of estrogen on progesterone metabolism. *Steroids 29:* 771, 1977.
63. Steinberger, E., Ficher, M. and Smith, K. D. An enzymatic defect in androgen biosynthesis in human testis: A case report and response to therapy. *Andrologia 6:* 59, 1974.
64. Rodriguez-Rigau, L. J., Tcholakian, R. K., Smith, K. D., and Steinberger, E. *In vitro* steroid metabolic studies in human testis. II. Metabolism of cholesterol, pregnenolone, progesterone, androstenedione and testosterone by testes of an estrogen-treated man. *Steroids 30:* 729, 1977.
65. Chowdhury, M., Tcholakian, R. K. and Steinberger, E. An unexpected effect of oestradiol-17β on luteinizing hormone and testosterone. *J. Endocrinol. 60:* 375, 1974.
66. Dörner, G., Stahl, F., Rohde, W. and Schnorr, D. An apparently direct inhibitory effect of oestrogen on the human testis. *Endokrinologie 66:* 221, 1975.
67. Rodriguez-Rigau, L. J., Tcholakian, R. K., Smith, K. D. and Steinberger, E. Effect of *in vivo* estrogen administration on *in vitro* steroid bioconversion in human testes. In Troen, P. and Nankin, H. R. (eds): The Testis in Normal and Infertile Men. New York, Raven, 1977, p. 457.
68. Doerr, P. and Pirke, K. M. Cortisol-induced suppression of plasma testosterone in normal adult males. *J. Clin. Endocrinol. Metab. 43:* 622, 1976.
69. Kreuz, L. E., Rose, R. M. and Jennings, J. R. Suppression of plasma testosterone levels and psychological stress. *Arch. Gen. Psych. 26:* 479, 1972.
70. Matsumoto, K., Takeyasu, K., Mizutani, S., Hamanaka, Y. and Uozumi, T. Plasma testosterone levels following surgical stress in male patients. *Acta Endocrinol.* (Copenhagen) *65:* 11, 1970.
71. Weinstein, R. L., Kelch, R. P., Jenner, M. R., Kaplan, S. L. and Grumbach, M. M. Secretion of unconjugated androgens and estrogens by the normal and abnormal human testis before and after human chorionic gonadotropin. *J. Clin. Invest. 53:* 1, 1974.
72. Scholler, R., Grenier, J., Roger, M. and Castanier, M. Levels of eight steroids in plasma after normal testis stimulation. *Ann. d'Endocrinol.* (Paris) *36:* 351, 1975.
73. Smith, K. D., Steinberger, E., and Perloff, W. H. Polycystic ovarian disease. *Am. J. Obstet. Gynecol. 93:* 994, 1965.

124

Disorders of Testicular Function (Male Hypogonadism)

Emil Steinberger

"Male hypogonadism" is the diagnostic term frequently used to describe disorders of testicular function associated with inadequate sperm production, or diminution of androgen secretion, or both. This term is also employed regardless of the primary site of the disorder, e.g., testicular disease, pituitary failure, or hypothalamic disorder. Its continuing use is probably unfortunate. It may create a misunderstanding of the disease process and its consequences in the patient's mind, and it may also interfere with the clarity of the clinician's diagnostic thinking. It is essential to differentiate between spermatogenic insufficiency which is not related to hormonal deficiency and that associated with disturbed pituitary or hypothalamic function or with primary Leydig cell failure. This is particularly important because of the recently developed forms of effective therapy for testicular dysfunction secondary to systemic hormonal disturbances.

To simplify the diagnostic approach, testicular disorders can be placed into three major categories: those associated with low, those with normal, and those with elevated gonadotropin levels. Recognizing the imperfection of such categorization and the overlapping that may occur, we shall attempt to place the various forms of testicular disorders into one of these categories.

TESTICULAR DISORDERS ASSOCIATED WITH LOW GONADOTROPIN LEVELS

Historically, testicular dysfunction associated with low or undetectable gonadotropin levels was thought to be due to primary pituitary disease. Recent advances in the understanding of the physiology of the releasing factors and the availability of LHRH for clinical use led to the consideration of the hypothalamus as well as the pituitary as the possible primary sites of the disorder. The end result of disease affecting either of those two organs is a subnormal level of circulating gonadotropins producing deficiency in both the endocrine (androgenic) and exocrine (spermatogenic) function of the testes. Different clinical states may result depending on several factors: the age of onset of the disorder (prepubertal or postpubertal), its severity, and the presence of selective or total pituitary deficiency. Consequently, in patients with clinical parameters of gonadotropin deficiency, the function of other pituitary hormones should always be investigated.

COMPLETE, SELECTIVE PREPUBERTAL GONADOTROPIN FAILURE—"HYPOGONADOTROPIC EUNUCHOIDISM"

Numerous authors[1–3] have described the syndrome of hypogonadotropic eunuchoidism, a failure of appropriate gonadotropin secretion prepubertally, at puberty, and in adulthood. Although it would be desirable to diagnose this condition prior to the onset of puberty in order to be able to institute therapy at the appropriate age, until recently the routinely available laboratory techniques were neither sufficiently sensitive nor specific for measurement of gonadotropin levels in prepubertal males. The development of radioimmunoassay techniques allowed demonstration of measurable gonadotropin levels in prepubertal individuals[4,5] and led to the discovery of characteristic nocturnal oscillations and elevation of plasma gonadotropin levels in males entering puberty (Fig. 124-1). This observation offered a valuable tool in the diagnosis of hypogonadotropic states in the developing male. Although it has been demonstrated that gonadotropins (Fig. 124-2) can be detected in the plasma and urine of prepubertal males,[4–6] measurement of gonadotropin levels in children is not helpful in establishing a diagnosis of hypogonadotropic state because of the extremely low concentrations normally present. Even in the adult, a diagnosis of a hypogonadotropic state on the basis of a single plasma gonado-

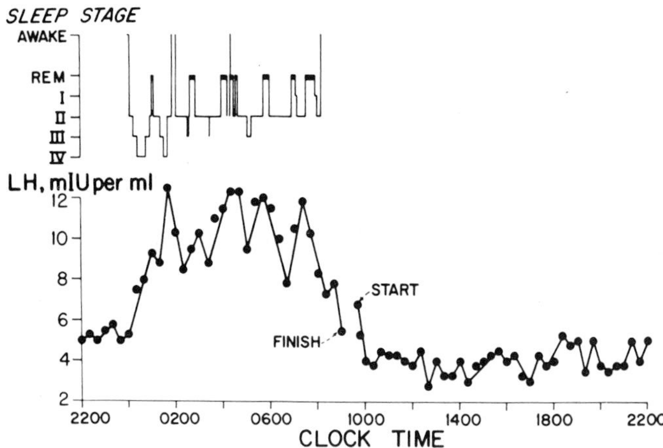

Fig. 124-1. Plasma LH concentration sampled every 20 minutes around the clock in early puberty. The sleep histogram is shown above the 8-hour period of nocturnal sleep. Sleep stages are awake, REM = –, stages I–VI by depth of line graph. Plasma LH concentration is expressed as mIU/ml 2d IRP-HMG. (Reprinted, by permission. From R. Boyar et al., *New England Journal of Medicine 287:* 582, 1972.)

tropin determination is difficult to establish. On frequent serial determinations, LH levels at some points may be barely at the sensitivity limits of the radioimmunoassay, and FSH is frequently undetectable in a considerable number of samples. Furthermore, in the adult male, gonadotropins show rapid oscillations of great magnitude within short periods of time (Fig. 124-3), precluding valid interpretations from a single sample determination of the hormone levels. To circumvent this difficulty, multiple sample techniques have been developed.[7,8]

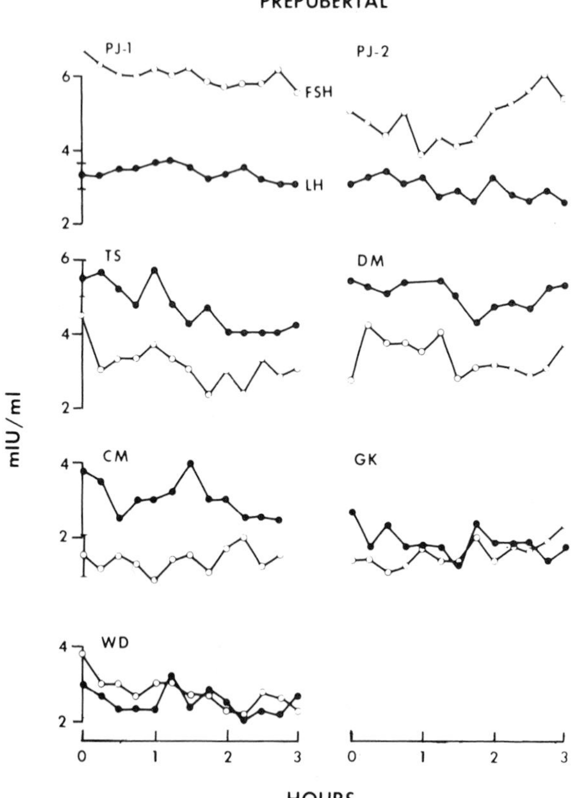

Fig. 124-2. Serum FSH (open circles) and LH (closed circles) levels in prepubertal children. The vertical bars represent ± SD of the mean of samples. SD's for LH and FSH are similar at the same level and only representative values are shown. (From A. Johanson, *Journal of Clinical Endocrinology and Metabolism 39:* 154, 1974.)

Because of the difficulty in utilizing plasma gonadotropin levels in the diagnostic workups of hypogonadotropic conditions, provacative function tests have been frequently employed. The clomiphene citrate (Clomid*) stimulation test is useful in certain circumstances. When the hypothalamic-pituitary axis is intact and the patient is beyond the prepubertal stage of development, administration of Clomid will result in an increase of gonadotropin secretion, probably by stimulating the release of LHRH. In prepubertal children, administration of Clomid results in suppression of gonadotropins.[9]

Although administration of LHRH should serve as a potentially useful test to demonstrate the intactness of pituitary gonadotropic function, it appears that it may not differentiate clearly between hypothalamic and pituitary disease.[10]

In patients with hypogonadotropic disorders, the characteristic clinical features of "eunuchoidism" (eunuchoid skeleton, high-pitched voice, small testes (1 × 2 cm) of normal consistency, lack of bitemporal scalp hair recession, sparse or absent pubic hair, and diminished body hair growth) do not become manifest until the age of puberty. Confirmation of a clinical impression of hypogonadotropic eunuchoidism can be achieved by appropriate laboratory studies, which may include measurement of waking and sleep gonadotropin levels, determination of plasma androgen levels, clomiphene citrate test, HCG stimulation tests, LHRH stimulation tests, and the microscopic study of testicular biopsy (see Chapter 123).

The etiology and pathophysiology of hypogonadotropic hypogonadism are unclear. It may encompass several different diseases or a spectrum of disorders with the common denominator of diminished or absent secretion of gonadotropins. Sex-chromosome-linked dominant inheritance has been suggested as the etiologic factor by some investigators,[11] while others consider it to be autosomal recessive.[12] Recently evidence was presented[13] suggesting that it is inherited as an autosomal dominant disorder (Fig. 124-4). Numerous reports in the literature demonstrate a familial occurrence of hypogonadotropic eunuchoidism and its association with other anomalies such as mental retardation, color blindness, syndactyly, nerve deafness, cerebellar ataxia, ichthyosis, harelip, cleft palate, unilateral cryptorchidism, and in particular, anosmia (for review, see ref. 14).

The association between hypogonadism and anosmia was first reported by Kallmann et al.;[15] hence, this syndrome is frequently referred to as Kallmann's syndrome. Hamilton et al.[16] evaluated olfactory acuity in a series of patients with hypogonadotropic hypogonadism utilizing a standardized force choice, three-stimulus sniff technique with vapors of pyridine, nitrobenzene, and thiophene.[17] As a result of this study, they decided to divide the hyposmic subjects into two groups: those who failed entirely to respond to the vapors at the primary olfactory area (hyposmia type I) and those who showed a diminished response (hyposmia type II). Since the two groups showed a different response to therapy, such diagnostic separation may be of benefit from a prognostic viewpoint.

The disorder is probably not due to pituitary disease. In most instances, no pituitary pathology can be detected. The patient's gonadotropin levels rise in response to administration of LHRH;[18] however, the short-term response to the releasing factor is abnor-

*Clomiphene citrate, Merrell-National Laboratories, Cincinnati, Ohio.

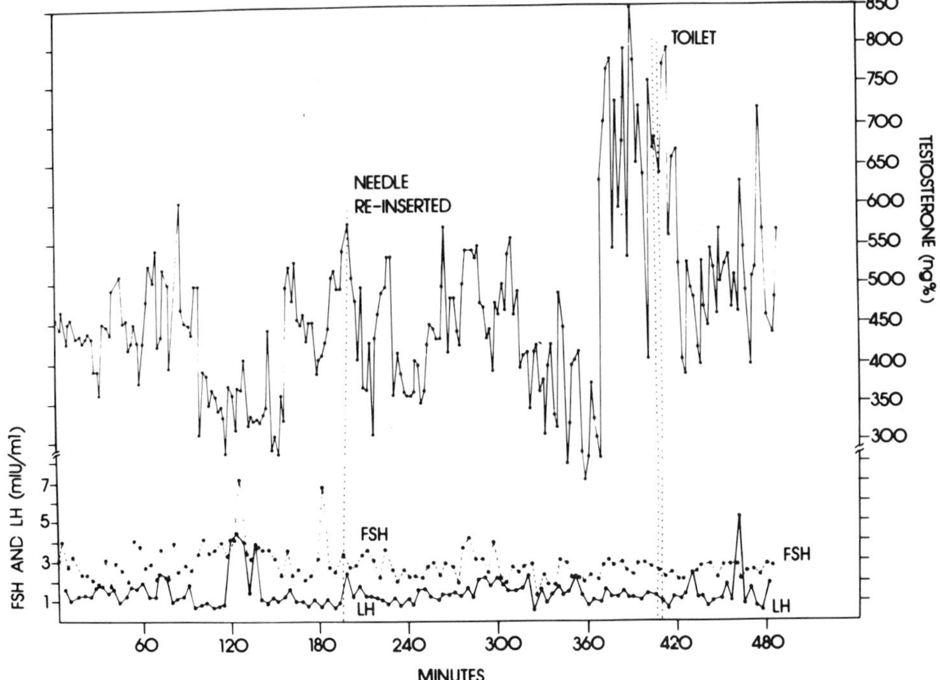

Fig. 124-3. Plasma levels of testosterone, FSH, and LH from blood samples taken every 2 minutes for 8 hours. (From K. D. Smith et al., *Fertility and Sterility 25:* 965, 1974.)

mal.[19] The reported instances of hypoplasia of the mammillary bodies, olfactory bulbs and tracts, hypothalamus, and the anterior portion of the white commissure suggest that Kallmann's syndrome is due to a congenital anomaly of the hypothalamus.[20,21]

Therapy

The choice of therapeutic methods should be indicated by the pathophysiology and diagnostic findings. Patients with normal olfactory acuity, selective gonadotropin failure, normal karyotype, and no evidence of organic lesions of the brain or the pituitary gland may respond to treatment with clomiphene citrate (Clomid). Response to therapy in these patients suggests that they suffer essentially with delayed puberty rather than with an irreversible state of hypogonadotropism. Although various doses of Clomid have been employed, it appears that the duration of treatment may be more important than the dose. Treatment with 50 mg of clomiphene citrate daily for a period of several months may result in adequate gonadotropin release and stimulation of testicular function including spermatogenesis. Monitoring gonadotropin levels early in therapy will provide information concerning the patient's response. Patients with Kallmann's syndrome, particularly with hyposmia type I, do not respond to Clomid administration, while patients with type II occasionally do.[16] Patients who do not respond to Clomid should be treated with a combination of gonadotropin preparations, human chorionic gonadotropin (HCG) and human pituitary (HPG) or menopausal (HMG) gonadotropin. Although a number of therapeutic regimens have been suggested, it appears that a 6- to 8-week treatment with HCG, 4000 IU twice weekly, followed by a combination of HCG (2000 IU) and HMG (75 IU FSH and 75 IU LH) twice weekly will induce rapid androgen production and subsequently complete spermatogenesis within 3 to 6 months.

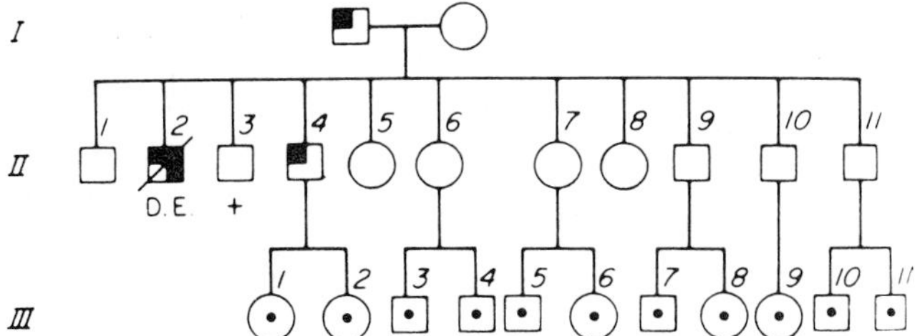

Fig. 124-4. Kindred 1 studied for mechanism of genetic transmission of hypogonadotropic eunuchoidism. Opaque area in upper left-hand corner depicts anosmia. Note *male* to *male* transmission. Opaque area entire right side depicts hypogonadism. Diagonal line indicates cryptorchidism. Central dot indicates prepubertal age. (From R. J. Santen and C. A. Paulsen, *Journal of Clinical Endocrinology and Metabolism 36:* 47, 1973.)

Since the basic defect in hypogonadotropic eunuchoidism appears to be the lack of appropriate LHRH secretion, therapy with this hormone should be the most logical approach to treatment of this disorder. Although optimistic reports have been published,[22] the efficacy of this form of treatment must receive further confirmation before it can be accepted.

Both clomiphene citrate and gonadotropin therapy aim to establish testicular function, including spermatogenesis. If spermatogenesis is not considered an important end point of therapy or if gonadotropins are not available, replacement therapy with androgens can be administered with a clear understanding on the part of the physician and the patient that this form of therapy will only stimulate appropriate somatic development, development of secondary sex characteristics, and development of libido and potency. Spermatogenic function of the testes will not be restored, and it may actually be affected adversely if later in life an attempt to stimulate it with gonadotropins is considered.

Only injectable androgens should be utilized, preferably the long-acting esters, e.g., testosterone enanthate. The latter can be administered at a dose of 200 mg at weekly intervals for 4 to 6 weeks or until definite signs of masculine development appear, at which time the dose can be diminished to a maintenance level of 200 mg every 3 to 4 weeks.

PARTIAL SELECTIVE PREPUBERTAL GONADOTROPIN FAILURE

This is a considerably more common condition than hypogonadotropic eunuchoidism and must be differentiated from "delayed puberty," which may present clinically with identical signs and symptoms. The clinical picture varies with each individual and with the degree of pubertal development at the time of examination. Pubertal development commences usually at the expected age and frequently may be associated with pubertal gynecomastia; however, it proceeds slowly, and the individual may never reach the adult state of gonadal development. The gonadotropins are either undetectable or in the "low" range. Testosterone levels do not reflect a pubertal spurt. The testes are beyond the prepubertal stage in their development and exhibit normal consistency. Testicular biopsy shows definite signs of initiation of the spermatogenic process. Response to clomiphene is useful as a diagnostic test to detect delayed puberty.

Therapy

If the response to clomiphene is positive, most likely the diagnosis of delayed puberty is correct. A therapeutic trial with clomiphene may actually induce puberty and thus serve as a diagnostic test to rule out delayed puberty. If no sustained or adequate response to clomiphene is obtained, one or more courses of HCG therapy may bring on completion of puberty and continuation of normal function after cessation of therapy. Each course of therapy consists of administration of 2000 IU HCG three times weekly for 8 weeks. Patients who do not assume spontaneous function after discontinuation of treatment suffer from permanent hypogonadotropism and may have to be managed therapeutically in the same fashion as those with complete selective gonadotropin failure.

SELECTIVE POSTPUBERTAL GONADOTROPIN FAILURE—"HYPOGONADOTROPIC HYPOGONADISM"

This is a rare condition of unknown etiology. Patients may complain of loss of libido and potency, diminution in the rate of beard growth, and a decrease in body hair. Gonadotropin and testosterone production is decreased. There is no clinical or laboratory evidence for a decline in the production of other pituitary hormones. No structural changes in the pituitary gland or the hypothalamus have been observed in these patients. Although a hypoandrogenic clinical picture is present, the patients are not eunuchoid, since skeletomuscular and sexual development was complete prior to the onset of the gonadotropic deficiency.

Therapy

If fertility is desired, therapy with HCG and HMG as described above should be effective. Otherwise, replacement therapy with long-acting androgens is indicated.

PREPUBERTAL PANHYPOPITUITARISM—"PITUITARY DWARFISM"

Lack of growth is the most dramatic clinical feature. The lesion responsible for this condition causes primarily a deficiency in growth hormone production but may also affect the production of gonadotropic, adrenocorticotropic, and thyrotropic hormones. During the prepubertal stages of the disease, the diagnosis is difficult to establish because of technical difficulties in measuring low gonadotropin levels in children. As the chronologic puberty approaches, deficiency in sexual development becomes evident.

It is of interest to note that in spite of gonadotropic and androgen deficiency these patients do not develop the skeletal changes (eunuchoid skeleton) characteristic of a low-androgen milieu. This probably results from the associated growth hormone deficiency.

The role of growth hormone in the expression of the LH effect on the testes remains unclear. It has been suggested on the basis of experiments in rats that growth hormone may enhance the response of developing testes to LH.[23] It has also been reported that patients with isolated growth hormone deficiency and apparently normal gonadotropin levels and gonadal function may exhibit inadequate development of the phallus. This finding was interpreted as suggestive of the possibility that growth hormone may be essential for normal effect of LH on androgen production by the developing human testes.[24] However, careful function studies in growth hormone deficient boys (bone age 5 to 12 years) failed to support the idea that growth hormone has a major permissive effect on Leydig cell function in man.[6]

Therapy

Similar to that described for hypogonadotropic eunuchoidism (p. 1549) and the appropriate replacement therapy for panhypopituitorism (see Chapter 18).

POSTPUBERTAL PANHYPOPITUITARISM

In this group of patients, great variability in the degree of hypogonadism can be observed, depending on the extent of gonadotropin loss. The condition can occur spontaneously (e.g., secondary to a pituitary tumor) or can be the result of medical intervention (e.g., secondary to therapeutic hypophysectomy). The gonadal changes are due to diminution in the circulating levels of gonadotropins, and the somatic manifestations are an expression of hypoandrogenicity. The most common presenting symptoms are loss of potency, varying degrees of libido changes, regression of secondary sex characteristics (beard, body hair, etc.), skin changes (wrinkling of facial skin), and muscle weakness. Secondary to a sudden cessation of pituitary function, e.g., complete hypophysectomy, loss of libido and potency may occur rapidly (in days or weeks). In patients with pituitary tumors the decline in sexual function may be gradual, extending over a period of months or years. However, the loss of sexual function frequently may be the earliest presenting complaint in patients with a pituitary tumor.

If the hypoandrogenic state is not corrected while the other trophic hormones are being replaced, bone changes and emotional disturbances may also develop. The microscopic picture of the testes varies greatly depending on the completeness of the hypogonadotropic state and its duration. Contrary to some opinions the seminiferous tubules do not regress to a prepubertal state but develop a pathological picture characterized by varying degrees of degeneration and disorganization of the seminiferous epithelium and thickening, fibrosis, and hyalinization of the walls of the seminiferous tubules. The Leydig cells become atrophic.

Therapy

If fertility is desired, gonadotropin therapy as described for hypogonadotropic eunuchoidism may be effective. Otherwise, testosterone enanthate, 200 mg every 3 weeks, will provide the necessary androgenic support. Appropriate replacement therapy with the other pituitary trophic hormones is to be administered as required (see Chapter 18).

THE FERTILE EUNUCH (ISOLATED LH DEFICIENCY, THE PASQUALINI SYNDROME)

In 1950, Pasqualini and Bur described a patient with eunochoid phenotype, normal testis size, and spermatogenesis.[25] This condition was subsequently described by a number of authors, and the term "fertile" eunuch was coined.[13,26–29] In these patients serum FSH is usually within normal range, while LH is decreased or undetectable, and testosterone levels are markedly depressed.[27,28] The spermatogenic activity may vary from several million spermatozoa per millimeter to azoospermia, but in all cases where biopsy was obtained, varying degrees of spermatogenesis were detected in the seminiferous tubules.

The pathophysiology is not entirely clear. Isolated deficiency of LH is the underlying etiologic factor as far as deficient testicular function is concerned. However, in view of the presence of spermatogenesis, it would be difficult to accept the possibility that production of testosterone is entirely curtailed. Most likely, normal levels of FSH and varying degrees of LH insufficiency still permit production of testosterone in the testes in quantities sufficient to maintain a degree of spermatogenic activity. Unfortunately, no studies on intratesticular levels of testosterone in these patients are available to clarify this question.

Therapy

Therapy with HCG is usually effective in stimulating androgen production and virilization as well as in improving sperm production.

THE PRADER-WILLI SYNDROME

This syndrome is characterized by hypotonia, hypomentia, hypogonadism, and obesity (HHHO syndrome). It is frequently associated with cryptorchidism. The original description of this syndrome was provided by Prader, Labhart, and Willi.[30] The disorder usually makes its appearance in infancy; the patients exhibit uncontrollable hyperphagia and impaired temperature regulation.

The etiology of hypogonadism in this syndrome is difficult to establish. It has been suggested that the hypogonadotropic state is responsible for the failure of the testes to develop and for the lack of development of secondary sex characteristics. Indeed, in some reports, deficiency of both LH and FSH has been demonstrated with good androgen response to HCG, suggesting impairment of Leydig cell function.[31] However, other authors reported normal[32,33] or even elevated[34,35] levels of gonadotropins in this syndrome. In patients with low gonadotropin levels, administration of clomiphene citrate induces a rise in both LH and FSH.[36,37] These observations suggest that the hypothalamic-pituitary axis in patients with Prader-Willi syndrome may be intact. Morphologic evaluation of the brain and the pituitary gland seems to support this conclusion. No microscopic changes could be detected in these structures.[32]

Therapy

The therapeutic approach toward hypogonadism in Prader-Willi syndrome is difficult to suggest in general terms. Those with low gonadotropin levels may respond to gonadotropin therapy or to administration of Clomid. Others may require androgen replacement therapy in order to stimulate the development of secondary sex characteristics.

THE LAURENCE-MOON-BIEDL SYNDROME

This syndrome of familial hypogonadism is associated with retarded growth, syndactyly or polydactyly, obesity, retinitis pigmentosa, and mental retardation. Little, if any, information is available concerning the pathophysiology of this disorder.[38] There appears to be a high rate of consanguinity (25 percent) among parents.

The etiology of gonadal lesions in the syndrome may also be protean. In some instances the classic features of hypogonadotropin hypogonadism are obvious; in other cases, evidence of primary testicular lesion is present.[39,40]

THE ALSTRÖM SYNDROME

Although apparently a separate entity, the Alström syndrome resembles in many respects the Laurence-Moon-Biedl syndrome. It is an autosomal recessive disorder associated with retinal degeneration, obesity, nerve deafness, nephropathy, and hypogonadism. It differs from the Laurence-Moon-Biedl syndrome in that it does not encompass mental retardation or polydactyly but includes a variety of metabolic disorders, e.g., hypertrigliceridemia, hyperuricemia, and acanthosis nigricans.

HYPERANDROGENIC DISORDER OF THE ADRENAL GLAND

Although this syndrome is due, not to primary hypofunction of the pituitary gland, but to the hyperfunction of the adrenal, it is included in this chapter because the diminution of testicular function is caused by low gonadotropin levels. The low levels of circulating gonadotropins result from the suppression of the pituitary gonadotropic function by androgens produced in the diseased adrenal gland. The details of the pathogenesis and pathophysiology as well as details of therapy of hyperandrogenic disorders of the adrenal gland are discussed in Chapter 97.

Hyperandrogenic function of the adrenal gland is most commonly caused by congenital or acquired adrenal hyperplasia and less frequently by adrenal tumors. The best documented cases of gonadal abnormalities are those associated with congenital rather than acquired adrenal hyperplasia. The virilizing types of congenital adrenal hyperplasias (type I—partial C-21 hydroxylase deficiency; type II—complete C-21 hydroxylase deficiency; type III—C-11 hydroxylase deficiency) are associated with hypogonadotropic hypogonadism. Types IV (3β-hydroxysteroid deficiency), V (17α-hydroxylase deficiency), and VI (cholesterol side chain cleaving enzyme deficiency) cause primary hypogonadism as a result of the inability of the Leydig cells to produce androgens because of the specific enzyme deficiency that the Leydig cells share in this condition with the adrenal cells. These disorders are not included in the category of hypogonadotropic hypogonadism.

In patients with congenital adrenal hyperplasia types I, II, and III, the fetal differentiation of the male gonads and the sex organs proceeds in a relatively uneventful fashion, although at birth the penis may be larger than normal. The youngsters, however, begin to exhibit pubertal changes within the first few years of life. The bone age is accelerated, the penis shows rapid development, and pubic and axillary hair develops. The testes, however, remain infantile in size and in microscopic appearance. Thus the patients exhibit the clinical signs and symptoms of precocious pseudopuberty. Plasma androgen levels are elevated, while gonadotropins are very low or undetectable. In some instances, bilateral adrenal rests may be present in the gonadal tissue, causing enlargement of the testis.[41] The testicular enlargement may be mistaken for testicular maturation (true precocious puberty) or testicular tumors.

Therapy

Therapy of the underlying pathological state, adrenal hyperplasia, with corticoids results in suppression of the excessive androgenic production by the adrenal gland and may permit development of normal testicular function including spermatogenesis.[42]

ESTROGEN-PRODUCING ADRENAL CARCINOMA

Suppression of pituitary gonadotropins by estrogens secreted by an adrenal carcinoma will result in spermatogenic arrest and cessation of Leydig cell function and thus of androgen production, in the male.[43]

Successful therapy of the neoplasm resulting in removal of the source of the estrogens will restore testicular function.

TESTICULAR DISORDERS ASSOCIATED WITH ELEVATED GONADOTROPIN LEVELS

FUNCTIONAL PREPUBERTAL CASTRATE SYNDROME ("ANORCHIA," "VANISHING TESTES," "FUNCTIONAL CASTRATE," "TESTICULAR AGENESIS")

Congenital absence of the testes is the basic feature of this disorder. The patients develop normally during childhood, including normal development of external genitalia. They fail to enter puberty and to develop secondary sex characteristics. If left untreated the typical eunuchoid phenotype results. This condition is associated with perhaps the highest plasma levels of gonadotropins of all testicular disorders and extremely low testosterone levels. The etiology of this condition is unclear (for review, see refs. 44 and 45). Although a genetic basis of "anorchia" is unlikely, and in most cases a normal karyotype has been reported, in some patients cytogenetic abnormalities have been detected.[45] The possibility of testicular destruction during fetal life secondary to viral or other infection of the fetus, vascular accidents, or torsion has been considered. The destruction of the testis must occur between the 7th to the 14th weeks of intrauterine life, because absence of the testes during earlier stages of fetal development would result in phenotypic abnormalities characterized by various degrees of female phenotype.[46]

The diagnosis is relatively simple in individuals of postpubertal age. The patient exhibits male phenotype with infantile external genitalia and a scrotum that is either empty or contains small tissue masses representing remnants of the wolffian ducts. No androgens are produced, since testes are absent, and pubertal changes fail to occur. The patient exhibits somatic signs of eunuchoidism as well as genital infantilism. However, in contradistinction to patients with hypogonadotropic eunuchoidism who are usually tall, functional castrates are usually of short stature. There are no congenital or cytogenetic abnormalities associated with this disorder, which helps to differentiate it from male Turner's syndrome.

The diagnosis of anorchia in a prepubertal individual cannot be made on a clinical basis. The absence of testes from the scrotum may be due to cryptorchidism, and even the most thorough surgical exploration may miss the testis. With the advent of sensitive techniques for the determination of plasma testosterone and gonadotropin levels the differentiation between cryptorchidism and anorchia in prepubertal boys became a much simpler and more reliable task. In normal prepubertal boys, gonadotropins, although usually detected, are generally low; in functional castrates, they are elevated. Both prepubertal and postpubertal cryptorchid testes respond to HCG with increased testosterone production. Thus, in a prepubertal functional castrate, failure to respond to stimulation with HCG by an increase in plasma testosterone levels is almost diagnostic for this condition.

Therapy

Replacement therapy with a long-acting parenteral preparation of testosterone as outlined above is mandatory. The treatment has to be continued for life to provide for proper sexual development and function and for the appropriate metabolic state.

TESTICULAR ECTOPIA

General Considerations

A disturbance in the descent of the testes, which normally occurs as part of their development, may result in either incomplete descent or translocation of the testes to sites other than the scrotum. If the testes fail to leave the abdominal cavity, they remain "hidden" in the abdomen; hence the term "cryptorchidism" [*kryptos* = hidden + *orchis* = testis (Greek)]. Consequently, while these testes are ectopic [*ectos* = outside + *topos* = place (Greek)], they are also "hidden." Once the testes leave the abdominal cavity, they can be seen and/or palpated; thus, they are no longer "cryptorchid." They may be retarded in their descent through the inguinal canal (inguinal testes or inguinal ectopic testes), or they may migrate into the suprapubic area (suprapubic or pubopenile ectopic testes), the femoral area (crural ectopic testes), or the perineum (perineal ectopic testes).

The incidence of testicular ectopia at birth is placed at approximately 10 percent and in adult man at about 0.4 percent.[47,48] Consequently most (96 percent) of the cases of testicular ectopia observed at birth are corrected spontaneously.

Etiologic Factors

The etiologic factors responsible for failure of or for inappropriate testicular descent are unclear. Although in a substantial number of patients, anatomical obstruction preventing normal descent has been demonstrated during surgery,[49] the cause of this abnormality has not been uncovered. It has been suggested that, in general, all cryptorchid testes have an abnormality of the germinal epithelium that is genetic in origin rather than due to increased temperature in the ectopic position.[48,50,51] If genetic abnormality is the primary underlying cause of germinal epithelium defects in all cases of ectopic testes, then therapy directed toward their placement in the scrotum (whether surgical or hormonal) should fail to restore spermatogenic function, but this is not the case. A possibility should then be considered that testicular ectopia has multiple etiologic factors, including a genetic factor. It is of particular importance to note that the incidence of ectopia in other gonadal disorders (e.g., Klinefelter's syndrome, Sertoli cell only syndrome, hypogonadotropic eunuchoidism, etc.) is relatively high,[52] emphasizing the importance of a complete workup, including cytogenetic evaluation, endocrine studies, and testicular biopsy (at the time of surgical correction) in patients with testicular ectopia.

Therapy

The therapy of testicular ectopia can be approached from either a surgical or a medical viewpoint or a combination of both. The question of medical versus surgical therapy has been discussed by many authors. In patients with unilateral cryptorchidism the chances of anatomical abnormality are higher than in bilateral, and the surgical approach is frequently utilized. It should be stressed, however, that even in cases of unilateral cryptorchidism, the patient may respond to hormonal therapy. Fundamentally, it is the end result of the therapy that must be employed to evaluate its efficacy. If success of therapy is judged by whether or not the testes end up in the scrotal position, then surgical intervention (orchidopexy) provides the most rapid and most effective therapy. If fertility is used as the criteria, the available information is not entirely adequate to draw a clear conclusion. Charny is pessimistic in regard to successful outcome of surgical therapy.[53] Others have published data demonstrating a relatively high frequency of fertility following orchidopexy.[52,54,55]

Surgical procedure is at times difficult. The possibility of interference with the blood supply, particularly in very young patients, is real. A lack of success may be due, in some patients, not so much to irreversibility of the germinal epithelium lesion, but to the surgical trauma, particularly trauma to the vasculature.

The usual approach to therapy of cryptorchidism involves a therapeutic trial of hormonal therapy. This should be attempted only under supervision of a therapist who is experienced in managing these patients. Of course, if successful, it will obviate the necessity for surgery. Second, it will stimulate some growth of the testes, particularly the cord and its vessels, possibly making the surgery easier. On the other hand, increased vascularity secondary to HCG administration may be disadvantageous to the surgical approach.

The age when therapeutic intervention is to be commenced has been a point of controversy. The opinions vary greatly. Some authors suggest that therapy be instituted before the age of 1 year,[56] while others suggest the age of 16.[57] Since 96 percent of all testicular ectopias present at birth correct themselves spontaneously during childhood, intervention prior to 1 year of age does not seem to be justified. The majority of authors consider the age of 5 to 7 as optimal for therapeutic intervention.

The increased incidence (40 times greater) of neoplasia in cryptorchid testes[58,59] stimulated an aggressive surgical approach to therapy. Some authors advocate orchiectomy when orchidopexy is impractical. It should be kept in mind, however, that translocation of the testis from its ectopic site to the scrotum (orchidopexy) apparently does not change the incidence of neoplastic transformation.[60,61] Some authors who observed neoplastic transformation in the testes following orchidopexy advocate orchiectomy as preventive therapy, especially if no improvement in spermatogenesis is noted within 2 years after bringing the testes into the scrotum.[62,63] This cautious approach should be tempered by the fact that the overall incidence of testicular cancer is very low (0.002 percent; thus, even a 40-fold increase brings the incidence to 0.08 percent, still an extremely low figure hardly justifying orchiectomy as therapy of choice for cryptorchidism. It must also be kept in mind that orchiectomy will require that the patient receive lifelong testosterone replacement therapy, which may carry a considerable risk of serious side effects.

Medical Therapy

It has been the experience that therapy with gonadotropins will induce the descent of cryptorchid testes in selected cases. HCG has been the most commonly employed gonadotropic preparation. There is no total agreement on the precise dosage, frequency, and duration of therapy. We feel that therapy should be individualized, and a careful follow-up is mandatory to prevent overtreatment. Administration of 2000 IU HCG three times weekly for a period of 6 weeks is the commonly used regimen. We frequently repeat this course of therapy at least once before resorting to surgery.

KLINEFELTER'S SYNDROME

As described by Klinefelter et al.,[64] this syndrome is characterized by pea-sized, very firm scrotal testes, gynecomastia (appearing at puberty), eunuchoidism, azoospermia, hyalinization of the seminiferous tubules, high gonadotropin levels, and low 17-ketosteroids. Subsequent to the original description of the syndrome, a number of other features were added and the original signs and symptoms clarified:

1. The protean clinical features of this syndrome were documented, particularly the variability of the presence of gynecomastia, female hair distribution, and light beard growth.[65]
2. Association with various other systemic disorders like diabetes mellitus (for review, see ref. 66) and mental disorders (for review, see ref. 67) were noted.
3. The genetic etiology of this condition was discovered.[68] Chromosomal analysis of somatic cells from patients with Klinefelter's syndrome revealed a karyotype of 47XXY as well as various combinations of poly-X and poly-Y complements, deletions, and mosaicism (for review, see ref. 14).
4. The concept of congenital absence (gonadal dysgenesis) of germ cells in testes from patients with Klinefelter's syndrome was challenged by studies demonstrating small areas of spermatogenesis in testes of men with positive sex chromatin[69] and disproven by finding spermatogenesis in testes of a patient with Klinefelter's syndrome and a 74XXY karyotype.[70]
5. The suggestion that testes of Klinefelter's syndrome patients are deficient in testosterone production has been defined both from quantitative[71] and pathophysiologic[72] viewpoints.

In adult men, diagnosis of Klinefelter's syndrome can be made in most cases with relative ease on the basis of clinical evaluation, and it can be confirmed by laboratory studies of chromosomes, gonadotropin levels, pattern of testosterone production, and the appearance of testicular biopsy. In prepubertal males the diagnosis cannot be made on a clinical basis and in many instances cannot even be suspected but can easily be diagnosed on the basis of the above-mentioned laboratory investigations.

Therapy

No form of therapy capable of inducing sperm formation is available. When adrogen deficiency is present, therapy with testosterone is recommended (Delatestryl, 200 mg every 3 weeks).

ULLRICH-TURNER'S SYNDROME (MALE TURNER'S SYNDROME)

This is a rare condition presenting with the phenotypic characteristics of Turner's syndrome: short stature, low-set ears, webbed neck, "shield" chest, cardiovascular anomalies, ocular anomalies, cubitus valgus, cryptorchidism, and clinical signs of diminished androgen function. Although most of these patients show normal karyotype, some exhibit various chromosomal abnormalities.[73] The testes reveal a picture ranging from various degrees of spermatogenic activity to complete fibrosis. In some cases, gynecomastia, lymphedema, and mental retardation may be present. The etiology of this syndrome is entirely unknown, and therapy is directed primarily toward correction of the hypoandrogenic state.

REIFENSTEIN'S SYNDROME

The phenotype of these patients resembles that of Klinefelter's syndrome patients (eunochoid build, small testes, azoospermia, gynecomastia, and hypospadias.[74] The testes show various degrees of spermatogenesis. The karyotype, however, is that of a normal male (46XY). The etiologic factors are unknown, and therapy involves correction of congenital anomalies and replacement therapy with androgens.

SERTOLI CELL ONLY SYNDROME (DEL CASTILLO SYNDROME)

This syndrome is characterized by azoospermia and elevated gonadotropin levels associated with normal androgenic function of the testes. There are no associated congenital abnormalities, and the karyotype is normal. The testes frequently are of normal size, but the seminiferous tubules contain only Sertoli cells. There is no peritubular fibrosis or hyalinization. Congenital absence of germ cells has been considered to be the etiologic factor.[75] No therapy is available to correct the aspermatogenic state.

THE XX SYNDROME

A group of phenotypic males with clinical characteristics resembling the Klinefelter's syndrome were shown to have 46XX karyotype.[76] These patients present with psychosexual male identification and relatively normal male body habitus. Usually the amount of body and pubic hair is less than average. The penis and scrotum are normal; the testes are small, and their histology resembles that in Klinefelter's syndrome. Testosterone levels are usually normal. The explanation for the XX complement of sex chromosomes is lacking. The possibility has been suggested that the short arms of the Y chromosome have translocated onto autosomes.

PURE GONADAL DYSGENESIS (XY TYPE), STREAK GONADS

The male pattern of sex chromosomes in these patients is associated with a eunuchoid female phenotype. None of the classic male marks of Turner's syndrome are present. Patients develop female sex characteristics and show typical streak gonads.[77] It has been postulated that the XY karyotype in these patients is due to deletion of the long arms of one of the X chromosomes.

CONGENITAL DEFICIENCIES OF STEROIDOGENIC ENZYMES

Congenital Adrenal Hyperplasias

Types IV, V, and VI of congenital adrenal hyperplasia (see p. 133) are associated with severe abnormalities of the reproductive tract because of the generalized inability of the steroidogenic tissues to synthesize androgens. Since in all three types no steroids capable of suppression of gonadotropin secretion are produced, these disorders should be associated with elevated gonadotropin levels. However, only sporadic case reports are available in the literature, none providing a careful evaluation of each of these syndromes in large groups of subjects. The available data strongly suggest that these syndromes can occur in pure and complete or in partial or mixed forms. All of them result in varying degrees of male pseudohermaphroditism.

Type IV: Deficiency of 3β-Hydroxysteroid Dehydrogenase and Δ^5-Δ^4 Isomerase Enzyme Complex. This form of congenital adrenal hyperplasia associated with male pseudohermaphroditism was described by Bongiovanni.[78] The enzymic block does not permit the formation of Δ^4 steroids, and thus neither corticoids nor androgens such as androstenedione or testosterone are formed. Formation of very weak androgens such as dihydroepiandrosterone and Δ^5-androstenediol is not curtailed. Patients exhibit normal male genital ducts and incomplete masculinization of the external genitalia.

Type V: Deficiency of 17α-Hydroxylase. Grumbach and Van Wyk[79] cite from the literature 3 cases of this enzymic deficiency occurring in the male. They were phenotypic females with male genital duct development, testes, female external genitalia, and vagina.

Type VI: Deficiency of Cholesterol Side Chain Cleaving Enzymes (Congenital Lipoid Adrenal Hyperplasia). These individuals exhibit at birth severe adrenal insufficiency and ambiguous genitalia (male pseudohermaphroditism).[79,80] The external genitalia are female, but the genital ducts are male. The karyotype is 46XY. The testes show thickening of basement membrane and diminution in the number of spermatogonia.[81]

Other Forms of Congenital Deficiency of Steroidogenic Enzymes Resulting in Male Pseudohermaphroditism But Not Associated with Adrenal Insufficiency

Deficiency in 17,20 Desmolase (Progesterone Side Chain Cleaving Enzyme). A familial form of male pseudohermaphroditism associated with partial deficiency of desmolase has been described.[82] Clinical signs of the disorder are ambiguous external genitalia, cryptorchid testes, and a 46XY karyotype. Since the defect results specifically in inadequate androgen formation and intact corticoid synthesis in the adrenals, androgen therapy at the appropriate time will permit normal development of secondary sex characteristics.

Deficiency in 17β-Hydroxysteroid Oxidoreductase. The 17β-hydroxysteroid oxidoreductase is responsible for conversion of the immediate precursor, androstenedione to testosterone. Partial block of this enzyme has been linked in the literature with male pseudohermaphroditism.[83,84] The external genitalia in these patients are either female or ambiguous. Usually testes are ectopic, and a blind vaginal canal is present. The karyotype is 46XY. Therapy depends on sex assigned at birth.

End-Organ Insensitivity to Androgens

Feminizing Testes (Complete Testicular Feminization). In this form of male pseudohermaphroditism the androgen target tissues are unable to respond to testosterone. It is unlikely that the condition is due to a steroidogenic defect in the formation of testosterone. It has been suggested that the insensitivity of the target cells to testosterone is due to deficiency of 5α-reductase, an enzyme that converts testosterone to dihydrotestosterone, the active androgen in the androgen target cell. Recent information suggests that the defect lies in the inability of the target cell to bind testosterone or, in other words, in defective androgen receptor mechanisms in the cell.[85] The patients affected by this disorder are genetic males (karyotype 46XY) with a female phenotype. They exhibit female secondary sex characteristics, including good breast development and female body contours. External genitalia are those of a female. There is normal development of the vulva. The vagina, however, ends in a blind pouch. There are no female internal sex organs. The testes, usually located in the labia majora, on microscopic examination reveal fetal appearance and are predisposed to malignancy.[86] There is no or only sparse development of axillary or pubic hair.[86,87] The disorder is either an X-linked recessive or male-limited autosomal dominant trait.[87,88] The plasma testosterone levels are within the range of normal adult males,[89] and the testicular tissue produces testosterone in vitro actually at a higher rate than normal.[90] Administration of testosterone to these patients fails to induce virilization.

Incomplete Testicular Feminization. In this variant of the syndrome, feminization is incomplete, and at puberty, signs of virilization become obvious: hirsutism, phallic enlargement, and labioscrotal fusion. It is assumed that this form of testicular feminization is due to a partial degree of insensitivity to androgens.[87,91]

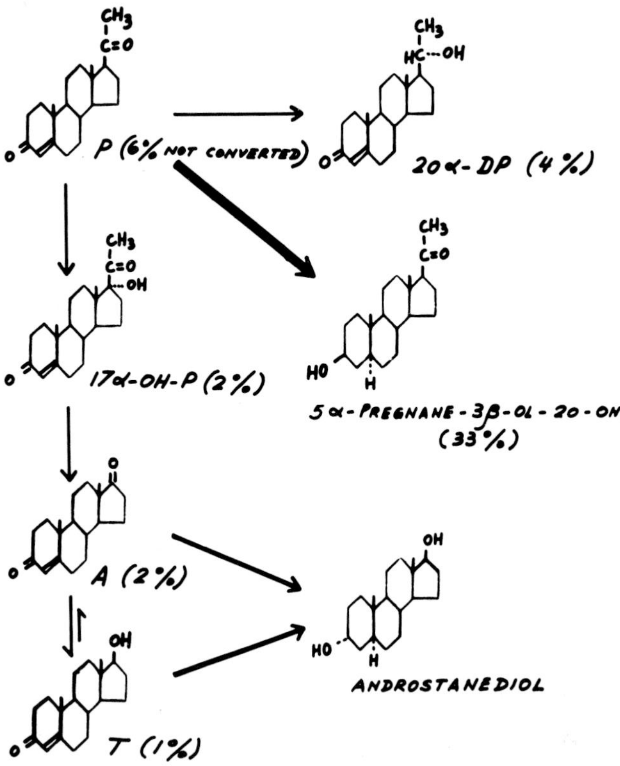

TESTICULAR DISORDERS ASSOCIATED WITH NORMAL GONADOTROPIN LEVELS

ADULT SEMINIFEROUS TUBULE FAILURE

In most instances the gonadotropin levels are within normal limits except when the damage to the seminiferous epithelium is extremely severe. In these individuals, FSH may be elevated.

Idiopathic

This diagnostic category probably contains various still unidentified pathological states. The patients usually present with a complaint of infertility. Seminal fluid examination reveals various degrees of oligospermia, and a testicular biopsy shows damage to the seminiferous epithelium. Clinically the Leydig cell function appears to be normal; however, in some of these patients, "low normal" levels of testosterone that could be augmented by treatment with gonadotropins[92] were detected.

Recently, abnormal steroidogenesis in testes of a patient with "idiopathic" adult seminiferous tubule failure has been demonstrated. Excessive 5α-reduction of the early steroidal precursors in the biogenetic pathway of androgens was detected. This abnormality reduced the capacity of the testes to secrete testosterone (Fig. 124-5). This abnormality was successfully treated with a combination of HCG and HMG.[93]

In general, however, no adequate form of therapy is available for this group of patients. A number of therapeutic modalities has been suggested, and a certain degree of success has been reported. Possibly the success in the limited number of patients has been due to chance, where in spite of the lack of a specific diagnosis, a specific form of therapy was administered with positive results.

Testosterone Rebound Therapy. Heckel et al.[94] suggested that in some patients improvement in spermatogenic function will result following suppression of spermatogenesis produced by administration of large doses of testosterone. While a certain number of patients may respond to this form of therapy, the majority does

Fig. 124-5. Steroid biosynthetic pattern found in testicular tissue obtained at biopsy. Numbers in parenthesis indicate percent conversion of ^{3}H-progesterone. P, progesterone; 20α-DP, 20α-dihydroprogesterone; 17α-OH-P, 17α-hydroxyprogesterone. A, androstenedione; T, testosterone. (From E. Steinberger et al., *Andrologia 6:* 59, 1974.)

not. No clear guidelines are available to preselect the "responders."

Low-Dose Testosterone Therapy. Low doses of testosterone have been advocated for therapy of oligospermia, an idea still reflected in the description of therapeutic indications for testosterone in the *Physicians' Desk Reference.*[95] No convincing clinical data, however, are available in support of the use of low doses of testosterone for stimulation of spermatogenesis. In fact, recent experimental data suggest that this form of therapy may not only be of no benefit, but may actually be detrimental.[72]

Human Gonadotropins. Some patients with low or "normal" levels of gonadotropins and oligospermia may respond to gonadotropin therapy.[96] The reason for inconsistency of the therapeutic response is unclear but probably relates to the inability to make a proper specific diagnosis and possibly to the lack of complete understanding of the response of the germinal epithelium to gonadotropic hormones.

Thyroid Hormone. Although L-triiodothyronine (Cytomel) has been suggested as a "specific" therapeutic agent in oligospermia,[97] no adequate evidence as to its effectiveness has been provided. This form of therapy is not indicated for correction of oligospermia unless definite evidence of hypothyroidism is present.

Miscellaneous Agents. The early claims for a beneficial effect of vitamins E and C on spermatogenesis in man are not supported by experimental evidence. Phenelzine (a monoamine oxidase inhibitor)[98] and perphenazine (Trilafan), a tranquilizer,[99] have been suggested to be effective for treatment of oligospermia. The experience with these drugs is too limited to warrant definite conclusions. Clomid (clomiphene citrate) has been reported to improve sperm production.[100] Again, the effect is not predictable, and no definite guidelines are available for patient selection. The drug probably exerts its effect by inducing increased gonadotropin secretion. More extensive evaluation will be in order before any conclusions about its efficiency can be made.[101]

POSTORCHITIS OLIGOSPERMIA

Mumps orchitis is the most common infection resulting in testicular damage. However, any infection that leads to testicular involvement and even distant infectious processes that may not involve the testis may also produce testicular damage.

Testicular damage secondary to mumps orchitis becomes clinically evident within a few weeks after the inflammatory process subsides. The testis may show varying degrees of atrophy, although the seminiferous tubules usually show patchy involvement. If the damage is severe, the gonadotropin levels may rise, although testosterone production remains normal. There is no specific form of therapy. Estrogen therapy during the acute stages of orchitis has been advocated to "place the germinal epithelium at rest," but there is no evidence that this form of therapy is actually effective.

OTHER CAUSES OF TESTICULAR DISORDERS

NEUROLOGIC DISEASE

Extensive lesions of the spinal cord are frequently associated with testicular dysfunction. In paraplegics, in addition to varying degrees of impotency and ejaculatory disturbances occurring in most patients, testicular damage has also been documented in over 50 percent of cases.[102,103] The microscopic lesions are limited primarily to the seminiferous epithelium, which shows spermatogenic arrest.[104] The Leydig cells appear to be unaffected, and androgen production is essentially unchanged. The etiology of seminiferous epithelium damage in paraplegics remains unclear. No direct relationship between the level of the cord lesion and the presence or the degree of spermatogenic arrest has been detected. Furthermore, no relationship between the degree of impotency, ejaculatory dysfunction, and spermatogenic damage has been noted.[104] The suggestion was made that disturbance in the temperature regulatory mechanism resulting from the neurologic lesion is responsible for the spermatogenic damage.[105] Sympathectomy affects scrotal skin and interferes with the sweating process;[106] in addition, the cremasteric reflex is lost. These changes may possibly interfere with the normal thermoregulatory mechanism of the scrotum. A neurologic deficit in the regulation of vascular tone may directly, or indirectly via the thermoregulatory mechanism, also be involved in the etiology of seminiferous epithelium damage. Vascular stagnation (both arterial and venous) secondary to the neurologic lesion with subsequent anoxia of the testicular parenchyma has been considered as another possible etiologic factor.[107]

Unquestionably both the character and the extent of testicular lesions vary in patients with neurologic disorders. Furthermore, spontaneous improvement following the acute episode may occur. Careful evaluation and prevention of exposure of the testes to temperature elevations are probably the only form of medical management currently available.

MYOTONIA DYSTROPHICA

In this familial disorder characterized by myopathy and myotonia, the patients are frequently affected by cataracts and frontal baldness. In addition, testicular damage has been observed in 80 percent of the cases.[108,109] Pubertal development is normal, and the only physical clues of testicular damage may be testicular atrophy, which occurs at varying times after puberty, and infertility. Although the microscopic appearance of the testis resembles at times the characteristic pattern found in testes of patients with Klinefelter's syndrome, cytogenetic abnormalities are not usually associated with this syndrome, and in some patients, varying degrees of spermatogenic activity can be observed.[108]

The patients do not exhibit signs of androgen deficiency. Whether testicular changes are the result of a primary testicular disorder or occur secondary to hypothalamic-pituitary dysfunction has been unclear until recently.[108] Studies of plasma gonadotropins utilizing radioimmunoassay in 39 adult patients with myotonia dystrophica demonstrated substantially elevated circulating levels of both LH and FSH,[110] which clearly indicated the existence of primary testicular disease in these patients. The underlying cause of the testicular damage remains unknown, however.

No known form of therapy for germinal epithelium damage is available.

PHYSICAL AND CHEMICAL AGENTS

Ionizing Radiation

Rugh and Grupp suggested that as a result of their extreme radiosensitivity, the testes could be used as a tissue dosimeter in cases of accidental exposure to ionizing radiation.[111] Indeed, the sensitivity of testes to irradiation was reported within 8 years[112] after the initial discovery of x-rays by Roentgen in 1895.[113] Although a considerable body of information has accumulated concerning the effects of ionizing radiation on the testes of subhuman species (for reviews, see Oakberg[114] and Ellis[115]), the information concerning the response of human testes to radiation remains scarce for obvious reasons. Most data are based on studies of rat and mouse testes. Microscopic studies of the testes suggest that the germinal elements are most sensitive to radiation, while the Sertoli cells and Leydig cells are relatively radioresistant. In rodents the B type spermatogonia and certain generations of type A spermatogonia are most radiosensitive, the spermatocytes less sensitive, and the spermatids most resistant of all the various types of germ cells.[116] This distribution of radiosensitivity among the various types of germ cells is responsible for the characteristic and orderly "maturation depletion" pattern of the regressive changes in the germinal epithelium after an acute exposure to radiation and for the orderly sequence of repopulation of the germinal epithelium occurring during the regeneration period.[117]

Although the basic characteristics of the response of the germinal epithelium to ionizing radiation is similar in all mammals, certain specific quantitative differences exist, particularly in the timing of postregression recovery and in the details of the effects on specific types of spermatogonia.[114,118] The experimental information obtained in man[118,119] reveals that doses as low as 15 R (local testicular irradiation) cause reduction in sperm count and that 100 R cause immediate morphologic damage to the sensitive types of germ cells. Chromosomal analysis of testicular tissue cultures from subjects exposed to 100 R revealed a significant increase in both stable and unstable chromosome aberrations but no chromatid changes.

Analogous to the lower species, the spermatogonia in human testes are the most sensitive and the spermatids the most radioresistant cell types in the germinal epithelium. Among the spermatogonia the B type are the most sensitive. Their precursors, the type A dark and pale spermatogonia, are somewhat less sensitive, while the daughter cells of type B spermatogonia, the preleptotene spermatocytes, are 10 times less sensitive. The spermatids are 40 times less sensitive to the effects of ionizing radiation in comparison to B type spermatogonia. These estimates were made simply on the basis of morphologically detectable changes in the cells and are not correlated necessarily with biochemical and particularly with genetic sensitivity of the germ cells to radiation

The latter is of particular concern and interest; however, no direct information regarding the mutogenic effects of ionizing radiation on germinal epithelium cells of the human testes, except for the limited cytogenetic studies mentioned above, is available.

In rodent testes the recovery of spermatogenesis following radiation-induced damage is fairly rapid and relatively uniform, particularly following irradiation with doses of 600 R or less. In man, repopulation is delayed for a considerable period of time and is unpredictable and erratic. The relative radioresistance of Leydig cells demonstrated in lower species[115,116] has also been shown in man. No significant changes in production of testosterone or estrogen were detected, although elevation of FSH levels was observed.[119]

The response of fetal or perinatal testes to ionizing radiation has been studied primarily in rodents. A marked radiosensitivity of gonocytes was noted.[120] Their sensitivity increases during fetal life and then decreases during the neonatal period.[121] Morphologic changes in Leydig cells[122] and diminished androgen secretion[123] have also been demonstrated in testes of immature animals exposed to ionizing radiation.

Incidence of testicular damage encountered in clinical practice resulting from accidental exposure to radiation has been extremely low,[124] the damage usually being attributed to a variety of industrial accidents. However, the application of ionizing radiation therapy for gonadal and extragonadal neoplasia may become a factor in the incidence of radiation-induced testicular damage. Unfortunately, no reliable form of medical therapy to prevent, protect, or treat germinal epithelium damage resulting from the exposure to ionizing radiation is available. Shielding the gonad during the administration of ionizing radiation is the only viable approach to prevention.

Heat

It was suspected as early as the 19th century that heat may be detrimental to the spermatogenic function of the testes.[125] Crew postulated that spermatogenic damage in cryptorchid testes is due to temperature elevation in the testicular parenchyma of the intraabdominal testes.[126] Fukui[127] and Moore[128] provided experimental evidence that elevation of testicular temperature produces germinal epithelium damage. These findings were subsequently confirmed and extended to most mammalian species, including man, by numerous investigators (for reviews, see refs. 124 and 129). Extensive quantitative studies in the rat demonstrated that certain segments of the meiotic prophase and early steps of spermatid development are most heat-sensitive.[130] Although in man no similar detailed studies of changes in the seminiferous epithelium are available, a large body of evidence has accumulated to support the conclusion that human testes are also heat-sensitive and respond to temperature elevation with spermatogenic damage.

The observation was made at the turn of the century that febrile illnesses in man (typhus, scarlet fever, etc.) are associated with testicular damage.[131,132] Definite clinical evidence linking fever and testicular damage has been provided in more recent reports[133,134] and experimental evidence based on the effect of artificially induced elevation of intratesticular temperature in man provided direct evidence for the detrimental effect of heat on human testes.[135–138] The sensitivity of human germinal epithelium to even slight elevation in temperature has been stressed by numerous authors.[139,140] Wearing tight clothing, "jockey" shorts, or athletic supporters has been implicated in induction of intratesticular hyperthermia with resulting oligospermia.[141]

Unfortunately, the available information concerning the possible role of slight changes in temperature in induction of oligospermia and infertility is too fragmentary to allow direct and specific clinical application. It is of interest to note, however, that it has been suggested that the changes in intratesticular temperature resulting from the adoption of Western mode of dress could be sufficient to induce an increased mutation rate that might imply genetic hazards 100 to 1000 times greater than those estimated from different sources of radiation to which man is currently exposed.[142]

Chemical Agents

Alkylating Agents. The damaging effects of alkylating agents on the testes were first demonstrated in studies of the effect of nitrogen mustard on neoplasia in the mouse.[143] Subsequently, Hendry et al.[144] observed testicular damage in rats and dogs treated with massive doses of synthetic alkylating agents, derivatives of ethyleneimine. Comprehensive investigations into the effects of one of the ethyleneimine derivatives, TEM (triethylenemelamine, 2,3,6-trisethyleneimino-s-triazine), revealed its specific effect on the testes.[145,146] In further studies, a complicated action of TEM on the various stages of the germ cell development was noted. Low doses (0.05 mg/kg) produced no morphologic effect but induced sterility, and high doses (0.2 mg/kg) produced specific destruction of type A spermatogonia with ensuing "maturation depletion" similar to that following the effects of ionizing radiation.[147,148] Literally dozens of various alkylating agents have been demonstrated subsequently to produce in the seminiferous epithelium of experimental animals specific lesions similar in general terms to those induced by TEM but varying in specific cellular sites of action.[149,150]

Other Chemical Agents. Numerous nonalkylating chemosterilants, antimetabolites, cytotoxic agents, pesticides, fungicides, antibiotics, narcotics, antitumor drugs, etc. have been reported to produce testicular damage (for reviews, see refs. 149–152).

The earliest observations of germinal epithelium damage were made incidentally during investigations on the anticancer properties of several toxic substances.[143,153] Nelson and his co-workers were the first to initiate systematic and comprehensive studies of the effects of various chemical agents on the testes and the fertility in the male. The initial group of chemical substances investigated were the nitrofurans, a class of heterocyclic antibacterial agents. A number of nitrofuran derivatives, including Furacin [5-nitro-2-furfuraldehyde-2-(2-hydroxyethyl) semicarbazone], Furadroxyl [5-nitro-2-furfuraldehyde-2-(2-hydroxyethyl) semicarbazone], Furadantin [N(5-nitro-2-furfurylidine)-1-aminohydantoin] and furazolidone [N(5-nitro-2-furfurylidine)-3-amino-2-oxazolidone], were investigated and all have shown a specific direct effect on the seminiferous epithelium, resulting in arrest of spermatogenesis at the pachytene stage of the development of the primary spermatocytes. These agents did not interfere with pituitary gonadotropic function or androgen production by the testes.[117,154–157] Similar effects on the male reproductive system were obtained in studies of several other classes of compounds, the thiophens,[158] substituted dichloroacetyl diamines,[159,160] and dinitropyrroles.[161,162]

Although most studies concerned with the effects of chemical agents on the testes have been performed in lower species, fragmentary information is also available concerning their effects in man. One of the nitrofurans, Furadantin, has been tested clinically. "Suggestive" effects on sperm counts were observed in 30 percent of the volunteers employed in this study, and 20 percent of biopsies obtained in these volunteers revealed signs of germinal epithelium damage.[163] The substituted dichloracetyl diamines were also tested clinically. These agents were shown to be highly effective in causing spermatogenic arrest and cessation of sperm production, but their Antabuselike side effects precluded the possibility of clinical application.[164]

Although numerous alkylating, cytotoxic, and other anticancer agents have been administered to men for cancer therapy, relatively few reports are available concerning the effect of these drugs on the reproductive system of the treated cancer patients. Most reports are single case studies or, at best, reports on small series of patients. Following the therapy of patients with cancer or nephrotic syndrome with mercaptopurine, cyclophosphamide, methotrexate, chlorambucil, nitrogen mustard, vincristine, or procarbazine, suppression of spermatogenesis has been noted; in many instances after cessation of therapy, patients experienced recovery of sperm production and in some cases recovery of fertility.[165–173]

The return of fertility in a segment of patients receiving this therapy could be interpreted in a positive way, but it should be tempered with a note of caution. Animal experiments provide evidence that these agents induce mutations in the stem cells of the germinal epithelium. These mutations are transferred to the offspring. Consequently, it is possible that a return of fertility in human males treated with these agents may result in introduction of mutant genes into the human genetic pool with totally unknown consequences for future generations.

A possibility has been raised that narcotic and psychedelic drugs may interfere with normal reproductive function in the male and even cause damage to the germ cells expressed by congenital anomalies in offspring.[174–176] The information on this topic is even more limited and more controversial than that on the effects of alkylating and cytotoxic agents. Clearly more intensive studies are indicated to clarify this extremely important question.

VASCULAR ABNORMALITIES

Interference with Normal Blood Supply

Unfortunately, there is available for obvious reasons only limited experimental information about the effects of interruption of blood supply to the human testes. In experimental animals, extensive studies have been conducted on this topic. Most data are available for the rat testes. In this species permanent interruption of the spermatic artery at a point along its course in the abdomen before it anastomoses with the vasal artery induces a rapid and complete degeneration of the testes.[177] The severity and degree of the damage and the extent of subsequent repair following temporary interruption of the blood supply is related to the duration of the ischemic episode. Complete interruption of the blood supply for up to 90 minutes produces no morphologic changes in spermatogenesis. With increased duration of ischemia, specific and characteristic changes take place in the seminiferous epithelium. After 120 minutes of ischemia, severe, generalized damage of all the germ cells in the seminiferous tubules is produced. It appears that cells engaged in DNA synthesis are most sensitive to ischemia.[178,179]

Vasoactive agents such as Apresoline also produce germinal epithelium damage.[180,181] It appears that ischemia produced by the vasoconstrictive action of these drugs is responsible for spermatogenic damage.

In man, interference with the blood supply may occur spontaneously as a result of testicular torsion. Clinical studies suggest that a 360° torsion of less than 12 hours duration may not produce necrosis of the testes, but the degree of spermatogenic impairment following such episodes may vary greatly.[182] It must be emphasized that in clinical conditions of testicular torsion, not only is the arterial blood supply compromised but also the venous drainage is interfered with. The latter will cause testicular congestion and damage to the parenchyma, because the testis is covered by a relatively inelastic membrane, while the seminiferous tubules are soft and easily compressed. Nevertheless, careful evaluation and every attempt to salvage testicular tissue is in order even if it is suspected that spermatogenic function may be lost. Conservation of androgen-producing capacity alone will be important to prevent the necessity of lifelong therapy with androgens.

The limited experimental studies in man suggested that interruption of the internal spermatic artery at the external inguinal canal for periods up to 15 days produces no damage to the testes. However, morphologic changes are observed in the seminiferous tubules after a 24-hour interruption of the blood supply of both the internal spermatic artery and the artery to the ductus deferens; after 5 days of blood flow interruption, necrosis of the testis occurs.[183]

Varicocele

It has been well over 400 years since the first mention of varicocele, "a compact pack of vessels filled with melancholic blood," was made.[184] This anomaly of testicular and vasal veins did not, however, achieve its notoriety until the second half of this century, when Tulloch[185] reported on the beneficial effects of varicocelectomy in infertile males. This operation was subsequently introduced in the United States by Charny[186] and popularized here by Dubin and Amelar.[187]

Varicocele is a condition in which the veins responsible for vascular drainage of the testicle become abnormally dilated. A varicocele occurring exclusively on the right side is suggestive of a pathological lesion involving the right retroperitoneal space or an intraperitoneal lesion in the vicinity of the drainage of the right internal spermatic vein into the vena cava. This condition will not be discussed here. A varicocele occurring on the left side, however, "appears to be related to either the congenital absence or incompetency of valves in the left internal spermatic vein. The unusually long length, erect posture of man, and right angle termination of the gonadal vein poorly enables the vein to resist incompetency and consequently retrograde flow."[188] It is the varicocele occurring on the left side that has been associated with disorders of testicular function. Although considerable evidence has accumulated suggesting a cause-and-effect relationship between the presence of varicocele and male infertility (for review, see refs. 189 and 190), the statistics on incidence of varicocele in infertile men are difficult to interpret because of the great variation in the type of patient population seen by different authors. The estimates range from 4.6 percent in a study of a group of 5000 patients[191] to 39.0 percent in a group of 1294.[192] Unfortunately, only scanty information is available for the incidence of varicocele in normal fertile male population. Clark[193] reported an incidence of varicocele in 8 percent of "normal" population, while Steeno et al.,[194] in a study of 894 males between the ages of 18 and 20, observed a 13.5 percent incidence. No information is available on the incidence of varicocele in men who recently fathered children. Similarly, there is no agreement as to the type of testicular function abnormality associated with varicocele. Although it appears that most infertile patients with varicocele have low sperm counts,[195] no similar studies have been made in men with varicocele who have fathered children.

MacLeod[196] suggested that infertile patients with varicocele exhibit a characteristic pattern of sperm morphology: an increased incidence of tapered, amorphous, and immature sperm; however, he later reported that 50 percent of men with varicocele do not demonstrate any abnormalities in their seminal fluid.[197] Other authors[190] in recent studies suggest that all infertile patients with varicocele exhibit morphologic abnormalities of spermatozoa but many show sperm counts within normal range.

Since, after ligation of varicocele for therapeutic purposes, only 50 to 80 percent of patients respond with changes in sperm count or sperm morphology,[196] the parameter frequently utilized in assessment of therapeutic success has been the pregnancy rate.[199] Recently, some authors reported no changes in seminal fluid characteristics subsequent to varicocele ligation but observed an increase in conception rate.[200] These observations suggest that another factor may be involved in the infertile couples in which the male suffers with varicocele, namely the "female factor" or the "couple" factor. In most of the above-cited studies, either no information is provided concerning the female partner and couple interaction or a statement is made that "no abnormality was present in the female." In a recent study of a group of infertile patients where both partners were followed by the same team of physicians, the males were either not treated or treated only by varicocele ligation, while the wives were carefully evaluated and an attempt was made to correct as much as possible the slightest reproductive system abnormality. In this study, the incidence of pregnancy in wives of men with varicoceles who were operated did not differ from those whose husbands were not operated.[201]

It appears that varicocele indeed may have an etiologic relationship to testicular abnormalities; a clear and specific relationship still has not been established. Similarly, a definite cause-and-effect relationship between correction of varicocele, improvement in seminal fluid characteristics, and increased incidence of pregnancy will require further investigation.

The mechanism by which varicocele produces testicular damage remains unclear. The earliest suggestions were that the dilated veins interfere with the cooling mechanism of the testes.[202] This hypothesis has been subsequently discarded.[203] However, it should be noted that recent preliminary experimental data have been presented in primates and strongly suggest that temperature elevation indeed may be an important etiologic factor.[204] An increase of adrenal steroids as a result of reflux from the adrenal vein was suggested but not supported by subsequent data.[205] Recently, Cohen et al.[206] suggested that increased concentrations of catecholamines in the spermatic vein may be the causative factor in spermatogenic damage in men with varicocele.

A considerable body of data has accumulated implicating the presence of varicocele in male infertility, but a review of the same data clearly indicates that a great deal of work will still be necessary to clarify the relationships between varicocele and testicular function, the mechanisms by which varicocele possibly produces testicular damage, and the role varicocele ligation plays in therapy.

REFERENCES

1. Heller, C. G. and Nelson, W. O., Classification of Male Hypogonadism and a Discussion of the Pathologic Physiology, Diagnosis and Treatment. *J. Clin. Endocrinol. 8:* 345, 1948.
2. Howard, R. P., Sniffen, R. C., Simmons, F. A., and Albright, F., Testicular Deficiency: Clinical and Pathologic Study. *J. Clin. Endocrinol. 10:* 121, 1950.
3. Albert, A., Underdahl, L. O., Greene, L. F., and Lorenz, N., Male Hypogonadism. IV. The Testis in Prepubertal or Pubertal Gonadotropic Failure. *Proc. Staff Meet. Mayo Clin. 29:* 131, 1954.
4. Burr, I. M., Sizonenko, P. C., Kaplan, S. L., and Grumbach, M. M., Hormonal Changes in Puberty. I. Correlation of Serum Luteinizing Hormone and Follicle Stimulating Hormone with Stages of Puberty, Testicular Size, and Bone Age in Normal Boys. *Pediatr. Res. 4:* 25, 1970.
5. Root, A. W., Moshang, T., Jr., Bongiovanni, A. M., and Eberlein, W. R., Concentrations of Plasma Luteinizing Hormone in Infants, Children and Adolescents with Normal and Abnormal Gonadal Function. *Pediatr. Res. 4:* 175, 1970.
6. Kulin, H. E. and Santen, R. J., Endocrinology of Puberty in Man, in Spilman, C. H., Lobl, T. J., and Kirton, K. T. (eds): Regulatory Mechanisms of Male Reproductive Physiology. Amsterdam, *Excerpta Medica,* 1976, p. 175.
7. Smith, K. D., Tcholakian, R. K., Chowdhury, M., and Steinberger, E., Rapid Oscillations in Plasma Levels of Testosterone, LH and FSH in Men. *Fertil. Steril. 25:* 965, 1974.
8. Goldzieher, J. W., Dozier, T. S., Smith, K. D., and Steinberger, E., Improving the Diagnostic Reliability of Rapidly Fluctuating Plasma Hormone Levels by Optimized Multiple-Sampling Techniques. *J. Clin. Endocrinol. Metab. 43:* 824, 1976.
9. Kulin, H. E., Grumbach, M. M., and Kaplan, S. L., Gonadal-Hypothalamic Interaction in Prepubertal and Pubertal Man: Effect of Clomiphene Citrate on Urinary Follicle-Stimulating Hormone and Luteinizing Hormone and Plasma Testosterone. *Pediatr. Res. 6:* 162, 1972.
10. Mortimer, C. H., Besser, G. M., McNeilly, A. S., Marshall, J. C., Harsoulis, P., Tunbridge, W. M. G., Gomez-Pan, A., and Hall, R., Luteinizing Hormone and Follicle Stimulating Hormone-Releasing Hormone Test in Patients with Hypothalamic-Pituitary-Gonadal Dysfunction. *Br. Med. J. 4:* 73, 1973.
11. Nawakowski, H. and Lenz, W., Genetic Aspects in Male Hypogonadism. *Recent Prog. Horm. Res. 17:* 53, 1961.
12. Ewer, R. W., Familial Monotropic Pituitary Gonadotropin Insufficiency. *J. Clin. Endocrinol. Metab. 28:* 783, 1968.
13. Santen, R. J. and Paulsen, C. A., Hypogonadotropic Eunuchoidism. I. Clinical Study of the Mode of Inheritance. *J. Clin. Endocrinol. Metab. 36:* 47, 1973.
14. Sparkes, R. S., Simpson, R. W., and Paulsen, C. A., Familial Hypogonadotropic Hypogonadism with Anosmia. *Arch. Intern. Med. 121:* 534, 1968.
15. Kallmann, F., Schonfeld, W. A., and Barrera, S. E., The Genetic Aspects of Primary Eunuchoidism. *Am. J. Ment. Defic. 48:* 203, 1944.
16. Hamilton, C. R., Henkin, R. I., Weir, G., and Kliman, B., Olfactory Status and Response to Clomiphene in Male Gonadotropin Deficiency. *Ann. Intern. Med. 78:* 47, 1973.
17. Marshall, J. R. and Henkin, R. I., Olfactory Acuity, Menstrual Abnormalities, and Oocyte Status. *Ann. Intern. Med. 75:* 207, 1971.
18. Kastin, A. J., Gual, C., and Schally, A. V., Clinical Experience with Hypothalamic Releasing Hormones. Part 2. Luteinizing Hormone-Releasing Hormone and Other Hypophysiotropic Releasing Hormones. *Recent Prog. Horm. Res. 28:* 201, 1972.
19. McNeilly, A. S., Anderson, D. C., Besser, G. M., Marshall, J. C., Harsoulis, P., Alexander, L., Ormston, B. J., Hall, R., and Collins, W., The Luteinizing Hormone (LH) and Follicle-Stimulating Hormone Response to Synthetic LH Releasing Factor in Man. *J. Endocrinol. 55:* xxiv, 1972.
20. De Morsier, G., Etudes sur les Dysraphies Crânio-Encéphaliques; Agénésie des Lobes Olfactifs (Télencéphaloschizis Latéral) et des Commissures Calleuse et Antérieure (Télencéphaloschizis Médian); La Dysplasie Olfacto-Génitale. *Schweiz. Arch. Neurol. Psychiatr. 74:* 309, 1954.
21. Gauthier, G., La Dysplasie Olfacto-Génitale (Agénésie des Lobes Olfactifs avec Absence de Développement Gonadique à la Puberté). *Acta Neuroveg. 21:* 345, 1960.
22. Mancini, R. E., in Hypothalamic Hypophysiotropic Hormones, Physiological and Clinical Studies. Proceedings of the Serono Research Foundation Conference, Acapulco, Mexico, 1972. Amsterdam, Excerpta Medica Foundation, 1973.
23. Lostroh, A. J., Hormonal Control of Spermatogenesis, in Spilman, C. H., Lobl, T. J., and Kirton, K. T. (eds): Regulatory Mechanisms of Male Reproductive Physiology. Amsterdam, *Exerpta Medica,* 1976, p. 13.
24. Tanner, J. M., Whitehouse, R. H., Hughes, P. C. R., and Vince, F. P., Effect of Human Growth Hormone Treatment for 1 to 7 Years on Growth of 100 Children, with Growth Hormone Deficiency, Low

Birthweight, Inherited Smallness, Turner's Syndrome and Other Complaints. *Arch. Dis. Child. 46:* 745, 1971.

25. Pasqualini, R. Q. and Bur, G., Sindrome Hipoandrogénico con Gametogenesis Conservada. Clasificación de la Insuficiencia Testicular. *Rev. Asoc. Méd. Argent. 64:* 6, 1950.
26. McCullagh, E. P., Beck, J. C. and Schaffenburg, C. A., A Syndrome of Eunuchoidism with Spermatogenesis, Normal Urinary FSH and Low or Normal ICSH ("Fertile Eunuchs"). *J. Clin. Endocrinol. 13:* 489, 1953.
27. Albert, A., Underdahl, L. O., Greene, L. F., and Lorenz, N., Male Hypogonadism. *Proc. Staff Meet. Mayo Clin. 30:* 31, 1955.
28. Faiman, C., Hoffmann, D. L., Ryan, R. J., and Albert, A., The Fertile Eunuch Syndrome: Demonstration of Isolated Luteinizing Hormone Deficiency by Radioimmunoassay Technique. *Mayo Clin. Proc. 43:* 661, 1968.
29. Santen, R. J. and Paulsen, C. A., Hypogonadotropic Eunuchoidism, II. Gonadal Responsiveness to Exogenous Gonadotropins. *J. Clin. Endocrinol. Metab. 36:* 55, 1973.
30. Prader, A., Labhart, A., and Willi, H. Ein Syndrom von Adipositas, Leinwuchs, Kryptorchismus and Oligophrenia nach Myatonie-artigen Zustanol im Neugeborenenalter. *Schweiz. Med. Wschr. 26:* 1260, 1956.
31. Hamilton, C. R., Scully, R. E., and Kliman, B., Hypogonadotropinism in Prader-Willi Syndrome. Induction of Puberty and Spermatogenesis by Clomiphene Citrate. *Am. J. Med. 52:* 322, 1972.
32. Zellweger, H. and Schneider, H. J., Syndrome of Hypotonia-Hypomentia-Hypogonadism-Obesity (HHHO) or Prader-Willi Syndrome. *Am. J. Dis. Child. 115:* 588, 1968.
33. Hoefnagel, D., Costello, P. J., and Hahtoum, K., Prader-Willi Syndrome. *J. Ment. Defic. Res. 11:* 1, 1967.
34. Prader, A., and Willi, H., Das Syndrom von Imbezillitat. Adipositas, Muskelhypotonie, Hypogenitalismus, Hypogonadismus und Diabetes Mellitus mit "Myatonie"—Anamnese. Verhand. 2. int. Kongr. psych. Entw.-Stör. Kindes-Alt., Vienna, 1961, Part I, p. 353.
35. Juul, J. and Dupont, A., Prader-Willi Syndrome. *J. Ment. Defic. Res. 11:* 12, 1967.
36. Bardin, C. W., Ross, G. T., and Lipsett, M. B., Site of Action of Clomiphene Citrate in Men: A Study of the Pituitary-Leydig Cell Axis. *J. Clin. Endocrinol. Metab. 27:* 1558, 1967.
37. Cargille, C. H., Ross, G. T., and Bardin, C. W., Clomiphene and Gonadotrophin in Men. *Lancet 2:* 1298, 1968.
38. Roth, A. A., Familial Eunuchoidism: The Laurence-Moon-Biedl Syndrome. *J. Urol. 57:* 427, 1947.
39. Oettlé, A. G., Rabinowitz, D., and Seftel, H. C. The Laurence-Moon Syndrome with Germinal Aplasia of the Testis. *J. Clin Endocrinol. Metab. 20:* 683, 1960.
40. Reinfrank, R. F. and Nichols, F. L., Hypogonadotrophic Hypogonadism in the Laurence-Moon Syndrome. *J. Clin. Endocrinol. Metab. 24:* 48, 1964.
41. Dahl, E. V. and Bahn, R. C., Aberrant Adrenal Cortical Tissue Near the Testis in Human Infants. *Am. J. Pathol. 40:* 587, 1962.
42. Wilkins, L. and Cara, J., Further Studies on the Treatment of Congenital Adrenal Hyperplasia with Cortisone. V. Effects of Cortisone Therapy on Testicular Development. *J. Clin. Endocrinol. 14:* 287, 1954.
43. Sohval, A. R. and Gabrilove, J. L., Testicular Histopathology in Feminizing Tumors of Adrenal Cortex. *J. Urol. 93:* 711, 1965.
44. Burns, E., Segaloff, A., Carrera, G. M., and Colbert, D. W., Congenital Absence of Gonads: Report of 2 Cases. *Trans. Amr. Assoc. Gen.-Urin. Surg. 54:* 53, 1962.
45. Abeyaratne, M. R., Aherne, W. A., and Scott, J. E. S., The Vanishing Testis. *Lancet 2:* 822, 1969.
46. Jost, A., Sur le Rôle des Gonades Foetales dans la Différenciation Sexuelle Somatique de l'Embryon de Lapin. *C. R. Assoc. Anat. 34:* 255, 1947.
47. Charny, C. W. and Wolgin, W., Cryptorchism. New York, Hoeber-Harper, 1957.
48. Ward, B. and Hunter, W. M., The Absent Testicle: A Report on a Survey Carried Out Among School Boys in Nottingham. *Br. Med. J. 5179:* 110, 1960.
49. de la Balze, F. A., Mancini, R. A., Arrillaga, F., Andrada, J. A., Vilar, O., Gurtman, A. I., and Davidson, O. W., Histologic Study of the Undescended Human Testis During Puberty. *J. Clin. Endocrinol. Metab. 20:* 286, 1960.
50. Engle, E. T., Atypical Cytology in Testes Biopsies. *J. Urol. 62:* 694, 1949.
51. Giarola, A., Protection of Reproductive Capacity as a Factor in Therapy for Undescended Testicle. *Fertil. Steril. 18:* 375, 1967.
52. Hortling, H., de la Chapelle, A., Johansson, C. J., Niemi, M., and Sulamaa, M., An Endocrinologic Follow-up Study of Operated Cases of Cryptorchidism. *J. Clin. Endocrinol. Metab. 27:* 120, 1967.
53. Charny, C. W., The Spermatogenic Potential of the Undescended Testis Before and After Treatment. *J. Urol. 83:* 697, 1960.
54. Gross, R. E. and Jewett, T. C., Jr., Surgical Experiences From 1222 Operations for Undescended Testis. *J.A.M.A. 160:* 634, 1956.
55. Scott, L. S., Delayed Treatment of Cryptorchidism with Subsequent Infertility. *Fertil. Steril. 18:* 782, 1967.
56. Thompson, W. O. and Heckel, N. J., Endocrine Treatment of Cryptorchidism. *J.A.M.A. 117:* 1953, 1941.
57. Drake, C. B., Treatment of Cryptorchidism. *J.A.M.A. 163:* 626, 1957.
58. Gilbert, J. B. and Hamilton, J. B., Incidence and Nature of Tumors in the Ectopic Testis. *Surg. Gynecol. Obstet. 71:* 731, 1940.
59. Campbell, H. E., The Incidence of Malignant Growth of the Undescended Testicle: A Reply and Reevaluation. *J. Urol. 81:* 663, 1959.
60. Gilbert, J. B., Development of Testicular Tumors After Orchidopexy. *J. Urol. 46:* 740, 1941.
61. Sumner, W. A., Malignant Tumor of Testis Occurring 29 Years After Orchiopexy. *J. Urol. 81:* 150, 1959.
62. Schwartz, J. W. and Reed, J. F., Pathology of Cryptorchidism. *J. Urol. 76:* 429, 1956.
63. Altman, B. L. and Malament, M., Carcinoma of the Testis Following Orchiopexy. *J. Urol. 97:* 498, 1967.
64. Klinefelter, J. F., Jr., Reifenstein, E. C., Jr., and Albright, F., Syndrome Characterized by Gynecomastia, Aspermatogenesis Without A-Leydigism and Increased Excretion of Follicle-Stimulating Hormone. *J. Clin. Endocrinol. 2:* 615, 1942.
65. Heller, C. G. and Nelson, W. O., Hyalinization of the Seminiferous Tubules Associated with Normal or Failing Leydig-Cell Function. A Discussion of Relationship to Eunuchoidism, Gynecomastia, Elevated Gonadotropins, Depressed 17-Ketosteroids and Estrogens. *J. Clin. Endocrinol. 5:* 1, 1945.
66. Nielsen, J., Johansen, K., and Yde, H., Frequency of Diabetes Mellitus in Patients with Klinefelter's Syndrome of Different Chromosome Constitutions and the XYY Syndrome. Plasma Insulin and Growth Hormone Level After a Glucose Load. *J. Clin. Endocrinol. 29:* 1062, 1969.
67. Haken, P. C. S., Clarke, M., and Breslin, M., Psychopathology in Klinefelter's Syndrome. *Psychosom. Med. 26:* 207, 1964.
68. Nelson, W. O., Evaluation of Testicular Function, in Reproduction and Sterility. Michigan State University, Centennial Symposium Report, 79, 1955.
69. Bunge, R. G. and Bradbury, J. T., Newer Concepts of the Klinefelter Syndrome. *J. Urol. 76:* 758, 1956.
70. Steinberger, E., Smith, K. D., and Perloff, W. H., Spermatogenesis in Klinefelter's Syndrome. *J. Clin. Endocrinol. Metab. 25:* 1340, 1965.
71. Lipsett, M. B., Davis, T. E., Wilson, H., and Canfield, C. J., Testosterone Production in Chromatin-Positive Klinefelter's Syndrome. *J. Clin. Endocrinol. Metab. 25:* 1027, 1965.
72. Steinberger, E., Smith, K. D., Tcholakian, R. K., Chowdhury, M., Steinberger, A., Ficher, M., and Paulsen, C. A., Steroidogenesis in Human Testis, in Mancini, R. E. and Martini, L. (eds): Male Fertility and Sterility, *Proceedings of Serono Symposia,* Vol. 5. New York, Academic Press, 1974, p. 149.
73. Chaves-Carballo, E. and Hayles, A. B., Ullrich-Turner Syndrome in the Male: Review of the Literature and Report of a Case with Lymphocytic (Hashimoto's) Thyroiditis. *Mayo Clin. Proc. 41:* 843, 1966.
74. Bowen, P., Lee, C. S., Migeon, C. J., Kaplan, N. M., Whalley, P. J., McKusick, V. A., and Reifenstein, E. C., Hereditary Male Pseudohermaphroditism with Hypogonadism, Hypospadias, and Gynecomastia: Reifenstein's Syndrome. *Ann. Intern. Med. 62:* 252, 1965.
75. Nelson, W. O. and Heller, C. G., Diseases of the Reproductive System. The Testis. *Annu. Rev. Med. 2:* 179, 1951.
76. De La Chapelle, A., Analytical Review: Nature and Origin of Males with XX Sex Chromosomes. *Am. J. Hum. Genet. 24:* 71, 1972.
77. Neuhauser, G. and Back, F., Zytogenetische Varianten des Ullrich Turner Syndroms. *Med. Klin. 63:* 836, 1968.
78. Bongiovanni, A. M., The Adrenogenital Syndrome with Deficiency

of 3β-Hydroxysteroid Dehydrogenase. *J. Clin. Invest. 41:* 2086, 1964.
79. Grumbach, M. M. and Van Wyk, J. J., Disorders of Sex Differentiation, in Williams, R. H. (ed): *Textbook of Endocrinology.* Philadelphia, W. B. Saunders Co., 1974, p. 423.
80. Prader, A. and Anders, G. J. P. A., Zur Genetik der Kongenitalen Lipoid-hyperplasie der Nebennieren. *Helvt. Paediatr. Acta 17:* 285, 1962.
81. Kirkland, R. T., Kirkland, J. L., Johnson, C. M., Horning, M. G., Librik. L., and Clayton, G. W., Congenital Lipoid Adrenal Hyperplasia in an Eight-Year-Old Phenotypic Female. *J. Clin. Endocrinol. Metab. 36:* 488, 1973.
82. Zachmann, M., Völlmin, J. A., Hamilton, W., and Prader, A., Steroid 17,20-Desmolase Deficiency: A New Cause of Male Pseudohermaphroditism. *Clin. Endocrinol. 1:* 369, 1972.
83. Saez, J. M., de Peretti, E., Morera, A. M., David, M., and Bertrant, J., Familial Male Pseudohermaphroditism with Gynecomastia Due to a Testicular 17-Ketosteroid Reductase Defect. I. Studies *in vivo. J. Clin. Endocrinol. Metab. 32:* 604, 1971.
84. Goebelsmann, Y., Horton, R., Mestman, J. H., Arce, J. J., Nagata, Y., Nakamura, R. N., Thorneycroft, I. H., and Mishell, D. R., Jr., Male Pseudohermaphroditism Due to Testicular 17βHydroxysteroid Dehydrogenase Deficiency. *J. Clin. Endocrinol. Metab. 36:* 867, 1973.
85. Wilson, J. D., Recent Studies on the Mechanism of Action of Testosterone. *N. Engl. J. Med. 287:* 1284, 1972.
86. Morris, J. M., The Syndrome of Testicular Feminization in Male Pseudohermaphrodites. *Am. J. Obstet. Gynecol. 65:* 1192, 1953.
87. Simmer, H., Pion, R. J., and Dignam, W. J., Testicular Feminization. Springfield, Ill., Charles C. Thomas, 1965.
88. Grumbach, M. M. and Barr, M. L., Cytologic Tests of Chromosomal Sex in Relation to Sexual Anomalies in Man. *Recent Prog. Horm. Res. 14:* 255, 1958.
89. Judd, H. L., Hamilton, C. R., Barlow, J. J., Yen, S. S. C., and Kliman, B., Androgen and Gonadotropin Dynamics in Testicular Feminization Syndrome. *J. Clin. Endocrinol. Metab. 34:* 229, 1972.
90. Steinberger, E., Ficher, M., and Smith, K. D., Relation of *in vitro* Metabolism of Steroids in Human Testicular Tissue to Histologic and Clinical Findings, in Rosemberg, E. and Paulsen, C. A. (eds): The Human Testis. New York, Plenum Publishing Corp., 1970, p. 439.
91. Rosenfield, R. L., Lawrence, A. M., Liao, S., and Landau, R. L., Androgens and Androgen Responsiveness in the Feminizing Testis Syndrome. Comparison of Complete and "Incomplete" Forms. *J. Clin. Endocrinol. Metab. 32:* 625, 1971.
92. de Kretser, D. M., Taft, H. P., Brown, J. B., Evans, J. H., and Hudson, B., Endocrine and Histological Studies on Oligospermic Men Treated with Human Pituitary and Chorionic Gonadotropins. *J. Endocrinol. 40:* 107, 1968.
93. Steinberger, E., Ficher, M., and Smith, K. D., An Enzymatic Defect in Androgen Biosynthesis in Human Testis: A Case Report and Response to Therapy. *Andrologia 6:* 59, 1974.
94. Heckel, N. J., Rosso, W. A., and Kestel, L., Spermatogenic Rebound Phenomenon After Testosterone Therapy. *J. Clin. Endocrinol. 11:* 235, 1951.
95. Physicians' Desk Reference (ed. 31). Oradell, N.J., Litton Publications Inc., 1977.
96. Lunenfeld, B., Goldman, B., and Ismajovich, B., Assessment of Results with Gonadotropic Therapy, in Rosemberg, E. (ed): Gonadotropins. Los Altos, Calif., Geron-X, 1968, p. 513.
97. Taymor, M. L. and Selenkow, H. A., Clinical Experience with L-Triiodothyronine in Male Fertility. *Fertil. Steril. 9:* 560, 1958.
98. Davis, J. T., Bridges, R. B., and Coniglio, J. G., Changes in Lipid Composition of the Mature Testis. *Biochem. J. 98:* 342, 1966.
99. Steward, B. H., The Infertile Male: A Diagnostic Approach. *Fertil. Steril. 19:* 110, 1966.
100. Jungck, E. M., Roy, S., Greenblatt, R. B., and Mahesh. V. B., Effect of Clomiphene Citrate on Spermatogenesis in the Human. *Fertil. Steril. 15:* 40, 1964.
101. Heller, C. G., Rowley, M. J., and Heller, G. V., Clomiphene Citrate: A Correlation of Its Effect on Sperm Concentration and Morphology, Total Gonadotropins, ICSH, Estrogen and Testosterone Excretion, and Testicular Cytology in Normal Men. *J. Clin. Endocrinol. Metab. 29:* 638, 1969.
102. Cooper, I. S., Rynearson, E. H., MacCarty, C. S., and Power, M. H., Metabolic Consequences of Spinal Cord Injury. *J. Clin. Endocrinol. 10:* 858, 1950.
103. Munro, D., Horne, H. W., and Paull, D. P., The Effect of Injury to the Spinal Cord and Cauda Equina on the Sexual Potency of Men. *N. Engl. J. Med. 239:* 903, 1958.
104. Stemmermann, G. N., Weiss, L., Auerbach, O., and Friedman, M., A study of the germinal epithelium in male paraplegics. *Am. J. Clin. Pathol. 20:* 24, 1950.
105. Bors, E., Engle, E. T., Rosenquist, R. C., and Holliger, V. H., Fertility in Paraplegic Males. *J. Clin. Endocrinol. 10:* 381, 1950.
106. Monro, P. A. G., Sympathectomy. London and New York, Oxford University Press, 1959.
107. Hodson, N., Sympathetic Nerves and Reproductive Organs in the Male Rabbit. *J. Reprod. Fertil. 10:* 209, 1965.
108. Drucker, W. D., Blanc, W. A., Rowland, L. P., Grumbach, M. M., and Christy, N. P., The Testis in Myotonic Muscular Dystrophy; A Clinical and Pathologic Study with a Comparison with the Klinefelter Syndrome. *J. Clin. Endocrinol. Metab. 23:* 59, 1963.
109. Rimoin, D. L. and Schimke, R. N., Genetic Disorders of the Endocrine Glands. St. Louis, C. V. Mosby Co., 1971.
110. Harper, P., Penny, R., Foley, T. P., Jr., Migeon, C. J., and Blizzard, R. M., Gonadal Function in Males with Myotonic Dystrophy. *J. Clin. Endocrinol. Metab. 35:* 852, 1972.
111. Rugh, R. and Grupp, E., X-irradiation Lethality Aggravated by Sexual Activity of Male Mice. *Am. J. Physiol. 198:* 1352, 1960.
112. Albers-Schoenberg, H. E., Über eine bisher unbekannte Wirkung der Röntgen strahlen auf den Organismus der Tiere. *Münch. Med. Wschr. 50:* 1859, 1903.
113. Röntgen, W. K., Sitzungsberichte der Würzburger Physikalischen-Medicinischen Gesellschaft, December 28, 1895. *Nature 53:* 274, 1895.
114. Oakberg, E. F., Mammalian Gametogenesis and Species Comparisons in Radiation Response of the Gonads, in: Effects of Radiation on Meiotic Systems. Vienna, International Atomic Energy Agency, 1968, p. 3.
115. Ellis, L. C., Radiation Effects, in Johnson, A. D., Gomes, W. R., and VanDemark, N. L. (eds): The Testis, vol. III. New York, Academic Press, 1970, p. 333.
116. Oakberg, E. F., Initial Depletion and Subsequent Recovery of Spermatogonia of the Mouse After 20 R of Gamma Rays and 100, 300, and 600 of X-ray. *Radiat. Res. 11:* 700, 1959.
117. Steinberger, E. and Nelson, W. O., Effect of Furadroxyl Treatment and X-irradiation on the Hyaluronidase Concentration of Rat Testis. *Endocrinology 60:* 105, 1957.
118. Rowley, M., Leach, D. R., Warner, G. A., and Heller, C. G., Effect of Graded Doses of Ionizing Radiation on the Human Testis. *Radiat. Res. 59:* 665, 1974.
119. Paulsen, C. A., The Study of Irradiation Effects on the Human Testis, Including Histologic, Chromosomal and Hormonal Aspects. Progress Report to Atomic Energy Commission Contract AT (45-1)-1781, 1966.
120. Hughes, G., Radiosensitivity of Male Germ Cells in Neonatal Rats. *Int. J. Radiat. Biol. 4:* 511, 1962.
121. Beaumont, H. M., Changes in the Radiosensitivity of the Testis During Foetal Development. *Int. J. Radiat. Biol. 2:* 247, 1960.
122. Erickson, B. H., Effects of Neonatal Gamma Irradiation on Hormone Production and Spermatogenesis in the Testis of the Adult Pig. *J. Reprod. Fertil. 8:* 91, 1964.
123. Wall, P. G., Effects of X-irradiation of Differentiating Leydig Cells of the Immature Rat. *J. Endocrinol. 23:* 291, 1961.
124. Steinberger, E. and Steinberger, A., Testis: Basic and Clinical Aspects, in Balin, H. and Glasser, S. (eds): Reproductive Biology, Amsterdam, *Excerpta Medica,* 1972, p. 144.
125. Felizet, G. and Branca, A., Histologie du Testicule Ectopique. *J. Anat. Physiol. (Paris) 34:* 589, 1898.
126. Crew, F. A. E., A suggestion as to the Cause of the Aspermatic Condition of the Imperfectly Descended Testis. *J. Anat. (Lond.) 56:* 98, 1922.
127. Fukui, N., On Action of Heat Rays Upon the Testicle: An Histological, Hygienic, and Endocrinological Study. *Acta Sch. Med. Univ. Kioto 6:* 225, 1923.
128. Moore, C. R., Properties of Gonads as Controllers of Somatic and Psychical Characteristics; Testicular Reactions in Experimental Cryptorchidism. *Am. J. Anat. 34:* 269, 1924.
129. VanDemark, N. L. and Free, M. J., Temperature Effects, in [John-

son, A. D., Gomes, W. R., and VanDemark, N. L. (eds)]: The Testis, vol. III. New York, Academic Press, 1970, p. 233.
130. Chowdhury, A. K. and Steinberger, E., A Quantitative Study of the Effect of Heat on Germinal Epithelium of Rat Testis. *Am. J. Anat. 115:* 509, 1964.
131. Cordes, H., Untersuchungen über den Einfluss acuter und chronischer Allgemeinerkrankungen auf die Testikel, speziell auf die Spermatogenese, sowie Beobachtungen über das Auftreten von Fett in den Hoden. *Arch. Pathol. Anat. Physiol. 151:* 402, 1898.
132. Koch, K., Zwischenzellen und Hodenatrophie. *Arch. Pathol. Anat. Physiol. 202:* 376, 1910.
133. MacLeod, J., Effect of Chicken-Pox and of Pneumonia on Semen Quality. *Fertil. Steril. 2:* 523, 1951.
134. Kar, J. K., Azoospermia. An Analysis of 42 Cases. *Int. J. Sexol. 7:* 42, 1955.
135. MacLeod, J. and Hotchkiss, R. S., The Effect of Hyperpyrexia Upon Spermatozoa Counts in Men. *Endocrinology 28:* 780, 1941.
136. Watanabe, A., The Effect of Heat on the Human Spermatogenesis. *Kyushu J. Med. Sci. 10:* 101, 1959.
137. Tokuyama, I., as cited by C. P. Leblond, E. Steinberger, and E. C. Roosen-Runge, in Hartman, G. C., (ed): Mechanisms Concerned with Conception. New York, Pergamon Press, 1963, p. 39.
138. Rock, J. and Robinson, D., Effect of Induced Intrascrotal Hyperthermia on Testicular Function in Man. *Am. J. Obstet. Gynecol. 93:* 793, 1965.
139. Davidson, H. A., Treatment of Male Subfertility. Testicular Temperature and Varicoceles. *Practitioner 173:* 703, 1954.
140. Robinson, D. and Rock, J., Intrascrotal Hyperthermia Induced by Scrotal Insulation: Effect on Spermatogenesis. *Obstet. Gynecol. 29:* 217, 1967.
141. Kapadia, R. N. and Phadka, A. M., Scrotal Suspenders and Subfertility. *J. Family Welfare 2:* 27, 1955.
142. Ehrenberg, L., von Ehrenstein, G., and Hedgren, A., Gonad Temperature and Spontaneous Mutation-Rate in Man. *Nature 180:* 1433, 1957.
143. Landing, B. H., Goldin, A., and Noe, H. A., Testicular Lesions in Mice Following Parenteral Administration of Nitrogen Mustards. *Cancer 2:* 1075, 1949.
144. Hendry, J. A., Homer, R. F., Rose, F. L., and Walpole, A. L., Cytotoxic Agents. III. Derivatives of Ethyleneimine. *Br. J. Pharmacol. 6:* 357, 1951.
145. Bock, M. and Jackson, H., The Action of Triethylenemelamine on the Fertility of Male Rats. *Br. J. Pharmacol. 12:* 1, 1957.
146. Jackson, H. and Bock, M., The Effect of Triethylenemelamine on the Fertility of Rats. *Nature 175:* 1037, 1955.
147. Steinberger, E., Nelson, W. O., Boccabella, A., and Dixon, W. J., A Radiomimetic Effect of Triethylenemelamine on Reproduction in the Male Rat. *Endocrinology 65:* 40, 1959.
148. Steinberger, E., A Quantitative Study of the Effect of an Alkylating Agent (Triethylenemelamine) on the Seminiferous Epithelium of Rats. *J. Reprod. Fertil. 3:* 250, 1962.
149. Fox, B. W. and Fox, M., Biochemical Aspects of the Actions of Drugs on Spermatogenesis. *Pharmacol. Rev. 19:* 21, 1967.
150. Jackson, H. and Schnieden, H., Pharmacology of Reproduction and Fertility. *Annu. Rev. Pharmacol. 8:* 467, 1968.
151. Steinberger, E., Potential Male Antifertility Agents, in McMahon, F. G. (ed): Endocrine Metabolic Drugs, vol. VI. Mount Kisco, N.Y., Futura Publishing Co., 1974, p. 33.
152. Gomes, W. R., Metabolic and Regulatory Hormones Influencing Testis Function, in Johnson, A. D., Gomes, W. R., and VanDemark, N. L. (eds): The Testis, vol. III. New York, Academic Press, 1970, p. 68.
153. Prior, J. T. and Ferguson, J. H., Cytotoxic Effects of a Nitrofuran on the Rat Testis. *Cancer 3:* 1062, 1950.
154. Nelson, W. O. and Steinberger, E., The Effect of Furadroxyl Upon the Testis of the Rat. *Anat. Rec. 112:* 367, 1952.
155. Nelson, W. O. and Steinberger, E., Effects of Nitrofuran Compounds on the Testis of the Rat. *Fed. Proc. 12:* 103, 1953.
156. Nelson, W. O., Steinberger, E., and Boccabella, A., Recovery of Spermatogenesis in Rats Treated with Nitrofurans. *Anat. Rec. 118:* 333, 1954.
157. Paul, H. E., Paul, M. F., Kopko, F., Bender, R. C., and Everett, G., Carbohydrate Metabolism Studies on the Testes of Rats Fed Certain Nitrofurans. *Endocrinology 53:* 585, 1953.
158. Steinberger, E., Boccabella, A., and Nelson, W. O., Cytotoxic Effects of 5-chlor-2-acetyl Thiophen (Ba 11044) on the Testis of the Rat. *Anat. Rec. 125:* 312, 1956.
159. Coulston, F., Beyler, A. L., and Drobeck, H. P., The Biologic Actions of a New Series of Bis(Dichloroacetyl)-Diamines. *Toxicol. Appl. Pharmacol. 2:* 715, 1960.
160. Nelson, W. O. and Patanelli, D. J., Chemical Control of Spermatogenesis, in Austin, C. R. and Perry, J. S. (eds): Agents Affecting Fertility. Boston, Little Brown, 1965, p. 78.
161. King, T. O., Berliner, V. R., and Blye, R. P., Pharmacology of 2,4-dinitropyrroles—A New Class of Anti-spermatogenic Compounds. *Biochem. Pharmacol. 12(Suppl.):* 69, 1963.
162. Patanelli, D. J. and Nelson, W. O., A Quantitative Study of Inhibition and Recovery of Spermatogenesis. *Recent Prog. Horm. Res. 20:* 491, 1964.
163. Nelson, W. O. and Bunge, R. G., Effect of Therapeutic Dosages of Nitrofurantoin (Furadantin) Upon Spermatogenesis in Man. *J. Urol. 77:* 275, 1957.
164. Heller, C. G., Moore, D. J., and Paulsen, C. A., Suppression of Spermatogenesis and Chronic Toxicity in Men by a New Series of Bis(Dichloroacetyl) Diamines. *Toxicol. Appl. Pharmacol. 3:* 1, 1961.
165. Sherins, R. J. and DeVita, V. T., Effect of Drug Treatment for Lymphoma on Male Reproductive Capacity. *Ann. Intern. Med. 79:* 216, 1973.
166. Richter, P., Calamera, J. C., Morgenfeld, M. C., Kierszenbaum, A. L., Lavieri, J. C., and Mancini, R. E., Effect of Chlorambucil on Spermatogenesis in the Human with Malignant Lymphoma. *Cancer 25:* 1026, 1970.
167. Kumar, R., Biggart, J. D., McEvoy, J. and McGeown, M. G., Cyclophosphamide and Reproductive Function. *Lancet 1:* 1212, 1972.
168. Miller, D. G., Alkylating Agents and Human Spermatogenesis, *J.A.M.A. 217:* 1662, 1971.
169. Cheviakoff, S., Calamera, J. C., Morgenfeld, M., and Mancini, R. E., Recovery of Spermatogenesis in Patients with Lymphoma after Treatment with Chlorambucil. *J. Reprod. Fertil. 33:* 155, 1973.
170. Penso, J., Lippe, B., Ehrlich, R., and Smith, F. G., Jr., Testicular Function in Prepubertal and Pubertal Male Patients Treated with Cyclophosphamide for Nephrotic Syndrome. *J. Pediatr. 84:* 831, 1974.
171. Buchanan, J. D., Fairley, K. F., and Barrie, J. U., Return of Spermatogenesis After Stopping Cyclophosphamide Therapy. *Lancet 2:* 156, 1975.
172. Hinkes, E. and Plotkin, D., Reversible Drug-Induced Sterility in a Patient with Acute Leukemia. *J.A.M.A. 223:* 1490, 1973.
173. Etteldorf, J. N., West, C. D., Pitcock, J. A., and Williams, D. L., Gonadal Function, Testicular Histology, and Meiosis Following Cyclophosphamide Therapy in Patients with Nephrotic Syndrome. *J. Pediatr. 88:* 206, 1976.
174. Berlin, C. M. and Jacobson, C. B., Psychedelic Drugs—a Threat to Reproduction? *Fed. Proc. 31:* 1326, 1972.
175. Cicero, T. J., Bell, R. D., Wiest, W. G., Allison, J. H., Polakoski, K., and Robins, E., Function of the Male Sex Organs in Heroin and Methadone Users. *N. Engl. J. Med. 292:* 882, 1975.
176. Jacobson, C. B. and Berlin, C. M., Possible Reproductive Detriment in LSD Users. *J.A.M.A. 222:* 1367, 1972.
177. Oettlé, A. G. and Harrison, R. G., Histologic Changes Produced in the Rat Testis by Temporary and Permanent Occlusion of the Testicular Artery. *J. Pathol. Bacteriol. 64:* 273, 1952.
178. Steinberger, E. and Tjioe, D. Y., Spermatogenesis in Rat Testes After Experimental Ischemia. *Fertil. Steril. 20:* 639, 1969.
179. Tjioe, D. Y. and Steinberger, E., A Quantitative Study of the Effect of Ischemia on the Germinal Epithelium of the Rat Testes. *J. Reprod. Fertil. 21:* 489, 1969.
180. Boccabella, A. V., Salgado, E. D., and Alger, E. A., Testicular Function and Histology Following Serotonin Administration. *Endocrinology 71:* 827, 1962.
181. Kormano, M., Karhunen, P., and Kahanpaa, K., Effect of Long-Term 5-Hydroxy-tryptamine Treatment on the Rat Testis. *Ann. Med. Exp. Biol. Fenn. 46:* 474, 1968.
182. Hellner, H., Die örtlichen Kreislaufstorungen des Hodens. *Beitr. Klin. Chirurgie 158:* 225, 1933.
183. Iwasita, K., Örtliche Blutzirkulationsstorung des Hodens. III. Mitteilung: Klinisch-experimentelle Beitrage zur Kenntnis des Einflusses der Samenstranggefäss-Absperrung auf den Hoden. *Z. Zellforsch. 45:* 126, 1939.
184. Pare, A., Quoted by W. S. Tulloch in Varicocele. *Proc. R. Soc. Med. 55:* 5, 1962.
185. Tulloch, W. S., Consideration of Sterility Factors in Light of Subsequent Pregnancies: Subfertility in Male. *Edinb. Med. J. 59:* 29, 1952.

186. Charny, C. W., Effect of Varicocele on Fertility. *Fertil. Steril. 13:* 47, 1962.
187. Dubin, L. and Amelar, R. D., Varicocelectomy as Therapy in Male Infertility: A Study of 504 Cases. *Fertil. Steril. 26:* 217, 1975.
188. Brown, J. S., Dubin, L., Becker, M., and Hotchkiss, R. S., Venography in the Subfertile Man with Varicocele. *J. Urol. 98:* 388, 1967.
189. Young, D. H., Influence of Varicocele on Spermatogenesis. *Br. J. Urol. 28:* 426, 1956.
190. Amelar, R. D. and Dubin, L., Male Infertility, Current Diagnosis and Treatment. *Urology 1:* 1, 1973.
191. Klosterhalfen, H. and Schirren, C., Uber die operative Wiederherstellung der Zengungsfähigkeit des Mannes. *Dtsch. Med. Wschr. 89:* 2234, 1964.
192. Dubin, L. and Amelar, R. S., Etiologic Factors in 1294 Consecutive Cases of Male Infertility. *Fertil. Steril. 22:* 469, 1971.
193. Clarke, B. G., Incidence of Varicocele in Normal Men and Among Men of Different Ages. *J.A.M.A. 198:* 1121, 1966.
194. Steeno, O., Knops, J., Declerck, L., Adimoelja, A., and van de Voorde, H., Prevention of Fertility Disorders by Detection and Treatment of Varicocele at School and College Age. *Andrologia 8:* 47, 1976.
195. Hammer, R., Studies on Impaired Fertility in Man. London, Oxford Press, 1954.
196. MacLeod, J., Seminal Cytology in the Presence of Varicocele. *Fertil. Steril. 16:* 735, 1965.
197. MacLeod, J., Further Observations on the Role of Varicocele in Human Male Infertility. *Fertil. Steril. 20:* 545, 1969.
198. Fernando, N., Leonard, J. M., and Paulsen, C. A., The Role of Varicocele in Male Fertility. *Andrologia 8:* 1, 1976.
199. Dubin, L. and Amelar, R. D., Varicocelectomy as Therapy in Male Infertility: A Study of 504 Cases. *J. Urol. 113:* 640, 1975.
200. Lindholmer, C., Thulin, L. and Eliasson, R., Semen Characteristics Before and After Ligation of the Left Internal Spermatic Veins in Men with Varicocele. *Scand. J. Urol. Nephrol. 9:* 177, 1975.
201. Smith, K. D., Rodriguez, L., and Steinberger, E., The Infertile Couple, Working with Them Together, in Cockett, A. T. K. and Urry, R. L. (eds): Male Infertility. Workup, Treatment and Research. New York, Grune & Stratton, 1977, p. 211.
202. Harrison, R. G., Functional Importance of the Vascularization of the Testis and Epididymis for the Maintenance of Normal Spermatogenesis. *Fertil. Steril. 3:* 366, 1952.
203. Stephenson, J. D. and O'Shaughnessy, E. J., Hypospermia and Its Relationship to Varicocele and Intrascrotal Temperatures. *Fertil. Steril. 19:* 110, 1968.
204. Alexander, N. J., Fertility and Antibody Levels in Rhesus Monkeys after Vasovasostomy. IX World Congress of Fertility and Sterility, April 12–16, 1977, Miami, Florida, p. 332.
205. Lindholmer, C., Thulin, L., and Eliasson, R., Concentrations of Cortisol and Renin in the Internal Spermatic Vein of Men with Varicocele. *Andrologie 5:* 21, 1973.
206. Cohen, M. S., Plaine, L., and Brown, J. S., The Role of Internal Spermatic Vein Plasma Catecholamine Determinations in Subfertile Men with Varicoceles. *Fertil. Steril. 26:* 1243, 1975.
207. Boyar, R., Finkelstein, J., Roffwarg, H., Kapen, S., Weitzman, E., and Hellman, L., Synchronization of LH Secretion with Sleep During Puberty. *N. Engl. J. Med. 287:* 582, 1972.
208. Johanson, A., Fluctuations of Gonadotropin Levels in Children. *J. Clin. Endocrinol. Metab. 39:* 154, 1974.

125

Male Infertility

Emil Steinberger

The available surveys suggest that 0.3 to 15 percent of all married couples encounter fertility problems. This figure, however, may be a gross underestimate. It is difficult to establish the incidence of infertility becuase the definition of the infertile state is subjective and relative, and it depends on what the physician or the couple feels is the time interval necessary for conception to occur. Some couples will consult a physician after several months of unsuccess; others may wait several years.

The incidence of "male infertility" as the cause of barren marriages has been variously quoted; the frequently mentioned figure is 50 percent.[1] Precise incidence rates are not easily obtainable, particularly since, in many instances, both partners are implicated. In the reports on the "male infertility" incidence, the evaluation of the fertility potential of the female partner is frequently not provided.

When examining the "male factor," the physician is concerned with evaluation of specific parameters of the male reproductive system function (both organic and psychologic) rather than with determination of an "absolute" fertility potential of the male partner, since the only direct and reliable approach to the assessment of an "absolute" fertility potential would be to mate the male partner with an "absolutely fertile" female. The latter is obviously impractical even if it were possible to determine the "absolute fertility" of the female.

As recently as the 1950s, the female was frequently considered the principal cause of the couple's infertility. Many textbooks dealing with infertility have focused on the female, ignoring for the most part the contribution of the male to this problem. As it became apparent that in a substantial number of barren couples an abnormality of the reproductive system could be detected in the male, a search for the "responsible partner" became the primary objective of the evaluation. Since the couple is commonly seen by two physicians practicing different specialties (gynecology and urology), communication problems render management of the couple difficult and produce less than optimal results.

In the past 15 years, physicians have become acutely aware of the shortcomings of the concept of a "partner-directed" approach, and a "couple-directed" approach to the management of infertility problems has been proposed.[2] This concept is supported by various investigators and practitioners dealing with disorders of the reproductive system.[3–5]

When evaluating a couple's fertility potential, the physician must not be unduly concerned with the absolute fertility potential of either partner but rather with the potential ability of the *couple* to produce offspring. In some instances the male partner may indeed be the primary cause of a couple's infertility, although his fertility potential might be adequate for fathering a child with a different, more fertile female partner. In such a case, although a definite defect in the male partner's reproductive system may be present, one may elect to treat the female partner vigorously, particularly if treatment of the male would involve lengthy and difficult procedures. Of course, the converse may also be the case. Consequently, the investigation and treatment of infertility must involve the couple rather than each partner separately. The couple should ideally be seen by a physician, or by a team of physicians, conversant with the various medical and surgical disciplines related to the disorders of the reproductive system in both sexes.

EVALUATION OF THE MALE

The initial evaluation of the male includes the following parameters: (1) the ability to produce a satisfactory ejaculate; (2) the ability to deliver the ejaculate at the appropriate time to the appropriate area of the female reproductive tract; and (3) the capacity of the spermatozoa to penetrate the ovulatory cervical mucus and retain adequate motility in it.

A thorough history may by itself provide the necessary clue to the presence of an etiologic factor responsible for one of the well-defined disorders affecting testicular function (Chapter 124): endocrine disorder (e.g., diabetes mellitus, pituitary disease, or thyroid disease), genetic-developmental disorders (e.g. Klinefelter's syndrome, cryptorchidism), neurologic disorders, sexual dysfunction, anatomical abnormalities (e.g., hypospadias), or gonadal damage secondary to exposure to toxic substances (alcohol, various chemicals, etc.) or to various forms of radiation (ionizing, diathermy, etc.).

The physical examination frequently yields information that may be directly supportive of a diagnostic clue found in the course of obtaining the history. During the physical examination, special attention is paid to the position of the testes in the scrotum and to their size and consistency (soft, unusually firm, irregular). The epididymis is examined for structural irregularities, indurations, cysts, etc. to detect a possible block. The pampiniform plexus is carefully examined with the patient standing and during the Valsalva maneuver in order to rule out the presence of a varicocele. The rectal examination is conducted to uncover prostatic or seminal vesicle disease (prostatitis or seminovesiculitis).

Regardless of findings obtained in the course of the history and physical examination, careful evaluation of the seminal fluid must be performed. A perfectly normal history and physical examination may be associated with severe abnormalities of the ejaculate. Evaluation of the ejaculate (see Chapter 123) is simple, but it requires considerable attention on the part of the physician to make it meaningful. Unless the seminal fluid is obtained by masturbation, the collection may be incomplete. The patient must be appropriately instructed to prevent this most common cause of erroneous results.

It is important for the physician to know what has been the customary frequency of the patient's ejaculatory activity in the immediate past, since it may seriously influence the sperm counts. Severe oligospermia has been reported to result from a high frequency of ejaculation.[6] In view of the documented variability in the quality of the ejaculate, particularly pronounced in patients with oligospermia, it is necessary to examine several ejaculates,[4–6] each produced after a 2- to 3-day abstinence period. These precautions must be taken under consideration before conclusions can be drawn concerning the qualitative and quantitative parameters of a patient's semen production.

Since this is the first time the term "oligospermia" is mentioned, a brief discussion of it is warranted. Although the meaning of the word "oligospermia" is clear, the point at which the diminished density of spermatozoa in an ejaculate (number of sperm per volume of semen) denotes oligospermia is more difficult to define. In the past, seminal fluid with density of spermatozoa of less than 60 million per milliliter was considered to constitute oligospermia.[7] Later a density lower than 40 million per milliliter was considered to be oligospermic,[8] and patients with such counts were regarded as subfertile or infertile. Some authors considered sperm counts of 20 million per milliliter or higher to be euspermic,[9] and such patients were classified as fertile. Recently, we had an opportunity to evaluate ejaculates from a large number of allegedly fertile males in the reproductive age who requested vasectomy for fertility control. More than 41 percent had counts of less than 40 million per milliliter, and 19 percent had less than 20 million per milliliter. This suggests that the point at which the sperm count should be considered oligospermic may have to be lowered even further, possibly to less than 10 million per milliliter.[10]

While it is difficult and at times impractical in the course of evaluating male fertility potential to follow a rigid outline, general guidelines can be suggested. They are summarized in Figures 125-1, 125-2, and 125-3.

Figure 125-1 is self-explanatory, requiring only a few comments. It should be reemphasized that regardless of the findings on history and physicial examination, serial evaluation of several seminal fluid specimens must be conducted, and even when no abnormality of the seminal fluid is detected, further procedures should be carried out, namely the postcoital test and, where indicated, the in vitro sperm penetration test. Analysis of the seminal fluid (see Chapter 123) may provide information suggestive of abnormalities in different segments of the reproductive tract: abnormal volume (high or low) suggests a disturbance in the secretory function of the seminal vesicles, and an absence of fructose suggests either a block of the ejaculatory ducts or a congenital absence of the seminal vesicles. Pus and bacteria are most frequently associated with prostatitis and seminovesiculitis. Teratospermia points toward an intratesticular abnormality, but severe oligospermia may be associated not only with testicular disease but also with partial obstruction of the epididymal duct (Fig. 125-2).

The presence of a classic endocrine (hypogonadotropic hypogonadism) or genetic (Klinefelter's syndrome, etc.) syndrome responsible for inadequate sperm production can be detected in most instances during history and physical examination. (The details of evaluation and management of these syndromes are discussed in Chapter 124.)

The initial endocrine studies involve the determination of plasma LH, FSH, and testosterone levels. When levels are found to be normal, scrotal exploration and testicular biopsy are performed in order to rule out: (1) epididymal and/or vas blocks;[11] (2) partial enzyme defect in androgen biogenetic pathways;[12] and (3) adult seminiferous tubule failure or other specific morphologically diagnosable abnormalities (e.g., Sertoli cell syndrome).

When plasma testosterone levels are low, an HCG stimulation test is performed to determine whether the testes are responsive to gonadotropin therapy. In case of poor or no response, replacement therapy with androgens is instituted to maintain proper androgenicity, but the fertility potential cannot be restored.

Selective elevation in plasma FSH levels indicates severe damage to the seminiferous epithelium,[13] for which no therapy is available at this time, and no further workup is indicated.

The procedures carried out as part of the scrotal exploration are summarized in Figure 125-3. Because of the increased awareness that abnormalities in the testes' excretory system, including complete or partial block of the epididymal duct, may lead to azoospermia or severe oligospermia, exploration of the scrotum, which permits adequate visualization of the testis, the epididymis, and the vas, becomes a procedure of choice to replace a simple

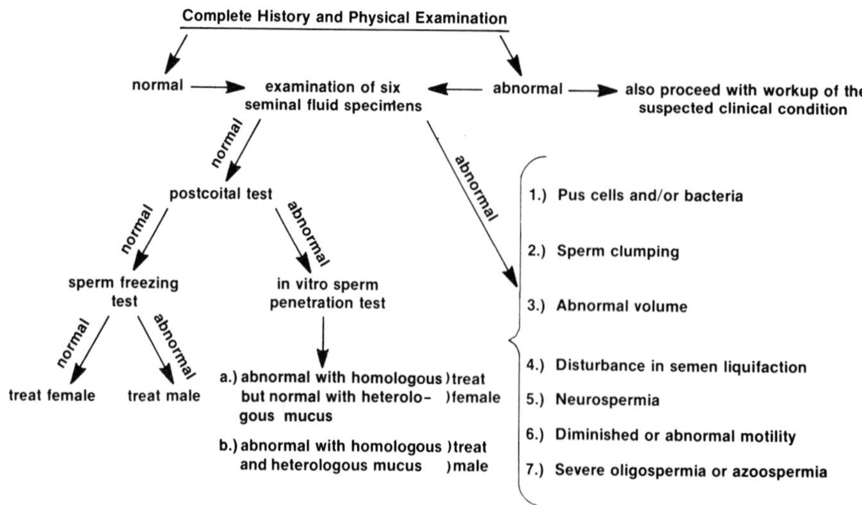

Fig. 125-1. Initial evaluation of the male reproductive system.

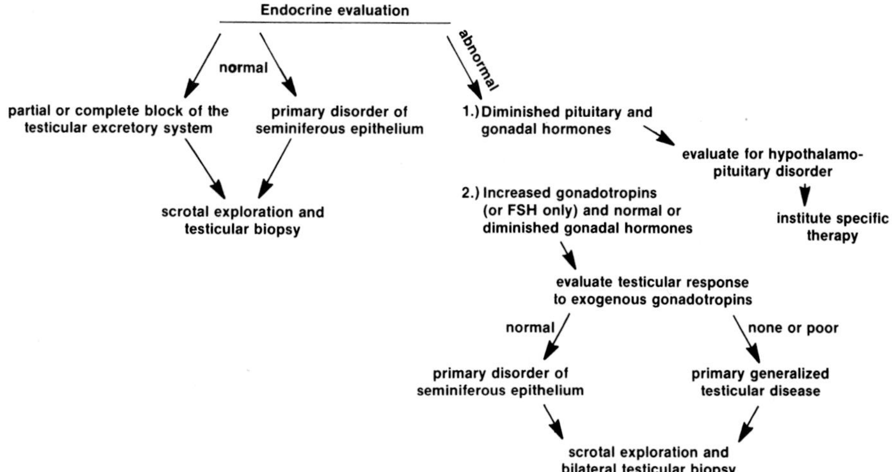

Fig. 125-2. Evaluation of patients with severe oligospermia or severe azoospermia (with normal Hx and Px).

biopsy performed through a small scrotal incision. Ligation of varicocele can be performed at the same time as the scrotal exploration. Some surgeons, however, prefer to repair an epididymal or vas block at a later time. Nevertheless, a diagnosis of a block, whether the block is repaired or not, is of utmost importance in order to spare the patient lengthy and expensive periods of medical therapy.

The evaluation of testicular biopsy includes morphologic, biochemical, and cytogenetic studies. It is imperative that appropriate techniques (see Chapter 123) for procurement of the biopsy be utilized and the tissue be adequately processed for morphologic studies;[14] otherwise, testicular biopsy may become a useless exercise. The microscopic examination of the tissue should be conducted by an experienced individual. When indicated, one of the quantitative techniques for evaluation of spermatogenesis[15,16] should be utilized. The recently developed techniques for evaluation of steroid biosynthetic pathways and steroid levels (see Chapter 123) in biopsies of testes, while requiring relatively sophisticated laboratory facilities, may be helpful not only in diagnosis of specific enzymic abnormalities in the androgen biogenetic pathways[17] but also in choice of successful therapy.[12]

Not all diagnostic procedures need to be carried out in each case. The selection of appropriate procedures will depend on the results of the diagnostic workup leading to the scrotal exploration and biopsy and on findings during surgery.

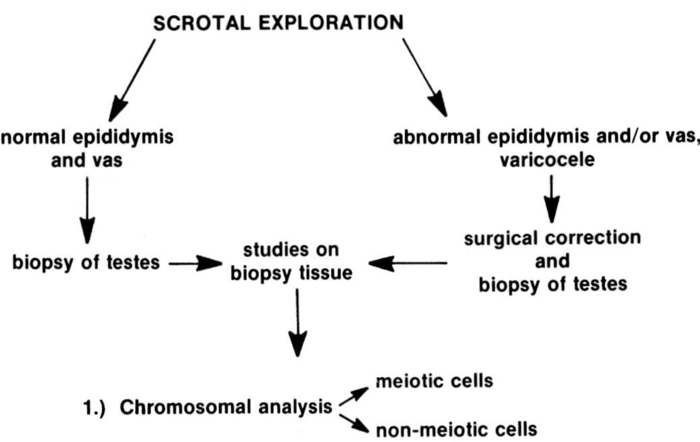

Fig. 125-3. Scrotal exploration.

THERAPY

The single most common abnormality associated with the contribution of the male to the couple's infertility is severe oligospermia or azoospermia. This may result from (1) an endocrine disorder of the hypothalamic-pituitary axis; (2) a block in the excretory ducts; (3) adult seminiferous tubule failure; (4) genetic abnormality; (5) postinfection damage; (6) specific but unexplained lesions, etc. (e.g., Sertoli cell only syndrome); or (7) intratesticular steroid pathway abnormalities.

Sperm production deficiency secondary to an endocrine disorder of the hypothalamic-pituitary axis is usually amenable to specific hormonal therapy discussed in Chapter 124. Blocked excretory ducts can be treated surgically. The scarred tissue causing the block is resected and appropriate anatomosis carried out. Although the general rate of success utilizing this approach is relatively low (10 to 30 percent), even in the hands of an experienced reproductive system surgeon, this is a worthwhile therapeutic procedure in properly selected patients.[11]

The most common cause of azoospermia or oligospermia is the adult seminiferous tubule failure. In most instances, it is of unknown etiology, and no adequate form of therapy is available.

In the past several years, a number of reports in the literature suggest a causal relationship between some cases of oligospermia, teratospermia, disturbances in sperm motility, diminished "fertility," and the presence of a varicocele. Similarly, numerous reports suggest improvement in the above-listed parameters subsequent to high ligation of the varicocele.[18] Although the efficacy of this form of therapy has not been demonstrated beyond doubt, varicocele ligation, when properly performed, is considered an appropriate form of therapy, since other forms of therapy provide even less satisfactory results. Since only a fraction of patients respond to varicocelectomy, it would be advantageous to be able to select the "responders" prior to surgery. So far, this has not been successful.[19]

A large body of literature concerning medical therapy of male infertility has accumulated (for a recent review, see ref. 20). A number of hormonal and nonhormonal agents have been hailed as effective forms of therapy. Among nonhormonal agents, phenelzine sulfate, vitamin E, vitamin C, arginine, and others have been advocated at one time or another. There is, however, no adequately documented evidence supporting the effectiveness of these agents.

One of the most common hormonal forms of therapy for the

past 30 years has been the thyroid hormone, particularly triiodothyronine (Cytomel). Unfortunately, the best evidence fails to support the effectiveness of thyroid hormone in therapy of testicular dysfunction or "male infertility" in euthyroid patients.

Adrenal corticoids have had a stormy history as therapeutic agents in the management of "male infertility," with strong proponents[21] and opponents.[22] Careful evaluation of the available data leads this author to the conclusion that empirical therapy of oligospermia with cortical steroids is not warranted.

Even greater controversy exists concerning the efficacy of Clomid* as an empirical form of therapy for oligospermia. Clomid induces an increase in gonadotropin production by the pituitary gland.[23] Although a number of authors reported significant improvement in a large proportion of treated patients with oligospermia,[24,25] others failed to observe any improvement.[26,27] Furthermore, suppression of spermatogenesis in normal men was reported after administration of high doses of Clomid.[28] The possibility exists that some patients with oligospermia may respond to a specific dose of Clomid. There is no adequate diagnostic procedure available at this time to select the "responders"; neither is sufficient information available concerning the effective dose. Consequently, Clomid should still be considered an experimental drug with a potential for becoming a part of the therapeutic armamentarium.

The effectiveness of gonadotropins in the therapy of adult seminiferous tubule failure has been difficult to evaluate. The disorder is a poorly delineated pathological state in a group of patients probably suffering with disorders of various etiology, all producing a common end result—oligospermia. The therapeutic agent (gonadotropins) is similarly poorly defined (different preparations varying in degree of purity and in FSH/LH ratios), not available in adequate amounts, and exceedingly expensive. In most reports dealing with gonadotropin therapy of oligospermia the patient treatment groups were made up randomly rather than selectively, making the analysis of the results difficult.[20] Nevertheless, the available data appear to be promising and suggest that a specific segment of this random population may indeed be amenable to gonadotropin therapy.[12]

Two forms of testosterone therapy have been attempted. In one, testosterone has been administered to "stimulate" spermatogenesis.[29] No adequate evidence is available in support of the idea that a testosterone injection in the suggested dosage range is beneficial therapy for any form of deficiency in sperm production. The other form of testosterone therapy involves administration of large doses of testosterone to suppress spermatogenesis,[30] since it has been reported that in some patients with oligospermia, improvement in sperm production occurs after cessation of testosterone treatment when recovery of the sperm production by the testes takes place.[31] This has been termed "testosterone rebound" therapy. It has been employed with varying degrees of success in the past 25 years.[32]

Recently, an orally active synthetic androgen, exhibiting little if any hepatotoxicity,[33] was reported to be effective in therapy of oligospermia.[34] The reports are not clearly documented, and its use effectiveness will have to await adequate confirmational studies.

In summary, the therapy of male infertility, particularly inadequate sperm production, is at best a difficult, tedious, and frequently unrewarding experience. When various forms of therapy (exclusive of surgery) are critically appraised, it appears that the empirical "shotgun" therapy with Cytomel, vitamin E, arginine, etc. has no place in a physician's therapeutic armamentarium at this time. Gonadotropin therapy, whether direct or indirect via Clomid, as well as androgen therapy, holds definite promise for a selected group of infertile males. The major question in the utilization of these forms of therapy lies in the ability to make a precise and specific diagnosis in order to uncover a "responsive" case. This hinges on the availability of sophisticated laboratory facilities and a properly trained physician for interpretation of the results. Unquestionably, further advances in our basic knowledge of the male reproductive system and development of simpler and more precise diagnostic techniques will result in marked improvement of therapeutic success.

*Clomiphene citrate, Merrell-National Laboratories, Cincinnati, Ohio.

REFERENCES

1. Murphy, D. P. and Torrano, E. F., Male Fertility in 3620 Childless Couples. *Fertil. Steril. 16:* 337, 1965.
2. Steinberger, E. and Steinberger, A., Testis: Basic and Clinical Aspects, in Balin, H. and Glasser, S. (eds): Reproductive Biology. Amsterdam, *Excerpta Medica,* 1972, p. 144.
3. Smith, K. D., Rodriguez, L., and Steinberger, E., The Infertile Couple, Working With Them as a Couple, in Cockett, A. T. K. and Urry, R. L. (eds): Male Infertility. Workup, Treatment and Research. New York, Grune & Stratton, 1977, p. 211.
4. Newton, J., Craig, S., and Joyce, D., The Changing Pattern of a Comprehensive Infertility Clinic. *J. Biosoc. Sci. 6:* 477, 1974.
5. Sherins, R. J., Clinical Aspects of Treatment of Male Infertility With Gonadotropins: Testicular Response of Some Men Given HCG With and Without Pergonal, in Mancini, R. E. and Martini, L. (eds): Male Fertility and Sterility, Proceedings of Serono Symposia, vol. 5. New York, Academic Press, 1974, p. 545.
6. Freund, M., Effect of Frequency of Emission on Semen Output and an Estimate of Daily Sperm Production in Man. *J. Reprod. Fertil. 6:* 269, 1963.
7. Meaker, S. R., Human Sterility. Baltimore, Williams and Wilkins, 1934.
8. American Fertility Society. How to Organize a Basic Study of the Infertile Couple. Monograph published by the American Fertility Society, Birmingham, Ala., 1971.
9. MacLeod, J. and Gold, R. Z., The Male Factor in Fertility and Infertility. II. Spermatozoon Counts in 1000 Men of Known Fertility and in 1000 Cases of Infertile Marriage. *J. Urol. 66:* 436, 1951.
10. Smith, K. D. and Steinberger, E., What is Oligospermia? In Troen, P. and Nankin, H. R. (eds): The Testis in Normal and Infertile Men. New York, Raven Press, 1977, p. 489.
11. Schoysman, R., Proceedings of the IX World Congress on Fertility and Sterility. Miami, Florida, April 1977.
12. Steinberger, E., Ficher, M., and Smith, K. D., An Enzymatic Defect in Androgen Biosynthesis in Human Testis: A Case Report and Response to Therapy. *Andrologia 6:* 59, 1974a.
13. Smith, K. D., Tcholakian, R. K., Chowdhury, M., and Steinberger, E., An Investigation of Plasma Hormone Levels Before and After Vasectomy. *Fertil. Steril. 27:* 145, 1976.
14. Rowley, M. J. and Heller, C. B., The Testicular Biopsy: Surgical Procedure, Fixation and Staining Technics. *Fertil. Steril. 17:* 177, 1966.
15. Steinberger, E. and Tjioe, D. Y., A Method for Quantitative Analysis of Human Seminiferous Epithelium. *Fertil. Steril. 19:* 960, 1968.
16. Rowley, M. J. and Heller, C. G., Quantitation of the Cells of the Seminiferous Epithelium of the Human Testis Employing the Sertoli Cell as a Constant. *Z. Zellforsch. Mikrosk. Anat. 115:* 461, 1971.
17. Steinberger, E., Smith, K. D., Tcholakian, R. K., Chowdhury, M., Steinberger, A., Ficher, M., and Paulsen, C. A., Steroidogenesis in Human Testes, in Mancini, R. E. and Martini, L. (eds): Male Fertility and Sterility, *Proceedings of Serono Symposia,* vol. 5. New York, Academic Press, 1974, p. 149.
18. Dubin, L. and Amelar, R. D., Varicocelectomy As Therapy in Male Infertility: A Study of 504 Cases. *Fertil. Steril. 26:* 217, 1975.
19. Fernando, N., Leonard, J. M., and Paulsen, C. A., The Role of Varicocele in Male Fertility. *Andrologia 8:* 1, 1976.
20. Steinberger, E., Medical Treatment of Male Infertility. *Andrologia 8(Suppl. 1):* 77, 1976.
21. Stewart, B. H. and Montie, J. E., Male Infertility: An Optimistic Report. *J. Urol. 110:* 216, 1973.

22. Mancini, R. E., Lavieri, J. C., Muller, F., Andrada, J. A., and Saraceni, D. J., Effect of Prednisolone Upon Normal and Pathologic Human Spermatogenesis. *Fertil. Steril. 17:* 500, 1966.
23. Bardin, C. W., Ross, G. T., and Lipsett, M. B., Site of Action of Clomiphene Citrate in Men: A Study of the Pituitary-Leydig Cell Axis. *J. Clin. Endocrinol. Metab. 27:* 1559, 1969.
24. Paulson, D. F., Wacksman, J., Hammond, C. B., and Wiebe, H. R., Hypofertility and Clomiphene Citrate Therapy. *Fertil. Steril. 26:* 982, 1975.
25. Reyes, F. I. and Faiman, C., Long-term Therapy With Low-dose Cisclomiphene in Male Infertility: Effects of Semen, Serum FSH, LH, Testosterone and Estradiol, and Carbohydrate Tolerance. *Int. J. Fertil. 19:* 49, 1974.
26. Dedes, M. and Da Rugna, D., Erfahrungen mit Clomiphenzitrat bei Fertilitätstörungen des Mannes. *Praxis (Schweiz. Rundschau Med.) 63:* 704, 1974.
27. Foss, G. L., Tindall, V. R., and Birkett, J. P., The Treatment of Subfertile Men With Clomiphene Citrate. *J. Reprod. Fertil. 32:* 167, 1973.
28. Heller, C. G., Rowley, M. J., and Heller, G. V., Clomiphene Citrate: A Correlation of Its Effect on Sperm Concentration and Morphology, Total Gonadotropins, ICSH, Estrogen and Testosterone Excretion, and Testicular Cytology in Normal Men. *J. Clin. Endocrinol. Metab. 29:* 638, 1969.
29. Physicians' Desk Reference. Oradell, N.J., Litton Industries, 1977, pp. 1417 and 1512.
30. Heller, C. G., Nelson, W. O., Hill, I. B., Henderson, E., Maddock, W. O., Jungck, E. C., Paulsen, C. A., and Mortimore, G. E., Improvement in Spermatogenesis Following Depression of the Human Testis with Testosterone. *Fertil. Steril. 1:* 415, 1950.
31. Heckel, N. J., Rosso, W. A., and Kestel, L., Spermatogenic Rebound Phenomenon After Testosterone Therapy. *J. Clin. Endocrinol. 11:* 235, 1951.
32. Rowley, M. J. and Heller, C. G., The Testosterone Rebound Phenomenon in the Treatment of Male Infertility. *Fertil. Steril. 23:* 498, 1972.
33. Giarola, A., Effect of Mesterolone on the Spermatogenesis of Infertile Patients, in Mancini, R. E. and Martini, L. (eds): Male Fertility and Sterility, *Proceedings of Serono Symposia,* vol. 5. New York, Academic Press, 1974, p. 479.
34. Mauss, J., Ergebnisse der Behandlung von Fertilitätstörungen des Mannes mit Mesterolon oder einem Plazebo. *Arzneim.-Forsch. 24:* 1338, 1974.

126

Functional Tumors of the Testis

Mortimer B. Lipsett

EPIDEMIOLOGY

Testicular tumors are relatively rare, accounting for about 2 percent of cancers in men.[1,2] However, they are the most common cancers of middle life in men. Epidemiologic differences have been noted. For example, the incidence of testicular cancer in the black population in this country and throughout the world is one-fifth that of the white population, and there has been an increasing incidence of testicular cancer reported from Denmark.[3] The reasons for these differences are unknown. A recent study[4] confirms the difference in incidence between white and nonwhite populations and also suggests that occupational differences may alter the frequency of testicular cancer.

Tumors of the testis originate from any tissue in the testis and are, therefore, quite diverse in structure and function. Germ cell neoplasms account for 97 percent of testicular tumors and are generally malignant, whereas tumors of the specialized gonadal stroma tend to be benign. Both cell types give rise to functional tumors. Bilateral testicular tumors are rare and are generally seminomas.[5] An abbreviated classification of testicular tumors adapted from Mostofi[6] is given in Table 126-1.

CLINICAL MANIFESTATIONS

The common presenting complaint is a testicular mass that is usually painless. When metastatic disease is present, the signs and symptoms depend on the location of the metastatic deposits. Functional tumors, however, may signal their presence by hormonal effects. Thus virilization in the child and gynecomastia and sterility in the adult may be the initial signs of the tumor. It should be noted that primary mediastinal germ cell tumors[7] may be similarly functional and resemble in every respect testicular germ cell tumors.

GERM CELL TUMORS

CLINICAL ASPECTS

There are clear differences in survival among the different histologic types of germ cell tumors. In the largest single series,[8] the 17-year survival of 834 men was 53 percent; of the men with seminoma, survival was 75 percent. None of the men with choriocarcinoma, either singly or in combination with other cancer types, was alive after 17 years. Survival rates for men with embryonal carcinoma or teratoma were 28 and 63 percent, respectively. In other studies[9,10] the high survival rates for men with seminoma were again confirmed with 3 and 5 years survivals of 81 and 95 percent. Removal and/or radiation of regional and para-aortic lymph nodes is necessary to achieve these high remission rates in seminoma. Seminoma of the testis is radiosensitive, and even radiotherapy of recurrent disease has proved efficacious in producing long remissions.

Germ cell tumors of the testis are yielding to chemotherapy. Mithramycin has been shown to be a uniquely effective single agent for therapy of germ cell tumors.[11] In 1960, however, the first report of the efficacy of combined drug therapy (actinomycin D, chlorambucil, methotrexate) appeared.[12] Subsequently there have been many reports of increasingly frequent long-term survivals of men with metastatic disease who have received combination chemotherapy.[13] A variety of protocols and combinations of chemotherapeutic agents have been used. The most important new therapeutic agent that has been introduced is cis-diaminedichloroplatinum(II) (DDP). This agent singly and in combination with other agents has given response rates from 40 to 90 percent.[14] An increasing number of these patients are apparently achieving complete and long-lasting remission.

HORMONES FROM TUMORS

HUMAN CHORIONIC GONADOTROPIN (HCG)

At this point, the word "functional" needs clarification. For purposes of this chapter, functional tumors are defined as those that secrete hormones or substances closely allied with them. For example, a tumor that secretes a fragment of HCG will be classified as functional.

Since the report of Zondek[15] in 1937, positive pregnancy tests have been associated with trophoblastic neoplasms. It has become clear, however, that this association is neither invariable nor exclusive.[16–21] There are several reasons for these discrepancies. The apparent low frequency of positive pregnancy tests in trophoblastic disease is undoubtedly due to the relative insensitivity of the

Table 126-1. Pathologic Classification of Testicular Tumors

Germ cell tumors
Seminoma
Choriocarcinoma
Embryonal cell carcinoma
Combination of the above
Teratoma
Tumors of specialized gonadal stroma
Leydig cell
Sertoli cell
Granulosa-theca cell
Mixed germ cell and stroma components
Gonadoblastoma
Tumors of adnexae and metastatic tumors

test. A positive pregnancy test, either biologic or immunologic, requires 500 IU of HCG per liter of urine, and normal subjects rarely excrete as much as 50 IU/liter. Thus there is a considerable range where the gonadotropin excretion may be abnormal but undetectable by usual pregnancy tests. With the development of a radioimmunoassay specific for plasma HCG,[22] the hormone has been found more frequently[23] than would have been predicted by studies using pregnancy tests. Since any HCG in plasma is abnormal and the lower limit of the assay is 1 ng/ml, this test facilitates detection of functional cancers. By contrast, a plasma HCG concentration of 100 ng/ml is necessary before the urine pregnancy test becomes positive.

The finding of positive pregnancy tests with HCG in the plasma of patients with embryonal carcinoma and seminomas may be due to either misclassification or the ectopic hormone syndrome. Testicular tumors are often mixed (i.e., contain two or more cell types), and the trophoblastic component may be but a small fraction of the total cell mass.[16] Random biopsy, therefore, may not discover the trophoblastic component. Or alternatively, the occurrence of HCG in nontrophoblastic tumors of the testis may be no different than its occurrence in nontesticular tumors;[23] i.e., it may be still another example of the production of polypeptide hormones by tumors derived from nonendocrine tissues.

The recent demonstration by Braunstein et al.[24] that HCG can be identified even in extracts of normal testis, albeit in low amounts, raises important questions about the significance of finding HCG in any testicular tumor. To muddy the waters still further, it has now been shown[25] that there is a gonadotropin in the pituitary gland and urine of normal subjects that cross-reacts with an antiserum highly specific for HCG. Thus the identification of HCG by immunologic criteria in cancer tissue, or for that matter in any tissue, is now moot and must await clarification.

As with other protein hormones, "unfinished" peptides can be secreted, and free subunits of HCG as well as altered forms or the molecule have been described in a male patient with embryonal cell carcinoma.[26] It is quite probable that some patients will be found who will secrete only subunits of HCG. This secretory activity will not be recognized by the usual pregnancy test, yet measurement of these subunits could serve as a marker for diagnosis and therapy.

HUMAN PLACENTAL LACTOGEN (HPL; CHORIONIC SOMATOMAMMOTROPIN)

Human placental lactogen is the prominent product of the placenta during the last half of pregnancy (Chapter 130). It has been found in men with trophoblastic cancers[27] and, interestingly, in some men with anaplastic carcinoma of the lung secreting large amounts of HCG.[27] Although HPL does not resemble HCG structurally, its secretion appears to follow that of HCG when the HCG secretion rate is high.

OTHER PROTEINS

Carcinoembryonic antigen and alpha-fetoprotein have been noted sporadically in association with teratomas. In systematic studies, Edsmyr et al.[28] and Perlin et al.[29] measured these two fetal protein markers and HCG in 11 men with advanced teratocarcinomas. Alpha-fetoprotein and HCG occurred together or independently, and increased levels of carcinoembryonic antigen were not necessarily associated with high levels of the other two. Braunstein et al.[20] similarly noted a discordance in the occurrence of HCG and alpha-fetoprotein. Whether this reflects survival of differing clones of cells or intrinsic variations of protein synthesis by a single cell type remains to be clarified.

ESTROGENS

In normal adult men, about one-third of plasma estradiol is secreted by the testis,[31] and the remainder is derived from plasma testosterone in peripheral tissues.[32] Estrogen excretion was increased in normal men by injection of HCG[33] and testicular secretion similarly increased. Thus the facile explanation for the high estrogen excretion of men with HCG-secreting neoplasms was stimulation of the Leydig cell. But Kirschner et al.[34] found that the Leydig cell was unresponsive to HCG in men with trophoblastic tumors, so other explanations were sought.

The synthesis of estrogen by the trophoblast from dehydroepiandrosterone sulfate, a normal plasma steroid, has been described in normal pregnancy (Chapter 133) and in women with trophoblastic tumors.[35] Similarly, men with metastatic trophoblastic disease were able to metabolize plasma dehydroepiandrosterone sulfate to estrogens.[36] Thus the tumor itself is responsible for the synthesis of estrogens from nonestrogenic precursors. It is almost certainly these estrogens, synthesized by the tumor, that are responsible for the gynecomastia associated with HCG-secreting tumors.

TUMORS OF THE SPECIALIZED GONADAL STROMA

INTERSTITIAL CELL TUMORS

The histogenesis and classification of tumors of the gonadal stroma have been discussed by Mostofi et al.[37] and Teilum.[38] The most common are the interstitial cell tumors. These tumors are generally benign and histologically resemble the normal interstitial cell. In the prepubertal child they cause virilization; in adults, gynecomastia is the frequent presenting complaint as a result of excessive estrogen production.

The children present the picture of macrogenitosomia praecox, the so-called infant Hercules. They are tall, well-muscled, and have early appearance of beard and mustache hair. Phallic growth is stimulated, but the testes remain small, since tubule growth is not increased because of suppression of FSH. The tumor is often palpable; occasionally it can only be discovered at surgical exploration.

The differential diagnosis should present no problems. The small testicular size in conjunction with virilization indicates androgen production from other than pituitary stimulation. Measurement of HCG will serve to rule out HCG-secreting germ cell tumors. Congenital adrenal hyperplasia is characterized by high urinary 17-ketosteroids and pregnanetriol with suppression by glucocorticoids. Patients with adrenal cancer almost always have a greatly increased excretion of 17-ketosteroids and a mass depressing the kidney. The 17-ketosteroid excretion of the boy with a benign interstitial cell tumor is above that of his normal counterpart but below that of adult men and is not suppressible by exogenous glucocorticoids.

The causes for the feminization that is the hallmark of the interstitial cell tumor in the adult are complex. In one carefully studied patient,[39] the tumor apparently secreted estradiol and was responsive to stimulation by HCG and suppression by fluoxymesterone. Since "hypervirilization" cannot be recognized in adult men, increased levels of testosterone resulting from an interstitial cell tumor would remain unsuspected in the adult.

Detailed biochemical investigation of these tumors[40–42] has shown that they possess the characteristic enzyme patterns of the normal Leydig cell but that 11β-hydroxylase activity characteristic of the adrenal cortex has also been noted.[41,42] This does not imply that adrenal cortical rest cells were present; rather, it seems more likely that tumorigenesis was accompanied by the appearance of the enzyme.

It is of interest that interstitial cell tumors in prepubertal boys are surrounded by tubules with advanced spermatogenesis.[43,44] This is one further piece of evidence for the hypothesis that high local concentrations of testosterone are necessary for spermatogenesis.

The malignant interstitial cell tumor is even rarer, only 15 having been described. Gynecomastia has often been a feature. An intensive study of one case[45] revealed that the tumor secreted androgens as well as some 11β-hydroxy-C_{19}-steroids. A detailed review of the endocrine behavior of these tumors has been presented.[46] There are no case reports of malignant interstitial cell tumors in childhood.

SERTOLI CELL TUMORS

These tumors are rare,[38] and the only evidence that they produce estrogen is the occasional observation of gynecomastia. In the dog, Sertoli cell tumors are more common; bioassayable estrogen was reported in one tumor[47] and accelerated estrogen synthesis in another.[48] The demonstration of estrogen secretion by a Sertoli cell tumor in man has not been made.

BILATERAL TUMORS OF CONGENITAL ADRENAL HYPERPLASIA

Enlargement of the testes in a man with untreated congenital adrenal hyperplasia has been reported, and 15 earlier cases were reviewed.[49] It is clear that the bilateral tumorous enlargement consisted of masses of cells morphologically resembling interstitial cells. Nevertheless, the tissue behaved as adrenal cortical tissue and was under ACTH control. It is important to recognize the syndrome to prevent bilateral orchiectomy.

REFERENCES

1. MacKay, E. N. and Sellers, A. H. A statistical review of malignant testicular tumours based on the experience of the Ontario Cancer Foundation Clinics, 1938–1961. *Can. Med. Assoc. J. 94:* 889, 1966.
2. Johnson, D. E. Testicular Tumors. Med. Exam. Pub. Co., Flushing, N.Y., 1972.
3. Clemmesen, J. A doubling in mortality from testis carcinoma in Copenhagen, 1943–1962. *Acta Pathol. Microbiol. Scand. 72:* 348, 1968.
4. Mustacchi, P. and Millmore, D. Racial and occupational variations in cancer of the testis: San Francisco, 1956–1965. *J. Natl. Cancer Inst. 56:* 717, 1976.
5. Morris, S. A., Vaughan, E. D. Jr., and Constable, W. C. Problems in management of primary bilateral germ cell testicular tumors: Report of 3 cases and review of the literature. *J. Urol. 115:* 566, 1976.
6. Mostofi, K. Testicular tumors. *Cancer 32:* 1186, 1973.
7. Martini, N., Golbey, R. B., Hajdu, S. I., et al. Primary mediastinal germ cell tumors. *Cancer 33:* 763, 1974.
8. Nefzger, M. D. and Mostofi, F. K. Survival after surgery for germinal malignancies of the testis I. Rates of survival in tumor groups. *Cancer 30:* 1225, 1972.
9. Lindsey, C. M. and Glenn, J. F. Germinal malignancies of the testis: Experience, management and prognosis. *J. Urol. 116:* 59, 1976.
10. Quivey, J. M., Fu, K. K., Herzog, K. A., et al. Malignant tumors of the testis: Analysis of treatment results and sites and causes of failure. *Cancer 39:* 1247, 1977.
11. Kennedy, B. J. Mithramycin therapy in advanced testicular neoplasms. *Cancer 26:* 755, 1970.
12. Li, M. C., Whitmore, W. F. Jr., Golbey, R., et al. Effects of combined drug therapy on metastatic cancer of the testis. *J.A.M.A. 174:* 1291, 1960.
13. Klepp, L., Klepp, R., Host, H., et al. Combination chemotherapy of germ cell tumors of the testis with vincristine adriamycin, cyclophosphamide, actinomycin D and medroxyprogesterone acetate. *Cancer 40:* 638, 1977.
14. Rozencweig, M., VonHoff, D. D., Slavik, M. et al. Cis-diaminedichloroplatinum(II): A new anticancer drug. *Ann. Intern. Med. 86:* 803, 1977.
15. Zondek, B. Gonadotropin hormone in the diagnosis of chorioepithelioma. *J.A.M.A. 108:* 607, 1937.
16. Dixon, F. J. and Moore, R. A. Tumors of the male sex organs, in Dixon, F. J. and Moore, R. A. (eds.): Atlas of Tumor Pathology, Section VIII, fasc. 32. Washington, D.C. Armed Forces Institute of Pathology, 1952.
17. Hurley, J. V. Testicular tumours, with especial reference to their association with urinary gonadotrophins. *Aust. N.Z. J. Surg. 31:* 180, 1962.
18. Hobson, B. M. The excretion of chorionic gonadotrophin by men with testicular tumours. *Acta Endocrinol. (Kbh) 49:* 337, 1965.
19. Horn, Y. and Hochman, A. End results in treatment of malignant testicular tumors. *Oncology 21:* 72, 1967.
20. Lindenmeyer, D., Horung, D., and Korner, F. Hormonal changes in urine and plasma in patients with various testicular tumours before and after treatment. *Urol. Int. 28:* 127, 1973.
21. Lindenmeyer, D., Horung, D., and Korner, F. Hormonal changes in urine and plasma in patients with various testicular tumours before and after treatment. *Urol. Int 28:* 135, 1973.
22. Vaitukaitis, J. L., Braunstein, G. D., and Ross, G. T. A radioimmunoassay which specifically measures human chorionic gonadotropin in the presence of human luteinizing hormone. *Am. J. Obstet. Gynecol. 113:* 751, 1972.
23. Braunstein, G. D., Vaitukaitis, J. L., Carbone, P. P., et al. Ectopic production of human chorionic gonadotrophin by neoplasms. *Ann. Intern. Med. 78:* 39, 1973.
24. Braunstein, G. D., Rasor, J., and Wade, M. E. Presence of chorionic-gonadotropin-like substance in normal testes. *N. Engl. J. Med. 293:* 1339, 1975.
25. Chen, H. C., Hodgen, G. D., Matsuura, S., et al. Evidence for a gonadotropin from nonpregnant subjects that has physical, immunological, and biological similarities to human chorionic gonadotropin. *Proc. Natl. Acad. Sci., USA 73:* 2885, 1976.
26. Vaitukaitis, J. L. Immunologic and physical characterization of human chorionic gonadotropin (hCG) secreted by tumors. *J. Clin. Endocrinol. 37:* 505, 1973.
27. Weintraub, B. D. and Rosen, S. W. Ectopic production of human chorionic somatomammotropin by nontrophoblastic cancers. *J. Clin. Endocrinol. 32:* 94, 1971.
28. Edsmyr, F., Wahren, B., and Silfversward, C. Usefulness of immunology and hormonal markers in the treatment of testis tumors. *Intern. J. Rad. Oncol. Biol. Phys. 1:* 279, 1976.
29. Perlin, E., Engeler, J. E., Jr., Edson, M., et al. The value of serial measurement of both human chorionic gonadotropin and alpha-fetoprotein for monitoring germinal cell tumors. *Cancer 37:* 215, 1976.
30. Braunstein, G., McIntire, R. and Waldmann, R. Discordance of human chorionic gonadotropin and alpha-fetoprotein in testicular terato carcinomas. *Cancer 31:* 1065, 1973.

31. Kelch, R. P., Jenner, M. R., Weinstein, R., et al. Estradiol and testosterone secretion in human, simian, and canine testes, by males with hypogonadism and in male pseudohermaphrodites with feminizing testis syndrome. *J. Clin. Invest. 51:* 824, 1972.
32. Longcope, C., Kato, T., and Horton, R. Conversion of blood androgen to estrogens in normal adult men and women. *J. Clin. Invest. 51:* 824, 1972.
33. Leach, R. B., Maddock, W. O., Tokuyama, I., et al. Clinical studies of testicular hormone production. *Recent Prog. Horm. Res. 12:* 377, 1956.
34. Kirschner, M. A., Wider, J. A., and Ross, G. T. Leydig cell function in men with gonadotropin-producing testicular tumors. *J. Clin. Endocrinol. 30:* 504, 1970.
35. Siiteri, P. K., and MacDonald, P. C. The utilization of circulating dehydroisoandrosterone sulfate for estrogen synthesis during human pregnancy. *Steroids 2:* 713, 1963.
36. Kirschner, M. A., Cohen, F. B., and Jespersen, D. Estrogen production and its origin in men with gonadotropin-producing neoplasma. *J. Clin. Endocrinol. 39:* 112, 1974.
37. Mostofi, F. K., Theiss, E. A., and Ashley, D. J. B. Tumors of specialized gonadal stroma in human male patients. *Cancer 12:* 944, 1959.
38. Teilum, G. Classification of testicular and ovarian androblastoma and Sertoli cell tumors. *Cancer 11:* 769, 1958.
39. Gabrilove, J. L., Nicolis, G. L., Mitty, H. A. et al. Feminizing interstitial cell tumor of the testis: Personal observations and a review of the literature. *Cancer 35:* 1184, 1975.
40. Savard, K., Dorfman, R. I., Baggett, B., et al. Clinical, morphological and biochemical studies on a malignant testicular tumor. *J. Clin. Invest. 39:* 534, 1960.
41. Smith, E. R., Breuer, H., and Schriefers, H. A. Study of the steroid metabolism of an interstitial-cell tumour of the testis. *Biochem. J. 93:* 583, 1964.
42. Wegienka, L. C. and Kolb, F. O. Hormonal studies of a benign interstitial cell tumour of the testis producing androstenedione and testosterone. *Acta Endocrinol. (Kbh). 56:* 481, 1967.
43. Gittes, R. F., Smith, G., Conn, C. A. et al. Local androgenic effect of interstitial cell tumor of the testis. *J. Urol. 104:* 774, 1970.
44. Steinberger, E., Root, A., Ficher, M. et al. The role of androgens in the initiation of spermatogenesis in man. *J. Clin. Endocrinol. 37:* 746, 1974.
45. Lipsett, M. B., Sarfaty, G. A., Wilson, H., et al. Metabolism of testosterone and related steroids in metastatic interstitial cell carcinoma of the testis. *J. Clin. Invest. 45:* 1700, 1966.
46. Ober, W. B., Kabakow, B., and Hecht, H. Malignant interstitial cell tumor of the testis: A problem in endocrine oncology. *Bull. N.Y. Acad. Med. 52:* 561, 1976.
47. Huggins, C. and Moulder, P. S. Estrogen production by Sertoli cell tumors of the testis. *Cancer Res. 5:* 510, 1945.
48. Pierrepoint, C. G., Galley, J. M., Griffiths, K. et al. Steroid metabolism of a Sertoli cell tumor of the testis of a dog with feminization and alopecia and of the normal canine testis. *J. Endocrinol. 38:* 61, 1970.
49. Fore, W. W., Bledsoe, T., Weber, D. M., et al. Cortisol production by testicular tumors in adrenogenital syndrome. *Arch. Intern. Med. 130:* 59, 1972.

127

Testicular Function in the Aging Male

Keith D. Smith

THE RELATIONS BETWEEN AGING AND TESTICULAR FUNCTION

Numerous investigations into the relationship between testicular function and advancing age have been reported. Early reports involved measurement of urinary 17-ketosteroids and urinary gonadotropins. With the development of sophisticated techniques for measurement of blood hormone levels, determination of concentrations of testosterone, estradiol, FSH, and LH in both peripheral and spermatic vein blood became possible. As early as 1958, Hollander and Hollander[1] demonstrated a decline in spermatic vein testosterone levels with increasing age. Although early studies of circulating testosterone levels in men of various ages suggested no correlation between testosterone and age,[2–4] in more recent reports the overall trend is of a gradual decline in the plasma testosterone level with increasing age. Although declining, the levels apparently remained within the normal male range (Fig. 127-1).[5–14]

Testosterone production rates have been related to aging by several investigators. This measure, the product of the metabolic clearance rate and the plasma level of testosterone, was also found to decrease with advancing age (Fig. 127-2).[3,5,15] The decline in the testosterone production rate, resulting predominantly from a decline in the metabolic clearance rate, could be detected at an earlier age than a decline in plasma testosterone levels.[3,5,15] This finding suggests that the effects of age on the systemic vascular system and on peripheral circulation may be an important factor in the observed decrease in testosterone production rates.

An elegant study of age-related changes in human testes obtained at autopsy of 121 men ranging in age from 14 to 73 yr has been reported.[16] Degenerative changes in the seminiferous tubules were noted to increase with age and to follow a distribution pattern closely related to regional blood supply. These changes were most severe in the distal areas of the arterial supply. Focal depletion of spermatogenesis and thickening of the basement membrane began in the fourth and fifth decades while Leydig cell pigmentation did not occur until later. Concurrent microangiographic studies of the testes revealed age-related vascular changes. These findings suggest that most of the testicular changes associated with aging may result from vascular involvement, rather than endocrine failure or primary testicular failure.

Free testosterone is thought to be the active form of this hormone in the circulation. Free testosterone also appears to decline with age, and its decline commences earlier than that of total blood testosterone levels (Fig. 127-3).[5,8,9,11,14,17,18] This suggests that the androgen binding protein in blood (TeBG) may increase with age. This possibility was supported by several investigators.[5,6,14] In addition to changes in circulating testosterone levels and production rates, a decreased response of Leydig cells to hCG stimulation has been noted with advancing age.[7–9]

Dihydrotestosterone (DHT) has been considered to be the metabolically active androgen in man. Only a few measurements of the levels of this androgen in blood in relation to aging have been reported. Horton *et al.*[12] noted higher DHT levels in older than younger men, while Hallberg *et al.*[14] found that both total and free DHT declined with increasing age.

Attempts to correlate changes in blood estrogen levels with age resulted in inconsistent findings. Longcope[7] found blood estradiol levels lower in older than younger men while the converse was noted by others.[6,9,14,19] To further confuse the issue, some investigators found no correlations between blood estradiol levels and age.[13,20] Rubens *et al.*[9] noted the percent free estradiol declined in blood with increasing age while total estradiol levels increased. Since estrogen elevates plasma sex steroid binding globulin, increased levels of this protein in aged men may result from rising blood estrogen levels.

Age-related changes in circulating gonadotropin levels have been reported. In most instances slight rises in blood LH levels, beginning somewhere after the age of 50, have been described.[8–11,13,14,17,21] However, the rises were gradual and in no way resembled the marked increases associated with menopause in the female. On the other hand, Haug *et al.*[20] were unable to find any correlation between serum LH levels and age. The relation between blood FSH levels and age is even less convincing. When elevation in blood FSH was noted with increasing age, it was usually of lesser magnitude than that of LH.[9–11,13,14] Several investigators were unable to find any age-related changes in blood FSH levels.[8,17,20] The response of LH and FSH to gonadotropin-releasing hormone (GnRH) was found to be greater in older than in younger men.[9] Conversely, Haug *et al.*[20] and Snyder *et al.*[17] noted a diminished response to GnRH as age increased.

There is a dearth of information on the effect of age on spermatogenesis. The numerous anecdotal accounts of paternity in elderly men are seldom supported by semen analyses. In the few instances where this has been evaluated, no significant relation between age and sperm count has been noted.[22,23] Seymour *et al.*[24] evaluated a semen sample in a 94-yr-old father of a newborn and noted normal motility and morphology of the spermatozoa and a sperm count of "65% of the customary number." Unfortunately, the customary number was not defined. Histologic sections of the

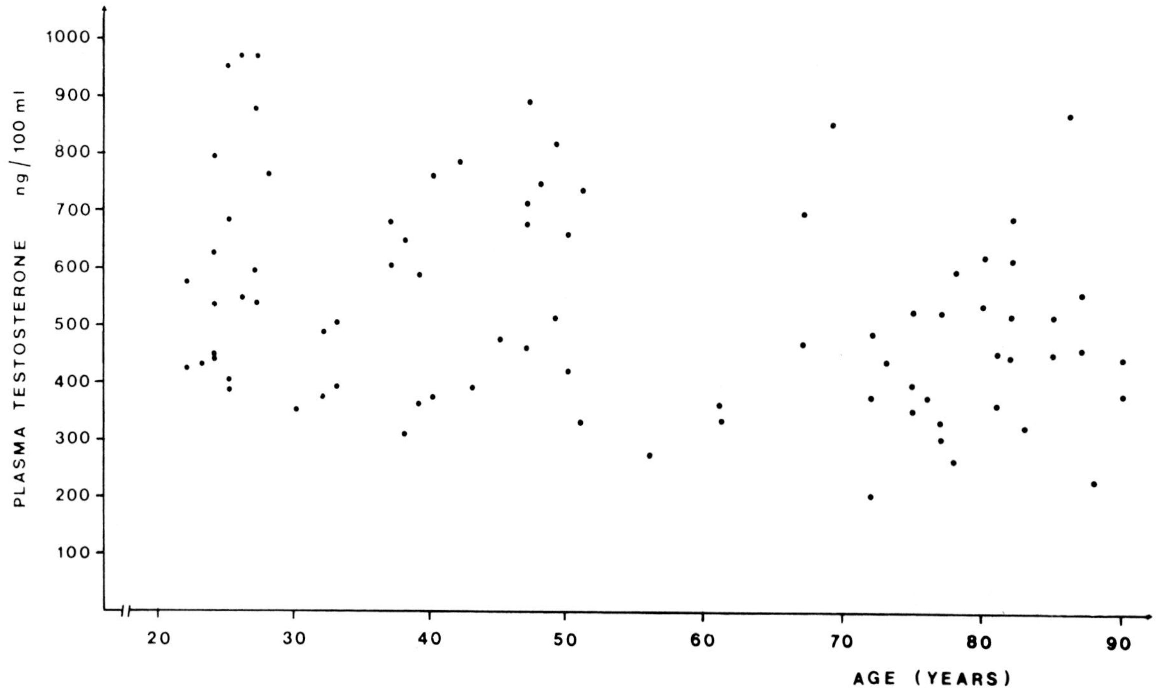

Fig. 127-1. Relation of circulating testosterone levels and age in 84 men aged 22 to 90. [From Pirke and Doerr: Acta Endocrinol. (Copenhagen) *74:* 792, 1973, with permission.]

testis of older men often show some tubules with deficient spermatogenesis while other tubules appear normal. In view of the apparent dependence of spermatogenesis on high local concentration of testosterone,[25] it is unlikely that spermatogenesis could continue in the presence of primary Leydig cell failure.

In summary, it would appear that some age-related changes in the pituitary-testicular axis do occur. Blood testosterone levels are lower in older than in younger men. Free testosterone is even lower, probably due to elevated sex steroid binding globulin. Sex steroid binding globulin elevations may result from increased blood estrogen levels. Blood LH levels are slightly higher with increasing age, and FSH changes are equivocal. Despite these changes, none of the hormone levels fall outside normal adult male ranges.

AGING AND PRIMARY TESTICULAR FAILURE

Although numerous studies suggest a relation between potency and age, a clear association between hormonal changes and potency is difficult to establish. Numerous studies of large populations of men have clearly demonstrated a gradual increase of impotence with age. A marked rise in incidence of impotence occurs between the ages of 50 and 60 yr (Fig. 127-4).[26–29] It is interesting to observe from the data in Figure 127-4 that it is also in this age group that free testosterone levels and testosterone production rates begin declining. This might suggest a cause-and-effect relationship. Such a conclusion, however, is probably erroneous. Not only are many other factors involved in modification of sexual behavior, but also in most instances of impotence in men of this age testosterone therapy is not effective.

The increasing frequency of impotence in aging men prompted innumerable efforts to relate this symptom to a physiologic phenomenon, a "male climacteric," rather than to any psychologic or pathologic process. Periodically, techniques to "rejuvenate" the aging male have been proposed and usually discarded. Steinach[30] postulated that ligation of the vas produced an atrophy of the germinal epithelium resulting in an overgrowth of Leydig cells and an increased production of testosterone which induced "rejuvenation." Neihaus[31] wrote glowingly of the results of ligation of the efferent ducts of the testes, a procedure purported not only to improve potency but also to relieve benign prostatic hypertrophy and stimulate cardiovascular function.

In the 1930s many investigators began to employ the newly identified male hormone, testosterone, for therapy of impotence, for rejuvenation of the aging male, and for the "male climacteric." Werner[32] promoted the effectiveness of testosterone esters to relieve declining potency and numerous other symptoms ascribed to the "male climacteric." Table 127-1 lists the order of frequency of symptoms noted by Werner in a study of 273 men. Treatment with testosterone propionate was instituted in 181 of these patients

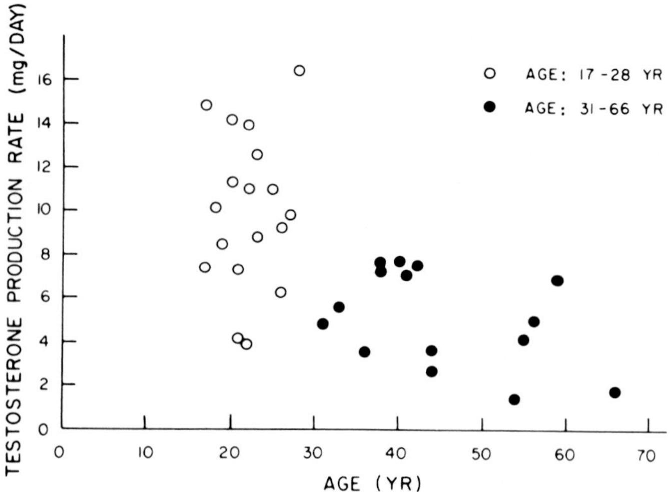

Fig. 127-2. Relation of testosterone production rate and age in 18 men aged 17 to 66. (From Persky *et al.*: Psychosom. Med. *33:* 265, 1971, with permission.)

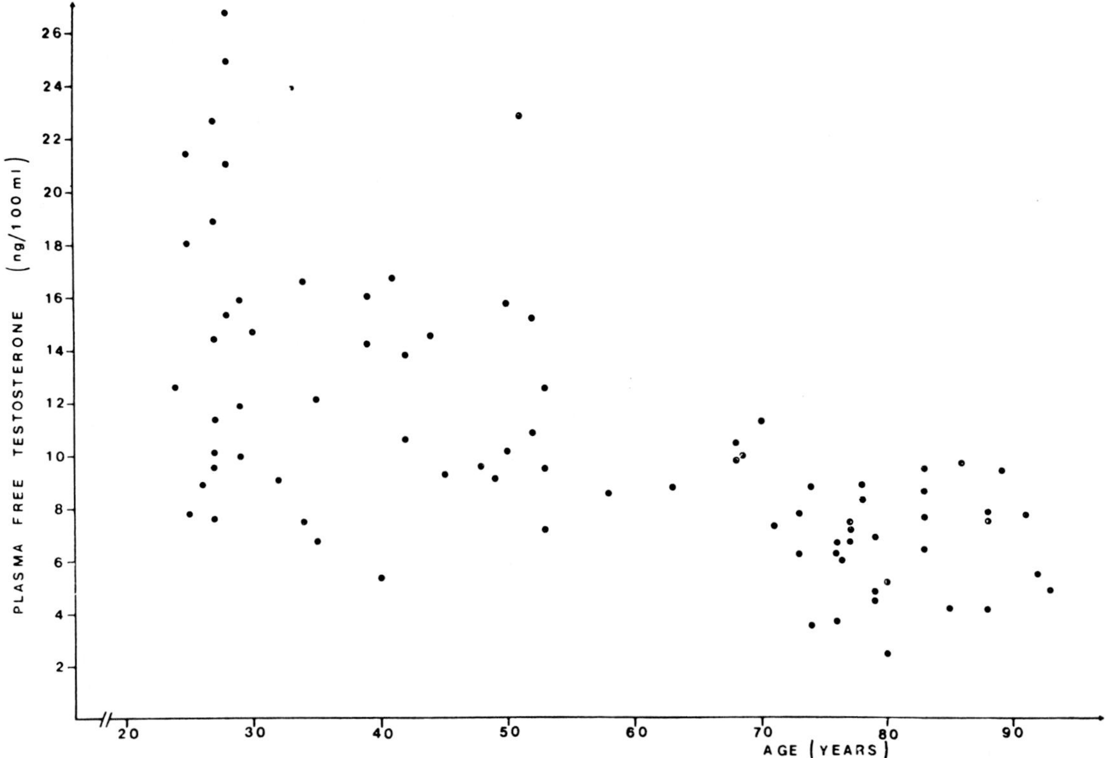

Fig. 127-3. Relation of circulating free testosterone levels and age in 82 men aged 22 to 93. [From Pirke and Doerr: Acta Endocrinol. (Copenhagen) *80:* 171, 1975, with permission.]

and symptomatic improvement was noted in 176. Other investigators, employing similar therapy, described varying results from complete success to total failure. A group of elderly men with a constellation of symptoms would simply be labeled diagnostically "male climacteric" and treated empirically on the assumption that their symptomatology was due to low testosterone levels. Thus, one of the problems facing the early investigators was lack of definition of the pathologic process and lack of appropriate diagnostic procedures.

The first objective approach to the diagnosis of the male climacteric was that of Heller and Myers in 1944,[33] who studied 38 men complaining of symptoms resembling female menopause. Urinary gonadotropins were normal in 15 and elevated in 23. Testosterone therapy was instituted in 9 men with normal and 20 men with elevated gonadotropins. All men in the latter group noted improvement, while none of the symptoms of the 9 men with normal gonadotropin levels were improved. These authors concluded that the male climacteric was a clinical entity that could be diagnosed by finding elevated urinary gonadotropins in men with appropriate symptoms and that would respond to testosterone therapy. They cautioned, however, that the condition was rare and should not be expected to occur in every male. It should be remembered that none of these investigators had the advantage of modern technology that would allow them to measure blood testosterone levels in their patients.

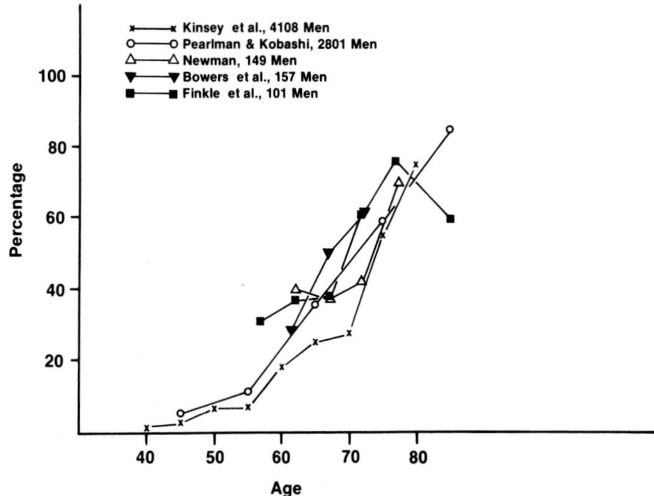

Fig. 127-4. Relation between the percent of men with impotence and age. (Plotted from the data reported by Pearlman and Kobashi: J. Urol. *107:* 298, 1972.)

Dorland's Medical Dictionary[34] defines climacteric as: "the syndrome of endocrine, somatic and psychic changes occurring at the termination of the reproductive period in the female" or accompanying "the *normal* diminution of sexual activity in the male." (Author's emphasis) Thus, by the dictionary's definition, the climacteric is a measurable endocrine and reproductive organ abnormality in the female but a nebulous, poorly defined symptom complex in the male. If a true male climacteric exists, it should be endocrinologically similar to the female climacteric. There is no evidence in the literature suggestive of a universally occurring, age-related, primary testicular failure associated with a relatively sudden cessation of testosterone production. However, as discussed earlier, some changes in hormone production in the male do occur as age increases.

To return to Dorland's definition of climacteric, in the female this condition is defined as occurring at the termination of the reproductive period. Thus, in the female the climacteric occurs when oogenesis and the associated hormone production ceases. This is a physiologic process that will occur in every woman over a

Table 127-1. Frequency of Symptoms in 273 Men with the Male Climacteric Syndrome

Symptom	Percent
Nervousness, subjective	90.5
Potency decreased or absent	90.1
Libido decreased or absent	80.5
Irritability	80.2
Fatigability and lassitude	80.2
Depression	77.2
Memory and concentration decreased	75.8
Sleep disturbed	59.3
Loss of interest	58.5
Ill at ease	56.4
Tachycardia, palpitation, and dyspnea	51.2
Excitability	49.0
Vertigo	46.5
Numbness and tingling	43.9
Occipitocervical aching	41.9
Fear	40.6
Worry, unnecessary	33.7
Cold hands and feet	32.9
Vague pains	32.9
Headache	31.8
Itching	31.8
Hot flushes	29.3
Loss of self confidence	27.1
Futility	27.1
Scotomas	26.0
Constipation	24.9
Unsociability	23.8
Obesity	21.5
Aching in the vertex	17.5
Sweating	17.9
Crying	15.3
Tinnitus	10.6
Thoughts of self destruction	7.4
Chilly sensations	6.2
Self accusations	2.4
Psychosis	2.4
Suicide attempted (2 patients)	

From Werner: J. Am. Med. Assoc. *132:* 188, 1946, with permission.

relatively limited age range. No evidence has been published of a similar age-defined decline in germ cell and androgen production in the testis.

An attempt to define the onset of a "normal" diminution of sexual activity in the male might suggest that the male climacteric begins in the late teens or early twenties. Kinsey[26] reported peak sexual outlets for men to be 3.2 to 4.8 weekly during the teens followed by a gradual decline to a mean of 1.8 weekly at 50, 1.3 weekly at 60, and 0.9 weekly at 70.

These considerations fail to support the conclusion that a physiologic state akin to female menopause occurs universally in men. Unquestionably, a diminution of testicular function with advanced age can be demonstrated. However, this change seems to occur parallel to diminution in the efficiency of function of other organs in the aging male. Premature cessation or significant diminution of testicular function undoubtedly occurs in some men, but in these instances it most likely is related to a specific pathologic process.

Premature cessation of testicular function associated with well-defined pathologic processes (e.g., orchitis, torsion of the testis, castration) is easily diagnosed and does not require further elucidation. The gradual cessation of testicular function in the aging male can proceed at various rates. In men with accelerated rates, it is important to diagnose this condition and treat it appropriately. Diagnosis presents a challenge to the physician since the symptoms have both emotional and organic components.

The most important screening test is semen analysis. The likelihood of finding testosterone levels below the normal range in patients with normal sperm output is remote (see Chapter 123). On the other hand, an equivocal result of semen analysis suggests the necessity of evaluation of the hypothalamic-pituitary-testicular axis. Borderline testosterone levels associated with relatively normal gonadotropin values can be further evaluated by hCG stimulation tests. A blunted response to hCG suggests failing Leydig cell function and the possibility of a beneficial response to therapy. Low testosterone levels associated with high gonadotropins are diagnostic of primary Leydig cell failure.

In the event the necessary tests cannot be performed, a therapeutic trial may be in order. Appropriate androgen therapy may be initiated and a placebo substituted at a later date. Alternatively, therapy may be instituted with a placebo that is subsequently replaced by an active androgen. A response to the androgen and a failure to respond to the placebo is suggestive of primary Leydig cell failure. A response to both placebo and androgen is suggestive of a psychologic rather than an endocrine etiology. A failure of response to either measure may indicate psychologic, neurologic, or vascular etiologies.

THERAPY OF PRIMARY TESTICULAR FAILURE

The goal of therapy is to provide testosterone replacement in an amount equivalent to the normal production rate of testosterone. Unfortunately, this cannot be accomplished easily with the currently available testosterone preparations. Effective preparations, devoid of hepatotoxicity or other metabolic side effects, must be administered parenterally. The available oral androgens are more useful as anabolic agents than as testosterone replacements. If they are given at high enough dosages to provide testosterone replacement therapy, undesirable side effects—e.g., cholestatic jaundice—may occur. Of the available parenteral preparations, testosterone propionate is relatively short-acting and requires at least weekly injections. Testosterone enanthate and testosterone cypionate are longer-acting and can usually be given at intervals of about 3 weeks. Since the goal of therapy is to provide an amount of testosterone equivalent to normal production rate without producing elevated blood testosterone levels, even the long-acting testosterone preparations are not ideal. For example, in order to achieve testosterone levels equivalent to the normal production rate, injections of 200 mg every 10 to 14 days are required.[35]

An alternative to the use of parenteral testosterone preparations is the use of silastic capsules containing one of the testosterone esters. These capsules could be implanted in the subcutaneous tissue at intervals of about every 6 months. Unfortunately, this therapeutic modality is still not available for routine use.

Whatever therapeutic regime is employed, it is important to monitor blood testosterone, FSH, and LH levels to be sure that the proper amount of hormone is being provided. In addition, attention should be given to red blood cell counts, hemoglobin levels, serum cholesterol, serum lipids, and liver enzymes. The prostate should be checked at intervals of every 3 to 6 months.

Finally, it must be remembered that although primary testicular failure results in deficient androgen production, an emotional overlay is almost always present. Sympathetic supportive psychotherapy is an essential part of therapy.

REFERENCES

1. Hollander, N. and Hollander, V. P. The microdetermination of testosterone in human spermatic vein blood. *J. Clin. Endocrinol. Metab. 18:* 966, 1958.
2. Coppage, W. S., Jr. and Cooner, A. E. Testosterone in human plasma. *N. Engl. J. Med. 273:* 902, 1965.
3. Kent, J. R. and Acone, A. B. Plasma testosterone levels and aging in males. In Vermeulen, A. and Exley, D. (eds.): Androgens in Normal and Pathological Conditions. Amsterdam, Excerpta Medica International Congress, Series 101, 1966, p. 31.
4. Gandy, H. M. and Peterson, R. E. Measurement of testosterone and 17-ketosteroids in plasma by the double isotope dilution derivative technique. *J. Clin. Endocrinol. Metab. 28:* 949, 1968.
5. Vermeulen, A., Rubens, R. and Verdonck, L. Testosterone secretion and metabolism in male senescence. *J. Clin. Endocrinol. Metab. 34:* 730, 1972.
6. Pirke, K. M. and Doerr, P. Age related changes and interrelationships between plasma testosterone, oestradiol and testosterone-binding globulin in normal adult males. *Acta Endocrinol. (Copenhagen) 74:* 792, 1973.
7. Longcope, C. The effect of human chorionic gonadotropin on plasma steroid levels in young and old men. *Steroids 21:* 583, 1973.
8. Nieschlag, E., Kley, H. K., Wiegelman, W., Solbach, H. G. and Krüskemper, H. L. Lebensalter und Endokrine Funktion der Testes des Erwachsenen Mannes (Age and endocrine function of the testes in adult men). *Dtsch. Med. Wochenschr. 98:* 1281, 1973.
9. Rubens, R., Dhont, M. and Vermeulen, A. Further studies on Leydig cell function in old age. *J. Clin. Endocrinol. Metab. 39:* 40, 1974.
10. Baier, H., Bird, G. and Weinges, K. F. Serum levels of FSH, LH and testosterone in human males. *Horm. Metab. Res. 6:* 514, 1974.
11. Stearns, E. L., MacDonnell, J. A., Kaufman, B. J., Padua, R., Lucman, T. S., Winter, J. S. D. and Faiman, C. Declining testicular function with age. Hormonal and clinical correlates. *Am. J. Med. 57:* 761, 1974.
12. Horton, R., Hsieh, P., Barberia, J., Pages, L. and Cosgrove, M. Altered blood androgens in elderly men with prostate hyperplasia. *J. Clin. Endocrinol. Metab. 41:* 793, 1975.
13. Greenblatt, R. B., Oettinger, M. and Bohler, C. S.-S. Estrogen-androgen levels in aging men and women: Therapeutic considerations. *J. Am. Geriatr. Soc. 24:* 173, 1976.
14. Hallberg, M. C., Wieland, R. G., Zorn, E. M., Furst, B. H. and Wieland, R. M. Impaired Leydig cell reserve and altered serum androgen binding in the aging male. *Fertil. Steril. 27:* 812, 1976.
15. Persky, H., Smith, K. D. and Basu, G. K. Relation of psychologic measures of aggression and hostility to testosterone production in man. *Psychsom. Med. 33:* 265, 1971.
16. Sasano, N. and Ichijo, S. Vascular patterns of the human testis with special reference to its senile changes. *Tohoku J. Exp. Med. 99:* 269, 1969.
17. Snyder, P. J., Reitano, J. F. and Utiger, R. D. Serum LH and FSH responses to synthetic gonadotropin-releasing hormone in normal men. *J. Clin. Endocrinol. Metab. 41:* 938, 1975.
18. Pirke, K. M. and Doerr, P. Age related changes in free plasma testosterone, dihydrotestosterone and oestradiol. *Acta Endocrinol. (Copenhagen) 80:* 171, 1975.
19. Kley, H. K., Nieschlag, E., Bidlingmaier, F. and Krüskemper, H. L. Possible age-dependent influence of estrogens on the binding of testosterone in plasma of adult men. *Horm. Metab. Res. 6:* 213, 1974.
20. Haug, E., Aakvaag, A., Sand, T. and Torjesen, P. A. The gonadotrophin response to synthetic gonadotrophin-releasing hormone in males in relation to age, dose, and basal serum levels of testosterone, oestradiol-17β and gonadotrophins. *Acta Endocrinol. (Copenhagen) 77:* 625, 1974.
21. Schalch, D. S., Parlow, A. F., Boon, R. C. and Reichlin, S. Measurement of human luteinizing hormone in plasma by radioimmunoassay. *J. Clin. Invest. 47:* 665, 1968.
22. MacLeod, J. and Gold, R. S. The male factor in fertility and infertility. II. Spermatozoon counts in 1000 men of known fertility and in 1000 cases of infertile marriage. *J. Urol. 66:* 436, 1951.
23. Smith, K. D. and Steinberger, E. What is oligospermia? In Troen, P. and Nankin, H. R. (eds.): The Testis in Normal and Infertile Men. New York, Raven, 1977, p. 489.
24. Seymour, F. I., Duffy, C. and Koerner, A. A case of authentic fertility in a man, aged 94. *J. Am. Med. Assoc. 105:* 1423, 1935.
25. Steinberger, E. Hormonal control of mammalian spermatogenesis. *Physiol. Rev. 51:* 1, 1971.
26. Kinsey, A. C., Pomeroy, W. B., Martin, C. E. and Gebhardt, P. H. Sexual Behavior in the Human Male. Philadelphia, Saunders, 1948, p. 226.
27. Finkle, A. L., Moyers, T. G., Tobenkin, M. I. and Karg, S. J. Sexual potency in aging males. I. Frequency of coitus among clinic patients. *J. Am. Med. Assoc. 170:* 1391, 1959.
28. Bowers, L. M., Cross, R. R., Jr. and Lloyd, F. A. Sexual function and urologic disease in the elderly male. *J. Am. Geriatr. Soc. 11:* 647, 1963.
29. Pearlman, C. K. and Kobashi, L. I. Frequency of intercourse in men. *J. Urol. 107:* 298, 1972.
30. Steinach, E. Biologic methods against the process of old age. *Med. J. Res. 125:* 77, 1927.
31. Neihaus, P. Modern views on hypertrophy of the prostate. *Lancet I:* 307, 1936.
32. Werner, A. A. The male climacteric. Report of two hundred and seventy-three cases. *J. Am. Med. Assoc. 132:* 188, 1946.
33. Heller, C. G. and Myers, G. B. The male climacteric, its symptomatology, diagnosis and treatment. Use of urinary gonadotropins, therapeutic test with testosterone propionate and testicular biopsies in delineating the male climacteric from psychoneurosis and psychogenic impotence. *J. Am. Med. Assoc. 126:* 472, 1944.
34. Dorland, W. A. N. The American Illustrated Medical Dictionary, 25th Edition. Philadelphia, Saunders, 1974, p. 327.
35. Steinberger, E. and Smith, K. D. Effect of chronic administration of testosterone enanthate on sperm production and plasma testosterone, FSH and LH levels. A preliminary evaluation of a possible male contraceptive. *Fertil. Steril. 28:* 1320, 1977.

128

Gynecomastia

Luis J. Rodriguez-Rigau
Keith D. Smith

Gynecomastia is defined as excessive development of the male mammary glands.[1] Macroscopically, it represents a concentric increase in glandular and stromal tissue. It is usually grossly evident (Fig. 128-1) and may vary in size from a small button of tissue to breasts indistinguishable from those of an adult female. It is usually bilateral, although unilateral gynecomastia is not infrequent.[2] Hypertrophy, inversion and retraction of the nipple are rare.

Histologically, gynecomastia results from both an increase of the stroma and some degree of proliferation of the ducts. The most important stromal changes are hypervascularity, fibroblastic proliferation, deposition of collagen fibers, and hyalinization. Proliferation of the ducts consists of an increase in their number and length and the formation of pseudolobules.

From a histopathologic point of view, three types of gynecomastia have been described[3]:

1. *Florid type:* The tissue contains an increased number of ducts, proliferation of ductal epithelium, periductal edema, and a highly cellular fibroblastic stroma accompanied by adipose tissue.
2. *Fibrous type:* The ducts are dilated in association with slight to moderate epithelial proliferation, absence of periductal edema and adipose tissue, and an almost acellular fibrous stroma.
3. *Intermediate type:* The tissue contains components of both histologic patterns.

It has been suggested that the above histologic patterns may reflect differences in the nature of the mammogenic stimulus operative in each case.[4,5] However, other investigators have failed to demonstrate a clear relation between the histologic appearance of the gynecomastia and the clinical condition with which it was associated.[3,6] These authors have suggested that the histologic features of gynecomastia undergo progressive changes with time, irrespective of etiology, and that the overall microscopic appearance depends on the duration of the disorder. Bannayan and Hadju[3] suggested that gynecomastia of less than 4 months' duration is typically of the florid type, while the fibrous type represents gynecomastia of 1 year or more duration. Thus, florid gynecomastia may regress or may progress to the fibrous type, which once established, seldom disappears.

Gynecomastia accounts for over 65 percent of male breast disorders.[7] It occurs predominantly during puberty and adolescence, in neonatal life, and during the "male climacteric" years. Pubertal gynecomastia has been reported to occur in over 60 percent of adolescent boys, with a peak incidence at the age of 14 and an average duration of 1 to 2 years.[8] In the majority of cases, this disorder is part of the physiologic process of puberty, and spontaneous regression is common. Even in this age group, however, enlargement of the breast may be indicative of an underlying disease, and careful evaluation should be routine.

The incidence of gynecomastia in adults has not been extensively studied. Webster[9] reported a frequency of 8 per 100,000 in navy hospital admissions during World War II. However, a higher incidence has been reported by other authors.[10] Gynecomastia appears to affect Caucasians predominantly.[3]

The pathophysiology of gynecomastia remains unclear. It has been associated with a wide variety of dissimilar causative factors (Table 128-1). Although the relationship between estrogen and breast development is well established, in most patients with gynecomastia an estrogen excess has not been demonstrated.[71–74] Caplan[75] suggested that the estrogen–androgen ratio could be more important than the absolute estrogen levels. In addition, it is possible that the original estrogen stimulus could have subsided at the time the hormone levels were obtained.[6] Consequently, normal estrogen levels may not exclude the possibility that either a transient estrogen elevation or an estrogen–androgen imbalance was the original stimulus to development of gynecomastia.

This theory is supported by the recent studies of Lee[76] and LaFranchi et al.,[77] who demonstrated transient elevations of serum estradiol levels in adolescents at the time of onset of breast hypertrophy. This elevation was detected when testosterone levels were not rising, resulting in a markedly increased estradiol–testosterone ratio. They suggested that this transient elevation of the estrogen–androgen ratio could trigger the initiation of breast enlargement. Once gynecomastia is established, it could regress, persist, or even become permanent without further hormonal stimulus.[78]

Consistently elevated estrogen levels have been found only in those patients with feminizing adrenal carcinoma[39] or Leydig-cell tumor of the testis.[38] In the presence of liver disease, it has been suggested that gynecomastia may be associated with elevated estrogen levels resulting from a defect in steroid conjugation by the liver.[54,55] However, others have been unable to confirm this hypothesis.[79,80]

The gynecomastia associated with nutritional deficiencies and "refeeding" following malnutrition was the subject of a considerable number of studies shortly after World War II. These studies were prompted by the observation of gynecomastia during the recovery of severely malnourished prisoners of war. Paulsen postulated that during the period of malnutrition, gonadotropin stimulation of the testes decreased; during the "refeeding" process, pituitary gonadotropins would increase, resulting in a "second puberty" manifested by enhanced testicular function and gynecomastia.[7] He further suggested that the same mechanism could

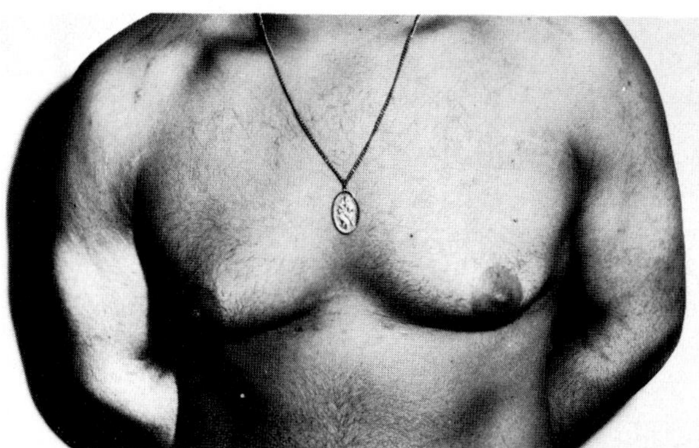

Fig. 128-1. Idiopathic gynecomastia in an 18-year-old male.

explain the gynecomastia associated with liver disease,[57] renal failure,[52] and other clinical conditions that result in generalized malnutrition.

Gynecomastia rarely develops in patients with hypogonadotropic hypogonadism. However, it has been reported to occur in many conditions with elevated gonadotropin levels (Klinefelter and Reifenstein syndromes, mumps orchitis, etc.). Possibly the increased levels of gonadotropins could lead to relative estrogen overproduction by the testis. A similar meçhanism could apply to the gynecomastia associated with bronchogenic carcinoma with ectopic production of gonadotropins[43] or testicular choriocarcinoma with secretion of chorionic gonadotropin.[36] Investigation of estrogen levels in most of these conditions, however, has failed to demonstrate significant abnormalities.[81] An investigation of estrogen-androgen ratios in these patients might be of benefit.

Table 128-1. Causes of Gynecomastia

I.	*Endocrine* 1. Testis: castration,[11] cryptorchidism,[12] Klinefelter's syndrome,[4] Reifenstein's syndrome,[13] male climacteric,[11] mumps orchitis,[14] hermaphroditism,[15] 2. Adrenal: Cushing's syndrome,[16] hyperplasia (11β-hydroxylase deficiency)[17] 3. Thyroid: hyperthyroidism,[18] hypothyroidism[19] 4. Parathyroid: hyperparathyroidism[20] 5. Hypothalamic: Albright's syndrome[21] 6. Pituitary: hyperprolactinemia[85,86]
II.	*Drug-induced* Estrogens,[22] androgens,[23] gonadotropins,[24] adrenal steroids,[25] digitalis,[26] methyl-dopa,[27] phenothiazines,[28] reserpine,[29] thiacetazone,[30] isoniazide,[31] cimetidine,[32] spironolactones,[33] methadone,[34] marihuana[35]
III.	*Tumoral* Testicular tumors (choriocarcinoma,[36] Sertoli cell tumor,[37] Leydig-cell tumor[38]), adrenal tumors[39] (adenoma, carcinoma), pituitary adenomas,[40] (eosinophilic, basophilic, chromophobe), choriocarcinoma (stomach,[41] retroperitoneal[42]), bronchogenic carcinoma,[43] paraganglioma,[44] gastric adenocarcinoma,[45] hepatic carcinoma,[46] lymphomas,[47] leukemias,[48] myeloma,[49] hypernephroma[50]
IV.	*Metabolic* 1. Renal: chronic pyelonephritis or glomerulonephritis,[51] renal failure,[52] chronic hemodialysis[53] 2. Hepatic: cirrhosis,[54] hemachromatosis,[54] hepatitis[55] 3. Nutritional: malnutrition,[56] "refeeding" following malnutrition,[57] following severe illness or extensive surgery,[58] chronic ulcerative colitis,[59] leprosy,[60] tuberculosis[61]
V.	*Developmental* Neonatal,[62] prepubertal,[63] pubertal[64]
VI.	*Other* Paraplegia,[65] muscular dystrophy,[66] mental deficiencies,[67] chromosomal abnormalities,[68] familial,[69] idiopathic[70]

Gynecomastia has been associated with both hypofunction and hyperfunction of the thyroid gland.[18,19] Since thyrotropin-releasing hormone (TRH) has been demonstrated to stimulate both TSH and prolactin release,[82] it has been postulated that increased prolactin could be the cause of gynecomastia in patients with primary hypothyroidism or secondary hyperthyroidism.[83] Klemm et al.[84] evaluated prolactin levels in patients with gynecomastia before and after stimulation with TRH. High prolactin levels and excessive response to TRH were found in 2 of the 10 patients studied. In one case, a pituitary adenoma was diagnosed, but in the other no sella turcica enlargement or other abnormality could be detected. Finally, hyperprolactinemia has also been observed in patients with galactorrhea in addition to gynecomastia[85,86] and in those with gynecomastia due to intake of tranquilizers.[87]

Frank et al.[88] and later Payne and Ryan[89] reported on the presence of human placental lactogen (HPL) in the serum of male subjects with testicular tumors and in testicular extracts of normal men. They postulated that HPL could be responsible for the gynecomastia of some men, particularly those with testicular tumors.

Finally, to explain the pathophysiology of gynecomastia in patients with normal hormonal levels, it was postulated that end-organ (breast) tissue metabolism could be altered in certain patients, predisposing them toward the development of gynecomastia despite a normal hormonal environment.[7] This could explain the cases of familial gynecomastia reported in the literature.[90,91] Miller et al.[92] reported deficiency of 3β-hydroxysteroid dehydrogenase in breast tissue of 6 patients with gynecomastia. This deficiency, by reducing the production of testosterone from dehydroepiandrosterone, could lead to a local tissue imbalance in the androgen–estrogen ratio. Rajendran et al.[93] studied the in vitro steroid biosynthetic potential of breast tissue from 7 patients with gynecomastia. Estrogens were formed from androgens in amounts comparable to female breast tissue. A marked reduction in serum estrogen levels in these patients followed surgical removal of the breast tissue. The authors postulated that aromatization of androgens in the breast tissue could be etiologically implicated in the development of gynecomastia.

In the adult patient, gynecomastia may be a manifestation of a serious underlying illness. It may receive the major emphasis by the patient or his physician, while more subtle manifestations of the underlying disease go unnoticed.[24] Consequently, all cases of gynecomastia call for a careful history and physical examination and appropriate laboratory evaluation. Particular attention should be directed to testes, adrenals, thyroid, liver, lungs, cardiovascular system, nutritional status of the patient, and history of drug intake. Since a number of therapeutic agents are known to produce gynecomastia (Table 128-1), the history of drug use must be carefully evaluated.

The differential diagnosis of gynecomastia includes such entities as lipoma, carcinoma, neurofibromatosis, diffuse increase in adipose tissue (obese patients), and leukemic infiltration.

The therapy of gynecomastia has not been very rewarding. When the offending agent can be identified (e.g., intake of sex steroids like birth control pills, glycosides, phenothiazine, etc.), termination of these agents, if feasible, may result in regression of breast development (Figs. 128-2 and 128-3). When the gynecomastia is a secondary manifestation of a serious underlying disorder (e.g., neoplasia, metabolic disturbance, etc.) the therapy directed toward the primary disease obviously takes precedence. In most cases, the breast enlargement is idiopathic in nature, and the only

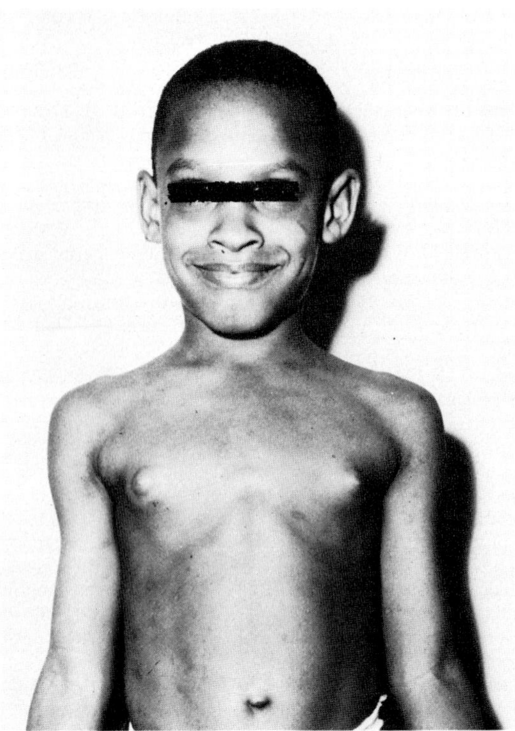

Fig. 128-2. Gynecomastia in a 7-year-old boy induced by surreptitious ingestion of mother's contraceptive pills.

therapeutic modality available is the surgical removal of the offending tissue.

In summary, gynecomastia can be associated with a large number of pathologic states. In some cases the pathophysiologic mechanisms for its development have been elucidated or postulated. In the majority of cases, however, the pathogenesis is poorly understood.

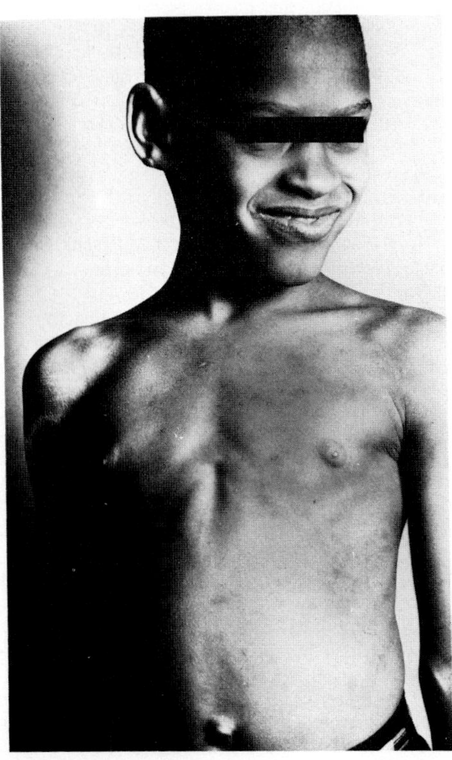

Fig. 128-3. Regression of the gynecomastia of the patient in Fig. 128-2 after discontinuation of the contraceptive pills.

REFERENCES

1. Dorland's Medical Dictionary, ed. 25. Philadelphia, W. B. Saunders, 1974, p. 673.
2. Sbar, S. Unilateral gynecomastia. *N. Engl. J. Med. 286:* 1367, 1972.
3. Bannayan, G. A. and Hadju, S. I. Gynecomastia: Clinicopathologic study of 351 cases. *Am. J. Clin. Pathol. 57:* 431, 1972.
4. Klinefelter, H. F., Reifenstein, E. C. and Albright, F. Syndrome characterized by gynecomastia, aspermatogenesis without A-Leydigism and increased excretion of follicle-stimulating hormone. *J. Clin. Endocrinol. 2:* 615, 1972.
5. Schwartz, I. S. and Wilens, S. L. The formation of acinar tissue in gynecomastia. *Am. J. Pathol. 43:* 797, 1963.
6. Nicolis, G. L., Modlinger, R. S. and Gabrilove, J. L. A study of the histopathology of human gynecomastia. *J. Clin. Endocrinol. Metab. 32:* 173, 1971.
7. Paulsen, C. A. The testis, in Williams, R. H. (ed.): Textbook of Endocrinology, ed. 5. Philadelphia, W. B. Saunders, 1974, p. 323.
8. Nydick, M., Bustos, J., Dale, J. H. and Rawson, R. W. Gynecomastia in adolescent boys. *JAMA 178:* 449, 1961.
9. Webster, G. V. Gynecomastia in the Navy. *Mil. Surgeon 95:* 375, 1944.
10. Giacobine, J. W. and Searle, N. B. Management of gynecomastia. *Am. J. Surg. 102:* 395, 1961.
11. Sirtori, C. and Veronesi, U. Gynecomastia. A review of 218 cases. *Cancer 10:* 645, 1957.
12. Sprung, M. Gynecomastia and cryptorchidism. *Vojnosanit Pregl. 31:* 402, 1974.
13. Bowen, P., Lee, C. S. N., Migeon, C. J., Kaplan, N. M., Whalley, P. J., McKusick, V. A. and Reifenstein, E. C. Hereditary male pseudohermaphroditism with hypogonadism, hypospadias and gynecomastia (Reifenstein's syndrome). *Ann. Intern. Med. 62:* 252, 1965.
14. Heller, C. G. and Nelson, W. O. Hyalinization of the seminiferous tubules associated with normal or failing Leydig-cell function. Discussion of relationship to eunuchoidism, gynecomastia, elevated gonadotropins, depressed 17-ketosteroids and estrogens. *J. Clin. Endocrinol. 5:* 1, 1945.
15. Summit, R. L. Differential diagnosis of genital ambiguity in the newborn. *Clin. Obstet. Gynecol. 15:* 112, 1972.
16. Migeon, C. J. and Gardner, L. I. Urinary estrogens in hyperadrenocorticism; influence of cortisone, compound F, compound B and ACTH. *J. Clin. Endocrinol. Metab. 12:* 1513, 1952.
17. Mclaren, N. K., Migeon, C. J. and Raiti, S. Gynecomastia with congenital virilizing adrenal hyperplasia (11β-hydroxylase deficiency). *J. Pediatr. 86:* 579, 1975.
18. Bercovici, J. P. and Mauvais-Jarvis, P. Hyperthyroidism and gynecomastia: Metabolic studies. *J. Clin. Endocrinol. Metab. 35:* 671, 1972.
19. Larsson, O., Sundbom, C. M. and Astedt, B. Gynecomastia and diseases of the thyroid. *Acta Endocrinol. 44:* 133, 1963.
20. Mollet, E. and Bittard, M. Hyperparathyroidism and gynecomastia. *Nouv. Presse Med. 1:* 1898, 1972.
21. Hall, R. and Warrick, C. Hypersecretion of hypothalamic releasing hormones: a possible explanation of the endocrine manifestations of polyostotic fibrous dysplasia (Albright's syndrome). *Lancet I:* 1313, 1972.
22. Hendrickson, D. A. and Anderson, W. R. Diethylstilbestrol-therapy gynecomastia. *JAMA 213:* 468, 1970.
23. McCullagh, E. P. and Rossmiller, H. R. Methyl testosterone androgenic effects and the production of gynecomastia and oligospermia. *J. Clin. Endocrinol. 1:* 496, 1941.
24. Wheeler, C. E., Cawley, E. P., Gray, H. T. and Curtis, A. C. Gynecomastia: A review and analysis of 160 cases. *Ann. Intern. Med. 40:* 985, 1954.
25. Edwards, R. A., Shimkin, M. B. and Shaver, J. S. Hypertrophy of the breasts due to injection of adrenal cortex in a man with Addison's disease. *JAMA 111:* 412, 1938.
26. LeWinn, E. B. Gynecomastia during digitalis therapy. *N. Engl. J. Med. 248:* 316, 1953.
27. AMA Council on Drugs. A new antihypertensive: methyldopa (Aldomet). *JAMA 186:* 504, 1963.

28. Morgolis, I. B. and Gross, C. G. Gynecomastia during phenothiazine therapy. *JAMA 199:* 942, 1967.
29. Robinson, B. Breast changes in the male and female with chlorpromazine or reserpine therapy. *Med. J. Aust. 2:* 239, 1957.
30. Chunhaswasdikul, B. Gynecomastia in association with administration of thiacetazone in the treatment of tuberculosis. *J. Med. Assoc. Thai. 57:* 323, 1974.
31. Bergogne-Berezin, E., Nouhouayi, A., Letonturier, P., Thibault, B. and Tourneur, R. Gynecomastia caused by isoniazid. Value of determination of the inactivation phenotype. *Nouv. Presse Med. 5:* 213, 1976.
32. Hall, W. H.: Breast changes in males on cimetidine. *N. Engl. J. Med. 295:* 841, 1976.
33. Sussman, R. M. Spironolactone and gynecomastia. *Lancet 1:* 58, 1963.
34. Thomas, B. L. Methadone-associated gynecomastia. *N. Engl. J. Med. 294:* 169, 1976.
35. Harmon, J. and Aliapoulios, M. Gynecomastia in marihuana users. *N. Engl. J. Med. 287:* 936, 1972.
36. Gilbert, J. B. Studies in malignant testis tumors; syndrome of choriogenic gynecomastia. *J. Urol. 44:* 345, 1940.
37. Teilum, G. Estrogen-producing Sertoli cell tumors of human testis and ovary. *J. Clin. Endocrinol. 9:* 310, 1949.
38. Dixon, F. J. and Moore, R. A. Testicular tumors and gynecomastia. *Cancer 6:* 427, 1953.
39. Gabrilove, J. L., Sharma, D. C., Wotiz, H. H. and Dorfman, R. I. Feminizing adrenocortical tumors in the male. A review of 52 cases including a case report. *Medicine 44:* 37, 1965.
40. Turkington, R. W. Secretion of prolactin by patients with pituitary and hypothalamic tumors. *J. Clin. Endocrinol. Metab. 34:* 159, 1972.
41. Uei, Y., Koketsu, M., Konda, C. and Kimura, K. Cytodiagnosis of hCG-secreting choriocarcinoma of the stomach. Report of a case. *Acta Cytol. (Baltimore) 17:* 431, 1973.
42. Flacherer, H. P. Primary retroperitoneal choriocarcinoma in a male. *Zentratbl. Allg. Pathol. 117:* 40, 1973.
43. Charles, M. A., Claypool, R., Schaef, M., Rosen, S. W. and Weintraub, B. D. Lung carcinoma associated with production of three placental proteins: Ectopic human chorionic gonadotropin, human chorionic somatomammotropin and placental alkaline phosphatase. *Arch. Intern. Med. 132:* 427, 1973.
44. Dell'Acqua, G. B. and Sensi, S. Paraneoplastic endocrine syndrome with a retroperitoneal paraganglioma. *Munch. Med. Wochenschr. 115:* 1171, 1973.
45. Rivadeneyra, J., Gonzalez-Angulo, A., Cortes-Gallegos, V., Padilla-Romo, I. and Aguilar-Parada, E. Gastric adenocarcinoma with trophoblastic differentiation and gonadotropin production. *Arch. Invest. Med. (Mex) 3:* 503, 1972.
46. Morrione, T. G. Effect of estrogens on the testis in hepatic insufficiency. *Arch. Pathol. 37:* 39, 1944.
47. Dexter, C. J. Benign enlargement of the male breast. *N. Engl. J. Med. 254:* 996, 1956.
48. Seligman, B. R., Rosner, F. and Solomon, R. B. Chronic myelogenous leukemia. Disseminated intravascular coagulation and chloromas containing sea-blue histocytes. *NY State J. Med. 75:* 1271, 1975.
49. Gault, J. E. Gynecomastia and multiple myeloma. *Med. J. Aust. 2:* 318, 1961.
50. Stokes, J. F. Unexpected gynecomastia. *Lancet II:* 911, 1962.
51. Schmitt, G. W., Shehacleh, I. and Sawin, C. T. Transient gynecomastia in chronic renal failure during chronic intermittent hemodialysis. *Ann. Intern. Med. 69:* 73, 1968.
52. Lindsay, R. M., Briggs, J. D., Luke, R. G., Boyle, I. T. and Kennedy A. C. Gynecomastia in chronic renal failure. *Br. Med. J. 4:* 779, 1967.
53. Freeman, R. M., Lawton, R. L. and Fearing, M. O. Gynecomastia: an endocrinologic complication of hemodialysis. *Ann. Intern. Med. 69:* 67, 1968.
54. Hall, P. F. Gynecomastia. Olebe, Australia, Australiasian Medical Publishing Co. Ltd., 1969, p. 104.
55. Zondek, B. and Black, R. Estrone clearance test in infectious hepatitis. *J. Clin. Endocrinol. 7:* 519, 1947.
56. Klatskin, G., Slater, W. T. and Humm, F. D. Gynecomastia due to malnutrition. I. Clinical studies. *Am. J. Med. Sci. 213:* 19, 1947.
57. Kark, R. M., Morey, G. R. and Paynter, C. R. Re-feeding (nutritional) gynecomastia in cirrhosis of the liver. I. Clinical considerations. *Am. J. Med. Sci. 222:* 154, 1951.
58. Hibbs, R. E. Gynecomastia associated with vitamin deficiency disease. *Am. J. Med. Sci. 213:* 176, 1947.
59. Kyle, L. H. Gynecomastia in association with chronic ulcerative colitis. *N. Engl. J. Med. 240:* 537, 1949.
60. Srinivasan, H. Surgical problems in leprosy. *J. Indian Med. Assoc. 61:* 406, 1973.
61. Molina, C., Aberkane, B. and Conguy-Douard, T. A. Les gynécomasties chez les tuberculeux pulmonaires. A propos de cinq observations. *Moroc. Med. 36:* 635, 1957.
62. Marrio, P. and Oddo, G. Gynecomastia in the newborn induced by maternal milk? An unusual complication of oral contraceptives. *Nouv. Presse. Med. 3:* 2579, 1974.
63. August, G. P., Chandra, R. and Hung, W. Prepubertal male gynecomastia. *J. Pediatr. 80:* 259, 1972.
64. Jung, F. T. and Shelflon, A. L. Mastitis, mazoplasia mastalgia and gynecomastia in normal adolescent male. *Ill. Med. J. 73:* 15, 1938.
65. Cooper, I. S., MacCarty, C. S. and Rynearson, E. M. Gynecomastia in paraplegic males. *J. Neurosurg. 7:* 364, 1950.
66. Clarke, B. G., Shapiro, S. and Monroe, R. G. Myotonia atrophilica with testicular atrophy: urinary excretion of interstitial-cell-stimulating (luteinizing) hormone, androgens and 17-ketosteroids. *J. Clin. Endocrinol. Metab. 16:* 1235, 1956.
67. Sareen, C. K., Ruvalcaba, R. M. and Kelley, V. C. Gynecomastia in the physically and mentally handicapped. *Am. J. Ment. Defic. 76:* 153, 1971.
68. Relider, H., Bruhl, P. and Seth, P. K. XX-male syndrome. Pathogenesis and aspects of diagnostic pitfalls. *Urologe A 14:* 182, 1975.
69. Edwards, J. A. and Bannerman, R. M. Familial gynecomastia. *Birth Defects 7:* 193, 1971.
70. Berger, A., Simma, W. and Fischer, P. Chromosomal sex determination in idiopathic gynecomastia. *Wien. Klin. Wochenschr. 84:* 699, 1972.
71. Jull, J. W. and Dossett, J. A. Hormone excretion studies of gynecomastia of puberty. *Br. Med. J. 2:* 795, 1964.
72. Bidlingmaier, F. and Know, D. Plasma testosterone and estrogens in pubertal gynecomastia. *Z. Kinderheilkd. 115:* 89, 1973.
73. Bidlingmaier, F., Wagner-Barnak, M., Butenandt, O. and Know, D. Plasma estrogens in childhood and puberty under physiologic and pathologic conditions. *Pediatr. Res. 7:* 901, 1973.
74. Wieland, R. G. Pituitary-gonadal function in pubertal gynecomastia. *J. Pediatr. 79:* 1002, 1971.
75. Caplan, R. M. Gynecomastia from a non-estrogenic anti-androgen. *J. Clin. Endocrinol. Metab. 27:* 1348, 1967.
76. Lee, P. A. The relationship of concentrations of serum hormones to pubertal gynecomastia. *J. Pediatr. 86:* 212, 1975.
77. LaFranchi, S. H., Parlow, A. F., Lippe, B. M., Coyotupa, J. and Kaplan, S. A. Pubertal gynecomastia and transient elevation of serum estradiol levels. *Am. J. Dis. Child. 130:* 927, 1975.
78. Wilkins, L. In: The Diagnosis and Treatment of Endocrine Disorders in Childhood and Adolescence, ed. 3. Springfield, Charles C Thomas, 1965, p. 207.
79. Glass, S. J., Edmondson, H. A. and Soll, S. N. Sex hormone changes associated with liver disease. *Endocrinology 27:* 749, 1940.
80. Rupp, J., Cantarow, A., Rakoff, A. E. and Paschkis, K. E. Hormone excretion in liver disease and in gynecomastia. *J. Clin. Endocrinol. 11:* 688, 1951.
81. Gabrilove, J. L., Nicolis, G. L. and Hausknecht, R. V. Urinary testosterone, oestrogen production rate and urinary oestrogen in chromatin positive Klinefelter's syndrome. *Acta Endocrinol. 63:* 499, 1970.
82. Jacobs, L. S., Snyder, P. F., Utiger, R. D. and Daughaday, W. H. Prolactin response to thyrotropin releasing hormone in normal subjects. *J. Clin. Endocrinol. Metab. 36:* 1069, 1973.
83. Fournier, P. J. R., Desjardins, P. D. and Friesen, M. G. Current understanding of human prolactin physiology and its diagnostic and therapeutic applications. A review. *Am. J. Obstet. Gynecol. 118:* 337, 1974.
84. Klemm, W., Rager, K., Gupta, D., Nolte, K., Bierich, J. R., Schindler, A. and Keller, E. Hyperprolactinemia in boys with gynecomastia. *J. Endocrinol. 67:* 56P, 1975.
85. Frantz, A. G., Kleinberg, D. L. and Noel, G. L. Studies on prolactin in man. *Recent Progr. Horm. Res. 28:* 527, 1972.
86. Volpe, R., Killinger, D., Bird, C., Clark, A. F. and Friesen, H. Idiopathic galactorrhea and mild hypogonadism in a young adult male. *J. Clin. Endocrinol. Metab. 35:* 684, 1972.
87. Turkington, R. W. Serum prolactin levels in patients with gynecomastia. *J. Clin. Endocrinol. Metab. 34:* 62, 1972.

88. Frantz, A. G., Rabkin, M. T. and Friesen, H. Human placental lactogen in choriocarcinoma of the male. Measurement by radioimmunoassay. *J. Clin. Endocrinol. Metab. 25:* 1136, 1965.
89. Payne, R. A. and Ryan, R. J. Human placental lactogen in the male subject. *J. Urol. 107:* 99, 1972.
90. Wallach, E. E. and Garcia, C. R. Familial gynecomastia without hypogonadism: a report of three cases in one family. *J. Clin. Endocrinol. Metab. 22:* 1201, 1962.
91. Rosewater, S., Gwinup, G. and Hamwi, G. J. Familial gynecomastia. *Ann. Intern. Med. 63:* 377, 1965.
92. Miller, W. R., McDonald, D., MacFayden, I., Roberts, M. M. and Forrest, A. P. M. Androgen metabolism in gynecomastia breast tissue. *Clin. Endocrinol. 3:* 123, 1974.
93. Rajendran, K. G., Shah, P. N., Bagli, N. P., Mistry, S. S. and Ghosh, S. N. Steroid biosynthetic potential of gynecomastia tissue in man. *Horm. Res. 6:* 329, 1975.

129

Synopsis of Diagnosis and Treatment of Male Reproductive System Disorders and Current Research Trends

Emil Steinberger

DIAGNOSIS AND TREATMENT

The time-honored approach to the diagnosis of testicular disorders calls for identification of three categories of patients: those with high, those with normal, and those with low gonadotropin levels. The introduction in the past several years of radioimmunoassay techniques for quantitation of gonadotropins offered markedly improved means for precise and sensitive measurement of these hormones in blood. The radioimmunoassay techniques provided the physician with a rapid and relatively simple tool for determining patients' gonadotropin levels and thus for classifying them into one of the three above-mentioned broad diagnostic categories early during the investigational process. This rather simple approach, however, provides only very crude diagnostic guidance. A number of specific disorders do not fit into a classification based solely on gonadotropin levels. Various testicular disorders resulting from genetic, neurologic, vascular, or environmental factors or induced by drugs or toxic substances have to be considered outside of this classification (see Chapter 124).

In view of this, and for the purpose of this summary, an attempt will be made to present a different classification of testicular disorders, one based on etiology and on the influence of environmental factors. As a unifying thought the therapeutic parameter will be utilized as the underlying and fundamental function.

DISORDERS OF TESTICULAR DYSFUNCTION RESPONSIVE TO ENDOCRINE THERAPY

The most clearly understood group of testicular disorders that are amenable to therapy is hypogonadotropic hypogonadism, or a variant of this condition (Chapter 124). The diagnosis of diminished gonadotropin production can now be made with a reasonable degree of certainty utilizing not only the measurement of peripheral gonadotropin levels but also a variety of function tests (see Chapter 123). A clear diagnosis of hypogonadotropism directs the physician toward specific therapy consisting of administration of the appropriate type and the appropriate amount of gonadotropins. This should result not only in restoration of the androgenic function of the testes but also in stimulation and, in some instances, adequate restoration of the spermatogenesis compatible with fertility (see Chapter 124). However, a careful clinical and laboratory evaluation including, where indicated, detailed genetic study is essential to make a precise diagnosis, since some conditions also associated with hypogonadotropism, frequently congenital in nature, may not respond to gonadotropic therapy (see Chapter 125). Similarly a number of hyperandrogenic disorders of the adrenal gland or estrogen-producing adrenal tumors can be associated with low gonadotropin levels (see Chapter 125) but will present different laboratory finding and will require a totally different therapeutic approach.

Patients with oligospermia associated with adult seminiferous tubule failure usually show normal plasma gonadotropin and testosterone levels. In some instances, however, "low-normal" testosterone levels have been observed and found to be associated with enzymic lesion in testicular steroidogenic pathways. Since these patients may respond to gonadotropic therapy with marked improvement in spermatogenesis, every effort should be made to detect this condition (see Chapter 124). Congenital deficiency in steroidogenic enzymes affecting all steroidogenic tissues (testes and adrenals) will also lead to lack of androgen production by the testes and result in severe hypogonadism. The appropriate adrenal replacement therapy will not restore either androgenic or spermatogenic function of the testes. In these patients, only androgen replacement therapy is effective. No therapy for stimulation of spermatogenic activity is available.

CONGENITAL AND GENETIC DISORDERS OF THE TESTES

Various syndromes associated with spermatogenic deficiency fall within the category of congenital and genetic disorders. Some represent various degrees of cytogenetically detectable abnormalities, e.g., Klinefelter's syndrome, Reifenstein's syndrome, the male Turner's syndrome, and pure gonadal dysgenesis (see Chapter 124). Characteristically, these conditions can be diagnosed clinically by an astute physician. Unfortunately, no therapy for spermatogenic failure is available. If hypoandrogenism is present, androgen replacement is indicated.

Congenital abnormalities include the functional prepubertal castrate syndrome or the "vanishing testes" syndrome and various forms of testicular ectopia (see Chapter 124). Therapy for functional castrates involves only androgen replacement. No consensus has been reached in regard to therapy of testicular ectopia. First, therapy depends greatly on the position of the testes. In patients with pubic, crural, or perineal testes, the only form of therapy is surgical. In patients with unilateral cryptorchidism, medical therapy can be attempted, but surgery is frequently required. In patients with bilateral cryptorchid testes, particularly if testes are in the inguinal canal, medical therapy is frequently effective and suggested as the initial approach. The age at which therapy should be commenced is also still a point of controversy. The majority of authors suggest 5 to 7 years as the optimal age.

NEUROMUSCULAR DISORDERS

A variety of myopathies and neuropathies are associated with gonadal lesions (Chapter 124). The pathophysiology is unclear. Frequently the gonadotropin levels are elevated, but plasma androgens are normal. If impotency is present, usually it is not secondary to endocrine deficiency.

In some patients with cord lesions, retrograde ejaculation is present. In most instances, however, the sperm production is also impaired. The mechanism involved in damage to seminiferous tubules in these patients is unclear.

ENVIRONMENTAL FACTORS

Both physical and chemical agents can induce serious and at times irreversible damage to the testes, particularly to the seminiferous epithelium. The best-known effects of physical agents are those of ionizing radiation and heat. When administered at a sufficiently high dose and for a sufficient length of time, both will induce an irreversible destruction of stem cells of the germinal epithelium, resulting in permanent cessation of spermatogenic activity. No form of therapy is available to reverse this condition. Short-term or low-dose exposure may be associated with restoration of spermatogenic activity after a suitable period of recovery. However, the possibility of permanent genetic damage has to be considered in such cases.

Pitifully little is known about the effects of chemical agents, pharmacologically active substances, and a variety of other substances present in the environment. The initial observations, in the early 1950s, of germinal epithelium damage after exposure to alkylating agents were incidental findings in studies of these substances as possible anticancer drugs. Subsequently, interest in alkylating, radiomimetic, and cytotoxic drugs was revived as a result of the search for a male contraceptive. The high toxicity of these agents very rapidly dampened this enthusiasm, however, and resulted in the cessation of investigations. We are now facing a situation where a large number of individuals are exposed to a variety of pharmacologic agents, including alkylating agents, organic substances in the form of pesticides and fungicides, etc. Similarly industrial workers, as well as other segments of the population, are exposed to substances that have totally unknown effects on the testes (see Chapter 124). The cytotoxic and alkylating agents have been shown to induce mutations in germ cells of mammals. It has also been shown that men treated with these agents for a variety of neoplasias respond with severe damage to the germinal epithelium, which, however, depending on the dose and the duration of treatment, may be reversible and may allow the individual to regain fertility. Consequently, children are fathered by men who may carry genetic mutations in their germ cells and thus may introduce mutant genes into the human genetic pool with unknown consequences for future generations.

VASCULAR DISTURBANCES

Recently a great deal of interest has centered upon the observation that varicocele is associated in an unusually high percentage of cases with male infertility. Numerous publications suggest that this vascular abnormality is indeed damaging to the function of the spermatogenic epithelium and is associated with defective spermatogenesis. Various reports also suggest that ligation of the varicocele may result in a significant improvement of testicular function and an increase in fertility potential. The mechanism by which varicocele produces the damage is still unclear; numerous factors, including increased temperature of the testes, toxic substances, and increased concentration of adrenal steroids or catecholamines, have been suggested as the cause. Although a great deal of information has accumulated in the literature associating varicocele with infertility and ligation of the varicocele with improvement of the infertile state, it appears that a considerable additional effort will have to be expended in order to clearly demonstrate the relation of varicocele to spermatogenic damage, the mechanism by which this damage occurs, and the therapeutic efficacy of the surgical intervention.

INFERTILITY

Male infertility may result from testicular dysfunction, loss of integrity of the ductal system, disorders of the sex accessories (prostate and seminal vesicles), congenital or acquired abnormalities of the phallus, or neuropsychiatric disturbances. Each of these areas must be investigated during the diagnostic evaluation of the infertile male. Since fertility requires the interaction of both the male and the female, a couple-directed approach toward the diagnosis and therapy of infertility is mandatory (see Chapter 125).

A careful history and physical examination frequently provides crucial clues toward the diagnosis of overt endocrine, genetic, developmental, or vascular etiology of the infertile state. The most important single laboratory investigation is the analysis of seminal fluid. When properly performed, it will provide all the necessary information in a large segment of male partners of the infertile couple (for details, see Chapter 123). The next single most important laboratory test in men with compromised sperm production is the determination of FSH levels (see Chapter 123). The presence of markedly elevated FSH levels signifies extremely severe and irreversible damage of the germinal epithelium and suggests that no further investigations are warranted. Subtle abnormalities of the hypothalamus-pituitary axis and Leydig cell function can be detected utilizing a variety of endocrine function tests (Chapter 123). Recently sophisticated tests of the androgen biogenetic pathway in testicular tissue obtained at biopsy became feasible. These laboratory tests permit detection of deficiency of specific steroidogenic enzymes and thus permit the establishment of a definitive diagnosis and specific therapy (see Chapter 123).

Considerable attention has been focused recently on immunologic aspects of male infertility. A variety of tests have been proposed. However, the results of these tests and their relationship to fertility are difficult to interpret. Probably, postcoital tests and investigation of the in vitro ability of spermatozoa to penetrate ovulatory cervical mucus provides all the necessary information concerning possible immunologic abnormality of the spermatozoa.

One of the more important recent diagnostic endeavors has been the recognition of epididymal blocks as a cause of azoospermia or severe oligospermia. The characteristic epididymal lesions associated with an epididymal block can easily be recognized during scrotal exploration. Application of advanced microsurgical techniques provides the possibility of correction of these lesions.

In summary, although remarkable advances were made in the past several years in the development of diagnostic techniques required for evaluation of male infertility, the therapeutic success has lagged seriously behind. The only available specific therapy is that directed toward gonadotropic or Leydig cell deficiencies. Most other forms of therapy, particularly numerous forms of empirical treatment, will require a great deal more investigation before they can be considered to be effective. Surgical correction of epididymal or vasal blocks will require further refinement of microsurgical techniques, and the possible beneficial effect of varicocele ligation will require additional studies before it can be considered as an important method in therapy of male infertility.

CURRENT RESEARCH TRENDS

Disorders of the male reproductive system, particularly testicular disorders, not only may affect the individual's fertility potential but may also produce a variety of systemic consequences, e.g., inappropriate somatic, emotional, and social development, when the disorder occurs in utero or prior to puberty, and a variety of emotional, metabolic, and reproductive abnormalities when it occurs in adult life. Except for fertility disturbances, which may be caused not only by testicular disorder but also by malfunction of the excretory ducts, sex accessory organs, the nervous system, the urethra, or the phallus, the systemic abnormalities are related primarily to testicular disorders and specifically to abnormalities in the Leydig cell function.

Testicular disorders were poorly understood until the multifaceted aspect of the pathophysiology of testicular disease was recognized. At present, we are still only at the threshold of understanding the etiologic factors and pathophysiology of most testicular disorders; however, sufficient progress has been made to permit fairly precise diagnostic evaluation of some patients with testicular dysfunction.

Elucidation of the details of the kinetics of human spermatogenesis permitted the development of techniques for quantitation of the spermatogenic process. Although this technique is still primarily a research procedure, it has already shed considerable light on the details of spermatogenic lesions and their relationship to sperm output and to endocrine parameters. A simplification of this technique, which will allow it to be performed routinely, should soon provide the clinician with an important tool for establishing a precise diagnosis, aid him in devising specific therapy, and help in clarifying the prognosis.

Elucidation of the details of hormonal control of spermatogeneis (Chapter 122) has led toward the evolution of rational therapy of germinal epithelium failure associated with hormonal deficiencies. The appreciation of quantitative hormonal relationships and their relation to the spermatogenic process has led to reevaluation of our concepts of hormonal therapy and its indications. The experimental data suggesting the requirement of FSH for completion of spermatogenesis stimulated drug manufacturers to develop gonadotropic preparations with high FSH activities. The discovery that completion of meiotic division requires extremely high local concentrations of testosterone has stimulated studies to devise techniques for creating such conditions. On the other hand, the appreciation of the fact that parenteral administration of available testosterone preparations will not produce sufficiently high intratesticular concentrations of testosterone suggested that this form of therapy cannot be effective in treatment of spermatogenic lesions (see Chapter 122).

Probably one of the most important areas of recent research that has had a direct impact on the diagnostic and therapeutic capabilities of the practicing physician deals with the evolution of our knowledge related to the synthesis, secretion, transport, metabolism, and the biochemical mechanisms of action of androgen. In addition to the development of analytical techniques for quantitation of androgens and their metabolites in blood, urine, and various tissues, a number of recently discovered fundamental concepts either already have found their way into the practitioners' therapeutic and diagnostic armamentarium or hold a promise to do so. The discovery of testosterone-binding globulin (TeBG) pointed to the fact that only a small fraction of total plasma testosterone, the fraction that is not bound to TeBG (free testosterone), is biologically active. The concept that testosterone is a "prohormone" which, at the site of its action (e.g., the prostate or hypothalamus), is converted to an "active" androgen (dihydrotestosterone, DHT) or is aromatized to estrogens not only provided an explanation for a variety of physiologic mechanisms but also provided the basis for appreciation of pathophysiology of a number of congenital abnormalities and metabolic disorders (see Chapter 120). The elucidation of steroid dynamics, development of techniques to measure steroid production rates, renal clearance rates, and details of peripheral metabolism of various gonadal steroids (Chapter 120) in turn permitted development of clinically useful diagnostic techniques. The investigation of molecular mechanisms of androgen action led to the discovery of specific cytoplasmic androgen receptors and to the appreciation of induction by androgens of the transcriptional processes in the nuclei of responsive cells leading to synthesis of specific proteins. This work clarified the pathophysiology of several genetic abnormalities of the reproductive tract, including testicular feminization, various forms of pseudohermophroditism, and various forms of abnormalities of the external genitalia (see Chapter 121). The elucidation of the details of androgen biogenetic pathways (Chapter 119) and its application to the study of testes with defective spermatogenesis holds particularly exciting promise to help the clinician in diagnosis and ultimately in the development of effective therapy of patients with compromised sperm production currently diagnosed as "adult seminiferous tubule failure" or "idiopatic oligospermia." This group of patients comprises probably the largest segment of men with infertility, and no specific form of therapy is available for them. Discovery of abnormalities in the androgen biogenetic pathways in testes of these patients permitted detection of specific steroid enzyme deficiences (Chapter 125). Thus, specific diagnosis could be established of deficiencies that respond to specific forms of therapy. The techniques for in vitro investigations of androgen biogenetic pathways are still restricted to research laboratories; however, simplification of these procedures should soon place them within the reach of well-equipped hospital laboratories (see Chapter 123).

One of the most active areas of investigation involves the elucidation of the molecular mechanisms related to hormonal control of spermatogenesis. As a result of these studies, the "stepchild" of the testes—the Sertoli cell—emerged as probably one of the most important cellular elements in the testes related to the effects of hormones or spermatogenesis. A specific binding protein (androgen binding protein, ABP) has been discovered in the Sertoli cells. Although its role is still unclear, it undoubtedly plays an important role in the function of seminiferous epithelium and maturation of spermatozoa in the epididymis. Not only is it a specific testicular protein, but apparently its synthesis is under FSH control. This is the first important biochemical end point of

FSH action discovered in the testes. The Sertoli cell not only is the exclusive site of ABP production but also appears to be the only cellular element in the seminiferous tubules effected directly by FSH (see Chapter 122). These studies are still only of theoretical importance, but unquestionably as the mechanisms of hormone action on seminiferous epithelium become better understood, important information will flow toward clarification of diagnostic techniques and development of new therapeutic approaches.

The current direction of research and its recent advances suggest a marked expansion of the diagnostic horizons. They promise to provide the clinician with tools for specific biochemical diagnoses of seminiferous tubule dysfunction, Leydig cell disease, or subclinical hypothalamic-pituitary insufficiency leading to testicular abnormality. The availability of specific diagnostic techniques should permit the development of rational therapy in patients with inadequate sperm production.

Endocrinology of Conception, Pregnancy, and Parturition

130

Conception, Gamete and Ovum Transport, Implantation, Fetal–Placental Hormones, Hormonal Preparation for Parturition, and Parturition Control

John E. Buster
John R. Marshall

Because of the broad scope of this chapter, it must be more of a general review than an in depth analysis. Although it will emphasize data derived from humans or primates, it must sometimes use data from other mammals simply because of the paucity of available information.

No biologic events can exceed the events considered in this chapter in long-term importance or effect. Endocrine factors always play important roles in the control of these events.

CONCEPTION

SPERM TRANSPORT

The process of conception in the female begins with sperm transport from the vagina to the site of conception in the distal portion of the fallopian tube. An excellent review of this subject is provided by Hafez.[1] The involved organs are lined by ciliated and secretory cells, both of which play an intimate part in the transport process and are exquisitely sensitive to estrogens and progestogens.

The cervix has three transport functions that relate to sperm: (1) rapid transport of sperm to the uterine cavity, (2) colonization of cervical crypts with sperm, and (3) slow prolonged release of sperm. Rapid transport occurs immediately after sperm are placed in the vagina. Within 5–15 min following vaginal deposition, motile spermatozoa can be found in the fallopian tubes; orgasm is not required[2–4] and does not appear to play a role in sperm transport.[5] This is demonstrated by artificial insemination, in which motile sperm are placed at the cervical os by mechanical means. Fertility rate is high and no orgasm occurs. Some spermatozoa find their way into the endocervical crypts (Fig. 130-1), which serve as reservoirs. Over the next several hours, many of these spermatozoa find their way into the upper tract. This mechanism provides a more long-term source for the continued presence of spermatozoa in the upper genital tract. The role of sperm motility is poorly understood. Since disease states exist of nonmotile sperm that are otherwise healthy and such men are infertile, it is known that sperm motility is necessary. However, transport in the rapid phase to the fallopian tubes is so rapid (5 min) and sperm movement is so slow (0.1–3 mm/min), that this movement cannot account for transport.

The presence of a clear, slightly alkaline, low-viscosity cervical mucus is essential for sperm transport through the cervix. Endocrine control of cervical mucus is mediated by estrogens and progestogens. Estrogens secreted during the late follicular phase stimulate the endocervical glands to produce mucus favoring sperm transport.[6] Progestogens change this mucus to a scanty, cellular, viscous barrier.[7] With the appearance of progesterone effects in the luteal phase, the mucus becomes thick and gummy and is poorly suited for sperm penetration and transport. Thus, maximal sperm transport occurs with peak levels of unopposed estrogen just prior to ovulation.[8]

The mucus is a hydrogel composed of water and solids and consists of both low- and high-viscosity fractions.[9] The low-viscosity fraction is composed of nonmucin proteins, salts, liquids, and carbohydrates, whereas the high-viscosity fraction is composed of mucins. Under estrogen stimulation the mucinous macromoles of the high-viscosity fraction form into cross-linked chains which form long, parallel, interconnected strands several millimeters in length (Fig. 130-2). This structure is thought to allow the low-viscosity material to flow in a directed manner while the high-viscosity mucus is fixed in the endocervical crypts. This macromo-

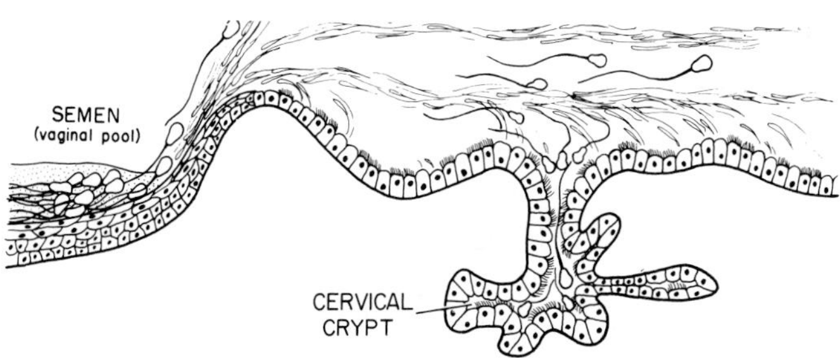

Fig. 130-1. Endocervical crypts acting as reservoirs for gradual release of spermatozoa into the upper genital tract. (Modified from Hafez and Kanagawa, In Hafez and Evans (eds.): Human Reproduction, Conception and Contraception, 1973. Courtesy of Harper & Row.)

lecular structure probably plays an important role in guiding the sperm along the endocervical canal into the endometrial cavity and into the endocervical crypts.

The endocervical mucus also fulfills a filtering function in that of all the materials contained in semen, only the normal, highly motile sperm pass through to progress to the upper genital tract.

SPERM CAPACITATION

In many species spermatozoa must undergo certain metabolic changes that occur in the female genital tract before they are able to fertilize the ovum.[10,11] The process seems to involve a sequential activation of a series of hydrolytic enzymes that allow the sperm to digest a passage through the cumulus oophorous, corona radiata, and zona pelucida. Capacitation seems to be unique to mammals and appears to be required by all species including primates and man.[12] In man the time required for capacitation appears to be 4–5 h[13] and can occur in the vagina, uterus, or oviduct.[14]

Estrogens do not appear to be required for capacitation to occur; the uteri of immature or oophorectomized rabbits are able to capacitate sperm with or without treatment with estrogens or gonadotropins.[15] Progesterone, however, demonstrates an anticapacitation effect in the uterus, though not in the oviduct.[14–16] Low doses of human chorionic gonadotropin (HCG) and luteinizing hormone (LH) enhance capacitation, whereas higher doses depress capacitation, probably through stimulation of the ovary to secrete progestogens.[17]

After capacitation, sperm oxygen consumption is increased.[18] The capacitation process appears to involve two distinct phases. The first phase appears to involve the removal of a "coating" or, perhaps, an inhibitor substance from enzyme receptor sites on the surface of the sperm. No structural changes are observable during this process. The second phase involves a morphologic change during which the acrosome is lost (Fig. 130-3). This apparently allows the acrosomal enzymes to come in contact with the materials surrounding the oocyte and allows penetration of the oocyte by the sperm. The latter phase has been termed the *acrosome reaction*.

SPERM TRANSPORT IN THE UPPER GENITAL TRACT

The mechanisms of sperm transport from the uterotubal junction to the distal portion of the fallopian tube are poorly understood. Tubal sperm transport appears to be regulated by two processes. One consists of a periodic ejection from the uterotubal junction, which Blandau has demonstrated to occur with the uterine contractions.[19] The other is transport of sperm through the oviduct, which is caused by peristaltic contractions at the time of ovulation, possibly enhanced by ciliary motion.[19]

While estrogens are known to increase and progestogens to inhibit[20–22] uterine contractions, the effect of steroids on sperm transport in the tubes is unknown.

GAMETE AND OVUM TRANSPORT

OVUM TRANSPORT THROUGH THE FALLOPIAN TUBE

After ovulation, delivery of the ovum to the endometrial cavity involves two distinct steps: (1) ovum pick-up by the fimbria from the surface of the ovary, and (2) transport of the egg mass through the tube.

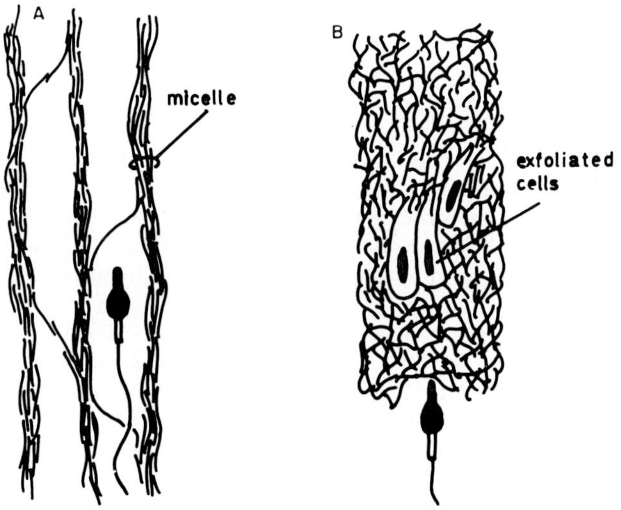

Fig. 130-2. Model of cervical mucus physical structure. A. Ovulatory or estrogenic type of secretions. Micellar structure is opened to sperm penetration. B. Luteal or progestogenic type secretions. There is a dense, disorganized micellar structure which is believed to act as a barrier to sperm penetration. (From Odeblad, E.: Acta Obstet. Gynec. Scand. *47* (Suppl) 1: 59–79, 1968 (Berlingska Boktryckeriet).)

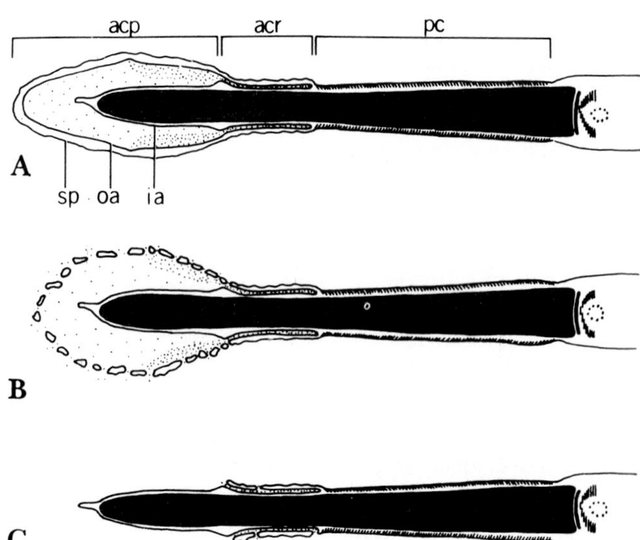

Fig. 130-3. Acrosomal reaction. Capacitated spermatozoa before (A), during (B), and after (C) acrosomal reaction. Acp, acrosomal cap region; acr, acrosomal collar region; ia, inneracrosomal membrane; oa, outeracrosomal membrane; pc, postnuclear cap region; sp, plasma membrane of the spermatozoon. (From Yanagimachi, R., and Noda, Y. D.: Am. J. Anat. *128:* 429–462, 1970 (Wistar Inst. Press).)

In the human, the oocyte is released from the ruptured follicle directly into the peritoneal cavity. Under the stimulatory effect of estrogen the fimbria move back and forth across the surface of the ovary. These movements, dramatically documented on a film by Blandau and Boling,[23] are affected by the combined muscular action of the wall of the fallopian tube, the infundibulopelvic ligament, uterovarian ligament, the meso tubarium, and the musculus attrahenstubae. Ovum pick-up is effected by the action of the cilia located on the fimbriated portion of the fallopian tube. Estrogen is the essential factor in inducing the muscular and ciliary activity required for egg pick-up. Without appropriate concentrations of estrogen, the fimbria are inactive and not closely applied to the ovarian surface.

Actual ovum pick-up is accomplished by the action of the cilia, which creates a flow of fluid into the fallopian tube. The cells of the cumulus are sticky and provide the means whereby the cilia are able to move the oocyte cell mass into the ostium of the fallopian tube. In the absence of this tacky cumulus, the cilia are ineffective in moving the ovum.[24] While estrogens are essential for the activity involved in transport, absolute concentrations seem to be less important than the decrease in estrogen concentration which occurs immediately following the midcycle LH peak and during the initial phase of egg transport.[24] Although progesterone probably takes part in the regulation of egg transport, its exact role is unclear. Progesterone levels begin to rise at about the time of ovulation. This information is interesting in light of the fact that progesterone administration increases the beating rate of the cilia by approximately 20 percent.[25]

Recent evidence suggests that prostaglandins may also play a role in oviductal motility and egg transport. E Series prostaglandins (PGE) relax while F series prostaglandins (PGF) stimulate muscular activity in the human oviduct.[26] These effects are modified by ovarian steroids, with progesterone increasing response to PGE_1 and decreasing response to $PGF_{2\alpha}$.[27] The preovulatory increase in estradiol concentration may stimulate $PGF_{2\alpha}$ synthesis in the oviductal tissue, with the peak value occurring when the tissue is most sensitive to stimulation by $PGF_{2\alpha}$.[28] Increased serum concentrations of progesterone may decrease the response to $PGF_{2\alpha}$ stimulation and increase the response to PGE_1.[27]

Once the ovum has been picked up, transport through the proximal two-thirds of the fallopian tube appears to be under the control of muscular contractions rather than ciliary action. For several hours after ovulation, the tube demonstrates an impressively complex pattern of segmental, pendular, peristaltic, and antiperistaltic contractions.[29] In addition, in some species the eggs are moved back and forth with a rotary motion that appears to be important in laying down an even coating of the mucopolysaccharides that are deposited on the eggs and form the tertiary membranes.[30]

In most mammalian species, fertilization occurs in the distal portion of the fallopian tube, and the zygote then rapidly moves into the ampullary portion of the tube, where it remains for approximately 3 days. In most species the isthmus of the tube serves as a physiologic sphincter, although no anatomic sphincter is demonstrable.[31,32] Control of both rate of transport through the ampullary portion of the tube and the isthmic sphincter are regulated by hormonal substances. Estrogen stimulates, whereas progesterone, in general, relaxes.[33,34] Both may act through prostaglandin intermediaries.[35–38] Data concerning the importance of an adrenergic isthmic sphincter and the importance of neurohypophyseal hormones are conflicting.[39]

In addition to their effects on motility, ciliary action, and ovum transport, estrogens and progesterone cause profound cyclic modifications in tubal histology and epithelial functions that are important to zygote viability. Estrogens cause an increase in height of the tubal epithelium,[40] while progesterone causes a secretory change, with the release of large amounts of PAS-reactive diastase-resistant material into the tubal lumen.[41–44] Estrogens increase, whereas progesterone decreases the rate of secretion of tubal fluid.[45,46] Tubal fluid is high in lactate and pyruvate, both of which are required for in vitro development of the zygote in experimental animals.[45,47] This fluid is also rich in bicarbonate, which is important in bringing about dispersion of the corona radiata cells from the ovum and probably facilitates conception.[47,48] Finally, tubal fluid appears to stimulate corona cell pseudopods, which normally extend into the zona pelucida, later to be withdrawn.[49,50]

PHARMACOLOGIC EFFECTS OF HORMONES

Virtually no information concerning the pharmacologic action of hormones on egg transport is available from humans. Virtually all of the work relating ovarian steroids to egg transport has been done in intact or oophorectomized animals receiving exogenous hormones. Using these models there are profound species differences, and it is therefore difficult to relate these studies directly to humans. Depending upon the animal and the dose, estrogen can either "lock" the tube, with resultant delayed transport, or can increase the rate of transport, with resultant premature passage of the oocyte into the endometrial cavity.[31,51–54] The effect of progestational steroids on egg transport is dependent upon the timing of administration of progestogens. When administered prior to ovulation, accelerated transport occurs.[55] When the same dose is given after ovulation, a marginal delay in transport is observed.[56] Pharmacologic administration of prostaglandins can also affect tubal egg transport.[28] Estrogens may enhance the effects of locally released norepinephrine by preventing inactivation.[57]

IMPLANTATION

Fertilization usually takes place in the distal third of the fallopian tube; however, under pathologic conditions, this process can also take place in the peritoneal cavity or in the ovary. The action of the tube on the egg mass gradually removes the corona radiata, making sperm penetration easier. Random movement brings the sperm and the egg into contact; there is no evidence of any trophic substance serving to attract the sperm to the egg. The zona pelucida can be entered at any point by the sperm. The hyaluronidase, or other enzymes such as acrosin, on the capacitated sperm head is thought to facilitate sperm penetration through the zona pelucida in all mammalian species as well as man.[58] The entire fertilizing sperm enters the ovum.[59] Thus, there is both a nuclear and cytoplasmic contribution to the zygote. Following sperm penetration, the fertilized ovum forms the second polar body. Nuclear material from sperm and ovum develop into male and female pronuclei, which meet and unite. Fusion of these haploid nuclei gives rise to a new individual with a diploid number of chromosomes. Subsequent divisions are mitotic.

The first mitotic cleavage occurs after approximately 30 h and gives rise to the two-cell zygote stage.[60] Subsequent cleavages occur at an accelerating rate as the resulting cells become smaller and smaller. The four-cell state occurs about 40 h following fertilization.[61] The morula appears at about 50–60 h, and the blastocyst appears 3–4 days following fertilization.[60]

On about the fourth day following ovulation the blastocyst, still encased in the zona pelucida, enters the endometrial cavity[62] and then begins to develop eccentrically within the zona. Approximately 5–6 days following fertilization, protoplasmic processes from the blastocyst cells grow through the zona pelucida, passing beyond its outer boundary.[62] About 6–6½ days following fertilization the blastocyst attaches to the uterine mucosa by means of these penetrations through the zona. The zona pelucida then disappears and the expanding conceptus settles into the endometrium.

That portion of the blastocyst which came to lie against the zona pelucida and which subsequently perforated through the zona constitutes that portion of the blastocyst destined to become trophoblastic cells. Those cells that are more internally located come to form the inner cell mass, that portion destined to become the embryo.

FETAL–PLACENTAL HORMONES

The placenta, and the fetus and placenta in cooperation, secrete a diverse profile of glycoprotein, protein, and steroid hormones into the maternal circulation. Concentrations of these hormones in peripheral blood change with increasing gestational age and fetoplacental maturity. Abnormally high or low concentrations occur in association with a variety of obstetric disorders.

PROTEIN AND GLYCOPROTEIN HORMONES

Origins and Mechanisms of Production

The pattern of pregnancy-related glycoprotein and protein hormones measurable in peripheral blood from implantation to parturition is determined largely by placental syncytiotrophoblast secretion into the intervillous space.[63–69] Relatively small but significant amounts of these hormones are secreted into the fetal circulation. Their production continues without immediate regard to fetal viability. Rate-modulating mechanisms are poorly understood.[68–74] Likewise, very little is known about the effects of placental glycoprotein and protein hormones secreted into the fetal circulation.[70,71] The list of known secreted placental proteins and glycoproteins is becoming increasingly lengthy and includes: HCG, human placental lactogen (HPL), human chorionic thyrotropin, pregnancy-specific β_1-glycoprotein, heat-stable alkaline phosphatase, and many others.[74,75] Only HCG and HPL, both readily measurable in peripheral blood by specific radioimmunoassay[76–80] have been investigated extensively.

HCG is a double-chained glycoprotein with a molecular weight of approximately 36,000–40,000.[81] The α chain is biochemically and immunologically similar to the α chain of the three pituitary glycoprotein hormones: LH, follicle-stimulating hormone (FSH), and thyroid-stimulating hormone.[81,82] The β chain is biochemically and immunologically unique, a feature which has been utilized to develop relatively specific radioimmunoassays for HCG and its β subunit.[76] The major role of HCG appears to be in the support of corpus luteum progesterone production, a function essential for maintenance of the pregnancy through the seventh week calculated from the last menstrual period of a 28-day cycle.[83,84] Its function(s) beyond the seventh week is not known.[68] Likewise, the mechanisms regulating its production and secretion by the placenta are not understood. The circulating half-life of HCG is a two-component disappearance curve: the first component is about 11 h, and the second component is about 23 h.[85]

HPL is a 190-amino acid polypeptide with a molecular weight of approximately 21,500.[86,87] Its molecular structure is similar to that of prolactin and growth hormone.[86,87] The major functions of HPL are probably involved with mobilization and metabolism of maternal fat stores.[88] Since HPL is an insulin antagonist, it appears to be involved with the regulation of maternal blood sugar levels so as to provide optimally for fetal caloric requirements.[88] This effect is undoubtedly a major factor in the diabetogenic effect of pregnancy. The mechanisms regulating its production and secretion by the placenta are poorly understood.[73] The circulating half-life of HPL is 12–25 min.[89]

Maternal Serum Concentrations in Normal and Diseased Pregnancies

HCG is first detectable in peripheral serum 7–12 days following a conceptual ovulation (days 21–26 of a 28-day cycle)[64,90,91] (Fig. 130-4). This corresponds closely to the penetration of the trophoblast-covered blastocyst into the endometrial stroma on the seventh postovulatory day and its subsequent direct apposition to the maternal circulation.[92] HCG levels rise logarithmically over the 10 days following implantation at a doubling time of 1.7 days.[65] Peak circulating concentrations vary around a mean of about 60,000 mIU/ml between 9 and 12 weeks.[93] This is followed by a fall to a plateau ranging from 12,000 to 28,000 mIU/ml between 16 and 30 weeks. There is then a small gradual second rise to about 45,000 mIU/ml at term.[93]

In women presenting with threatened abortion, serum HCG concentrations generally correlate well with the ultimate outcome. In one investigation HCG concentrations exceeding 18,600 mIU/ml, measured at the time of initial evaluation, were associated with a favorable outcome.[94] Values of less than 10,600 mIU/ml were, with unusual exceptions, associated with ultimate abortion of the pregnancy.[94]

In women afflicted with untreated gestational trophoblastic neoplasms, HCG concentrations are generally greater than 320,000 mIU/ml. HCG levels in this range strongly support this diagnosis, provided that the sample is obtained after the 14th week of amenorrhea.[95] Since, with normal pregnancy the highest HCG concentrations are observed between the 9th and 12th weeks and may occasionally reach or exceed 320,000 mIU/ml, serum HCG concentrations measured prior to the 14th week are not diagnostic. HCG measurements are frequently utilized as a tumor marker to indicate whether residual tumor is present following surgical or chemotherapeutic treatment. Specific β-subunit radioimmunoassays for HCG, which show less cross-reactivity with LH, are particularly suited to this purpose when HCG concentrations fall into the pituitary LH range and persistent HCG activity may

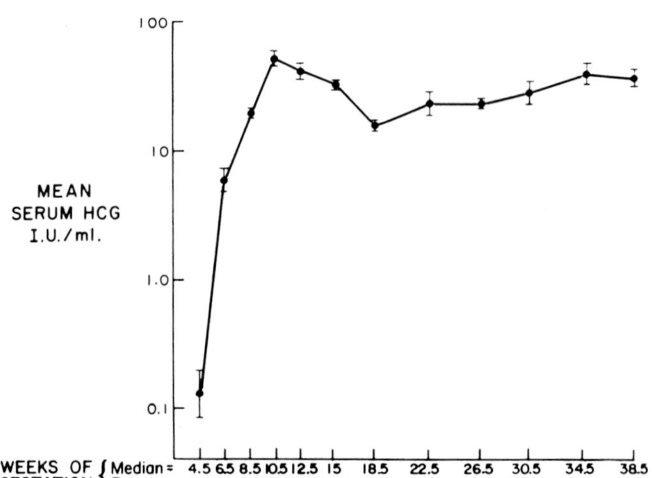

Fig. 130-4. Serum HCG concentrations from conception until term. Mean ± SEM. (From Goldstein et al.: Am. J. Obstet. Gynecol. *102:* 110–114, 1968.

otherwise be masked. Remission is considered obtained when HCG is repeatedly undetectable by a β-subunit assay over 3 consecutive weeks. The remission is considered permanent if HCG remains undetectable after 5 yr.[96]

HPL is first detectable during the 5th–6th week of pregnancy[80] (Fig. 130-5). HPL concentrations rise gradually from approximately 0.2 μg/ml between 7 and 10 weeks to a plateau ranging from approximately 6.0 to 10.0 μg/ml beginning at 34 weeks and persisting until term.[79,93,97] From 30 weeks on there are few normal values of less than 4.0 μg/ml.[96]

In women presenting with threatened abortion in whom abortion does not subsequently occur, the rise in HPL concentrations characteristic of the first trimester continues with little deviation. In cases in which abortion does occur, HPL is very low and correlates well with the outcome if the sample is obtained at 9 weeks or after.[98,99]

In women afflicted with trophoblastic disease, HPL concentrations consistently fall within a range of less than 10 percent of the normal level for the estimated gestational age of the pregnancy.[93] The reasons for low HPL concentrations are unknown but may be related to trophoblastic immaturity and to a deficiency of the more sophisticated enzyme systems necessary to produce this hormone.[93] Unusually high HCG levels associated with very low HPL levels after 8 weeks gestational age strongly suggest the diagnosis of trophoblastic disease.[93]

In women pregnant in the third trimester in whom there is need to assess fetal well being, HPL concentrations may be of significant predictive value in the assessment of hypertensive toxemia and dysmaturity–postmaturity syndromes but are of no value in the management of diabetes and Rh sensitization.[97] After 30 weeks, concentrations of less than 4 ng/ml ("fetal danger zone"[97]) are an indication of serious fetal compromise.[97]

STEROID HORMONES

Origins and Mechanisms of Production

Steroid hormones measurable in maternal blood from implantation to parturition arise from multiple maternal and fetal–placental sources. The relative contributions of maternal adrenals, ovaries, liver, and fetus–placenta to circulating maternal concentrations of certain steroids shift sharply during the first trimester from maternal origins to fetal–placental origins.

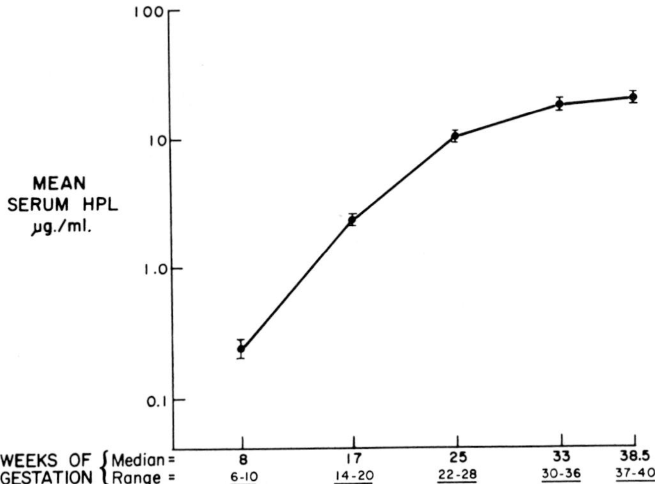

Fig. 130-5. Serum HPL levels in normal pregnancy from first trimester until term. Mean ± SEM. (Modified from Saxena et al.: Am. J. Obstet. Gynecol. *102:* 120, 1968.)

First Trimester. Immediately following conception, the major source of circulating sex steroids is the corpus luteum, which, supported by rising HCG levels, continues to function well past its normal 14-day life span. The corpus luteum remains as a major source of circulating maternal sex steroids through approximately 12–13 weeks.[19,100] After the 7th week, however, the placenta assumes an increasingly important quantitative role in the production and secretion of steroid hormones (the luteoplacental shift), which continues until the time of parturition. This is substantiated by reports that surgical luteectomy prior to the 7th week almost invariably results in abortion, while after the 7th week such surgery does not disturb the pregnancy.[83,84] These findings illustrate the important functional autonomy acquired by the conceptus following the 7th week as it becomes increasingly efficient in steroid hormone production.

Second and Third Trimesters. During the second and third trimesters of pregnancy, the profile of steroid hormone levels measured in the maternal circulation is the result of a series of complex interactions centered on the placenta, with precusor exchanges involving the fetal adrenals and liver and maternal adrenals and liver.

The *placenta* becomes the single most important production source of C_{18} and C_{21} sex steroids in both fetal and maternal circulations. At term, it secretes them in strikingly large amounts. The placenta is an imcomplete steroidogenic organ in that many of the enzyme systems needed to produce steroid hormones from simple two-carbon acetate are not present. The placenta can extract, however, the necessary precursors and intermediates from either the fetal or maternal circulations.

The *fetal adrenal cortex* ultimately differentiates into a thick inner (fetal) zone and a thin outer (definitive) zone. The original elements of the fetal zone first appear at about 35 days (dated from the last menstrual flow) and are steroidogenically active by 50 days.[101] The definitive zone first appears at about 50 days,[101] but it is not substantially involved in steroidogenesis until well into the second trimester,[102] in rough temporal association with development of the hypothalamus and hypophyseal portal vascular systems.[103] Since there is a functioning fetoplacental circulation by 4 weeks,[92] the steroids produced by the fetal cortex are presented to the placenta as soon as the former is hormonally active. The fetal zone is the major source of C_{19} steroids until birth. After birth, with removal of the placenta, the fetal zone undergoes atrophy.

The fetal circulation contains a substantial preponderance of sulfoconjugated Δ^5C_{21} steroids—e.g., pregnenolone sulfate (Δ^5P-S), 17α-hydroxypregnenolone sulfate (17-Δ^5P-S)—and Δ^5C_{19} steroids—e.g., dehydroepiandrosterone sulfate (D-S) and 16α-hydroxydehydroepiandrosterone sulfate (16-D-S). A circulating fetal hormone profile, shifting heavily toward Δ^5 sulfoconjugates rather than Δ^4 steroids, is apparently the result of a fetal adrenal zone 3β-hydroxysteroid dehydrogenase enzyme deficiency combined with a very active fetal sulfokinase system.[74,75] The fetal regulation of its own adrenal cortical function probably involves ACTH, prolactin, and perhaps other fetal trophic hormones.[70,71,104–109] Prior to 20 weeks, the fetal cortex will develop normally in the absence of ACTH, as it does in the anencephalic.[108] HCG, fetal prolactin, or other trophic hormones must therefore be of some significance in its initial development.[109] Beyond 20 weeks, ACTH apparently has both maintenance and regulatory roles, as has been demonstrated by studies on both normal and anencephalic pregnancies in the third trimester.[108] In addition, it appears that the fetal adrenal may function in secretory bursts similar to the adult since fetal scalp levels of Δ^5 P-S and D-S fluctuate considerably but in parallel during the stress of normal labor.[110]

The *maternal adrenal cortex* is a major source of precursors for placental steroidogenesis, particularly D-S. Approximately 30 percent of the daily maternal production of D-S is extracted by the placenta and converted to estradiol (E_2).[111] In addition, the maternal adrenal cortex secretes a considerable quantity of cortisol, which, after oxidation of the 11-hydroxyl group (11β-hydroxysteroid dehydrogenase) by the placenta, enters the fetal circulation predominantly as cortisone.[112] The physiologic importance of this exchange is not understood.

The *fetal liver* is the major source of circulating fetal cholesterol since transfer from the maternal circulation is probably minimal.[113] Fetal liver cholesterol may be an important substrate in fetal adrenal steroidogenesis. Under conditions of fetal malnutrition, depleted fetal cholesterol stores may be a rate-limiting factor in the adrenal production of Δ^5 steroid sulfoconjugates.[114] In addition, the fetal liver has a very active 16α-hydroxylase system, and is therefore quantitatively important in the 16α-hydroxylation of a variety of C_{18}, C_{19}, and C_{21} steroids.[74,75] The measurement of maternal levels of 16α-hydroxylated placental steroids, e.g., estriol (E_3) and estetrol (E_4), have been investigated clinically as indicators of fetal well being since they are derived largely from circulating fetal 16α-hydroxylated precursors.

The *maternal liver* is the major source of circulating maternal cholesterol, the single most important precursor in placental progesterone production.[74,75,115] It is also a minor source of 16α-hydroxylated steroid sulfoconjugates.[111,116] Finally, the maternal liver clears and conjugates placental steroids, which then become highly water soluble and are easily excreted through the maternal kidneys.[117]

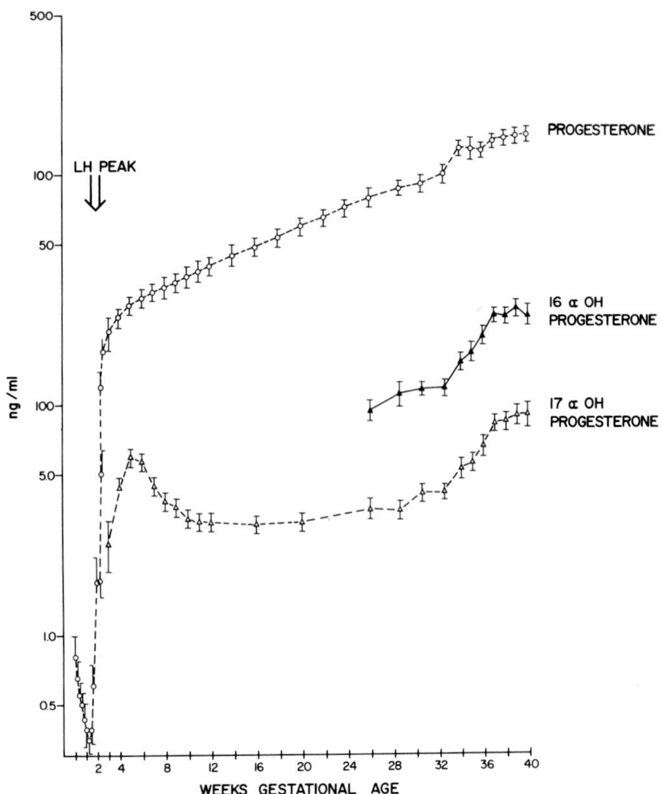

Fig. 130-6. Mean concentrations ± SEM of progesterone, 16α-hydroxyprogesterone, and 17α-hydroxyprogesterone from the first trimester until term. Data were compiled from several reports.[100,118,119,126] Gestational ages are calculated from the last menstrual flow.

Maternal Serum Concentrations in Normal and Diseased Pregnancies

C_{21} Steroids. *Serum progesterone* (P) concentrations are less than 1 ng/ml during the follicular phase of the normal menstrual cycle (Fig. 130-6). In a conceptual cycle, P concentrations rise to 1–2 ng/ml on the day of the LH peak, rise again sharply to a plateau of 10–35 ng/ml over the subsequent 7 days, fluctuate generally within the limits of this plateau through the 10th week (dated from the last menstrual flow), and then show a sustained rise which continues until term; at term P concentrations range from 100 to 300 ng/ml.[118,119] As mentioned previously, P originates almost entirely from the corpus luteum prior to 5–6 weeks gestational age. The luteoplacental shift occurs soon after the 7th week. After 12 weeks, the placenta is the major source of P[100] (Fig. 130-7). The placenta contains all of the enzyme systems necessary to produce P from circulating maternal cholesterol and is minimally dependent upon fetal steroidogenesis.[74,75,115] For these reasons, P concentrations in maternal serum reflect upon corpus luteum steroidogenesis during the first 5–6 weeks, a mixture of corpus luteum and placental steroidogenesis through the 12th week, and then primarily placental steroidogenesis from the 12th week until term.

In women presenting with threatened spontaneous abortion in the first trimester, P concentrations measured at the time of initial evaluation correlate roughly with ultimate prognosis. Approximately 80 percent of those with P less than 10 ng/ml will abort.[94]

In women pregnant with hydatidiform moles, P concentrations are significantly elevated above normal levels for comparable gestational age. This disparity is particularly pronounced between the 10th and 20th weeks. Blood HCG levels greater than 320,000 mIU/ml after 14 weeks of amenorrhea, combined with an elevated P concentration, are indicative of a hydatidiform mole.[95]

In women whose pregnancies are complicated by rhesus isoimmunization, P concentrations are elevated approximately two-fold above values from normal pregnancies of comparable gestational age. This elevation may be related to a 2–3-fold increase in placental mass associated with erythroblastosis.[120] Higher P concentrations have been associated with a less favorable prognosis.[120]

Serum 17α-hydroxyprogesterone (17-P) concentrations are less than 0.5 ng/ml during the follicular phase of the normal menstrual cycle. In a conceptual cycle, 17-P concentrations rise to about 1 ng/ml on the day of the LH peak, fall slightly for about 1 day, rise again over the subsequent 4–5 days to a level of 1–2 ng/ml, and then increase gradually to a mean of approximately 2 ng/ml (luteal phase levels) at the end of 12 weeks; this level remains relatively stable until about the 32nd week, when there begins an abrupt sequential rise to a mean of approximately 7 ng/ml at 37 weeks, which persists until term[100,118,119] (Fig. 130-6). The rise beginning at 32 weeks correlates strikingly with the activity of fetal maturational processes known to begin at this time.

17-P originates predominantly from the corpus luteum during the first trimester of pregnancy[100,121] (Fig. 130-8). The ovaries continue to be a source of 17-P throughout pregnancy. During the third trimester, however, the placenta, utilizing fetal precursors, secretes increasing amounts of 17-P and is probably the major source of this hormone at term.[122]

In women undergoing spontaneous abortion, falling concentrations of 17-P parallel falling concentrations of P.[123] Although speculative, it is possible that 17-P levels may provide information in assessing the mechanism of abortions due to corpus luteum dysfunction. Up through the time of the luteoplacental shift, at about 7 weeks, 17-P levels reflect primarily on corpus luteum steroidogenesis.[100,121]

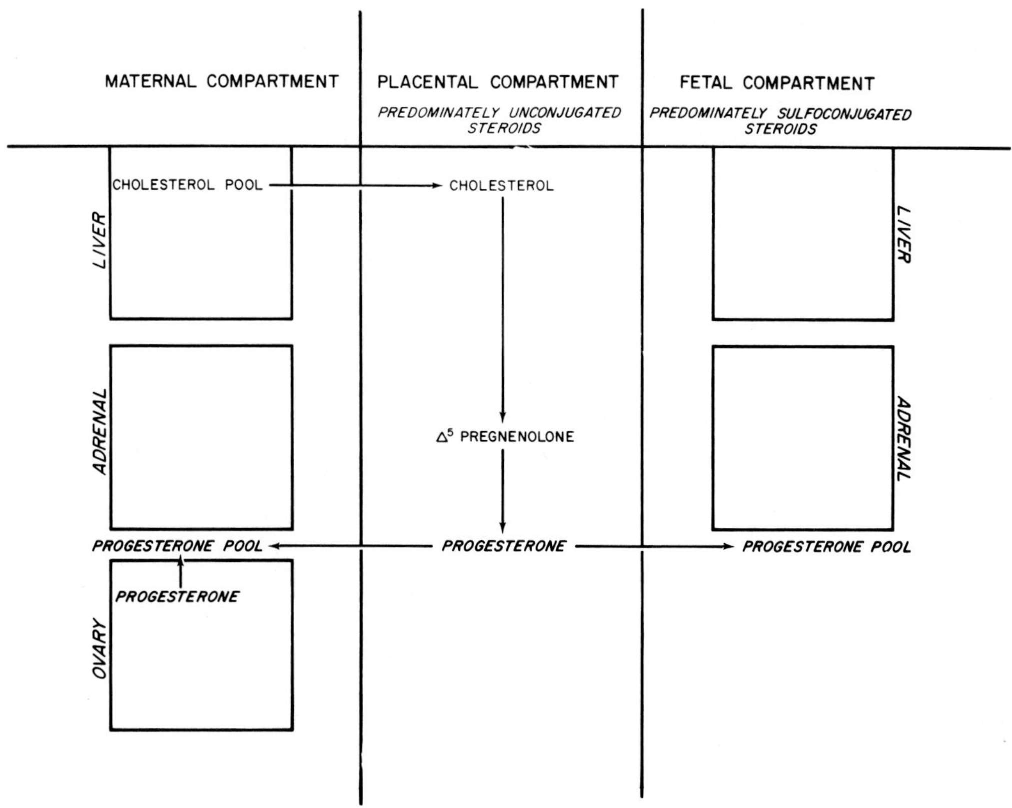

Fig. 130-7. Anatomic compartmentalization of progesterone production. Although several pathways other than the ones depicted are known to exist, the extraction and conversion of cholesterol from the maternal pool is believed to be a major source of fetal placental progesterone production.[75,115]

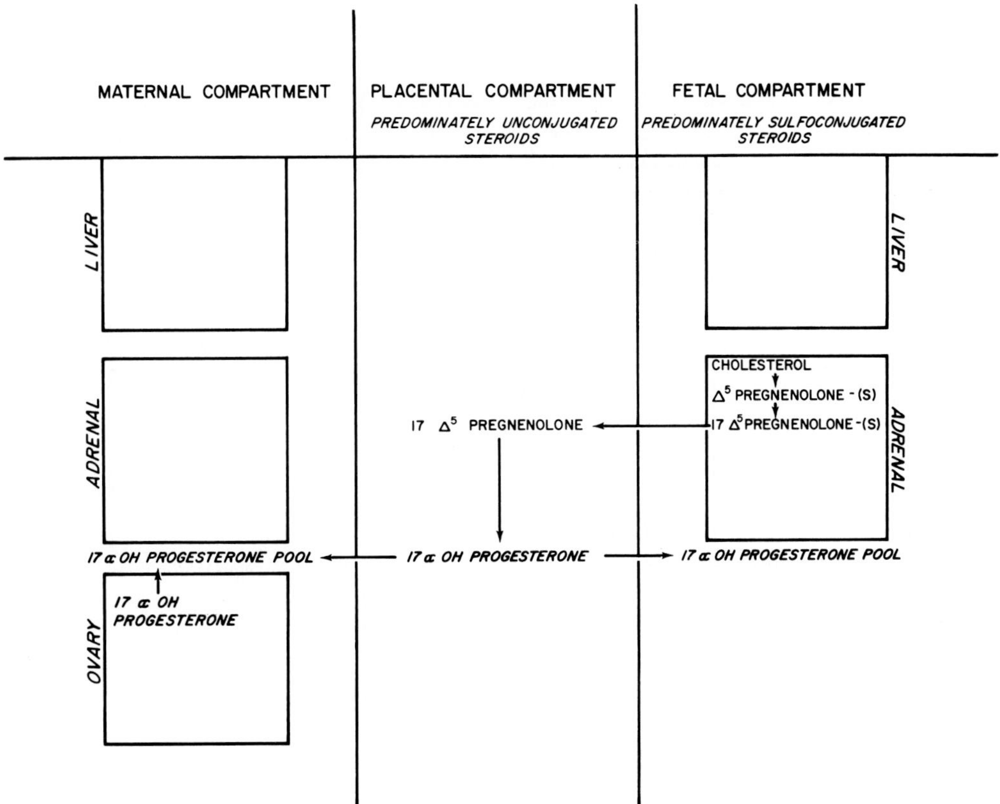

Fig. 130-8. Anatomic compartmentalization of 17α-hydroxyprogesterone production. The corpus luteum is the major source of 17α-hydroxyprogesterone during the first trimester. The fetus and placenta in cooperation are believed to secrete the great bulk of this steroid during the third trimester. Although several known alternate pathways are not depicted, the suppression of 17α-hydroxyprogesterone concentrations by intravenous maternal cortisol infusion during the third trimester indicates that a major pathway is from fetal adrenal cholesterol through the Δ^5C_{21} sulfoconjugates to 17-Δ^5 pregnenolone sulfate. 17-Δ^5 pregnenolone sulfate is converted to 17α-hydroxyprogesterone by placental 3β-hydroxysteroid dehydrogenase and Δ^{4-5} isomerase systems.[74,75,122,126]

Serum 16α-hydroxyprogesterone (16-P) concentrations fluctuate around a mean of 0.5 ng/ml during the follicular phase of the normal menstrual cycle and rise significantly to a mean of 1.2 ng/ml during the luteal phase.[124] 16-P levels rise gradually with increasing gestational age, until about the 32nd week; then an abrupt continuous sequential rise begins from a mean of about 12 ng/ml (32 weeks) to about 25 ng/ml at 37 weeks, which persists until term (Fig. 130-6). The overall pattern of 16-P levels from 32 weeks to term is nearly identical to 17-P and is therefore associated temporally with the activation of fetal maturational processes during the third trimester.

Sources of 16-P have been studied only superficially but are probably predominantly fetoplacental throughout later pregnancy[125,126] (Fig. 130-9). While there is a highly significant third trimester association between rising levels of 16-P and 17-P, it is possible that the measurement of these two hormones provides data about fetal steroidogenic activities that are related but reflect very different mechanisms of regulation.[126] It has been shown that large maternal intravenous doses of cortisol produce an abrupt and precipitus drop in maternal levels of 17-P but affect 16-P very little.[126] It therefore appears that the availability of placental 16-P precursors, unlike that of 17-P precursors, is not directly regulated by the fetal adrenal or fetal pituitary adrenal feedback loops. Data available from second-trimester isotope studies and third-trimester concentration gradient measurements indicate that the major pathway in the production of 16-P centers around 16α-hydroxylation of placental Δ^5 pregnenolone by the fetal liver.[74,75] The final steps probably involve conversion of 16-Δ^5P-S of fetal liver origin to 16-P by the placenta, which then secretes this steroid into the maternal and fetal circulations[74,75] (Fig. 130-9).

The relationship of 16-P concentrations to fetal well being is unknown. 16-P concentrations correlate closely with unconjugated E_3, which is believed to reflect upon fetal condition with considerable accuracy (see below).[125] The use of 16-P concentrations as a peripheral circulating marker of the fetal maturation process has been suggested.[126]

C_{19} Steroid. Serum D-S levels fluctuate widely around a mean of 1600 ng/ml through the normal menstrual cycle. In pregnancy, with advancing gestational age, D-S levels decrease. At term, they fluctuate around a mean of 800 ng/ml[128,129] (Fig. 130-10).

D-S originates almost entirely from the maternal adrenal cortex, where its secretion pattern is regulated by maternal ACTH.[116] In nongravid women, D-S is cleared by the liver and kidney and excreted into the urine with the various other 17-ketosteroids.[116] In pregnancy, there is a progressive increase in the metabolic clearance rate of D-S (MCR_{D-S}), which rises some 6–10-fold above nonpregnant levels (about 7 liters/24 h).[109] This increase in MCR_{D-S} is related in large part to irreversible placental extraction of D-S with ultimate conversion through intermediates to placental estrogens. The increase in MCR_{D-S} is probably the cause of lower D-S levels during pregnancy. In this regard, it is interesting that falling maternal D-S levels plot almost identically to the log reciprocal of rising maternal E_2 levels (Fig. 130-10),[129] and the rate of this conversion rises with advancing gestational age in association with increasing placental mass.[130]

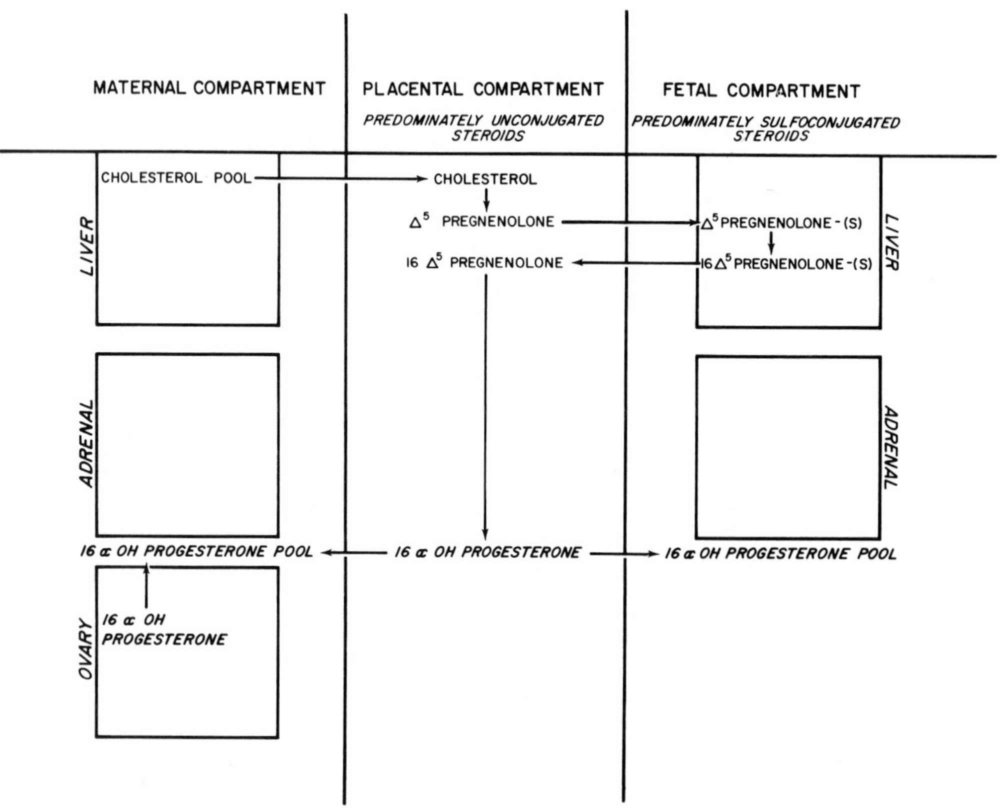

Fig. 130-9. Anatomic compartmentalization of 16α-hydroxyprogesterone production. The bulk of circulating maternal 16α-hydroxyprogesterone probably originates from the maternal ovary during early first trimester but shifts progressively toward fetal–placental production during later pregnancy. Although many pathways are probably involved with the production of 16α-hydroxyprogesterone and are not depicted here, the nonsuppressibility of circulating maternal 16α-hydroxyprogesterone after a maternal intravenous infusion of cortisol implies that the production of this steroid by the fetus and placenta is not dependent upon fetal ACTH regulation. Available data as a whole indicate that the predominant pathways involve fetal liver 16α-hydroxylation of placental Δ^5 pregnenolone, completely bypassing fetal adrenal conversion of cholesterol to Δ^5 pregnenolone, a major site of ACTH steroidogenic regulation.[102,124–127,151,185]

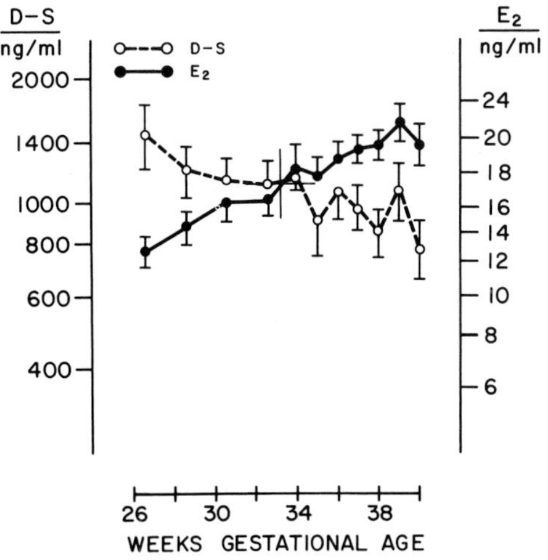

Fig. 130-10. Maternal D-S (DHEA-S) and E_2 (estradiol) concentrations (ng/ml) from 26 weeks to term. Mean ± SEM was calculated from 19 normal subjects sampled serially. Increasing MCR_{D-S} is probably the cause of falling D-S levels with increasing gestational age.[109,128,129] Gestational ages are calculated from last menstrual flow. Falling D-S and rising E_2 concentrations probably reflect upon increasing placental conversion of D-S to estradiol with advancing gestational age and increasing placental mass.[129,130]

There is evidence to indicate that the efficiency with which the placenta extracts circulating maternal D-S and converts it to estrogens becomes impeded early in the course of disorders associated with impaired placental function.[131–133] One approach to this problem has involved the measurement of MCR_{D-S} in pregnancies at risk for toxemia. MCR_{D-S} increases at a subnormal rate long before the onset of hypertension and proteinuria.[131] MCR_{D-S} may be an indicator of uteroplacental perfusion,[131–133] and, if so, suggests that a defect in uteroplacental perfusion regulation may be a major factor leading to toxemia.

Another approach to this problem has involved the administration of a large maternal intravenous dose of D-S with serial measurement of postinfusion D-S levels combined with simultaneous measurement of D-S placental end products, e.g., unconjugated dehydroepiandrosterone (D), estrone (E_1), and E_2. Even in the second trimester, with an intact functioning placenta, the half-life of the D-S dose is significantly shorter than when the placenta is removed.[134] In addition, with the placenta intact, there is a striking and abrupt rise in serum levels of unconjugated D, E_1, and E_2 that does not occur when the placenta is removed. These data indicate that the D-S dose is being extracted and converted to various unconjugated end products by the placenta in measurable amounts.[134] This test has been refined by use of serial E_4 measurements to monitor the response to D-S.[135] E_4 (see below) is formed from circulating fetal 15α-hydroxylated precursors. Following intravenous infusion of D-S, E_4 levels rise gradually beginning at 1 h and reaching maximum levels at 4 h. In order for this to occur the D-S must either cross or be converted in the placenta in order to be 15α-hydroxylated to a circulating fetal E_4 precursor. Such a test has a theoretical advantage of assessing both the fetal and placental metabolism of the D-S load.[135]

The clinical utility of these tests has been under study by many investigators.[135–138] They may prove useful in the early diagnosis of placental insufficiency states[135–138] and in vivo definition of congenital placental enzyme deficiencies.[134–136]

C_{18} Steroids. Serum unconjugated E_1 concentrations are less than 0.1 ng/ml during the follicular phase and may reach 0.3 ng/ml during the luteal phase of a normal menstrual cycle. Following a conceptual cycle, E_1 levels remain within the luteal phase range through 6–10 weeks. Subsequently there is a gradual increase to a range of approximately 2–30 ng/ml at term (Fig. 130-11).[100,119,139]

E_1 originates primarily from maternal sources (ovaries, adrenals, peripheral conversion) for the first 4–6 weeks. After this time, the placenta secretes increasing quantities of E_1, which it converts from circulating maternal and fetal D-S. After the first trimester, the placenta is the major source of circulating E_1 (Fig. 130-12).[100]

Unconjugated E_1 levels probably reflect upon the same metabolic processes involved with the production of unconjugated E_2. Individual variation and range of values for unconjugated E_1 are so wide, however, that its concentrations have not been studied extensively in diseased pregnancies.[139]

Serum E_2 concentrations are less than 0.1 ng/ml during the follicular phase and may reach 0.15 ng/ml during the luteal phase of a normal menstrual cycle. Following a conceptual cycle, E_2 closely parallels the pattern described for E_1, with a gradual increase to a range of 6–40 ng/ml[118,139] at term (Fig. 130-11).

E_2 originates almost exclusively from the maternal ovaries for the first 5–6 weeks. After this time, the placenta secretes increasing quantities of E_2, which it converts from circulating maternal and fetal D-S. After the first trimester, the placenta is the major source of circulating E_2.[100] At term, approximately equal amounts of placental E_2 are converted from circulating maternal D-S and fetal D-S (Fig. 130-12).[140,141]

In women presenting with threatened first-trimester abortion, E_2 concentrations measured at the time of initial evaluation correlate roughly with ultimate prognosis. Approximately 90 percent of those in whom E_2 is less than 0.4 ng/ml will abort.[94]

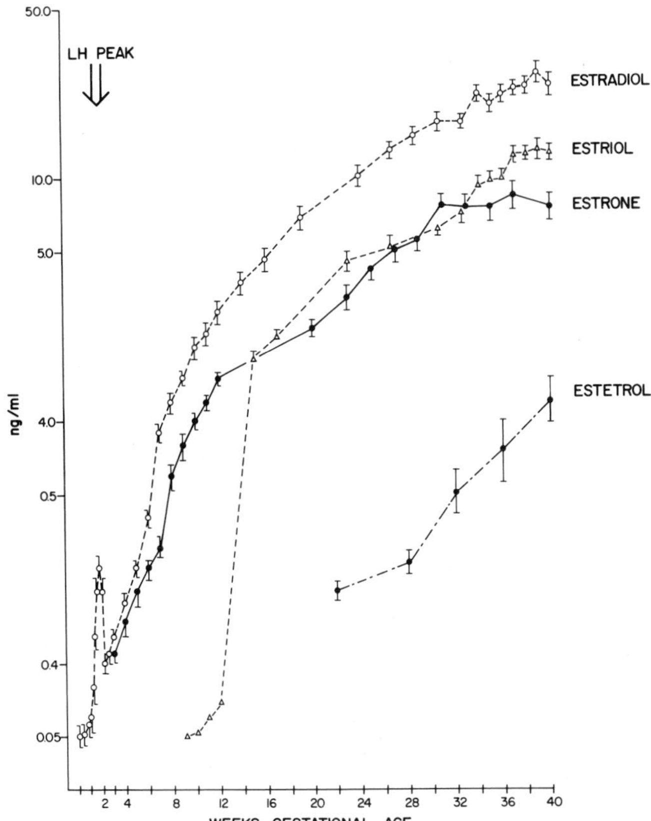

Fig. 130-11. Mean concentrations ± SEM of estrone, estradiol, estriol, and estetrol from early first trimester until term. Data were compiled from several different reports.[100,118,119,129,155] Gestational ages are calculated from the last menstrual flow.

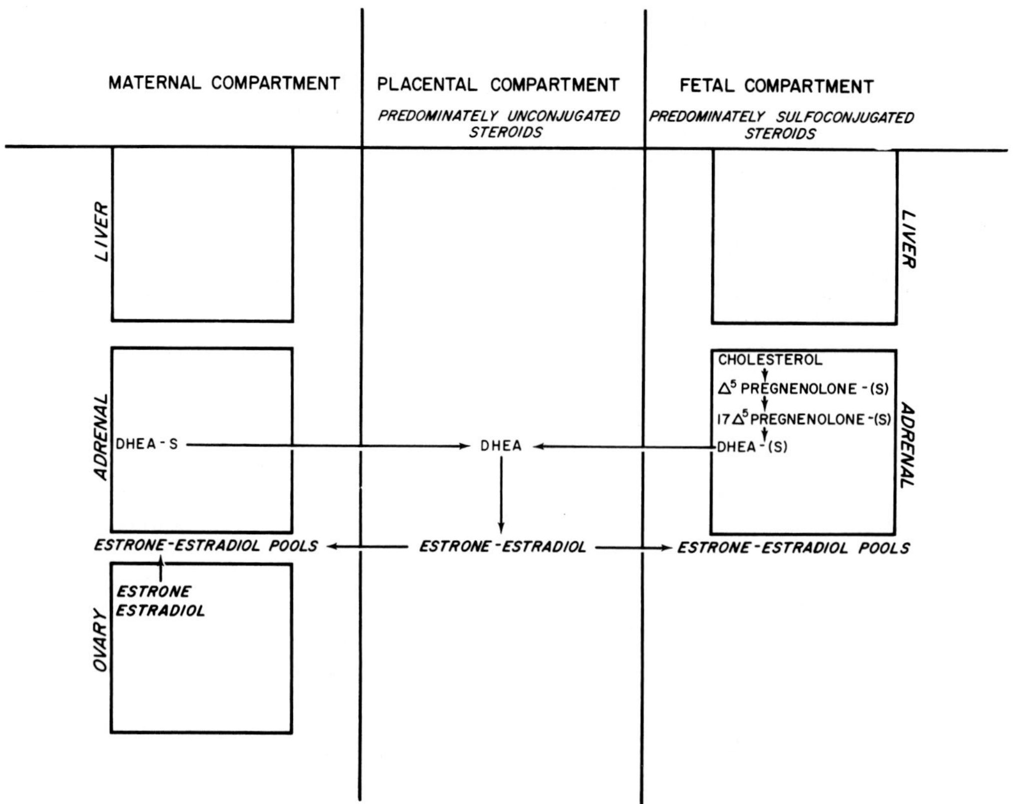

Fig. 130-12. Anatomic compartmentalization of estrone and estradiol production. During the first trimester the corpus luteum is the major source of circulating maternal estrone and estradiol. Progressing through the second into the third trimester the placenta becomes the major source of these two steroids. At term, the placenta extracts D-S (DHEA-S) from both maternal and fetal circulations and, via placental hydrolysis and aromatization, converts this steroid to estrone and estradiol, which is secreted into both the maternal and the fetal circulations for further metabolism.[74,75,108]

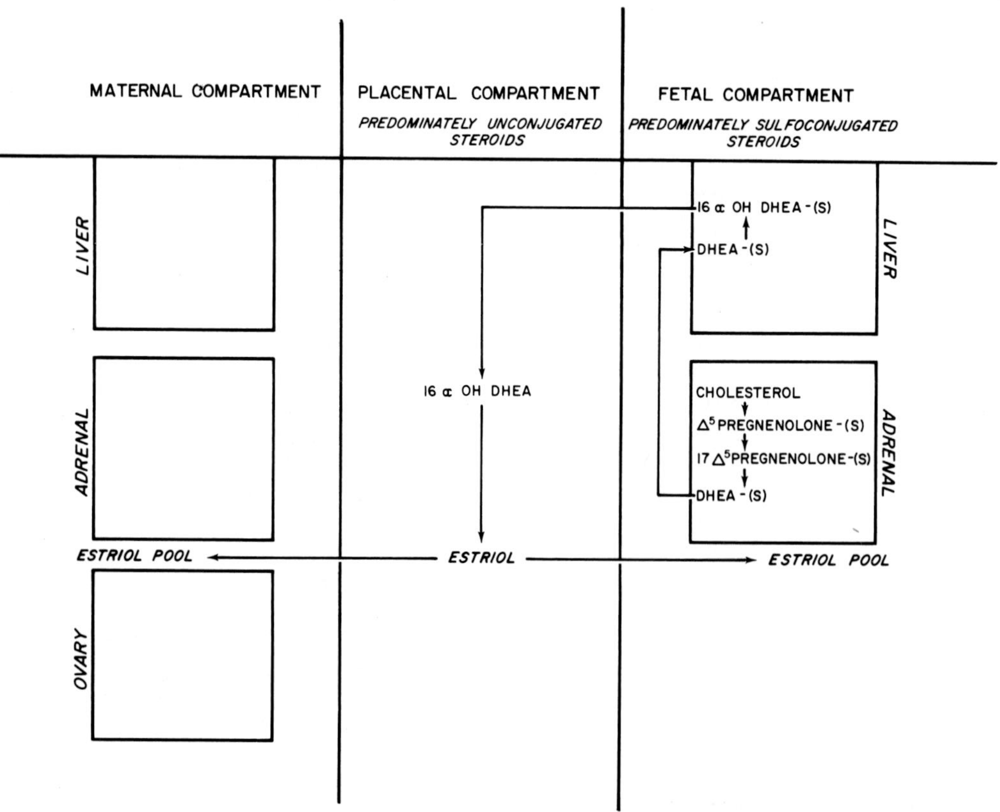

Fig. 130-13. Anatomic compartmentalization of estriol production. The major precursor to estriol production by the placenta is believed to be fetal 16α-hydroxydehydroepiandrosterone sulfate [16α-OH DHEA-(S)]. 16α-hydroxylation of D-S is believed to be a fetal liver steroidogenic activity with minimal activity involving the fetal adrenal and some activity involving the maternal liver. Circulating maternal estriol levels are suppressible by maternal intravenous cortisol infusion, implying a significant role of fetal ACTH regulation in a conversion of fetal adrenal cholesterol to Δ^5 pregnenolone and subsequent intermediates.[75,104,108,151]

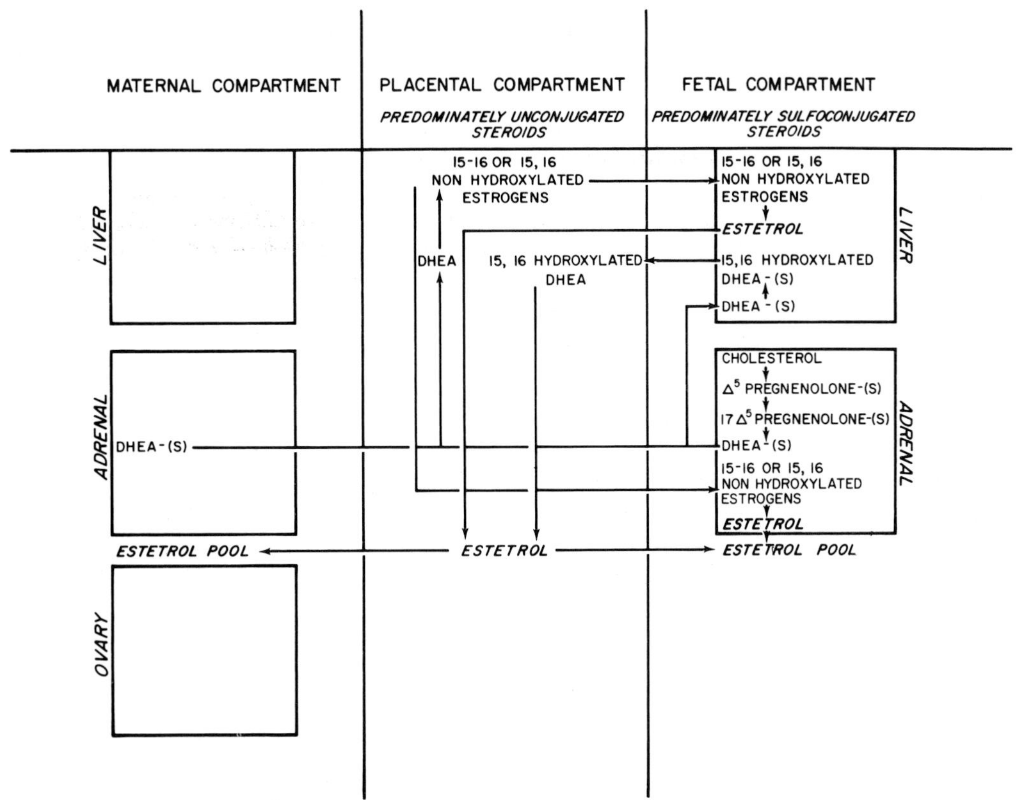

Fig. 130-14. Anatomic compartmentalization of estetrol production. The quantitative importance of pathways depicted is not known. The 15, 16-hydroxylated neutral steroids and 15, 16 or 15-16 nonhydroxylated estrogens are believed to be major contributors. D-S [DHEA-(S)] of fetal adrenal origin is probably quantitatively the major estetrol precursor, however, D-S of maternal adrenal origin may be a significant contributor.[135,154]

In the assessment of fetal well being during the third trimester, E_2 concentrations show a rough correlation with the clinical situation. Although original reports were promising,[141] other recent studies indicate a considerable overlap between normal and abnormal values.[142] In addition, E_2 fluctuates frequently to misleadingly low concentrations.[143] Since nearly half of E_2 secreted at term is converted by the placenta from maternal D-S, it is possible that undulations in maternal adrenal D-S production may explain, in part, this lack of correlation.

Serum unconjugated E_3 is undetectable at a sensitivity of 0.01 ng/ml in nonpregnant women. E_3 is first detectable at a sensitivity of 0.05 ng/ml at 9 weeks[100] and then increases gradually to a range of approximately 6–24 ng/ml at term (Fig. 130-11).[144] There is a particularly sharp rise, as well as scattering of values, between 35–40 weeks (Fig. 130-11).[139,144]

Unconjugated E_3 originates almost exclusively from the placenta.[117,145] It is produced chiefly from placental conversion of fetal 16-D-S.[74,75,114] The appearance of unconjugated E_3 in maternal serum at 9 weeks corresponds closely to increasing steroidogenic development of the fetal adrenal cortex.[71,143] Its continued production is therefore dependent upon the presence of a living fetus (Fig. 130-13).

Changes in unconjugated E_3 concentrations reflect upon fetal death, fetal anomalies, hydatidiform mole, and fetoplacental well being during the third trimester.

Fetal death at any time in the second or third trimester produces a striking drop in unconjugated E_3 concentrations within 1–2 h following demise.[144] Within 4–6 h following death, concentrations are consistently less than 1 ng/ml in the second trimester and less than 2.5 ng/ml in the third trimester.[110,144]

Fetal anomalies associated with adrenal hypoplasia, e.g., anencephaly, are associated with low concentrations of unconjugated E_3.[144] For this reason, evaluation of unexplained low unconjugated E_3 levels should include ultrasonography or x-ray.

Hydatidiform moles are associated with low concentrations of unconjugated E_3.[144] Presumably, this occurs secondary to the absence of a fetal adrenal and liver and the consequent deficiency of fetal 16α-hydroxylated sulfoconjugated precursors.

Deteriorating fetoplacental health during the third trimester is associated with falling unconjugated E_3 concentrations. The weight of available data indicates that placental secretion of E_3 is related to many factors, including fetal size and fluctuations in fetoplacental oxygen tension. The former has been documented.[147] The latter is strongly suggested by the known rate-limiting effects of fetal precursor availability on placental E_3 biosynthesis,[148] the decreased availability of fetal precursors in growth-retarded newborns,[149,150] and the established observation that steroidogenic pathways involved with the fetal biosynthesis of these precursors are dependent on availability of molecular oxygen.[151] Furthermore, published clinical experience with urinary E_3 and serum E_3 measurements shows best correlations with various hypoxia and malnutritive "placental insufficiency" disorders such as pregnancy-induced hypertension, idiopathic intrauterine growth retardation and postdatism—less so with diabetic embryopathy.[152] The major clinical value of E_3 determinations has been in the assurance of fetal well being and in the prevention of unnecessary obstetric intervention.[152] Each patient, however, requires sampling on multiple occasions in order to establish a trend. Attempts to construct a statistical "fetal danger zone" applicable to all pregnancies have been disappointing.[142]

Serum unconjugated E_4 levels are undetectable at a sensitivity of 0.05 ng/ml in nonpregnant women. Unconjugated E_4 levels rise with increasing gestational age to a range of approximately 1–4 ng/ml during the third trimester (Fig. 130-11).[153]

Unconjugated E_4 originates almost exclusively from the placenta. It is produced chiefly from placental conversion of circulating fetal 15α-hydroxylated derivatives of E_2, E_3, and D-S (Fig. 130-14).[154] Its continued production is therefore dependent upon the presence of a living fetus.

Unconjugated E_4 concentrations reflect upon fetal death, fetal anomalies, and molar pregnancies, as do unconjugated E_3 levels. In the assessment of fetoplacental well being, preliminary studies suggest that unconjugated E_4 does not correlate any better, if as well, with the clinical situation than does E_3.[154,155] The measurement of E_4 in combination with a loading intravenous dose of D-S, as was described previously, has been promising.[135]

PARTURITION

In a normally progressing human pregnancy, fetal preparation for parturition is nearly complete by 34–36 weeks gestational age (dated from last menstrual period). Delivery at any time from this point to 40 weeks is generally productive of a newborn free of the hazards of prematurity. A multiplicity of interdependent hormonal events involving both mother and fetus regulate the final maturation process, culminating in the events surrounding labor and delivery.

HORMONAL PREPARATION FOR PARTURITION: FETAL MATURATION AND ITS REGULATION

At approximately 34–36 weeks, there is a striking increase in fetal exposure to endogenous glucocorticoids. This observation is supported by reports indicating a sharp rise in amniotic fluid cortisol in samples obtained after 34 weeks as opposed to samples obtained between 20 and 34 weeks[156] (Fig. 130-15). A sharp third trimester rise in cord levels of cortisol and cortisone confirm that similar changes occur in the fetal circulation with statistically significant correlations.[157] This corticoid rise is probably mediated almost entirely in the fetal compartment since most circulating fetal cortisol (biologically the most active corticoid) is believed to be of fetal origin[157] Presumably, the fetal adrenal is producing increasing amounts of corticoid in response to fetal ACTH. However, it is likely that there is an intrinsic increase in fetal adrenal sensitivity of ACTH since circulating fetal ACTH levels fall rather than rise at this time (Fig. 130-15).[158] Augmented adrenal sensitivity to ACTH with increasing gestational age has been clearly documented in the fetal lamb model and may involve a facilitating effect of fetal prolactin.[159,160]

The corticoid rise is associated with the induction of enzyme systems catalyzing the production of pulmonary surfactant and the storage of glycogen in the fetal liver, skeletal, and cardiac muscle.[161–164] Both events occur approximately concomitantly at 34–36 weeks. The increase in pulmonary surfactant is essential for alveolar stability and, when not present in adequate amounts, results in widespread atelectasis and respiratory distress after birth.[162] Glycogen stores are the major source of carbohydrates for modulation of blood sugar levels during the early hours of extrauterine life. They are also directly related to the ability of the fetus to withstand hypoxia during labor.[161,162]

The central regulator of the third trimester maturational sequence is unknown. Extrapolation from in vitro and animal investigation combined with associations evident from human studies permit the generalizations that are summarized in Fig. 130-15: (1) Rising levels of fetal prolactin activate fetal adrenal receptor sites,[105,165] stimuate increasing fetal adrenal growth rate,[105] and

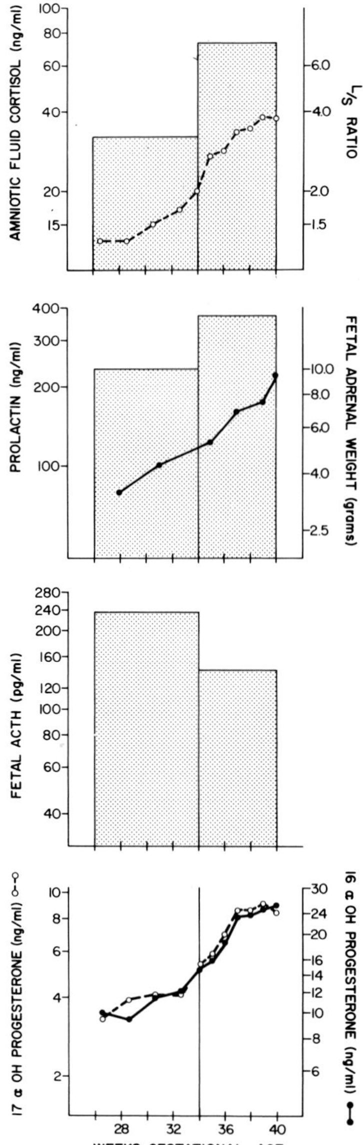

Fig. 130-15. Hormonal interrelationships of fetal maturation regulation from 26 weeks until term. At 34 weeks there is an abrupt rise in amniotic fluid and circulating fetal cortisol, a mechanism believed to be the final common pathway through which fetal maturational processes are regulated. There is an associated abrupt rise in the lecithin/sphingomyelin ratio,[162–164] a marker of fetal pulmonary surfactant maturation. In common with the rise in fetal cortisol is an increase in circulating prolactin levels. This is associated with an increase in fetal adrenal mass, increased storage of steroid precursors, and increasing sensitivity of the fetal adrenal to ACTH. Circulating levels of fetal ACTH fall abruptly at 34 weeks and remain at lower levels until term. The suppression of fetal ACTH may reflect upon a negative feedback mechanism mediated through cortisol. There is an abrupt rise in circulating maternal concentrations of 16α-hydroxyprogesterone and 17α-hydroxyprogesterone beginning at 34 weeks, in striking association with the above intrauterine hormonal and maturational processes. Maternal 17α-hydroxyprogesterone concentrations are corticosteroid suppressible and would therefore appear to reflect upon accelerated fetal adrenal steroidogenic activity. Maternal concentrations of 16α-hydroxyprogesterone are not corticosteroid suppressible and are not directly dependent upon fetal adrenal ACTH-regulated steroidogenesis; therefore they may reflect more upon the induction of fetal liver 16α-hydroxylase enzyme activity, which in turn may be modified by increasing fetal cortisol production.[105,122,136,156–158,162–164]

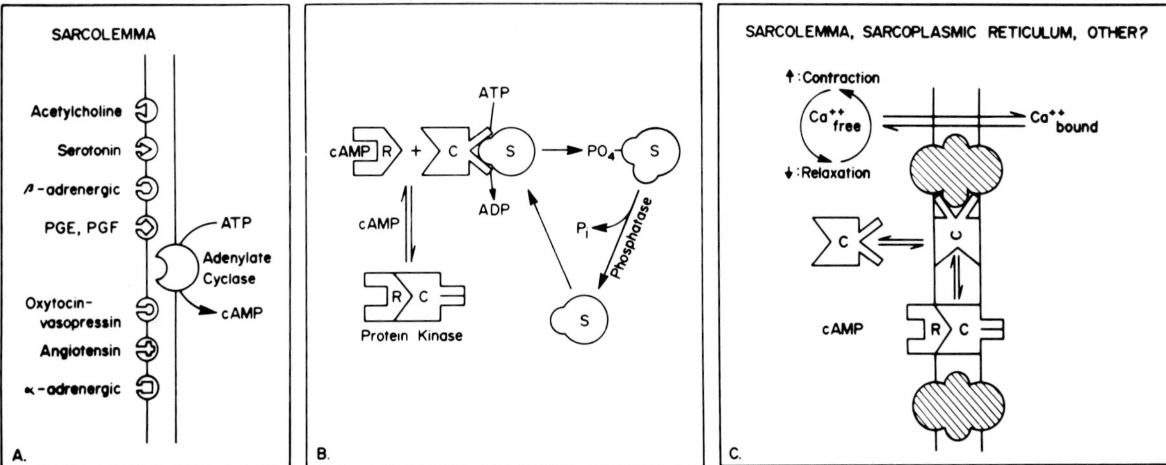

Fig. 130-16. Possible mechanisms through which the myometrial adenylate cyclase system regulates contractility. A. cAMP levels elevated by β-adrenergic stimulation of adenylate cyclase in the sarcolemma are modified by a variety of active agents in a process mediated by their specific membrane receptors. B. cAMP activates cytosol protein kinase by binding to the regulatory subunit (R), liberating free catalytic subunit (C), which then phosphorylates specific protein substrates (S), altering their activity or function. C. In myometrial smooth muscle cells, free catalytic subunits translocate to cell membranes, where they are incorporated through hydrophobic interactions. Increased phosphorylation of specific membrane proteins by the newly acquired protein kinase molecules in some manner increases Ca^{++} transport activity, lowering the free:bound ratio of intracellular Ca^{++}, causing inactivation of actomyosin Ca^{++} sensitive ATPase and hence relaxation. (From Korenman and Krall: Biol. Reprod. *16:* 1, 1977.

facilitate steroidogenesis, resulting in increasing fetal cortisol (and other corticoids?) production. (2) Rising fetal corticoid levels activate diverse fetal maturational processes, including pulmonary surfactant, as indicated by rising amniotic fluid lecithin/sphingomyelin ratios.[162–164] (3) Rising fetal corticoid levels also suppress fetal pituitary ACTH.[158] (4) Rising maternal circulating concentrations of 16-P and 17-P result from placental passage/production of these steroids, whose precursors may be directly involved with increasing fetal corticoid production or are the result of steroidogenic pathways stimulated by fetal corticoids.[126]

HORMONAL REGULATION OF LABOR

The present level of knowledge does not permit a unified construct that clearly binds the multiplicity of fetal and maternal regulatory mechanisms that trigger the onset of labor in the human. The weight of available data, however, indicates that the final common pathway leading to myometrial irritability, contractility, and actual labor is directed through mechanisms modulating myometrial adenylate cyclase and intracellular Ca^{++} sequestration.[166] Through a series of complex interactions beginning with cell membrane receptor binding by hormones or other regulatory substances, cAMP levels are either increased or suppressed, eventuating through several steps to increased intracellular sequestration of Ca^{++} ↑ (cAMP) with relaxation or Ca^{++} liberation ↓ (cAMP) with contraction. Known intermediate details of this process have been reviewed in depth[166] (Fig. 130-16). Major effectors interacting with specific cAMP-modulating receptors include the prostaglandins and their intermediates, oxytocin, and catecholamines. Each of these is reviewed below under fetal or maternal factors in parturition control.

Fetal Factors

These factors include fetal membrane and decidual prostaglandin synthesis, fetal steroids, and fetal oxytocin.

Prostaglandins. Prostaglandins exert both a sensitizing and myometrial stimulating effect through their specific surface receptors.[166] The prostaglandin sequence beginning with arachadonic acid–enriched phospholipids is outlined in Figure 130-17. Arachadonic acid, the common progenitor to the various prostaglandins and their intermediates, resides in cell membranes of the amnion, chorion, and deciduum, primarily in the 2-acyl position of the ubiquitous glycerophospholipids (Fig. 130-18).[167–170] Bound as an

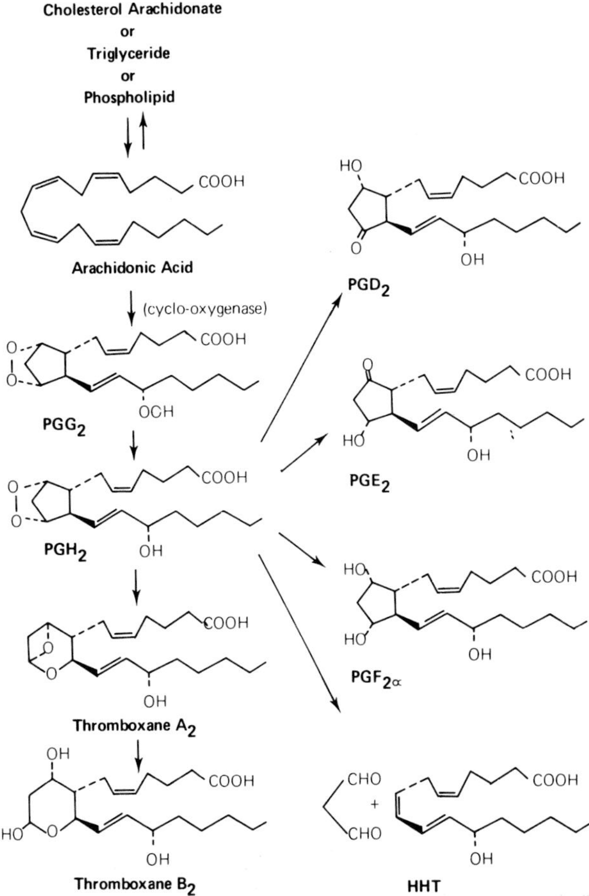

Fig. 130-17. Arachadonic acid cascade. (Modified from Ramwell et al.: Biol. Reprod. *16:* 70, 1977.)

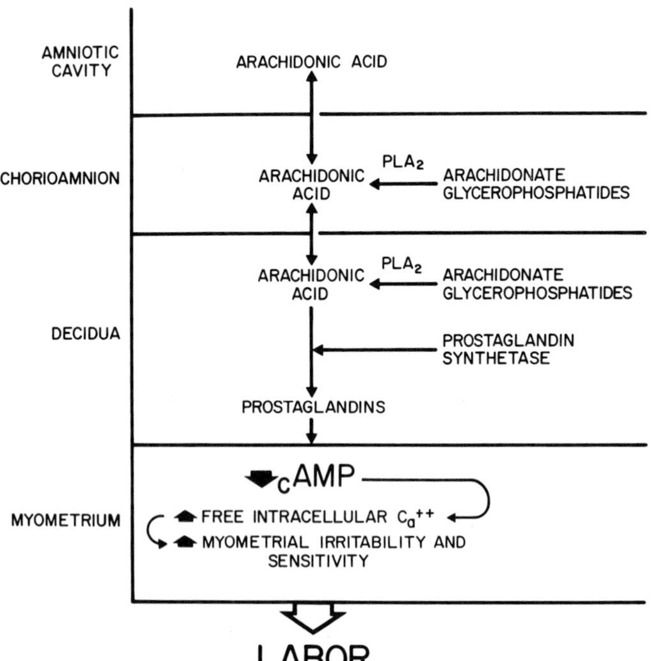

Fig. 130-18. Anatomic compartmentalization of phospholipids and prostaglandin synthesis in fetal membranes and decidua. The final common pathway for uterine contractility is mediated through cAMP. Prostaglandins are believed to suppress intracellular cAMP levels, which, through intermediate steps, lead to increased intracellular unbound Ca^{++} and myometrial contraction PLA_2: phospholipase A_2.

arachadonate-2-glycerophophatide, arachadonic acid is released into the prostaglandin sequence by the lysosomal enzyme phospholipase A_2 (PLA_2).[167,171,172] PLA_2 activity is greatest in the amnion and decidua and is contained by the lysosomal stability of these tissues,[167] a stability believed to be maintained in part by P and disrupted by E_2.[167,173] PLA_2 activity is increased by any mechanical, toxic, or hormonal factor that disrupts the integrity of lysosomal membranes. Once arachadonic acid is liberated, it is acted upon quickly by cyclooxygenase to form the PGG_2 and PGH_2 endoperoxides (Fig. 130-17), which themselves, though short lived, may be biologically active prior to their transformation to the classical E and F series prostaglandins.[168] PLA_2 activity is believed to be the major rate-limiting factor[167,168,171,172] and may be a major regulatory point in the initiation of parturition. During labor there is a marked elevation of amniotic fluid arachadonic acid, PGE, and $PGF_{2\alpha}$, presumably from retrograde movement of these substances from fetal membranes and decidua.[169] Prostaglandins secreted into the maternal circulation are cleared by the lungs and are therefore not detected at elevated levels in the peripheral circulation.[168] The anatomic compartmentalization of these processes is depicted in Figure 130-18.

Fetal Steroids. By strong inference from animal data and as suggested by the tendency of anencephalic pregnancies to labor either too early or too late, it is likely that the fetal hypothalamic–pituitary–adrenal axis is at least a fine modulator in the timing of human parturition. In human studies, there is no characteristic shift of maternal steroid concentrations just prior to or during labor.[167] The demonstration of a P-binding substance[173] in the chorioamnion, a protein which competes for P and may labilize lysosomal stability, provides a steroid-mediated mechanism that would not be measurable as a change in circulating concentrations in either mother or fetus. Animal models describing fetal steroidal modulation of parturition have been reviewed widely.[174–177] The extension of these models to man is very uncertain.[184]

Fetal Oxytocin. Fetal oxytocin concentrations measured after vaginal delivery exceed those measured in newborns delivered by cesarean section.[178] Oxytocin from the fetal side is transferred into the maternal circulation[179] and could be important in initiating and/or maintaining labor. This is implied from studies in fetal lambs showing that oxytocin infusion on the fetal side stimulates uterine contractions.[180]

Maternal Factors

Maternal Oxytocin. Hormonal events within the uterus cause it to become increasingly sensitive to the maternal influences of oxytocin with increasing gestational age. Oxytocin sensitivity is practically nil until approximately 20 weeks, at which time it increases progressively to plateau at 36 weeks, until just prior to labor, when it increases again.[181] Maternal oxytocin is released in spurts once labor is started. The further labor has progressed, the greater the spurt frequency.[182,183] Oxytocin acts directly on myometrial receptors to produce its depolarizing effect, possibly via adenylate cyclase suppression, and is therefore presumably complimentary to prostaglandins.[166] Maternal oxytocin may be involved with maintenance of established labor.

Maternal Catecholamines. Maternal catecholamines reach myometrial α and β receptors both by the circulation and neuronal transmission. Catecholamine receptors are copious throughout the myometrium, but the exact role of catecholamines in modulating parturition is unknown.[166]

REFERENCES

1. Hafez, E. S. E. Gamete transport. In Hafez, E. S. E., and Evans, T. N. (Eds.): Human Reproduction: Conception and Contraception. New York, Harper & Row, 1973, p. 85.
2. Rubenstein, B. B., Strauss, H., Lazarus, M. L., and Hankin, H. Sperm survival in women. *Fertil. Steril. 2:* 15, 1951.
3. Masters, W. H., and Johnson, V. E. Human Sexual Response. Boston, Little, Brown, 1966.
4. Masters, W. H., and Johnson, V. E.: Uterine response and sperm migration. In Human Sexual Response. Boston, Little, Brown, 1966.
5. Sobrero, A. J. Sperm migration in the female. *J. Sex. Res. 3:* 319, 1967.
6. Cohen, M. R., Stein, I. F., and Kaye, B. M. Spinnbarkeit: A characterization of cervical mucus, significance at ovulation time. *Fertil. Steril. 3:* 201, 1952.
7. Moghissi, K. S. Cyclic changes of cervical mucus in normal and progestin treated women. *Fertil. Steril. 17:* 663, 1966.
8. Sobrero, A. J. Sperm migration in the female genital tract. In Hartman, C. G. (ed.): Mechanisms Concerned with Conception. New York, MacMillan, 1963, p. 173.
9. Odeblad, E. The physics of the cervical mucus. *Acta Obstet. Gynecol. Scand. 38* [*Suppl. 1*]: 44, 1959.
10. Chang, M. C. Fertilizing capacity of spermatozoa deposited into the fallopian tubes. *Nature* 168: 697, 1951.
11. Austin, C. R. Observations on the penetration of the sperm into the mammalian egg. *Aust. J. Sci. Res. 4B:* 581, 1951.
12. Dukelow, W. R., and Fujimoto, S. Capacitation of sperm. In Behrman, S. J., and Kistner, R. W. (eds.): Progress in Infertility, 2nd ed. Boston, Little, Brown, 1975, p. 745.
13. Seitz, H. M., Rocha, G., Brackett, B. G., and Mastroianni, L. Maturation and cleavage of human ova in vitro. In Proceedings of the Third Annual Meeting of the Society for the Study of Reproduction. New York, Academic, 1970, p. 16.

14. Bedford, J. M. Experimental requirement for capacitation and observations on ultrastructural changes in rabbit spermatozoa during fertilization. *J. Reprod. Fertil.* [*Suppl*] *2:* 35, 1967.
15. Bedford, J. M. The influence of oestrogen and progesterone on sperm capacitation in the reproductive tract of the female rabbit. *J. Endocrinol. 46:* 191, 1970.
16. Chang, M. C. Capacitation of rabbit spermatozoa in the uterus with special reference to the reproductive phases of the female. *Endocrinology 63:* 619, 1958.
17. Soupart, P. Effects of human chorionic gonadotropin on capacitation of rabbit spermatozoa. *Nature 212:* 408, 1966.
18. Hamner, C. E., and Williams, W. L. Effect of the female reproductive tract on sperm metabolism in the rabbit and fowl. *J. Reprod. Fertil. 5:* 143, 1963.
19. Blandau, R. J. Gamete transport in the female mammal. In Greep, R. O., Astwood, E. B., and Geiger, S. R. (eds.): Handbook of Physiology, section 7, vol. 2. Baltimore, Waverly, 1973. p. 153.
20. Carsten, M. E. Regulation of myometrial composition, growth, and activity. In Assali, N. S. (ed.): Biology of Gestation, vol. 1. New York, Academic, 1969, p. 355.
21. Kao, C. Y. Ionic basis of electrical activity in uterine smooth muscle. In Wynn, R. M. (ed.): Cellular Biology of the Uterus. Amsterdam, North-Holland, 1967, p. 386.
22. Csapo, A. I. The four direct regulatory factors of myometrial function. In Wolstenholme, G. E. W., and Knight, J. (eds.): Progesterone: Its Regulatory Effect on the Myometrium. London, Churchill, 1969, p. 13.
23. Blandau, R. J., and Boling, J. L. An experimental approach to the study of egg transport through the oviduct of mammals. In Segal, S. J., Crozier, R., Corfman, P., and Condliffe, P. (eds.): The Regulation of Mammalian Reproduction. Springfield, Ill., Thomas, 1972.
24. Blandau, R. J. Gamete transport—comparative aspects. In Hafez, E. S. E., and Blandau, R. J. (eds.): The Mammalian Oviduct. Chicago, University of Chicago Press, 1969, p. 129.
25. Borell, V., Nilsson, O., and Westman, A. Ciliary activity in the rabbit fallopian tube during oestrus and after copulation. *Acta Obstet. Gynecol. Scand. 36:* 22, 1957.
26. Coutinho, E. M., and Maia, M. S. The contractile response of the human uterus, fallopian tubes and ovary to prostaglandins in vivo. *Fertil. Steril. 22:* 539, 1971.
27. Spilman, C. H. Oviduct response to prostaglandins. Influence of estradiol and progesterone. *Prostaglandins 7:* 465, 1974.
28. Spilman, C. H., and Harper, M. J. R. Effects of prostaglandins on oviductal motility and egg transport. *Gynecol. Invest. 6:* 186, 1875.
29. Asdell, S. A. Spermatozoan and ovum transport through the oviduct. *Zooiatria 3:* 1, 1961.
30. Greenwald, G. S. Endocrine regulation of the secretion of mucin in the tubal epithelium of the rabbit. *Anat. Rec. 130:* 447, 1958.
31. Greenwald, G. S. A study of the transport of ova through the rabbit oviduct. *Fertil. Steril. 12:* 80, 1961.
32. Lisa, J. R., Gioia, J. D., and Rubin, I. C. Observations on the interstitial portion of the fallopian tube. *Surg. Gynecol. Obstet. 99:* 159, 1954.
33. Harper, M. J. R. Hormonal control of transport of eggs in cumulus through the ampulla of the rabbit oviduct. *Endocrinology 78:* 568, 1966.
34. Greenwald, G. S. In vivo recording of intraluminal pressure changes in the rabbit oviduct. *Fertil. Steril. 14:* 666, 1963.
35. Salomy, M. and Harper, M. J. R. Cyclical changes of oviduct motility in rabbits. *Biol. Reprod. 4:* 185, 1971.
36. Spilman, C. H., and Harper, M. J. R. Effect of prostaglandins on oviduct motility in estrous rabbits. *Biol. Reprod. 9:* 36, 1973.
37. Spilman, C. H. Oviduct motility in the rhesus monkey. Spontaneous activity and response to prostaglandins. *Fertil. Steril. 25:* 935, 1974.
38. Spilman, C. H., Forbes, A. D., and Norland, J. F. Oviduct motility during the rhesus monkey menstrual cycle. Effect of prostaglandins. *Biol. Reprod. 9:* 68, 1973.
39. Brundin, J. Hormonal regulation of egg transport through the mammalian oviduct. In Behrman, S. J., and Kistner, R. W. (eds.): Progress in Infertility, 2nd ed. Boston, Little, Brown, 1975, p. 119.
40. Novak, E., and Everett, H. S. Cyclic and other variations in the tubal epithelium. *Am. J. Obstet. Gynecol. 16:* 499, 1928.
41. Fredricsson, B. Histochemistry of the oviduct. In Hafez, E. S. E., and Blandau, R. J. (eds.): The Mammalian Oviduct. Chicago, University of Chicago Press, 1969.
42. Velardo, J. T., and Rosa, C. G. Histochemistry of enzymes in the female genital system. In Granmann, W., and Neumann, K. (eds.): Handbuch der Histochemie, vol. 7, part 3. Stuttgart, Gustav Fischer, 1963.
43. Bjorkman, N., and Fredricsson, B. Ultrastructural features of the human oviduct epithelium. *Int. J. Fertil. 7:* 259, 1962.
44. Nilsson, O., and Reinius, S. Light and electron microscopic structure of the oviduct. In Hafez, E. S. E., and Blandau, R. J. (eds.): The Mammalian Oviduct. Chicago, University of Chicago Press, 1969.
45. Mastroianni, L., Jr., and Wallach, R. C. Effect of ovulation and early gestation on oviduct secretions of the rabbit. *Am. J. Physiol. 200:* 815, 1961.
46. Hamner, C. E., and Fox, S. B. Biochemistry of oviductal secretions. In Hafez, E. S. E. and Blandau, R. J. (eds.): The Mammalian Oviduct. Chicago, University of Chicago Press, 1969, p. 333.
47. Mastroianni, L., Jr., and Estheshamzadeh, J. Corona cell dispersing properties of rabbit tubal fluid. *J. Reprod. Fertil. 8:* 145, 1964.
48. Stambaugh, R., Noriega, C., and Mastroianni, L., Jr. Biocarbonate ion: the corona cell dispersing factor in tubal fluid. *J. Reprod. Fertil. 18:* 51, 1969.
49. Harper, M. J. K. Factors influencing sperm penetration of rabbit eggs in vivo. *J. Exp. Zool. 173:* 47, 1970.
50. Odor, D. L. Electron microscopic studies on ovarian oocytes and in fertilized tubal ova in the rat. *J. Biophys. Biochem. Cytol. 7:* 567, 1960.
51. Burdick, H. O., and Pincus, G. The effect of oestrin injections upon the developing ova of mice and rabbits. *Am. J. Physiol. 111:* 201, 1935.
52. Yanagimachi, R., and Sato, A. Effects of a single oral administration of ethinyl estradiol on early pregnancy in the mouse. *Fertil. Steril. 19:* 787, 1968.
53. Humphrey, K. W. The effects of oestradiol 3, 17β on tubal transport in the laboratory mouse. *J. Endocrinol. 42:* 17, 1968.
54. Noyes, R. W., Adams, C. E., and Walton, A. The transport of ova in relation to the dosage of oestrogen in ovariectomized rabbits. *J. Endocrinol. 18:* 108, 1959.
55. Chang, M. C. Effects of progesterone and related compounds on fertilization, transportation, and development of rabbit eggs. *Endocrinology 81:* 1251, 1967.
56. Pauerstein, C. J., Fremming, B. D., and Martin, J. E. Influence of progesterone and alpha adrenergic blockade upon tubal transport of ova. *Gynecol. Invest. 1:* 257, 1970.
57. Coutinho, E. M. Oviductal motility and secretory functions. In Greep, R. O. (ed.): Reproductive Physiology. London, Butterworths; Baltimore, University Park Press, 1974.
58. Stambaugh, R., and Buckley, J. Comparative studies of the acrosomal enzymes of rabbit, rhesus monkey, and human spermatozoa. *Biol. Reprod. 3:* 275, 1970.
59. Zamboni, L. Mishell, D. R., Jr., Bell, J. H., and Baca, M. Fine structure of the human ovum in the pronuclear stage. *J. Cell Biol. 30:* 579, 1966.
60. Hertig, A. T., Rock, J., Adams, E. C., and Mulligan, W. J. On the preimplantation stages of the human ovum: a description of four normal and four abnormal specimens ranging from the second to the fifth day of development. *Contrib. Enbryol. 35:* 199, 1954.
61. Doyle, L. L., Lippes, J., Winters, H. S., and Margolis, A. J. Human ova in the fallopian tube. *Am. J. Obstet. Gynecol. 95:* 115, 1966.
62. Shettles, L. B. Fertilization and early development from the inner cell mass. In Philipp, E. E., Barnes, J., and Newton, M. (eds.): Scientific Foundations of Obstetrics and Gynecology. Philadelphia, Davis, 1970, p. 134.
63. Midgely, A. R., Jr., and Pierce, G. B., Jr. Immunohistochemical localization of human chorionic gonadotropin. *J. Exp. Med. 115:* 289, 1962.
64. Catt, K. J., Dufau, M. L., and Vaitukaitis, J. L. Appearance of HCG in pregnancy plasma following the initiation of implantation of the bastocyst. *J. Clin. Endocrinol. Metab., 40:* 537, 1975.
65. Marshall, J. R., Hammond, C. B., Ross, G. T., et al. Plasma and urinary chorionic gonadotrophin during early human pregnancy. *Obstet. Gynecol. 32:* 760, 1968.
66. Thiede, H. A., and Choate, J. W. Chorionic gonadotrophin localization in the human placenta by immunofluorescent staining. II. Demonstration of HCG in the trophoblast and amnion epithelium of immature and mature placentas. *Obstet. Gynecol. 22:* 433, 1963.
67. Sciarra, J. J., Kaplan, S. L., and Grumbach, M. M. Localization of anti-human growth hormone serum within the human placenta: evidence for a human chorionic "growth hormone—prolactin." *Nature 199:* 1005, 1963.
68. Van Leusden, A. J. Chorionic gonadotrophin in pathological preg-

nancy. In Klopper, A. (ed.): Plasma Hormone Assays in Evaluation of Fetal Well Being. New York, Churchill Livingstone, 1976, p. 48.

69. Josimovich, J. B. Placental protein hormones in pregnancy. *Clin. Obstet. Gynecol. 16:* 46, 1973.

70. Lauritzen, C. H., and Lehmann, W. D. Levels of chorionic gonadotrophin in the newborn infant and their relationship to adrenal dehydroepiandrosterone. *J. Endocrinol 39:* 173, 1967.

71. Johannisson, E. The foetal adrenal cortex in the human. Its ultrastructure at different stages of development and in different functional states. *Acta Endocrinol. (Kbh.)* [*Suppl.*] *130:* 1, 1968.

72. McNeilly, A. S., Gardner, J., Bradford, D., and Chard, T. Control of placental hormonal release by "mass action" feedback. *Nature (in press)*

73. Boime, I., Smith, D., and Szcesna, E. The membrane dependent cleavage of the human placental lactogen precursor. *Gynecol. Invest. 8:* 1977, Abstract 7.

74. Diczfalusy, E. Endocrine functions of the human fetus and placenta. *Am. J. Obstet. Gynecol. 119:* 419, 1974.

75. Diczfalusy, E. Steroid metabolism in the foeto-placental unit. In Pecile, A., and Fenzi, C. (eds.): The Foeto-Placental Unit. Amsterdam, Excerpta Medica, 1969, p. 65.

76. Vaitukaitis, J., Braunstein, G. D., and Ross, G. T. A radioimmunoassay which specifically measures human chorionic gonadotrophin in the presence of human luteinizing hormone. *Am. J. Obstet. Gynecol. 113:* 751, 1972.

77. Saxena, B. N., and Landesman, R. The use of a radioreceptor assay of human chorionic gonadotropin for the diagnosis and management of ectopic pregnancy. *Fertil. Steril. 26:* 397, 1975.

78. Yen, S. S. C., Pearson, O., and Rankin, J. S. Radioimmunoassay of serum chorionic gonadotrophin and placental lactogen in trophoblastic disease. *Obstet. Gynecol. 32:* 86, 1968.

79. Letchworth, A. T. Human placental lactogen assay as a guide to fetal well being. Klopper, A. (ed): Plasma Hormone Assays in Evaluation of Fetal Well Being. New York, Churchill Livingstone, 1976, p. 147.

80. Saxena, B. N., Refetoff, S., Emerson, K., and Selenkow, A. J. Rapid radioimmunoassay for human placental lactogen. *Am. J. Obstet. Gynecol. 101:* 874, 1968.

81. Bahl, O. P., Carlsen, R. B., Bellisario, R., and Swaminathan, L. Human chorionic gonadotropin: amino acid sequence of the α and β subunits. *Biochem. Biophys. Res. Commun. 48:* 416, 1972.

82. Morgan, F. J., Kammerman, S., and Canfield, R. E. Studies on the structure and activity of HCG. In Saxena, B. N., Beling, C. G., and Gandy, H. M. (eds.): Gonadotropins. New York, Wiley–Interscience, 1972, p. 211.

83. Csapo, A. I., Pulkkinen, M. O., and Wiest, W. G. Effects of luteectomy and progesterone replacement in early pregnant patients. *Am. J. Obstet. Gynecol. 115:* 759, 1973.

84. Csapo, A. I., Pulkkinen, M. O., and Kaihola, H. A. The effect of estradiol replacement therapy on early pregnant luteectomized patients. *Am. J. Obstet. Gynecol. 117:* 987, 1973.

85. Yen, S. S. C., Llerena, O., Little, B., and Pearson, O. H. Disappearance rates of endogenous luteinizing hormone and chorionic gonadotropin in man. *J. Clin. Endocrinol. 28:* 1763, 1968.

86. Friesen, H. G. Purification of a placental factor with immunologic and chemical similarity to human growth hormone. *Endocrinology 76:* 369, 1965.

87. Li, C. H., Dickson, J. S., and Chung, D. Amino acid sequence of HCS. *Arch. Biochem. Biophys. 155:* 95, 1973.

88. Yen, S. S. C. Endocrine regulation of metabolic homiostasis during pregnancy. *Clin. Obstet. Gynecol. 16:* 130, 1973.

89. Pavlov, C., Chard, T., and Letchworth, A. T. Circulating levels of HCG in late pregnancy: disappearance from the circulation after delivery, variation during labour, and circadian variation.*J. Obstet. Gynecol. Br. Commonw 79:* 629, 1972.

90. Wide, L. Early diagnosis of pregnancy. *Lancet 2:* 863, 1969.

91. Mishell, D. R., Nakamura, R. M., Barberia, J. M., et al. Initial detection of human chorionic gonadotropin in serum in normal gestation. *Am. J. Obstet. Gynecol. 118:* 990, 1974.

92. Boving, B. G., and Larson, J. F. Implantation. In Hafez, E. S. E., and Evans, T. N. (eds.): Human Reproduction, Conception and Contraception. New York, Harper & Row, 1973, p. 133.

93. Saxena, B. N., Goldstein, D. P., Emerson, K., and Selenkow, A. J. Serum placental lactogen levels in patients with molar pregnancy and trophoblastic tumors. *Am. J. Obstet. Gynecol. 102:* 115, 1968.

94. Nygren, K. G., Johansson, E. D. B., and Wide, L. Evaluation of the prognosis of threatened abortion, from peripheral plasma levels of progesterone, estradiol, and human chorionic gonadotrophin. *Am. J. Obstet. Gynecol. 116:* 922, 1973.

95. Teoh, E. S., Das, N. P., Dawood, M. Y., et al. Serum progesterone and serum chorionic gonadotrophin in hydatidiform mole and choriocarcinoma. *Acta Endocrinol. 70:* 791, 1972.

96. Pastorfide, G. B., Goldstein, D. P., and Kosasa, T. S. The use of a radioimmunoassay specific for human chorionic gonadotropin in patients with molar pregnancy and gestational trophoblastic disease. *Am. J. Obstet. Gynecol. 120:* 1025, 1974.

97. Spellacy, W. N. Human placental lactogen in high risk pregnancy. *Clin. Obstet. Gynecol. 16:* 298, 1973.

98. Gartside, M. W., and Tindall, B. R. The prognostic value of human placental lactogen (HPL) levels in threatened abortion. *Br. J. Obstet. Gynecol. 82:* 303, 1975.

99. Niven, P. A. R., Landon, J., and Chard, T. Placental lactogen levels as a guide to outcome of threatened abortion. *Br. Med. J. 3:* 799, 1972.

100. Tulchinsky, D., and Hobel, C. J. Plasma human chorionic gonadotrophin, estrone, estradiol, estriol, progesterone, and 17α-hydroxyprogesterone in human pregnancy: III. Early normal pregnancy. *Am. J. Obstet. Gynecol 117:* 884, 1973.

101. Jirasek, J. E. Morphological and histochemical analysis of the development of adrenals and gonads in man. In Gual, C. (ed.): Progress in Endocrinology. International Congress Series No. 184, Amsterdam, Excerpta Medica, 1969, p. 1100.

102. Reynolds, J. W. Adrenal cortical function: transition from fetus to newborn. In: Perinatal Endocrinology. Meade-Johnson Symposium on Perinatal and Developmental Medicine, No. 8. December 1975, p. 23.

103. Fisher, D. A. Thyroid physiology in the perinatal period. In: Perinatal Endocrinology. Meade-Johnson Symposium on Perinatal and Developmental Medicine, No. 8. December, 1975, p. 38.

104. Simmer, H. H., Tulchinsky, D., Gold, E. M., et al. On regulation of estrogen production by cortisol and ACTH in human pregnancy at term. *Am. J. Obstet. Gynecol. 119:* 283, 1974.

105. Winters, A. J., Colston, C., MacDonald, P. C., and Porter, J. C. Fetal plasma prolactin levels. *J. Clin. Endocrinol. Metab. 41:* 626, 1975.

106. Lis, M., Gilardeau, C., and Chretien, M. Effect of prolactin on corticosterone production by rat adrenals. *Clin. Res. 21:* 1027, 1973.

107. Witorsch, R. J., and Kitay, J. I. Pituitary hormones affecting adrenal 5α-reductase activity: ACTH, growth hormone and prolactin. *Endocrinology 91:* 764, 1972.

108. Simmer, H. H. Disorders of placental endocrine functions. In Assali, N. S. (ed.): Pathophysiology of Gestation, Vol. 2. New York, Academic Press, 1972, p. 77.

109. Serron-Ferre, M., Lawrence, C. C., and Jaffe, R. Role of HCG in the regulation of the fetal zone of the human fetal adrenal gland. *Gynecol. Invest. 8:* 1977, abstract 87.

110. Buster, J. E. Unpublished observations.

111. Gant, N. F., Madden, J. D., Siiteri, P. K. et al. A sequential study of the metabolism of hydroisoandrosterone sulfate in primigravid pregnancy. In Scow, R. O. (ed.): Endocrinology. Proceedings of the Fourth International Congress of Endocrinology, Washington, D.C. Amsterdam, Excerpta Medica, 1972, p. 1026.

112. Murphy, B. E. P., Clark, S. J., Donald, I. R., et al. Conversion of maternal cortisol to cortisone during placental transfer to the human fetus. *Am. J. Obstet. Gynecol. 118:* 538, 1974.

113. Spellacy, W. N., Ashbacher, L. V., Harris, G. K., et al. Total cholesterol content in maternal and unbilical vessels in term pregnancies. *Obstet. Gynecol. 44:* 661, 1974.

114. Liggins, G. C. Endocrinology of the foeto-maternal unit. In Shearman, R. P. (ed.): Human Reproductive Physiology. Oxford, Blackwell, 1972, p. 138.

115. Hellig, H., Lefebvre, Y., Gattereau, D., and Bolte, E. Placental progesterone production in the human. In Pecile, A., and Fenzi, C. (eds.): The Foeto-Placental Unit. Amsterdam, Excerpta Medica, 1969, p. 152.

116. Baulieu, E. E., Corpechot, C., Dray, F., et al. An adrenal secreted "androgen:" dehydroisoandrosterone sulfate: its metabolism and a tentative generalization on the metabolism of other steroid conjugates in man. *Recent Prog. Horm. Res. 21:* 411, 1965.

117. Kirdani, R. Y., Sampson, D., Murphy, G. P., et al. Studies on phenolic steroids in human subjects: XVI. Role of the kidney in the disposition of estriol. *J. Clin. Endocrinol. Metab. 34:* 546, 1972.

118. Abraham, G. E., Odell, W. D., Swerdloff, R. S., et al. Simultaneous radioimmunoassay of plasma FSH, LH, progesterone, 17-hydroxyprogesterone, and estradiol-17β. *J. Clin. Endocrinol. Metab. 34:* 312, 1972.
119. Tulchinsky, D., Hobel, C. J., Yeager, E., et al. Plasma estrone, estradiol, estriol, progesterone and 17-hydroxyprogesterone in human pregnancy, I. Normal pregnancy. *Am. J. Obstet. Gynecol. 112:* 1095, 1972.
120. Tulchinsky, D., Hobel, C. J., Yeager, E., et al. Plasma estradiol, estriol and progesterone in human pregnancy, II. Clinical applications in Rh-isoimmunization disease. *Am. J. Obstet. Gynecol. 113:* 766, 1972.
121. Yoshimi, R., Strott, C. A., Marshall, J. R., et al. Corpus luteum function in early pregnancy. *J. Clin. Endocrinol. Metab. 29:* 225, 1969.
122. Tulchinsky, D., and Simmer, H. H. Source of plasma 17α-hydroxyprogesterone in human pregnancy. *J. Clin. Endocrinol. Metab. 35:* 799, 1972.
123. Tulchinsky, D., Karow, W. G., Gentry, W. et al. Plasma steroids in pregnancy. Proceedings of the International Symposium on Clinical Applications of Hormone Assays in Pregnancy. Fresnes, France, 1973.
124. Abraham, G. E., Samojlik, E., Kyle, F. W., et al. Radioimmunoassay of plasma 16α-hydroxyprogesterone. *Anal. Lett. 6:* 675, 1973.
125. Abraham, G. E., and Samojlik, E. Correlation between plasma unconjugated estriol and 16α-hydroxyprogesterone during human pregnancy. *Obstet. Gynecol. 44:* 767, 1974.
126. Buster, J. E., Chang, R. J., Preston, D. L., et al. Interrelationships of circulating maternal steroid concentrations in normal third trimester pregnancies. I: C_{21} steroids. (submitted for publication).
127. Chang, R. J., and Abraham, G. E. Serum concentrations of 16α-hydroxyprogesterone on maternal and fetal circulations. (submitted for publication).
128. Buster, J. E., and Abraham, G. E. Radioimmunoassay of plasma dehydroepiandrosterone sulfate. *Anal. Lett. 5:* 543, 1972.
129. Buster, J. E., Chang, R. J., Preston, D. L., et al. Interrelationships of circulating maternal steroid concentrations in normal third trimester pregnancies. II: C_{18} and C_{19} steroids. (submitted for publication).
130. MacDonald, P. C., and Siiteri, P. K. Origin of estrogen in women pregnant with an anencephalic fetus. *J. Clin. Invest. 44:* 465, 1965.
131. Gant, N. E., Hutchinson, H. T., Siiteri, P. K., and MacDonald, P. C. Study of the metabolic clearance of dehydroisoandrosterone sulfate in pregnancy. *Am. J. Obstet. Gynecol. 111:* 555, 1971.
132. Gant, N. E., Madden, J. D., Siiteri, P. K., and MacDonald, P. C. The metabolic clearance of dehydroisoandrosterone sulfate. III. *Am. J. Obstet. Gynecol. 123:* 159, 1975.
133. Gant, N. E., Hutchinson, H. T., Siiteri, P. K., and MacDonald, P. C. Study of the metabolic clearance of hydroisoandrosterone sulfate in pregnancy. IV. *Am. J. Obstet. Gynecol. 124:* 143, 1976.
134. Buster, J. E., Abraham, G. E., Kyle, F. W., et al. Serum steroid levels following a large intravenous dose of steroid sulfate precursor during the second trimester of human pregnancy. I. Dehydroepiandrosterone sulfate. *J. Clin. Endocrinol. Metab. 38:* 1031, 1974.
135. Tulchinsky, D. The value of estrogen assays in obstetric disease. In Klopper, A. (ed.): Plasma Hormone Assays in Evaluation of Fetal Well Being. New York, Churchill-Livingstone, 1976, p. 72.
136. Lauritzen, G., Strecker, J., and Lehmann, W. D. Dynamic test of placental function: some findings on the conversion of DHEA-S to oestrogens. In Klopper, A. (ed.): Plasma Hormone Assays in Evaluation of Fetal Well Being. New York, Churchill-Livingstone, 1976, p. 113.
137. Klopper, A., and Jandial, V. The conversion of dehydroepiandrosterone to estrogen—a dynamic placental function test. *Eur. J. Obstet. Gynecol. Reprod. Biol. 5:* 93, 1975.
138. Crabben, van der, H., Kaiser, E., and Warner, C. The placenta function test by dehydroepiandrosterone sulfate, an estrogen precursor. Second International Congress on Perinatal Medicine, London, 1971. Basel, Karger, 1971, p. 94.
139. Lindberg, B. S., Johansson, E. D. B., and Nilsson, B. A. Plasma levels of nonconjugated estrone, estradiol-17β, and estriol during uncomplicated pregnancy. *Acta Obstet. Gynecol. Scand.* [*Suppl*] *32:* 21, 1974.
140. Siiteri, P. K., and MacDonald, P. C. Placental estrogen biosynthesis during human pregnancy. *J. Clin. Endocrinol. Metab. 26:* 751, 1966.
141. Tulchinsky, D., and Korenman, S. G. The plasma estradiol as an index of fetoplacental function. *J. Clin. Invest. 50:* 1490, 1971.
142. Lindberg, B. S., Johansson, E. D. G., and Nilsson, B. A. Plasma levels of nonconjugate oestradiol-17β and oestriol in high-risk pregnancies. *Acta Obstet. Gynecol. Scand.* [*Suppl*] *32:* 37, 1974.
143. Townsley, J. D., Gartmen, L. J., and Crystle, C. D. Maternal serum 17β-estradiol levels in normal and complicated pregnancies: a comparison with other estrogen indices of fetal health. *Am. J. Obstet. Gynecol. 115:* 830, 1973.
144. Tulchinsky, D., Hobel, C. J., and Korenman, S. G. A radioligand assay for plasma unconjugated estriol in normal and abnormal pregnancies. *Am. J. Obstet. Gynecol. 111:* 311, 1971.
145. Klopper, A., Masson, G., Campbell, D., et al. Estriol in plasma: a conpartmental study. *Am. J. Obstet. Gynecol. 117:* 21, 1973.
146. Tulchinsky, D., and Abraham, G. E. Radioimmunoassay of plasma estriol. *J. Clin. Endocrinol. Metab. 33:* 775, 1971.
147. Loriaux, D. L., Ruder, H. J., Knab, D. R., et al. Estrone sulfate, estrone, estradiol, and estriol plasma levels in human pregnancy. *J. Clin. Endocrinol. Metab. 35:* 887, 1972.
148. Crystle, C. D., Dubin, N. H., Grannis, G. F., et al. Investigation of precursor availability in the regulation of estrogen synthesis in normal human pregnancy. *Obstet. Gynecol. 42:* 718, 1973.
149. Reynolds, J. W., and Mirkin, B. L. Urinary steroid levels in newborn infants with intrauterine growth retardation. *J. Clin. Endocrinol. Metab. 36:* 576, 1973.
150. Turnipseed, M. R., Bentley, K., and Reynolds, J. W. Serum dehydroepiandrosterone sulfate in premature infants and infants with intrauterine growth retardation. (submitted for publication).
151. McKerns, K. W. Steroidogenesis and metabolism in the adrenal cortex. In McKerns, K. W. (ed.): Steroid Hormones and Metabolism. New York, Appleton-Century-Crofts, 1969, p. 9.
152. Buster, J. E., and Ostergard, D. R. Current status of plasma estriol in the assessment of pathological pregnancies. *Obstet. Gynecol Dig. 15:* 33, 1973.
153. Fishman, J., and Buzik, H. Radioimmunoassay of 15α-hydroxyestriol in pregnancy plasma. *J. Clin. Endocrinol. Metab. 35:* 892, 1972.
154. Sciarra, J. J., Tagatz, G. E., Notation, A. D., et al. Estriol and estetrol in amniotic fluid. *Am. J. Obstet. Gynecol. 118:* 626, 1974.
155. Tulchinsky, D., Frigolatto, F. D., Ryan, K. J., and Fishman, J. Plasma estetrol as an index of fetal well being. *J. Clin. Endocrinol. Metab. 40:* 560, 1975.
156. Fencl, M., and Tulchinsky, D. Concentrations of cortisol in amniotic fluid during pregnancy. *N. Engl. J. Med. 292:* 133, 1975.
157. Murphy, B. E. P., Patrick, J., and Denton, R. L. Cortisol in amniotic fluid during human gestation. *J. Clin. Endocrinol. Metab. 40:* 164, 1975.
158. Winters, A. J., Oliver, C., Colston, C., et al. Plasma ACTH levels in the human fetus and neonate as related to jet age and parturition. *J. Clin. Endocrinol. Metab. 39:* 269, 1974.
159. Wintour, E. M., Brown, E. J., Denton, D. A., et al. The ontogeny and regulation of corticosteroid secretion by the ovine foetal adrenal. *Acta Endocrinol. 79:* 301, 1975.
160. Madill, D., and Bassett, J. M. Corticosteroid release by adrenal tissue from foetal and newborn lambs in response to corticotrophin stimulation in a perfusion system in vitro. *J. Endocrinol. 58:* 75, 1973.
161. Liggins, G. C. Endocrinology of the foeto-maternal unit. In Shearman, R. P. (ed.): Human Reproductive Physiology. Oxford, Blackwell, 1972, p. 138.
162. Brown, B. J., Gabert, A. J., and Stenchever, M. A. Respiratory distress syndrome, surfactant biochemistry, and acceleration of fetal maturity: a review. *Obstet. Gynecol. Surv. 30:* 71, 1975.
163. Gluck, L., and Kulovich, M. V. Lecithin/sphingomyelin ratios in amniotic fluid in normal and abnormal pregnancy. *Am. J. Obstet. Gynecol. 115:* 539, 1973.
164. Donald, I. R., Freeman, R. K., Goebelsmann, U., et al. Clinical experience with the amniotic fluid lecithin/sphingomyelin ratio. *Am. J. Obstet. Gynecol. 115:* 547, 1973.
165. Turkington, R. W., Frantz, W. L., and Majumder, G. C. Effector–receptor relations in the action of prolactin. In Pasteels, J. L., and Robyn, C. (eds.): Prolactin: Proceedings of the International Symposium on Human Prolactin, Brussels, June 12–14, 1973, p. 25.
166. Korenman, S. G., and Krall, J. R. The role of cyclic AMP in the regulation of smooth muscle cell contraction to uterus. *Biol. Reprod. 16:* 1, 1977.
167. Liggins, G. C., Forster, C. S., Grieves, S. A., and Schwartz, A. I. Control of parturition in man. *Biol. Reprod. 16:* 39, 1977.

168. Ramwell, P. W., Leovey, E. M. K., and Sintetos, A. L. Regulation of the arachidonic acid cascade. *Biol. Reprod. 16:* 70, 1977.
169. MacDonald, P. C., Schultz, F. M., Duenhoelter, J. H., et al. Initiation of human parturition. I. Mechanisms of action of arachidonic acid. *Obstet. Gynecol 44:* 629, 1974.
170. Schwarz, B. E., Schultz, F. M., MacDonald, P. C., et al. Initiation of human parturition. III. Fetal membrane content of prostaglandin E_2 and $F_{2\alpha}$ precursor. *Obstet. Gynecol. 46:* 564, 1975.
171. Schultz, F. M., Schwarz, B. E., MacDonald, P. C., et al. Initiation of human parturition. II. Identification of phospholipase A_2 in fetal chorio-amniotic and uterine decidua. *Am. J. Obstet. Gynecol. 123:* 650, 1975.
172. Schwarz, B. E., Schultz, F. M., MacDonald, P. C., et al. Initiation of human parturition. IV. Demonstration of phospholipase A_2 in the lysosomes of human fetal membranes. *Am. J. Obstet. Gynecol. 125:* 1089, 1976.
173. Schwarz, B. E., Mylowich, L., Johnston, J. M., et al. Initiation of human parturition. V. Progesterone binding substance fetal membranes. *Obstet. Gynecol. 48:* 685, 1976.
174. Thorburn, G. D., Challis, J. R., and Currie, W. B. Control of parturition in domestic animals. *Biol. Reprod. 16:* 18, 1977.
175. Lanman, J. T. Parturition in nonhuman primates. *Biol. Reprod. 16:* 28, 1977.
176. Liggins, G. C. Fetal influences on myometrial contractility. *Clin. Obstet. Gynecol. 16:* 148, 1973.
177. Nathanielsz, P. W. In Fetal Endocrinology: An Experimental Approach. Amsterdam, Elsevier/North Holland, 1976.
178. Chard, T., Hudson, C. N., Edwards, C. R. W., and Boyd, N. R. H. The release of oxytocin and vasopressin by the human fetus during labour. *Nature 234:* 352, 1971.
179. Dawood, M. Y., Wang, C. F., Gupta, R., and Fuchs, F. Fetal contribution of oxytocin in human parturition. *Gynecol. Invest. 8,* 1977, Abstract 39.
180. Nathanielsz, P. W., Comline, R. S., and Silver, M. Uterine activity following intravenous administration of oxytocin in the foetal sheep. *Nature 243:* 417, 1973.
181. Quilligan, E. J. Maternal factors influencing the onset of labor. *Clin. Obstet. Gynecol. 16:* 150, 1973.
182. Gibbens, D., Boyd, N. R. H., and Chard, T. Spurt release of oxytocin during human labor. *J. Endocrinol. 53:* 185, 1972.
183. Chard, T. The posterior pituitary and induction of labor. In Klopper, A., and Gardner, J. (eds.): Endocrine Factors of Labor. Cambridge, Cambridge University Press, 1973, p. 61.
184. Chang, R. J., Buster, J. E., Blakely, J. L., et al. Simultaneous comparison of Δ^5-3β-hydroxysteroid levels in the fetoplacental circulation of normal pregnancy in labor and not in labor. *J. Clin. Endocrinol. Metab. 42:* 744, 1976.
185. Solomon, S., Bird, C. E., Ling, W., Iwamiya, M., and Young, P. C. M. Formation and metabolism of steroids in the fetus and placenta. *Recent. Prog. Horm. Res. 43:* 297, 1967.

131

Lactation and Galactorrhea

Cesare Aragona
Henry G. Friesen

MORPHOLOGIC AND FUNCTIONAL DEVELOPMENT OF THE BREAST

MORPHOLOGIC DEVELOPMENT OF THE BREAST (MAMMOGENESIS)

The mammary gland, which is derived from the ectoderm, first is evident in the 4-mm embryo as a mammary band from which the mammary crest or milk line develops. After several modifications, the epithelial nodule is recognizable buried in mesenchyme. In the 120–150-mm embryo, secondary epithelial buds develop, forming cellular cords that lengthen and bifurcate and give rise, by reabsorption of the internal cells, to the excretory and lactiferous ducts of the mammary gland. The human mammary gland is a compound tubuloalveolar gland, consisting of 15–25 irregular lobes radiating from the mammary papilla or nipple. The lobes are separated by a layer of dense connective tissue and are embedded in an abundance of adipose tissue. Each lobe is subdivided into a series of lobules from which emerge lactiferous ducts lined by stratified squamous epithelium. Loose intralobular connective tissue surrounds the system of ducts, permitting greater distensibility as the epithelial portion of the gland develops during pregnancy and lactation.

At birth, the mammary structures are still rudimentary, but, in some newborns, particularly prematures, a slight degree of secretory function is observed ("witch's milk") within a few days after birth. When this occurs the mammary gland appears enlarged and the epithelial ducts expand into milk sinuses. Secretory activity results from high prolactin levels in the newborn. Subsequently, the breast enters a quiescent state. With the onset of puberty in the female, the areola enlarges and becomes more pigmented and further growth occurs. These changes are related to the onset of estrogen and progesterone secretion by the ovary.

There is, in fact, considerable variation in the development of mammary gland function among different species, acinar development being more pronounced in species with a long progestational phase. In species with short estrus cycles (e.g., mouse and rat) in which the follicular phase of the cycle is predominant and the luteal phase almost nonexistent, only the duct system develops and, in these species, complete development of the mammary gland occurs only in pregnancy. In species with a long luteal phase such as primates, mammary development during each menstrual cycle is considerable and, in a limited sense, is similar to the changes occurring during pregnancy.

BREAST CHANGES DURING THE MENSTRUAL CYCLE

During each menstrual cycle, cyclic proliferative changes and active growth of duct tissues occur; these changes progress during the follicular and periovulatory phases, reach a maximum in the late luteal phase, and then regress. Histologic examinations of the normal breast reveal that after puberty mammary development consists of a slow progressive increase in glandular tissue brought about by epithelial out-growths which lengthen, hollow out, and form further subdivisions of the ducts. The complex groupings of ductules, surrounded by loose and delicate stroma, thus form rudimentary lobules. In the mammary gland it is difficult to distinguish alveolar from epithelial cells of intralobular ducts, since both are lined by a single layer of epithelium and are capable of secretion. Normal growth goes no further in nonpregnant subjects, and it is generally agreed that true alveoli are not usually present until the third month of pregnancy.

Thus, between puberty and adult life, a limited development of the mammary gland occurs which is accompanied by cyclic changes, but complete development of mammary function occurs only in pregnancy.

BREAST CHANGES DURING PREGNANCY

The development of the human mammary gland during pregnancy has been reviewed elsewhere.[1] At the beginning of pregnancy, there is rapid growth and branching from terminal portions of the gland, at least in part at the expense of interstitial adipose tissue. Increased vascularity accompanies the infiltration of interstitial tissue by lymphocytes, eosinophils, and plasma cells. True glandular acini, the basic components of a functional mammary gland, appear at the beginning of the third month. The hollow alveolus is lined by a single layer of myoepithelial cells. The highly branched myoepithelial cells enclose the glandular alveolus in a loosely meshed network surrounded by capillaries, with the lumen of the alveolus connected to an intralobular duct. In the second trimester of pregnancy, alveolar secretion begins and then increases further during the third trimester. In the last month of pregnancy, the enlargement of the breast results largely from hypertrophy of parenchymal cells and distension of the alveoli with a hyaline, eosinophilic secretion termed *colostrum*.

HORMONAL EFFECTS ON MAMMARY GROWTH AND FUNCTION

There is a vast literature dealing with the hormonal control of mammary growth and function. In these studies, attempts have been made to establish the simplest hormonal combinations required for duct and lobuloalveolar growth, principally using hypophysectomized, adrenalectomized, and oophorectomized rats. Using these animals Lyons et al.,[2] in their classic experiments, demonstrated that a large number of hormones were involved including six pituitary hormones; prolactin, ACTH, growth hormone, thyrotropin (TSH), follicle-stimulating hormone (FSH), and luteinizing hormone (LH). In addition, the placenta secretes a prolactin-like hormone. Moreover, steroid hormones from the ovary and adrenal plus thyroid and insulin are involved in mammary growth and function. However, in several cases (TSH, FSH, and LH) the hormones listed do not act directly on the gland; their effects result from the secretion of hormones from target glands which they stimulate. Despite the fact that these classic studies were performed on rats, the conclusions derived from these experiments very frequently have been applied to many species, including humans.

Studies by Topper[3] and Turkington[4] in cultured mouse mammary glands have demonstrated that three hormones, prolactin, insulin, and hydrocortisone, are required for mammary growth and function. Insulin alone results in the multiplication of epithelial cells and formation of lobuloalveolar architecture. However, for complete cytologic and functional differentiation of the epithelial cells in preparation for secretion of specific milk products, a combination of hydrocortisone, insulin, and prolactin are required. It has also been demonstrated that human placental lactogen exhibits a prolactin-like effect on mammary glands in this system. These studies in rodent mammary glands illustrate the complexity of the mechanisms involved in mammary growth and function. It must be emphasized, however, that only limited studies of hormonal effects on human breast tissue have been performed and precise mechanisms by which these effects are mediated are virtually unknown.

The role of ovarian hormones in mammogenesis in women is clearly established on clinical grounds because gonadal failure in the prepubertal period results in an absence of mammary gland development. However, once mammary development is complete, oophorectomy has a much less obvious effect. Among the ovarian hormones, estrogens appear to be associated with the proliferation of the ductal system, as pointed out in the classic studies of Folley[5] and Meites[6] in the rat and mouse and by others[7] in women. Progesterone, on the other hand, appears to be necessary for complete mammogenesis, in animal models as well as in women. Clinical reports of enlargement of the breast in women on oral contraceptives provide additional evidence for the role of sex steroids on the human mammary gland. During pregnancy, progesterone, estradiol, estrone, and estriol blood concentrations increase markedly, indicating an increased production of these steroids by the fetal–placental unit.[8]

An increase of plasma cortisol also occurs due to the increase in cortisol-binding globulin (transcortin) which accompanies the increases in estrogen secretion. Furthermore, high levels of human chorionic gonadotropin (HCG), prolactin, and placental lactogen (HPL) are found, and, more recently, the presence of a corticotropinlike placental hormone has been reported.[9] It is likely that all these hormonal factors, summarized in Figure 131-1, work in concert to produce the mature alveolar system in human mammary glands.

HORMONES AND LACTATION

We have considered briefly the hormones that are involved in the development of the mammary gland. We propose now to consider the hormones that are necessary for lactation and to review the mechanisms by which they extend their effects. Unfortunately, much of our knowledge is derived from studies in species other than the human, and hence we are forced to extrapolate from this knowledge to the human; in so doing, the reader should appreciate that this extension may not always be warranted. Folley, along with Lyons and his colleagues, were among the first to stress that lactation results from the interaction of many hormones acting on the breast. The list includes many if not all of the hormones listed in the previous section.

PROLACTIN

Of all the hormones necessary for lactation, none is more important than prolactin. As outlined in Chapter 15, human prolactin was identified as a separate pituitary hormone only recently;[10,11] however, since that time considerable information has accumu-

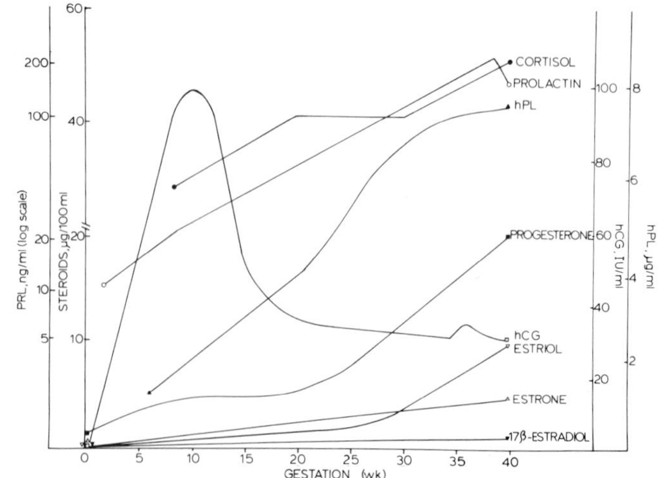

Fig. 131-1. Serum concentrations of prolactin, HPL, HCG, cortisol, progesterone, estriol, estrone, 17β-estradiol during pregnancy. (Values obtained from various sources in the literature.)

lated about the physiologic and pharmacologic factors controlling its secretion. These studies are reviewed in Chapter 15. In this section we propose to review the role of human prolactin in lactation.

During pregnancy there is a gradual and progressive increase in serum prolactin concentrations from a mean of 7–10 ng/ml before pregnancy until term, when values average 200 ng/ml in maternal serum. In the postpartum period in women who are not breast feeding, prolactin concentrations gradually decrease to nonpregnant levels by 3–6 weeks. In women who breast feed the pattern of prolactin secretion varies during the postpartum period.[12] In the first 1–2 weeks, basal prolactin values are elevated, ranging from 50 to 200 ng/ml; with each episode of breast feeding serum prolactin values increase slightly, reaching maximal values at 30 min. In an intermediate phase lasting from 2 weeks until approximately 3 months postpartum, basal prolactin levels are still slightly elevated; with each period of breast feeding, serum prolactin increases to a much greater extent than in the first phase. It is common to see 10- and 20-fold increases over basal values 30 min after the onset of breast feeding. In the final phase, which begins approximately 2–3 months postpartum, basal prolactin concentrations may be within the range seen in nonpregnant subjects and breast feeding may produce no change or only minor increases in serum prolactin, and yet as much as a liter or more of milk is produced daily.

With the use of a pharmacologic agent (2 Br-α-ergocryptine; CB-154) that specifically inhibits prolactin secretion, it has been possible to clarify the role of this hormone in human lactation.[13] When CB-154 is administered in the immediate postpartum period, the elevated prolactin concentrations decline within hours to nonpregnant values and breast engorgement and lactation is abolished. This clinical experiment demonstrates that prolactin is essential for the initiation of lactation. Presumably, in women with Sheehan's syndrome, lactation does not occur because prolactin disappears from the circulation after pituitary infarction in the immediate postpartum period. On the other hand, if estrogens are used to suppress lactation and breast engorgement in the postpartum period, serum prolactin values are actually raised slightly above those seen in nursing subjects, but, of course, no milk is formed. These observations demonstrate that the action of prolactin at the breast is inhibited by high concentrations of estrogens. It is likely that the same mechanism is responsible for preventing milk formation during pregnancy. Similar interaction may account for the initiation of lactation. With the rapid decline in estrogens in the immediate postpartum period, the inhibitory effects of steroids are removed, allowing prolactin to act unimpeded on the fully developed and primed mammary gland. Administration of CB-154 at any period postpartum is completely effective in inhibiting lactation in women. Indeed, when all available milk is removed with a breast pump after lactation is well established postpartum, if CB-154 is administered, 4–6 h later no further milk is obtainable, indicating that prolactin is essential for milk formation and that the duration of action of prolactin is relatively brief.

Quite possibly, the surge of prolactin secretion which follows each episode of suckling serves to stimulate maximal milk formation and readies the breast for the next feed. Similarly, in monkeys a single large increase in serum prolactin produces histologically recognizable lactational changes in the mammary gland within hours. It is clear from anecdotal accounts that breast engorgement and milk formation can occur with surprising rapidity after a variety of events, including surgical procedures, or more gradually after repeated nipple stimulation, as occurs in "wet nurses," some of whom have been in the postmenopausal age group. It is assumed that these events are accompanied by increases in serum prolactin, but thus far no systematic studies have been conducted.

In most species, prolactin is essential for the onset of lactation, but there are considerable species differences. In the cow, for example, prolactin is critical for the initiation of lactation, whereas subsequently, when serum prolactin concentrations are reduced with CB-154, milk yield declines only 10–20 percent. Thus far, there have been very few studies in which attempts have been made to determine whether milk yield and the concentration of prolactin values can be correlated. However, in one study no correlation of basal prolactin values with milk yield was found, but there appeared to be a positive correlation between the magnitude of the increase in prolactin following breast feeding and milk yield. Others have attempted to increase milk production with the use of agents which increase serum prolactin such as thyrotropin-releasing hormone (TRH). While milk yield was not increased, fat and protein content were raised. Similar studies with TRH in cows failed to produce any effect on milk yield and composition. Moreover, older studies with exogenous administration of prolactin to cows also failed to demonstrate any striking effects on milk production. It appears, therefore that prolactin plays an important, indeed critical, role in the initiation of lactation in many species, including humans, but its role in maintaining lactation is more variable. In women the secretion of prolactin in the postpartum period varies, gradually declining. Nevertheless, the low levels in serum late in the postpartum period remain critical for the maintenance of lactation.

It is generally accepted that, in mammals, one of the principal target tissues for prolactin is the mammary gland. The direct effects and mechanism of action of prolactin on mammary gland differentiation, growth, and function have been examined extensively in animal models. Recent observations support the hypothesis that prolactin, like other polypeptide hormones, exerts its effect on mammary cells without entering the cytoplasm of the target cell (Fig. 131-2). Prolactin covalently linked to Sepharose is biologically active in terms of stimulating RNA synthesis in mouse mammary epithelial cells, and hence it is suggested that prolactin initiates its effect by an action on the cell membrane because it is presumed that the Sepharose–prolactin complexes do not enter the cells. Others using autoradiographic techniques have shown that ^{125}I-prolactin is localized on the surface of epithelial cells. In addition to binding to membrane preparations isolated from mammary glands, ^{125}I-prolactin also binds with high affinity to similar preparations obtained from different tissues of many species. These specific hormone-binding sites in tissue membranes are generally held to be hormone receptors. However, it must be

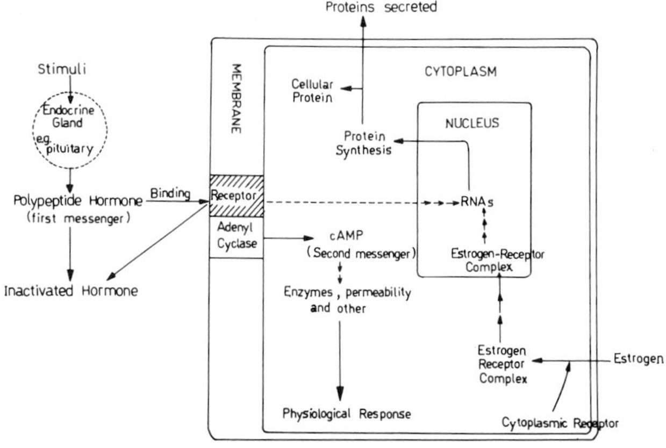

Fig. 131-2. Postulated mechanism of action of hormone at receptor level.

appreciated that some experts feel that not all binding sites are receptors.

The characterization and significance of prolactin receptors is under very active investigation. These discrete entities are proteolipids that are located in the plasma membranes of target cells. They bind prolactin with a high degree of affinity and specificity and it is presumed that those cells that contain prolactin receptors are target cells for the hormone. If the prolactin receptors are biologically significant, it should be possible to inhibit the action of prolactin by blocking its receptors. With the production of antisera to purified prolactin receptors, the stimulation of milk protein synthesis (casein) by prolactin was completely inhibited in rabbit mammary tissue in vitro, providing direct confirmation of the hypothesis that prolactin receptors are critically involved in mediating the action of this hormone. With antisera to rabbit mammary gland prolactin receptors one can inhibit prolactin binding in membrane preparations from other tissues and even from other species. These results demonstrate that prolactin receptors in different tissues and species are immunochemically related.

Since prolactin receptors are critically involved in mediating the action of prolactin, their number may also regulate the action of prolactin. Several studies dealing with the prolactin receptor in the female rat liver as a model system have demonstrated that the number of prolactin receptors are modulated by a variety of factors such as age, sex, hormones, and dietary factors. Figure 131-3 summarizes the results of some of these studies. Thus it is apparent that a certain hormonal environment is required for the maintenance or the induction of prolactin receptors and that continuous active protein synthesis is essential for the maintenance of membrane receptors whose rapid turnover may have an important role in modulating hormone action. From such considerations it follows that the biologic response may result from the interaction of the hormone with its receptor. Figure 131-4 schematically illustrates this relationship.

Unlike other polypeptide hormones (e.g., TSH and glucagon), it has not been possible to demonstrate that prolactin activates adenylate cyclase or any membrane-bound enzyme. Although the immediate biochemical event that follows the interaction of prolactin with membrane receptors has not been recognized, some of the changes that are produced by prolactin in the mammary gland include formation of cAMP-dependent protein kinase and cAMP-binding protein. Nuclear protein phosphorylation secondary to the activation of protein kinase may lead to gene activation, and thus

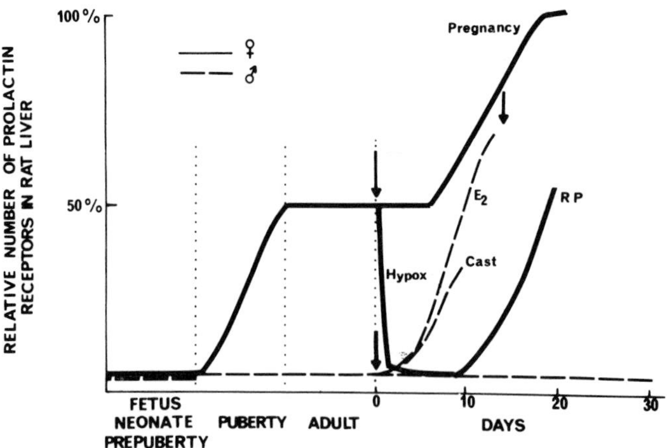

Fig. 131-3. Relative activity of prolactin receptor in rat liver in several physiologic and experimental conditions. In prepubertal rats binding is low in males and females. The receptor levels increase at the time of puberty in female rats, and pregnancy causes a further increase in number of receptors. In male rats, treatment with estrogen leads to an induction of prolactin receptors in the liver so that the number of receptors reaches, if not exceeds, that found in the female; castration has a smaller but definite effect. The pituitary gland appears to have a critical role in the induction of the receptor since, following hypophysectomy in female rats, the prolactin receptors disappear rapidly and implantation of pituitaries into the kidney capsule results in the secretion of prolactin, which presumably is the factor responsible for the induction and maintenance of the prolactin receptor. Arrows indicate the beginning of treatment. E_2, estradiol; RP, renal pituitary transplant.

to the stimulation of transcription. This is followed by the synthesis of a number of species of RNA that are essential for ribosome formation and milk protein synthesis, including the necessary enzymes involved in this process. Recently it has also been reported[14] that prolactin produces major increases in ornithine decarboxylase, an enzyme which regulates polyamine synthesis (spermine and spermidine). Several studies implicate polyamines in the stabilization of polynucleic acids and ribosome structure and therefore suggest a role for ornithine decarboxylase in the regulation of protein synthesis and growth.

It must be emphasized that this scheme of the mechanism of action of prolactin is an oversimplified picture of a very complex mechanism which has been studied largely in mammary gland explants and organ culture systems derived principally from ro-

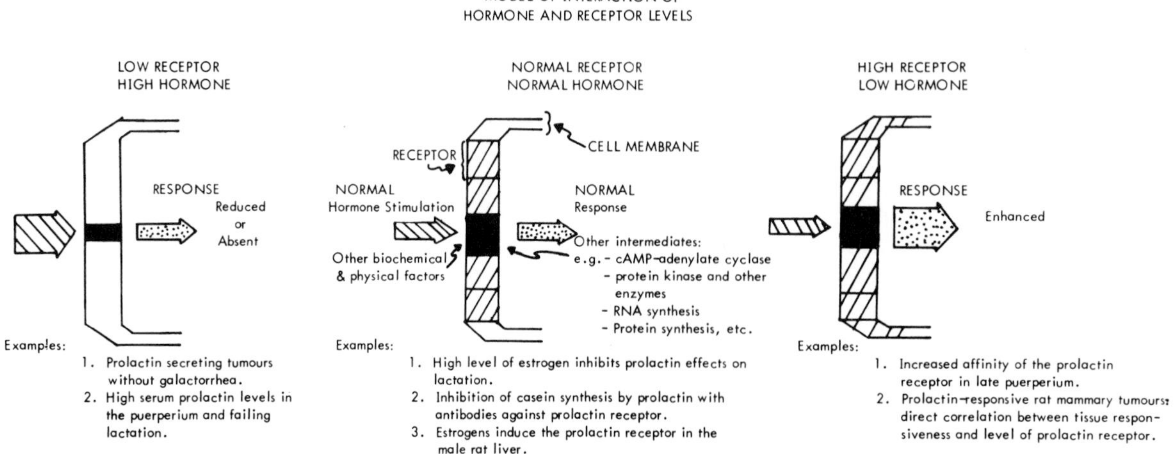

Fig. 131-4. Model of interaction of hormone and receptor levels. The biologic response results from the interaction of the hormone with the receptor. Variations in either hormone or receptor parameter may lead to an altered response.

dents. It is obvious that further studies are required to elucidate the roles and the precise mechanism of action of the various hormones involved in human mammary gland development and function.

In addition to stimulating milk protein synthesis, prolactin also affects enzymes involved in fat synthesis in mammary and adipose tissues. In the former lipoprotein lipase is activated, while in adipose tissues it is inhibited. As a result, the hydrolysis of circulating lipoproteins is preferentially redirected toward the mammary gland, thereby providing the necessary substrates for the synthesis of triglycerides by mammary tissue.

Prolactin is also known to affect sodium and water transport in a number of tissues. Whether it plays any role in determining electrolyte transport and ionic composition of milk is unknown.

HUMAN GROWTH HORMONE (HGH) AND HUMAN PLACENTAL LACTOGEN (HPL)

These two hormones, although chemically and functionally different from prolactin, exhibit overlapping effects in a number of assay systems. Both hormones produce very comparable lactational changes in the rabbit mammary gland, cause luteotropic effects in rats, and stimulate proliferation of the pigeon crop sac epithelium. Despite these similarities, important differences remain, the principal one being that HPL has very little somatotropic activity. It is unlikely that HGH plays an important role in breast development and lactation in humans since HGH secretion is suppressed during the latter half of pregnancy. The strongest evidence against an important role for HGH in mammary function stems from the clinical observation that patients with a genetic deficiency of HGH appear to have normal breast development and a few of these patients appear to lactate normally. It is possible, however, that HGH may play a permissive role in augmenting milk production. Lyons, for example, found that HGH administration enhanced milk yield, as judged by an accelerated weight gain of infants whose mothers were treated with HGH.

The role of HPL in breast development remains speculative. HPL concentrations gradually increase throughout the first two trimesters of pregnancy, reaching average concentrations of 5–8 μg/ml, and these values are maintained throughout the last trimester. Following delivery, HPL disappears rapidly and generally is undectectable 24 h later. Although HPL is a potent lactogen when tested in a number of assay systems, it is secreted at a time when the lactogenic response of the breast to prolactin is inhibited by high levels of estrogens. However, it is possible that HPL as well as prolactin acts to facilitate mammary growth and development. In the rat placental lactogen levels can be reduced progressively by selective fetectomy performed during pregnancy. It is possible to demonstrate that, when there is a major decrease in placental lactogen, mammary development and subsequent lactation in the postpartum period are seriously impaired. Whether HPL similarly affects the human breast remains uncertain. One possible mechanism by which HPL and prolactin might facilitate growth of the mammary gland during pregnancy is that prolactin, and possibly HPL, stimulates the formation of estrogen receptors in the cytoplasm, thereby perhaps increasing the responsiveness of the gland to this growth stimulant.

THYROID HORMONES

Thyroid hormones are important for adequate milk secretion. In rats, the degree of lactation is directly related to thyroid secretion, while large doses of thyroid depress milk yield in both rats and rabbits. In cows and goats, thyroid hormones are galactopoietic, and clinical observations in humans also suggest a beneficial effect of thyroid hormones on lactation. On the other hand, hypothyroidism in human subjects may be associated with galactorrhea. In this situation treatment with thyroid reverses both symptoms. As mentioned in Chapter 12, TRH stimulates the secretion of both TSH and prolactin in normal subjects, and in hypothyroid individuals there is an even greater release of TSH and prolactin.

INFLUENCE OF PARATHYROIDS

Removal of parathyroids from lactating animals depresses lactation. In cows, despite the large amounts of calcium secreted in milk, parathyroid gland activity appears to be depressed at the height of lactation.

INSULIN AND SERUM GROWTH FACTORS

Early studies indicated that insulin is necessary for the proper function of the mammary gland. Injections of insulin increase milk yield in lactating rats, while in goats and cows similar treatment decreases milk yield. The importance of insulin in humans is unknown, but recent evidence has demonstrated the presence of large numbers of specific insulin-binding sites in human mammary glands. The precise role which insulin plays in stimulating mammary function has not been defined. It is likely, however, that insulin stimulates glucose entry into the cell and accelerates lipogenesis. In addition, in tissue culture of mouse and rat mammary epithelial cells, insulin at high concentrations acts as a mitogen. Serum contains a number of factors which stimulate mammary epithelial cell replication. These factors have some of the characteristics of somatomedin or nonsuppressible insulinlike activity, but in other respects are different.

Epidermal growth factor (EGF), a single-chain polypeptide isolated from the male mouse submaxillary gland, causes epithelial cells of mouse mammary glands and mammary carcinomas to proliferate in organ culture. The presence of immunoreactive EGF in serum of pregnant women has been reported,[15] and recently human EGF has been detected in human urine using a radioreceptor assay. In addition, there may be a specific serum mammary growth factor which may be of considerable importance in regulating cell replication in the mammary gland.

OXYTOCIN

There is evidence that oxytocin may exert a galactopoietic action in some species, including the goat, sheep, and rat. One possible explanation for this effect stems from the fact that oxytocin stimulates the release of prolactin from the anterior pituitary; second, oxytocin minimizes inhibitory pressures within alveoli; and third, oxytocin increases the supply of nutrients to the alveolar cells by increasing the permeability of membranes. In humans there is no evidence for any galactopoietic action of oxytocin; its only role appears to be in the milk ejection reflex, but even here the evidence is conflicting.

ESTROGEN AND PROGESTERONE

Oophorectomy has no detrimental effects on established lactation and in some instances ovarian suppression stimulates milk secretion. Galactopoietic effects of estrogens, particularly in farm animals, have been reported. Estrogens stimulate prolactin release in humans, but in large amounts they exert an inhibitory effect on lactation, probably by a direct action on the mammary gland. Thus estrogens appear to be important in modulating the responsiveness of the mammary gland to lactogenic hormones.

The role of specific estrogen receptors in mediating the action of estrogens in target organs has received considerable attention in recent years. Specific protein receptors for 17β-estradiol sedimenting at 8–9 S have been described in the cytoplasmic fraction from a variety of breast carcinomas, both of animal and human origin. However, there is a lack of evidence of a comparable estrogen receptor in the normal mammary gland, in spite of the well-accepted responsiveness of this tissue to estrogens. On the other hand, specific estrogen-binding proteins with high specificity and affinity for 17β-estradiol have been found in the cytoplasmic and nuclear fractions of lactating mammary gland of the rat[16] and mouse.[17] In most steroid-receptor systems, the hormone initially interacts with the receptor molecule in the cytoplasm and is subsequently translocated to the nucleus. In the lactating mammary gland it has been suggested that the nuclear localization of the hormone is dependent on an initial interaction of the hormone with the cytoplasmic receptors.

We have already discussed the influence of estrogens on prolactin receptors; in the rat, both in vitro[18] and in vivo,[19] estrogen receptors appear to be modulated by prolactin. Thus the interactions of these hormones are complex at the target tissue level.

Apart from its role in mammogenesis, there is lack of evidence of any influence of progesterone in human lactation. In rats there is evidence of an inhibitory effect of large doses of progesterone on lactose content in the mammary gland. Elevated progesterone concentrations inhibit lactalbumin synthesis in mouse mammary gland explants, and it is postulated that lactogenesis in the rat is triggered by the removal of a progesterone block on the secretory activity of the mammary alveolar cells. The fact that high doses of progestogens administered to women have little effect on the amount of milk or the duration of lactation suggests that progesterone has a minor role in human lactation.[20]

ADRENAL STEROIDS

The adrenal cortex exerts an unquestionable effect on milk secretion in experimental animals. Early in 1941, when Folley and Young suggested that a lactogenic complex of anterior pituitary hormones was necessary to bring about the initiation of lactation, prolactin and ACTH were recognized to be the most important hormones. Subsequently, the effects of ACTH on the initiation of lactation were attributed to glucocorticoid secretion. In several species, such as the rat, mouse, and goat, adrenal steroids are essential for the induction and maintenance of milk secretion. The functional activity of corticosteroids is dependent on the level of cortisol-binding globulin (CBG). In the rat there is a precipitous decrease in CBG activity early in lactation, accompanied by an increase in corticosterone levels. Thus, corticosteroid activity is maximal and, together with prolactin, may initiate full lactation. However, the role of adrenal steroids in human lactation is still unknown and it may be misleading to make any assumptions from the data in rats.

LACTATION

INITIATION

There is considerable variation among different species in the time when milk can first be detected in mammary alveoli during pregnancy. In ruminants very considerable quantities of milk may be produced before parturition, and, indeed, milk production continues uninterrupted during the early stages of pregnancy. In the rat and rhesus monkey copious milk secretion does not occur until 2 days after parturition. Similarly, in humans the alveoli become distended with colostrum in the last third of pregnancy but mammary secretion does not appear until 3–4 days after childbirth. There are numerous theories concerning the possible involvement of endocrine mechanisms in the initiation of lactation. Recently it has been suggested that the secretory activity of the alveolar epithelium during pregnancy is inhibited by steroids from the fetal placental unit which exert an inhibitory effect directly on mammary epithelial cells, rendering them less responsive to lactogenic hormones. The observations that serum prolactin levels reach their peak shortly before delivery, when no lactation occurs, and that estrogen treatment inhibits puerperal lactation in the presence of elevated serum prolactin, support this hypothesis.[13,21] At parturition a fall in the concentration of steroids in blood permits the mammary gland to respond to the "lactogenic complex."

EFFECT OF SUCKLING ON PROLACTIN AND OXYTOCIN

The mechanisms involved in the maintenance of milk production have been defined in part. One of the most potent factors favoring the establishment of lactation is nipple stimulation. There are many anecdotal reports in which nonpregnant women have been able to produce an adequate supply of milk within a few days of taking a baby to the breast. When the newborn suckles, a complex chain of events is initiated. A neural stimulus is transmitted to the brain, where it results in the secretion of prolactin and oxytocin. The exact anatomic pathways that mediate the release of prolactin and oxytocin have not been defined in humans, but some experimental data is available in animals. The relationship between suckling and prolactin release was suggested as early as 1957 by Grosvenor and Turner.[22] They reported that in the rat a significant decrease of pituitary prolactin occurred after suckling. Subsequently others noted the disappearance of prolactin granules under the same conditions using electron microscopic techniques. With the availability of specific and sensitive radioimmunoassays, increases in serum prolactin with suckling have been observed in cows, goats, sheep, and humans. When nursing women were allowed to hold their infants but not to breast feed, prolactin did not increase despite the occurrence of the milk let-down reflex. The application of a breast pump at regular periods of breast feeding caused prolactin elevations similar in timing and magnitude to those occurring during suckling; hence it is concluded that neither psychic factors associated with expectation of nursing, nor the presumed release of oxytocin as evidenced by milk let-down are effective in stimulating the release of prolactin.[23] On the other hand, in a recent study Bunner and Vanderlaan[24] investigated the maternal plasma prolactin concentration in relation to nursing episodes throughout a 24-h period with blood samples every 30 min. They found that prolactin does not have any consistent, immediate relationship to nursing episodes! These findings, which were obtained in four women, if confirmed by other investigators, will provide further evidence of how limited our knowledge of the physiology of human lactation is.

The milk ejection caused by posterior pituitary extracts was first observed in 1910 in lactating goats. Both posterior pituitary hormones, oxytocin and vasopressin, cause milk ejection, but oxtocin is five times more active than vasopressin. Oxytocin exerts a direct effect on the myoepithelial elements surrounding the alveoli of the breast, causing them to contract and force milk into the mammary ducts, where it is more readily available to the suckling infant. The symptoms of milk let-down occur more frequently in successful breast feeders, whereas incomplete let-down is frequently found in unsuccessful breast feeders. Although suckling is the primary stimulus in the milk ejection reflex, it may be conditioned by factors such as the sight of the baby, scheduled time of feeding, and breast preparation. Pain, distraction, embarrassment, and anesthetics tend to inhibit the reflex.

Caldeyro Barcia and his colleagues[1] have carried out extensive studies on the milk let-down reflex in humans. They catheterized human mammary ducts and measured intraductal pressure under various physiologic circumstances. The injection of oxytocin and suckling of the nipple on the opposite breast or dilation of the cervix produced a marked increase in ductal pressure. The rhythmic contraction induced by suckling was closely mimicked by successive intravenous injections of oxytocin given at frequent intervals in an appropriate dose, while a continuous intravenous infusion or a single intravenous or intramuscular injection of a high dose of oxytocin evoked nonphysiologic responses, suggesting that oxytocin release occurs in repeated spurts in women. It is estimated that the intermittent release of 1 and 10 mU oxytocin would stimulate the rhythmic contractions observed during breast feeding.

More recently, serum oxytocin concentrations have been determined during periods of breast feeding in both animals and humans. Present assay methods are not sufficiently sensitive to measure basal circulating oxytocin. However, during milking or breast feeding, frequent, rapid intermittent spurts of oxytocin are detected in plasma. These spurt discharges of oxytocin also occur during the resting phase but with a reduced frequency.

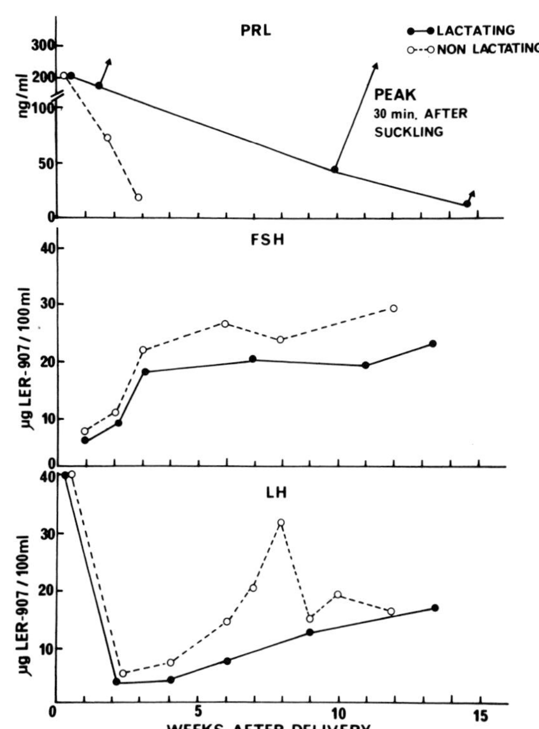

Fig. 131-5. Simplified representation of serum concentrations of prolactin, FSH, and LH in lactating and nonlactating women during the puerperium.

ENDOCRINE CHANGES IN THE PUERPERIUM

In the puerperium, major physical, psychologic, and hormonal adjustments take place. Hormones produced by the fetal–placental unit disappear rapidly. The endocrine changes that occur in women who are breast feeding are different from those in women who are not. The changes in serum prolactin and oxytocin that occur after suckling have already been outlined. In this section, the effect of breast feeding on ovarian function will be considered in more detail.

FSH and LH have been measured in the postpartum period[25,26] and attempts have been made to correlate such changes with ovulation and the return of menses (Fig. 131-5). FSH, which is almost undetectable during late pregnancy and the first week postpartum, returns to normal levels after 7–18 days and thereafter remains relatively high during the period of hyperprolactinemia. In the first week LH levels appear to be high, but these apparently high concentrations for the most part are due to the cross-reaction of HCG in the radioimmunoassay. Following clearance of HCG basal LH levels are low compared to levels observed during a normal menstrual cycle.* Furthermore, the normal episodic LH fluctuations which occur during normal menstrual cycles are absent in the first 2 weeks postpartum.[27] Thus the occurrence of the first postpartum ovulation is preceded by LH levels increasing to normal values, the occurrence of LH fluctuations, and finally, the LH ovulatory peak.

Serum estradiol and progesterone levels decline within a few days following delivery to low values, and these patterns parallel those previously reported for urinary estrogen and pregnanediol secretion in the postpartum period. Since estradiol levels remain low for a longer period in women who breast feed successfully, it appears that the ovarian response to endogenous FSH levels, which are in the normal range, is subnormal. One possible cause for ovarian unresponsiveness is the elevated prolactin levels in women who are breast feeding. The apparent refractoriness to endogenous gonadotropins in lactating women agrees with the finding of an inadequate response to exogenous gonadotropin stimulation. In one study,[28] as much as 2000 IU HCG was given to lactating subjects from day 5 to day 20 postpartum, and in inadequate response in terms of urinary estrogens, pregnanediol, and endometrial biopsy was observed. In recent studies carried out in our laboratory, we have found that patients in the immediate postpartum period (first week) fail to respond to gonadotropin-releasing hormone (LHRH) with an increase in LH and FSH, and that the period of unresponsiveness is more prolonged in women who are breast feeding. These observations suggest that the periodic bursts of prolactin release that follow suckling may have an important inhibitory effect on the hypothalamic–pituitary gonadal axis. However, in one study of nonlactating women, the effect on gonadotropins of ethinyl estradiol administered from day 10 to day 14 of the puerperium was examined. It was concluded by these investigators that in the postpartum period the hypothalamic–pituitary system is capable of responding appropriately to the positive feedback of exogenous estrogen stimulation. The recovery of pituitary ovarian function following delivery appears analogous to the recovery of the pituitary adrenal system following glucocorticoid suppression, in which adrenal responsiveness lags behind the recovery of pituitary function.

The time of the occurrence of the first ovulation after childbirth is influenced by breast feeding: the longer the duration and intensity of breast feeding, the longer the delay in the onset of ovulation. An average of 49 days (SD ± 12) to the first postpartum ovulation was found by Peres et al.[29] in women in whom lactation

*Specific β-chain radioimmunoassays for LH that do not cross-react with HCG show that LH concentrations are suppressed in the immediate postpartum week and throughout pregnancy.

was suppressed immediately postpartum. In lactating women the first ovulation occurred on average at 112 days (SD ± 71), with no ovulation before day 35. Thus it appears that breast feeding does not provide an absolute protection against pregnancy, since some women do ovulate despite lactation. Furthermore, it must be pointed out that in some lactating women, endometrial biopsies revealed changes compatible with the secretory phase at the 49th postpartum day, and yet these individuals failed to menstruate until 10 weeks later. Thus the synchronization of ovulation and menstruation and the recovery of fertility in the postpartum period require further investigation.

CLINICAL ASPECTS OF LACTATION

COMPOSITION OF COLOSTRUM AND MILK

Colostrum

In the last weeks of pregnancy and in the first few days postdelivery, a small amount of fluid usually can be expressed from the mammary gland. This opalescent fluid, which is small in volume, yellowish in color, and contains fat globules, is known as *colostrum*. Microscopic examination of this fluid reveals multinucleated cells loaded with particles of fat. These "foam cells" are derived from alveolar and ductal cells which have been shed into the lumen. Colostrum contains about 8 percent protein, including lactalbumin and lactoglobulin, but it contains little or no casein, fat, and lactose.

Milk

Usually, 2–4 days after delivery colostrum is replaced by milk. Physicochemically milk is an emulsion of fat in water and the relative proportion of each component varies throughout a period of breast feeding. This fact was appreciated as early as 1473, when wet nurses were advised to first milk the breast to drain the watery fluid before allowing the infant to nurse. Together with water and fat droplets in suspension (3–4 percent), milk contains 1 percent proteins (casein, lactalbumin, and lactoglobulin), 7 percent lactose, electrolytes in solution, minerals, and vitamins. A comparison of the composition of human and cow's milk can be found elsewhere.[30] Human milk contains over 100 known constituents and additional components are constantly being identified.

Evidence is accumulating of the great importance of a balanced diet for optimal nutrition of the infant. Although there is very little difference between the caloric energy provided by human and cow's milk (about 70 kcal/100 ml), there must be an overall balance of nutrients as well as of individual constituents in the infant's diet. One example which illustrates this point is the fact that infantile tetany is reported to occur almost exclusively in formula-fed babies.[31,32] This results from the very different calcium and phosphorous content which is found in human milk as compared to various formulas which are widely utilized. Furthermore, formula-fed infants seem more susceptible to infection in infancy, including gastroenteritis, recurrent respiratory infection, and a variety of viral diseases. This problem is especially acute in underdeveloped countries where hygienic measures are not widely employed.

Specific properties of human milk that increase resistance to infection have in fact been reported.[33] One of these is a nitrogen-containing polysaccharide which favors the growth of *Lactobacillus bifidus*. The presence of this organism confers a protective effect against invasive enteropathogenic organisms, such as *Escherichia coli*. Furthermore, antibodies (IgA), lysozyme (300 times more than in cow's milk), and interferon produced by the lymphocytes of the milk itself may also have a protective effect.

Milk, by itself, combined with fetal stores and sunlight, is usually adequate to sustain growth and nutrition in the infant for 4–6 months. At the end of the first week postpartum, 550 ml milk/day are produced, and by 2–3 weeks this increases to 800 ml/day, with maximal rates as great as 1.5–2 liters/day.

MATERNAL DIETARY REQUIREMENTS FOR MILK PRODUCTION AND COMPOSITION

In order to avoid major depletion of maternal tissue reserves, the diet of the lactating woman must be adequate. Within reason, she may eat her usual diet, but the ingestion of meat, fish, and eggs is important, and fresh fruit, green vegetables, and salads are recommended. Fluid intake should be liberal. Supplemental iron is often prescribed and, during lactation, there should be an adequate dietary intake of calcium. Recommended daily caloric intake as well as useful information with regard to the composition of human and cow's milk may be found elsewhere.[30] Many attempts have been made to assess the effects of maternal food restriction on lactation. It is generally agreed that lactation persists despite severe malnutrition, however, with extreme maternal deprivation the protein and fat content of human milk is lower. Severe dehydration also decreases milk yield.

The fat content in milk over a 24-h period is relatively constant, but a diurnal variation has been reported, with minimal values occurring in the first morning feeding and the highest at midmorning. These changes are not influenced by the mother maintaining a uniform distribution of calories and fat intake over a 24-h period. Dietary fat composition, however, does influence the types of fatty acids that are found in milk.

There is a considerable difference in the fat content of the initial and final phase of milk produced with each breast feeding, with higher concentrations in the latter. It has been suggested[34] that these changes in biochemical composition of human milk during the feed are associated with development of an appetite control mechanism in breast-fed babies. The change in milk composition is a cue for the baby to stop feeding. No such cue would be received by a bottle-fed baby because neither taste nor flavor alters during the feed.

There is little correlation between the prepregnant size of the breast and the amount of milk produced postpartum. On the contrary, milk production is closely related to the extent of mammary gland development during pregnancy and also seems to depend on proper antenatal and immediate postnatal breast stimulation. Problems resulting from inverted nipples or poor nipple protrusion usually resolve spontaneously during pregnancy. In the last weeks of gestation, pregnant women may express colostrum from the nipples twice a day and it may be a helpful exercise if the patient learns how to empty the breast manually antepartum before the breasts become engorged and painful.

In the first few hours postpartum, the newborn may be nursed at each breast for 3 min at intervals of 4 h. Thereafter, each period of suckling is increased 1 min each day. Toward the end of the first week, regular breast feeding periods at 4-h intervals are generally established. In the first week of lactation, the newborn often cannot empty the breast adequately and manual expression or pumping is necessary to maintain and increase milk secretion. Pumping also relieves breast tenderness and pain caused by the engorged milk-filled mammary glands. After 7–10 days, when breast feeding is well established, not more than 10 min on each breast should be allowed because the available milk is removed in this period and excessive suckling can injure the areolae and nipples. Both breasts should be suckled at each nursing period; areolae and nipples should be cleaned with a nonirritant sterile solution before and after nursing, and nipples should be covered with a sterile pad during nursing-free intervals.

In recent decades, the decline in lactation which began in the Western world has spread to less-developed parts of the world, initially involving the elite and, subsequently, the general population in urban areas. In the developed countries, a variety of factors, both social and economic, have contributed to the "epidemiology of lactation failure." No reliable statistics exist about the proportion of women who breast feed their babies today and the length of time they continue to do so, but in the United States it has been reported that 80–90 percent of infants are entirely formula-fed. There has also been an interesting reversal in the usual social class bias regarding lactation. Until recently, artificial feeding was favored by the upper social classes, whereas now these groups most favor breast feeding.

A final cautionary note must be added about drug ingestion and breast feeding. It has become apparent that a number of drugs should not be given to the mother while she is nursing. These include atropine, anticoagulants, antithyroid drugs, antimetabolites, cathartics (excluding senna), dihydrotachysterol, iodides, narcotics, radioactive preparations, bromides, ergot, tetracyclines, and metronidazole (Flagyl).

A group of drugs widely used during breast feeding are oral contraceptives, but before considering them it may be more useful to consider the general problem of contraception in the postpartum period. In the past, breast feeding was perhaps the principal means by which child spacing was attempted; however, it is evident that the protection against a new pregnancy was quite inadequate. More reliable contraception can be provided by intrauterine devices (IUD) or oral agents. The IUD has the advantage of not interfering with lactation; however, it must be pointed out that the rate of expulsion of the IUD may be rather high. (Contraception is discussed in detail in Chapter 112.)

Previously, when contraceptives containing large amounts of estrogens and progestagens were used, breast feeding was inhibited. However, with the lower steroid content of oral contraceptives currently in use, lactation is only slightly diminished (especially when the oral agents are started after lactation is well established). These compounds may alter some aspects of blood-clotting mechanisms, but they do not interfere with uterine involution to any significant degree. On the other hand, there is evidence that steroids may increase iron absorption, resulting in greater requirements for folic acid, vitamin B_{12}, pyridoxine, and tryptophan. Finally, it should be recognized that the mammary gland excretes steroids and their metabolites in milk. Because of this fact, oral contraceptives generally are not recommended when the mother is breast feeding.

DISTURBANCES OF LACTATION

Engorgement

This common complication, which usually affects both breasts, generally occurs between days 2 and 4 postpartum. The condition results from milk retention and vascular and lymphatic stasis accompanied by edema of the tissues. During this period, the breasts become firm, tense, and swollen, and the areolae become edematous, resulting in less nipple protrusion, which makes it difficult for the infant to suckle. Although there may be considerable local discomfort, systemic symptoms apart from slight temperature elevation are uncommon. A much less pronounced degree of engorgement may occur after weaning.

Agalactia

This is the complete absence of lactation and is rare. It is, of course, the hallmark of patients who suffer from Sheehan's syndrome (postpartum pituitary necrosis) and results from prolactin deficiency.

Failing Lactation

In humans, very little is known about the reasons for failing lactation, and only empirical approaches have been used to correct or reverse the process. A decline in milk yield is most frequently encountered early in breast feeding. Some estimates indicate that five of six failures have occurred by the end of the third month and a high proportion of these have already taken place by the sixth week. In one study of 1100 patients with this problem, in 40 percent no recognized cause for the failure could be identified.[35] In this circumstance, one must resort to formula feeding.

Attempts to increase milk yield with hormonal therapy date back to 1896, when it was reported that thyroid extracts increased milk yield both in women and in cows. More recently, HGH preparations have been used to increase milk yield, but neither treatment has general application. Pharmacologic agents including phenothiazines and TRH have been shown to increase serum prolactin concentrations, and attempts have been made to enhance milk production in both animals and humans with TRH. Current studies have determined that oral TRH, 5 mg every 12 h, stimulates milk secretion without causing any endocrine dysfunction.[36]

In some conditions it is inadvisable for the mother to breast feed. These include: the presence of serious systemic disease such as tuberculosis, heart disease, or mental disturbances; the ingestion of certain drugs (e.g., antithyroid drugs, diuretics) that are excreted in the milk and could have a deleterious effect on the newborn; and local conditions of the breast such as severe engorgement, mastitis, abscess, etc. In addition, various conditions affecting the baby, such as prematurity, cleft palate, mental deficiency, etc., also constitute reasons not to breast feed.

SUPPRESSION OF LACTATION

Prior to the introduction of estrogens to suppress lactation, a variety of empirical measures were tried, including the application of breast binders along with restriction of fluid intake, and the use of laxatives and diuretics. At times, the treatment was worse than the problem because, despite the application of all these measures, the breasts became engorged and painful. Suppression of lactation with estrogens began in the late 1930s. A variety of estrogen preparations are currently used. A common practice is to give ethinyl estradiol (0.25 mg) three times daily for 5 days, or longer if necessary. Quinestrol (2 mg) orally or a single intramuscular injection of estradiol valerate (10 mg) is almost always successful in preventing secretion provided these agents are given within 6 h of delivery. Good results have also been reported with chlorotrianisene. With any of these regimens a failure rate of 10–20 percent is frequently observed. Estrogens are most effective when administered a few hours after delivery, and it is desirable to achieve high plasma concentrations initially and subsequently to decrease the levels gradually in order to avoid delayed engorgement. A longer list of steroids which have been used to suppress postpartum lactation, their dose, and relative effectiveness can be found elsewhere.[37]

The inhibitory action of estrogen on lactation appears to be exerted at the mammary gland by blocking the action of prolactin. In addition, estrogen may potentially interfere with proper uterine involution. For some patients, the administration of estrogens enhances the risk of thromboembolic complications in the puerperium. More recently, an ergot alkaloid preparation, CB-154, has been used to inhibit lactation. This agent specifically suppresses prolactin secretion and inhibits postpartum breast engorgement as well as established lactation.

GALACTORRHEA SYNDROMES

Galactorrhea is the secretion of milk from the breast under nonphysiologic circumstances. The amount of milk secreted varies greatly, ranging from as little as a drop, which can be expressed manually, to continuous copious and spontaneous milk leakage. It is important to remember that a small amount of serous fluid can often be expressed from the breasts of multipara and this finding by itself should not be interpreted as galactorrhea. Hippocrates observed centuries ago that "if a woman is not with child, nor has brought forth, have milk, her menses are obstructed." If amenorrhea accompanies galactorrhea, it generally indicates that a more extensive disturbance of hypothalmic–pituitary function exists.

Three eponymic designations of amenorrhea and galactorrhea have been recognized: the Chiari-Frommel, Argonz del Castillo, and Forbes-Albright syndromes. In 1855, Chiari described the onset of galactorrhea and amenorrhea which followed parturition. Several decades later, Frommel reported the same entity, and the syndrome is now known as the Chiari-Frommel syndrome. It is characterized by the postpartum onset of amenorrhea, galactorrhea, and hyposecretion of gonadotropins and estrogens. Another classic description by Ahumada and del Castillo in 1932 and by Argonz and del Castillo in 1953 outlined a similar symptom complex, consisting of amenorrhea and galactorrhea which developed without any direct relation to pregnancy. In 1954 Forbes and Albright reported that, of 15 patients who developed spontaneous lactation, amenorrhea, and decreased levels of total urinary gonadotropins (mouse uterine weight method), 7 had an enlargement of the sella turcica and a pituitary tumor.

The medical literature is replete with examples that demonstrate that the classification of galactorrhea based on eponyms is somewhat artificial. In the same patient, galactorrhea may or may not develop in the postpartum period, and a pituitary tumor may be demonstrable months or years later. Hence, at first, such patients would be classified as Chiari-Frommel or Argonz and del Castillo, and subsequently as Forbes-Albright. We therefore suggest that an etiologic classification is preferable (Table 131-1). When one examines the etiologic classification, it is helpful to ask whether there is an absolute increase in serum prolactin concentration or an abnormal prolactin secretory response following the administration of provocative or inhibitory agents. This approach is also useful because when galactorrhea is accompanied by grossly elevated concentrations of serum prolactin it is more likely that a serious underlying disorder is present. Contrariwise, when no abnormality of prolactin secretion is evident, it is more likely that galactorrhea represents a fairly benign symptom.

Table 131-1. Classification of the Galactorrhea Syndromes

I. Galactorrhea associated with disorders of the hypothalamic–pituitary axis
- A. Organic
  1. Hypothalamus: infiltrative or degenerative processes
     - a. Tumors: primary or secondary (craniopharyngiomas are the most common example of the first variety)
     - b. Infiltrative: histiocytosis x
     - c. Degenerative: postencephalitic; posttraumatic fracture of the base of the skull; embolism of hypothalamic area
  2. Pituitary stalk lesion
  3. Pituitary lesion
     - a. Prolactin-secreting tumors
     - b. Acromegaly
     - c. Cushing's syndrome
     - d. "Empty sella" syndrome
- B. Functional
  1. Pregnancy related (Chiari-Frommel syndrome)
  2. Pharmacologic agents and galactorrhea
     - a. Hormones: sex steroids, i.e., estrogens (e.g., while on or after withdrawal of oral contraceptives)
     - b. Psychotropic agents [e.g., chlorpromazine, reserpine, and methyldopa (Aldomet)]
  3. Galactorrhea and other disorders: local factors such as mechanical stimulation of the nipple or areola (e.g., excessive suckling); disturbances of the chest wall; surgery, particularly in the thoracic region (e.g., pneumonectomy, thoracoplasty, cardiac surgery), cervical spinal lesions; herpes zoster; burns of chest

II. Galactorrhea associated with thyroid disorders

III. Galactorrhea and adrenal disorders: adrenal insufficiency and adrenal carcinoma

IV. Ectopic production of prolactin

V. Idiopathic

CLASSIFICATION OF GALACTORRHEA

GALACTORRHEA AND HYPOTHALAMIC DISORDERS

Organic

Galactorrhea associated with hypothalamic lesions, regardless of whether it results from an infiltrative or degenerative process, is usually accompanied by a modest elevation of serum prolactin. This increase probably results from the loss of prolactin-inhibitory factor (PIF), which normally suppresses the secretion of prolactin by the pituitary. The precise nature of PIF remains unclear. Until recently, most of the evidence suggested that PIF was a peptide, but some new experiments suggest that dopamine may be an equally good candidate. A more extensive discussion of the hypothalamic control of prolactin secretion is found in Chapter 15. A mechanism leading to an elevated serum prolactin concentration and galactorrhea in patients after stalk section of the pituitary is related to the interruption of the portal blood flow and the delivery of PIF to the pituitary.

Pituitary Lesions. Prolactin-secreting pituitary tumors are the most common endocrine tumors of the pituitary gland, accounting for 25–30 percent of all pituitary tumors. Only one-third of the prolactin-secreting tumors produce galactorrhea. In some patients with nonfunctioning chromophobe adenomas of the pituitary gland, expansion of the tumor into the median eminence also leads to elevated serum prolactin values because of destruction of the inhibitory areas controlling prolactin secretion. In a study of 15 patients with pituitary tumors, 5 had prolactin levels greater than 200 ng/ml, and in larger series values of above 500 ng/ml have been common.[37a] If the concentration of prolactin is between 30 and 200 ng/ml, the values are not diagnostic of a prolactin-secreting tumor, because involvement of the hypothalamus by any tumor may lead to a deficiency of PIF secretion, resulting in modest elevations of serum prolactin as well. Serum prolactin concentrations greater than 200 ng/ml are most frequently associated with a primary prolactin-secreting tumor.

Abnormal Lactation and Acromegly. Galactorrhea is seen in a variable proportion of patients with acromegaly. In one study[37b] of 19 cases of acromegaly, it was found that, with the exception of a single case, all had serum prolactin levels in the normal range. In this situation it is likely that the intrinsic lactogenic effect of HGH is responsible for the lactation. On the other hand, other authors report that 20–40 percent of patients with active acromegaly also hypersecrete prolactin.[37c]

Functional

Those patients in whom no organic defect of the hypothalamic–pituitary–prolactin axis can be identified are classified as cases of "functional" galactorrhea. Patients with a primary organic disease such as hypothyroidism may also have a functional disturbance of the hypothalamic control mechanism regulating prolactin secretion.

Pregnancy-Related Galactorrhea. As was discussed earlier, galactorrhea that arises in relation to pregnancy and is associated with amenorrhea has been referred to as the Chiari-Frommel syndrome. Normally there is a major increase in prolactin-secreting cells during pregnancy, which gradually involute postpartum. If the involutionary process fails to progress normally, presumably hyperprolactinemia might persist. However, very little is known about the precise mechanism leading to the hyperprolactinemia and galactorrhea. In some patients, perhaps 10 percent, the syndrome is self-limiting, whereas in others galactorrhea persists for years. In a significant percentage of these patients, conclusive evidence of a pituitary tumor emerges eventually, and indeed, some investigators feel that a substantial proportion of these patients harbor a microadenoma which enlarges very slowly.

Pharmacologic Agents and Galactorrhea

Oral contraceptives. There are no adequate data on the occurrence of secondary amenorrhea in the normal population, nor on its incidence in women who have stopped treatment with oral contraceptives. Rice-Wray et al.[38] found that 2.8 percent of their patients failed to menstruate for periods of 3–12 months after cessation of oral contraceptives. This complication after discontinuing oral contraceptives seems more common among patients who had oligomenorrhea prior to treatment. In 10–20 percent of these patients who develop amenorrhea, galactorrhea occurs as well.

The influence of prolonged estrogen and progestagen therapy is believed to alter the hypothalamic–pituitary–prolactin axis, but the precise mechanism remains obscure. In general, basal prolactin levels in women taking contraceptives are in the normal range, but there are conflicting reports about the average mean concentrations. In most studies, no differences or only very minor elevations were found.

In patients with amenorrhea-galactorrhea, serum prolactin concentrations are usually modestly elevated. In some patients with normal serum prolactin and galactorrhea, menses resumed when prolactin levels were reduced with CB-154, suggesting that galactorrhea and amenorrhea are both prolactin dependent. It is most important to remember that patients with prior menstrual irregularities are more prone to develop postpill amenorrhea-galactorrhea, and indeed it is wise to forewarn patients of this possibility.

Psychotropic agents. These include reserpine, methyldopa, phenothiazines (such as chlorpromazine, trifluoperazine, thioridazine, pericyazine, and fluphenazine), and phenothiazine derivatives (such as amitriptyline and imipramine). All these drugs are commonly associated with elevated prolactin values and galactorrhea. These elevated levels persist for periods of 2–3 weeks after termination of therapy. The cause of the elevated prolactin concentrations is due to a reduction in the biogenic amines in the hypothalamus. The latter either directly (e.g., dopamine) or indirectly (via PIF) inhibit the secretion of prolactin by the pituitary.

GALACTORRHEA AND OTHER DISORDERS

Mechanical stimulation of the nipple or the areolae or disturbances of the chest wall have resulted in galactorrhea. It is postulated that stimulation of the fourth, fifth, and sixth intercostal nerves may trigger a neural reflex arc resulting in increased prolactin secretion. A persistent stimulation of the reflex arc by excessive suckling as well as a variety of pathologic events such as scarring, herpes zoster, or burns of the chest wall, etc., can lead to the same result.

Abnormal Lactation Associated with Disorders of the Thyroid

Juvenile hypothyroidism occasionally is associated with galactorrhea and precocious sexual maturation. Galactorrhea and hypothyroidism are actually more common in adults and, in some cases, amenorrhea is present as well. Although most patients with hypothyroidism respond to TRH with an exaggerated increase in prolactin, only a few have elevated basal serum prolactin concentrations or galactorrhea, but, of course, all have elevated serum TSH concentrations. Careful dose–response studies in humans have shown that TRH always stimulates both TSH and prolactin secretion. The selective increase in serum TSH in patients with hypothyroidism implies that there is no absolute increase in the secretion of TRH, but that in hypothyroid subjects the pituitary thyrotrope is peculiarly sensitive to the effect of TRH. Indeed, recent direct measurements of TRH secretion reveal no increase of TRH secretion in hypothyroidism. Replacement therapy with thyroid leads to a normalization of the elevated serum prolactin as well as of the pituitary hyperresponsiveness to TRH, and galactorrhea usually disappears concurrently over a period of several weeks.

There have been occasional reports of galactorrhea and hyperthyroidism, but we are unaware of any prolactin measurements in this situation. We have studied one man who developed galactorrhea following therapy for hyperthyroidism. Upon investigation, this patient was found to have a pituitary prolactin-secreting tumor. Presumably, when he was hyperthyroid, prolactin secretion by the tumor was sufficiently inhibited, and only as he became euthyroid did the prolactin-secreting tumor become evident.

Galactorrhea and Adrenal Disorders

There are several isolated reports of galactorrhea developing in patients with adrenal disorders. One patient with adrenal insufficiency whom we studied presented with galactorrhea, amenorrhea, and elevated serum prolactin and ACTH concentrations. When the diagnosis was made and replacement therapy with corticoids was initiated, both the amenorrhea and galactorrhea disappeared. This case provides evidence that some milk secretion is possible in the virtual absence of adrenal steroids. On the other hand, galactorrhea has been reported to occur rarely in patients with Cushing's syndrome. In most of these patients, no plausible mechanism for the galactorrhea can be postulated. Most patients receiving large doses of steroids in fact have a somewhat diminished increase in serum prolactin after TRH administration.

Ectopic Production of Prolactin

Turkington has reported the ectopic production of prolactin in one patient with a bronchogenic carcinoma and in several patients with galactorrhea and a hypernephroma.[39]

Idiopathic

In order to establish the etiology of galactorrhea, all possibilities must be considered. With a careful history and appropriate laboratory examination, it is possible to make a definite diagnosis in about 50–70 percent of patients. However, there is a residual group of patients in whom no cause for galactorrhea can be established; hence they are classified as idiopathic. In patients with high prolactin levels without any other symptom, hypothalamic dysfunction with altered feedback response may be postulated. On the other hand, in those patients with galactorrhea and prolactin levels in the normal range it may be speculated that there is an altered responsiveness of the breast. It is becoming apparent, in fact, that to assess the overall biologic effect of a hormone, at least two factors appear to be important: the hormone concentration and the target tissue responsiveness. While much of our effort thus far has been concentrated on measuring hormone levels, we anticipate that the studies of hormone receptors (e.g., prolactin, insulin, steroids) as an index of tissue responsiveness will provide new insight and will increase our rudimentary understanding of the factors leading to galactorrhea.

CLINICAL ASPECTS OF GALACTORRHEA

In patients with galactorrhea, the abnormal breast discharge may be the sole symptom or it may be accompanied by other clinical features. A normal or abnormal menstrual and obstetric history may precede the onset of galactorrhea. Patients may be unaware of any breast discharge or may complain of fullness of the breast, tenderness, moisture, or staining of the brassiere with milk. The discharge may be unilateral or bilateral. Upon examination, the breast usually appears normal. Rarely one may encounter swollen, tender breasts giving rise to a picture indistinguishable from postpartum breast engorgement. Spontaneous milk discharge may be present or milk may be expressed from one or both nipples. The abnormal breast discharge appears as a white, thick, milky secretion or as a milklike fluid. There are both qualitative and quantitative differences between secretions occurring in patients with galactorrhea and normal lactation, with the former exhibiting a higher protein and fat and lower lactose content. In breast biopsies in cases of galactorrhea, histologic changes consistent with lactation have been noted, with the exception that in mammary lobules only some of the acini exhibit this change; many acini are small and fail to reveal any secretory changes. If amenorrhea is present, it is usually associated with minimal pelvic abnormalities, although vaginal examination may reveal hypoestrogenic effects.

LABORATORY STUDIES OF GALACTORRHEA

Laboratory studies are designed to establish the etiology of the galactorrhea. It is important to identify a pituitary tumor or organic lesion which may give rise to galactorrhea, and therefore one must be aware of all the various causes of galactorrhea listed in this section. In general, therefore, the laboratory studies one requests are determined by one's clinical suspicion. First of all, it is helpful to determine serum prolactin concentrations under basal conditions. Figure 131-6 shows the basal prolactin values in 65 patients with galactorrhea of diverse etiology. It is apparent that many patients have values in the normal range. If the values are greater than 200 ng/ml, and certainly if they are in excess of 500 ng/ml, a primary prolactin-secreting pituitary tumor is almost certain. If the values are less than 20 ng/ml, a pituitary tumor is most unlikely and, indeed, the finding suggests that no well-defined organic lesion of the hypothalamus or pituitary will be found. When prolactin values are between 20 and 200 ng/ml, any of the possibilities listed in Table 131-1 must be considered.

The diagnosis of microadenomas of the pituitary gland is being made with increasing frequency. In this case the most helpful diagnostic features are slightly elevated serum prolactin plus an abnormality of the sella turcica, which may be evident only after tomography of the sella turcica. Among patients with elevated serum prolactin concentrations, even if no evidence of pituitary enlargement can be detected radiologically, it is conceivable, and indeed probable, that a certain number will ultimately prove to have pituitary tumors. What is not clear is the exact percentage.

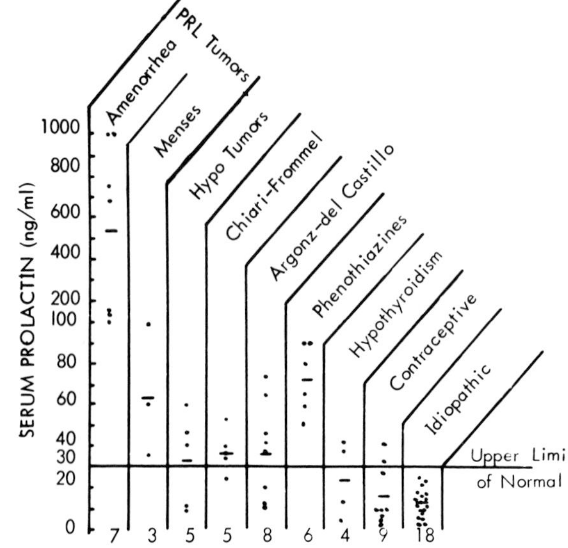

Fig. 131-6. Serum prolactin levels in patients with galactorrhea of diverse etiology.

However, case reports in the literature attest to the very slow growth of some of these tumors over a period of several decades.

In addition to tests of prolactin secretion, other endocrine studies of pituitary function are indicated if there is a suspicion of a pituitary lesion. This could include measurement of serum HGH, TSH, ACTH, and gonadotropins (LH and FSH) under basal and stimulated conditions. If amenorrhea is present, it may be helpful to determine ovarian function under basal conditions as well as after provocative stimuli. Endometrial biopsy may be useful in the assessment of amenorrhea, and in some cases the administration of progestational agents is helpful in assessing whether there is sufficient estrogen secretion to induce withdrawal bleeding.

A number of stimulation and inhibition tests have been described for the functional evaluation of prolactin secretion. Although these tests have provided interesting information, they have not been as helpful as was hoped initially in distinguishing between an organic and a functional disorder leading to hyperprolactinemia. The nature of the tests and the expected responses are considered in detail in Chapter 15.

THERAPY OF GALACTORRHEA

The therapy of patients with galactorrhea depends on the etiology. Treatable lesions should not be missed. The importance of diagnosing an organic lesion such as a pituitary tumor is obvious.

If a primary prolactin-secreting tumor is diagnosed in a patient with galactorrhea, several modalities of therapy are available: surgery, radiation therapy, or medical treatment. If there is visual field impairment, surgical removal of the tumor is mandatory. We personally favor the transphenoidal approach because of the lower morbidity and the excellent results which are possible, especially in patients with microadenomas. If the adenoma is small, it usually can be removed selectively, leaving the residual normal pituitary tissue intact.[40] Within hours after removal of the adenoma, prolactin levels are in the normal range, galactorrhea disappears within several days, and menses resume within 1–2 months. This is the optimal result. When the tumors are larger and have extended beyond the sella turcica, such favorable results are rare and usually prolactin values remain persistently elevated and the galactorrhea and amenorrhea also persist. The unsatisfactory results in the treatment of large tumors underscore the importance of early diagnosis and treatment.

Radiation therapy has been tried in the past in patients with amenorrhea–galactorrhea and a pituitary tumor. In some, symptoms were alleviated, leading one to assume that previously elevated prolactin values had decreased to the normal range. However, most of these reports antedate the availability of reliable prolactin assays. It would be very desirable to carry out a prospective study to see the extent to which elevated serum prolactin values are reduced by conventional radiotherapy. It is likely that after radiotherapy with high-voltage radiation or with heavy particles serum prolactin concentrations are more likely to decrease as compared to any changes after conventional radiotherapy, but the data is simply not available as yet.

In patients in whom no organic disorder can be identified, therapy in the past has been empirical and often unsatisfactory. Nevertheless, the objective is clear: namely, to terminate galactorrhea, reestablish menses, and, in some cases, induce ovulation and pregnancy. Fortunately, in occasional patients the syndrome disappears spontaneously, especially in those patients in whom the syndrome appeared postpartum or postpill. In a few patients, the administration of estrogen or progestogens will prevent the abnormal lactation, probably by an inhibitory effect exerted at the level of the breast. Treatment with clomiphene and gonadotropins has been advocated in some patients because galactorrhea may disappear once ovulation has been induced. However, in general, the results with these agents have been unsatisfactory.

More recently, more success has been obtained with drugs that specifically lower the level of serum prolactin. L-Dopa administered orally (0.5 g 4–5 times a day) was the first drug to be used to inhibit galactorrhea and induce normal menses. However, in our experience, the short duration of action of the drug necessitates frequent administration and makes its general use somewhat impractical. Moreover, serum prolactin levels are rarely suppressed uniformly throughout a 24-h period.

A more promising agent is the ergot alkaloid CB-154. This drug is remarkably effective in lowering prolactin either in functional disorders or in cases of pituitary tumors. CB-154, unlike L-dopa, has a long duration of action (12–16 h) and, hence, can be given only 2–3 times per day and still effectively inhibit prolactin secretion. Again, whereas the effect of L-dopa on prolactin diminishes with time (days), the effect of CB-154 persists as long as the drug is given. The drug has been used in several hundred patients with amenorrhea–galactorrhea and elevated prolactin values with almost uniformly successful results. Hyperprolactinemia usually disappears in a matter of days, followed by cessation of galactorrhea; within 1–2 months, a resumption of menses is noted.

CB-154 has proved equally effective in the treatment of patients with functional amenorrhea–galactorrhea and hyperprolactinemia, and patients with proven microadenoma and the same symptoms (Fig. 131-7).[41] In a few patients with amenorrhea-galactorrhea and normal prolactin levels, CB-154 has been able to restore menses and cause the disappearance of galactorrhea. Therefore, it would appear that in some patients, even though prolactin values are in the normal range, they are sufficiently high to inhibit the normal function of the hypothalamic pituitary–gonadal axis as well as to stimulate milk formation in the breast. In a number of patients, the restoration of normal menses has been followed by pregnancy. In general, as soon as the diagnosis of pregnancy is established, CB-154 is discontinued to minimize the likelihood of congenital abnormalities. Fortunately, none have been noted in patients who have been treated with CB-154 thus far.

Some concern has been expressed that, if patients with microadenomas become pregnant, the high estrogen levels may act to promote tumor growth, and could lead to chiasmatic compression and visual field defects. However, the numbers of pregnancies occurring in patients who have been on CB-154 and have microadenomas is still relatively small. The most disappointing aspect of treatment with CB-154 as well as with L-dopa is that, although the amenorrhea–galactorrhea and hyperprolactinemia can be corrected when patients are taking these agents, upon discontinuation the complete disorder tends to recur fairly soon. Hence, the underlying abnormality appears to persist and the reversal is probably due to the selective inhibition of prolactin secretion. In view of this transitory effect, one can well question whether treatment is warranted as the risk of chronic treatment with CB-154 is not known. The risk must be balanced against the benefit—a return of menses and the cessation of galactorrhea, which in some cases is little more than a nuisance. It is our recommendation that CB-154 is especially useful in the treatment of amenorrhea–galactorrhea if the patient is anxious to become pregnant because menses and fertility frequently can be restored.

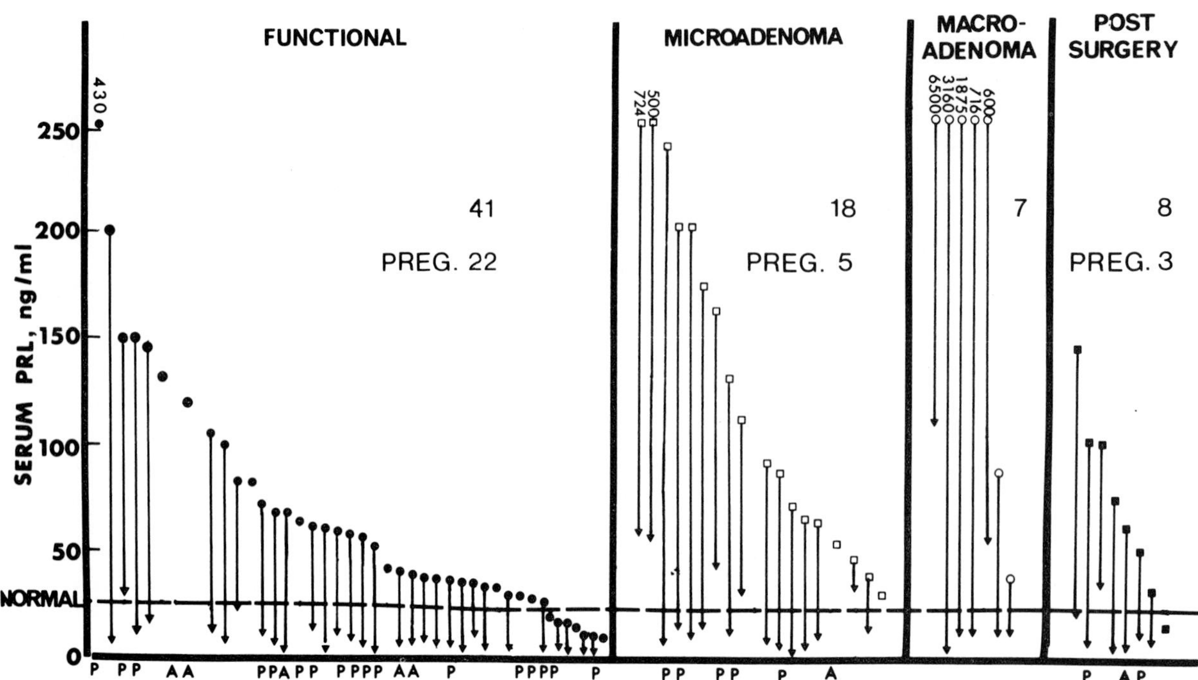

Fig. 131-7. Serum prolactin values before and during therapy of patients with bromocryptine (CB-154). The pretreatment value of each patient is indicated by the symbol at the top of each vertical line and the lowest recorded value during treatment by the arrow at the bottom of each line. In a few patients only pretreatment values were available. The upper limit of normal is indicated by the horizontal line above the abscissa. "P" indicates the patient was pregnant at the time of analysis. "A" indicates the patient aborted. Data from Friesen and Tolis.[41]

The side effects of treatment with CB-154 are relatively minor. Nausea and vomiting occur; they are dose dependent and are more prominent in the initial stages of therapy. An occasional patient becomes hypotensive, especially with the initial dose, and this must be watched for carefully.

The therapy of patients in which galactorrhea is secondary to other causes depends on the underlying disease. Patients with hypothyroidism require thyroid, while patients with adrenal insufficiency are treated with steroids, and so on. In summary, the etiology underlying the development of amenorrhea–galactorrhea dictates the treatment. Of greatest importance is the exclusion of an underlying pituitary tumor. It is recognized that a significant percentage of patients with so-called "functional" disorders in reality harbor prolactin-secreting microadenomas. In approximately half the patients who present with galactorrhea, prolactin values are in the normal range. This constellation of findings strongly suggests a benign disorder, the exact nature of which remains unknown. In the majority of these patients, an adequate explanation and reassurance is all that is required. It is evident that our knowledge of the regulation of normal mammary function is still rudimentary and that much remains to be learned in patients with abnormalities of lactation.

REFERENCES

1. Cowie, A. T., Tindal, J. S.: The Physiology of Lactation. London, Edward Arnold, 1971, p. 107.
2. Lyons, W. R., Li, C. H., Johnson, R. E.: The hormonal control of mammary growth and lactation. *Recent. Prog. Horm. Res. 14:* 219, 1958.
3. Topper, Y.: Multiple hormone interactions in the development of mammary gland in vitro. *Recent. Prog. Horm. Res. 26:* 287, 1970.
4. Turkington, R. W.: Molecular biological aspects of prolactin, in Wolstenholme, G. E. W., Knight, J. (eds.): Lactogenic Hormones. Edinburgh, Livingstone, 1972, p. 111.
5. Folley, S. J.: Endocrine control of the mammary gland. II. Lactation. *Br. Med. Bull. 5:* 135, 1948.
6. Meites, J.: Maintenance of the mammary lobulo-alveolar system in rats after adreno-orchidectomy by prolactin and growth hormone. *Endocrinology 76:* 1220, 1965.
7. Huseby, R. A., Thomas, L. B.: Histological and histochemical alterations in the normal breast tissues of patients with advanced breast cancer being treated with estrogenic hormones. *Cancer 7:* 54, 1954.
8. Diczfalusy, E.: Endocrine functions of the human fetoplacental unit. *Fed. Proc. 23:* 791, 1964.
9. Genazzani, A. R., Fraiolif, F., Hurlimann, J., et al.: Immunoreactive ACTH and cortisol plasma levels during pregnancy. Detection and partial purification of corticotropin-like placental hormone: the human chorionic corticotropin (HCC). *Clin. Endocrinol. 4:* 1, 1975.
10. Hwang, P., Guyda, H., Friesen, H. G.: Purification of human prolactin. *J. Biol. Chem. 274:* 1955, 1972.
11. Lewis, U. J., Singh, R. N. P., Seavey, B. K.: Problems in the purification of human prolactin, in Boyns, A. R., Griffiths, K. (eds.): Prolactin and Carcinogenesis. Cardiff, Wales, Alpha Omega Alpha, 1972, p. 4.
12. Tyson, J. E., Hwang, P., Guyda, H., et al.: Studies of prolactin secretion in human pregnancy. *Am. J. Obstet. Gynecol. 113:* 14, 1972.
13. Brun, Del Re, R., del Pozo, E., De Grandi, P., et al.: Prolactin inhibition and suppression of puerperal lactation by Br-ergocryptine (CB-154): a comparison with estrogen. *Obstet Gynecol. 41:* 884, 1973.
14. Richards, J. F.: Ornithine decarboxylase activity in tissues of prolactin-treated rats. *Biochem. Biophys. Res. Commun. 63:* 292, 1975.
15. Ances, I. G.: Serum concentrations of epidermal growth factor in human pregnancy. *Am. J. Obstet. Gynecol. 115:* 357, 1973.
16. Gardner, D. G., Wittliff, J. L.: Specific estrogen receptors in the lactating mammary gland of the rat. *Biochemistry 12:* 3090, 1973.
17. Shyamala, G., Nandi, S.: Interaction of 6,7-^{3}H-17βestradiol with the mouse lactating mammary tissue in vivo and in vitro. *Endocrinology 91:* 861, 1972.

18. Leung, B. S., Sasaki, G. H.: Prolactin and progesterone effect on specific estradiol binding in uterine and mammary tissues in vitro. *Biochem. Biophys. Res. Commun. 55:* 1180, 1973.
19. Costlow, M. E., Buschowra, R. A., Chamness, G. C., et al.: Autoregulation of prolactin receptors. Program of the 57th Annual Meeting of the Endocrine Society, 1975, p. 79, abstract 58.
20. Karim, M., Ammar, R., Elmahgoub, S., et al.: Injected progestogen and lactation. *Br. Med. J. 1:* 200, 1971.
21. Bruce, J. O., Ramirez, V. D.: Site of action of the inhibitory effect of estrogen upon lactation. *Neuroendocrinology 6:* 19, 1970.
22. Grosvenor, C. E., Turner, C. W.: Release and restoration of pituitary lactogen in response to nursing stimuli in lactating rats. *Proc. Soc. Exp. Biol. Med. 96:* 723, 1957.
23. Noel, G. L., Suh, H. K., Frantz, A. G.: Prolactin release during nursing and breast stimulation in postpartum and non-postpartum subjects. *J. Clin. Endocrinol. Metab. 38:* 413, 1974.
24. Bunner, D. L., Vanderlaan, W. P.: Prolactin level in lactating women. *Clin. Res. 23:* 387A, 1975.
25. Said, S. A. H., Wide, L.: Serum levels of FSH and LH following normal parturition. *Acta Obstet. Gynecol. Scand. 52:* 361, 1973.
26. Reyes, F. I., Winter, J. S. D., Faiman, C.: Pituitary–ovarian interrelationships during the puerperium. *Am. J. Obstet. Gynecol. 114:* 589, 1972.
27. Bohnet, H. G., Dahlen, H. G., Schneider, H. P. G.: Hyperprolactinemia and pulsatile LH fluctuation. *Acta Endocrinol.* [*Suppl. 184*] *75:* 109, 1974.
28. Zarate, A., Canales, E. S., Soria, J., et al.: Ovarian refractoriness during lactation in women: effect of gonadotropin stimulation. *Am. J. Obstet. Gynecol. 112:* 1130, 1972.
29. Perez, A., Vela, P., Masnick, G. S., et al.: First ovulation after childbirth: the effect of breast-feeding. *Am. J. Obstet. Gynecol. 114:* 1041, 1972.
30. Vorherr, H.: To breast-feed or not to breast-feed? *Postgrad. Med. J. 51:* 127, 1972.
31. Oppe, T. E., Redstone, D.: Calcium and phosphorus levels in healthy newborn infants given various types of milk. *Lancet 1:* 1045, 1968.
32. Baum, D., Cooper, L., Davies, P. A.: Hypocalcaemic fits in neonates. *Lancet 1:* 598, 1968.
33. Jelliffe, D. B.: Unique properties of human milk (remarks on some recent developments). *J. Reprod. Med. 14:* 133, 1975.
34. Hall, B.: Changing composition of human milk and early development of an appetite control. *Lancet 1:* 779, 1975.
35. Robinson, M.: Failing lactation. *Lancet 1:* 66, 1943.
36. Tyson, J. E., Zanartu, J., Perez, A., et al.: Puerperal lactation in response to oral TRH. *Clin. Res. 23:* 243A, 1975.
37. Vorherr, H.: Suppression of postpartum lactation. *Postgrad. Med. J. 52:* 145, 1972.
37a. Friesen, H., Hwang, P., Tolis, G., Tyson, J., Myers, R.: in Boyns, A. R., Griffiths, K. (eds.): Prolactin and Carcinogenesis. Cardiff, Wales, Alpha Omega Alpha, 1972, pp. 64–80.
37b. Frantz, A., Kleinberg, D. L., Noel, G.: Studies on prolactin in man. *Recent. Prog. Horm. Res. 28:* 527, 1972.
37c. Jacobs, L. S., Daughaday, W. H.: Human prolactin. in Pasteels. J. L., Robyn, C. (eds.): *Excerpta Medica,* Amsterdam, 1973, pp. 189–205.
38. Rice-Wray, E., Correu, S., Gorodovsky, J., et al.: Return of ovulation after discontinuance of oral contraceptives. *Fertil. Steril. 18:* 212, 1967.
39. Turkington, R. W.: Ectopic production of prolactin. *N. Engl. J. Med. 285:* 1455, 1971.
40. Hardy, J., Beauregard, H., and Robert, F.: Prolactin secreting pituitary adenomas: Transsphenoidal microsurgical treatment. In Robyn, C., and Harter, M. (eds.): Progress in Prolactin Physiology and Pathology. Elsevier North Holland Biomedical Press, 1978, pp. 361–370.
41. Friesan, H., Tolis, G.: The use of bromocryptine in the galactorrhea amenorrhea syndromes: the Canadian Cooperative Study. *Clinical Endocrinol. 6* (Suppl.): 91–99, 1977.

132

Gestational Neoplasms

Donald P. Goldstein

INTRODUCTION

This summary of the current status of the epidemiology, classification, morphology, endocrinology, and management of gestational neoplasms is based on the experience accumulated at the New England Trophoblastic Disease Center between July 1965 and December 1977, during which time 901 patients were admitted for treatment (Table 132-1). Seventy-one percent of these patients were diagnosed as having molar pregnancy. Of the remaining 29 percent, slightly more than half had no evidence of metastases. An overall cure rate of 93 percent was achieved.

DEFINITION OF TERMS

Gestational neoplasms is the term used to describe a group of biologically and morphologically interrelated tumors that arise from pregnancy. They most commonly follow molar pregnancy but may also develop as a consequence of a term delivery, abortion, or ectopic gestation. Morphologically, two distinct histologic entities exist: hydatidiform mole, which develops only after molar pregnancy, and choriocarcinoma (CCA), which can occur following any type of gestation. When the antecedent pregnancy is molar, the tumor that develops may be either locally invasive or metastatic hydatidiform mole or CCA. When the disease follows an ectopic pregnancy, abortion, or term delivery, it may metastasize early because of the advanced degree of malignancy (choriocarcinoma). Difficulty is frequently encountered in establishing a precise morphologic diagnosis. Patients are thus classified clinically as having nonmetastatic disease if the tumor is confined to the uterus, and metastatic if the tumor has spread beyond the uterine fundus.

INCIDENCE AND ANTECEDENT PREGNANCIES

The incidence of gestational neoplasms as related to the various types of pregnancies is illustrated in Fig. 132-1. In the United States, CCA follows term delivery in approximately 1 of 150,000 live births; spontaneous abortion in approximately 1 of 15,000 live births; ectopic pregnancy in approximately 1 of 5000 live births; and molar pregnancy in approximately 1 of 1500 live births. Both molar pregnancy and its sequelae are more common in other parts of the world, particularly the Far East. In this hospital, invasive mole develops in approximately 14 percent of all patients with an antecedent molar pregnancy, and metastatic spread occurs in approximately 4 percent. It is equally important to be aware of the often obscure interrelationship that exists between nonmolar pregnancy and gestational neoplasms. Most clinicians readily establish a diagnosis of gestational neoplasm when persistent uterine enlargement, irregular vaginal bleeding, a persistently positive pregnancy test, and pulmonary lesions follow molar pregnancy. However, this diagnosis is frequently overlooked, at least initially, when the antecedent pregnancy is nonmolar and somewhat remote in time. When there is a delay in diagnosis, patients frequently present with far-advanced trophoblastic neoplasm, often relatively resistent to chemotherapy.

Although there are a number of studies suggesting either a viral, nutritional, or genetic etiology for gestational neoplasms, the true cause of this condition remains obscure.

CLASSIFICATION

Patients with gestational neoplasms can be divided into five classes on the basis of the morphologic diagnosis, antecedent pregnancy, and extent and duration of disease (Fig. 132-2). A thorough pretreatment evaluation should be carried out in each new patient, including a complete history, physical and neurologic examination, review of the available histopathology, baseline HCG determination, determination of peripheral blood counts including the platelet count, evaluation of hepatic and renal function, stool guaiac tests, and a chest x-ray. Intravenous pyelography should be performed if a pelvic mass is present or if the patient has undergone major pelvic surgery. Electroencephalography and CAT and liver scanning should be obtained if any evidence of metastatic disease is present on the initial work-up or if there is a histopathologic diagnosis of CCA. Hepatic and pelvic arteriography may be useful in selected cases. A complete work-up of the GI tract is mandatory if occult or frank blood is detected. A diagnostic curettage should be carried out for a more precise morphologic diagnosis if one has not been performed during the previous month. When this information is obtained, it is possible to make an accurate judgment as to which therapeutic class a specific patient should be placed in and ultimately on which class to base therapy.

Class 1 (molar pregnancy) includes all patients with molar pregnancy. The class is further subdivided into group a, evacuation with prophylactic chemotherapy, and group b, evacuation without prophylactic chemotherapy.

Class 2 (low-risk nonmetastatic neoplasm) includes all patients with persistent trophoblastic tissue localized to the uterus but without clinical, radiologic, or morphologic evidence of deep myometrial invasion. Histologically, this persistent tissue could be either hydatidiform mole (group a) or, very rarely, CCA (group b).

Class 3 (high-risk nonmetastatic neoplasm) includes patients with clinical, radiologic, and morphologic evidence of deep myometrial invasion. Although the histologic diagnosis is usually invasive mole (group a), invasive CCA (group b) may be present in a small percentage.

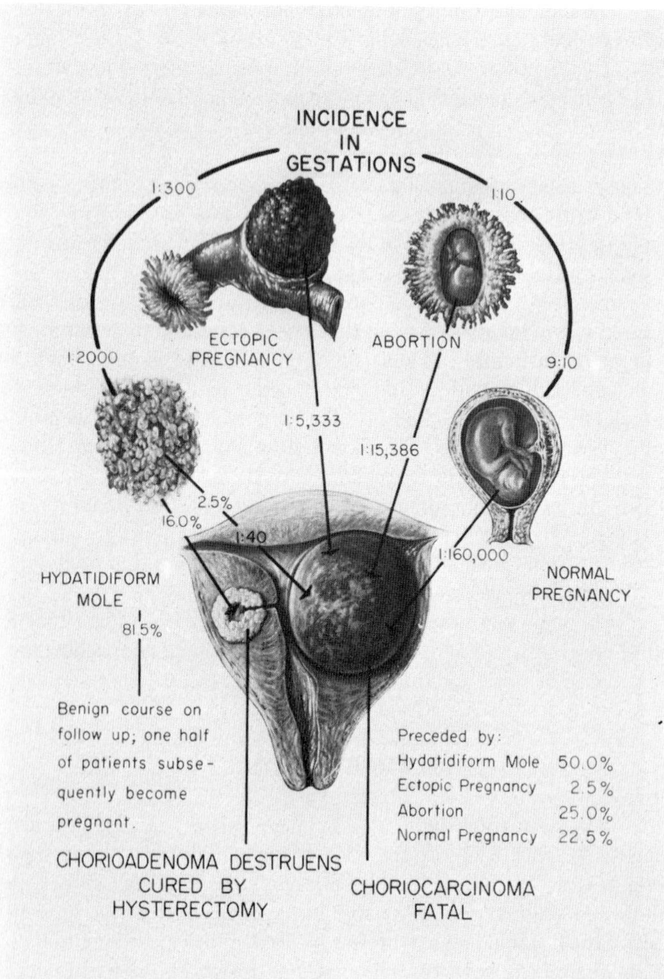

Fig. 132-1. Interrelationships of pregnancies and gestational neoplasms (from Hertig and Mansell[1]).

Table 132-1. Summary of Clinical Material (New England Trophoblastic Disease Center, July 1, 1965–December 31, 1977)

Total number of patients admitted	901
Total number of patients with molar pregnancy	638 (71%)
Uncomplicated	527 (82%)
Complicated	112 (18%)
Total number of patients with gestational trophoblastic neoplasms	262 (29%)*
Nonmetastatic	154 (59%)
Metastatic	108 (41%)
Remissions	244 (93%)
Deaths	14 (5%)
Alive with disease (AWD)	4 (2%)

*Includes patients who developed complications following evacuation of a molar pregnancy.

Class 4 (low-risk metastatic neoplasm) includes metastatic disease less than 4 months from termination of the antecedent pregnancy or the onset of symptoms and an HCG titer of less than 100,000 IU/liter (or its equivalent). Furthermore, these patients have no evidence of brain, liver, renal, splenic, or bowel metastases. Histologically, one may encounter either hydatidiform mole (group a) or CCA (group b).

The final group of patients, *Class 5* (high-risk metastatic neoplasm), includes those in whom the duration of the disease is greater than 4 months from the termination of the antecedent pregnancy or the onset of symptoms and the gonadotropin titer is greater than 100,000 IU/liter (or its equivalent). CCA is the only histologic diagnosis encountered in this group. A high percentage of these patients also have brain, liver, bowel, renal, or splenic lesions that are associated with an unfavorable response to chemotherapy.

This revised classification schema developed in 1970 at the New England Trophoblastic Disease Center is a modification of the original NIH clinical classification adopted officially for worldwide use at the Bagua conference held in the Philippines in 1966. It incorporates important observations made since then by Ross et al.[2] and by Hammond and Parker,[3] who suggested that patients with metastatic disease need to be separated into good and poor prognosis categories because of lower survival figures in those patients with brain and hepatic metastases, HCG titers over 100,000 IU/liter, and a duration of disease over 4 months from the onset of symptoms. Similarly, patients with nonmetastatic disease respond differently to similar chemotherapeutic protocols, depending upon the presence of local invasion and the morphology of the tumor. The NETDC classification has proven extremely helpful in that it permits optimal therapeutic protocols to be utilized for each type of patient encountered, thus individualizing treatment.

PATHOLOGIC CONSIDERATIONS

HYDATIDIFORM MOLE

Gestational neoplasms begin in the placenta at the site of the most primitive of human cells, the trophoblasts (cytotrophoblasts and syncytiotrophoblasts). In hydatidiform mole, fetal vascularity is frequently lost, and the villi become swollen (hydropic). In addition, the trophoblastic cells surrounding the villi show varying degrees of proliferation. The fetus generally undergoes death and

THERAPEUTIC CLASSIFICATION OF GESTATIONAL TROPHOBLASTIC NEOPLASMS (NETDC)

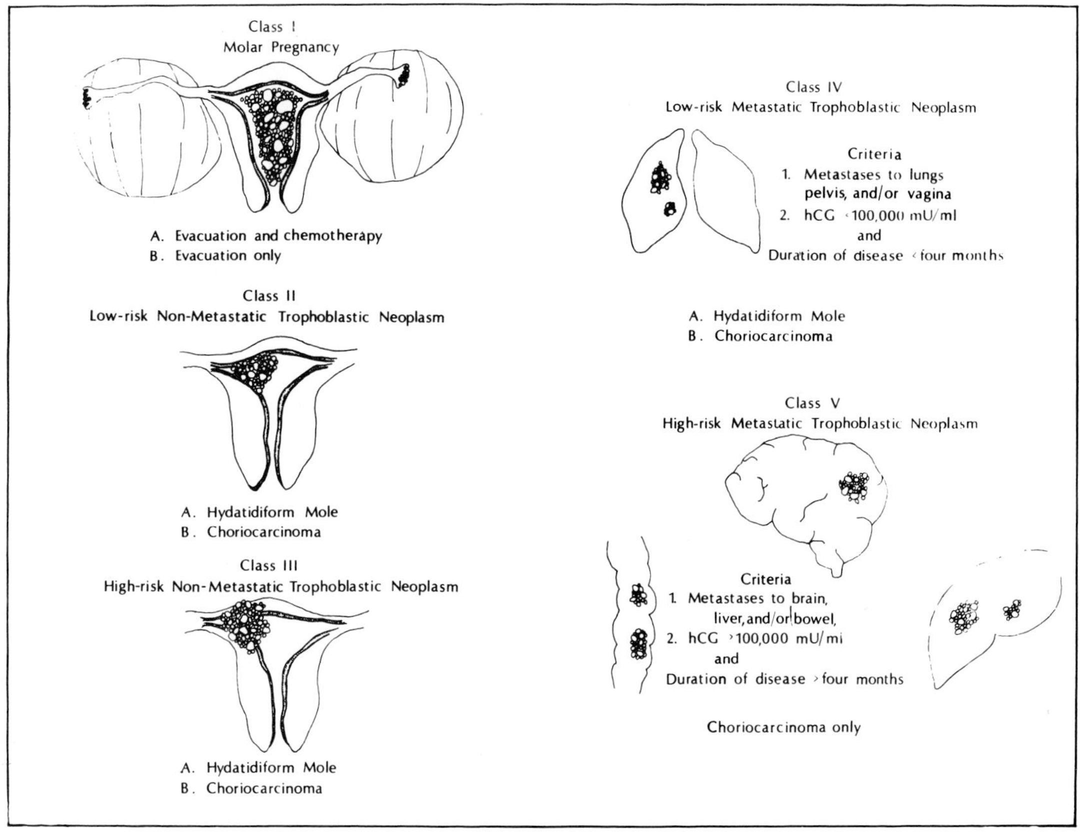

Fig. 132-2. NETDC therapeutic classification.

deterioration but can usually be identified, along with residual membranes, if the entire specimen is examined carefully. Theca lutein cysts frequently accompany molar pregnancy and other types of gestational neoplasms and represent the end result of overstimulation of the ovaries due to high levels of chorionic gonadotropin produced by the proliferating trophoblastic cells. The cystic ovaries generally regress over the succeeding 2 to 3 months following evacuation in parallel with HCG regression.

Molar disease can be grouped into six distinct groups based on specific morphologic criteria, with group I representing the most benign-appearing trophoblastic cells and group VI representing the most malignant. This grouping correlates well with the ultimate clinical outcome. The criteria used to establish the severity of the disease includes the degree of hyperplasia of the individual trophoblastic cells, the number of mitotic figures present, and the atypia noted (Table 132-2).[4] If left untreated, invasive mole can cause

Table 132-2. Hydatidiform Mole Classification

Group	Name	Histologic Criteria	Number of Cases	Number of Malignancies
I	Benign	None to slight hyperplasia of the trophoblast	22	0
II	Probably benign	Slight to moderate hyperplasia	30	2
III	Possibly benign	Hyperplasia with slight anaplasia	33	4
IV	Possibly malignant	Moderate anaplasia with hyperplasia	59	10
V	Probably malignant	Marked anaplasia with hyperplasia	39	20
VI	Malignant	Exuberant trophoblastic growth (variable mitotic activity) with marked anaplasia and often evidence of endometrial invasion	17	17
Total			200	53

Source: From A. T. Hertig and H. Mansell, *in* Atlas of Tumor Pathology. Washington, D.C., Armed Forces Institute of Pathology, 1956.

difficulty in one of two ways—either by perforating through the full thickness of the uterine wall, leading to massive intraperitoneal hemorrhage, or by eroding into uterine vessels, leading to vaginal bleeding which can be life-threatening.

CHORIOCARCINOMA

CCA represents the more malignant histologic type of gestational neoplasm and consists of sheets of pure cytotrophoblasts and syncytiotrophoblasts, which either locally invade the uterine wall or spread extensively via the bloodstream. CCA is characterized by a very anaplastic type of trophoblastic tissue that has lost its ability to recapitulate its normal pathophysiologic function, that is, the formation of villus structures (Fig. 132-3). CCA can be both highly destructive locally in the uterus or widely metastatic.

Table 132-3. Metastatic Sites in 100 Patients with Gestational Neoplasms and Their Relative Frequency

Lungs	85
Pelvis	13
Vagina	12
Brain	9
Liver	6
Bowel	3
Other	3
Undetermined*	8

*Persistent HCG elevation following hysterectomy.

METASTATIC SITES

Table 132-3 lists the most common metastatic sites and their relative frequency of occurrence. Following hysterectomy, patients may occasionally present with an elevated gonadotropin level but with no demonstrable metastases despite thorough evaluation. If left untreated, however, these patients will ultimately develop clinically demonstrable lesions.

The *lungs* are the most common site of metastatic disease, particularly when CCA is present. Metastases to the lungs occur in three characteristic patterns: the so-called ping-pong or snowball pattern, which is usually scattered throughout both lung fields but may also be solitary (Fig. 132-4); enlargement in the hilar area; and miliary spread throughout both lung fields. Lung lesions, in general, may respond quite well to chemotherapy regardless of their size and pattern, although, because of the formation of scar tissue, the larger lesions may persist on x-ray for months after gonadotropin remission is achieved and the patient's chemotherapy is discontinued. Although pulmonary lesions occasionally undergo necrosis during chemotherapy and cause pleural irritation, rarely do they hemorrhage sufficiently to necessitate thoracotomy. It is wise to avoid any attempts at surgical extirpation of solitary lesions as primary therapy because at thoractotomy, numerous smaller satellite lesions are usually present that are undetected roentgenologically.[5]

The *vagina* is the second most common location for metastatic spread. Vaginal lesions may be present either suburethrally, where they frequently cause a foul-smelling purulent discharge, or as a highly vascular implant on the anterior or posterior fornix near the cervix, which may bleed spontaneously and require suturing.

The *liver* may be involved with either one or more scattered nodules or diffusely with smaller lesions. Liver metastases are almost always seen only in patients with late disease and are associated with an extremely poor prognosis. The liver scan is a useful tool for diagnosis, but unfortunately small, scattered lesions are often missed by this technique. Hepatic angiography appears to be a more accurate technique for identifying the presence of hepatic spread.

Brain lesions are encountered almost exclusively in those cases where there has been a delay in making a diagnosis, such as after term delivery. Patients with cerebral metastases frequently die of hemorrhage before adequate treatment can be instituted. Brain scan, electroencephalography, and careful neurologic examination are successful in detecting approximately 95 percent of cerebral lesions, but the other 5 percent can remain silent until

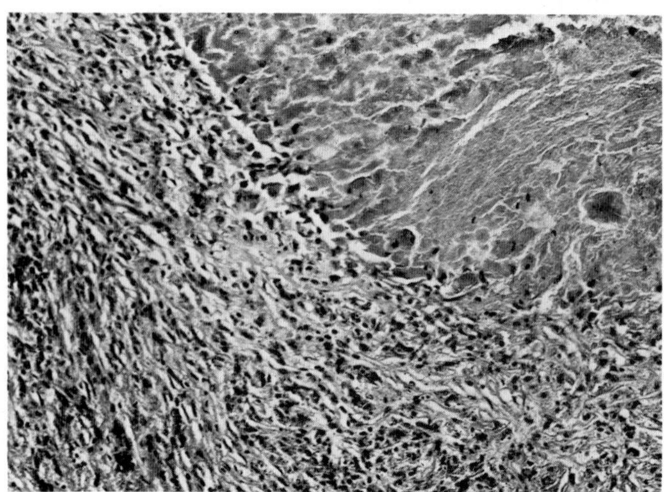

Fig. 132-3. Choriocarcinoma (Microscopic).

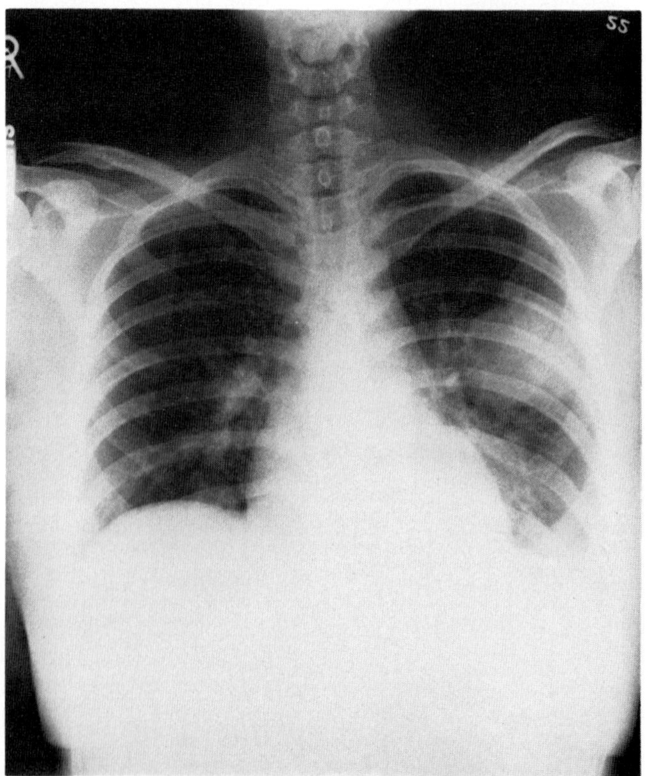

Fig. 132-4. Chest x-ray showing typical pattern of chest metastases.

hemorrhage suddenly develops. CAT scanning has proved extremely valuable in the detection of early asymptomatic metastases. Also, Bagshawe has reported that cerebral lesions are invariably associated with markedly elevated HCG levels in the cerebrospinal fluid.[6] These diagnostic techniques may prove lifesaving in the 5 percent of patients whose tumor is otherwise undetectable.

Occasionally, *bowel* lesions develop, usually silently. These are also associated with a poorer prognosis. Since they do not respond to chemotherapy and require surgical resection, careful guaiac screening with radiologic backup must be used conscientiously in all patients in whom bowel lesions are likely to be present. Sudden massive gastrointestinal bleeding requiring multiple transfusions may occur, especially after chemotherapy-induced pancytopenia. These patients are frequently poor surgical candidates for emergency bowel surgery.

ENDOCRINE ASPECTS

During the past two decades, there has been a rapid proliferation of sensitive, specific, quantitative radioimmunoassays that are capable of detecting a wide variety of polypeptide and steroidal hormones in minute aliquots of body fluids. This capability has provided new insights into the metabolic and endocrine events that are associated with gestational neoplasms. It is also noteworthy that the endocrine capabilities of gestational neoplasms is in part responsible for the excellent results that have been achieved during this same time span with chemotherapy.

PEPTIDE HORMONES

Human Chorionic Gonadotropin

Structure. Human chorionic gonadotropin (HCG) is a glycoprotein produced by all trophoblastic tissue regardless of whether it arises from pregnancy or de novo from the ovary or some extragonadal site. It consists of two polypeptide chains attached to a carbohydrate moiety, with a total molecular weight of approximately 30,000. The polypeptide portion accounts for 66 percent of the molecular weight, and the carbohydrate content represents the remainder. Amino acid analysis reveals remarkably high values for proline, cystine, and serine, with no free -SH groups. The molecule is unique in its high sialic acid content, and the varying potency estimates and heterogeneity of isolated preparations have been attributed to alterations in the sialic content during purification. The function of the carbohydrate portion of the molecule is unknown, but it appears to be essential for biologic activity, since enzymatic removal of sialic acid abolishes the hormone's biologic properties.

It has recently been shown that many of the polypeptide hormones of the placenta and pituitary gland share similar immunologic characteristics, which seem to be related to their configuration. These hormones are constructed of two polypeptide chains, alpha and beta, with an attached carbohydrate. Immunologic and biologic specifity seems to be conveyed by the beta chain. This unusual feature has permitted the development of highly specific assay techniques that are now in wide clinical use.

Biologic Effects. The biologic effects of HCG and its function in pregnancy are not completely understood, but its major role appears to be its function as a luteotropin. HCG can stimulate and prolong the otherwise transient existence of the corpus luteum, thereby assuring a continued supply of ovarian progesterone until the placenta itself can secrete this steroid, which is essential for the maintenance of pregnancy. This transition from ovarian to placental progesterone source occurs at about 6 to 8 weeks of gestation. Other functions for HCG that have been postulated but not confirmed include tropic actions on the placenta itself and on the fetal adrenals and gonads. In common with HLH, it causes luteinizing of ovarian follicular and interstitial cells, induces ovulation of follicles primed by follicle-stimulating hormone (HFSH), and causes stimulation of the interstitial cells and testosterone synthesis by the testis (Table 132-4). The mechanism of its actions has not been established with certainty.

Measurement. Requirements for the assay of HCG depend on the nature of the clinical or research application. Pregnancy tests requiring a simple yes or no answer can be performed using rather gross qualitative systems. Measurement of HCG for describing the endocrine dynamics of reproduction or in the management of patients with trophoblastic disease require assays of higher specificity and sensitivity (Table 132-5).

Bioassay. Biologic assays of HCG depend upon the measurement of the response of the ovary or testis of the experimental animal (usually rats, mice, or toads) to the gonadotropin. These include the primary response of increase in ovarian weight or hyperemia and the secondary response of increase in size of secondary sex organs produced by the increased steroidogenesis in gonadotropin-stimulated gonads. The latter tests include measurement of increases in weight of uterine, prostatic, or total male accessory reproductive organs. Expulsion of ova or sperm from amphibia is also utilized for HCG bioassay.

Bioassay methods (with the exception of the mouse uterine weight test) by their very nature are relatively insensitive, with the lower limits of sensitivity approximately 2000–3000 IU/liter of urine (or its equivalent). This limits their usefulness in the management of patients with chorionic tumors to those with very high HCG levels, such as patients with unevacuated molar pregnancy or those with extensive disease. By and large, the bioassays have been replaced by simpler, more accurate, and less expensive immunologic methods.

Immunoassay. The capacity of HCG and other protein hormones to evoke a specific antibody response upon injection into animals has been utilized to prepare antisera for use in immunologic assays. For the assay of HCG to be specific, either an antigen of highest possible purity must be available or the beta subunit fragment must be used. Although the purest antigens now used are still not completely homogeneous on immunoelectrophoresis, they can be employed for practical purposes. Antisera to HCG cross-react with human pituitary luteinizing hormone (HLH) and human pituitary thyrotropin (HTSH) because the two molecules share immunologic determinants of the alpha chain.

Table 132-4. Biological Actions of HCG

Male
Gynecomastia
Testicular tubular atrophy
Hyperplasia of interstitial cells
Female
Galactorrhea
Theca luteinization
Arias-stella reaction

Table 132-5. HCG Assays: Past and Present

Test	End Point	Time Involved	Approximate Sensitivity
Ascheim-Zondek	Hemorrhagic follicles and corpora lutea in immature mice (urine)	5 days	3–5 IU/ml
Friedman	Ovulation in rabbits (urine)	24–46 hours	3–5 IU/ml
Kupperman	Hyperemia in rate ovaries (serum)	2 hours	3–5 IU/ml
Hogben	Ovulation by the toad (urine)	24 hours	3–5 IU/ml
Gaili Mainini	Expulsion of sperm from male amphibia (urine)	2 hours	3–5 IU/ml
Latex slide test	Immunologic agglutination of latex particle on a slide (urine)	2 minutes	3–5 IU/ml
Hemagglutination	Inhibition of hemagglutination reaction (urine)	2 hours	0.75 IU/ml
Radioimmunoassay	Competitive binding of labeled antigen (serum)	18 hours	0.005 IU/ml
Radioreceptor assay	Binding of HCG-LH to specific sites on bovine corpora lutea or cells	1 hour	0.001 IU/ml

The three general types of immunologic assays now available for the measurement of HCG are (1) agglutination inhibition, which depends on the ability of HCG to inhibit the agglutination reaction between HCG-coated red cells and HCG antisera; (2) complement-fixation tests, which rely on the utilization of complement in antigen-antibody interaction; and (3) radioimmunoassays, which depend upon competition of the antigen to be measured with radioactively labeled HCG for sites on the antibody. With the exception of the newly developed beta subunit radioimmunoassay, the immunoassays share the same limitations as the bioassays with respect to the lack of specificity and sensitivity. The lower limit of sensitivity of the agglutination-inhibition and complement fixation immunoassays is approximately 750–2000 IU/liter of urine (or its equivalent). This makes them satisfactory for use in the diagnosis of molar pregnancy and in most cases of chorionic tumors, but they are not sufficiently sensitive for use in monitoring the patient's response to therapy or for follow-up when the HCG level regresses toward the normal range of endogenous HLH.

Radioimmunoassay. During the past 10 years, great advances have been made in the measurement of HCG by highly sensitive, specific, and quantitative radioimmunoassays that use serum, plasma, or urine. These assays have virtually replaced the other immunoassay methods. Initially, radioimmunoassays for HLH were used to measure HCG by virture of the immunologic cross-reaction that exists between these two polypeptide hormones. The difficulty encountered with this approach became apparent when the HCG titer dropped to the range of endogenous HLH levels, and it was assumed that this meant that all residual trophoblastic tumor tissue was eradicated. This has been shown not to be the case by the frequency, at least by present standards, of relapse, which occurred in approximately 10 percent of the patients.

This limiting factor was overcome by the development of the beta subunit radioimmunoassay by Vaitukaitis et al.,[7] which permits specific measurement of HCG in the presence of HLH. The availability of this new tool provides the ideal technique for use in the measurement of HCG for all phases of management of chorionic tumor patients—diagnosis, monitoring of therapy, and follow-up.

Radioreceptor Assay. In 1977, Dawood and co-workers reported on still another technique for measuring HCG based on the immunologic cross-reaction between HLH and HCG.[8] This assay utilizes binding sites of membranes prepared from bovine corpora lutea, which have been demonstrated to have a greater affinity for HLH than HCG. These workers have reported detection of HCG as early as day 18, that is, 4 days after conception, suggesting the preimplantation production of HCG. The application of this assay to the early diagnosis of pregnancy, to ectopic pregnancy, and in patients with trophoblastic neoplasms is currently being assessed.

Application of Assays to Management of Gestational Neoplasms. Hertz et al. should be credited with having introduced the concept that the measurement of HCG is the single most important test for the diagnosis, monitoring of therapy, and follow-up of patients with chorionic tumors.[9] Originally this was carried out by the use of the mouse uterine weight bioassay, one of the semiquantitative methods that measured HCG together with human follicle-stimulating hormone (HFSH) and HLH. For the reasons outlined above, radioimmunoassay is used almost exclusively at this time.

Molar Pregnancy. Serial, quantitative measurement of HCG is absolutely required for the proper management of patients with molar pregnancy, not only for diagnosis but also, and more importantly, as the only accurate method of determining whether or not an individual patient will develop proliferative trophoblastic sequelae. This concept is relatively new and, unfortunately, is often overlooked by clinicians. One of the reasons for the laxity in HCG follow-up of patients with molar pregnancy is the lack of understanding of how the available assays for HCG can be used to identify problem patients.

Patients with molar pregnancy normally produce large quantities of HCG, at least as much as is produced in normal pregnancy for the corresponding gestational age. In about one-third of cases, the amount of HCG produced markedly exceeds the normal amount.[10] This finding is used as one of the presumptive signs in diagnosis. When the HCG level is in this range, it is possible to use any of the bioassay or immunoassay methods with reliability; the ultrasensitive and more specific radioimmunoassay methods are not required. In a small number of patients with molar pregnancy, however, the amount of HCG produced is in the lower limits of normal or well below the usual range for normal pregnancy, analogous to the situation that exists with missed abortion and intrauterine fetal death. The molar pregnanices characterized by a low HCG output are generally quite benign in that the trophoblastic elements show minimal hyperplasia and atypia. Rarely do they lead to proliferative complications such as local invasion and metastases.

The diagnosis of molar pregnancy is usually made by a constellation of signs, symptoms, and laboratory and radiographic studies rather than on the basis of a single HCG determination. In order to use the HCG level for diagnosis, it is generally necessary to obtain serial values over a few weeks. The peak excretion of HCG in normal pregnancy occurs generally at 10 to 12 weeks, gestational age. After that time there is a significant drop in HCG secretion by the placenta. In most patients with molar pregnancy, the HCG level fails to plateau following the end of the first trimester or rises markedly in association with proliferation of the trophoblastic cell mass and the uterine enlargement that results. Curry et al. have shown that when this occurs together with theca-lutein cyst formation, the patient is in greater danger of developing malignant sequelae.[11]

Accurate quantitative measurement of HCG secretion is far more important once the molar pregnancy is evacuated, and the clinician must determine whether the particular patient will be one of the 14 to 18 percent who ultimately develop a chorionic tumor requiring additional therapy. Our studies of over 900 patients with molar pregnancy and gestational tumors show clearly that the only accurate means of making this determination and assessing the malignant potential of hydatidiform mole is by following the regression of the HCG titer serially at weekly or biweekly intervals until the titer either reaches normal levels or plateaus and becomes reelevated, in which case residual tumor is present.

Ideally, HCG levels should be determined by the most accurate, sensitive, and specific method available. If radioimmunoassay is unavailable, then immunoassays or bioassays can be substituted. When the HCG level drops to the lower limits of sensitivity of the assay being used, the clinician must seek a laboratory capable of performing the most sensitive bioassay, namely the mouse uterine weight test, or one set up to carry out radioimmunoassay.

Studies utilizing the beta subunit radioimmunoassay show that rapid regression of HCG levels usually occurs within 30 days in patients in whom evacuation was by total abdominal hysterectomy and within 40 days following suction evacuation (Fig. 132-5).[12] Complete disappearance of HCG occurs at an average of 90 ± 15 days following suction curettage and 55 ± 12 days following abdominal hysterectomy regardless of whether or not the ovaries are removed. The discrepancy between the disappearance time of HCG after suction evacuation and abdominal hysterectomy probably reflects more complete removal of the trophoblastic cell mass by the latter operation.

Serum levels of HCG persist longer when assayed by the specific beta subunit radioimmunoassay method than by the less-specific radioimmunoassay technique, which measures both HLH and HCG simultaneously. In this situation, the low level of HCG overlaps with physiologic levels of HLH, giving a false impression that all HCG-producing trophoblastic tissue is eradicated. In most instances, this finding is of little practical importance, since the drop in the HCG titer to this low level indicates that remission has occurred. Occasionally, however, the HCG titer becomes reelevated, and treatment is required. For this reason, a single titer in the normal range, regardless of the assay method used, cannot be relied upon as an infallible indication of remission. To circumvent this problem, we recommend that the following protocol be adhered to rigidly in the follow-up of all patients with molar pregnancy after evacuation, regardless of the histologic appearance of the tissue or the benignity of the postevacuation course of the patient.

1. HCG level should be obtained weekly and chest x-ray studies, monthly following evacuation.
2. Therapy should be withheld if the HCG level regresses serially.
3. After the HCG level is normal for 3 consecutive weeks, it should be tested monthly for 6 consecutive months.
4. Patients should be instructed to avoid pregnancy during the entire follow-up period. Birth control pills are permitted.
5. Follow-up may be discontinued after 6 consecutive months of normal HCG levels. Pregnancy is permitted thereafter.
6. The patient should be treated for chorionic tumor if the serum HCG level plateaus for more than 2 consecutive weeks, or if it rises, or if metastases occur.

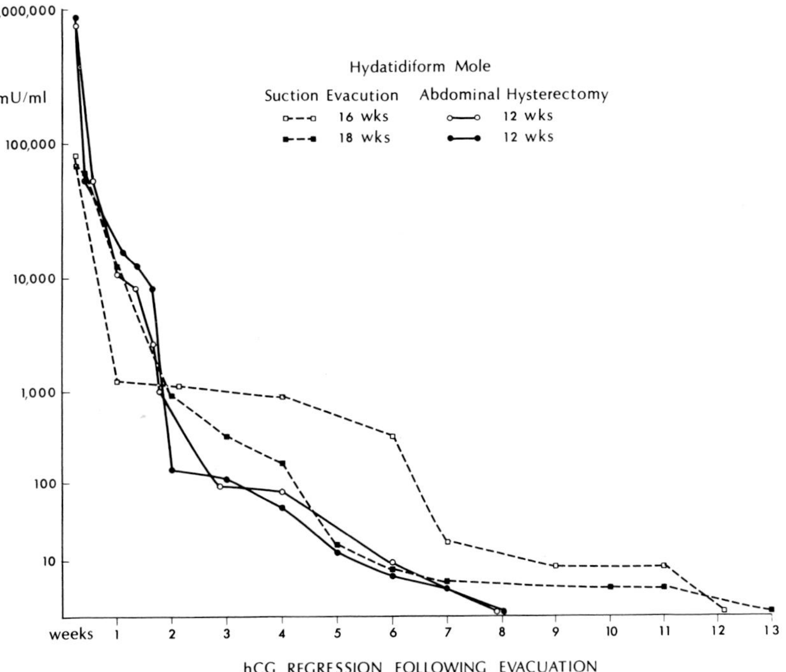

Fig. 132-5. Regression curve of HCG following evacuation of molar pregnancy.

If patients with molar pregnancy are followed according to these guidelines, women who are destined to develop a chorionic tumor will be identifiable within a few weeks. No longer is it appropriate to apply the rule that patients are considered to have a chorionic tumor if the HCG level is still elevated after 60 days. With the beta subunit assay, patients are encountered who require 90 days or longer for complete regression of the HCG level. The pattern of HCG regression has been shown to be more important than the actual time it takes for regression to occur.

Gestational Neoplasms. It is impossible to adequately treat patients with gestational chorionic tumors without having available a reliable, sensitive, and ideally, a specific assay for HCG, since it has been amply demonstrated that the HCG level is the most accurate indication of the amount of viable trophoblastic tumor tissue present. This is true because, for example, the pulmonary nodule seen on the chest x-ray film or the adnexal mass palpated at pelvic examination may be made up largely of either adjacent normal tissue or necrotic tumor, and the amount of viable trophoblastic tissue present is minimal. In the past, the philosophy of treatment was to administer courses of chemotherapy as close together as toxicity permitted and to continue treatment until the HCG level was normal for 3 consecutive weeks, at which time the patient was thought to be in remission. In some centers, in an attempt to reduce the 10 percent incidence of relapse that was associated with this treatment regimen, additional courses of chemotherapeutic agents were administered even after the HCG level was normal. This treatment protocol usually required a rather prolonged period of hospitalization because of the severity of the toxic manifestations that invariably followed the relatively frequent (every 7 to 15 days) administration of potent oncolytic agents.

Since the development of the beta subunit radioimmunoassay, it has been possible to modify this traditional treatment regimen and to use the new and specific assay technique to guide treatment on the basis of growth and regeneration of chorionic tumor tissue. Serum HCG levels are determined weekly after each course of treatment, and therapy is withheld as long as the HCG level is regressing, regardless of how long a time that may entail. Patients are usually discharged from the hospital shortly after peak toxicity and are followed on an outpatient basis with physical examination and laboratory studies, including complete blood counts and liver function tests. Therapy is withheld as long as the HCG level is regressing serially. If the titer values drop to normal and remain normal for 3 consecutive weeks, then no subsequent therapy is administered, and the patient is followed monthly for 6 months and bimonthly for another 6 months.

Careful contraception is advised, and birth control pills are usually prescribed. The patient is re-treated if the HCG level plateaus for more than 2 consecutive weeks or if it rises during or after treatment. Re-treatment occurs on an inpatient or outpatient basis, depending on the clinical condition of the patient and the extent of her toxic reaction to the chemotherapeutic agent being utilized.

The patient is considered to be in complete sustained remission, which means cured for all practical purposes, if the HCG levels remain normal for 1 year. No relapses have been observed at this center in over 350 patients after 12 consecutive months of normal HCG titers. Since institution of the beta subunit radioimmunoassay for HCG, no relapse has been observed in patients treated at our center if the HCG level has been normal for 3 consecutive months. The patient is allowed to become pregnant after 1 year of follow-up.

This change to a less-intensive mode of therapy has been made possible by the availability of sensitive and specific assays for the measurement of HCG, which reliably guide the clinician in evaluating the status of the patient at any given time. Without such a specific cell marker, it could not be possible to administer oncolytic agents on the basis of tumor growth and regression, but instead, administration would have to be on a more empiric basis. The marked reduction in the duration of hospitalization, the total drug dose required to induce remission, and the toxicity that has resulted from this new therapeutic approach, is a welcome relief for patients and their families and is of particular importance to the oncologist because it has been achieved without sacrificing overall effectiveness.

Nongestational Chorionic Neoplasms. Mixed or pure chorionic tumors arising de novo in both males and females from the ovary, testis, and, occasionally, extragonadal regions also produce HCG. Tumors of the following sites have been reported either with elevated gonadotropin titers and found to contain choriocarcinoma or as abberrant production but with the possibility that choriocarcinoma elements might have been present: ovary (dysgerminoma, primary choriocarcinoma, teratoma, undifferentiated), testes (seminoma, embryonal carcinoma, teratocarcinoma, choriocarcinoma, liposarcoma), fallopian tube, breast, mediastinum or thymus, kidney, urinary bladder, liver, stomach, small intestine, colon, rectum, esophagus, pancreas, retroperitoneum, lung, pineal, posterior cranial fossa, pituitary region, sacrococcygeus, insulinoma, skin (melanoma), and adrenal gland.[13]

In managing patients with these tumors, the measurement of HCG is equally important in diagnosis, in monitoring the effectiveness of treatment, and in follow-up. Unfortunately, the results of treatment in this group of patients are not as favorable as in the group with chorionic tumors of gestational origin. Nonetheless, the guidelines for use of various endocrine assays are similar.

Aberrant Production by Nontrophoblastic Neoplasms. Reports of aberrant gonadotropin are largely anecdotal, relying upon nonspecific "pregnancy test" or other assays that do not separate FSH, HLH, HCG, or their subunits. Nevertheless, there is clear evidence that many tumors can synthesize some type of gonadotropic hormone.

Clinical Features. The patient may present with precocious puberty, uterine bleeding, gynecomastia, other evidence of increased sex steroid production or a positive pregnancy test in a male or nongravid female. A positive immunoassay and gynecomastia in a male have been reported presaging the diagnosis of a bronchogenic carcinoma as long as a year before the diagnosis was firmly established. No reports of women complaining of breast changes in such conditions were found in review. While breast hypertrophy may be produced by HCG tumors or HCG administration, there is as yet no evidence that these hormones can cause a breast response directly. Rather, the gynecomastia is attributed to secondary stimulation, the tumor HCG causing excess elaboration of sex steroids from the gonads, adrenal, or both. When a patient presents with evidence of estrogen excess, gonadotropin-producing tumors need to be considered in addition to the usual steroid secreting neoplasms.

Tumors Described. Cancers of the following tissues appear to represent bona fide examples of aberrant gonadotropin secretion, with or without associated clinical effects, although descriptions of the type of gonadotropin and firm proof of production may be incomplete; skin (melanoma), hemopoietic system (acute lymphatic leukemia, acute myelogenous leukemia, chronic myelogenous leukemia, multiple myeloma, adrenal cortex (carcinomas), breast (carcinoma), kidney (renal cell carcinoma), liver (hepatoma, hepatoblastoma), lung (epidermoid, anaplastic oat cell, adenocarcinoma), stomach (carcinoma), and ovary ("germ cell," dysgerminoma). Occasionally, a "pure" dysgerminoma producing gonadotropins has occurred coincident with an intrauterine pregnancy.[14]

It has been postulated that luteinization of ovarian stroma in the presence of metastatic or primary ovarian cancer results from the aberrant production of minute quantities of gonadotropin which exert a powerful local influence. However, a change in avidity for the uptake of circulating gonadotropins in tumor involved ovaries could also explain this picture.

Human Placental Lactogen

The isolation in 1962 of a distinct new placental hormone culminated more than 30 years of scattered observations on the isolation of lactogenic and growth hormone—like principles from the human placenta. Although it has been variously called human placental lactogen (HPL), chorionic-growth-hormone-prolactin, purified placental protein, and human chorionic somatomammotropin (HCS), this hormone has now been established as a single substance with lactogenic, luteotropic, and growth activities that is produced by trophoblastic cells of the normal placenta as well as by trophoblastic tumor tissue. Indeed, it may account for some of the hitherto unexplained metabolic alterations of pregnancy. HPL has been characterized as having a molecular weight of 30,000–38,000, with an amino acid composition remarkably similar to that of human pituitary growth hormone. Analysis suggests that HPL is a dimer of two polypeptide chains of equivalent weight (19,000) held together loosely by hydrogen binding without interchain disulfude links. No carbohydrate moiety has been identified.[15]

Methods of Assay. Biologic assays are available for the measurement of each of the biologic actions of the hormone on the basis of its prolactin, luteotropic, and growth hormonelike activities. Since HPL was first detected and identified by immunologic means, however, sensitive and specific readioimmunoassays were readily available for its measurement in normal pregnancy and later in abnormal pregnancy, including molar pregnancy, and in chorionic tumors. Early work in radioimmunoassay was confused by the immunologic cross-reaction of pituitary growth hormone with HPL, but this problem was largely overcome by preparation of purified antigens and by recognition of the fact that HPL is present in serum at many times the concentration of growth hormone.

The half-life of HPL in plasma is about 20 minutes, which explains its rapid disappearance after delivery. Levels in serum are detectable early in pregnancy and rise progressively to 2–10 μg/ml at term, with disappearance from plasma within 4 hours post partum.[16]

Clinical Application of Assays.

Molar Pregnancy. HPL has been shown to be present in varying concentrations in the serum and plasma of patients with unevacuated molar pregnancy, the concentration depending upon the gestational age of the molar pregnancy and, to some degree, on its histologic characteristics. In general, the HPL levels range from 0.014 to 0.36 μg/ml, which is 10 to 100 times less than the normally expected levels for the corresponding gestational age. A single HPL determination in this low range, however, does not indicate a diagnosis of molar pregnancy with certainty, because in some instances the HPL level in a patient with molar disease overlaps the low level of HPL seen in patients with missed abortion or intrauterine fetal death. Serum HPL levels are useful in diagnosis of molar pregnancy when they are used together with the HCG level in establishing a so-called HCG/HPL ratio. High HCG levels in conjunction with low HPL values suggest molar pregnancy or a chorionic tumor. This comparison proved valuable in the diagnosis of molar pregnancy before techniques such as ultrasound and amniography were used extensively.[17]

Another interesting application of the HPL test is in helping to assess the malignant potential of a hydatidiform mole. If one correlates serum HPL activity with the histologic grade of the evacuated molar specimen and curettings, using the criteria established by Hertig and Sheldon,[4] it appears that the HPL level correlates well with the length of gestation (in weeks) and the histologic evidence of malignancy but not at all with the biologic activity of the trophoblastic tumor cells as reflected in the HCG level (Fig. 132-6). As a matter of fact, the correlation is inverse, meaning that the more malignant the tissue appears to the pathologist, the lower the HPL value is likely to be. This correlation is sufficiently consistent so that it might be used in selecting high-risk patients for postevacuation chemotherapy, in addition to other newly established criteria, such as uterine enlargment and the presence of theca-lutein cysts.[17]

Regression of circulating levels of HPL occurs within hours after evacuation of a molar pregnancy because of its short half-life, similar to the situation that occurs following normal delivery. This is true even when there is rather prolonged regression of the HCG titer. For this reason it is not possible to use the HPL regression curve in assessing the potential of the patient's molar pregnancy to develop proliferative trophoblastic sequelae.

Gestational Neoplasms. Approximately 50 percent of patients with either metastatic or nonmetastatic chorionic tumors have detectable amounts of HPL in plasma or serum, the range being

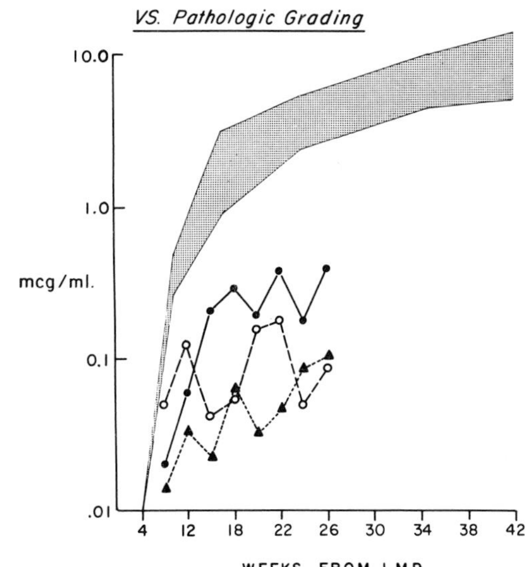

Fig. 132-6. HPL levels in patients with molar pregnancy.

0.004–400 μg/ml[18] (Table 132-6). As a general rule, patients with a more malignant type of tumor, i.e., choriocarcinoma as compared with hydatidiform mole, will have either undetectable or barely detectable values, while the more benign-appearing (and biologically acting) type of tumor will have higher HPL values. These levels are independent of the HCG level and the location of the tumor, since choriocarcinoma in the uterus is associated with the same low or barely detectable levels as choriocarcinoma anywhere else in the body.

Nongestational Chorionic Neoplasms. Males and females with nongestational chorionic tumors have also been found to have low but detectable amounts of HPL. These values are similar to those noted in patients with gestational choriocarcinoma and suggest a biologic and metabolic relationship between these two types of chorionic tumors even though they are derived from different types of tissue and respond rather differently to treatment. Since nongestational chorionic tumors manufacture and secrete HCG more efficiently than HPL, the assay of HCG is more important as a test for the presence of disease and its response to treatment.

Human Molar Thyrotropin

A number of investigators have shown that thyroid function tests performed on normally pregnant women suggest a mild hyperthyroid state when compared with nonpregnant controls. Most of these changes, however, can be explained without concluding that there is an increased production of thyroid hormone per se. Studies show that the increased serum concentrations of thyroxine (T_4) and triiodothyronine (T_3) during pregnancy occur as a consequence of an estrogen-induced increase in thyroid binding-globulin (TBG) rather than as a direct increase in production of T_4 or T_3.[19] Normal levels of free T_4; which probably represents the biologically active portion of circulating thyroid hormone, have been reported during normal pregnancy. The increased thyroid uptake of radioactive iodine noted in pregnancy has been attributed to a decreased serum iodide concentration that results from increased renal iodide loss. Finally, while variable levels of total biologic thyrotropic (TSH) activity have been reported in pregnancy, the values are probably not significantly different from levels found in the nonpregnant state. While subtle clinical findings of mild hyperthyroidism may be present in normally pregnant women, it is unusual to find significant hyperthyroid changes.

In contradistinction to normal pregnancy, there have been numerous reports of patients with unevacuated hydatidiform mole who had significant laboratory and clinical evidence of hyperthyroidism.[20] The laboratory findings in these patients disappeared within days following evacuation of the mole even though the clinical finding persisted for weeks. Furthermore, these changes often appeared to be accompanied to toxemiclike symptoms. Indeed, in a few patients similar to those mentioned above, the circulating TSH level was found to be increased. In 1960, Dowling et al. referred to several patients with unevacuated molar pregnancy who had only laboratory evidence of hyperthyroidism, but none was clinically hyperthyroid.[21] In one of the most complete studies of this phenomenon, Galton et al. reported that in 20 women with unevacuated molar pregnancy, almost all had significant elevation of thyroid function tests that cleared rapidly with evacuation of the mole.[19] None of these patients was clinically hyperthyroid.

Table 132-6. Serum HPL Levels in 23 Patients with Gestational Neoplasms

Diagnosis	Number of Patients	Mean ± S.D. (μg/ml)	Range (μg/ml)
Invasive mole	11	0.34 ± 0.08	0.72–0.02
Nonmetastatic choriocarcinoma	3	0.092 ± 0.03	0.27–0.01
Metastatic choriocarcinoma	9	0.086 ± 0.04	0.34–0.01

Abnormalities in thyroid function tests have also been reported in patients with chorionic tumors, either gestational or nongestational. In 1963, Odell et al. reported 7 patients with elevated thyroid function tests out of 94 patients with metastatic trophoblastic disease.[22] In these patients, clinical hyperthyroidism was either not present or minimal, and the thyroid gland was normal in size. The laboratory indices showed that increased thyroid function rapidly disappeared with chemotherapy. This report also demonstrated that plasma TSH levels were significantly elevated in 2 patients studied extensively; assay of the tumor from these 2 patients revealed TSH activity greater than that of equivalent amounts of blood by the McKenzie mouse bioassay.

Herschman was able to obtain a large amount of serum and molar tissue from a patient with hyperthyroidism associated with hydatidiform mole.[20] In these studies, he was able to carry out extensive characterization of a biologically active thyrotropin from these materials and compare it with other human thyrotropins, including those from the pituitary gland and normal placenta. He found that bioassay of the serum gave a response that was longer in duration than that of pituitary TSH but shorter than that of the long-acting thyroid stimulator (LATS) of Graves' disease. In these studies, antibodies to either bovine or human TSH failed to neutralize the biologic activity of serum or of an extract of the tumor. In addition, the serum and the extract of the tumor showed no cross reactivity in the radioimmunoassay for bovine TSH and had only minimal cross-reactivity in this type of assay for human TSH. In contrast, a thyrotropin extracted from human placenta, called human chorionic thyrotropin, cross-reacted completely in a radioimmunoassay for bovine TSH but not in an assay for human TSH.

Herschman has also shown using extraction studies that trophoblastic TSH seems to be of higher molecular weight than pituitary TSH and that fractions that had molar TSH activity were devoid of IgG, giving evidence that trophoblastc TSH is not LATS, which is an IgG. This trophoblastic thyrotropin was identical, in both biologic and immunologic activity and in molecular size, with the thyrotropic substance obtained from women with normal pregnancy and from one of our male patients with choriocarcinoma arising in the testis who developed hyperthyroidism during a relapse in his disease. This at least suggests that trophoblastic "TSH" is the same as or similar to human chorionic thyrotropin and that patients with molar pregnancy and chorionic tumors are producing larger quantities than are normally pregnant women.

This picture becomes confused by more recent data from Herschman's group, suggesting that the thyrotropin state seen in patients with molar pregnancy and trophoblastic neoplasms may in fact be caused by the intrinsic thyrotropic activity of HCG itself. This observation notwithstanding, it seems reasonable to assume that, in some patients at least, a thyrotroxic state can be induced by a thyrotropic substance produced by the trophoblastic cells, the nature of which has not been fully defined.

Clinical Application of Studies. Galton et al. reported the laboratory and clinical findings in a group of patients before and after removal of the molar gestation.[19] Prior to molar evacuation, all patients had moderately to greatly elevated values for thyroidal radioactive iodine uptake, serum protein-bound iodine (PBI), and absolute iodine uptake. Values for serum PBI and serum T_4 were consistently very greatly increased, averaging more than twice those found in normal pregnancy. On the other hand, the maximum binding capacity of TBG was variably affected and ranged between the values found in normal controls and those in normal pregnancy. Values for the absolute concentration of free T_4 in serum were, on the average, only moderately elevated, since the proportion of free T_4 was moderately low, although not as low as in normal pregnancy. Sera from patients with molar pregnancy contained high levels of TSH activity, as assessed in the McKenzie mouse bioassay system. Despite these evidences of increased thyroid function and hypersecretion of T_4, patients with molar pregnancy were neither goitrous nor overly thyrotoxic. Galton et al. concluded that in patients with molar pregnancy, thyroid function and T_4 secretion are stimulated, often greatly so, by an unusual thyroid stimulator that is demonstrable in the blood and that is probably of molar origin.

All the patients reported above with either hydatidiform mole or metastatic trophoblastic disease and the hyperthyroid syndrome had very high levels of HCG. These quantities of HCG are distinctly above the average produced by patients with normal pregnancy and other less far-advanced cases of chorionic tumor. Plasma TSH levels, by bioassay, have been measured in a number of these patients and have been found to be consistently elevated. This raises the question of whether or not HCG has an intrinsic TSH-like activity. Huge amounts of HCG from normal pregnancy have been assayed by three different bioassay techniques—the McKenzie mouse assay, Bakke's in vitro assay, and Bates' day-old chick assay—and no intrinsic TSH-like activity could be detected. Recently, however, Kenimer et al.[22] have studied the same problem using a more sensitive and specific techniques and have concluded that HCG has some limited intrinsic TSH activity (on a 1:4000 ratio basis).[23]

In light of all this clinical and laboratory work, it seems fair to say that nearly all women with unevacuated mole pregnancy have laboratory evidence of increased thyrotropin function when the HCG levels are markedly elevated (greater than 500,000 IU/liter or its equivalent), although only 5 to 6 percent are clinically hyperthyroid. Treatment is molar evacuation, although a few patients may present with frank thyroid storm, which requires vigorous therapy to stabilize the individual before evacuation can be carried out. We have used beta-adrenergic blocking agents for this purpose, particularly when toxemia accompanied the thyrotoxicosis.

Patients with chorionic tumors, either gestational or nongestational, have much less chance of having both laboratory and clinical findings of hyperthyroidism than do patients with primary molar pregnancy, unless the HCG level is quite high. When this complication does occur in patients with chorionic tumors, institution of appropriate chemotherapy usually is followed by rapid resolution of the hyperthyroid state, even if the disease later becomes refractory to treatment and relapse occurs. Relapse in the hyperthyroid state is much more rare, although it does occur. Supportive treatment with sedation and beta-adrenergic blocking agents is also indicated in this group of patients.

STEROID HORMONES

Estrogens

The origins of the extremely high amounts of estrogen excreted by the normally pregnant female have recently been delineated and the significance of the fractions with regard to assessing female well-being are now appreciated. It is now accepted that estrogen synthesis from cholesterol or acetate does not occur in the normal placenta. Hormonally inactive steroids, however, such as dehydroepiandrosterone (DHEAS) from fetal and maternal adrenals, may be converted to estrogens by the placenta. Approximately 90 percent of estriol (E_3) is derived from the fetoplacental unit in normal pregnancy. In the earlier phases of pregnancy, a fetal contribution might be present, but it is more likely that a maternal adrenal source of precursor is utilized. Thus far, it has not been shown that the ovaries produce significant amounts of E_3 in either the nonpregnant or the normal pregnant state. However, maternal liver will convert to E_3 some of the estriol (E_2) secreted by the ovary, irrespective of ovarian stimulation by such agents as HCG.

Early studies of urinary estrogens determined in small numbers of patients with molar pregnancies showed diminished levels or levels consistent with the nonpregnant range. Additional studies found that there was a tendency for E_3 excretion in patients with molar pregnancy and choriocarcinoma to be less than that in normal pregnancy. This was confirmed by Barlow et al.,[23] who showed that in only 4 of the 12 women with chorionic tumors was the infused ^{3}H-DHEAS converted into estrogen, and although total estrogen levels may be in the normal range, E_3 levels are low.[24] In contrast, DHEAS infused into a patient with hydatidiform mole was converted to estrogenic steroids and could account for as much as 50 percent of the estrogen secreted. It thus appears that even in the absence of the fetus, as is usually the situation in molar pregnancy, the neoplastic trophoblastic tissue retains the ability of normal trophoblastic tissue to convert steroid hormone precursors to estrogenic substances.

Dawood et al[24] have recently shown that serum E_2 levels in patients with molar pregnancy are significantly higher than those in normal pregnancy of corresponding gestation, and one of a large group of patients with molar pregnancy had E_2 levels within the nonpregnant range.[25] This increased E_2 is postulated to be derived from one of two possible sources in molar pregnancy: the hyperstimulated ovary seen associated with molar pregnancy via the Δ^4 pathway from progesterone to androstenedione and then to E_2, or via the Δ^5 pathway from pregnenolone to dehydroepiandrosterone and then to E_2. The low level of E_2 found after aborted molar pregnancy suggests that the abnormal trophoblastic tissue produces (or converts) E_2. Thus the elevated E_2 level in molar pregnancy is contributed by the trophoblastic tissue and also by the hyperstimulated ovary.

Information on patients with choriocarcinoma is scant. In women with gestational choriocarcinoma the total urinary estrogens have been found in the range of nonpregnant females or slightly above normal. Barlow et al.[23] showed that only 4 of the 12 women with malignant trophoblastic disese converted the infused ^{3}H-DHEAS into estrogen at the rates of 1.6, 0.9, 2.0, and 24.8 percent (Table 132-7).[24] Again, those were studies based on urinary excretion. It is not known whether the smaller conversion rate is

Table 132-7. Estradiol/Estriol Production Rates in Patients with Normal and Molar Pregnancy and CCA

Subject	PR* E_2(μg/D)	PR$^+$ E_3(μg/D)	% Conversion E_2 to E_3
Normal pregnancy (5 weeks)	842	214	7.9
Normal pregnancy (9 weeks)	1519	374	8.6
Normal pregnancy (14 weeks)	2913	2158	31.3
Hydatidiform Mole (16 weeks)	1335	152	5.1
Choriocarcinoma	1394	173	10.8

*PR-E_2—production rate of estradiol.
†PRE_3—production rate of estriol.

due to a relatively deficient aromatizing system or whether this is simply due to the small amount of active trophoblastic tissue available. Pattillo et al.[25] demonstrated estrogen synthesis by malignant trophoblastic cell cultures when incubated with either ^{3}H-androstenedione or ^{3}H-DHEAS.[26] In a male choriocarcinoma patient of MacDonald and Siiteri, 3.7 percent of injected DHEAS was converted to E_2 and E_1 (compared to 0.2 percent normal male conversion rate) and the urinary production rate of E_1 was tenfold greater than in normal males. Neither production rates based on plasma studies nor measurements of plasma estrogen concentrations have been done in patients with malignant trophoblastic disease.

Progesterone

It has been well established that the normal placenta produces significant quantities of progesterone and its metabolite, pregnanediol. Several recent studies in patients with molar pregnancy have shown elevated serum progesterone levels measured by competitive protein-binding radioimmunoassay[27] These studies show that serum progesterone values are consistently higher in molar pregnancies between the twelfth and twentieth week of gestation than in normal pregnancies of a corresponding gestational age. In addition, patients with theca-lutein cysts were found to have progesterone levels higher than patients without cystic ovaries. This suggests that a relationship may exist between HCG and progesterone metabolism because theca-lutein cysts are almost always present in the group of patients with elevated HCG levels.

There are conflicting reports in the literature regarding progesterone production in patients with chorionic tumors. Ishizuka et al.[28] reported decreased levels after chemotherapy in patients with a good response to chemotherapy and increased amounts in patients who ultimately were shown to respond poorly to drug therapy.[28] Measurements of plasma progesterone in patients with metastatic disease have not been found to be higher than luteal phase levels. No production rate studies are available. Urinary excretion of pregnanediol correlates well with HCG excretion in intact molar pregnancy. In choriocarcinoma there seems to be a discrepancy between high HCG and low steroid hormone levels. It is possible that steroidogenesis is impaired in trophoblastic tumor tissue. Little is known regarding what portion of progesterone is derived from the ovaries, although recent studies suggest that theca-lutein cysts of patients with molar pregnancy are the principal source of progesterone and 17 α-hydroxyprogesterone.

Abnormal trophoblastic tissue is known to contain large amounts of progesterone, and incubation studies have shown that it can convert pregneninolone (Pe) into progesterone very efficiently. Furthermore, Frandsen and Stakemann[28] reported urinary pregnanediol to be at nonpregnancy level in 3 patients,[29] but Brown et al. found it to be below luteal phase level and observed an increased amount with the first chemotherapeutic treatment.[30]

MOLAR PREGNANCY

DIAGNOSIS

The diagnosis of molar pregnancy can be made on the basis of presumptive, probable, and positive criteria (Table 132-8).

Table 132-8. Diagnostic Criteria of Molar Pregnancy

Presumptive signs
Vaginal bleeding
Excessive uterine size
Anemia
Toxemia of pregnancy
Hyperemesis
Hyperthyroidism
Trophoblastic embolization
Absent fetal heart tone
Absent fetal skeleton on x-rays
Probable signs
Elevated chorionic gonadotropin levels
Decreased chorionic somatomammotropin levels
Decreased estriol excretion and production rates
Decreased progesterone levels and pregnanediol excretion
Abnormal urinary and vaginal cytology
Changes in other biochemical studies
Theca lutein cysts
Positive signs
Amniography
Ultrasonsography
Pelvic arteriography
Spontaneous passage of vesicles
Vaginal wall metastases
Transabdominal needle biopsy

Presumptive Signs

Irregular painless bleeding occurs almost universally and ranges in character from dark brown, the so-called prune juice discharge, to bright red. The bleeding usually begins shortly after the first missed period and consists of either spotting or hemorrhaging. Cramps occur when molar tissue has begun or is about to be passed spontaneously. The uterus is found to be enlarged beyond dates in slightly over half the patients. The size of the uterus generally correlates with the proliferative potential of the trophoblastic tissue and the height of the HCG titer, two of the criteria cited by Hammond and associates as being of prognostic importance in molar disease.

Nausea and vomiting occur more frequently than in normal pregnancy and, in general, are much more severe and intractable. Toxemia of pregnancy, which develops in the first or early second trimester, is virtually pathognomonic of this disease. Hyperthyroidism manifested clinically by diffuse enlargement of the thyroid gland, tachycardia, warm skin, and occasionally weight loss may be caused by the production of molar thyrotropin by the proliferating trophoblastic cells. When excess thyroid hormone activity is suspected, a thyroid profile should be obtained to confirm the diagnosis. When hyperthyroidism is present, thyroid storm may develop at the time of evacuation unless special measures are adopted. This syndrome is limited almost exclusively to patients with large moles in whom the HCG level is markedly elevated, generally over 1 million IU/liter, and for this reason some investigators question the importance of molar thyrotropin and implicate HCG, which does exhibit some thyrotropic activity as described above.

Acute pulmonary complications develop in a small number of patients as a result of trophoblastic embolization to the pulmonary artery bed. Patients develop varying degrees of shortness of breath, tachypnea, cyanosis, hemoptysis, tachycardia, and right heart failure. This condition usually becomes apparent shortly after evacuation but Kohorn et al.[30] have reported that symptoms may be elicited prior to that time.[31] Blood gases show decreased Po_2, and chest x-rays show diffuse bilateral infiltration. Complete resolution of these pulmonary lesions generally occurs spontaneously within 72 to 96 hours following the onset of symptoms (Fig. 132-7). Roentgenographic signs should not be confused with either pulmonary embolism, which occurs rarely with this disease,

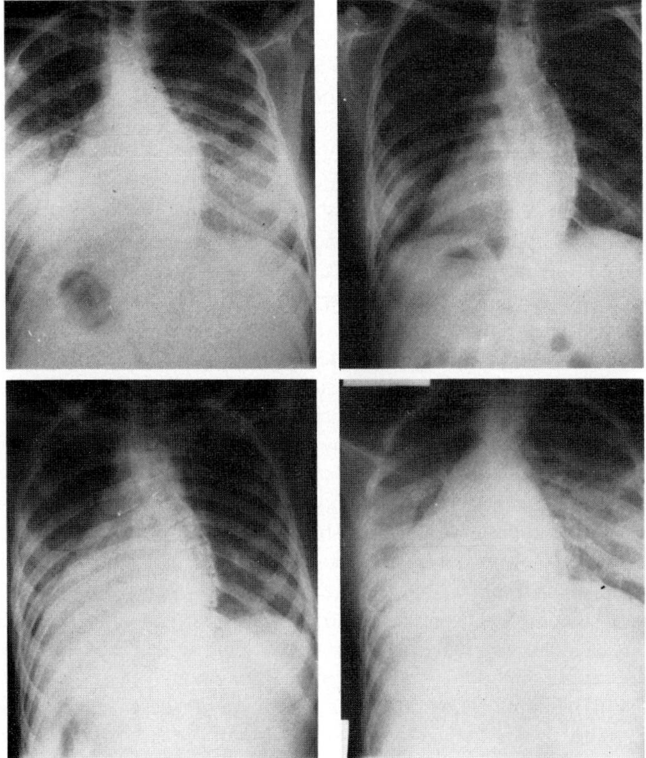

Fig. 132-7. Chest x-rays showing trophoblastic embolization with spontaneous recovery in 72 hours.

or with lung metastases, which are encountered on occasion in patients with unevacuated moles. As is the case with hyperthyroidism, the condition occurs more commonly in patients with excessive uterine enlargement and markedly elevated levels of HCG.

Other presumptive signs of molar pregnancy include absent fetal heart tones and movement despite an enlarging uterus and absence of a fetal skeleton in uteri larger than 16 weeks' gestational age. In the differential diagnosis of molar pregnancy, the clinician must include multiple gestation, enlarging uterine leiomyomas with threatened miscarriage, and inaccurate menstrual dates.

Probable Signs

The increased number of proliferating trophoblastic cells of a molar pregnancy produce larger quantities of HCG than are seen at the corresponding gestational age in a normal single pregnancy. Rarely does the HCG level in patients with a single or multiple pregnancy exceed 100,000 IU/liter after the twelfth week of pregnancy.[32] Molar pregnancy, in contrast, is frequently associated with much higher HCG levels. Where the trophoblastic cell mass is smaller and the uterine growth pattern is consistent with or smaller than dates, as is the case in approximately 50 percent of patients, the level of HCG is usually equal to or lower than that seen in a normal gestation of the corresponding gestational age.

The presence of theca-lutein cysts can be detected by palpation in approximately 40 percent of patients with molar pregnancy. Ultrasonic detection of enlarged cystic ovaries at the time of diagnostic scanning indicates that theca-lutein cysts are probably more common than appreciated by palpation alone because of the difficulties inherent in detecting minimal ovarian enlargement when the uterus is larger than 20 weeks in size. Theca-lutein cyst formation is almost exclusively limited to those patients in whom the HCG level is markedly elevated, which also correlates with the presence of excessive uterine enlargement.

Positive Signs

An attempt should be made to make a positive diagnosis of molar pregnancy when this condition is suggested by the presence of one or more probable or presumptive signs and before spontaneous passage of vesicles occur. Two relatively recent techniques have made early diagnosis or molar pregnancy a reality—amniography and ultrasonsography.

Definitive diagnosis of molar pregnancy prior to evacuation can be accomplished by *amniography,* which consists of the injection of radiopaque material into the uterine cavity. Patients are prepared for this procedure by routine catheterization of the urinary bladder, by obtaining a preliminary radiograph of the abdomen, and by testing for sensitivity to the contrast medium. The lower abdomen is surgically prepped and draped. A No. 18 spinal needle with stylet is introduced transabdominally into the uterine cavity at a point in the midline 3–5 cm below the umbilicus. After aspiration to verify intrauterine location of the needle, 15–20 ml of radiopaque materials are injected rapidly. The needle is then withdrawn, and anteroposterior and lateral radiographs are taken immediately. A "honeycombed" pattern is consistent with a diagnosis of molar pregnancy (Fig. 132-8). Satisfactory radiographs have been obtained in 227 women with suspected molar pregnancy, 220 of whom had the condition. The remaining 7 patients were found to have normal single or multiple pregnancies, missed abortions, and ovarian cysts with coexisting normal intrauterine pregnancies. To our knowledge, there have been no reports of untoward effects on either mother or fetus from this procedure when properly executed.

Ultrasonic scanning of the uterus is the second technique that reliably yields a positive diagnosis of molar pregnancy after the twelfth week of gestation. The main advantage of this technique is that is is noninvasive and nonradiographic. The use of the newly introduced Real-Time Equipment quite clearly reveals the vesicular nature of the mole (Fig. 132-9). Ultrasound can also detect the presence of theca-lutein cysts that may not be palpable by pelvic examination. Occasionally, false-positive sonograms are encountered because of the presence of an intrauterine pregnancy in a leiomyomatous uterus or a missed abortion. For this reason, it has been our practice to utilize amniography in conjunction with ultrasonography when the uterus is sufficiently large to permit insertion of a needle transabdominally. On rare occasion, ultrasound examination of a patient suspected of having a molar pregnancy reveals a sac and normal fetal structures that subsequently disappear, re-

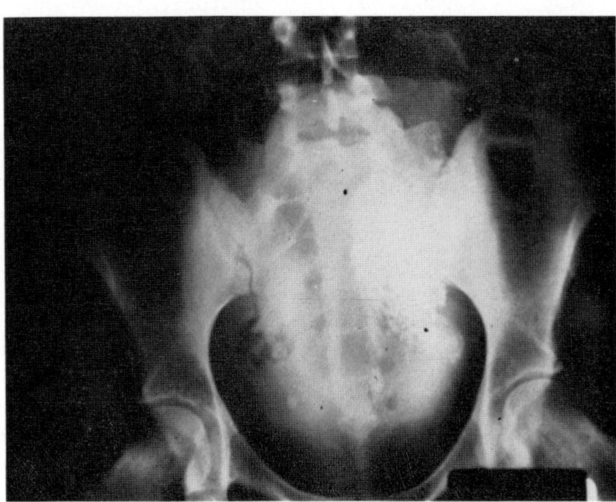

Fig. 132-8. Amniogram showing molar pregnancy in situ.

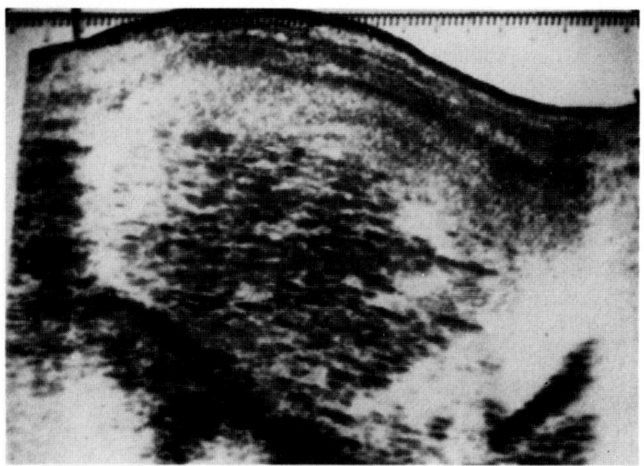

Fig. 132-9. Ultrasound showing molar pregnancy in situ.

vealing a true mole. One can only surmise that this represents the rare finding of a molar pregnancy in transition. Serial sonography may, therefore, be worthwhile when a definitive diagnosis of a mole is not made initially and the clinical signs and symptoms persist.

Pelvic angiography, though available in most modern x-ray departments, is potentially hazardous and yields little additional information, although Cockshott and co-workers[32] feel that the malignant potential of the mole can be ascertained by the use of this technique.[33]

The presence of vaginal wall metastases places the patient in a more advanced classification, which makes the use of chemotherapy at the time of evacuation essential. Careful search for other possible metastatic sites should also be carried out when such a lesion is present. Biopsy of a vaginal wall lesion for diagnostic purposes may lead to excessive hemorrhage and should only be undertaken in the operating room with blood available. The use of deep mattress sutures is extremely helpful in controlling bleeding. Rarely, hypogastric artery ligation is required. Transuterine biopsy for diagnosis using a Vim-Silverman needle is reported but has not been utilized on this service.

The vigorous pursuit of a positive diagnosis of molar pregnancy in patients with probable and presumptive signs is warranted because early diagnosis and evacuation is associated with reduced morbidity with respect to blood loss, infection, toxemia, hyperemesis, and hyperthyroidism. There is no evidence, however, that early diagnosis and evacuation reduces the incidence of proliferative trophoblastic sequelae, which is more dependent on the biological potential of the tumor.

EVACUATION

Once a positive diagnosis of molar pregnancy is made, the patient should be thoroughly evaluated with respect to anemia, hyperthyroidism, toxemia, and renal function. A baseline chest x-ray must be obtained to rule out pulmonary metastases. A careful physical examination is of primary importance in determining the presence of metastases to nonpulmonary sites which may occur, albeit rarely, prior to evacuation. Anemia may be severe enough to necessitate transfusion with packed cells. Toxemia may require either sedation or the introduction of diuretics and antihypertensive agents in the pre-, intra-, and postevacuation periods. Hyperthyroidism should be treated with beta-adrenergic blocking agents such as propranolol to reduce the likelihood of thyroid storm induced by anesthesia. Molar thyrotropin has a short half-life, and therefore the danger of storm is more or less over within 36 hours after evacuation. Hyperemesis should be controlled by antiemetics, and any electrolyte imbalance should be corrected.

The selection of the method of evacuation depends on the patient's plans for future childbearing. Suction evacuation followed by sharp curettage is the preferred technique in patients who desire preservation of reproduction function.

When the uterus is empty, pelvic examination should be performed to determine the presence of theca-lutein cysts. These usually regress over a period of about 3 months following evacuation. Occasionally either torsion or spontaneous hemorrhage into the cyst or rupture into the peritoneal cavity occurs, and the patient develops signs of an acute abdominal catastrophe requiring surgical intervention. Abdominal hysterotomy for the evacuation of a molar pregnancy is now considered an obsolete procedure and should be utilized only when the suction apparatus is unavailable or experience with its use is limited.

If the diagnosis of a mole is made at the time of spontaneous expulsion, suction evacuation should be carried out immediately using the same technique. If the diagnosis of molar pregnancy is made by the pathologist after a curettage for what was thought to be an incomplete, therapeutic, or missed abortion, and the initial curettage has been adequate, no further curettement is necessary, but careful gonadotropin follow-up is mandatory.

In patients who no longer desire to preserve reproductive function, abdominal hysterectomy with the molar pregnancy in situ appears to be the optimal method of evacuation, providing the clinician has experience with the gravid hysterectomy technique. Otherwise, the patient's best interest is served by performing a suction curettage and tubal ligation followed by careful gonadotropin follow-up. Hysterectomy with the mole in situ virtually eliminates any possibility of the patient developing proliferative trophoblastic sequelae of either the nonmetastatic or metastatic type. The ovaries can be preserved even when theca-lutein cysts are present, but it may be wise to decompress the multiloculated cysts by puncture aspiration.

ROLE OF PROPHYLACTIC CHEMOTHERAPY

There has been considerable interest in the use of prophylactic chemotherapy at the time of evacuation of molar pregnancy in an attempt to reduce the incidence of trophoblastic sequelae.[33] The results of a program recently completed at the New England Trophoblastic Disease Center have been analyzed and demonstrate a clear difference in the prognosis of a patient with molar pregnancy when evacuated under a course of prophylactic chemotherapy using actinomycin D versus evacuation without chemotherapy (Table 132-9). A complication rate of 18 percent was noted in 402 untreated cases of molar pregnancy, whereas a complication rate of 4 percent was noted in a matched group of 237 patients who were evacuated during a course of actinomycin D therapy. No metastases were encountered in the treated group, whereas in the untreated group, 5 percent of patients developed extrauterine spread. Toxic side effects of the 5-day course of actinomycin D have been minimal and do not appear to pose a serious problem. There is some controversy regarding the wisdom of pretreating all patients with molar pregnancy, particularly when adequate HCG follow-up is available. However, in those parts of the world where molar pregnancy is more common (such as in the Far East), or in patients in whom proliferative trophoblastic complications are more likely to occur and where HCG follow-up is less than optimal, the use of adjunctive chemotherapy offers improved long-term results.

Table 132-9. Class I. Molar Pregnancy (New England Trophoblastic Disease Center, July 1, 1965–December 31, 1977)

Results	Number of Patients (%)	
	A (Evac. and CT)*	B (Evac. only)†
Normal involution	228 (96%)	330 (82%)
Proliferative trophoblastic sequelae		
Nonmetastatic	9 (4%)	52 (13%)
Metastatic	0	20 (5%)
Totals	237 (100%)	402 (100%)

*Suction evacuation (or hysterectomy) with prophylactic actinomycin D.
†Suction evacuation (or hysterectomy) only.

Table 132-10. Subsequent Pregnancies in 527 Patients with Uncomplicated Moles

Outcome	Number
Term delivery	296
Still birth	2
Premature delivery	44
Spontaneous abortion	
First trimester	85
Second trimester	6
Therapeutic abortion	12
Ectopic	4
Repeat Moles	6
Total number of pregnancies	455
	No./Deliveries
Congenital Malformations	18/342 (5%)
Major obstetrical complications	48/342 (14%)

*Four patients had three consecutive molar pregnancies.

FOLLOW-UP

All patients with molar pregnancy, regardless of whether or not prophylactic chemotherapy is utilized, must be followed closely after evacuation with quantitative HCG determinations, since this has proved to be the only technique that will accurately detect those patients who are likely to develop proliferative trophoblastic sequelae from those who will run a benign postevacuation course. Ideally, HCG measurement should be carried out on serum using the beta subunit radioimmunoassay, which is capable of assaying HCG quantitatively from very high levels down to extinction. When this assay is unavailable, however, the radioimmunoassay for luteinizing hormone may be substituted, providing pituitary suppression by progestational agents is carried out to reduce the level of endogenous luteinizing hormone, which could give the impression that low levels of HCG persist. The quantitative immunoassay performed on a 24-hour urine specimen is adequate for the diagnosis of molar pregnancy and for follow-up immediately after evacuation when the HCG level is still quite elevated. However, this technique cannot be used when the HCG level drops below 2000 IU/liter, at which point a serum radioimmunoassay is needed.

SUBSEQUENT PREGNANCY

One concern of patients who have experienced a molar pregnancy, particularly those without children, is that they will have difficulty with subsequent pregnancies. Table 132-10 summarizes the outcome of subsequent pregnancies in a series of 629 patients. The ultimate outlook for a successful gestation is excellent. There does, however, appear to be a slightly higher incidence of spontaneous miscarriage in the first postmolar pregnancy, both in patients who received prophylactic chemotherapy and in untreated controls, as well as an increased incidence of recurrent moles. The high incidence of recurrent moles in this relatively small group of patients raises the question of some common but as yet obscure etiological factor.

NONMETASTATIC GESTATIONAL NEOPLASMS

CLASS 2 (LOW-RISK NONMETASTATIC DISEASE)

Class 2 constitutes a small group of women with uterine subinvolution, persistent vaginal bleeding, and elevated HCG levels without evidence of deep myometrial invasion. The majority of the cases follow evacuation of a molar pregnancy and result from a small amount of residual molar tissue in the uterine cavity (group a); rarely CCA is found (group b). Treatment is based on the desire of the patient to preserve the uterus for future childbearing (Table 132-11). If preservation of the uterus is the goal, then therapy should consist of chemotherapy, either methotrexate (MTX) with citrovorum factor (CF) rescue or actinomycin D. MTX should be avoided in any patient with laboratory evidence of liver function abnormality because of its marked hepatotoxicity at the dose utilized. Under these circumstances, actinomycin D is used instead, since this drug is not associated to any significant degree with hepatocellular dysfunction. When patients no longer desire to preserve fertility, total abdominal hysterectomy should be carried out, with or without bilateral salpingo-oophorectomy. Surgery should be performed on the third day of an adjunctive course of either MTX or actinomycin D. Table 132-12 summarizes the overall results of therapy in 48 patients who were treated for Class 2 disease between 1965 and 1977. All patients are in complete remission, and 28 pregnancies have already been reported without an increased incidence of major obstetrical problem or congenital abnormalities. Patients in this group generally require only a single course of chemotherapy or hysterectomy because of the minimal and superficial nature of their tumor process (Fig. 132-10).

CLASS 3 (HIGH-RISK NONMETASTATIC DISEASE)

Class 3 constitutes a larger group of patients who present with uterine enlargement, persistent vaginal bleeding, ovarian cysts, elevated HCG levels, and evidence of deep myometrial invasion by pelvic arteriography, curettage, and/or clinical examination. The majority of these cases follow evacuation of a molar pregnancy and have an histologic diagnosis of invasive mole (group a) rather than CCA (group b).

Table 132-11. Class II. Low-Risk Nonmetastatic Gestational Neoplasms NETCD Recommended Treatment Protocol

Preservation of fertility
1. Single agent CT:
   Low dose MTX with CFR
   ACT-D
2. Curettage during course

Sacrifice of fertility
1. TAH w/wo BSO
2. Adjunctive single-agent CT

HCG follow-up
- Weekly until normal for 3 consecutive weeks
- Monthly until normal for 6 consecutive months

Table 132-12. Class II. Low-Risk Nonmetastatic Gestational Neoplasms (New England Trophoblastic Disease Center, July 1, 1965–December 31, 1977)

	Remissions/Total Number of Patients (% Remissions)	
Therapy	Hydatidiform A (Mole)	B (CCA)
1° MTX*	24/24 (100)	6/6 (100)
1° ACT-D*	11/11 (100)	1/1 (100)
1° Hysterectomy†	3/3 (100)	3/3 (100)
Totals	38 (100)	10 (100)

*One course only.
†Adjunctive chemotherapy used.

The therapy selected for these patients is also based on the patient's desire to preserve fertility, inasmuch as the results of both chemotherapy and surgery are comparable (Table 132-13). The younger patients who wish to preserve reproductive function should be treated sequentially with MTX with CF rescue and actinomycin D.

Response to therapy is monitored by weekly serum HCG titers, and the subsequent course of therapy is administered on the basis of the HCG regression curve. If remission is attained with one or more courses of the initial agent, no further therapy is required. However, if the HCG titer plateaus despite two consecutive courses or rises during or after a course of treatment, the second agent is begun and continued until remission is achieved (Fig. 132-11).

Table 132-13. Class III. High-Risk Nonmetastatic Gestational Neoplasms NETDC Recommended Treatment Protocol

Preservation of fertility
1. Sequential single-agent CT:*
   Low dose MTX with CFR and ACT-D
2. Curettage during initial course
3. Hypogastric arterial infusion (when indicated)
4. Local resection (when indicated)

Sacrifice of fertility
1. TAH w/wo BSO
2. Adjunctive single-agent CT

HCG follow-up
- Weekly until normal × 3 consecutive weeks
- Monthly until normal × 6 consecutive months
- Bimonthly until normal × 12 months

*Administered on basis of HCG response.

When patients do not desire to preserve fertility, the treatment of choice is total abdominal hysterectomy with or without bilateral salpingo-oophorectomy. Surgery should be performed on the third day of an adjunctive course of either MTX or actinomycin D using the same dose schedule. Studies show that there is no increase in postoperative morbidity when adjunctive therapy is used, providing good surgical technique and sound principles of wound closure are followed.

Table 132-14 summarizes the overall results of therapy in 115 patients who were treated for Class 3 disease between 1965 and 1977. All but 1 patient are in complete remission. Analysis of the 71 subsequent pregnancies reveal no increased incidence of congenital malformations or major obstetrical complications. In most instances, complete remission was accomplished with either MTX or actinomycin D. Twenty-five cases, however, required the use of both agents administered sequentially. Hysterectomy was performed in 11 instances electively because the patients did not desire to undergo prolonged drug therapy for the purpose of preserving fertility.

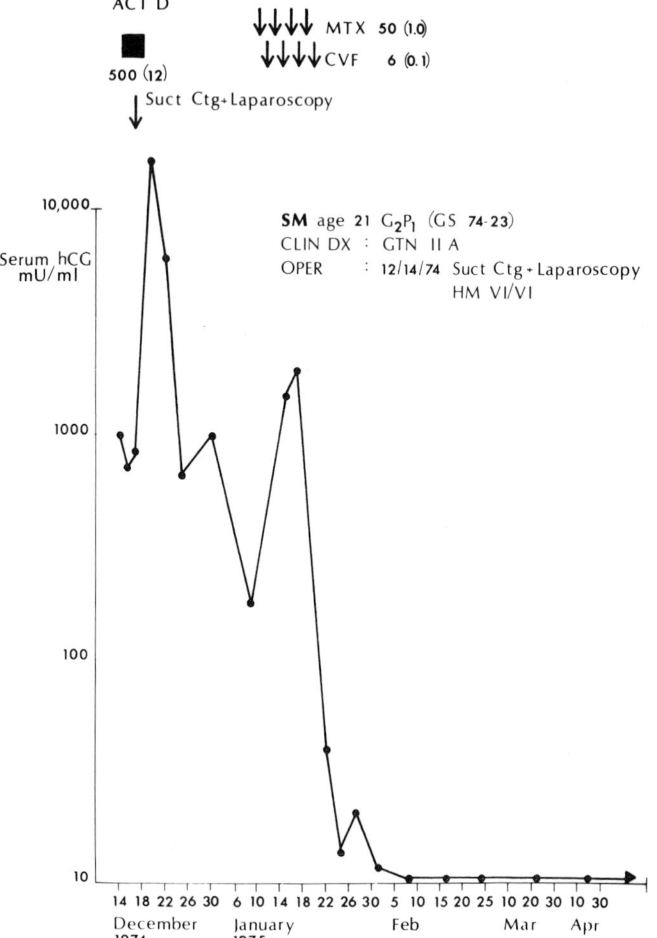

Fig. 132-10. HCG regression curve in patient being treated for low-risk nonmetastatic disease (Class 2).

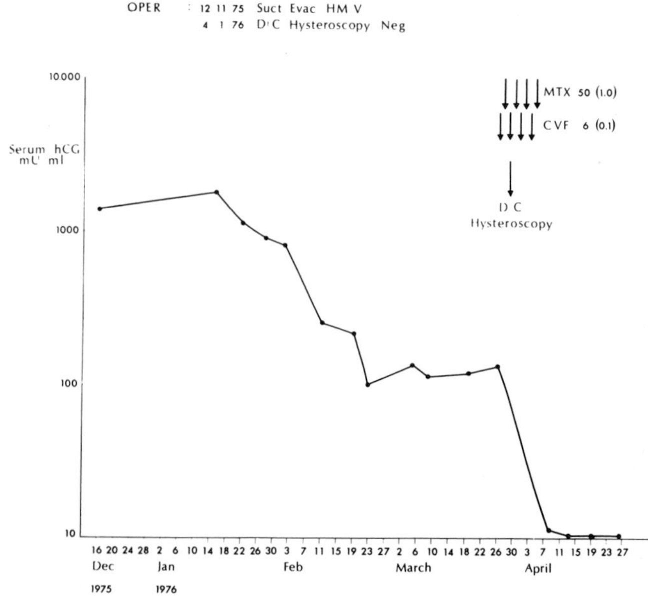

Fig. 132-11. HCG regression curve in patient being treated for high-risk nonmetastatic disease (Class 3).

Table 132-14. Class III. High-Risk Nonmetastatic Gestational Neoplasms (New England Trophoblastic Disease Center, July 1, 1965–December 31, 1977)

Remission Therapy	Remission/Total Number of Patients (% Remission) A (Hydatidiform Mole)	B (CCA)
1° MTX	42/53 (79)	9/15 (60)
1° ACT-D	23/33 (72)	3/3 (100)
Sequential MTX or ACT-D	20/20 (100)	5/5 (100)
1° Hysterectomy*	7/7 (100)	4/4 (100)
Totals*	93/93 (100)	21/22† (100)

*Adjunctive chemotherapy used.
†1 Patient AWD.

In rare instances, particularly where excessive toxicity to systemic chemotherapy is encountered, it may be necessary to employ hypogastric arterial infusion in order to deliver an adequate dose of drug and avoid serious system toxicity.

METASTATIC GESTATIONAL NEOPLASM

CLASS 4 (LOW-RISK METASTATIC DISEASE)

Class 4 constitutes a group of patients who present with demonstrable metastases to the lungs, vagina, pelvis, and/or other organs exclusive of the brain, liver, kidney, spleen, and/or bowel. The duration of disease is less than 4 months from the termination of the antecedent pregnancy or the onset of symptoms, and the HCG level is less than 100,000 IU/liter, or its equivalent, depending upon the assay utilized.

Despite the presence of metastatic disease, the known histologic diagnosis in the majority of Class 4 patients is hydatidiform mole (group a) rather than CCA (group b). It should be emphasized that the initial work-up specifically excludes all attempts at obtaining a precise morphologic diagnosis if this requires more than a curettage or vaginal biopsy. Thus, many patients grouped into the hydatidiform mole category may indeed have CCA in a metastatic site.

The therapy selected for this group of patients in contrast to those in Classes 2 and 3 is chemotherapy regardless of the patient's desire to preserve fertility (Table 132-15). After initial evaluation the patient should be treated primarily with sequential MTX with CF rescue and actinomycin D. The same principles apply to monitoring the response to therapy in Class 4 patients as was outlined above in the section describing the management of Class 2 and 3 disease. Subsequent courses of the primary drug are administered on the basis of the HCG regression curve, rather than on the subsidence of toxic manifestations. If remission is obtained with one or more successive courses of the primary agent, no further therapy is required. However, if the HCG level plateaus despite two successive courses of the initial agent, or rises during or after a course of treatment, then the initial agent should be discontinued and the second agent employed until either remission is achieved or resistance to the second agent is encountered (Fig. 132-12).

Table 132-15. Class IV. Low-Risk Metastatic Gestational Neoplasms NETDC Recommended Treatment Protocol

Primary therapy
1. Sequential single agent CT:*
   Low dose MTX with CFR, and ACT-D
2. Curettage optimal

Secondary therapy (for resistent cases)
1. Triple therapy:*
   Low dose MTX with CFR
   Cyclophosphamide
2. High dose MTX with CFR (SFCI)*
3. ITMA (Bagshawe)*

Hysterectomy for uterine enlargement, infection or bleeding only

HCG follow-up
- Weekly until normal × 3 consecutive weeks
- Monthly until normal × 6 consecutive months
- Bimonthly until normal × 12 months
- Every 6 months until normal × 5 years

*Administered on basis of HCG response.

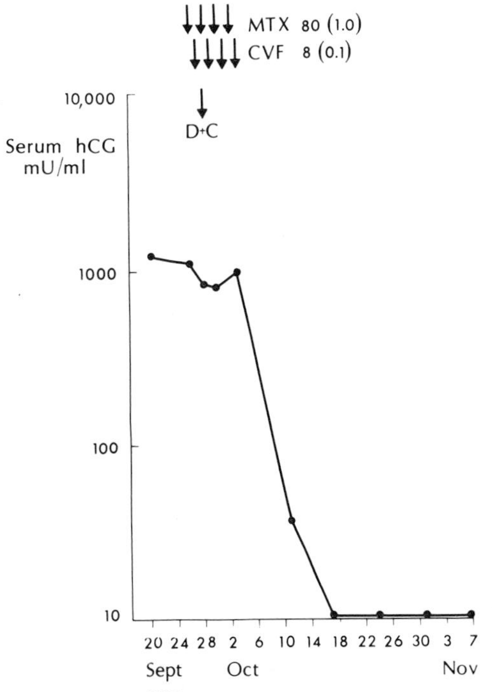

Fig. 132-12. HCG regression curve in patient being treated for low-risk metastatic disease.

Patients who develop resistance to both MTX with CF rescue and actinomycin D are started on triple therapy. Hysterectomy is performed only if there is evidence of significant residual tumor.

Table 132-16 summarizes the overall results of therapy and the type of therapy required for remission in 72 patients who were treated for Class 4 disease between 1965 and 1977. All patients are in complete remission. Analysis of the 23 subsequent pregnancies reveal no increased congenital malformations or obstetrical complications. Complete remission was accomplished with single agent therapy in 27 out of 40 patients with a histologic diagnosis of hydatidiform mole and in 14 out of 28 patients with CCA. The remaining patients required either sequential therapy with MTX and actinomycin D, triple therapy, or high-dose MTX/CF rescue. A higher percentage of patients with a known histologic diagnosis of hydatidiform mole achieved remission with single-agent therapy than did those with CCA, presumably because of the greater degree of malignancy and thus resistance in the latter.

CLASS 5 (HIGH-RISK METASTATIC DISEASE)

Class 5 constitutes a group of patients who present with demonstrable metastases in the brain, liver, kidney, spleen and/or bowel, with a duration of disease greater than 4 months from termination of the antecedent pregnancy or the onset of symptoms and with HCG levels greater than 100,000 IU/liter (or its equivalent, depending upon the assay utilized). Since this group yields the poorest survival, it is fortunate that it comprises the smallest number of patients. Most have had an antecedent term pregnancy after which the diagnosis of gestational neoplasm was missed when the symptoms first developed. All the patients in this group have been found to have CCA; therefore, no breakdown into groups a or b is made.

When the existence of this high-risk type of patient was first delineated, the mortality approached 100 percent despite the use of conventional sequential therapy followed by triple therapy. The most common cause of death in this group was found to result from hemorrhage from cerebral or hepatic metastases. The subsequent addition of whole-head irradiation (as adjunct to actinomycin D therapy) when cerebral lesions were diagnosed improved survival by 50 percent in that small subgroup of Class 5 patients. Actinomycin D was selected as the treatment of choice to use with whole head irradiation because of its ability to cross the blood-brain barrier. Liver metastases are less satisfactorily managed. A significant advance was made when Hammond and Parker bypassed conventional sequential therapy and promptly commenced primary head irradiation when cerebral metastases were encountered and suggested that radiation therapy to the liver might also be useful.[3]

On the basis of this background information, the therapy selected for this group of patients is as follows: After initial evaluation the patient is treated primarily with triple therapy (Table 132-17). Hysterectomy is also required more commonly because of the high incidence of residual tumor, in contrast to the situation that exists in Class 4 patients, in whom residual uterine tumor is unusual. Adjunctive whole-head irradiation is employed immediately if cerebral metastases are identified or even strongly suspected but not proven, because the danger of death from intracerebral hemorrhage is high and usually fatal when it occurs. When hepatic lesions are proven by liver scan, arteriography, and/or surgery, one of three courses of action may be employed: (1) systemic therapy may be started because of diffuse metastatic disease and the hepatic lesion dealt with later if no response is noted; (2) local irradiation may be used as an adjunct to chemotherapy, as in the case with cerebral lesions; or (3) hepatic artery infusion may be employed without systemic therapy using the triple-therapy regimen, particularly if the hepatic metastases is present without other demonstrable lesions. If intraperitoneal hemorrhage develops from a hepatic lesion, surgery must be performed in an attempt to stop the bleeding by local suturing or even by hepatic artery ligation. Bowel lesions should be resected when diagnosed by stool guaiac tests and localized by roentgenologic

Table 132-16. Class IV. Low-Risk Metastatic Gestational Neoplasms (New England Trophoblastic Disease Center, July 1, 1965–December 31, 1977)

Remission Therapy	Remissions/Total Number of Patients (% Remissions) A (Hydatidiform Mole)	B (CCA)
1° MTX	15/20 (75)	8/14 (57)
1° ACT-D	12/20 (60)	6/14 (42)
Sequential MTX or ACT-D	13/15 (87)	10/14 (71)
2° Triple TX	1/1 (100)	3/3 (100)
2° HD MTX-CFR	1/1 (100)	1/1 (100)
Totals	42/42 (100)	28/28 (100)

Table 132-17. Class V. High-Risk Metastatic Gestational Neoplasms NETDC Recommended Treatment Protocol

Primary therapy
1. Triple therapy*
   Low dose MTX with CFR
   ACT-D
   Cyclophosphamide
2. High dose MTX with CFR (SFCI)*

Subsequent therapy
1. ITMA (Bagshawe)*
2. Experimental protocols.*

Special therapy
1. Brain metastases: whole-head irradiation—3000 rads
2. Liver metastases: infusion therapy, irradiation
3. Bowel metastases: surgery
4. Uterine enlargement or bleeding: surgery

HCG follow-up
Weekly until normal × 3 consecutive weeks
Monthly until normal × 12 consecutive months
Every 6 months until normal × 5 years

*Administer courses on basis of HCG response.

Table 132-18. Class V. High-Risk Metastatic Gestational Neoplasms

Remission Therapy* (Total Number of Patients, 29)		
< 1975		
1° MTX	0	6/20 (30%)
1° ACT-D (LD)	4	
Sequential MTX or ACT-D	1	
2° Triple TX	1	
2° HD MTX w CFR	0	
3° Experimental protocols	0	
>1975		
1° Triple TX	2	6/9 (66.6%)
1° HD MTX w CFR	2	
1° HD ACT-D	1	
2° ITMA	1	
Totals		
Remissions	12/29	(41.3%)
Deaths	14/29	(48.2%)
Alive with disease	3/29	(10.3%)

*X-ray therapy and surgery utilized when indicated.

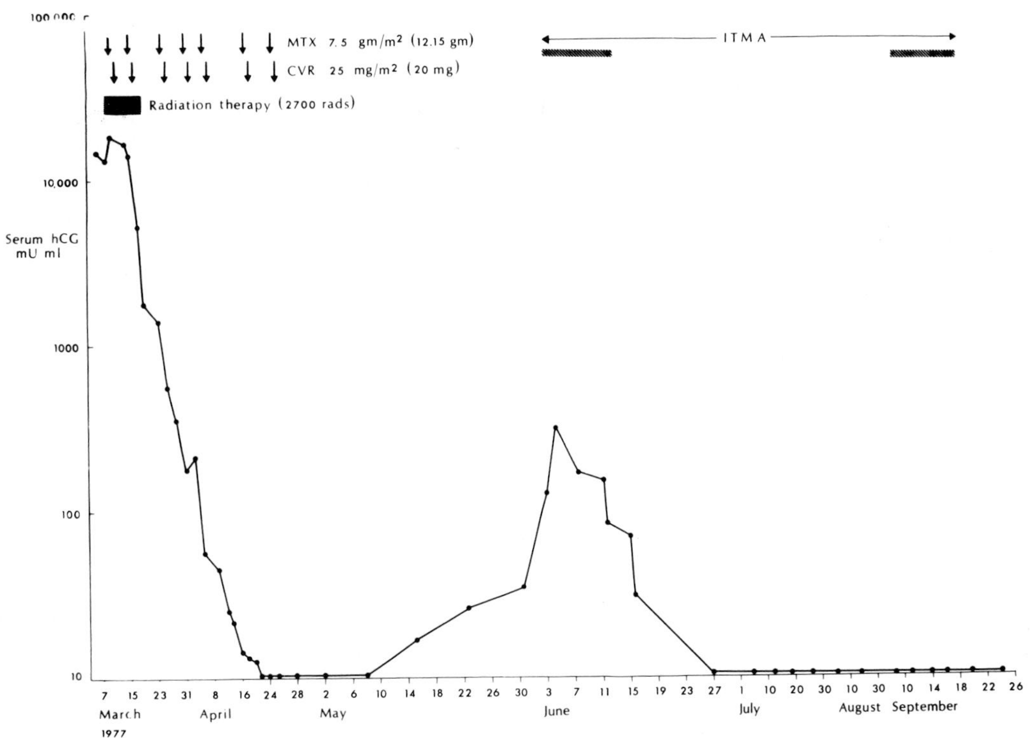

Fig. 132-13. HCG regression curve in a patient with high-risk gestational neoplasms.

study of the gastrointestinal tract. Splenic and renal metastases encountered more commonly in this group of patients with far-advanced disease generally respond to systemic therapy and do not require special treatment techniques.

If resistance to primary therapy is encountered, then intensive multiple-agent treatment must be employed. Both primary and secondary treatment is administered on the basis of serum HCG levels as in the other classes (Fig. 132-13).

Table 132-18 summarizes the results obtained in 29 patients with Class 5 gestational neoplasm between 1965 and 1977. The results are shown in two time periods (<1975 and >1975), which reflects the fact that in 1975, more intensive therapy was used

Table 132-19. Summary of Remission Therapy (New England Trophoblastic Disease Center, July 1, 1965–December 31, 1977)

Class	Therapy	Remission/Total	Number of Patients (%)
I A	Evacuation and CT	228/237	(96)
B	Evacuation only	330/402	(82)
II A/B	Single agent CT w/wo hysterectomy	48/48	(100)
III A/B	Sequential CT, or single-agent CT/hysterectomy	114/115 (AWD—1)	(99)
*IV A/B	1° Sequential CT 2° Triple tx or HDMTX w CFR	70/70	(100)
†*V <1975	1°Sequential CT 2° Triple tx or HD MTX w CFR	12/29 (AWD—3)	(41)
>1975	1° Triple tx, HDMTX-CFR or ACT-D 2° ITMA 3° Experimental protocols		
Totals		Remissions	
	1°	744/901	(82.5)
	2° 3 °	137/901	(15.2)
	Failures	14/901	(1.5)
	Alive with disease	4/899	(0.4)

*Hysterectomy, when indicated.
†Radiotherapy, when indicated.

primarily after single-agent or lower dose treatment was shown to be ineffective. It appears that there has been some improvement in cure rates although the numbers are still small. The three pregnancies that occurred in this group of patients represent a significant achievement in modern oncology, since all offspring that went to term were normal and the pregnancies uncomplicated.

SUMMARY

The treatment of gestational neoplasms has changed dramatically from primarily surgical to primarily medical over the past 20 years. This change has occurred as a result of a number of factors unique to gestational neoplasms, including the findings that trophoblastic neoplasms are exquisitely sensitive to chemotherapeutic agents and always produce HCG, which serves as a cell marker. Complete remission can be achieved in virtually all patients by utilizing these two principles (Table 132-19). In the majority of patients, a normal reproductive career may be anticipated once the disease is eradicated, thus permitting gestational neoplasms to be designated as God's first cancer and man's first cure.

REFERENCES

1. Hertig, A. T. and Mansell, H.: Tumors of the female sex organs. Part I. Hydatidiform mole and choriocarcinoma. *In* Atlas of Tumor Pathology. Washington, D.C., Armed Forces Institute of Pathology, 1956.
2. Ross, G. T., Goldstein, D. P., Hertz, R., Lipsett, M. B., and Odell, W. D.: Sequential use of methotrexate and actinomycin D in the treatment of metastatic choriocarcinoma and related trophoblastic disease in women. *Am. J. Obstet. Gynecol. 93:* 223–229, 1965.
3. Hammond, C. G. and Parker, R. T.: Diagnosis and treatment of trophoblastic disease. *Obstet. Gynecol. 34:* 132, 1970.
4. Hertig, A. T. and Sheldon, W. H.: Hydatidiform mole—pathologicoclinical correlation of 200 cases. *Am. J. Obstet. Gynecol. 53:* 1–36, 1947.
5. Shirley, R. L., Goldstein, D. P. and Collins, J. J., Jr.: The role of thoracotomy in the management of patients with chest metastases from gestational trophoblastic disease. *J. Thorac. Cardiovasc. Surg. 63:* 545–550, 1972.
6. Bagshawe, K. D.: Risk and prognostic factors in trophoblastic disease. *Cancer 38:* 1373, 1976.
7. Vaitukaitis, J. L., Braunstein, G. D., and Ross, G. T.: A radioimmunoassay which specifically measures human chorionic gonadotropin in the presence of human luteinizing hormone. *Am. J. Obstet. Gynecol. 113:* 751, 1972.
8. Dawood, M. Y., Saxens, B. B., and Landesian, R.: Human chorionic gonadotropin and its subunit in hydatidiform mole and choriocarcinoma. *Obstet. Gynecol. 50:* 172, 1977.
9. Hertz, R., Lewis, J., Jr., and Lipsett, M. B.: Five years' experience with the chemotherapy of metastatic choriocarcinoma and related trophoblastic tumors in women. *Am. J. Obstet. Gynecol. 82:* 631–640, 1961.
10. Wide, L. and Hobson, B.: Imunological and biological activity of human chorionic gonadotropin in urine and serum of pregnant women and women with a hydatidiform mole. *Acta Endocrinol. 54:* 105, 1967.
11. Curry, S. L., Hammond, C. B., Tyrey, L., Creasman, W. T., and Parker, R. T.: Diagnosis, management and long-term follow-up of patients with hydatidiform mole. *Obstet. Gynecol. 45:* 1, 1975.
12. Goldstein, D. P. and Kosasa, R. S.: The subunit radioimmunoassay for hCG-clinical application. *In* Progress in Gynecology, M. L. Taymor and T. H. Green, Jr. (eds.). New York, Grune and Stratton, 1975, chap. 3, pp. 145–184.
13. Goldstein, D. P.: Endocrine assay in chorionic tumors. *Clin. Obstet. Gynecol. 18:* 41–60, 1975.
14. Goldstein, D. P., Kosasa, R. S., and Skarin, A. T.: Clinical application of a specific radioimmunoassay for human chorionic gonadotropin in trophoblastic and non-trophoblastic tumors. *Surg. Gynecol. Obstet. 138:* 747, 1974.
15. Beal, P. and Doughaday, W. H.: Human placental lactogen: Studies of its acute metabolic effects and disposition in normal man. *J. Clin. Invest. 46:* 103, 1966.
16. Saxena, B. N., Goldstein, D. P., Emerson, K., Jr., and Selenkow, H. A.: Serum placental lactogen levels in patients with molar pregnancy and trophoblastic tumors. *Am. J. Obst. Gynec. 102:* 115–121, 1968.
17. Saxena, B. N., Emerson, K., Jr., and Selenkow, H. A.: Serum placental lactogen (HPL) levels as an index of placental function. *N. Engl. J. Med. 281:* 225, 1969.
18. Goldstein, D. P.: Serum placental lactogen activity in patients with molar pregnancy and trophoblastic tumors. A reliable index of malignancy. *Am. J. Obstet. Gynecol. 110:* 583, 1971.
19. Galton, M. A., Ingbar, S. H., Jimenez-Fonseca, J., and Hershman, J. M.: Alterations in thyroid hormone economy in patients with hydatidiform mole. *J. Clin. Invest. 50:* 1345, 1971.
20. Herschman, J. M.: Hyperthroidism induced by trophoblastic thyrotropin. *Mayo. Clin. Proc. 47:* 913, 1972.
21. Dowling, J. T., Ingbar, S. H., and Freinkel, W.: Iodine metabolism in hydatidiform mole and choriocarcinoma. *J. Clin. Endocrinol. Metab. 20:* 1, 1960.
22. Odell, W. B., Bates, R. W., and Rivlin, R. S.: Increased thyroid function without clinical hyperthyroidism in patients with choriocarcinoma. *J. Clin. Endocrinol. Metab. 23:* 658, 1963.
23. Kenimer, J. G., Herschman, J. M., and Higgins, H. P.: The thyrotropin in hydatidiform moles is human chorionic gonadotropin. *J. Clin. Endocrinol. Metab. 35:* 482, 1975.
24. Barlow, J. J., Goldstein, D. P., and Reid, D. E.: A study of in vivo estrogen biosynthesis and production rates in normal pregnancy, hydatidiform mole, and choriocarcinoma. *J. Clin.,Endocrionol. Metab. 27:* 1928, 1967.
25. Dawood, M. Y., Ratnam, S. S., and Teoh, E. S.: Serum estradiol-17 and serum human chorionic gonadotropin in patients with hydatidiform moles. *Am. J. Obstet. Gynecol. 119:* 904, 1974.
26. Patillo, R., Gey, G. O., and Delfs, E.: The hormone-synthesizing trophoblastic cell in vitro: A model for cancer research and placental hormone synthesis. *Ann. N.Y. Acad. Sci. 172:* 288, 1971.
27. Dawood, M. Y.: Progesterone concentrations in the serum of patients with intact and aborting hydatidiform moles. *Am. J. Obstet. Gynecol. 119:* 911, 1974.
28. Ishizuka, N.: Chemotherapy of trophoblastic neoplasia. *World Obstet.-Gynecol. 15:* 69, 1963.
29. Frandsen, V. A. and Staakeiarn, G.: The site of production of estrogenic hormones in human pregnancy. II. Experimental investigations of the role of the fetal adrenal. *Acta Endocrinol. 43:* 184, 1963.
30. Brown, J. B., Beidser, N. A., and Smith, M. A.: Excretion of urinary estrogens in pregnant patients treated with cortisone and its analogues. *J. Obstet. Gynaecol. Br. Commonw. 75:* 819, 1966.
31. Kohorn, E. I., McGinn, R. C., Gee, J. B. L., Goldstein, D. P., and Osathanondh, R.: Pulmonary embolization of trophoblastic tissue in molar pregnancy. *Obstet. Gynecol. 51:* 165–205, 1978.
32. Brody, S. and Cartlstrom, G.: Human chorionic gonadotropin in abnormal pregnancy. Serum and urinary findings using various immunoassay techniques. *Acta Obstet. Gynecol. Scand. 44:* 32, 1965.
33. Cockshott, W. P., Evans, K. T., and Hendrickse, J. P. de V:: Arteriography of trophoblastic tumors. *Clin Radiol. 15:* 1, 1964.

133

Fetal Endocrinology: Endocrine Disease and Pregnancy

Delbert A. Fisher

INTRODUCTION

During the past three decades, our understanding of fetal endocrine physiology has expanded rapidly. The pioneering work of Dr. Alfred Jost has been extended by numerous investigators and more recently by the availability of radiolabeled hormones and a variety of sensitive and specific hormone radioimmunoassay procedures. These techniques have been applied to studies of aborted human fetuses, as well as normal newborn infants, and to acute and chronic studies of fetuses of several mammalian and primate species. Finally, careful observation of the fetal pathophysiology associated with endocrine diseases in human pregnancy has continued to provide important clues and correlative data with which to construct working models of fetal endocrine ontogenesis and metabolism. The data and our models remain incomplete in many details, but the larger picture of fetal autonomy proposed by Dr. Jost has been substantiated.[1–3]

PLACENTAL TRANSFER OF HORMONES

Much work has been conducted regarding the transfer of hormones across the placental "barrier," and it is now clear that this barrier is essentially absolute for polypeptide hormones and relative for steroid hormones.

POLYPEPTIDE HORMONES

Fetal pituitary gland function has been studied in several species[1–3] by cytologic methods, measurements of hormone content, experimental removal of the fetal pituitary, and hormone injections into normal or pituitary-deprived fetuses. These data suggest that the placenta is impermeable to growth hormone (GH), ACTH, gonadotropins, and thyrotropin (TSH). Recent direct studies confirm the absence of significant placental transfer of growth hormone,[4–6] TSH,[7] ACTH,[8–11] and luteinizing hormone (LH).[12,13] There is less information regarding posterior pituitary peptides and the available evidence is contradictory.

There is some placental transfer of oxytocin, at least in the guinea pig and sheep.[14,15] However, available evidence in the sheep and man suggest minimal transfer of vasopressin.[16,17] Placental transfer of insulin and glucagon[18–22] and of parathyroid hormone and calcitonin[23,24] also are minimal. Finally, the absence of plasma renin in the anephric fetus, in contrast to the normal fetus, suggests that the placenta also is impermeable to this hormone.[25] Thus, it seems that the placenta of all species studied is essentially impermeable to polypeptide hormones, with the possible exception of the smallest, the posterior pituitary hormones with molecular weights approximating 1100.

STEROID HORMONES

The placenta has been considered to be generally permeable to the transfer of adrenal corticosteroids.[26–30] While direct measurements are not available in the human, average maternal–fetal and fetal–maternal transfer rates of cortisol in sheep near term are 0.63 and 1.18 mg/day, respectively (SD is 13 percent for both estimates).[26,29] From these data it is estimated that 0.9 and 77 percent of the respective mean daily secretion rates of cortisol in the ewes and fetuses (66.7 and 1.54 mg/day, respectively) are cleared by the placenta each day. The placenta also is permeable to aldosterone and progesterone, as well as to androgenic and estrogenic steroids.[31–34] However, any placental transfer of estrogens or progesterone is diminished in importance in human pregnancy by the fact that the placenta also synthesizes large quantities of these hormones. Diczfalusy and Mancuso[32] and others have shown that the placenta is capable of synthesizing estrogens from fetal adrenal steroid precursors, especially dehydroepiandrosterone sulfate and 16-hydroxydehydroepiandrosterone, but cannot manufacture estrogens de novo from progesterone or pregnenolone. Progesterone is formed largely from blood-borne cholesterol.[32,35]

THYROID HORMONES

Courrier and Aron, in 1929,[36] were the first to study placental transfer of thyroid hormones. Because they observed that large amounts of animal thyroid failed to alter fetal thyroid gland morphology in pregnant bitches and guinea pigs, they concluded that thyroid hormones did not cross the placental barrier. Extensive studies by numerous investigators in many species since that time have confirmed this conclusion.[37–43] Very little hormone traverses the placenta at physiologic serum concentrations; at high blood levels more transfer may occur. For example, in the rat, guinea pig, rabbit, and monkey,[37–39,43] the maternal–fetal equilibrium distribution of labeled T_4 administered to pregnant mothers is about 20/1.

In the monkey, increasing the maternal serum T_4 concentration 300 percent does not measurably alter fetal serum T_4 or inhibit T_4 synthesis by the fetal thyroid gland.[43] In the sheep, fetal surgical thyroidectomy leads to rapid disappearance of T_4 from fetal blood and marked increase in fetal serum TSH concentrations.[38,41] Kinetic studies of placental transfer in normal sheep indicate net maternal–fetal transfer of 0.6 μg T_4 and 0.7 μg T_3 daily. These amounts represent less than 7 percent of total daily T_4 equivalent of iodothyronine turnover in the euthyroid fetus and about 0.1 and 1 percent, respectively, of mean maternal T_4 and T_3 turnover rates.[41]

In man the results are essentially similar. There are marked baseline maternal–fetal serum concentration gradients of T_4 and free T_4 prior to 35–40 weeks, at which time the gradient seems to reverse.[38,44] Fetal serum T_3 and free T_3 levels are low throughout gestation so that a marked maternal–fetal gradient exists throughout gestation.[42] Little or no placental transfer of labeled T_4 occurs early in gestation,[45] and although some placental transfer of labeled thyroid hormones is observed at term,[46,47] the extent is limited. Loading of pregnant women near term or during labor with large quantities of T_4 (1500–8000 μg) or T_3 (300 μg) leads to minimal maternal–fetal hormone transfer. Only about 1 percent of the 8000-μg T_4 load reaches the fetus and the chronic 300 μg/day T_3 dose reduces serum T_4 levels minimally and inconsistently.[48,49] Keynes reported that administration of 500 μg T_4 daily to a pregnant woman on propylthiouracil did not prevent goiter in the fetus.[50] Carr et al.,[51] after administering 1400 mg dessicated thyroid daily to a pregnant woman, observed a cord blood BEI of only 4.5 μg/100 ml in an infant shown to have a small residual of functioning thyroid tissue.

CATECHOLAMINES

Understanding of placental transfer of catecholamines is limited. There is some evidence, however, to suggest that epinephrine and norepinephrine can traverse the placental barrier. Maternal injection of norepinephrine produces transient fetal bradycardia[52] and maternal epinephrine infusion results in fetal tachycardia, cardiac irregularity, and an increase in fetal blood sugar concentration.[53] The observation that radiolabeled d,l-norepinephrine activity appears in fetal blood after maternal injection[54] suggests that these fetal effects are due, at least in part, to placental passage of the hormones.

SUMMARY

The general pattern of placental permeability to hormones is summarized in Table 133-1; the molecular weight, lipid solubility, and mode of action in regard to cell membrane binding are shown for the several hormone species. As can be observed, placental transfer relates more to molecular weight than to the other listed characteristics. Studies in a variety of species, particularly rabbits, have indicated that the placenta is more permeable to lipid-soluble than to lipid-insoluble substances and that placental permeability to lipid-insoluble molecules decreases with increasing molecular weight.[55] The data regarding placental transfer of hormones is in general agreement with these results. It should be pointed out, however, that the lipid solubility of the hormones listed is relatively minimal as contrasted with acetylene, which was used in the rabbit studies. Thus, it is not clear to what extent placental permeability to hormones relates to lipid solubility in contrast to molecular weight.

Placental transfer is listed as all or none in Table 133-1, whereas progressively increasing permeability with decreasing molecular weight is likely. Relative permeability data related to free hormone concentration differences across the placenta are not available. Nonetheless, the minimal placental permeability to thyroid hormones and relatively greater permeability to steroid hormones suggests that the threshold molecular weight for significant hormone transfer at physiologic concentrations is in the range of 350–800.

ONTOGENESIS OF FETAL HORMONE SYSTEMS

GENERAL

Hormone systems can be classified in two major groups, as shown in Table 133-2. The neuroendocrine transducer systems transduce or convert neural into endocrine information. Three such mechanisms have been identified: (1) the hypothalamic–anterior pituitary system, (2) the hypothalamic–posterior pituitary system, and (3) the autonomic nervous system. In addition to the

Table 133-1. Patterns of Placental Hormone Transfer as Related to Molecular Weight, Lipid Solubility, and Mode of Action

			Mode of Action		
Hormone Species	Approximate Molecular Weight	Lipid Solubility	Cell Membrane Receptor Binding	Intracellular Protein Receptor Binding	Placental Transfer
Polypeptide hormones	1100–30,000	—	Yes	No	No
Thyroid hormones	800	±	No	Yes	No
Steroid hormones	350	±	No	Yes	Yes
Catecholamines	180	–	Yes	No	Yes

Table 133-2. Types of Endocrine Systems

Neuroendocrine transducer systems
Hypothalamus–anterior pituitary–target organs
Hypothalamus–posterior pituitary
Sympathetic nervous system
Autonomous endocrine systems
Endocrine pancreas (insulin–glucagon)
Parathyroid gland–thyroid C cells (parathyroid hormone–calcitonin)

neuroendocrine systems, at least two autonomous endocrine systems are known: (1) the insulin–glucagon and (2) the parathyroid hormone–calcitonin systems. In these systems, hormone secretion is largely regulated by local glandular substrate feedback mechanisms.

During fetal life neither the neuroendocrine transducer systems nor the autonomous endocrine systems seem to be of vital importance to survival or growth. The maternal–placental unit provides a constant supply of growth and energy substrates, provides regulation of water and electrolyte metabolism, maintains respiratory and excretory functions, and controls body temperature within narrow limits. Growth of the fetus seems to be predominantly controlled by inherent genetic or tissue factors rather than pituitary or placental hormones. Certain aspects of fetal metabolism may be influenced, however, by fetal or placental hormones, and fetal pituitary target organ function (particularly the adrenal glands and gonads) may be hormone dependent.

The events of parturition abruptly terminate this period of dependent development and precipitate a series of profound metabolic stresses; extrauterine survival requires autonomous thermogenesis and alimentation as well as autonomous respiratory and excretory activities, which are largely dependent upon the functional capacity of the endocrine systems. The neuroendocrine transducer systems appear to be well developed at birth and function smoothly to defend against the stresses of extrauterine exposure. The autonomous endocrine systems, however, regulating blood sugar and calcium levels, are relatively less mature and/or are suppressed in utero. Thus abnormalities related to stabilization of blood sugar and serum calcium concentrations are relatively frequent in the early neonatal period.

ONTOGENESIS OF NEUROENDOCRINE TRANSDUCER SYSTEMS

Adenohypophyseal and Neurohypophyseal Systems

The human fetal pituitary gland, including both the adenohypophysis and neurohypophysis, is embryologically intact by 11–12 weeks. By this time the buccal connection (Rathke's pouch) is obliterated by the developing sphenoid bone and the pituitary gland becomes partially encapsulated within the sella turcica. Capillaries in the mesenchymal tissue surrounding the developing pituitary and the developing diencephalon form a neurohemal complex which may provide for the transfer of neurohumors. The primary plexus of the pituitary portal blood vascular system develops at 14–15 weeks and continuity of the primary and secondary plexus of the system probably is completed by 19–21 weeks. There is parallel development of the hypothalamic nuclei and the median eminence and supraoptic tract are identifiable by 20–21 weeks. Thus, by midgestation the fetal hypothalamic–pituitary complex is well developed.[56]

By 8–10 weeks of gestation, the fetal hypothalamus contains significant concentrations of thyrotropin-releasing hormone (TRH), gonadotropin-releasing hormone (GnRH), and growth hormone release–inhibiting hormone (SRIH). Mean concentrations approximate 5 pg/mg tissue for TRH, 1.5 pg/mg for GnRh, and 15 pg/mg for SRIH between 8 and 24 weeks.[56]

Secretory granules have been identified within anterior pituitary cells by 10–12 weeks. In addition, GH, FSH, LH, TSH, ACTH, prolactin (PRL), oxytocin, vasotocin (AVT), and vasopressin (AVP) can be identified in significant concentrations in pituitary tissue at this time.[38,56–64] Table 133-3 summarizes changes in hormone content in the pituitary gland throughout gestation. Serum hormone concentration changes with gestational age are summarized in Table 133-4. Hormone concentrations within the pituitary increase progressively, whereas concentrations in fetal serum tend to peak near midgestation and decrease progressively toward term.

There is heterogeneity of pituitary GH and PRL with regard to molecular size. The proportions of "little," "big," and "big-big" GH in the fetal pituitary have been reported to be 85–95 percent, 5–10 percent, and minimal and variable, respectively, by Kaplan et al.[56] "Little", "big," and "big-big" PRL concentrations in the fetal pituitary were 82–95 percent, 1–15 percent, and 1–8 percent, respectively.[56] These data were derived using saline extracts, so that the likelihood of solvent-mediated hormone aggregation was minimal but enzymatic cleavage of prohormones could occur.

These authors also studied pituitary and serum gonadotropins in the fetus. These are glycopeptides composed of two different subunit peptide chains, designated α and β. It was noted that the α subunits of LH and FSH predominanted both in the fetal pituitary and in fetal serum. β Subunits of these hormones usually were not detected. Moreover, the α subunit concentrations usually exceeded intact hormone levels in both pituitary and serum of the fetus.[56] The significance of the latter observations is not clear. Elevated serum levels of α chains of FSH or LH in adults have been observed in states of hypersecretion, suggesting that α subunit predominance in the fetus may reflect relatively high secretion

Table 133-3. Human Fetal Mean Pituitary Hormone Content

Gestational Age (weeks)	Mean Pituitary Weight (mg)	GH (ng)	PRL (ng)	LH (ng)		FSH (ng)		TSH (mU)	ACTH (mU)	AVP (mU)	Oxytocin (U)
				M	F	M	F				
10–14	3.4	0.44	4.1	21	88	1.8	7.4	0.21	—	0.07	—
15–19	6.7	9.2	14.8	165	797	13	316	0.69	496	0.25	12
20–24	16.0	59.4	405	490	3940	51	3726	3.3	—	1.0	33
25–29	36.4	256	542	1222	4983	149	5789	—	—	1.5	110
30–34	49.7	578	872	—	2353	—	2010	10.0	—	—	—
35–40	99.1	675	2039	1590	—	361	—	—	—	4.65	250

Data from Kaplan et al.,[56] Levina,[57] Fukuchi et al.,[59] and Pavlova et al.[64]

Table 133-4. Hormone Concentrations in Human Fetal Serum

Gestational Age (weeks)	GH (ng/ml)	PRL (ng/ml)	LH (ng/ml) M	LH (ng/ml) F	FSH (ng/ml) M	FSH (ng/ml) F	TSH (μU/Ml)	ACTH (pg/ml)
10–14	65	25			10	15		
15–19	115	17		12			2.4	249
20–24	132	18	7		17	24	9.6	
25–29	54							
30–34	43	208						
35–40	35	268	Und*	Und*	1.8	1.8	8.9	143

*Undetectable.
Data from Winters et al.,[11] Fisher et al.,[38] Kaplan et al.,[56] and Allen et al.[65]

rates of the hormones. This hypothesis would be compatible with the high serum levels of intact hormone measured in fetal serum.

These events suggest a pattern of development of hypothalamic–anterior pituitary function as outlined in Table 133-5. The postulated maturation of higher nervous system (CNS) inhibition of hypothalamic activity[56] is based on the observations that GH secretion in the newborn period is not readily suppressed with glucose, that there is no sleep-induced rise in serum GH in the newborn, and that there seems to be a progressive maturation of inhibitory electrical activity in the neocortex during the latter half of gestation. The low levels of serum GH and TSH in the anencephalic infant support the view that anterior pituitary hormone secretion is dependent on an intact hypothalamus (Table 133-6).

The late increase in fetal serum PRL concentrations (Table 133-4) does not seem to be dependent on hypothalamic function since serum PRL concentrations in cord blood of normal and anencephalic infants are similar[56] (Table 133-6). Rather, the increase in fetal serum PRL has been postulated to be due to the progressive increase in maternal–fetal estrogen levels. Whether progressive modulation of prolactin-inhibitory hormone secretion plays a role is not clear. There is considerable indirect evidence that negative feedback control of TSH, ACTH, FSH, and LH secretion develop during the last half of gestation.[56] The control systems for TSH and ACTH secretion seem to be mature or largely so at birth. However, the neuroendocrine control systems for GH, FSH, and LH continue to mature during the early weeks,

Table 133-5. Postulated Maturation of Fetal Hypothalamic–Pituitary System

First trimester
- Low rate of synthesis and secretion of anterior pituitary hormones.
- Hypothalamic hormones may reach pituitary gland by diffusion and stimulate hormone secretion.
- *or* Anterior pituitary hormone secretion may be autonomous.

Second trimester
- With mature hypothalamus and intact hypophyseal–portal blood vascular system, unrestrained release of growth hormone releasing hormone (GRH), corticotropin releasing hormone (CRH), gonadotropin releasing hormone (GnRH), and thyrotropin releasing hormone (TRH) lead to intense stimulation of GH, ACTH, FSH, LH, and TSH secretion.

Third trimester
- Progressive modulation of anterior pituitary hormone secretion correlates with brain maturation and may relate in part to development of higher central nervous system inhibition of hypothalamic hormone secretion.
- Progressive maturation of negative feedback control systems for ACTH, TSH, LH, and FSH secretion.

Data from Kaplan et al.[56] and Fisher et al.[38]

months, and years of extrauterine life[56] (see section on Adaptation to Extrauterine Life: Other Hormone Adaptations).

There is relatively little information regarding maturation of fetal neurohypophyseal function. It is of interest that recently the fetal pituitary early in gestation has been shown to contain AVT, a peptide important in control of water metabolism in amphibians, but not previously believed present in mammals.[63] Pituitary AVT content seems to decrease progressively with increasing gestational age, whereas AVP and oxytocin concentrations increase progressively (Table 133-3). The AVT/AVP content ratio in pituitary tissue thus decreases progressively with increasing fetal age.[63] The significance of fetal AVT is not known; perhaps it has no functional significance but represents another example of the concept of "ontogeny recapitulating phylogeny."

Fetal serum AVP concentrations are easily measurable during the last half of gestation and there is evidence that they increase in response to hypertonic saline.[17] Fetal serum concentrations also increase in association with or in response to parturition: cord blood concentrations are high after vaginal delivery, but not after cesarean section delivery.[16] It is not yet clear whether this response is evoked by the stress of vaginal delivery on the fetus or whether it represents stimulation of fetal neurohypophyseal hormone (oxytocin) release by stimuli other than stress as a part of the labor process. The ability of the newborn infant to respond to isotonic dextran or to hypertonic saline with appropriate alterations in kidney free water clearance suggests that both volume and osmolar control systems for modulation of AVP secretion are largely mature at birth.[67] Immature renal function rather than limitation in AVP secretory capacity accounts for the limited concentrating capacity (about 600 mOsm/liter) of the newborn infant.[17,67]

Autonomic Nervous System

By 6–7 weeks gestation the primordia of the sympathetic trunk ganglia have taken definite form and have become linked by longitudinal nerve cords destined to become the sympathetic trunks. The primordia of the prevertebral plexuses and the terminal sympathetic ganglia also have begun to organize. The preaortic sympathetic primordia at this time are composed of primitive sympathetic neurons and chromaffin cells which proceed to condense into chains of cell masses along the abdominal aorta.[68] By 10–12 weeks the paired adrenal medullary masses are well developed, as are numerous extramedullary paraganglia derived from the preaortic cell masses and scattered throughout the abdominal and pelvic sympathetic plexuses.[68,69] Most of the chromaffin tissue in the fetus is represented in these extramedullary, paraaortic paraganglia, which may reach a maximum size of 2–3 mm in diameter by 28 weeks gestation, after which time they slowly regress.[69] The largest of the paraganglia, the organs of Zukerkandl,

Table 133-6. Pituitary Hormone Concentrations in Human Anencephalic Serum at Term

No. of Infants	Hormone	Approx. Mean Serum Concentration: Anencephalic	Normal
9	GH (ng/ml)	7	34
5	HPL (ng/ml)	10	168
3	FSH (ng/ml)	< 1	1.8
3	LH (ng/ml)	< 1	Und*
4	TSH (μU/ml)	Und*	9
2	ACTH (pg/ml)	10	143

*Undetectable.
Data from Kaplan et al.,[56] Allen et al.,[65] and Hayek et al.[66]

are located near the origin of the inferior mesenteric arteries. These enlarge progressively until by term they measure 10–15 mm in length; after birth they gradually atrophy, disappearing completely by 2–3 yr of age. The adrenal medullae are histologically somewhat immature at birth. but resemble the adult gland by about 1 yr of age.[69]

Catecholamines can be identified in fetal chromaffin tissue by 10–15 weeks gestation and concentrations increase progressively to term.[70,71] Both epinephrine and norepinephrine are present in adrenal medullary tissue, but norepinephrine predominates in the organs of Zuckerkandl and the smaller paraganglial tissue. This difference presumably relates to the effect of adrenal cortical hormone on the final step in epinephrine synthesis, the methylation of norepinephrine to epinephrine. The activity of the enzyme phenylethanolamine-N-methyl transferase, which catalyzes this step, is stimulated by adrenal glucocorticoids.[72] The unique location of the adrenal medulla provides high local concentrations of glucocorticoids, favoring epinephrine synthesis. Fetal hypophysectomy reduces adrenal medullary epinephrine content in rats and ACTH restores this activity.[73] The ontogenesis of fetal chromaffin tissue is summarized in Figure 133-1.

Development of control of catecholamine secretion in autonomic and extramedullary chromaffin tissues is not entirely understood. The capacity to secrete epinephrine seems to relate to the

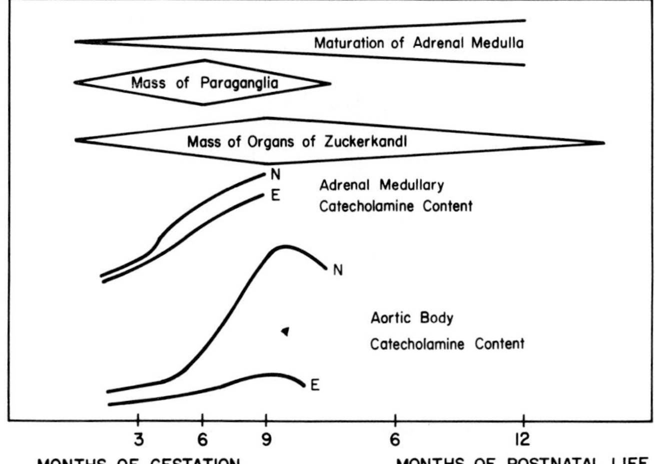

Fig. 133-1. Maturation of chromaffin tissue in the human fetus. Adrenal medulla is relatively immature at birth. Paired organs of Zuckerkandl make up the largest mass of chromaffin tissue in the newborn. Adrenal medullae produce and secrete both epinephrine (E) and norepinephrine (N), whereas the aortic bodies, including the paraganglia and the organs of Zuckerkandl, secrete predominantly norepinephrine.

maturation of the adrenal gland and the development of adrenal splanchnic innervation. The norepinephrine cells of the fetal adrenal medulla can respond directly to asphyxia with norepinephrine secretion long before the splanchnic innervation develops, and the extrame dullary norepinephrine cells presumably respond similarly.[74,75] In the sheep fetus, the response to asphyxia appears early in gestation and falls off near term. The adult type of CNS response to asphyxia is mediated by splanchnic nerves and is not observed in this species until near term.[74]

There is little information regarding source or concentrations of circulating catecholamines in the fetus. Basal plasma catecholamine levels are very low in the fetal sheep,[75] perhaps because of the relatively high and stable environmental temperature and the weightlessness characterizing the intrauterine environment. There are no studies of the control systems for catecholamine secretion in the human fetus. The human newborn is capable of responding to hypoglycemia and to cold exposure with increased epinephrine secretion,[68] presumably via CNS-mediated splanchnic stimulation of the adrenal medulla. The large mass of paraganglionic tissue is not innervated[76] and probably releases norepinephrine in response to direct stimuli, including asphyxia, but asphyxia has not been shown to stimulate norepinephrine in the newborn infant.

ONTOGENESIS OF AUTONOMOUS ENDOCRINE SYSTEMS

Insulin–Glucagon System

The pancreas is identifiable by 4 weeks of gestation in the human fetus, and it synthesizes proinsulin, insulin, and glucagon by 7–10 weeks (Table 133-7).[77–80] By midgestation insulin and glucagon concentrations within the pancreas of the fetus exceed adult pancreatic concentrations.[79,80] Fetal pancreatic tissue also is a rich source of somatostatin,[81,82] a fact of interest since this hypothalamic tetradecapeptide is known to be capable of inhibiting both insulin and glucagon secretion.[83]

While fetal pancreatic hormone concentrations are high, secretion is obtunded. Insulin release from the fetal rat pancreas in vitro in response to glucose or pyruvate is minimal, but can be markedly enhanced by the addition of theophylline, a phosphodiesterase inhibitor, or by glucagon or dibutyryl cAMP, both of which raise intracellular cAMP levels.[77,84–86] Secretion can be inhibited by oliogomycin[84] and stimulated by arginine and certain cations such as potassium and barium.[85,86] These observations suggest that in the fetus, as in the adult, insulin release from the pancreas is an energy-dependent process requiring the accumulation of both cAMP and a product or products of the intermediatry metabolism of glucose and/or pyruvate. There is much less information regarding control of fetal pancreatic glucagon release, but it is known that arginine or alanine stimulates glucagon release from the fetal pancreas in vitro.[78]

Insulin release in vivo in fetal mammals is quite variable, and there are species differences.[87] However, in studies preceding

Table 133-7. Mean Insulin and Glucagon Concentrations in Human Fetal Pancreas

Gestational Age (weeks)	Insulin (μU/mg)	Glucagon (ng/mg)
7–10	333	4.0
11–15	1190	9.7
16–25	4170	66.0

Data from Schaeffer et al.[77]

hysterotomy in pregnant women, glucose or arginine have not been observed to provoke insulin secretion near midgestation.[22,88] Near term, prior to the onset of labor, serum insulin levels in the human fetus are relatively unresponsive to high glucose concentrations.[89] Similar observations have been made in the fetal monkey near term.[21,90] Moreover, as in the in vitro studies, glucagon or theophylline were observed to augment the insulin response to glucose in the fetal monkey.[90] The glucagon secretion response also appears to be obtunded in vivo, as in vitro. Hyperglycemia does not suppress fetal plasma glucagon levels in rats, monkeys, or lambs,[91–93] and acute hypoglycemia does not evoke glucagon secretion in the rat fetus.[93]

These studies suggest that the obtunded insulin and glucagon secretion responses in the fetus are related to a deficient capacity of the fetal pancreatic islet cells to generate cAMP and/or to rapid cAMP destruction by phosphodiesterase. A 2–3-fold increase in islet cell cAMP has been observed in newborn rats during the first 72 h, in keeping with this hypothesis.[94] In addition, theophylline or glucagon in pharmacologic doses increases insulin secretion in the newborn human infant.[95] Thus, the newborn pancreatic islet cells are relatively immature at birth with regard to their capacity to secrete hormone. The relatively rapid maturation of responsiveness to glucose in the neonatal period in both premature and mature infants suggests that this obtunded state might be a secondary result of the relatively stable fetal serum glucose levels maintained by placental transfer of maternal glucose, rather than a primary temporally fixed maturation process.

Parathyroid Hormone–Calcitonin System

The parathyroid glands are derived from the paired third and fourth pharyngeal pouches. These pouches are identifiable on the lateral wall of the pharyngeal gut by 4–5 weeks gestation. The third pouches are destined to form the thymus and inferior parathyroid glands and the fourth pouches the superior parathyroid glands.[87] The fifth pharyngeal pouches form the paired ultimobranchial bodies, which are incorporated into the thyroid gland during embryogenesis as the parafollicular C cells, the calcitonin-secreting cells.[87] The parathyroid glands develop embryologically between 5 and 12–14 weeks and increase from a diameter of less than 0.1 mm at 14 weeks to some 1–2 mm at birth. Adult glands measure 2–5 mm in width and 3–8 mm in length.[87] Near term, fetal parathyroid cells are composed largely of inactive chief cells and a few intermediate chief cells containing occasional secretion granules. Active chief cells are not observed.[96] There are no data regarding parathyroid hormone (PTH) content of fetal or newborn parathyroid glands, but recent data indicates that C cells are prominent in the neonatal thyroid gland and that the calcitonin content is as high as 540–2100 mU/g tissue, values as much as 10 times those observed in the normal adult gland.[97]

Information regarding function of the fetal parathyroid glands or thyroid C cells is limited. Scothorne[98] has studied the effect of human fetal parathyroid glands explanted to chick chorioallantoic membrane adjacent to neonatal rat parietal bone. Resorption of the fetal bone was observed in preparations containing glands from 12–13-week fetuses, suggesting that such glands contain PTH. Recent studies have shown that the fetal sheep can increase serum PTH concentrations in response to a fall in serum calcium induced by EDTA.[99] This stimulus also resulted in a prompt increase in renal phosphate clearance, suggesting that the increased fetal serum PTH levels evoked a renal response. Littledike et al.[100] have studied the fetal response to calcium infusion in the sheep and shown that the third trimester fetus can respond promptly with increased serum calcitonin levels to hypercalcemia. Thus the fetal sheep parathyroid gland, like that of the fetal rat, seems capable of hormone secretion. This also appears to be true for the calcitonin-secreting C cells.

In humans the fetus at term has low circulating concentrations of PTH and relatively high levels of calcitonin,[101,102] and the PTH response to hypocalcemia is obtunded.[101] Presumably this is due to the prevailing high levels of total and ionized calcium maintained in fetal blood by active placental transport from maternal blood.[103] The postulated status of the PTH–calcitonin system is shown in Figure 133-2. The high levels of fetal serum calcium are thought to suppress parathyroid function and stimulate calcitonin secretion. This would tend to promote calcium–phosphorus deposition in fetal bone, but obtunds the transition of the fetus to autonomous extrauterine existence as the placental supply of maternal calcium is removed.

SUMMARY

Table 133-8 summarizes the state of endocrine function in the fetus. As indicated in the foregoing discussion, the fetus functions autonomously with regard to all of the listed hormones except cortisol and perhaps catecholamines, which have been shown to cross the placental barrier. Basal secretion rates for all of the anterior pituitary hormones probably are relatively high near the end of the second trimester, perhaps falling off during the third trimester as feedback inhibitory control is established. However, quantitative studies have not been conducted. Since serum ACTH and TSH levels are normal or increased in the face of normal or increased cortisol and T_4 concentrations, the sensitivity of feedback for these systems probably is not normal in utero. Both systems are suppressible in the newborn but the sensitivity of feedback control relative to the adult is not clear. By 1 month of age ACTH and TSH feedback control probably are similar to the adult. Serum FSH and LH concentrations also are high at midgestation in the face of very high serum estrogen levels, but are suppressed near term. There is evidence that the sensitivity of estrogen feedback in inhibition of gonadotropin secretion in the newborn is greater than the sensitivity in the adult.[56] Thus the rates of maturation of feedback control systems for anterior pituitary hormone secretion appear to differ. Both insulin and glucagon secretion are suppressed in the fetus, probably because there is little variation in fetal blood sugar levels. The high fetal serum

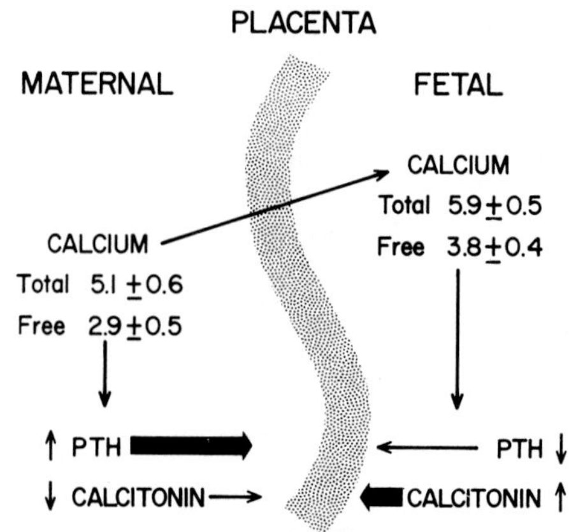

Fig. 133-2. Postulated maternal–fetal parathyroid hormone (PTH)–calcitonin interrelationships. Maternal serum calcium is "pumped" across the placenta, maintaining relatively high fetal serum calcium concentrations which inhibit PTH secretion and stimulate calcitonin. Maternal PTH secretion is stimulated near term by slight reductions in "free" calcium concentrations coincident with increased fetal calcium deposition.

Table 133-8. Summary of Endocrine Functions in the Fetus

Hormone	Neuroendocrine Transducer: Basal Secretion	Neuroendocrine Transducer: Feedback Control	Gland Function	Tissue Response
GH	Prob I	—	—	Prob D
PRL	Prob I	—	—	Prob N
ACTH	Prob I	Yes	—	N
FSH–LH	Prob I	Yes	—	N
TSH	Prob I	Yes	—	N
AVP	Prob N		—	N
Cortisol	—	—	I	N
Thyroid hormones	—	—	I	N
Catecholamines	Prob D	—	Prob D	N
Insulin	—	—	D	Prob N
Glucagon	—	—	D	Prob D
PTH	—	—	D	D
Calcitonin	—	—	I	Prob N

N, normal; I, increased; D, decreased; Prob, probably.

calcium concentrations suppress fetal parathyroid gland function and stimulate the thyroid C cells.

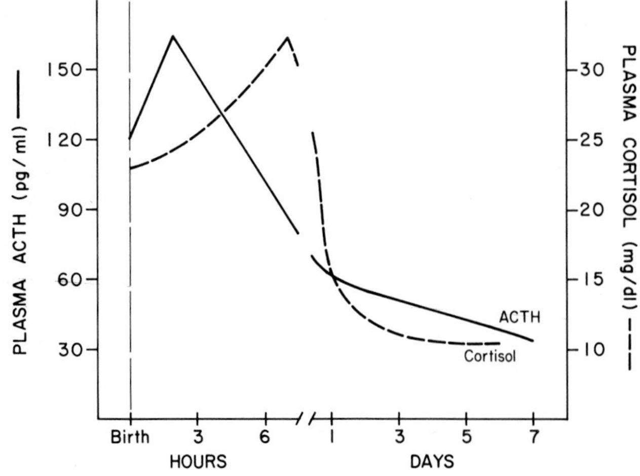

Fig. 133-3. Pituitary (ACTH) adrenal responses to delivery of the human fetus. Cord serum ACTH concentrations are relatively high but increase further in response to the "stress" of extrauterine exposure. The ACTH stimulus increases adrenal cortisol secretion and produces a transient increase in serum cortisol concentration persisting for 2–3 days. (Data from Winters et al.[11] and Reynolds.[105]

ADAPTATION TO EXTRAUTERINE LIFE

GENERAL

Survival of the newborn infant in the extrauterine environment requires prompt transition from placental respiration to air breathing. In addition, a series of metabolic stresses, including hypothermia, hypoglycemia, and hypocalcemia must be defended. Successful defense requires effective function of the neuroendocrine transducer systems regulating secretion of ACTH, TSH, and catecholamines and transition of the autonomous endocrine systems from a milieu of substrate sufficiency to one of substrate insufficiency. In addition, alterations in the secretion patterns of other anterior pituitary hormones (GH, PRL, FSH, and LH) occur with transition from intrauterine to extrauterine existence. These changes are summarized in Figures 133-3 to 133-7.

ADRENAL RESPONSE

Figure 133-3 summarizes the nonspecific "stress" response characterized by ACTH stimulation of adrenal cortisol secretion.[104,105] The critical nature of this response is demonstrated by the fact that anencephalic infants survive the first few hours of extrauterine exposure only if given exogenous glucocorticoid.[56] In the normal newborn infant cord blood ACTH concentrations are elevated, averaging about 120 pg/ml.[11] With parturition there is a surge in plasma ACTH followed by a slow fall during the first day of extrauterine life. This ACTH surge is followed by an increase in serum cortisol concentrations. Reported concentrations have varied somewhat, but most authors agree that serum cortisol in the newborn peaks within the first 12 h gradually falling to baseline within 72 h.[105]

NEONATAL THERMOGENESIS

Figure 133-4 summarizes the catecholamine, TSH, and thyroid hormone secretion responses observed in the newborn. A surge in catecholamine release is reflected in a sharp rise in urinary excretion of epinephrine and norepinephrine in the immediate newborn period.[106,107] This surge presumably is stimulated by extrauterine cooling and is associated with stimulation of cell membrane β-adrenergic receptors of brown fat cells. Lipolysis is stimulated and increases in blood glycerol and free fatty acid (FFA) levels occur in association with augmented, fatty acid–fueled, thermogenesis within brown fat.[108,109] The catecholamine surge is shown in Figure 133-4 as reflected in plasma FFA levels since plasma catecholamine concentration data are not available.

The serum TSH concentration is observed to increase within the first 30 min after birth from a mean of 11 to a mean of about 85 μU/ml; the level falls gradually to baseline by 24–48 h.[87,110,111] This TSH surge also is stimulated by extrauterine cooling and is followed by marked increases in serum T_4 and T_3 concentrations, both peaking at about 24 h.[110] There is evidence to support the view that this transient hyperthyroid state significantly potentiates catecholamine thermogenesis.[111] Thus, the unique brown fat supply of the newborn and the integrated catecholamine–thyroid hormone secretory surges mediated by the neuroendocrine transducer

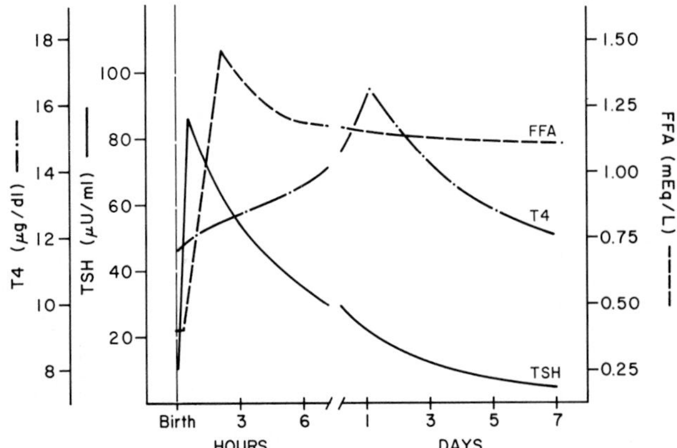

Fig. 133-4. Stimuli for neonatal nonshivering thermogenesis in the newborn infant. Serum free fatty acid (FFA) concentrations are shown as a reflection of catecholamine release, which occurs very early after birth, presumably stimulated by neonatal cooling. Cooling also evokes a TSH surge maximal at 30 min. This in turn stimulates thyroid secretion of T_4 and T_3. The catecholamines stimulate thermogenesis in brown fat tissue, and this thermogenesis is potentiated by the transient hyperthyroxinemia. (Data from Keele and Kay,[108] Erenberg et al.,[110] and Sack et al.[115])

systems provide for the augmented nonshivering thermogenesis critical for survival of the fetus in the extrauterine environment.[87,108–111]

CALCIUM HOMEOSTASIS

Figure 133-5 summarizes the changes in the PTH–calcitonin system associated with removal of the placental calcium supply. There is a fall in serum calcium concentration, which in the full-term infant is modest (11.3–9.5 mg/dl) and nadirs at 24–48 h. Under similar circumstances in the child or adult a prompt increase in PTH secretion would increase calcium mobilization from bone and serum calcium concentrations would return promptly to baseline. In the newborn, however, the parathyroid glands, chronically suppressed in utero, show a delayed response, so that the hypocalcemia is accentuated and prolonged.[101] In premature or small for gestational age newborns, early hypocalcemia may be much more marked and prolonged and the incidence of symptomatic hypocalcemia is much greater.[87] Calcitonin concentrations are high in cord blood at birth[102] and fall in response to the fall in serum calcium concentration during the newborn period.

Calcium homeostasis in the newborn also is limited by the low level of glomerular filtration which limits phosphate excretion and predisposes to hyperphosphatemia and hypocalcemia.[87] This can be aggravated by the ingestion of cow's milk, which has a high phosphorus/calcium concentration ratio. In addition, renal responsiveness to PTH is limited in the newborn during the first few days of life.[87] These limitations in renal function and in renal PTH response, like the parathyroid secretory response, are more marked in the premature and undergrown newborn and contribute to the increased tendency to hypocalcemia in such infants. PTH secretion and calcium homeostasis probably are normal or nearly so within 1–2 weeks in full-term infants and by 2–4 weeks of age in premature infants.[101]

GLUCOSE HOMEOSTASIS

Figure 133-6 graphically shows the alterations in glucose homeostasis in the newborn infant. The abrupt curtailment of placental glucose leads to a prompt reduction in blood glucose in the newborn infant. This provokes a significant rise in plasma glucagon concentration maximal within 2 h of birth.[112] Plasma insulin levels are low and remain so. The early increase in plasma glucagon may be conditioned or provoked by umbilical cord cutting, possibly mediated by catecholamines.[112] In addition, neonatal cooling and the hypoglycemia per se act as stimuli for catecholamine release. In turn, both epinephrine and norepinephrine stimulate glucagon release and tend to inhibit insulin.[113]

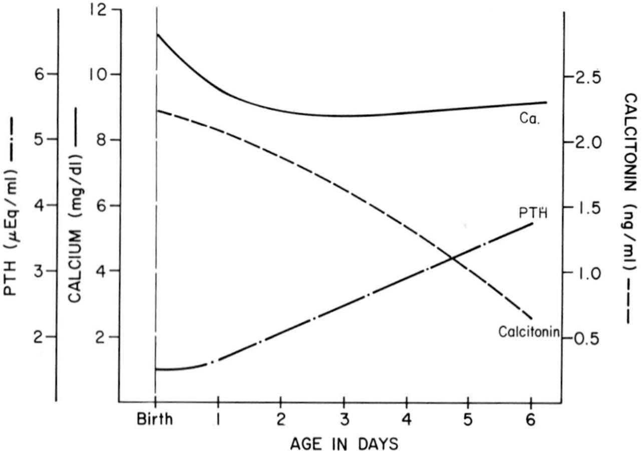

Fig. 133-5. Calcium homeostasis in the newborn infant. With the advent of parturition and elimination of the transplacental calcium supply, serum calcium falls in the early neonatal period. This results in a fall in serum calcitonin concentrations, but the parathyroid hormone response is delayed 2–3 days. As a result mild hypocalcemia persists several days. (Data from David and Anast[101] and Samaan et al.[102]

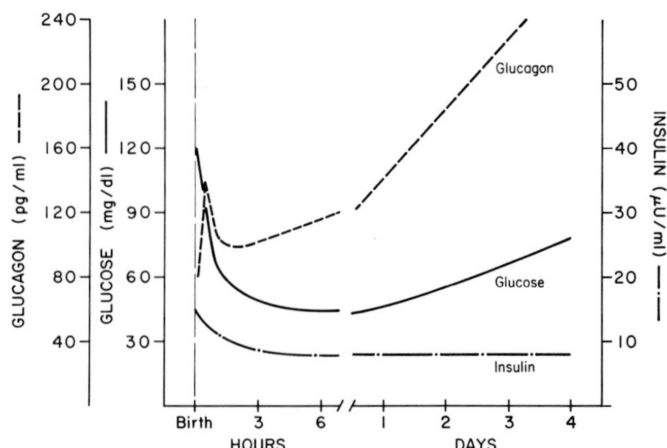

Fig. 133-6. Glucose homeostasis in the newborn infant. Abrupt curtailment of maternal glucose results in a rapid fall in blood glucose concentration in the newborn. This and other stimuli, including umbilical cord cutting and catecholamine secretion, provoke an early increase in glucagon release, but this is limited in extent. In spite of the low plasma insulin concentrations, blood glucose remains low during the first 24 h. Both plasma glucagon and glucose concentrations increase progressively during the first 3–4 days. Cord blood insulin concentrations are low and remain low during the first few days of life. (Data from Sperling et al.[112])

This early glucagon surge is limited in extent and duration and blood glucose, glucagon, and insulin concentrations remain relatively stable between 2 and 24 h. The glucose levels, although stable, are low and provide a continuing stimulus to glucagon release, as do catecholamines (Fig. 133-4). As a result of these chronic stimuli during the first 3–4 days of life, there is a progressive increase in the circulating concentration of pancreatic glucagon as pancreatic secretory capacity progressively matures.[113] This increase correlates with a slow rise in blood glucose to normal concentrations. The early glucagon surge and the catecholamine surge rapidly deplete tissue glycogen stores, so that the slow increase in blood glucose after 24 h is due largely to progressive maturation of hepatic gluconeogenic capacity under the stimulus of the high and increasing glucagon/insulin ratio.[113]

Feeding further promotes these changes. Protein intake stimulates release of gut glucagon[112] and the increased blood amino acid levels tend to stimulate pancreatic glucagon secretion. There is evidence to suggest that low blood glucose associated with increased amino acid levels provokes glucagon release, whereas high blood glucose with increased blood amino acid concentrations favors insulin release.[112] Thus the ingestion of colostrum with its high concentration of amino acid or the feeding of artificial milk in the presence of the low blood glucose concentrations acts as a potentiating stimulus for glucagon release during the early hours and days of life. Feeding also provides carbohydrate substrate (glucose or lactose) directly.

In the healthy term newborn glucose homeostasis is achieved within 5–7 days. In the premature infant or the small for gestational age infant, the rise of blood glucose to normal levels may require 1–2 weeks. In the latter infants glucagon does not seem to be the limiting factor nor does cortisol or GH;[87] rather glycogen reserves and hepatic gluconeogenesis seem relatively impaired.[87,113]

OTHER HORMONE ADAPTATIONS

Figure 133-7 summarizes the changes in GH, PRL, FSH, and LH occurring in the neonatal period and during infancy. Blood GH levels are high at birth, averaging about 40 ng/dl,[56,114] and remain elevated for a period of several days. The pattern of change is observed in both term and premature infants, indicating that the mechanism relates more to extrauterine exposure than to gestational age.

Cord blood PRL concentrations also are elevated and increase further during the first 30–60 min after birth in association with the TSH surge (Fig. 133-4). The parallel increases in TSH and PRL presumably are mediated by cold-stimulated TRH release.[115] Serum PRL levels thereafter decrease rapidly, so that concentrations are within the normal range for infants by 1 week of age.[116] This rapid fall presumably relates to the rapid decrease in plasma estrogen concentrations in the newborn as the placental source of estrogen is removed.[56]

Serum FSH and LH concentrations are unmeasurable at birth, presumably because of the high levels of circulating estrogens. As the estrogen level falls during the first 1–2 days of extrauterine life, serum gonadotropin concentrations increase progressively to peak values at 1–2 months of age.[117] There are differences in male and female infants not shown in Figure 133-7, where combined mean values are shown. FSH levels are higher in female infants, peaking at 2–3 months and falling slowly to prepubertal concentrations by 4 y of age; values in males peak at 1–3 months and fall to low levels by 4 months.[117] In males LH concentrations peak at a higher mean level than in female infants; values peak at 1 month and fall to low levels by 4 months.[117]

FETAL COMPLICATIONS OF MATERNAL DISEASE

MATERNAL THYROTOXICOSIS

Pregnancy seems not to alter thyroid homeostasis in any major way, but a number of minor changes in selected thyroid function parameters occur. There is an increase in serum concentrations of TBG with a reciprocal reduction in thyroxine-binding prealbumin. These changes occur early in gestation (4–8 weeks), presumably secondary to the increased estrogen secretion which stimulates hepatic production of thyroxine binding globulin (TBG).[118] The increased TBG level increases the extrathyroidal pool of T_4 and T_3 and increases serum concentrations of these hormones, but the concentrations of free T_4 and free T_3 in maternal serum appear to be unchanged throughout most of gestation.[118,119] Serum TSH concentrations measured by a specific human pituitary TSH radioimmunoassay also are similar in nonpregnant women and pregnant women after 10–12 weeks gestation.[119]

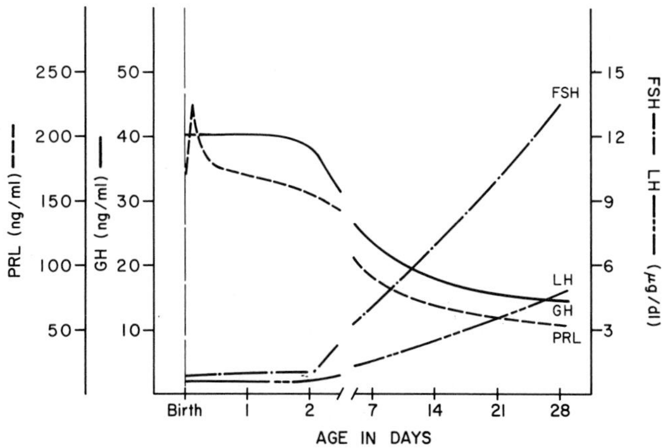

Fig. 133-7. Serum levels of pituitary growth hormone, prolactin, and gonadotropin during the early neonatal period. Growth hormone concentrations are elevated in cord blood but gradually fall during the first week of life. Cord blood prolactin levels also are high, and a further increase is observed during the first hour of life in association with the TSH surge (see Fig. 133-4). Thereafter prolactin levels gradually fall. Serum FSH and LH concentrations are low in cord blood and gradually increase during the first weeks of extrauterine life, presumably in response to removal of the estrogen inhibition. (Data from Cornblath et al.,[114] Sack et al.,[115] Guyda and Friesen,[116] and Winter et al.[117])

In addition, the placenta produces two chorionic hormones which have thyroid-stimulating bioactivity. The first, human chorionic gonadotropin (HCG), is produced in greatest concentrations during the first half of gestation. Serum concentrations peak at 2–3 months at levels of 50–150 U/ml. Such levels of HCG have an inherent thyroid-stimulating activity equivalent to 25–75 μU/ml of pituitary TSH.[119] Normal serum levels of pituitary TSH average about one-tenth of these concentrations (<10 μU/ml). The placenta also produces a human chorionic thyrotropin (HCT) in small amounts. Most placental extracts contain less than 10 mU HCT, but values as high as 10–20 units have been observed.[118] Whether HCT circulates in significant concentrations is not known since it is not possible to separate the TSH, HCG, and HCT bioactivity, and an adequately specific HCT radioimmunoassay has not been developed. However, the similarity of circulating free T_4 and pituitary TSH concentrations in pregnant and nonpregnant women suggests that HCT does not exert a major physiologic role during human pregnancy. Finally, there is suggestive evidence for some enlargement of the maternal thyroid gland and an increase in thyroid radioiodine uptake during gestation,[118,120] but these changes, perhaps due to some increase in renal iodide excretion,[121] seem to be variable and of questionable physiologic impact.[118]

Thyrotoxicosis occurs in only 1 of 1500 pregnancies and diagnosis may be difficult. Normally there is an increase in metabolic rate and a mild state of hypermetabolism accompanying euthyroid pregnancy. This, with the increase in serum thyroid hormone concentrations, particularly if associated with some thyroid enlargement, may confuse the diagnosis, especially in mild cases. In vitro tests of thyroid function must be accompanied by an assessment of TBG levels to estimate the free T_4 or free T_3 index.

The maternal thyrotoxic state usually does not harm the fetus; thyroid hormones do not cross the placenta. However, maternal weight loss should be prevented, for it may lead to fetal malnutrition. Maternal hypothyroidism also is undesirable since it compromises placental blood supply and fetal nutrition. In addition, circulating maternal thyroid-stimulating immunoglobulins can cross the placental barrier near term and may produce neonatal thyrotoxicosis.[122] The major risk to the fetus is the possibility of fetal *hypothyroidism* produced as a result of maternal treatment: either ablation of the fetal thyroid secondary to therapeutic radioiodine or hypothyroidism produced secondary to placental transfer of antithyroid drugs. Several instances of ablation of the fetal thyroid gland have been reported after radioiodine treatment of maternal thyrotoxicosis during the second trimester of gestation,[44,118] and it is now recognized that radioiodine therapy is contraindicated during pregnancy.

Iodides, propylthiouracil, and methimazole appear to cross the placental barrier without difficulty. Therefore, treatment of the pregnant woman with these antithyroid drugs carries some risk of fetal goiter and/or hypothyroidism.[87,118] When such therapy is utilized, doses should be kept to the minimum necessary to control the maternal hyperthyroid state. When this is done, the risk of fetal goiter probably is no more than 1–2 percent. Concomitant maternal treatment with T_4 has been recommended to prevent subtle maternal hypothyroidism.[118]

Surgery also is an acceptable alternative treatment for maternal thyrotoxicosis during pregnancy. Usually it is postponed until the second trimester, and antithyroid drug therapy is used to control the disease during the first half of the gestational period. T_4 replacement has been suggested postoperatively to minimize the risk of maternal hypothyroidism. Propranolol may be useful in preparing the pregnant thyrotoxic subject for surgery, but this drug does not control the hypermetabolic state, and if used near term it may affect uterine contractions and produce depression of the neonate.[118]

Most physicians prefer to use antithyroid drugs with or without added T_4 and to follow the thyrotoxic pregnant woman carefully. Iodide usually is not necessary and increases the risk of fetal goiter. The propylthiouracil dose should be kept below 300 mg/day if possible. The newborn should be examined carefully at birth and cord blood obtained for measurement of serum T_4 and TSH concentrations. The serum T_4 should exceed 7 μg/dl and TSH should be less than 20 μU/ml, although 2–3 percent of normal infants have values as high as 60 μU/ml. Neonatal hypothyroidism due to propylthiouracil is transient, lasting 1–2 weeks, and in the absence of signs or symptoms or a large goiter probably does not require treatment.

Neonatal Graves' disease may occur in the newborn of a mother with the disease. In most instances the disease is transient, lasting 1–3 months, in which case it is believed to be the result of transplacental passage of the long-acting thyroid stimulator, an immunoglobulin known to be capable of stimulating the thyroid gland. More recently other thyroid-stimulating immunoglobulins (TSI) have been described in Graves' disease and these, too, presumably can cross the placenta and stimulate the fetal thyroid gland.[122] The sex ratio for infants with neonatal Graves' disease is 1/1 in contrast to the 6–8/1 predominance of involved females with adult-onset disease. This fact also favors a TSI etiology.

In many instances the neonatal disease lasts many months, in which case a TSI etiology is unlikely.[123] The etiology of the disease in these cases is not clear. A hereditary predisposition is likely.[123] In either instance, neonatal Graves' disease may be difficult to diagnose. Clinical manifestations and goiter may be minimal at birth and become marked during the second week of life, after the infant has been discharged from the nursery. The delayed signs and symptoms may result from transplacental antithyroid drug which has suppressed thyroid function in the fetus. Neonatal Graves' disease carries a mortality approximating 20 percent and thus requires vigorous therapy with iodides and propylthiouracil. All infants of women with Graves' disease should be carefully evaluated at birth and carefully followed during the neonatal period to prevent prolonged hypothyroidism and provide early treatment of neonatal Graves' disease.

CUSHING'S SYNDROME AND PREGNANCY

The coexistence of Cushing's syndrome and pregnancy also is uncommon, in part because pregnancy is uncommon in women with the disease. Early in the disease 30 percent of patients are amenorrheic, and with advanced disease amenorrhea is present in 50–75 percent. The outcome of pregnancy in 26 cases reported between 1952 and 1972 and collated by Grimes et al.[124] is shown in Table 133-9. Fifty-three percent of these pregnancies resulted in spontaneous abortion, premature delivery, or stillbirth. Only 42 percent of the women delivered term infants; thus, the prognosis for a normal pregnancy is poor.

Table 133-9. Prognosis for Pregnancy in Active Cushing's Syndrome

	No. of Pregnancies	Percent of Pregnancies
Spontaneous abortion	4	15
Therapeutic abortion	1	4
Premature delivery	6	23
Stillbirth	4	15
Term birth	11	42
Total	26	99

Data from review of literature reported by Grumes et al.[124]

The diagnosis of Cushing's syndrome in the pregnant woman, like the diagnosis of Graves' disease, is complicated by the alterations in hormone metabolism normally occurring during gestation. Pregnancy increases the circulating concentrations of corticosteroid-binding globulin and thus increases serum cortisol concentrations. This effect is related to increased hepatic production of corticosteroid-binding globulin stimulated by the increased estrogen production during pregnancy. Cortisol secretion is not increased during pregnancy and the circulating level of free cortisol is essentially unchanged. Aldosterone secretion, in contrast, is increased in association with increased plasma renin activity, but clinical evidence of aldosterone hypersecretion (hypertension and hypokalemia) is not seen.[124]

The most reliable approach to diagnosis is the urinary excretion of 17-hydroxycorticosteroids before and during dexamethasone suppression. Early diagnosis and therapy are extremely important to minimize fetal risk. If surgical treatment is indicated, postoperative management includes corticosteroid replacement therapy to prevent adrenal insufficiency. Other therapeutic approaches should include consideration of preventing maternal adrenal insufficiency, which can significantly impair placental function and fetal nutrition. Supplemental steroid treatment also may be necessary during the stress of labor and delivery.

Other possible fetal risks of maternal Cushing's syndrome include virilization, anomalies, and fetal adrenal suppression with neonatal adrenal insufficiency. Fetal virilization has been reported in association with virilizing adrenal tumors but has not been reported with Cushing's syndrome. Corticosteroids have produced cleft palate and other anomalies in animals, but no increased incidence of fetal anomalies has been observed in man secondary to corticosteroid excess.[124,125] Since ACTH does not cross the placental barrier and steroid hormones cross easily, the high maternal corticosteroid levels can suppress fetal ACTH secretion during the last trimester of gestation and result in adrenal insufficiency in the newborn. However, this complication appears to be uncommon.[126]

Exogenous corticosteroid medication can produce Cushing's syndrome, but in this instance, too, the risk to the fetus appears to be minimal. Maternal estriol excretion and cord blood levels of estriol precursors tend to be reduced when doses of steroids in excess of 75 mg/day are given,[105] but neonatal adrenal insufficiency is not seen and postnatal excretion of cortisol metabolites is normal.[127] Thus routine corticosteroid treatment of the newborn of women with Cushing's syndrome or women given exogenous corticosteroid during pregnancy is not indicated. However, the attending physician should be aware of the possibility and recognize the clinical features of adrenal insufficiency in the newborn.[126]

HYPERPARATHYROIDISM AND PREGNANCY

Friderichsen, in 1938,[128] first described the occurrence of tetany in the newborn of a mother with undiagnosed hyperparathyroidism. In the intervening years many similar cases have been described. Many cases of hyperparathyroidism in adults are subclinical and a variety of factors may exacerbate such latent disease. These include bed rest, surgery, dehydration, infection, palpation of the neck, and pregnancy.[87,129,130] Increased maternal PTH secretion occurs regularly during the last trimester of normal pregnancy. During this period the fetal need for calcium is maximal and maternal serum PTH concentrations increase measurably.[131] When there is coexistent parathyroid hyperplasia or adenoma, this added stress may precipitate signs and symptoms. Clinical manifestations in the pregnant woman with hyperparathyroidism include renal calculi, skeletal disease, and hyperemesis gravidarum. Symptoms and signs may present early in gestation, later in gestation, or in some instances in the postpartum period.[130] Neonatal tetany may be the first clue to the maternal disorder. The mother in all reported cases has had hypercalcemia and hypophosphatemia, and a parathyroid adenoma was found in each instance in which surgery was performed.[87]

There is a high incidence of spontaneous abortion, stillbirth, and neonatal death associated with maternal hyperparathyroidism.[130,132] The risk of perinatal death and neonatal tetany have been considered to be as high as 25 and 50 percent, respectively.[129] The 50 percent incidence of marked hypocalcemia in the infant of the hyperparathyroid mother is believed to be due to suppression of the fetal parathyroid glands by the prolonged intrauterine hypercalcemia. Once removed from the hypercalcemic environment, the infant has an absolute or relative hypoparathyroidism such that he cannot maintain his serum calcium concentration in the absence of exogenous calcium infusion. Hypomagnesemia also may occur and may contribute to the inhibition of PTH secretion as well as its renal effect.[87,129] Renal immaturity and the high-phosphate diet when cow's milk is fed potentiate hyperphosphatemia and hypocalcemia. The hypocalcemia usually responds to administration of calcium salts over periods of a few days to 2 weeks. Studies of urinary phosphate excretion have indicated that 3 months may be required for the parathyroid glands of the newborn to regain normal function.[129] After cessation of treatment most infants have remained asymptomatic without residual sequelae.

HYPOPARATHYROIDISM AND PREGNANCY

Hypoparathyroidism during pregnancy is uncommon and in most instances probably is not associated with fetal or newborn morbidity.[133] However, there are a few instances of fetal–newborn hyperparathyroidism reported in association with maternal hypoparathyroidism.[134–136] In these rare cases, the mothers, where documented, had persistent hypocalcemia but there was a tendency to amelioration of the maternal hypoparathyroid state during the pregnancy.[134] The infants' birth weights ranged from 1000 to 2400 gm and gestational age from 28 to 40 weeks.

The infant reported by Gerloczy and Farkas in 1953, as quoted by Bronsky et al.,[135] was born with persistent hypotonia and hypercalcemia and had marked and generalized bone demineralization with subperiosteal bone resorption. She also had persistent vomiting, failed to thrive, and died of pneumonia at 47 days. The twin infants reported by Landing and Kamoshita[136] died within 30 h, with hyaline membrane disease. Both had marked bone changes (osteitis fibrosa) and parathyroid hyperplasia. The few other cases had minimal neonatal morbidity; bone roentgenograms, however, revealed skeletal changes of osteitis fibrosa cystica.

Serum PTH levels have not been measured in such infants, but it has been postulated that fetal parathyroid hyperplasia and PTH hypersecretion result from the persistent maternal (and fetal) hypocalcemia. The fetal hyperparathyroidism results in failure of normal fetal bone calcification and/or, near term, in bone demineralization. It is of interest that most of the infants with hyperparathyroid bone disease and without symptoms have had normal serum calcium concentrations: 7.9–10.6 mg/dl measured on days 1–27.[136] This "relative hypocalcemia" may be due to amelioration of the PTH hypersecretion during the neonatal period. The bone lesions disappear within a few months.[136]

DIABETES MELLITUS AND PREGNANCY

The prevalence of overt diabetes mellitus during gestation approximates 1 in 350 pregnancies.[137,138] However with careful screening, using diagnostic glucose tolerance tests, many patients with gestational diabetes and minimal clinical symptoms can be detected, so that the total incidence of insulin-dependent and gestational diabetes mellitus increases to 1–2.5 percent of all pregnancies.[138]

Pregnancy in women with gestational or insulin-dependent diabetes mellitus is associated with an increased incidence of fetal wastage and congenital anomalies,[137,138] and with increased neonatal mortality and morbidity.[137–139] These risks are related directly to the duration and lack of control of the maternal disease.[138]

The clinical manifestations of severe diabetes mellitus in the mother are similar to those in the nonpregnant diabetic individual. In many instances of gestational diabetes, however, the diagnosis can be difficult because in normal pregnancy there is a tendency to decreased glucose tolerance, increased levels of fasting and stimulated serum insulin, and insulin resistance.[87,137,138] These changes are most striking late in gestation and probably are attributable to the antiinsulin effects of chorionic somatomammotropin, estrogens, and progestins secreted by the placenta.[87,138] The added stress of insulin resistance of pregnancy may precipitate gestational diabetes mellitus in genetically predisposed women with marginal reserve insulin secretory capacity.

Clinical features suggesting gestational diabetes include a family history of diabetes mellitus, prior delivery of a baby weighing 4000 g, or more, or a prior unexplained stillbirth, neonatal death, or major fetal anomaly. Maternal obesity or clinical hydramnios also are suggestive. The presence of glucose in a second fasting urine specimen and/or a blood sugar of 130 mg/dl or greater 1 h after a 50-g oral glucose load are useful screening procedures but are not diagnostic. The final diagnosis must be based on an abnormal glucose tolerance test. An oral glucose tolerance test is best performed during the third trimester when insulin antagonism is most likely to precipitate glucose intolerance. Two or more blood glucose (Somogyi-Nelson venous) values equal to or greater than 90 mg/dl fasting, 165 mg/dl at 1 h, 145 mg/dl at 2 h, or 125 mg/dl at 3 h are considered indicative of abnormal glucose intolerance during pregnancy.[140] Thirty-five percent of patients fulfilling these criteria will eventually manifest overt (nonpregnancy) diabetes.[138,141]

The newborns of women with diabetes mellitus appear obese and plethoric, are large for gestational age, and have visceromegaly involving the heart, liver, and spleen. The increase in body weight is due both to increased carcass mass and to increased body fat content.[142,143] There is also hypertrophy and hyperplasia of the fetal pancreatic islets, which contain increased amounts of insulin. Such infants respond in utero to glucose with an adult-type insulin response.[89,112] Cord blood insulin levels also tend to be higher than levels in normal infants.[112,144] This state of functional hyperinsulinism presumably results in the increased body fat, the increase in selected organ size, and the increased body size of the infant of the mother with diabetes mellitus.

In the neonatal period these infants manifest an increased tendency to severe hypoglycemia. About 50 percent of offspring of insulin-treated mothers manifest blood sugar levels below 20 mg/dl within 1–3 h after birth, and low values may persist several hours in the absence of treatment. Moreover, the expected increase in plasma FFA concentrations is obtunded,[87,112] the increase in glucagon secretion is suppressed,[122,145] and urinary excretion of catecholamines is relatively decreased.[106] Thus, the present view is that prolonged maternal (and fetal) hyperglycemia results in pancreatic islet cell hyperplasia and hyperfunction and that the hyperinsulinemia and hyperglycemia suppress pancreatic islet α cell function.[146] The combined hyperinsulinemia and hypoglucagonemia results in profound neonatal hypoglycemia, which may be aggravated by decreased catecholamine secretion. Sulfonylurea administration to gestationally diabetic women as treatment for hyperglycemia also may potentiate neonatal hypoglycemia and produce intractable hypoglycemia which requires concentrated glucose infusions and even exchange transfusion.[147]

This sequence of events can be minimized by strict control of abnormal blood sugar levels in pregnant women.[138,148] The perinatal mortality rate shows an inverse correlation with mean maternal blood glucose concentration, declining from 23.6 percent when mean blood sugar exceeds 150 mg/dl to 3.8 percent with values below 100 mg/dl.[149] Intensive approach to strict regulation by a specialized internist–obstetrician–pediatrician team has been advocated for the insulin-dependent diabetic.[138] This approach and avoidance of premature delivery is said to reduce perinatal mortality to less than 3 percent.[138] Maintenance of euglycemia can sometimes be accomplished by diet alone in the gestational diabetic woman, but normalization of blood sugar levels usually requires insulin. Normalization of blood sugar levels in this group of pregnant women reduces perinatal mortality to less than 1 percent.[138,150]

REFERENCES

1. Jost, A. Anterior pituitary function in foetal life. In Harris, G. W., and Donovan, B. T. (eds.): *The Pituitary Gland,* vol. 2. London, Butterworths, 1966, p. 299.
2. Jost, A., and Picon, L. Hormonal control of fetal development and metabolism. In: *Advances in Metabolic Disorders,* Vol. 4. New York, Academic, 1970, p. 123.
3. Jost, A. Hormones in development; past and prospects. In Hamburgh, M., and Barrington, E. J. W. (eds.): *Hormones in Development.* New York, Appleton-Century-Crofts, 1971, p. 1.
4. Gitlin, D., Kumate, J., and Morales, C. Metabolism and maternofetal transfer of human growth hormone in the pregnant woman at term. *J. Clin. Endocrinol. Metab. 25:* 1599, 1965.
5. Laron, A., Pertzelan, A., Mannheimer, S., Goldman, J., and Guttman, S. Lack of placental transfer of human growth hormone. *Acta Endocrinol. 53:* 687, 1966.
6. King, K. C., Adam, P. A. J., Schwartz, R., and Teramo, K. Human placental transfer of human growth hormone. *Pediatrics 48:* 534, 1971.
7. Erenberg, A., and Fisher, D. A. Thyroid hormone metabolism in the foetus. In: *Foetal and Neonatal Physiology.* Cambridge, Cambridge University Press, 1973, p. 508.
8. Kittinger, G. W., Beamer, N. B., Hagemenas, F., et al. Evidence for autonomous pituitary adrenal function in the near-term fetal rhesus. *Endocrinology 91:* 1037, 1972.
9. Jones, C. T., Luther, E., Ritchie, J. W. K., and Worthington, D. The clearance of ACTH from the plasma of adult and fetal sheep. *Endocrinology 96:* 233, 1974.
10. Miyakawa, I., Ikeda, I., and Maeyama, M. Transport of ACTH across human placenta. *J. Clin. Endocrinol. Metab. 39:* 440, 1974.
11. Winters, A. J., Oliver, C., Colston, C., MacDonald, P. C., and Porter, J. C. Plasma ACTH levels in the human fetus and neonate as related to age and parturition. *J. Clin. Endocrinol. Metab. 39:* 269, 1974.
12. Foster, D. L., Cruz, T. A. C., Jackson, G. L., Cook, B., and Nalbandov, A. V. Regulation of luteinizing hormone in the fetal and neonatal lamb. III. Release of LH by the pituitary in vivo in response to crude ovine hypothalamic extract or purified porcine gonadotrophin releasing factor. *Endocrinology 90:* 673, 1972.
13. Foster, D. L., Karsch, F. J., and Nalbandov, A. V. Regulation of luteinizing hormone (LH) in the fetal and neonatal lamb. II. Study of placental transfer of LH in the sheep. *Endocrinology 90:* 589, 1972.
14. Burton, A. M., Illingworth, D. V., Challis, J. R. G., and McNeilly, A. S. Placental transfer of oxytocin in the guinea pig and its release during parturition. *J. Endocrinol. 60:* 499, 1974.
15. Noddle, B. A. Transfer of oxytocin from the maternal to the fetal circulation in the ewe. *Nature 203:* 414, 1964.
16. Chard, T., Hudson, C. N., Edwards, C. R. W., and Boyd, N. R. H. The release of oxytocin and vasopressin by the human foetus during labour. *Nature 234:* 352, 1971.
17. Weitzman, R. E., Fisher, D. A., Robillard, J., et al. Arginine vasopressin response to an osmotic stimulus in the fetal sheep. *Pediatr. Res. 12:* 35, 1978.
18. Sperling, M. A., Erenberg, A., Fiser, R. H., Oh, W., and Fisher, D. A. Placental transfer of glucagon in sheep. *Endocrinology 93:* 1435, 1973.
19. Adam, P. H. J., King, K., Schwartz, R., and Teramo, K. Human placental barrier to ^{125}I-glucagon early in gestation. *J. Clin. Endocrinol. Metab. 34:* 772, 1971.
20. Wolf, H., Sabata, V., Frerichs, H., and Stubbe, P. Evidence for impermeability of the human placenta for insulin. *Horm. Metab. Res. 1:* 224, 1969.
21. Mintz, D. H., Chez, R. A., and Horger, E. O. Fetal insulin and growth hormone in the subhuman primate. *J. Clin. Invest. 48:* 176, 1969.
22. Adam, P. A. J., Teramo, K., Raiha, N., Gitlin, D., and Schwartz, R. Response to acute elevation of the fetal glucose concentration and placental transfer of human insulin I^{131}. *Diabetes 18:* 409, 1969.
23. Alexander, D. P., Button, H. G., Nixon, D. A., et al. Calcium, parathyroid hormone and calcitonin in the foetus. In: *Foetal and Neonatal Physiology.* Cambridge, Cambridge University Press, 1973, p. 421.
24. Garel, J. M., Milhaud, G., and Sizonenko, P. Thyrocalcitonine et barrière placentaire chez le rat. *C. R. (Paris) 269:* 1785, 1969
25. Symonds, E. M., and Furler, I. Plasma renin levels in the normal and anephric fetus at birth. *Biol. Neonate 23:* 133, 1973.
26. Beitins, I. Z., Kowarski, A., Shermeta, D. W., DeLemos, R. A., and Migeon, C. J. Fetal and maternal secretion rate of cortisol in sheep: diffusion resistance of the placenta. *Pediatr. Res. 4:* 129, 1969.
27. Dixon, R., Hyman, A., Gurpide, E., et al. Foeto-maternal transfer and production of cortisol in the sheep. *Steroids 16:* 771, 1970.
28. Drost, M., Kumagai, L. F., and Guzman, M. Sequential foetal–maternal plasma cortisol levels in sheep. *J. Endocrinol. 56:* 483, 1973.
29. DiStefano, J. J. III, Durango, A. R., Jang, M., et al. Estimates and estimation errors of hormone secretion, transport and disposal rates in the maternal–fetal system. *Endocrinology 93:* 324, 1973.
30. Bashore, R. A., Smith, F., and Gold, E. M. Placental transfer and metabolism of 4-^{14}C cortisol in the pregnant monkey. *Nature 228:* 774, 1970.
31. Boyard, F., Ances, I. G., Tapper, A. J., et al. Transplacental passage and fetal secretion of aldosterone. *J. Clin. Invest. 49:* 1389, 1970.
32. Diczfalusy, E., and Mancuso, S. Oestrogen metabolism in pregnancy. In Klopper, A., and Diczfalusy, E. (eds.): *Foetus and Placenta.* Oxford, Blackwell, 1969, p. 191.
33. Solomon, S., and Friesen, H. G. Endocrine relations between mother and fetus. *Ann. Rev. Med. 19:* 399, 1968.
34. Smith, W., and Adams, N. Transplacental influence of androgen upon ovulatory mechanisms in the rat. *J. Endocrinol. 48:* 477, 1970.
35. Ryan, K. J. Steroid hormones in mammalian pregnancy. In: *Handbook of Physiology,* section 7, vol. 2, part 2, Female Reproductive System. Baltimore, American Physiological Society 1973, p. 285.
36. Courrier, R., and Aron, M. Sur le passage de l'hormone thyroidienne de le mère au foetus à travers le placenta. *C. R. Soc. Biol. 100:* 839, 1929.
37. Josimovich, J. B. Passage of hormones through the placenta. In: *Handbook of Physiology,* section 7, vol. 2, part 2, Female Reproductive System. Baltimore, American Physiological Society 1973, p. 277.
38. Fisher, D. A., Dussault, J. H., Sack, J., and Chopra, I. J. Ontogenesis of hypothalamic–pituitary–thyroid function and metabolism in man, sheep and rat. *Recent Prog. Horm. Res. 33:* 59, 1977.

39. Geloso, J. P., Hemon, P., Legrand, J., Legrand, C., and Jost, A. Some aspects of thyroid physiology during the perinatal period. *Gen. Comp. Endocrinol. 10:* 191, 1968.
40. Hopkins, P. S., and Thorburn, G. D. Placental permeability to maternal thyroxine in sheep. *J. Endocrinol. 49:* 549, 1971.
41. Erenberg, A., Omori, K., Oh, W., and Fisher, D. A. The effect of fetal thyroidectomy on thyroid hormone metabolism in maternal and fetal sheep. *Pediatr. Res. 7:* 870, 1973.
42. Fisher, D. A., Dussault, J. H., and Lam, R. W. Serum and thyroid gland triiodothyronine in the human fetus. *J. Clin. Endocrinol. Metab. 36:* 397, 1973.
43. Pickering, D. E. Thyroid physiology in the developing monkey fetus. *Gen. Comp. Endocrinol. 10:* 182, 1965.
44. Van Herle, A. J., Young, R. T., Fisher, D. A., Uller, R. P., and Brinkman, C. R. Intrauterine treatment of a hypothyroid fetus. *J. Clin. Endocrinol. Metab. 40:* 474, 1975.
45. Osorio, C., and Myant, N. B. Thyroid hormones in pregnancy *Br. Med. Bull. 16:* 159, 1960.
46. Grumbach, M. M., and Werner, S. C. Transfer of thyroid hormones across the human placenta at term. *J. Clin. Endocrinol. Metab. 16:* 1392, 1956.
47. Kearns, J. E., and Hutson, W. Tagged isomers and analogues of thyroxine; their transmission across the human placenta and other studies. *J. Nucl. Med. 4:* 453, 1963.
48. Fisher, D. A., Lehman, H., and Lackey, C. Placental transfer of thyroxine. *J. Clin. Endocrinol. Metab. 24:* 393, 1964.
49. Raiti, S., Holyman, C. B., Scott, R. L., and Blizzard, R. M. Evidence for the placental transfer of triiodothyronine in human beings. *N. Engl. J. Med. 277:* 456, 1967.
50. Keynes, G. Obstetrics and gynaecology in relation to thyroxicosis and myesthenia gravis. *J. Obstet. Gynecol. 59:* 173, 1952.
51. Carr, E. A., Beierwaltes, W. H., Raman, G., et al. The effect of maternal thyroid function on fetal thyroid function and development. *J. Clin. Endocrinol. Metab. 19:* 1, 1959.
52. Beard, R. W. Response of the human foetal heart and maternal circulation to adrenaline and noradrenaline. *Br. Med. J. 1:* 443, 1962.
53. Zuspan, F. P., Whaley, W. H., Nelson, G. H., and Ahlquist, R. P. Placental transfer of epinephrine. I. Maternal–fetal metabolic alterations of glucose and nonesterified fatty acids. *Am. J. Obstet. Gynecol. 95:* 284, 1966.
54. Sandler, M., Ruthven, C. R. J., Contractor, S. F., et al. Transmission of noradrenaline across the human placenta. *Nature 197:* 598, 1963.
54a. Cosmi, E. V., and Condorelli, S. Passaggio transplacentare delle catecholamine nella pecord. *Acta Anaesth. Ital. 24:* 43, 1973.
55. Faber, J. J. Diffusional exchange between foetus and mother as a function of the physical properties of the diffusing materials. In: *Foetal and Neonatal Physiology.* Cambridge, Cambridge University Press, 1973, p. 306.
56. Kaplan, S. L., Grumbach, M. M., and Aubert, M. L. The ontogenesis of pituitary hormones and hypothalamic factors in the human fetus: maturation of central nervous system regulation of anterior pituitary function. *Recent Prog. Horm. Res. 32:* 161, 1976.
57. Levina, S. E. Endocrine features in development of human hypothalamus, hypophysis and placenta. *Gen. Comp. Endocrinol. 11:* 151, 1968.
58. Gitlin, D., and Biassucci, A. Ontogenesis of immunoreactive growth hormone, follicle-stimulating hormone, thyroid-stimulating hormone, luteinizing hormone, chorionic prolactin, and chorionic gonadotropin in the human conceptus. *J. Clin. Endocrinol. Metab. 29:* 926, 1969.
59. Fukuchi, M., Inoue, T., Abe, H., and Kumahara, Y. Thyrotropin in human fetal pituitaries. *J. Clin. Endocrinol. Metab. 31:* 565, 1970.
60. Kaplan, S. L., Grumbach, M. M., and Shepard, T. H. The ontogenesis of human fetal hormones. I. Growth hormones and insulin. *J. Clin. Invest. 51:* 3080, 1972.
61. Fisher, D. A. Fetal maternal thyroid relationships. In: International Congress Series, No. 273. Amsterdam, *Excerpta Medica,* 1973, p. 1045.
62. Aubert, M. L., Grumbach, M. M., and Kaplan, S. L. The ontogenesis of human fetal hormones. III. Prolactin. *J. Clin. Invest. 56:* 155, 1975.
63. Skowsky, W. R., and Fisher, D. A. Fetal neurohypophyseal arginine vasopressin and arginine vasotocin in man and sheep. *Pediatr. Res. 11:* 627, 1977.
64. Pavlova, E. B., Pronina, T. S., and Skebelskaya, Y. B. Histostructure of adenhypophysis of human fetuses and contents of somatotropic and adrenocorticotropic hormones. *Gen. Comp. Endocrinol. 10:* 269, 1968.
65. Allen, J. P., Cook, D. M., Kendall, J. W., and McGilvra, R. Maternal–fetal ACTH relationship in man. *J. Clin. Endocrinol. Metab. 37:* 23, 1973.
66. Hayek, A., Driscoll, S. G., and Warshaw, J. B. Endocrine studies in anencephaly. *J. Clin. Invest. 52:* 1636, 1973.
67. Fisher, D. A., Pyle, H. R., Jr., Porter, J. C., Beard, A. G., and Panos, T. C. Control of water balance in the newborn. *Am. J. Dis. Child. 106:* 137, 1963.
68. Greenberg, R. E. The physiology and metabolism of catecholamines. In Gardner, L. I. (ed.): *Endocrine and Genetic Diseases of Childhood.* Philadelphia, Saunders, 1969, p. 762.
69. Coupland, R. E. The prenatal development of the abdominal para-aortic bodies in man. *J. Anat. 86:* 357, 1952.
70. Greenberg, R. E., and Lind, J. Catecholamines in tissues of the human fetus. *Pediatrics 77:* 904, 1961.
71. Niemineva, K., and Pekkarinen, A. The noradrenaline and adrenaline content of human fetal adrenal glands and aortic bodies. *Ann. Med. Exp. Biol. Fenn. 30:* 234, 1952.
72. Wurtman, R. J. Control of epinephrine synthesis in the adrenal medulla by the adrenal cortex: hormonal specificity and dose response characteristics. *Endocrinology 79:* 608, 1966.
73. Margolis, E. L., Roffi, J., and Jost, A. Norepinephrine methylation in fetal rat adrenals. *Science 154:* 275, 1966.
74. Comline, R. S., and Silver, M. Development of activity in the adrenal medulla of the foetus and newborn animal. *Br. Med. Bull. 22:* 16, 1966.
75. Jones, C. T., and Robinson, R. O. Plasma catecholamines in foetal and adult sheep. *J. Physiol. 248:* 15, 1975.
76. Muscholl, E., and Vogt, M. Secretory responses of extramedullary chromaffin tissue. *Br. J. Pharmacol. Chemother. 22:* 193, 1964.
77. Schaeffer, L. D., Wilder, M. L., and Williams, R. H. Secretion and content of insulin and glucagon in human fetal pancreatic slices in vitro. *Proc. Soc. Exp. Biol. Med. 143:* 314, 1973.
78. Rastogi, G. K., Latarte, J., and Fraser, T. R. Proinsulin content of pancreas in human fetus of healthy mothers. *Lancet 1:* 7, 1970.
79. Steinke, J., and Driscoll, S. G. The extractable insulin content of pancreas from fetuses and infants of diabetic and control mothers. *Diabetes 14:* 573, 1965.
80. Assan, R., and Boillot, J. Pancreatic glucagon and glucagon-like material in tissues and plasmus from human fetuses 6–26 weeks old. In: *Metabolic Processes in the Fetus and Newborn Infant.* Baltimore, Williams & Wilkins, 1971, p. 218.
81. Polak, J. M.,Pearse, A. G. E., Crimelius, L., Bloom, S. R., and Arimura, A. Growth hormone release inhibiting hormone in gastrointestinal and pancreatic D-cells. *Lancet 1:* 1220, 1975.
82. Vale, W. Personal communication.
83. Vale, W., Brazeau, P., Rivier, C., et al. Somatostatin. *Recent Prog. Horm. Res. 31:* 365, 1975.
84. Lambert, A. E., Junod, A., Stauffacher, W., Jeanrenaud, B., and Renold, A. E. Organ culture of fetal rat pancreas. I. Insulin release induced by caffeine and by sugars and some derivatives. *Biochem. Biophys. Acta 184:* 529, 1969.
85. Heinze, E., and Steinke, J. Insulin secretion during development: response of isolated pancreatic islets of fetal, newborn and adult rats to theophylline and arginine. *Horm. Metab. Res. 4:* 234, 1972.
86. Ashworth, M. A., Leach, F. M., and Melner, R. D. G. Development of insulin secretion in the human fetus. *Arch. Dis. Child. 48:* 151, 1973.
87. Fisher, D. A. Endocrine physiology I and II. In Smith, C. A., and Nelson, N. M. (eds.): *The Physiology of the Newborn Infant,* 4th ed. Springfield, Ill., Thomas, 1976, p. 554.
88. King, K. C., Butt, J., Raivo, K., et al. Human maternal and fetal insulin response to arginine. *N. Engl. J. Med. 285:* 607, 1971.
89. Oakley, N. W., Beard, R. W., and Turner, R. C. Effect of sustained maternal hyperglycemia on the fetus in normal and diabetic pregnancies. *Br. Med. J. 1:* 466, 1972.
90. Chez, R. A., Mintz, D. H., and Hutchinson, D. H. Effect of theophylline on glucagon and glucose-mediated plasma insulin responses in subhuman primate fetus and neonate. *Metabolism 20:* 805, 1971.
91. Chez, R. A., Mintz, D. H., and Epstein, M. F. Glucagon metabolism in non-human primate pregnancy. *Am. J. Obstet. Gynecol. 120:* 690, 1974.
92. Fiser, R. H., Jr., Erenberg, A., Sperling, M. A., Oh, W., and Fisher, D. A. Insulin–glucagon substrate interrelations in the fetal sheep. *Pediatr. Res. 8:* 951, 1974.

93. Girard, J. R., Kervran, A., Soufflet, E., and Assan, R. Factors affecting the secretion of insulin and glucagon by the rat fetus. *Diabetes 23:* 310, 1974.
94. Mintz, D. H., Levey, G. S., and Schenk, A. Adenosine 3′5′-cyclic monophosphate and phosphodiesterase activities in isolated fetal and neonatal rat pancreatic islets. *Endocrinology 92:* 614, 1973.
95. Grasso, S., Messina, A., Saporito, N., and Reitano, G. Effect of theophylline glucagon and theophylline plus glucagon on insulin secretion in the premature infant. *Diabetes 19:* 837, 1970.
96. Nakagami, K., Yamazaki, Y., and Tsunoda, Y. An electron microscopic study of the human fetal parathyroid gland. *Z. Zellforsch. Mikrosk. Anat. 85:* 89, 1968.
97. Wolfe, H. J., DeLellis, R. A., Voelkel, E. F., and Tashjian, A. H., Jr. Distribution of calcitonin-containing cells in the normal neonatal human thyroid gland: a correlation of morphology and peptide content. *J. Clin. Endocrinol. Metab. 41:* 1076, 1975.
98. Scothorne, R. J. Functional capacity of the fetal parathyroid glands with reference to their clinical use as homografts. *Ann. N.Y. Acad. Sci. 120:* 669, 1964.
99. Smith, F. G., Jr., Alexander, D. P., Britton, A. G., Buckle, R. M., and Nixon, D. A. Parathyroid hormone in fetal and adult sheep. The effect of hypocalcemia. *J. Endocrinol. 53:* 339, 1972.
100. Littledike, E. T., Arnaud, C. D., and Whipp, S. C. Calcitonin secretion in ovine, procine and bovine fetuses. *Proc. Exp. Biol. Med. 139:* 428, 1972
101. David, L., and Anast, C. S. Calcium metabolism in newborn infants. *J. Clin. Invest. 54:* 287, 1974.
102. Samaan, N. A., Anderson, G. D., and Adam-Mayne, M. E. Immunoreactive calcitonin in the mother, neonate, child, and adult. *Am. J. Obstet. Gynecol. 121:* 622, 1975.
103. Delavoria Papadoulos, M., Battaglia, F. C., Bruns, P. D., and Meschia, G. Total, protein bound and ultrafilterable calcium in maternal and fetal plasmas. *Am. J. Physiol. 213:* 363, 1967.
104. Cacciari, E., Cicognani, A., Pirazzoli, P., et al. Plasma ACTH values during the first seven days of life in infants of diabetic mothers. *J. Pediatr. 87:* 943, 1975.
105. Reynolds, J. W. Feto-placental and neonatal steroid endocrinology. In Smith, C. A., and Nelson, N. M. (eds): *The Physiology of the Newborn Infant,* 4th ed. Thomas, Springfield, Ill., 1976, p. 664.
106. Light, I. H., Sutherland, J. M., Loggie, J. M., and Gaffney, T. E. Impaired epinephrine release in hypoglycemic infants of diabetic mothers. *N. Engl. J. Med. 277:* 394, 1967.
107. Stern, L., Ramos, A., and Leduc, J. Urinary catecholamine excretion in infants of diabetic mothers. *Pediatrics 42:* 598, 1968.
108. Keele, D. K., and Kay, J. L. Plasma free fatty acid and blood sugars levels in newborn infants and their mothers. *Pediatrics 37:* 597, 1966.
109. Sinclair, J. C. Metabolic rate and temperature control. In Smith, C. A., and Nelson, N. M. (eds.): *The Physiology of the Newborn Infant,* 4th ed. Springfield, Ill., Thomas, 1976, p. 354.
110. Erenberg, A., Phelps, D. L., Oh, W., and Fisher, D. A. Total and free thyroxine and triiodothyronine concentrations in the newborn period. *Pediatrics 53:* 211, 1974.
111. Fisher, D. A., and Sack, J. Thyroid function in the neonate and possible approaches to newborn screening for hypothyroidism. In Fisher, D. A., and Burrow, G. N. (eds.): *Perinatal Thyroid Function and Disease.* New York, Raven, 1975, p. 197.
112. Sperling, M. A., De Lamater, P. V., Phelps, D., et al. Spontaneous and amino acid stimulated glucagon secretion in the immediate postnatal period: relation to glucose and insulin. *J. Clin. Invest. 53:* 1159, 1974.
113. Sperling, M. A. Insulin and glucagon in fetal and neonatal physiology. In Stave, U. (ed.): *Perinatal Physiology.* New York, Plenum, (in press).
114. Cornblath, M., Parker, M. L., Reisner, S. H., Forbes, A. E., and Daughaday, W. H. Secretion and metabolism of growth hormone in premature and full term infants. *J. Clin. Endocrinol. Metab. 25:* 209, 1965.
115. Sack, J., Fisher, D. A., and Wang, C. C. Serum thyrotropin, prolactin and growth hormone levels during the early neonatal period in the human infant. *J. Pediatr. 89:* 298, 1976.
116. Guyda, H. J., and Friesen, H. G. Serum prolactin levels in humans from birth to adult life. *Pediatr. Res. 7:* 534, 1973.
117. Winter, J. S. D., Faiman, C., Hobson, W., Prasad, A. V., and Reyes, F. I. Pituitary gonadal relations in infancy. I. Patterns of serum gonadotropin concentrations from birth to four years of age in man and chimpanzee. *J. Clin. Endocrinol. Metab. 40:* 545, 1975.
118. Selenkow, H. A. Therapeutic considerations for thyrotoxicosis during pregnancy. In Fisher, D. A., and Burrow, G. N. (eds.): *Perinatal Thyroid Physiology and Disease.* New York, Raven, 1975, p. 145.
119. Hershman, J. M., Kenimer, J. G., Higgins, H. P., and Patillo, R. A. Placental thyrotropins. In Fisher, D. A., and Burrow, G. N. (eds.): *Perinatal Thyroid Physiology and Disease.* New York, Raven, 1975, p. 11.
120. Pochin, E. E. The iodine uptake of the human thyroid throughout the menstrual cycle and in pregnancy. *Clin. Sci. 11:* 441, 1952.
121. Dowling, J. T., Hutchinson, D. L., Hindle, W. R., and Kleeman, C. R. Effects of pregnancy on iodine metabolism in the primate. *J. Clin. Endocrinol. Metab. 21:* 779, 1961.
122. Fisher, D. A. Pathogenesis and therapy of neonatal Graves' disease. *Am. J. Dis. Child. 130:* 133, 1976.
123. Hollingsworth, D. R., and Mabry, C. C. Congenital Graves' disease. In Fisher, D. A., and Burrow, G. N. (eds.): *Perinatal Thyroid Function and Disease.* New York, Raven, 1975, p. 163.
124. Grimes, E. M., Fayez, J. A., and Miller, G. L. Cushing's syndrome and pregnancy. *Obstet. Gynecol. 42:* 550, 1973.
125. Bongiovanni, A. M., and McPadden, A. J. Steroids during pregnancy and possible fetal consequences. *Fertil. Steril. 11:* 181, 1960.
126. Kreiner, K., and DeVaux, W. D. Neonatal adrenal insufficiency associated with maternal Cushing's syndrome. *Pediatrics 47:* 516, 1971.
127. Kulin, H. E., Metzl, K., and Peterson, R. Urinary tetrahydrocortisone and tetrahydrocortisol in infants born of mothers with corticosteroids during pregnancy. *J. Pediatr. 69:* 648, 1966.
128. Friderichsen, C. Hypocalcemie bei einern Brustkind und Hypercalcemie bei der Mutter. *Monatsschr. Kinderheilkd. 75:* 146, 1938.
129. Butler, O. S., Levi, J., Greif, E., et al. Prolonged neonatal parathyroid suppression. *Arch. Surg. 106:* 722, 1973.
130. Pederson, N. T., and Permin, H. Hyperparathyroidism and pregnancy. *Acta Obstet. Gynecol. Scand. 54:* 281, 1975.
131. Cushard, W. G., Creditor, M. A., Canterbury, J. M., and Reiss, E. Physiologic hyperparathyroidism in pregnancy. *J. Clin. Endocrinol. Metab. 34:* 767, 1972.
132. Ludwig, G. D. Hyperparathyroidism in relation to pregnancy. *N. Engl. J. Med. 267:* 637, 1962.
133. Anderson, G. W., and Musselman, L. The treatment of tetany in pregnancy: with a brief review of the literature. *Am. J. Obstet. Gynecol. 43:* 547, 1942.
134. Aceto, T., Butt, R. E., Bruck, E., Schultz, R. B., and Perez, Y. R. Intrauterine hyperparathyroidism: a complication of untreated maternal hypoparathyroidism. *J. Clin. Endocrinol. Metab. 26:* 487, 1966.
135. Bronsky, D., Kiamko, R. T., Moncada, R., and Rosenthal, I. M. Intrauterine hyperparathyroidism secondary to maternal hypoparathyroidism. *Pediatrics 42:* 606, 1968.
136. Landing, B. H., and Kamoshita, S. Congenital hyperparathyroidism secondary to maternal hypoparathyroidism. *J. Pediatr. 77:* 842, 1970.
137. Spellacy, W. N. Diabetes mellitus complicating pregnancy. *Mod. Med. 37:* 91, 1969.
138. Rodman, H. M., Gyves, M. T., Fanaroff, A. A., and Merkatz, I. R. The diabetic pregnancy as a model for modern perinatal care. In New, M. I., and Fiser, R. H., Jr. (eds.): *Diabetes and Other Endocrine Disorders During Pregnancy.* New York, Liss, 1976, pp. 13–32.
139. Dekaben, A., and Baird, R. The outcome of pregnancy in diabetic women. I. Fetal wastage, mortality and morbidity in offspring of diabetic and control mothers. *J. Pediatr. 55:* 563, 1959.
140. O'Sullivan, J. B., and Mahan, C. Criteria for the oral glucose tolerance test in pregnancy. *Diabetes 13:* 278, 1964.
141. O'Sullivan, J. B. Gestational diabetes: unsuspected, asymptomatic diabetes in pregnancy. *N. Engl. J. Med. 264:* 1082, 1961.
142. Osler, M., and Pedersen, J. The body composition of infants of diabetic mothers. *Pediatrics 26:* 985, 1960.
143. Fee, B. A., and Weil, W. B., Jr. Body composition of infants of diabetic mothers by direct analysis. *Ann. N.Y. Acad. Sci. 110:* 869, 1963.
144. Pildes, R. S., Hart, R. T., Warrner, R., and Cornblath, M. Plasma insulin response during oral glucose tolerance tests in newborn of normal and gestationally diabetic mothers. *Pediatrics 44:* 76, 1969.
145. Bloom, S. R., and Johnston, D. I. Failure of glucagon release in infants of diabetic mothers. *Br. Med. J. 4:* 453, 1972.
146. Massi-Benedetti, F., Falorni, A., Luyckx, A., and Lefebvre, P.

Inhibition of glucagon secretion in the human newborn by simultaneous administration of glucose and insulin. *Horm. Metab. Res. 6:* 392, 1974.

147. Adam, P. A. J., and Schwartz, R. Diagnosis and treatment: should oral hypoglycemic agents be used in pediatric and pregnant patients? *Pediatrics 42:* 819, 1968.

148. Persson, B., Gentz, J., and Kellum, M. Metabolic observations of infants of strictly controlled diabetic mothers. *Acta Paediatr. Scand. 62:* 465, 1973.

149. Karlsson, K., and Kjellmer, I. The outcome of diabetic pregnancies in relation to the mother's blood sugar level. *Am. J. Obstet. Gynecol. 112:* 213, 1972.

150. O'Sullivan, J. B., Charles D., Mahan, C. M., and Dandrow, R. V. Gestational diabetes and perinatal mortality rate. *Am. J. Obstet. Gynecol. 116:* 901, 1973.

134

Synopsis of Diagnosis and Treatment

William D. Odell

Chapters 130 to 133 present data and concepts related to the physiology and pathophysiology of pregnancy. Drs. Marshall and Hobel (Chapter 130) describe the present concepts in the human of conception, implantation function of the fetal–placental unit, and parturition. Dr. Goldstein (Chapter 132) describes current concepts of diagnosis and therapy of gestational trophoblastic neoplasms. These neoplasms at times appear in a highly malignant form and, without therapy, lead to death in a few months. Within the past 20 years, even metastatic trophoblastic neoplasms have proved curable by appropriate therapy in established centers. Dr. Fisher (Chapter 133) describes the development of the endocrinology of the fetus and its relation to the maternal system. Here, too, within the past 10 years, concepts of placental transport of peptide hormones and the thyronines have changed, modifying treatment of disorders. For example, prior to about 1965, it was believed that triiodothyronine (T_3) and thyroxine (T_4) were transported from maternal to fetal blood. Some individuals advocated treatment of maternal thyrotoxicosis by using antithyroid durgs in large doses plus T_3. The latter was supposed to ensure fetal thyroid hormonal status. It now appears clear that T_3 passes the placental barrier poorly, while antithyroid drugs pass well—thus, present beliefs dictate treatment with the smallest dose of antithyroid drugs (if drugs are selected as therapy over surgery) required to control the disease. This is another example of changing concepts of medicine in this brief period of 10 years.

Another example arises in Chapter 131 by Dr. Friesen. Prior to about 1970, it was felt that prolactin-secreting pituitary adenomas were relatively rare and that patients with galactorrhea-amenorrhea syndromes usually *did not* have an adenoma. Techniques of x-ray interpretation have changed rapidly, and the recognition of more subtle abnormalities, coupled to new pituitary microsurgical techniques, has revealed that many, possibly most, patients with galactorrhea syndromes have microadenomas. This rapid advance in clinical disease recognition has been made feasible largely because of isolation, purification, and development of assays for human prolactin, work in large part stemming from Dr. Friesen's efforts.

Once again, the reader is cautioned that if these chapters were written 10 years ago, they would have not included much of what is recorded today. Ten years from this reading, much of this material will be changed and shown to be wrong.

Diffuse Hormonal Systems

135

Hormones of the Gastrointestinal Tract

Bernard M. Jaffe

INTRODUCTION

Gastrointestinal function is modulated by a complex series of hormonal interrelationships. Although initially only three gastrointestinal hormones were recognized, during the past few years a number of new peptides have been discovered and each ascribed to a specific endocrine cell. Since these endocrine cells are widely distributed throughout the enteric mucosa, the gastrointestinal tract has recently been recognized as a major endocrine system. Further recognition of numerous interrelationships with hormones of the conventional endocrine glands has heightened interest in the humoral aspects of the gastrointestinal tract. This chapter will attempt to survey pertinent recent aspects of the physiology and pathophysiology of the gastrointestinal hormones, concentrating particularly on the newly recognized gastrointestinal peptides.

Grossman[1] hypothesized that a number of gastrointestinal hormones acted on a single receptor with two interacting sites. This hypothesis suggested that on the basis of site-specific affinity the hormones could be divided into two structurally related groups—gastrinlike [gastrin and cholecystokinin–pancreozymin (CCK-PZ)] and secretinlike [secretin, glucagon, vasoactive intestinal peptide (VIP), and gastric inhibitory polypeptide (GIP)]. It further predicted that all target end organs that reacted to one of these hormones would also react to all the others. Simultaneous action of two (or more) hormones on the same site would produce either competitive augmentation or inhibition, whereas interaction of two or more hormones with both sites would result in noncompetitive augmentation or inhibition. It would thus become critical to evaluate not only the action of the hormones themselves, but also the efficacy of these actions as well. Although there has been no direct substantiation of this hypothesis, it has provided a useful framework for the study of the gastrointestinal hormones.

Since the development of gastrin radioimmunoassays, there has been a spurt in the understanding of the physiology of this peptide hormone. These advances have recently been reviewed in detail.[2–5] Accordingly, the physiology and pathophysiology of gastrin will be discussed only in the context of the Zollinger-Ellison syndrome. Since radioimmunoassay systems for secretin and CCK-PZ have not been generally available, there has been relatively slower progress in the understanding of the physiologic role of these hormones. The available information on these compounds has been reviewed,[6–10] and consequently these peptide hormones will be discussed only by comparing their actions and chemical structures with those of gastrin and VIP–GIP. This chapter will concentrate on the newer and "candidate" hormones of the gastrointestinal tract[11] and on the recent developments in the pathophysiology of the Zollinger-Ellison and watery diarrhea–hypokalemia–achlorhydria (WDHA) syndromes.

NEWER GASTROINTESTINAL HORMONES

VASOACTIVE INTESTINAL POLYPEPTIDE (VIP)

Chemistry

Bayliss and Starling[12] noted in 1902 that intestinal extracts possess vasodepressor activity. Since that time, a number of vasoactive compounds have been isolated from the gastrointestinal tract, including histamine, prostaglandins, substance P,[13] secretin, and CCK-PZ. Said and Mutt[14] described the isolation of a new vasodepressor peptide from hog intestine. The compound was initially shown to increase femoral and splanchnic artery blood flow while producing a substantial fall in systemic arterial pressure. The peptide was prepared from a methanolic extract of porcine small intestine purified by two successive steps of ion-exchange chromatography on carboxymethylcellulose (first in 0.0125 M phosphate buffer eluted with 0.2N HCl and then in 0.1M ammonium bicarbonate), countercurrent distribution (using a 200-tube transfer in 1-butanol and 0.1M ammonium bicarbonate), and gel filtration on Sephadex G-25 (0.2M acetic acid).[15] The purified product was distinguished from prostaglandins, bradykinin, and histamine by its actions on a number of smooth muscle strips in cascade,[16] from secretin and glucagon by its amino acid composition (the absence of glycine and the presence of isoleucine), and from CCK-PZ by the fact that the latter compound is not extracted into methanol. The amino acid sequence of the vasoactive intestinal polypeptide (VIP) was determined,[17,18] and the compound was synthesized.[19]

Pure porcine VIP is a polypeptide consisting of 28 amino acids with a calculated molecular weight of 3381. The N- and C-terminal residues are histidine and asparagine, respectively. The structure of VIP (shown in Table 135-1) shows a remarkable number of similarities with the structures of porcine glucagon and secretin. Amino acid residues 1, 2, 6, and 7 are common to both glucagon and secretin; residues 3, 12, 13, 14, and 23 are shared with secretin, and residues 10 and 28 are shared with glucagon. Although 11 of the 28 (39 percent) amino acid residues in VIP are common to either glucagon or secretin, all but one of the positions of identity are in the N-terminal (1–14) portion of the molecule, resulting in a unique C-terminal end. Furthermore, comparing the structures of porcine VIP and glucagon, 10 nonconservative transformations are evident, in positions 3 (Glu–Gln), 8 (Asp–Ser), 9 (Asn–Asp), 14 (Arg–Leu), 15 (Lys–Asp), 17 (Met–Arg), 18 (Ala–Arg), 20 (Lys–Gln), 21 (Lys–Asp), and 28 (Asn–Asp).

Structure–Function Relationships

Bodanszky and colleagues[20] synthesized a number of fragments of the VIP molecule. Although Makhlouf et al.[21] demonstrated that VIP fragments 1–8, 18–28, 15–28, and 14–28 did not stimulate pancreatic or biliary secretion, Schebalim et al.[22] noted that the C-terminal 14–28 fragment induced a 20 mg/dl rise in blood sugar and stimulated intestinal secretion with one-tenth the potency of the native molecule. In the studies of Bodanszky et al.,[20] VIP 7–28 possessed up to 15 percent of the biologic activity of VIP in causing hypotension and tracheal and gastric relaxation; shorter compounds had less than 2 percent of the biologic activity.

Although VIP shares structural similarities with both secretin and glucagon, it has a unique spectrum of actions. Mutt and Said[18] postulated that residues 10 and 28 are critical for determining the specific biologic activity. In addition to the specificity of the linear structure of VIP, its spatial configuration differs from that of both secretin and glucagon. By studying the ORD spectra of these peptides in water, Bodanszky et al.[23] noted that VIP behaved like a molecule with 20 percent helix and 80 percent random coil; this is in contrast with the moderate helical character of secretin and the virtual absence of helicity in glucagon. The study of both linear and spatial structures is relevant only when considered in terms of receptor site specificity, since it is the receptor which determines the biologic activity. The VIP receptors in the liver, pancreas, and fat cell membranes have been carefully studied.[24–28] Binding to these receptors was not inhibited even by large quantities of glucagon, but was competitively inhibited by secretin at concentrations 100 times that of VIP. In liver plasma membranes VIP had a very high affinity for adenyl cyclase (half-maximal activity is achieved by 2×10^{-10} M), but VIP stimulated this enzyme to only one-fourth the maximal activity stimulated by glucagon. In fat cell membranes, VIP was 30 times more potent in stimulating adenyl cyclase activity than was glucagon. In both membrane systems, secretin behaved much like VIP. Because of the similarity of their effect on the adenyl cyclase system and the results of the binding studies, it has been postulated that VIP and secretin share common (or very closely related) receptors that are quite different from those of glucagon.

Distribution and Cells of Origin

VIP is widely distributed in the gastrointestinal tract. Using a specific radioimmunoassay for VIP, Bloom et al.[29] reported that in monkeys the largest amounts of VIP were in the colon (235 ± 84 μg) and ileum (105 ± 23 μg), with lesser amounts in the gastric fundus, duodenum, and jejunum. In the dog intestinal tract, the concentrations of VIP were highest in the ileum (35 ng/mg protein), followed by the jejunum (15 ng/mg) and duodenum (5 ng/mg).[30] Polak et al.[31] utilized immunohistochemistry and electron microscopy to study the VIP cells in the gastrointestinal tract of a number of species. The data on the distribution of cells substantiated the radioimmunoassay findings. VIP cells were usually pyramidal rather than oval and frequently had long apical processes extending toward the lumena of glands; they have tentatively been identified as H cells.[32] Recently, Bryant et al.[33] reported that brain tissue from humans as well as from mice, rats, and pigs contained significant amounts of VIP. In the rat, the highest concentrations were in the hemisphere (27.5 ± 6.4 pmole/g) and brainstem (4.0 ± 1.0 pmole/g). Similar concentrations were detected in human brain (compared to 136 ± 27 pmole/g in human colon). Immunohistochemical techniques were utilized to demonstrate specific VIP staining in nerve fibers in the pancreas, salivary gland, and myenteric plexus of the distal intestine. The data suggested that VIP may have a dual role, as gastrointestinal hormone and as neurotransmitter.

Actions

Cardiorespiratory Effects. VIP was initially recognized and named because of its potent vasodepressor activity.[15] Intraarterial infusions of VIP (40 ng/kg) increased femoral artery flow by 50 percent while doses of 400 ng/kg tripled systemic blood flow, an

Table 135–1. Comparative Structures of Secretinlike Peptide Hormones

	1	2	3	4	5	6	7	8	9	10	11	12	13	14	15	16	17	18	19	20	21	22
VIP	His	Ser	Asp	Ala	Val	Phe	Thr	Asp	Asn	Tyr	Thr	Arg	Leu	Arg	Lys	Gln	Met	Ala	Val	Lys	Lys	Tyr
Secretin	His	Ser	Asp	Gly	Thr	Phe	Thr	Ser	Glu	Leu	Ser	Arg	Leu	Arg	Asp	Ser	Ala	Arg	Leu	Gln	Arg	Leu
Glucagon	His	Ser	Gln	Gly	Thr	Phe	Thr	Ser	Asp	Tyr	Ser	Lys	Tyr	Leu	Asp	Ser	Arg	Arg	Ala	Gln	Asp	Phe
GIP	Tyr	Ala	Glu	Gly	Thr	Phe	Ile	Ser	Asp	Tyr	Ser	Ile	Ala	Met	Asp	Lys	Ile	Arg	Gln	Gln	Asp	Phe

	23	24	25	26	27	28	29	30	31	32	33	34	35	36	37	38	39	40	41	42	43
VIP	Leu	Asn	Ser	Ile	Leu	Asn	NH_2														
Secretin	Leu	Gln	Gly	Leu	Val	NH_2															
Glucagon	Val	Gln	Trp	Leu	Met	Asp	Thr														
GIP	Val	Asn	Trp	Leu	Leu	Ala	Gln	Gln	Lys	Gly	Lys	Lys	Ser	Asp	Trp	Lys	His	Asn	Ile	Thr	Gln

effect which persisted for 27 min. Intravenous infusions (400 ng/kg) lowered systemic blood pressure by 15 mm Hg, while cardiac output increased by 43 percent. These effects were more consistent with a primary inhibitory effect on peripheral resistance. Similar observations were made in the splanchnic, coronary, and pulmonary circulations. Infusions of VIP at doses of 0.04-0.4 μg/kg/min increased the flow in the hepatic artery by 41 percent and in the portal vein by 15 percent; superior mesenteric artery flow was decreased by 5 percent.[34] As will be discussed below, caval infusions were more effective in inducing changes in both splanchnic flow and resistance than were infusions in the portal circulation.[14] In canine studies, Yoshida et al.[35] reported that at doses that were too small to affect either blood flow or blood pressure, VIP increased coronary flow; at 2 μg/kg it stimulated flow by an average of 69.5 percent. In addition, VIP had a positive inotropic effect on cardiac muscle in vivo and in vitro, the magnitude of which was comparable to that of glucagon.[36] Finally, studies by Said and Kitamura[37] demonstrated that VIP decreased peripheral vascular resistance in isolated perfused canine lungs in which pulmonary arterial hypertension had been induced either by ventilation with 8 percent 0_2 or with infusion of histamine.

VIP has been shown to have very potent effects on the lungs. In addition to dilating pulmonary vessels, VIP relaxed isolated guinea pig trachea.[38] This bronchodilator effect was shown to significantly (> 25 percent) antagonize the constrictive effects of histamine and prostaglandin $F_{2\alpha}$ ($PGF_{2\alpha}$) on pulmonary resistance and compliance.[39] In addition, VIP has been shown to augment alveolar and minute ventilation by 30 percent, increasing both rate and tidal volume. This increase was shown to be abolished by chemoreceptor denervation, suggesting that respiratory augmentation is attributable to chemoreceptor stimulation.[15]

Metabolic Effects. The metabolic effects of VIP are similar to those of glucagon, both compounds causing lipolysis and glycogenolysis. In isolated fat cells from rat epididymal fat pads, VIP significantly stimulated lipolysis (D_{50} of 26.3 ng/ml).[40] This effect was shown to be mediated via the adenyl cyclase system. VIP stimulated adenyl cyclase activity and lipolysis in rat epididymal fat cells; in fat cells from chicken gizzard fat, VIP stimulated neither adenyl cyclase nor lipolytic activity.

The glycogenolytic and hyperglycemic effects of VIP have been demonstrated in vivo and in vitro.[41] In dogs, intravenous infusion of VIP (3.6 μg/kg) increased blood sugar by an average of 21.7 percent, and in this regard demonstrated 33.5 percent of the activity of glucagon. In experiments utilizing rabbit liver slices in vitro, VIP had 60 percent of the glycogenolytic activity of glucagon. VIP was shown to release insulin by two mechansims, an indirect one resulting from hyperglycemia and a direct incretic effect (demonstrated in vitro),[42] in the presence of glucose.[42] As is discussed in the section dealing with the WDHA syndrome, intravenous infusion of VIP in dogs caused slight hypercalcemia.[21]

Hematopoietic System. Band and Chang recently demonstrated that VIP (4–8 μg/ml) inhibits ADP- and collagen-induced platelet aggregation (quoted in ref. 43).

Gastrointestinal Tract. VIP is a potent inhibitor of all gastric functions. Intravenous infusion of this peptide (0.5– 8 μg/kg/hr) inhibited gastric acid secretion stimulated by pentagastrin, histamine,[44,45] and a meal.[46] In addition, VIP inhibited gastric pepsin secretion (by 75 percent) and motility[45] and substantially reduced the serum gastrin response to a meal.[46] The competitive nature of the inhibition of gastric acid secretion as well as the inhibition of both histamine-stimulated acid secretion and gastric pepsin secretion are all unique characteristics of VIP.

In its actions on the pancreas, VIP is a partial agonist of the effects of secretin. Intravenous infusion of VIP in dogs[21,45] and cats[47] stimulated pancreatic secretion of water and bicarbonate. The responses occurred within 5 min and were short lived (about 15 min). Given as a background to increasing amounts of secretin, VIP increased the submaximal responses by as much as 70 percent but did not augment the maximal response to secretin. In its actions on the pancreas, VIP was approximately one-sixth to one-fourth as potent as secretin. VIP did not stimulate pancreatic enzyme secretion (although it increased enzyme output by stimulating flow). The pancreatic effects of VIP appear to be mediated via the adenyl cyclase system.[24,48] VIP was shown to relax the isolated guinea pig gallbladder and to counteract the contractile effect of CCK-PZ.[49] Infusion of large amounts of VIP augmented bile flow in dogs, but this effect was almost certainly pharmacologic.[34]

In contrast to its actions on the stomach, VIP was shown to be a potent stimulant of intestinal secretion.[50] The peptide evoked a stimulatory response within 5 min after starting an intravenous infusion (13 μg/min). The effect was considerably greater in the ileum than in the jejunum. In this action, VIP was considerably more potent than either glucagon or secretin. In this regard, glucagon was a partial agonist with an efficacy of 0.55. The intestinal secretory effect appeared to be mediated by the adenyl cyclase system. Schwartz et al.[51] demonstrated that in rabbit ileal mucosa in vitro, VIP (0.1–2.0 μg/ml) stimulated cAMP production. When added to the serosal side of an Ussing chamber containing rabbit ileal mucosa, VIP (2 μg/ml) stimulated secretion of sodium and chloride and increased the short-circuit current. Although these studies suggested that the intestinal effects of VIP were predominantly secretory, Jaffer et al.[52] demonstrated that VIP also caused contraction of duodenal and ileal smooth muscle in vitro.

The actions of VIP are summarized in Table 135-2 and can be compared to those of secretin (Table 135-3) and glucagon (Table 135-4). The gastrointestinal effects of VIP have been reviewed by Makhlouf and Said.[53]

Table 135-2. Effects of Vasoactive Intestinal Polypeptide

Effects of Vasoactive Intestinal Polypeptide
Cardiorespiratory
Decreased peripheral resistance
Increased systemic, splanchnic, coronary, and pulmonary arterial flow
Systemic hypotension
Increased cardiac output
Positive inotropic effect
Bronchodilitation
Stimulation of respiration
Metabolic
Lipolysis
Glycogenolysis and hyperglycemia
Insulin release
Hypercalcemia
Hematopoietic
Inhibition of platelet aggregation
Gastrointestinal
Inhibition of gastric acid and pepsin secretion
Inhibition of gastric motility
Inhibition of gastrin release
Stimulation of pancreatic bicarbonate and water secretion
Augmentation of bile flow
Intestinal secretion of volume and electrolytes

Table 135-3. Biologic Actions and Release of Secretin

Actions
Stimulates contraction of
Gallbladder
Pyloric sphincter
Inhibits contraction of
Lower esophageal sphincter*
Stomach*
Intestine*
Stimulates water–electrolyte secretion of
Pancreas*
Liver*
Brunner's glands
Inhibits water–electrolyte secretion of stomach
Inhibits water–electrolyte absorption of
Intestine
Gallbladder
Stimulates secretion of enzymes in
Stomach
Pancreas*
Stimulates secretion of insulin**
Inhibits secretion of
Gastrin
Glucagon
Stimulates lipolysis
Increases
Heart rate
Stroke volume
Stimulates blood flow in
Superior mesenteric artery
Femoral artery
Pancreas
Small intestine
Inhibits blood flow in
Hepatic artery
Gastric mucosa
Inhibits gastrin-induced parietal cell hyperplasia
Release
Hydrochloric acid* (as of 1976 the only known physiologic substance)
Food (data contradictory)
Protein†
Fat†
Vagus†
Local neural mechanisms†

*Physiologic.
†Possible.

Table 135-4. Biologic Actions of Glucagon

Stimulates water–electrolyte secretion in
Liver
Brunner's glands
Inhibits water–electrolyte secretion in
Pancreas
Stomach
Inhibits enzyme secretion of pancreas
Stimulates secretion of insulin
Stimulates lipolysis, glycogenolysis, and gluconeogenesis
Inhibits contraction of
Stomach
Intestine
Sphincter of Oddi
Increases
Heart rate
Stroke volume
Increases blood flow in
Superior mesenteric artery
Femoral artery
Small intestine
Decreases blood flow in
Hepatic artery
Gastric mucosa

Release

Very little is known about the mechanisms of release of VIP. In a preliminary canine study, Ebeid et al.[54] reported that calcium infusion increased peripheral concentrations of radioimmunoassayable VIP. VIP levels increased within 3 min and had returned to basal levels within 30 min. There are as yet no data on the possible VIP response to a meal.

Inactivation

By monitoring the stimulation of pancreatic secretion, femoral and splanchnic blow flows, and systemic blood pressure, several studies[14,47,55] demonstrated that infusion of VIP into the portal vein evokes significantly smaller responses than systemically administered peptide. Since these studies implicated the liver in its inactivation, the peripheral levels of VIP have been studied in a number of patients with cirrhosis and resultant portosystemic shunts. Since VIP reproduces some of the symptoms of cirrhosis, including peripheral vasodilitation, glucose intolerance, and hyperventilation, it was suggested that VIP which gained access to the systemic circulation might be implicated in the etiology of these abnormalities. Unfortunately, the data have been inconsistent. Said et al.[56] reported elevated peripheral VIP levels in cirrhotic patients. In the studies of Ebeid et al.[57] cirrhotics had higher levels of VIP following creation of a portocaval shunt (168 ± 29 pg/ml) than preoperatively (94 ± 18 pg/ml); 4 patients with hepatic insufficiency had significantly elevated levels, 302 ± 68 pg/ml). On the other hand, Elias et al.[58] reported normal levels of VIP in 44 patients with liver disease (20 ± 8 pg/ml versus controls 18 ± 9 pg/ml), including subgroups of patients with surgical protocaval shunts (21 ± 10 pg/ml), natural shunts (21 ± 9 pg/ml), and hepatic encephalopathy (20 ± 8 pg/ml).

Conclusions

The hormonal status of VIP is still uncertain. The peptide has been localized to a specific intestinal cell, its spectrum of action has been delineated, and it has been potentially implicated in the etiology of the WDHA syndrome (see below). However, there have been no data which demonstrate that VIP is released following a physiologic stimulus such as a meal. The effects of VIP have been elucidated by experiments utilizing exogenous VIP; there have been none performed in which endogenous VIP has been shown to elicit any response. These experiments are critical before VIP can be classified as a hormone. As a "candidate hormone," VIP awaits a physiologic assignment.

GASTRIC INHIBITORY POLYPEPTIDE (GIP)

Chemistry

According to the description of Kosaka and Lim,[59] enterogastrone is a hormone that is released from the mucosa of the duodenum by fat or products of the digestion of fat and its primary function is the inhibition of gastric acid secretion and motility. Evidence for such an inhibitor was initially presented by Ewald and Boas;[60] these investigators demonstrated that the addition of olive oil to a meal depressed gastric acid secretion in human subjects. Later studies by Pavlov,[61] Farrell and Ivy,[62] and Feng et al.[63] substantiated the concept, implicated the duodenum, and noted that the humoral factor also inhibited gastric motility and pepsin secretion. The recent finding by Brown and Pederson that 10 percent pure porcine CCK-PZ contained potent enterogastrone activity,[64] and that this activity was independent of CCK-PZ (i.e., it had no effect on gall bladder contraction or on pancreatic enzyme secretion),[65] has led to the subsequent isolation and characterization of gastric inhibitory polypeptide (GIP).[66]

GIP has been purified from 10 percent pure porcine CCK-PZ by absorption to alginic acid followed by chromatography on carboxymethylcellulose and Sephadex G-25.[67] The pure preparation contained 2 IDU of CCK-PZ activity/mg and was very susceptible to degradation by trypsin. The absence of proline served to distinguish this peptide from CCK-PZ, as did the high concentration of glutamine and the lysine:arginine ratio. Pure porcine GIP is a polypeptide consisting of 43 amino acids with a calculated molecular weight of 5105.[68] The N- and C-terminal residues are tyrosine and glutamine, respectively. The structure of GIP (Table 135-1) shows a remarkable number of similarities with the structures of porcine glucagon and secretin; of the first 26 amino acid residues, 15 are shared in glucagon and 9 in secretin. Comparing the structures of porcine secretin and GIP, four nonconservative transformations[69] are evident, in positions 12 (Arg–Ile), 14 (Arg–Met), 16 (Ser–Lys), and 21 (Arg–Asp). The C-terminal heptadecapeptide sequence is unique among gastrointestinal hormones and contains four basic (lysines) and only one acidic (Asp) residue.

Structure–Function Relationships

Despite considerable structural similarity to secretin, glucagon, and VIP, very few comparative studies on the effects of these peptides have been performed. Consequently, as of now, it is impossible to ascribe specific functions to specific portions of the GIP molecule. The entire peptide sequence appears to be necessary for physiologic action; molecular fragments produced by cleavage with trypsin and cyanogen bromide (1–14 and 15–43) were incapable of stimulating insulin release.[70] Brown et al. [71,72] have recently provided evidence for molecular heterogeneity of GIP. Fractionation of circulating immunoreactive GIP (released by a mixed meal) on Sephadex G-50 yielded a major peak corresponding to that of ^{125}I-GIP, as well as a peak of larger molecular weight (and unknown physiologic importance).

Distribution and Cells of Origin

Brown et al.[71,72] and O'Dorisio et al.[73] demonstrated that concentrations of immunoreactive GIP were highest in acid–alcohol extracts of mid- and distal duodenum and jejunum. GIP was measured in lower concentrations in extracts of the gastric antrum, proximal duodenum, and ileum, but could not be identified in the colon, gastric fundus, or esophagus. Using immunofluorescence, histochemistry, and electron microscopy, Polak et al.[74] localized GIP cells in the midzone of the glands of the canine and human duodenum and to a lesser degree, jejunum. The GIP cell, now recognized as the K cell,[75] contains the hormone in characteristic 300-nm granules with electron-dense cores surrounded by less dense matrices.

Actions

GIP is a potent inhibitor of gastric acid secretion.[76] In canine experiments, infusions of GIP, 4 μg/kg/hr, produced a mean 40 percent inhibition of gastric acid secretion stimulated by histamine to 60 percent of maximum. This degree of inhibition is similar to that induced by fat in the duodenum.[77] Neither secretin nor CCK-PZ inhibit histamine-stimulated gastric acid secretion. GIP was similarly effective in inhibiting acid secretion stimulated by pentagastrin (1 μg/kg/hr caused 75 percent inhibition) and by insulin (4 μg/kg/hr caused 45 percent inhibition). Gastric pepsin secretion stimulated by histamine, pentagastrin, and insulin were similarly suppressed. GIP also inhibited gastric motility[68,72,78] and the meal-stimulated release of antral gastrin.[46,79] The infusions of exogenous GIP which have been shown to inhibit gastric secretory activity result in serum GIP levels comparable to those observed following a mixed meal.[70] The experiments of Brown and co-workers provided even more potent evidence that GIP plays a physiologic role in the control of gastric acid secretion; in these studies, gastric secretion was inhibited by endogenous GIP, liberated by duodenal irrigation with corn oil and glucose.[71]

Since impure preparations of CCK-PZ have been shown to stimulate insulin secretion and improve glucose tolerance during glucose administration,[80] Dupre et al.[81] studied the effects of exogenous pure GIP on insulin secretion in human volunteers. At a rate of 1 μg/min, infusions of GIP augmented serum GIP levels to 1.0 ng/ml (the peak postcibal GIP levels), suggesting that the dose chosen was physiologic. GIP administered in saline had no significant effect on either serum insulin or on plasma glucose concentrations. On the other hand, compared to the infusion of glucose alone, simultaneous administration of GIP and glucose doubled the rate of insulin secretion and decreased the plasma glucose concentrations by one-third, significantly improving the glucose tolerance curve. In dogs, infusion of graded doses (0.25, 0.5 and 1.5 μg/kg) of GIP (without glucose) resulted in dose-related increases in serum insulin levels and decreases in plasma glucose concentrations.[70] The insulinotropic action was further documented by the demonstration that GIP stimulated insulin release from perfused rat islets in vitro.[82,83] Recent experiments have suggested that GIP also releases glucagon from the rat pancreas in vivo and in vitro.[71] These observations are consistent with the postulate that GIP might be involved in the enteroinsular axis, the mechanism by which gastrointestinal hormones mediate the increased insulin response to oral administration of glucose.[84,85]

In dogs prepared with Thiry-Vella loops of jejunum and ileum, infusion of GIP (9 μg/min) caused profound and significant increases in secretory volume from both segments of the small intestine.[50] Neither secretin nor the active C-terminal fragment of CCK-PZ stimulated secretion of intestinal succus. Since large quantities of GIP were utilized in these studies, it is uncertain whether the effect is physiologic or pharmacologic in nature. GIP did not influence secretion from the pancreas, biliary tract, or Brunner's glands.[71]

Release

In order to measure endogenous concentrations of GIP, Kuzio et al.[86] developed a radioimmunoassay for this peptide. The assay system, which does not cross-react with any gastrointestinal hormone, utilizes guinea pig antibodies to porcine GIP and ^{125}I-porcine GIP. Fasting serum levels of GIP in 48 normal subjects averaged 237 ± 14 pg/ml. Following a standard breakfast, concentrations of GIP increased to more than 1200 pg/ml at 45 min, and, demonstrating a second peak at 120 min, remained elevated for 4 h. In attempting to interpret the biphasic pattern of GIP release following feeding, Brown[87] noted that only the second peak was identified in volunteers who ingested a fat suspension (Lipomul). Cleator and Gourley[88] also studied the effects of feeding on serum immunoreactive GIP levels. After a standard breakfast GIP increased from a mean baseline level of 410 ± 23 pg/ml to a peak of 3.5 ± 1.1 ng/ml 2 h later, and declined slowly over the subsequent 3 h. Since nothing is known about the circulating half-life of GIP, it was impossible to determine if the prolonged postcibal response was due to very slow inactivation of the peptide or to continuous stimulation of GIP release from the small intestine. The magnitude of the response to a mixed meal was greater than the response to any of its components which have been shown to release GIP, particularly fat, glucose, and amino acids.

O'Dorisio et al.[89] administered 50 ml of corn oil intraduodenally to 4 dogs with gastric and duodenal fistulas. GIP levels increased to a mean peak of 2525 pg/ml 60 min later; this release of GIP was associated with a 90 percent inhibition of pentagastrin-stimulated gastric acid secretion. Falco et al.[90] administered 67 g of corn oil to 10 normal human volunteers. From a mean fasting GIP level of 272 pg/ml, serum GIP levels increased within 15 min, peaked at 60 min (1345 ± 291 pg/ml), and declined very slowly, remaining significantly elevated at 180 min. Despite the pronounced release of GIP, there were no changes in either blood glucose or serum insulin levels. The absence of an insulinotropic effect of endogenous GIP raised serious question as to the role of GIP in the enteroinsular axis. However, Brown et al.[71] and Crockett et al.[91] recently demonstrated that endogenous GIP liberated by corn oil was capable of potentiating the release of insulin in human subjects; sequential administration of 25 g of glucose intravenously and 67 g of corn oil orally resulted in augmented insulin secretion and accelerated disposal of glucose. These studies implicate GIP in the enteric control of insulin secretion.

Oral glucose has been shown to be a potent stimulant of endogenous GIP release. Cataland et al.[92] demonstrated that ingestion of 75 g of glucose by 21 normal volunteers resulted in a rapid (less than 5 min) release of immunoreactive GIP, which peaked at 30 min. Basal levels (319 ± 18 pg/ml) increased to a mean maximum of only 747 ± 59 pg/ml, considerably lower than the peak levels achieved after a mixed meal. Release of insulin was augmented; insulin levels peaked at 85 ± 10 μU/ml (from a mean basal level of 11 ± μU/ml). Although intravenous infusion of a comparable amount of glucose resulted in a significantly higher blood glucose level, it did not stimulate release of GIP; insulin release peaked more rapidly (10 min) but at a much lower average level (32 ± 8 μU/ml). These studies demonstrated that GIP release did not depend on only the blood glucose concentration. This concept was supported by the studies of Andersen et al.[93] utilizing the glucose clamp technique. In the hyperglycemic and euglycemic clamps, oral glucose stimulated immunoreactive GIP release.

Abnormalities in oral glucose tolerance have been associated with abnormalities in GIP release. Adult-onset diabetics have normal basal GIP levels, but in response to an oral glucose load, they release significantly more immunoreactive GIP (peak 1400 pg/ml) than do normal controls (peak 750 pg/ml).[71,94] Similarly, patients with chronic pancreatitis (pancreatic diabetics) hyperrespond to a 50-g oral glucose load.[95] In 10 patients previously treated by vagotomy and pyloroplasty, rapid gastric emptying resulted in an earlier and more substantial release (peak at 15 min, 1510 ± 134 pg/ml) of GIP as well as insulin.[96] The exaggerated insulin release may be partially responsible for late hypoglycemia in some patients with the dumping syndrome.

Duodenal perfusion with glucose resulted in dose-dependent stimulation of endogenous GIP and inhibition of gastric acid secretion.[71,89]

Since intraduodenal amino acids have been shown to be insulinotropic, Thomas et al.[97] studied the GIP response to amino acids in 10 normal adults. Introduodenal amino acids stimulated significantly more GIP (integrated GIP secretion 13 ng/min/ml) and insulin (integrated insulin secretion 5 mU/min/ml) than did intravenous amino acids, despite the fact that the parenteral amino acids resulted in a higher mean peak α-amino nitrogen concentration. In more selective studies, these investigators were able to distinguish between amino acids that stimulate CCK-PZ (valine, tryptophan, phenylalanine, methionine) and trypsin release and those that stimulate release of GIP and insulin.[98] In contrast to amino acids, protein did not result in release of GIP.[88]

The actions and mechanisms of release of GIP are summarized in Table 135-5.

Inactivation and Catabolism

O'Dorisio et al.[99] recently provided evidence for renal inactivation of GIP. Sixteen uremic patients had significantly higher basal GIP levels than did normal controls (1006 ± 145 versus 132 ± 31 pg/ml). In addition, in the uremics, the GIP response to a meal was of greater magnitude and duration. After liberation of GIP by intraduodenal glucose, canine renal venous concentrations of GIP were 40 percent lower than arterial levels.

Conclusions

It is relatively certain that GIP is a classical hormone. It has been localized to a specific intestinal cell and shown to be released by fat, glucose, and amino acids. Endogenous GIP released by either fat or glucose inhibits gastric acid secretion and augments the insulin response to glucose. There are some problems, however. As Grossman has noted, for equal rises in serum immunoreactive GIP levels, exogenous hormone produces less inhibition of gastric acid secretion than does oral fat and releases less insulin than does oral glucose. Two possible explanations have been proposed: either the circulating form of the molecule and the compound purified from the intestinal mucosa are not identical, or, alternatively, GIP is neither the only incretin released by glucose nor the only enterogastrone released by fat. Answers to questions such as these should be forthcoming with continued research.

MOTILIN

Brown et al.[100] noted that perfusion of the canine duodenum either with an alkaline buffer or with a solution of pancreatic juice resulted in increased gastric motility (increased frequency and

Table 135-5. Biologic Actions and Release of GIP

Actions
Inhibition of
Gastric acid secretion
Gastric pepsin secretion
Gastric motility
Gastrin release
Stimulation of
Intestinal secretion
Insulin release
Glucagon release
No effect on
Pancreatic secretion
Biliary secretion
Brunner's glands secretion
Release
Standard meal
Oral glucose
Oral amino acids
Oral fat
Not released by
Alcohol
Meat extract (protein)
Acid in duodenum (presumed)

amplitude of contractions). Two possible explanations were entertained—release of a stimulatory agent or suppression of release of an inhibitory factor. The former possibility was substantiated by the subsequent observation that Boots pancreozymin stimulated the motility of denervated gastric pouches.[101] Fractionation of this pancreozymin preparation on Sephadex G-75 resulted in a fraction which stimulated gastric motility but did not stimulate protein release from the cat pancreas.[102] Starting with a side fraction in the purification of secretin from hog small intestinal mucosa, Brown and associates[103,104] utilized successive chromatography on carboxymethylcellulose, Sephadex G-25, TEAE-cellulose, and Sephadex G-25 to purify "motilin." The resultant peptide stimulated gastric motility and pepsin secretion but had no effect on acid secretion from fundic pouches. Purified motilin has a molecular weight of 2700 and consists of 22 amino acids. Its amino acid sequence, Phe–Val–Pro–Ile–Phe–Thr–Tyr–Gly–Glu–Leu–Gln–Arg–Met–Gln–Glu–Lys–Glu–Arg–Asn–Lys–Gly–Gln[11,104,105] is quite different from that of any other known gastrointestinal hormone.

The actions of motilin and a synthetic analogue, norleucine-13-motilin,[106] have been studied in a number of species. The predominant effect is on contractility of the smooth muscle of the gastrointestinal tract. In vitro, intestinal and gastric smooth muscle strips from man and rabbit (but not from dog, rat, or guinea pig) were contracted by norleucine-13-motilin in concentrations as low as 2×10^{-9} M;[107,108] these effects were not blocked by hexamethonium (ganglionic blockade), tetrodotoxin (axonal conduction blockade), or atropine (anticholinergic), but were inhibited by theophyllinelike drugs and inhibitors of calcium transport. Smooth muscle preparations from the uterus, gallbladder, and vascular system were unresponsive to motilin. In in vivo studies, motilin (0.1 ng/kg/hr) increased the tone of the antrum, fundus, duodenum, and lower esophageal sphincter,[109–111] stimulated gastric pepsin secretion,[112] and inhibited gastric protein synthesis.[113] Despite the increased gastric tone, norleucine-13 motilin slowed gastric emptying in man,[112] presumably because it simultaneously slowed propagation of antral electrical impulses.[114]

Using immunofluorescence, histochemistry, and electron microscopy, Pearse et al.[115] and Polak et al.[116] have localized motilin within the enterochromaffin (EC) cells. Motilin-containing EC cells were most numerous in the duodenum and upper jejunum, in which the pyramidal shaped cells were located in the lower portion of the mucosa with the hormone granules primarily on the basement membrane side. All motilin–EC cells were argyrophil and 85 percent were argentaffin. EC cells in the stomach and colon contained no motilin. This distribution of motilin was supported by studies in which immunoreactive motilin concentrations were measured in extracts of canine gastrointestinal mucosa.[117]

In the dog, alkalinization of the duodenum with 0.3M Tris buffer resulted in release of radioimmunoassayable motilin into the circulation. Basal levels averaged 294 ± 44 pg/ml; levels rose to 498 ± 100 pg/ml at 2 min and 916 ± 96 pg/ml at 5 min. This release of motilin was associated with a fivefold increase in motility. In man, duodenal alkalinization did not result in motilin release; on the contrary, within 3 min after duodenal *acidification* with 50 ml of 0.1N HCl, motilin levels rose 60 percent (from a mean basal value of 25 pmol/liter) and remained significantly elevated for 45 min.[118] The duration of the elevation of plasma motilin levels is somewhat difficult to interpret since the pancreaticoduodenal secretion must have neutralized the acid within a few minutes and the half-life of motilin has been shown to be 4.5 min.[119]

At present, it is impossible to adequately assess the physiologic importance of motilin. The apparent threshhold pH at which motilin is released from the canine small intestine, 8.5, is higher than the usual physiologic range. In human studies, elevations of gastric pH and diversion of gastric acid from the duodenum have been shown to stimulate gastric motility;[120,121] however, in man, recent studies have demonstrated that motilin is released following duodenal acidification (rather than alkalinization) and slows gastric emptying. At this time, there is no evidence that motilin plays a significant role in the phsyiologic control of gastric emptying. Since motilin causes contraction of both the stomach and the colon, an alternative possibility is that motilin mediates the gastrocolic reflex. Whether or not motilin plays a physiologic role in gastrointestinal function remains to be clarified.

MAMMALIAN AND AVIAN PANCREATIC POLYPEPTIDES

As byproducts in the purification of insulin and glucagon, two laboratories independently isolated homologous pancreatic polypeptide hormones.[122,123] Purified sequentially by acid–alcohol extraction, gel filtration, ion-exchange chromatography using DEAE-cellulose, and droplet countercurrent distribution,[124] the 4200 molecular weight peptides have been sequenced as shown in Table 135-6. The avian and mammalian peptides have signficant structural homology, with 16 common amino acid residues. The similarities among the four mammalian peptides are even more striking, with variations only in positions 2, 6, and 23. The C-terminal tyrosine amide is critical for biologic activity.[125]

It has been very difficult to evaluate the biologic role of bovine pancreatic polypeptide (BPP), since for all actions studied, both stimulatory and inhibitory responses have been demonstrated.[126,127] In the nonsecreting dog, BPP (20–100 μg/kg/hr) stimulated gastric acid secretion from both vagally innervated and denervated portions of the stomach; on the other hand, in the presence of spontaneous or pentagastrin-stimulated acid secretion, BPP (40–50 μg/kg/hr) was a potent inhibitor. Given by slow intravenous infusion, BPP (5–10 μg/kg/hr) caused relaxation of the pylorus, pyloric sphincter, duodenum, ileocecal sphincter, and descending colon; larger doses (50–100 μg/kg/hr) caused increased motility. The gallbladder, choledochus, and pancreas were quite sensitive to BPP. At 0.125–5.0 μg/kg/hr, BPP relaxed the gallbladder and increased choledochal tone without altering bile flow. The effect of BPP on pancreatic secretion of water and bicarbonate was complex and dose related. Secretin-stimulated pancreatic secretion was augmented by low (0.0125–0.025 μg/kg) and inhibited by high (1–5 μg/kg) doses of BPP; intravenous infusions of BPP caused a biphasic response—initial stimulation with subsequent inhibition. Finally, pancreatic enzyme and protein secretion were suppressed by BPP.

The spectrum of actions of avian pancreatic polypeptide (APP) is somewhat clearer, as both metabolic and gastric effects have been described.[128,129] In 6-week-old chickens, intravenous injection of APP (100 μg/kg) caused profound hepatic glycogen depletion and hypoglycerolemia, paradoxically, without altering plasma glucose levels. At considerably lower doses (6.25 μg/kg) APP caused several-fold increases in proventricular ("gastric") volume, acid, pepsin, and total protein secretion; this action was of greater magnitude and duration than the effect of pentagastrin. APP did not influence the rates of bile, pancreatic, or gizzard secretion and did not alter cardiovascular dynamics. Unfortunately, to date, there are no data on the spectrum of actions of the human pancreatic polypeptide (HPP).

Pancreatic APP concentrations have been measured in a number of avian species.[130] In all species examined, including pidgeon,

Table 135–6. Structure of Pancreatic Polypeptides

	1	2	3	4	5	6	7	8	9	10	11	12	13	14	15	16	17	18
Bovine	Ala	Pro	Leu	Glu	Pro	Gln	Tyr	Pro	Gly	Asp	Asp	Ala	Thr	Pro	Glu	Gln	Met	Ala
Human	Ala	Pro	Leu	Glu	Pro	Val	Tyr	Pro	Gly	Asp	Asp	Ala	Thr	Pro	Glu	Gln	Met	Ala
Ovine	Ala	Ser	Leu	Glu	Pro	Gln	Tyr	Pro	Gly	Asp	Asp	Ala	Thr	Pro	Glu	Gln	Met	Ala
Porcine	Ala	Pro	Leu	Glu	Pro	Val	Tyr	Pro	Gly	Asp	Asp	Ala	Thr	Pro	Glu	Gln	Met	Ala
Avian	Gly	Pro	Ser	Gln	Pro	Thr	Tyr	Pro	Gly	Asp	Asp	Ala	Pro	Val	Glu	Asp	Leu	Ile

	19	20	21	22	23	24	25	26	27	28	29	30	31	32	33	34	35	36
Bovine	Gln	Tyr	Ala	Ala	Gln	Leu	Arg	Arg	Tyr	Ile	Asn	Met	Leu	Thr	Arg	Pro	Arg	Tyr-NH_2
Human	Gln	Tyr	Ala	Ala	Asp	Leu	Arg	Arg	Tyr	Ile	Asn	Met	Leu	Thr	Arg	Pro	Arg	Tyr-NH_2
Ovine	Gln	Tyr	Ala	Ala	Glu	Leu	Arg	Arg	Tyr	Ile	Asn	Met	Leu	Thr	Arg	Pro	Arg	Tyr-NH_2
Porcine	Gln	Tyr	Ala	Ala	Glu	Leu	Arg	Arg	Tyr	Ile	Asn	Met	Leu	Thr	Arg	Pro	Arg	Tyr-NH_2
Avian	Arg	Phe	Tyr	Asp	Asn	Leu	Gln	Gln	Tyr	Leu	Asn	Val	Val	Thr	Arg	His	Arg	Tyr-NH_2

goose, guinea foul, duck, spoonbill, owl, and hawk, significant APP-like immunoreactivity was demonstrated. Among chickens, pancreatic APP concentrations were highest in 19-day embryos (13 mg/100 g) and somewhat less in day-old chicks (6 mg/100 g); in older animals, pancreatic concentrations averaged 3–4 mg/100 g. No APP was detected in extracts of chicken heart, gizzard, liver, spleen, small intestine, or proventriculus. Using immunofluorescent techniques, Larsson et al.[131] localized APP within polygonal or spindle-shaped cells distributed throughout the exocrine pancreas. The APP cells contained cytoplasmic peptide-containing granules, were distinct from the A, B, and D islet cells, and had the capacity to take up and decarboxylate L-dopa. In contrast to the distribution of APP, HPP has been localized within cells on the periphery of the islets; only very few HPP cells were noted within the exocrine parenchyma and the relatively small ducts.[132]

Radioimmunoassay systems have been utilized to demonstrate postcibal release of pancreatic polypeptide in birds[133] and man.[134–136] Basal levels of HPP averaged 50 ± 3 pg/ml. Release of pancreatic polypeptide was stimulated better by protein and dilute acid than by fat or carbohydrate. Partial pancreatectomy markedly reduced both fasting APP levels and the humoral response to feeding.[133] In man, the postcibal HPP response was biphasic: 20–30 min following a meal, serum levels of HPP increased from 48 ± 5 to 385 ± 55 pmol/liter and reached a later 4-h plateau of 300 ± 50 pmol/liter.[136] Fourteen patients with duodenal ulcer disease had elevated basal HPP levels (110 ± 40 pmol/liter). Following vagotomy, the HPP response to a meal was virtually abolished, suggesting that release of the peptide was under neural control.

In a recent study, Polak et al.[137] demonstrated high tissue (20/33) and plasma (18/28) levels of HPP in patients with pancreatic APUDomas. HPP immunofluorescent cells were located among clusters of cells producing other hormones and were numerous in both primary and metastatic tumor tissue. The role of HPP in these tumors is not clear.

In summary, homologous mammalian and avian polypeptides have been purified from the pancreas, localized to a specific immunofluorescent cell, and shown to be released following a protein meal. The physiologic role of these peptides remains to be elucidated. They remain peptide hormones without known effects.

BOMBESIN

Erspamer and Melchiorri[138] have carefully screened extracts of the skin of 500 species of frogs for biologically active peptides. They have described four families of peptides—the bombesinlike, the physaelaminlike, the caeruleinlike, and the bradykininlike peptides. The family of bombesinlike peptides (Table 135-7) has received considerable attention recently because of potent effects on the gastrointestinal tract. A number of investigators have proposed that bombesin may play a physiologic role in mammals, mediating the release of gastrin from the antrum. The recent reports that human antra contain immunoreactive bombesinlike material[139–141] supports this possibility.

Bombesin is a tetradecapeptide which has been extracted from the skins of two European frogs, *Bombina bombina* and *Bombina variegata*. The frog skins contain 200–700 μg of bom-

Table 135-7. Structure of Bombesinlike Peptides

	1	2	3	4	5	6	7	8	9	10	11	12	13	14
Bombesin	Pyroglu	Glu	Arg	Leu	Gly	Asn	Gln	Trp	Ala	Val	Gly	His	Leu	Met NH_2
Alytesin	Pyroglu	Gly	Arg	Leu	Gly	Thr	Gln	Trp	Ala	Val	Gly	His	Leu	Met NH_2
Ranatensin				Pyroglu	Val	Pro	Gln	Trp	Ala	Val	Gly	His	Phe	Met NH_2
Litorin						Pyroglu	Gln	Trp	Ala	Val	Gly	His	Phe	Met NH_2

besin/g wet weight. In purifying bombesin, methanolic abstracts were subjected to chromatography on alkaline alumina columns, followed by elution with descending concentrations of ethanol. The C-terminal heptapeptide was found to be the smallest analogue which demonstrated any bombesinlike activity; the C-terminal nonapeptide is as active as the entire molecule.[142] The analogues, litorin, alytesin, and ranatensin, have similar effects on smooth muscle strips.[143,144] Bombesin has both gastrointestinal and extraintestinal actions, which are summarized in Table 135-8 and described below.

The primary gastrointestinal action is stimulation of gastrin release and gastric acid secretion. Intravenous infusion (50–200 ng/kg/hr) and subcutaneous injection (5–30 ng/kg) of bombesin stimulated gastric acid secretion (but not pepsin secretion) in dogs with Heidenhain pouches and gastric fistulas.[145] The acid secretory response was virtually totally abolished by atropine (0.2 mg/kg) and substantially inhibited (50 percent) by hexamethonium (5 mg/kg). Infusions of bombesin (0.1–1.0 μg/kg/hr) stimulated release of immunoreactive gastrin;[141,146–148] following a 60-min infusion, gastrin levels rose from 68 ± 10 to 289 ± 17 pg/ml. Gastrin release was directly related to the bombesin dose. Gastrin levels fell after the infusion was stopped and reached basal levels within 60 min. At the peak of bombesin infusion, feeding did not augment the gastrin response. The acid secretory response and the release of gastrin were both significantly delayed and inhibited (almost 40 percent) by acidification of the antrum. Antrectomy suppressed (by 80–90 percent) the secretory and gastrin responses to bombesin infusion. Atropine, secretin, and metiamide reduced the gastric acid secretory response to bombesin but did not significantly affect the release of gastrin from the antrum. During bombesin infusin, little gastrin (see below) was released almost immediately and peaked rapidly, whereas levels of big gastrin rose more slowly but were sustained. These effects were confirmed in human experiments[149,150] which demonstrated that bombesin liberated only antral (not duodenal) gastrin.

Bombesin infusions in dogs and normal humans were shown to cause gallbladder contraction and decrease the opening pressure of the ampulla of Vater.[151–154] Secretion of an enzyme-rich bicarbonate-poor pancreatic fluid was stimulated as well.[155] These effects were not abolished by antrectomy, suggesting that bombesin also releases CCK-PZ.[151] Bombesin-induced release of immunoreactive CCK-PZ was recently documented,[7] and release of secretin was disproved.[156,157]

Bombesin has gastrin-independent effects on intestinal motility. The myoelectrical effects reported by Caprilli et al.[158] included an increase in the pacesetter potential in the antrum, duodenum, jejunum, and ileum, reduction in the propagation velocity of the pacesetter potential, abolition of spikes in the duodenum and jejunum (but not in the antrum or ileum), "electrical disorganization" in the duodenum (a characteristic electrical pattern with irregular sequences of small and slow potentials), and no consistent effect on the colon. The motility counterpart was total inhibition of duodenal and jejunal motility (preceded in the duodenum by a short stimulation) and contraction of the pyloric–antral region and the ileocecal valve; after cessation of the bombesin infusion, motor activity rebounded, producing motor hyperactivity and acceleration of intestinal transit.[159,160]

The extragastrointestinal effects of bombesin included hypertension due to contraction of vascular muscle,[161] contraction of urinary tract and bronchial smooth muscle,[162,163] and an antidiuretic effect on the kidney which proceeded in some infusions to complete cessation of urine flow.[164]

Polak et al.[140] have recently studied the distribution of immunoreactive bombesin cells in the human gastrointestinal tract. The cells (probably H cells) were noted throughout the length of the gastrointestinal tract (but not in the pancreas) but were most concentrated in the duodenum. In a single tumor which caused the Zollinger-Ellison syndrome but was found to be devoid of gastrin, bombesinlike immunoreactivity was detected. These observations suggest that bombesin or a bombesinlike peptide may play a physiologic role in man, mediating the release of gastrin from the antrum. The confirmation of this hypothesis awaits the development of radioimmunoassay systems sensitive enough to measure changes in serum bombesin levels during physiologic events that increase gastrin release and gastric acid secretion.

Table 135-8. Biologic Actions of Bombesin

Stimulation of antral gastrin release
Stimulation of gastric acid secretion
Contraction of the gallbladder
Stimulation of pancreatic secretion of water and enzymes
Stimulation of CCK-PZ release
Inhibition of intestinal myoelectric activity
Inhibition of intestinal motility
Hypertension
Contraction of urinary and bronchial smooth muscle
Antidiuretic effect on the kidney

SECRETIN AND CCK-PZ UPDATED

Secretin

Since two major actions of secretin are the stimulation of pancreatic bicarbonate secretion and the inhibition of acid secretion, it has long been assumed that secretin plays a postcibal role in controlling pancreatic exocrine and gastric secretory function. This assumption has been challenged by recent experiments that have attempted to correlate changes in pancreatic and gastric secretion with alterations in circulating levels of immunoreactive secretin. Rhodes and colleagues[164a] have utilized secretin infusions to demonstrate that increments in plasma secretin as small as 20 pg/ml were sufficient to increase pancreatic bicarbonate output by 10-fold. However, attempts by several investigators to demonstrate meal-stimulated increases in circulating secretin have consistently failed. Secretin release has been demonstrated following acidification of the duodenum to a luminal pH below 3.5[164b–164d] Under normal circumstances, feeding does not lower the intraduodenal pH below 4.5, however, it does result in stimulation of pancreatic bicarbonate secretion. Abolition of HCl-induced secretin release by somatostatin does not totally suppress stimulation of pancreatic exocrine secretion.[164e] Duodenal acidification has been shown to suppress gastric acid secretion, but this inhibitory effect could not be reproduced by infusions of secretin, which resulted in plasma secretin levels considerably higher than those observed after intraduodenal acid.[164b] Furthermore, the studies of Ward and Bloom were unable to establish any relationship between secretin levels and rates of gastric secretion.[164b] Vagotomy has been shown to abolish the gastric inhibitory response to duodenal acidification[164f] but not to suppress HC1-induced secretin release.[164g] On the basis of these observations, it is difficult to ascribe a major physiologic role to secretin. One possible explanation is a synergistic effect of secretin plus cholecystokinin or VIP, in which case minute amounts of postprandial secretin might have potent actions.

Another role ascribed to secretin has been the modulation of intestinal glucose- and amino acid-induced insulin release.[164h]

However, irrigation of the duodenum with a number of sugars, amino acids, and fatty acids failed to increase peripheral secretin levels.[164i,j]

New roles for secretin have been proposed. Henry and colleagues suggested that since secretin levels rose progressively with starvation, the lipolytic action of this peptide may play a protective role by providing nutrition.[164k] Straus and associates have implicated secretin in the pathogenesis of pancreatitis; they demonstrated that ingestion of ethanol, known to cause spasm in the sphincter of Oddi, caused a substantial increase in plasma secretin.[164l] In coeliac disease, postcibal pancreatic exocrine secretion is diminished, presumably due to failure of duodenal secretin release. Depressed secretin responsiveness to duodenal acidification has been documented in adults and children with coeliac disease[164] but concentrations of intestinal S cells[164n,o] have been described as both abnormally low[164m] and high.[164p] Failure of secretin release has also been implicated in the pathogenesis of duodenal ulcer disease, and the beneficial effects of carbenoxylone on ulcer healing have been ascribed to augmented secretin release.[164q] However, in two comparative studies,[164g,r] duodenal ulcer patients and normal controls released similar amounts of secretin in response to duodenal acidification,[164r] thus nullifying this hypothesis on the etiology of peptic ulcer disease.

The biologic half-life of secretin is quite short, in the range of 3 min.[164s] The evidence as to the major site of inactivation of secretin is contradictory. Chey and colleagues[164t] noted that secretin administered via the portal vein produced less inhibition of gastric acid secretion than did identical infusions via the systemic route; furthermore, in isolated perfused rat livers, CCl_4 treatment prolonged the biologic activity of secretin threefold. Similar observations were made by Kolts and associates,[164u] who reported significant prolongation of the immunologic half-life of exogenous secretin in cirrhotic adults. In contrast, Curtis and co-workers[164v] did not demonstrate hepatic uptake or catabolism of either exogenous or endogenous secretin but did document a major catabolic role for the kidney. The discrepancies in these studies may be explained by differences in radioimmunoassay antibody specificity in terms of the portions of the secretin molecule recognized. This is complicated by recent descriptions of at least one larger circulating molecular form of secretin.[164w,x]

CCK-PZ

Postcibal release of CCK-PZ has been demonstrated by a number of investigators. Milk[164y] and fatty meals[164z,aa] were shown to be potent stimulants of CCK-PZ release, and the response to a mixed meal (166 g carbohydrate, 59 g protein, 9 g fat) persisted for more than 4 h. In addition to the normal responses, a number of abnormalities in release of CCK-PZ have been described. Diabetics and patients with duodenal ulcer disease had early, short-lived responses.[164bb] In the latter group of patients, treatment with metiamide (an H_2 receptor antagonist) lowered basal levels of immunoreactive CCK-PZ, suggesting that basal rates of CCK-PZ secretion may depend upon stimulation of duodenal and jejunal mucosa by secreted gastric acid;[164cc] in contrast, Bilroth II gastrectomy has been shown to impair postcibal CCK-PZ release.[164dd] Patients with the Zollinger-Ellison syndrome have markedly elevated basal levels of CCK-PZ, but no correlation has been established with levels of serum gastrin.[164bb]

Patients with exocrine pancreatic insufficiency have CCK-PZ levels one-hundred-fold elevated above the normal range ($>$ 50 pg/ml).[164y] The presumed explanation for this abnormality is failure of trypsin-mediated feedback inhibition of CCK-PZ release. The elevated CCK-PZ levels may explain a number of abnormalities in patients with pancreatitis and exocrine deficiency, including accelerated gastric emptying and increased concentrations of intestinal mucosal enzymes.

Patients with coeliac disease have been shown to have both impaired release of CCK-PZ as well as decreased reponsiveness to endogenous and exogenous hormone. These observations have been substantiated by recent radioimmunoassay studies;[164ee] 9 of 10 patients studied had elevated basal levels of CCK-PZ (mean coeliac 1081 ± 250; normal 68 ± 28 pg/ml). They did not yet have tonic gallbladder contractions. Following a fatty meal, CCK-PZ levels rose only about one-fifth as much as normal and gallbladder emptying was markedly delayed and reduced.

CCK-PZ has also been implicated in the control of appetite[164ff] and of gastric emptying.[164gg] Excessive circulating concentrations of CCK-PZ may cause irritable bowel symptoms as well as functional dyspepsia.[164hh,ii]

CCK-PZ is produced in the I cells[164jj] particularly prevalent in the duodenal and jejunal mucosa.[164aa] The hormone has a short biologic half-life of about 3 min.[164bb] It is largely taken up and metabolized by the kidney.[164bb]

ENDOCRINE ABNORMALITIES

ZOLLINGER-ELLISON SYNDROME

Although a number of reports had identified patients with peptic ulcer disease, gastric acid hypersecretion, and non-beta islet cell tumors,[165–167] Zollinger and Ellison[168] first proposed that the islet cell tumors produced an ulcerogenic hormone which mediated the symptoms of the peptic ulcer. Using a dog bioassay, Gregory et al.[169] and Grossman et al.[170] reported that ulcerogenic tumors contained a gastrinlike material. A subsequent report[171] documented that the amino acid composition of the secretagogue from an extract of Zollinger-Ellison tumor was identical to that of gastrin. The role of gastrin in the ulcerogenic syndrome was confirmed by the studies of McGuigan and Trudeau[172] which demonstrated that patients with the Zollinger-Ellison syndrome had markedly elevated serum levels of immunoreactive gastrin. The availability of gastrin radioimmunoassay systems has dramatically improved the clinician's ability to diagnose the Zollinger-Ellison syndrome; as a result, the spectrum of the disease has broadened considerably. Although only about 1000 well-documented cases have been reported, the frequency of diagnosis of this syndrome has increased and it is now estimated that it accounts for almost 1 percent of operative cases of peptic ulcer disease. In the following section, the clinical manifestations of the Zollinger-Ellison syndrome and recent observations on the hormone, gastrin, will be summarized.

Clinical Features

The triad initially characterized by Zollinger and Ellison[168] included recalcitrant peptic ulcer disease, gastric acid hypersecretion, and islet cell tumors. Diarrhea, steatorrhea, and multiple endocrine abnormalities have each been reported with sufficient frequency to warrant inclusion in the list of the primary clinical characteristics.

Sixty percent of the reported patients have been male.[173] Although the majority of patients have been diagnosed between the third and fifth decades, the syndrome has been described in patients ranging from 7 to 90 years old.[174,175] Eighty percent of the patients were symptomatic for more than 1 yr before the diagnosis was established.

In their review of 244 patients, Ellison and Wilson[173] reported that 93 percent of the patients had peptic ulcer disease, while 7 percent had diarrhea alone (30 percent had both ulcers and diarrhea). In this series, pain was the most consistent symptom, attributable to acute perforation of an ulcer in 18 percent, to chronic ulceration in 74 percent, and to diarrhea in 15 percent; additional complaints included diarrhea (36 percent), vomiting (26 percent), melena (22 percent) and hematemesis (19 percent). In a series of 25 patients, Way et al.[176] reported that 90 percent had abdominal pain; in this group of patients, the ulcers were particularly virulent, causing serious hemorrhage in 40 percent and perforation in 36 percent.

In 65 percent of Zollinger-Ellison patients, the initial ulcer was in the duodenal bulb;[173] gastric ulcers were relatively uncommon, accounting for only 7 percent of the total. Multiple ulcers have been reported in up to 20 percent of patients.[177] In 20–26 percent of patients, ulcers were located in ectopic locations, i.e., the distal duodenum and proximal jejunum.[173,178,179]

Hypersecretion of gastric acid is a characteristic of the ulcerogenic syndrome and until the development of gastrin radioimmunoassays was the mainstay for diagnosis. Collective experience has shown that abnormalities in gastric acid secretion may be suggestive of, but are rarely diagnostic of, the Zollinger-Ellison syndrome. In patients with intact stomachs, four parameters have been characterized:

One-Hour Basal Acid Secretion >15 meq. In the experience of Aoyagi and Summerskill,[180] 68 percent of patients with the Zollinger-Ellison syndrome had basal secretory volumes that exceeded 15 meq/h. In 10 Zollinger-Ellison patients, basal acid secretion ranged from 15–76 and averaged 34.3 ± 8.7 meq/h.[181] Kaye et al.[182] and Bernades et al.[183] reported a false-positive rate of 10 percent among patients with uncomplicated peptic ulcer disease.

Overnight Basal Acid Secretion >100 meq. In the collective review of Ellison and Wilson,[173] 74 percent of Zollinger-Ellison patients had overnight gastric outputs exceeding this limit. However, in the experience of Bernardes et al.,[183] 8.5 percent of 495 duodenal ulcer patients also secreted at least 100 meq in a nocturnal 12-h collection.

Ratio of Basal Acid Output to Maximally Stimulated Acid Output (BAO/MAO) >0.6. This parameter, suggested by Marks et al.,[184] is based upon the concept that Zollinger-Ellison patients are constantly stimulated by circulating gastrin to a level significantly higher than "basal." However, Aoyagi and Summerskill[180] and Sanchez et al.[185] reported that one-third to one-half of Zollinger-Ellison patients had BAO/MAO ratios of less than 0.6.

BAC(Concentration)/MAC >0.6. Ruppert et al.[186] reported that 9 of 9 Zollinger-Ellison patients had BAC/MAC ratios exceeding this value. However, Winship[187] noted that 6 of 39 normal subjects had ratios that exceeded 0.6; Kaye et al.[182] reported up to 18 percent false-positives, suggesting that this criterion lacked specificity. Although Lewin et al.[188] proposed that combinations of criteria were useful in diagnosing the Zollinger-Ellison syndrome, false-positives and false-negatives as well as variability in measurements of gastric secretion[189] preclude their use as definitive diagnostic criteria.

Diarrhea has been reported in 16–81 percent of patients with the Zollinger-Ellison syndrome.[173,190,191] In 18 percent diarrhea was the initial complaint, preceding the onset of ulcer pain; in 7–16 percent diarrhea was the major manifestation of the abnormality. Half the patients described by Ellison and Wilson[173] had six or more bowel movements per day as well as hypokalemia ($K < 2.9$ meq/liter), but it is impossible to be certain if or how many of these patients had the WDHA syndrome. In general, hypokalemia is unusual (one-third of patients);[192] 75 percent of the patients have had daily fecal outputs of 1000 cc or less, and only 26.5 percent have described more than 10 stools per day.[193] The diarrhea associated with ulcerogenic tumors has been aborted by continuous aspiration of gastric secretion or by total gastrectomy.[194–198] The final characteristic of the diarrhea associated with islet cell tumors is the frequent (>80 percent) association with steatorrhea.[193]

Pluriglandular involvement has been reported in 10–40 percent of patients with the Zollinger-Ellison syndrome.[173,176,199] The distribution of organ involvement in two large series is summarized in Table 135-9.[200,201] In the series reported by Ballard et al.,[200] the clinical features included hyperparathyroidism in 87 percent, peptic ulcer disease in 56 percent, hypoglycemia in 36 percent, chromophobe adenoma in 28 percent, acromegaly in 19 percent, diarrhea in 13 percent, and Cushing's syndrome and hyperthyroidism in 2 percent each. In related findings, islet cell tumors have been shown to secrete a number of hormones, including gastrin, ACTH, MSH,[202] gastrin and insulin,[203] and gastrin and serotonin.[204] The most common (20 percent) endocrinopathy reported in patients with the Zollinger-Ellison syndrome has been hyperparathyroidism.[205] Calcium has been shown to release antral[206] as well as tumor gastrin (see below), and elevated levels of gastrin have been reported in patients with hyperparathyroidism (even in non-Zollinger-Ellison patients).[207] Since hyperparathyroid patients have higher basal acid secretory rates and incidences of peptic ulcer disease,[208] it sometimes may be difficult to diagnose the Zollinger-Ellison syndrome in patients with primary hyperparathyroidism.

Diagnosis

The diagnosis of the Zollinger-Ellison syndrome depends on the clinical features plus additional data relating to gastric acid secretion (which has been described above), radiography, pancreatic angiography and scanning, and measurements of circulating levels of gastrin.

Characteristic radiographic abnormalities have been described in patients with the Zollinger-Ellison syndrome.[209–212] The findings are due to gastric hypersecretion and therefore are only positive in patients with florid manifestations of the syndrome; on the other hand, they have also been observed in patients with other hypersecretory states. Characteristically, the stomach has large rugal folds due to mucosal hyperplasia and edema; in addition it is frequently atonic with sluggish peristalsis and contains large amounts of secretions. In addition to being the most common site for ulcers, the duodenum is dilated and manifests "duodenitis" with edema, irregularity, and blunted valvulae conniventes. The latter observations are characteristic for the jejunum which, in addition, is hypermotile.

Table 135-9. Distribution (%) of Endocrine Gland Involvement in MEA Type I

	Ballard et al.[200]	Crozier et al.[201]
Parathyroid	88	88
Pancreas	85	84
Pituitary	65	51
Adrenals	19	42
Thyroid	19	27

The rate of success in diagnosing ulcerogenic tumors by angiography has been less than 50 percent. Although there have been isolated successes,[213–215] failure has been more common,[176,216] and at least one false-positive has been reported.[217] Pancreatic scanning with selenomethionine has also generally been disappointing.[218]

The diagnosis of the Zollinger-Ellison syndrome is best made by measuring elevated levels of circulating gastrin. Biologic assay systems have proven unsuccessful, lacking both sensitivity and specificity; initial optimism in using the rats' stomach bioassay to diagnose hypergastrinemia[219] has waned due to high incidences of false-positive and false-negative determinations.[220,221]

The critical determination in confirming the diagnosis of the Zollinger-Ellison syndrome is the circulating level of immunoassayable gastrin. Early reports using this technique[172,222,223] suggested that these patients had levels of serum gastrin elevated at least 10-fold above normal (>100 pg/ml). Further experience has, on the other hand, demonstrated that there is a wide range of abnormal levels. Among 15 proven cases described by Thompson et al.,[198] 3 had levels of 500–1000 pg/ml and the remainder had levels that exceeded 1 ng/ml. In patients with gastric hypersecretion and serum gastrin levels that exceed 500 pg/ml, the diagnosis of ulcerogenic tumor is clear and no further diagnostic evaluation is necessary. In equivocal cases with intermediate gastrin levels (<500 pg/ml), two stimulation tests have been extremely useful—calcium infusion and secretin injection.

Trudeau and McGuigan[224] reported that a patient with the Zollinger-Ellison syndrome had an exaggerated response to calcium infusion; levels of serum gastrin varied directly with those of calcium. Basso and Passaro[225] noted that as a result of release of gastrin from tumors, calcium-stimulated gastric acid secretion equaled or exceeded the maximal acid response to betazole. On the basis of these observations, the exaggerated acid secretory and the gastrin responses following calcium infusion (4mg/kg/hr) have been successfully utilized to confirm the diagnosis of Zollinger-Ellison syndrome.[226–228]

Secretin, a known inhibitor of gastric acid secretion and gastrin release, has been shown to have a paradoxical stimulatory effect in patients with ulcerogenic tumors.[229–233] The gastrin-releasing effect is maximal 2–10 min after the intravenous injection of secretin (2 U/kg) and is mediated by a hypercalcemia response. Similar observations have been described following administration of glucagon.[234,235]

Deveney et al.[236] thoroughly evaluated the usefulness of calcium and secretin in confirming the diagnosis of the Zollinger-Ellison syndrome. All 17 patients with histologically confirmed ulcerogenic tumors had calcium-induced increases in serum gastrin that exceed 450 pg/ml; with this test, false-positive responses were noted in 4 of 30 peptic ulcer patients; in addition, it was impossible to evaluate intermediate changes (increases of 150–450 pg/ml). Secretin injection was more specific. In 17 Zollinger-Ellison patients secretin injection resulted in increased gastrin levels (more than 100 pg/ml) within 10 min, whereas this response was not reported in any of 24 subjects with uncomplicated duodenal ulcer. In addition to increased specificity, the secretin challenge is quicker (<30 min) and safer.

It was initially postulated that hypergastrinemic Zollinger-Ellison patients could not release additional gastrin following a meal. Although one study confirmed this hypothesis,[237] it was dispelled by the reports of Greider et al.,[238] who observed postcibal gastrin release in a number of Zollinger-Ellison patients.

In addition to elevated serum gastrin levels, Zollinger-Ellison patients have been reported to have increased circulating concentrations of calcitonin[239] and parathyroid hormone.[240]

In addition to the Zollinger-Ellison syndrome, several other causes of peripheral hypergastrinemia have been described, but these are not associated with hypersecretion of gastric acid. The differential diagnosis for patients with peripheral hypergastrinemia must consider pernicious anemia,[241] chronic atrophic gastritis,[242,243] chronic renal failure,[244] gastric carcinoma,[245] pheochromocytoma,[246] vitiligo,[247] rheumatoid arthritis,[248] and excluded gastric antrum.[249]

Treatment

It has only recently been recognized that medical therapy plays a role in the management of patients with the Zollinger-Ellison syndrome. Antacids,[250] anticholinergics,[251] combinations of antacids and anticholinergics,[252] gastric irradiation,[253] and H_2 receptor antagonists[254] have all proven useful in managing gastric hypersecretion. Streptozotocin has been utilized to control the growth of malignant gastrinomas.[255,256] Nonetheless, the mainstay of therapy remains surgical ablation of acid-secreting tissue.

In a recent review of 624 patients from the Zollinger-Ellison registry,[257] the sites of the primary lesions were pancreas 426 (68 percent), duodenum 103 (17 percent), islet cell hyperplasia 40 (6 percent), and metastatic without defined primary 55 (9 percent). Primary gastric ulcerogenic tumors have been extraordinarily rare.[258] Optimal surgical management of ulcerogenic tumors varies with the primary site.

Pancreatic islet cell tumors are best treated by total gastrectomy, with or without resection of the tumor. This is supported by data on the distribution of the lesions as well as past experience. Fifty-nine percent of ulcerogenic tumors have been malignant; among these, approximately 80 percent have metastasized by the time the diagnosis has been made.[257] Of the 35 percent of the lesions that were benign, less than half (16 percent) were both single and not associated with islet cell hyperplasia. Thus, among all ulcerogenic tumors, only one in six was subject to cure by local pancreatic resection. Among the 426 pancreatic tumors, only 109 (25 percent) were single (including benign and localized malignant tumors). Based only on the distribution of lesions, the likelihood for success by resection of the ulcerogenic tumor is small. Ellison and Wilson[173] reported in 1964 that 50 percent of the patients treated by subtotal gastrectomy were dead, as were 75 percent of the patients subjected to vagotomy and drainage; on the other hand, 19 of 22 patients treated by total gastrectomy were alive. Similar observations were made in a series of children, all of whom (7/7) were alive following total gastrectomy and only one-fourth of whom (2/8) survived lesser gastric procedures.[259] Total gastrectomy has been shown to improve survival in Zollinger-Ellison patients.[260] Among 267 patients with known metastatic disease, 137 had total gastrectomies; cumulative survival rates for these patients were 75 percent at 1 yr, 55 percent at 5 yrs, and 42 percent at 10 yrs. The 30 patients treated by less than total gastrectomy fared considerably worse, with 51 percent survival at 1 yr, 25 percent at 5 yrs, and only 18 percent at 10 yrs; tumor-related deaths were twice as frequent in the latter group. In the subgroup of patients with hepatic metastases, similar observations were recorded; 5-yr survivals were 42 percent in the total gastrectomy group versus 7 percent in the less than total gastrectomy group.

The causes of death among 561 patients with Zollinger-Ellison syndrome were analyzed by Fox et al.[257] (Table 135-10). Although total gastrectomy had a slightly higher operative mortality rate, it prevented death from peptic ulcer disease and halved the tumor-

Table 135-10. Causes of Death in Patients with Zollinger-Ellison Syndrome

	Total Gastrectomy	Less Than Total Gastrectomy
Total patients	268	293
Alive	187 (70%)	127 (43%)
Died from		
Ulcer disease	0	83
Postop. complication	41	28
Tumor progression	16	33
Miscellaneous	23	22

related mortality rate. Nonetheless, among the 561 patients, progressive tumor growth resulted in the death of 49 patients, 10 percent of the total group. Friesen[261] reported tumor regression following total gastrectomy in two patients with proven metastatic islet cell carcinomas. Serum gastrin levels have been reported to fall by approximately 50 percent following total gastrectomy.[262] Sanzenbacher et al.[263] and Zollinger et al.[264] have recently suggested that following total gastrectomy the response to calcium infusion has significant prognostic implications, with persistent postoperative responses signifying persistent tumor and portending a poor prognosis. Thus, postoperative gastrin measurements have proven useful in following patients, even after total gastrectomy.

Duodenal islet cell tumors represent 10–18 percent of ulcerogenic tumors.[190,209,257] In the most recent data, these lesions have accounted for 103 of 800 cases (13 percent). For this subgroup of patients, the need for total gastrectomy has been less well documented. Oberhelman and Nelson[265] have successfully treated 8 patients by resecting the duodenal tumors. Similar success has been reported by Jaffe et al.,[266] Goldgraber,[267] Scobie and Beetham,[268] Ragins and Del Guercio,[269] Guida et al.,[270] and Singleton et al.[194] In the series reported by Weichert et al.,[271] 4 out of 8 patients required total gastrectomy because of the extent of disease. Of the 4 treated by duodenal resection and subtotal gastrectomy, 2 died in the immediate postoperative period due to ulcer complications; at autopsy both of these patients were shown to have had residual tumor. Fischer and Hicks[272] and Thistlethaite and Horwitz[273] also reported failure of local resection due to the presence of unsuspected residual or metastatic tumor. The risk of local resection was emphasized by the collected findings in 103 patients with duodenal islet cell tumors.[257,274] Only 48 patients (47 percent) had isolated duodenal tumors; the remaining patients had duodenal islet cell carcinomas with metastases (26 patients), both duodenal and pancreatic tumors (24 patients), and combined duodenal tumor–pancreatic islet hyperplasia (5 patients). Despite the anatomic distribution, in the author's experience, if no metastatic or pancreatic tumor is apparent, local duodenal resection is safe and the result can be monitored using postoperative levels of serum gastrin.

Hyperplasia of the gastrin-producing cells was first proposed as a cause of a Zollinger-Ellison–like syndrome by Berson and Yalow,[237] who described duodenal ulcer patients whose postprandial gastrin levels exceeded 1 ng/ml. On the basis of an immunohistochemical study of 8 hypergastrinemic patients, Polak et al.[275] suggested that there were two different types of Zollinger-Ellison syndrome. In cases associated with either a gastrinoma or islet cell hyperplasia (type 2), the histories were long, gastrin levels were high, and antral G cells were histochemically normal. In the newer variant, type 1, the histories were short, the serum gastrin levels were very high, and the pancreas had no tumors and only minimal (if any) islet cell hyperplasia; the critical observation was that the antral G cells were profoundly hyperplastic, and the antrum was reported to be the site of excess gastrin production.

In type 1, the syndrome should be readily manageable by antrectomy alone. Cowley et al.[276] described 1 patient with immunofluorometrically confirmed G cell hyperplasia whose serum gastrin level fell from 8300 to 50 pg/ml and whose gastric acid secretory rate was lowered by 92 percent following antrectomy and pancreatic biopsy. Similar patients were described by DiMagno and Go[277] and Ganguli et al.[278] Straus and Yalow[279] studied 11 patients with fasting hypergastrinemia and antral G cell hyperplasia. In contrast to the marked gastrin responses to calcium and secretin, they noted exaggerated gastrin responses following standard high-protein test meals. On this basis, they suggested that the meal challenge was the optimal way to differentiate between Zollinger-Ellison types 1 and 2. The concept of G cell hyperplasia as a cause of a Zollinger-Ellison–like syndrome is still somewhat in question. Currently, this symptom complex is considered by most investigators as a rare (3 of more than 400 peptic ulcer patients in the study of Hansky[280]) variant of peptic ulcer disease.

Pathophysiology

The mechanisms for gastric acid hypersecretion, diarrhea, and steatorrhea have been carefully studied and recently reviewed.[193,205] The abnormalities will be discussed under the following categories: upper gastrointestinal tract, proximal small intestine, and distal ileum and colon. All the abnormalities have been ascribed to hypersecretion of gastrin by ulcerogenic tumors.

Upper Gastrointestinal Tract. Massive gastric hypersecretion is one of the hallmarks of the Zollinger-Ellison syndrome. The two predominant mechanisms involved are elevated circulating levels of gastrin and gastric mucosal hyperplasia with increased parietal cell mass, both of which result in high basal as well as histamine-stimulated acid secretion. As will be discussed below, non-beta islet cell tumors have been shown to release biologically active forms of gastrin; removal of these tumors has resulted in prompt cessation of gastric basal hypersecretion.[281] Johnson et al.[282,283] have demonstrated that gastrin has a trophic effect on the gastric mucosa in vivo and in vitro. Continuous stimulation of the mucosa by tumor-released gastrin can account for increased parietal cell activity, measured both by augmented rates of maximally stimulated cell acid secretion as well as by assessments of parietal cell density and mass.[284]

The volume and composition of the fluid leaving the duodenal-jejunal junction both under basal conditions[285] and under conditions simulating a meal[196] clearly demonstrate that patients with the Zollinger-Ellison syndrome have marked pancreatic hypersecretion of water and electrolytes and partial neutralization of acid.[286] Pancreatic hypersecretion has been demonstrated in a number of Zollinger-Ellison patients, both in the basal and stimulated states,[287,288] A number of factors may be involved in the pancreatic hypersecretion, including the effect of gastrin itself on pancreatic secretion, pancreatic hyperplasia as the result of the trophic effect of gastrin on the pancreas,[289] and the release of secretin and CCK-PZ by duodenal acidification. Hypersecretion of the Brunner's glands and biliary tract has also been suggested.[290] The fact that the luminal secretions of the upper jejunum have lower pH than normal (frequently as low as 2.0) implies that the stimulation of pancreatic, duodenal, and biliary secretion is inadequate to fully neutralize the amount of acid produced by the stomach.

Proximal Small Intestine. The proximal small intestine bears the brunt of gastric acid hypersecretion. Nasogastric suction has been shown to abort the diarrhea.[194–196] The importance of H^+ (as compared to volume) in the causation of diarrhea was illustrated in the studies of Haubrich et al.;[291] The reinstallation into the duodenum of aspirated and neutralized gastric secretion did not cause diarrhea. The low jejunal pH has been implicated in a number of abnormalities. Adibi et al.[292] demonstrated that jejunal acidification markedly suppressed the leucine-stimulated jejunal absorption of water and electrolytes. Although some studies have suggested that gastrin causes increased intestinal motility,[293,294] the weight of the evidence is that the hypermotility characteristic of the Zollinger-Ellison syndrome[209,295] is caused by the large volume of acid that reaches the small intestine. Acid-induced morphologic changes in the jejunum were reported by Shimoda and Rubin.[252] Repeated biopsies in a single patient revealed abnormal villi, cellular infiltration of the lamina propria, and submucosal hemorrhage and edema. Electron microscopy demonstrated that the tips of the villi resembled gastric mucosal cells and that some of the Brunner's gland cells had some of the characteristics of parietal cells. The overall picture was that of "gastric metaplasia."

Some of the causes of malabsorption and steatorrhea can also be ascribed to intestinal acidification. Shimoda and Rubin[252] have demonstrated that lipases (secreted in normal amounts by the pancreas) were inactivated at low duodenal pH; neutralization of the duodenal contents normalized hydrolysis of fats to free fatty acids and resulted in increased absorption of fats by uninjured villi. Bile salts, particularly conjugates with glycine, have pKa values of 4.0; at lower pH, bile salts are precipitated, making them unavailable for micelle formation, and contributing to the malabsorption of fat.[296,297] Intestinal malabsorption of sugars has been shown to be suppressed at acid pH.[298] Protein malabsorption, also produced by intestinal acidification,[209] has been ascribed to a specific mucosal defect.[299]

In addition to the effects of intestinal acidification, gastrin itself has been shown to have a potent effect, inhibiting the intestinal absorption of water and electrolytes.[300] Since total gastrectomy almost always cures the diarrhea without significantly affecting serum gastrin levels, the role of gastrin itself must be relatively small.

Distal Ileum and Colon. The only significant abnormality reported in the distal intestinal tract is the malabsorption of vitamin B_{12}.[193]

In summary, the diarrhea in Zollinger-Ellison patients is caused by a number of coexisting factors, including increased intestinal motility, small intestinal mucosal damage, acidification of the duodenum and proximal jejunum, and decreased intestinal absorption of water and electrolytes. The same factors have been implicated in the malabsorption of fats, sugars, proteins, and vitamin B_{12}.

Chemistry of Gastrin

The gastrin molecules initially isolated by Gregory[301] were a pair of heptadecapeptides which differed only in the presence (gastrin II) or absence (gastrin I) of sulfate on the tyrosine residue in position 12. Heptadecapeptide pairs isolated from antra of hogs, dogs, cats, sheep, cows, and humans[302] differed from each other only in minor (one codon triplet) substitutions in one or two residues (table 135-11). The molecules were characterized by a strongly negative character due to four or five sequential glutamic acid residues (positions 6–10). The C-terminal tetrapeptide moiety was found to possess all the biologic activities of the 17-amino acid molecule.[303]

Berson and Yalow[304–306] compared the endogenous forms of gastrin with the heptadecapeptide molecules and found a larger and more basic form of gastrin in tissue and plasma. The larger molecular form, "big gastrin," was shown to exist in sulfated and nonsulfated forms and to be converted to the heptadecapeptide form ("little gastrin") by the action of trypsin (acting at the Lys–Lys sequence, residues 16 and 17; Table 135-11). Conversion of big gastrin (G-34) to little gastrin (G-17) occurs in the G cell, since G-17 is the storage form. There is no evidence that little gastrin can be conjugated to the N-terminal heptadecapeptide to form big gastrin.

Walsh et al.[307] studied the relative potencies of big and little gastrins. Under steady conditions, molar concentrations of endogenous G-34 had to be five times as great as those of G-17 in order to produce the same biologic effects. In terms of exogenous doses (produced by infusions), the longer half-life of big gastrin afforded it slightly greater potency than that of G-17.

In addition to G-17 and G-34, both larger and smaller molecular forms have been described. Yalow and colleagues[308–310] reported that in normal subjects the major fraction of immunoreactive gastrin was larger than G-34. This molecular form, "big-big gastrin," was shown to have little if any biologic activity, to have a half-life of about 90 min, not to be released following a meal, and to be convertible to both G-34 and G-17 by trypsin. Rehfeld et al.[311] have also isolated a compound larger than big gastrin, but smaller than the big-big form. There are no data evaluating the biologic activity of this molecular form, component 1. Minigastrin,[312] consisting of 4–17 amino acid residues of G-17, exists in sulfated and nonsulfated forms, has almost the same potency as little gastrin, and is biologically active for a short time (half-life <2 min).[313]

All five of the molecular forms have been isolated in patients with ulcerogenic tumors.[312,314,315] In addition, an inactive fragment corresponding to amino residues 1–13 of G-17 has been isolated from the serum of patients with the Zollinger-Ellison syndrome.[316] Creutzfeldt et al.[199] reported that there is great variability in the distribution of forms of gastrin in tissue and plasma from patients with ulcerogenic tumors. In general, tumors contained mostly little gastrin (the storage form), while plasma contained primarily big gastrin. Some of the characteristics of the molecular forms of gastrin are summarized in Table 135-12.

As stated above, the C-terminal tetrapeptide amide, common to all active forms of gastrin, possesses the full range of physiologic actions of the parent molecule. The structure–function relationships of this portion of the molecule have been carefully studied.[317–319] Biologic activity increases with increased chain length. The amide group is absolutely necessary for activity and substitutions for aspartic acid and methionine result in inactive compounds. A synthetic pentapeptide (Table 135-11) is quite active and has become the standard stimulant for maximal secretion of gastric acid.

CCK-PZ shares the C-terminal tetrapeptide amide with gastrin. Although the two peptides have overlapping spectra of actions (Tables 135-13 and 135-14), CCK-PZ has greatly increased potency for the actions on the gallbladder and pancreas. The specificity of action is dependent upon the sulfated tyrosine in position 27. Although gastrins I and II are equally effective peptides, desulfated CCK-PZ is virtually inactive. Caerulein, a derivative of the skin of *Hyla caerulea,* has a CCK-PZ–like spectrum of actions.

Table 135-11. Structure of Gastrin and Gastrin-Related Molecules

Gastrin-34 Man (MW 3839)	1 2 3 4 5 6 7 8 9 10 11 12 13 14 15 16 17 18 19 20 21 22 23 24 25 26 27 28 29 30 31 32 33 34 Pyroglu Leu Gly Pro Gln Gly His Pro Ser Leu Val Ala Asp Pro Ser Lys Lys Gln Gly Pro Trp Leu Glu Glu Glu Glu Glu Ala Tyr Gly Trp Met Asp Phe-NH_2
Gastrin-17-I Man (MW 2096)	1 2 3 4 5 6 7 8 9 10 11 12 13 14 15 16 17 Pyroglu Gly Pro Trp Leu Glu Glu Glu Glu Glu Ala Tyr Gly Trp Met Asp Phe-NH_2
Gastrin-17-II Man (MW 2176)	Pyroglu Gly Pro Trp Leu Glu Glu Glu Glu Glu Ala Tyr (SO_3H) Gly Trp Met Asp Phe-NH_2
Gastrin-17 Hog	Pyroglu Gly Pro Trp Met Glu Glu Glu Glu Glu Ala Tyr (SO_3H) Gly Trp Met Asp Phe-NH_2
Gastrin-17 Dog	Pyroglu Gly Pro Trp Met Glu Glu Ala Glu Glu Ala Tyr Gly Trp Met Asp Phe-NH_2
Gastrin-17 Cow and sheep	Pyroglu Gly Pro Trp Val Glu Glu Glu Glu Ala Ala Tyr Gly Trp Met Asp Phe-NH_2
Gastrin-17 Cat	Pyroglu Gly Pro Trp Leu Glu Glu Glu Glu Ala Ala Tyr Gly Trp Met Asp Phe-NH_2
Gastrin-13-I Man	Trp Leu Glu Glu Glu Glu Glu Ala Tyr Gly Trp Met Asp Phe-NH_2
Pentapeptide	t-Boc-B Ala Trp Met Asp Phe-NH_2
CCK-PZ - 33 Man (MW 3918)	1 2 3 4 5 6 7 8 9 10 11 12 13 14 15 16 17 18 19 20 21 22 23 24 25 26 27 28 29 30 31 32 33 Lys Ala Pro Ser Gly Arg Val Ser Met Ile Lys Asn Leu Gln Ser Leu Asp Pro Ser His Arg Ile Ser Asp Arg Asp Tyr (SO_3H) Met Gly Trp Met Asp Phe-NH_2
Caerolein (MW 1352)	1 2 3 4 5 6 7 8 9 10 Pyroglu Glu Asp Tyr Thr Gly Trp Met Asp Phe-NH_2

Table 135-12. Characteristics of Molecular Forms of Gastrin

	Big-Big	Component 1	Big	Little	Mini
Molecular weight	10,000	5000	3900	2100	1700
Half-life (min)	90?	—	15.8	3.2	1.8
Potency					
Endogenous	0	0	0.17	1.0	0.8
Exogenous	0	0	1.1	1.0	0.8
Percent in plasma					
Fasting		(75)	15	10	<1
Postprandial		(20)	55	25	<1
Gastrinoma	9	<2	58	27	5
Percent in Tissue					
Antrum			10–20	80–90	
Duodenum			50	50	
Gastrinoma	0	<5	20	70	5

Recently, a gastrinlike compound has been discovered in the central nervous system of vertebrates.[320] The role of this compound is largely unknown.

PEPTIC ULCER DISEASE

Although patients with duodenal ulcer disease have increased rates of gastric acid secretion and gastrin is a potent stimulant of acid secretion, it has been very difficult to implicate gastrin in the etiology of duodenal ulcer disease. Patients with duodenal ulcer disease have fasting gastrin levels indistinguishable from those of controls.[321–323] Berson and Yalow[324] suggested that normal gastrin levels were inappropriately high for the degree of hypersecretion and proposed that this represented a failure of feedback inhibition in duodenal ulcer patients. This hypothesis has yet to be proved. Attempts to correlate gastrin levels with rates of acid secretion have failed in patients who secreted more than 10 meq/h.[325,326]

Duodenal ulcer patients have been shown to hyperrespond to a protein meal[321–323] as well as to calcium infusion.[206] Two possible explanations have been proposed. The first is that the antrum and duodenum of patients with duodenal ulcer disease contain more gastrin than do those of normal controls. This possibility has been ruled out by studies that reported normal tissue levels of gastrin in ulcer patients.[278] The second possibility is that release of gastrin at low intragastric pH is inhibited less in ulcer patients than in controls; data from a recent study have supported this possibility.[327]

Patients with duodenal ulcer disease have increased parietal cell masses and, therefore, higher maximal acid secretory rates. Since gastrin is the only compound with a specific trophic effect on gastric mucosa,[328] it is not unlikely that gastrin is involved in the pathogenesis of duodenal ulcer disease, at least by stimulating the mass and density of the parietal cell area.

WDHA SYNDROME

Priest and Alexander[329] emphasized the association of pancreatic islet cell tumors and diarrhea. The syndrome became more clearly defined by Verner and Morrison,[330] who noted that hypokalemia was a prominent feature and that peptic ulceration was conspicuously absent. Murray et al.,[331] as well as Espiner and Beaven,[332] noted the association with achlorhydria and suggested that tumors might be secreting a gastric secretory inhibitor. This concept was supported by subsequent studies which demonstrated normal parietal cells despite the presence of achlorhydria.[333] Recognizing the similarities of the syndrome with cholera and the etiologic role of the pancreas, Matsumoto et al.[334] proposed that the syndrome be called *pancreatic cholera*. Marks et al.[335] suggested the designation *WDHA (Watery diarrhea, hypokalemia, achlorhydria)* syndrome. Verner and Morrison[336] have recently suggested the modification *WDHH*, suggesting that hypochlorhydria was more common than achlorhydria. For purposes of this discussion, the designations *Verner-Morrison syndrome, WDHA syndrome,* and *pancreatic cholera* will be used interchangeably.

To date, approximately 75 cases of WDHA syndrome have been described. The clinical manifestations of this syndrome have been quite well characterized and reviewed recently.[337] Although there has also been considerable progress in understanding the pathophysiology of this symptom complex,[338] no single hormonal mediator has been implicated in its etiology. The discussion that follows will present clinical features first, followed by the pathophysiologic aspects of the problem.

Clinical Features

The WDHA syndrome is typically a disease of middle-aged females. Sixty-five percent of the reported patients have been women. The patients have ranged in age from 17 to 72 and averaged 47 yr of age.[336] In most patients symptoms were present for 3–4 yr before the diagnosis was established.

The hallmark of the syndrome is watery diarrhea. In one-half

Table 135-13. Biologic Actions and Release of Gastrin

Actions
- Stimulates contraction of
  - Lower esophageal sphincter*
  - Stomach
  - Intestine
  - Gallbladder
- Inhibits contraction of
  - Sphincter of Oddi
  - Pylorus
- Stimulates water–electrolyte secretion of
  - Stomach*
  - Pancreas
  - Liver
  - Brunner's glands
- Inhibits water–electrolyte absorption of intestine
- Stimulates enzyme secretion of
  - Stomach
  - Pancreas*
- Stimulates secretion of
  - Secretin
  - Insulin
- Stimulates release of histamine
- Stimulates histadine decarboxylase
- Stimulates amino acid uptake of gastric mucosa
- Stimulates growth of gastric mucosa
- Stimulates blood flow in
  - Superior mesenteric artery
  - Gastric mucosa
  - Pancreas
  - Small intestine
- Lowers blood pressure

Release
- L-Amino acids*
- Vagal stimulation*
- Distention of stomach*
- Calcium
- Epinephrine
- Hypoglycemia
- Food, protein particularly*
- Bombesin

*Physiologic.

Table 135-14. Biologic Actions and Release of Cholecystokinin

Actions
Stimulates contraction of
Gallbladder
Intestine
Pyloric sphincter
Quiet stomach
Inhibits contraction of
Lower esophageal sphincter
Sphincter of Oddi
Active stomach
Stimulates water–electrolyte secretion of
Pancreas
Stomach
Liver
Brunner's glands
Inhibits absorption of small bowel water–electrolyte
Stimulates enzyme secretion of
Pancreas
Stomach
Stimulates secretion of
Insulin
Glucagon
Stimulates
Amino acid uptake by pancreas
Growth of pancreas
Lowers systolic arterial pressure
Increases
Superior mesenteric artery flow
Pancreatic blood flow
Small intestinal blood flow
Release
L-Amino acids
Fatty acids
Hydrochloric acid
Food
Saline purgatives
Bombesin

the patients the diarrhea is intermittent;[193] during the quiescent periods, the stools decrease in volume and assume a semisolid consistency. With the progression of the disease, particularly when the syndrome is caused by malignant tumors, the diarrhea becomes sustained. During active phases of the disease, patients describe profuse watery diarrhea commonly necessitating more than 10 movements per day. The daily stool volumes have ranged from 3 to 10 liters and averaged 4.6 liters.[336] The stool has the appearance of weak tea and is extremely rich in electrolytes, particularly potassium and bicarbonate. Daily fecal losses of potassium are in the order of 200–400 meq, and this loss is responsible for a characteristic hypokalemia (mean 2.2 meq/liter) associated with lethargy, nausea, vomiting, crampy abdominal pain, and muscular weakness. Fecal secretion of bicarbonate results in metabolic acidosis, and arterial pH as low as 7.1 has been described. The dehydration, weight loss, and electrolyte depletion are very difficult to treat and have been responsible for the deaths of 7 patients (almost 10 percent of the reported cases).[329,330,339–342]

Despite massive diarrhea, steatorrhea is uncommon. Of 22 patients described by Rambaud and Matuchansky,[193] 19 had normal fecal fat excretion; mild steatorrhea has been described in only 4 patients.[340,343–345] In addition, abnormalities in the D-xylose and Schilling tests, as well as in small bowel biopsies, have been reported in one patient each.[193] Cessation of the diarrhea has consistently followed resection of benign adenomas. Other factors shown to have a mollifying effect on the diarrhea include adrenal steroids and pregnancy. Adrenal steroid therapy improved the diarrhea of 7 of 12 reported patients.[329,333,334,346–349] In one patient, a remission of the syndrome occurred during pregnancy,[343] and in another, a severe exacerbation of diarrhea occurred 2½ weeks following delivery.[350]

Although the first patient described by Priest and Alexander[329] developed a superficial gastric ulcer while receiving adrenal corticosteroids, peptic ulceration has not been a feature of WDHA syndrome. Rather gastric acid hyposecretion has been characteristic of this syndrome. Basal achlorhydria was described in 59 percent of the patients tested, and half of these did not respond to histamine.[336] Examination of a compilation of reported patients[336,351] revealed achlorhydria in 14 and hypochlorhydria in 16 of 54 patients. Among 13 patients in whom gastric secretory studies were performed both before and after resection of an adenoma, 8 developed rebound hypersecretion;[333,334,336,350,352,353] several of these patients developed peptic ulcers, one of which required vagotomy for control. Gastric biopsies have demonstrated normal parietal cells, even in achlorhydric patients.[334,352,354] De Muro et al.[355] demonstrated that hypokalemia suppressed gastric secretion, and in 1 patient potassium replacement increased the rate of acid secretion. Nonetheless, it is clear that hypokalemia alone is not responsible for the hyposecretion; many patients have been described in whom hypochlorhydria persists despite normokalemia. Finally, decreased secretion of gastric intrinsic factor and pepsin have been corrected by resection of a diarrheagenic tumor.[356] These data are all consistent with tumor secretion of a gastric secretory inhibitor.

Hyperglycemia has been reported in 16 of 31 patients. The etiology of this abnormality is either hypokalemia[357,358] or a diabetogenic effect of the secreted hormone. In support of the latter possibility, dissection of the tumor produced an increased blood sugar level in 1 patient.[332] Following resection of islet cell tumors, glucose tolerance tests have returned to normal.[346,359,360]

Hypercalcemia has been another common manifestation of the WDHA syndrome. Serum calcium determinations were abnormal in 18 of 37 patients.[336] Parathyroidectomy has proven to be ineffective in controlling tumor-induced hypercalcemia.[329,330,361] On the other hand, in at least 7 patients hypercalcemia has been cured by resection of pancreatic adenomas.[331,332,335,343,346,353,361] Tetany has been described in 4 hypercalcemic patients.[330,361–363] Hypomagnesemia is thought to be the cause of the tetany, which is worsened by the administration of potassium during attempts to correct hypokalemia.

Flushing has been reported in 14 patients. The cause of these episodes of erythema and urticaria is unknown. Serotonin cannot be implicated in the majority of cases, although 2 patients have been shown to have high circulating levels of serotonin.[364,365]

A number of uncommon manifestations have also been reported. Three patients have manifested severe congestive heart failure, presumably due to hypokalemia-induced myocardial damage.[353,366] Uremia, the cause of death in a number of patients, has been ascribed to hypokalemic vacuolar tubular nephropathy.[367] Finally, psychosis has been reported in 3 patients.[341,353,368] The clinical manifestations of the WDHA syndrome are summarized in Table 135-15.

The diagnosis of WDHA syndrome must be suspected in any patient who manifests watery diarrhea and hypokalemia, particularly when associated with achlorhydria, hyperglycemia, hypercalcemia, or flushing. However, establishing the diagnosis is still quite difficult. Despite considerable progress, there is still no specific blood hormone analysis that is diagnostic; this will be discussed in

Table 135-15. Clinical Manifestations of the WDHA Syndrome

Symptom	Incidence (%)
Watery diarrhea	100
Hypokalemia	100
Hypo- or achlorhydria	59
Hypoglycemia	53
Flushing	19
Tetany	5
Congestive heart failure	3
Psychosis	3

detail in the following section. Although selenomethionine (^{75}Se) scans and celiac arteriograms have been useful in localizing pancreatic tumors in some patients,[330,343,353,369] the definitive diagnostic maneuver remains the exploratory laparotomy.

Pancreatic tumors were demonstrated in 43 of 55 reported patients.[337] Of these 43 tumors, 23 were benign adenomas. Although 7 patients died of complications of the diarrhea before the diagnosis was established (benign tumors were disclosed at autopsy),[329,330,340–342,344] resection of benign islet cell tumors cured the symptoms of the WDHA syndrome in the remaining 16. In all 20 patients who had malignant islet cell tumors, metastases were demonstrated at the time of diagnosis. Several of these patients had temporary remissions following palliative resection of malignant lesions. As mentioned above, corticosteroids (but not other hormones[340]) have been useful in controlling diarrhea in patients whose tumors could not be completely removed.[354] With rare exceptions, radiation therapy and chemotherapy with 5-fluorouracil have not been beneficial.[370,371] In a recent report, intraarterial infusions of streptozocin produced dramatic remissions in 2 patients.[372] Eleven patients with pancreatic cholera did not have discrete pancreatic tumors, but hyperplasia of the non-beta islet cell tissue was demonstrated;[336] 8 of these patients were cured by pancreatic resection.[350,359,361,373,374] The frequency of islet cell hyperplasia (20 percent of reported cases) necessitates distal pancreatectomy for biopsy if a pancreatic neoplasm is not discovered at the time of exploratory laparotomy. Until recently the pancreas has been implicated in all cases of WDHA syndrome, whether due to carcinoma, adenoma, or hyperplasia. Fausa et al.[375] first described the cure of WDHA syndrome following removal of a retroperitoneal ganglioneuroma. Of 30 patients described by Said and Faloona,[376] 5 were shown to have bronchogenic carcinomas (squamous cell), and a pheochromocytoma and ganglioneuroblastoma were reported in 1 patient each. It appears, therefore, that extrapancreatic causes of WDHA syndrome are not rare and this possibility must be carefully considered in the diagnostic work-up of all patients with watery diarrhea.

Pathophysiology

The abnormalities in the WDHA syndrome will be discussed under three anatomic categories—the upper gastrointestinal tract, the small bowel, and the colon. The pathophysiology of the syndrome has recently been described in detail.[338]

Upper Gastrointestinal Tract. Although histamine-fast achlorhydria has been reported in only 30 percent of the patients,[336] gastric hyposecretion has been the general rule. The typical characteristics of this syndrome have included depressed basal gastric acid secretion with a relatively normal response to pentagastrin. Nonetheless, the diagnosis of the WDHA syndrome cannot be ruled out by high basal acid secretion in single determinations. Possible explanations for this phenomenon include elevations in serum gastrin (reported in 4 of 17 patients[377]) and in urinary gastric secretagogue activity.[338]

There has been considerable disagreement as to the status of pancreatic exocrine secretion in patients with the WDHA syndrome. The majority of patients have had normal basal pancreatic secretion as well as normal responses to injected secretin.[335,338,352,366,373] However, extracts of some (but not all) diarrheagenic tumors have been shown to stimulate pancreatic secretion of water and electrolytes.[369] Schmitt et al.[365] have reported an unusual patient in whom pancreatic secretion was maximal under basal condition (i.e., there was no secretory response to injected secretin) and diarrhea was controlled by continuous aspiration of duodenal contents. These observations implied that pancreatic secretion played a significant role in the pathogenesis of diarrhea in this patient.

Characteristic biliary tract abnormalities have included a dilated gallbladder[334,338,360,369] containing bile with increased concentrations of bicarbonate and chloride and decreased levels of bile acids (cholic, chemodeoxycholic, and deoxycholic acids). Hepatic bile flow has been slightly increased.

In the overwhelming majority of patients, moderate abnormalities in gastric, pancreatic, and biliary secretions do not significantly contribute to the diarrhea. This has been substantiated by the observation in one carefully studied patient that the volume and composition of the fluid leaving the fourth portion of the duodenum was normal.[338]

Small Intestine. The predominant abnormality in the WDHA syndrome has been localized to the small intestine; it is characterized by the failure of absorption or by active secretion of water and electrolytes. Despite normal intestinal transit times, the volume of secretions leaving the terminal ileum has been approximated at almost 10 times normal. The electrolyte concentrations in the jejunum have been shown to be normal except for slightly increased potassium and markedly augmented bicarbonate, resulting in abolition of the normal proximal-distal intestine HCO_3 concentration gradient. Despite normal intestinal absorption of leucine and glucose, these compounds do not stimulate jejunal absorption of water or sodium.[378] The end result of these abnormalities is significant luminal loss of water and electrolytes, particularly potassium and bicarbonate. These anomalies have been reproduced by a tumor extract.[379]

Colon. In contrast to the small intestine, the colon has been shown to absorb 75–80 percent of luminal water, sodium, chloride, and bicarbonate. In a patient reported in detail,[338] the colon absorbed more sodium and water than the maximal theoretical capacities of this organ.[380] The most likely explanation for this excessive absorption is secondary aldosteronism.[381,382] Aldosterone has been shown to stimulate colonic absorption of water and sodium but to have little effect on the human small bowel.[383] The aldosterone effect on the colon has been shown to promote massive colonic secretion of potassium (along with chloride as the anion)[384] and result in hypokalemia. In at least 2 patients, elevated urinary excretion of tetrahydroaldosterone (80 and 180 μg/24 h; control, less than 60 μg/24 h) has been documented.[338,370]

The result of these upper and lower intestinal abnormalities (summarized in Fig. 135-1) is excretion of large volumes of watery (secreted by the small intestine) stool containing high concentrations of bicarbonate (secreted by the jejunum) and potassium (secreted by the colon).

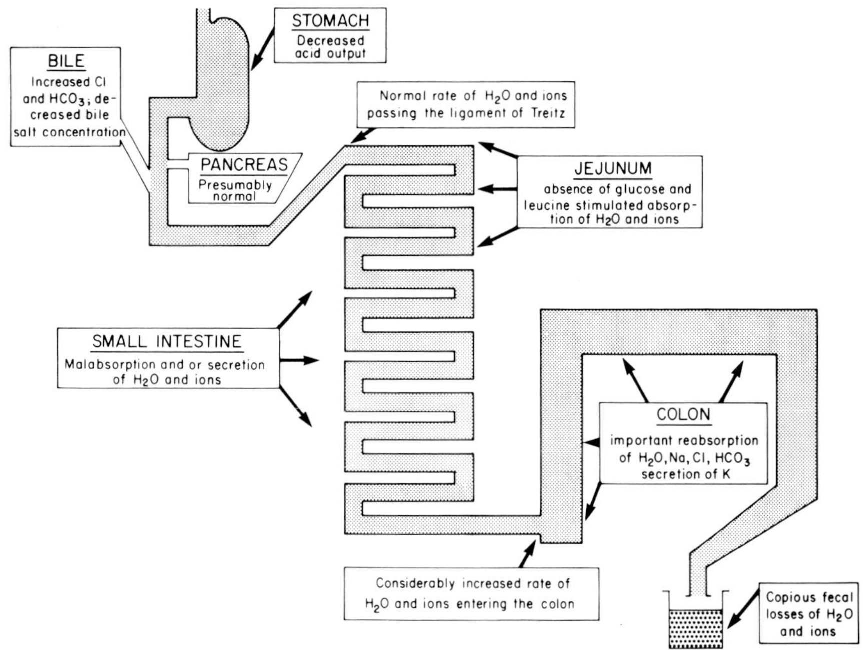

Fig. 135-1. Pathophysiologic abnormalities in the WDHA syndrome. (From Rambaud et al.: Pancreatic cholera: studies on tumoral secretions and pathophysiology of diarrhea. *Gastroenterology 69:* 110, 1975. Copyright 1975, The Williams and Wilkins Co., Baltimore.)

Humoral Mediator

There is till considerable question as to the mediator(s) of the WDHA syndrome. A number of hormones have been nominated as candidate mediators. In this section, the evidence implicating and ruling out each of the possible mediators will be reviewed.

Barbezat and Grossman[385] have postulated that the combination of gastrin and glucagon is responsible for the WDHA syndrome. Although glucagon inhibits gastric acid secretion and motility,[386,387] increases blood glucose levels, and stimulates intestinal motility,[50] it has been shown to cause hypocalcemia[388] and inhibit pancreatic exocrine function.[389] Although gastrin stimulates intestinal secretion[390] and bile flow,[391,392] its pancreatic effect[393] causes hypoglycemia, and the peptide causes hypocalcemia[394] and obviously stimulates gastric acid secretion. Although occasional elevations of these peptides have been reported,[365,377] the overwhelming evidence has ruled out these peptides, alone or in combination, as the major mediators of the WDHA syndrome.

Serotonin, implicated in the diarrhea of the carcinoid syndrome,[395,396] has been suggested as a possible mediator in the WDHA syndrome. Increased urinary excretion of 5-HIAA has been reported in a number of patients.[332,365,370] In addition to causing diarrhea, serotonin has been shown to inhibit gastric acid secretion[397,398] and cause flushing, both common characteristics of the WDHA syndrome. However, the evidence has largely excluded serotonin as the major humoral agent in this syndrome. A number of studies have reported normal urinary excretion rates of 5-HIAA.[331,333,334,339,352,353,356,366] Although serotonin induces diarrhea, its effect is largely due to an increase of intestinal tone and motility,[399] presumably by reducing the intraluminal pressure threshhold for intestinal peristalsis[400] rather than by inhibiting intestinal absorption of water and electrolytes. Steatorrhea and shortened transit times, common features in the serotonin-mediated carcinoid syndrome, are very unusual in pancreatic cholera.[193] Finally, serotonin inhibits pancreatic secretion.[401]

Zollinger et al.[369] suggested that secretin or a secretinlike hormone is responsible for the diarrhea in the WDHA syndrome. This suggestion was based on the operative findings in 2 patients of tensely distended gallbladders and continuous refilling of the duodenum with secretions. Chemical analysis of the bile revealed elevated concentrations of bicarbonate and chloride with decreased concentrations of bile salts, findings consistent with a secretin effect. Extracts of hepatic metastases from 1 patient stimulated the rate of pancreatic flow as well as the bicarbonate concentration; extracts of the second tumor were inactive in the biologic assay system. Using the same tumor extracts, Tompkins et al,[402] demonstrated a potent secretinlike choleretic effect, increasing the flow of bile with elevated concentrations of chloride and bicarbonate. In agreement with the studies of Wormsley,[403] secretin infusion produced severe diarrhea. Sanzenbacher et al.[404] utilized intestinal perfusion techniques with a triple lumen tube to demonstrate that in man secretin stimulated intestinal secretion of water and electrolytes in sufficient quantities to reproduce losses noted in the WDHA syndrome.

Positive bioassays[356,365,405] and radioimmunoassays[354,365] for secretin have been reported. Secretin has an appropriate spectrum of action, causing intestineal secretion,[406,407] inhibiting acid secretion,[408] and producing hypercalcemia. Nonetheless, recent evidence has suggested that secretin is probably not the diarrheagenic hormone. On a pathophysiologic basis, the large majority of patients have had normal basal pancreatic secretory function and normal stimulation with exogenous secretin.[335,352,366,373] In addition, immunoreactive secretin levels have been normal in most patients with this syndrome[377] (S. Bloom, personal communication; G. Boden, personal communication).

Infusions of prostaglandin E (PGE) can reproduce all the symptoms of the WDHA syndrome, including secretory diarrhea,[409,410] hypochlorhydria,[411] flushing,[412] hypercalcemia,[413] and hyperglycemia,[414] Sandler et al.[415] and Schmitt et al.[365] each reported high (bioassayable and radioimmunoassayable) prostaglandin levels in a patient with this syndrome. Jaffe and Condon[377] have recently reported that 8 (including 3 with normal levels of VIP) of 21 patients with the WDHA syndrome had elevated peripheral plasma levels of PGE. The mean level for all the patients was 993 ± 490 pg/ml, compared to control data, 272 ± 18 pg/ml. In

Table 135-16. Spectrum of Action of Possible Mediators of the WDHA Syndrome

	Serotonin	Gastrin	CCK-PZ	Glucagon	Secretin	VIP	GIP	PGE
Stimulates intestinal secretion	—	—	+	+	+	+	+	+
Inhibits gastric acid	+	—	+	+	+	+	+	+
Inhibits gastric pepsin	+	—	—	+	+	+	+	+
Hyperglycemia		±	±	+	±	+	—	+
Hypercalcemia		—	—	—	+	+		+
Vasodilitation	+	+	+			+		+
Increases pancreatic secretion	—	+	+	—	+	+	—	—
Stimulates adenyl cyclase				+	+	+		+
Choleresis		+	+	+	+	+	—	

1 patient, circulating concentrations of PGE were elevated before both resection of the primary tumor (9939 pg/ml) and a subsequent extirpation of a solitary hepatic metastasis (1063 pg/ml); following resections, levels returned to normal. The consistent variation of PGE levels with the presence and absence of symptoms implied that PGE was involved in the etiology of at least this patient's diarrhea. On the contrary, 13 of 21 patients in this study and several others[356,372] had normal levels of PGE, excluding the possibility that PGE is the sole mediator of this syndrome.

Currently, the greatest attention has been directed to VIP. The spectrum of actions of this compound (see earlier discussion of VIP) is perfectly consistent with the possibility that it may be the diarrheagenic hormone. Bloom et al.[416] first reported elevated levels of VIP in the plasma (1030–1390 pg/ml; control <100 pg/ml) and tumor from 5 patients with the WDHA syndrome. Isolated reports promptly verified these observations.[338,349,365,375,417,418] Said and Faloona[376] have recently reported that immunoreactive VIP concentrations were elevated in 26 of 28 plasma samples and 13 of 13 WDHA tumor extracts. VIP levels were elevated in patients with pancreatic neoplasms as well as those with islet cell hyperplasia and ectopic (lung and adrenal) malignancies. Following successful alleviation of the symptoms (surgical resection of adenomas or steroid/streptozotocin control of the diarrhea), VIP levels fell in 5 of 5 patients; following subtotal pancreatectomy for islet cell hyperplasia, plasma VIP levels remained elevated in 3 patients, 2 of whom remained symptomatic. In Bloom and Polak's series,[419] 17 patients were found to have plasma VIP levels ranging from 200 to 2000 pg/ml (mean normal 20 pg/ml); 10 tumors contained 1–100 μg/g of tumor. In contrast to the report of Said and Faloona,[376] several patients with islet cell hyperplasia were shown to have normal levels of VIP; these patients were classified as having "pseudo Verner-Morrison syndrome." Despite the apparent solidarity of these observations, it is clear that VIP is probably not the sole mediator of the WDHA syndrome. A number of cases have been reported in which patients with the WDHA syndrome associated with pancreatic malignancies had normal plasma levels of VIP.[372,377,420]

On the basis of the conflicting observations described above, the most plausible explanation is that the WDHA syndrome is not a uniform entity, but rather a heterogenous mixture of diarrheagenic syndromes caused by a number of humoral mediators (Table 135-16). This is quite consistent with the concept that diarrheagenic tumors are APUDomas (see below) possessing the potential to synthesize and release a spectrum of active peptides and amines.

APUDomas

The APUD cells constitute a group of diversified cells that are specialized for the production of polypeptides and amines.[421,422] The characteristics of the APUD system are listed in Table 135-17. The name was derived from two of these characteristics—*a*mine *p*recursor *u*ptake and *d*ecarboxylation.

In the gastrointestinal tract, the majority of APUD cells possess long apical processes which reach the gland lumens. The microvilli at the luminal tips of the cells may serve a sensory function, responding to alterations in the contents of the glands. The pancreatic APUD cells probably respond both to variations in blood glucose levels as well as secreted gastrointestinal polypeptide hormones. Although histologic studies have revealed no nerve endings on the APUD cells, their proximity to vagal nerve fibers suggests that their function may be influenced by nervous stimuli.

The concept specifies that the APUD cells have a common origin, predominantly from the embryonic neural crest.[423] It further implies that the cells retain some totipotentiality and can, under certain circumstances, synthesize "ectopic" amine or polypeptide products. The functional gastrointestinal APUD cells, their polypeptide products, and their distribution are summarized in Table 135-18.

The term APUDoma was coined by Szijj et al.[424] and is currently used to describe a variety of functioning and nonfunctioning tumors of endocrine cell origin. Welbourn et al.[421] have divided APUDomas into two groups: orthoendocrine (secreting normal cell products) and paraendocrine (secreting amines or polypeptides that are foreign to the specific cells involved but normally synthesized by other APUD cells) syndromes. Examples of orthoendocrine APUD syndromes include the Zollinger-Ellison syndrome (gastrinoma), the WDHA syndrome (VIPoma), and the carcinoid syndrome (serotoninoma); an example of a parendocrine APUD syndrome is the ectopic ACTH syndrome.

APUDomas may be solitary or multiple. Solitary APUDomas (one cell type) may secrete one or more hormonal products. An example of the latter situation, combined insulinoma-gastrinoma, was described by Heitz et al.[425] Multiple APUD syndromes have been subdivided into two groups. The first, MEA I, includes abnormalities related particularly to the islets, intestines, adrenals, and pituitary.[426] A familial variant of this syndrome, Werner's syndrome,[427] has been shown to be transmitted as an autosomal dominant characteristic. The second multiple endocrinopathy, MEA II, includes medullary carcinomas of the thyroid, pheo-

Table 135-17. APUD Characteristics

Fluorogenic amine content
Amine precursor uptake
Amino acid decarboxylase
High content of side-chain carboxyl groups (masked metachromasia)
High content of α-glycerophosphate dehydrogenase
High content of nonspecific esterases/cholinesterases
Ultrastructure (endocrine granules)
Specific immunofluorescence and immunoelectrocytochemistry

Table 135-18. Gastrointestinal Hormone-Producing Cells

Peptide	Cell Type	Distribution Major	Distribution Minor
Gastrin	G	Antrum Duodenum	Jejunum
Secretin	S	Duodenum Jejunum	Ileum
CCK-PZ	I	Duodenum Jejunum	Ileum
GIP	K	Duodenum Jejunum	Ileum
Motilin	EC	Duodenum Jejunum Ileum	
VIP	H	Ileum Colon	Jejunum Duodenum Fundus
Bombesin(-like)	H	Fundus Antrum Duodenum	Jejunum Ileum

chromocytomas, carcinoids, and fibromatosis (Sipple's syndrome[428]). The only abnormality common to both syndromes is hyperparathyroidism, probably a secondary phenomenon.

In addition to providing accurate pathologic descriptions, the APUD cell concept is a useful conceptual model. It facilitates the understanding and organization of a number of related and unrelated endocrine anomalies.

REFERENCES

1. Grossman, M. I. Gastrin, Cholecystokinin, and Secretin Act on One Receptor. *Lancet 1:* 1088, 1970.
2. Walsh, J. H., and Grossman, M. I. Gastrin. *N. Engl. J. Med. 292:* 1324, 1377, 1975.
3. Hansky, J. Clinical Aspects of Gastrin Physiology. *Med. Clin. North Am. 58:* 1217, 1974.
4. Walsh, J. H. Clinical Significance of Gastrin Radioimmunoassay. *Semin. Nucl. Med. 5:* 247, 1975.
5. Thompson, J. C. Gastrin and Gastric Secretion. *Ann. Rev. Med. 20:* 291, 1969.
6. Grossman, M. I. Spectrum of Biological Actions of Gastrointestinal Hormones, in S. Andersen (ed.): *Frontiers in Gastrointestinal Hormone Research.* Stockholm, Almquist and Wiksell, 1970, p. 17.
7. Rayford, P. L., Miller, T. A., and Thompson, J. C. Secretin, Cholecystokinin, and Newer Gastrointestinal Hormones. *N. Engl. J. Med. 294:* 1093, 1157, 1976.
8. Bloom, S. R. Hormones of the Gastrointestinal Tract. *Br. Med. Bull. 30:* 62, 1974.
9. Hubel, K. A. Secretin: A Long Progress Note. *Gastroenterology 62:* 318, 1972.
10. Ondetti, M. A., Rubin, B., Engel, S. L., Plusec, J., and Sheehan, J. T. Cholecystokinin–Pancreozymin: Recent Developments. *Am. J. Dig. Dis. 15:* 149, 1970.
11. Grossman, M. I. Candidate Hormones of the Gut. *Gastroenterology 67:* 730, 1974.
12. Bayliss, W. M., and Starling, E. H. The Mechanism of Pancreatic Secretion. *J. Physiol. 28:* 325, 1902.
13. Von Euler, U. S., and Gaddum, J. H. An Unidentified Depression Substance in Certain Tissue Extracts. *J. Physiol. 72:* 74, 1931.
14. Said, S. I., and Mutt, V. Potent Peripheral and Splanchnic Vasodilator Peptide from Normal Gut. *Nature 225:* 863, 1970.
15. Said, S. I., and Mutt, V. Polypeptide with Broad Biological Activity: Isolation from Small Intestine. *Science 169:* 1217, 1970.
16. Piper, P. J., Said, S. I., and Vane, J. R. Effects of Smooth Muscle Preparations of Unidentified Vasoactive Peptides from Intestine and Lung. *Nature 225:* 1144, 1970.
17. Said, S. I., Mutt, V. Isolation from Porcine Intestinal Wall of a Vasoactive Octacosapeptide Related to Secretin and to Glucagon. *Eur. J. Biochem. 28:* 199, 1972.
18. Mutt, V., and Said, S. I. Structure of the Porcine Vasoactive Intestinal Octacosapeptide. *Eur. J. Biochem. 42:* 581, 1974.
19. Bodanszky, M., Klausner, Y. S., Lin, C. Y. Mutt, V., and Said, S. I. Synthesis of the Vasoactive Intestinal Peptide (VIP). *J. Am. Chem. Soc. 96:* 4973, 1974.
20. Bodanszky, M., Klausner, Y. S., and Said, S. I. Biological Activities of Synthetic Peptides Corresponding to Fragments of and to the Entire Sequence of the Vasoactive Intestinal Peptide. *Proc. Natl. Acad. Sci. U.S.A. 70:* 382, 1973.
21. Makhlouf, G. M., Said, S. I., and Yau, W. M. Interplay of Vasoactive Intestinal Peptide (VIP) and Synthetic VIP Fragments with Secretin and Octapeptide of Cholecystokinin (Octa-CCK) on Pancreatic and Biliary Secretion. *Gastroenterology 67:* 737, 1974.
22. Schebalim, R., Said, S. I., and Makhlouf, G. M. Interplay of Glucagon, Vasoactive Intestinal Polypeptide (VIP) and Synthetic Fragments of VIP in Intestinal Secretion. *Clin. Res. 22:* 368A, 1974.
23. Bodanszky, M., Bodanszky, A., Klausner, Y. S., and Said, S. I. A Preferred Conformation in the Vasoactive Intestinal Peptide (VIP). Molecular Architecture of Gastrointestinal Hormones. *Bioorganic Chem. 3:* 133, 1974.
24. Christophe, J., Conlon, T. P., and Gardner, J. D. Initial Step in the Action of Vasoactive Intestinal Peptide (VIP): Specific Binding to Plasma Membrane Receptors. *Clin. Res. 23:* 392A, 1975.
25. Bataille, D., Rosselin, G., and Freychet, P. Interactions of Glucagon, Gut Glucagon, Vasoactive Intestinal Polypeptide, and Secretin with Their Membrane Receptors. *Isr. J. Med. Sci. 11:* 687, 1975.
26. Bataille, D., Freychet, P., and Rosselin, G. Interactions of Glucagon, Gut Glucagon, Vasoactive Intestinal Polypeptide, and Secretin with Liver and Fat Cell Plasma Membranes: Binding and Specific Sites and Stimulation of Adenylate Cyclase. *Endocrinology 95:* 713, 1974.
27. Desbuquois, B. The Interacton of Vasoactive Intestinal Polypeptide and Secretin with Liver-Cell Membranes. *Eur. J. Biochem. 46:* 439, 1974.
28. Desbuquois, B., Laudat, M. H., and Laudat, Ph. Vasoactive Intestinal Polypeptide and Glucagon: Stimulation of Adenylate Cyclase Activity via Distinct Receptors in Liver and Fat Cell Membranes. *Biochem. Biophys. Res. Commun. 53:* 1187, 1973.
29. Bloom, S. R., Bryant, M. G., and Polak, J. M. The Distribution of Gut Hormones. *Gut 16:* 821, 1975.
30. Tai, H. H., Roth, F. L., and Chey, W. Y. Radioimmunoassay of Vasoactive Intestinal Polypeptide (VIP): Development and Its Application to Studies of Distribution and Heterogeneity of VIP in the Gastrointestinal Tract. *Gastroenterology 70:* 960, 1976.
31. Polak, J. M., Pearse, A. G. E., Garand J-C., and Bloom, S. R. Cellular Localization of a Vasoactive Intestinal Peptide in the Mammalian and Avian Gastrointestinal Tract. *Gut 15:* 720, 1974.
32. Solcia, E., Polak, J. M., Buffa, R., Capella, C., and Pearse, A. G. E. Endocrine Cells of the Intestinal Mucosa, in J. C. Thompson (ed.): *Gastrointestinal Hormones.* Austin, University of Texas Press, 1975, pp. 155–168.
33. Bryant, M. G., Polak, J. M., Modlin, I., et al. Possible Dual Role for Vasoactive Intestinal Peptide as Gastrointestinal Hormone and Neurotransmitter Substance. *Lancet 1:* 991, 1976.
34. Thulin, L. Effects of Gastrointestinal Polypeptides on Hepatic Bile Flow and Splanchnic Circulation. *Acta Chir. Scand.* [Suppl.]*441:* 5, 1973.
35. Yoshida, T., Geumei, A. M., and Said, S. I. Vasoactive Intestinal Peptide: A Potent Coronary Vasodilator. *Clin. Res. 22:* 58A, 1974.
36. Said, S. I., Bosher, L. P., Spath, J. A., and Kontos, H. A. Positive Inotropic Action of Newly Isolated Vasoactive Intestinal Polypeptide (VIP). *Clin. Res. 20:* 29, 1972.
37. Said, S. I., and Kitamura, S. Vasoactive Polypeptide Dilates Pulmonary Vessels During Alveolar Hypoxia, Histamine Infusion, or Air Breathing. *Fed. Proc. 30:* 380, 1971.
38. Said, S. I., Kitamura, S., Yoshida, T., Preskitt, J., and Holden, L. D. Humoral Control of Airways. *Ann. N.Y. Acad. Sci. 221:* 103, 1974.
39. Hara, N., Geumei, A., Chijimatsu, Y., and Said, S. I. Vasoactive Intestinal Peptide Aerosol Protects Against Histamine and Prostaglandin $F_{2\alpha}$-Induced Bronchoconstriction. *Clin. Res. 23:* 347A, 1975.

40. Fransden, E. K., and Moody, A. J. Lipolytic Action of a Newly Isolated Vasoactive Intestinal Polypeptide. *Horm. Metab. Res. 5:* 196, 1973.
41. Kerins, C., and Said, S. I. Hyperglycemic and Glycogenolytic Effects of Vasoactive Intestinal Polypeptide. *Proc. Soc. Exp. Biol. Med. 142:* 1014, 1973.
42. Schebalin, R., Brooks, A. M., Said, S. I., and Makhlouf, G. M. The Insulinotropic Effect of Vasoactive Intestinal Peptide (VIP): Direct Evidence from *in Vitro* Studies. *Gastroenterology 66:* 772, 1974.
43. Said, S. I. Vasoactive Intestinal Polypeptide (VIP). Current Status, in J. C. Thompson (ed.): *Gastrointestinal Hormones.* Austin, University of Texas Press, 1975, pp. 591–597.
44. Schorr, B. A., Said, S. I., and Makhlouf, G. M. Inhibition of Gastric Secretion by Synthetic Vasoactive Intestinal Peptide (VIP). *Clin. Res. 22:* 23A, 1974.
45. Konturek, S., Thor, P., Dembinski, A., and Krol, R. Vasoactive Intestinal Peptide: Comparison with Secretin for Potency and Spectrum of Physiologic Action, in J. C. Thompson (ed.): *Gastrointestinal Hormones.* Austin, University of Texas Press, 1975, pp. 611–633.
46. Villar, H. V., Fender, H. R., Rayford, P. L., Ramas, N. I., and Thompson, J. C. Inhibiton of Gastrin Release and Gastric Secretion by GIP and VIP, in J. C. Thompson (ed.): *Gastrointestinal Hormones.* Austin, University of Texas Press, 1975, pp. 467–473.
47. Konturek, S. J., Domschke, S., Domschke, W., et al. Comparison of Vasoactive Intestinal Peptide and Secretin in Pancreatic Stimulation and Hepatic Inactivation in Cats. *Gastroenterology 70:* 903, 1976.
48. Robberecht, P., Deschodt-Lanckman, M., DeNeef, P., Borgeat, P., and Christophe, J. In Vivo Effects of Pancreozymin, Secretin, Vasoactive Intestinal Polypeptide and Pilocarpine on the Levels of Cyclic AMP and Cyclic GMP in the Rat Pancreas. *FEBS Lett. 43:* 139, 1974.
49. Said, S. I., and Makhlouf, G. M. Vasoactive Intestinal Polypeptide: Spectrum of Biological Activity, in W. Y. Chey and F. B. Brooks (eds.): *Endocrinology of the Gut.* Thorofare, N.J., Charles B. Slack, 1974, pp. 83–87.
50. Barbezat, G. O., and Grossman, M. I. Intestinal Secretion: Stimulation by Peptides. *Science 174:* 422, 1971.
51. Schwartz, C. J., Kimberg, D. V., Sheerin, H. E., Field, M., and Said, S. I. Vasoactive Intestinal Peptide Stimulation of Adenylate Cyclase and Active Electrolyte Secretion in Intestinal Mucosa. *J. Clin. Invest. 54:* 536, 1974.
52. Jaffer, S. S., Farrar, J. T., Yau, W. M., and Makhlouf, G. M. Mode of Action and Interplay of Vasoactive Intestinal Peptide (VIP), Secretin and Octapeptide of Cholecystokinin (Octa-CCK) on Duodenal and Ileal Muscle *in Vitro. Gastroenterology 66:* 716, 1974.
53. Makhlouf, G. M., and Said, S. I. The Effect of Vasoactive Intestinal Peptide (VIP) on Digestive and Hormonal Function, in J. C. Thompson (ed.): *Gastrointestinal Hormones.* Austin, University of Texas Press, 1975, pp. 599–610.
54. Ebeid, E. M., Murray, P., Soeters, P. B., and Fischer, J. E. Release of Vasoactive Intestinal Peptide (VIP) by Calcium Infusions. *Am. J. Surg. 133:* 140, 1977.
55. Kitamura, S., Yoshida, T., and Said, S. I. Vasoactive Intestinal Polypeptide Inactivation in Liver and Potentiation in Lung of Anesthetized Dogs. *Proc. Soc. Exp. Biol. Med. 148:* 25, 1975.
56. Said, S. I., Faloona, G. R., Deon, H., Unger, R. H., and Siegel, S. R. Vasoactive Intestinal Polypeptide: Elevated Levels in Patients with Hepatic Cirrhosis. *Clin. Res. 22:* 367A, 1974.
57. Ebeid, A. M., Murray, P., Soeters, P. B., and Fischer, J. E. The Effect of Portal Systemic Shunt and Hepatic Insufficiency on Plasma Levels of Vasoactive Intestinal Peptide. *Gastroenterology 70:* 958, 1976.
58. Elias, E., Mitchell, S. J., and Bloom, S. R. Vasoactive Intestinal Peptide in Cirrhosis. *Lancet 2:* 1312, 1975.
59. Kosaka, T., and Lim, R. K. S. On the Mechanism of the Inhibition of Gastric Secretion by Fat. *Chin. J. Physiol. 4:* 213, 1930.
60. Ewald, C. A., and Boas, J. *Virchows Arch. Pathol. 104:* 271, 1886. (cited by Gregory, R. A. Secretory Mechanisms of the Gastrointestinal Tract. New York, Edward Arnold, 1962, p. 118).
61. Pavlov, I. P. The Work of the Digestive Glands, 2nd ed. (Transl. W. H. Thompson) London, Charles Griffin, 1910.
62. Farrell, J. I., and Ivy, A. C. Studies on the Motility of the Transplanted Gastric Pouch. *Am. J. Physiol. 76:* 227, 1926.
63. Feng, T. P., Hou, H. C., and Lim, R. K. S. On the Mechanism of the Inhibiton of Gastric Secretion by Fat. *Chin. J. Physiol. 3:* 371, 1929.
64. Brown, J. C. and Pederson, R. A. A Multiparameter Study on the Action of Preparations Containing Cholecystokinin–Pancreozymin. *Scand. J. Gastroenterol. 5:* 537, 1970.
65. Brown, J. C., Pederson, R. A., Jorpes, E., and Mutt, V. Preparation of Highly Active Enterogastrone. *Can. J. Physiol. Pharmacol. 47:* 113, 1969.
66. Brown, J. C., and Dryburgh, J. R. Chemistry of Gastric Inhibitory Polypeptide (GIP) and Motilin, in W. Y. Chey and F. P. Brooks (eds.): *Endocrinology of the Gut.* Thorofare, N.J., Charles B. Slack, 1974, pp. 14–21.
67. Brown, J. C., Mutt, V., and Pederson, R. A. Further Purification of a Polypeptide Demonstrating Enterogastrone Activity. *J. Physiol. 209:* 57, 1970.
68. Brown, J. C., and Dryburgh, J. R. Gastric Inhibitory Polypeptide II: The Complete Amino Acid Sequence. *Can. J. Biochem. 49:* 867, 1971.
69. Bodanszky, M. The Secretin Family and Evolution, in J. C. Thompson, (ed.): *Gastrointestinal Hormones.* Austin, University of Texas Press, 1975, pp. 507–518.
70. Pederson, R. A., Schubert, H. E., and Brown, J. C. The Insulinotropic Action of Gastric Inhibitory Polypeptide. *Can. J. Physiol. Pharmacol. 53:* 217, 1975.
71. Brown, J. C., Dryburgh, J. R., Ross, S. A., and Dupre, J. Identification and Actions of Gastric Inhibitory Polypeptide. *Recent Prog. Horm. Res. 31:* 487, 1975.
72. Brown, J. C., Dryburgh, J. R., Moccia, P., and Pederson, R. A. The Current Status of GIP, in J. C. Thompson (ed.): *Gastrointestinal Hormones.* Austin, University of Texas Press, 1975, pp. 537–547.
73. O'Dorisio, T. M., Crockett, S. E., Mazzaferri, E. L., et al. Canine Gastric Inhibitory Polypeptide (GIP): Immunologic Characterization, Gastrointestinal Localization, and Response to Intraduodenal Glucose. *Clin. Res. 22:* 605A, 1974.
74. Polak, J. M., Bloom, S. R., Kuzio, M., Brown, J. C., and Pearse, A. G. E. Cellular Localization of Gastric Inhibitory Polypeptide in the Duodenum and Jejunum. *Gut 14:* 284, 1973.
75. Buffa, R., Polak, J. M., Pearse, A. G. E., et al. Identification of the Intestinal Cell Storing Gastric Inhibitory Peptide. *Histochemistry 43:* 249, 1975.
76. Pederson, R. A., and Brown, J. C. Inhibition of Histamine-, Pentagastrin-, and Insulin-Stimulated Gastric Secretion by Pure Gastric Inhibitory Polypeptide. *Gastroenterology 62:* 393, 1972.
77. Johnson, L. R., and Grossman, M. I. Effects of Fat, Secretin, and Cholecystokinin on Histamine-Stimulated Gastric Secretion. *Am. J. Physiol. 216:* 1176, 1969.
78. Catresana, M., Lee, K. Y., and Chey, W. Y. Actions of Synthetic Porcine Motilin, Octapeptide of Cholecystokinin (CCK), Gastric Inhibitory Polypeptide (GIP) and Secretin on Myoelectric Activity of Gastric Antrum and Duodenum. *Fed. Proc. 35:* 218, 1976.
79. Rayford, P. L., Villar, H. V., Reeder, D. D., and Thompson, J. C. Effect of GIP and VIP on Gastrin Release and Gastric Secretion. *Physiologist 17:* 319, 1974.
80. Dupre, J., Curtis, J. D., Unger, R. H., Waddell, R. W., and Beck, J. C. Effects of Secretin, Pancreozymin, or Gastrin on the Response of the Endocrine Pancreas to Administration of Glucose or Arginine in Man. *J. Clin. Invest. 48:* 745, 1969.
81. Dupre, J., Ross, S. A., Watson, D., and Brown, J. C. Stimulation of Insulin Secretion by Gastric Inhibitory Polypeptide in Man. *J. Clin. Endocrinol. Metab. 37:* 826, 1973.
82. Tze, W. T. Gastric Inhibitory Polypeptide (GIP): A Potent Stimulator of Insulin Release. *Gastroenterology 68:* 621, 1975.
83. Schauder, P., Brown, J. C., Frerichs, H., and Creutzfeldt, W. Gastric Inhibitory Polypeptide: Effect of Glucose-Induced Insulin Release from Isolated Rat Pancreatic Islets *in Vitro. Diabetologia 11:* 483, 1975.
84. Creutzfeldt, W. Gastrointestinal Hormones and Insulin Secretion. *N. Engl. J. Med. 288:* 1238, 1973.
85. Rehfeld, J. F. Gastrointestinal Hormones and Insulin Secretion. *Scand. J. Gastroenterol. 7:* 289, 1972.
86. Kuzio, M., Dryburgh, J. R., Malloy, K. M., and Brown, J. C. Radioimmunoassay for Gastric Inhibitory Polypeptide. *Gastroenterology 66:* 357, 1974.
87. Brown, J. C. "Enterogastrone" and Other New Gut Peptides. *Med. Clin. North Am. 58:* 1347, 1974.

88. Cleator, I. G. M., and Gourley, R. H. Release of Immunoreactive Gastric Inhibitory Polypeptide (IR-GIP) by Oral Ingestion of Food Substances. *Am. J. Surg. 130:* 128, 1975.

89. O'Dorisio, T. M., Martin, E. W. Jr., Thomford, N. R., Mazzaferri, E. L., and Cataland, S. Endogenous Gastric Inhibitory Polypeptide (GIP) Release and Acid Secretion (AS). *Clin. Res. 23:* 483A, 1975.

90. Falco, J. M., Crockett, S. E., Cataland, S., and Mazzaferri, E. L. Gastric Inhibitory Polypeptide (GIP) Stimulated by Fat Ingestion in Man. *J. Clin. Endocrinol. Metab. 41:* 260, 1975.

91. Crockett, S. E., Cataland, S., Falko, J. M., and Mazzaferri, E. L. The Insulinotropic Effect of Endogenous Gastric Inhibitory Polypeptide in Normal Subjects. *J. Clin. Endocrinol. Metab. 42:* 1098, 1976.

92. Cataland, S., Crockett, S. E., Brown, J. C., and Mazzaferri, E. L. Gastric Inhibitory Polypeptide (GIP) Stimulation by Oral Glucose in Man. *J. Clin. Endocrinol. Metab. 39:* 223, 1974.

93. Andersen, D. K., Brown, J. C., Tobin, J. D., and Andres, R. The Role of Gastric Inhibitory Polypeptide (GIP) in the Augmentation of Glucose-Stimulated Insulin (IRI) Release. *Clin. Res. 23:* 589A, 1975.

94. Ross, S. A., Brown, J. C., Dryburgh, J., and Dupre, J. Hypersecretion of Gastric Inhibitory Polypeptide in Diabetes Mellitus. *Clin. Res. 21:* 1029, 1973.

95. Botha, J. L., Vinik, A. I., and Brown, J. C. Gastric Inhibitory Polypeptide (GIP) in Chronic Pancreatitis. *J. Clin. Endocrinol. Metab. 42:* 791, 1976.

96. Thomford, N. R., Sirinek, K. R., Crockett, S. E., Mazzaferri, E. L., and Cataland, S. Gastric Inhibitory Polypeptide: Response to Oral Glucose After Vagotomy and Pyloroplasty. *Arch. Surg. 109:* 177, 1974.

97. Thomas, F. B., Mazzaferri, E. L., Crockett, S. E., et al. Stimulation of Secretion of Gastric Inhibitory Polypeptide and Insulin by Intraduodenal Amino Acids. *Gasterenterology 70:* 523, 1976.

98. Thomas, F. B., Sinar, D., Mazzaferri, E. L., et al. Selective Release of Gastric Inhibitory Polypeptide in Man by Intraduodenal Amino Acids. *Gastroenterology 70:* 943, 1976.

99. O'Dorisio, T. M., Sirinek, K. R., Pace, W. G., Mazzaferri, E. L., and Cataland, S. Basal and Postcibal Serum Gastric Inhibitory Polypeptide Concentrations in Patients with Chronic Renal Failure. *Gastroenterology 70:* 924, 1976.

100. Brown, J. C., Johnson, L. P., and Magee, D. F. Effect of Duodenal Alkalinization on Gastric Motility. *Gastroenterology 50:* 333, 1966.

101. Brown, J. C. Presence of a Gastric Motor-Stimulating Property in Duodenal Extracts. *Gastroenterology 52:* 225, 1967.

102. Brown, J. C., and Parkes, C. O. Effect of Fundic Pouch Motor Activity of Stimulatory and Inhibitory Fractions Separated from Pancreozymin. *Gastroenterology 53:* 731, 1967.

103. Brown, J. C., Mutt, V., and Dryburgh, J. R. The Further Purification of Motilin, a Gastric Motor Activity Stimulating Polypeptide from the Mucosa of the Small Intestine of Hogs, *Can. J. Physiol. Pharmacol. 49:* 399, 1971.

104. Brown, J. C., Cook, M. A., and Dryburgh, J. R. Motilin, a Gastric Motor Activity-Stimulating Polypeptide: Final Purification, Amino Acid Composition, and C-Terminal Residues. *Gastroenterology 62:* 401, 1972.

105. Brown, J. C., Cook, M. A., and Dryburgh, J. R. Motilin, a Gastric Motor Activity Stimulating Polypeptide: The Complete Amino Acid Sequence. *Can. J. Biochem. 51:* 533, 1973.

106. Wunsch, E., Brown, J. C., Deimer, K.-H., et al. Zur Synthese von Norleucin-13-Motilin. *Z. Naturforsch. 28c:* 235, 1973.

107. Shubert, E., Mitznegg, P., Strunz, U., et al. Influence of the Hormone Analogue 13-Nle-Motilin and of 1-Methyl-3-Isobutylxanthine on Tone and Cyclic 3′-, 5′-AMP Content of Antral and Duodenal Muscles in the Rabbit. *Life Sci. 16:* 263, 1975.

108. Strunz, U., Domschke, W., Mitznegg, P., et al. Analysis of the Motor Effects of 13-Norleucine Motilin on the Rabbit, Guinea Pig, Rat, and Human Alimentary Tract *in Vitro. Gastroenterology 68:* 1485, 1975.

109. Jennewein, H. M., Hummelt, H., Siewert, R., and Waldeck, F. The Motor-Stimulating Effect of Natural Motilin on the Lower Esophageal Sphincter, Fundus, Antrum and Duodenum in Dogs. *Digestion 13:* 246, 1975.

110. Gutierrez, J. G., Thanik, K. D., Chey, W. Y., and Yajima, H. The Effect of Motilin on the Lower Esophageal Sphincter of the Opossum. *Gastroenterology 70:* 958, 1976.

111. Rosch, W., Lux, G., Domschke, S., et al. Effect of 13-Nle-Motilin on Lower Esophageal Sphincter Pressure (LESP) in Man. *Gastroenterology 70:* 931, 1976.

112. Ruppin, H., Domschke, S., Domschke, W. et al. Effects of 13-Nle-Motilin in Man—Inhibition of Gastric Evacuation and Stimulation of Pepsin Secretion. *Scand. J. Gastroent. 10:* 199, 1975.

113. Mitznegg, P., Domschke, W., Domschke, S., et al. Protein Synthesis in Human Gastric Mucosa: Effects of Pentagastrin, Secretin and 13-Nle-Motilin. *Acta Hepatogastroenterol. 22:* 333, 1975.

114. Green, W. E. R., Ruppin, H., Wingate, D. L., et al. Direct Effects of 13-Nle-Motilin on Canine Gastric and Duodenal Motility. *Gastroenterology 70:* 890, 1976.

115. Pearse, A. G. E., Polak, J. M., Bloom, S. R., et al. Enterochromaffin Cells of the Mammalian Small Intestine as the Source of Motilin. *Virchows Arch.* [*Cell Pathol.*] *16:* 111, 1974.

116. Polak, J. M., Pearse, A. G. E., and Heath, C. M. Complete Identification of Endocrine Cells in the Gastrointestinal Tract Using Semithin Thin Sections to Identify Motilin Cells in Human and Animal Intestine. *Gut 16:* 225, 1975.

117. Dryburgh, J. R., and Brown, J. C. Radioimmunoassay for Motilin. *Gastroenterology 68:* 1169, 1975.

118. Mitznegg, P., Domschke, W., Wunsch, E. et al. Release of Motilin After Duodenal Acidification. *Lancet 1:* 888, 1976.

119. Mitznegg, P., Bloom, S. R., Domschke, W., et al. Disappearance Half Time of Exogenous and Endogenous Motilin in Man. *Naunyn-Schmiedebergs Arch. Pathol.*[*Suppl.*]*293:* R63, 1976.

120. Shay, H., and Gershon-Cohen, J. Experimental Studies in Gastric Physiology in Man: The Mechanism of Gastric Evacuation in Man: The Mechanism of Gastric Evacuation After Partial Gastrectomy as Demonstrated Roentgenologically. *Am. J. Dig. Dis. Nutr. 2:* 608, 1935.

121. Thomas, J. E., Crider, J. O., and Mogan, C. J. A Study of Reflexes Involving the Pyloric Sphincter and Antrum and their Role in Gastric Evacuation. *Am. J. Physiol. 108:* 683, 1934.

122. Lin, T. M., and Chance, R. E. Spectrum Gastrointestinal Actions of a New Bovine Pancreas Polypeptide (BPP). *Gastroenterology 62:* 852, 1972.

123. Kimmel, J. R., Pollock, H. G., and Hazelwood, R. L. A New Pancreatic Polypeptide Hormone. *Fed. Proc. 30:* 1318, 1971.

124. Kimmel, J. R., Hayden, L. J., and Pollock, H. G. Isolation and Characterization of a New Pancreatic Polypeptide Hormone. *J. Biol. Chem. 250:* 9369, 1975.

125. Lin, T. M., Evans, D. C., and Chance, R. E. Action of a Bovine Pancreatic Polypeptide (BPP) on Pancreatic Secretion in Dogs. *Gastroenterology 66:* 852, 1974.

126. Lin, T. M., and Chance, R. E. Bovine Pancreatic Polypeptide (BPP) and Avian Pancreatic Polypeptide (APP). *Gastroenterology 67:* 737, 1974.

127. Lin, T. M., and Chance, R. E. Gastrointestinal Actions of a New Bovine Pancreatic Polypeptide (BPP), in J. C. Thompson (ed.): *Gastrointestinal Hormones.* Austin, University of Texas Press, 1975, pp. 143–145.

128. Hazelwood, R. L., Turner, S. D., Kimmel, J. R., and Pollock, H. G. Spectrum Effects of a New Polypeptide (Third Hormone?) Isolated from the Chicken Pancreas. *Gen. Comp. Endocrinol. 21:* 485, 1973.

129. Hazelwood, R. L. The Avian Endocrine Pancreas. *Am. Zool.* **13:** *699, 1973.*

130. Langslow, D. R., Kimmel, J. R., and Pollock, H. G. Studies of the Distribution of a New Avian Pancreatic Polypeptide and Insulin Among Birds, Reptiles, Amphibians and Mammals. *Endocrinology 93:* 558, 1973.

131. Larsson, L-I., Sundler, F., Hakanson, R., Pollock, H. G., and Kimmel, J. R. Localization of APP, a Postulated New Hormone, to a Pancreatic Endocrine Cell Type. *Histochemistry 42:* 377, 1974.

132. Larsson, L.-I., Sundler, F., and Hakanson, R. Immunohistochemical Localization of Human Pancreatic Polypeptide (HPP) to a Population of Islet Cells. *Cell Tissue Res. 156:* 167, 1975.

133. Kimmel, J. R., and Pollock, H. G. Factors Affecting Blood Levels of Avian Pancreatic Polypeptide (APP), a New Pancreatic Hormone. *Fed. Proc. 34:* 454, 1975.

134. Floyd, J. C., Jr., Chance, R. E., Hayashi, M., Moon, N. E., and Fajans, S. S. Concentrations of a Newly Recognized Pancreatic Islet Polypeptide in Plasma of Healthy Subjects and in Plasma and Tumors of Patients with Insulin-Secreting Islet Cell Tumors. *Clin. Res. 23:* 535A, 1975.

135. Floyd, J. C., Jr., Fajans, S. S., and Pek, S. Regulation in Healthy Subjects of the Secretion of a Newly Recognized Pancreatic Islet Polypeptide. *Clin. Res. 24:* 485A, 1976.
136. Schwartz, T. W., Stadil, F., Chance, R. E., et al. Pancreatic-Polypeptide Response to Food in Duodenal-Ulcer Patients Before and After Vagotomy. *Lancet 1:* 1102, 1976.
137. Polak, J. M., Adrian, T. E., Bryant, M. G., et al. Pancreatic Polypeptide in Insulinomas, Gastrinomas, VIPomas and Glucagonomas. *Lancet 1:* 328, 1976.
138. Erspamer, V., and Melchiorri, P. Active Polypeptides of the Amphibian Skin and Their Synthetic Analogues. *Pure Appl. Chem. 35:* 463, 1973.
139. Walsh, J. H., and Holmquist, A. L. Radioimmunoassay of Bombesin Peptides: Identification of Bombesin-Like Immunoreactivity in Vertebrate Gut Extracts. *Gastroenterology 70:* 948, 1976.
140. Polak, J. M., Hobbs, S., Bloom, S. R., Solcia, E., and Pearse, A. G. E. Distribution of a Bombesin-Like Peptide in Human Gastrointestinal Tract. *Lancet 1:* 1109, 1976.
141. Erspamer, V., and Melchiorri, P. Actions of Bombesin on Secretions and Motility of the Gastrointestinal Tract, in J. C. Thompson (ed.): *Gastrointestinal Hormones.* Austin, University of Texas Press, 1975, pp. 575–589.
142. Broccardo, M., Erspamer, G. F., Melchiorri, P., Negri, L., and De Castiglione, R. Relative Potency of Bombesin-Like Peptides. *Br. J. Pharmacol. 55:* 221, 1975.
143. Clineschmidt, B. V., Geller, R. G., Govier, W. C., Pisano, J. J., and Tanimura, T. Effects of Ranatensin, a Polypeptide from Frog Skin, on Isolated Smooth Muscle. *Br. J. Pharmacol. 41:* 622, 1971.
144. Endean, R., Erspamer, V., Erspamer, G. F., et al. Parallel Bioassay of Bombesin and Litorin, a Bombesin-Like Peptide from the Skin of Litoria Aurea. *Br. J. Pharmacol. 55:* 213, 1975.
145. Bertaccini, G., Erspamer, V., and Impicciatore, M. The Actions of Bombesin on Gastric Secretion of the Dog and the Rat. *Br. J. Pharmacol. 49:* 437, 1973.
146. Bertaccini, G., Erspamer, V., Melchiorri, P., and Sopranzi, N. Gastrin Release by Bombesin in the Dog. *Br. J. Pharmacol. 52:* 219, 1974.
147. Basso, N., Improta, G., Melchiorri, P., and Sopranzi, N. Gastrin Release by Bombesin in the Antral Pouch Dog. *Rendic. Gastroenterol. 6:* 95, 1974.
148. Impicciatore, M., Debas, H., Walsh, J. H., Grossman, M. I., and Bertaccini, G. Release of Gastrin and Stimulation of Acid Secretion by Bombesin in Dog. *Rendic. Gastroenterol. 6:* 99, 1974.
149. DelleFave, G. F., Corazziari, E., Melchiorri, P., et al. Effects of Bombesin on the Gastrinaemic Levels and Gastric Acid Secretion in Man. *Rendic. Gastroenterol. 5:* 239, 1973.
150. Basso, N., Lezoche, E., Materia, A., Giri, S., and Speranza, V. Effect of Bombesin on Extragastric Gastrin in Man. *Am. J. Dig. Dis. 20:* 923, 1975.
151. Erspamer, V., Improta, G., Melchiorri, P., and Sopranzi, N. Evidence of Cholecystokinin Release by Bombesin in the Dog. *Br. J. Pharmacol. 52:* 227, 1974.
152. Erspamer, V., Melchiorri, P., and Sopranzi, N. Effects of Bombesin (BBS) on Gastrinoemia, Gastric, Pancreatic, and Biliary Secretion and on Gallbladder Motor Activity in the Dog. *Rendic. Gastroenterol. 5:* 240a, 1973.
153. Corazziari, E., DelleFave, G. F., Melchiorri, P., and Torsoli, A. Effects of a New Polypeptide, Bombesin, on Gall Bladder and Duodeno-Jejunal Junction Mechanical Activity in Man. *Rendic. Gastroenterol. 5:* 140, 1973.
154. Corazziari, E., Torsoli, A., Melchiorri, P., and DelleFave, G. F. Effect of Bombesin on Human Gall Bladder Emptying. *Rendic. Gastroenterol. 6:* 52, 1974.
155. Basso, N., Giri, S., Improta, G., et al. External Pancreatic Secretion After Bombesin in Man. *Gut 16:* 994, 1975.
156. Villar, H. V., Llanos, O. L., Rayford, P. L., and Thompson, J. C. Effect of Bombesin on Circulating Levels of Secretin Before and After Antrectomy. *Gastroenterology 70:* 947, 1976.
157. Fender, H. R., Curtis, P. J., Rayford, P. L., Reeder, D. D., and Thompson, J. C. Effect of Bombesin on Gastrin and Secretin and on Gastric and Pancreatic Secretion. *Physiologist 18:* 212, 1975.
158. Caprilli, R., Melchiorri, P., Improta, G., Vernia, P., and Frieri, G. Effects of Bombesin and Bombesin-Like Peptides on Gastrointestinal Myoelectric Activity. *Gastroenterology 68:* 1228, 1975.
159. Bertaccini, G., Impicciatore, M., Molina, E., and Zappia, L. Action of Bombesin on Human Gastrointestinal Motility. *Rendic. Gastroenterology 6:* 45, 1974.
160. Corazziari, E., Torsoli, A., DelleFave, G. F., Melchiorri, P., and Habib, F. I. Effects of Bombesin on the Mechanical Activity of the Human Duodenum and Jejunum. *Rendic. Gastroenterol. 6:* 55, 1974.
161. Erspamer, V., Melchiorri, P., and Sopranzi, N. The Action of Bombesin on the Systemic Arterial Blood Pressure of Some Experimental Animals. *Br. J. Pharmacol. 45:* 442, 1972.
162. Impicciatore, M., and Bertaccini, G. The Bronchoconstrictor Action of the Tetradecapeptide Bombesin in the Guinea-Pig. *J. Pharm. Pharmacol. 25:* 872, 1973.
163. Erspamer, V., Erspamer, G. F., Inselvini, M., and Negri, L. Occurrence of Bombesin and Alytesin in Extracts of the Skin of Three European Discoglossid Frogs and Pharmacological Actions of Bombesin on Extravascular Smooth Muscle. *Br. J. Pharmacol. 45:* 333, 1972.
164. Erspamer, V., Melchiorri, P., and Sopranzi, N. The Action of Bombesin on the Kidney of the Anaesthetized Dog. *Br. J. Pharmacol. 48:* 438, 1973.
164a. Rhodes, R. A., Tai, H-H, and Chey, W. Y. Observations on Plasma Secretin Levels by Radioimmunoassay in Response to Duodenal Acidification and to a Meat Meal in Humans. *Dig. Dis. 21:* 873, 1976.
164b. Ward, A. S., and Bloom, S. R. The Role of Secretin in the Inhibition of Gastric Secretion by Intraduodenal Acid. *Gut 15:* 889, 1974.
164c. Rayford, P. L., Curtis, P. J., Fender, H. R., and Thompson, J. C. Plasma Levels of Secretin in Man and Dogs—Validation of a Secretin Radioimmunoassay. *Surgery 79:* 658, 1976.
164d. Boden, G., and Chey, W. Y. Preparation and Specificity of Antiserum to Synthetic Secretin and Its Use in a Radioimmunoassay (RIA). *Endocrinology 92:* 1617, 1973.
164e. Boden, G., Sivitz, M. C., Owen, O. E., Essa-Koumar, N., and Landor, J. H. Somatostatin Suppresses Secretin and Pancreatic Exocrine Secretion. *Science 190:* 163, 1975.
164f. Ward, A. S. The Effect of Vagotomy on the Inhibition of Gastric Secretion by Intraduodenal Acid. *Br. J. Surg. 61:* 698, 1974.
164g. Ward, A. S., and Bloom, S. R. Effect of Vagotomy on Secretin Release in Man. *Gut 16:* 951, 1975.
164h. Chisholm, D. J., Young, J. D., and Lazarus, L. The Gastrointestinal Stimulus to Insulin Release. *J. Clin. Invest. 48:* 1453, 1969.
164i. Boden, G., Essa, N., Owen, O. E., and Reichle, F. A. Effects of Intraduodenal Administration of HCl and Glucose on Circulating Immunoreactive Secretin and Insulin Concentrations. *J. Clin. Invest. 53:* 1185, 1974.
164j. Boden, G., Essa, N., and Owen, O. E. Effects of Intraduodenal Amino Acids, Fatty Acids, and Sugars on Secretin Concentrations. *Gastroenterology 68:* 722, 1975.
164k. Henry, R. W., Flanagan, R. W. J., and Buchanan, K. D. Secretin—A New Role for an Old Hormone. *Lancet 2:* 202, 1975.
164l. Straus, E., Urbach, H.-J., and Yalow, R. S. Alcohol-Stimulated Secretion of Immunoreactive Secretin. *N. Engl. J. Med. 293:* 1031, 1975.
164m. Rhodes, R. A., Chey, W. Y., Tai, H. H., and Escoffery, R. Impaired Release of Secretin in Celiac Sprue. *Clin. Res. 23:* 578A, 1975.
164n. Bussolati, G., Capella, C., Solcia, E., Vassallo, G., and Vezzadini, P. Ultrastructural and Immunofluorescent Investigations on the Secretin Cell in the Dog Intestinal Mucosa. *Histochemie 26:* 218, 1971.
164o. Polak, J. M., Coulling, I., Bloom, S., and Pearse, A. G. E. Immunofluorescent Localization of Secretin and Enteroglucagon in Human Intestinal Mucosa. *Scand. J. Gastroenterol. 6:* 739, 1971.
164p. Polak, J. M., Pearse, A. G. E., Van Noorden, S., Bloom, S. R., and Rossiter, M. A. Secretin Cells in Coeliac Disease. *Gut 14,* 870, 1973.
164q. Rooney, P. J., Sturrock, R., Hayes, J. R., et al. Effect of Carbenoxolone Upon Immunoreactive Secretin in Patients with Rheumatoid Arthritis. *Lancet 1:* 592, 1974.
164r. Cano, R., Bloom, S. R., and Isenberg, J. I. Pancreatic Bicarbonate Secretion and Serum Secretin in Response to Graded Amounts of Duodenal Acidification in Duodenal Ulcer and Normal Subjects. *Gastroenterology 68:* 870, 1975.
164s. Curtis, P. J., Fender, H. R., Rayford, P. L., and Thompson, J. D.

Disappearance Half-Time of Endogenous and Exogenous Secretin in Dogs. *Gut 17:* 595, 1976.

164t. Chey, W. Y., Hendricks, J., and Lorber, S. H. Inactivation of Secretin by the Liver. *Clin. Res. 19:* 389, 1971.

164u. Kolts, B. E.., Fabri, P. J., and McGuigan, J. E. The Half-Life of Exogenous Secretin in Cirrhosis. *Gastroenterology 70:* 903, 1976.

164v. Curtis, P. J., Fender, H. R., Rayford, P. L., and Thompson, J. C. Catabolism of Secretin by the Liver and Kidney. *Surgery 80:* 259, 1976.

164w. Straus, E., Urbach, H., and Yalow, R. S. Secretin RIA—Methodology and Application to Studies of Distribution and Molecular Forms of Secretin in Tissues. *Proc. Endocrinol. Soc.* 185, 1975.

164x. Boden, G., Murthy, N. S., and Silver, E. "Big" Secretin. *Clin. Res. 23:* 245A, 1975.

164y. Harvey, R. F., Dowsett, L., Hartog, M., and Read, A. E. A Radioimmunoassay for Cholecystokinin–Pancreozymin. *Lancet 2:* 826, 1973.

164z. Young, J. D., Lazarus, L., and Chisholm, D. J. Radioimmunoassay of Pancreozymin Cholecystokinin in Human Serum. *J. Nucl. Med. 10:* 743, 1969.

164aa. Reeder, D. D., Becker, H. D., Smith, N. J., Rayford, P. L., and Thompson, J. C. Measurement of Endogenous Release of Cholecystokinin by Radioimmunoassay. *Ann. Surg. 178:* 304, 1973.

164bb. Thompson, J. C., Fender, H. R., Ramus, N. I., Villar, H. V., and Rayford, P. L. Cholecystokinin Metabolism in Man and Dogs. *Ann. Surg. 182:* 496, 1975.

164cc. Spence, R. W., Celestin, L. R., and Harvey, R. F. Effect of Metiamide on Basal and Stimulated Serum Cholecystokinin Levels in Duodenal Ulcer Patients. *Gut 17:* 920, 1976.

164dd. Del Mazo, J., Goldstein, R., Sundy, M., and Davidson, P. Serum Levels of Cholecystokinin–Pancreozymin in Patients with Partial Gastrectomy and Gastrojejunostomy and in Chronic Pancreatitis Patients. *Gastroenterology 70:* 957, 1976.

164ee. Low-Beer, T. S., Harvey, R. F., Davies, E. R., and Reed, A. E. Abnormalities of Serum Cholecystokinin and Gallbladder Emptying in Celiac Disease. *N. Engl. J. Med. 292:* 961, 1975.

164ff. Dafny, N., and Jacobson, E. D. Cholecystokinin and Central Nervous Regulation of Appetite, in J. C. Thompson (eds.): *Gastrointestinal Hormones.* Austin, University of Texas Press, 1975, p. 643.

164gg. Debas, H. T., Farooq, O., and Grossman, M. I. Inhibition of Gastric Emptying Is a Physiological Action of Cholecystokinin. *Gastroenterology 68:* 1211, 1975.

164hh. Nebel, O. T., and Castell, D. O. Lower Esophageal Sphincter Pressure Changes After Food Ingestion. *Gastroenterology 63:* 778, 1972.

164ii. Harvey, R. F., and Read, A. E. Effect of Cholecystokinin on Colonic Motility and Symptoms in Patients with the Irritable-Bowel Syndrome. *Lancet 1:* 1, 1973.

164jj. Polak, J. M., Bloom, S. R., Rayford, P. L., et al. Identification of Cholecystokinin-Secreting Cells. *Lancet 2:* 1016, 1975.

164kk. Owyang, C., Ng, P. Y., Go, V. L. W., and Reilly, W. Cholecystokinin—Metabolic Clearance and Tissue Distribution. *Gastroenterology 70:* 925, 1976.

165. Strom, R. A Case of Peptic Ulcer and Insulinoma. *Acta. Chir. Scand. 104:* 252, 1952.

166. Sailer, S., and Zinninger, M. Massive Islet Tumor of the Pancreas Without Hypoglycemia. *Surg. Gynecol. Obstet. 82:* 301, 1946.

167. Forty, F., and Barrett, G. M. Peptic Ulceration of the Third Portion of the Duodenum Associated with Islet-Cell Tumours of the Pancreas. *Br. J. Surg. 40:* 60, 1952.

168. Zollinger, R. M., and Ellison, E. H. Primary Peptic Ulcerations of the Jejunum Associated with Islet Cell Tumors of the Pancreas. *Ann. Surg. 142:* 709, 1955.

169. Gregory, R. A., Tracy, H. J., French, J. M., and Sircus, W. Extraction of a Gastrin-Like Substance from a Pancreatic Tumor in a Case of Zollinger-Ellison Syndrome. *Lancet 1:* 1045, 1960.

170. Grossman, M. I., Tracy, H. J., and Gregory, R. A. Zollinger-Ellison Syndrome in a Bantu Woman, with Isolation of a Gastrin-Like Substance from the Primary and Secondary Tumors. II. Extraction of a Gastrin-Like Activity from Tumors. *Gastroenterology 41:* 87, 1961.

171. Gregory, R. A., Tracy, H. J., Agarwal, K. L., and Grossman, M. I. Aminoacid Constitution of Two Gastrins Isolated from Zollinger-Ellison Tumour Tissue. *Gut 10:* 603, 1969.

172. McGuigan, J. E., and Trudeau, W. L. Immunochemical Measurement of Elevated Levels of Gastrin in the Serum of Patients with Pancreatic Tumors of the Zollinger-Ellison Variety. *N. Engl. J. Med. 278:* 1308, 1968.

173. Ellison, E. H., and Wilson, S. D. The Zollinger-Ellison Syndrome; Reappraisal and Evaluation of 260 Registered Cases. *Ann. Surg. 160:* 512, 1964.

174. Cathcart, R. S., III, Webb, C. M., and Otherson, H. B., Jr. Zollinger-Ellison Syndrome in a Seven-Year Old Boy: A Case Report. *Surgery 66:* 401, 1969.

175. Ellison, E. H., and Wilson, S. D. Ulcerogenic Tumor of the Pancreas. *Proc. Clin. Cancer 3:* 225, 1967.

176. Way, L., Goldman, L., and Dunphy, J. E. Zollinger-Ellison Syndrome: An Analysis of Twenty-Five Cases. *Am. J. Surg. 116:* 293, 1968.

177. Bonfils, S., and Bernades, P. Zollinger-Ellison Syndrome: Natural History and Diagnosis. *Clin. Gastroenterol. 3:* 539, 1974.

178. Hallenbeck, G. A. The Zollinger-Ellison Syndrome. *Gastroenterology 54:* 426, 1968.

179. Zollinger, R. M. Reflections on the Ulcerogenic Syndrome. *Am. Surg. 33:* 610, 1967.

180. Aoyagi, T., Summerskill, W. H. J. Gastric Secretion with Ulcerogenic Islet Cell Tumor. *Arch. Intern. Med. 117:* 667, 1966.

181. Thompson, J. C., Reeder, D. D., Villar, H. V., and Fender, H. R. Natural History and Experience with Diagnosis and Treatment of the Zollinger-Ellison Syndrome. *Surg. Gynecol. Obstet. 140:* 721, 1975.

182. Kaye, M. D., Rhodes, J., and Beck, P. Gastric Secretion in Duodenal Ulcer with Particular Reference to the Diagnosis of Zollinger-Ellison Syndrome. *Gastroenterology 58:* 476, 1970.

183. Bernades, P., Mignon, M., Bensalem, R., et al. Discriminative Interest of the Study of Basal Acid Secretion and Pepsin Acid Correlation in Zollinger-Ellison Syndrome and Peptic Ulcer. *Digestion 9:* 1, 1973.

184. Marks, I. N., Selzer, G., Louw, J. H., and Bank, S. Zollinger-Ellison Syndrome in a Bantu Woman with Isolation of a Gastrin-Like Substance from the Primary and Secondary Tumors. I. Case Report. *Gastroenterology 41:* 77, 1961.

185. Sanchez, R. E., Longmire, W. P., Jr., and Passaro, E. Jr. Acid Secretion and Serum Gastrin Levels in the Zollinger-Ellison Syndrome. *Calif. Med. 116:* 1, 1972.

186. Ruppert, R. D., Greenberger, N. J., Beman, F. M., and McCullough, F. M. Gastric Secretion in Ulcerogenic Tumors of the Pancreas. *Ann. Intern. Med. 67:* 808, 1967.

187. Winship, D. H. Problems in the Diagnosis of Zollinger-Ellison Syndrome by Analysis of Gastric Secretion, in L. Demling and R. Ottenjahn (eds.): *Non-Insulin-Producing Tumors of the Pancreas.* Stuttgart, Thieme, 1969, pp. 129–140.

188. Lewin, M. R., Stagg, B. H., and Clark, C. G. Gastric Acid Secretion and Diagnosis of Zollinger-Ellison Syndrome. *Br. Med. J. 2:* 139, 1973.

189. Winship, D. H., and Ellison, E. H. Variability of Gastric Secretion in Patients With and Without the Zollinger-Ellison Syndrome. *Lancet 1:* 1128, 1967.

190. Christlieb, A. R., and Schuster, M. M. Zollinger-Ellison Syndrome. *Arch. Intern. Med. 114:* 381, 1964.

191. Bonfils, S., and Bader, J. P. The Diagnosis of Zollinger-Ellison Syndrome with Special Reference to the Multiple Endocrine Adenomas. *Prog. Gastroenterol. 2:* 332, 1970.

192. Zollinger, R. M., and Grant, G. N. Ulcerogenic Tumor of the Pancreas. *J.A.M.A. 190:* 181, 1964.

193. Rambaud, J. C., and Matuchansky, D. Diarrhoea and Digestive Endocrine Tumors. *Clin. Gastroenterol. 3:* 657, 1974.

194. Singleton, J. W., Kern, F., Jr., and Waddell, W. R. Diarrhea and Pancreatic Islet Cell Tumor: Report of a Case with a Severe Jejunal Mucosal Lesion. *Gastroenterology 49:* 197, 1965.

195. Deleu, J. Tytgat, H., Van Goidsenhoven, G. E. Diarrhea Associated with Pancreatic Islet Cell Tumors. *Am. J. Dig. Dis. 9:* 97, 1964.

196. Soergel, K. H. Mechanism of Diarrhea in the Zollinger-Ellison Syndrome, in L. Demling and R. Ottenjann (eds.): *Non-Insulin-Producing Tumors of the Pancreas—Modern Aspects of Zollinger-Ellison Syndrome and Gastrin.* Stuttgart, Thieme, 1969, pp. 152–164.

197. Edmeads, J. G., Matthews, R. E., McPhedran, N. T., and Ezrin, C. Diarrhea Caused by Pancreatic Islet Cell Tumours. *Can. Med. Assoc. J. 86:* 847, 1962.

198. Thompson, J. C., Reeder, D. D., and Bunchman, H. H. Clinical Role of Serum Gastrin Measurements in the Zollinger-Ellison Syndrome. *Am. J. Surg. 124:* 250, 1972.
199. Creutzfeldt, W., Arnold, R., Creutzfeldt, C., and Track, N. S. Pathomorphologic, Biochemical, and Diagnostic Aspects of Gastrinomas (Zollinger-Ellison Syndrome). *Hum. Pathol. 6:* 47, 1975.
200. Ballard, H. S., Frame, B., and Hartsock, R. J. Familial Multiple Endocrine Adenoma–Peptic Ulcer Complex. *Medicine 43:* 481, 1964.
201. Crosier, J. C., Azerad, E., and Lubetzki, J. L'Adenomatose Polyendocrinienne (Syndrom de Werner). A Propos d'Une Observation Personelle. Revue de la Litterature. *Sem Hop Paris 47:* 494, 1971.
202. Law, D. H., Liddle, G. W., Scott, H. W. Jr., and Tauber, S. D. Ectopic Production of Multiple Hormones (ACTH, MSH, and Gastrin) by a Single Malignant Tumor. *N. Engl. J. Med. 273:* 292, 1965.
203. Shieber, W. Insulin-Producing Zollinger-Ellison Tumor. *Surgery 54:* 448, 1963.
204. Block, M. A., Kelly, A. R., and Horn, R. C., Jr. Elevation of Multiple Humoral Substances in Zollinger-Ellison Syndrome. *Arch. Surg. 98:* 734, 1969.
205. Isenberg, J. I., Walsh, J. H., and Grossman, M. I. Zollinger-Ellison Syndrome. *Gastroenterology 65:* 140, 1973.
206. Reeder, D. D., Becker, H. D., and Thompson, J. C. Effect of Intravenously Administered Calcium on Serum Gastrin and Gastric Secretion in Man. *Surg. Gynecol. Obstet. 138:* 847, 1974.
207. Dent, R. I., James, J. H., Wang, C. W., et al. Hyperparathyroidism: Gastric Acid Secretion and Gastrin. *Ann. Surg. 176:* 360, 1972.
208. Barreras, R. F., and Donaldson, R. M., Jr. Role of Calcium in Gastric Hypersecretion, Parathyroid Adenoma and Peptic Ulcer. *N. Engl. J. Med. 276:* 1122, 1967.
209. Christoforidis, A. J., and Nelson, S. W. Radiological Manifestations of Ulcerogenic Tumors of the Pancreas. *J.A.M.A. 198:* 511, 1966.
210. Zboralske, F. F., and Amberg, J. R. Detection of the Zollinger-Ellison Syndrome: The Radiologist's Responsibility. *Am. J. Roentgenol. 104:* 529, 1965.
211. Weber, J. M., Lewis, S., and Heasley, K. H. Observations on Small Bowel Pattern Associated with the Zollinger-Ellison Syndrome. *Am. J. Roentgenol. 82:* 973, 1959.
212. Amberg, J. R., Ellison, E. H., Wilson, S. D., and Zboralske, F. F. Roentgenographic Observation in the Zollinger-Ellison Syndrome. *J.A.M.A. 190:* 185, 1964.
213. Moritz, M., Kahn, P. C., Callow, A. D., and Levitan, R. Unusual Clinical Manifestations and Angiographic Findings in a Patient with the Zollinger-Ellison Syndrome. *Ann. Intern. Med. 71:* 1133, 1969.
214. Clemett, A. R., and Park, W. M. Arteriographic Demonstration of Pancreatic Tumor in the Zollinger-Ellison Syndrome. *Radiology 88:* 32, 1967.
215. Fontaine, R., Kieny, R., and Lang, G. Decouverte par l'Angiographie Selective d'une Tumeur Ulcerogene du Pancreas a Symptomatologie Atypique. *Mem. Acad. Chir. 91:* 896, 1965.
216. Ludin, H., Enderlin, F., and Fahrlander, H. J. Failure to Diagnose Zollinger-Ellison Syndrome by Pancreatic Angiography. Report of a Case. *Br. J. Radiol. 39:* 494, 1966.
217. Korobkin, M. T., Palubinskas, A. J., and Glickman, M. G. Pitfalls in Arteriography for Islet-Cell Tumors of the Pancreas. *Radiology 100:* 319, 1971.
218. Malmed, R. N., Agnew, J. E., and Bouchier, I. A. The Normal and Abnormal Pancreatic Scan. *Quant. J. Med. 37:* 607, 1968.
219. Moore, F. T., Murat, J. E., Endahl, G. L., Baker, J. L., and Zollinger, R. M. Diagnosis of Ulcerogenic Tumor of the Pancreas by Bioassay. *Am. J. Surg. 113:* 735, 1967.
220. Thomson, C. G., Cleator, I. G. M., and Sircus, W. Experience with a Rat Bioassay in the Diagnosis of the Zollinger-Ellison Syndrome. *Gut 11:* 409, 1970.
221. Wilson, S. D., Mathison, J. A., Schulte, W. J., and Ellison, E. H. The Role of Bioassay in the Diagnosis of Ulcerogenic Tumors. *Arch. Surg. 97:* 437, 1968.
222. Friesen, S. R., Bolinger, R. E., Pearse, A. G. E., and McGuigan, J. E. Serum Gastrin Levels in Malignant Zollinger-Ellison Syndrome After Total Gastrectomy and Hypophysectomy. *Ann. Surg. 172:* 504, 1970.
223. Passaro, E., Jr., Basso, N., Sanchez, E. R., and Gordon, H. E. Newer Studies in the Zollinger-Ellison Syndrome. *Am. J. Surg. 120:* 138, 1970.
224. Trudeau, W. L., and McGuigan, J. E. Effects of Calcium on Serum Gastrin Levels in the Zollinger-Ellison Syndrome. *N. Engl. J. Med. 281:* 862, 1969.
225. Basso, N., and Passaro, E. Jr. Calcium-Stimulated Gastric Secretion in the Zollinger-Ellison Syndrome. *Arch. Surg. 101:* 399, 1970.
226. Morrow, D. J., and Passaro, E., Jr. Calcium Infusion Test Before and After Total Gastrectomy in the Zollinger-Ellison Syndrome. *Am. J. Surg. 129:* 62, 1975.
227. Kolts, B. E., Herbst, C. A., and McGuigan, J. E. Calcium and Secretin-Stimulated Gastrin Release in the Zollinger-Ellison Syndrome. *Ann. Intern. Med. 81:* 758, 1974.
228. Schwartz, D. L., White, J. J., Saulsbury, F., and Haller, J. A., Jr. Gastrin Response to Calcium Infusion: An Aid to the Improved Diagnosis of Zollinger-Ellison Syndrome in Children. *Pediatrics 54:* 599, 1974.
229. Isenberg, J. I., Walsh, J. H., Passaro, E. Jr., Moore, E. W., and Grossman, M. I. Unusual Effect of Secretin on Serum Gastrin, Serum Calcium and Gastric Acid Secretion in a Patient with Suspected Zollinger-Ellison Syndrome. *Gastroenterology 62:* 626, 1972.
230. Korman, M. G., Soveny, C., and Hansky, J. Paradoxical Effect of Secretin on Serum Immunoreactive Gastrin in the Zollinger-Ellison Syndrome. *Digestion 8:* 407, 1973.
231. Bradley, E. L., III, Galambos, J. T., Lobley, C. R., and Chan, Y-K. Secretin–Gastrin Relationships in Zollinger-Ellison Syndrome. *Surgery 73:* 550, 1973.
232. Schrumpf, E., Petersen, H., Berstad, A., Myren, J., and Rosenlund, B. The Effect of Secretin on Plasma Gastrin in the Zollinger-Ellison Syndrome. *Scand. J. Gastroenterol. 8:* 145, 1973.
233. Bali, J. P., Balmes, J. L., Fournajoux, J., Cayrol, B., and Khazrai, H. Effects of Secretin on Immuno-Reactive Serum Gastrin in Two Cases of Zollinger-Ellison Syndrome. *Digestion 7:* 277, 1972.
234. Korman, M. G., Soveny, C., and Hansky, J. The Effect of Glucagon on Serum Gastrin II. Studies in Pernicious Anemia and the Zollinger-Ellison Syndrome. *Gut 14:* 459, 1973.
235. Becker, H. D., Reeder, D. D., and Thompson, J. C. Effect of Glucagon on Circulating Gastrin. *Gastroenterology 65:* 28, 1973.
236. Deveney, C., Way, L., Deveney, K., Jones, S., and Jaffe, B. Calcium and Secretin Tests in Diagnosis of Gastrinoma. *Gastroenterology 70:* 968, 1976.
237. Berson, S. A., and Yalow, R. S. Radioimmunoassay in Gastroenterology. *Gastroenterology 62:* 1061, 1972.
238. Greider, M. H., Rosai, J., and McGuigan, J. E. The Human Pancreatic Islet Cells and Their Tumors. II. Ulcerogenic and Diarrheagenic Tumors. *Cancer 33:* 1423, 1974.
239. Sizemore, G. W., Go, V. L. W., Kaplan, E. L., et al. Relations of Calcitonin and Gastrin in the Zollinger-Ellison Syndrome and Medullary Carcinoma of the Thyroid. *N. Engl. J. Med. 288:* 641, 1973.
240. Jaffe, B. M., Peskin, G. W., and Kaplan, E. L. Serum Levels of Parathyroid Hormone in the Zollinger-Ellison Syndrome. *Surgery 74:* 621, 1973.
241. McGuigan, J. E., and Trudeau, W. L. Serum Gastrin Concentrations in Pernicious Anemia. *N. Engl. J. Med. 282:* 358, 1970.
242. Ganguli, P. C., Cullen, D. R., and Irvine, W. J. Radioimmunoassay of Plasma Gastrin in Pernicious Anemia, Achlorhydria Without Pernicious Anemia, Hypochlorhydria, and in Controls. *Lancet 1:* 155, 1971.
243. Korman, M. G., Strickland, R. G., and Hansky, J. Serum Gastrin in Chronic Gastritis. *Br. Med. J. 2:* 16, 1971.
244. Korman, M. G., Laver, M. C., and Hansky, J. Hypergastrinemia in Chronic Renal Failure. *Br. Med. J. 1:* 209, 1972.
245. McGuigan, J. E., and Trudeau, W. L. Serum and Tissue Gastrin Concentrations in Patients with Carcinoma of the Stomach. *Gastroenterology 64:* 22, 1973.
246. Hayes, J. R., Kennedy, T. L., Ardill, J., Shanks, R. G., and Buchanan, K. D. Stimulation of Gastrin Release by Catecholamines. *Lancet 1:* 819, 1972.
247. Howitz, J., and Rehfeld, J. F. Serum-Gastrin in Vitiligo. *Lancet 1:* 831, 1974.
248. Rooney, P. J., and Dick, W. C. Hypergastrinemia in Rheumatoid Arthritis. *Br. Med. J. 4:* 298, 1973.
249. Korman, M. G., Scott, D. F., Hansky, J., and Wilson, H. Hyper-

gastrinemia Due to an Excluded Gastric Antrum: A Proposed Method for Differentiation from the Zollinger-Ellison Syndrome. *Aust. N.Z. J. Med. 3:* 266, 1972.

250. Shuster, F., and Alexander, H. C. Antacid Relief of Diarrhea in Zollinger-Ellison Syndrome. *J.A.M.A. 208:* 2162, 1969.

251. Lawrie, R., Hunt, J. N., and Williamson, A. W. R. Treatment of Zollinger-Ellison Syndrome. *Lancet 1:* 203, 1966.

252. Shimoda, S. S., and Rubin, C. R. The Zollinger-Ellison Syndrome with Steatorrhea. I. Anticholinergic Treatment Followed by Total Gastrectomy and Colonic Interposition. *Gastroenterology 55:* 695, 1968.

253. Bank, S., Marks, I. N., and Searly, R. Malignant Zollinger-Ellison Syndrome in a Bantu Woman with a Prolonged Remission After Gastric Radiotherapy. *Gut 6:* 279, 1965.

254. Richardson, C. T., and Walsh, J. H. The Value of a Histamine H_2-Receptor Antagonist in the Management of Patients with the Zollinger-Ellison Syndrome. *N. Engl. J. Med. 294:* 133, 1976.

255. Hayes, J. R., O'Connell, N., O'Neill, T., Fennelly, J. J., and Weir, D. G. Successful Treatment of a Malignant Gastrinoma with Streptozotocin. *Gut 17:* 285, 1976.

256. Stadil, F., Stage, G., Rehfeld, J. F., Efsen, F., and Fischerman, K. Treatment of Zollinger-Ellison Syndrome with Streptozotocin. *N. Engl. J. Med. 294:* 1440, 1976.

257. Fox, P. S., Hofmann, J. W., Wilson, S. D., and De Cosse, J. J. Surgical Management of the Zollinger-Ellison Syndrome. *Surg. Clin. North Am. 54:* 395, 1974.

258. Royston, C. M. S., Brew, D. S. J., Garnham, J. R., Stagg, B. H., and Polak, J. The Zollinger-Ellison Syndrome Due to an Infiltrating Tumour of the Stomach. *Gut 13:* 638, 1972.

259. Wilson, S. D., Schulte, W. J., and Meade, R. C. Longevity Studies Following Total Gastrectomy in Children with the Zollinger-Ellison Syndrome. *Arch. Surg. 103:* 108, 1971.

260. Fox, P. S., Hofmann, J. W., DeCosse, J. J., and Wilson, S. D. The Influence of Total Gastrectomy on Survival in Malignant Zollinger-Ellison Tumors. *Ann. Surg. 180:* 558, 1974.

261. Friesen, S. R. Effect of Total Gastrectomy on the Zollinger-Ellison Tumor: Observations by Second-Look Procedures. *Surg. 62:* 609, 1967.

262. Passaro, E., Jr., and Gordon, H. E. Malignant Gastrinoma Following Total Gastrectomy. *Arch. Surg. 108:* 444, 1974.

263. Sanzenbacher, L. J., King, D. R., and Zollinger, R. M. Prognostic Implications of Calcium-Mediated Gastrin Levels in the Ulcerogenic Syndrome. *Am. J. Surg. 125:* 116, 1973.

264. Zollinger, R. M., Martin, E. W. Jr., Carey, L. C., Sparks, J., and Minton, J. P. Observations on the Postoperative Tumor Growth Behavior of Certain Islet Cell Tumors. *Ann. Surg. 184:* 525, 1976.

265. Oberhelman, H. A., Jr., and Nelson, T. S. Surgical Consideration in the Management of Ulcerogenic Tumors of the Pancreas and Duodenum. *Am. J. Surg. 108:* 132, 1964.

266. Jaffe, B. M., Peskin, G., and Kaplan, E. L. Diagnosis of Occult Zollinger-Ellison Tumors by Gastrin Radioimmunoassay. *Cancer 29:* 694, 1972.

267. Goldgraber, M. D. Steatorrhea: A Clinical–Pathologic Correlation. *Isr. Med. J. 22:* 156, 1963.

268. Scobie, B. A., and Beetham, D. T. Zollinger-Ellison Syndrome due to Duodenal Ectopic Islet Cell Tumour. *N.Z. Med. J. 65:* 979, 1966.

269. Ragins, H. D., and Del Guercio, L. R. M. Bioassay of the Serum in Zollinger-Ellison Syndrome. *Arch. Surg. 98:* 94, 1969.

270. Guida, P. M., Todd, J. E., Moore, S. W., and Beal, J. M. Zollinger-Ellison Syndrome with Interesting Variations. *Am. J. Surg. 112:* 807, 1966.

271. Weichert, R. F., III, Roth, L. M., Krementz, E. T., Hewitt, R. L., and Drapanas, T. Carcinoid–Islet Cell Tumors of the Duodenum. *Am. J. Surg. 121:* 195, 1971.

272. Fisher, E. R., and Hicks, J. Further Pathologic Observations on the Syndrome of Peptic Ulcer and Multiple Endocrine Tumors. *Gastroenterology 38:* 458, 1960.

273. Thistlethaite, J. R., and Horwitz, A. Ulcerogenic Islet Cell Tumors of the Pancreas. *Postgrad. Med. 24:* 599, 1958.

274. Hofmann, J. W., Fox, P. S., and Wilson, S. D. Duodenal Wall Tumors and the Zollinger-Ellison Tumors. Surgical Management. *Arch. Surg. 107:* 334, 1973.

275. Polak, J. M., Stagg, B., and Pearse, A. G. E. Two Types of Zollinger-Ellison Syndrome: Immunofluorescent, Cytochemical and Ultrastructural Studies of the Antral and Pancreatic Gastrin Cells in Different Clinical States. *Gut 13:* 501, 1972.

276. Cowley, D. J., Dymock, I. W., Boyes, B. E., et al. Zollinger-Ellison Syndrome Type I: Clinical and Pathological Correlations in a Case. *Gut 14:* 25, 1973.

277. Di Magno, E. P., and Go, V. L. W. Malabsorption Secondary to Antral Gastrin-Cell Hyperplasia. *Mayo Clin. Proc. 49:* 727, 1974.

278. Ganguli, P. C., Polak, J. M., Pearse, A. G. E., Elder, J. B., and Hegarty, M. Antral–Gastrin-Cell Hyperplasia in Peptic-Ulcer Disease. *Lancet 1:* 583, 1974.

279. Straus, E., and Yalow, R. S. Differential Diagnosis in Hyperchlorhydric Hypergastrinemia. *Gastroenterology 66:* 867, 1974.

280. Hansky, J. Antral–Gastrin-Cell Hyperplasia in Peptic Ulcer Disease. *Lancet 1:* 1344, 1974.

281. Rawson, A. B., England, M. T., Gillam, G. G., French, J. M., and Stammers, F. A. R. Zollinger-Ellison Syndrome with Diarrhoea and Malabsorption. Observations on a Patient Before and After Pancreatic Islet-Cell Tumour Removal without Resort to Gastric Surgery. *Lancet 2:* 131, 1960.

282. Johnson, L. R., Aures, D.,and Hakanson, R. Effect of Gastrin on the *in vivo* Incorporation of [^{14}C] Leucine into Protein of the Digestive Tract. *Proc. Soc. Exp. Biol. Med. 132:* 996, 1969.

283. Johnson, L. R., Aures, D., and Yuen, L. Pentagastrin Induced Stimulation of the *in vitro* Incorporation of [^{14}C] Leucine into Protein of the Gastrointestinal Tract. *Am. J. Physiol. 217:* 251, 1969.

284. Sum, P., and Perey, B. J. Parietal-Cell Mass (PCM) in a Man with Zollinger-Ellison Syndrome. *Can. J. Surg. 12:* 285, 1969.

285. Bramwell, H., and French, A. B. Physiologic Response to Gastric Acid Hypersecretion in Zollinger-Ellison Syndrome. *Am. J. Dig. Dis. 13:* 191, 1968.

286. Soergel, K. H. Flow Measurements of Test Meals and Fasting Contents in the Human Small Intestine, in L. Demling and R. Ottenjahn (eds.): *Gastrointestinal Motility*. Stuttgart, Thieme, 1971, pp. 81–92.

287. Dreiling, D. A., and Greenstein, A. Pancreatic Function in Patients with the Zollinger-Ellison Syndrome. Observations Concerning Acid–Bicarbonate Secretion. *Med. Chir. Dig. 1:* 1, 1972.

288. Petersen, H., Myren, J., and Liavag, I. Secretory Response to Secretin in a Patient with Diarrhoea and the Zollinger-Ellison Pattern of Gastric Secretion. *Gut 10:* 796, 1969.

289. Mayston, P. D., and Barrowman, J. A. The Influence of Chronic Administration of Pentagastrin upon the Rat Pancreas. *Q. J. Exp. Physiol. 56:* 113, 1971.

290. Shimoda, S. S., Saunders, D. R., and Rubin, C. E. The Zollinger-Ellison Syndrome with Steatorrhea. II. The Mechanism of Fat and Vitamin B_{12} Malabsorption. *Gastroenterology 55:* 705, 1968.

291. Haubrich, W. S., O'Neil, F. S., and Block, M. A. Observations on Steatorrhea Associated with Gastric Hypersecretion and Pancreatic Islet Cell Neoplasm. *Ann. Intern. Med. 56:* 302, 1962.

292. Adibi, S. A., Ruiz, C., Glaser, P., and Fogel, M. R. Effect of Intraluminal pH on Absorption Rates of Leucine, Water, and Electrolytes in Human Jejunum. *Gastroenterology 63:* 611, 1972.

293. Logan, C. J. H., and Connell, A. M. The Effect of a Synthetic Gastrin-Like Pentapeptide on Intestinal Motility in Man. *Lancet 1:* 996, 1966.

294. Smith, A. N., and Hogg, D. Effect of Gastrin II on the Motility of the Gastrointestinal Tract. *Lancet 1:* 403, 1966.

295. Shafer, W. H., McCormack, L. J., and Hoerr, S. O. Non-Beta Islet-Cell Carcinoma of the Pancreas, with Flushing Attacks and Diarrhea. Report of a Case. *Cleve. Clin. Q. 32:* 13, 1965.

296. Hoffman, A. F. A Physicochemical Approach to the Intraluminal Phase of Fat Absorption. *Gastroenterology 50:* 56, 1966.

297. Go, V. L. M., Poley, J. R., Hofmann, A. F., and Summerskill, W. H. J. Disturbances in Fat Digestion Induced by Acidic Jejunal pH due to Gastric Hypersecretion in Man. *Gastroenterology 58:* 638, 1970.

298. Goldenberg, G. J., and Cummins, A. J. The Effect of pH on the Absorption Rate of Glucose in the Small Intestine of Human. *Gastroenterology 45:* 189, 1963.

299. Mansbach, C. M., Wilkins, R. M., Dobbins, W. O., and Tyor, M. P. Intestinal Mucosal Function and Structure in the Steatorrhea of Zollinger-Ellison Syndrome. *Arch. Intern. Med. 121:* 487, 1968.

300. Moshal, M. G., Broitman, S. A., and Zamcheck, N. Gastrin and Absorption. A Review. *Am. J. Clin. Nutr. 23:* 336, 1970.

301. Gregory, R. A. Gastrin—The Natural History of a Peptide Hormone. *Harvey Lect. 64:* 121, 1968.

302. Bentley, P. H., Kenner, G. W., and Sheppard, R. C. Structures of Human Gastrins I and II. *Nature 209:* 583, 1966.

303. Tracy, H. J., and Gregory, R. A. Physiological Properties of a Series of Synthetic Peptides Structurally Related to Gastrin I. *Nature 204:* 935, 1964.
304. Berson, S. A., and Yalow, R. S. Nature of Immunoreactive Gastrin Extracted from Tissues of Gastrointestinal Tract. *Gastroenterology 60:* 215, 1971.
305. Yalow, R. S., and Berson, S. A. Size and Charge Distinctions Between Endogenous Human Plasma Gastrin in Peripheral Blood and Heptadecapeptide Gastrins. *Gastroenterology 58:* 609, 1970.
306. Yalow, R. S., and Berson, S. A. Further Studies on the Nature of Immunoreactive Gastrin in Human Plasma. *Gastroenterology 60:* 203, 1971.
307. Walsh, J. H., Debas, H. T., and Grossman, M. I. Pure Human Big Gastrin: Immunochemical Properties, Disappearance Half Time, and Acid-Stimulating Action in Dogs. *J. Clin. Invest. 54:* 477, 1974.
308. Yalow, R. S., and Berson, S. A. And Now "Big, Big" Gastrin. *Biochem. Biophys. Res. Commun. 48:* 391, 1972.
309. Yalow, R. S., and Wu, N. Additional Studies on the Nature of Big Big Gastrin. *Gastroenterology 65:* 19, 1973.
310. Straus, E., and Yalow, R. S. Studies on the Distribution and Degradation of Heptadecapeptide, Big and Big Big Gastrin. *Gastroenterology 66:* 936, 1974.
311. Rehfeld, J. F., Stadil, F., and Vikelsoe, J. Immunoreactive Gastrin Components in Human Serum. *Gut 15:* 102, 1974.
312. Gregory, R. A., and Tracy, H. J. Isolation of Two Minigastrins from Zollinger-Ellison Tumour Tissue. *Gut 15:* 683, 1974.
313. Debas, H. T., Walsh, J. H., and Grossman, M. I. Pure Human Minigastrin: Secretory Potency and Disappearance Rate. *Gut 15:* 686, 1974.
314. Gregory, R. A., and Tracy, H. J. Isolation of Two "Big Gastrins" from Zollinger-Ellison Tumour Tissue. *Lancet 2:* 797, 1972.
315. Rehfeld, J. F., and Stadil, F. Gel Filtration Studies on Immunoreactive Gastrin in Serum from Zollinger-Ellison Patients. *Gut 14:* 369, 1973.
316. Dockray, G. J., and Walsh, J. H. Amino Terminal Gastrin Fragment in Serum of Zollinger-Ellison Syndrome Patients. *Gastroenterology 68:* 222, 1975.
317. Morley, J. S. Structure–Function Relationships in Gastrin-Like Peptides. *Proc. R. Soc.* [*Biol.*] *170:*97, 1968.
318. Trout, H. H., III, and Grossman, M. I. Penultimate Aspartyl Unnecessary for Stimulation of Acid Secretion by Gastrin-Related Peptide. *Nature* [*New Biol*] *234:* 256, 1971.
319. Debas, H. T., and Grossman, M. I. Active Analogs of the C-Terminal Tripeptide of Gastrin. *Gastroenterology 66:* 836, 1974.
320. Vanderhaeghen, J. J., Signeau, J. C., and Gepts, W. New Peptide in the Vertebrate CNS Reacting with Antigastrin Antibodies. *Nature 257:* 604, 1975.
321. Walsh, J. H., and Grossman, M. I. Circulating Gastrin in Peptic Ulcer Disease. *Mt. Sinai J. Med. 40:* 374, 1973.
322. Korman, M. G., Soveny, C., and Hansky, J. Serum Gastrin in Duodenal Ulcer. *Gut 12:* 899, 1971.
323. Trudeau, W. L., and McGuigan, J. E. Serum Gastrin Levels in Patients with Peptic Ulcer Disease. *Gastroenterology 59:* 6, 1970.
324. Berson, S. A., and Yalow, R. S. Gastrin in Duodenal Ulcer. *N. Engl. J. Med. 284:* 445, 1971.
325. Trudeau, W. L., and McGuigan, J. E. Relations Between Serum Gastrin Levels and Rates of Gastric Hydrochloric Acid Secretion. *N. Engl. J. Med. 284:* 408, 1971.
326. Gedde-Dahl, D. Radioimmunoassay of Gastrin: Fasting Serum Levels in Humans with Normal and High Gastric Acid Secretion. *Scand. J. Gastroenterol. 9:* 41, 1974.
327. Walsh, J. H., Richardson, C. T., and Fordtran, S. pH Dependence of Acid Secretion and Gastrin Release in Normal and Ulcer Subjects. *J. Clin. Invest. 55:* 462, 1975.
328. Johnson, L. R. Gut Hormones on Growth of Gastrointestinal Mucosa, in Chey, W. Y., and Brooks, F. P. (eds.). *Endocrinology of the Gut.* Thorofare, N.J., Slack, 1974, pp. 163–177.
329. Priest, W. M., and Alexander, M. K. Islet Cell Tumor of the Pancreas with Peptic Ulceration, Diarrhea and Hypokalemia. *Lancet 2:* 1145, 1957.
330. Verner, J. V., and Morrison, A. B. Islet Cell Tumor and a Syndrome of Refractory Watery Diarrhea and Hypokalemia. *Am. J. Med. 25:* 374, 1958.
331. Murray, J. S., Paton. R. R., and Pope, C. E. II Associated with Flushing and Diarrhea. *N. Engl. J. Med. 264:* 436, 1961.
332. Espiner, E. A., and Beaven, D. W. Nonspecific Islet-Cell Tumor of the Pancreas with Diarrhea. *Q. J. Med. 31:* 447, 1962.
333. Hindle, B., McBrien, D. J., and Cramer, B. Watery Diarrhea and an Islet Cell Tumor. *Gut 5:* 359, 1964.
334. Matsumoto, K. K., Peter, J. B., Schultze, R. G., Hakim, A. A., and Franck, P. T. Watery Diarrhea and Hypokalemia Associated with Pancreatic Islet Cell Adenoma. *Gastroenterology 50:* 231, 1966.
335. Marks, I. N., Bank, S., and Louw, J. H. Islet Cell Tumor of the Pancreas with Reversible Watery Diarrhea and Achlorhydria. *Gastroenterology 52:* 695, 1967.
336. Verner, J. V., and Morrison, A. B. Non-B Islet Cell Tumors and the Syndrome of Watery Diarrhea, Hypokalemia and Hypochlorhydria. *Clin. Gastroenterology 3:* 595, 1974.
337. Verner, J. V., and Morrison, A. B. Endocrine Pancreatic Islet Cell Disease with Diarrhea. *Arch. Intern. Med. 133:* 492, 1974.
338. Rambaud, J. C., Modigliani, R., Matuchansky, C., et al. Pancreatic Cholera. *Gastroenterology 69:* 110, 1975.
339. Telling, M., and Smiddy, F. G. Islet Cell Tumors of the Pancreas with Intractable Diarrhoea. *Gut 2:* 12, 1961.
340. Parkins, R. A. Severe Watery Diarrhea and Potassium Depletion Associated with an Islet-Cell Tumor of the Pancreas. *Br. Med. J. 2:* 356, 1961.
341. Martini, G. A., Strohmeyer, G., Haug, P., and Gusek, W. Inselzelladenom des Pankreas mit Urtikarielleum Exanthem Durchfallen, Sowiekalium ant Eiweissverlust uber den Darm. *Dtsch. Med. Wochenschr. 89:* 313, 1964.
342. Gutch, C. F., and Kisner, P. Islet Cell Tumor, Diarrhea, and Hypopotassemia. *Nebr. State Med. J. 47:* 119, 1962.
343. Goulon, M., Mercier, J. N., Reilly, J., and LaPorte, A. Carcinome Langerhansien Responsable d'Hypersecretion Gastrique Acid, de Diarrhee Chronique, d'Hypokaliemie Severe avec Paralysies et d'Hypoglycemie. *Sem. Hop. Paris 36:* 812, 1960.
344. Moldawer, P. M., Nardi, G. L., and Raker, J. W. Concomitance of Multiple Adenomas of the Parathyroids and Pancreatic Islets with Tumor of the Pituitary: A Syndrome with Familial Incidence. *Am. J. Med. Sci. 222:* 190, 1954.
345. Scudamore, H. H., McConahey, W. M., and Priestley, J. T. Nontropical Sprue and Functioning Islet-Cell Adenoma of the Pancreas: Report of a Case. *Ann. Intern. Med. 49:* 909, 1958.
346. Chears, W. C., Jr., Thompson J. E., Hutcheson, J. B., and Patterson, C. O. Pancreatic Islet Cell Tumor with Severe Diarrhea. *Am. J. Med. 29:* 529, 1960.
347. Knappe, V. G., Fleming, F., Stobbe, H., and Wendt, T. Pankreasinselzelladenom mit der Trias Diarrhoe, Hypokaliamie, und Hyperglykamie. *Dtsch. Med. Wochenschr. 91:* 1224, 1966.
348. Smith, R. The Zollinger-Ellison Syndrome. *Ann. R. Coll. Surg. Engl. 37:* 160, 1965.
349. Seif, F. J., Sadowski, P., Heni, F., et al. Das Vasoaktive Intestinale Polypeptid beim Verner-Morrison Syndrome. *Dtsch. Med. Wochenschr. 100:* 399, 1975.
350. Sircus, W., Brunt, P. W., Walker, R. J., et al. Two Cases of Pancreatic Cholera with Features of Peptide-Secreting Adenomatosis of the Pancreas. *Gut 11:* 197, 1970.
351. Verner, J. V. Clinical Syndromes Associated with Non-Insulin Producing Tumors of the Pancreatic Islets, in L. Demling and R. Ottenjahn (eds.): *Non-Insulin Producing Tumors of the Pancreas.* Stuttgart, Thieme, 1969, pp. 165–186.
352. Gjone, E., Fretheim. B., Nordoy, A., Jacobsen, C. D., and Elgjo, K. Intractable Watery Diarrhea, Hypokalemia and Achlorhydria Associated with Pancreatic Tumors Containing Gastric Secretory Inhibitory. *Scand. J. Gastroenterol. 5:* 401, 1970.
353. Lopes, V. M., Reis, D. D., and Cunha, A. B. Islet Cell Adenoma of the Pancreas with Reversible Watery Diarrhea and Hypokalemia. *Am. J. Gastroenterol. 53:* 17, 1970.
354. Kraft, A. R., Tompkins, R. K., and Zollinger, R. M. Recognition and Management of the Diarrheal Syndrome Caused by Non-Beta Islet Cell Tumors of the Pancreas. *Am. J. Surg. 119:* 163, 1970.
355. De Muro, P., Rownski, P., Calaresu, I., and Fragui, A. The Importance of Potassium in the Mechanism of Gastric Hydrochloric Acid Secretion. *Acta Med. Scand. 170:* 403, 1961.
356. Andersson, H., Dotevall, G., Fagerberg, G., et al. Pancreatic

Tumor with Diarrhea, Hypokalemia, and Hypochlorhydria. *Acta Chir. Scand. 138:* 102, 1972.
357. Conn, J. W. Hypertension, the Potassium Ion and Impaired Carbohydrate Tolerance. *N. Engl. J. Med. 273:* 1135, 1965.
358. Mondon, C. E., Burton, S. D., Grodsky, G. M., and Ishida, T. Glucose Tolerance and Insulin Response of Potassium-Deficient Rat and Isolated Liver. *Am. J. Physiol. 215:* 779, 1968.
359. Hess, W. Dearrhoen mit Hypokaliamie, Pradiabetes und Subacitat: Ein Neues Syndrom bei Uberfunktion des Inselapparetes. *Helv. Chim. Acta 35:* 87, 1968.
360. Zenker, R., Forrell, M. M., and Erpenbeck, R. Zum Kenntnis eines Seltenen Durch ein Pankreasadenom Verursachten Krankeitsyndroms. *Dtsch. Med. Wochenschr. 91:* 634, 1966.
361. Brown, C. H., and Crile, G., Jr. Pancreatic Adenoma with Intractable Diarrhea, Hypokalemia, and Hypercalcemia. *J.A.M.A. 190:* 30, 1963.
362. Koenen-Schmahling, B., Hartwick, G., and Dittrich, H. Verner-Morrison Syndrome: A Case Report. *Munch. Med. Wochenschr. 112:* 98, 1970.
363. Stoker, D. J., and Wynn, V. Pancreatic Islet Cell Tumor with Watery Diarrhea and Hypokalemia. *Gut 11:* 911, 1970.
364. Gloor, V. F., Pletscher, A., and Hardmeier, T. Metastasierendes. Inselzelladenom des Pancreas mit 5-Hydroxytryptamin und Insulinproduktion. *Schweiz Med. Wochenschr. 94:* 1476, 1964.
365. Schmitt, M. G., Jr., Soergel, K. H., Hensley, G. T., and Chey, W. Y. Watery Diarrhea Associated with Pancreatic Islet Cell Carcinoma. *Gastroenterology 69:* 206, 1975.
366. Classen, M., Gail, K., Breining, H., and Demling, L. Verner-Morrison Syndrome. *Dtsch. Med. Wochenschr. 97:* 277, 1972.
367. Relman, A. S., and Schwartz, W. B. The Nephropathy of Potassium Depletion: A Clinical and Pathological Entity. *N. Engl. J. Med. 255:* 195, 1956.
368. Pabst, K., Kummerle, F., Hennekenser, H. H., and Mappes, G. Beitrag zum Krankheitsbild des Verner-Morrison Syndroms. *Dtsch. Med. Wochenschr. 94:* 9, 1969.
369. Zollinger, R. M., Tompkins, R. K., Amerson, J. R., et al. Identification of the Diarrheagenic Hormone Associated with Non-Beta Islet-Cell Tumours of the Pancreas. *Ann. Surg. 168:* 502, 1968.
370. Cerda, J. J., Raffensberger, E. C., and Rawnsley, H. M. Cholera-Like Syndrome and Pancreatic Islet Cell Tumors. *Med. Clin. North Am. 54:* 567, 1970.
371. Moore, F. T., Nadler, H., Radefeld, D. A., and Zollinger, R. M. Prolonged Remission of Diarrhea due to Non-Beta Islet Cell Tumor of the Pancreas by Radiotherapy. *Am. J. Surg. 115:* 845, 1968.
372. Kahn, C. R., Levy, A. G., Gardner, J. D., et al. Pancreatic Cholera: Beneficial Effects of Treatment with Streptozotocin. *N. Engl. J. Med. 292:* 941, 1975.
373. Jacobs, W. H., Halperin, P., and Mantz, F. A. Watery Diarrhea and Hypokalemia due to Non-Beta Islet Cell Hyperplasia of the Pancreas. *Am. J. Gastroenterol. 15:* 333, 1972.
374. Leger, L., Bertola, J., and Riberi, A. M. Hyperplasia Adenomatusa del Pancreas Endocrino y Dolores. *Prensa Med. Argent. 49:* 1715, 1962.
375. Fausa, O., Fretheim, B., Elgjo, K., Semb, L. S., and Gjone, E. Intractable Watery Diarrhoea, Hypokalaemia, and Achlorhydria Associated with Non-Pancreatic Retroperitoneal Neurogenous Tumour Containing Vasoactive Intestinal Peptide (VIP). *Scand. J. Gastroenterol. 8:* 713, 1973.
376. Said, S. I., and Faloona, G. R. Elevated Plasma and Tissue Levels of Vasoactive Intestinal Polypeptide in the Watery Diarrhea Syndrome due to Pancreatic Bronchogenic and Other Tumors. *N. Engl. J. Med. 293:* 155, 1975.
377. Jaffe, B. M., and Condon, S. Prostaglandins E and F in Endocrine Diarrheagenic Syndromes. *Ann. Surg. 184:* 516, 1976.
378. Rambaud, J. C., Bitoun, A., Matuchansky, C., Modigliani, R., and Bernier, J.-J. Etude de l'Absorption Jejunale et Ileale de l'Eau et des Electrolytes dans un Cas de Syndrome de Verner-Morrison; Effet du Glucose. *Biol. Gastroenterol. 5:* 627c, 1972.
379. Gardner, J. D., and Cerda, J. J. *In vitro* Inhibition of Intestinal Fluid and Electrolyte Transfer by a Non-Beta Islet Cell Tumor. *Proc. Soc. Exp. Biol. Med. 123:* 361, 1966.
380. Devroede, G. J., and Phillips, S. J. Studies of the Perfusion Technique for Colonic Absorption. *Gastroenterology 56:* 92, 1969.
381. Levitan, R., and Inglefinger, F. J. Effect of d-Aldosterone on Salt and Water Absorption from the Intact Human Colon. *J. Clin. Invest. 44:* 801, 1965.
382. Edmonds, C. J. Effect of Aldosterone on Mammalian Intestine. *J. Steroid Biochem. 3:* 143, 1972.
383. Ricour, C., Millot, M., and Balsan, S. Sodium Conservation after Total or Subtotal Colonic Resection in Children. *Scand. J. Gastroenterol. 8:* 743, 1973.
384. Rambaud, J. C., Matuchansky, C., Modigliani, R., et al. Etude de l'Absorption Colique de l'Eau et des Electrolytes dans un Cas de Syndrome de Verner-Morrison. *Biol. Gastroenterol. 5:* 626c, 1972.
385. Barbezat, G. O., and Grossman, M. I. Cholera-Like Diarrhea Induced by Glucagon Plus Gastrin. *Lancet 1:* 1026, 1971.
386. Melrose, A. G. The Effect of Glucagon on Gastric Secretion in Man. *Gut 1:* 142, 1960.
387. Mayer, J., and Sudsaneh, S. Mechanism of Hypothalmic Control of Gastric Contractions in the Rat. *Am. J. Physiol. 197:* 274, 1959.
388. Birge, S. J., and Avioli, L. V. Glucagon-Induced Hypocalcemia in Man. *J. Clin. Endocrinol. Metab. 29:* 213, 1969.
389. Dyck, W. P., Toxler, E. C., Jr., Lasater, J. M., and Hightower, N. C., Jr. Influence of Glucagon on Pancreatic Exocrine Secretion in Man. *Gastroenterol. 58:* 532, 1970.
390. Gingell, J. C., Davies, M. W., and Shields, R. Effect of a Synthetic Gastrin-Like Pentapeptide upon the Intestinal Transport of Sodium Potassium, and Water. *Gut 9:* 111, 1968.
391. Zaterka, S., and Grossman, M. I. The Effect of Gastrin and Histamine on Secretion of Bile. *Gastroenterol. 50:* 500, 1966.
392. Saubermann, A., and Silen, W. Gastrin: A Stimulant of Hepatic Bile Secretion. *Surg. Forum 18:* 296, 1967.
393. Lernmark, A., Hellman, B., and Coore, H. G. Effects of Gastrin on the Release of Insulin *in Vitro*. *J. Endocrinol. 43:* 371, 1969.
394. Cooper, C. W., Schwesinger, W. H., Mahgoub, A. M., and Ontjes, D. A. Thyrocalcitonin: Stimulation of Secretion by Pentagastrin. *Science 172:* 1238, 1971.
395. Misiewicz, J. J., Waller, S. L., and Eisner, M. Motor Responses of Human Gastrointestinal Tract to 5-Hydroxytryptamine *in Vivo* and *in Vitro*. *Gut 7:* 208, 1966.
396. Kaplan, E. L., Jaffe, B. M., and Peskin, G. A New Provocative Test for the Diagnosis of the Carcinoid Syndrome. *Am. J. Surg. 123:* 173, 1972.
397. Haverback, B. J., Bogdanski, D., and Hogben, C. A. M. Inhibition of Gastric Acid Secretion in the Dog by the Precursor of Serotonin, 5-Hydroxytryptophan. *Gastroenterology 34:* 188, 1958.
398. Black, J. W., Fisher, E. W., and Smith, A. N. The Effects of 5-Hydroxytryptamine on Gastric Secretion in Anesthetized Dogs. *J. Physiol. 141:* 27, 1958.
399. Haverback, B. J., and Davidson, J. D. Serotonin and the Gastrointestinal Tract. *Gastroenterology 35:* 570, 1958.
400. Bulbring, E., and Lin, R. C. Y. The Effect of Intraluminal Application of 5-Hydroxytryptamine and 5-Hydroxytryptophan on Peristalsis: The Local Production of 5-HT and Its Release in Relation to Intraluminal Pressure and Propulsive Activity. *J. Physiol. 140:* 381, 1958.
401. Hudock, J. J., Khentigan, A., Venamee, P., and Lawrence, W., Jr. The Effect of Serotonin and Serotonin Antagonists on External Pancreatic Secretion in Dogs. *J. Surg. Res. 3:* 307, 1963.
402. Tompkins, R. K., Kraft, A. R., and Zollinger, R. M. Secretin-Like Choleresis Produced by a Diarrheogenic Non-Beta Islet Cell Tumor of the Pancreas. *Surgery 66:* 131, 1969.
403. Wormsley, K. G. Response to Secretin in Man. *Gastroenterology 54:* 197, 1968.
404. Sanzenbacher, L. J., Mekhjian, H. S., King, D. R., and Zollinger, R. M. Studies on the Potential Role of Secretin in the Islet Cell Tumor Diarrheogenic Syndrome. *Ann. Surg. 176:* 394, 1972.
405. Cleator, J. G. M., Thomson, C. G., Sircus, W., and Coombes, M. Bio-Assay Evidence of Abnormal Secretin-Like and Gastrin-Like Activity in Tumour and Blood in Cases of "Choleraic Diarrhoea." *Gut 11:* 206, 1970.
406. Hubel, K. A. Effects of Secretin and Glucagon in Intestinal Transport of Ions and Water in the Rat. *Proc. Soc. Exp. Biol. Med. 139:* 656, 1972.
407. Mekhjian, H., King, D., Sanzenbacher, L., and Zollinger, R.

Glucagon (GI) and Secretin (Se) Inhibit Water and Electrolyte Transport in the Human Jejunum. *Gastroenterology 62:* 782, 1972.

408. Greenlee, H. B., Longhi, E. H., Guerrero, J. D., et al.: Inhibitory Effect of Pancreatic Secretin on Gastric Secretion. *Am. J. Physiol. 190:* 396, 1957.

409. Horton, E. W., Main, I. H. M., Thompson, C. F., and Wright, P. M. Effect of Orally Administered Prostaglandin E_1 on Gastric Secretion and Gastrointestinal Motility in Man. *Gut 9:* 655, 1968.

410. Matuchansky, C., and Bernier, J.-J. Effect of Prostaglandin E_1 on Glucose, Water and Electrolyte Absorption in the Human Jejunum. *Gastroenterology 64:* 1111, 1973.

411. Robert, A., Nezamis, J. E., and Phillips, J. P. Inhibition of Gastric Secretion by Prostaglandins. *Am. J. Dig. Dis. 12:* 1073, 1967.

412. Nakano, J., and McCurdy, J. R. Cardiovascular Effects of Prostaglandin E_1. *J. Pharm. Exp. Ther. 156:* 538, 1967.

413. Franklin, R. B., and Tashjian, A. H., Jr. Intravenous Infusion of Prostaglandin E_2 Raises Plasma Calcium Concentration in the Rat. *Endocrinology 97:* 240, 1975.

414. Robertson, R. P., Gavareski, D. J., Porte, D., Jr., and Bierman, E. L. Prostaglandin (PG)E_1: Inhibition of Glucose-Stimulated Insulin Secretion in the Intact Dog. *Clin. Res. 21:* 635, 1973.

415. Sandler, M., Karim, S. M. M., and Williams, E. D. Prostaglandins in Amine–Peptide-Secreting Tumors. *Lancet 2:* 1053, 1968.

416. Bloom, S. R., Polak, J. M., and Pearse, A. G. E. Vasoactive Intestinal Peptide and Watery Diarrhea Syndrome. *Lancet 2:* 14, 1973.

417. Graham, D. Y., Johnson, C. D., Bentlif, P. S., and Kelsey, J. R., Jr. Islet Cell Carcinoma, Pancreatic Cholera, and Vasoactive Intestinal Peptide. *Ann. Intern. Med. 83:* 782, 1975.

418. Swift, P. G. F., Bloom, S. R., and Harris, F. Watery Diarrhea and Ganglioneuroma with Secretion of Vasoactive Intestinal Peptide. *Arch. Dis. Child. 50:* 896, 1975.

419. Bloom, S. R., and Polak, J. M. The Role of VIP in Pancreatic Cholera, in J. C. Thompson (ed.): Gastrointestinal Hormones. Austin, University of Texas Press, 1975, pp. 635–642.

420. Ebeid, A. M., Murray, P., Hirsch, H., Wesdorp, R. I. C., and Fischer, J. E. Radioimmunoassay of Vasoactive Intestinal Peptide. *J. Surg. Res. 20:* 355, 1976.

421. Welbourn, R. B., Pearse, A. G. E., Polak, J. M., Bloom, S. R., and Joffe, S. N. The APUD Cells of the Alimentary Tract in Health and Disease. *Med. Clin. North Am. 58:* 1359, 1974.

422. Pearse, A. G. E., and Polak, J. M. Endocrine Tumours of Neural Crest Origin: Neurolophomas, APUDomas and the APUD Concept. *Med. Biol. 52:* 3, 1974.

423. Weichert, R. F., III. The Neural Ectodermal Origin of the Peptide-Secreting Endocrine Glands. *Am. J. Med. 49:* 232, 1970.

424. Szijj, T., Czapo, Z., Lasslo, F. A., and Kovacks, K. Medullary Cancer of the Thyroid Gland Associated with Hypercorticism. *Cancer 24:* 167, 1969.

425. Heitz, P. H., Steiner, H., Halter, F., Egk, P., and Kapp, J. P. Multihormonal Amyloid-Producing Tumour of the Islets of Langerhans in a Twelve Year Old Boy. *Virchows Arch.[Pathol. Anat.]353:* 312, 1971.

426. Friesen, S. R., Hermreck, A. S., and Mantz, F. A. Glucagon, Gastrin, and Carcinoid Tumors of the Duodenum, Pancreas, and Stomach: Polypeptide "Apudomas" of the Foregut. *Am. J. Surg. 127:* 90, 1974.

427. Werner, F. Genetic Aspects of Adenomatosis of Endocrine Glands. *Am. J. Med. 16:* 363, 1954.

428. Sipple, J. H. Association of Pheochromocytoma with Carcinoma of the Thyroid Gland. *Am. J. Med. 31:* 163, 1961.

136

Kallikreins (Kininogenases) and Kinins*

Melville Schachter
Susanne Barton

KALLIKREIN-KININOGEN-KININ SYSTEM

KALLIKREINS (KININOGENASES) AND KININS

The kallikreins, or kininogenases, are a group of similar proteolytic enzymes, viz., serine proteases, with a marked substrate specificity. They are present in many glands as well as in body fluids—e.g., blood, lymph and urine. They have similar pharmacologic actions on blood vessels and smooth muscles in vivo. These actions are for the most part indirect, being due to the rapid enzymic cleavage of specific substrates, kininogens, present in plasma and lymph, resulting in the release of kinin, a peptide, that produces the effects. There are a growing number of these peptides which are closely related in structure, the prototype being a nonapeptide called bradykinin. Bradykinin and other kinins are inactivated by chymotrypsin, carboxypeptidases, and other peptidases present in plasma and many organs. The kallikrein-kinin system therefore is in many ways analogous to the renin-angiotensin system.

The discovery of kallikreins can be regarded as having begun in 1926 with the observations of Frey and Kraut[1,2] that human urine contained a thermolabile, nondialysable substance that produced a prolonged arterial hypotension in the dog on intravenous injection. Intensive research on kallikrein was pursued by Eugen Werle of Munich and his colleagues[3–6,23] from 1930 until his death in 1975. The early workers, seeking the source of the protein vasodepressor substance discovered in urine, found a similar substance in the pancreas[2,7] and in blood plasma.[8] They concluded, therefore, that this substance discovered in the urine circulated as a hormone in the blood after having originated in the pancreas. They named it kallikrein, from the Greek *kallikreas,* another term for *pancreas*. Since Frey, Kraut, and Werle regarded it as an activatable circulating vasodilator hormone, they also referred to it as "Kreislaufhormon". They called its inactive precursor kallikreinogen (now prekallikrein). It is interesting that more than 50 years later, as discussed subsequently in this chapter, the renal kallikrein-kinin system is being considered as a possible opposing mechanism to the renin-angiotensin system in the regulation of arterial blood pressure and sodium balance.

A significant further discovery was made in 1937 by Werle *et al.*[9] when they found that the addition of kallikrein to human serum caused the rapid appearance of a substance that contracted isolated smooth muscles. They named it substance DK, a designation meant to indicate this pharmacologic property—viz., *Darm-Kontrahierende* Substanz. This was the first clear demonstration that a smooth-muscle-stimulating substance was released from an inactive precursor and by an enzymic action; the results of the original experiment are shown in Fig. 136–1. This demonstration preceded by 2 yr the analogous observation that renin owed its pharmacologic activities to its ability to release a peptide from an inactive precursor in plasma.[10,11] Werle and Hambuechen[12] in 1943 drew the correct analogy between the *indirect* hypertensive and hypotensive actions of renin and kallikrein, respectively. In 1948, Werle and Berek[13] suggested that substance DK should be renamed kallidin, and that its precursor (or substrate for kallikrein) should be called kallidinogen. In 1949 Rocha e Silva, Beraldo, and Rosenfeld[14] described the release of an active peptide by trypsin and snake venoms from a substrate belonging to the globulin fraction of plasma. They named the active peptide bradykinin. It soon became clear that this trypsin-bradykininogen-bradykinin system was very similar to the kallikrein-kallidinogen-kallidin system. Schachter and colleagues[15–18] subsequently discovered that peptides closely resembling, if not identical with, bradykinin and kallidin existed in a *free form* in wasp and hornet venom. They suggested that these peptides and those released from a substrate in mammalian plasma by various enzymes all possessed a significantly similar structure and they therefore introduced the generic term kinin for them. This suggestion was made on the basis of a comparative study of the pharmacologic and chemical properties of various "kallidins," "bradykinins," and "wasp kinins." The suggested term kinin became justified by the subsequent proof of the chemical structure of many of these peptides, all of which have been shown to contain a basic prototypal amino acid sequence (see Refs. 22 and 29) (Fig. 136–2). The terms kininogenase and kinino-

*Dedicated respectfully to the memory of Eugen Werle (1902–1975), distinguished scientist, scholar and pioneer of the kallikrein-kininogen-kinin system.

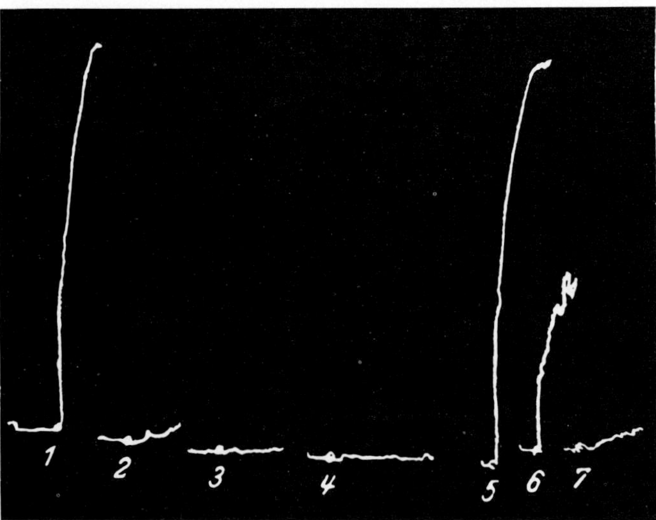

Fig. 136-1. Original record obtained by Werle, Göetze, and Keppler in 1937 showing that a preparation of salivary kallikrein release a "kinin" (subs DK) from human serum which contracts the isolated guinea-pig ileum. The "kinin" is gradually inactivated after its release. Trace shows isotomic contractions of ileum. 1. serum + kallikrein, 2. serum, 3. kallikrein, 4. dialysed submaxillary gland extract, 5. serum + kallikrein—1-min incubation 6. serum + kallikrein—10 min incubation 7. serum + kallikerin—16 min incubation. (From Werle *et al. Biochem Z. 289:* 217, 1937, with permission.)

gen were introduced in 1961 when a new and potent kallikrein-like enzyme was discovered in the accessory sex glands of the guinea-pig.[19] The term kininogenase-kininogen-kinin system now has extensive usage, and at least for the time being, is a useful terminology.[20]

The results of investigations since 1950 (see Refs. 4, 21, 22, and 23) have resulted in significant modification of some of the earlier views. Thus, it is now established that the original kallikreins, like other newly discovered kininogenases, are not identical molecules as originally assumed, nor are they derived from a parent molecule. They are, however, sufficiently similar to be classified as a generic group. Like trypsin and other proteases, they may occur in multiple forms in some tissues. For example, four chemically distinguishable although immunologically identical

Kinin		Nonapeptide Sequence										Source
Bradykinin		Arg-	Pro-	Pro-	Gly-	Phe-	Ser-	Pro-	Phe-	Arg		
Kallidin	Lys-	–	–	–	–	–	–	–	–	–		Kininogen
	Met-Lys-	–	–	–	–	–	–	–	–	–		
Bradykinin		Arg-	Pro-	Pro-	Gly-	Phe-	Ser-	Pro-	Phe-	Arg		
Thr^6- Bradykinin		–	–	–	–	–	Thr	–	–	–		Frog Skin
Val^1 – Thr^6- Bradykinin		Val	–	–	–	–	Thr	–	–	–		
Bradykinyl – Glycyl - - - -		–	–	–	–	–	–	–	–	–	-Gly- Lys- Phe- His	
etc.		–	–	–	–	–	–	–	–	–	-Val- Ala- Pro- Ala- Ser	
etc.		–	–	–	–	–	–	–	–	–	-Ile- Tyr	
etc.		–	–	–	–	–	Thr	–	–	–	-Ile- Ala- Pro- Glu - Ile- Val	
	Pyr-Thr-Asn-$(Lys)_3$-Leu-Arg-Gly-	–	–	–	–	–	–	–	–	–		
	Thr-Ala-$(Thr)_2$-$(Arg)_3$-Gly-*	–	–	–	–	–	–	–	–	–		Wasp Venom
	Ala- Arg-	–	–	–	–	–	–	–	–	–		

Fig. 136–2. Amino acid sequence of 12 known slightly different kinins, of which 10 have a common nonapeptide sequence which is shown in the middle block; the two with minor substitutions in this sequence are Thr^6-bradykinin and Val^1-thr^6-bradykinin, both found in skin of different species of frog. The nonapeptide bradykinin and six other variants have been isolated from frog skin. [Adapted from Schachter,[22] Pisano,[29] and Nakajima, 1976 (see Ref. 131).]

kallikreins have been isolated from rat urine,[24] and multiple forms have been described in the submaxillary glands of the rat[25] and in the submaxillary gland[26] and pancreas of the pig.[27]

Kininogenases are now classified as serine proteases, which along with the early kallikreins include enzymes like trypsin, chymotrypsin, elastase, thrombin, fibrinolysin, the $C\bar{1}$ esterase component of complement, and others.[28] All these enzymes appear to have histidine, serine, and aspartic acid forming the significant spatial configuration of the active site. The different serine proteases vary in their substrate specificities and, in general, the kallikreins are highly specific, their only substrates being one or two kininogens in plasma which are hydrolysed to yield a kinin. There appear to be some distinctions in specificity between the different kallikreins and, in general, those of glandular origin yield mainly the decapeptide kallidin (or lysyl-bradykinin), whereas plasma kallikrein, trypsin, fibrinolysin, and snake venoms yield the nonapeptide bradykinin (Fig. 136–2).[22,29] Thus far the kallikreins, or kininogenases, are for the most part relatively similar basic glycoproteins, with molecular weights between 25,000 and 40,000.[22,29,30] A significant exception appears to be plasma kallikrein, which has a reported mol wt of at least 100,000 and exists in at least three forms in human plasma as inactive precursors, or prekallikreins.[31,32] All the kallikreins and kininogenases thus far studied hydrolyse various synthetic amino acid esters, α-*N*-benzoyl-*L*-arginine ethyl ester (BAEe) most effectively of all. This hydrolysis is the basis of the chemical assay. The bioassay of kininogenases measures the release of kinin by the latter's hypotensive action in vivo or by its contraction of smooth muscle in vitro.

The available evidence indicates that the kallikreins or prekallikreins in the salivary glands and pancreas are present in granules, which, like trypsinogen, are secreted into the lumen.[33–36] There is recent evidence, however, that in the cat[37,38] submaxillary kallikrein is present in granules that are present in the striated ducts rather than in the acinar cells. In the cat these are located in the apical region of the duct cells, apparently for secretion into the duct lumen, and are primarily mobilized by stimulation of the sympathetic rather than by the parasympathetic nerve supply. However, the kininogenase in the coagulating gland of the guinea-pig, called CGK (coagulating gland kininogenase), is present largely or entirely in the cytosol.[39] In the rat kidney cortex it appears to be a component of the membranes constituting part of the microsomal fraction of homogenates.[40] Renin, however, sediments in the heavy nuclear and mitochondrial fractions of the same homogenates. It is apparent that the kininogenases do not have a common subcellular location in different tissues.

PREKALLIKREINS (PREKININOGENASES) AND NATURAL KALLIKREIN INHIBITORS

Kininogenases present in plasma, pancreas, intestine, and colon are present in an inactive form, whereas those in the salivary gland and accessory sex glands of the guinea-pig appear to be present only in an active form.[4,22,29] There seem to be different views as to whether renal kininogenase is present only in an active[29] or in both forms.[41,42] The renal kininogenases appear to be identical with, and probably are the source of, those in urine.[43] Other enzymes, apparently kininogenases, which have received little attention, have been described in nerve, brain, bronchial mucosa, and other tissues, mostly in an inactive form. Pancreatic and plasma kallikrein are readily activated by changes in pH, by organic solvents and by trypsin or enterokinase (see Ref. 22). The inactivating component of the prekallikrein molecule is small, and contrary to the early assumptions is not identical with any of the large-molecular circulating inhibitors. The latter may be regarded (like the circulating antithrombins) as homeostatic agents which neutralize any excess of activated kininogenase. The kininogenases, like other serine proteases such as thrombin, plasmin, trypsin, and others, are susceptible to various inhibitors of animal and plant origin. The broad subject of protease inhibitors is discussed in detail in recent reviews.[44,45] Here, only the major naturally occurring inhibitors of kallikrein present in mammalian tissues are discussed.

Studies of inhibitors of kallikrein and other proteases have recently led to the merging of what appeared to be different problems. Thus, a kallikrein inhibitor described in bovine organs (tissue inhibitor) in 1930 by Kraut, Frey, and Werle,[46] and a trypsin inhibitor discovered in 1936 by Kunitz and Northrop,[47] were studied independently by different research groups for over 30 years. It has now emerged that these inhibitors are, in fact, the same compound.[48,49] The kallikrein inhibitor occurs only in cattle and in other ruminants and has not been found in organs of other mammals. It is most conveniently extracted from lung and parotid gland. Kunitz, in his pioneer studies on the inhibitor of trypsin, also prepared the inhibitor from bovine pancreas. Although for many years Kunitz's inhibitor was thought to be present in other mammals, including man, this is not the case, and it too is presently only in bovine organs. This common inhibitor of kallikrein and trypsin is, in fact, a polyvalent protease inhibitor. Curiously enough, the pancreas of man and other mammals, including cattle, also contains a specific trypsin inhibitor which is distinct from the polyvalent inhibitor. The amino acid sequences of these compounds have recently been established. The molecular weight of the polyvalent inhibitor is 6500, whereas that of the specific trypsin inhibitor is slightly less. Commercial preparations of the polyvalent inhibitor (Trasylol, Zymofren, Iniprol, etc.) are prepared either from bovine lung or parotid gland.

During the early studies on kallikrein, it was soon found that the serum or plasma of mammals had the ability to "inactivate" various kallikreins. Much of the subsequent work on these inhibitors has been done with human plasma (see Refs. 4, 22, and 50). Recently, four known large-molecular circulating proteins have been identified with the kininogenase inhibitors. These are the $C\bar{1}$ esterase inhibitor, α_2-macroglobulin, α_1-antitrypsin, and antithrombin III (see Refs. 45).[51–55] The genetic absence or defect in one or other of these circulating inhibitors, as well as the specific absence of prekallikrein, kininogen, and of plasma kininase, have recently been reported in man. Some of these conditions are discussed later in this chapter.

KININS, KININOGENS, KININASES, AND KININ POTENTIATORS (BPF)

When it became apparent in 1937 that the pharmacologic actions of the kallikreins were due to the release of kinin, it became important to prepare a substrate, preferably free of prekallikrein, inhibitors of kallikrein, and of kininases. Werle achieved this in the same year[9] by simply heating plasma or serum for 1 to 3 h at 56 to 60 C. Other crude but simple and effective substrates for measuring kininogenase by bioassay soon became available. Diniz and Carvalho[56] developed a method for the quantitative determination of kininogen in plasma which has since been used extensively. Early studies on the activation of the plasma kininogenase-kininogen-kinin system led to the suggestion that mammalian plasmas contain more than one kininogen, and the inference that different kininogenases had preferential specificities for kininogen I or II. Despite some disagreements about details, it is currently held that kininogens are acidic glycoproteins and that most mammals contain more than one in their plasma. These are designated as high-molecular and low-molecular weight forms, HMW and LMW kininogens, respectively. These have now been isolated from various species and the HMW and LMW forms of bovine origin have molecular weights of 76,000 and 48,000, respectively.[57–59] The kinin moiety is in the internal portion of the chain in HMW kininogen, whereas in the LMW form it is located at the carboxyl terminal end of the chain. Various molecular forms of human kininogen have also been isolated.[60–64] Recently, reports have appeared of inherited kininogen deficiency in man. These are discussed in the next section.

A brief review of the history of kinins has already been given. Fig. 136–2 shows the kinins whose structures have now been established. As is evident in the figure, some kinins are split off from plasma kininogen by the action of different kininogenases, whereas some occur in nature in a free, or pre-formed and active form. In almost every instance, however, they share the common nonapeptide sequence called bradykinin. In two exceptions, thr^6-bradykinin and val^1-thr^6-bradykinin, there are minor substitutions in the common nonapeptide chain (see Refs. 22, 29, 65, and 131). The comparative or evolutionary significance of the kininogenases and kinins is very interesting but remains obscure. There are, however, some interesting speculations.[28,66] The kinins released by the different kininogenases in mammals are mainly bradykinin and lysyl-bradykinin (or kallidin). The highest concentrations of kinins exist in the venoms of certain Hymenoptera, particularly in the wasp, but also in the hornet, and relatively large amounts are found in the skin of certain amphibia (see Refs. 22, 29, and 65).

The major mammalian kinis have essentially the same pharmacologic properties and there appear to be only quantitative differences in their relative potencies in different biologic tests (see Refs. 4, 22, 67, and 68). All are hypotensive and contract most isolated smooth muscle preparations but relax the rat duodenum; they increase capillary permeability, produce pain when applied to a blister base on human skin,[17] and in the guinea-pig cause a bronchoconstriction that is specifically antagonized by salicylates and related compounds.[69–71] More recently, interesting and possibly significant actions of kinins have been found—e.g., natriuretic activity, stimulation of prostaglandin synthesis, enhancement of sperm motility, and the stimulation of cell proliferation. These and other new findings are discussed later in this chapter. Most of the kinins shown in Fig. 136–2 have been synthesized along with many analogues.[72–74] The search for a specific antibradykinin compound has not yet succeeded, and despite some early encouragement, potential antagonists thus far tend themselves to possess kinin activity and are surprisingly unpredictable in their antibradykinin activity. The chemistry of structure-activity relationships of kinins is discussed in articles by Stewart *et al.*[73,74]

A kinin-inactivating enzyme in plasma was also discovered in 1937 by Werle *et al.*[9] when they discovered the kinin-releasing action of kallikrein (Fig. 136–1). It was later noted that kinin (or substance DK) was inactivated at different rates by sera or lymph of different mammals and that serum of the guinea-pig was particularly effective.[12,75] Later, the properties and specificities of different kininases were established. Thus, a plasma carboxypeptidase which hydrolyses the Phe^8-Arg^9 bond of bradykinin releasing the C-terminal arginine, has been purified and named kininase I (previously known as carboxypeptidase N).[76,77] Another plasma kininase, kininase II, splits the Pro^7-Phe^8 site of bradykinin, releasing the dipeptide Phe-Arg. It has recently been shown that kininase II is identical with the angiotensin I-converting enzyme.[78,79] Thus, and perhaps it deserves emphasis, the same enzyme that *activates* the decapeptide angiotensin I *inactivates* bradykinin. Further, this enzyme, or a very closely related group of dipeptide hydrolases, occurs not only in plasma but in high concentrations in lung, kidney, and other tissues.[78,79] The physiologic significance of the widespread distribution of these enzymes in relation to inactivation and release of vasoactive peptides is interesting, but currently obscure. Chymotrypsin is also an effective kininase and was the first pure enzyme to help characterize kinins. It splits the Phe^8-Arg^9 bond of bradykinin rapidly and the Phe^5-Ser^6 more slowly. Trypsin does not inactivate bradykinin but releases the N-terminal lysine from lys-bradykinin and the met-lys dipeptide from metkallidin (see Refs. 4 and 22). There are a large number of kinin-inactivating enzymes of diverse animal origin including bacterial kininases (see Ref. 76).

Kininases may be inhibited to a varying degree both in vitro and in vivo, and thus enhance the effects of kinins. Werle *et al.*[9] used cysteine for this purpose, particularly in vivo, because of its relative nontoxicity. Compounds of different nature are also effective inhibitors in vitro—e.g., mercaptoethanols, 2-3 dimercaptopropanol (BAL), *o*-phenanthroline, 8-OH quinoline, and a variety of other compounds, most of which are metal binding agents and effectively bind the metal co-factor of these enzymes (see Refs. 4, 22, and 76). Natural and synthetic small peptides have also been found to be effective kininase inhibitors. Examples of naturally occurring peptides with this action are fibrinopeptides[80] and peptides in snake venoms.[81-83] These peptides inhibit kininase II and possibly kininase I as well, thus potentiating the action of kinins, and are therefore also designated as BPFs (bradykinin potentiating factors). They also inhibit the hydrolysis of angiotensin I since, as previously discussed, the angiotensin I-converting enzyme and kininase II are the same enzyme. Recently a number of these peptides originally isolated from snake venoms have been synthesized.[83-85] Two of these, a penta- and a nonapeptide, have already been studied experimentally, and are known in the literature as SQ 20475 (BPF_{5a}) and SQ 20881 (BPF_{9a}), respectively. These synthetic inhibitors are substrate competitors and act largely, or in part, by inhibiting the hydrolysis of bradykinin and angiotensin I.[84] Their possible usefulness in the analysis of physiologic and pathologic processes as well as in therapy is apparent, and relevant studies are currently being made. Thus, the nonapeptide SQ 20881 has failed to potentiate nerve-induced vasodilatation in the salivary gland experimentally, indicating that kinins are not involved in the accompanying glandular hyperaemia.[86,87] On the other hand, by inhibiting the converting enzyme, it reduces the effect of angiotensin I in animals and man,[88,89] and in experimental renovascular hypertension in rats.[90,91] In recent interesting studies, Miller *et al.*[92] studied the effect of BPF-nonapeptide during hypertension induced by renal artery constriction in the conscious dog. They found that the hypertension could be prevented by BPF-nonapeptide in the early stages of hypertension when plasma renin levels were elevated. Later, the plasma renin levels returned to normal, hypertension persisted, and BPF was now ineffective in reducing it. These are interesting observations for the analysis of the genesis and stages of development in hypertension of different origins. Further studies are desirable in the search for a therapeutic use for these synthetic BPF-peptides.

SOME RECENT AREAS OF DEVELOPMENT IN THE KALLIKREIN-KININ SYSTEM

The period 1925 to 1950 had a steady and extensive development of the kallikrein-kinin system by Werle and his colleagues, which received little or no general attention. The period 1950 to 1965, however, saw a wide interest develop in the subject, and the new methods in peptide and protein chemistry soon led to the isolation and synthesis of several kinin peptides, kinin potentiators, kininogens, kininogenases, and kininases, as well as of the inhibitors of the latter two enzymes. Recently, from 1970 onwards, a rather new and productive phase seems to be developing. Thus, inherited deficiencies of specific components of the human plasma kallikrein system have been described, and the latter has been shown to be interrelated with the blood coagulating system. Kallikreins are now known to have natriuretic effects, and possible interrelationships of the renal kallikrein-kinin and renin-angiotensin systems are currently being explored in physiology and in experimental and clinical hypertension. Recent studies on a kininogenase in sperm and observations on cyclic variations in plasma kininogen concentrations have suggested a new possible role of kininogenases in reproduction. Also, kinins and prostaglandins appear to have interrelated metabolic actions. Finally, kininogenases and kinins have been reported to have mitogenic or proliferative effects on cells. These recent developments are discussed below.

PLASMA KALLIKREIN-KININ SYSTEM

An observation that suggested some link between plasma kallikrein and blood coagulation was made by Keele and his colleagues in 1957, who found that human plasma released a kinin (PPS, "pain-producing substance") on contact with glass (see Ref. 93). Margolis[94] subsequently found that the plasma of a patient with Hageman trait, whose blood does not clot in glass despite no abnormal tendency to bleeding,[95] failed to release a kinin on glass contact. In 1961, Schachter and his colleagues,[96] in a study of plasma kallikrein, plasmin, and kinin release, suggested "that those individuals deficient in the so-called Hageman Factor (HF) in their plasma may in fact be deficient in the inactive kallikrein precursor". This proposition has turned out to be close to the truth with the discovery in 1973 by Wuepper of an inherited deficiency of plasma prekallikrein, or Fletcher factor,[97] which, like Hageman and Christmas factors, was named after the patient in whom it was discovered by Hathaway *et al.* in 1965.[98] This deficiency was found to be associated with a prolonged blood thromboplastin formation. Although distinct from Hageman factor, like HF-deficient plasma, plasma deficient in Fletcher factor failed to generate kinin on contact with kaolin or glass, and the patients also had neither coagulation defects in vivo nor other haemostatic problems.[97] It has also been shown that HF activates both Fletcher factor and PTA (clotting factor XI).[99,100] These findings are illustrated in Fig. 136–3, which shows some of the relationships between the kallikrein-kinin system in plasma and the intrinsic blood coagulation system. In this scheme, HF (factor XII) occupies a central role, linking both systems. Fig. 136–3 also shows a new significant property of kallikrein—viz., its marked ability to activate pre-HF, thus providing a positive feedback system for maintained HF formation.[101-104] Further, individuals with prekallikrein (Fletcher factor) deficiency have defects in coagulation (intrinsic system), in fibrinolysis, in kinin generation, and in the chemotactic properties of their plasma in vitro. All these defects are corrected by the addition of prekallikrein.[105] The correction of these defects by pure prekallikrein is held to be due to the marked ability of kallikrein to activate pre-HF,[101-106] as illustrated in Fig. 136–3. Fig. 136–3 also shows that plasmin, like kallikrein, is activated by HF (or by fragments of pre-HF derived during its activation).[107] This explains older observations of a fibrinolytic defect in HF-deficient plasma.[108,109] Again plasmin, like kallikrein, is a positive-feedback agent or amplifying system for HF-dependent pathways (Fig. 136–3).[107] Recently, evidence of a *negative* control mecha-

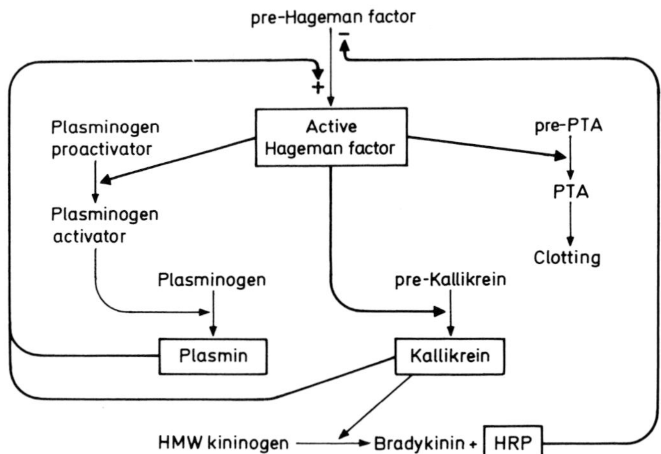

Fig. 136–3. Diagram showing interrelationship between plasma kallikrein and blood coagulating systems. [From Katori *et al.*: In Haberland, G. L. (eds): Kininogenases 3, International Symposium of Academic Science and Literature, Mainz, February 1975. New York, Schattauer, 1975, p. 11, with permission.]

nism for HF has also been suggested. Suzuki and colleagues have shown that plasma kallikrein releases, in addition to bradykinin, two peptide fragments from pure bovine HMW-kininogen.[58,59] One of these peptides has unusual features and has been designated as HRP (histine-rich peptide). It consists of 41 residues with serine and arginine at the NH_2 and COOH end of the molecule, respectively. It is very basic and contains 11 residues of both histidine and glycine and seven residues of lysine, so that these three amino acids alone constitute about 70 percent of the molecule, which has a molecular weight of 4584. HRP has little or no kinin-like activity. However, even in low concentrations it inhibits the activation of pre-Hageman factor by glass insofar as it prevents activation of prekallikrein, and inhibits clotting and the generation of kinin.[110] Suzuki and his colleagues suggest, therefore, that HRP, in contrast to kallikrein and plasmin, which facilitate HF-dependent pathways, acts as a negative-feedback agent on pre-HF, an action appropriate for the final product of a biochemically complex and possibly physiologically significant "cascade" system (Fig. 136–3). Finally, purified fractions of plasma kallikrein and plasminogen activator indicate that both are effective chemotactic agents for human leucocytes,[111] suggesting a possible link between clotting, kallikrein, and inflammation.

The above observations on plasma kallikrein also show that at least some physiologically significant actions of a kininogenase—for example, the activation of pre-HF—are unrelated to the release of a kinin. This liklihood has previously been expressed by Schachter *et al.*[17,39,112] For example, "Indeed, like that of the kininogenase, trypsin, their (kininogenases) physiological significance may even be unrelated in some instances to their ability to release a kinin."[39]

Fletcher trait, or the absence of prekallikrein, is now one of a number of inherited deficiencies in the kallikrein-kinin system of plasma; indeed, a very similar condition called Fitzgerald trait has recently been described,[113] and further studies are required to definitely distinguish it from Fletcher factor deficiency. A deficiency of one of the circulating kallikrein inhibitors—viz., the C$\bar{1}$ esterase inhibitor—was first demonstrated in 1962[114] in hereditary angioedema. This, and subsequent studies,[115] indicate that the absence of this inhibitor results in the ineffective inhibition of excess plasma kallikrein, resulting in bouts of spreading subcutaneous edema. The latter is probably due to kinin released locally in amounts sufficient to increase the concentration of the circulating peptide. Several other deficiencies in the plasma kallikrein-kinin system have recently been described. One of these is apparently due to a hereditary deficiency of kininase I and is characterized by episodes of excessive orthostatic falls in pulse pressure accompanied by facial erythema, ecchymoses, and other cutaneous vascular manifestations. These episodes are accompanied by elevated plasma kinin concentrations. The patients are reported to have normal concentrations of plasma prekallikrein, but those of kininase I are below normal. It is suggested that the latter deficiency is causally related to the condition described as "hyperbradykininism, a new orthostatic syndrome."[116] A case of auto-DNA sensitization associated with episodes of painful cutaneous areas followed by edema and ecchymotic lesions has also been attributed to hyperbradykininism, again thought to be due to decreased kininase activity.[117] In support of this hypothesis, subcutaneous perfusates were found to contain apparently excessive concentrations of bradykinin, and the acute cutaneous episodes were reduced in severity by Trasylol, the polyvalent kallikrein-trypsin inhibitor. The authors suggest that the vascular reactions in AES and DNA-S may be associated with a kininase deficiency or defect. Further studies are required since the evidence necessary to prove an etiologic role for kininase deficiency in these conditions is still meagre.

Finally, an apparent specific deficiency of HMW-kininogen has recently been described—viz., Flaujeac trait.[118] A similar condition has been independently described as William's trait.[119] Whether kininogen has biologic significance other than serving as a substrate for kininogenases remains to be determined. Its hereditary absence in man should help provide an answer to this question.

RENAL KALLIKREIN, HYPERTENSION, PROSTAGLANDINS

Kallikrein was originally described briefly in kidney tissue by Werle,[120,121] who concluded that it was either present or formed in the tubules. A tubular location, at least as the major source of renal kallikrein, has since been supported by other investigators.[122,123] The intraarterial injection of bradykinin produces a diuresis and an increased excretion of sodium from the homolateral but not from the contralateral kidney.[124,125] The concentration of kallikrein in the kidney of the dog and other mammals decreases from the outer to the inner cortex, and the medulla and papilla contain very little.[123,126] Subcellularly, in distinction from renin, which is located almost entirely in the mitochondrial and nuclear fractions of rat kidney cortex,[40] the kallikrein has been reported by different workers to be in the lysosomal[42] or microsomal[40] fractions of homogenates, respectively.

Excellent evidence that the urinary kallikreins are derived unchanged from ones synthesized in the kidney has recently been presented. Nustad *et al.*[24] have demonstrated that the urine and kidney of the rat both contain four kallikreins. In each case they were indistinguishable from one another in their biologic activity and in their immunologic properties but behaved slightly differently in electrofocusing and disc gel electrophoresis.[24] Those in urine, however, were indistinguishable from those in the kidney. Further, the same radioactive kallikreins were isolated from rat kidney slices incubated with [^{3}H]-*L*-leucine, indicating that the kidney is the site of their synthesis.[127]

Recently, the urinary excretion of kallikrein has been measured in hypertension in man and experimental animals. It has been found to be subnormal in patients with essential or renovascular (stenosis) hypertension (see Ref. 131);[128–130] also in SH (spontaneous hypertensive) rats and in rats made hypertensive by experimental renal stenosis (see Refs. 131 to 133). In contrast, it is increased in primary aldosteronism, in patients and animals receiving sodium-retaining steroids, and in patients with phaeochromocytoma (see Refs. 129 to 131). As might be expected from the increased excretion in primary aldosteronism, aldosterone appears to regulate kallikrein secretion in normal subjects. Thus, normal subjects show increased kallikrein excretion in response to a low-sodium intake, to a high-potassium intake, or to administration of the synthetic mineralocorticoid, fludrocortisone. Correspondingly, kallikrein excretion falls after administration of the antagonist, spironolactone.[130]

McGiff *et al.* first reported that kinins activate the prostaglandin-synthesizing system in the kidney. From this and other observations indicating a biochemic interrelationship between kinins and prostaglandins, they further conclude that prostaglandins mediate some and modulate other actions of kinin, which is released intrarenally.[134a,b] Nasjletti and Colina-Chourio come to the same conclusion from studies on the isolated perfused rabbit kidney, and suggest that "a coupling of kinins and prostaglandins intrarenally may be directed towards the facilitation of salt and water excretion.[135]

Despite their complexity, these recent observations suggest that renal kallikrein may be of significance in electrolyte and water balance. The fact that injection of antibody against bradykinin inhibits natriuresis induced by an infusion of isotonic saline[136] supports the hypothesis that the kallikrein-kinin system participates physiologically in regulating sodium excretion by the kidney. The observation of Werle *et al.*[137] that the kininogen concentration of plasma rises to a mean value that is 3.5 times the normal (in some cases 7 times) 72 h after bilateral nephrectomy suggests that there is a constant consumption of plasma kininogen by renal kininogenase. A similar increase occurs in concentrations of plasma angiotensinogen.[138]

KALLIKREINS, KININS, AND REPRODUCTION

It has been known for some time that changes in the concentrations of all components of the plasma kallikrein-kininogen-kinin system occur in women and animals during the estrous and menstrual cycles, pregnancy, and parturition.[120,139–142] In general, the plasma kininogen concentrations rise two- to fourfold during pregnancy and rapidly fall to normal after parturition. Melmon *et al.*[143] have suggested that plasma prekallikrein is activated at birth and that the released kinin mediates the neonatal vascular changes—viz., dilatation of the pulmonary vasculature and constriction of the umbilical vessels and of the ductus arteriosus. Because of the cyclic variations in kininogen concentrations, it has also been suggested that kinins may be involved in ovulation as well as in parturition (see Ref. 141). At present all these possibilities must be regarded as speculative.

The presence of a potent kininogenase in the coagulating, prostate and other accessory sex glands of the guinea-pig has been known since 1961. It was also noted that the prostate of man and other mammals failed to contain significant amounts of such an enzyme.[19] Recently, however, a kininogenase with the specificity and potency of trypsin has been shown by Fritz *et al.* to be present in human and other mammalian spermatozoa. This enzyme, named *acrosin,* is thought to be located in the inner, and its inhibitors near the outer, acrosomal membrane (see Ref. 45).[144,145] Fritz suggests that the main functions of acrosin may be to increase sperm motility and to digest a path through the zona pellucida of the ovum and so facilitate sperm penetration. Pancreatic killikrein has recently been studied in this respect both in vitro and in vivo, and has been reported not only to enhance sperm motility, presumably via release of kinin, but also to increase the sperm count of ejaculates.[146–148] Finally, successful clinical results have been claimed in the treatment of male infertility following injections of pancreatic kallikrein.[148,149] These results should be regarded with interest and caution.

KALLIKREIN AND CELL PROLIFERATION

In a recent series of publications,[150–152] Rixon and Whitfield have presented evidence that kinins, released from injured tissues, may function as local growth control agents or "wound hormones," initiating tissue regeneration. They find that bradykinin markedly increases the mitosis rate of rat thymus lymphocytes in vitro and that the injection of pancreatic kallikrein into rats causes a marked stimulation of DNA synthesis and mitosis in the bone marrow.[152] They conclude that this mitogenic action of kallikrein is probably indirect—i.e., through the liberation of kinins. Mandel *et al.*[153] have reported that the systemic administration of kallikrein exerts a very favorable effect on survival of x-irradiated animals and on the recovery of radiodermatitis produced by local irradiation; also, that kallikrein promotes regeneration of bone marrow after whole-body irradiation. The significance of these dramatic results awaits further investigations.

FURTHER PHYSIOLOGIC AND PATHOPHYSIOLOGIC CONSIDERATIONS

Physiologic

Numerous symposia and reviews on kallikreins and kinins since 1960 have repeatedly speculated on the physiologic role of these enzymes and of the peptides they release (see Refs. 6, 21, 22, 23, 45, 75, 76, 112, and 131). The fact remains, however, that 50 years since its discovery, when it was considered to be a circulating hormone involved in vascular regulation—viz., a *Kreislaufhormon*—its possible role in vascular physiology has not been established with any more certainty. The most persistent claim for a physiologic role of kallikreins and kinins has been that they are mediators of functional hyperaemia in glands and other organs.[154,155] This view is not universally accepted, and evidence in disagreement with the hypothesis has been presented for the salivary[156] and sweat glands.[157] Nonetheless, the ready releasability of kinins by kininogenases from their ubiquitous precursors does mean that their participation in vascular or other physiologic events must always be borne in mind. Figure 136–4 illustrates the main components, activators, inhibitors, and various other factors relevant to the kallikrein-kinin system.

The recent developments in our knowledge of the kininogenases of plasma, kidney, and sex glands have been specifically discussed earlier in this chapter. Their possible importance in blood coagulation-injury-repair events, electrolyte and fluid balance, and in reproductive processes respectively are definite possibilities. Further investigations in these areas are to be awaited with interest.

Pathophysiologic

The temptation to implicate kininogenases and kinins in different pathologic processes has been a strong one, and they have been suggested as etiologic or contributory factors in many diverse

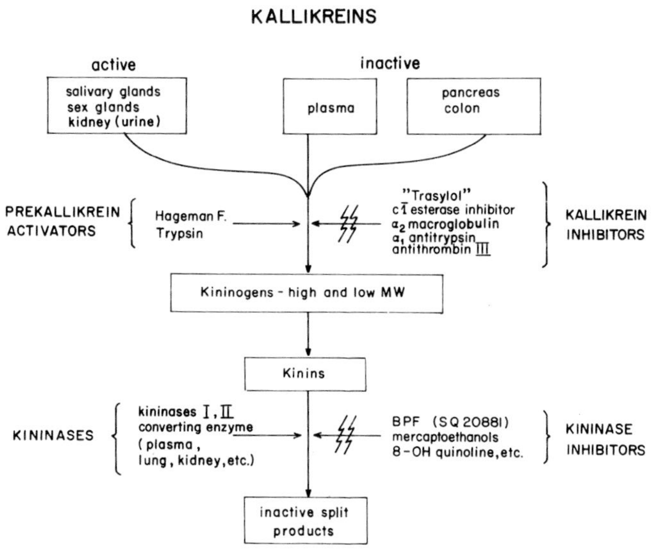

KALLIKREINS

active: salivary glands, sex glands, kidney (urine)
inactive: plasma; pancreas, colon

PREKALLIKREIN ACTIVATORS: Hageman F., Trypsin
KALLIKREIN INHIBITORS: "Trasylol", $C\bar{1}$ esterase inhibitor, α_2 macroglobulin, α_1 antitrypsin, antithrombin III

Kininogens - high and low MW

Kinins

KININASES: kininases I, II, converting enzyme (plasma, lung, kidney, etc.)
KININASE INHIBITORS: BPF (SQ 20881), mercaptoethanols, 8-OH quinoline, etc.

inactive split products

Fig. 136–4. Diagram of main components of kallikrein-kinin system.

conditions—e.g., migraine and other neurologic conditions, vasovagal syncope, shock (hemorrhagic, endotoxic, etc.), dumping syndrome, pancreatitis, diverse arthritides, certain transfusion reactions, burns, protozoal infections, and liver cirrhosis.[22,76,158] A primary involvement of kininogenases is probably not clearly established in any of these conditions and it is probable that their role is secondary or of minor importance to the significant pathologic processes in most of them.

However, in some cases of carcinoid syndrome and in hereditary angioedema (see Ref. 22) and possibly in hyperbradykininism associated with a hereditary kininase deficiency,[116] there is quite clear evidence that an excess of liberated kinin contributes in a significant way to the clinical signs and symptoms. Hereditary angioedema and the hyperbradykininism syndrome have been discussed under the section *Plasma Kallikrein-Kinin System.* The carcinoid system is dealt with in detail in Chapter 138.

Recently, in a controlled trial of 105 patients with acute pancreatitis treated with the polyvalent kallikrein-trypsin inhibitor, Trasylol, a significant beneficial effect of the inhibitor was observed. According to Trapnell,[131] the usual tendency for mortality to rise with age was abolished in the treated group. The recent purification of this and other kininogenase inhibitors should encourage therapeutic trials where inhibition of kininogenase and other proteolytic activity is desired.

GENERAL CONSIDERATIONS

In a symposium on kininogenases and kinins held in 1968, the Introduction to the symposium ended as follows: "It seems that the biological significance of the kinins and of the endogenous agents which release them is far from clear. Their major significance may well lie in a biological system which, for the present, is not apparent to us."[159] Since then, interesting new properties of these substances have been described—e.g., natriuretic activity, involvement in blood coagulation, enhancement of sperm motility, stimulation of cell proliferation, and others. It is begining to appear that kininogenases do not have a *specific* physiologic function. Themselves a large group of enzymes, the kininogenases belong to the wider group of serine proteases, and it would seem likely that they, like other serine proteases, have a common and primitive ancestral origin as have the kinins (Fig. 136–2) which they release. It seems reasonable to conclude, therefore, that they have evolved to participate in *a wide diversity of comparative biologic activities* (see Ref. 28).

The development of our knowledge of kininogenases and kinins has been an at times confusing but always intriguing and challenging subject. There is little doubt, however, that our accumulating biochemic and biologic information is leading us to exciting and clearer interpretations of the significance of these substances.

ADDENDUM: NOTE ADDED IN PROOF

Since this chapter was completed, kallikrein has been specifically and more precisely located in several organs of different mammals by immunofluorescence microscopy. In the submandibular and other salivary glands the enzyme seems confined to the apical regions of duct cells only, and to be secreted into the lumen. There is no evidence of its presence in significant amounts in the acinar cells or interstitial tissues of the rat,[160,161] cat[162,163] and guinea-pig.[164] Similar studies on the rat pancreas, however, demonstrate its presence in the acinar rather than in the duct cells.[165] In this organ it probably co-exists in acinar secretory granules together with the other serine proteases like trypsin. In the coagulating gland of the guinea-pig it appears to be soluble in the cytoplasm rather than in secretory granules or other organelles and to be present in all the secretory cells.[164] The different cellular and subcellular locations in different organs indicate different functions for the various kallikreins.

ACKNOWLEDGMENTS

It is a pleasure to acknowledge helpful discussions and correspondence with Dr. Marion Webster, Dr. K.F. Austen, Dr. C.G. Cochrane, Dr. R. G. Geller, Dr. S. Iwanaga, Dr. A. P. Kaplan, Dr. J. J. Pisano, Dr. T. Suzuki and Dr. KD. Wuepper.

REFERENCES

1. Frey, E. K.: Zusammenhange Zwischen Herzarbeit und Nierentätigkeit. *Arch Klin Chir 142:* 663, 1926.
2. Frey, E. K., Kraut, H.: Ein neues Kreislaufhormon und seine Wirkung. *Arch Exp Pathol Pharmakol 133:* 1, 1928.
3. Frey, E. K., Kraut, H., Werle, E.: Kallikrein (Padutin). Stüttgart Enke, 1950.
4. Frey, E. K., Kraut, H., Werle, E.: Das Kallikrein-Kinin System und seine Inhibitoren. Stüttgart, Enke, 1968.
5. Werle, E.: History of kallikrein and some aspects of its chemistry and physiology. In Haberland, G. L., Rohen, J. W. (eds): Kininogenases. International Symposium, Mainz, Germany. New York, Schattauer, 1973, p 7.
6. Werle, E.: In Pisano, J. J., Austen, F. K. (eds): Chemistry and Biology of the Kallikrein-Kinin System in Health and Disease. Washington DC, US Govt Printing Office, 1976.
7. Kraut, H., Frey, E. K., Werle, E.: Der Nachweis eines Kreislaufhormons in der Pankreasdrüse. *Z Physiol Chem 189:* 97, 1930.
8. Kraut, H., Frey, E. K., Werle, E.: Über den Nachweis und des Vorkommen des Kallikreins im Blut. *Z Physiol Chem 222:* 73, 1933.
9. Werle, E., Götze, W., Keppler, E.: Über die Wirkung des Kallikreins auf den isolierten Darm und über eine neue darmkontrahierende Substanz. *Biochem Z 289:* 217, 1937.
10. Braun-Menendez, E. J., Fasciolo, J. C., Leloir, L. F., Munoz, J. M.: The substance causing renal hypertension. *J Physiol (London) 98:* 283, 1940.

11. Page, I. H., Helmer, O. M.: Crystalline pressor substance, angiotensin, resulting from reaction between renin and renin activator. *J Exp Med 72:* 29, 1940.
12. Werle, E., Hambuechen, R.: Zur Kenntnis der blutdrucksendkenden und spasmolytischen Wirkung des Kallikreins und der Substanz Dk. *Arch Exp Pathol Pharmakol 201:* 311, 1943.
13. Werle, E., Berek, U.: Zur Kenntnis des Kallikreins. *Angew Chem 60A:* 53, 1948.
14. Rocha e Silva, M., Beraldo, W. T., Rosenfeld, G.: Bradykinin, a hypotensive and smooth muscle stimulating factor released from plasma globulin by snake venoms and by trypsin. *Am J Physiol 156:* 261, 1949.
15. Jaques, R., Schachter, M.: The presence of histamine, 5-hydroxytryptamine and a slow contracting substance in wasp venom. *Br J Pharmacol 9:* 53, 1954.
16. Schachter, M., Thain E. M.: Chemical and pharmacological properties of the potent, slow-contracting substance (kinin) in wasp venom. *Br J Pharmacol 9:* 352, 1954.
17. Holdstock, D. J., Mathias, A. P., Schachter, M.: A comparative study of kinins, kallidin and bradykinin. *Br J Pharmacol 12:* 149, 1957.
18. Bhoola, K. D., Calle, J. D., Schachter, M.: Identification of acetylcholine, 5-hydroxytryptamine, histamine and a new kinin in hornet venom (*V crabro*). *J Physiol (London) 159:* 167, 1961.
19. Bhoola, K. D., May May Yi, R., Morley J, Schachter, M.: Release of kinin by an enzyme in the accessory sex glands of the guinea-pig. *J Physiol (London) 163:* 269, 1962.
20. Webster, M. E.: Appendix. Report of the Committee on Nomenclature for Hypotensive Peptides. In Erdös, E. G., Back, N., Sicuteri, F. (eds): Hypotensive Peptides, New York, Springer, 1966, p. 648.
21. Schachter, M.L Kinins—a group of active peptides. *Ann Rev Pharmacol 4:* 281, 1964.
22. Schachter, M.: Kallikreins and Kinins. *Physiol Rev 49:* 510, 1969.
23. Vogel, R., Werle, E., Zickgraf-Rudel, G.: Neuere Aspecte der Kininforschung. *Z Klin Chem Klin Biochem 8:* 177, 1970.
24. Nustad, K., Pierce, J. V.: Purification of rat urinary kallikreins and their specific antibody. *Biochem 13:* 2312, 1974.
25. Ekfors, T. O., Reikkinen, P. J., Malmirarjo, T., Hopsu-Havu, V. K.: Four isozymic forms of a peptidase resembling kallikrein purified from a rat submandibular gland. *Z Physiol Chem 348:* 111, 1967.
26. Fiedler, F., Müller, B., Werle, E.: Charakterisierung verschiedener Schweinekallikreine mittels Diisopropylfluorophosphat. *Hoppe-Seyler's Z Physiol Chem 351:* 1002, 1970.
27. Fiedler, F., Hirschauer, C., Werle, E.: Characterization of pig kallikreins A and B. *Hoppe-Seyler's Z Physiol Chem 346:* 1879, 1975.
28. Stroud, R. M.: A family of protein-cutting proteins. *Sci Am* July 1974, p 74.
29. Pisano, J. J.: Chemistry and biology of the kallikrein-kinin system. In Reich, E., Rifkin, D. B., Shaw, E. (eds): Cold Spring Harbour Conference on Cell Proliferation, Vol 2, Cold Spring Harbour Laboratory, 1975, p 199.
30. Suzuki, T., Takahashi, H., Kimiya, M., Horiuchi, K., Nagasawa, S.: Protein components which relate to the kinin-releasing system in bovine plasma. In Back, N., Sicuteri, F., (eds): Advances in Experimental Medicine and Biology, vol. 21. New York, Plenum, 1972, p 77.
31. Colman, R. W., Mattler, L., Sherry, S.: Studies on the prekallikrein (kallikreinogen)-kallikrein enzyme system of human plasma. I. Isolation and purification of plasma kallikreins. *J Clin Invest 48:* 11, 1969.
32. Sampaio, C., Wong, S-C., Shaw, E.: Human plasma kallikrein purification and preliminary characterization. *Arch Biochem Biophys 165:* 133, 1974.
33. Dorey, G., Bhoola, D.: I. Ultrastructure of acinar cell granules in mammalian submaxillary glands. *Z Zellforsch 126:* 320, 1972.
34. Bhoola, K.: The subcellular distribution of pancreatic kallikrein. *Biochem Pharmacol 18:* 2279, 1969.
35. Chiang, T. S., Erdös, E., Miwa, I., Tague, L. L., Coalson, J. J.: Isolation from a salivary gland of granules containing renin and kallikrein. *Circ Res 23:* 507, 1968.
36. Erdös, E. G., Tague, L. L., Miwa, I.: Kallikrein in granules of the submaxillary gland. *Biochem Pharmacol 17:* 667, 1968.
37. Barton, S., Sanders, E. J., Schachter, M., Uddin, M.: Autonomic nerve stimulation, kallikrein content and acinar cell granules of the cat's submandibular gland. *J Physiol 251:* 363, 1975.
38. Garrett, J. R., Kidd, A.: Effects of nerve stimulation and denervation on secretory material in submandibular striated duct cells of cats, and the possible role of these cells in the secretion of salivary kallikrein. *Cell Tissue Res 161:* 71, 1975.
39. Barton, S. C., Schachter, M.: Subcellular location of the kininogenase in the coagulating gland of the guinea-pig. *Biochem Pharmacol 22:* 1121, 1973.
40. Nustad, K., Rubin, I.: Subcellular localization of the renin and kininogenase in the rat kidney. *Br J Pharmacol 40:* 326, 1970.
41. Werle, E., Vogel, R.: Über die Freisetzung einer Kallikreinartigen Substanz aus Extracten verschiender organe. *Arch Int Pharmacodyn 131:* 257, 1961.
42. Carvalho, I. F. de, Diniz, C. R.: Kinin-forming enzyme (kininogen) in the rat kidney. *Ann NY Acad Sci 116:* 912, 1964.
43. Nustad, K., Pierce, J. V., Vaaje, K.: Synthesis of kallikreins by rat kidney slices. *Br J Pharmacol 53:* 229, 1975.
44. Vogel, R., Trautschold, I., Werle, E.: Natürliche Proteinasen-Inhibitoren. Stüttgart, Thieme, 1966.
45. Proteases and Biological Control. Reich, E., Rifkin, B. D., Shaw, E. (eds): Cold Spring Harbour Conference on Cell Proliferation, vol 2. Cold Spring Harbour Laboratory, 1975.
46. Kraut, H., Frey, E. K., Werle, E.: Über die Inaktivierung des Kallikreins. *Z Physiol Chem 192:* 1, 1930.
47. Kunitz, M., Northrop, J. H.: Isolation from beef pancreas of crystalline trypsinogen, trypsin, a trypsin inhibitor, and an inhibitor-trypsin compound. *J Gen Physiol 19:* 991, 1936.
48. Anderer, F. A., Hornle, S.: Struktur untersuchungen am Kallikrein-Inaktivator aus Rinderlunge. I. Molekulargewicht, Endgruppenanalyse und Aminosaüre-Zusammensetzung. *Z Naturforsch 206:* 457, 1965.
49. Kassel, B., Radicevic, V., Ansfield, M. S., Laskowski, M.: The basic trypsin inhibitor of bovine pancreas. IV. The linear sequence of the 58 amino acids. *Biochem Biophys Res Commun 18:* 255, 1965.
50. Vogel, R., Werle, E.: Kallikrein Inhibitors. In Erdös, E. G., Wilde, A. F. (eds): Handbook of Experimental Pharmacology: Bradykinin, Kallidin and Kallikrein, vol. XXV. New York, Springer, 1970, p 213.
51. Gigli, I., Mason, J. W., Colman, R. W., Austen, K. F.: Interaction of plasma kallikrein with the $C\bar{1}$-inhibitor. *J Immunol 104:* 574, 1970.
52. McConnel, D. J.: Inhibitors of kallikrein in human plasma. *J Clin Invest 51:* 1611, 1972.
53. Fritz, H., Wunderer, G., Kummer, K., Heimburger, N., Werle, E.: α_1-Antitrypsin und $C\bar{1}$-Inaktivator: Progressiv-Inhibitoren für Serumkallikreine von Mensch und Schwein. *Z Physiol Chem 353:* 906, 1972.
54. Lahiri, B., Rosenberg, R., Talamo, R. C., Mitchell, B., Bagdasarian, A., Coleman, R. W.: Antithrombin III: An inhibitor of human plasma kallikrein. *Fed Proc 33:* 642, 1974.
55. Bagdasarian, A., Lahiri, B., Talamo, R. C., Wong, P., Coleman, R. W.: Immunochemical studies of plasma kallikrein. *J Clin Invest 54:* 1444, 1974.
56. Diniz, C. W., Carvalho, I. F. de: A micromethod for determination of bradykininogen under several conditions. *Ann NY Acad Sci 104:* 77, 1963.
57. Komiya, M., Kato, H., Suzuki, T.: Bovine plasma kininogens. III. Structural comparison of high molecular weight and low molecular weight kininogens. *J Biochem 76:* 833, 1974.
58. Han, Y. N., Komiya, M., Iwanaga, S., Suzuki, T.: Studies on the primary structure of bovine high molecular-weight kininogen. *J Biochem 77:* 55, 1975.
59. Han, Y. N., Komiya, M., Kato, H., Iwanaga, S., Suzuki, T.: Primary structure of bovine high molecular weight kininogen: Chemical compositions of kinin-free kininogen and peptide fragments released by plasma kallikrein. *FEBS 57:* 254, 1975.
60. Pierce, J. V.: Structural features of plasma kinins and kininogens. *Fed Proc 27:* 52, 1968.
61. Pierce, J. V.: Purification of mammalian kallikreins, kininogens and kinins. In Erdös, E. G., Wilde, A. F. (eds): Handbook of Experimental Pharmacology: Bradykinin, Kallidin and Kallikrein, vol XXV. New York, Springer, 1970, p 21.
62. Habermann, E.: Kininogens. In Erdös, E. G., Wilde, A. F. (eds):

Handbook of Experimental Pharmacology: Bradykinin, Kallidin and Kallikrein, vol XXV. New York, Springer, 1970, p 250.
63. Spragg, J., Austen, K. F.: Preparation of human kininogen-II. Enzymatic digestion and modification. *Biochem Pharmacol 23:* 781, 1974.
64. Habal, F. M., Movat, H. Z., Burrowes, C. E.: Isolation of two functionally different kininogens from human plasma: Separation from proteinase inhibitors and interaction with plasma kallikrein. *Biochem Pharmacol 23:* 2291, 1974.
65. Ishikawa, O., Yasuhara, T., Nakajima, T., Tachibana, S.: On the biological active peptide in the skin of *Rana rugosa*. The 12th Symposium on Peptide Chemistry, Kyoto, 1974.
66. Dunn, R. S., Perks, A. M.: Comparative studies of plasma kinins: The kallikrein-kinin system in poikilotherm and other vertebrates. *J Gen Comp Physiol 26:* 165, 1975.
67. Schachter, M., Morley, J.: Biologically active polypeptides. In Bacharach, A. L., Laurence., D. R. (eds): Evaulation of Drug Activities: Pharmacometrics, vol 2. New York, Academic, 1964, p 627.
68. Trautschold, I.: Assay methods in the kallikrein system. In Erdös, E. G., Wilde, A. F. (eds): Handbook of Experimental Pharamcology: Bradykinin, Kallidin and Kallikrein, vol XXV. New York, Springer, 1970, p 52.
69. Collier, H. O. J., Holgate, J. H., Schachter, M., Shorley, P. G.: The bronchoconstrictor action of bradykinin in the guinea-pig. *Br J Pharmacol 15:* 290, 1960.
70. Bhoola, K. D., Collier, H. O. J., Schachter, M., Shorley, P. G.: Action of some peptides on bronchial muscle. *Br J Pharmacol 19:* 190, 1962.
71. Collier, H. O. J.: Kinins and ventilation of the lungs. In Erdös E. G., Wilde, A. F. (eds): Handbook of Experimental Pharmacology: Bradykinin, Kallidin and Kallikrein, vol XXV. New York, Springer, 1970, p 409.
72. Schröder, E.: Structure activity relationships of kinins. In Erdös, E. G., Wilde, A. F. (eds): Handbook of Experimental Pharmacology: Bradykinin, Kallidin and Kallikrein, Vol XXV. New York, Springer, 1970, p 324.
73. Brady, A. H., Ryan, J. W., Stewart, J. M.: Circular dichroism of bradykinin and related peptides. *Biochem J 121:* 179, 1971.
74. Stewart, J. M.: Structure-activity relationships among the kinins. In Margoulies, M., Greenwood, F. C. (eds): Structure-Activity Relationships of Protein and Polypeptide Hormones. Amsterdam, *Excerpta Medica,* 1971, p 23.
75. Schachter, M.: Some properties of kallidin, bradykinin and wasp venom kinin. In Schachter, M. (ed): Polypeptides which Affect Smooth Muscles and Blood Vessels, London, Pergamon, 1960, p 232.
76. Erdös, E. G.: Enzymes that inactivate vasoactive peptides. In Brodie, B. B., Gillette, J. (eds): Handbook of Experimental Pharmacology, new series, vol XXVIII/2. New York, Springer, 1971, p 620.
77. Osima, G., Kato, J., Erdös, E. G.: Subunits of human plasma carboxypeptides N (kininase I: anaphylatoxin inactivator). *Biochem Biophys Acta 365:* 344, 1974.
78. Igic, R., Sorrels, K., Nakajima, T., Erdös, E. G.: Identity of kininase II with an angiotensin I converting enzyme. In Back, N., Sicuteri, F. (eds): Vasopeptides: Chemistry, Pharmacology and Pathophysiology, New York, Plenum, 19 , p 149.
79. Erdös, E. G.: Angiotensin I converting enzyme. *Circ Res 36:* 247, 1975.
80. Gladner, J. A., Murtaugh, P. A., Folk, J. E., Laki, K.: Nature of peptides released by thrombin. *Ann NY Acad Sci 104:* 47, 1963.
81. Ferreira, S. H., Rocha e Silva, M.: Potentiation of bradykinin and eledoisin by B.P.F. (bradykinin potentiating factor) from *B. jararaca* venom. *Experientia 21:* 347, 1965.
82. Kata, H., Suzuki, T.: Structure of bradykinin potentiators isolated from snake venoms. *J Jpn Biochem Soc 40:* 574, 1968.
83. Stewart, J. M., Ferreira, S. H., Greene, L. G.: Bradykinin potentiating peptide Pca-Lys-Trp-Ala-Pro. *Biochem Pharmacol 20:* 1557, 1971.
84. Kato, J, Suzuki, K., Okada, K., Kimura, T., Sakakibara, S.: Structure of potentiator A, one of the five bradykinin potentiating peptides from the venom of *A. halysblomhoffii. Experimentia 29:* 574, 1973.
85. Stewart, J. M., Freer, R. J.: Inhibitors of the pulmonary destruction of bradykinin in the rat. In Peeters, H. (ed): Protides of the Biological Fluids, 20th Colloquium, Oxford, New York, Pergamon, 19 , p 331.
86. Schachter, M., Barton, S., Karpinski, E.: Sympathetic vasocilatation in the submaxillary gland and its enhancement after chronic parasympathetic denervation. *Experientia 29:* 1498, 1973.
87. Schachter, M., Barton, S., Karpinski, E.: Analysis of vasodilatation in the submaxillary gland using potentiators of acetylcholine and kinins. *Experientia 29:* 973, 1973.
88. Bianchi, A., Evans, D. B., Cobb, M., Peschka, M. T., Schaeffer, T. R., Laffen, R. J.: Inhibition by S.Q. 20881 of vasopressor response to angiotensin I in conscious animals. *Eur J Pharmacol 23:* 90, 1973.
89. Collier, J. G., Robinson, B. R., Vane, J. F.: Reduction of pressor effects of angiotensin I in mouse by synthetic nonapeptide (BPP_{5a}or SQ20881) which inhibits converting enzyme. *Lancet 1:* 72, 1973.
90. Kreiger, E. M., Salgado, H. C., Assan, C. J., Greene, L. G., Ferreira, S. H.: Potential screening test for detection of overactivity of reninangiotensin system. *Lancet 1:* 269, 1971.
91. Engel, S. L., Schaeffer, T. R., Waugh, M. H., Rubin, B.: Effects of the nonapeptide SQ 20,881 on blood pressure of rats with experimental renovascular hypertension. *Proc Soc Exp Biol Med 143:* 483, 1972.
92. Miller, E. D., Samuels, A. I., Haber, E., Barger, A. C.: Inhibition of angiotensin conversion and prevention of renal hypertension. *Am J Physiol 228:* 448, 1975.
93. Keele, C. A.: Formation of pain-producing polypeptide (PPS) from plasma. In Schachter, M. (ed): Polypeptides which Affect Smooth Muscles and Blood Vessels, London, Pergamon, 1960, p 253.
94. Margolis, J.: Activation of plasma by contact with glass: Evidence for a common reaction which releases plasma kinin and initiates coagulation. *J Physiol 144:* 1, 1958.
95. Ratnoff, O. D., Calopy, J. E.: A familial haemorrhagic trait associated with a deficiency of a clot-promoting fraction of plasma. *J Clin Invest 34:* 602, 1955.
96. Bhoola, K. D., Calle, J. D., Schachter, M.: The effect of bradykinin, serum kallikrein and other endogenous substances on capillary permeability in the guinea-pig. *J Physiol 152:* 75, 1960.
97. Wuepper, K. D.: Prekallikrein deficiency in man. *J Exp Med 138:* 1345, 1973.
98. Hathaway, W. E., Belhassen, L. P., Hathaway, H. S.: Evidence for a new plasma thromboplastin factor. I. Case report, coagulation studies and physico-chemical properties. *Blood 26:* 521, 1965.
99. Kaplan, A. P., Austen, K. F.: A prealbumin activator of prekallikrein. II. Derivation of activators of prekallikrein from active Hageman factor by digestion with plasmin. *J Exp Med 133:* 696, 1971.
100. Burrowes, C. E., Movat, H. Z., Soltay, M. J.: The kinin system in human plasma. VI. The action of plasmin. *Proc Soc Exp Biol Med 138:* 959, 1971.
101. Cochrane, C. G., Revak, S. D., Wuepper, K. D., Johnston, A., Morrison, D. C., Ulevitch, R.: Activation of Hageman factor and the kinin-forming, intrinsic clotting, and fibrinolytic systems. In Raspe, E. (ed): Advances in the Biosciences 12, Schering Symposium on Immunopathology, Yugoslavia, May 28 1973, Vieweg. New York, Pergamon, p 237.
102. Kaplan, A. P.: The Hageman factor dependent pathways of human plasma. *Microvasc Res 8:* 97, 1974.
103. Cochrane, C. G., Revak, S. D., Wuepper, K. D.: Activation of Hageman factor in solid and fluid phases. A critical role of kallikrein. *J Exp Med 138:* 1565, 1973.
104. Cochrane, C. G., Revak, S. D., Aikin, B. S., Wuepper, K. D.: The structure and activation of Hageman factor. In Lepow, I., Ward, P. (eds): Inflammation: Mechanisms and Control. New York, Academic, 1970, p 119.
105. Weiss, A. S., Gallin, J. A., Kaplan, A. P.: Fletcher factor deficiency. A diminished rate of Hageman factor activation caused by absence of prekallikrein, with abnormalities of coagulation, fibrinolysis, chemotactic activity, and kinin generation. *J Clin Invest 53:* 622, 1974.
106. Kay, A. B., Kaplan, A. P.: Chemotaxis and haemostasis. *Br J Haematol 31:* 417, 1975.
107. Kaplan, A. P., Austen, K. F.: The fibrinolytic pathway of human plasma (isolation and characterization of the plasminogen proactivator). *J Exp Med 136:* 1378, 1972.
108. Niewiarowski, S., Prou-Wartelle, O.: Role du facteur contact (fac-

teur Hageman) dans la fibrinolyse. *Thromb Diath Haemorrh 6:* 411, 1961.
109. Iatridis, S. G., Ferfuson, J. H.: Plasminoplastin generation test of normal, HF⁻, PTA⁻, X⁻, PTC⁻ and AHF⁻ platelet-poor plasmas: Evidence that only HF⁻ plasma has an abnormal fibrinolytic activity *Nature (London) 207:* 1404, 1965.
110. Katori, M., Iwanaga, S., Komiya, M., Han, Y. N., Suzuki, T., Oh-Ishi, S.: Structure and a possible physiological function of a fragment, "histidine-rich peptide" released from bovine plasma high molecular weight kininogen by plasma kallikrein. In Haberland, G. L., Rohen, J. H., Blumel, G., Huber, P. (eds): Kininogenases 3, International Symposium of Academic Science and Literature at Mainz, February 1975. New York, Schattauer, 1975, p 11.
111. Kaplan, A. P., Goetze, E. J., Austen, K. F.: The fibrinolytic pathway of human plasma. II. The generation of chemotaxic activity by activation of plasminogen proactivator. *J Clin Invest 52:* 2591, 1973.
112. Schachter, M.: Pharmacologically active peptides. In Robson, J. M., Stacey, R. S. (eds): Recent Advances in Pharmacology. London, Churchill, 1962, p 162.
113. Sato, H., Ratnoff, O. D., Waldmann, R., Abraham, J.: Deficiency of a hitherto unrecognized agent, Fitzgerald factor, participating in surface-mediated reactions of clotting, fibrinolysis, generation of kinins, and of the property of diluted plasma enhancing vascular permeability (PF/Dil). *J Clin Invest 55:* 1082, 1975.
114. Landerman, N. S., Webster, M. E., Becker, E. L., Ratcliffe, H. E.: Hereditary angioneurotic oedema. II. Deficiency of inhibitor for serum globulin permeability factor and/or plasma kallikrein. *J Allergy 33:* 330, 1962.
115. Donaldson, V. H.: Mechansims of activation of C$\bar{1}$ esterase in hereditary angioneurotic edema plasma in vitro: role of Hageman factor, clot-promoting agent. *J Exp Med 127:* 411, 1968.
116. Streeten, D. H. P., Kerr, C. B., Prior, J. C., Dalakos, T. H.: Hyperbradykininism: A new orthostatic syndrome. *Lancet 18:* 1048, 1972.
117. Leiba, H., Almog, C., Kaufman, S., Edery, H.: Possible role of bradykinin in a patient with recurrent cutaneous ecchymoses (DNA sensitization). *Isr J Med 8:* 67, 1972.
118. Wuepper, K. D., Miller, D. R., Lacombe, M. J.: Flaujeac trait: Deficiency of human plasma kininogen. *Fed Proc 34:* 859, 1975.
119. Coleman, R. W., Bagdasarian, A., Talamo, R. C., Seavey, M. Scott, C. F., Kaplan, A. P.: Williams trait: Combined deficiency of plasma plasminogen proactivator, kininogen, and a new procoagulant factor. *Fed Proc 34:* 859, 1975.
120. Werle, E.: Kallikrein and kallidin. In Schachter, M. (ed): Polypeptides which Affect Smooth Muscles and Blood Vessels, London, Pergamon, 1960, p 199.
121. Werle, E., Vogel, R.: Über die Kallikrein Ausscheidumg im Harn nach experimenteller Nierenschädigung. *Arch Int Pharmacodyn 126:* 171, 1960.
122. Barton, S., Schachter, M.: Kininogenase in kidney after ligation of the ureter and after experimental aortic stenosis. *Experientia 30:* 1289, 1974.
123. Carretero, O. A., Scicli, A. G.: Renal kallikrein: Its localization and possible role in renal function. *Fed Proc 35:* 194, 1976.
124. Webster, M. E., Gilmore, J. P.: Influence of kallidin-10 on renal function. *Am J Physiol 206: 714, 1964.*
125. Barraclough, M. A., Mills, I. H.: Effect of bradykinin on renal function. *Clin Sci 28:* 69, 1965.
126. Furtado, M. R. F.: Kinins and the kidney. *Cienc Cult (Maracaibo) 23:* 497, 1971.
127. Nustad, K., Vaaje, K., Pierce, J. V.: Synthesis of kallikreins by rat kidney slices. *Br J Pharmacol 53:* 229, 1975.
128. Margolius, H. S., Geller, R. G., Pisano, J. J., Sjoesrma, A.: Altered urinary kallikrein excretion in human hypertension. *Lancet 2:* 1063, 1971.
129. Margolius, H. S., Geller, R. G., de Jong, J. J., Pisano, J. J., Sjoersma, A.: Urinary kallikrein excretion in hypertension. *Circ Res 31:* 125, 1972.
130. Margolius, H. S., Horwitz, D., Pisano, J. J., Keiser, H. R.: Relationships among urinary kallikrein, mineralocorticoids and human hypertensive disease. *Fed Proc 35:* 203, 1976.
131. Symposium. Chemistry and Biology of the Kallikrein-Kinin System in Health and Disease. Pisano, J. J., Austen, K. F. (eds): Washington DC, US Govt Printing Office, 1976.
132. Croxatto, H. R., San Martin, M.: Kallikrein-like activity in the urine of renal hypertensive rats. *Experientia 26:* 1216, 1970.
133. Keiser, H. R., Geller, R. G., Margolius, H. S., Pisano, J. J.: Urinary kallikrein in hypertensive animal models. *Fed Proc 35:* 199, 1976.
134a. Terragno, N. A., Lonigro, A. J., Malik, K. V., McGiff, J. C.: The relationship of the renal vasodilator action of bradykinin to the release of a prostaglandin E-like substance. *Experientia 28:* 437, 1972.
134b. McGiff, J. C., Itskovitz, H. D., Terragno, A., Wong, PY-K.: Modulation and mediation of the action of the renal kallikrein-kinin system by prostaglandins. *Fed Proc 35:* 175, 1976.
135. Nasjletti, A., Colina-Chourio, J.: Interaction of mineralocorticoids, renal prostaglandins and the renal kallikrein-kinin system. *Fed Proc 35:* 189, 1976.
136. Marin-Grez, M.: The influence of antibodies against bradykinin on isotonic saline diuresis in the rat: Evidence for kinin involvement in renal function. *Pflügers Arch 350:* 231, 1974.
137. Werle, E., Leysath, G., Schmal, A.: Über das verhalten des Kininogenspiegels nach Nieren und nach nebennierenextirpation bei der Ratte. *Z Physiol Chem 349:* 107, 1968.
138. Blaquier, P.: Kinetic studies on renin-angiotensinogen reaction after nephrectomy. *Am J Physiol 208:* 1083, 1965.
139. Werle, E., Preisser, F.: Entstehung von z ei die glatte Muskulatur erregenden Substanzen in Milch. *Naturwissenschaften 43:* 376, 1956.
140. McCormick, J. T., Senior, J.: Plasma kinin and kininogen levels in the female rat during the oestrous cycle, pregnancy, parturition and the puerperium. *Br J Pharmacol 50:* 237, 1974.
141. McDonald, M., Perks, A. M.: Plasma bradykininogen and reproductive cycles: Studies during the oestrous cycle and pregnancy in the rat, and in the human menstrual cycle. *Can J Zool 54:* 941, 1976.
142. Senior, J., Whalley, E. T.: Plasma kininogen during the oestrous cycle, early pregnancy and pseudopregnancy in the rat. *J Physiol 256:* 167, 1976.
143. Melmon, K. L., Cline, M. J., Hughes, T., Mies, A. S.: Kinins, possible mediators of neonatal circulatory changes in man. *J Clin Invest 47:* 1295, 1968.
144. Fritz, H.: The kallikrein-kinin system in reproduction—biochemical aspects. In Haberland, G. L., Rojen, J. W., Schirren, C., Huber, P. (eds): Kininogenases 2, International Symposium of Academic Science and Literature, Mainz. New York, Schattauer, 1975, p 9.
145. Palm, S., Fritz, H.: Components of the kallikrein-kinin system in human midcycle cervical mucus and seminal plasma. In Haberland, G. L., Rohen, J. W., Schirren, C., Huber, P. (eds): Kininogenases 2, International Symposium of Academic Science and Literature, Mainz. New York, Schattauer, 1975, p 17.
146. Schill, W., Haberland, G. L.: Kinin-induced enhancement of sperm motility. *Hoppe-Seyler's Z Physiol Chem 335:* 229, 1974.
147. Schill, W. G.: Influence of the kallikrein-kinin system on human sperm motility in vitro. In Haberland, G. L., Rohen, J. W., Schirren, C., Huber, P. (eds): Kininogenases 2, International Symposium of Academic Science and Literature, Mainz. New York, Schattauer, 1975, p 129.
148. Ishigami, J., Kamidono, S.: Clinical experiences with kallikrein in male infertility. In Haberland, G. L., Rohen, J. W., Schirren, C., Huber, P. (eds): Kininogenases 2, International Symposium of Academic Science and Literature, Mainz. New York, Schattauer, 1975, p 155.
149. Fromatin, M., Perin, G., Gautier, D., Thabut, A.: Treatment of oligoasthenospermias with kallikrein. In Haberland, G, L., Rohen, J. W., Schirren, S., Huber, P. (eds): Kininogenases 2, International Symposium of Academic Science and Literature, Mainz. New York, Schattauer, 1975, p 151.
150. Perris, A. D., Whitfield, J. F.: The mitogenic action of bradykinin on thymic lymphocytes and its dependence on calcium. *Proc Soc Exp Biol Med 130:* 1198, 1969.
151. Rixon, R. H., Whitfield, J. F., Bayliss, J.: The stimulation of mitotic activity in the thymus and bone marrow of rats by kallikrein. *Horm Metab Res 3:* 279, 1971.
152. Rixon, R. H., Whitfield, J. F.: Kallikrein, kinin and cell proliferation, In Haberland, G. L., Rohen, J. W. (eds): Kininogenases, 1st Symposium on Physiological Properties and Pharmacological Rationale. New York, Schattauer, 1971, p 131.
153. Mandel, P., Rodesch, J., Mantz, J. M.: The treatment of experimental radiation lesions by kallikrein. In Haberland, G. L., Rohen, J. W. (eds): Kininogenases, 1st Symposium on Physiologi-

cal Properties and Pharmacological Rationale. New York, Schattauer, 1971, p 171.
154. Hilton, S. M.: Plasma kinin and blood flow. In Schachter, M. (ed): Polypeptides which Affect Smooth Muscles and Blood Flow. London, Pergamon, 1960, p 258.
155. Hilton, S. M.: The physiological role of glandular kallikreins. In Erdös, E. G., Wilde, A. F. (eds): Handbook of Experimental Pharmacology, vol XXV. New York, Springer, 1970, p 389.
156. Schachter, M.: Vasodilatation in the submaxillary gland of the cat, rabbit and sheep. In Erdös, E. G., Wilde, A. F. (eds): Handbook of Experimental Pharmacology, vol XXV. New York, Springer, 1970, p 400.
157. Frewin, D. B., McConnell, D. J., Downey, J. A.: Is a kininogenase necessary for human sweating? *Lancet 2:* 744, 1973.
158. Kellermeyer, R. W., Graham, R. C., Jr.: Kinins—possible physiologic and pathologic roles in man. *N Engl J Med 279:* 754, 802, 859, 1968.
159. Schachter, M.: Introduction to kinins: A group of vasoactive peptides. *Fed Proc 27:* 49, 1968.
160. Ørstavik, T. B., Brandtzaeg, P., Nustad, K., Halvorsen, K. M.: Cellular localization of kallikreins in rat submandibular and sublingual salivary glands. *Acta Histochem 54:* 183, 1975.
161. Brandtzaeg, P., Gautvik, K. M., Nastad, K., Pierce, J. V.: Rat submandibular gland kallikreins: Purification and cellular localization. *Br J Pharmacol 56:* 155, 1976.
162. Hojima, Y., Maranda, B., Moriwaki, C., Schachter, M.: Direct evidence for the location of kallikrein in the striated ducts of the cat's submandibular gland by the use of specific antibody. *J Physiol* (London) *268:* 793, 1977.
163. Maranda, B., Rodrigues, J. A. A., Schachter, M., Shnitka, T. K., Weinberg, J.: Studies on kallikrein in the duct systems of the salivary glands of the cat. *J Physiol* (London) *276:* 321, 1978.
164. Schachter, M., Maranda, B., Moriwaki, C.: Localization of kallikrein in the coagulating and submandibular glands of the guinea-pig. *J Histochem Cytochem* April, 1978.
165. Nustad, K., Ørstavik, T. B., Gautvik, K. M., Pierse, J. V.: Glandular kallikreins. *Gen Pharmacol 9:* 1, 1978.

137

Prostaglandins and Humoral Regulation

Peter W. Ramwell
Elizabeth M. K. Leovey

In 5 years time probably as much as one-third of the contents of the unofficial pharmacopeias will be found to involve prostaglandins synthesis or metabolism in one form or another. The speed at which the field is moving since the original description of the molecular structure makes difficult the development of a reasonable perspective. We have avoided the cataloging and tabulation of the innumerable endocrine studies, for they are often derived with data from one species employing massive doses of only one or two prostaglandins, at a time when many prostanoate structures are still awaiting identification and characterization. The key question is how to identify which of the multitude of animal in vitro and in vivo observations may have pragmatic significance to the patient. This conservative approach may be prudent since in the 5 years' time referred to above, a new chapter may bear scant relationship to what is written now.

INTRODUCTION

Prostaglandins are important for the endocrinologist because they are not only highly active substances but, in contrast with classical hormones, are present in all cells of the human body with few exceptions; this situation obtains since they are quickly and easily made by microsomes. Thus the mature human erythrocyte which does not possess microsomes does not make prostaglandins. The rate-limiting step in prostaglandin synthesis is usually the availability of *free* arachidonic acid which is the most abundant precursor. This highly unsaturated, fatty acid and its own precursor, linoleic acid, constitute the dietary essential fatty acids. There is little doubt now remaining that this dietary *essentiality* is linked directly to the role of these highly unsaturated fatty acids as prostaglandin precursors.

A variety of peroxides are formed by oxygenases which incorporate molecular oxygen into arachidonic acid, which by itself is inactive. In contrast, the different oxygenated derivatives of arachidonic acid are active. Samuelsson has shown that by far the most potent compounds spring from the formation of a unique endoperoxide that yields a veritable cascade of prostanoate and nonprostanoate compounds which, because of the catholic nature of their properties, prompted us earlier to coin the phrase "wide spectrum of biological activity" (Fig. 137-1).

Some of the prostanoate compounds, for example those of the PGE class (see below), not only release hormones such as prolactin and growth hormones but mimic many of the trophic hormones themselves (TSH, LH, ACTH) and in addition contract or relax all four types of smooth muscle. Since there are qualitative differences between individuals of the PGE class, the neophyte's despair is understandable when he masters the properties of the PGE, PGF, PGB, and PGA classes only to discover that he then has to master the properties of the PGDs, which are currently only just beginning to be studied. Subsequently, he learns that an even newer group of prostaglandins have been discovered—namely, the PGI_2 or prostacyclins—which pose an even greater threat in that they promise to permutate the individuals of some of the other classes.

However, the speed with which the field is moving means that not all the compounds of the classes described above, which have been identified by rigorous structural analysis, have necessarily been synthesized. Moreover where a synthesis has been described it may not be sufficiently convenient to produce large enough quantities so as to make the compounds freely available. Where purity, stability, and uniformity of compounds is an FDA requisite prior to clinial testing then the supply position is exacerbated accordingly.

ARACHIDONATE SYSTEMS

Clearly, effort must be made to obtain a comprehensive profile of the endocrinologic properties of all the compounds. In this respect, great care must be exercised with respect to species differences. For example, $PGF_2\alpha$ is luteolytic in most species but not in women. Another and parallel approach is to study the pathophysiologic problems from the point of view of the regulation

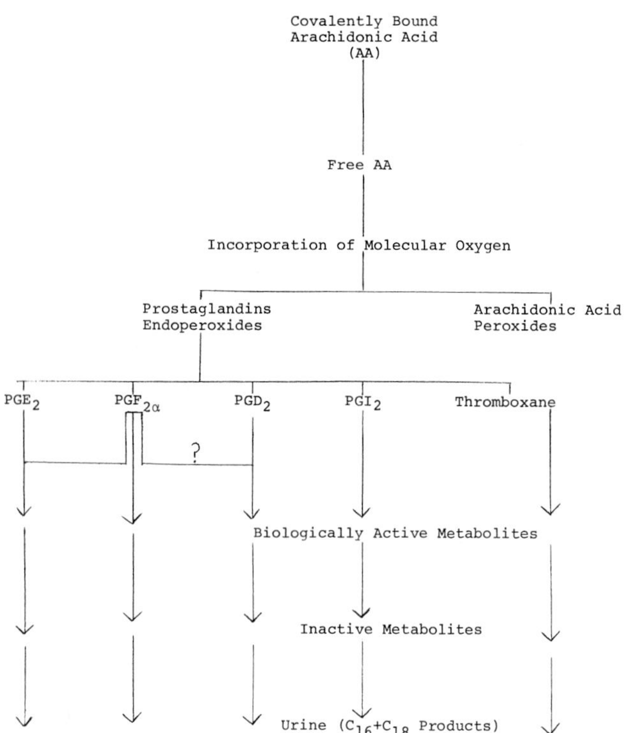

Fig. 137-1. Simplified diagram of the main components of the catabolism of arachidonic acid.

of arachidonate which is the rate-limiting step initiating this complex multibranching cascade of compounds. Thus the myometrial synthesis of oxytocic prostaglandins by the uterus at term is recognized to be a critical step in parturition. This synthesis is blocked by aspirin, and in consequence birth will be delayed. Some studies indicate that both arachidonic acid and phospholipase A_2 content increase in the chorioamniotic membrane during gestation, and that as progesterone falls at the end of the third semester it permits calcium activation of the phospholipase which in turn releases the prostaglandin precursors. Studies of the effect of arachidonate to initiate labor have been successful but dissection is necessary to elucidate which elements of the cascade are formed in sufficient quantities to mediate delivery.

Another example is in Bartter's syndrome (see below), which can be considered simplistically as a problem in an arachidonic acid system. Thus arachidonic acid releases renin from the juxtaglomerular apparatus (JGA) as does PGE_2 and PGD_2. The former is blocked by aspirin or indomethacin but not the latter two. These nonsteroidal, antiinflammatory drugs have been used successfully to reduce the hyperreninemia observed in the syndrome. It will be of interest to inquire into the turnover rates of arachidonic acid in the systemic and renal circulations and in the JGA itself.

However, a knowledge of the precise prostanoate and nonprostanoate compounds released when the cascade is initiated is needed, which means that more convenient methods of quantitative analysis need to be developed for clinical application. Thus in those neoplastic hypercalcemias that are responsive to indomethacin,[1] it is unlikely that components of the PGE series that contain powerful bone-resorbing agents is the primary prostaglandin class since they are so easily removed from plasma by a single transit through the lung. Clearly, the identity of the prostanoate compounds released must be matched with knowledge derived from the systematic testing for bone-resorbing properties of the individual elements of the cascade.

As indicated earlier, many of the prostaglandins have not been systematically tested. Thus, the PGE and PGF series have been generally employed, since they are available in milligram quantities. In most endocrine tissues they have been found to elevate cyclic AMP and GMP levels, respectively. The PGD compounds are also formed in abundance from the same precursor but have not been widely tested due to lack of supplies and to a mistaken assumption of their lack of activity. Moreover, it might well be that none of these three classes are significant because their common endoperoxide precursor or another product such as PGI_2, or thromboxane A_2, may have the major role.

The development of synthetic prostaglandin analogs is of considerable interest to the clinician since they have longer duration of activity due to decreased metabolism and greater intrinsic potency and hence more specifity. Thus a series of methylated PGE compounds have been used to inhibit gastric acid secretion and promote ulcer healing in man. One of these long-acting compounds has also been found not only to inhibit melanoma in tissue culture but also in vivo in a mouse model by Jaffe and Santoro.[2]

In summary, the current approach to understanding the clinical problems is based on isolation, identification, synthesis, and biologic characterization of the prostanoate and nonprostanoate compounds involved in a particular tissue. The use of FDA-approved and therefore readily available inhibitors of the prostaglandin pathway has been a major step in the identification of clinically significant arachidonic-acid–prostaglandin systems.

SIGNIFICANCE OF ARACHIDONIC ACID

The question arises as to the initiating role of arachidonic acid in pathophysiology. Prostaglandins do not appear to be stored. Increased prostaglandin release, which occurs in many situations, is a reflection of prior arachidonic acid release. However, although prostaglandins have been measured in many of these circumstances, the same cannot be said for arachidonic acid. The occurrence of this acid in the plasma as a free acid, as an ester of cholesterol, or in its key location in the 2 position of phospholipids is well known. What is not generally appreciated is that arachidonic acid is unique in that it has a high turnover rate in human plasma and it appears to be regulated in a completely different manner from the other fatty acids which respond, all in concert, to feeding, starvation, and to nicotinic acid.

DIETARY SOURCES

Diets dieficient in arachidonic acid, or its precursor, linoleic acid (Fig. 137-2), are well known to cause poor growth, skin disorders, and decreased fertility in animals. Some carnivores, such as cats, cannot convert linoleic acid to arachidonic acid by chain elongation and desaturation, and therefore require arachidonate to be present in their diet. Deficiency syndromes are clearly observed in patients and especially children who have diets lacking these two fatty acids. The diet has to be substantially deficient since the characteristic infant eczema is easily eliminated if linoleate is added to the diet in sufficient quantities to make up 1 percent of the total calories consumed. Holman[3] has recently reviewed the subject and has given an excellent account of the biochemic mechanisms involved. A useful clinical test for deficiency is to take serum and to determine the ratio of the abnormal fatty acid (5,8,11-eicosatrienoic acid) that is formed in the absence

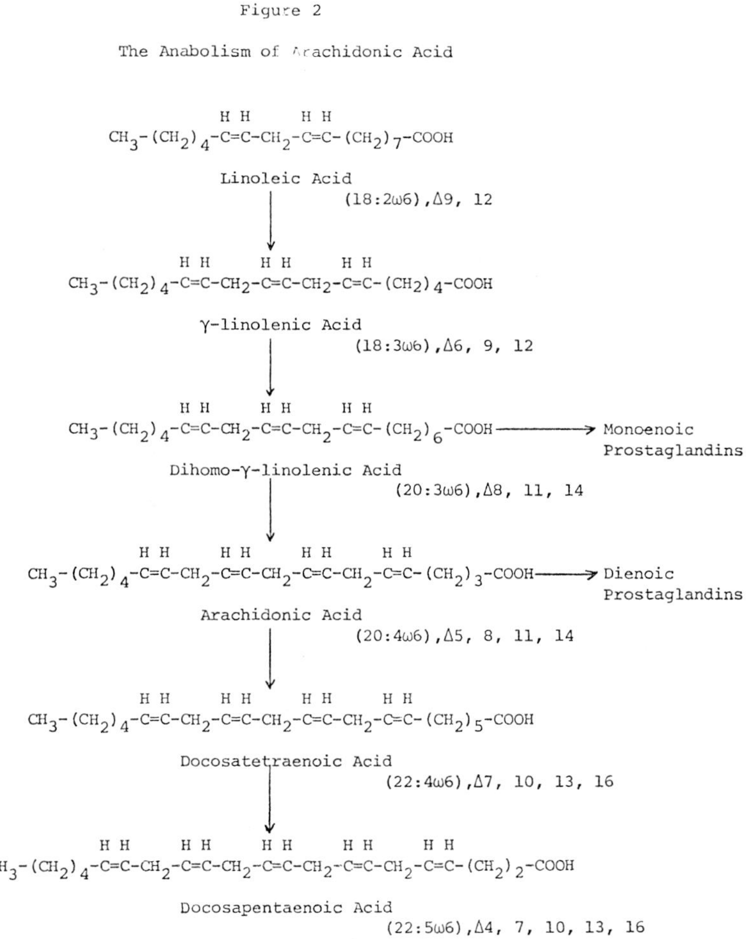

Fig. 137-2. Two types of nomenclature are used. The first figure in parentheses refers to carbon chain length, the next figures give the degree of unsaturation, and ω6 refers to the carbon from the methyl end at which the double bond conjugation begins. In contrast, the Δ nomenclature refers to the position of each double bond where numbering begins from the carboxylic group. The trienoic prostaglandins are derived from Δ5,8,11,14,17-eicosapentaenoic acid which is not synthesized from linoleic acid.

of linoleate, to that of the tetraenoic arachidonate (i.e., the triene/tetraene ratio). There is evidence to indicate that new-born children are relatively deficient in essential fatty acids and that the serum rapidly approaches normal values in breast-fed babies in contrast to those fed cow milk. Other routes of administration have been tested with success. Noteworthy is the rubbing of sunflower seed oil, which contains primarily linoleic acid, into the skin of babies receiving long-term intravenous feeding of fat-free preparations. This procedure reversed both the dermatitis which is characteristic of the deficiency and also improved the "triene/tetraene ratio." This dermal application of linoleate may have other consequences since the feeding of linoleate appears to decrease platelet aggregability.[4] Decreased aggregation may be due to the relative accumulation of homogamma linoleic acid which is the product created prior to further desaturation to arachidonate (Fig. 137-2). Homogamma linoleic acid is known to inhibit platelet aggregation in vivo and is presumably due to the formation of the monoenoic prostaglandins PGE, which is a powerful stabilizer of platelets. Confusingly, arachidonic acid itself, when added to platelet-rich plasma, is an aggregator of platelets in that it yields prostaglandins endoperoxides from which thromboxane is quickly made, and this compound, as its name implies, is a powerful aggregator of platelets. There are, however, other explanations possible since linoleic acid inhibits the metabolism of arachidonate by the cycloxygenase. In addition PGI_2, a potent anti-aggregator of platelets,[5] is formed by the endothelium. The effect of dietary manipulation upon the relative production of PGI_2 versus thromboxanes requires study. Clearly, we are just beginning to understand how to manipulate prostaglandins by withholding or feeding suitable precursors. However, we are not fully cognizant of the dynamics of the metabolic fatty acid pathways involved and even less so of the dynamics of the subsequent prostaglandin metabolic pathways. Nevertheless, this type of approach to modifying platelet aggregation is valuable since it will help serve as a model in manipulating hormone secretion or action.

TISSUE SOURCES

The free arachidonate concentration in humans is low (3 μg/ml) and independent of the total FFA level.[6] The feeding of ethyl arachidonate to men for 2 to 3 weeks increased the percentage of arachidonate in the triglycerides, phospholipids, and cholesterol esters but not the plasma-free arachidonate.[1] In man at rest the fractional turnover rate of arachidonate is higher (50 percent) than that of oleate, but during exercise the arterial concentration and turnover rate of arachidonate did not change while the arterial concentration of oleate decreased 10 percent and the fractional turnover rate increased 90 percent. No significant net transport of arachidonate could be detected between muscle tissue, lungs, the kidney, and the liver.[7] Interestingly, the fractional turnover rate on a weight basis[8] was higher (40 percent) for women although the arterial concentrations of arachidonate were not significantly different. Probably little arachidonic acid is metabolized by β oxidation, chain elongation, or autoxidation. Incorporation into the phospholipid, triglyceride, and cholesterol esters occurs but the main catabolic route may be via peroxidation and endoperoxidation. Lipoxygenases, such as mammalian lipoxygenase, catalyze oxidation of polyunsaturated fatty acids. The hydroperoxides break down to other products, one of which—malonaldehyde—is also a breakdown product of the prostaglandin endoperoxide. Interestingly, nonenzymatic autoxidation of arachidonic acid can occur and produce endoperoxide products which transform into a number of possible prostaglandin-like isomers,[9] of which less than 1 percent are biologically active.

Free arachidonate is necessary for formation of the prostaglandins since neither methyl arachidonate nor 1-stearoly-2-arachidonly-lecithin serve as precursors.[10] Phospholipase A_2 is significant in this respect due to the high abundance of arachidonate in the 2 position of phospholipids. The treatment of isolated tissues with phospholipase A_2 results in a dramatic increase in prostaglandin production. Bull seminal vesicles form significant quantities of prostaglandins only after the addition of phospholipase A_2.[11] Human seminal plasma is rich in prostaglandins and the predominant acylhydrolase is phospholipase A_2.[12] Similarly, the phospholipases observed in chorioamnion and decidua, which contain arachidonate,[13,14] are thought to initiate parturition by the release of arachidonate which yields the oxytocic prostanoate compounds. Aggregating agents stimulate phospholipase A_2 in platelets.[15,16] TSH will stimulate phospholipase A_2 to effect prostaglandin formation in thyroid.[17] Other acylhydrolases may be involved in arachidonate release. Thus lipoprotein lipase has been suggested by Shemesh *et al.*[18] as the acylhydrolase that frees arachidonate from plasma lipoprotein for use by the bovine corpus luteum. Moreover, in rat kidney not only will phospholipases[19] liberate arachidonate for prostaglandin synthesis but so will triglyceride lipase,[20] since the triglycerides of rat kidney are unusual in containing high amounts of arachidonate.

PROSTAGLANDIN STRUCTURES

The archidonic acid metabolites called prostaglandins (PG) possess the prostanoic acid skeleton. The carbon numbering starts at the acid end. All naturally occurring prostaglandins have a *trans* double bond between C-13 and C-14. Further unsaturations occur between C-5 and C-6 and between C-17 and C-18 and are in the *cis* conformation. The degree of unsaturation is denoted by a numerical subscript after an indication of the class of prostaglandin. The classes vary in substitution on the five-membered ring. Thus the PGEs are β hydroxy ketones having a carbonyl function at C-9 and a hydroxyl group at C-11. The PGDs, in contrast to PGEs, have the ring substituents inverted—i.e., they now possess C-11 carbonyl and C-9 hydroxyl. The PGFs are more polar and have hydroxyls at both C-9 and C-11 positions. The α indicates the orientation of the C-9 hydroxyl group, which can also be β to yield compounds with different properties. The PGA class are dehydration products of the PGE series and have a carbonyl at C-9 and as a consequence of the dehydration have a double bond between C-10 and C-11. This double bond may rearrange between C-8 and C-12 to form the PGB class which is relatively inactive. Prostaglandin I_2 has, in addition to the five membered ring, another ring formed by linking the C-9 oxygen substituent to C-6. If other groups are present on the prostanoic skeleton these are referred to the carbon with which they are associated and to the identity of the group itself, 15-keto-PGF$_2\alpha$.

BIOSYNTHESIS

After Bergstrom *et al.*[21,22] isolated and elucidated the structure of PGF_1 and PGE_1, arachidonic acid was demonstrated[23,24] to be the precursor of the dienoic series of the prostaglandins. From $^{18}O_2$ studies,[25] and the isolation of both 12-hydroxy-8-cis, 10-cis-hepta-decadienoic acid (HHT) and malonaldehyde, the endoperoxide PGH_2 was postulated. The endoperoxide, PGG_2, and PGH_2 (Fig. 137-3) were eventually isolated and partially characterized[26] as highly unstable materials ($t_{1/2}$ in saline approximately 5 min). This work was performed on seminal vesicles.

In contrast, when arachidonate is incubated with platelets,[27] little prostaglandin E and F are formed. The three major products are HHT, HETE (12-hydroxy-5-*cis,* 8-*cis,* 10-*trans,* 14-*cis*-eicosatetraenoic acid) and TXB_2 (or thromboxane B_2, PHD) which is the hemiacetal derivative of 8-(1-hydroxy-3-oxopropyl)-9, 12L-dihydroxy-5-*cis,* 10-*trans*-heptadecadienoic acid. HETE is a leucotactic agent, and is formed not via the cyclooxygenase endoperoxide pathway at all but by a lipoxygenase,[28] a new arachidonic acid metabolic pathway resembling nonenzymatic peroxidation or autoxidation. This pathway may be important in that it is not blocked by aspirin but is blocked by the arachidonic acid analog—namely, 5,8,11,14,-eicosatetraynoic acid (Roche)—which was originally tested, interestingly enough, in treating acne.

Thromboxane B_2 was formed when PGG_2 or PGH_2 was incubated with platelets, and there were indications of another endoperoxide metabolite. The intermediate in this conversion of the endoperoxides was trapped, and a product that was substituted at the hemiacetal of thromboxane B_2 was obtained. From this and other data, thromboxane A_2 was postulated. It has a short half-life of approximately 30 sec in aqueous solutions.

Another product of endoperoxide metabolism has just been elucidated. Initially, 6-keto-PGF$_1\alpha$ was observed as an endoperoxide product of rat stomach fundus and of sensitized guinea pig lung challenged with antigen.[29] Subsequently, Vane et al[5] observed a potent anti-aggregatory substance produced from arachidonic acid by aortic microsomes which degraded to 6-keto-PGF$_1\alpha$. The active substance PGI_2 was rapidly characterized and its structure elucidated.[30] It may be the vasodilator product of arachidonate which has eluded characterization for years and is commonly observed when arachidonate is infused systematically. Whether still other endoperoxide metabolites exist may be a very important consideration.

METABOLISM

The lifetime in biologic systems of the prostaglandins E_2, $F_2\alpha$, D_2, and PGI_2 is short due to rapid metabolism. PGE_2 can undergo both enzymatic and nonenzymatic dehydration to PGA_2, which rearranges first to an intermediate PGC and finally to PGB. The biologic significance of this conversion is still a matter of debate. However, the first step in the major pathway of PGE and PGF metabolism is the conversion of the C-15 hydroxy by C-15-

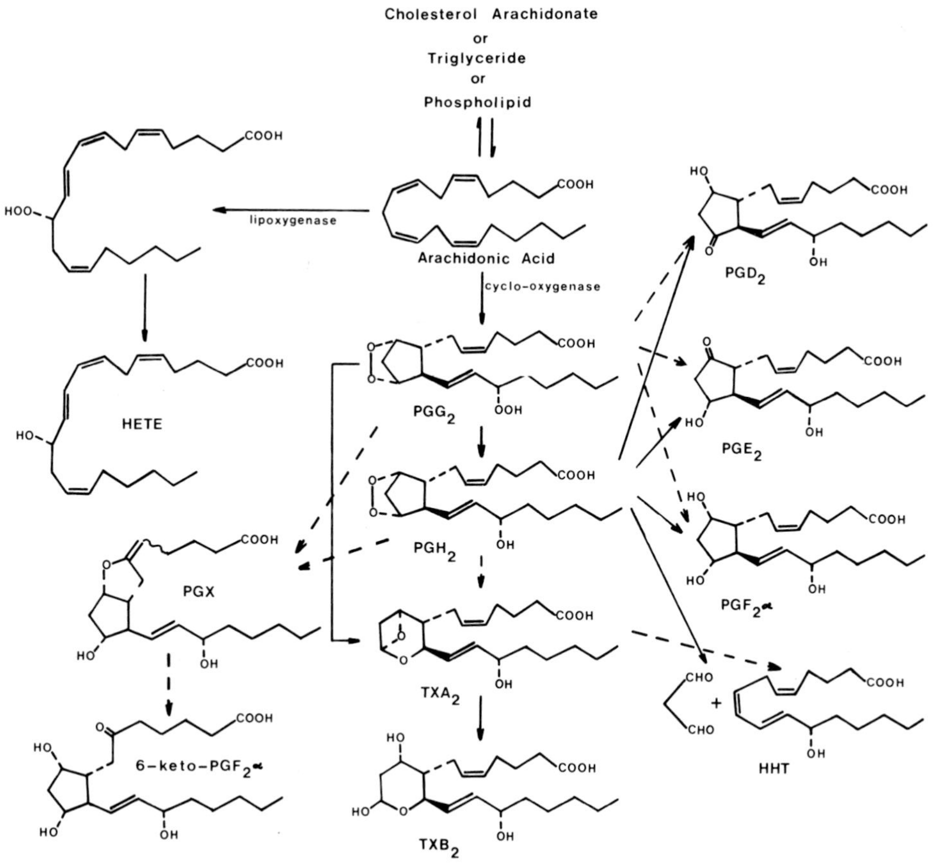

Fig. 137-3. The metabolism of arachidonic acid. Two pathways of arachidonic acid metabolism are shown: the lipoxygenase and the cyclooxygenase. Reactions that go through intermediates are shown with dashed arrows. The new prostaglandin PGX and its decomposition product are drawn.

hydroxyprostaglandin dehyrogenase (PGDH), which is present in all tissues and especially the placenta, to afford 15-keto-PGE_2 and 15-keto-$PGF_2\alpha$. This product, 15-keto-$PGF_2\alpha$, is not observed because of its rapid conversion by a Δ^{13} reductase to 13,14-dihydro-15-keto-$PGF_2\alpha$. The 15-keto-PGE_2 metabolite undergoes the same conversion. A further transformation of the 13,14-dihydro-15-keto derivatives is reduction of the 15-keto to yield 13,14-dihydro-PGE_2 and 13,14-dihydro-$PGF_2\alpha$, respectively, both of which have approximately the same biologic activity as their PGE_2 precursor in platelets[31] and as their $PGF_2\alpha$ precursor in the human uterus.[32] In general, the metabolites of the prostaglandins are less potent than their PGE_2 or PGF_2 precursor. In some species, PGE_2 can be converted to $PGF_{2\alpha}$ by a 9-ketoreductase which complicates attempts to monitor the production of PGE_2.

Thromboxane B_2, the metabolite of TXA_2 also undergoes metabolism somewhat like PGEs and PGFs to form 15-keto-TXB_2, 15-keto-13,14-dihydro-TXB_2, 2,3-dinorthromboxane-B_2 and 11-keto-TXB_2. All of these undergo further β and ω oxidation steps. PGI_2 metabolism has been complicated by its apparent stability upon passage through lungs. The nonenzymatic decomposition product is 6-keto-PGF_1 α which is formed when PGI_2 is extracted into organic solvents. How extensively this decomposition occurs biologically, has not been ascertained at the present. Prostacyclin can be a substrate for 15-PGDH to yield 6,15-diketo-$PGF_1\alpha$. Observed natural metabolites are 4,13-diketo-7,9-dihydroxy-dinorprostan-1,18-dioic acid and 4,13-diketo-7,9-dihydroxytetra-norprostan-1,16-dioic acid.

EXCRETION

The major urinary metabolites—PGE_2 (7α-hydroxy-5,11-diketotetranorprostane-1,16-dioic acid) and $PGF_2\alpha$ (5α,7α-dihydroxy-11-ketotetranorprostane-1,16-dioic acid)—are formed by β oxidation and ω oxidation steps. At present the best method of following 24-h prostaglandin production is to extract urine for these metabolites and to measure them by radio-immunoassay or by mass spectrometry. Numerous other products and intermediates have been postulated and elucidated by Samuelsson *et al.*[33] Thus any measurement of 24-h production should also include measurement of the product of thromboxane B_2 and PGI_2 once these are better characterized.

DRUG AND HORMONAL CONTROL OF THE ARACHIDONATE-PROSTAGLANDIN CASCADE

The precursors of the mono and trienoic prostaglandins—namely, homogamma linoleic and the eicosapentaenoic acids—are far less abundant in man than arachidonate. Therefore, our emphasis will be placed on the latter precursor. However one should not assume that the same metabolic sequence or similar biologic properties apply to the metabolites of all three precursors. For example, although all three precursors yield endoperoxides and prostaglandins, it is doubtful that PGG_1 yields a thromboxane A_1 and a PGI can not be produced from dinono-δ-linolenic acid.[34]

CONTROL OF ARACHIDONATE

There is evidence both from the sex difference in the turnover of plasma arachidonate measured by Hagenfeldt and from the estrogen-induced changes in plasma arachidonate observed by Lyman[35] that genodal steroids regulate arachidonate. Male animals are far more subject to the effect of arachidonate in inducing a hypoxic response to pulmonary platelet aggregation than females. This effect is promoted by androgen in females or castrates and is blocked by aspirin.[36] However the precise mechanisms of action of genodal steroids on arachidonate anabolism or catabolism is obscure since there are so many potential sites of action—including stimulation or inhibition of enzyme synthesis (see below).

As far as arachidonate is concerned, mepacrine and cloroquine inhibit release.[37] Furosemide (and possibly similar diuretics) cause an immediate increase in plasma arachidonate which results in renin release and prostaglandin production.[38] Earlier it was thought that furosemide exerted some of its diuretic effects or caused renin release by inhibiting the activity of the key metabolizing enzyme—namely, prostaglandin 15-dehydrogenase. Now it appears that in addition, furosemide increases prostaglandin synthesis. Whatever the mechanism, the fact remains that clinical doses of indomethacin reduce the effectiveness of furosemide as a diuretic. This situation probably applies in part to treatment with large doses of aspirin.

Gryglewski and co-workers[39] have suggested that the glucocorticoids may exert their antiinflammatory actions by preventing the acylhydrolases coming into contact with the phospholipid substrate—i.e., glucocorticoids may act by stabilizing lysosomal and cell membranes to prevent release of enzymes. Other workers, notably Piper[40] and Chang,[41] do not agree, and suggest that the steroids prevent prostaglandin release from cells. Both views are not incompatible. Tashjian[42] has explored the effects of hydrocortisone on mouse fibrosarcoma cells and concludes that the steroid inhibits prostaglandin formation. Also he finds that although the prostaglandin content of the cell is normal, the content in the tissue culture medium is reduced.

Inhibition of release of free arachidonate induced by serum has been demonstrated by Hong and Levine[43] with hydroxycorticosteroids and other steroid antiinflammatory drugs in transformed mouse fibroblasts that contain ^{14}C-arachidonic acid incorporated in the phospholipids. Indomethacin effected only a slight reduction in the release of radioactive material. Estradiol 17β and dehydroisoandrosterone produced no significant reduction of release. The potency of the steroid antiinflammatory drug appeared to determine the extent of inhibition.

CONTROL OF CYCLOOXYGENASE

The regulation of this enzyme is not clearly understood although the effects of cofactors such as catecholamines, glutathione, ascorbic acid, and metals have been described in modifying total synthesis and the direction of synthesis between the different prostaglandins. With the elucidation of the new prostaglandin pathways, some of the work needs to be repeated, and in consequence it will not be discussed further.

Estrogen both in vivo and in vitro increase prostaglandin synthesis in the uterus. The in vitro data with uterine microsomes suggests a direct effect on the enzyme rather than on an acyl hydrolase. Similar data with estrogen was obtained by Goldberg and Ramwell[44] in platelet membranes. In the presence of an excess of arachidonate, they showed in addition that androgen inhibits synthesis of PGE_2 or $PGF_2\alpha$. Synthesis of the enzyme itself is under hormonal control in the different target tissues of the genodal steroids.

The inhibitory role of the nonsteroidal antiinflammatory drug is well known by now. There are a variety of mechanisms for inhibiting the cyclooxygenase enzyme[45] ranging from substrate analogs such as acetylenic acids, oleic acid, reversible and nonreversible inhibitors to metal complexing agents.

A wide variety of antiinflammatory drugs—arylpyrazolones, arylacetic acids, arylamino benzoic acids, hydroxybenzoates, etc.[45–47]—have been tested. Aspirin, indomethacin, medofenamate, and ibuprofen are the most popular. Inhibition of the cyclooxygenase results in reduced prostaglandin synthesis, and in platelets a shift is observed of the arachidonate to the lipoxygenase path of the cascade which results in HETE formation.[26] The kinetics and cofactor requirements of this system and the effects of drugs have been extensively studied. Inhibition results vary from system to system, species to species, and from in vitro to in vivo.[48] Both aspirin and indomethacin are irreversible inhibitors, possibly modifying the enzyme by acylation. The important thing to bear in mind is that this enzyme complex undergoes very rapid turnover. A second point is that the spectrum of products formed varies with the enzyme source, concentration of substrate, and according to Nugteren[49] it varies with species, which may explain the variation in inhibition alluded to above.

CONTROL OF 9-KETOREDUCTASE

The interconversion of prostaglandins is of considerable interest. PGEs and PGDs are vasodilators and, in contrast to $PGF_2\alpha$, release renin. Weber *et al.*[38] have shown that salt loading increases the proportion of $PGF_2\alpha$ found and that it also stimulates 9-ketoreductase in both renal medulla and cortex. McGiff and his colleagues[50] have effectively coupled the kallikrein-kinin and prostaglandin systems by their studies on the effects of bradykinin and angiotensin on prostaglandin synthesis. Cyclic GMP and AMP, like $PGF_2\alpha$ and PGE_2, are known to be vasoconstrictor and vasodilator, respectively. McGiff *et al.* have shown that the venoconstrictor effects of bradykinin may be mediated by stimulating cycle GMP, which in turn stimulates the 9-ketoreductase to convert PGE_2 (and PGD_2, presumably) to $PGF_2\alpha$. Thus several elements of a control system are apparent.[51]

CONTROL OF 15-DEHYDROGENASE

This enzyme is widely distributed and is located in different forms in lung and placenta. In the lung it has a key role in markedly reducing pulmonary transit of the prostaglandins. The enzyme content appears to be increased by progesterone, for in pregnant animals the systemic response to intravenous prostaglandins, as opposed to intraarterial administration, is markedly attenuated.[52] In addition, Blackwell and Flower[53] have measured enzyme activity in pregnant and nonpregnant animals and confirm these observations. The enzyme has a short half-life and synthesis is easily prevented by cycloheximide, etc. At least one antifertility drug is thought to act by inhibiting PGDH so that endogenous $PGF_2\alpha$ builds up and promotes luteolysis.[54] Whether such a drug can promote luteolysis in women will be interesting since $PGF_2\alpha$ so far has been ineffective. This is in contrast to tests in subprimates where $PGF_2\alpha$ has been remarkably successful. Several products are now commerically available for cycling cattle and horses. The vaginal and oral use of $PGF_2\alpha$ in women at term to promote delivery has proved to be successful. Vaginal pessaries of $PGF_2\alpha$ have a significant role in delivery of the dead fetus in the third trimester when oxytocin is not very effective.

CONTROL OF THROMBOXANE SYNTHETASE

Thromboxane A_2 is produced from the prostaglandins endoperoxides in brain, lung, platelets, and umbilical vessels. However, thromboxane A_2 is not synthesised in kidney. It is a powerful vasoconstrictor and was originally termed "rabit aorta contracting substance" due to its high potency on spiral strips when compared with the prostaglandins or endoperoxides. Undoubtedly the generation of thromboxane A_2 by platelets will mean that great attention will be paid to this compound since it is also a coronary vasoconstrictor. Several drugs inhibit the enzyme—namely, benzydamine and imidazole.[55]

CONTROL OF PROSTACYCLIN SYNTHETASE

Gryglewski et al[56] have tested possible prostacyclin synthetase inhibitors. The most effective was 15-hydroperoxy arachidonic acid (15-HPAA, actually 5-cis,8-cis,11-cis,13-transeicosatetraenoic acid. Other long chain fatty acid hydroperoxide fatty acids also inhibit this synthetase.[57]

PROSTAGLANDINS AS LOCAL HUMORS

The prostaglandin system has great significance in medicine since it forms one of only a few families of compounds that possess many members exhibiting high biologic activity. They are simpler than the steroids or peptides but their spectrum of activity is wider. They may be evolutionary more primitive molecules than the peptides. Every cell type responds in a specific manner to prostaglandins of a particular class. For example, both PGE_1 and PGE_2 increase progesterone synthesis and cyclic AMP in corpea lutea. There are some exceptions to this rule, as in platelets where PGE_1 and PGE_2 both increase cyclic AMP but have opposite effects on platelet fragility.

In spite of the flexibility and freedom of rotation of parts of the molecule, there is a remarkable degree of stereo specificity in the biologic activity of the different isomers of the same prostaglandin. Thus $PGF_2\alpha$, which has five assymetric centers and two double bonds, has the potential for 2^7 or 128 potential stereoisomers.[56] $PGF_2\beta$ relaxes airways in contrast to $PGF_2\alpha$ which is a branchoconstrictor. Specific binding sites have been isolated for PGE_1, PGE_2, $PFG_1\alpha$, and $PGF_2\alpha$ from different tissues.

One of the significant problems in early discussions of the putative humoral role of prostaglandins was that they are probably not vital for life,[59] Tissue cultures completely deficient in essential fatty acids grow and metabolize satisfactorily. However, neither do the properties with respect to contact inhibition change.[60] There is evidence that labor is prostaglandin-mediated, and one can envisage the oxytocic prostaglandins as working locally. As Karim first showed, uterine venous prostaglandin levels are elevated in parturition. Prostaglandins probably have a local humoral role in blood vessels as we envisaged in 1966,[61] and more recently as proposed by Wong and McGiff.[50] They may regulate flow in the ductus arteriosus, which can be closed with aspirin and kept patent with PGE_1.[62] The nonprostanoate compound, thromboxane A_2, probably helps control bleeding from umbilical vessels since this structure is particularly rich in the potent vasoconstrictor. The role of prostaglandins in treating the infant exzema syndrome associated with essential fatty acid deficiency is becoming clear. In the rat model, Ziboh and Hsia[63] successfully used topical prostaglandins to alleviate the symptoms.

It is unlikely that the presence of arachidonic acid in the 2 position of phospholipids contributes significantly to cell function other than providing a rapidly mobilizing source of prostaglandin precursor. Recent studies by Russell and Deykin[64] indicate that the dynamics of arachidonic acid incorporation and transfer between specific phospholipids in platelet membranes prior to and following challenge is complex. Our original views are largely unchanged in that we regard prostaglandins as modulators or amplifiers and attentuators of hormone action. The fact that we could increase basal cyclic AMP levels in isolated fat cells by inhibiting prostaglandin synthesis[65] added weight to our belief that in fat tissue, prostaglandins served to promote homeostasis by acting as negative-feedback regulators of lipolysis.[66] An interesting situation exists in gastric mucosa where we[67] and Robert[68] describe in rat and dog, respectively, the inhibition of gastric secretion with PGE_1. By inhibiting prostaglandin synthesis we succeeded in showing that although the basal acid secretion was increased, the response to pentagastrin was of the same order as in the untreated animals. Moreover, the degree of inhibition by exogenous PGE_1 of this evoked response of acid was the same in both prostaglandin-deficient and normal animals. These studies indicate that the endogenous prostaglandins may regulate the functional "setting" of a tissue.

It may be useful to the clinical endocrinologist to conclude with a conjectural analysis of the effect of cyclooxygenase inhibitors in Bartter's syndrome. In Figures 137-4 and 137-5 and Table 137-1 are the data obtained by Norby *et al.*[69] in the successful treatment of a 22-month-old girl with 100 mg/kg aspirin. The data are essentially self-explanatory. This situation, as mentioned earlier, may be considered as an arachidonic acid syndrome since we know that arachidonic acid yields at least two products that promote renin release—namely, PGE_2 and PGD_2.[70] A variety of nonsteroidal antiinflammatory drugs have been found effective, and in consequence the probability is good that the reduction in renin is due to decreased conversion of arachidonate. The biochemic lesion may therefore be due to (1) increased release of arachidonate, (2) decreased metabolism by PGDH, or (3) decreased metabolism by 9-ketoreductase. The first possibility requires identification of the arachidonate precursor since it may not necessarily be phospholipid because arachidonate is abundant in renal triglyceride. If β agonists and cyclic AMP increase renin

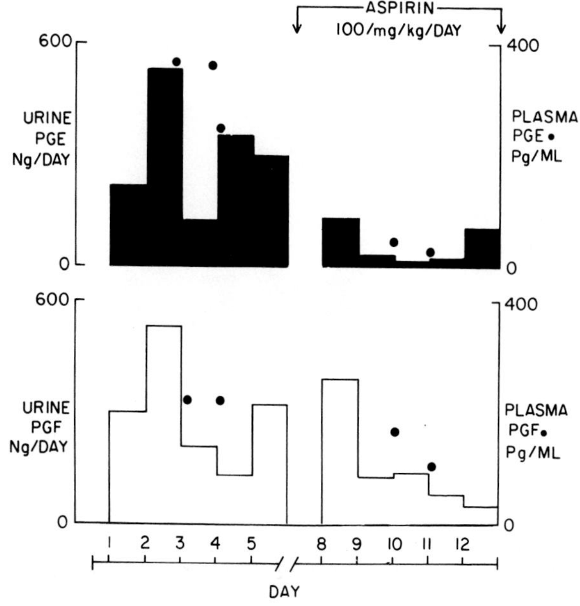

Fig. 137-4. Acute effect of aspirin on urine and plasma prostaglandins.

Table 137-1. Effect of Aspirin in Bartter's Syndrome

	Weight (kg)	Serum-Potassium (mmol/l)	Plasma-Renin Activity (ng/ml/m)	Urine-Aldosterone (μg/day)	Serum-Salicylate (mg/dl)	Urine-PGE (ng/day)	Urine-PGF (ng/day)	Plasma-PGE (pg/ml)	Plasma-PGF (pg/ml)
Control period Mean ± (SEM)	7.0 ± 0.2	2.9 ± 0.1	83 ± 13	14 ± 2	0	225 ± 56	252 ± 59	293 ± 69	218 ± 21
Aspirin-therapy period Mean ± (SEM)	8.0 ± 0.1	3.6 ± 0.1	20 ± 5	6 ± 2	15.8 ± 1.5	25 ± 4	99 ± 11	23 ± 5	110 ± 12
p	<0.1	<0.01	<0.01	<0.01	—	<0.01	>0.05	<0.01	<0.01

release, then it is possible that the cyclic AMP may activate the lipase to release arachidonate. The second possibility is of interest if progesterone treatment increases PGDH synthesis in humans. The third possibility is intriguing if $PGF_2\alpha$ inhibits renin release as described by Weber *et al.*[38] or if it is a significant pathway for reducing PGE_2 and PGD_2 levels. Behind all this conjecture lurks the likely role of the other prostanoate and nonprostanoate compounds and the effects on the system of the kinins as described earlier.[50]

CLINICAL CHEMISTRY

There is an increasing demand for analysis of blood and urine to indicate whether basal levels of the prostaglandins are elevated or whether treatment with cyclooxygenase inhibitors are successful. The question is what to analyze. Clearly it is desirable to be able to gain an idea of the total amount of arachidonate entering the cyclooxygenase pathway. For clinical studies it is possible to answer many questions by concentrating on estimating blood and urine metabolite levels. This approach markedly reduces the number of compounds. The position is still complex since the metabolites of the thromboxane and prostacyclin pathways are still being characterized.

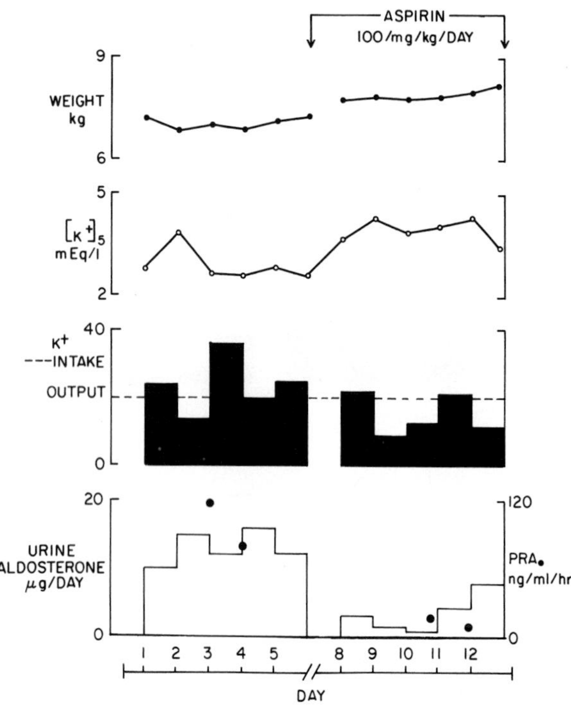

Fig. 137-5. Effect of aspirin on plasma-renin activity, aldosterone excretion, and potassium balance.

The most practical procedure at present is to measure $PGF_2\alpha$ in the urine by radio-immunoassay. The levels may not necessarily be accurate but will provide a rank order. The amounts observed largely reflect renal synthesis of prostaglandins, and if a cyclooxygenase inhibitor is given orally or systemically then the changes in production of renal prostaglandins will reflect changes in total body synthesis.

More ambitiously, it is desireable to be able to "profile" the prostanoate and nonprostanoate compounds in the venous drainage of a tumor or kidney. At present only two methods approach practicality—namely, radio-immunoassay and mass spectrometry.[71] For clinical studies, both methods require extraction and separation of the prostaglandins. Both procedures require a large number of specific antibodies for the prostanoate and nonprostanoate compounds and their ultimate metabolites or a similar number of deuterated reference compounds as internal standards for mass spectrometry.

Investigators can make a dramatic contribution by developing a less laborious method of profiling the innumerable compounds. One approach may be to make derivatives of the prostaglandins, thromboxanes, and their metabolites and to use the powerful discriminating properties of high-pressure liquid chromatography to thus obtain a profile of the arachidonate metabolites.

We have omitted many areas of prostaglandin involvement in endocrinology, neuroendocrinology, and sympathetic transmitter regulation. However, we hope that by concentrating on a few examples it has been possible to engender a sense of perspective and a strategy for research in what is at this time a bewilderingly complex mosaic.

ACKNOWLEDGMENTS

We are especially grateful for the assistance of Anthony Sintetos and for support from ONR, NIH, and the Washington Heart Association.

REFERENCES

1. Seyberth, H. W., Segre, G. V., Morgan, J. L., Sweetman, B. J., Potts, J. T., and Oates, J. A.: Prostaglandins as mediators of hypercalcemia associated with certain types of cancer. *N Eng J Med 293:* 1278, 1975.
2. Jaffe, B. M., and Santoro, M. G: Prostaglandins and cancer. In Ramwell, P. W. (ed): *Prostaglandins,* vol 3. New York, Plenum, 1977, p 329.
3. Holman, R. T.: Significance of essential fatty acids in human nutrition. In Paoletti, R., Porcellati, G., and Jacini, G.: *Lipids,* vol 1. New York, Raven, 1976, p 215.
4. O'Brien, J. R., Etherington, M. D., Jamieson, S., Vergroesen, A. J., and Ten Hoor F.: Effect of a diet of polyunsaturated fats on some platelet-function tests. *Lancet 2:* 995, 1976.

5. Moncada, S., Needleman, P., Bunting S., and Vane, J. R.: An enzyme isolated from arteries transforms prostaglandin endoperoxides to an unstable substance that inhibits platelet aggregation. *Nature 263:* 663, 1976.
6. Hagenfeldt, L.: The concentration of individual free fatty acids in human plasma and their interrelationships. *Ark Kemi 29:* 57, 1968.
7. Hagenfeldt, L., and Wahren, J.: Turnover of plasma-free arachidonic and oleic acids in resting and exercising human subjects. *Metabolism 24:* 799, 1975.
8. Hagenfeldt, L., Hagenfeldt, K., and Wennmalm, A.: Turnover of plasma free arachidonic and oleic acids in men and women. *Horm Metab Res 7:* 467, 1975.
9. Pryor, W. A., Stanley, J. P., and Blair, E.: Autoxidation of polyunsaturated fatty acids: II. A suggested mechanism for the formation of TBA-reactive materials from prostaglandin-like endoperoxides. *J Lipid Res 11:* 370, 1976.
10. Vonkeman, H., and Van Dorp, D. A.: The action of prostaglandin synthetase on 2-arachidonyl-lecithin. *Biochim Biophys Acta 164:* 430, 1968.
11. Kunze, H., and Vogt, W.: Significance of phospholipase A for prostaglandin formation. *Ann NY Acad Sci 180:* 123, 1972.
12. Kunze, H., Nahas, H., and Wurl, M.: Phospholipases in human seminal plasma. *Biochim Biophys Acta 348:* 35, 1974.
13. Grieves, S. A., and Liggins, G. C.: Phospholipase A activity in human and ovine uterine tissues. *Prostaglandins 12:* 229, 1976.
14. Schwarz, B. E., Schultz, F. M., MacDonald, P. C., and Johnston, J. M.: Initiation of human parturition: IV. Demonstration of phospholipase A_2 in the lysosomes of human fetal membranes. *Am J Obset Gynecol 125:* 1089, 1976.
15. Schoene, N. W., and Iacono, J. M.: Phospholipase A_2 activity in lysed human blood platelets. *Fed Proc 33:* 685, 1974.
16. Bills, T. K., Smith, J. B., and Silver, M. J.: Metabolism of ^{14}C-arachidonic acid in human platelets. *Biochim Biophys Acta 424:* 303, 1976.
17. Haye, B., Champion, S., and Jacquemin, C.: Stimulation by TSH of prostaglandin synthesis in pig thyroid. In Samuelsson, B., Paoletti, R. (eds): *Advances Prostaglandin and Thromboxane Research,* vol 1. New York, Raven, 1976, p 29.
18. Shemesh, M., Bensadoun, A., and Hansel, W.: Lipoprotein lipase activity in the bovine corpus luteum during the estrous cycle and early pregnancy. *Proc Soc Exp Biol Med 151:* 667, 1976.
19. Kalisker, A., and Dyer, D. C.: *In vitro* release of prostaglandins from the renal medulla. *Eur J Pharm 19:* 305, 1972.
20. Danon, A., Chang, L. C. T., Sweetman, B. J., Nies, A. S., and Oates, J. A.: Synthesis of prostaglandins by the rat renal papilla *in vitro. Biochim Biophys Acta 388:* 71, 1975.
21. Bergstrom, S., and Sjovall, J.: The isolation of prostaglandin E from sheep prostate glands. *Acta Chem Scand 14:* 1701, 1960.
22. Bergstrom, S., and Sjovall, J.: The isolation of prostaglandin E from sheep prostate glands. *Acta Chem Scand 14:* 1693, 1960.
23. Van Dorp, D. A., Beerthuis, R. K., Nugteren, D. H., and Vonkeman, H.: The biosynthesis of prostaglandins. *Biochim Biophys Acta 90:* 204, 1964.
24. Bergstrom, S., Danielsson, H., and Samuelsson, B.: The enzymatic formation of prostaglandin E_2 from arachidonic acids. *Biochim Biophys Acta 90:* 207, 1964.
25. Samuelsson, B.: On the incorporation of oxygen in the conversion of 8,11,14 eicosatrienoic acid to prostaglandin E_1. *J Am Chem Soc 87:* 3011, 1965.
26. Hamberg, M., Svensson, J., Wakabayashi, T., and Samuelsson, B.: Isolation and structure of two prostaglandin endoperoxides that cause platelet aggregation. *Proc Natl Acad Sci USA 71:* 345, 1974.
27. Hamberg, M., and Samuelsson, B.: Prostaglandin endoperoxides. Novel transformations of arachidonic acid in human platelets. *Proc Natl Acad Sci USA 71:* 3400, 1974.
28. Nugteren, D. H.: Arachidonate lipoxygenase in blood platelets. *Biochim Biophys Acta 380:* 299, 1975.
29. Dawson, W., Boot, J. R., Cockerill, A. F., Mallen, D. N. B., and Osborne, D. J.: Release of novel prostaglandins and thromboxanes after immunological challenge of guinea pig lung. *Nature 262:* 699, 1976.
30. Johnson, R. A., Morton, D. J., Kinner, J. H., Gorman, R. R., Mcguire, J. C., Sun, F. F., et al: The chemical structure of prostaglandin X (prostacyclin). *Prostaglandins 12:* 915, 1976.
31. Westwick, J.: The effect of pulmonary metabolites of prostaglandins E_1, E_2 and $F_2\alpha$ on ADP-induced aggregation of human and rabbit platelets. *Br J Pharmacol 58:* 297P, 1976.
32. Bydeman, M., Green, K., Toppozada, M., Wiqvist, N., and Bergstrom, S.: The influence of prostaglandin metabolites on the uterine response to $PGF_2\alpha$. A clinical and pharmacokinetic study. *Life Sci 14:* 521, 1974.
33. Samuelsson, B., Granstrom, E., Green, K., Hamberg, M., and Hammarstrom, S.: Prostaglandins. *Ann Rev Biochem 44:* 669, 1975.
34. Needleman, P., Minkes, M., and Raz, A.: Thromboxanes: Selective biosynthesis and distinct biological properties. *Science 193:* 163, 1976.
35. Lyman, R. L.: Endocrine influences on the metabolism of polyunsaturated fatty acids. *Prog Chem Fats Other Lipids 9:* 195, 1968.
36. Uzunova, A. D., Ramey, E. R., and Ramwell, P. W.: Arachidonate-induced thrombosis in mice: effects of gender or testosterone and estradiol administration. *Prostaglandins 13:* 995, 1977.
37. Gryglewski, R. J.: Prostaglandins and prostaglandin synthesis inhibitors in etiology and treatment of inflammation. VI *Int Cong Pharmacol,* 1975, pp 151–160.
38. Weber, P. C., Larsson, C., and Scherer, B.: PGE-9-ketoreductase as a mediator of salt-intake related prostaglandin-renin interaction. *Nature 266:* 65, 1977.
39. Gryglewski, R. J., Panczenko, B., Korbut, R., Grodzinska, L., and Ocetkiewicz, A.: Corticosteroids inhibit prostaglandin release from perfused mescenteric blood vessels of rabbit and from perfused lungs of sensitized guinea pig. *Prostaglandins 10:* 343, 1975.
40. Lewis, G. P., and Piper, P. J.: Inhibition of release of prostaglandins as an explanation of some of the actions of anti-inflammatory corticosteroids. *Nature 254:* 308, 1975.
41. Chang, J., Lewis, G. P., and Piper, P. J.: The effects of anti-inflammatory steroids on levels of prostaglandins in adipose tissue *in vitro. J Pharmacol 56:* 342P, 1976.
42. Tashjian, A. H., Jr, Voelkel, E. F., McDonough, J., and Levine, L.: Hydrocortisone inhibits prostaglandin production by mouse fibrosarcoma cells. *Nature 258:* 739, 1975.
43. Hong, S. L., and Levine, L.: Inhibition of arachidonic acid release from cells as the biochemical action of anti-inflammatory corticosteroids. *Proc Natl Acad Sci USA 73:* 1730, 1976.
44. Goldberg, V., and Ramwell, P. W.: Effects of steroids on $PGE_2\alpha$ and $PGF_2\alpha$ synthesis in rat platelets. *Br J Pharmacol* (submitted).
45. Lands, W. E. M., and Rome, L. H.: Inhibition of prostaglandin biosynthesis. In Karim, S. (ed): *Prostaglandins: Chemical and Biochemical Aspects,* vol 1. Baltimore, University Park Press, 1976, p 87.
46. Shen, T. Y., Ham, E. A., Cirillo, V. J., and Zanetti, M.: Structure activity relationship of certain prostaglandin synthetase inhibitors. In Robinson, J. H., Vane, J. R. (eds): *Prostaglandins Synthetase Inhibitors.* New York, Raven, 1974, p 19.
47. Gryglewski, R. J.: Structure-activity relationships of some prostaglandin synthetase inhibitors. In Robinson, J. H., Van, J. R. (eds): *Prostaglandin Synthetase Inhibitors.* New York, Raven, 1974, p 35.
48. Flower, R. J., and Vane, J. R.: Some pharmacologic and biochemical aspects of prostaglandin biosynthesis and its inhibition. In Robinson, H. J., Vane, J. R. (eds): *Prostaglandin Synthetase Inhibitors.* New York, Raven, 1974, p 9.
49. Nugteren, D. H.: Arachidonate lipoxygenase. In Silver, J., Smith, J. B., Cosis, J. J. (eds): *Prostaglandins in Hematology.* Cochecton Center, New York, Spectrum, 1977, p 11.
50. Wong, P. Y-K., and McGiff, J. C.: Enzymatic regulation of prostaglandin levels in blood vessels: Relationship to cyclic GMP. *Fed Proc* (in press).
51. Flamenbaum, W., and Kleinman, J. G.: Prostaglandins and renal function or "a trip down the rabbit hole." In Ramwell, P. W. (ed): *Prostaglandins,* vol 3. New York, Plenum, 1977, p 267.
52. Bedwani, J. R., and Marley, P. B.: Increased inactivation of prostaglandin E_2 by the rabbit lung during pregnancy. *Br J Pharmacol 50:* 459, 1974.
53. Blackwell, G. J., and Flower, R. J.: Effects of steroid hormones on tissue levels of prostaglandin 15-hydroxydehydrogenase in the rat. *Br J Pharmacol* 343P, 1975.
54. Carminati, P., Luzzani, F., Soffientini, A., and Lerner, L. J.: Effect of pregnancy terminating compounds on prostaglandin metabolism in the rat. V. *International Congress of Endocrinology,* abstracts, p. 165, 1976.
55. Needleman, P., Moncada, S., Raz, A., Ferrendelli, J. A., and Minkes, M.: Application of immidazone as a selective thromboxane synthetase inhibitor in human platelets. *Proc Natl Acad Sci USA* (in press).
56. Gryglewski, R. J., Bunting, S., Moncada, S., Flower, R. J. , and Vane, J. R.: Arterial walls are protected against deposition of platelet

thrombi by a substance (prostaglandin X) which they make from prostaglandin endoperoxides. *Prostaglandins 12:* 685, 1976.
57. Leovey, E. M. K.: 1977 winter prostaglandin conference. *Prostaglandins 14:* 181, 1977.
58. Andersen, N. H., and Ramwell, P. W.: Biological aspects of prostaglandins. *Arch Int Med 133:* 30, 1974.
59. Ramwell, P. W., and Shaw, J. E.: Biological significance of the prostaglandins. *Recent Prog Horm Res 26:* 139, 1970.
60. Bailey, J. M., and Dunbar, L. M.: Essential fatty acid requirements of cells in tissue culture: A review. *Exp Mol Pathol 18:* 142, 1973.
61. Ramwell, P. W., Shaw, J. E., and Jessup, R.: Spontaneous and evoked release of prostaglandins from frog spinal cord. *Am J Physiol 211:* 998, 1966.
62. Coeani, F., Olley, P. M., and Bodach, E.: Prostaglandins: A possible regulator of muscle tone in the ductus arteriosus. In Samuelsson, B., Paoletti, R. (eds): *Advances in Prostaglandin and Thromboxane* Research, vol 1. New York, Raven, 1976, p 417.
63. Ziboh, V. A., and Hsia, S. L.: Effects of prostaglandin E_2 on rat skin: Inhibition of sterol ester biosynthesis and clearing of scaly lesions in essential fatty acid deficiency. *J Lipid Res 13:* 458, 1972.
64. Russell, F. A., Deykin, D.: The effect of thrombin on the uptake and transformation of arachidonic acid by human platelets. *Am J Hematol 1:* 59, 1976.
65. Shaw, J. E., Jessup, S. J., and Ramwell, P. W.: Prostaglandin-adenyl cyclase relationships. In Greengard, P., Robison, G. A., Paoletti, R. (eds): *Advances in Cyclic-Nucleotide Research,* vol 1. New York, Raven, 1972, p 479.
66. Shaw, J. E., and Ramwell, P. W.: Release of prostaglandin from rat epididymal fat pad on nervous and hormonal stimulation. *J Biol Chem 243:* 1498, 1968.
67. Shaw, J. E., and Ramwell, P. W.: Inhibition of gastric secretion in rats by prostaglandin E_1. In Ramwell, P. W., Shaw, J. E. (eds): *Prostaglandin Symposium of the Worcester Foundation for Experimental Biology.* New York, Interscience, 1958, p 47.
68. Robert, A.: Antisecretory property of prostaglandins. In Ramwell, P. W., Shaw, J. E. (eds): *Prostaglandin Symposium of the Worcester Foundation for Experimental Biology.* New York, Interscience, 1958, p 47.
69. Norby, L., Lentz, R., Flamenbaum, W. and Ramwell, P.: Prostaglandins and aspirin therapy in Barter's syndrome. *Lancet 2*(7986): 604, 1976.
70. Bolger, P. M., Shea, P. T., Ramwell, P. W., Eisner, G., and Slotkoff, L. M.: Renal effects of prostaglandin D_2 (PGD_2). *Fed Proc* (submitted).
71. Salmon, J. A., and Kraim, S. M. M.: Methods for analysis of prostaglandins. In Karim, S. M. M. (ed): *Prostaglandins: Chemical and Biochemical Aspects.* Baltimore, University Park Press, 1976.

138

The Carcinoid Syndrome

D. G. Grahame-Smith

The term karzenoide (carcinoid) was first used by Oberndorfer[1] to describe a group of intestinal tumors which grew more slowly and ran a more benign course than more common intestinal adenocarcinomas. It was shown[2] that these tumors probably derived from the Kultschitzky cells of the intestinal mucosa; and because these cells and many of the tumors stained with silver stains, the tumors came to be called argentaffinomas. Between 1952 and 1954 it was realized that carcinoid tumors were associated sometimes with a recognizable syndrome of clinical symptoms and signs.[3–6] Because of this distinct clinical picture, it is possible to spot case reports fitting the carcinoid syndrome in the literature prior to 1952.[7–9] Although the syndrome has been variously called carcinoidosis or argentaffinosis, the term carcinoid syndrome has now come into general use. In addition it is now recognized that the syndrome may occur occasionally in association with tumors that are not argentaffinomas or even strictly carcinoid in type.

5-Hydroxytryptamine (5-HT) was first found in a carcinoid tumor by Lembeck,[10] and for several years the flushing, diarrhea, valvular lesions, and bronchoconstriction found in the carcinoid syndrome were thought to be due to the secretion of this substance by the tumor. This is probably not true, and matters have now become much more complicated with the realization that tumors associated with the carcinoid syndrome may produce kallikrein which leads to the production of bradykinin, sometimes histamine, and perhaps prostaglandins. In fact the endocrine potential of the gastrointestinal tract and the demonstration of the secretion of polypeptides such as motilin and vasoactive intestinal peptide (VIP) promises to make matters even more complicated.[11] This humoral complexity is matched by the recognition of the variability of the presentation of the syndrome; and although flushing, diarrhea, and valvular lesions of the heart form the cardinal manifestations of the syndrome, the differing quality and incidence of these symptoms led Sjoerdsma and Melmon[12] to speak of "the carcinoid spectrum."

To make any sense of the pathogenesis of the manifestations of the carcinoid syndrome it is necessary to try and link together our understanding of the cell of origin, its pathologic setting in the tumor, the secretory potentiality of the tumor, the biochemistry and pharmacology of the substances released, and the way that they produce the clinical manifestations. Understanding of these matters helps one to approach therapy in a rational way. A comprehensive review of the carcinoid syndrome has been published recently.[13]

CELL OF ORIGIN

In recent years[11] it has been demonstrated that the mammalian gastrointestinal tract and pancreas contain at least 13 ultrastructurally and cytochemically distinguishable endocrine cells. These have been called the APUD cell series (amine content and/or amine precursor uptake and decarboxylation). It is thought that many of these cells derive from the neuroectoderm of the neural crest. The enterochromaffin cell from which carcinoid tumors derive is one of the cell series. These cells may be recognized by their ultrastructural characteristics and by their cytochemic and histochemic properties. Williams and Sandler[14] and Pariente *et al.*[15] have attempted to correlate the embryologic derivation of tumors producing the carcinoid syndrome with their histochemic properties of functional activity (Table 138-1). This classification

Table 138-1. Characteristics of Carcinoid Tumors Derived from Different Divisions of the Embryonic Gut

	Fore-gut	Mid-gut	Hind-gut
Histologic structure	Tendency to be trabecular; may differ widely from classical pattern	Characteristic	Tendency to be trabecular
Argentaffin and diazo reactions	Usually negative	Positive	Often negative
Association with the carcinoid syndrome	Frequent	Frequent	None
Tumor 5-HT content	Low	High	Not detected
Urinary 5-HIAA	High	High	Normal
5-HTP secretion	Frequent	Rare	Not detected
Metastases to bone (usually osteoblastic) and skin	Common	Unusual	Common
Association with other endocrine secretion	Frequent	Not described	Not described

From Williams and Sandler: *Lancet 1:* 238, 1963; and Pariente *et al.*: *Presse Med. 75:* 221, 1967, with permission.

takes as its reference point the ileal tumor which derives from the mid-gut since this is most common and fairly predictable in its behavior. The tumors classified as arising from the embryonic fore-gut include bronchial, pancreatic, and gastric tumors. Mid-gut tumors usually arise in the ileum. Hind-gut tumors arise in the rectum and colon.

This classification is useful in indicating that carcinoid tumors are neither structurally nor functionally homogeneous. The different histochemic reactions probably reflect important differences in cell function, and although the enterochromaffin cell system has a common parent cell, the cells in different sites differentiate structurally and functionally. But by consideration of the embryonic derivation of the cell of origin the structure and function of the tumors can be partly systematized.

Apart from the bronchial, pancreatic, biliary tract, and gastrointestinal tumors, the carcinoid syndrome may also be associated with ovarian tumors.[16,17] Such ovarian tumors are usually teratomas containing argentaffin cell tissue.

Moertel *et al.*[18] and Cohen *et al.*[19] report cases of the carcinoid syndrome associated with medullary carcinomas of the thyroid. Medullary thyroid carcinomas arise from the parafollicular cell system of the thyroid,[20] and this cell system contains 5-hydroxytryptamine. Medullary thyroid carcinomas may secrete not only 5-hydroxytryptamine but also calcitonin and prostaglandins.[21]

Carcinoid tumors have also been described as arising from the cervix uterae[22] and the testis.[23–25]

GENERAL PATHOLOGY

Although there is an extensive literature describing the overall pathology of gastrointestinal carcinoid tumors, there does not appear to be any pathologic feature—except that of definite malignancy and metastatic spread—that distinguishes carcinoid tumors not causing the syndrome from those that do. McDonald[26] reviewed 418,116 surgical specimens and 16,401 autopsies; 356 gastrointestinal carcinoid tumors were found, but only in 4 cases was this associated with the syndrome. Moertel and his colleagues[27] found 14 cases of the syndrome amongst 209 cases of small intestinal carcinoid tumors. Sanders and Axtell[28] found 77 cases of the syndrome in 2502 reports of gastrointestinal carcinoid tumors. These series represent an incidence of 1 to 7 cases of the syndrome for every 100 cases of gastrointestinal carcinoids.

Sanders[29] reviewed 3633 cases of reported gastrointestinal carcinoid; in Table 138-2 is shown the incidence of gastrointestinal carcinoids at various sites of the gastrointestinal tract and their association with the syndrome. It can be seen that the most common site for tumors associated with the syndrome is the small bowel, usually the ileum, but that the most common site for carcinoid tumors is the appendix, though these are rarely associated with the carcinoid syndrome.

Moertel *et al.*[30] found that the carcinoid tumor was the commonest tumor of the ileum, with the lower ileum being the area most frequently involved.

The primary tumor is often less than 1.5 cm in diameter and not often larger than 3.5 cm. Carcinoid tumors of the ileum are frequently multiple. The primary lesion is firm and its cut surface is yellowish. It invades first the submucosal layers into the mucosal layer and then involves the peritoneum and mesentery. There is often considerable fibrotic reaction around the tumor. It is very likely that the tumor produces a substance that stimulates fibroblastic growth, and frequently if intestinal obstruction occurs it is found to be due to the stenosis caused by the fibrotic reaction. The tumor frequently spreads to mesenteric lymph nodes, and their mass may predispose to volvulus. Infarction of segments of the small intestine may occur[31] and may be due either to obstruction of mesenteric vessels by the mass of metastatic lymph nodes, fibrotic reaction, or to an elastic vascular sclerosis of mesenteric blood vessels.[32]

With gastrointestinal tumors it appears that hepatic metastases are almost essential for the appearance of the syndrome. There are two possible reasons for this. First, when the tumor products drain into the portal venous system the liver probably effectively metabolizes and therefore inactivates them. Hepatic metastases, however, drain their products into the systemic circulation via the hepatic veins, thus avoiding hepatic inactivation. Secondly, there may be an effect of sheer tumor mass in that gastrointestinal tumors are usually small and the amount of humoral material they

Table 138-2. Incidence of G.I. Carcinoids and Association with Syndrome

	No. Patients	Syndrome
Esophagus	1	0
Stomach	98	7
Duodenum	80	1
Small bowel	992	39
Meckel's diverticulum	46	6
Appendiceal	1609	2
Cecum and ascending colon	59	3
Left colon	35	0
Rectum	706	0
Gallbladder	7	0

From Sanders, R. J.: *Carcinoids of the Gastrointestinal Tract.* Springfield, Ill., Thomas, 1973.

secrete is likely to be much less than that secreted by a large mass of tumor so often found in the liver. Hepatic metastases may be multiple and fairly small or they may be few and massive. The latter may be amenable to hepatic surgery. Large hepatic metastases frequently undergo necrosis producing clinical symptoms. In Table 138-3 is shown the distribution of metastases from gastrointestinal carcinoid tumors.[33] Sandler[34] has pointed out that carcinoids arising from fore-gut and hind-gut embryonic structures more commonly give rise to bony metastases than those arising from mid-gut derivatives.

HISTOLOGIC APPEARANCE

If ileal tumors are taken as most typical, then the tumor is composed of small polygonal or round cells having basophilic nuclei. The cells occur in clusters, cords, or in an alveolar pattern.[35] The structural appearance is usually sufficient to recognize a carcinoid tumor but several histochemic reactions are available for complete recognition.[29,35]

APPENDICEAL CARCINOID TUMORS

Although malignant appendiceal carcinoids can produce the carcinoid syndrome, the association is rare.[36] The low incidence of metastases from appendiceal carcinoids and their infrequent association with the carcinoid syndrome may be due to the fact that because of obstructive appendicitis leading to removal of the tumor, metastatic spread and the carcinoid syndrome are avoided.

GASTRIC CARCINOID TUMORS

Christodoulopoulos and Klotz[37] reviewed 79 cases of gastric carcinoid tumors and found 5 cases of the carcinoid syndrome. By the time the syndrome presents in association with gastric carcinoid tumors, metastases to the liver are invariably present. Epigastric pain, anorexia, weight loss, and gastrointestinal bleeding may be present as symptoms of the primary tumor itself. The tumors are often multiple. Gastric carcinoids frequently show unusual histochemic reactions, and are clinically associated with "geographical" flushing and paroxysmal headache. The tumors often produce histamine, and 5-hydroxytryptophan and 5-hydroxytryptamine are often found in the urine in addition to 5-hydroxyindoleacetic acid.

BRONCHIAL CARCINOIDS

The pathology of this type of tumor is rather complex.[13] The main point is that the bronchial carcinoid tumor should be distinguished from bronchial neoplasms of the salivary gland type—so-called adenoid cystic carcinomas (cylindromas) and muco-epidermoid tumors.

Table 138-3. Distribution of Metastases from Gastrointestinal Carcinoid Tumors

Organ	No. Cases	Organ	No. Cases
Lymphatics	180	Omentum	6
Liver	137	Brain	6
Mesentery	99	Spleen	5
Peritoneum	52	Adrenal	4
Bone	11	Mediastinum	3
Lungs	10	Kidney	2
Pancreas	10	Thyroid	2
Ovary	9	Testis	1
Skin	7	Gallbladder	1

From Davies, A. J.: *Ann. R. Coll. Surg. Engl. 25:* 277, 1959, with permission.

By the time these tumors produce the carcinoid syndrome, distant metastases are usually present, though this is not invariably the case.[38]

Bronchial carcinoids usually arise from the mucosa of major segmental bronchi, lobar, or main bronchi. The morphologic pattern is more variable than that of the gastrointestinal carcinoids. Recent studies by Bensch and his colleagues[39–41] have led to the proposal that bronchial carcinoid tumors spring from enterochromaffin cells lying in the bronchial mucosa. There are certain similarities between the ultrastructural appearances of bronchial carcinoids and oatcell carcinomas of the bronchus; and the proposal has been put forward that bronchial carcinoids and oatcell carcinomas are, on the one hand, rather benign, and on the other, anaplastic highly malignant forms of the same tumor type. Bronchial carcinoids are associated with the carcinoid syndrome, and oatcell carcinomas of the bronchus may also cause the carcinoid syndrome.[13]

BIOCHEMISTRY

5-HYDROXYTRYPTAMINE

Following Lembeck's[10] demonstration of 5-hydroxytryptamine (5-HT) in a carcinoid tumor it was shown that whole-blood 5-HT concentrations were raised in the carcinoid syndrome[42] and that there was an increase in urinary excretion of 5-hydroxyindoleacetic acid (5-HIAA).[43] Increased synthesis and metabolism of 5-HT remains the most important diagnostic biochemic feature of the carcinoid syndrome.

5-HT is synthesized in the carcinoid tumor by two enzymatic steps. First, tryptophan is 5-hydroxylated to form 5-hydroxytryptophan (5-HTP),[44,45] and then this is decarboxylated to form 5-HT by aromatic L-amino acid decarboxylase (Fig. 138-1).[46] In tumors arising from the bronchus, pancreas, and gastric mucosa there may be a relative lack of 5-HTP decarboxylase or some fault in the biochemic organization of the cell whereby the tumor fails to decarboxylate all the 5-HTP formed. The tumor then contains and releases 5-HTP and 5-HT and the urine then contains 5-HTP, 5-HT, and 5-HIAA. This can be an important diagnostic point in picking up a carcinoid tumor arising from an embryonic fore-gut derivative or an atypical tumor. Most carcinoid tumors, however—particularly ileal tumors—synthesize 5-HT completely. The tumors and their metastases contain large amounts of 5-HT.[47]

There appears to be no fixed relationship between the concentration of 5-HT in the tumor and the degree of increase in urinary 5-HIAA. The importance of 5-HT in producing the symptoms of the carcinoid syndrome is still uncertain, but 5-HT is undoubtedly released from the tumor because blood 5-HT levels are usually raised. This rise in blood 5-HT levels is mainly due to a rise in the amount of 5-HT bound to blood platelets and not to a great rise in free-plasma 5-HT levels.

It does not appear that in the majority of patients 5-HT is paroxysmally released during flushing.[48] 5-HT released from hepatic metastases into the hepatic veins will be largely taken up by the lung,[49] and the ability of the lung to take up 5-HT varies.[50] This presumably may alter the amount of 5-HT entering the systemic circulation, and thus the rate of release of 5-HT from the tumor, the extent of its tissue inactivation, and platelet binding may go some way to explain the variability of the involvement of 5-HT in the production of symptoms. The 5-HT released is oxidatively deaminated to 5-HIAA, which is excreted in the urine. 5-HIAA

Tryptophan

Tryptophan 5-hydroxylase

5HTP

5HTP Decarboxylase

5HT

Monoamine oxidase

5HI-acetaldehyde

Aldehyde dehydrogenase

5HIAA

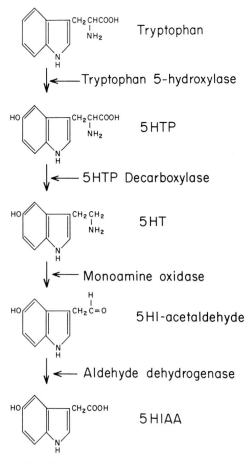

Fig. 138-1. Synthesis of metabolism of 5-HT.

may also be produced within the tumor. Urinary 5-HIAA reflects, therefore, not only circulating 5-HT oxidatively deaminated outside the tumor but also 5-HIAA produced in and released from the tumor. A minor route of 5-HT metabolism is its conversion to 5-hydroxytryptophol.[51] Conversion through this route is increased by ethanol ingestion, but the clinical significance of this is not known.

Normal urinary 5-HIAA excretion is unusual in the carcinoid syndrome but it can occur.[34] Urinary 5-HIAA excretion is raised but the degree of rise is variable from patient to patient and the amount excreted varies from time to time within the patient. Dreux *et al.*[52] found that blood 5-HT levels may be a more sensitive index to the presence of a secreting carcinoid tumor. The estimation of blood 5-HT levels is not easy, and at the moment urinary 5-HIAA estimations are generally available in most clinical laboratories.

BRADYKININ

The studies of Robertson *et al.*,[48] Levine and Sjoerdsma,[53] and Oates *et al.*[54] left little doubt that 5-HT was not the sole cause of carcinoid flushing. Oates and his colleagues found that carcinoid tumors contained the enzyme kallikrein and that blood bradykinin levels increased during a flush. Melmon *et al.*[55] showed that carcinoid kallikrein when incubated with purified human kininogen produced lysyl-bradykinin, which would be converted in the circulation to bradykinin (Fig. 138-2). In some patients who flush it would appear that kallikrein is released paroxysmally from the tumor into the circulation where it acts to convert kininogen to

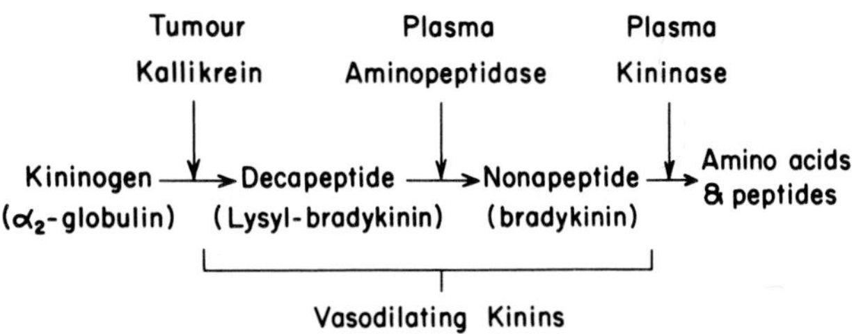

Fig. 138-2. Synthesis and metabolism of bradykinin.

lysyl-bradykinin, which is then converted to bradykinin. These polypeptides produce vasodilatation. Bradykinin is inactivated by uptake into tissues by plasma aminopeptidases.

There are several points, however, that suggest that other tumor products may be released to cause flushing. Not all patients have increases in plasma bradykinin during a flush.[56,57] Intravenous bradykinin, in most carcinoid patients, does not produce precisely the quality of the spontaneous flush.[13]

Histamine, particularly in those patients with gastric carcinoid tumors, gives rise to very vivid red and patchy flushing (geographical). Several investigators[13] have found increased histamine and histamine metabolite urinary excretion, particularly in patients with gastric carcinoid tumors. Histamine is produced by the decarboxylation of histidine. Normal gastric mucosa contains histidine decarboxylase, and this may be the reason why gastric carcinoids are particularly prone to increased histamine production.

Although a role for prostaglandins in the carcinoid syndrome has been invoked,[21] the evidence for this at the moment is minimal.[58] The other polypeptides known to be present in the gut which need investigation in regard to their role in the carcinoid syndrome are motilin, vasoactive intestinal peptide, and substance P.

CLINICAL PRESENTATION

The chief symptoms and signs of the carcinoid syndrome are shown in Table 138-4. Flushing appears to be the most common symptom, with diarrhea next. Cardiac valvular lesions are common, but wheezing is generally rarer than indicated by Thorsen.[59] The different combinations and variable quality of these major features and their association with less common symptoms com-

Table 138-4. Clinical Manifestations of the Carcinoid Syndrome

Total number of cases*		79
Male	48	
Female	29	
Age at presentation		
Male		18–80
Female		33–80
Flushing		74
Diarrhea		68
Asthma		18
Edema		52
Heart lesions		41
Pellagra-like skin lesions		5
Peptic ulcers		5
Arthralgia		6

From Thorson, A.: *Acta Med. Scand. 334:* Suppl. 7, 1958, with permission.
*Sex of the patient is not given.

prise the carcinoid spectrum. Differences from one patient to another in the quality of the syndrome probably reflect the capacity of the tumor to produce different quantities and types of hormones and the variation of the patient's response to them.

OCCURRENCE

Linnell and Mänsson[60] estimated that "at a rough guess it [the carcinoid syndrome] might occur once or twice every ten years in the population of Malmö [230,000 inhabitants]." There appears to be no sex difference in the incidence, and the age range varies widely—in my own patients from 18 to 76 yr. The age of presentation, however, is little guide to the age of initial occurrence of the tumor. It is not unusual to get the history of a small bowel tumor being removed 10 to 15 yr before presentation of the syndrome. Many carcinoid tumors, particularly ileal tumors, are very slow growing and it seems that only when a considerable mass of tumor draining its secretory products into the systemic circulation is present that the syndrome presents itself.

FLUSHING

There are four types of flushing[13,61]:

1. A diffuse erythematous flush in the normal flushing area—i.e., the face, neck, and upper anterior chest—though on occasions more widespread and involving the whole body. This type of flushing is usually paroxysmal, the flush being of 2 to 5 min duration. Between flushes the patient may look quite normal.
2. This flush has a violaceous tinge to it. It affects the same areas but lasts longer than type 1. Facial color is often permanently increased and the facial skin may become severely cyanotic. These patients often show dilated cutaneous facial veins and telangiectases, suffused conjuctivae, and watering eyes.
3. A third type of flushing occurs in association with bronchial carcinoid tumors. Flushes often last up to several hours and sometimes days. The flushed skin is red, and often the whole body skin is flushed. Lacrimation is profuse and the conjunctival mucosa is red. Hypotension and tachycardia may be present. Facial skin may become edematous and the normal facial creases become exaggerated into deep folds. Some patients complain of enlargement of the parotid and submaxillary salivary glands. During this flushing diarrhea frequently worsens.
4. The flush found in association with gastric carcinoid tumors is bright red and patchy (geographical), usually most evident around the root of the neck, and is thought to be due to histamine release.

Experience now indicates that the flushing described under item 1 is distinct from the flushing described under item 2 and is not merely a forerunner of it.

Often there is a simple relationship of meal times to the occurrence of flushing, and it may be precipitated in individual patients by certain foods, such as cheese and salty bacon. Alcohol in any form often provokes flushing as does excitement or anxiety. The degree of flushing is extremely variable.

Biochemic Pharmacology of Flushing

As previously stated, 5-HT is not thought to be a main factor in the etiology of the flushing,[48] and in many but not all cases bradykinin seems to be implicated.

Flushing may be provoked by the intravenous injection of small quantities of certain catecholamines. It is believed[57] that the catecholamines, noradrenaline and adrenaline, when injected, circulate to the tumor to release kallikrein and perhaps other flush-provoking materials from the tumor. The flush-provoking action of noradrenaline, adrenaline, and dopamine is blocked by α-adrenergic blocking agents.

Flushing after alcohol is more delayed than after iv catecholamines. When flushing is provoked by alcohol it may be very severe and prolonged. This action of alcohol is also blocked in some patients by α-adrenergic blocking agents.[57] It has been suggested that alcohol releases an endogenous catecholamine that circulates to the tumor to release kallikrein. In some patients with a history of alcohol-induced flushing it appears that whereas the first alcoholic drink produces flushing, further alcohol after a short period of time does not produce flushing and a rest period from alcohol is necessary before its flush-provoking activity returns.

DIARRHEA

Diarrhea may occur without flushing, and flushing may occur without diarrhea, and the relationship between diarrhea and flushing is variable. Often there is no definite temporal relationship between diarrhea and flushing, and the striking dissociation in many patients and diarrhea leads to the conclusion that these two symptoms are probably not due to the same humoral secretion. Occasionally diarrhea may be associated with intestinal obstruction by the primary tumor, but this is unusual. In most cases the diarrhea seems to be due to a humoral mechanism. It may vary from one urgent and explosive stool daily to the passage of fluid stools, as much as 20 times a day. Usually diarrhea appears to be due to increased intestinal motility. The involvement of humoral secretions which might increase intraluminal gut water has not yet been demonstrated in the carcinoid syndrome, as it has in the WDHA syndrome (pancreatic cholera).[62]

Indirect evidence points to 5-HT being responsible in some way for the diarrhea. Methysergide, a 5-HT antagonist, is often effective in combating the diarrhea and *p*-chlorophenylalanine, which by blocking tryptophan hydroxylase may prevent they synthesis of 5-HT in the tumor, is also sometimes effective in controlling diarrhea.[63] Misiewicz *et al.*[64] have shown that the pattern of intestinal motility induced by 5-HT is not unlike that seen in the carcinoid syndrome.

MALABSORPTION AND THE CARCINOID SYNDROME

Although reported, this is uncommon.[13] Melmon *et al.*[65] found no abnormality of the jejunal mucosa on biopsy, and although previous ileal resection is often raised as a possible cause, this does not seem to be the only factor. Lymphatic obstruction by tumor or fibrosis might theoretically be causative. There has, however, been striking improvement of malabsorption when methysergide is given, suggesting that 5-HT is in some way involved.[65] Malabsorption should always be considered in the carcinoid syndrome, particularly in relation to the cachexia that sometimes occurs. It may also be another factor involved in the production of pellagra-like skin lesions which are otherwise thought to be due to nicotinamide deficiency induced by tryptophan deficiency arising from the utilization of tryptophan by the tumor in making 5-hydroxyindoles. These pellagra-like skin lesions may respond to treatment with nicotinamide.

ABDOMINAL PAIN

Among the causes of abdominal pain in the carcinoid syndrome are peptic ulceration,[26] intestinal obstruction due to intestinal stenosis caused by the tumor or associated fibrosis, "colicky" pain associated with increased intestinal motility and diarrhea, pain arising from necrosis of hepatic metastases, and pain arising from intestinal segmental infarction.

Pain arising from hepatic metastases is very common. Awareness of the clinical picture helps in diagnosis. The surface of the liver, which is often grossly enlarged, is usually tender over a small area; and as this tenderness and pain occurs, the symptoms of either flushing or diarrhea increase and wane as the pain disappears. During these episodes of tumor necrosis the urine may contain an excess of 5-hydroxyindole metabolites. Occasionally the necrosing metastases can be localized by physical examination, and this localization matched with the location of the metastases on a hepatic scan. Although abdominal pain is most usual from hepatic metastases, a metastasis necrosing high in the right lobe of the liver may produce pleuritic pain and a basal pleural effusion of bronchopneumonia. Occasionally tumor metastases may necrose through the liver capsule and release their contents into the intraabdominal cavity. This may lead to severe peritoneal pain.

RESPIRATORY SYMPTOMS

Mattingly and Sjoerdsma[66] found asthma and respiratory distress in about 20 percent of their cases. Respiratory symptoms present in two ways. Hyperventilation is common during flushing and it may be due to 5-HT release.[48] The asthmatic component occurs usually on a background of chronic bronchitis, emphysema, and chronic airways obstruction, and may become measurably worse during a flush. Bronchoconstriction may be seen during anesthesia, and Mengel[67] states that intravenous methysergide may be effective in overcoming this. Subcutaneous adrenaline should never be given to relieve the asthma of the carcinoid syndrome since this may worsen the symptomatology.

FIBROSIS AND THE CARCINOID SYNDROME

Peritoneal fibrosis, pleural adhesions, and constrictive pericarditis have been reported.[13] Retroperitoneal fibrosis may occasionally produce ureteric obstruction and obstructive renal failure.

CARDIAC LESIONS

The most comprehensive study of carcinoid heart disease is that of Roberts and Sjoerdsma.[68] The essential lesion consists of focal or diffuse deposits of fibrous tissue on the luminal surface of the internal elastic lamina of the heart valves and chambers. The deposits form whitish-yellow glistening smooth coatings on the endocardium; the right side of the heart is much more commonly involved than the left. The fibrosis affects the pulmonary valve, usually producing pulmonary stenosis, and also the tricuspid valve, with most commonly tricuspid incompetence though tricuspid functional stenosis may be present. Fibrous deposits are frequently present in the right atrium, on the internal linings of the great veins, and the coronary sinus. Fibrous tissue may also coat the right ventricle, though most commonly it caps the papillary muscles and involves the chordae tendiniae. Usually when lesions on the left side of the heart occur they are accompanied by lesions on the right. However, Von Bernheimer and his colleagues[38] described a nonmetastatic bronchial carcinoid tumor accompanied by fibrous lesions on the intima of the pulmonary veins and lesions of the mitral and aortic valves without any apparent involvement of the right side of the heart.

The precise cause of the cardiac lesions is unknown. The predominance of right-sided lesions with gastrointestinal carcinoids accompanied by hepatic metastases indicates that some substance released from hepatic metastases into the hepatic veins travels to the right side of the heart, causes damage in the valves, and is then probably removed during passage through the lungs. In patients with bronchial carcinoid tumors or lung metastases from gastrointestinal carcinoid tumors, the left-sided lesions are presumably due to substances draining directly into the pulmonary veins and into the left side of the heart, thus avoiding inactivation by the lungs. There is little evidence from which to identify the agents responsible.[13]

CARCINOID HEART DISEASE

The signs of carcinoid heart disease vary considerably from patient to patient, and within patient, depending not only upon the extent of the fibrotic lesions but also on the hemodynamic state which varies with the degree of flushing. The most common and striking sign is abnormal jugular venous pulsation indicating tricuspid valve disease. Tricuspid systolic murmurs indicate tricuspid incompetence, and tricuspid diastolic murmurs, usually becoming most obvious during flushing, may indicate tricuspid stenosis. There is great variation in the quality of these murmurs. The systolic murmur of pulmonary stenosis is usually of low intensity, though harsh in quality. Right-ventricular hypertrophy frequently occurs in association with tricuspid and pulmonary lesions.

The development of the right-sided cardiac lesions is of interest. Frequently the patient presents with fully developed cardiac lesions. On the other hand, one sometimes observes the development of cardiac disease over several years. The degree of functional cardiac impairment varies. Some patients with very severe valvular lesions have little functional impairment for many years and then deteriorate quickly. Perhaps individual myocardial function and the degree of intermittent or permanent increase in cardiac output caused by vasodilation are the variables determining the degree of myocardial failure. Congestive cardiac failure is common. There are no specific features on X-ray or electrocardiography that point to carcinoid heart disease.

PREGNANCY AND THE CARCINOID SYNDROME

Reddy *et al.*[69] reported five pregnancies in women with the carcinoid syndrome; in all cases labor was premature, the fetus was stillborn or died after birth, and in 1 case multiple congenital abnormalities were present. 5-Hydroxytryptamine is toxic to the fetus and placenta of pregnant animals.[70]

MENTAL CHANGES

The occurrence of psychiatric disturbances in the carcinoid syndrome is disputed. Although 5-HT is a central neurotransmitting agent, 5-HT in the circulating blood does not cross the blood-brain barrier easily and would not be expected to cause mental disturbance.

However, personal observation of 2 cases of the carcinoid syndrome who presented in the late stage of their illness with intermittent stupor, confusion, and hallucinations and the report by Lehmann[71] of a patient with mental disturbance and stupor suggest that occasionally disturbances of the mental state and consciousness may occur. Lehmann[71] observed that iv and oral L-tryptophan reversed the mental disturbances, suggesting that tryptophan deficiency (perhaps causing brain 5-HT deficiency) was responsible.

PEYRONIE'S DISEASE

Bivens *et al.*[72] reported 2 cases of Peyronie's disease accompanying the carcinoid syndrome.

ARTHROPATHY

Thorson[59] described arthralgia occurring in the carcinoid syndrome, and recently Plonk and Feldman[73] observed stiffness in the hand joints, pain on hand movements, and pain on releasing grip in 3 out of 5 consecutive patients. X-rays of the hands showed loss of bone density in the juxta-articular areas of the phalanges, multiple cystic areas in the phalanges, and erosions of the interphalangeal joint surfaces.

DIAGNOSIS

DEMONSTRATION OF TUMOR GROWTH

Primary ileal tumors are often small, impalpable, and difficult to demonstrate on routine barium studies. Cope and Warwick[74] have dealt in detail with the role of radiology in the detection of carcinoid tumors of the gastrointestinal tract.

Commonly the liver is enlarged and palpable, but occasionally it is not. Radioscanning of the liver is very useful in demonstrating metastatic growth and in giving information about feasibility of partial hepatectomy. When hepatic metastases have been proved and no primary tumor can be found clinically and radiologically in the abdomen, chest, and rarer sites such as the ovary and testis, then it is probable that a primary intraabdominal tumor is present. Then the question arises as to whether to attempt to demonstrate this by laparotomy.

Anesthesia can be risky in patients with the carcinoid syndrome, and bronchial constriction and hypotensive collapse may occur. If the syndrome is present, flushing can be provoked, and there is an increased excretion of 5-hydroxyindole metabolites in the urine, then in my view the only justification for laparotomy would seem to be either to avert or treat intestinal obstruction, or to remove an appreciable amount of functioning tumor mass from the liver or from elsewhere. Ileal primaries producing the carcinoid syndrome can occasionally be associated with large intraabdominal lymph node metastatic growth, and removal of functional tumor tissue from extrahepatic sites within the abdomen can lead to improvement.

FLUSH PROVOCATION

In about one-third of patients alcohol will produce flushing. A measure of whisky or 10 cc of ethanol in 15 cc of orange juice is usually effective.

Flushes are usually provoked in the carcinoid syndrome with intravenous catecholamines, and this provocation may be successful even in patients who do not complain of spontaneous flushing. Noradrenaline or adrenaline are administered intravenously in amounts not greater than 15 to 20 μg of adrenaline. The details of the administration of catecholamines and the time sequence of flushing are very important in establishing the diagnosis, and are described in detail elsewhere.[13] Great care should be taken in provoking a flush with catecholamines in any patient who has a past history of cardiac arrhythmia, heart failure, or asthma.

BIOCHEMIC DIAGNOSIS

QUANTITATIVE ESTIMATIONS OF URINARY 5-HIAA

The chemical methods have been described in detail by Udenfriend *et al.*[75] with modifications by McFarlane *et al.*[76] Urinary 5-HIAA excretion does not exceed 10 mg/24 h in normal subjects. Urinary 5-HIAA excretion exceeding 30 mg/day can be quickly picked up by the screening test described by Udenfriend and his colleagues. False-positives may occur in patients taking chlorpromazine and eating many bananas (which contain 5-HT). Urinary 5-HIAA excretion may be moderately raised in idiopathic steatorrhea.

QUALITATIVE ANALYSIS OF URINARY 5-HYDROXYINDOLES

In typical cases of the carcinoid syndrome, particularly those with ileal tumors, only an excess of 5-HIAA is visible on paper chromatograms of unextracted urine.[77] 5-HTP and 5-HT as well as 5-HIAA may appear when an atypical tumor is present—i.e., bronchial, pancreatic, or gastric. Estimations of plasma and whole-blood 5-HT levels may be diagnostic, particularly in those patients with normal or only slightly raised urinary 5-HIAA excretion. The measurement of blood bradykinin levels is not widely available and is generally not of diagnostic value.

PROGNOSIS

The rate of growth of primary ileal tumors and their hepatic secondaries is often very slow. Patients may live for many years troubled by pharmacologic effects of the tumor's secretion. Some ileal tumors and certainly bronchial and pancreatic tumors have a much worse prognosis. The development of marked cardiac lesions and the development of congestive cardiac failure worsens the prognosis. The metabolic effects of severe diarrhea, general weakening caused by recurrent flushing, and the cachexia associated with malignant disease often combine to produce a complex state of affairs which results in death. Urinary 5-HIAA excretion is little guide to prognosis. These are only general observations and there is a great deal of variability.

TREATMENT

SURGICAL

Bronchial or ovarian primaries without secondaries should be removed and may lead to a cure.[16] If an ileal or other gastrointestinal primary is present and accompanied by secondary growth, removal is indicated if the primary is large, causing mechanical obstruction or local effects, or if operation is being undertaken for removal of secondary growth. Apart from hepatic surgery, abdominal exploration is sometimes worthwhile since tumor growth in abdominal lymph nodes and large ovarian metastases can occasionally be removed with symptomatic improvement.[78]

But perhaps surgical treatment produces best results when hepatic metastases are removed from the liver. By utilizing liver radioscanning and coeliac angiography it is possible to see whether

(1) there are large hepatic metastases which might be shelled out or (2) the metastases are mainly confined to one lobe of the liver, in which case a right or left partial hepatectomy may be performed. On occasions this can produce a very worthwhile remission of the symptoms of the syndrome. Removal of hepatic metastases is also advocated in those patients whose abdominal pain can be ascribed to necrosing secondaries in the liver. Reviews of the place of surgery in the treatment of carcinoid syndrome are available.[13,79,80]

CYTOTOXIC DRUG THERAPY

Mengel and Shaffer[81] feel that cytotoxic drug therapy is beneficial only when there is evidence of rapid tumor growth and that a combination of cyclophosphamide and methotrexate is the most effective chemotherapy. They produced significant liver shrinkage in 24 of 41 patients treated. David *et al.*[82] produced tumor regression, as measured by reduction in liver size, by using either 5-fluorouracil, streptozotocin, or a combination of 5-fluorouracil with streptozotocin. However, some patients had evidence of tumor regression without a decreased output of 5-HIAA.

It is important to note that cytotoxic drug therapy may produce a severe flare-up of symptoms as the tumor necroses. At this point in time cytotoxic drug therapy should probably be confined to patients having very significant symptoms producing disability in whom surgery is not indicated and in whom tumor growth is fairly rapid.[83] Murray-Lyon *et al.*[84] reported 3 cases of mid-gut carcinoids treated by regional perfusion of the liver with 5-fluorouracil. They suggest that 5-fluorouracil should be first infused into the hepatic artery to decrease the function of hepatic metastases prior to ligation of the hepatic artery. After ligation of the hepatic artery, infusion of 5-fluorouracil into a tributary of the portal vein is carried out to treat any areas of surviving tissue. In 2 of the 3 patients remissions of the carcinoid syndrome were achieved for 5 months with recurrence of minor symptoms at 12 and 16 months.

PHARMACOLOGIC THERAPY

A scheme of the pharmacology of the carcinoid syndrome, indicating points of pharmacologic attack, is shown in Figure 138-3.

INHIBITION OF SYNTHESIS

5-HT

α-Methyl dopa. Occasionally α-methyl dopa, which partially inhibits the conversion of 5-HTP to 5-HT, relieves flushing, but whether this is due to the inhibition of the synthesis of 5-HT or to an interference with the action of catecholamines to release flush-provoking substances from the tumor cells is unknown. It is worth trying α-methyl dopa in those patients with the cyanotic type of flush, particularly if accompanied by hyperventilation. Doses of 2 g/day may be effective.

Parachlorophenylalanine (PCP)

Engleman *et al.*[63] showed that PCP was an effective inhibitor of 5-HT synthesis in the carcinoid syndrome. It acts by blocking the conversion of tryptophan to 5-hydroxytryptophan. It has little effect upon flushing but it can relieve the diarrhea and occasionally improves the patient's appetite, vigor and well-being.[13] The drug is not generally available; but if used, doses of up to 4 g/day may be necessary.

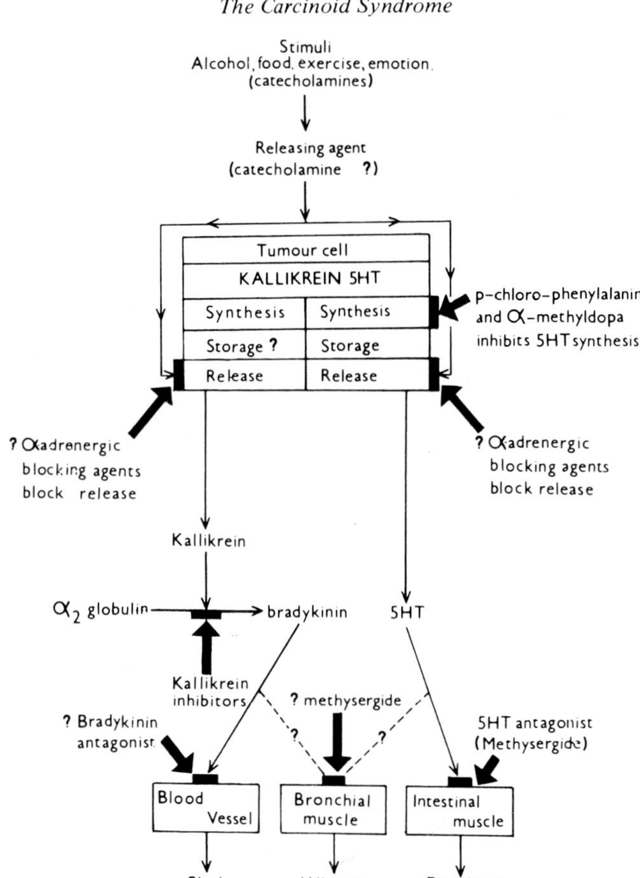

Fig. 138-3. Scheme of the pharmacology of the carcinoid syndrome. Central to this scheme is the tumor cell synthesizing kallikrein and 5-HT (serotonin). The tumor stores and releases these substances with presumably production of the main symptoms as shown toward the bottom of the scheme. Stimuli, probably through the mediation of a catecholamine, cause release of materials from the tumor, and the action of these catecholamines may be blocked by α-adrenergic blocking agents. On the other hand, one can inhibit synthesis of 5-HT most effectively with parachlorophenylalanine and less effectively with α-methyldopa. Kallikrein inhibitors so far have not been useful in preventing the production of bradykinin in this syndrome. Methysergide is the most effective treatment of the diarrhea in the carcinoid syndrome and must at present be presumed to act by antagonizing 5-HT. No effective bradykinin antagonist is yet known. It may be that methysergide blocks the action of 5-HT to produce bronchoconstriction. The thick black arrows leading to black blocks indicate theoretical sites of attack with various forms of therapy.

Kallikrein and Bradykinin

TRASYLOL, a commercial kallikrein inhibitor, will inhibit carcinoid tumor kallikrein in vitro.[55] However infusion of large amounts of trasylol failed to prevent spontaneous flushing and flushing induced by catecholamines in patients with the carcinoid syndrome.[85] At the moment trasylolo has little place in the treatment of the carcinoid syndrome.

PREVENTION OF THE RELEASE OF ACTIVE SUBSTANCES FROM THE TUMOR

α-Adrenergic Blocking Agents

The effect of catecholamines, certain foods, excitement, exercise, and alcohol can in some patients be inhibited by administration of phenoxybenzamine 10 to 20 mg t.i.d. per os with a resultant

Table 138-5. Details of Cases Relating Carcinoid Tumors, the Carcinoid Syndrome, and Insulin Production

Tumor Type	Argent-Affinity	Carcinoid Syndrome	Hypo-glycemia	Hyper-insulinism	Tumor Insulin	Pancreatic Insulin	Tumor 5-Hydroxy-indoles	Urinary 5-Hydroxy-indoles
Pancreatic islet cell adenoma + multiple ileal carcinoids	±	−	+	+	NT	NT	NT	Normal
Pancreatic islet cell	±	Diarrhea	−	NT	+	+	5-HT+	NT
Pleomorphic pancreatic? islet cell	−	+	+	NT	−	NT	−	+
Bronchial carcinoid	−	+	+	+	+	+	NT	NT
Pancreatic adenocarcinoma (? type)	−	+	+	+	NT	NT	NT	5-HT+
Malignant ileal argentaffinoma	+	+	+	+	+	NT	5-HT+	5-HIAA+

NT: not tested; +: present; −: absent; 5-HT: 5-hydroxytryptamine; 5-HIAA: 5-hydroxyindoleacetic acid.
For references see Grahame-Smith, D. G.: *The Carcinoid Syndrome*. London, Heinemann, 1972.

diminution in the frequency and severity of flushing attacks. The side-effects of phenoxybenzamine such as dizziness and nasal obstruction limit its use, and not infrequently patients become refractory to its effect.[13]

INHIBITION OF THE PHARMACOLOGIC ACTION OF ACTIVE SUBSTANCES RELEASED FROM THE TUMOR

Methysergide

This drug is frequently effective in treating the diarrhea of the carcinoid syndrome.[86] Its effect is obvious within a day or so. Dosages vary from 3 to 8 mg daily given in three divided doses. Little or no effect upon flushing is noted. Side-effects of this drug noted in relation to its use in the treatment of migraine[87] include vascular spasm, retroperitoneal fibrosis, and cardiac valvular fibrosis, the latter two being reminiscent of the spontaneous fibrotic tendency seen in the carcinoid syndrome. The risk of these toxic effects must be weighed against its potential benefit.

Cyproheptadine, or a new 5-HT antagonist BC105 (a benzocycloheptothiozine derivative)[88] may also be effective in controlling diarrhea. Chlorpromazine is occasionally useful in diminishing the flushing attacks, and in flushing caused by bronchial tumors dramatic improvement may ensue from the use of prednisone in dosages of 20 mg/day. Nicotinamide should be used for the treatment of pellagra-like skin lesions. Heart failure should be treated by conventional therapy, and resistant edema often responds to spironolactone. Wheezing, if disabling, is best treated with a salbutamol aerosol, which does not provoke flushing.

ECTOPIC HORMONE PRODUCTION

Apart from producing 5-HT and kallikrein, carcinoid tumors may, on occasion, produce other hormones.[13] Carcinoids of foregut derivation have been implicated in the production of Cushing's syndrome and removal of a bronchial carcinoid has led to remission of the etopic ACTH syndrome.[89] Hyperpigmentation is occasionally seen in the carcinoid syndrome, but it is uncertain whether this is due to excess MSH production. Oatcell carcinomas of the bronchus may produce the carcinoid syndrome, and the relationship of bronchial carcinoid tumors to oatcell carcinomas of the bronchus has already been mentioned. No definite evidence is available for the production of parathyroid hormone, antidiuretic hormone, or gonadotrophins by a carcinoid tumor.

The association of the carcinoid syndrome with pancreatic tumors and with insulin production is an intriging one, and the relevant data are set out in Table 138-5.

REFERENCES

1. Oberndorfer, S. Karizinoide: Tumoren des Dunndarms. *Frankf. Z. Pathol. 1:* 426, 1907.
2. Masson, P. Carcinoids (argentaffin-cell tumours) and nerve hyperplasia of appendicular mucosa. *Am. J. Pathol. 4:* 181, 1928.
3. Biorck, G., Axen, O., and Thorson, A. H. Unusual cyanosis in a boy with congenital pulmonary stenosis and tricuspid insufficiency. Fatal outcome after angiocardiography. *Am. Heart J. 44:* 143, 1952.
4. Thorson, A., Biorck, G., Bjorkman, G., and Waldenstrom, J. Malignant carcinoid of the small intestine with metastases to the liver, valvular disease of the right side of the heart (pulmonary stenosis and tricuspid regurgitation with septal defects), peripheral vasomotor symptoms, bronchoconstriction and an unusual type of cyanosis: a clinical and pathologic syndrome. *Am. Heart J. 47:* 795, 1954.
5. Isler, P., and Hedinger, C. Metastasierendes Dunndarmcarcinoid mit schweren, vorwiegend das rechte Herz betrefferden Klappenfehlern und Pulmonalstenose—Ein eigenartiger Symptomenkomplex? *Schweiz. Med. Wochenschr. 83:* 1953.
6. Rosenbaum, F. F., Santer, D. G., and Claudon, D. B. Essential telangiectasia, pulmonic and tricuspid stenosis and neoplastic liver disease. A possible new clinical syndrome. *J. Lab. Clin. Med. 42:* 941, 1953.
7. Cassidy, M. A. Abdominal carcinomatosis with probable adrenal involvement. *Proc. R. Soc. Med. 24:* 139, 1930.
8. Millman, S. Tricuspid stenosis and pulmonary stenosis complicating carcinoid of the intestine with metastases to the liver. *Am. Heart J. 25:* 391, 1943.
9. Currens, J. H., Kinney, T. D., and White, P. D. Pulmonary stenosis with intact interventricular septum: report of eleven cases. *Am. Heart J. 30:* 491, 1945.
10. Lembeck, F. 5-hydroxytryptamine in a carcinoid tumour. *Nature (London) 1972:* 910, 1953.
11. Pearse, A. G. E. The endocrine cells of the G.I. tract: Origins, morphology and functional relationships in health and disease. *Clin. Gastroenterol. 3:3:* 491, 1974.
12. Sjoerdsma, A., and Melmon, K. L. The carcinoid spectrum. *Gastroenterology 47:* 104, 1964.

13. Grahame-Smith, D. G. *The Carcinoid Syndrome*. London, Heinemann, 1972.
14. Williams, E. D., and Sandler, M. The classification of carcinoid tumours. *Lancet 1:* 238, 1963.
15. Pariente, R., Even, P., and Brouet, G. Etude ultrastructurale des carcinoides bronchiques; II Discussion. *Presse Med. 75:* 221, 1967.
16. Waldenstrom, J. Clinical picture of carcinoidosis. *Gastroenterology 35:* 565, 1958.
17. Chatterjee, K., and Heather, J. C. Carcinoid heart disease from primary ovarian tumours. *Am. J. Med. 45:* 643, 1968.
18. Moertel, C. G., Beahrs, O. H., Woolner, L. B., and Tyce, G. M. 'Malignant carcinoid syndrome' associated with non-carcinoid tumours. *N. Engl. J. Med. 273:* 244, 1965.
19. Cohen, S. L., MacIntyre, I., Grahame-Smith, D. G., and Walker, G. J. Alcohol-stimulated calcitonin release in medullary carcinoma of the thyroid. *Lancet ii:* 1172, 1973.
20. Williams, E. D. 5-hydroxyindoles and the thyroid. *Adv. Pharmacol. 6B:* 151, 1968.
21. Sandler, M., Karim, S. M. M., and Williams, E. D. Prostaglandins in amine-peptide-secreting tumours. *Lancet 2:* 1053, 1968.
22. Driessens, J., Clay, A., Adenio, L., and Demaille, A. Tumeur cervico-uterine et syndrome biologique de carcinoidose. *Arch. Anat. Pathol. Semaine. Hop. 12:* 200, 1964.
23. Brown, N. J. The pathology of testicular tumours. Miscellaneous tumours of mainly epithelial type. *Br. J. Urol. 36:* Suppl. 70, 1964.
24. Dockerty, M. B., and Scheifley, C. H. Metastasing carcinoid. Report of an unusual case with episodic cyanosis. *Am. J. Clin. Pathol. 25:* 770, 1955.
25. Simon, H. B., McDonald, J. R., and Culp, O. S. Argentaffin tumour (carcinoid) occurring in benign cystic teratoma of testicle. *J. Urol. 72:* 892, 1954.
26. MacDonald, R. A. Study of 356 carcinoids of the gastrointestinal tract: Report of four new cases of the carcinoid syndrome. *Am. J. Med. 21:* 867, 1956.
27. Moertel, C. G., Sauer, W. G., Dockerty, M. B., and Baggenstoss, A. H. Life history of the carcinoid tumour in the small intestine. *Cancer 14:* 901, 1961.
28. Sanders, R. J., and Axtell, H. K. Carcinoids of the gastrointestinal tract. *Surg. Gynecol. Obstet. 199:* 369, 1964.
29. Sanders, R. J. *Carcinoids of the Gastrointestinal Tract*. Springfield, Ill., Thomas, 1973.
30. Moertel, C. G., Dockerty, M. B., and Baggenstoss, A. H. Multiple primary malignant neoplasms. I, II and III. *Cancer 14:* 221, 231, 238, 1961.
31. Murray-Lyon, I. M., Rake, M. O., Marshale, A. K., and Williams, R. Malignant carcinoid tumour with gangrene of the small intestine. *Br. Med. J. 4:* 770, 1973.
32. Anthony, P. P., and Drury, R. A. B. Elastic vascular sclerosis of mesenteric blood vessels in argentaffin carcinoma. *J. Clin. Pathol. 23:* 110, 1970.
33. Davies, A. J. Carcinoid tumours (Argentaffinomata). *Ann. R. Coll. Surg. Engl. 25:* 277, 1959.
34. Sandler, M. 5-hydroxyindoles and the carcinoid syndrome. *Adv. Pharmacol. 6B:* 127, 1968.
35. Martin, E. D., and Potet, F. Pathology of endocrine tumours of the G.I. tract. *Clin. Gastroenterol. 3:3:* 511, 1974.
36. Marincek, B. Zur Frage metastasierender Appendix karzinoide mit Karzinoidsyndrom. *Schweiz. Med. Wochenschr. 103:* 1641, 1973.
37. Christodoulopoulos, J. B., and Klotz, A. P. Carcinoid syndrome with primary carcinoid tumour of the stomach. *Gastroenterology 40:* 429, 1961.
38. Von Bernheimer, H., Ehnriger, H., Heistracher, P., Kraupp, P., Lachnit, V., Obiditsch-Mayer, I., and Wenzl, M. Biologisch aktives, nicht metastasiergendes Bronchuscarcinoid nit Linksherzsyndrom. *Wien. Klin. Wochenschr. 72:* 867, 1960.
39. Bensch, K. G., Gordon, G. B., and Miller, L. R. Studies on bronchial counterpart of the Kultschitzky (argentaffin) cell and innervation of bronchial glands. *J. Ultrastruct. Res. 12:* 668, 1965a.
40. Bensch, K. G., Gordon, G. B., and Miller, L. R. Electron microscopic and biochemical studies on the bronchial carcinoid tumour. *Cancer 18:* 592, 1965b.
41. Bensch, K. G., Corrine, B., Pariente, R., and Spencer, H. Oat cell carcinoma of the lung: Its origin and relationship to bronchial carcinoid. *Cancer 22:* 1163, 1968.
42. Pernow, B., and Waldenstrom, J. Determination of 5-hydroxytryptamine, 5-hydroxyindole acetic acid and histamine in thirty three cases of carcinoid tumours (argentaffinoma). *Am. J. Med. 23:* 16, 1957.
43. Page, I. H., Corcoran, A. C., Udenfriend, S., Sjoerdsma, A., and Weissbach, H. Argentaffinoma as an endocrine tumour. *Lancet 1:* 198, 1955.
44. Grahame-Smith, D. G. Tryptophan hydroxylation in carcinoid tumours. *Biochem. Biophys. Acta 86:* 176, 1964.
45. Grahame-Smith, D. G. The biosynthesis of 5-hydroxytryptamine in carcinoid tumours and intestine. *Clin. Sci. 33:* 147, 1967.
46. Langemann, V. H. Amino acid decarboxylase and amino oxidase in carcinoid tumour. In Lewis, G. P. (ed.): *5-Hydroxytryptamine*. New York, Macmillan (Pergamon), 1958, p. 159.
47. Gowenlock, A. H., and Platt, D. S. The clinical chemistry of carcinoid tumours. In "the clinical chemistry of monoamines" Varley, H., Gowenlock, A. H. (eds.), vol. 2. New York, Elsevier, 1962, p. 140.
48. Robertson, J. I. S., Peart, W. S., and Andrews, T. M. The mechanism of facial flushes in the carcinoid syndrome. *Q. J. Med. 21:* 103, 1962.
49. Vane, J. R. Release and fate of vasoactive hormones in the circulation. *Br. J. Pharmacol. 35:* 209, 1969.
50. Davis, V. E. Discussion of the role of 5-hydroxyindoles in the carcinoid syndrome. *Adv. Pharmacol. 6B:* 143, 1968.
51. Davis, V. E., Brown, H., Huff, J. A., and Cashaw, J. L. The alteration of serotonin metabolism to 5-hydroxytryptophol by ethanol ingestion in man. *J. Lab. Clin. Med. 69:* 132, 1967.
52. Dreux, C., Bousquet, B., and Halter, D. L'exploration biochimique des tumeurs carcinoides. *Ann. Biol. Clin. (Paris) 31:* 283, 1973.
53. Levine, R. J., and Sjoerdsma, A. Pressor amines and the carcinoid flush. *Ann. Int. Med. 58:* 818, 1963.
54. Oates, J. A., Melmon, K., Sjoerdsma, A., Gillespie, L., and Mason, D. T. Release of a kinin peptide in the carcinoid syndrome. *Lancet 1:* 514, 1964.
55. Melmon, K., Lovenberg, W., and Sjoerdsma, A. Identification of lysyl-bradykinin as the peptide formed *in vitro* by carcinoid tumour kallikrein. *Clin. Chim. Acta 12:* 292, 1965.
56. Oates, J. A., Pettinger, W. A., and Doctor, R. B. Evidence for the release of bradykinin in the carcinoid syndrome. *J. Clin. Invest. 45:* 173, 1966.
57. Adamson, A. R., Grahame-Smith, D. G., Peart, W. S., and Starr, M. Pharmacological blockade of carcinoid flushing provoked by catecholamines and alcohol. *Lancet 2:* 293, 1969.
58. Feldman, J. M., Plonk, J. W., and Cornette, J. C. Serum prostaglandin $F_2\alpha$ concentration in the carcinoid syndrome. *Prostaglandins 7:* 501, 1974.
59. Thorson, A. Studies on carcinoid disease. *Acta Med. Scand. 334:* Suppl. 7, 1958.
60. Linell, F., and Mänsson, K. On the prevalence and incidence of carcinoids in Malmo. *Acta Med. Scand. 179:* Suppl. 377, 1966.
61. Grahame-Smith, D. G. The carcinoid syndrome. *Am. J. Cardiol. 21:* 376, 1968.
62. Ramaud, J. C., and Matuchansky, C. Diarrhoea and digestive endocrine tumours. *Clin. Gastroenterol. 3:3:* 657, 1974.
63. Engleman, K., Lovenberg, W., and Sjoerdsma, A. Inhibition of serotonin synthesis by parachlorophenylalanine in patients with the carcinoid syndrome. *N. Engl. J. Med. 277:* 1103, 1967.
64. Misiewicz, J. J., Waller, S. L., and Eisner, M. Motor responses of the human gastrointestinal tract to 5-hydroxytryptamine *in vivo* and *in vitro*. *Gut 7:* 208, 1966.
65. Melmon, K. L., Sjoerdsma, A., Oates, J. A., and Laster, L. Treatment of malabsorption and diarrhoea of the carcinoid syndrome with methysergide. *Gastroenterology 48:* 18, 1963.
66. Mattingly, T. W., and Sjoerdsma, A. The cardiovascular manifestations of functioning carcinoid tumours. *Mod. Concepts Cardiovasc. Dis. 25:* 7, 1956.
67. Mengel, C. E. Therapy of the malignant carcinoid syndrome. *Ann. Int. Med. 62:* 587, 1965.
68. Roberts, W. C., and Sjoerdsma, A. The cardiac disease associated with the carcinoid syndrome (carcinoid heart disease). *Am. J. Med. 36:* 5, 1964.
69. Reddy, D. V., Adams, F. H., and Baird, C. Teratogenic effects of serotonin. *J. Paediatr. 63:* 394, 1963.
70. Southgate, J., and Sancler, M. 5-hydroxyindole metabolism in pregnancy. *Adv. Pharmacol. 6A:* 179, 1968.
71. Lehmann, J. Mental disturbances followed by stupor in a patient with carcinoidosis. *Acta Psychiatr. Scand. 42:* 153, 1966.
72. Bivens, C. H., Marecek, R. L., and Feldman, J. M. Peyronie's disease—A presenting complaint of the carcinoid syndrome. *N. Engl. J. Med. 289:* 844, 1973.
73. Plonk, J. W., and Feldman, J. M. Carcinoid arthropathy. *Arch. Int. Med. 134:* 651, 1974.

74. Cope, V., and Warwick, F. The role of radiology in the detection of endocrine tumours in the G.I. tract. *Clin. Gastroenterol. 3:3:* 621, 1974.
75. Udenfriend, S., Weissbach, H., and Brodie, B. B. Assay of serotonin and related metabolites, enzymes and drugs. *Methods Biochem. Anal. 6:* 95, 1958.
76. Macfarlane, P. S., Dalgliesh, C. C., Dutton, R. W., Lennox, B., Nyhus, L. M., and Smith, A. N. Endocrine aspects of argentaffinoma. *Scot. Med. J. 1:* 148, 1956.
77. Jepson, J. B. Paper chromatography of urinary indoles. *Lancet 2:* 1009, 1955.
78. Sauer, W. G., Dearing, W. H., and Flock, E. V. Diagnosis and clinical management of functioning carcinoids. *J. Am. Med. Assoc. 168:* 139, 1958.
79. Malafosse, M. Carcinoid tumours: Surgical problems. *Clin. Gastroenterol. 3:3:* 711, 1974.
80. Zeegen, R., Rothwell-Jackson, R., and Sandler, M. Massive hepatic resection for the carcinoid syndrome. *Gut 10:* 617, 1969.
81. Mengel, C. E., and Shaffer, R. D. The carcinoid syndrome. In Holland, J. F., Frei, E. (eds): *Cancer Medicine,* chap. 24. Philadelphia, Lea & Febiger, 1973, p. 10.
82. Davis, Z., Moertel, C. G., and McIlrath, D. C. The malignant carcinoid syndrome. *Surg. Gynecol. Obstet. 137:* 637, 1973.
83. Carter, S. K., and Broder, L. E. The cytostatic therapy of secretory tumours of the G.I. tract. *Clin. Gastroenterol. 3:3:* 733, 1974.
84. Murray-Lyon, I. M., Dawson, J. L., Parsons, V. A., Rake, M. O., Blendis, L. M., Laws, J. W., and Williams, R. Treatment of secondary hepatic tumours by ligation of hepatic artery and infusion of cytotoxic drugs. *Lancet 2:* 172, 1970.
85. Grahame-Smith, D. G., Peart, W. S., and Ferriman, D. G. Carcinoid syndrome. *Proc. R. Soc. Med. 58:* 701, 1965.
86. Peart, W. S., and Robertson, J. I. S. The effect of a serotonin antagonist (UML 491) in carcinoid disease. *Lancet 2:* 1172, 1961.
87. Graham, J. R. Methysergide for the prevention of headache. Experience in five hundred patients over three years. *N. Engl. J. Med. 270:* 67, 1964.
88. Loong, S. C., Lance, J. W., and Rawle, K. C. T. The control of flushing and diarrhoea in carcinoid syndrome by an antiserotin agent, BC 105. *Med. J. Aust. B5:* 845, 1968.
89. Liddle, G. W., Nicholson, W. E., Island, D. P., Orth, D. N., Abe, K., and Lowder, S. C. Clinical and laboratory studies of ectopic humoral syndromes. *Recent Prog. Horm. Res. 25:* 283, 1969.

139

Ectopic Hormone Syndromes and Multiple Endocrine Neoplasia

Louis M. Sherwood
Victor E. Gould

INTRODUCTION

Systemic manifestations of malignant disease which are independent of the tumor or its metastatic lesions have been of considerable interest to clinicians for years. With increasing recognition of malignant disorders and the shift in hospital populations to include more patients with cancer, there is even greater interest in early recognition of extratumor manifestations. This subject has been the basis of a number of reviews[1] and of an extensive recent conference.[2] A number of synonymous terms refer to this fascinating group of disorders, including ectopic hormone syndromes, endocrine phenocopies, paraendocrine tumors, paraneoplastic syndromes, and production of hormones by nonendocrine tumors. The term "ectopic" refers to the production of proteins by tissues not normally known to produce them. Other terms refer to the production of a clinical syndrome by the tumor which mimics one of the common endocrine or metabolic disorders. It is appropriate to include in this discussion the multiple endocrine neoplasia syndrome, since many aspects of the embryogenesis and development of the ectopic hormone syndrome are parallel. Although this chapter will deal primarily with those products of tumors that produce biochemic or clinical endocrine disorders, there are a number of extraneoplastic manifestations (not yet proven to be due to a hormone) which are of general importance and which will also be discussed.

Malignant tumors may be associated with a variety of clinical manifestations of primary, secondary, or tertiary nature. The tumor itself, depending on the organ or site of origin, may lead to clinical suspicion because of presenting symptoms such as gastrointestinal bleeding, cough, or dysphagia. Secondly, it is not uncommon for tumors to present to the clinician as a metastatic lesion well before evidence of a primary tumor is even detected. Examples include hepatomegaly due to carcinoma of the colon, abnormal behavior or neurologic disorders due to brain metastases from carcinoma of the lung or breast, a skeletal fracture due to a metastatic lesion, or cord compression from metastatic tumor to the extradural space. Thirdly, a malignant disorder may present one of a variety of extraneoplastic manifestations which could be due to the production of protein hormones, tumor antigens, enzymes, or other substances. In some instances, the association is based on clinical or empirical observations without definitive documentation of production of a normal or abnormal substance by the tumor itself.

PARANEOPLASTIC SYNDROMES NOT YET PROVEN TO BE DUE TO A HORMONE OR TUMOR PROTEIN

Although a major emphasis of this chapter is the ectopic hormone syndrome, there are many extraneoplastic manifestations of importance that may be proven at a later date to have a humoral basis.

FEVER

Patients with malignant disorders are candidates for episodic fever. Because of their debilitated physical condition and exposure to radiotherapy and potent cytotoxic chemotherapeutic agents, patients are susceptible to infection or drug reaction, common and well-known causes of fever. In some cases, necrosis of tumor or hemorrhage into the tumor is believed to cause fever. There are, nevertheless, instances in which fever associated with a tumor has not been due to infection or tumor necrosis and yet is related to the tumor itself. Bodel and Atkins[3,4] provided evidence for experimental production of fever from pyrogens. In an animal model, they described the production of endogenous leukocyte pyrogens by polymorphonuclear leukocytes, monocytes, peritoneal and alveolar macrophages, as well as phagocytic cells of the reticuloendothelial system of liver, spleen, and lymph nodes. Lymphocytic cells do not apparently produce pyrogen. Activators such as endotoxins of gram-negative bacteria, viruses, particles that can be phagocytized, and pyrogenic steroids may provoke the release of endogenous pyrogens. Likewise, antigen-antibody complexes also function as activators of the system, possibly by releasing a non-pyrogenic intermediate substance such as a lymphokine, which activates the release of leukocyte pyrogen.

The situation in man is not quite so clear, and circulating endogenous pyrogens have not been demonstrated often in human blood during febrile episodes. However, pyrogen was extracted from renal carcinoma tissue in two febrile patients and not from normal kidney by Rawlins *et al.*[5] Human leukocytes incubated in vitro do not release pyrogen spontaneously unless activated. Therefore, human tumor cells have been incubated in vitro, and the supernatant fluid used to stimulate pyrogen release in animals. Bodel and Atkins[3,4,6] were able to demonstrate this phenomenon with clear cell carcinoma of the kidney where both tumor and capsule incubated in vitro produced a pyrogen that caused fever in rabbits. Similar studies were done with spleen and lymph nodes from patients with Hodgkin's disease. The generation of fever in these animal models did not always correlate, however, with the presence of fever in the patients. In some cases it is believed that tumor antigens associated with antibody complexes might have served as activators for the release of endogenous pyrogen. Although futher studies of tumor-associated pyrogens need to be performed, it is clear that some tumors can produce proteins that cause pyrogenic reactions in experimental animals and man, while in other cases, tumor-associated products (e.g., antigens) might stimulate inflammatory cells of the host to release endogenous pyrogen. These experimental observations suggest an etiologic basis for episodes of fever that occur frequently in patients with Hodgkin's disease, renal cell carcinoma, and other disorders and in whom infection, tissue necrosis, abnormalities in liver function, or drug reaction cannot be implicated to explain the fever.

WEIGHT LOSS AND OTHER METABOLIC CHANGES

Extreme weight loss and cachexia are frequent findings in patients with widespread malignancy. Anorexia, change in taste for food, decreased intake, emotional depression, and multiple drug therapy are often described as factors directly related to weight loss and cachexia. Nevertheless, decreased food intake and anorexia cannot account completely for the progressive cachexia of these patients as evidenced by experimental studies in animals using forced feeding, paired feeding, and caloric restriction.[7] Likewise, clinical observations suggest that hyperalimentation results in only transient improvement of nutritional status which cannot be maintained for long periods. Forced feeding in some cases actually has a detrimental effect.[8]

Since the normal mechanisms for controlling appetite and hunger are quite complex, it is difficult to determine how tumor factors might have an effect on these processes. Regulation of hunger involves a central control system in the brain, with specific areas in the hypothalamus controlling satiety and feeding. Some of the factors include reflexes generated from the gastrointestinal tract (e.g., gastric contractions); thermal factors related to the specific dynamic action of food substances; concentrations of hormones such as insulin, growth hormone, glucagon, and some of the gut hormones; glucose, lipid, and other metabolic products in blood; osmoregulatory factors; and a variety of evironmental and emotional factors related to normal appetite mechanisms. Therefore, the disruption of these mechanisms in the patient with malignancy can be complex and multifactorial. Nevertheless, there is evidence for peptides in the urine of fasted animals which are believed to have anorexic properties.[9] These substances have also been found in the urine of patients with malignant neoplasms,[10] and although it has been speculated that the tumor could produce such a peptide, there is as yet no confirmatory evidence. Likewise, there are humoral factors apparently generated during the fed state that can suppress food intake when infused into hungry animals.[11,12] Theologides[7,13] proposed that tumors might produce anorexia or cachexia because of peptides or other substances which could modulate the activity of various enzymes (activating or inactivating them in host tissues). Alterations in metabolic patterns of the host would disrupt homeostatic mechanisms. If host metabolism were chaotic, nutritional substances normally used for body growth would be used principally to support growth of the tumor.

A variety of metabolic abnormalities have been described in patients with malignant disorders. It is well known that patients with malignancy have a high rate of anerobic glycolysis.[14,15] If anerobic glycolysis is used as a principal means of energy production by tumors, formation of ATP would be much less than it would be from aerobic glycolysis. Anerobic glycolysis is a relatively inefficient pathway of energy production, and it produces large quantities of lactic acid. Although some lactic acid can be metabolized to water and carbon dioxide, most of it is regenerated to glucose via the Cori cycle (lactate is not excreted or oxidized in the Krebs cycle). Furthermore, there is an increased mobilization of protein to amino acids from steroids and other factors contributing to gluconeogenesis. Energy required for the regeneration of glucose from lactate leads to increasing demands on host energy resources. The tumor thus utilizes glucose for its own needs at the expense of loss of energy from the host, an efficient way of producing a thermodynamically cachexic state. One theoretical approach, therefore, is to provide more efficient energy utilization by using inhibitors of gluconeogenesis (such as inhibiting conversion of oxalacetate to phosphoenolpyruvate or pyruvate to oxalacetate[15]).

Many of the adaptive mechanisms which are normally observed in an individual during starvation or semistarvation seem impaired in the patient with uncontrolled malignant growth.[16] There is failure to reduce caloric expenditure, a continued utilization of amino acids and lactate for gluconeogenesis, and an inability to oxidize exogenous glucose normally. Nevertheless, the malignant tumor which usually makes up less than 5 percent of the total body mass manages to maintain its rate of growth. There are many questions that remain to be answered about the cachexia of malignancy. A variety of host and tumor factors are involved, but there is a possibility that specific proteins will be identified that are actually produced by the cancer and lead to alterations in host metabolism.[9,10] This is a promising area for future investigation, but at present very little definitive information exists.

ABNORMAL IMMUNOLOGIC FUNCTION AND CONNECTIVE TISSUE DISORDERS

Malignant disorders have been associated with a wide variety of immunologic syndromes (involving both excessive and impaired immune response) as well as connective tissue disorders. These vary from disorders associated with a clone of immunoglobulin-producing cells (some of which may have antibody characteristics) to connective tissue disorders such as dermatomyositis believed to be related to tumor antigens. It is beyond the scope of this chapter to discuss tumor immunology and current theories related to the development of tumors through blocking antibodies. On the other hand, it is pertinent to describe briefly a few of the immune syndromes that may be associated with malignant disorders. Specific production of tumor proteins such as carcinoembryonic antigen and alpha-fetoprotein will be discussed later.

Some malignant disorders are associated with failure of cell-mediated and/or humoral immunity. These observations may be complicated by the use of radiotherapy and immunosuppressive and cytotoxic agents in the treatment of cancer. As early as the first part of the century, Reed noted cutaneous anergy (negative tuberculin reactions in patients with advanced Hodgkin's disease).[17] More recently it has been appreciated that there is a generalized deficiency of cell-mediated immunity in Hodgkin's disease.[18] The lymphocytes of these patients respond poorly to in vitro stimulation by phytohemagglutinin,[19] and skin allografts are tolerated much better than in normal subjects.[20] Humoral immune responses may also be impaired in Hodgkin's disease, with hypogammaglobulinemia being a feature of advanced Hodgkin's disease.[21] In general the degree of immunologic impairment tends to correlate with the extent and the histology of the disease.[22] Although some patients who have positive responses to skin tests and other tests of cellular immune function tend to have a better prognosis, this is a controversial area. Recent studies evaluating immune function in patients with lymphoid malignancies indicate many immunologic disturbances similar to those noted earlier in Hodgkin's disease.[22] Such observations have led to the use of BCG and other agents to stimulate immune responses.

Of interest is the observation that patients with malignancy may have a factor in plasma that suppresses immunologic activity. A recent report by Glasgow *et al.*[23] examined 53 patients with malignant disease for hypersensitivity to skin antigen and 2,3-dinitrochlorobenzene. Of 41 patients with negative skin tests, 66 percent had immunosuppressive factors in serum. Most of the activity was found in a peak of protein on gel filtration with a molecular weight less than 10,000 daltons. Other chemical studies suggested that the factor was a peptide and that it suppressed human lymphocytes in vitro and the plaque-forming response to sheep erythrocytes. It principally suppressed cellular immune mechanisms and was not antigen-specific.[23] This factor had no resemblance to blocking factors found in the serum of patients with malignancies by Sjogren and others.[24] It would be intriguing if the tumor cell were responsible for the production of this abnormal protein, but there is no evidence for this as yet.

At the other extreme are hyperimmune phenomena which have been associated with malignancy. A variety of connective tissue disorders—e.g., polymyositis, dermatomyositis, scleroderma, and hypertrophic osteoarthropathy—have been noted.[25] The pathogenesis of polymyositis and dermatomyositis is of considerable interest in relation to current theories of immune function. The disorder of skin and muscle that occurs in individuals with tumors appears to be similar to that in patients without tumors, but there is a higher incidence of malignancy in older individuals who have dermatomyositis. On the other hand, children and young adults seem to have no increased association. Furthermore, there are a number of reports suggesting a regression of the connective disorder after resection of the tumor. This is particularly exciting in view of the considerable evidence that dermatomyositis is an autoimmune disorder.[25–30]

Polymyositis has been produced in guinea pigs by immunization with homogenized rabbit skeletal muscle and the use of Freund's adjuvant,[26,27] and it is believed that the animal model has some resemblance to human disease. Studies of human dermatomyositis show evidence for cytotoxic lymphocytes in vitro, specific transformation of lymphocytes in response to muscle antigens, cytotoxicity of lymphocytes for muscle cells in tissue culture, and specific release of lymphotoxin from lymphocytes on contact with muscle antigen.[28–30] Relatively few studies of patients with both dermatomyositis and malignancy have been performed, but the immunologic findings in those few cases seem similar. The obvious question is whether there is a cross-reacting antigen between muscle and the tumor so that the development of antibodies to a tumor antigen precipitates muscle destruction through the production of cytotoxic lymphocytes. An alternate theory is that a tumor enzyme or other secretory product could modify muscle, perhaps during invasion, and stimulate production of antibodies against muscle.[28–30] Other immunologic explanations are possible as well. It is likely that there are patients with tumors who do not present the clinical manifestations of dermatomyositis of polymyositis but who have muscle antibodies in their serum or whose lymphocytes can be demonstrated to be cytotoxic for muscle tissue.

If a parallelism is to be drawn between such immune phenomena and the humoral syndromes associated with cancer, it is likely that biochemical and immunologic evidence will be present in many patients who do not necessarily manifest clinical syndromes. It is in these areas that the usefulness of humoral or immune markers for malignancy might lead to earlier diagnosis. Other antibodies against tissues have been described in a wide variety of patients with malignant disease, particularly with the technique of immunofluorescence.[25] Antibodies to smooth muscle using an immunofluorescence technique were detected in nearly 70 percent of patients with cancer. Such antibodies are not specific, however, since they have also been found in patients with liver disease and other disorders.[25]

NEUROLOGIC DISORDERS

A wide variety of neurologic and neuromuscular disorders have been described in association with malignancy. These syndromes have been appreciated since the early part of the century and were popularized by Brain.[31] Patients with malignant disease often have neurologic findings that cannot be attributed directly to metastatic lesions in the central or peripheral nervous system. These syndromes include peripheral neuropathy (both sensory and motor), radiculopathy, degeneration of the dorsal roots, myelopathic disorders, cerebellar degeneration, and a myasthenia gravis-like syndrome. It is important to recognize these disorders since they often cause disability which is far in excess of the neoplastic disease itself.[32] The abnormalities may also precede the more direct effects of the malignancy so that recognition can lead to early diagnosis. If they are recognized as complications of the neoplasm, unnecessary neurosurgery or other therapeutic maneuvers can also be avoided. Although the reports in the literature consider principally the peripheral neuropathy and myelopathy, central nervous system complications can be significant. In an extensive study of 250 males with bronchogenic carcinoma and 250 females with breast cancer, 16 percent of the men and 4.4 percent of the women had neurologic or muscular signs.[33] Of these patients, only 7 had involvement of the central nervous system while the rest had peripheral nerve and muscular dysfunction. The same authors subsequently expanded their series to over 1400 patients with various types of malignancy.[34] Of this group, 162 had some form of neuromyopathy and 41 had manifestations in the central nervous system (11 motor neuron, 15 myelopathic, 15 cerebellar). One must be cautious, however, in ascribing these abnormalities to the malignancy since other causes of neuropathy can occur in these patients. For example, in males with carcinoma of the lung, there may be a history of ethanol intake which could cause a peripheral neuropathy otherwise ascribed to the malignancy.[32] The types of disorders encountered clinically are described below:

Cerebral

Dementia is one of the most common of the cerebral complications and was noted by Brain[35] in 14 of 43 patients with neurologic complications and by Posner[36] in a significant number of patients. The abnormalities involve a spectrum from confusion to severe organic brain syndrome with loss of memory and cerebral function; they may develop acutely or over a long period of time. Pathologic abnormalities may or may not be found at postmortem examination, but these sometimes include degenerative changes in the hippocampus and amygdaloid.[37,38]

Brain Stem

A variety of brain stem abnormalities including ophthalmoplegia, bulbar palsy, ataxia, vertigo, and nystagmus may be observed. Optic neuritis is also occasionally found in association with extensive demyelination.[38]

Cerebellar Disorders

Degeneration of the cerebellum is said to be one of the more frequent central nervous system complications of malignancy.[38] The signs are usually bilateral and symmetric, and involve ataxia of the extremities, tremors of intention, and dysarthria which may be severe; it is unusual to find vertigo or nystagmus. The course is usually severe, and the patient may become completely disabled. Pathologically there may be degeneration of the Purkinje fibers with perivascular inflammation and accompanying degeneration of brain stem nuclei; cord signs may be associated.

Myelopathic Disorders

These may involve large tract and/or motor neuron degeneration, sometimes resembling amyotrophic lateral sclerosis and subacute necrosis. Norris[39] noted some form of malignancy in approximately 10 percent of 130 patients with amyotrophic lateral sclerosis. Subacute necrosis of the cord occurs as a rapidly ascending motor and sensory paralysis to the thoracic cord level. At autopsy there may be degeneration of both white and gray matter.[40]

Neuromuscular and Muscular Disorders

Myasthenia gravis-like syndromes have been reported in patients with carcinoma and are frequently given the eponym Eaton-Lambert syndrome.[41] The myasthenia may be mild or have a typical onset like myasthenia gravis, but many of the patients have symptoms in the extremities before bulbar muscles are affected, making it somewhat different from classical myasthenia. Likewise, the responses to medication are much more variable than in the classical disease, and there is a marked sensitivity to curare-like medication. Weakness is often most marked in the pelvic and thigh muscles, although some of the patients have difficulty in swallowing. In the cases described by Eaton and Lambert,[41] there was a strong male predominance. Definite findings were noted by these authors on electromyographic testing, and many abnormalities were present only on electromyography. Most of the reported cases of the syndrome have been associated with pathology in the chest, particularly bronchogenic carcinoma of the small cell or oat cell type, although the association of myasthenia and thymoma is well known. Myasthenia has also been associated with lymphosarcoma and lymphoma, as well as carcinoma of the pancreas, breast, prostate, ovary, thyroid palate, cervix, kidney, and rectum.[32,41] Although there is an overlap between classical myasthenia gravis and the Eaton-Lambert syndrome, they can be distinguished by some of the electromyographic features and by the fact that classical myasthenia usually presents with bulbar symptoms and is not usually associated with the depression of reflexes common in patients with carcinoma.[32]

Peripheral Nerve Disorders

Peripheral neuropathy is probably the most frequent of the neurologic syndromes associated with malignancy.[42] The neuropathic disorders are sometimes associated with myelopathy and signs in the central nervous system. Many of the myopathic disorders are associated with considerable involvement of the peripheral nerves as well, and may have an abnormal electromyogram even if it is not expected clinically. Neuropathy may take the form of either a mild symmetric sensory disease which occurs late in the course of a malignant disorder or an acute and severe sensory and motor myopathy that may occur early in the disease and progress to severe paralysis. The latter type may be noted before the presence of the neoplasm is even recognized, and it occasionally remits.[32,42] Protein concentration in the cerebrospinal fluid may be elevated, suggesting pathology at the root, and there is occasionally pleocytosis. The peripheral nerves may show loss of both myelin and axon, although the myelin loss usually predominates and degeneration of the dorsal root ganglia has been detected. Removal of the tumor generally causes no improvement in the peripheral neuropathy.

Theories about the etiology of the neurogenic syndromes are multiple, and the actual relationship between underlying neoplasm and neurologic disturbance is unclear. Theories include infectious, metabolic, toxic, and autoimmune etiologies as well as nutritional deficiences. [32,38] The multifocal leukoencephalopathy frequently associated with Hodgkin's disease and other tumors has been ascribed in some cases to a Papova virus (on the basis of electron microscopic and tissue culture evidence).[43] Likewise, in some of the dementias, there may be evidence for viral encephalitis. In disorders associated with metabolic derangements such as hypercalcemia or hypokalemia, a basis for some of the neurologic or muscular abnormalities is present. There is evidence for toxin production by some tumors, as well as evidence for autoimmune mechanisms. Wilkinson and Zeromski[44] noted antibodies against brain in the sera of patients with carcinomatous neuromyopathy. One could postulate cross-reactivity between the tumor antigen and the nervous system, producing a model similar to allergic encephalomyelitis. Nutritional deprivation and cachexia could also be used to explain some of the neurologic abnormalities, particularly if one postulates that metabolic disorders might affect the nervous system as well. These syndromes represent an interesting group of disorders that are frequently associated with malignancy. Their exact etiology remains unexplained, but their importance in terms of patient disability is considerable.

VASCULAR DISORDERS

A variety of vascular disorders may be associated with malignancy, but the two principal ones recognized are migratory thrombophlebitis and marantic (or nonbacterial) endocarditis. Malignant disease may be associated with an increased tendency both for thrombosis and hemorrhage. Slichter and Harker[45] studied 77 patients with malignancy, some of whom were receiving antithrombotic therapy including anticoagulants and/or platelet-function inhibitors. In general, they noted decreased survival of ^{51}Cr-labeled platelets and ^{125}I fibrinogen. These hemostatic changes were related to the extent of the malignant process and tended to regress somewhat with therapy. Requirement for transfusion was most often present when platelets were decreased. Possible causes for the low platelet count included decreased production, increased destruction, or a combination of factors. They tried to isolate these factors from chemotherapy and concluded that a failure of platelet production was the principal cause of thrombocytopenia in malignancy.

The same authors studied a number of patients having venous thromboembolism associated with solid tumors or Hodgkin's disease. These individuals were characterized by increased platelet and fibrinogen consumption up to four times the normal.[46] They speculated that the circulating platelets were removed directly by reacting with tumor tissue surfaces (presumably because of inadequate or abnormal endothelialization of the blood-tumor interface), and that fibrinogen might be consumed as a result of platelet or surface initiation of fibrin formation. Fibrinogen but not platelet survival was improved with heparin therapy. Several patients treated with dipyridamole and/or aspirin showed improvement in platelet and fibrinogen survival. Although these inhibitors prevent tumor-induced consumption of platelet and fibrinogen, they probably would not provide helpful therapy for bleeding problems because they cause platelet dysfunction. Furthermore, platelet consumption is a less important cause of thrombocytopenia than impaired production or increased pooling. The patients with cancer-associated venous thromboembolism may be benefited by heparin or coumadin therapy but not by inhibitors of platelet function.

There is interesting evidence that mucin-producing tumors may be associated with increased intravascular coagulation.[47] Entrance of mucus derived from the adenocarcinoma into the circulation is believed to act as a stimulus to coagulation, and there is a higher incidence of postoperative deep-vein thrombosis in these patients. Crude tumor extracts containing partially purified mucin activated factor X and coagulation activity, while inactivation of thromboplastic activity could be produced by the removal of sialic acid with neuraminidase.[47,48] The actual incidence of deep-vein thrombosis in association with carcinoma is not known. In general, the chances of finding a malignancy in a patient with clinical deep-vein thrombosis are small, but some of the newer techniques used to diagnose deep-vein thrombosis (such as radioactive fibrinogen scanning) turn up a much higher incidence of thrombosis than has previously been suspected. This is particularly true in patients with malignant disease who undergo surgery.

In patients with widespread neoplastic disease, microangiopathic hemolytic anemia may result from diffuse fibrin deposition. These patients may have several clotting defects, and this has been noted particularly in patients with promyelocytic leukemia and adenocarcinoma of the prostate.[48] The most likely cause of intravascular coagulation is contact of circulating blood with thromboplastic substances produced by the neoplastic cells. In some cases, heparin therapy may reverse some of the hemostatic problems.

The etiology of marantic endocarditis is a complete enigma, and there is no information available on the pathogenesis. Theoretically tumors produce substances that cause thrombosis or other changes on the endocardium or on heart valves.

DERMATOLOGIC DISORDERS

There is an interesting association between neoplastic disorders and dermatologic lesions. A number of abnormalities are related to genetic endocrine disorders (such as Sipple's syndrome), but others seem to be associated with malignant disease. The association with dermatomyositis has already been described and may involve bluish-red discoloration around the face, neck, chest, and extremities, as well as heliotrope discoloration of the eyes. Of considerable interest is the entity acanthosis nigricans, a velvety, verrucous and hyperpigmented lesion that occurs frequently in body folds such as the axilla. It may also be associated with increased keratin production of the palms and soles. There is a significant association of acanthosis with visceral malignancy. The two manifestations usually occur simultaneously, although the dermatologic lesion may precede the cancer by a considerable period of time.[49] Recently an unusual syndrome of marked resistance to insulin has been described in patients with acanthosis by Kahn *et al.*[50] These patients do not have an associated malignancy nor do those with acanthosis and other similar metabolic disorders such as lipoatrophic diabetes (Chapter 89).

Other dermatologic abnormalities associated with malignant tumors include erythema gyratum repens (an unusual zebra-like abnormality noted most prominently on the back) and ichthyosis, which may be present in patients with reticuloendotheliosis or carcinoma.[51] A number of bullous abnormalities have been associated with tumors. These include dermatitis herpetiformis and bullous pemphigoid, a disorder in which antibody to basal lamina in the skin can be demonstrated.[51] An association between glucagon-producing tumors and a necrolytic bullous skin disease has also been noted.[52] A number of patients with lymphoma and other malignancies have herpes zoster, and the disseminated form has been noted in some patients on immunosuppressive therapy.[51]

The dermatologic manifestations associated with the carcinoid syndrome have been described elsewhere in this volume and will not be reviewed here. In addition, external manifestations in Gardner's syndrome and Peutz-Jeghers syndrome have been noted.

Evidence supporting the association of dermatologic lesions with visceral malignancy is as follows[51]:

1. Specific activity of the tumor that causes the dermatologic lesion (e.g., flushing associated with carcinoid)
2. A genetic relationship between the dermatologic abnormality and malignancy (Gardner's syndrome)
3. Dermatologic abnormalities caused by autoimmune disorders (dermatomyositis or bullous pemphigoid)
4. Simultaneous onset of the dermatologic abnormality and the malignancy
5. Remission of the dermatologic abnormality after removal or cure of the tumor

RENAL DISORDERS

There is an interesting association between malignancy and immune disease of the kidney. Bilateral renal vein thrombosis and amyloidosis can be complications of malignancy or myeloma-like syndromes. Lee *et al.*[53] reported an 11 percent incidence of carcinoma in 101 patients presenting with the nephrotic syndrome. Eight of the patients showed evidence of membranous glomerulonephritis, 1 patient had lobular glomerulonephritis, and another had only minimal abnormalities. These included tumors of the bronchus, cervix, ovaries, kidneys, and oropharynx. In addition, patients with lymphoma and leukemia have been reported to have nephrotic syndrome in association with these diseases without evidence of invasion of the renal parenchyma.[53–55] Not infrequently, treatment of the lymphoma or Hodgkin's disease with immunosuppressive drugs or radiation resulted in remission of lymphoma as well as the nephrotic syndrome. This association suggests a strong relationship, based on evidence that nephrotic syndrome frequently results from the deposition of antigen-antibody complexes on the basal lamina. It was postulated and then proven that renal biopsies from patients with carcinoma and the nephrotic syndrome would have deposition of IgG and IgM on the basal lamina by immunofluorescence;[55] an identical antigen was then obtained from a lung tumor extract and from elution of the involved glomerulus. This association proved a direct relationship between the synthesis of tumor antigens and associated circulating immune complexes which deposit in the kidney.

A wide variety of other renal problems may be seen in association with malignant tumors. These include problems related to mechanical compression or obstruction of the genitourinary tract, infection associated with obstruction, renal failure associated with hypercalcemia and hyperuricemia, renal tubular acidosis, and nephrogenic diabetes insipidus noted in hyperglobulinemic states.

SUMMARY

The various tumor-related syndromes described in this section represent systemic manifestations and organ-specific manifestations associated with malignancy. In most instances, a definite association between production of a protein by the tumor and these manifestations has not been proven. Suggestive evidence has been provided in the case of pyrogen production, anorexigenic peptides, tumor antigens which produce immune complex disease, and thromboplastic substances which lead to accelerated coagulation. Precise characterization or purification of these tumor proteins has not yet been accomplished. In the ectopic hormone syndromes, on the other hand, more readily definable products have been associated with tumors and have caused clinical syndromes that duplicate in many respects the abnormalities produced by endocrine hyperplasia or an endocrine tumor. In the section that follows, major emphasis will be placed on the endocrine and metabolic syndromes related to ectopic hormone production. Prior to a detailed description of these syndromes, however, an introductory section will deal with the importance of these syndromes and some of the theories concerning their pathogenesis.

GENERAL ASPECTS OF THE ECTOPIC HORMONE SYNDROMES

SIGNIFICANCE

The ectopic hormone syndromes are of considerable interest not only to the clinician and pathologist but also to the developmental biologist and molecular biologist.[1,2] For the clinician, they represent a fascinating spectrum of endocrine and biochemical disorders assocaited with malignant disease. It is important to emphasize that these are being identified with increasing frequency as clincial problems; they are not medical curiosities! As the number of patients with malignant disease occupying hospital beds increases, greater recognition is being given to the elaboration by tumors of humoral and other proteins. The concepts of tumor markers and of earlier diagnosis of malignant disease are important areas of future research in clinical medicine. The tumors are of considerable interest to the pathologist because of the association of the specific histologic types with discrete clinical syndromes and because of the identification with the electron microscope of secretory granules in many of the tumors.[56] To the developmental biologist and molecular biologist the tumors are extremely important because they may hold the key to a better understanding of normal embryologic and ontogenetic phenomena. Subsequent sections will review data from the embryologic literature which bear on these clinical syndromes and which may provide clues for the clinical investigator and the embryologist in pursuit of ties between basic biology and the clinical problems.

Of considerable interest to the clinician is the idea that elaboration of a humoral or protein substance may provide a clue to the presence of a neoplasm while it is still resectable and before metastases appear. Occasionally this can be a frustrating search, as evidenced by the study of Rudnick and Odell[57] of a male patient with an elevated concentration of chorionic gonadotropin and no obvious testicular neoplasm. There was no evidence for a tumor in this patient until metastases suddenly appeared. At postmortem examination, a microscopic neoplasm was found in the testis which was producing the gonadotropic substance. As there is increasing recognition of a variety of substances produced by tumors, one may look forward to a time in the not-too-distant future when individuals above a certain age may be screened for a variety of hormonal and antigenic substances in pursuit of asymptomatic neoplasms. Moreover, evidence derived from experimental models and clinical sources indicates that dysplastic nonneoplastic cells may develop structural and functional alterations in their secretory apparatus, suggesting the possibility of diagnosing and monitoring preneoplastic changes through laboratory determinations of secretory products.[58,59]

At times, the metabolic and hormonal effects of the tumor hormone may be more devasting to the patient than the neoplasm itself. This may be particularly true of the severe hypokalemia and weakness associated with an ACTH-producing tumor, severe and life-threatening hyponatremia in the inappropriate ADH syndrome, and a life-threatening hypercalcemia in those tumors associated with ectopic production of parathyroid hormone or other hypercalcemic substances. The persistence or regression of the metabolic manifestations following surgery, radiotherapy, or chemotherapy is of considerable importance to the clinician, since the metabolic manifestations are frequently associated with the presence of tumor.

In patients who present with tumors and associated endocrine manifestions, it is extremely important to determine whether the tumor itself is responsible or whether there is a concomittant endocrine disorder. Endocrine or metabolic disorders that are not rare may coexist with neoplastic disease and present a somewhat confusing picture (e.g., hyponatremia, hypercalcemia). For example, one of the authors (L.M.S.) recently observed a patient with severe hypercalcemia who had bony metastases due to carcinoma of the breast and severe Paget's disease of bone. Despite the fact that the patient had two well-recognized causes for hypercalcemia, she also had an elevated level of parathyroid hormone in the blood by radioimmunoassay and persistent hypophosphatemia. Neck exploration revealed a large parathyroid adenoma which was removed, and the patient's hypercalcemia was corrected.

DOCUMENTATION

A variety of indirect as well as direct methods have been utilized to document the presence of the ectopic hormone syndrome. In many cases the observations are empiric and based on clinical phenomena, but recently more direct chemical or immunologic data have been available to provide accurate documentation. Under each of the hormonal syndromes to be detailed, specific evidence for the methods of documentation will be provided, but basic principles covering all ectopic hormone syndromes are reviewed below. Evidence for the existence of an ectopic hormone syndrome is generally provided by one or more of the following pieces of evidence.[1,2]

1. Recognition of a known clinical endocrine syndrome in the presence of a malignant neoplasm. One must be careful to exclude a coexisting disorder of an endocrine gland (see above)
2. Biochemical manifestations suggestive of production of a hormone or its effects in the presence of a neoplasm (e.g., a high serum calcium or low serum sodium in the presence of a lung tumor)
3. Disappearance or remission of endocrine or metabolic abnormalities after surgery, radiotherapy, or chemotherapy
4. Reappearance of endocrine or biochemical abnormalities associated with recurrence of the tumor
5. Measurement of increased levels of circulating hormones in the blood or urine
6. Extraction of hormone from tumor tissue
    a. Measurement of hormonal activity by a variety of bioassay techniques
    b. Measurement of hormonal activity by one or more immunologic or radioimmunoassay methods
    c. Biochemical and physiologic characterization of tumor peptides
7. An arteriovenous difference in hormone concentration across the tumor bed, with a higher concentration in the venous circulation
8. Evidence for synthesis of hormone by the tumor in vitro (e.g., continuous release of hormone in tissue culture or the incorporation of radioactive amino acids into labeled hormone)

PATHOGENESIS

There is much speculation and little solid evidence concerning the pathogenesis of tumor-associated hormone syndromes. It has been popular to characterize them as tumors whose cells have dedifferentiated and consequently regained the capability to produce proteins characteristic of a less-well-differentiated or embryonic state. Tissue that might at an early stage form neural plate, for example, at a later stage might be more restricted in development and exclusively become lens tissue. In vitro experiments that have been done with tumor tissue co-cultured with embryonic tissue showed that embryonic tissue could induce organization in some of the tumors. For example, Ellison *et al.*[60] were able to show that an undifferentiated rat renal tumor co-cultivated with the dorsal spinal cord from mouse embryo produced differentiated kidney tubules. There may be close correspondence between these inductive mechanisms and the development of tumors. It has been suggested, for example, that neoplastic transformation might be a pathologic counterpart of normal differentiation and might arise by a misprogramming of gene activity by epigenetic mechanisms.[61] The ectopic production of hormones or similar proteins by tumors would be examples of the dedifferentiation of tumor cells and the acquisition (or regaining) of previous competence followed by misprogramming and abnormal activation of genes.

This can be broken down further by suggesting that the ectopic hormone syndrome can be categorized into one of three groups.[62] The first group of tumors would have acquired previous competence such as those endodermal derivatives that synthesize hormones characteristic of other endodermal tissues. A second group would be mesodermal derivatives that would have had to undergo more extensive differentiation than the first group. Third would be a group of ectodermal or mesodermal tumors that have become labile enough as a result of dedifferentiation to acquire the functions of endodermally derived glands. A corollary of this hypothesis is that one may be able to predict the likelihood of an ectopic endocrinopathy occurring with certain neoplasms. The observations to support this model are based on observed interactions between embryonic tissues and tumor cells in tissue culture.

THE APUD CONCEPT AND ITS IMPLICATIONS

More specific relationships of hormone production and the neuroectoderm have been suggested by a number of authors. The notion of a complex endocrine system comprising isolated cells scattered throughout the gastrointestinal tract and related viscera is not new; Feyrter originally presumed it to be of endodermal derivation and suggested that the alimentary tract was one diffuse endocrine organ.[63] However, solid evidence pointing to the existence of a neuroectodermally derived endocrine system whose essential function was amine and/or peptide production has accumulated only within the last decade.

The basic features shared by these cells are cytochemical and ultrastructural. Properties of these cells include high levels of amine precursors such as 5-hydroxytryptophan (5-HT), α-glycerophosphate dehydrogenase, esterase, and cholesterase, etc.[64,65] Additional properties were subsequently described, and the acronym APUD (amine precursor uptake and decarboxylation) was introduced by Pearse and colleagues.[66,67] The essential feature of these cells is their capability to take up substances like dopa or 5-HT, decarboxylate them, and subsequently produce biogenic amines which can be demonstrated in tissue sections by formalin-induced fluorescence. The amines presumably can be utilized as building blocks for the production of more complex peptides.

At the electron microscopic level, APUD cells display prominent rough endoplasmic reticulum and Golgi complex, and are generally rich in free ribosomes. However, their most characteristic feature is the consistent presence of round secretory granules which display an inner core of variable electron density, a pale surrounding halo and a single encompassing membrane (Figs. 139-1 and 139-2). The diameter of the granules varies considerably but falls mostly within the 100-to-250-mμ range and is often fairly uniform within a given cell type. The electron density and configuration of the core also vary greatly, but they may be quite characteristic as exemplified by the paracrystalline profiles seen in nonneoplastic pancreatic β cells and in some of their tumors as well.

The experimental methods used to show the migration of APUD cells from their origin in neural crest through the mesoderm to their final destination in the primitive intestine include the following:

1. Neural crest cell identification with tritiated thymidine incorporation
2. Grafting of neural crest elements between two related but morphologically distinct avian species
3. Formalin-induced fluorescence of biogenic amine-producing neural crest cells

These methods were applied and embryos sacrificed at sequential developmental phases, leading to the demonstration of neural crest derivation and APUD characteristics of numerous cells populating the gastrointestinal tract and related tissues.[68–70] The APUD system includes all peptide-producing cells of the stomach, duodenum, intestine, pancreatic islets, adrenal medulla, extra-drenal paraganglia cells, adenohypophysis, parafollicular thyroid cells, and melanoblasts.[71] Additional cells with APUD characteristics were found in the respiratory tree and the gastrointestinal and urogenital tracts, although their secretory products and function remain unclear.[69,71,72] The parathyroid chief cells pose an important hurdle; although they produce a peptide hormone and display secretory granules, their cytochemical characteristics differ from the APUD-type cells.[71,73] However, other investigators have strongly advocated the inclusion of the parathyroids within the APUD system.[74]

Predictably, the introduction of the APUD concept has resulted in considerable controversy since its acceptance would imply revisions in long-held notions of embryology, pathology, etc. A taxonomic proliferation has already occurred, and generic terms to designate APUD-cell-derived neoplasms such as *Apudoma,*[75,76] *Neurolophoma,*[71] and *Neuroendocrinoma*[77,78] have been introduced. Neoplasms that would be included under such umbrella terms include islet cell tumors, carcinoid, pheochromocytoma, ganglioneuroma, neuroblastoma, paraganglioma, medullary carcinoma of the thyroid, bronchial neuroendocrinoma (carcinoid), oat cell carcinoma of the lung, and some thymomas. Certain poorly understood "undifferentiated" neoplasms of the gastrointestinal tract, mediastinum, etc., which display typical neurosecretory granules under the electron microscope may be shown to contain considerable quantities of vanillylmandelic acid (VMA) and 5-HIAA. Clinically active and inactive tumors may display granules indistinguishable from each other (Figs. 139-1 and 139-2), and from those of normal endocrine cells (Fig. 139-3).

Although the precise number is not clear, only a portion of the above-mentioned neoplasms are associated with clinically obvious hormonal syndromes. This could be explained quantitatively or on

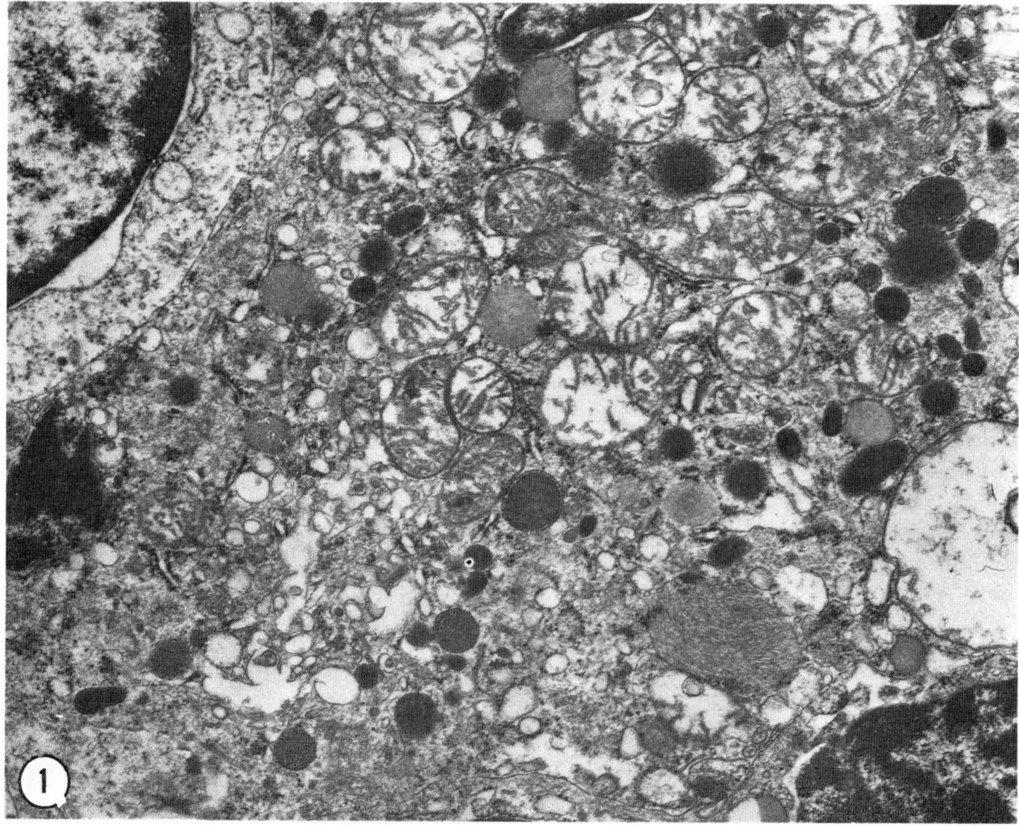

Fig. 139-1. Cushing's syndrome associated with pulmonary oat cell carcinoma in a 67-yr-old male. Electron micrograph of two adjacent neoplastic cells. Note prominent secretory granules with rather dense core. (22,500×)

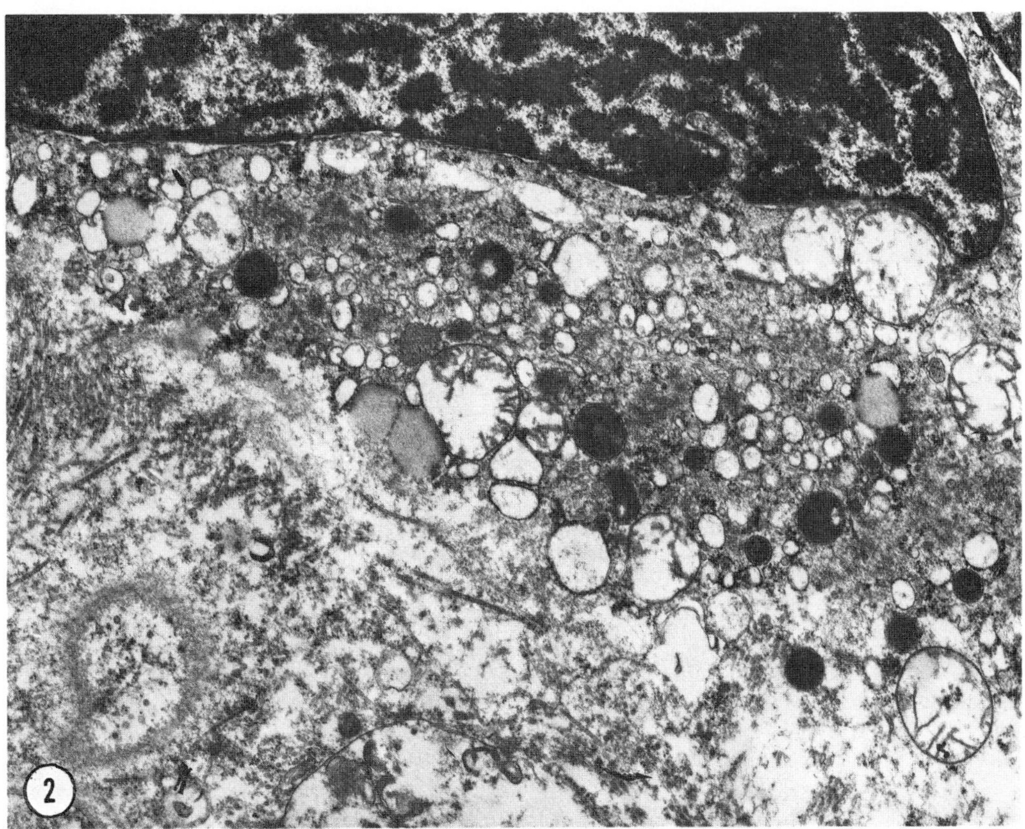

Fig. 139-2. Pulmonary oat cell carcinoma not associated with any detectable hormonal syndrome in a 73-yr-old male. Electron micrograph shows secretory granules which do not seem to differ greatly from those seen in Figure 139-1. (22,500×)

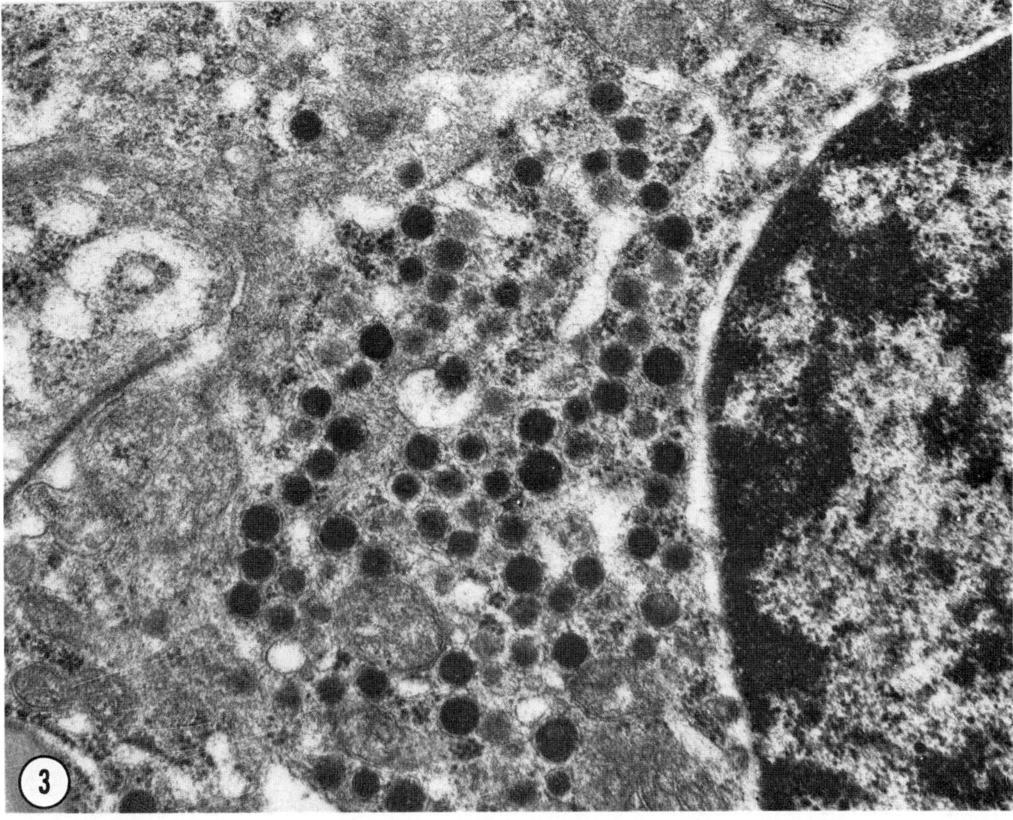

Fig. 139-3. A 22-yr-old male, known to have been in good health, died shortly after sustaining severe thoracoabdominal trauma. Electron micrograph is of acidophilic cell of anterior hypophysis. Note abundant secretory granules morphologically similar to those of Figures 139-1 and 139-2. (20,700×)

the basis of aberrations in the secretory apparatus of the neoplastic cells. Production of biologically active or inactive materials might be represented by recognizable but highly variable secretory granules and biochemic manifestations (Fig. 139-4). In this regard, it is possible that some of these tumors may be able to complete the hormonal synthetic process to the prohormone level (proinsulin, big ACTH, etc.), but they lack the crucial enzyme-converting systems necessary to yield fully active biologic hormones.[56] However, even the presence of mature granules (and presumably active hormone) within tumor cells does not guarantee a clinically recognizable hormonal syndrome. The tumor cells might have a deficient microtubular-filamentary apparatus, preventing effective ejection of the secretory materials from the cells.[78]

Both benign and malignant tumors may display chromosomal anormalities which could result in alterations in the appropriate expression of gene function. Therefore, structurally and functionally abnormal secretory activity on the part of tumors is hardly surprising. If one considers that most, if not all, previously mentioned tumors may actually derive from the same neuroectodermal cell line, many of their puzzling features become clarified:

1. The cytochemical commonality of the APUD cells (normal as well as neoplastic) and their similar biosynthetic pathways would explain the secretion of more than one hormone by a single tumor. This multiple secretory activity may be synchronous or asynchronous and may or may not be reflected in clinically detectable hormonal syndromes. [79]
2. The widespread distribution of APUD cells, could indicate that a number of hormone-secreting tumors derived from them and generally felt to be "ectopic" (i.e., ACTH-producing oat cell carcinoma of the lung) may be so in terms of normal differentiated cell function, but not so from the viewpoint of histogenesis.
3. Some neuroendocrine-type neoplasms (pheochromocytomas) may occur in association with important developmental anomalies of the neural crest such as von Recklinghausen's and Hirschsprung's diseases. This association has led to the term "neurocristopathy."[80]
4. Finally, the APUD concept may be useful in explaining the pathogenesis of the multiple endocrine neoplasia syndrome. Thus, if one accepts the common embryogenetic derivation of the APUD cells and suggests the possible incorporation of a tumorigenic factor into the genome of their common neuroectodermal precursor, a rational, although speculative, pathogenesis is suggested.[77] Alternatively, stimulatory and inhibitory relationships and feedback mechanisms among the various components of the APUD system may play an important role in the development of multiple endocrine neoplasia syndromes.

The APUD system may have developed from primitive neural transmitter cells, these simple elements having migrated from their original location to populate other organs and tissues as environmental requirements changed. While their basic cytochemical makeup and capability to synthesize biogenic amines remained unchanged, some components of the system acquired the capacity to produce more complex peptides.[71] Given this premise, neoplas-

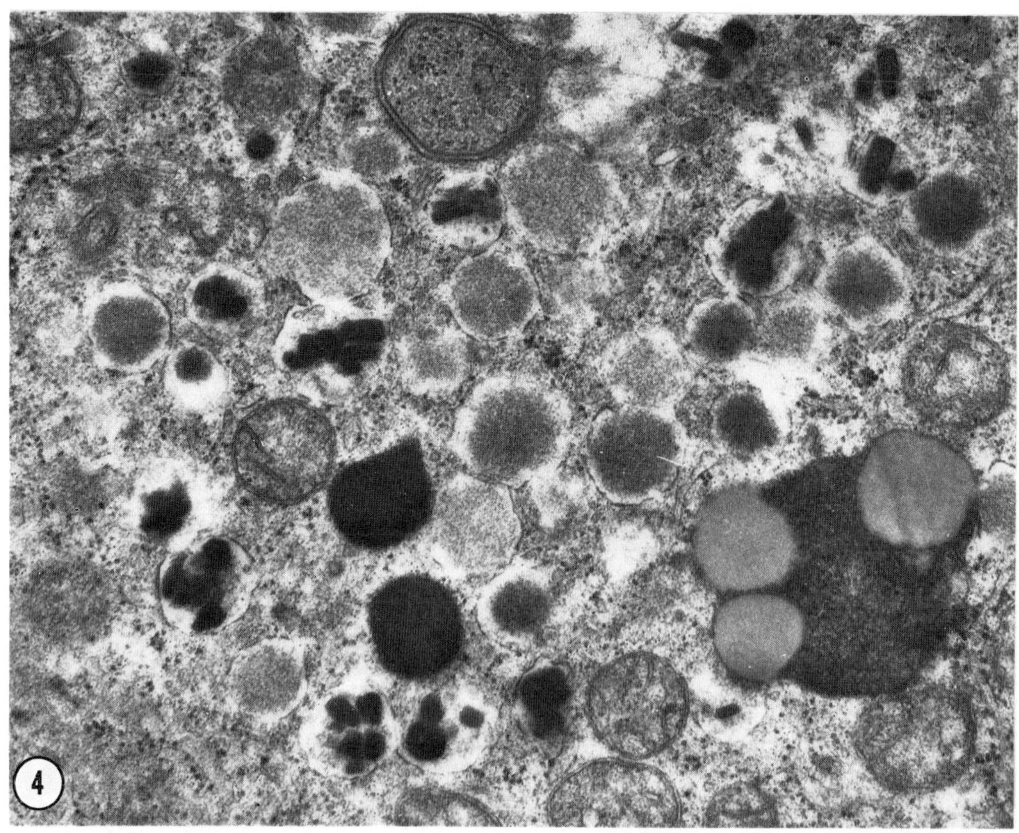

Fig. 139-4. This 52-yr-old female had mild, occasional episodes of hypoglycemia for several years. Small islet cell adenoma in the tail of the pancreas. Electron micrograph depicts numerous secretory granules of varying density, some of which show obvious paracrystalline profiles. (72,500×)

tic transformation of these cells may result in severe structural and functional changes in the secretory apparatus; as a result neoplastic APUD cells may:

1. Remain similar to the cells from which they are derived and synthesize and secrete an active hormone(s)
2. Produce a hormone, but fail to release it
3. Revert to the secretion of simpler amines
4. Evolve to produce more complex peptides not normally secreted by the cells from which they derive
5. Develop more than one secretory pattern
6. Produce aberrant materials which will be biologically inactive[78]

LIMITATIONS OF THE APUD CONCEPT

The APUD concept has stimulated interest and research, offering a rational, but speculative, explanation for many obscure features of tumor-associated hormone production. However, many aspects of abnormal endocrine activity related to tumors remain unclear, and it seems unlikely that the APUD concept will completely resolve the problem. Even if all current APUD-related ideas are accepted, many neoplasms associated with abnormal peptide material cannot be included within the system. Examples of these would include the hypoglycemia associated with some hepatomas and sarcomas and the hypercalcemia reported with a host of highly variable tumors (see below). It is likely that some cells (and therefore the tumors derived from them) may be excluded from the APUD system by further investigations while other elements may be included. Moreover, some premises basic to the APUD concept have now been challenged. Recent experiments involving ablation of the ectoderm in rat embryos failed to prevent the appearance of pancreatic β cells, reopening the question of their embryogenesis.[81] Investigations involving heterologous grafts provided negative data regarding origin of some of the intestinal endocrine cells from neuroectoderm.[82] Alternatively, one might speculate that neuroectodermal cells migrated toward and populated the primitive gut far earlier than previously suspected. Possibly, APUD characteristics may not be the exclusive domain of neuroectodermal cells, and could be generated by endodermal cells. As our knowledge of embryology and physiology increases, rigid notions attributing a specific function to cells of precise embryonal derivation have been shown to be mistaken (e.g., not only mesenchymal cells but also various epithelial cells are capable of collagen synthesis[83]).

CLINICAL COUNTERPART OF THE APUD HYPOTHESIS

Weichert[74] presents an extensive series of arguments to support his theory for a common origin of the ectopic hormone syndromes and multiple endocrine neoplasia. Based on similarities in their development, histologic and biochemical capabilities, the frequent production of ectopic hormone syndromes in association with foregut derivatives, and the development of multiple endocrine neoplasia in the same glands, he suggests their origin from common neuroectodermal cell precursors. Some of the evidence he cites is as follows: Common characteristics can be noted in tumors of all of the foregut derivatives, and they have many similiarities histochemically to carcinoid tumors. Argentaffin cells have been described along the entire alimentary tract from mouth to anus, but they are most common in the duodenum, appendix, Meckel's diverticulum, and terminal ileum. Islets of tissue have been described not only in their classical location in the foregut but also extending into the exocrine system, emphasizing the migration of these cells in the budding and branching of the primordial endodermal cell cords. Cells of the neurogenic system which can give rise to carcinoid tumors are carried into the endodermal primordial pancreas during development and can be traced to the site of the islets. Occasional argentaffin cells are left behind in the ducts and acini, and can be transformed into hormone-producing tumor tissue. The parathyroid, thymus, and ultimobranchial body developed similarly, but have no remaining connection with the gastrointestinal tract. Weichert[74] argues further that if hormone-secreting cells are argentaffin in nature, then functioning islet cell tumors could be expected to appear wherever argentaffin cells are found. Islet cell tumors producing a variety of hormones such as insulin, gastrin, glucagon, and secretin have been reported from the lung, stomach, pancreas, duodenum, and biliary tree. Furthermore, carcinoid tumors associated with serotonin production have also been described in the same sites. These cells have the ability to produce both hormones and serotonin and its precursors.

Carcinoid tumors may have their origins in the foregut, midgut, or hindgut, and may be associated with a variety of syndromes.[74] Foregut carcinoids (e.g., gastric) tend to produce an atypical carcinoid syndrome in which 5-hydroxytryptophan rather than serotonin is produced, while midgut carcinoids frequently produce the typical carcinoid syndrome and serotonin. Hindgut carcinoids are not generally active. These differences in characteristics are thought to be caused by the presence of serotonin and its precursors, while the pheochromocytoma is dependent on the presence of catecholamines. In some cells of the gut (enterochromaffin cells), there is both an argentaffin and chromaffin reaction, suggesting that these cells may contain both catecholamines and serotonin. Likewise these overlapping chemical aspects have been identified in endocrine organs including the pituitary gland, pancreas, and thyroid. Some cells that do not stain with silver may be related to the argentaffin cell but are merely going through a clear cell cycle. The changes in hormone synthesis and secretion by various tumors that seem to be initially unrelated also support this argument. Production of ACTH, for example, can be associated with brochogenic carcinoma, thymic tumors, oat cell carcinoma, anaplastic carcinoma of the pancreas, thyroid carcinoma, and carcinomas of the gastrointestinal tract. There are many histologic similarities among carcinoid, oat cell, and thymic tumors, and carcinoid has frequently been confused with the oat cell carcinoma histologically. The bronchogenic tumor is a foregut derivative containing cells with APUD characteristics, and it can produce almost all of the polypeptide hormones.

Levine and Metz[84] have taken a somewhat different approach to classifying the ectopic hormone-producing tumors. They feel that the concept of totipotentiality of cells is unproductive since there is no way to prove or disprove it. Rather, they noted the association of hormone production with specific tumor cell types and focused on selective aspects of derepression rather than it being a random process. After a careful review of the literature, they concluded that almost all known ectopic hormone-producing tumors could be classified into one of two major groups (group I and group II), with the remainder described as transitional since they had characteristics of both groups. Their classification and system analysis was based on considerations of developmental biology, histology, and ultrastructure as well as hormone-producing capabilities.

The tumors defined in group I have characteristics similar to those defined by Weichert.[74] These are the cells designated as APUD cells and appear to be biochemically related to those having embryologic origin in the neural crest.[69] All of the tumors in this group have the ability to synthesize and secrete all of the other hormones characteristic of group I but not group II, with rare exception. They suggest that group I tumors are derived from neural crest cells which traveled through the primitive endoderm and in which migratory cells became incorporated into the bronchial tree, pancreatic anlagen, and various derivatives of the branchial arches. Although these cells earlier in their development seemed to lack differentiated secretory capacity, they can be identified by histochemical techniques as precursors of secretory cells. They tend to assume basal location and are organized into glands and follicles. Eventually they develop mature secretory cells with granules. The authors argue that the common embryologic ancestry probably accounts for their shared secretory potential and that the differences that might occur among group I cells could be due to different tissue environments in which they come to rest, origins in different parts of the neural crest with exposure to different inducers, or different amounts of time in the neural crest prior to migration into the endoderm. These cells which contain biologically active aromatic amines; such as dopamine, serotonin, and histamine; show marked metachromasia with acridine dyes or toluidine blue, and have a high content of substances giving specific cytochemical characteristics such as α-glycerophosphate menadione reductase and other enzymes responsible for the argyrophilic characteristics. The enzymes are thought to participate in generating lipid for the membranes of the secretory granules. The tumors in this group include the foregut carcinoid, oat cell carcinoma, pancreatic islet cell tumor, tumors of pancreatic and biliary ducts, thyroid medullary carcinoma, and malignant epithelial thymoma. The hormones produced by tumors of group I include insulin, calcitonin, ACTH, melanocyte-stimulating hormone, vasopressin, gastrin, glucagon, secretin, and various biogenic amines and precursors including serotonin, histamine and the catecholamines.

The tumors classified in group II include hepatoma, cholangioma, Wilms' tumor, hypernephroma, adrenal cortical tumor, nongerminal gonadal tumor, vascular tumor, connective tissue and mesodermal tumor, reticuloendothelial tumor, squamous cell lung carcinoma, gastrointestinal tumors (excluding tumors of group I), and melanoma. Hormones of placental origin (particularly those associated with glycoprotein hormones) and fetal antigens such as α feto-globulin and placental-type enzymes are exclusively associated with group II tumors. The characteristic secretory granules noted in group I tumors are not classically noted in the group II tumors, but there may be a heterogenous group of cellular inclusion bodies suggesting secretory activity. Very few tumors of this group have been well studied ultrastructurally in cases where they were thought to be producing hormone. The authors argue that the unifying characteristics of the group II tumors, despite their heterogeneity, are primarily in the hormones secreted which include parathyroid hormone, erythropoietin, gonadotropins, human placental lactogen, prolactin, growth hormone, insulin-like activity, renin, and thyrotropin. The authors believe that they result from a more primitive kind of differentiation than the tumors of group I.

In the third group, Levine and Metz[84] have classified transitional tumors such as the pheochromocytoma, paraganglioma, neuroblastoma, and ganglioneuroma. While these tumors have in common with group I a derivation from the neural crest, they proceed directly from the neural crest to ultimate locations in the adrenal medulla and sympathetic ganglia without traversing the endoderm of the gastrointestinal tract. These tumors have been characterized as transitional because of the hormones they secrete. They definitely produce some of the group I hormones such as ACTH, MSH, and biogenic amines, and probably insulin, calcitonin, glucagon, and secretin. Secretion of group II hormones such as insulin-like activity and placental lactogen have been well documented, and there is evidence for production of parathyroid hormone and erythropoietin as well. Clearly they do not fit satisfactorily into the other groups and have therefore been listed as transitional. They may coexist with a tumor in group I in families that have multiple neoplasms. The melanoma is also classified as a transitional tumor by these authors because it occasionally produces not only the hormones of group I but also parathyroid hormone, gonadotropins, and erythropoietin.

Levine and Metz[84] support their system by indicating the very unusual crossovers that occur between the groups of tumors they have defined. There has been no difinite documentation of release of a group I hormone by a group II tumor, and there are only scarce reports of release of group II hormones by group I tumors. A major problem the authors noted in making their classification was the kind of information that was readily available in the literature. In many cases the diagnosis and reporting of the ectopic syndrome has been based on clinical criteria with only limited or entirely speculative chemical information. There are a large number of isolated case reports, some of which may, in fact, be inaccurate. Some of the assays for hormones have been too insensitive, and some of the immunoassays may have been misleading. Additionally, there may be inhibitors present in tumors which could interfere with bioassay effects,and some of the tumors may have been nonhomogeneous or only intermittently secreting.

One additional theory is the "sponge theory" in which it has been argued that tumors do not secrete the hormone in question but merely have the capacity to absorb large quantities. This hypothesis would be inconsistent with the appearance of a clinical syndrome in the face of a high level of the hormone or appropriate antigen or enzyme in the blood. There is no good evidence that the so-called "sponge theory" has validity, and it is not given wide credence at the present time.

The pathogenesis of the ectopic hormone syndrome is still unclear. Although the general theory of derepression associated with neoplasia is widely held and the development of characteristics of a former state of cellular differentiation presumed, the nonrandom nature of the process, the association of histologic types with specific hormone production, and the association with cells having APUD characteristics makes the phenomenon seem less random.[1] At present, there is no additional solid information available on the pathogenesis of these syndromes, except that more sensitive assays and careful evaluations have provided evidence that ectopic hormone production may be a much more common phenomenon in maliganant disorders than appreciated previously. There is at least one experimental animal system that might be used to provide further data.[85] This is the so-called GPL syndrome, which is associated with alterations in granulopoiesis, thrombopoiesis, and lipid mobilization in certain inbred strains of mice. Further studies of this system and others may shed additional light on these abnormalities.

It is extremely important that the extopic hormones be purified and characterized biochemically, so that it can be determined whether they exist in the same biochemical form as their counterparts in the endocrine gland. Also, careful analysis of the tumor tissue, including ultrastructural studies and biochemical characterization, is essential.[78] Our understanding of the ectopic syndromes will be furthered by basic developments in developmental biology and biochemistry which provide new evidence concerning the nature of epigenetic mechanisms, phase-active genomes, and the entire process of cell differentiation. For these reasons, the ectopic hormone syndromes are of broad interest to both the clinician and the basic scientist. The remainder of the chapter will deal with specific hormonal syndromes reported in the literature.

ECTOPIC ACTH SYNDROME

HISTORICAL ASPECTS

In 1928, a pathologist in London described the first ectopic hormone syndrome, although the author was not aware of the nature of the disorder at the time.[86] In his report, Brown described an obese, pigmented, and plethoric 45-yr-old woman with polydipsia, anorexia, weakness, blurred vision, baldness, hirsutism, and purpura. Laboratory studies showed polycythemia, hyperglycemia, and a normal sella turcica on skull x-ray. At autopsy the patient had a 1-cm oat cell carcinoma of the lung and enlarged adrenal glands. This patient was reported several years before the description of Cushing's syndrome, and association of the tumor with adrenal hyperplasia was not recognized. In the 50 years hence, more than 200 patients with adrenal hyperplasia in association with tumors have been reported.[87]

The term "ectopic ACTH syndrome" was first defined by Meador *et al.*,[88] who demonstrated the presence of ACTH-like activity in extracts of nonendocrine tumors associated with Cushing's syndrome. Further studies by Liddle *et al.*[89] showed similarities between ACTH extracted from tumors and the hormones from pituitary glands in tests of biologic activity, chromatographic behavior, and physical and chemical properties.

TUMOR TYPES

The ectopic ACTH syndrome has been associated principally with tumors of the lung, thymus, and pancreas. The following tumors account for the majority of cases[87]:

1. Oat cell carcinoma of lung, 60 percent
2. Thymic tumors, 15 percent
3. Pancreatic carcinoma (usually islet cell), 10 percent
4. Bronchial adenoma (carcinoid type), 4 percent
5. The remaining 11 percent include pheochromocytoma, medullary carcinoma of the thyroid, various neurogenic tumors, tumors of the parotid, ovary, prostate, and kidney. More rarely, carcinoma of the breast, esophagus, colon, gallbladder, testis, or uterus may be responsible.

On the basis of recent radioimmunoassay studies, Gewirtz and Yalow[90] have suggested that ectopic ACTH production was even more widespread than appreciated clinically. In the tumors and plasma of patients with carcinoma of the lung without clinical Cushing's syndrome, they noted significant quantities of ACTH. Extracts from 14 of 15 lung carcinomas in patients without clinical Cushing's syndrome contained immunoreactive ACTH. No ACTH was found in extracts of control lung tissue distant from the tumor site, normal liver tissue, or lymph nodes; liver metastases from the tumors contained ACTH. These tumors contained almost exclusively "big" ACTH, which eluted in the void volume of a Sephadex G-50 column. Nonpulmonary tumors rarely contained ACTH except for islet cell tumors and one of the two Zollinger-Ellison tumors. Although the quantities of ACTH present (5 to 55 ng/g wet weight) were lower than those found in patients with the clinical ectopic ACTH syndrome (1.75 to 2.5 μg/g), they were definitely significant. A total of 53 percent of 83 patients with carcinoma of the lung had plasma ACTH concentrations in the afternoon greater than 150 pg/ml. Most of the patients with values under 150 were patients who had received radiation therapy or chemotherapy. Elevation to 150 pg/ml was also noted in 31 percent of 25 patients with chronic obstructive pulmonary disease, 28 percent of 25 patients with other severe lung disease, and 10 percent of 33 control patients. ACTH in the plasma of patients with carcinoma, as well as chronic obstructive lung disease, was principally big-ACTH.

The presence of big-ACTH in association with nonneoplastic pulmonary disease suggested that dysplastic neuroendocrine cells in the bronchi may also be capable of abnormal secretory activity; ultrastructural evidence to that effect has recently been reported.[59]

BIOCHEMICAL AND PHYSIOLOGICAL CHARACTERISTICS OF ECTOPIC ACTH

1. Bioassay—Ectopic ACTH extracted from nonpituitary tumors from patients with the clinical syndrome has been indistinguishable from the pituitary hormone in a number of bioassays.[88,89] The following assay characteristics of ectopic ACTH are also noted for the pituitary hormone:
   a. Stimulation of adrenal hyperplasia
   b. Stimulation of cortisol secretion, and 17-keto-steroid excretion in man
   c. Stimulation of corticosterone secretion in the rat
   d. Parallel dose-response curves for production of cyclic AMP and steroids
   e. Melanocyte-stimulating activity in the frog skin, both in vitro and in vivo
   f. In vitro release of free fatty acids from adipose tissue
2. Chromatographic characteristics and physical/chemical properties of ectopic and pituitary ACTH[89] are as follows:
   a. Extractable from tumor tissue with glacial acetic acid and precipitated with acetone and ether from acetic acid
   b. Adsorbed to cation exchanger (IRC-50) from dilute acetic acid and eluted with 50-percent acetic acid
   c. Absorbed to oxycellulose from dilute acetic acid and eluted with 0.1 N HCl
   d. Similar behavior in countercurrent distribution systems
   e. Separable from MSH on SE-sephadex column
   f. Inactivated by trypsin and chymotrypsin and quite labile in unheated human plasma
   g. Stable in acid and quite labile in alkali
   h. Can be dialyzed only at acid pH after being added to plasma
   i. Inactivated by hydrogen peroxide which oxidizes methionine residues
   j. Inactivated by periodate

Definitive information on the amino acid sequence of ectopic ACTH is not yet available. Upton and Amatruda[91] purified ACTH from at least three separate tumors. Although the ectopic hormone behaved chromatographically identically to pituitary ACTH, different amino acid compositions were noted. Of interest was the fact that threonine and isoleucine were present in the ectopic hormone despite their absence in human pituitary ACTH. Minor contamination of the preparation could also account for these results, however. Of interest was that ACTH activity was also noted in fractions of higher molecular weight.[91]

3. Immunologic Assays—Antibodies to the pituitary hormone have been shown to neutralize the activity of ectopic ACTH.[89] More specific studies of the characteristics of the ectopic molecule have been done with antisera

directed against the amino (N)-terminal or carboxyl (C)-terminal portions of the molecule.[92] Similar cross-reactivity of ectopic ACTH N-terminal and C-terminal antisera was noted, but there was an excessive amount of C-terminal reactivity. Whether this resulted from a fragment of degraded hormone or an entirely separate biologically inactive peptide molecule could not be determined. Biologic activity was generally in good agreement with N-terminal activity. Ratcliffe *et al.*[93] also showed dissociation between N-terminal and C-terminal activity.

4. "Big" ACTH (pro-ACTH)—A form of ACTH considerably larger than the 39 amino acid pituitary peptide ("little" ACTH) has been described by Yalow and Berson[94,95] as the predominant form of ACTH in the plasma of patients with the ectopic syndrome. Big-ACTH had minimal biologic activity but could be converted to active or "little" ACTH by trypsinization.[96] On gel filtration (Sephadex G50) big-ACTH eluted right after the void volume, while little-ACTH eluted much later. Normal pituitary ACTH was predominantly in the little form, with a small peak at the position of big-ACTH. This was in striking contrast to tumor extracts from patients with and without Cushing's syndrome which contained predominantly big-ACTH with an elution peak of immunoreactive hormone right after the void volume. In a carcinoma of the lung, the primary tumor contained 60 percent or more big-ACTH, the lymph node metastasis 75 percent or more, and liver metastasis 80 percent or more.[95] In other tumors, the range of big-ACTH was between 35 and 70 percent. The striking finding was the ubiquitous presence of immunoreactive ACTH in both primary and metastatic tumors of patients without clinical evidence of ectopic Cushing's syndrome, whereas the incidence of ACTH in tumors other than those of the lung was much lower. Control studies showed no evidence for other peptide hormones such as growth hormone, parathyroid hormone, and gastrin. The suggestion that ACTH production by lung tumors might be much more common than previously appreciated has also been made by Knight *et al.*[97] and Hauger-Klevene.[98]

   Excessive quantities of big-ACTH in the tumor tissue could result from deficiencies in the enzyme responsible for converting "big" hormone to "little," abnormalities in the packaging of precursor or enzyme, or other factors in the tissue which could act as inhibitor of conversion.[96] Big-ACTH is also the predominant form of the hormone in the circulation of these patients and excludes the possibility that preferential release of "little" hormone is an etiologic factor in the identification of "big" hormone tissue extracts. Orth *et al.*[99] did not find evidence of big-ACTH in their studies, but their extraction techniques and cation-exchange chromatography procedures may have excluded big-ACTH from the preparation. Furthermore, there is some question whether their antisera were capable of recognizing the "big" form of the hormone. The association of ACTH with lung tumors, regardless of histologic type, does not exclude the notion that neuroendocrine bronchial cells are responsible for the production of the hormonal material. Dysplastic bronchial cells are frequently encountered in lungs with carcinomas of most if not all variants, and such dysplastic cells have proven capable of aberrant secretory activity.[59,90] These intriguing observations suggest that serum assays, particularly those combined with gel filtration, might be potentially useful as a tumor screening procedure.[94–96] And since dysplastic changes in the bronchial mucosa also had increased production of ACTH, screening of serum from individuals with precancerous lesions might prove useful as an early diagnostic aid.[59,90,96] The lack of clinical Cushing's syndrome in the majority of patients with ectopic ACTH productions can readily be explained by the fact that these tumors largely produce and contain big-ACTH, which has minimal or no biologic activity and is a glycoprotein.

   In a more recent report from the same investigators, Ayvazian *et al.*[100] noted increased concentration of ACTH in the plasma of 21 of 24 patients with untreated lung cancer, and the hormone was detectable in extracts of tumor or bronchial washings from the remaining three. Elevations were found in only 10 of 38 treated patients. In the 5 patients who had prolonged survival, there was low plasma ACTH after surgery, or the patients had no elevations in ACTH before therapy. All carcinomatous tissue, primary and metastatic, from lung carcinoma patients had ACTH, while normal lung or tumors metastatic to the lung did not contain ACTH. In a group of patients with chronic obstructive lung disease who had moderately elevated concentrations of ACTH, 3 patients with the highest hormone concentrations subsequently developed carcinoma. The survival of most of the patients was less than 14 months, and the authors suggested that the tumors must be large, have a higher than minimally detectable hormone concentration, or be more active in secretion than the normal pituitary gland for elevated concentrations of hormone to become detectable.[100] This reduces the likelihood that the tumor marker characteristics of the hormone assay would lead to earlier diagnosis. On the other hand, the assay may be useful in determining the efficacy of treatment. Furthermore, the presence of big-ACTH in bronchial washings may eliminate the necessity to do thoracotomy for diagnostic biopsy. This may help to differentiate between primary and metastatic lesions to the lungs. Recent studies by Odell et al[100a] have confirmed the results of Gerwirtz and Yalow[90] and suggested, moreover, that ACTH may be present in a wide variety of nonpulmonary neoplasms as well.

5. Peptides with Corticotropin-Releasing Factor (CRF) Activity—Although Upton and Amatruda[91] recently described the presence of peptides with CRF-like activity in the tumors of patients with ectopic ACTH syndrome, a variety of indirect observations had suggested that such peptides might be found. Christy[101] described 2 patients with ectopic ACTH syndrome who responded to the adrenal inhibitor metyrapone, suggesting that such tumors enhanced pituitary ACTH secretion by "unknown means." Landon *et al.*[102] noted stimulation of steroid production by vasopressin and hypoglycemia in a patient with the ectopic ACTH syndrome and suggested that CRF peptides might be released. Two patients with ACTH-producing carcinoids were shown to respond to metyrapone and partly to suppression by dexamethasone.[103] In the report by Upton and Amatruda,[91] four peptides with CRF-like activity were identified, two each from pancreatic tumors and an oat cell carcinoma of the

lung. The peptides were purified to homogeneity and were shown to be devoid of direct adrenal-stimulating activity. Their ACTH-releasing activity in the rat was comparable to vasopressin, but there was no antidiuretic activity. Amino acid analyses indicated that the peptides were different from ACTH. Their findings have helped to explain the response of some patients with the ectopic syndrome to metyrapone, and suggest that these tumors produce factors that not only stimulate the adrenal gland but also cause secretion of ACTH from the normal pituitary (Fig. 139-5). Two of the peptides were active in vivo and in vitro, and the other two only in vivo. Imura *et al.*[104] recently studied six tumors from patients with the ACTH syndrome and found CRF-like activity in all of them. These studies were performed by an in vitro pituitary incubation method, but the details were not described, and controls for vasopressin activity were not provided.

6. Production of ACTH in vitro—Hirata *et al.*[105] recently performed extensive studies in vitro on tumor tissues from 4 patients with ectopic ACTH syndrome. These included three tumors of the lung (two malignant carcinoids and an undifferentiated carcinoma) and a tumor of the stomach (malignant carcinoid). All but one of the patients lacked classical features of Cushing's syndrome and showed, instead, muscle weakness, edema, hypertension, hypokalemia, and glycosuria. Variable responses in the physiologic activity of these tumors were noted during incubations in vitro. Release of ACTH by one or more of the tumors in response to extracts of rat median eminence, norepinephrine, cyclic AMP, and dibutyryl cyclic AMP were noted. In one tumor, biogenic amines, norepinephrine, and serotonin caused increased production of tissue cyclic AMP without increasing the release of ACTH. These findings led to speculation on the possible dissociation of adenyl cyclase receptors and hormone release or altered tumor receptors as suggested by Shorr *et al.*[106,107] Incorporation of radioactive amino acids into two tumors showed that the labeled hormone was predominantly or exclusively big-ACTH.[105] This protein was devoid of biologic activity but could be converted to little-ACTH by trypsin.

The variable responses of the tumors to regulators of adenyl cyclase production and hormone release suggest that some of our concepts of tumor autonomy in the ectopic ACTH syndrome may have to be revised. Production of CRF-like material by ectopic tumors suggests that normal hypothalamic and pituitary functions can be modulated by the tumor, whereas the findings in the in vitro studies suggest regulation by the tumor itself. The response to dexamethasone or metyrapone by tumors may be more common than already suggested. Because of the infrequent application of the radioimmunoassay for ACTH to serum measurements in such patients in response to stimulators or suppressors of ACTH secretion, further investigation is needed. In recent studies involving short-term culture studies of human placental fragments, Genazzani *et al.*[108] suggested the production of a protein with ACTH-like immunoreactivity in the radioimmunoassay but with a different standard curve. Whether this material (human chorionic corticotrophin) has a molecular weight similar to big-ACTH was not determined.

CLINICAL CHARACTERISTICS

Most patients with the ectopic ACTH syndrome do not have the classical clinical features of Cushing's syndrome.[89] Even though they have very high levels of ACTH and cortisol in the blood, the signs and symptoms may be subtle. It has been argued that the excess cortisol must be present for several years in order to produce the classical physical abnormalities of Cushing's syndrome; furthermore, the catabolic effects of malignant tumors (see above) may also be responsible for aspects of the clinical presenta-

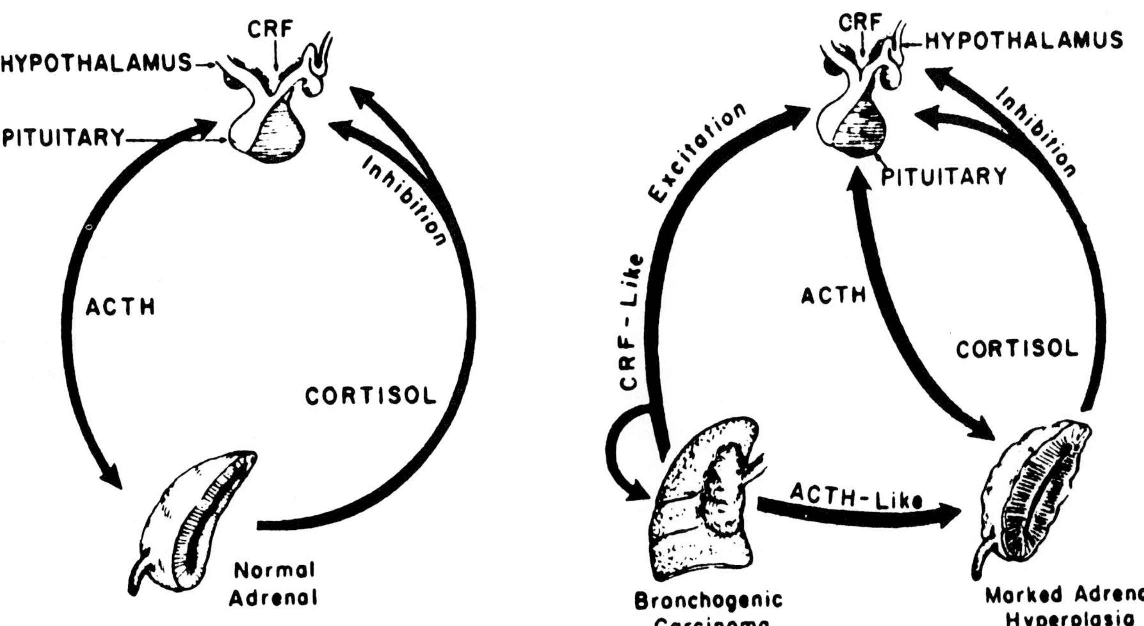

Fig. 139-5. Comparison of the normal feedback relation (left-hand side) with an ectopic ACTH-producing neoplasm (right-hand side). (From Amatroda, T. T., and Upton, G. Evidence for the presence of tumor peptides with corticotropin-releasing-factor-like activity in the ectopic ACTH syndrome. New Engl. J. Med. 285: 419, 1971. Reprinted, by permission.)

tion. Common among the major physical abnormalities in patients with this disorder are the following:

1. Weight loss, in contrast to classical Cushing's syndrome in which weight gain, centripetal obesity, and livid striae are common
2. Generalized muscle weakness, related to hypokalemic alkalosis, steroid myopathy, and carcinomatous neuropathy and/or myopathy
3. Hyperpigmentation, related to high levels of ACTH as well as tumor production of MSH
4. More frequent appearance in males, in contrast to pituitary Cushing's disease which is more common in women
5. Peripheral edema, related to mineralocorticoid effects of cortisol
6. Hypertension
7. Polyuria, polydipsia, and other manifestations of glucose intolerance
8. Hirsutism and acne in some cases
9. Pulmonary congestion
10. Lymphadenopathy or evidence of obstruction of superior vena cava
11. Signs and symptoms of lung or other tumors including metastatic disease

LABORATORY DIAGNOSIS OF ECTOPIC ACTH SYNDROME

1. Routine laboratory tests
   a. Unexplained hypokalemic alkalosis, particularly when observed in the absence of diuretics, is more common than in patients with pituitary Cushing's disease and suggests ectopic Cushing's syndrome or primary aldosteronism.
   b. Abnormal glucose tolerance.
2. Hormonal measurements
   a. Elevated levels of plasma cortisol without diurnal variation.
   b. Elevated levels of urinary 17-hydroxysteroids and 17-ketosteroids and urinary free cortisol. Extraordinarily high levels of both 17-hydroxy and 17-ketosteroids are noted due to the very high levels of ACTH. The selective increases of 17-ketosteroids, which tend to be noted in adrenal carcinoma, are not noted in this syndrome.
   c. Hyperresponsiveness to ACTH administration.
   d. Response to metyrapone: not usually present but several reports have appeared in the literature (see above).
   e. Dexamethasone suppression (both low-dose and high-dose) is usually absent. Because of CRF-like peptide production, partial suppression might theoretically occur in some. This has been noted particularly with thymomas and bronchial carcinoids.[101–103,109,110]
   f. Elevated plasma ACTH: although measurable in only a few laboratories, elevated immunoassayable ACTH is the hallmark of the diagnosis. Simple elevation of ACTH, however, does not differentiate absolutely between ectopic and Cushing's disease due to pituitary hormone excess. The levels of the ACTH in the ectopic syndrome are, in general, higher than those in pituitary disease. With the recent studies of Gewirtz and Yalow,[96] elevation of the ACTH both in the blood and in the tumor tissue, particularly of the "big" variety, is a much more frequent hallmark of the disorder than previously suspected. Increases may be noted even in patients without clincial or biochemical evidence of Cushing's syndrome. The degree and frequency of elevation of "big" ACTH in the serum and tumors of patients with both pulmonary and nonpulmonary tumors needs much additional study.
   g. Increased secretion of 5-hydroxyindoleacetic acid: oat cell carcinoma may be extremely difficult to distinguish from carcinoid tumors. A number of tumors have been reported in which production of serotonin as well as ectopic ACTH has been described.[111] This has been particularly true for the bronchial carcinoids and medullary carcinoma of the thyroid.
   h. Occasionally the presence of the syndrome is detected clinically or biochemically even before the tumor becomes apparent in the patient. Since the most likely cause is an oat cell carcinoma of the lung, such a tumor may appear at a later date than the clinical syndrome. Careful examination of chest radiographs and tomograms looking for mediastinal widening, atelectasis, and abnormal densities should be performed. In some cases where the disease was thought to be pituitary in origin, bilateral adrenalectomy was done, with the malignant tumor appearing at a much later date.[112]
   i. Electron microscopy of ACTH-producing tumors shows neurosecretory-type granules and similarities to the carcinoid.[113–116]

THERAPY OF ECTOPIC ACTH SYNDROME

Therapy for patients with the ectopic ACTH syndrome is complex and depends principally on the underlying tumor. Since the most common cause of the syndrome is oat cell carcinoma, the prognosis is usually extremely poor. There have been recent advances in the chemotherapy of this disorder with combination chemotherapy, but the prognosis nonetheless remains grim. A similar outlook is present in those patients with islet cell carcinomas or malignant thymomas, although occasional surgical cures have been described. The prognosis is usually better for patients with pheochromocytoma, paraganglioma, thymoma, or bronchial carcinoid.[89,112,116]

In some cases the major clinical manifestations of the tumor are due to hypercorticism and its effects such as hypokalemia, muscle weakness, and diabetes. Administration of oral or intravenous potassium, sodium restriction, and the administration of spironolactone may be helpful. One might consider bilateral total adrenalectomy in patients where a more favorable prognosis warranted the procedure. Under exceptional circumstances, a primary malignant neoplasm producing ACTH might be removed successfully by surgery.[117] This would also be true for the more benign tumors associated with the disorder. Normally, however, some form of medical management of adrenal steroid production is necessary and can be performed with one or more inhibitors of adrenal steroid biosynthesis or cytolytic therapy. The agents include metyrapone (which blocks the 11-β hydroxylase enzyme converting 11-deoxycortisol to cortisol), aminoglutethimide (which blocks the conversion of cholesterol to pregnenolone) or *o.p.'*, DDD which is an adrenal cytolytic agent. Successful use of metyrapone in the management of ectopic ACTH has been described.[118–120] Double blockade with aminoglutethimide[121,122] in combination with metyrapone may be even more effective. The simultaneous use of *o,p*[1] DDD and the other two agents will result in cytolytic activity while steroid hormone production is being inhibited.

ECTOPIC PRODUCTION OF MELANOCYTE-STIMULATING HORMONE

Hyperpigmentation is a common clinical manifestation in patients with chronic and debilitating illness, especially in gastrointestinal disorders such as sprue, adenocarcinoma, Whipple's disease, etc. Increased pigmentation in these disorders has not been associated clearly with ectopic production of peptides that increase melanocyte activity. On the other hand, the hyperpigmentation frequently associated with the ectopic ACTH syndrome has been, at least in part, associated with the production of melanocyte-stimulating hormone (MSH or MSH-like activity) by the tumors.[89,123] Hyperpigmentation can be produced by large quantities of ACTH because of homologies between the amino terminal end of the ACTH molecule and MSH, as demonstrated clearly by Lerner and McGuire.[124] The same cell that produces ACTH in the normal pituitary is also responsible for producing β-MSH.[125] Shimizu *et al.*[126] demonstrated that tumors contain more MSH activity than can be accounted for by their content of ACTH alone, and that tumor MSH can be separated from ACTH.[127] Extensive studies of the MSH content of tumors were performed by Abe *et al.*[128,129] who noted that less than 5 percent of the biologic MSH-like-activity of human pituitary glands was due to α-MSH and that the tumors also contained a minority of their MSH as α-MSH. Abe *et al.*[129,130] showed that over 95 percent of the biologically active MSH in human pituitary glands and serum was due to β-MSH or a related peptide. Extracts of 11 tumors from patients with the ectopic ACTH syndrome contained material immunologically identical to β-MSH. Some of the biologic MSH-like activity in the tumors could not be accounted for by material identical to β-MSH;[125] this was later shown to be due to ACTH fragments, as both N-terminal and C-terminal fragments in tumor extracts were described by Orth.[125] It is apparent that ectopic tumors may not only produce ACTH and β-MSH but also fragments. Whether the fragments are produced spontaneously or are due to degradation by enzymes will require further studies involving protein synthesis. Isolated production of MSH by tumors has not been reported, and the hyperpigmentation associated with chronic nonmalignant disease has been shown not to be due to MSH.[128,129] Some of the β-MSH activity being measured in the pituitary and plasma may be material of higher molecular weight than the native hormone.[131,132] The normal pituitary gland synthesizes the molecule β-lipotropin (β-LPH) which has 91 amino acids[133] and γ-lipotropin (γ-LPH), which is identical to the 1-58 portion of β-LPH. Since β-MSH corresponds to a sequence in the lipotropin molecule, and since all three peptides have melanotropic properties, antibodies directed against MSH might be measuring other peptides as well. Whether β-MSH in man is derived from cleavage of larger peptides or might be a degradation product of larger molecules during extraction is not yet clear, but the recent studies of Gilkes *et al.*[134] suggest strongly that most of what has been measured heretofore as β-MSH is actually lipotropin activity. Recent studies[134a] suggest that a larger precursor molecule containing the sequence of ACTH as well as lipotropin may be the initial synthetic product in normal tissues as well as tumors. Although specific antibodies to lipotropin molecules have been developed, gel-filtration analyses of immunoreactive components in serum need to be performed. Elevated levels of lipotropin have also been noted by Gilkes *et al.*[134] in the ectopic ACTH syndrome. Hyperpigmentation of Addison's disease has been shown to be largely due to β-MSH or lipotropin.[129] Although metastases to the adrenal gland are not uncommon, the development of hypoadrenalism and secondary increases in ACTH and β-MSH due to metastatic disease are unusual. No satisfactory explanation for the hyperpigmentation in other tumor syndromes is yet available.

ECTOPIC PITUITARY AND PLACENTAL HORMONES

GROWTH HORMONE

Ectopic production of growth hormone (HGH) is one of the less frequently documented hormonal syndromes. Since major fluctuations in plasma HGH in response to exercise, dietary intake and sleep, etc. are observed, it may be difficult to differentiate clinically between HGH production from tumors and increases in secretion related to normal physiologic events.[135] Steiner *et al.*[136] first showed elevated circulating levels of HGH in a patient with a lung tumor; following surgical resection of the adenocarcinoma, immunoreactive HGH in plasma fell from 38 to 3 ng/ml. The patient's symptoms rapidly disappeared but the tumor was not analyzed for growth hormone. Cameron *et al.*[137] reported a similar patient in whom HGH was not elevated, but it failed to suppress normally. The physiologic abnormality was still present after partial resection of an undifferentiated adenocarcinoma of the lung, but the osteoarthropathy was improved. With immunofluorescent antibodies, the tissue showed reactivity for both HGH and human placental lactogen (HPL). Only one of three patients with hypertrophic osteoarthropathy described by DuPont *et al.*[138] had elevated levels of growth hormone. Increased growth hormone concentrations in 7 of 18 bronchogenic and 5 of 8 gastric adenocarcinomas have been reported by Beck and Burger.[139]

More convincing documentation was suggested by the work of Greenberg *et al.*,[140] who showed that growth hormone could be synthesized and secreted from a poorly differentiated large-cell lung tumor in tissue culture, and that there was disappearance of an elevated plasma level of HGH and hypertrophic osteoarthropathy after surgical resection. Cells were maintained in continuous culture for 4 months, and synthesis of HGH in vitro was documented by incorporation of radioactive amino acids into a protein which had similar chromatographic and molecular-weight characteristics to HGH. Release of hormone from the cultured cells was stimulated by activators of the adenyl cyclase system.[140] Whether hypertrophic osteoarthropathy is related directly to HGH or might be associated with some other peptide or substance produced by the tumor is not yet clear. Since the clinical and radiologic manifestations of hypertrophic osteoarthropathy are different from the pure growth hormone excess noted in acromegaly, its relationship has not yet been documented.[141] The tumor concentration of HGH was 190 ng/g compared with adjacent nontumorous lung of 60 ng/g. This is the only report of an ectopic tumor that produced HGH in culture,[140] although both human and animal pituitary tumors have been demonstrated to produce growth hormone continuously in cell culture. There is some evidence that certain tumors may actually stimulate pituitary growth hormone release.[2]

HUMAN PLACENTAL LACTOGEN

Human placental lactogen (HPL) [or human chorionic somatomammotropin (HCS)] is a protein hormone produced by the trophoblastic layer of the placenta which is closely related to HGH in its biologic and immunologic properties,[143] as well as its amino acid sequence.[144] It is representative of the structural homologies that are extensive between placental and pituitary hormones: pituitary ACTH with human chorionic corticotropin; pituitary thyroid stimulating hormone with human chorionic thyrotropin; luteinizing hormone with human chorionic gonadotropin; pituitary growth hormone and prolactin with human placental lactogen. In 1968, Grumbach *et al.*[145] reported increased concentrations of HPL (normally only a female hormone during pregnancy) in the serum of a male with gynecomastia and an anaplastic large cell carcinoma of the lung. The patient's tumor had previously been reported to contain gonadotropin by bioassay.[146] Weintraub and Rosen[147] noted that 11 of 128 patients with nontrophoblastic tumors had elevated levels of HPL. Seven of 64 patients with lung tumors had increased HPL in sera; and of these 7, 5 patients had gynecomastia and increased secretion of estradiol. Of the 5 patients with gynecomastia, 4 also had evidence of increased production of chorionic gonadotropin. In 89 nonneoplastic sera studied by Weintraub and Rosen[147] and in other sera studied by Payne and Ryan,[148] no HPL was noted. Thus, the presence of this protein in nonpregnant serum was truly indicative of a hormone-producing hormone. In some cases, Weintraub and Rosen[147] were only able to detect HPL in the serum after concentration by affinity chromatography. In their normal subjects, even affinity chromatography provided no evidence for the peptide hormone, indicating concentrations of less than 0.002 ng/ml. Of the patients with nontrophoblastic tumors, HPL was detected in 7 with lung tumors (4 undifferentiated, 1 oat cell, 1 adenocarcinoma, and 1 epidermoid tumor) and 1 each with lymphoma, pheochromocytoma, hepatoma, and hepatoblastoma. The series was biased in terms of patients who had gynecomastia; the only other individuals having elevated values of HPL in blood consisted of both male and female patients with trophoblastic tumors. In patients with nontrophoblastic tumors, HPL concentration varied from 0.007 to 14 ng/ml, in the patients with trophoblastic tumors from 3 to 180 ng/ml, and in normal third trimester subjects from 2 to 7 μg/ml. There was a reasonable correlation between the level of HPL in patients with trophoblastic tumors and therapy. The hormone in tissue extracts and plasma behaved identically in the radioimmunoassay to native HPL, but the level was well below that required for lactogenic or somatotropic assay activity in most bioassay systems. The presence of ectopic HPL has been shown to be associated with the production of other placental proteins, such as chorionic gonadotropin and placental alkaline phosphatase. [149,150] The concordance of these three markers in indicating the presence of cancer was described by Sussman *et al.*, [149] who studied sera from 8 patients with nontrophoblastic malignancy. Three sera contained all three marker proteins, three sera contained two of the three markers (alkaline phosphatase and HCG or HCG and HPL), and two sera contained only one marker (alkaline phosphatase or HPL). Concordance of biochemical markers and clinical responses were noted, however, when this was studied in detail.[149,150]

Evidence has accumulated recently that there is a big form of HPL in placental tissue and in the blood of pregnant women[151,152] that is closely related to "big" forms of HGH and prolactin. Further studies have shown this larger material to be a disulfide dimer of the native molecule.[151,152] This may not be a true precursor hormone, but its significance needs to be determined. Further studies of ectopic tumors that produce HPL will have to be examined carefully for the presence of larger forms of the molecule in tumor tissue extracts and in blood.

PROLACTIN

Only in recent years has definite evidence been established for the presence of a distinct prolactin molecule in human pituitary glands and blood.[153] Turkington[154] demonstrated elevated concentrations of prolactin in the serum of a man with undifferentiated carcinoma of the lung and a woman with galactorrhea who had renal cell carcinoma. Following therapy with radiation and nephrectomy, respectively, serum concentrations of prolactin by radioimmunoassay decreased. The renal cell carcinoma was shown to produce prolactin in tissue culture, which was verified by bioassay and neutralized by prolactin antibodies. Measurements of prolactin in the serum of 20 additional patients with carcinoma of the lung failed to show any increase. Rees *et al.*[155] have also identified immunoreactive prolactin in a bronchogenic tumor. A further search for estopic tumors producing prolaction will be initiated as the use of the radioimmunoassay for human prolactin is extended.

GLYCOPROTEIN HORMONES

Gonadotropins

The clinical association between tumors of the lung and gynecomastia was first described[156] in 1915; and ectopic production of gonadotropin has now been associated with abnormalities of the breast. Furthermore, a number of boys with precocious puberty secondary to production of a luteinizing hormone (LH)-like substance have been described by McArthur *et al.*[157] These patients all had other associated abnormalities such as spina bifida occulta and hemihypertrophy of the tongue and extremities. Hepatomegaly in these individuals was assocaited with accelerated growth and virilization, and increased LH activity was demonstrated. At autopsy, the liver revealed a tumor or hepatoblastoma, and the testes showed proliferation of Leydig cells. Ectopic hormone production in these patients could not be suppressed with estrogen therapy.

Gynecomastia is frequently found in adults with malignant disease, especially when they have liver disease or are receiving drugs such as chlorpromazine, digitalis, reserpine, or spironolactone.[157] Gynecomastia has been associated with carcinoma of the lung and sometimes in association with hypertrophic pulmonary osteoarthropathy. Increased estrogen production was reported in 10 patients with carcinoma of the lung,[42] and this may be related to the production of gonadotropin by lung tumors.[146] The presence of increased gonadotropin and gynecomastia may even antedate the appearance of the lung tumor.[158] In this patient, gynecomastia was felt to be due to gonadotropin production with secondary increases in estrogen production. A low content of gonadotropin was measured in the pituitary at autopsy, supporting the concept that gonadotropin production occurred from the tumor.

Faiman *et al.*[161] reported a step up in the arteriovenous concentrations for follicle-stimulating hormone (FSH) across an adenocarcinoma of the lung, providing direct evidence for production of the hormone by the tumor. Although precocious puberty in boys and gynecomastia in men have been the principal syndromes associated with ectopic gonadotropin secretion, levels of chorionic gonadotropin in excess of levels found in the first trimester of pregnancy have been documented in patients without any clinical manifestations.[162] In addition to carcinoma of the lung and hepatoblastoma, tumors of the testis, ovary, pineal gland, mediastinum, adrenal, breast, bladder, and melanoma may be associated with ectopic gonadotropin production.[1,163,164] Two types of gonadotropins are produced by the normal pituitary, FSH, and LH. These glycoprotein hormones have recently been shown to consist of both α and β subunits. The α subunit appears to be similar or identical in these two gonadotropins and thyroid-stimulating hormone, and only slightly modified in human chorionic gonadotropin (HCG). Immunologically, the α subunits are indistinguishable. The β subunit, on the other hand, is different and accounts for hormonal specificity.[165] Assays not only for the intact hormone, but also for the α and β subunits, have been developed and are used in screening as tumor markers (see below). Production of ectopic FSH by tumors is uncommon but has been described by Rosen *et al.*[160]

Estrogen production in men with gonadotropin-producing neoplasms has recently been studied by Kirschner *et al.*[166] Urinary estradiol production rates were elevated in six men with gonadotropin-producing tumors (four with choriocarcinoma and two with tumors of stomach and lung) and were correlated with gonadotropin and tumor mass. The origin of the elevated estradiol was determined by administering dehydroepiandrosterone sulfate (DHEA) intravenously and determining conversion to estradiol; radioactive DHEA was also incubated with tumor tissue. Gonadotropin-producing tumors could convert DHEA sulfate directly to estradiol, indicating that they behave like normal trophoblastic tissue. These findings provide an additional indication that the tumor behaves like placental tissue in that it can carry out the same biochemical function. Other possibilities were that the gonadotropin could stimulate enzyme induction in the testes at the site of estrogen formation or that the gonadotropin could stimulate testicular secretion of estrogen. The latter two were ruled out except for the small possibility that some of the estrogen might be coming from the testis. Trophoblastic tumors also perform many of the same biochemical functions as normal placenta such as secretion of HCG and its β subunit, secretion of HPL, and production of alkaline phosphatase.

Human Chorionic Gonadotropin (HCG)

Chorionic gonadotropin is very closely related biochemically and biologically to LH in the pituitary gland and has been well-recognized as a marker of certain ectopic tumors. Chorionic gonadotropin is generally present in tumors that have trophoblastic characteristics. The giant cell tumors of the lungs, which have been associated with chorionic HCG production, have some histologic similarities to choriocarcinoma.[167] With specific radioimmunoassays which are designed to look at immunologic characteristics of the β subunit, it is now possible to differentiate FSH, LH, and HCG production. This was not previously possible with the use of bioassays, and some of the reports in the literature are confused by these factors. As emphasized by Rudnick and Odell,[57] pregnancy tests should not be used to diagnose and follow the progress of patients with gonadotropin-producing neoplasms since their sensitivity is adequate for pregnancy but not for the ectopic tumor state. A variety of lung tumors can be associated with gonadotropin production including the well-differentiated epidermoid carcinoma, poorly differentiated carcinoma, oat cell tumor, and bronchiolar carcinoma.[168]

Recently, ectopic production of the isolated β subunit of HCG has been described using specific subunit radioimmunoassays.[169,170] Material identical to this protein was found in the serum (300 ng/ml) and tumor extract from a patient with a pancreatic adenocarcinoma.[169] Although it appeared to be heterogeneous, it had β-subunit activity in several assays. No evidence of complete HCG or α subunit was detectable in serum or tumor extracts by radioimmunoassay or bioassay. The patient described demonstrated isolated polypeptide subunit formation, a situation analogous to the dissociated production of α or β chains of hemoglobin in thalassemia or light chains in patients with amyloidosis. The free α and β subunits have little or no biologic activity.[165] Rabson *et al.*[171] described a bronchogenic tumor associated with ectopic production of biologically active HCG in which clonal strains from the tumor in tissue culture produced varying quantities of the subunits.[172] Braunstein *et al.*[173] studied 443 patients with nonneoplastic disorders with a radioimmunoassay measuring both the β subunit and HCG. In these sera he detected neither of these antigens except from three female blood bank donors in whom the possibility of pregnancy could not be excluded. The evidence for isolated β-subunit production implies that the α and β subunits are independently transcribed, but little is known about the mechanism of normal subunit production and assembly to form a complete molecule. Braunstein *et al.*[173] identified HCG-like material in over 7 percent of a large number of sera of patients with malignancy, and they were not able to exclude the possibility that the β subunit was being measured in some. Recent studies by Franchimont[174] and by Rosen and Weintraub[175] suggest that the α subunit may be present in higher-than-normal concentrations in the sera of certain cancer patients. However, unlike the β subunit of HCG, the α and β subunits of LH, FSH, and TSH may not be specific cancer markers since they are components of normally circulating hormones and could be released from normal pituitary or from the peripheral metabolism of the hormone. The patient described by Rosen and Weintraub[176] was a 27-yr-old female with a malignant gastric carcinoid which contained extremely high concentrations of material resembling the α subunit in its immunologic and biologic properties. Isolated production of the α subunit was not accompanied by comparable amounts of β subunit or the complete hormone. This particular tumor also had high concentrations of parathyroid hormone and calcitonin. Significant elevations of α subunit were also noted in 3 of 24 additional patients with carcinoid tumors and 3 of 106 patients with bronchogenic carcinoma. The possibility that isolated subunit production may be a significant tumor marker has been emphasized by a number of workers.[175,176,176a] Kahn et al[126a] noted that the presence of HCG or one of its subunits, particularly α in plasma, was correlated closely with malignancy in islet cell tumors.

Braunstein *et al.*[177] recently described in normal human testis a material that was immunologically related to HCG and could be adsorbed on concanavalin A. Thus, the fetal tissue responsible for production of the hormone during pregnancy may not be suppressed completely in the adult. This provides a plausible explanation for testicular tumors giving rise to HCG, but does not clarify why other tumors may produce these hormones ectopically. Adenocarcinoma of the stomach, ovary, pancreas, and hepatomas are the tumors most commonly associated with ectopic HCG secretion, with the incidence of ectopic HCG secretion ranging between 17 and 40 percent in these selected tumor types.[173,177–181] Yoshimoto et al [177a] reported the widespread appearance of HCG in extracts of carcinoma of the colon, lung, pancreas, and stomach as well as its presence in normal liver and colon (in a form containing little or no carbohydrate). Ectopic hormone synthesis could be a much more prevalent phenomenon than previously appreciated.[100a]

THYROTROPIN (TSH)

Trophoblastic tumors have been associated with a mild form of hyperthyroidism characterized by tachycardia, skin changes, widened pulse pressure, tremor, and goiter.[163,182,183] Odell *et al.*[182] showed that the tumor hormone reacted in bioassays similar to TSH, but that it had little activity in the human radioimmunoassay. Hershman and Starnes[184] described a purified hormone from normal placenta and termed it human placental thyrotropin (HCT), while Hennen[185] isolated a TSH-like factor from an epidermoid carcinoma and noted similarities to TSH by bioassay and immunoassay. A pleural mesothelioma in another patient was shown to be associated with hyperthyroidism.[186] Hershman *et al.*[187] recently showed that HCT and tumor TSH are similar but not exactly identical. Interestingly, HCT reacts poorly in the human TSH immunoassay but reacts reasonably well with antisera against bovine TSH. Although the hyperthyroidism is usually mild, the patients reported by Hershman *et al.*[187] had severe hyperthyroidism, which was improved rapidly after evacuation of the hydatidiform mole. Whether the patients with trophoblastic tumors truly have ectopic syndromes is questionable, but the patients with mesothelioma and epidermoid carcinoma of the lung fit that category. The molar thyrotropin described by Hershman *et al.*[187] was higher in molecular weight than chorionic thyrotropin, had a longer duration of action, and was immunologically different. Testicular choriocarcinoma in association with hyperthyroidism has been described.[188] It has been suggested that chorionic thyrotropin may in fact be HCG.

VASOPRESSIN (ADH)

The association of malignant disease and inappropriate secretion of antidiuretic hormone (ADH) is now recognized frequently. A possible connection between the tumor and production of ADH was described by Winkler and Cranshaw[189] when they noted increased excretion of sodium in some cases of lung cancer, but no definite suggestion of a hormonal link was made. In 1957, Schwartz and colleagues[190] reported 2 patients with bronchogenic tumors who excreted concentrated urine containing large quantities of sodium despite the fact that they had severe hyponatremia. The authors suggested correctly that the water and electrolyte disorder was due to inappropriate secretion of ADH, but they suggested that the tumor stimulated secretion of ADH by the posterior pituitary. Additional data concerning the relationship to the tumor was provided by Thorn and Transbol[191] who showed the presence of large quantities of antiduiretic hormone in the urine of such a patient. Definitive evidence was provided by Amatruda *et al.*,[192] who showed evidence of ADH-like material in extracts of an oat cell carcinoma. Subsequently, a number of workers have reported ADH in extracts of tumor with values ranging from 4 to 750 μU/mg dry tumor.[193–196] In 1967, Bartter and Schwartz[197] reported an additional 12 patients with the hyponatremic syndrome and indicated that an ADH-like substance in tumor extract behaved in the immunoassay like vasopressin. Most of the reports are from carcinoma of the lung (particularly oat cell carcinoma)., but the syndrome has also been described in duodenal and pancreatic carcinoma.[89] Twenty-eight of 38 reported cases have been oat cell carcinoma of the lung, 7 being due to anaplastic carcinoma. The other 3 cases have been mucin-secreting adenocarcinomas of the lung and pancreas.[1,89]

The concentrations of ectopic ADH have been too small to permit purification and structural characterization, but the hormone behaves immulogogically like arginine vasopressin and indirect evidence suggests that it is very similar to the human hormone.[196] Certain properties of ectopic ADH make it similar to pituitary ADH,[89] as follows:

1. Inactivation by thioglycolate which disrupts the disulfide bond
2. Persistence of biologic activity similar to arginine vasopressin after the purification procedure
3. Similar behavior chromatographically on IRC-resin
4. Affinity for neurophysin
5. Susceptibility to inactivation by oxytocinase
6. Immunologic similarities to arginine vasopressin
7. Inactivation by vasopressin antibodies
8. Synthesis of vasopressin by bronchogenic carcinoma in vitro[198]

Release of ADH by tumor tissue in culture has also been described by Martin *et al.*[199] in an anaplastic carcinoma of the uterus from a patient with hyponatremia.

Since extraction of ADH from the tumors has been obtained and the hormone synthesized in vitro in tumor tissue by at least two investigators, it is clear that tumor production of hormone is at least one mechanism that accounts for the inappropriate ADH syndrome. However, a number of other causes exist:

1. Metastases to the hypothalamus stimulating the production of ADH[200]
2. A mediastinal or thoracic tumor affecting volume receptors and stimulating ADH secretion
3. Renal tubular defects in association with tumors, leading to natriuresis[201]
4. Central nervous system infections such as tuberculosis, basilar meningitis, or complicating tumors
5. Cerebrovascular disease
6. Subdural hematoma
7. Systemic illnesses such as polyneuritis, systemic lupus erythematosus, and pulmonary infection
8. Administration of certain drugs such as chlorpropamide, tolbutamide, vincristine, and morphine
9. Excessive use of cigarettes (?bronchial epithelial dysplasia)
10. Pain, trauma, and emotional stress

These and other factors must all be considered in the patient with malignancy who is noted to have inappropriate ADH secretion.[202] The hallmarks of the syndrome are hyponatremia, persistently concentrated urine in the face of hyponatremia, a low BUN, and the absence of peripheral edema. Although the syndrome is characterized by excessive secretion of ADH, it will not be expressed unless there is intake of significant water parenterally or orally. In a patient who has excessive secretion of hormone, the syndrome is not demonstrable clinically when fluid intake is restricted. Administration of diphenylhydantoin (500 mg iv in 5 min) has been shown to correct the inappropriate antidiuresis of many disorders, but it has no effect when it is due to a neoplasm. Therapy for the inappropriate ADH syndrome is usually accomplished by fluid restriction below 1 liter (for more severe cases below 500 mgl/day). Fluid restriction does not remove the source of the ADH, but it controls the clinical manifestations. The actual quantity of fluid retained in these patients is approximately 3 to 4 liters.

The clinical findings in the severe syndrome include symptoms of water intoxication and complications such as anorexia, nausea, vomiting, headache, fatigue, confusion, pseudobulbar palsy, and ultimately coma if the serum sodium is low enough.[197] Although treatment by fluid restriction is usually successful, hypertonic saline may occasionally be helpful in severely hyponatremic states. Hantman *et al.*[203] suggested that intravenous furosemide with hypertonic saline may produce negative water balance while conserving sodium and potassium. Other recent approaches to the treatment of inappropriate ADH syndrome include the use of lithium[204] and dimethylchlortetracycline.[205]

Hamilton *et al.*[206] reported that neurophysin may be produced by some tumors from patients with the syndrome. Neurophysin is a normal protein component of the posterior hypothalamus which is responsible for binding oxytocin and vasopressin, and its release is elevated by stimuli that caused the release of two hormones.[207,208]

PLACENTAL ENZYMES

Tumor proteins may not lead to any clinical or biochemical abnormality in the patient but may be useful as a marker for disease. This is characteristic of proteins such as enzymes or antigens produced by tumor tissue which give a clue to the presence of a neoplasm, but do not cause any clinical manifestations. The alkaline phosphatase enzyme of the placenta not normally found in adult men or nonpregnant women has been well described in a number of tumors by Stolbach *et al.*[209] The tumors producing ectopic alkaline phosphatase were primarily from the lung,[209] but other tumors were also reported. The alkaline phosphatase produced by the ectopic tumor tends to be the placental-type enzyme, which is heat-stable and can be distinguished as a separate enzyme. In 50 nonneoplastic sera, no evidence of placental alkaline phosphatase was identified by Sussman *et al.*[149] With increasing testing for various proteins by tumors, it is likely that the usefulness of such disease markers will be extended.

TUMORS AND HYPOGLYCEMIA—ECTOPIC PRODUCTION OF HYPOGLYCEMIC SUBSTANCES

Although the association of tumors with hypoglycemia is well documented, the pathogenesis of the hypoglycemia in these patients is not so clear. There are two major causes of fasting hypoglycemia associated with tumors: (1) insulin production by islet cell tumors, and (2) production of hypoglycemia from extrapancreatic tumors by other mechanisms. Although they may be clinically indistinguishable, separation can often be achieved by various laboratory studies and measurements. Other factors associated with fasting hypoglycemia include severe liver disease, hypopituitarism, hypothyroidism, hypoadrenalism, and decreased glucagon reserve. Islet cell tumors will not be discussed except in relation to multiple endocrine neoplasia (see below). The extrapancreatic tumors associated with hypoglycemia can be separated into several groups which will be defined below. To date, more than 180 such patients have been reported.[1,210]

1. Large mesenchymal or mesodermal tumors in the abdomen and thorax (42 percent): These tumors may be retroperitoneal, intraperitoneal, or intrathoracic. They are frequently large and include fibrosarcomas, mesotheliomas, neurofibromas, neurofibrosarcomas, spindle cell sarcomas, rhabdomyosarcomas, and leiomyosarcomas. They range in weight from 800 to 10,000 g, are frequently benign, and symptoms are alleviated by their removal.
2. Hepatocellular carcinoma or hepatoma (22 percent)
3. Adrenal cortical cell carcinoma (9 percent)
4. Pancreatic and bile duct (10 percent)
5. Miscellaneous tumors of lung and ovary, neuroblastoma, hemangiopericytoma and Wilm's tumor (17 percent)

Very few of these patients have had increases in serum insulin reported, although there are occasional reports.[211–215] In the patient reported by Unger *et al.*[212] immunoreactive insulin and glucagon were demonstrated at autopsy in the tumor, but there was no evidence confirming hypoglycemia during life. The report by Saeed *et al.*[213] suggested the presence of insulin or insulin-like activity on immunofluorescent staining of the tumors. Shames *et al.*[214] showed evidence of a bronchial carcinoid tumor which was histologically very similar to an islet cell tumor of the pancreas and may have been histologically related. The more recent report of Lyall *et al.*[215] showed no evidence of immunoreactive insulin in extracts of the tumors and no β-type secretory granules, but the patient had a clear increase of insulin in the basal state. Following removal of the tumor, glucose returned to normal and the authors suggested the possibility that the tumor might be stimulating insulin and possibly suppressing glucagon secretion. Recent ultrastructural studies of several retroperitoneal sarcomas associated with hypoglycemia failed to reveal secretory granules. Thus, there is no definite evidence that the hypoglycemia associated with extrapancreatic tumors is due to insulin production.

On the other hand, these tumors can clearly produce insulin-like activity (ILA), which can be demonstrated by stimulation of glucose uptake in vitro in bioassays using rat diaphragm or adipose tissue.[210] Insulin activity in serum normally consists of both immunoreactive insulin (which can be neutralized by specific antibodies) and nonsuppressible insulin-like activity (NSILA-s) which is capable of accomplishing in vitro biologic effects and cannot be neutralized by insulin antibodies. The latter substance is immunologically distinct from insulin and probably represents a different peptide or peptides.[216] There is recent evidence suggesting that NSILA-s may be related to one or more of the somatomedin peptides that are produced in the liver of animals in response to growth-hormone administration. The possibility that NSILA was related to somatomedins was suggested when it was noted that somatomedin could be extracted from plasma by an acid ethanol extraction method similar to that used for purification of NSILA-s.[217] Purification of the somatomedins has been recently accomplished[218] (see Chapter 140).

Megyesi *et al.*[219] recently developed a radioreceptor assay for NSILA-s and suggested increases in the concentration of this substance in the serum and tumor extracts of patients with the extrapancreatic hypoglycemic syndrome. Somatomedins increase the degradation of ^{14}C-glucose to carbon dioxide in epididymal fat pads and are antilipolytic substances. Marks *et al.*[210] extracted no insulin but found increased ILA in the serum of patients with Hodgkin's lymphoma, amelanotic melanosarcoma, and a fibrosarcoma. Additional studies concerning the nature of the peptide or peptides produced by these tumors clearly need to be done, but the recent studies suggesting production of NSILA-s somatomedins are highly suggestive and need to be continued.

It is likely that no single mechanism accounts for the hypoglycemia tumor syndrome. Various mechanisms may be responsible in patients with different tumors. Table 139-1 lists the possible causes of hypoglycemia in these patients.

Some years ago, Unger reviewed possible tumor mechanisms causing hypoglycemia[220] and suggested that evidence for overutilization of glucose by the tumors was limited. There is evidence for a high rate of glycolysis by tumors, and the large size

Table 139-1. Possible Causes of Hypoglycemia in Patients with Tumors

1. Production of insulin by the tumor
2. Production of NSILA-s or another somatomedin by tumor
3. Excessive glucose consumption by the tumor because of size
4. Production of metabolites which interfere with gluconeogenesis (e.g., tryptophan)
5. Acquired glycogen storage disease—noted with hepatocellular carcinoma
6. Malnutrition
7. Chemotherapy
8. Release of an insulin-secreting substance from the tumor
9. Suppression of counter-regulatory hormones or mechanisms

of such tumors could possibly contribute to excessive glucose utilization. Attempts have been made to answer the question by August and Hiatt,[221] who found an arteriovenous difference of 41 mg/100 ml across the tumor bed, but a glucose infusion was running at the time of measurement. Butterfield[222] noted no measurable glucose difference across a tumor bed. Critical review of the literature suggests that glucose utilization by the tumor itself in the absence of deficient counter-regulatory mechanisms is probably not sufficient to account for hypoglycemia,[220] particularly since the compensatory response by the normal liver is capable, at least temporarily, of a fivefold increase in glucose production. McFadzean and Yeung[223] made observations on the etiology of hypoglycemia with heptocellular carcinoma. They divided their patients with hypoglycemia and hepatocellular carcinoma into two groups, one of which seemed to have abnormally stable glycogen in liver tissue. They suggested from their histologic and other observations that an acquired form of glycogen storage disease due to mechanical and other factors in the liver might be part of the hypoglycemic syndrome.

The differential diagnosis between islet cell tumors and nonislet tumors is not difficult. The hallmark of the islet cell tumor is the presence of fasting hyperinsulinemia and/or proinsulinemia in the presence of low blood sugar. Plasma free fatty acids and lactate tend to be elevated in patients with extrapancreatic tumors, while they are correspondingly low in patients with islet cell tumors. The prognosis in these patients is generally related to the tumor type. The large retroperitoneal mesenchymal tumors, although huge, are often slowly growing and tend to be of a relatively low order of malignancy.

Amelioration of the hypoglycemia may result from partial or complete resection. Agents such as diazoxide, which may be extremely useful in treating islet cell tumors,[224] are of limited use in the nonpancreatic tumors. Sometimes these patients require, during the hypoglycemic attacks, continuous intravenous and oral glucose. The symptoms they manifest are related to the acuteness and severity of the hypoglycemia. Occasionally high doses of glucocorticoids to stimulate gluconeogenesis, long-acting glucagon, and streptozotocin may be helpful.

ECTOPIC PRODUCTION OF PARATHYROID HORMONE AND OTHER CALCIUM-MOBILIZING SUBSTANCES

The association of malignant disease with hypercalcemia is well recognized, frequent, and often of clinical importance. A number of potential mechanisms are responsible for this metabolic abnormality:

1. Direct invasion of bone by tumor: Particularly true of tumors that metastasize commonly to bone such as carcinoma of the lung, breast, kidney, and thyroid; prostatic carcinoma that metastasizes to bone usually causes osteoblastic metastases which are not associated with hypercalcemia
2. Production of parathyroid hormone (PTH) or PTH-like substance by tumor
3. Production of other bone-mobilizing substances such as prostaglandin or osteoclast activating factor
4. Coexistence of tumor with primary hyperparathyroidism: A disorder with a prevalence rate[225] of almost 1 per 1000
5. Coexistence with another cause of hypercalcemia: Vitamin D intoxication, sarcoid, hyperthyroidism, immobilization, adrenal insufficiency, etc
6. Administration of estrogen or androgen to a patient with carcinoma of breast metastatic to bone

The differential diagnosis of hypercalcemia of unknown etiology can usually be accomplished on clinical grounds. The principal difficulty at times is in differentiating between primary hyperparathyroidism and a latent malignant disorder. Osteolytic lesions must be greater than 1 cm in size to be observed radiographically.[226] The accuracy of diagnosis is improved markedly with isotopic bone scans, and core bone marrow biopsy may be a significant aid in diagnosing metastatic disease to bone. Compounding this difficulty in differential diagnosis at times is the frequency of hyperparathyroidism, which may coexist with other causes of hypercalcemia.

The association of malignancy and PTH production by tumors was first suggested in a discussion by Albright in a clinicopathologic conference at the Massachusetts General Hospital.[227] The patient was a 51-yr-old male with renal cell carcinoma associated with hypercalcemia and hypophosphatemia. Neck exploration revealed three normal parathyroid glands, and a large osteolytic lesion in the ileum was irradiated with improvement in the serum calcium and phosphorus. Although bioassay tests at that time were negative, it was suggested by Albright that the tumor might be exerting its metabolic effects by producing a PTH-like substance.[227] Plimpton and Gellhorn [228] popularized the association when they reported 10 additional patients with tumors and hypercalcemia. Four patients had renal cell carcinoma, and in 3 patients resection of the tumors was associated with return of the serum calcium to normal. Connor *et al.*[229] described 2 patients with lung cancer and hypercalcemia, one of whom developed hypercalcemia associated with tumor recurrence.

The first evidence for ectopic production of a PTH-like substance was suggested by Goldberg *et al.*,[230] who reported a positive assay for PTH in a renal carcinoma and its metastases, using the indirect technique of complement fixation inhibition.[231,232] More definitive evidence using a radioimmunoassay for PTH was provided by Sherwood *et al.*,[233] who quantitated the presence of a PTH-like substance in four carcinomas of the lung, an undifferentiated parotid tumor, an adrenal carcinoma, and a histiocytic lymphoma (reticulum cell sarcoma). PTH in these tumors varied from 0.75 to 8.93 ng bovine equivalent per gram dry weight, and the molecular weight of the tumor hormone by sucrose density gradient analysis was similar to that of bovine PTH. In a report by Knill-Jones *et al.*[234] an arteriovenous gradient of PTH across the tumor bed of a carcinoma of the bile ducts was demonstrated. The elevated concentrations of hormone in blood fell to normal after partial hepatectomy. The increased concentration in hepatic veins confirmed the production of hormone by the tumor.

Although an increase in immunoreactive PTH in blood suggests the presence of an ectopic hormone producing tumor, it does not differentiate readily production of hormone by the tumor from coexistent hyperparathyroidism unless selective catheterization across a tumor bed is done. A recent study by Riggs *et al.*[235] suggests that the hormone produced by ectopic tumors may be less immunoreactive than the hormone produced by normal parathyroid glands. Using their radioimmunoassay, they suggest that primary hyperparathyroidism and ectopic hyperparathyroidism can be differentiated. The differences in activity of the two substances in their assay could be related to:

1. Production of an altered polypeptide by the tumor
2. Secretion of an intermediate form or precursor from the tumor tissue
3. Abnormal metabolism of the hormone in serum or tissues
4. Release of additional factors which might affect the radioimmunoassay

More detailed studies of 6 patients with ectopic hyperparathyroidism[236] examined the molecular weight of immunoreactive serum fractions on gel filtration. They accounted for the decreased immunoreactivity of PTH in the blood of patients with the ectopic syndrome by identifying smaller quantities of carboxyl-terminal fragments in these patients in comparison with patients with primary hyperparathyroidism. Carboxyl-terminal fragment(s) have recently been shown to be the major form of circulating PTH.[237] Although the carboxyl-terminal fragment is not biologically active, Benson *et al.*[238] suggested that there was enough intact hormone circulating to account for the production of hypercalcemia. They also suggested the possibility that there might be even larger forms of hormone in the blood of patients with the ectopic syndrome. Elevated levels of PTH in patients with malignancy and hypercalcemia occurred with high frequency in these studies. This data must be reexamined in relation to new evidence suggesting that production of calcium-mobilizing substances other than PTH by such tumors may be common.

With the use of selective catheterization it is possible to determine the site of production of PTH when hypercalcemia and elevated levels of PTH are present. It was useful in identifying a renal cell carcinoma as the source of PTH production in a study by Blair *et al.*[239] The application of selective catheterization for patients with primary hyperparathyroidism has been well recognized.[240,241] Additional confirmation that ectopic tumors produce PTH was provided by the in vitro studies of Tashjian,[142] who showed that a tumor associated with ectopic PTH production released the hormone for months in tissue culture. Hartman *et al.*[242] showed that a squamous cell carcinoma synthesized a peptide similar to but not necessarily identical with human PTH.

Although the association of tumor with hypercalcemia in the absence of skeletal metastasis suggests the presence of PTH production by the tumor,[243] recent studies suggest that this is not always the case. One of the authors (LMS)[244] discussed a patient with squamous cell carcinoma of the lung associated with hypercalcemia. The patient had no skeletal metastasis on radiographic as well as postmortem examination, but the hypercalcemia could not be explained by the presence of PTH or a related substance in the tumor. Possibilities included destruction of tumor hormone in the postmortem tissue or the presence of some other substance which might be responsible for the association. Subsequently, Powell *et al.*[245] described 11 patients with tumors associated with hypercalcemia, low serum phosphorus, and the absence of demonstrable bony metastases. In these patients, therapy with surgery, radiation, or chemotherapy reversed the hypercalcemia. Bone resorption was subsequently demonstrated in tumor extracts from 3 patients using an in vitro mouse calvarium bioassay. Despite the evidence for a bone-mobilizing substance in tumor tissue, all radioimmunoassays for PTH or related substances were negative in extracts of the tumor and in the peripheral blood.

The nature of bone-mobilizing substances in these tumors is now becoming more clear, as recent evidence suggests that tumors may be producing active prostaglandins. This is consistent with observations in an experimental model in a mouse sarcoma in which Tashjian and his colleagues provided substantial evidence to support this hypothesis.[246]

The first clinical evidence for production of prostaglandins by a tumor was provided by Brereton *et al.*[247] when they described a patient with hypernephroma and hypercalcemia who responded to treatment with indomethacin. Elevated concentrations of prostaglandins E and F were identified in metastases to the liver from the tumor. Robertson *et al.*[248] reported a patient with hypernephroma and hypercalcemia, elevated concentrations of PGE in plasma, and low levels of PTH. Ito *et al.*[249] described a third patient with hypernephroma who had hypercalcemia responsive to indomethacin, but there were no measurements of prostaglandin. More extensive documentation was provided by Seyberth *et al.*,[250] who examined 29 patients with solid tumors, 14 of whom had hypercalcemia. In their control group were 6 patients with hypercalcemia and malignant hematologic disorders and 6 patients with primary hyperparathyroidism. Elevated levels of PGE_M, a metabolite of prostaglandin E_1 and E_2, were noted in the urine of 12 of 14 hypercalcemic patients, and there were only modest elevations in 7 of the 15 patients with a normal serum calcium. No abnormalities in the metabolite were found in control subjects, and PTH in the patients with hypercalcemia was undetectable. A variable response was noted in response to treatment of hypercalcemia with inhibitors of prostaglandin synthesis. The patients examined included 10 with carcinoma of the lung, 2 with adenocarcinoma of the pancreas, and 2 with adenocarcinoma of unknown etiology. Although these studies did not establish clearly whether the tumor or some other tissue was the source of the prostaglandin, they confirmed the relationship between hypercalcemia and postaglandin production. Further studies are necessary to establish more definitively this relationship.

In addition to the mouse sarcoma, an experimental tumor in the rabbit (VX_2 carcinoma) regularly induces hypercalcemia in the absence of bony metastases. In this animal model, thyroparathyroidectomy does not effect the ability of the tumor to induce and maintain hypercalcemia, and evidence has now accumulated that the VX_2 tumor produces a prostaglandin that is responsible for the hypercalcemia.[246,251] Evidence to support the etiology of hypercalcemia from prostaglandins in these animal models is the presence of hypercalcemia in the absence of metastases, the increased content of bone-resorbing activity and PGE_2 in tumor tissues, the release of PGE_2 and bone-resorbing activity into tissue culture media from these tumors, decreases in production of prostaglandin in cell culture and in vivo with indomethacin, parallel decreases in calcium and PGE_2 with indomethacin, increased concentrations of PGE_2 in tumor venous drainage, and production of hypercalcemia by infusion of prostaglandins.

A new bone-resorbing factor called osteoclast-activating factor (OAF) has been obtained from human lymphocytes by Luben *et al.*[252] This substance is a soluble mediator of resorption which has been identified in supernatant fluid from peripheral human leukocytes grown in tissue culture in the presence of antigen or phytomitogen. In an organ culture bioassay system, both stimulated actively osteoclastic resorption from fetal rat bones. It is of low molecular weight (less than 25,000) but has not yet been purified to homogeneous form; it may actually exist in two molecular forms. Activity has also been found in supernatant fluid from cultured lymphoid cell lines in patients with multiple myeloma, Burkitt's lymphoma, and one malignant lymphoma, but not from normal subjects or patients with other neoplasms.[253] The activity could be distinguished from prostaglandins PTH, and vitamin D-like compounds, and was sensitive to inhibition by glucocorticoids. Thus, it appears that hypercalcemia in patients with multiple myeloma and certain lymphomas might be explainable on this basis rather than PTH or prostaglandins.

On clinical grounds alone it may be extremely difficult to differentiate among patients with malignancy and hypercalcemia to determine whether they are producing PTH, prostaglandin, OAF, or even other substances. The suggestion several years ago that certain tumors might be associated with production of vitamin D-like osteolytic sterols has not held up to further scrutiny. The only discriminatory clinical features are the relationship of OAF production to myeloma and lymphoma, and prostaglandins to renal and lung tumors, although they have been reported with a wide variety of other neoplasms. Definite response of hypercalcemia to indomethacin or aspirin therapy also points to prostaglandin production.

Clinical observations that support the concept of production of hypercalcemia by a tumor substance are as follows:

1. Absence of skeletal metastases
2. Hypophosphatemia (does not differentiate from primary hyperparathyroidism)
3. Normal parathyroid glands at surgery or at postmortem
4. Return to normocalcemia after surgical extripation, radiation therapy, or chemotherapy
5. Recurrence of hypercalcemia associated with tumor recurrence

Specific measurements of PTH or one of the other substances is necessary in order to make more definitive determinations. Radioimmunoassays for the prostaglandins have now become available, and the PTH assay is reasonably well established. A radioimmunoassay for OAF will depend on purification of the substance.

The following tumors have been associated with ectopic production of PTH, although it has not been confirmed by immunoassay in all:

1. Lung: squamous cell carcinoma
2. Genitourinary: renal cell, bladder, testis, penis, adrenal, ovary, uterus, including cervix, vulva, breast, lymphoma
3. Gastrointestinal: colon, esophagus, pancreas, liver, and biliary
4. Parotid
5. Melanoma and other epidermoid

Lafferty[243] suggested certain features that may be helpful in differentiating patients with primary hyperparathyroidism from those with ectopic production of bone-mobilizing substances. These are general points and not by any means precise. The patient with severe hypercalcemia is more likely to have a malignancy, and the presence of alkaline phosphatase elevation in the absence of radiologic changes suggestive of osteitis fibrosa cystica also suggest a malignant cause.

The management of hypercalcemia can be divided into the management of acute hypercalcemic crisis and the elimination of etiologic factors responsible for chronic hypercalcemia.

ECTOPIC PRODUCTION OF CALCITONIN

The radioimmunoassay for calcitonin in serum has recently been developed, and Silva *et al.* reported 2 patients with ectopic secretion of calcitonin from oat cell carcinoma of the lung.[254] In 1 case production of calcitonin was documented by a high level of calcitonin (5400 pg/ml) present in the thymic vein draining the tumor. A high concentration of hormone was noted in the other tumor (200 ng/g wet weight of tissue). Both patients had normal serum calcium concentrations despite the production of calcitonin by the tumor. This is not dissimilar from patients with medullary carcinoma of the thyroid who produce large amounts of calcitonin, but generally have a normal serum calcium.[255] Other patients with ectopic production of calcitonin have been described in more recent reports.[256–258] In some cases of lung carcinoma, it has not been clear whether the calcitonin is being produced by the tumor or normal thyroid tissue. Ectopic production of calcitonin may be more common than previously appreciated.

ECTOPIC PRODUCTION OF ERYTHROPOIETIN

The kidney is known to be the principal source of erythropoietin, the hormone that stimulates red blood cell production. A variety of benign as well as malignant disorders of the kidney may be associated with increased production of erythropoietin; these include hypernephroma and benign conditions such as renal cysts and hydronephrosis. Elevated erythropoietin associated with non-neoplastic renal disease also suggests that dysplastic cells may be capable of hormon production. Strictly speaking, production of erythropoietin by a renal tumor is not an ectopic syndrome but rather a manifestation of the normal function of the organ. In other situations, ectopic production of this hormone may be associated with lesions such as cerebellar hemangioblastoma (21 percent), uterine fibroma (6 percent), adrenal cortical tumors (3 percent), ovarian neoplasms (3 percent), hepatomas (3 percent), and pheochromocytoma (1 percent).[1] More than half of the patients with excess erythropoietin production have malignant renal tumors or benign renal conditions.[259] Polycythemia occurs in 2 to 5 percent of patients with renal neoplasms and 9 to 20 percent of patients with cerebellar hemangioblastomas. Recent studies involving the synthesis and release of erythropoietin in vitro by renal tumors have confirmed the production of this hormone by renal tumors.[260] The production of hormone by the tumor does not necessarily correspond to polycythemia in the patient, as the presence of a malignancy may interfere with the polycythemic response. Detection of elevated levels of erythropoietin has depended principally on somewhat cumbersome bioassay techniques, as availability of purified hormones with development of a radioimmunassay for this substance has not yet been feasible on a large scale. With the potential development of radioimmunoassay for erythropoietin, it is likely that larger numbers of patients with excess erythropoietin will be described. Like other ectopic syndromes, detection of a biochemical marker may or may not be associated with physiologic effects in the patient. In addition to secretion of erythropoietin by tumors, it is also probable that some tumors produce thrombopientin[261] and also possibly leukopoietin or colony-stimulating factor.

MISCELLANEOUS SYNDROMES ASSOCIATED WITH ECTOPIC HORMONE PRODUCTION

RENIN-SECRETING TUMORS

A number of patients have been reported who have had hypertension associated with production of renin by tumors. These have principally been tumors of the kidney, particularly tumors of the juxtaglomerular apparatus. Wilm's tumor, and renal cell carcimona, but it has also been described in at least 1 patient with oat cell carcinoma of the lung.[262–265] Since the juxtaglomerular cell is normally the site of origin for renin, this could not be considered a truly ectopic syndrome; when produced form clear cell carcinoma or tumors outside the kidney, the designation of ectopic syndrome would be justified. Although some of these patients had severe hypertension, hypokalemia, increased peripheral vein renin activity, and secondary aldosteronsim, this is by no means consistent; in some patients, only mild hypertension has been noted. Intravenous pyelography has not always shown the tumors because of their small size, and selective arteriography as well as renal vein renin assays to show the step-up in production of renin in the kidneys may be necessary. The differential diagnosis for the patient with hypertension requires excluding malignant hypertension or renal vascular hypertension, which would also be associated with excessive amounts of renin. Increased production of renin has been shown by these tumors in vitro in tissue culture. Recent studies of renin in normal and tumor tissues has shown the presence of a higher molecular weight form of renin which is much less active biologically and which is present in some human plasmas, tumor extracts, and amniotic fluid, but not in normal plasma or kidney extracts. It is believed that some tumors may be associated with the production primarily of the larger form of renin.[266]

PRODUCTION OF PROSTAGLANDIN

In the section on hypercalcemia and tumors, production of prostaglandin E by animal and human tumors was described. In a recent report, production of prostaglandin A from an anaplastic renal tumor was associated with antihypertensive activity.[267] This patient developed severe hypertension after removal of the tumor and developed hemiparesis 1 yr after operation. Preoperatively, elevated levels of PGA (8.05 ng/ml) were found in the plasma, which were markedly reduced postoperatively to the normal range. It is likely that this and other instances of prostaglandin production by tumors may be associated with ectopic syndromes. With increased availability of the radioimmunoassays for prostaglandins A, E, and F, further syndromes are likely to be reported.

OSTEOMALACIA AND HYPOPHOSPHATEMIA

More than 30 patients have been reported who have had profound hypophosphatemia associated with tumors, and these are frequently associated with osteomalacia.[268] These patients had profound phosphaturia which was the cause of the osteomalacia and was reversible by removal of the tumor. Normal concentrations of parathyroid hormone have been found, and these tumors have included mesenchymomas, pleomorphic sarcomas, neurofibromas, sclerosing or cavernous hemangiomas, and a giant cell tumor of the rib. The etiology of the phosphaturia is uncertain, but a recent study suggests the possibility of decreased renal 1-α hydroxylase activity.[268a]

FETAL PROTEINS

Production of proteins normally found in fetal life has been associated with certain neoplasms.[269] The two principal antigens have been α fetoprotein associated with liver tumors and carcinoembryonic antigen associated with carcinoma of the bowel. Neither antigen has proven to be completely specific, and a discussion of their significance is beyond the scope of this chapter.

NERVE GROWTH FACTOR AND EPIDERMAL GROWTH FACTOR

A nerve growth factor which has prominent effects on sympathetic and sensory ganglia is produced by the normal mouse. Neuroblastoma cells in the mouse have been shown to produce nerve growth factor, and it is likely that certain human tumors if examined might do the same.[270] The same may be true of epidermal growth factor, whose structure is known but whose function is uncertain.

ALTERED HORMONE RECEPTORS

In addition to producing abnormal protein substances, a tumor might develop abnormal protein receptors in the course of its growth and development. This situation has been identified in an adrenal tumor of the rat which developed receptors to inappropriate hormones. In addition, to responding to ACTH, the adenyl cyclase enzyme of the rat adrenal tumor was stimulated by thyrotropin, luteinizing hormone, follicle-stimulating hormone and β-adrenergic agonists.[106,107]

MULTIPLE HORMONE PRODUCTION

Many of the patients described in the literature have had production of more than one ectopic hormone by a single tumor. These have been outlined in some detail in the sections dealing with specific neoplasm. In addition to ACTH, some tumors, for example, may produce melanocyte-stimulating hormone, gastrin, glucagon, parathyroid hormone, antidiuretic hormone, serotonin, and/or epinephrine.[271] Moreover, the production of multiple hormones may be asynchronous,[33] and individual hormone production may be periodic.

MULTIPLE ENDOCRINE NEOPLASIA

The popular designation of multiple endocrine adenomatosis (MEA) should be abandoned in favor of the term multiple endocrine neoplasia (MEN) since many neoplasms in the various groups are capable of clinically malignant behavior by pathologic criteria (medullary carcinomas of the thyroid, islet cell carcinomas, etc.).[78] The multiple endocrine neoplasia syndromes are familial disorders associated with pluriglandular abnormalities. They are included in a chapter on ectopic hormone syndromes since they have relationships with the ectopic syndromes, particularly with regard to their possible derivation from neuroectodermal cells. Since some aspects of individual hormone syndromes will be reviewed in other chapters, the descriptions here will focus on general and genetic aspects rather than on all aspects of the diagnosis and management of particular endocrine disorders.

EMBRYOLOGY

The organs involved in the multiple endocrine neoplasia syndromes include the pituitary, parathyroid, thyroid, pancreas, adrenal, and nervous system. In an earlier section, there was extensive discussion of the potential neuroectodermal origin of peptide-secreting endocrine glands. Although the membership of the parathyroid in the APUD system remains controversial, the proposal of Weichert[74] for the common origin of these endocrine glands is useful in explaining many aspects of the multiple endocrine neoplasis syndrome. The capacity of widely scattered neuroendocrine cells to develop peptide hormone-producing tumors makes it tempting to speculate that multiple endocrine neoplasia could be a dysplastic development of the neuroectoderm. The occasional association of neuroendocrine neoplasms with diseases such as von Recklinghausen's and Hirschsprung's has been discussed previously. With the caveats suggested earlier for the origin of all peptide-secreting cells from neuroectoderm, reservations concerning this hypothesis must be maintained. Nevertheless, the consistency of endocrine patterns makes such a proposal of potential interest.

The more common variety of the syndrome (type I) involves lesions of the anterior pituitary gland, parathyroid, and pancreatic islet, and, less commonly, other sites. The carcinoid syndrome can also be associated with this abnormality. Type II multiple endocrine neoplasia, or that associated with pheochromocytoma and medullary carcinoma of the thyroid, is more logically explained on a neuroectodermal basis. The adrenal medulla is clearly of neural crest origin, and the studies of Pearse[67,69] strongly suggest the neuroectodermal origin of the cells that give rise to the calcitonin-secreting medullary carcinoma of the thyroid. Weichert[74] suggested that the neuroectodermal origin of type II gives support to the concept that all peptide-secreting endocrine glands involved in the genetic syndromes are of neuroectodermal origin.

The pituitary gland is derived from two separate primordia, the posterior portion being an outgrowth of the diencephalon which becomes the hypothalamus and is of neuroectodermal origin. The anterior pituitary, on the other hand, is derived from Rathke's pouch which is not endoderm from the foregut but ectoderm anterior to the stomal plate.[74] This does not relate the anterior pituitary clearly to neural crest tissue but does not preclude the presence of neuroectodermal cells derived from another site. The origin of pancreatic islet cells from neuroectoderm has been open to question by recent embryologic findings.[81,82]

The genetic aspects and site of origin of the endocrine disorders in these syndromes have been well defined. The disorders are inherited by an autosomal dominant mode of an inheritance with a high degree of penetrance, variable expressivity, and pleiotropic expression in multiple organs. Manifestions in any individual family tend to be similar.

HISTORICAL ASPECTS

The disorder was first appreciated by pathologists in 1903 when Erdheim[272] discussed a patient with acromegaly who on postmortem examination was found to have four enlarged parathyroid glands in addition to an eosinophilic tumor of the pituitary. The association with pituitary adenomas was recorded by Cushing and Davidoff in 1927.[273] Clinical descriptions of multiple endocrine "adenomas" were initiated by Rossier,[274] who reported a family in which both male and female members had evidence of pluriglandular disease and peptic ulceration. The authors suggested the possibility of a familial disease at that time, but they did not have definitive evidence. A similar clinical report was made by Shelburn and McLaughlin.[275]

The modern era of interest in multiple endocrine adenomatosis includes reports of families by Wermer[276] and Moldawer *et al.*[277] Wermer first proposed that the syndrome was a genetic disorder and suggested a dominant autosomal gene with a high degree of penetrance. Although originally thought to be a separate disorder, the Zollinger-Ellison syndrome or association of peptic ulcer with non-β islet cell tumor is now thought to be a variant of type I multiple endocrine neoplasia.[278] Zollinger-Ellison syndrome and multiple endocrine neoplasia are therefore phenotypic variants of the same pleiotropic gene.

CLINICAL DISORDERS

Although the original reports were of disorders primarily of the pituitary, parathyroid, and islet cell, it has now become clear that there is more than one genetic disorder associated with endocrine tumors. Steiner *et al.*[279] suggested classification into two types based on clinical criteria. This classification is now generally held, although additional variants have recently been suggested. Since the affected organs may show abnormalities which include hyperplasia, adenoma, or carcinoma, Steiner *et al.*[78,279] have suggested the term multiple endocrine neoplasia (MEN), rather than multiple endocrine adenomatosis.

MULTIPLE ENDOCRINE NEOPLASIA, TYPE I

MEN, type I, includes patients whose manifestations involve principally the parathyroid glands, pancreatic islets, and pituitary, although disorders of the adrenal and thyroid glands and bronchial and intestinal carcinoid tumors and lipomas have been included in the syndrome. The clinical presentation and manifestations are protean, depending on the organs involved and whether or not the adenomas are functioning. An extensive review of 85 patients published by Ballard *et al.*[280] provides much of our current knowledge concerning the occurrence of various abnormalities. The following disorders were present in the 85 patients in their review:

1. Parathyroid gland hyperfunction in 74 of 85 patients (84 percent) was the most frequent endocrine disorder. In more than half, chief cell hyperplasia affected multiple parathyroid glands. This contrasted sharply with the low incidence of multiple parathyroid gland involvement in primary hyperparathyroidism. Renal and bone complications were infrequent.
2. Pituitary lesions were reported in 55 of 85 patients (64.9 percent), with the clinical picture generally being pituitary hypofunction and less commonly acromegaly (15 patients).
3. Pancreatic tumors were described in 69 patients (81.2 percent), were almost always multiple, and involved both β and non-β cells. About 36 percent of patients with pancreatic tumors had hypoglycemia, while other patients had atypical ulcer disease or watery diarrhea.
4. Adrenal cortex was involved in 31 patients (37.6 percent) and included cortical adenomas, hyperplasia, multiple adenomas, and nodular hyperplasia, although clinical findings were few. In only one instance was there evidence of hyperaldosteronism, and there was no Cushing's syndrome in this series.
5. Thyroid disease were present in 15 patients (18.8 percent) and included 2 patients with thyrotoxicosis and 1 patient with thyroid carcinoma. In the other patients, there were nonfunctioning adenomas, colloid goiter, or Hashimoto's thyroiditis. Simultaneous occurrence of pituitary and thyroid disease occurred in 12 of 15 patients.
6. Interstitial cell tumor of the testis was noted in 1 patient. Gonadal insufficiency was present in patients with pituitary disease.
7. Peptic ulcer was documented in 49 of 85 patients (57.6 percent), was multifocal in more than half, and often atypical in location. Complications of ulcers occurred in over 70 percent of patients. Complex ulcer disease was more common in patients with non-β-cell pancreatic tumors, and gastric acid hypersecretion was documented in many. Symptoms of peptic ulcer and its complications were more common than any of the endocrine manifestations in the clinical presentation of these patients.
8. Diarrhea was present in 11 patients who had large watery stools. Steatorrhea was present in 4.
9. Bronchial carcinoids were described in 4 patients.
10. Lipomas, frequently multicentric, were present in 11 patients.

The frequent case reports that appeared in the period 1950 to 1970 clearly established the close relationship between the Zollinger-Ellison syndrome and endocrine neoplasia. Between 20 and 40 percent of patients with Zollinger-Ellison syndrome have evidence of multiple endocrine tumors of a familial nature.[280] Extensive descriptions of the pathology of the tumors are given in the Ballard report and are not pertinent to the current discussion. Wermer[281] described the disease spanning several generations and proposed that the genetic mechanism was an autosomal dominant gene with mosaic pleiotropism. According to his proposal, the multiple organs, although different in function and structure, exhibit similar abnormalities of adenomatous or excessive growth, and he suggested that the cells of these organs have a specific factor that makes them responsive to the mutant change. In the series of Ballard *et al.*, [280] 33 patients came to autopsy, the most frequent cause being complications of peptic ulcer, but others died of hypoglycemic coma, pancreatic or brain surgery, carcinomatosis (islet cell), or metabolic abnormalities. In the Ballard series, the most frequent combinations included 22 patients with parathyroid, pancreatic, and piutitary disease with peptic ulcer, 14 patients with parathyroid and pancreatic disease with peptic ulcer, 12 patients with parathyroid, pancreatic, and pituitary disease, 11 patients with pituitary and pancreatic disease, and 10 patients with parathyroid and pituitary disease.

Depending on the functional state of the endocrine tissues in multiple endocrine neoplasia, patients may have hypopituitarism, acromegaly, hypogonadism, hyperparathyroidism, hypoglycemia, Cushing's syndrome, hyperthyroidism, carcinoid syndrome, and atypical or severe peptic ulcer disease. Glandular involvement may be simultaneous or it may asynchronously involve different tissues over the span of many years. The patients with Zollinger-Ellison syndrome have been shown to produce gastrin from the tumor. This was first identified in tumor tissue extract by Gregory,[282] but elevated levels of gastrin by radioimmunoassay in these patients were finally demonstrated.[283] Patients under 10 yr of age tend not to be affected with the manifestations of the syndrome.[284]

Interrelationships of hypergastrinemia and hyperparathyroidism have been noted in that individuals with the two disorders tend to secrete more gastrin when they have hyperparathyroidism.[285] In the series by Snyder *et al.*,[286] 14 of 46 patients had elevated levels of gastrin. Six of the patients had intractable peptic ulcer, while 8 had asymptomatic elevations and 12 of the patients with hypergastrinemia had a history of findings compatible with hyperparathyroidism. It was the recommendation of the authors that parathyroid surgery should precede surgical treatment for the ulcer disease, which in many cases means total gastrectomy.[286] Attempts to remove non-β islet cell tumors are only rarely successful.[287] In one interesting recent report[288] it appeared that gastrin production might be coming from parathyroid tissue. A recent follow-up report of 26 patients with Zollinger-Ellison syndrome treated by total gastrectomy showed good results even when metastatic tumor was present.[288] Zollinger-Ellison syndrome is ordinarily not familial, but when present the patient should be examined for other endocrine tumors, and relatives should be examined for the presence of familial disease. The islet cell tumors in these patients tend to grow extremely slowly, and therefore patients may survive for many years even with metastatic disease.[289] Evidence has been provided that the gastrin produced by Zollinger-Ellison tumors may in some cases be predominantly big gastrin.[290,291] Recent use of cimetione and other H_2 blockers has facilitated medical treatment of the ulcer disease.

A comprehensive review of the problems associated with management of patients with islet cell tumors has recently been published.[292] The authors reviewed the tumors of three cells, the β cell giving rise to insulinoma, the non-β cell producing Zollinger-Ellison syndrome, and other tumors associated with pancreatic cholera which may be producing a secretin-like peptide. They emphasize that total gastric resection is the treatment of choice for the Zollinger-Ellison syndrome while a direct resection of tumor is the major form of therapy for other islet cell neoplasms. Current management of patients with malignant islet cell disease includes the use of chemotherapeutic agents such as streptozotocin and L-asparaginase. Said and Faloona[293] recently developed a radioimmunoassay which reportedly measures vasoactive intestinal peptide (VIP), which they have studied in patients with pancreatic cholera or watery diarrhea. VIP was suspected as the hormone producing this syndrome since it stimulates intestinal secretion of water and electrolytes, enhances production of cyclic AMP, inhibits gastric acid secretion, dilates blood vessels, and elevates the serum calcium. In their studies, 26 of 28 patients with watery diarrhea had elevated levels of VIP, and increased amounts were found in 13 tissue extracts. However, others have not yet confirmed their findings. A fourth type of islet cell tumor has been described in association with glucagon production, mild diabetes, and a curious bullous necrolytic rash whose etiology is unclear.[52] A fifth type producing somatostatin has also been described in two patients.[293a,b] (For further discussion of endocrine tumors of gastrointestinal origin see Chapter 135.)

MULTIPLE ENDOCRINE NEOPLASIA, TYPE II

A second group of familial multiple endocrine disorders has been characterized by the association of a different set of tumors. This syndrome is distinct from MEN, type I, and tends to include tumors of the thyroid (medullary thyroid carcinoma), pheochromocytoma (singular, bilateral, or multiple), and parathyroid glands (chief cell hyperplasia).

In 1961, Sipple[294] noted the association of pheochromocytoma with carcinoma of the thyroid. In a subsequent report, Williams [295] identified 15 patients in the literature, added 2 of his own, and demonstrated that the thyroid cancer was a unique type known as medullary or solid type cancer which contained amyloid stroma. Subsequently, more than 250 patients with medullary carcinoma have been reported, and there have been a number of cases involving combinations of medullary cancer with other endocrine abnormalities. [255,296] Some of these reports have involved the association of thyroid cancer and pheochromocytoma with parathyroid hyperplasia, mucosal neuromas, Marfan's syndrome, and megacolon.

Steiner *et al.*[279] suggested that this group of patients be classified as MEN, type II, and in their report described a kindred which had 25 patients with pheochromocytoma, 5 with medullary thyroid carcinoma, 2 with parathyroid hyperplasia, and 1 with Cushing's syndrome. This group of disorders is genetically distinct from MEN, type I. Steiner *et al.*[279] reviewed 85 reported cases of familial pheochromocytoma, 20 of whom had hyperparathyroidism. MEN, type II, is also inherited as an autosomal dominant with high penetrance and variable expressivity, although many patients with nonfamilial disease have been described. The pheochromocytomas are characteristically bilateral and multiple, and have been described in up to 70 percent of patients with the familial syndrome. In patients with medullary thyroid carcinoma and pheochromocytoma, over 70 percent had bilateral pheochromocytoma whether the patients had sporadic or familial disease. Although familial pheochromocytoma is less common than the sporadic disease, families of patients who present with the disorder should be investigated for the possibility of a genetic syndrome. The manifestations of the adrenal tumor tend to occur in the third and fourth decades of life, and the disease in the familial variety occurs with about equal frequency in both sexes. Both sustained and intermittent hypertension has been noted, although the intermittent variety is more common. Neurofibromatosis and von Hippel-Lindau disease have been noted in association with both familial and sporadic pheochromocytoma.

Medullary carcinoma of the thyroid produces the hormone calcitonin and will not be discussed further as it is reviewed in another chapter. The diagnosis of medullary carcinoma has been facilitated markedly by the use of the radioimmunoassay for calcitonin, particularly after the infusion of calcium or gastrointestinal hormones. [297] Even microscopic tumors may be picked up by the calcitonin assay, which has had a high rate of success in detecting affected relatives of patients with medullary carcinoma of the thyroid. The technique has even been of value in picking up premalignant hyperplastic changes in the thyroid gland.[298] These changes were multicentric but demonstrated as an anatomically restricted increase in C-cell numbers. In addition to calcitonin, medullary carcinoma of the thyroid has been shown to produce histaminase, prostaglandins, serotonin, and an ACTH-like substance.[299] In the family described by Keiser *et al.*,[296] 25 patients had medullary carcinoma of the thyroid, 16 had parathyroid disease, 11 had pheochromocytoma and 6 patients had all three diseases. The screening procedure used by this group included measurement of calcium, phosphorus, alkaline phosphatase, histaminase, and calcitonin, 24-h urine collection for catecholamine metabolites; and measurement of calcitonin under basal conditions and after calcium infusion. Only individuals above 5 yr were screened, although the syndrome was not present in any under 5 yr. In the patients with pheochromocytoma and parathyroid hyperplasia or adenoma, thyroid carcinoma was uniformly present; if pheochromocytoma and hyperparathyroidism were present, there was a high likelihood of bilateral pheochromocytomas (84 percent).

Considerable attention has been focused on the fact that this group of patients also has neurologic abnormalities which include mucosal neuromas, marfanoid habitus, hyperplastic corneal nerves, and sometimes intestinal disorders such as ganglioneuromatosis and megacolon. It has been suggested recently by at least two authors that a third group of patients with multiple endocrine neoplasia be defined, variously called type III,[300] or multiple endocrine adenomatosis, type IIB.[301] The patients with the MEN, type IIB or III syndrome would be characterized as those with medullary thyroid carcinoma, pheochromocytoma, and associated abnormalities such as mucosal neuromas and hyperplastic corneal nerves.[301,302] It has become apparent from further familial studies that the syndrome of neuromas with pheochromocytoma and thyroid cancer is a distinct nosologic entity. The hallmark of this group is the presence of the neurologic abnormalities and the *very low* incidence of parathyroid disease (parathyroid disease being much more common in Sipple's syndrome or type IIA).

Patients with MEN, type III, when reviewed in 1975, consisted of 41 patients of whom 19 were male and 22 female.[300] About half showed the complete syndrome of multiple neuromas, bumpy lips, pheochromocytoma, and medullary carcinoma; 7 percent showed neuroma and pheochromocytoma and medullary carcinoma; and the remainder had a combination of neuromas, bumpy lips, and thyroid carcinoma. The most interesting and unusual manifestation were the neuromas, which appeared in all 41 subjects and were largely around the lips, tongue, and eyelids. Microscopically, the neuromas are due to masses of convoluted nerves surrounded by a thick perineurium without a capsule. They have much less connective tissue than the neurofibromas classically found in von Recklinghausen's disease. Because of the presence of neuromas, both lips are frequently diffusely enlarged and "bumpy." The abnormalities may be present at birth and may also be associated with thickened eyelids. Slit-lamp examination of the cornea may show hypertrophied corneal nerves. Involvement of the gastrointestinal tract with individual neuromas or diffuse intestinal ganglioneuromatosis was detected by surgery, rectal biopsy, or postmortem examination in 14 patients. Some had persistent diarrhea, but other gastrointestinal disorders included diverticulosis, megacolon, intestinal hypertrophy, and abnormal gastric motility. The diarrhea of patients with medullary carcinoma of the thyroid is complex and could conceivably involve neuromatous involvement of bowel or possibly the production of serotonin, prostaglandin, or other components. Marfanoid habitus was noted in 26 patients. It was characterized by a slender body build with a small amount of body fat and poor development of musculature. The extremities were long and thin, and increased joint flexibility was noted. Other abnormalities such as kyphosis, pectus abnormality of the chest, pes cavus, and high arched palate may be noted. None of the patients had ectopia lentis or aortic aneurysms in contrast to true Marfan's syndrome, and some had marked muscular wasting suggestive of myopathy. Like patients with MEN, type II, these patients may have decreased intradermal response to histamine, suggesting histaminase production.[301,302]

The low incidence of parathyroid disease is characteristic of MEN, type III. Whereas this occurred in over 50 percent of people with MEN, type II, only 1 patient of 41 had parathyroid disease in the series by Khairi *et al.*[300] This tends to refute the concept that calcitonin is a cause of the parathyroid hyperplasia. This was also established in the genetic studies by Melvin *et al.*,[297] who showed that some family members had normal circulating levels of calcitonin associated with parathyroid hyperplasia (suggesting parathyroid disease as an independent genetic variable). Type III is also inherited as a dominant trait, although the majority of individuals with this syndrome have been reported as isolated cases. Of interest is the recent observation that calcitonin may occasionally be produced both from mucosal neuromas and from pheochromocytomas in patients with MEN, type II or III.[302]

ACKNOWLEDGMENT

The expert technical assistance of Mrs. Nicolina Keil Litteria in the preparation of this chapter is gratefully appreciated.

REFERENCES

1a. Amatruda, T. T., Jr. Non-endocrine secreting tumors. In Bondy, P. K. (ed.): Duncan's Diseases of Metabolism. New York, Academic, 1973, pp. 1629–1650.

1b. Odell, W. D. Humoral manifestations of non-endocrine neoplasms In William's Textbook of Endocrinology. Williams, R. H. (ed.) New York, Saunders, 1974, pp. 1105–1116.

1c. Bower, B. F., and Gordan, G. Hormonal effects of non-endocrine tumors. *Ann. Rev. Med. 16:* 83, 1965.

1d. Lipsett, M. D., Odell, W. D., Rosenberg, L. E., and Waldman, T. A. Humoral syndromes associated with non-endocrine tumors. *Ann. Int. Med. 61:* 733, 1964.

2. Hall, T. C. (ed.) Paraneoplastic syndromes. *Ann. N.Y. Acad. Sci. 230:* 1, 1974.

3. Bodel, P. T., and Atkins, E. Human leukocyte pyrogen producing in rabbits. *Proc. Soc. Exp. Biol. Med. 139:* 690, 1972.

4. Atkins, E., Feldman, J. D., Francis, L., and Hursh, E. Studies on the mechanisms of fever accompanying delayed hypersensitivity. The role of the sensitized lymphocyte. *J. Exp. Med. 135:* 1113, 1972.

5. Rawlins, M. D., Luff, R. H., and Cranston, W. I. Pyrexia in renal carcinoma. *Lancet 1:* 1371, 1970.

6. Bodel, P. Tumors and fever. *Ann. N.Y. Acad. Sci. 230:* 6, 1974.
7. Theologides, A. The anorexia-cachexia syndrome: A new hypothesis. *Ann. N.Y. Acad. Sci. 230:* 14, 1974.
8. Terepka, A. R., and Waterhouse C. Metabolic observations during the forced feeding of patients with cancer. *Am. J. Med. 20:* 225, 1956.
9. Stevenson, J. A. F., Box, B. M., and Szlavko, A. J. A fat mobilizing and anoretic substance in the urine of fasting rats. *Proc. Soc. Exp. Biol. Med. 116:* 424, 1964.
10. Rudman, D., Del Rio, A. E., Garcia, L. A., Barnett, J., Howard, C. H., Walker, W., and Moore G. Isolation of two lipolytic pituitary peptides. *Biochemistry 9:* 99, 1970.
11. Davis, J. G. Food intake following broad mixing of hungry and satiated rats. *Psychol. Sci. 3:* 177, 1965.
12. David, J. D., Gallagher, R. J., and Ladore, R. S. Inhibition of food intake by humoral factor. *J. Comp. Physiol. Psych. 67:* 407, 1969.
13. Theologides, A. Pathogenesis of cachexia cancer. A review on the hypothesis. *Cancer 29:* 484, 1972.
14. Gold, J. Metabolic profiles in human solid tumors. *Cancer Res. 26:* 695, 1966.
15. Gold, J. Cancer cachexia and gluconeogeneis. *Ann. N.Y. Acad. Sci. 230:* 103, 1974.
16. Waterhouse, C. How tumors affect metabolism. *Ann. N.Y. Acad. Sci. 230:* 86, 1974.
17. Reed, D. M. On the pathological changes in Hodgkin's disease with special reference to its relations to tuberculosis. *Johns Hopkins Rep. 10:* 133, 1902.
18. Aisenberg, A. C. Studies on delayed hypersensitivity in Hodgkin's disease. *J. Clin. Invest. 41:* 1964, 1972.
19. Hersh, E. M., and Oppenheim, J. J. Impaired *in vitro* lymphocyte transformation in Hodgkin's disease. *N. Engl. J. Med. 273:* 1006, 1965.
20. Keller, W. D., Lamb, D. L., and Varco, R. L. Investigation of Hodgkin's disease with respect to the problems of homotransplantation. *Ann. N.Y. Acad. Sci. 87:* 187, 1960.
21. Ultmann, J. E., Cunningham, J. K., and Gellhorn, A. The clinical picture of Hodgkin's disease. *Cancer Res. 26:* 1047, 1966.
22. Harris, J., and Copeland, D. Impaired immuno-responsiveness in tumor patients. *Ann. N.Y. Acad. Sci. 230:* 56, 1974.
23. Glasgow, A. H., Nimberg, R. B., Menzoian, J. O., Saporoschetz, I., Cooperband, S. R., Schmid, K., and Mannick, J. A. Association of anergy with an immunosuppressive peptide fraction in patients with cancer. *N. Engl. J. Med. 291:* 1263, 1974.
24. Sjogren, H. O. , Hellstrom, I., Bansal, S. C., and Hellstrom, K. E. Suggestive evidence that the "blocking antibodies" of tumor bearing individuals may be antigen-antibody complex. *Proc. Natl. Acad. Sci. U.S.A. 68:* 1372, 1971.
25. Friou, G. J. Current knowledge and concepts of the relationship of malignancy, auto-immunity, immunologic disease. *Ann. N.Y. Acad. Sci. 230:* 23, 1974.
26. Dawkins, R. L., Eghtedari, A., and Holborow, E. J. Antibodies to skeletal muscle demonstrated by immunofluorescence in experimental autoallergic myositis. *Clin. Exp. Immunol. 9:* 329, 1971.
27. Morgan, G. E., Peter, J. B., and Newbould, B. B. Experimental allergic myositis in rats. *Arthritis Rheum. 14:* 599, 1971.
28. Currie, S., Saunder, M., and Knowles, M. Immunological aspects of polymyositis: The *in vitro* activity of lymphocytes on incubation with muscle antigen and with muscle cells in culture. *Q. J. Med. 157:* 63, 1971.
29. Dawkins, R. L., and Mastaglia, F. L. Cell mediated cytotoxicity to muscle in polymyositis. *N. Engl. J. Med. 288:* 434, 1973.
30. Johnson, R. L., Fink, C. W., and Ziff, M. Lymphotoxin formation by lymphocytes and muscle in polymyositis. *J. Clin. Invest. 51:* 2435, 1972.
31. Brain, W. R., and Norris, F., Jr. Remote Effects of Cancer on the Nervous System. New York, Grune & Stratton, 1965.
32. Tyler, H. R. Paraneoplastic syndromes of nerve, muscle and neuromuscular junction. *Ann. N.Y. Acad. Sci. 230:* 348, 1974.
33. Croft, P. B., and Wilkinson, M. Carcinomatous neuromyopathy: Incidence in patients with carcinoma of the lung and breast. *Lancet 1:* 184, 1963.
34. Croft, P. B., and Wilkinson, M. The incidence of carcinomatous neuromyopathy in patients with various types of carcinoma. *Brain 88:* 427, 1965.
35. Brain, W. R. The neurological complications of neoplasms. *Lancet 1:* 179, 1963.
36. Posner, J. B. Neurological complications of systemic cancer. *Med. Clin. N. Am. 55:* 625, 1971.
37. Wilner, E. C., and Brody, J. A. An evaluation of the remote effects of cancer on the nervous system. *Neurology 18:* 1120, 1968.
38. Joynt, R. J. The brain's uneasy peace with tumors. *Ann. N.Y. Acad. Sci. 230:* 342, 1974.
39. Norris, F., Jr. Prognosis in amyotrophic lateral sclerosis. *Trans. Am. Neurol. Assoc. 96:* 290, 1971.
40. Mancall, E. L., and Rosales, R. K. Necrotizing myelopathy associated with visceral carcinoma. *Brain 87:* 639, 1964.
41. Eaton, L. M., and Lambert, E. H. Electromyography and electric stimulation of nerves in diseases of motor unit. *J. Am. Med. Assoc. 163:* 1117, 1957.
42. Croft, P. B., Urich, A., and Wilkinson, M. Peripheral neuropathy of sensorimotor type association with malignant disease. *Brain 90:* 31, 1967.
43. Richardson, E. P., Jr. Our evolving understanding of progressive multifocal leukoencephalopathy. *Ann. N.Y. Acad. Sci. 230:* 358, 1974.
44. Wilkinson, P. C., and Zeromski, J. Immunofluorescent detection of antibodies against neurones in sensory carcinomatous neuropathy. *Brain 88:* 529, 1965.
45. Slichter, S. J., and Harker, L. A. Hemostasis in malignancy. *Ann. N.Y. Acad. Sci. 230:* 252, 1974.
46. Harker, L. A., and Slichter, S. J. Platelet and fibrinogen consumption in man. *N. Engl. J. Med. 287:* 999, 1972.
47. Pineo, G. F., Brain, M. C., Gallus, A. S., Hirsh, J., Hatton, M. W. C., and Regoeczi, E. Tumors, mucus production and hypercoagulability. *Ann. N.Y. Acad. Sci. 230:* 262, 1974.
48. Goodnight, S. H., Jr. Bleeding and intravascular clotting in malignancy: A review. *Ann. N.Y. Acad. Sci. 230:* 271, 1974.
49. Curth, H. O. Cutaneous manifestations associated with malignant internal disease, In Fitzpatrick, C. B., Arndt, K. A., Claude, W. H., Jr., *et al.* (eds.): *Dermatology in Internal Medicine*. New York, McGraw-Hill, 1971.
50. Kahn, C. R., Flier, J. S., and Bar, R. S. The syndromes of insulin resistance and acanthosis nigricans. Insulin-receptor disorders in man. *N. Engl. J. Med. 294:* 739, 1976.
51. Curth, H. O. How and why the skin reacts. *Ann. N.Y. Acad. Sci. 230:* 435, 1974.
52. Mallinson, C. N., Bloom, S. R., Warin, A. P., Salmon, P. R., and Cox, B. A. Glucagonoma syndrome. *Lancet 2:* 1, 1974.
53. Lee, J. C., Yamauchi, H., and Hopper, J. The association of cancer and the nephrotic syndrome. *Ann. Int. Med. 64:* 41, 1966.
54. Plager, J., and Stutzman, L. Acute nephrotic syndrome as a manifestation of active Hodgkin's disease. *Am. J. Med. 50:* 56, 1971.
55. Loughridge, L. W., and Lewis, M. G. Nephrotic syndrome in malignant disease of non-renal origin. *Lancet 1:* 256, 1971.
56. Gould, V. E., and Benditt, E. P. Ultrastructural and functional relationships of some human endocrine tumors. In Sommers, S. C. (ed.): *Pathology Annual*. New York, Appleton-Century-Crofts, 1973, pp. 205–230.
57. Rudnick, P., and Odell, W. D. In search of a cancer. *N. Engl. J. Med. 284:* 405, 1971.
58. Chejfec, G., and Gould, V. E. Malignant gastric neuroendocrinomas: Ultrastructural and biochemical characterization of their secretory activity. *Hum. Pathol. 8:* 443, 1977.
59. Gould, V. E., Sommers, S. C., and Terzakis, J. A. Ultrastructure of Neuroendocrine cells in normal and dysplastic bronchi. *Am. J. Pathol. 90:* 49, 1978.
60. Ellison, M. L., Ambrose, E. J., and Easty, G. C. Differentiation in a transplantable rat tumor maintained in organ culture. *Exp. Cell. Res. 55:* 198, 1968.
61. Sherbert, G. V. Epigenetic processes and their relevance to the study of neoplasms. *Adv. Cancer Res. 13:* 97, 1970.
62. Sherbert, G. V., Epigenetic mechanisms and paraneoplastic phenomena. *Ann. N.Y. Acad. Sci. 230:* 516, 1974.
63. Feyrter, F. Die peripheren endoKrinen (paraKrinen) Drüsen, In Kaufmann-Staemler, F., DeGuyter, G. (eds.): *Lehrbuch der speziellen pathologischen Anatome*. Berlin, 1969, vol. VII, p. 12.
64. Pearse, A. G. E. Common cytochemical properties of cells making polypeptide hormones with particular reference to calcitonin and the thyroid C cells. *Vet. Rec. 79:* 587–590, 1966.
65. Pearse, A. G. E. 5-Hydroxytryptophan uptake by dog thyroid C cells and its possible significance in polypeptide hormone production. *Nature 211:* 598, 1966.
66. Pearse, A. G. E. Common cytochemical and ultrastructural characteristics of cells producing hormones (the APUD series) and their relevance to thyroid and ultimobranchial cells and calcitonin. *Proc. R. Soc. B 170:* 71, 1968.

67. Pearse, A. G. E. The cytochemistry and ultrastructure of polypeptide hormone-producing cells (the APUD series) and embryologic, physiologic and pathologic implications of the concept. *J. Histochem. Cytochem. 17:* 303, 1969.
68. Le Dourain, N., and LeLievre, C. Demonstration de l'origine neural des cellules a calcitonine du corps ultimobranchial chez l'embryon du poulet. *C. R. Acad. Sci. Ser. D* Paris *270:* 2857, 1970.
69. Pearse, A. G. E., and Polak, J. M. Neural crest origin of the endocrine polypeptide (APUD) cells of the gastrointestinal tract and pancreas. *Gut 12:* 783, 1971.
70. Pearse, A. G. E. and Polak, J. M. Demonstration of the neural crest origin of type I (APUD) cells in the avian carotid body using a cytochemical marker system. *Histochemie 34:* 191, 1973.
71. Pearse, A. G. E. The APUD cell concept and its implications in pathology. In Sommers, S. C. (ed.): *Pathology Annual.* New York, Appleton-Century-Crofts, 1974, pp. 27–41.
72. Pearse, A. G. E., and Polak, J. M. Cytochemical evidence for the neural crest origin of mammalian ultimobranchial C cells. *Histochemistry 27:* 96, 1971.
73. Pearse, A. G. E. The APUD concept and its implications in pathology (Addendum). In Sommers, S. C. (ed.): *Endocrine Pathology Decennial.* New York, Appleton-Century-Crofts, 1975, pp. 162–163.
74. Weichert, R. F., III. The neural ectodermal origin of the peptide secreting endocrine glands. *Am. J. Med 49:* 232, 1970.
75. Fiesen, S. R., Hermreck, A. S., and Mantz, F. A. Glucagon, gastrin and carcinoid tumors of the duodenum, pancreas and stomach: Polypeptide apudomas of the foregut. *Am. J. Surg. 127:* 90, 1974.
76. Szijj, I., Csapo, Z., Lazlo, R. A., *et al.* Medullary cancer of the thyroid gland associated with hypercorticism. *Cancer 24:* 167, 1969.
77. Gould, V. E., and Benditt, E. P. Ultrastructural and functional relationships of some human endocrine tumors (Addendum). In Sommers, S. C. (ed.): *Endocrine Pathology Decennial.* New York, Appleton-Century-Crofts, 1975, pp. 190–193.
78. Gould, E. Neuroendocrinomas: APUD cell system neoplasms and their aberrant secretory activities. In Sommers, S. C. (ed.): *Pathology Annual.* New York, Appleton-Century-Crofts, 1977.
79. Hammar, S., and Sale, G. Multiple hormone producing islet cell carcinomas of the pancreas: A morphologic and biochemical investigation. *Hum. Pathol. 6:* 349, 1975.
80. Bolande, R. P. The neurocristopathies: A unifying concept of diseases arising in neural crest maldevelopment. *Hum. Pathol. 5:* 409, 1974.
81. Pictet, R. L., Rall, L. B., Phelp, P., and Rutter, W. The neural crest and the origin of the insulin-producing and other gastrointestinal hormone-producing cells. *Science 191:* 191, 1976.
82. Le Douarin, N. M., and Teillet, M. A. The migration of neural crest cells to the wall of the digestive tract in amion embryo. *J. Embryol. Exp. Morphol. 30:* 31, 1973.
83. Gould, V. E., and Battifora, H. The origin and significance of the basal lamina and some interstitial fibrillar components in epithelial neoplasms. In Sommers, S. C. (ed.): Pathology Annual. New York, Appleton-Century-Crofts, 1976.
84. Levine, R. J., and Metz, S. A. A classification of ectopic hormone-producing tumors. *Ann. N.Y. Acad. Sci. 230:* 533, 1974.
85. Liebelt, R. A., Gehring, G., Del Monte, L., Schuster, G., and Uebect, A. G. Paraneoplastic syndromes in experimental animal model systems. *Ann. N.Y. Acad. Sci. 230:* 547, 1974.
86. Brown, W. H. A case of pluriglandular syndrome: Diabetes in bearded women. *Lancet 2:* 1022, 1928.
87. Amatruda, T. T., and Upton, G. V. Hyperadrenocorticism and ACTH-releasing factor. *Ann. N.Y. Acad. Sci. 230:* 168, 1974.
88. Meador, C. K., Liddle, G. W., Island, D. P., Nicholson, W. E., Lucas, C. P., Nuckton, J. G., and Leutscher, J. A. Cause of Cushing's syndrome in patients with tumors arising from "nonendocrine" tissue. *J. Clin. Endocrinol. 22:* 693, 1962.
89. Liddle, G. W., Nicholson, W. E., Island, D. P., Orth, D. N., Abe, K., and Lowder, S. C. Clinical and laboratory studies of ectopic humoral syndromes. *Rec. Prog. Horm. Res. 25:* 283, 1969.
90. Gewirtz, G., and Yalow, R. S. Ectopic ACTH production in carcinoma of the lung. *J. Clin. Invest. 53:* 1022, 1974.
91. Upton, G. V., and Amatruda, T. T., Jr. Evidence for the presence of tumor peptides with corticotropin-releasing-factor-like activity in the ectopic ACTH syndrome. *N. Engl. J. Med. 285:* 419, 1971.
92. Orth, D. N., Island, E. P., Nicholson, W. E., Abe, K., and Woodham, J. P. ACTH radioimmunoassay: Interpretation and comparison with bioassay and clinical application. In Hayes, R. L., Goswitz, R. A., and Murphy, B. E. P. (eds.): Radioisotopes in Medicine. Washington, D.C., Atomic Energy Commission, 1968.
93. Ratcliffe, J. G., Knight, R. A., Besser, G. M., Landon, J., and Stansfeld, H. G. Tumor and plasma ACTH concentrations in patients with and without the ectopic ACTH syndrome. *Clin. Endocrinol. 1:* 27, 1972.
94. Yalow, R. S., and Berson, S. A. Size, heterogeneity of immunoreactive human ACTH in plasma and in extracts of pituitary glands and ACTH-producing thymoma. *Biochem. Biophys. Res. Commun. 44:* 439, 1971.
95. Yalow, R. S., and Berson, S. A. Characteristics of "big ACTH" in human plasma and pituitary extracts. *J. Clin Endocrinol. Metab. 36:* 415, 1973.
96. Gewirtz, G., Schneider, B., Krieger, D. T., and Yalow, R. S. "Big ACTH": Conversion to biologically active ACTH by trypsin. *J. Clin. Endocrinol. Metab. 38:* 227, 1974.
97. Knight, R. A., Ratcliffe, J. G., and Besser, G. M. Tumor ACTH concentrations in ectopic ACTH syndrome and in control tissues. *Proc. R. Soc. Med. 64:* 1266, 1971.
98. Hauger-Klevene, J. H. Asymptomatic production of ACTH: Radioimmunoassay in squamous cell, oat cell and adenocarcinoma of the lung. *Cancer 22:* 1262, 1968.
99. Orth, D. N., Nicholson, W. E., Mitchell, W. M., Island, D. P., and Liddle, G. W. Biologic and immunologic characterization and physical separation of ACTH and ACTH fragments in ectopic ACTH syndrome. *J. Clin. Invest. 52:* 1756, 1973.
100. Ayvazian, L. S., Schneider, B., Gewirtz, G., and Yalow, R. S. Ectopic production of big ACTH in carcinoma of the lung. *Am. Rev. Resp. Dis. 111:* 279, 1975.
100a. Odell, W., Wolfsen, A., Yoshimoto, Y., Weitzman, R., Fisher, D., and Hirose, S. Ectopic peptide synthesis: A universal concomittant of neoplasia. *Trans. Assoc. Amer. Phys. 90:* 204, 1977.
101. Christy, N. P. Adrenal corticotropic activity in the plasma of patients with Cushing's syndrome associated with pulmonary neoplasm. *Lancet 1:* 85, 1961.
102. Landon, J., James, V. H. T., and Peart, W. S. Cushing's syndrome associated with "corticotropin"-producing bronchial neoplasm. *Acta Endocrinol. 56:* 321, 1967.
103. Strott, C. A., Nugent, C. A., and Tyler, F. H. Cushing's syndrome caused by bronchial adenomas. *Am. J. Med. 44:* 97, 1968.
104. Imura, H., Matsukura, S., Yamamota, H., Hirata, Y., Nakai, Y., Endo, J., Tanaka, A., and Nakamura, M. Studies on ectopic ACTH-producing tumors: II. Clinical and biochemical features of 30 cases. *Cancer 35:* 1430, 1975.
105. Hirata, Y., Yamamoto, H., Matsukura, S., and Imura, H. *In vitro* release and biosynthesis of tumor ACTH in ectopic ACTH producing tumors. *J. Clin. Endocrinol. Metab. 41:* 106, 1975.
106. Schorr, I., and Ney, R. L. Abnormal hormone responses of an adrenocortical cancer adenyl cyclase. *J. Clin. Invest. 50:* 1295, 1971.
107. Schorr, I., Hinshaw, H. T., Cooper, M. A., Mahaffee, D., and Ney, R. L. Adenyl cyclase hormone responses of certain human endocrine tumors. *J. Clin. Endocrinol. Metab. 34:* 447, 1972.
108. Genazzani, A. R., Hurlimann, J., Fioretti, P., and Felber, J. P. *In vitro* synthesis of an ACTH-like hormone and human chorionic somatomammotrophin by placental and amniotic cells. *Experientia 30:* 430, 1974.
109. Manson, A. M., Ratcliffe, J. G., and Buckle, R. M. ACTH secretion by bronchial carcinoid tumors. *Clin. Endocrinol. 1:* 3, 1972.
110. Miura, K., Sasaki, C., Katsuhima, I., Ohtomo, T., Sato, S., Demura, H., Torikai, T., and Sasano. N. Pituitary-adrenal-cortical studies in a patient with Cushing's syndrome induced by thymoma. *J. Clin Endocrinol. Metab. 27:* 631, 1967.
111. Horai, T., Nishihara, H., Tateishi, R., Matsuda, N., and Hattori, N. Oat cell carcinoma of the lung simultaneously producing ACTH and serotonin. *J. Clin. Endocrinol. Metab. 37:* 212, 1973.
112. Pimstone, B. L., Uys, C. J., and Vogelpoel, L. Studies in a case of Cushing's syndrome due to ACTH-producing thymic tumor. *Am. J. Med. 53:* 521, 1972.
113. Hattori, S., Matsuda, M., and Tatershi, R. Oat cell carcinoma of the lung. Clinical and morphological studies in relation to its histogenesis. *Cancer 30:* 1014, 1972.
114. Corrin, G., and McMillian, M. Fine structure of an oat cell carcinoma of the lung associated with ectopic ACTH syndrome. *Br. J. Cancer 24:* 755, 1970.
115. Bensch, K. G., Corrin, B., Pariente, R., and Spencer, H. Oat cell

carcinoma of the lung. Its origin and relationship to bronchial carcinoid. *Cancer 22:* 1163, 1968.

116. Mason, A. M. S., Ratcliffe, J. G., Buckle, R. M., and Mason, A. S. ACTH secretion by bronchial carcinoid tumors. *Clin. Endocrinol 1:* 3, 1972.
117. Sachs, B. A., Becker, N., Bloomberg, A. E., and Grunwald, R. P. Cure of ectopic ACTH syndrome secondary to adenocarcinoma of the lung. *J. Clin. Endocrinol Metab. 30:* 590, 1970.
118. Orth, D. N., and Liddle, G. W. Results of treatment in 108 patients with Cushing's syndrome. *N. Engl. J. Med. 285:* 243, 1971.
119. Coll, R.,Horner,I., Kraiem, Z.,and Gafni, J. Successful metyrapone therapy of the ectopic ACTH syndrome. *Arch. Int. Med. 121:* 549,1968.
120. Carey, R. M., Orth, D. N., and Hartmann, W. H. Malignant melanoma with ectopic production of adrenal corticotropic hormone: Palliative treatment with inhibitors of adrenal steroid biosynthesis. *J. Clin. Endocrinol. Metab. 36:* 482, 1973.
121. Gorden, P., Becker, C. E., Levey, G. S., and Roth, J. Efficacy of amino-glutethimide in the ectopic ACTH syndrome. *J. Clin. Endocrinol Metab. 28:* 921, 1968.
122. McMillan, M., and Maisey, M. N. Effects of aminoglutethimide in a case of ectopic ACTH syndrome. *Acta Endocrinol. 64:* 676, 1970.
123. Liddle, G. W., Givens, J. R., Nicholson, W. E., and Island, D. P. The ectopic ACTH syndrome. *Cancer Res. 25:* 1057, 1965.
124. Lerner, A. B., and McGuire, J. S. Melanocyte-stimulating hormone and adrenal corticotropic hormone: Their relation to pigmentation. *N. Engl. J. Med 270:* 539, 1964.
125. Orth, D. N. Ectopic Adrenocorticotrophic and Melanocyte-Stimulating Hormones. Endocrinology, Proceedings of the IVth International Congress. Amsterdam, *Excerpta Medica,* 1973, pp. 1205–1210.
126. Shimizu, N., Ogata, E., Nicholson, W. E., Island, D. P., Ney, R. L., and Liddle, G. W. Studies on the melanotrophic activity of human plasma and tissues. *J. Clin. Endocrinol. Metab. 25:* 984, 1965.
127. Island, D. P., Shimizu, N., Nicholson, W. E., Abe, K., Ogata, E., and Liddle, G. W. Methods for separating small quantities of MSH and ACTH with good recovery of each. *J. Clin. Endocrinol. Metab. 25:* 975, 1965.
128. Abe, K., Nicholson, W. E., Liddle, G. W., Orth, D. N., and Island, D. P. Normal and abnormal regulation of beta-MSH in man. *J. Clin. Invest. 48:* 1580, 1969.
129. Abe, K., Nicholson, W. E., Liddle, G. W., Island, D. P., and Orth, D. N. Radioimmunoassay of beta-MSH of human plasma and tissues. *J. Clin. Invest. 46:* 1509, 1967.
130. Shapiro, M., Nicholson, W. E., Orth, D. N., Mitchell, W. M., and Liddle, G. W. Differences between ectopic MSH and pituitary MSH. *J. Clin. Endocrinol. Metab. 33:* 377, 1971.
131. Scott, A. P., and Lowry, P. J. Adrenocorticotrophic and melanocyte-stimulating peptides in the human pituitary. *Biochem. J. 139:* 593, 1974.
132. Bloomfield, G. A., Scott, A. P., Lowry, P. J., Gilkes, J. J. H., and Rees, L. H. A reappraisal of human beta MSH. *Nature 252:* 492, 1974.
133. Li, C. H., Barnafi, L., Chretien, M., and Chung, D. Isolation and amino-acid sequence of beta LPH from sheep pituitary glands. *Nature 208:* 1093, 1965.
134. Gilkes, J. J., Bloomfield, G. A., Scott, A. P., Lowry, P. R., Ratcliffe, J. G., Landon, J., and Rees, L. H. Development and validation of a radioimmunoassay for peptides related to beta melanocyte-stimulating hormone in human plasma: Lipotropins. *J. Clin Endocrinol. Metab. 40:* 450, 1975.

134a. Roberts, J. L., and Herbert, E. Characterization of a common precursor to corticotropin and β-lipotropin. *Proc. Nat. Acad. Sci. USA 74:* 5300, 1977.

135. Krieger, D. T., and Glick, S. M. Sleep EEG stages and plasma growth hormone concentration in states of endogenous and exogenous hypercortisolemia of ACTH elevation. *J. Clin. Endocrinol. Metab. 39:* 986, 1974.
136. Steiner, H., Dahlback, O., and Waldenstarm, J. Ectopic growth hormone production and osteoarthropathy in carcinoma of the bronchus. *Lancet 1:* 783, 1968.
137. Cameron, D. P., Burger, H. G., DeKretzer, D. M., Catt, K. J., and Best, J. B. On the presence of immunoreactive growth hormone in a bronchogenic carcinoma. *Austr. Ann. Med. 18:* 143, 1969.
138. Dupont, B., Hoyer, I., Borgeskov, F., and Nerup, J. Plasma growth hormone and hypertrophic osteoarthropathy in carcinoma of the bronchus. *Acta Med. Scand. 188:* 25, 1970.
139. Beck, C., and Burger, H. G. Evidence for the presence of immunoreactive growth hormone in cancers of the lung and stomach. *Cancer 30:* 75, 1972.
140. Greenberg, P. B., Beck, C., Martin, T. J., and Burger, H. G. Synthesis and release of human growth hormone from lung carcinoma in cell culture. *Lancet 1:* 350, 1972.
141. Hammarsten, J. F., and O'Leary, J. The features and significance of hypertrophic osteoarthropathy. *Arch. Int. Med. 99:* 431, 1957.
142. Tashjian, A. H., Jr. Animal cell cultures as a source of hormone. *Biotechnol. Bioeng. 11:* 109, 1969.
143. Josimovich, J. B., and McLaren, T. A. Presence in the human placenta and term serum of a highly lactogenic substance immunologically related to pituitary growth hormone. *Endocrinology 71:* 209, 1962.
144. Sherwood, L. M., Handwerger, S., McLaurin, W. D., and Lanner, M. Amino acid sequence of human placental lactogen. *Nature 233:* 59, 1971.
145. Grumbach, M. M., Kaplan, S. L., Sciarra, J. J., and Burr, I. M. Chorionic growth hormone prolactin secretion, disposition, biologic activity in man and postulated function as "growth hormone" of the second half of pregnancy. *Ann. Acad. Sci. 148:* 501, 1968.
146. Fusco, F. D., and Rosen, S. W. Gonadotropin-producing anaplastic large cell carcinoma of the lung. *N. Engl. J. Med 275:* 507, 1966.
147. Weintraub, B. D., and Rosen, S. W. Ectopic production of human chorionic somatotropin by non-trophoblastic cancers. *J. Clin. Endocrinol. Metab. 32:* 94, 1971.
148. Payne, R. A., and Ryan, R. J. Human placental lactogen in the male subject. *J. Urol. 107:* 99, 1972.
149. Sussman, H. H., Weintraub, B. D., and Rosen, S. W. Relationship of ectopic placental alkaline phosphatase to ectopic chorionic gonadotropin and placental lactogen. *Cancer 33:* 820, 1974.
150. Muggia, F. M., Rosen, F. W., Weintraub, B. O., and Hansen, H. H. Ectopic placental proteins in non-trophoblastic tumors. *Cancer 36:* 1327, 1975.
151. Schneider, A. B., Kowalski, K., and Sherwood, L. M. "Big" human placental lactogen: Disulfide linked peptide chains. *Biochem. Biophys. Res. Commun. 64:* 717, 1975.
152. Schneider, A. B., Kowalski, K., and Sherwood, L. M. Identification of "big" human placental lactogen in placenta and serum. *Endocrinology 97:* 1364, 1975.
153. Sherwood, L. M. Human prolactin. *N. Engl. J. Med. 284:* 774, 1971.
154. Turkington, R. W. Ectopic production of prolactin. *N. Engl. J. Med. 285:* 1455, 1971.
155. Rees, L. H., Bloomfield, G. A., Rees, G. M., Corrin, B., Franks, L. M., and Ratcliffe, J. G. Multiple hormones in a bronchial tumor. *J. Clin. Endocrinol. Metab. 38:* 1090, 1974.
156. Locke, E. A. Secondary hypertrophic osteoarthropathy and its relationship to clubbed fingers. *Arch. Int. Med. 15:* 659, 1915.
157. McArthur, J. W., Toll, G. D., Russfield, A. B., Reiss, A. M., Quinby, W. C., and Baker, W. H. Sexual precocity attributable to ectopic gonadotropin secretion by hepatoblastoma. *Am. J. Med. 54:* 390, 1973.
158. Treves, N. Gynecomastia—The origins of mammary swelling in the male: An analysis of 406 patients with breast hypertrophy, 525 with testicular tumors and 13 with adrenal neoplasms. *Cancer 11:* 1083, 1958.
159. Ginsburg, J., and Brown, J. B. Increased estrogen excretion in hypertrophic pulmonary osteoarthropathy. *Lancet 2:* 1274, 1961.
160. Rosen, W. S., Becker, C. E., Schlaff, S., Easton, J., and Gluck, M. C. Ectopic gonadotropin production before clinical recognition of bronchogenic carcinoma. *N. Engl. J. Med. 279:* 640, 1968.
161. Faiman, C., Colwell, J. A., Ryan, R. J., Hershman, J. M., and Shields, T. W. Gonadotropin secretion from a bronchogenic carcinoma. Demonstration by radioimmunoassay. *N. Engl. J. Med. 277:* 1395, 1967.
162. Vaitukaitis, J. L. Immunologic and physical characterization of human chorionic gonadotropin (HCG) secreted by tumors. *J. Clin. Endocrinol. Metab. 37:* 505, 1973.
163. Castleman, B., Scully, R. E., and McNeely, B. U. Case records of the Massachusetts General Hospital. *N. Engl. J. Med. 286:* 594, 1972.
164. Castleman, B., Scully, R. E., and McNeely, B. U. Case records of the Massachusetts General Hospital. *N. Engl. J. Med. 286:* 713, 1972.
165. Pierce, J. G. Subunits of pituitary thyrotropin—Their relationship to other glycoprotein hormones. *Endocrinology 89:* 1331, 1971.

166. Kirschner, M. A., Cohen, F. B., and Jespersen, D. Estrogen production and its origin in men with gonadotropin-producing neoplasms. *J. Clin. Endocrinol. Metab. 39:* 112, 1974.
167. Dailey, J. E., and Marcuse, P. M. Gonadotropin secreting giant cell carcinoma of the lung. *Cancer 24:* 388, 1969.
168. Cottrell, J. C., Becker, K. L., Matthews, M. J., and Moore, C. Histology of gonadotropin secreting bronchogenic carcinoma. *Am. J. Clin. Pathol. 52:* 720, 1969.
169. Weintraub, B. D., and Rosen, S. W. Ectopic production of the isolated beta subunit of human chorionic gonadotropin. *J. Clin. Invest. 52:* 3135, 1973.
170. Rayford, P. L., Vaitukaitis, J. L., Roth, G. T., Morgan, M. J., and Canfield, R. E. The use of specific antisera to characterize biologic activity of HCG-beta subunit preparations. *Endocrinology 91:* 144, 1972.
171. Rabson, A. S., Rosen, S. W., Tashjian, A. W., Jr., and Weintraub, B. D. Production of human chorionic gonadotropin *in vitro* by cell line derived from a carcinoma of the lung. *J. Natl. Cancer Inst. 50:* 669, 1973.
172. Tashjian, A. H., Jr., Weintraub, B. D., Barowsky, N. J., Rabson, A. S., and Rosen, S. W. Subunits of human chorionic gonadotropin: Unbalanced synthesis and secretion by clonal cell strains derived from a bronchogenic carcinoma. *Proc. Natl. Acad. Sci. U.S.A. 70:* 1419, 1973.
173. Braunstein, G. D., Vogel, G. L., Vaitukaitis, J. L., and Ross, G. T. Ectopic production of human chorionic gonadotropin in Ugandan patients with hepatocellular carcinoma. *Cancer 32:* 223, 1973.
174. Franchimont, P., Gaspard, U., Rueter, A., and Heynen, T. Polymorphism, protein and polypeptide hormones. *Clin. Endocrinol. 1:* 315, 1972.
175. Rosen, S. W., and Weintraub, B. D. Ectopic production of the isolated alpha subunit of the glycoprotein hormones: A quantitative marker in certain cases of cancer. *N. Engl. J. Med. 290:* 1441, 1974.
176. Weintraub, B. D., and Rosen, S. W. Competitive radioassays and "specific" tumor markers. *Metabolism 22:* 1119, 1973.
176a. Kahn, C. R., Rosen, S. W., Weintraub, B. D., Fajans, S. S., and Gordon, P. Ectopic production of chorionic gonadotropin and its subunits by islet-cell tumors. *New Eng. J. Med. 297:* 565, 1977.
177. Braunstein, G. D., Rasor, J., and Wade, M. E. Presence in normal human testes of a chorionic-gonadotropin-like substance distinct from human luteinizing hormone. *N. Engl. J. Med. 293:* 1339, 1975.
177a. Yoshimoto, Y., Wolfsen, A. R., and Odell, W. D., Human chorionic gonadotropin-like substance in nonendocrine tissues of normal subjects. *Science 197:* 575, 1977.
178. Vaitukaitis, J. L. Peptide hormones, as tumor markers. *Cancer 37:* 567, 1976.
179. Golde, D. W., Schambelan, M., Weintraub, B. D., and Rosen, S. W. Gonadotropin-secreting renal carcinoma. *Cancer 33:* 1018, 1974.
180. Rosen, S. W., Weintraub, B. D., Vaitukaitis, J. L., Sussman, H. H., Hershman, J. M., and Muggia, F. M. Placental proteins and their subunits as tumor markers *Ann. Int. Med. 82:* 71, 1975.
181. Vaitukaitis, J. L. Human chorionic gonadotropin as a tumor marker. *Ann. Clin. Lab. Sci. 4:* 276, 1974.
182. Odell, W. D., Bates, R. W., Rivlin, R. S., Lipsett, M. B., and Hertz, R. Increased thyroid function without clinical hyperthyroidism in patients with choriocarcinoma. *J. Clin. Endocrinol. Metab. 23:* 658, 1963.
183. Hershman, J. M., and Higgins, H. P. Hydatidiform mole—A cause of clinical hyperthyroidism. Two cases with evidence that the molar tissue secreted a thyroid stimulator. *N. Engl. J. Med. 284:* 573, 1971.
184. Hershman, J. M., and Starnes, W. R. Extraction and characterization of thyrotropic material in the human placenta. *J. Clin. Invest. 48:* 923, 1969.
185. Hennen, G. Characterization of a thyroid stimulating factor in a human cancer tissue. *J. Clin. Endocrinol. 27:* 610, 1967.
186. Devroede, G. J., and Tirol, A. F. Giant pleural mesothelioma associated with hypoglycemia and hyperthyroidism. *Am. J. Surg. 116:* 130, 1968.
187. Hershman, J. M., Higgins, H. P., and Starnes, W. R. Differences between thyroid stimulator in hydatidiform mole and human chorionic thyrotropin. *Metabolism 19:* 735, 1970.
188. Steigbigel, N. H., Oppenheim, J. J., and Fishman, L. M. Metastatic embryonal carcinoma of the testis associated with elevated plasma, TSH-like activity and hyperthyroidism. *N. Engl. J. Med. 271:* 345, 1964.
189. Winkler, A. W., and Cranshaw, O. S. Chloride depletion conditions other than Addison's disease. *J. Clin. Invest. 17:* 1, 1938.
190. Schwartz, W. B., Bennett, W., Curelop, E. S., and Bartter, F. C. A syndrome of renal sodium loss and hyponatremia probably resulting from inappropriate secretion of antidiuretic hormone. *Am. J. Med. 23:* 529, 1957.
191. Thorn, N. E., and Transbol, I. Hyponatremia and bronchogenic carcinoma associated with renal excretion of large amounts of antidiuretic material. *Am. J. Med. 35:* 257, 1963.
192. Amatruda, T. T., Jr., Mulrow, P. J., Gallagher, J. C., and Sawyer, W. H. Carcinoma of the lung with inappropriate antidiuresis: Demonstration of antidiuretic hormone-like activity in tumor extract. *N. Engl. J. Med. 269:* 544, 1963.
193. Bower, B. F., Mason, D. M., and Forsham, P. H. Bronchogenic carcinoma with inappropriate antidiuretic activity in plasma and tumor. *N. Engl. J. Med. 271:* 934, 1964.
194. Vorherr, H., Massry, S., Utiger, R., and Kleeman, C. Antidiuretic principle in malignant tumor extract from patients with inappropriate ADH syndrome. *J. Clin. Endocrinol. 28:* 162, 1968.
195. Utiger, R. D. Inappropriate antidiuresis and carcinoma of the lung: Detection of vasopressin in tumor extracts by immunoassay. *J. Clin. Endocrinol. 26:* 970, 1966.
196. Sawyer, W. H. Pharmacological characteristics of the antidiuretic principle and bronchogenic carcinoma for a patient with hyponatremia. *J. Clin. Endocrinol. 27:* 1497, 1967.
197. Bartter, S. C., and Schwartz, W. B. The syndrome of inappropriate secretion of antidiuretic hormone. *Am. J. Med. 42:* 790, 1967.
198. George, J. M., Capen, C. C., and Phillips, A. S. Biosynthesis of vasopressin *in vitro* and ultrastructure of a bronchogenic carcinoma. *J. Clin. Invest. 51:* 141, 1972.
199. Martin, T. J., Greenberg, P. B., Beck, C., and Johnston, C. I. Synthesis of Peptide Hormones by Human Tumors in Cell Cultures. Endocrinology Proceedings of the IV International Congress. Amsterdam, *Excerpta Medica,* 1973, pp. 1198–1204.
200. Olson, D. R., Buchan, G. C., and Porter, G. A. Inappropriate antidiuretic hormone secretion. *Arch. Int. Med. 124:* 741, 1969.
201. Rees, T., Rosalki, S. D., and MacLean, A. D. W. Hyponatremia, impaired renal tubular function and carcinoma of bronchus. *Lancet 2:* 1005, 1960.
202. Fichman, M. P., and Bethune, J. E. The role of adrenal corticoids in the inappropriate antidiuretic hormone syndrome. *Ann. Int. Med. 68:* 806, 1968.
203. Hantman, D., Rossier, B., Zohlman, R., and Schrier, R. Rapid correction of hyponatremia in a syndrome with inappropriate secretion of antidiuretic hormone. *Ann. Int. Med. 78:* 870, 1973.
204. White, M. G., and Fetner, C. D. Treatment of the syndrome of inappropriate secretion of antidiuretic hormone with lithium carbonate. *N. Engl. J. Med. 292:* 390, 1974.
205. Cherill, D. A., State, R. M., Birge, J. R., and Senger, I. Demeclocycline treatment in the syndrome of inappropriate antidiuretic hormone secretion. *Ann. Int. Med. 83:* 654, 1975.
206. Hamilton, D. P. N., Upton, G. V., and Amatruda, T. T., Jr. Evidence of the presence of neurophysin in tumors producing the syndrome of inappropriate antidiuresis. *J. Clin. Endocrinol. 35:* 764, 1972.
207. Robinson, A. G., Zimmerman, hE. A., and Frantz, A. G. Physiologic investigation of posterior pituitary binding proteins neurophysin I & neurophysin II. *Metabolism 20:* 1148, 1971.
208. Hamilton, B. P. Presence of neurophysin proteins in tumors associated with the syndrome of inappropriate ADH secretions. *Ann. N.Y. Acad. Sci. 248:* 153, 1975.
209. Stolbach, L. L., Krant, M. J., and Fishman, W. H. Ectopic production of an alkaline phosphatase isoenzyme in patients with cancer. *N. Engl. J. Med. 281:* 757, 1969.
210. Marks, L. J., Steinke, J., Podolsky, S., and Egdahl, R. H. Hypoglycemia associated with neoplasia. *Ann. N.Y. Acad Sci. 230:* 147, 1974.
211. Oleesky, S., Bailey, I., Samols, E., and Bilkus, D. A fibrosarcoma with hypoglycemia and a high serum insulin level. *Lancet 2:* 378, 1962.
212. Unger, R. H., Lochner, J., and Eisentraut, A. M. Identification of insulin and glucagon in bronchogenic metastasis. *J. Clin. Endocrinol. 24:* 823, 1964.
213. Saeed, S. M., Fine, G., and Horn, R. C., Jr. Hypoglycemia associated with extrapancreatic tumors. Immunofluorescent study. *Cancer 24:* 158, 1969.
214. Shames, J. M., Dhurandhar, N. R., and Blackard, W. T. Insulin

secreting bronchial carcinoid tumor with widespread metastases. *Am. J. Med. 44:* 632, 1968.
215. Lyall, S. S., Marieb, N. J., Wise, J. K., Cornog, J. L., Neville, E. C., and Felig, P. Hyperinsulinemic hypoglycemia associated with a neurofibrosarcoma. *Arch. Int. Med. 135:* 865, 1975.
216. Jakob, A., Hauri, C., and Froesch, E. R. Non-suppressible insulin-like activity in human serum III: Differentiation of two distinct molecules with non-suppressible ILA. *J. Clin. Invest. 47:* 2678, 1968.
217. Hall, K., and Uthne, K. Some biological properties of purified sulfation factor (SF) from human plasma. *Acta Med. Scand. 190:* 137, 1971.
218. VanWyk, J. J., Underwood, L. E., Hintz, R. L., Clemmons, D. R., Voina, S. J., and Weaver, R. P. The somatomedins: A family of insulinlike hormones under growth hormone control. *Recent Prog. Horm. Res. 30:* 259, 1974.
219. Megyesi, K., Kahn, C. R., Roth, J., and Gorden, P. Circulating NSILA-s in man. *J. Clin. Endocrinol. Metab. 41:* 475, 1975.
220. Unger, R. H. The riddle of tumor hypoglycemia. *Am. J. Med. 40:* 325, 1966.
221. August, J. T., and Hiatt, H. H. Severe hypoglycemia secondary to non-pancreatic fibrosarcoma with insulin activity. *J. Int. Med. 258:* 17, 1958.
222. Butterfield, W. J., Kinder, C. H., and Mahler, R. S. Hypoglycemia associated with sarcoma. *Lancet 1:* 703, 1960.
223. McFadzean, A. J., and Yeung, R. T. Further observations on hypoglycemia and hepatocellular carcinoma. *Am. J. Med. 47:* 220, 1969.
224. Graber, A. L., Porte, D., Jr., and Williams, R. H. Clinical use of diazoxide and mechanisms for its hypoglycemic effects. *Diabetes 15:* 143, 1966.
225. Boonstra, C. E., and Jackson, C. E. Hyperparathyroidism detected by routine serum calcium analysis: Prevalance in a clinic population *Ann. Int. Med. 63:* 468, 1965.
226. Bachman, A. L., and Sproul, E. E. Correlation of radiographic and autopsy findings in suspected metastasis in the spine. *Bull. N.Y. Acad. Sci. 31:* 146, 1955.
227. Albright, F. A. Case records: Massachusetts General Hospital #27, 461. *N. Engl. J. Med. 225:* 789, 1941.
228. Plimpton, C. H., and Gellhorn, A. Hypercalcemia in malignant disease without evidence of bone destruction. *Am. J. Med. 21:* 750, 1956.
229. Connor, T. B., Thomas, W. C., Jr., and Howard, J. E. Etiology of hypercalcemia associated with lung carcinoma. *J. Clin. Invest. 35:* 697, 1956.
230. Goldberg, M. F., Tashjian, A. H., Jr., Order, S. E., and Dammin, G. J. Renal adenocarcinoma containing a parathyroid hormone-like substance and associated with marked hypercalcemia. *Am. J. Med. 36:* 805, 1964.
231. Tashjian, A. H., Jr., Levine, L., and Munson, T. L. Immunochemical identification of parathyroid hormone in non-parathyroid neoplasms associated with hypercalcemia. *J. Exp. Med. 119:* 467, 1964.
232. Munson, T. L., Tashjian, A. H., Jr., and Levine, L. Evidence of parathyroid hormone in non-parathyroid tumors associated with hypercalcemia. *Cancer Res. 25:* 1062, 1965.
233. Sherwood, L. M., O'Riordan, J. L., Aurbach, G. D., and Potts, J. T., Jr. Production of parathyroid hormone by non-parathyroid tissue. *J. Clin. Endocrinol. 27:* 140, 1967.
234. Knill-Jones, R. P., Buckle, R. M., Parsons, V. Calne, R. Y., and Williams, R. Hypercalcemia and increased parathyroid hormone activity in a primary hepatoma: Studies before and after hepatic transplantation. *N. Engl. J. Med. 282:* 704, 1970.
235. Riggs, B. L., Arnaud, C. D., Reynolds, J. C., and Smith, L. H. Immunologic differentiation of primary hyperparathyroidism due to non-parathyroid cancer. *J. Clin. Invest. 50:* 2079, 1971.
236. Benson, R. C., Riggs, B. L., Pickard, B. M., and Arnaud, C. D. Immunoreactive forms of circulating parathyroid hormone in primary and ectopic hyperparathyroidism. *J. Clin. Invest. 54:* 175, 1974.
237. Segre, G. V., Habener, J. F., Powell, D., Tregear, G. W., and Potts, J. T., Jr. Parathyroid hormone in human plasma: Immunochemical characterization and biological implications. *J. Clin. Invest. 51:* 3163, 1972.
238. Benson, R. C., Riggs, B. L., Pickard, B. M., and Arnaud, C. D. Radioimmunoassay of parathyroid hormone in hypercalcemic patients with malignant disease. *Am. J. Med. 56:* 821, 1974.
239. Blair, A. J., Jr., Hawker, C. D., and Utiger, R. D. Ectopic hyperparathyroidism in a patient with metastatic hypernephroma. *Metabolism 22:* 147, 1973.
240. Powell, D., Shimkin, P. M., Doppman, J. L., Wells, S., Aurbach, G. D., Marx, S. J., Ketcham, A. S., and Potts, J. T., Jr. Primary hyperparathyroidism: Preoperative tumor localization and differentiation between adenoma and hyperplasia. *N. Engl. J. Med. 286:* 1169, 1972.
241. Eisenberg, H., Pallotta, J., and Sherwood, L. M. Selective arteriography, venography and venous hormone assay in diagnosis and localization of parathyroid lesions. *Am. J. Med. 56:* 810, 1974.
242. Hartman, C. R., MacGregor, R. R., Chu, L. L. H., McGregor, D. H., Cohn, D., and Hamilton, J. Evidence for the biosynthesis of PTH-like peptides by a human squamous cell carcinoma. Abstract of the Endocrine Society, 57th Meeting, New York, #2, 1975.
243. Lafferty, F. W. Pseudohyperparathyroidism. *Medicine 45:* 247, 1966.
244. Sherwood, L. M. Case records of the Massachusetts General Hospital. *N. Engl. J. Med. 284:* 839, 1971.
245. Powell, D., Singer, F. R., Murray, T. M., Minkin, C., and Potts, J. T., Jr. Non-parathyroid humoral hypercalcemia in patients with neoplastic diseases. *N. Engl. J. Med. 289:* 176, 1973.
246. Tashjian, A. H., Jr. Tumor humors and the hypercalcemias of cancer. *N. Engl. J. Med. 290:* 905, 1974.
247. Brereton, H. D., Halushka, P. V., Alexander, R. W., Mason, D. M., Keiser, H. R., and DeVita, V. T., Jr. Indomethacin-responsive hypercalcemia in a patient with renal cell adenocarcinoma. *N. Engl. J. Med. 291:* 83, 1974.
248. Robertson, R. P., Baylink, D. J., Marini, J. J., and Adkison, H. W. Elevated prostaglandins and suppressed parathyroid hormone associated with hypercalcemia and renal cell carcinoma *J. Clin. Endocrinol. Metab. 41:* 164, 1965.
249. Ito, H., Sanada, T., Katayama, T., and Shimazaki, J. Indomethacin-responsive hypercalcemia. *N. Engl. J. Med. 293:* 558, 1975.
250. Seyberth, H. W., Segre, G. V., Morgan, J. L., Sweetman, B. J., Potts, J. T., Jr., and Oates, J. A. Prostaglandins as mediators of hypercalcemia associated with certain types of cancer. *N. Engl. J. Med. 293:* 1278, 1975.
251. Voelkel, E. F., Tashjian, A. H., Jr., Franklin, R., Wasserman, E., and Levine, L. Hypercalcemia and tumor-prostaglandin: The VX_2 carcinoma model in the rabbit. *Metabolism 24:* 973, 1975.
252. Luben, R. A., Mundy, G. R., Trummel, C. L., and Raisz, L. G. Partial purification of osteoclast-activating factor from phytohemagglutinin-stimulated human leukocytes. *J. Clin. Invest. 53:* 1473, 1974.
253. Mundy, G. R., Luben, R. A., Raisz, L. G., Oppenheim, J. J., and Buell, D. N. Bone-resorbing activity in supernatants from lymphoid cell lines. *N. Engl. J. Med. 290:* 867, 1974.
254. Silva, O. L., Becker, K. L., Primack, A., Doppman, J., and Snider, R. H. Ectopic secretion of calcitonin by oat-cell carcinoma. *N. Engl. J. Med. 290:* 1122, 1974.
255. Melvin, K. E. W., Tashjian, A. H., Jr., and Miller, H. H. Studies in familial medullary thyroid carcinoma. *Recent Prog. Horm. Res. 28:* 399, 1972.
256. Whitelaw, A. L., and Cohen, S. L. Ectopic production of calcitonin. *Lancet 2:* 44, 1973.
257. Silva, O. L., Becker, K. L., Primack, A., Doppman, J. L., and Snider, R. H. Increased serum calcitonin levels in bronchogenic cancer. *Chest 69:* 495, 1976.
258. Deftos, L., McMillan, P. J., Sartiano, G. P., Abuid, J., and Robinson, A. G. Simultaneous ectopic production of parathyroid hormone and calcitonin. *Metabolism 25:* 543, 1976.
259. Lipsett, M. B., Odell, W. D., Rosenberg, L. E., and Waldmann, T. A. Humoral syndromes associated with non-endocrine tumors. *Ann. Int. Med. 61:* 733, 1964.
260. Sherwood, J. B., and Goldwasser, E. Erythropoietin production by human renal carcinoma cells in monolayer culture. *Endocrinology 99:* 504, 1976.
261. Levin, J., and Conley, C. L. Thrombocytosis associated with malignant disease. *Arch. Int. Med. 114:* 497, 1964.
262. Robertson, P. W., Klidjian, A., Harding, L. K., Walters, G., Lee, M. R., and Robb-Smith, A. H. T. Hypertension due to renin-secreting renal tumor. *Am. J. Med. 43:* 963, 1967.
263. Eddy, R. L., and Sanchez, S. A. Renin-secreting renal neoplasms and hypertension with hypokalemia. *Ann. Int. Med. 75:* 725, 1971.
264. Hollifield, J. W., Page, D. L., Smith, C., Michelakis, A. M., Staab, E., and Rhamy, R. Renin-secreting clear cell carcinoma of the kidney. *Arch. Int. Med. 135:* 859, 1975.

265. Hauger-Klevene, J. H. High plasma renin activity in an oat cell carcinoma: A renin-secreting carcinoma. *Cancer 26:* 1112, 1970.

266. Day, R. P., Luetscher, J. A., and Gonzalez, E. M. Occurrence of big renin in human plasma, amniotic fluid and kidney extracts. *J. Clin. Endocrinol. Metab. 40:* 1078, 1975.

267. Zusman, R. M., Snider, J. J., Cline, K., Caldwell, B. V., and Speroff, L. Antihypertensive function of a renal cell carcinoma. *N. Engl. J. Med. 290:* 843, 1974.

268. Stanbury, S. W. Osteomalacia. *Clin. Endocrinol. Metab. 1:* 239, 1972.

268a. Drezner, M. I. C., and Feinglos, M. N. Osteomalacia due to a 1α,25-dihydroxycholecalciferol deficiency. *J. Clin. Invest. 60:* 1046, 1977.

269. Hirai, H., and Alpert, E. (eds.) Carcinofetal proteins. Biology and chemistry. *Ann. N.Y. Acad. Sci. 259:* 1, 1970.

270. Murphy, R. A. Pantazis, N. J., Arnason, B. W., and Young, M Secretion of a nerve growth factor by mouse neuroblastoma cells in culture. *Proc. Natl. Acad. Sci. 72:* 1895, 1975.

271. O'Neal, L. W., Kipnis, D. M., Luse, S. A., Lacy, D. E., and Jarett, L. Secretion of various endocrine substances by ACTH secreting tumors. *Cancer 21:* 1219, 1968.

272. Erdheim, J. Aur Normalen und Pathologischen Histologie der glandula Thyroidia, Parathyroidia und Hypophysis. *Beitr. Pathol. Anat. Allg. Pathol. 33:* 158, 1903.

273. Cushing, H., and Davidoff, L. M. The pathological findings in 4 autopsy cases of acromegaly with a discussion of their significance. *Monograph 22.* New York, The Rockefeller Institute for Medical Research, 1927.

274. Rossier, P. H., and Dressler, M. Familiare Erkrankung innerskretorischer Drusen Kombiniert Mit Ulcuskrankheit. *Schweiz Med. Wochenschr. 20:* 95, 1939.

275. Shelburn, S. A., and McLaughlin, C. S. Jr. Coincidental adenomas of islet cells, parathyroid glands and pituitary gland. *J. Clin. Endocrinol. 5:* 232, 1945.

276. Wermer, P. Genetic aspects of adenomatosis of the endocrine glands. *Am. J. Med. 16:* 363, 1954.

277. Moldawer, M. P., Nardi, G. L., and Raker, W. Concomitance of multiple adenomas of the parathyroids: A syndrome with familial incidence. *Am. J. Med. Sci. 228:* 190, 1954.

278. Zollinger, R. M., and Ellison, E. H. Primary peptic ulceration associated with islet cell tumors of the pancreas. *Ann. Surg. 142:* 709, 1955.

279. Steiner, E. L., Goodman, A. D., and Powers, S. R. Study of a kindred with pheochromocytoma, medullary thyroid carcinoma, hyperparathyroidism and Cushing's disease. Multiple endocrine neoplasia, type II. *Medicine 45:* 371, 1968.

280. Ballard, H. S., Frame, B., and Hartsock, R. J. Familial multiple endocrine adenoma—peptic ulcer complex. *Medicine 43:* 481, 1964.

281. Wermer, P. Endocrine adenomatosis and peptic ulcer in a large kindred. *Am. J. Med. 35:* 205, 1963.

282. Gregory, R. A., Tracy, H. J., French, J. M., and Sircus W. Extraction of gastrin-like substance from pancreatic tumor in a case of Zollinger-Ellison syndrome. *Lancet 1:* 1045, 1960.

283. McGuigan, J. E., and Trudeau, W. L. Immunochemical measurement of elevated levels of gastrin in the serum of patients with pancreatic tumors of the Zollinger-Ellison variety. *N. Engl. J. Med. 278:* 1308, 1968.

284. Johnson, G. J., Summerskill, W. H. J., Anderson, V. E., and Keating, F. R., Jr. Clinical and genetic investigation of a large kindred with multiple endocrine adenomatosis. *N. Engl. J. Med. 277:* 1379, 1967.

285. Trudeau, W. L., and McGuigan, J. E. Effects of calcium on serum gastrin levels in the Zollinger-Ellison syndrome. *N. Engl. J. Med. 281:* 862, 1969.

286. Snyder, N., Scurry, M., and Hughes, W. Hypergastrinemia in familial multiple endocrine adenomatosis. *Ann. Int. Med. 80:* 321, 1974.

287. Ellison, E. H., and Wilson, S. D. Ulcerogenic tumor of the pancreas. *Prog. Clin. Cancer 3:* 225, 1967.

288. Cassar, J., Polak, J. M., and Cooke, W. M. Possible parathyroid origin of gastrin in a patient with multiple endocrine adenopathy, type I. *Br. J. Surg. 62:* 313, 1975.

289. Cameron, A. J., and Hoffman, H. N. Zollinger-Ellison syndrome: Clinical features and long term follow-up *Mayo Clin. Proc. 49:* 44, 1974.

290. Gregory, R. A., and Tracy, H. J. Isolation of two big gastrins from Zollinger-Ellison tumor tissue. *Lancet 2:* 797, 1972.

291. Yalow, R. S., and Berson, S. A. And now "big, big" gastrin. *Biochem. Biophys. Res. Commun. 48:* 391, 1972.

292. Schein, P. S., DeLellis, R. A., Kahn, C. R., Groden, P., and Kraft, A. R. Islet cell tumors: Current concepts and management. *Ann. Int. Med. 79:* 239, 1973.

293. Said, S. I., and Faloona, G. R. Elevated plasma and tissue levels of vasoactive interstitial polypeptide in the watery diarrhea syndrome due to pancreatic bronchogenic and other tumors. *N. Engl. J. Med. 293:* 155, 1975.

293a. Ganda, O. P., Weir, G. C., Soeldner, J. S., Legg, M. A., Chick, W. L., Patel, Y. C., Ebeid, A. M., Gabbay, K. A., and Reichlin, S. C. "Somatostatinoma": A somatostatin-containing tumor of the endocrine pancreas. *New Engl. J. Med. 296:* 963, 1977.

293b. Larsson, L. I., Holst, J. J., Kuhl, C., Lundquist, G., Hirsch, M. A., Ingemanssun, S., Lindkaer-Jensen, S., Rehfeld, J. F., and Schwartz, T. W. Pancreatic somatostatinoma. *Lancet 1:* 666, 1977.

294. Sipple, J. H. The association of pheochromocytoma with carcinoma of the thyroid. *Am. J. Med. 31:* 163, 1961.

295. Williams, E. D. A review of 17 cases of carcinoma of the thyroid and pheochromocytoma. *J. Clin. Pathol. 18:* 288, 1965.

296. Keiser, H. R., Beaven, M. A., Doppman, J., Wells, S., Jr., and Buja, L. M. Sipple's syndrome: Medullary thyroid carcinoma, pheochromocytoma, and parathyroid disease. *Ann. Int. Med. 78:* 561, 1973.

297. Melvin, K. E. W., Miller, H. H., and Tashjian, A. H., Jr. Early diagnosis of medullary carcinoma of the thyroid gland by means of calcitonin assay. *N. Engl. J. Med. 285:* 1115, 1971.

298. Wolfe, H. J., Melvin, K. E. W., Cervi-Skinner, S. J., Alsaadi, A. A., Juliar, J. F., Jackson, C. E., and Tashjian, A. H., Jr. C-cell hyperplasia preceding medullary thyroid carcinoma. *N. Engl. J. Med. 289:* 437, 1973.

299. Baylin, S. B., Beaven, M. A., Engelman, K., and Sjoerdsma, A. Elevated histaminase activity in medullary carcinoma of the thyroid gland. *N. Engl. J. Med. 283:* 1239, 1970.

300. Khairi, M. R. A., Dexter, R. N., Burzynski, N. J., and Johnston, C. C., Jr. Mucosa, neuroma, pheochromocytoma and medullary thyroid carcinoma, multiple endocrine neoplasia, type 3. *Medicine 54:* 89, 1975.

301. Block, M. B., Roberts, J. P., Kadair, R. G., Seyfer, A. E., Hull, S. F., and Nofeldt, F. D. Multiple endocrine adenomatosis, type IIB. *J. Am. Med. Assoc. 234:* 710, 1975.

302. Voelkel, E. F., Tashjian, A. H., Jr., Davidoff, F. F., Cohen, R. B., Perlia, C. P., and Wurtman, R. J. Concentrations of calcitonin and catecholamines in pheochromocytomas, mucosal neuroma and medullary thyroid carcinoma. *J. Clin. Endocrinol. Metab. 37:* 297, 1973.

140

Peptide Growth Factors

Judson J. Van Wyk
Raymond L. Hintz

INTRODUCTION

DEFINITION

A "growth factor" may be broadly defined as any substance that can stimulate cells to divide or to increase in size. Although many classic hormones, nutrients, and other substances satisfy this definition, this chapter will be restricted to a group of more recently recognized peptide growth factors that are powerful stimulants of cell growth in vitro. The physiological role of most of these substances is not yet known. Many of them are responsive to alterations in the levels of established hormones and may ultimately be proven to mediate some of their actions at the cellular level. The potency of these substances in in vitro systems suggests that they are well suited to exercise a crucial role in the processes of differentiation, growth, organ regeneration, wound healing, and tumorigenesis. At the very least, these peptide growth factors can serve as instruments for expanding our understanding of the molecular process involved in the regulation of cell growth.

Although many external signals are capable of triggering the secretion of differentiated cell products without stimulating cell division, mitogenic agents frequently stimulate both types of response in susceptible cells. As an example of this dual role, adrenocorticotropin (ACTH) normally stimulates adrenocortical cells to enlarge, synthesize new protein, and elaborate glucocorticoids. However, under special circumstances, ACTH is also believed to stimulate adrenal cells to proliferate. The nature of the response elicited in the target cell may be at least partially dependent on the phase of the cell cycle at the time of stimulation.

Supported by USPHS Research Grants AM 01022 (JJVW) and AM 19168 (RLH). J. J. Van Wyk is a recipient of Research Career Award #4 KO6 AM14115 from the National Institutes of Health

RELATION OF GROWTH FACTORS TO THE CELL CYCLE

In Figure 140-1 are diagrammatically represented the generally accepted five stages of the life cycle of a typical mammalian cell. The fully mature cell in G_0 is not committed to division. G_1 is a growth phase preparatory to S. S is the phase in which synthesis of DNA and replication of the chromosomes occur. G_2 represents a phase in which further protein synthesis takes place before mitosis can occur in M. Following mitosis, the daughter cells may either reenter the cycle or become "resting" G_0 cells. Certain cells, e.g., mature neurons, seem permanently locked in G_0, having lost their ability to divide. Others are either continually dividing or can divide in response to appropriate stimulation.[1] The major control point of this process seems to be at the transition from G_0 to G_1. Characterizing this transition are a group of metabolic events that have been collectively called a "positive pleiotypic response."[2]

Peptide growth factors have in common the capacity to elicit a "positive pleiotypic response" in responsive cells. Some of these growth factors have a high degree of selectivity for certain cell types and stimulate them both to divide and to synthesize highly specific cell products. Other growth factors are able to stimulate DNA synthesis and mitosis in a wider range of cell types but are less apt to stimulate these cells to function in a differentiated manner.

Many nonspecific stimuli such as proteolytic enzymes, plant lectins, and changes in the ionic environment are capable of eliciting renewed mitosis in cells that have grown to confluency in tissue culture. This mitogenic effect is presumed to result from alterations of the cell membrane. Thus the demonstration that a putative growth factor is capable of eliciting a pleiotypic response under the artificial conditions of cell culture need not necessarily imply a physiological role for that substance in vivo.

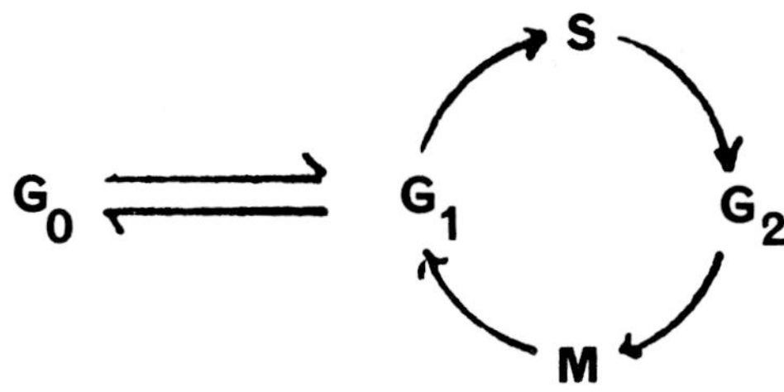

Fig. 140-1. Diagrammatic representation of the mammalian cell cycle.

CYCLIC NUCLEOTIDES AND CELL GROWTH

Although a number of peptide growth factors have now been shown to interact with cell membrane receptors in the same fashion as classic peptide hormones, the subsequent intracellular events leading to cell division are less well understood than those leading to differentiated cellular responses. Recent research has suggested that alterations in cyclic nucleotides may be involved in the transmission of pleiotypic signals. A variety of mitogenic agents have been used to show that transition from G_0 to G_1 is associated with a fall in intracellular cAMP.[3,4] It was hypothesized that a decrease in cAMP within the cell initiated or permitted cell division. Consistent with this concept is the finding that cell proliferation is inhibited by cAMP and its dibutyryl analogue. On the other hand, cGMP has, under certain circumstances, been shown to promote cell division,[5] and at least one mitogenic agent has been reported to stimulate a rapid, transient increase in cGMP levels within the cell.[6] cGMP has also been shown to stimulate protein and RNA synthesis in cell-free systems.[7] However, a recent study has cast doubt on any role of cGMP as an effector of cell division.[8] Other factors that may be involved and need further elucidation include the role of calcium,[9] other divalent cations, and intracellular polyamines.[10]

As noted above, some adult cells never divide, some are continually renewing, and others need specific stimuli for division. Similarly, cells in fetal life differ markedly from adult cells in their capacity to divide. It is not known whether these differences are attributable to the prevalence of receptors for mitogenic signals or whether subsequent events in the pleiotypic response govern the ability to respond to these signals. Finally, it has been postulated that negative controls on cell growth may be exercised by external inhibitors that oppose the action of growth factors. The term "chalone" has been applied by Bullough to this hypothetical group of substances.[11]

THE SOMATOMEDIN GROUP OF SERUM GROWTH FACTORS

HISTORY OF "SULFATION FACTOR" AND "SOMATOMEDIN"

Endocrinologists became interested in peptide growth factors when Salmon and Daughaday established that normal serum contained a factor that promoted the incorporation of $^{35}SO_4$ into costal cartilage explants of hypophysectomized rats.[12] They showed that this "sulfation factor" was dependent on growth hormone but distinct from it and proposed that the induction of this substance was responsible for the skeletal effects of growth hormone. In addition, this factor was later shown to stimulate the incorporation of thymidine into DNA[13] and uridine into RNA[14] and to stimulate the conversion of proline to hydroxyproline[15] in cartilage. It was also shown to have marked insulinlike actions in extraskeletal tissues[16] and to stimulate the proliferation of cultured HeLa cells.[17] In 1972, because of these diverse effects, the operational designation "sulfation factor" was replaced by the more general designation "somatomedin."[18] Many laboratories have subsequently confirmed the growth hormone dependency of serum somatomedin levels both in humans and in experimental animals. Furthermore, under a wide range of clinical conditions, plasma "sulfation factor activity" often correlates better with linear growth rates than do direct measurements of growth hormone itself.

It is increasingly recognized that the substance or substances in serum that stimulate cartilage growth share certain common properties with a larger group of peptide growth factors described by workers in other disciplines. Many of these other factors are also related in one way or another to insulin. Although some of these factors have been found to be growth-hormone-dependent and others androgen-dependent, the hormonal control mechanisms for the majority of them have not been studied. It is far from clear how many such growth factors exist, how they are formed, and what, if any, is their physiological role. These emerging parallelisms and the growing belief that many of these growth factors may be linked in some type of familial relationship have inevitably led to confusion concerning whether the term "somatomedin" should be broadened to include all growth-hormone-dependent growth factors or whether the term should be more restricted in its usage.

To avoid ambiguity, the term "somatomedin" will be used here to include only those growth factors found in plasma that (1) are under growth hormone control, (2) have insulinlike properties, and (3) promote the incorporation of sulfate in cartilage. Four substances that fulfill all three criteria have been isolated from plasma in pure or relatively pure form: somatomedin-A,[19] somatomedin-C,[20] NSILA-S (nonsuppressible insulinlike activity—soluble),[21] and MSA (multiplication stimulating activity).[22] Although published reports reveal these substances to be remarkably similar in their chemical and biological properties, their identity with one another has not been established.

Somatomedin-A and somatomedin-C were isolated in different laboratories using different modifications of the original sulfation factor assay to guide purification. Nonsuppressible insulinlike activity and multiplication stimulating activities, however, have different histories and only later were recognized as somatomedins. The convergence of these different lines of investigation therefore requires a brief explanation.

NONSUPPRESSIBLE INSULINLIKE ACTIVITY (NSILA)

In 1962, Leonard et al. reported that 90 percent of the insulinlike activity of serum measured by bioassay could not be neutralized by antibodies against insulin.[23] This excess has come to be known as "nonsuppressible insulinlike activity" (NSILA). Froesch and his co-workers in Zurich showed that there were at least two components of NSILA. Eighty percent of the total activity was precipitated by acid-ethanol and was designated NSILA-P. NSILA-P is a molecule of about 100,000 daltons which has so far resisted further purification and characterization.[24] The 20 percent of total NSILA that was soluble in acid ethanol was designated NSILA-S. Two closely related substances have now been purified to homogeneity and designated NSILA I and NSILA II.[24a] The amino acid sequence of these peptides reveals a high degree of correspondence with the B chain of insulin.[24b]

The original NSILA assay depended on the degradation of glucose by rat epididymal fat pads in the presence of insulin antibody.[25] More recently, NSILA-S has been shown to be a potent stimulator of DNA synthesis and cell replication in fibroblast cultures and to stimulate $^{35}SO_4$ incorporation into proteoglycans of cartilage.[26] Plasma levels of NSILA-S were found by Froesch to be growth-hormone-dependent.[27] Hence, NSILA-S fulfills the strictest requirements of a somatomedin.

MULTIPLICATION STIMULATING ACTIVITY (MSA)

The nature of the factor or factors in serum that are required for cell multiplication has intrigued cell biologists from the earliest days of tissue culture. Apart from the intrinsic importance of this question, the goal of perpetuating diploid mammalian cell lines in fully defined media cannot be realized so long as serum (traditionally calf serum) is required for cell replication.

Attempts to identify the nature of the mitogenic factor or factors in calf serum met with limited success until 1972, when Pierson and Temin reported a 6000-fold purification of "multiplication stimulating activity" (MSA) from calf serum. The active substance proved to be a small insulinlike peptide with a molecular weight of about 6000 daltons.[22,28] Dulak and Temin have subsequently isolated four similar peptides with MSA activity from the medium of certain rat liver cells that had been initially cloned on the basis of their ability to proliferate in the absence of serum.[29] MSA from this conditioned medium is designated CRL-MSA. These observations suggest that at least a portion of serum MSA arises in the liver.

MSA also stimulates sulfate incorporation into cartilage[20] and binding to the somatomedin-C receptor in cell membrane preparations. More recently, Cohen et al. have shown that MSA from rat serum is growth hormone dependent[30] and thus also fulfills all the requirements for a somatomedin.

CHEMISTRY OF THE SOMATOMEDINS

Since no enriched tissue sources have been found for the four substances fulfilling the criteria of somatomedins, it has been necessary to isolate them from large quantities of plasma. For this reason, purification of sufficient quantities for complete characterization has been difficult. All four substances are heat-stable peptides with molecular size estimates ranging between 6000 daltons for serum MSA and 8500 daltons for CRL-MSA. Available information on their respective electrical charge properties and amino acid compositions, however, suggests significant differences. It is unlikely that the question of identity or lack of identity between these substances will be resolved until amino acid sequences are known and sufficient quantities of each peptide, of unassailable purity, are available for side-by-side comparison.

In native plasma, most of the somatomedin activity is associated with large proteins that appear to have molecular weights ≧60,000 daltons. Less than 5 percent of the total activity is identifiable in the peptide fraction below 10,000 daltons. Evidence has been presented by Hintz for somatomedin-C[31] and by Zapf for NSILA-S[32] that the large molecular weight form is composed of the active peptide reversibly bound to a large carrier protein. Cohen and Nissley have made observations that suggest that MSA in rat plasma is also associated with carrier proteins.[33]

The concentrations of somatomedin in serum are several orders of magnitude higher than those that are characteristic of other peptide hormones. The somatomedins also have longer disappearance rates from blood, with half-times measured in hours rather than in minutes. These differences between peptide hormones and somatomedins may be accounted for by the fact that peptide hormones circulate as free peptides without a carrier protein; the level of *free* somatomedin in circulating blood is probably not much different from other potent hormones.

BIOLOGICAL ACTIONS OF THE SOMATOMEDINS

Actions in Cartilage

The primary action of somatomedin on cartilage is probably to promote protein synthesis, the step that appears to be rate limiting in the synthesis of sulfur-containing glucosaminoglycans. Somatomedin also stimulates RNA and DNA synthesis. Although it was originally anticipated that different growth factors might stimulate the synthesis of differentiated cell products and DNA, this has not proven to be the case. As shown in Figure 140-2, pure somatomedin-C fully replicates the action of serum in stimulating both the incorporation of $^{35}SO_4$ into proteoglycans and ^{3}H-thymidine into DNA.

Insulinlike Actions

Hall and Uthne showed that during successive stages of purification, sulfation factor activity in cartilage paralleled insulinlike activity in epididymal fat pads.[16] In virtually every in vitro system studied, somatomedin mimics the action of insulin. In adipose tissue, it stimulates glucose oxidation and lipid synthesis and inhibits epinephrine-induced lipolysis.[34] In muscle, it stimulates protein synthesis and membrane transport of amino acids and glucose. Kostyo and Uthne showed that the action of somatomedin in muscle is prompt, like insulin, rather than delayed, like growth hormone.[35] In several systems, the actions of somatomedin and insulin were additive when both substances were present in subsaturating concentrations.[36]

An explanation for the insulinlike properties of somatomedin was forthcoming when Hintz et al.[37] demonstrated that somatomedin can effectively compete with ^{125}I-insulin for binding to the insulin-binding site of cell membranes from liver, adipose tissue, and cartilage. Similar binding to the insulin receptor has been shown for NSILA-S,[27] somatomedin-A,[38] and MSA.[20] These observations imply a structural as well as a functional homology between the somatomedins and insulin. This is further borne out by the observation of D'Ercole et al.[39a] and Burghen et al.[39b] that both somatomedin-C and NSILA-S are powerful inhibitors of insulin degradation by the so-called insulin specific protease.

The concentrations of somatomedin required to elicit insulinlike responses in isolated tissues approximate the concentrations of somatomedin found in native plasma and thus are much higher than the concentrations of free somatomedin that might be freely available to tissue sites. For this reason, somatomedin may be of

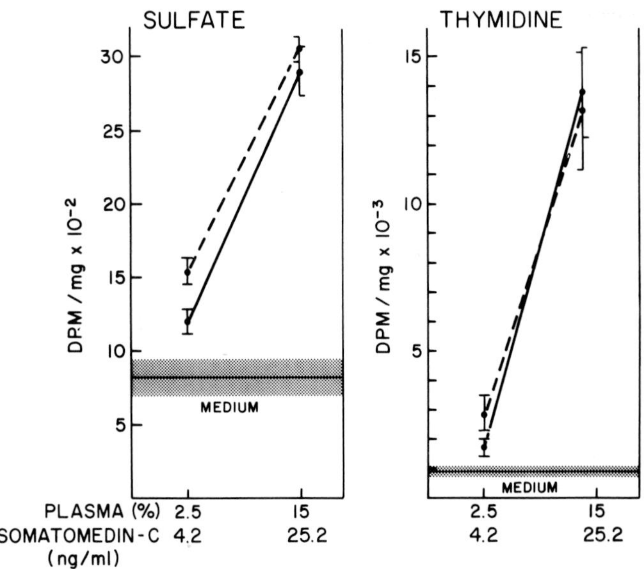

Fig. 140-2. Comparison of dose response curves to pure somatomedin-C (●----●) and pooled plasma from normal adult males (●——●) in standard cartilage assay for somatomedin activity. The uptakes of $^{35}SO_4$ and ^{3}H-thymidine per milligram (±SEM) are plotted on the ordinates of the left- and right-hand panels, respectively and the test concentrations of plasma and somatomedin-C on the abscissae. Uptakes were measured in costal cartilage segments from hypophysectomized rats.

minor physiological importance in the in vivo regulation of carbohydrate metabolism. At least it can be said that the "normal" concentrations of somatomedin found in the plasma of diabetic patients fail to protect them against carbohydrate intolerance! Although Froesch et al. found that injections of NSILA-S depress glucose levels in dogs,[27] they likewise concluded that at physiological levels, NSILA-S has little effect on glucose homeostasis. Megyesi, however, found a group of patients in whom hypoglycemia could be correlated with exceedingly high levels of NSILA-S.[39] These patients had mesenchymal tumors that presumably secreted NSILA-S ectopically.

Effect of Somatomedin and Insulin on Growth

Since insulin is only weakly active in sulfation factor and cell culture assays, it may be inferred that the growth-promoting action of the somatomedins is probably not due to their insulinlike properties. A better explanation for the unique growth promoting properties of somatomedin was provided by the finding that many cell types possess a specific high affinity receptor for somatomedin-C.[40,44] A similar unique receptor has been subsequently demonstrated for NSILA-S,[41,42] somatomedin-A,[43] and CRL-MSA.[43a] The somatomedin-C receptor is 50 to 100 times more sensitive to somatomedin-C than is the insulin receptor; furthermore, the affinity of insulin for the somatomedin receptor is about 1000 times less than that of somatomedin-C.[44] The binding ratios of the two substances to their respective receptors compare favorably with their relative biological potencies in assays that are specific for either growth promotion or insulinlike activity. These findings suggest that insulin is probably not a primary growth stimulant at physiological concentrations except to the extent that is necessary to preserve metabolic homeostasis. At very high levels, however, insulin can mimic the action of somatomedin in vitro and may also do so in vivo.

In addition to its effect on cartilage, somatomedin-C stimulates thymidine incorporation and increases mitotic rate in chick fibroblasts, rat liver cells, and ovarian tumor cells.[44] NSILA-S and MSA are likewise potent mitogenic agents for fibroblasts. Although insulin also stimulates DNA synthesis in many cell culture systems, it is not usually capable of stimulating mitosis except at exceedingly high dosages.

The cellular mechanisms by which somatomedin stimulates cell division are poorly understood. Pastan[45] and others have shown that the rate of cell proliferation in cultured cells is inversely related to cyclic AMP production. Thus it is of interest that Tell et al.[46] found that somatomedin inhibits hormonally induced increases of adenylate cyclase in several cell types. They found that somatomedin inhibits adenylate cyclase stimulation by epinephrine in lymphocytes and fat cells, in cartilage cells by parathyroid hormone, and in liver membranes by prostaglandin, PGE_1. Hepp and Renner have found that NSILA-S has a similar effect in adipose tissue.[47]

The exquisite sensitivity of somatomedin receptors to competition by unlabeled somatomedin has permitted the development of radioreceptor assays capable of measuring the somatomedins in unextracted plasma.[40] Using these assays, it has been possible to confirm the growth hormone dependency of the somatomedins (Fig. 140-3).

It is not yet clear whether there is one somatomedin receptor to which all the somatomedins bind or whether there are several different types of receptors; the available data suggest that there may be a single "growth receptor" that recognizes all the somatomedins, although not necessarily to the same extent. This would explain why the four members of the somatomedin family give nearly identical responses in all of the biological systems tested so far (Table 140-1).

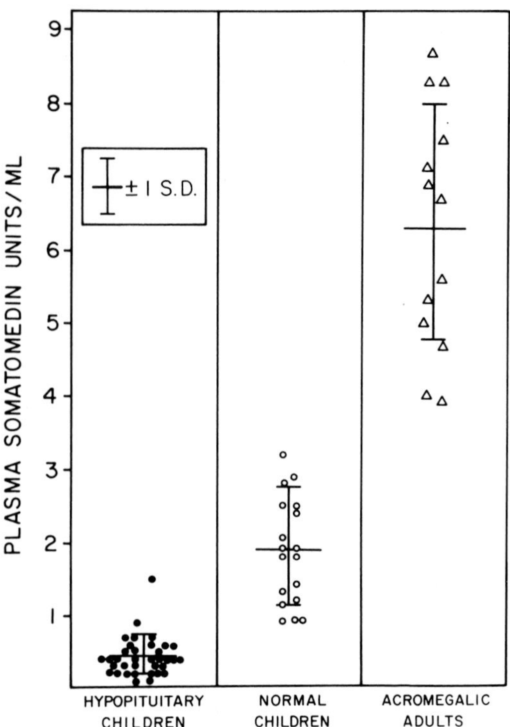

Fig. 140-3. Plasma somatomedin levels determined by the competitive placental membrane binding assay in 35 hypopituitary children, 19 normal children, and 12 adults with acromegaly. Determinations were run in duplicate at plasma concentrations ranging between 1 μl/ml (in acromegalics) and 20 μl/ml (in hypopituitary children). The somatomedin activity in each sample was determined by comparison with the normal plasma pool standard. The mean somatomedin values ± 1 SD are indicated for each group. (Reproduced, with permission, from J. J. Van Wyk and L. E. Underwood, *Annual Review of Medicine 26:* 427–441, 1975.)

Further evidence for the existence of at least two populations of naturally occurring somatomedins has come from the observations of Furlanetto et al., using a highly specific radioimmunoassay for somatomedin-C.[40a] Comparison of results obtained with the two assay systems reveal that the receptor assay detects both neutral and basic forms of somatomedin in human serum, whereas most of the somatomedin detected by the radioimmunoassay is basic. Furthermore, by the radioimmunoassay technique, hypopituitary patients have nearly undetectable concentrations of somatomedin-C, whereas by the radioreceptor assay and by most bioassays the concentrations in the serum of hypopituitary patients are about 40 percent of normal values. This implies that serum contains forms of somatomedin that are less growth-hormone-dependent than is somatomedin-C. More extensive reviews of the somatomedins and related peptides are provided in references 48 and 44a.

OTHER PEPTIDE GROWTH FACTORS DESCRIBED IN SERUM

The diversity of the other serum proteins and peptides that have been reported to have mitogenic activity is illustrated by the examples shown in Table 140-2. None of these factors has been reported to influence sulfate uptake in cartilage. They range from a

Table 140-1. Summary of Properties Common to the Somatomedin Group of Peptides

	Somatomedin-A	Somatomedin-C	NSILA-S	MSA
1. Peptide of ~ 7000 daltons	+	+	+	+
2. Transported in plasma on large carrier protein	+	+	+	+
3. Isoelectric point of free peptide	Neutral	Basic	Basic	Neutral
4. Growth-hormone-dependent	+	+	+	+
5. Insulinlike and cross-reacts with insulin receptor	+	+	+	+
6. Inhibits insulin degradation	NR	+	+	NR
7. Active in cartilage "sulfation factor" assays	+	+	+	+
8. Mitogenic for multiple cell types	+	+	+	+
9. Separate receptor distinct from insulin receptor	+	+	+	+
10. Inhibits adenylate cyclase	+	+	+	NR

NR = not reported.

tripeptide[49,50] to a macroglobulin of 640,000 daltons, which is reported to be complexed with insulin.[55] Many different cell culture assay systems have been used to detect these substances, and only rarely has the activity of these factors been reported in multiple cell lines and under different culture conditions. For this reason, the same factor may well have been described under several names. Although it is beyond the scope of this chapter to review the many serum proteins and peptides that have been described as mitogenic agents, several warrant special emphasis.

SOMATOMEDIN-B

Somatomedin-B is the designation given a serum peptide that induces thymidine incorporation in cultures of human glial-like cells but which is inactive in sulfation factor assays. It is present in acid-ethanol extracts of Cohn fraction IV and was discovered during the purification of human plasma for somatomedin activity.[19] Somatomedin-B is an acidic peptide with a molecular weight of 5400 daltons.[51] Uthne showed by bioassay and Yalow by radioimmunoassay that this peptide is partially growth hormone dependent.[52] Although it thus qualified as a somatomedin under the broad definition in use at that time, its lack of activity in cartilage assays excludes it from the somatomedin group of peptides as defined in this chapter. Furthermore, no cross-reaction has been found between somatomedin-B and either somatomedin-A or somatomedin-C in either radioimmunoassays or radioreceptor assays. It is of interest that the antibody to somatomedin-B fails to detect this peptide in serum from any subprimate species.

THROMBIN AND PLATELET GROWTH FACTOR

In many cell culture systems, serum is 5 to 10 times more mitogenic than an equivalent concentration of plasma from the same species. For this reason, attention has been focused on chemical products released during blood coagulation. Bovine thrombin is one such substance that stimulates contact-inhibited cells to undergo renewed proliferation.[56] This property is shared by many proteolytic enzymes and other substances and presumably results from alteration of membrane proteins. It is now clear, however, that a mitogen released from lysed platelets during blood coagulation accounts for most of the differences between serum and plasma.

Rutherford and Ross[57a] have shown that the platelet growth factor is a basic peptide of about 13,000 and that it possesses chemical and biological properties similar to those of the fibroblast growth factor isolated by Gospodarowicz (vide infra). Harker et al. have postulated that the agglutination and lysis of platelets on fatty plaques is responsible for the proliferative changes in the smooth muscle of arterial walls in atherosclerosis.[57b]

ERYTHROPOIETIN

Erythropoietin is an example of a mitogen specific for a highly specialized cell type. It causes red blood cell precursors to divide and differentiate into more mature erythroid cells capable of synthesizing hemoglobin. Plasma erythropoietin is a sialoprotein with a molecular weight reported to be 46,000 daltons.[58] This may be a dimer, since urinary erythropoietin has a molecular weight of about 23,000 daltons.[59] Erythropoietin is diminished in hypopitu-

Table 140-2. Partial List of Mitogenic Peptides and Proteins Described in Serum (None of these substances stimulate $^{35}SO_4$ incorporation by cartilage)

		Molecular Weight	Chemical Characteristics	Assay
Tripeptide Pickart and Thaler[49,50]		300	Gly-lys-his	Liver cells (rat)
Somatomedin-B Uthne[19,51]		5,400	Acidic	Gliallike cells (human)
Calf serum mitogen Houck and Cheng[53,54]		120,000	Sialoprotein	Diploid fibroblasts (human)
Calf serum factors Frank et al.[55]	S_1	640,000	α_2-Macroglobulin: insulin complex	Embryo fibroblasts (rat)
	S_2	26,000	β-Globulin	
Thrombin Chen and Buchanan[56]		38,000	Proteolytic enzyme	Embryo fibroblasts (chick)
Platelet factor Kohler and Lipton[57] Rutherford and Ross[57a]		13,000?	basic peptide	3T3 fibroblasts (mouse)
Erythropoietin Goldwasser and Kung[58] Dorado et al.[59]		23,000	Sialoprotein	$^{59}Fe \rightarrow$ erythrocytes (hypox rat)

itarism and, like the somatomedins, is responsive to growth hormone;[60] however, it is much more responsive to androgen administration.[61]

GROWTH FACTORS ISOLATED FROM MAMMALIAN TISSUES

Growth factors that have been isolated from tissue sources have been purified in much larger quantities than those found primarily in blood and urine. For this reason, more is known about their chemical and biological properties. Some of these tissue growth factors are listed in Table 140-3. They are classified here separately from serum factors solely for convenience rather than on the basis of any fundamental chemical or biological difference; indeed, some, if not all, of these substances are present in blood and urine and account for a portion of the mitogenic activity of these fluids.

NERVE GROWTH FACTOR (NGF)

Over two decades ago, it was discovered that extracts of snake venom or mouse salivary glands, when injected into the yolk of developing chick embryos, stimulated enlargement of sensory and sympathetic ganglia.[62] This activity, termed nerve growth factor (NGF), was subsequently found to stimulate sympathetic and sensory ganglia in newborn mammals as well as the growth of sympathetic ganglia in organ culture.[63,64] NGF is believed to have little, if any, mitogenic activity for other cell types. Although NGF is primarily a highly specific differentiating agent that exercises its primary role during fetal development, it also serves a maintenance function, since degeneration of sympathetic ganglia has been described following the administration of NGF antibodies to mature animals.[64] In addition to reptile venom and mouse submaxillary glands, NGF is produced by glioma cells[66] and chick fibroblast cultures.[67]

Purification of NGF has been achieved using mouse submaxillary glands as the source.[68,69] This single 118 amino acid polypeptide chain with three intrachain disulfide bonds is usually isolated as a dimer with a molecular weight of 26,000 daltons.[70] A comparison of the amino acid sequence of NGF with that of proinsulin reveals about 70 percent homology, thus suggesting an evolutionary relationship.[71] This ancestral relationship is very similar to that which has been postulated for somatomedin.

Nerve growth factor, like other peptide growth factors and peptide hormones, appears to exert its action through a highly specific cell membrane receptor.[70] This was elegantly demonstrated by Frazier, who showed that NGF, insolubilized by attachment to sepharose, retained its full biological activity in vitro.[72] Receptors for NGF have been identified recently in brain tissue and in a variety of peripheral organs in addition to nerve ganglia.[73] Although the significance of these receptors in brain and extraneural tissue is not known, it is possible that NGF will prove to have a broader role in development than is now apparent.[70]

EPIDERMAL GROWTH FACTOR (EGF)

The epidermal growth factor, discovered in male mouse salivary gland extracts by Cohen in 1962, induces premature eruption of the incisors and early opening of the eyelids in newborn mice.[74] Cohen has found that EGF occurs natively as a prohormone which, like proinsulin, is cleaved by an arginine esterase to a smaller peptide of 6000 daltons.[71,72] The amino acid sequence of EGF has been fully established and, unlike NGF, does not show any homology for insulin.[77]

Although EGF, like NGF, influences differentiation of specialized cells in early life, it is less restricted in its action and stimulates mitogenic activity in fibroblasts, epithelial cells, and mammary cells.[78] It acts primarily on cells of ectodermal origin and a few cell types of mesodermal origin. It is not active on cells of entodermal origin. Topical application of EGF to corneal wounds significantly hastens healing.[79] EGF has been shown to have specific cell surface receptor sites[80,81] and, like insulin and the somatomedins, inhibits hormonally stimulated adenylate cyclase.[82]

Salivary glands from adult male mice contain about 1000 ng/mg of wet tissue, whereas salivary glands from female mice or castrate male mice contain less than one-tenth of this amount. The physiological significance of these extremely high concentrations in adult male mice is still obscure. Salivary gland EGF is highly androgen-dependent, and the rise of immunoreactive EGF in female and castrate male glands following testosterone administration constitutes one of the most sensitive and specific in vivo assays for androgenic activity.[83,84] It is therefore surprising that the levels of EGF in plasma and urine are approximately the same in adult male, castrate male, and female mice.[85] The administration of adrenergic agents or stimulation of sympathetic ganglia causes a striking release of EGF from the salivary glands, with the rise in plasma concentration proportional to the salivary store.[85]

The presence of EGF in humans was first described by Ances,[86] who found that blood and urine from pregnant women contained a substance that cross-reacted with mouse EGF. Human EGF was subsequently isolated from the urine of pregnant women, using anti-mEGF as an immunoabsorbent.[87,88] Human EGF equals mEGF in mitogenic activity and in radioreceptor assays using ^{125}I-mEGF but is recognized relatively poorly by antibodies raised against mEGF. This may be accounted for by significant differences in the amino acid composition of EGF from the two species.[88] More recently, it was pointed out that the amino acid sequence -hEGF is very similar, if not identical, to urogastrone, a peptide that inhibits gastric secretion and protects against peptic ulcers.[88a]

Table 140-3. Partial List of Peptide Growth Factors Isolated from Tissues (References given in text)

	Source	Molecular Weight	Actions
Nerve growth factor	Salivary gland (male mouse)	26,000 (dimer)	Development of sympathetic and sensory neurons
	Snake venom	(Homologous with proinsulin)	
Epidermal growth factor	Salivary gland (male mouse)	6,400	Early tooth eruption and eyelid opening (mouse)
	Human pregnancy urine		Mitogen for fibroblasts, epithelial cells, and others
Ovarian growth factor	Pituitary	13,400 (basic)	Ovarian tumor cell survival
Fibroblast growth factor	Brain; pituitary	13,300 (basic)	Mitogen for 3T3 cells; frog limb regeneration
Myoblast growth factor	Brain	?	Proliferation of myoblasts in low-density cultures
Thymosin	Thymus	12,200	Proliferation of T lymphocytes Immunologic competence

OVARIAN GROWTH FACTOR (OGF)

The ovarian growth factor, a peptide of 13,000 daltons, was discovered by Gospodarowicz following his observation that crude gonadotropins, but not pure FSH or LH, stimulated the proliferation of cloned ovarian cells. By fractionating bovine pituitary glands, he was successful in isolating OGF, which was present as a contaminant in NIH standard gonadotropin and thyrotropin preparations.[89] Subsequent studies suggest that OGF functions primarily as a survival factor and that its apparent growth-promoting activity is attributable to postponement of cell death.[90]

FIBROBLAST GROWTH FACTOR (FGF)

During the course of studies with the ovarian growth factor, Gospodarowicz found that pituitary and brain extracts contain a closely related fibroblast growth factor (FGF) which, together with small amounts of glucocorticoid, is able to fully replicate the action of serum on the proliferation of many cell lines of entodermal and mesodermal origin.[91] Although FGF is a powerful mitogen for many cell lines, it usually does not provide a complete signal for cell division unless the medium is fortified with serum or other hormones such as dexamethasone or insulin.[92] FGF has no effect on epithelial cells or transformed fibroblasts.[93] In combination with serum, FGF is a potent mitogen for normal adrenocortical cells,[93a] granulosa cells,[93b] and luteal cells.[93c]

Both brain FGF and pituitary FGF are basic peptides of 13,000 daltons and differ only slightly in their amino acid composition. Although the ovarian growth factor is of the same molecular size, it is easily separated from the FGFs on gel electrophoresis.[94]

Antoniades and Scher have isolated a mitogenic peptide from whole clotted blood that has many properties similar to FGF.[94a] This peptide (pI = 9.4, mol. wt. = 13,500 daltons) is believed to originate in platelets, since by radioimmunoassay its concentration is much higher in serum from whole clotted blood than in serum from platelet-poor plasma.[94b] Although the identity of the platelet factor with FGF remains to be established, human pituitary extracts contain high concentrations of material that cross-reacts with antibodies raised against the mitogen isolated from serum.

Gospodarowicz has demonstrated that FGF has the capacity to induce partial limb regeneration in adult frogs after amputation.[94] Application of FGF to the stump site stimulates large numbers of undifferentiated blastemal cells which are then followed by the appearance of large sheets of differentiated cartilage and muscle. Since similar regeneration of amputated frog legs can be brought about by enriching the nerve supply with nerve grafts,[95] it is possible that FGF mediates this neurotropic effect.

MYOBLAST GROWTH FACTOR (MGF)

Recently, Gospodarowicz and his co-workers have demonstrated a third type of mitogenic peptide in brain and pituitary extracts. This myoblast growth factor (MGF) promotes the proliferation of myoblasts in low-density culture in the presence of 10 percent serum.[96] MGF appears chemically distinct from FGF, since it is a neutral peptide rather than basic.

THYMOSIN

Finally, thymosin is a highly specific growth and differentiating substance for thymus-dependent lymphoid cells.[97] Thymosin was isolated from bovine thymic tissue and found to be a peptide of 12,200 daltons containing a high content of dicarboxylic amino acids.[98] A role for thymosin in the development and acceleration of the maturation of lymphoid cells has been demonstrated in a wide variety of in vitro and in vivo model systems. The absence of thymosin may explain both the growth arrest after neonatal thymectomy and the dwarfism that characterizes the genetically athymic nude mouse. White has offered the tentative suggestion that thymosin is related to the somatomedin family of growth factors and may be influenced by growth hormone and thyrotropic hormone.[97]

CONCLUSION

This brief synopsis of the rapidly growing literature on peptide growth factors is reminiscent of the confusion that attended the early descriptive phases of endocrinology. It is obvious from the long list of dissimilar substances that can stimulate DNA synthesis and mitosis in fibroblasts that this property by itself is insufficiently specific to suggest any basis for further classification.

Out of this group there does emerge, however, a group of discrete peptides that strike a repetitive note. These are the smaller proteins and peptides that exhibit unique actions in specialized cell types. Many of these growth factors possess pronounced insulin-like properties, suggesting some ancestral relationship to insulin. Many of the better-studied factors have been found to be responsive to their anabolic hormones.

Although it may be premature to consider any of these growth factors as hormones or even as mediators of hormone action, the biological potency of these substances suggests that they may eventually prove to be constituents of an important part of the regulatory system that governs cell growth, cell differentiation, wound healing, organ regeneration, and possibly neoplastic growth. Recognition of this class of peptide growth factors is still very recent, however, and much needs to be learned before its position in the hierarchy of cell control mechanisms is established.

REFERENCES

1. Goss, R. T.: The strategy of growth, in Tier, H., Rytomea, T. (eds): Control of Cellular Growth in Adult Organisms. New York, Academic Press, 1967, pp 3–25.
2. Hershko, A., Mamont, P., Shields, R., et al: Pleiotypic response. *Nature (New Biol) 232:* 206–211, 1971.
3. Otten, J., Johnson, G. S., Pastan, I.: Regulation of cell growth by cyclic adenosine 3′,5′-monophosphate. Effect of cell density and agents which alter cell growth on cycline adenosine 3′,5′-monophosphate levels in fibroblasts. *J Biol Chem 247:* 7082–7087, 1972.
4. Frank, W.: Cyclic 3′,5′ AMP and cell proliferation in cultures of embryonic rat cell. *Exp Cell Res 71:* 238–241, 1972.
5. Hadden, J. W., Hadden, E. M., Haddox, M. K., et al: Guanosine 3′,5′ cyclic monophosphate: A possible intracellular mediatror of mitogenic influences in lymphocytes. *Proc Natl Acad Sci USA 69:* 3024–3027, 1972.
6. Seifert, W. E., Rudland, P. S.: Possible involvement of cyclic GMP in growth control of cultured mouse cells. *Nature 248:* 138– 140, 1974.
7. Mendelson, I. S., Anderson, M. D.: Rat mammary gland nuclear RNA polymerases in late pregnancy and lactation. *Biochim Biophys Acta 299:* 576–587, 1973.
8. Miller, Z., Lovelace, E., Gallo, M., Pastan, I.: Cyclic guanosine monophosphate and cellular growth. *Science 190:* 1213–1215, 1975.
9. von Humgen, K., Roberts, S.: Catecholamine and Ca^{++} activation of adenyl cyclase systems in synaptosomal fractions from rat cerebral cortex. *Nature (New Biol) 242:* 58–60, 1973.
10. Don, S., Weiner, H., Bachrach, U.: Specific increase in polyamine levels in chick embryo cells transformed by Rous sarcoma virus. *Cancer Res 35:* 194–198, 1975.
11. Bullough, W. S.: Chalone control systems, in LaBue, J., Gordon, A. S. (eds): Humoral Control of Growth and Differentiation. New York, Academic Press, 1973.
12. Salmon, W. D. Jr., Daughaday, W. H.: A hormonally controlled serum factor which stimulates growth. *J Lab Clin Med 49:* 825–836, 1957.

13. Daughaday, W. H., Reeder, C. J.: Synchronous activation of DNA synthesis in hypophysectomized rat cartilage by growth hormone. *J Lab Clin Med 68:* 357–368, 1967.

14. Salmon, W. D. Jr., DuVall, M. R.: A serum factor with sulfation factor activity simulates *in vitro* incorporation of leucine and sulfate into protein polysaccharide complexes, uridine into RNA and thymidine into DNA of costal cartilages from hypophysectomized rats *in vitro. Endocrinology 86:* 721–727, 1970.

15. Daughaday, W. H., Mariz, I. K.: Conversion of proline-U-C14 to labelled hydroxy-proline by rat cartilage *in vitro:* Effects of hypophysectomy, growth hormone, and cortisol. *J Lab Clin Med 59:* 741–752, 1962.

16. Hall, K., Uthne, K.: Some biological properties of purified sulfation factor from human plasma. *Acta Med Scand 190:* 137–143, 1971.

17. Salmon, W. D. Jr., Hosse, B. R.: Stimulation of HeLa cell growth by a serum factor with sulfation factor activity. *Proc Soc Exp Biol Med 136:* 805–808, 1971.

18. Daughaday, W. H., Hall, K., Raben, M. S., et al: Somatomedin: Proposed designation for sulfation factor. *Nature 235:* 107, 1972.

19. Uthne, K.: Human somatomedins: Purification and some studies on their biological actions. *Acta Endocrinol Suppl 175:* 1–35, 1973.

20. Van Wyk, J. J., Underwood, L. E., Hintz, R. L.: The somatomedins: A family of insulinlike hormones under growth hormone control. *Recent Prog Horm Res 30:* 259–295, 1974.

21. Oelz, O., Froesch, E. R., Bunzli, H. F., Humbel, R. E., Ritschard, W. J.: In Handbook of Physiology-Endocrinology 1. Bethesda, *Am Physiol Soc,* 1972, pp 685–702.

22. Pierson, R. W. Jr., Temin, H. M.: The partial purification from calf serum of a fraction with multiplication stimulative for chicken fibroblasts in cell culture and with non-suppressible insulin-like activity. *J Cell Physiol 79:* 319–329, 1972.

23. Leonards, J. R., Landau, B. P., Bartsch, G.: Assay of insulin-like activity with rat epididymal fat pad. *J Lab Clin Med 60:* 552–570, 1962.

24. Jakob, A., Hauri, C. H., Froesch, E. R.: Non-suppressible insulin-like activity in human serum 3. Differentiation of two distinct molecules with nonsuppressible ILA. *J Clin Invest 47:* 2678–2688, 1968.

24a. Rinderknecht, E., Humbel, R. E.: Polypeptides with nonsuppressible insulinlike and cell-growth promoting activities in human serum: Isolation, chemical characterization, and some biological properties of forms I and II. *Proc Natl Acad Sci, USA 73:* 2365–2369, 1976.

24b. Rinderknecht, E., Humbel, R. E.: Amino-terminal sequences of two polypeptides from human serum with nonsuppressible insulin-like and cell-growth promoting activities: Evidence for structural homology with insulin B chain. *Proc Natl Acad Sci, USA 73:* 4379–4381, 1976.

25. Froesch, E. R., Burgi, H., Ramseier, E. B., et al: Antibody-suppressible and nonsuppressible insulin-like activities in human serum and their physiologic significance. An insulin assay with adipose tissues of increased precision and specificity. *J Clin Invest 42:* 1816–1834, 1963.

26. Zingg, A. E., Froesch, E. R.: Effects of partially purified preparations with nonsuppressible insulin-like activity (NSILA-S) on sulfate incorporation into rat and chicken cartilage. *Diabetologia 9:* 472–476, 1973.

27. Froesch, E. R., Schlumpf, U., Heimann, R., Eigenmann, E., Zapf, J.: In Luft, R., Hall, K., (eds): Advances in Metabolic Disorders, vol 8. New York, Academic Press, 1975, pp 237–245.

28. Temin, H. M., Pierson, R. W., Jr., Dulak, N. C.: In Rothblat, G. H., Cristofalo, V. S. (eds): Growth, Nutrition and Metabolism of Cells in Culture. New York, Academic Press, 1972, pp 50–81.

29. Dulak, N. C., Temin, H. M.: A partially purified polypeptide fraction from rat liver cell conditioned medium with multiplication stimulating activity for embryo fibroblasts. *J Cell Physiol 81:* 153–160, 1973.

30. Cohen, K. L., Short, P. A., Nissley, S. P.: Growth hormone-dependent serum stimulation of DNA synthesis in chick embryo fibroblasts in culture. *Endocrinology 96:* 193–198, 1975.

31. Hintz, R. L., Orsini, E. M., Van Camp, M. G.: Evidence for a somatomedin binding protein in plasma. *The Endocrine Society,* 1974.

32. Zapf, J., Waldvodel, M., Froesch, E. R.: Specific binding of nonsuppressible insulin-like activity to chicken embryo fibroblasts and to a solubilized fibroblast receptor. *Arch Biochem 168:* 638–645, 1975.

33. Cohen, K. L., Nissley, S. P.: The serum half-life of somatomedin: Dependence on growth hormone stimulation. *Clin Res 23:* A317, 1975.

34. Underwood, L. E., Hintz, R. L., Voina, S. J., et al: Human somatomedin, the growth hormone dependent sulfation factor is anti-lipolytic. *Endocrinol Metab 35:* 195–198, 1972.

35. Uthne, K., Reagan, C. R., Gimple, L. P., et al: Effects of human somatomedin preparations on membrane transport and protein synthesis in the isolated rat diaphragm. *Endocrinol Metab 39:* 548–554, 1974.

36. Clemmons, D. R., Hintz, R. L., Underwood, L. E., et al: Common mechanism of actions of somatomedin and insulin on fat cells. Further evidence. *Isr J Med Sci 10:* 1254–1262, 1974.

37. Hintz, R. L., Clemmons, D. R., Underwood, L. E., et al: Competitive binding of somatomedin to the insulin receptors of adipocytes, chondrocytes and liver membranes. *Proc Natl Acad Sci USA 69:* 2351–2353, 1972.

38. Takano, K., Hall, K., Fryklund, L., et al: The binding of insulin and somatomedin A to human placental membrane. *Acta Endocrinol 80:* 14–31, 1975.

39. Megyesi, K., Kahn, C. R., Roth, J., et al: Hypoglycemia in association with extrapancreatic tumors: Demonstration of elevated plasma NSILA-S by a new radioreceptor assay. *J Clin Endocrinol Metab 38:* 931–934, 1974.

39a. D'Ercole, A. J., Decedue, C. J., Furlanetto, R. W., Underwood, L. E., Van Wyk, J. J.: Evidence that somatomedin-C is degraded by the kidney and inhibits insulin degradation. *Endocrinology 101:* 247–259, 1977.

39b. Burghen, G. A., Duckworth, W. C., Kitabchi, A. E., Solomon, S. S., and Poffenbarger, P. L.: Inhibition of insulin degradation by nonsuppressible insulin-like activity. *J Clin Invest 57:* 1089–1092, 1976.

40. Marshall, R. N., Underwood, L. E., Voina, S. J., Foushee, D. B., Van Wyk, J. J.: Characterization of the insulin and somatomedin-C receptors in human placental cell membranes. *J Clin Endocrinol Metab 39:* 283–292, 1974.

40a. Furlanetto, R. W., Underwood, L. E., Van Wyk, J. J., D'Ercole, A. J.: Estimation of somatomedin-C levels in normals and patients with pituitary disease by radioimmunoassay. *J Clin Invest 60:* 648–657, 1977.

41. Zapf, J., Zumstein, P., Froesch, E. R.: NSILA-S, epinephrine-stimulated lypolysis and cAMP release in rat adipose tissue. *Experientia 30:* 694, 1974.

42. Megyesi, K., Kahn, C. R., Roth, J., et al: Circulating NSILA-S in man: Basal and stimulated levels and binding to plasma components. *Clin Res 23:* A388, 1975.

43. Hall, K., Takano, K., Fryklund, L.: Radioreceptor assay for somatomedin-A. *J Clin Endocrinol Metab 39:* 973–976, 1974.

43a. Rechler, M. M., Podskalny, J. M., Nissley, S. P.: Interaction of multiplication stimulating activity with chick embryo fibroblasts demonstrates a growth receptor. *Nature 259:* 134–136, 1976.

44. Van Wyk, J. J., Underwood, L. E., Baseman, J. B., et al: Advances in Metabolic Disorders, vol 8. New York, Academic Press, 1975, pp 128–150.

44a. Van Wyk, J. J., Underwood, L. E.: The somatomedins and their actions, in Litwack, G. (ed): Biochemical Actions of Hormones, vol V. New York, Academic Press, 1977.

45. Pastan, I. H., Johnson, C. S., Anderson, W. B.: Role of cyclic nucleotides in growth control. *Annu Rev Biochem 44:* 491–522, 1975.

46. Tell, G. P., Cuatrecasas, P., Hintz, R. L., et al: Somatomedin: inhibition of adenylate cyclase activity in subcellular membranes of various tissues. *Science 180:* 312–315, 1973.

47. Hepp, K. D., Renner, R.: Insulin action on the adenyl cyclase system: Antagonism to activation by lipolytic hormones. *Fed Eur Biochem Soc Lett 20:* 191–194, 1973.

48. Luft, R., Hall, K.: Somatomedins and Some Other Growth Factors, vol 8. New York, Academic Press, 1975.

49. Pickart, L., Thaler, M. D.: Tripeptide in human serum which prolongs survival of normal liver cells and stimulates growth in neoplastic liver. *Nature (New Biol) 243:* 85–87, 1973.

50. Thaler, M. M., Pickart, L.: Stimulation of oxidative metabolism by growth factor from human serum. *Fed Proc 33:* 1344, 1974.

51. Sievertsson, H., Fryklund, L., Uthne, K., et al: Advances in Metabolic Disorders, vol 8. New York, Academic Press, 1975, pp 47–60.

52. Yalow, R., Hall, K., Luft, R.: Radioimmunoassay of somatomedin-B. Application to clinical and physiologic studies. *J Clin Invest 55:* 127–137, 1975.

53. Houck, J. C., Cheng, R. F.: Isolation, purification, and chemical characterization of the serum mitogen for diploid human fibroblasts. *J Cell Physiol 81:* 257–270, 1973.

54. August, G. P., Cheng, R. F., Hung, W., et al: Fibroblast proliferative activity in the sera of growth hormone deficient patients. *Horm Metab Res 5:* 340–341, 1973.
55. Renner, R., Hepp, K. D., Veser, J., et al: Effect of the growth stimulating serum proteins S1 and S2 on isolated fat cells of the rat. *Exp Cell Res 85:* 426–430, 1974.
56. Chen, L. B., Buchanan, J. M.: Plasminogen-independent fibrinolysis by proteases produced by transformed chick embryo fibroblasts. *Proc Natl Acad Sci USA 72:* 1312–1316, 1975.
57. Kohler, N., Lipton, A.: Platelets as a source of fibroblast growth-promoting activity. *Exp Cell Res 87:* 297–301, 1974.
57a. Rutherford, R. B., Ross, R.: Platelet factors stimulate fibroblasts and smooth muscle cells quiescent in plasma serum to proliferate. *J Cell Biol 69:* 196–203, 1976.
57b. Harker, L. A., Ross, R., Slichter, S. J., Scott, C. R.: Homocystine-induced arteriosclerosis: The role of endothelial cell injury and platelet response in its genesis. *J Clin Invest 58:* 731–741, 1976.
58. Goldwasser, E., Kung, C. K. H.: Purification of erythropoietin. *Proc Natl Acad Sci USA 68:* 697–698, 1971.
59. Dorado, M., Espada, J., Langton, A., et al: Molecular weight estimation of human erythropoietin by SDS-polyacrylamide gel electrophoresis. *Biochem Med 10:* 1–7, 1974.
60. Jepson, J. H., McGarry, E. E.: Hemopoiesis in pituitary dwarfs treated with human growth hormone and testosterone. *Blood 39:* 229–248, 1972.
61. Alexanian, R.: Erythropoietin and erythropoiesis in anemic man following androgens. *Blood 33:* 564–572, 1969.
62. Levi-Montalcini, R., Meyer, H., Hamburger, V.: *In vitro* experiments on effects of mouse sacromas 180 and 37 on spinal and sympathetic ganglia of chick embryo. *Cancer Res 14:* 49–57, 1954.
63. Levi-Montalcini, R., Angeletti, P. U.: Essential role of the nerve growth factor in the survival and maintenance of dissociated sensory and sympathetic embryonic nerve cells *in vitro*. *Develop Biol 7:* 653–659, 1963.
64. Levi-Montalcini, R.: The nerve growth factor. *Ann NY Acad Sci 118:* 149–170, 1964.
65. Levi-Montalcini, R., Angeletti, P. U.: Nerve growth factor. *Physiol Rev 48:* 534–569, 1968.
66. Longo, A. M., Penhoet, E. E.: Nerve growth factor in rat glioma cells. *Proc Natl Acad Sci USA 71:* 2347–2349, 1974.
67. Young, M., et al: Secretion of nerve growth factor by primary chick fibroblast cultures. *Science 187:* 361–362, 1975.
68. Bocchini, V., Angeletti, P. U.: The nerve growth factor: Purification as a 30,000-molecular-weight protein. *Proc Natl Acad Sci USA 64:* 787–794, 1969.
69. Angeletti, R. H., Bradshaw, R. A., Wade, R. D.: Subunit structure and amino acid composition of mouse submaxillary gland nerve growth factor. *Biochemistry 10:* 463–469, 1971.
70. Angeletti, R. H., Bradshaw, R. A., Frazier, W. A.: Advances in Metabolic Disorders, Vol 8. New York, Academic Press, 1975, pp 285–299.
71. Frazier, W. A., Angeletti, R. H., Bradshaw, B. A.: Nerve growth factor and insulin. *Science 176:* 482–488, 1972.
72. Frazier, W. A., Boyd, L. F., Bradshaw, R. A.: Interactions of nerve growth factor with surface membranes: Biological competence of insolubilized nerve growth factor. *Proc Natl Acad Sci USA 70:* 2931–2935, 1973.
73. Frazier, W. A., Boyd, L. F., Szutowicz, A.: Specific binding sites for ^{125}I-nerve growth factor in peripheral tissues and brain. *Biochem Biophys Res Commun 57:* 1096–1103, 1974.
74. Cohen, S.: Isolation of a mouse submaxillary gland protein accelerating incisor eruption and eyelid opening in the newborn animal. *J Biol Chem 237:* 1555–1562, 1962.
75. Taylor, J. M., Cohen, S., Mitchell, W. M.: Epidermal growth factor: high and low molecular weight forms. *Proc Natl Acad Sci USA 67:* 164–171, 1970.
76. Taylor, J. M., Mitchell, W. M., Cohen, S.: Characterization of the high molecular weight form of epidermal growth factor. *J Biol Chem 249:* 3198–3203, 1974.
77. Savage, C. R., Inagami, T., Cohen, S.: The primary structure of epidermal growth factor. *J Biol Chem 247:* 7612–7621, 1972.
78. Cohen, S., Taylor, J. M.: Epidermal growth factor: Chemical and biological characterization. *Recent Prog Horm Res 30:* 533–550, 1974.
79. Ho, P. C., Davis, W. H., Elliott, J. H., et al: Kinetics of corneal epithelial regeneration and epidermal growth factor. *Invest Ophthalmol 13:* 804–809, 1974.
80. O'Keefe, E., Hollenberg, M. D., Cuatrecasas, P.: Epidermal growth factor. Characteristics of specific binding in membranes from liver, placenta, and other target tissues. *Arch Biochem 164(2):* 518–526, 1974.
81. Carpenter, G., Lembach, K. J., Morrison, M. M., et al: Characterization of the binding of ^{125}I-labeled epidermal growth factor to human fibroblasts. *J Biol Chem 250:* 4297–4304, 1975.
82. Hollenberg, M. D., Cuatrecasas, P.: Epidermal growth factor: Receptors in human fibroblasts and modulation of action by cholera toxin. *Proc Natl Acad Sci USA 70:* 2964–2968.
83. Byyny, R. L., Orth, D. N., Cohen, S.: Radioimmunoassay of epidermal growth factor. *Endocrinology 90:* 1261–1266, 1972.
84. Barthe, P. L., Bullock, L. P., Mowszowicz, I., et al: Submaxillary gland epidermal growth factor: A sensitive index of biologic androgen activity. *Endocrinology 95:* 1019–1025, 1974.
85. Byyny, R. L., Orth, D. N., Cohen, S., et al: Epidermal growth factor: Effects of androgens and adrenergic agents. *Endocrinology 96:* 776–782, 1974.
86. Ances, I. G.: Serum concentrations of epidermal growth factor in human pregnancy. *Am J Obstet Gynecol 115:* 357–362, 1973.
87. Starkey, R. H., Cohen, S., Orth, D. N.: Epidermal growth factor: Identification of a new hormone in human urine. *Science 189:* 800–802, 1975.
88. Cohen, S., Carpenter, G.: Human epidermal growth factor: Isolation and chemical and biological properties. *Proc Natl Acad Sci USA 72:* 1317–1321, 1975.
88a. Gregory, H.: Isolation and structure of urogastrone and its relationship to epidermal growth factor. *Nature 257:* 325–327, 1975.
89. Gospodarowicz, D., Jones, K. L., Sato, G.: Purification of a growth factor for ovarian cells from bovine pituitary glands. *Proc Natl Acad Sci USA 71:* 2295–2299, 1974.
90. Nishawaki, K., Armelin, H. A., Sato, G.: Control of ovarian cell growth in culture by serum and pituitary factors. *Proc Natl Acad Sci USA 72:* 483–487, 1975.
91. Gospodarowicz, D.: Localisation of a fibroblast growth factor and its effect alone and with hydrocortisone on 3T3 cell growth. *Nature 249:* 123–127, 1974.
92. Holley, R. W., Kierman, J. A.: Control of the initiation of DNA synthesis in 3T3 cells: Serum factors. *Proc Natl Acad Sci USA 71:* 2908–2911, 1974.
93. Rudland, P. S., Seifert, W., Gospodarowicz, D.: Growth control in cultured mouse fibroblasts: Induction of the pleiotypic and mitogenic responses by a purified growth factor. *Proc Natl Acad Sci USA 71:* 2600–2604, 1974.
93a. Gospodarowicz, D., Ill, C. R., Hornsby, P. J., Gill, G. N.: Control of bovine adrenal cortical cell proliferation by fibroblast growth factor. Lack of effect of epidermal growth factor. *Endocrinology 100:* 1080–1089, 1977.
93b. Gospodarowicz, D., Ill, C. R., Birdwell, C. R.: Effects of fibroblast and epidermal growth factors on ovarian cell proliferation *in vitro*. I. Characterization of the response of granulosa cells to FGF and EGF. *Endocrinology 100:* 1108–1120, 1977.
93c. Gospodarowicz, D., Ill, C. R., Birdwell, C. R.: Effects of fibroblast and epidermal growth factors on ovarian cell proliferation *in vitro*. II. Proliferative response of luteal cells to FGF but not EGF. *Endocrinology 100:* 1121–1128, 1977.
94. Gospodarowicz, D., Rudland, P., Lindstrom, J., et al: Advances in Metabolic Disorders, vol 8. New York, Academic Press, 1975, pp 302–335.
94a. Antoniades, H. N., Stathacos, D., Scher, C. D.: Isolation of a cationic polypeptide from human serum that stimulates proliferation of 3T3 cells. *Proc Natl Acad Sci USA 72(7):* 2635–2639, 1975.
94b. Antoniades, H. N., Scher, C. D.: Growth factors derived from human serum, human platelets, and human pituitary: Properties and immunologic cross reactivity, in Sanford K (ed): Decennial Review Conference on Cell, Tissue, and Organ Culture, *Monograph Series of J Natl Cancer Inst,* 1977, (in press).
95. Singer, M.: Neurotrophic control of limb regeneration in the newt. *Ann NY Acad Sci 228:* 308–322, 1974.
96. Gospodarowicz, D., Weseman, J., Moran, J.: Presence in brain of a mitogenic agent promoting proliferation of myoblasts in low density culture. *Nature 256:* 216–219, 1975.
97. White, A., Goldstein, A. L.: Advances in Metabolic Disorders, vol 8. New York, Academic Press, 1975, pp 359–374.
98. Goldstein, A. L., Zatz, A., Hardy, M. M., et al: Purification and biological activity of thymosin, a hormone of the thymus gland. *Proc Natl Acad Sci USA 69:* 1800–1803, 1972.

Integrated Hormonal Control Systems

141

Endocrine and Metabolic Aspects of Fuel Homeostasis in the Fetus and Neonate

Morey W. Haymond
Anthony S. Pagliara

During the transition from intrauterine to extrauterine life a variety of metabolic changes and adaptations occur in fuel homeostasis. These adaptations allow the fetus to convert from a state in which he is totally dependent on maternal fuel sources delivered intravenously, to a state in which he relies on alimentation and his own endogenous substrates for the maintenance of normal cellular function and growth.

This chapter will deal with (1) placental transport and fetal storage of substrate (i.e., fat, glycogen, and protein), (2) the development of certain key enzymatic and hormonal systems that modulate substrate mobilization, interconversions, and utilization, and (3) how defects in normal development of these systems may result in pathology. It is recognized that a variety of inborn errors in metabolism (synthetic and catabolic disorders of amino acids, glycoproteins, and lipids) represent defects that may effect fuel homeostasis; it is beyond the scope of this chapter to consider this material. Since the most common defect resulting from abnormalities in fuel regulation in the neonatal period is hypoglycemia, primary attention will be given to factors affecting glucose homeostasis.

PLACENTAL TRANSPORT OF METABOLIC FUELS AND NUTRIENTS

The placenta has both endocrine and transport functions. The former is dealt with in Chapter 133. Normal fetal growth and development is wholly dependent upon the placenta for respiration, nutrition, and excretion. Unless the transplacental lifeline to the fetus can be established early and effectively maintained, pregnancy will terminate with absorption or expulsion of the embryo. Numerous substances are transferred from the maternal to the fetal circulation, and in regards to all aspects of energy metabolism the fetus is solely dependent on maternal sources. Physiologic or pathologic abnormalities inherent within the mother, fetus, or placenta may act to limit the availability of various substances for normal fetal development which in turn results in fetal wastage or neonatal defects. Since placental transport is intimately involved with normal fetal metabolism and development, certain selected aspects underlying this process will be considered briefly; the interested reader is referred to the excellent review by Longo for a more detailed discussion.[1]

TYPES OF PLACENTAL TRANSPORT

In contrast to the belief of early investigators that the placenta is simply a passive, semipermeable membrane, it has been clearly demonstrated that transfer of substances by this organ occurs by several different mechanisms including simple diffusion, active transport, facilitated diffusion, pinocytosis, and bulk flow.

Simple diffusion is the movement of a molecular species from an area of high concentration to one of low concentration, which is in response to either a chemical or electrochemical gradient due to charged ionic particles. Simple diffusion is a passive process which does not require energy; movement continues until equilibrium is obtained. Factors affecting rate of movement include molecular size, electrical charge, and lipid solubility.

Facilitated diffusion is the movement of molecules across a membrane from an area of higher concentration to one of lower concentration but differs from simple diffusion in that transfer is faster than would be predicted on a physical-chemical basis, there is decreased transport at high concentrations (saturation), and substances with similar molecular configurations are competitive inhibitors of transport.[2] This form of transport differs from active transport in that movement of substances does not occur against a gradient, and since no energy is required cannot be "poisoned" by metabolic inhibitors. The simplest hypothesis which would explain this type of transport is that a given substance combines with a "carrier" in the membrane, and this carrier-substrate complex crosses the membrane at a faster rate than the substrate alone.[1]

Active transport is the process in which energy is expended and results in "uphill" transport of a substance against an electrochemical gradient. Experimental evidence suggests that a membrane "carrier" that is linked to an ATP energy source combines chemically with the substrate. Characteristics of this type of transport include competition from molecules of similar species, inhibition of transport by metabolic poisons, and saturation kinetics.[1]

Micropinocytosis is a process in which specific extracellular macromolecules are taken up into the cell by the pinching off of small vesicles from the plasma membrane, allowing specific proteins to be removed from a solution containing a variety of proteins. Electron microscopic studies of the placenta have demonstrated micropinocytotic vesicles containing material that histologically resembles protein.[3]

PLACENTAL TRANSPORT OF SPECIFIC SUBSTANCES

The means of transport differs for various substances, and for some, more than one mode exist. Processes involved in transport of several compounds from mother to fetus which are important in fetal metabolism and development are summarized in Table 141-1.

Gases

The respiratory gases (O_2, CO_2) and the metabolically inert gases cross the placental barrier by simple diffusion.[4,5] The placental exchange of O_2 is determined by (1) the placental diffusing capacity in which O_2 diffuses from a high partial pressure in maternal blood to a lower partial pressure in fetal blood, (2) the uterine and umbilical arterial O_2 tensions, (3) the characteristics of the maternal and fetal oxyhemoglobin saturation curves, (4) the maternal and fetal placental hemoglobin flow rates, (5) the pattern of maternal to fetal blood flows, and (6) the amount of CO_2 exchanging. In a normal 3-kg fetus, the rate of fetal O_2 utilization is approximately 14 to 15 ml/min, the supply of O_2 in reserve is about 30 ml, and no mechanisms are available by which the fetus can increase its O_2 stores. Placental diffusing capacity will be decreased in clinical conditions that thicken the placental membranes or decrease the surface area of exchange, such as placental infarctions, diabetes mellitus, toxemia of pregnancy, other hypertensive disorders, syphilis, and erythroblastosis.[1]

Water and Electrolyte Transfer

Although a large number of studies have been performed relevant to water transport across the placenta, to date the exact mechanisms are not known. During the course of gestation there is a net increase of 4000 ml of water within the uterus, of which 3000 to 3200 ml are distributed through placental and fetal tissues and 500 to 1000 ml are present in amniotic fluids. In vivo and in vitro studies demonstrate that both the amnion and chorion are freely permeable to water. There are no quantitative data on the amount of water movement due to simple diffusion nor is there evidence to indicate that water is either secreted by the membranes or crosses by active transport. The most likely cause of large water movement is via bulk flow due to a hydrostatic pressure gradient between maternal and fetal blood. Only small or intermittant hydrostatic gradients could be responsible for movement of large amounts of water from maternal to fetal circulation.[1]

Early studies by Flexner and co-workers demonstrated that large quantities of sodium and other electrolytes cross the placenta.[6–8] It is generally assumed that sodium, potassium, and other univalent ions cross by simple diffusion and some may also cross by "solvent drag."

The concentrations of calcium, iron, iodine, and phosphate [1,9–11] in fetal blood are elevated as compared to those found in the maternal circulation, and it has been assumed that these ions are actively transported by the placenta.

Table 141-1. Transplacental Transport Mechanisms of Various Substances

	Diffusion	Facilitated Transport	Active Transport	Bulk Flow	Pinocytosis
Gasses					
O_2, CO_2, N_2, CO	+				
Ions					
Na^+, K^+, Cl^+	+				
Ca^{++}, Fe^{++}, PO_4, I			+		
Free amino acids			+		
Glucose		+			
Free fatty acids	+				
Steroids					
Estrogen	+				
Progesterone	+				
Cortisol	+				
Proteins					
Albumin					+
7S γ_2 globulins					+
19S macroglobulins					+
Fibrinogen					+
Transferin					+
Water				+	

Amino Acids, Polypeptides, and Proteins

It is well established that the free α-amino nitrogen concentration is higher in fetal than in maternal extra- and intracellular fluids in pregnant women, the rhesus monkey, sheep, rodents, and dogs, and it has been shown that each individual amino acid contributes differently to the high fetal:maternal ratio.[12,13] The normal fetal:maternal ratio varies from about 1.2 to 4.0, with a mean of 1.8.[14] Amino acid transport across the placenta demonstrates all the characteristics of active transport including (1) competition between certain amino acids such as histidine and glycine for the transport process,[15] (2) saturation of the transport process by high concentrations of amino acids,[16] and (3) inhibition of transport by metabolic inhibitors.[12]

Placental transfer of the polypeptide hormones is considered in detail in Chapter 133. Polypeptides cross the placenta poorly if at all, and for all practical purposes the fetus is dependent upon its own production and secretion. The majority of evidence is consistent with a placental barrier to the transport of the two polypeptides of major interest in this chapter—insulin[16,17] and glucagon.[18]

Although albumin, 7S γ_2-globulin and its F and S fragments, 19S macroglobulin, fibrinogen, transferrin, and acid glycoproteins have been demonstrated to cross the placenta by pinocytosis, the fetus probably synthesizes the vast majority of its structural and enzymatic proteins from amino acids derived from the maternal circulation.[1]

Lipid Transport

Placental transport of lipids has recently been reviewed by Robertson and Sprecher.[19] Fetal fat is the product of synthesis from carbohydrate and acetate and from free fatty acids transferred across the placenta. Free fatty acids exchange rapidly across the placenta by simple diffusion.[20,21] There appears to be no difference in total amount of fatty acid transferred regardless of degree of saturation, carbon chain length, or whether the fatty acid is given singly or in combination with other fatty acids in studies utilizing the perfused guinea pig placenta.[20]

Unlike free fatty acids, very little or no transport of complex lipids (e.g., cholesterol, phospholipids, or triglycerides) occurs across the guinea pig placenta[20] while in the fetal rat maternal cholesterol accounts for only 10 to 20 percent of the total fetal cholesterol pool.[22] Fetal cholesterol is lower than maternal concentrations, and this is considered to be related to the low β-lipoprotein content of fetal plasma. In contrast, α-lipoprotein content is the same in both maternal and fetal blood.[23] The cause of the low fetal β-lipoprotein could be a result of placental impermeability or catabolism of the β-lipoprotein-cholesterol complex.

As considered in Chapter 133, estrogens, progesterone, and cortisol readily cross the placenta. Besides transport, the placenta plays an active role in enzymatically altering the steroid structure, and such alteration may play a major role in the transport process. The placenta also converts inactive steroid precursors (i.e., cholesterol, pregnenolone, and dehydroepiandrosterone) to progesterone and estrogen.

Carbohydrate Transport

Glucose is considered by most to be the primary fetal fuel, although this concept has been challenged recently (see below). In man this concept is dependent upon the demonstration in the fetus of glycogen in a variety of tissues, of glucose in the circulating plasma, and indirect measurement of the respiratory quotient. Quantitatively there is a maternal-to-fetal transfer of approximately 6 mg. glucose/min/kg fetal weight,[1] or in a 3-kg fetus at term 26 gm of glucose/24 h. This represents only 34 cal/kg body weight/24 h and therefore would account for approximately one-third to one-quarter of the necessary calories for growth and development.

The physiologic events governing transport of carbohydrates are complex and must take into account the presence of amniotic, fetal, and maternal pools. Data obtained by several investigators[24–26] strongly suggest that the mechanism by which transport occurs is by facilitated diffusion. The evidence in support of this type of transport includes (1) the lack of transport against a gradient,[25,26] (2) a faster rate of transport than can be accounted for by passive diffusion alone,[25] (3) competition by other hexoses with D-glucose for transport, including evidence that D-glucose is transported more rapidly than the L-isomer,[27] (4) the more rapid transport of glucose (an aldohexose) than fructose (a ketohexose),[26] and (5) the more rapid transfer of D-xylose than the L-isomer.[2]

Maternal and fetal glucose concentrations are similar in early gestation.[17,27,28] At term a concentration gradient across the placenta from maternal artery to umbilical vein of about 10 to 30 percent has been repeatedly observed. The variability in this gradient is most likely related to the stress of delivery, and may reflect increased glucose utilization by the fetus.

The placenta synthesizes large amounts of glycogen from maternal glucose. The role, if any, of this glycogen in transport and metabolism is unknown. Placental glycogen concentration changes during pregnancy, and is highest at 8 weeks. This gradually declines until 18 to 20 weeks, and is maintained at a level of 15 to 20 mg/100 mg dry weight until term. There is continuous exchange between maternal glucose, placental glycogen, and fetal glucose.[29] At the present time there is no clear explanation of either the role or necessity of placental glycogen in the face of normal concentrations of maternal blood glucose; however, in unusual situations of substrate limitation to the fetus (i.e., placental anoxia or maternal hypoglycemia) this may be an important energy reserve.

In the human fetus a small amount of fructose (5 mg/100 ml) is present. Fetal fructose is produced by the placenta from glucose.[30] In sheep, although maternal levels of fructose are low, the fetal or newborn lamb has high plasma levels which disappear slowly after birth. Since the placenta of ungulates contains only small amounts of glycogen, it has been suggested that this may be an important source as a reserve nutrient for these species.[29]

Recent studies by Battaglia and associates[31,32] utilizing the nonstressed chronic catheterized sheep preparation have demonstrated that glucose is not the sole substrate for fetal energy requirements. These findings strongly challenge previously accepted dogma that glucose is the primary fuel in the human fetus.

In very elaborate and sophisticated studies, these investigators determined that total fetal oxygen consumption could be accounted for by glucose, amino acids, and lactate in the ratio of 2:1:1 in late gestation. Fructose, free fatty acids, and glycerol accounted for negligible amounts of the oxygen consumed. Further, they have demonstrated that of the substrates transported, 41 and 63 percent of the carbon and nitrogen, respectively, are retained for growth. These data underscore the importance of normal placental function, since alterations in the transport of a diverse group of substrates by a variety of mechanisms may have adverse affects on fetal growth and development.

ENDOCRINE CONTROL OF SUBSTRATE FLOW AND UTILIZATION

Unlike the adult, hormonal signals for control of substrate flow and utilization along metabolic pathways in the fetus and newborn are not well delineated. There are numerous unanswered questions: At what stage of fetal development does hormonal control become important in regulation of energy processes? Since the polypeptide hormones (insulin, glucagon, growth hormone) cannot be detected in the fetus prior to 8 to 10 weeks of gestation and there is no good evidence that these hormones can be transplacentally transported, are fetal biosynthetic processes at this stage of development under the control of hormonal factors other than those customarily associated with normal metabolism and growth in the neonate and child? When and how does hormonal control become established? Finally, once hormonal secretion is established, are these secretions necessary for the regulation of substrate metabolism in the developing fetus? Before considering some of the above questions, a brief review of endocrine control of metabolism in the growing child and adult is indicated.

ENDOCRINE CONTROL OF FUEL METABOLISM IN THE ADULT

Insulin is the predominant hormone regulating the blood glucose, since it is the only hormone whose direct action is to decrease the influx and accelerate the efflux of glucose from the vascular space. Insulin stimulates the transmembrane movement of glucose into skeletal and cardiac muscle and adipose tissue and the conversion of glucose to glycogen and triglyceride, as well as the intracellular transport of amino acid into tissues and their incorporation into protein.[33] The hormone, at even low concentrations, is a potent inhibitor of lipolysis.[34] The net effect of these actions on peripheral tissues is to accelerate glucose disappearance from the blood and to decrease the supply of gluconeogenic substrates (i.e., glycerol and amino acids) presented to the liver. In concert with these peripheral actions, insulin stimulates hepatic glycogen synthesis, impairs glycogenolysis, and markedly depresses hepatic gluconeogenesis. Current information suggests that these hepatic effects reflect an action of the hormone on the adenyl-cyclase–cyclic-nucleotide-phosphodiesterase system resulting in a decrease in the cellular concentration of cyclic AMP.[35] This action would result in activation of glycogen synthetase, inhibition of the phosphorylase system, and decreased activity of the gluconeogenic enzymes.

It is now recognized that the plasma glucose level is not the only determinant of insulin release, but that secretion is influenced by a variety of nutritional and humoral factors. A number of amino acids are capable of either directly stimulating insulin release from the β-cell or potentiating the effect of glucose on hormone secretion (see Chapter 76). Furthermore, the oral ingestion of glucose and protein provokes the secretion of enteric factors, which themselves stimulate insulin release.[36] Under normal circumstances, insulin secretion is primarily observed only during periods of nutrient ingestion; only minimal quantities need be secreted during fasting to prevent the development of unrestrained ketoacidosis. In all species thus far examined, plasma insulin falls to very low levels during caloric restriction: values below 5 to 10 μU/ml are routinely noted in man under these circumstances.[37,38]

Opposed to the hypoglycemic effects of insulin are the actions of adrenocorticotropic hormone (ACTH), cortisol, glucagon, epinephrine, and growth hormone. The net effect of these hormones is to increase the ambient blood glucose level by (1) inhibiting glucose uptake by muscle (i.e., epinephrine, cortisol, and growth hormone), (2) increasing endogenous gluconeogenic amino acid supply by mobilization from muscle (i.e., cortisol), (3) activating lipolysis and providing increased free fatty acids as a source of energy and glycerol for gluconeogenesis (i.e., epinephrine, glucagon, growth hormone, ACTH, and cortisol), (4) inhibiting insulin secretion from the pancreas (i.e., epinephrine), (5) acutely activating glycogenolytic and gluconeogenic enzymes (i.e., epinephrine and glucagon),[39] and (6) chronically inducing gluconeogenic enzyme synthesis (i.e., glucagon and cortisol).[40]

DEVELOPMENT OF FETAL AND NEONATAL HORMONE SECRETION

Growth and development of the fetus requires a complex system of regulatory controls. A great deal of evidence exists, that the endocrine system becomes active in early fetal life (see Chapter 133). The role of some of these organs and their secretions in normal development is clear, while in other cases the hormones are known to be present in both fetal tissues and blood but there is only a limited knowledge of their function. Further, it is not necessary to assume *a priori* that the presence of a hormone in utero dictates the same function or degree of activity observed for that hormone in the child or adult. For example, Jost and Jacquot have demonstrated that animals deprived of growth hormone and thyroid-stimulating hormone by decapitation in utero grow normally.[41] Similarly, infants with hypothalamic or pituitary hypoplasia generally are of normal weight and length at birth.[42] Shortly after birth, however, deficiencies of pituitary function become obvious when the infant fails to grow and develop normally. Similarly, although it is not clear whether insulin and/or glucagon are absolutely necessary for maintenance of fetal glucose homeostasis and the secretogogues controlling release in utero are not necessarily the same as in the adult, it is quite clear from observations in the infant of the diabetic mother and the infant born with transient diabetes that postnatal control of insulin release must develop rapidly.

FETAL PANCREATIC INSULIN AND GLUCAGON

Two successive generations of islets have been described in the developing human pancreas.[43,44] The first generation, observed at the 8th week, grows out from solid cords of cells which will form the primitive pancreatic tubules; the second generation begins to develop at the 3rd month of gestation and is formed from acinar cells, or from cells of the pancreatic ductules. The first generation progressively involutes after the 3rd month.

At 8 to 9 weeks gestation β cells and α^1 and α^2 cells, the latter containing glucagon,[45,46] can be seen with the electron microscope. In fetal life α cells are more numerous than the β cells. The number of β cells progressively increases and in the term fetus the ratio is 1:1 as compared to the human adult in whom the $\alpha{:}\beta$ cell ratio is 1:3 to 1:9.[47]

β cells containing distinct aldehyde-fuchsin-positive granules have been observed during the 3rd month, and secretory granules by the 4th or 5th month of gestation.[47] Immunoreactive insulin is not detectable in pancreatic extracts of the 35-mm fetus, but is present in the 80-to-300-mm crown-rump-size fetus (approximately 3 months gestation). Total pancreatic insulin content increases during pregnancy from 6.3 $\pm$ 1.1U/g between 20 and 32 weeks to 12.7 $\pm$ 3.2 U/g between 34 and 40 weeks as compared to 2.1 $\pm$ 0.3 U/g in the adult pancreas.[48]

Assan and Boillot[49] have determined the immunoassayable glucagon content of the human fetal pancreas between 6 and 26 weeks gestation. Glucagon is first detected at the end of the 8th week and demonstrates a logarithmic increase through 26 weeks, the duration of the study. The concentrations reached at this period are much higher than those found in the adult pancreas. Similar studies in the rat have shown that the maximum concentration of glucagon per gram of pancreas is attained around the 2nd week of gestation, then decreases to adult values.[50]

CONTROL OF FETAL AND NEONATAL INSULIN AND GLUCAGON SECRETION

Numerous studies of fetal plasma insulin responses to a glucose load have yielded conflicting results in the same as well as in different species.[50–56] A combination of factors most likely account for the discrepant results: species differences, the type of infusion (i.e., acute or chronic), the route of administration (i.e., fetal versus maternal infusion), and the age of the fetus.

In vitro studies with cultured explants of rat fetal pancreas[57] and 12-week-old human pancreas[58] have demonstrated that glucose and tolbutamide are poor stimulators of insulin release; however, in the presence of caffeine, insulin secretion is markedly potentiated by both agents. Milner *et al.*,[59] utilizing incubated pancreatic pieces from human fetuses of 12 to 24 weeks gestation, demonstrated that both glucose and tolbutamide were ineffective as insulin secretogogues, while agents considered to increase intracellular levels of 3′,5′-cyclic adenosine monophosphate (i.e., glucagon, theophylline, and dibutyrl cyclic adenosine monophosphate) stimulated insulin release in the presence or absence of glucose. The amino acids leucine and arginine differed from glucose in that each stimulated insulin release alone; however, the pattern of release differed between the two: arginine consistently stimulated insulin release from the pancreas of larger fetuses (e.g., >200 g), whereas leucine was more predictably effective from the pancreas of a fetus weighing less than 200 g. These data make it possible to speculate on the times in fetal life when different stimuli of insulin release become effective. At 12 to 14 weeks the β cell is capable of releasing insulin to substances that work via generation of cyclic AMP either by stimulating plasma membrane adenyl cyclase (e.g., glucagon) or by increasing intracellular concentrations of this nucleotide through inhibition of phosphodiesterase (e.g., caffeine and theophylline). At this early stage in development, leucine also stimulates insulin release. At 18 to 20 weeks arginine becomes an effective stimulus, but glucose does not result in significant insulin secretion until approximately the 24th week of fetal life.

In agreement with the above in vitro studies are the observations obtained in the primate fetus near term, which show that induction of fetal hyperglycemia is ineffective in elevating plasma insulin levels,[55] while glucagon injected directly into the fetus is associated with an increase.[60] Furthermore, theophylline, in concentrations that are ineffective alone in mediating insulin secretion, potentiates fetal insulin responses to glucagon and results in insulin secretion to glucose stimulation. Insulin secretion is also stimulated by the dibutyrl derivative of cyclic 3′,5′-adenosine monophosphate and tolbutamide. Following birth, the fetal pancreatic β-cell responses rapidly change and glucose becomes the primary secretogogue.[55,60]

In premature newborns, both theophylline and glucagon[61] are potent insulinogenic secretogogues, whereas glucose alone has little or no effect.[62,63] In contrast to glucose, administration of arginine[62] or a mixture of naturally occurring amino acids[63] results in insulin secretion. Both arginine or the mixture of amino acids in low concentrations, which individually have little or no effect on insulin release, act synergistically when administered in combination with glucose.

In the normal full-term human, several studies have shown that the fetal and newborn pancreas react sluggishly, if at all, to hyperglycemia.[64,65] Intravenous glucose given to the mother during the second stage of labor results in maternal hyperglycemia, a rapid and appropriate rise in maternal plasma insulin (Fig. 141-1), and a fall in free fatty acid concentration.[64] The maternal hyperglycemia is reflected in the fetal serum glucose concentration (Fig. 141-1), but this change has no effect on fetal serum insulin for the first 30 min, and only subsequently results in a small increase in plasma insulin.

At birth the maternal supply of glucose to the fetus ceases abruptly and the neonatal blood glucose concentration, which is normal by adult standards, declines to a mean level of 50 mg/100ml by 2 h of age. Subsequently, this level rises and is stabilized at approximately 70 mg/100 ml by the 3rd day of life.[66] Unstimulated, postabsorptive plasma insulin concentrations from birth through 7 days of age are relatively stable.[67,68] During this time interval there is a decreased rate of glucose disappearance following intravenous glucose administration, which is correlated with a reduced and delayed rate of insulin secretion. By the 3rd to 7th day of life, the glucose assimilation coefficient (K_t) increases toward that observed in older children and adults. Provided portal vein blood is

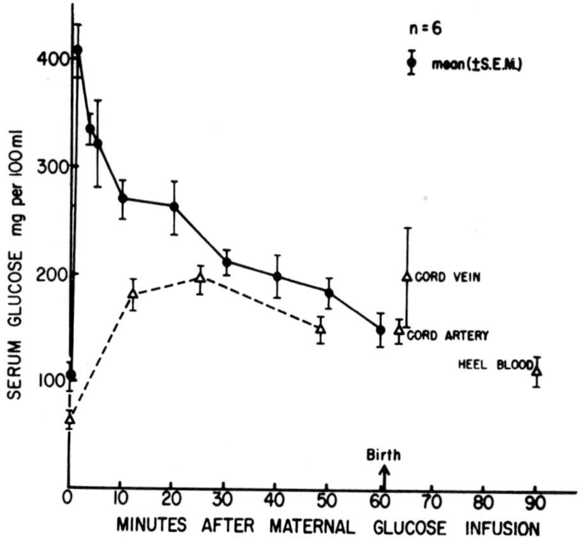

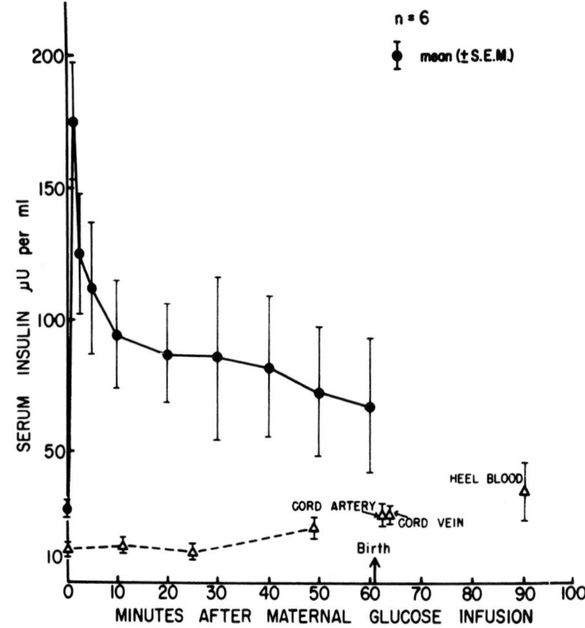

Fig. 141-1. Maternal (•) and fetal (Δ) serum glucose and immunoreactive insulin concentrations after injection of glucose (0.5 g/kg body wt) in the mother. (From Tobin, J.D., Roux, J.F., Soeldner, J.S.: Pediatrics *44*:668, 1969, with permission.)

sampled by umbilical vein catheter, both first and second phases of insulin release to intravenous glucose challenge have been observed; the total amount of insulin released during the first phase increases from day 1 to day 7. Similar to intravenous glucose, oral glucose challenge also results in a delayed release of insulin.[69,70]

As discussed in Chapter 79, the concept that glucagon plays an important role in fuel metabolism in the adult is well accepted. Glucagon is a potent stimulus of gluconeogenesis, is suppressed by high blood glucose concentrations, and stimulated by hypoglycemia and amino acids. Whether this hormone is of major importance in fetal and neonatal fuel homeostasis is presently being actively investigated.

Recent in vitro studies[71] utilizing the splenic lobe of newborn rat pancreas have demonstrated that glucagon release is not modified by changes in glucose concentrations. Similar to the β cell, the fetal α-cell secretion of glucagon to amino acid stimulation is potentiated by factors that elevate intracellular cyclic AMP. Investigations utilizing the chronically catheterized sheep fetus have also demonstrated that plasma glucagon concentrations are independent of acute changes in circulating blood glucose and are unresponsive to alanine stimulation.[72] Subsequent studies in this model have shown that theophylline administered along with alanine produces marked augmentation of glucagon secretion.[73] When fetal hyperglycemia or hypoglycemia is produced by infusing the pregnant rat with glucose or insulin, appropriate fetal insulin responses are observed without changes in circulating fetal glucagon. In contrast to these acute manipulations, chronic hypoglycemia induced either by fasting pregnant rats for 96 h or by inducing intrauterine growth retardation of the fetus results in marked elevations of fetal glucagon.[50]

Little information is available relevant to glucagon release in the human fetus except for the study by Assan and Boillot,[49] in which basal plasma glucagon concentrations in three fetuses (15,-25, and 26 weeks gestation) were in the range found in adults. Intraperitoneal injection of arginine in the 25-week fetus had no effect on glucagon release, and similarly no change in concentration occurred from basal levels over a 4-h period of observation in the 26-week fetus. However, in the term infant shortly after birth, arginine[74] and alanine[75] stimulated glucagon secretion.

In the human infant during the immediate postnatal period a significant increase in plasma glucagon occurs which is closely correlated with the characteristic fall in plasma glucose during the first 2 h of life. Despite the persistence of relative hypoglycemia, glucagon levels remain stable and do not significantly change between 2 and 24 h of life. A further significant elevation in plasma glucagon occurs from day 1 to day 3 of life, associated with the return of glucose to what is considered in the older child to be euglycemic levels. This change occurs simultaneously with the establishment of a routine feeding pattern.

As discussed in detail in Chapter 147, alanine, besides stimulating glucagon secretion, is considered to be a principal gluconeogenic precursor. Constant infusion of this amino acid for 30 min into normal 1-h-old infants increases plasma glucagon threefold but is ineffective in increasing plasma glucose. These observations suggest that gluconeogenesis from alanine is not established normally in utero or immediately after birth.[75] In older normal neonates, alanine would appear to be utilized for gluconeogenesis.[76]

In summarizing and integrating the information elaborated above, it would appear reasonable to suggest that

1. Carbohydrate metabolism in utero is not dependent on fetal insulin or glucagon and is dependent on maternal production and supply of glucose.
2. If insulin secretion does occur there is no reason, *a priori,* for the secretogogues to be those characteristic of adults. Since the fetus is growing rapidly, release of insulin by amino acids with subsequent amino acid uptake and protein synthesis would be a more appropriate role for insulin than the control of glucose homeostasis. Conversely, release of glucagon, a catabolic hormone, by amino acids would be counterproductive.
3. The adenyl-cyclase–cyclic-AMP system would appear to be of primary importance in both insulin and glucagon release. This system may provide a regulatory mechanism in modulating release of both hormones in utero and following birth. One might speculate that the "maturity" of this enzyme system, including the membrane-bound adenyl cyclase and cytosol phosphodiesterase, parallels the maturity of the fetus and infant.

HEPATIC ENZYME SYSTEMS AND SUBSTRATE REGULATION

Throughout gestation the fetus is dependent solely upon maternal supply and placental transfer of nutrients to meet the cellular metabolic demands for differentiation and growth. At the time of delivery the fetal organism loses its constant source of intravenous substrates and must be metabolically prepared to enter its first fast. To maintain normal cellular metabolism and anabolic growth, the newborn, like the older child and adult, must meet at least three requirements: (1) have adequate stores of hepatic glycogen, muscle protein, and fat from which substrates can be mobilized, (2) have or rapidly acquire the enzymatic capacity to release, interconvert, and utilize these substrates, and (3) release regulatory hormones in an appropriate manner to modulate enzyme induction, substrate mobilization, and peripheral utilization of metabolic fuels. Since the liver plays a central role in regulation of substrate interconversions, primary attention will be given to its role in fetal and neonatal glucose homeostasis.

The orchestration of these various interacting processes is manifested by a fall in plasma glucose following delivery and subsequent recovery. This fall in plasma glucose is associated with increased concentrations of cortisol, glucagon, and presumably epinephrine, and a subsequent rise in plasma free fatty acids and ketone bodies.[68,77,78] A failure in substrate delivery, interconversion, or utilization could lead to cellular dysfunction, hypoglycemia, central nervous system (CNS) symptoms, and, if sustained or profound, could result in permanent CNS damage or death.

One of the primary differences between the fetus and older child or adult is the absence or very low activities of a number of key hepatic enzymes (particularly gluconeogenic enzymes) necessary for fuel homeostasis in the fasting state.[79] Teleologically there is no need for hepatic gluconeogenesis in a fetus receiving constant "hyperalimentation." The appropriate temporal induction or activation of these enzymes may involve one or more mechanisms: transcription and/or translation from DNA or RNA, respectively, to form the nascent enzyme peptides, or allosteric activation of preexisting enzymes by changes in co-factors or intracellular substrate concentrations. The induction of these enzymes may involve genetically predetermined factors, the maturity of the organism, or differentiation of cellular sensitivity to circulating hormones or substrates, or some combination of these factors. It is not the purpose of this chapter to evaluate in depth these various possibilities; the interested reader is referred to a recent review.[79]

The majority of data on substrates and enzymic systems have

been derived from the rat and a variety of lower mammalian species, and much less (in comparison) from subhuman primates and man. Patterns of enzyme activities and substrate availability are similar in many species, despite the marked variability in relative maturity of these organisms at the time of delivery. For this reason, although caution should be applied, analogies from the rat or other mammalian species to man may provide a framework upon which to examine the human situation.

HEPATIC GLYCOGEN SYNTHESIS AND GLYCOGENOLYSIS

In the older child and adult, hepatic stores of glycogen are accumulated during periods of caloric (carbohydrate) intake, and constitute approximately 5 percent of the weight of the liver. Hepatic stores are slowly hydrolyzed 2 to 4 h following a meal to provide a readily releasable but limited supply of glucose during a period of time when hepatic gluconeogenic activity is sharply increasing and thus stabilizes a smooth transition from the fed to fasted state.[33,80] Before considering the unique metabolic situation of the fetus and neonate, a brief review of normal glycogen metabolism in the child and adult is indicated.

Glycogen Synthesis

Glucose is converted to uridine diphosphoglucose (UDPG) by the consecutive actions of glucokinase (or hexokinase), phosphoglucomutase, and UDPG pyrophosphorylase. Hepatic glycogen synthetase (UDP-glucose-glycogen glucosyl transferase) transfers a glucose residue from UDPG to an outer chain of glycogen in an α1,4 linkage. When the peripheral chain of glycogen reaches a length of 7 to 21 glycosyl units, a second enzyme, amylo-(1,4 → 1,6) glucan transferase (brancher enzyme), transfers a number of 1,4 linked glycosyl units from the end of a glycogen chain to another portion of the molecule in an α1,6 linkage (Fig. 141-2). Glycogen synthetase exists in an active dephosphorylated (glycogen synthetase *a*) and an inactive phosphorylated (glycogen synthetase *b*) form. Although a great deal of research has been carried out in an attempt to define the mechanisms that control the relative concentrations of these two forms of enzyme, no clear mechanisms have emerged.[81] Control of glycogen synthetase activity is mediated, at least in part, by factors altering intracellular second messenger (cyclic AMP) concentrations. Glucagon and epinephrine stimulate adenylate cyclase activity, increasing cyclic AMP, and activate a protein kinase which phosphorylates glycogen synthetase *a* to the inactive *b* form and therefore inhibits glycogen formation (Fig. 141-3). Insulin stimulates the conversion of the inactive (*b*) form to the active form (*a*), which results in the well-recognized activity of insulin, glycogen accumulation. In the liver this is not affected by substrate flux secondary to increased glucose uptake since glucose transport is not insulin-dependent. Insulin activation of hepatic glycogen synthetase can occur independent of intracellular concentrations of adenyl nucleotides and may be activating the glycogen synthetase *b* phosphatase directly.[81] Conversely, insulin may inactivate phosphorylase *a*, resulting in a net increase in glycogen stores.

Glycogenolysis

Phosphorylase is the rate-limiting enzyme that initiates glycogenolysis and catalyzes the cleavage of α1,4 glucosyl units. Although this enzyme can catalyze both glycogen degradation and synthesis in vitro, its specific function in vivo is glycogenolysis. Phosphorylase hydrolyzes successive glucose residues until four glucosyl units remain at each branch; the resultant glycogen molecule is termed a phosphorylase "limit dextrin"(Fig. 141-2b). Phosphorylase action can proceed no further until the α1,4-linked trisaccharide is removed from the α1,6-linked glucose by oligo (1,4 → 1,4)-glucan transferase enzyme. The α1,6 glucosyl unit is then removed as free glucose by amylo-1,6 glucosidase. These two enzymes [amylo-1,6 glucosidase and oligo (1,4 → 1,4)-glucan transferase] are termed the debrancher enzyme since the two enzymatic functions have not been separated.

The control mechanisms regulating the relative amounts of active and inactive phosphorylase are shown in Fig. 141-3. Activation of the membrane-bound adenyl cyclase by glucagon or epinephrine initiates a cascade of reactions resulting in the activation of phosphorylase. The series of reactions can be summarized as follows: (1) the increased intracellular concentration of cyclic AMP activates a protein kinase, which (2) phosphorylates dephosphophosphorylase *b* kinase to the active *a* form, which (3) catalyzes the phosphorylation of inactive phosphorylase *b* to the active *a* form. The inactivation of phosphorylase *a* is catalyzed by a highly specific phosphatase (Fig. 141-3). It would appear that a reciprocal activation and inactivation of glycogen synthetase and phosphorylase systems is mediated via a cyclic-AMP-dependent protein kinase as well as by insulin itself.[81]

FETAL AND NEONATAL GLYCOGEN METABOLISM

It is well documented that hepatic stores of glycogen are assimilated rapidly during the last third of gestation in all mammalian species examined including man (Figs. 141-4, 141-5).[82,83] In the human fetus hepatic glycogen is detectable as early as 8 to 10 weeks of gestation,[29,84] which of necessity implies the presence of hepatic glycogen synthetic enzymes. This early presence of hepatic glycogen differs from lower mammalian species (rat, rabbit, dog, and guinea pig) in which the fetal liver is devoid of glycogen until just prior to term.[82]

Phosphorylase is present in the preimplantation morula stage of the embryo,[85] but whether this cellular phosphorylase activity is maintained in the differentiating liver remains unknown. Following differentiation of the liver, phosphorylase activity in the rat is detectable prior to accumulation of hepatic glycogen.[82] However, even following the appearance of hepatic glycogen, phosphorylase would appear to have little role in maintenance of fetal plasma glucose, since glucose-6-phosphatase, a key enzyme necessary for glucose production from glycogen and gluconeogenesis, does not appear until the 19th to 20th day of gestation.[86]

Although the rate-limiting enzyme systems necessary for both hepatic glycogen synthesis and glycogen degradation are present prior to the accumulation of glycogen,[87] the mechanism by which glycogen accumulation occurs, as well as the source of substrate, remains somewhat vague. During the period of rapid glycogen accumulation, increases in hepatic glycogen synthetic enzymes occur.[82] Utilizing labeled incubation studies, the source of substrate for glycogen is most likely glucose, and not pyruvate, in the rat. However, in the guinea pig, incorporation of ^{14}C-labeled glucose, pyruvate, and fructose was found to be low even near term, at a time when hepatic glycogen stores were rapidly increasing.[87]

A variety of factors have been shown to alter fetal hepatic glycogen content. Jost and co-workers [41,88] provided the first evidence that fetal endocrine function was necessary for normal enzymic differentiation of the liver. In utero fetal decapitation of rabbits prevented the accumulation of glycogen and the increase in enzymes necessary for glycogen formation.[41,88,89] Treatment of the fetus with glucocorticoids corrected this abnormality.[89] In rats,

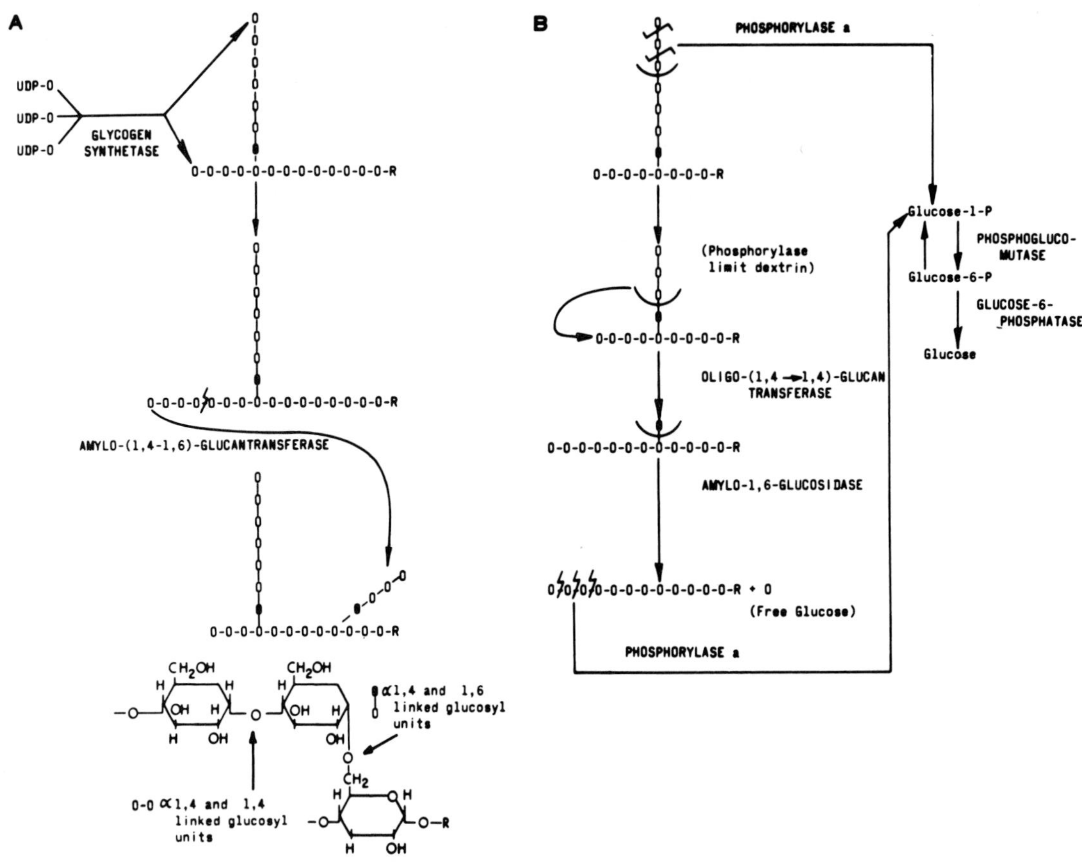

Fig. 141-2. A: synthesis of glycogen; B: degradation of glycogen; O: glucosyl monomer; UDP-O: uridine diphosphoglucose. (From J. Pediatr. *82* 2:365, 1973, with permission.)

both fetal decapitation and maternal adrenalectomy are necessary to create similar findings.[90] Treatment of the normal rat fetus with glucocorticoids results in glycogen accumulation at an earlier time in gestation.[79] Thus it would appear that glucocorticoids are involved in fetal glycogen metabolism. Catecholamines are known to have dramatic effects on glycogen metabolism in older children and adults by altering both hepatic glycogen synthetase and phosphorylase activities. Accumulation of epinephrine in the fetal adrenal gland is apparently controlled by the pituitary since decapitation depletes adrenal epinephrine. ACTH or cortisone treatment of the fetus restores these concentrations by increasing the activity of phenylethanol amino *N*-methyl transferase, the enzyme necessary for conversion of norepinephrine to epinephrine.[91,92]

Hepatic phosphorylase and glucose-6-phosphatase are neces-

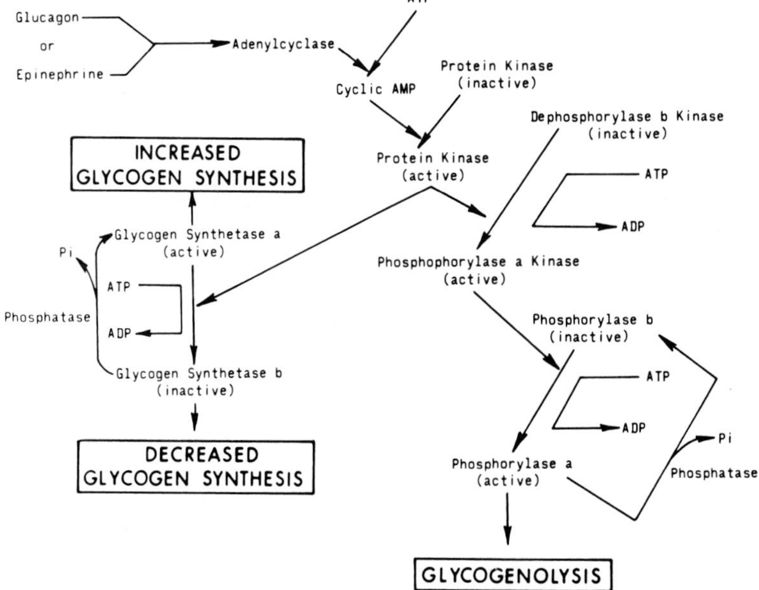

Fig. 141-3. Schematic representation for activation and deactivation of phosphorylase and glycogen synthetase. (From J. Pediatr. *82* Pt 2: 365, 1973, with permission.)

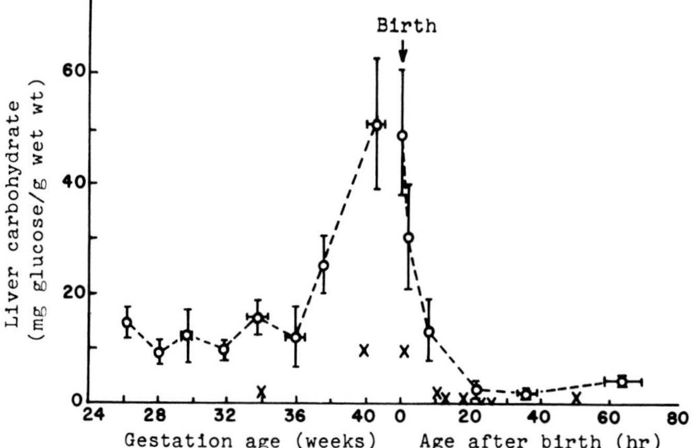

Fig. 141-4. Liver carbohydrate (CHO) concentrations in human fetuses during the last trimester and in babies after birth. The data were derived from autopsies performed on 15 fresh stillbirths, 32 babies 4 h old, and 40 babies up to 70 h old of > 37 weeks gestation. Dashed line: accumulation of liver CHO before birth and disappearance after birth; open circles (O): values in babies of normal birth weight for gestation; crossed lines (X): values of individual babies of low birth weight for gestation. (From Shelley, J.H., Neligan, G.A. Br. Med. Bull. *22*:34, 1966, by permission of the Medical Department, the British Council.)

sary for hydrolysis of glycogen and release of glucose into the systemic circulation. The activity of rat hepatic glucose-6-phosphatase is very low until the 19th to 20th day of gestation at which time its activity increases rapidly,[86] whereas phosphorylase activity, as already discussed, is detectable as early as the 17th day of gestation.[82] Adrenalectomy in adult rats is known to inhibit phosphorylase activity and glycogenolysis to cyclic AMP stimulation, and in newborn rats results in a 30-percent decrease in phosphorylase activity.[93] How much of the increase in phosphorylase activity is activation of existing enzyme or de novo synthesis is not clear. In contrast, the mechanism of normal induction of fetal glucose-6-phosphatase is dependent upon de novo protein synthesis. Intrauterine injection of glucagon or thyroxine results in a prompt (3-h) increase in the activity of glucose-6-phosphatase, whereas similar injections of these hormones with actinomycin D results in no

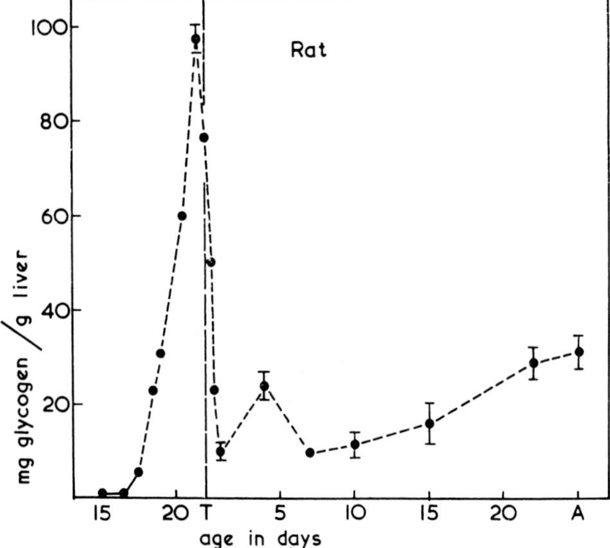

Fig. 141-5. Neonatal rat liver glycogen content. T: term; A: adult. Limits of ± SEM are shown where they are large enough to be drawn (From Ballard, F.J., Oliver, I.T.: Biochem. Biophys. Acta *71*:578, 1963, with permission.)

increase.[79] In utero fetal decapitation also prevents the normal increase in glucose-6-phosphatase.[89]

In contrast to the in vitro enzymatic data, in vivo stimulation with glucagon or dibutyryl cyclic AMP has little effect on mobilization of hepatic glycogen and elevation of plasma glucose until several hours following parturition.[93] Two explanations for this refractory period have been suggested including incomplete postnatal induction of glycogenolytic enzymes and end-organ resistance to hormonal stimulation. Recent investigations in the rat have demonstrated low adenylate cyclase responsiveness of fetal hepatic membranes to glucagon stimulation. Adenylate cyclase activity increases to adult levels only following 30 days of extrauterine life. Similarly, hormone-binding studies with fetal hepatic membranes showed decreased binding of both insulin and glucagon when compared to hepatic membranes of adult controls. Insulin binding reached mature values by 20 days of fetal life, whereas glucagon binding did not attain adult levels until the 30th postnatal day.[94] The demonstration of significant insulin binding, which is relatively unopposed by glucagon binding, may have physiologic importance for rapid fetal growth and protection from in utero fetal catabolism.

If one can equate the relative amounts of hepatic membrane-bound hormone to biologic activity, glycogen accumulation would be favored and gluconeogenesis inhibited despite significant concentrations of plasma insulin and glucagon in the fetus. Similarly, this could explain the refractory response of glycogen and plasma glucose to pharmacologic doses of glucagon in the early postnatal period,[93] as well as the apparent dichotomy of rising glucagon concentrations in the presence of a falling plasma glucose following delivery in the neonate.[74,95]

Hepatic Gluconeogenesis

Following brief periods of caloric deprivation, new glucose must be formed from other substrates to sustain primary glycolyzing tissues. This involves the interconversion of a variety of three carbon substrates or their precursors (lactate, pyruvate, glycerol, alanine, and other amino acids) to glucose. Three organs (liver, kidney, and intestine) have the enzymatic capability of converting these potential gluconeogenic substrates to free glucose. Little is known of the magnitude of intestinal contribution to glucose production in the fasted state. Liver is the major organ of gluconeogenesis in both man and a variety of animal models, [80,96] whereas kidney becomes an important gluconeogenic organ after prolonged fasting.[33]

Both in vivo and in vitro studies indicate that gluconeogenic amino acids play the dominant quantitative role as glucose precursors. When livers from fasted rats are perfused with mixtures of lactate, glycerol, and amino acids in physiologic concentrations, over 50 percent of the glucose formed is derived from amino acids.[96,97] In the fasted adult approximately 50 percent of net glucose production is derived from amino acid precursors, 30 percent from lactate (i.e., Cori cycle), and 10 percent from glycerol (i.e., lipolysis).[80] Of the various gluconeogenic amino acids, alanine is quantitatively the most important. Transhepatic catheterization studies in man indicate that in excess of 50 percent of glucose derived from gluconeogenic amino acids is formed from alanine (or approximately 25 percent of hepatic gluconeogenesis).[80]

Glutamine is another potential gluconeogenic substrate and, along with alanine, represents a significant portion of total amino acid efflux from skeletal muscle during fasting.[98] The quantitative contribution of glutamine to hepatic and renal gluconeogenesis has not been as clearly defined as that of alanine. Muscle is the major

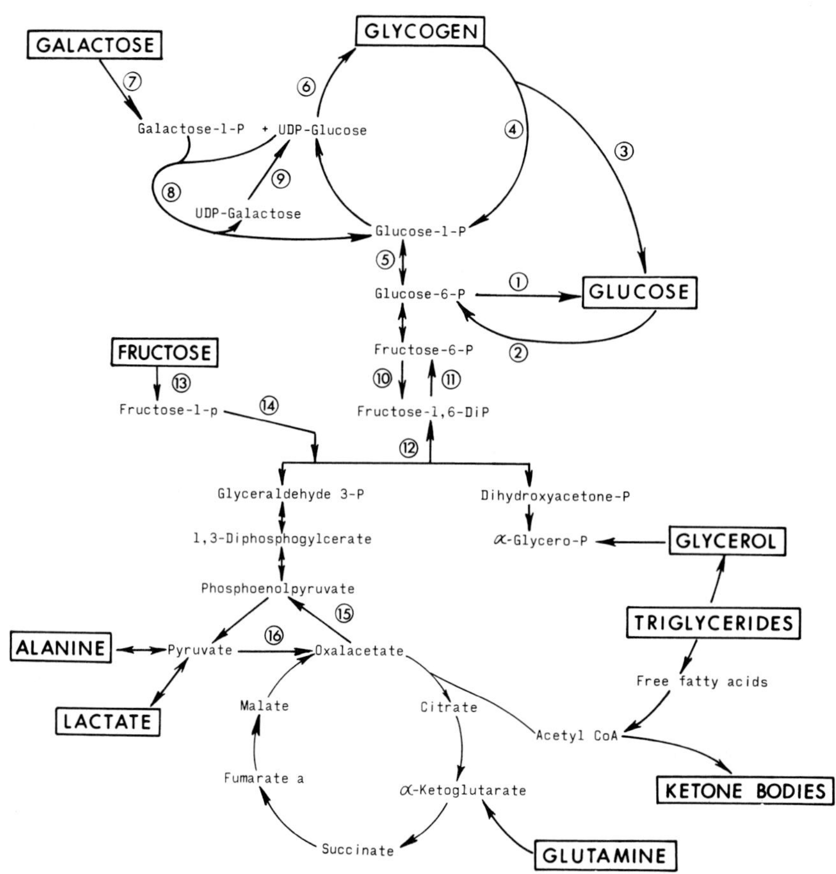

Fig. 141-6. Metabolic pathways involved in glycogen synthesis and degradation and gluconeogenesis. Key enzymes are designated by number. (1) glucose-6-phosphatase, (2) glucokinase, (3) amylo-1,6-glucosidase, (4) phosphorylase, (5) phosphoglucomutase, (6) glycogen synthetase, (7) galactokinase, (8) galactose-1-phosphate uridyl transferase, (9) uridine diphosphogalactose-4-epimerase, (10) phosphofructokinase, (11) fructose-1,6-diphosphatase, (12) fructose-1,6-diphosphate aldolase, (13) fructokinase, (14) fructose-1-phosphate aldolase, (15) phosphoenolpyruvate carboxykinase, (16) pyruvate carboxylase. Adapted from Dekaban and Baird: J. Pediatr. *55:* 563, 1959, with permission.

source of glutamine synthesis, and the intestinal tract rather than the liver may be the primary site of splanchnic glutamine uptake.[99]

Since alanine constitutes only 6 to 7 percent of the amino acid composition of skeletal muscle, [100] the major source of alanine efflux represents interconversion of amino acids derived from protein catabolism and pyruvate, an intermediate of glucose catabolism within the myocyte. In vitro incubation studies of the epitroclaris muscle of rats would support this concept.[101] A variety of regulatory mechanisms have been implicated in the control of protein catabolism within the myocyte: (1) circulating hormones (e.g., epinephrine, insulin, and glucocorticoids),[102–105] (2) circulating substrates (e.g., β-hydroxybutyrate),[106] and (3) neuronal factors.[107]

Within the hepatocyte substrates are converted to glucose via a functional reversal of the glycolytic pathway. Three unidirectional glycolytic enzymatic steps are bypassed by four key rate-limiting gluconeogenic enzymes: glucose-6-phosphatase, fructose-1,6-diphosphatase, phosphoenolpyruvate carboxykinase, and pyruvate carboxylase (Fig. 141-6).

Pyruvate carboxylase, a CO_2 fixing mitochondrial enzyme, converts pyruvate to oxaloacetate. This is the initial step in gluconeogenesis from pyruvate, lactate, or alanine. Phosphoenolpyruvate carboxykinase catalyzes the conversion of oxaloacetate to phosphoenolpyruvate. In rat this enzyme is found in the cytosol, whereas in man, guinea pig, and pig [108] it is present in both the cytosol and the mitochondria.

The conversion of fructose-1,6-diphosphate to fructose-6-phosphate is catalyzed by fructose-1,6-diphosphatase. This is a cytosolic enzyme and is involved in glucose formation from lactate, pyruvate, and amino acids as well as glycerol and fructose (Fig. 141-6).

Glucose-6-phosphatase hydrolyzes glucose-6-phosphate to glucose and is the final enzymatic step by which the liver releases free glucose derived from either glycogenolysis or gluconeogenesis. Its complete absence precludes glucose release by either of these important mechanisms with the exception of 8 percent of hepatic glycogen, which can be converted directly to free glucose by amylo-1,6 glucosidase (see above). This enzyme, glucose-6-phosphatase, is bound to microsomal membranes; little is known about the mechanisms by which its activity is regulated.

Net hepatic glucose production is the result of a balance between glycolysis and gluconeogenesis. In in vitro rat studies, the overall rate of glycolysis is one to two orders of magnitude lower than the maximal activities of the two rate-limiting enzymes, phosphofructokinase and pyruvate kinase. This implies that the activities of these enzymes operate in a "steady-state" situation at substrate concentrations far from equilibrium for the individual reaction, or have activities suppressed by metabolic effectors (Table 141-2).[109] A variety of substrates common to both glycolysis and gluconeogenesis affect the glycolytic rate: increased by 5′-AMP, 3′5′-cyclic AMP, P_i, NH_3, and FDP, and decreased by ATP and citrate. A prime example of this mutual control is the effect of increased intracellular concentrations of 5′-AMP, which inhibits fructose-1,6-diphosphatase activity and increases the activity of phosphofructokinase. The activities of unidirectional gluconeogenic enzymes are considerably higher than the maximal activity of phosphofructokinase, a primary control point for glycolysis (Table 141-2). Therefore during states of glucose need, metabolic effectors modulate these enzyme systems resulting in net glucose formation.

When the organism is in a "gluconeogenic posture" (fasting, diabetes), hepatic fatty acid oxidation is taking place which has three primary effects on gluconeogenesis: (1) provides the energy necessary for gluconeogenesis, (2) produces pyridine nucleotides necessary for ketogenesis and gluconeogenesis, and (3) increases acetyl CoA, an obligate activator of pyruvate carboxylase. Phosphoenolpyruvate carboxykinase has no known metabolic effectors, but increased synthesis of enzyme can be stimulated by glucocorticoids.

The primary control mechanisms for gluconeogenesis would appear to be in the first steps of substrate conversion.[109] In starvation or alloxan diabetes pyruvate is preferentially converted through the first two enzymatic steps [pyruvate carboxylase and phosphoenolpyruvate carboxykinase (PEPCK)] of gluconeogenesis and away from the citric acid cycle. This situation is reversed with refeeding or insulin administration. Glucocorticoids positively affect gluconeogenesis between pyruvate and the triose phosphates, and this effect may be due to de novo synthesis of PEPCK. The effect of glucagon on gluconeogenesis is considered to be at the level of pyruvate carboxylase. This is based on several observations:

1. In the perfused rat liver glucagon stimulates glucose synthesis from lactate and pyruvate but not from oxaloacetate.
2. The ratio of hepatic concentrations of pyruvate and oxaloacetate is altered by glucagon administration, an effect that is antagonized by insulin. This latter observation may result from increased generation of cyclic AMP since cyclic AMP mimics the action of glucagon and decreased concentrations of cyclic AMP are observed following insulin administration.[109]
3. Finally, hepatic gluconeogenesis is affected by substrate delivery rates. The fasted state is associated with increased flux of amino acids and lactate from muscle, and glycerol from fat tissues. In hepatic perfusion studies, saturation of gluconeogenic capacity is not achieved until lactate and amino acids are supplied in concentrations 50-fold greater than physiologic levels.[96] In this same context, studies in man and laboratory animals have demonstrated that the availability of an adequate supply of substrate represents a rate-limiting factor for gluconeogenesis.[33,37,110–113]

FETAL AND NEONATAL GLUCONEOGENESIS

Throughout gestation glucose is transported rapidly across the placenta so that fetal glucose approximates the maternal concentrations. As a result the fetus is protected from catabolic processes, such as gluconeogenesis, during the period of most rapid growth. Very little is known about the timing or mechanisms of induction of hepatic gluconeogenesis in the human fetus, and once again inference must be made from studies in various lower mammalian species.

There is considerable evidence in the literature from a variety of species that the enzymes necessary for gluconeogenesis have very low or absent activities in early and mid-gestation.[79] During the latter portion of gestation there is some increase in one or more

Table 141-2. Maximal Catalytic Capacities of Hepatic Enzymes Unique to Glycolysis and Gluconeogenesis

Glycolysis (μmol/min/g wet wt, 37 C)		Gluconeogenesis (μmol/min/g wet wt, 37 C)	
Phosphofructokinase	3.3	Pyruvate carboxylase	7.7
Pyruvate kinase	50.0	Phosphoenolpyruvate carboxykinase	6.7
Glycolysis (μmol glucose utilized)	0.2	Fructose-1,6-diphosphatase	15.0

Adapted from Coleman: In Bondy, P. K. (ed.): Diseases of Metabolism, ed. 6. Philadelphia, Saunders, 1969, p. 89, with permission.

of the key rate-limiting gluconeogenic enzyme(s) prior to parturition. However, in every species examined, at least one enzyme maintains low activity in utero until the immediate postnatal period.[79,114–118] This functional block in gluconeogenesis is further supported by in vitro liver-slice studies in which there is minimal conversion of labeled lactate, pyruvate, or alanine to glucose.[82,119,120]

A number of factors have profound effects on enzyme activities in the fetal and neonatal liver. Glucose-6-phosphatase activity is known to be extremely low during gestation in the rat and increases somewhat during the last 2 to 3 days prior to parturition, with a marked increase following delivery.[79,86] Early induction of this enzyme can be accomplished by premature delivery, intrauterine treatment of the fetus with glucagon, thyroxine or epinephrine, and cyclic AMP.[79] Decreased activity has been observed with postmaturity, intrauterine fetal decapitation, and intrauterine administration of glucose or actinomycin D.[79] Although the above situations may be artificial and pharmacologic, several conclusions are warranted: (1) increased activity of glucose-6-phosphatase requires a translational or transcriptional step; (2) at least one stimulus for increased enzyme activity and/or synthesis is cyclic AMP, since hormones that stimulate this nucleotide, as well as cyclic AMP itself, increase enzyme activity; and (3) glucose appears to be a potent effector of protein synthesis. Whether this effect is mediated by glucose directly, via insulin, or via other mechanisms, remains unknown. The mechanisms through which thyroxine or fetal pituitary hormones effect the induction of glucose-6-phosphatase are unknown, but these hormones may play a permissive role.

In most animal species fructose-1,6-diphosphatase and pyruvate carboxylase have low fetal activities which rapidly increase prior to delivery. Since the activities of these two enzymes are increasing prior to parturition, they would not appear to be rate-limiting.

In contrast, in most species, phosphoenolpyruvate carboxykinase would appear to be the last rate-limiting gluconeogenic enzyme induced in fetal or neonatal liver. This is demonstrated most clearly in the crossover studies of Ballard,[121] in which there was a marked increase in substrate concentrations just proximal to PEPCK (Fig. 141-7). In the rat, induction of PEPCK has many parallels to that of glucose-6-phosphatase but the mechanisms have been more precisely defined. The activity of this enzyme is not only inhibited by actinomycin D but by puromycin and amino acid analogs.[122] Therefore, de novo protein synthesis is necessary for induction. Cyclic AMP, dibutyl cyclic AMP, epinephrine, and glucagon stimulate the activity of this enzyme in vivo in rats,[122,123] and in vitro in rats[124] and human fetal liver.[125] Protection of the animal from hypoglycemia by glucose injection at the time of delivery as well as the administration of a variety of substrates (i.e., lactate, pyruvate, glycerol, galactose, fructose, mannose, and ribose) inhibited its induction.[122] Therefore it has been speculated that the substrates that inhibit enzyme activity may be operative

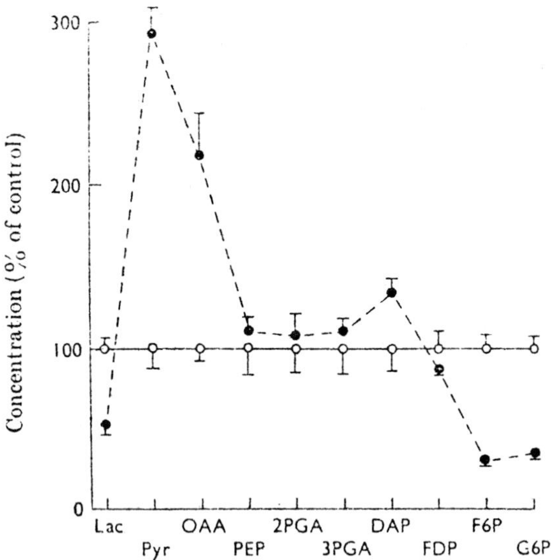

Fig. 141-7. Crossover plot comparing the concentrations of gluconeogenic intermediates in livers of 1 hr old rats (·) with the respective compounds in livers of fetal rats (○). Values shown are the means ± SEM for 8 to 10 determinations. Abbreviations used and the concentrations of each intermediate in fetal liver are: lactate (Lac), 5.74 μmol/g; pyruvate (Pyr), 0.074 μmol/g; oxaloacetate (OAA), 0.0075 μmol/g; phosphoenolpyruvate (PEP), 0.033 μmol/g; 2-phosphoglycerate (2PGA), 0.012 μmol/g; 3-phosphoglycerate (3PGA), 0.82 μmol/g; dihydroxyacetone phosphate (DAP), 0.12 μmol/g; fructose 1,6-diphosphate (FDP), 0.0059 μmol/g; fructose 6-phosphate (F6P), 0.113 μmol/g; glucose-6-phosphate (G6P), 0.406 μmol/g. (From Ballard, F.J.: Biochem J. *124*:265, 1971, with permission.)

by inhibiting endogenous glucagon secretion. Such a unifying theory is highly speculative since a number of these substrates (lactate, pyruvate, galactose, and fructose) have no effect on glucagon secretion from the in vitro perfused rat pancreas (see Chapter 76). Since simultaneous or subsequent injection of animals with glucose and glucagon resulted in increased enzyme activity, the inhibitory effect of glucose on PEPCK would not appear to be at the protein synthetic level.

Both epinephrine and norepinephrine stimulate PEPCK activity in the neonatal rat.[122] This implies that the autonomic nervous system may have a role in the induction of this enzyme. It has been established that vagal stimulation in adult rats results in an increase in hepatic output of glucose and a remarkable increase in glucose-6-phosphatase activity.[126] It would be difficult to conceive that the "trauma" of delivery and readjustment of a variety of physiologic parameters to extrauterine life would not be associated with a marked increase in epinephrine secretion and autonomic nervous system activity. The precise role of the autonomic nervous system in hepatic enzyme induction must await further studies.

The increased activity of PEPCK in man is even more complex than the rat model, since two gene loci are most likely involved, one for mitochondrial and the other for cytosolic enzyme. If the induction of PEPCK in man is similar to that in the pig, the primary increase in activity in the neonatal liver would be in the mitochondrial fraction.[108]

An additional rate-limiting factor which must be considered in the establishment of neonatal gluconeogenesis is tissue oxygenation. Hypoxemia even in the face of maximal glucagon stimulated PEPCK activity is associated with suppressed gluconeogenesis.[127] Since gluconeogenesis is an energy-requiring process, concentrations of high-energy phosphates become rate-limiting. Birth is associated with some degree of hypoxemia in all mammals whether due to delivery of the intact fetal placental unit as in the rat, or compromised blood flow to the infant with cord compression as he passes through the birth canal, or in conditions in which decreased fetal oxygenation is due to maternal or placental pathology (e.g., toxemia, maternal hypertension, long-standing maternal diabetes).

Normal fetal liver has a highly reduced redox potential and relatively low concentrations of ATP, a condition resembling hypoxemia in older animals and not favorable for gluconeogenesis.[121] Since hypoxemia in the adult is a potent stimulus for glycogenolysis and glycolysis, the observation of increased hepatic glycogen stores in the fetus at term would appear paradoxical. In the rat, immediately following delivery, there is increased activity of TCA cycle enzymes,[79] a fall in ADP and AMP, and increasing ATP concentrations,[121] conditions favorable for gluconeogenesis.

In summary, following delivery and with improved oxygenation the newborn of every mammalian species experiences a fall in plasma glucose during the early hours of life. Glucose subsequently rises even in the absence of oral alimentation and is associated with a decrease in hepatic glycogen and an increase in gluconeogenic enzyme activity. This period of "physiologic" hypoglycemia is associated with the secretion of a variety of hormones (glucagon, cortisol, growth hormone, and presumably epinephrine and norepinephrine), but whether their secretion is the result of the hypoglycemia or secondary to the stress of delivery or to extrauterine life remains to be determined.

The activity and regulation of gluconeogenesis in the newborn is more complex than that for mature animals. It involves not only the relative rates and controls of glycolysis and gluconeogenesis as described above but the induction of one or more key rate-limiting enzymes in gluconeogenesis (PEPCK and glucose-6-phosphatase), as well as improvement in systemic oxygenation. The complexity of the integration of these various processes is most appropriately demonstrated by the absence of a glucose or lactate response to infused alanine in normal human infants at 1 h of age,[75] but a rise in glucose to administered alanine by 24 h of age.[76] These data would imply that although alanine is utilized in the early minutes of extrauterine life, it is not contributing substantially to gluconeogenesis nor does it appear to be accumulating behind a functional enzyme block. Following 1 h of age, plasma free fatty acids rise, which contribute to ketogenesis, resulting in an increased hepatic concentration of acetyl CoA, an obligatory requirement for the activation of the first rate-limiting enzyme in gluconeogenesis, pyruvate carboxylase.

FATTY ACID AND KETONE BODY METABOLISM

The majority of fat stores in the fetus are accumulated during the last 5 weeks of gestation (Fig. 141-8).[130] Following delivery, the respiratory quotient of the newborn falls from 1.0 to 0.7 in the first days of life.[128] This would imply conversion from glucose (or glycolytic) metabolism to fatty acid metabolism. The human neonate has two types of fat stores; a unilocular white adipose tissue composed of cells with single fat vacuoles and a multilocular brown adipose tissue containing multi-vacuolated cells. Both are sensitive to circulating norepinephrine and other liplytic hormones (i.e., growth hormone, cortisol, and glucagon) and are innervated by syumpathetic fibers. The primary difference in the two tissues is their response to stimulation. In white fat, hydrolyses of stored triglycerides results in the release of free fatty acids and glycerol, whereas in brown fat, fatty acids are oxidized within the adipocyte, the primary result being the generation of heat. The brown color is due to the high mitochondrial content and capillaries. Since the neonate does not respond to hypothermia with shivering, as in

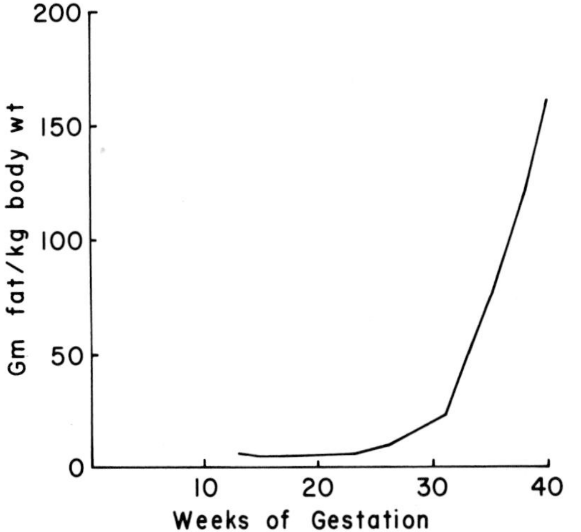

Fig. 141-8. Human fetal fat content (g/kg body wt) throughout gestation. (From Shaffer, A.J., Avery, M.E.: Diseases of the Newborn, ed 3. Philadelphia, Saunders, 1971, p. 21, with permission.)

the older child and adult, the brown fat plays a primary role in thermal homeostasis.[129]

In the fetus and the normal neonate immediately following delivery, circulating concentrations of free fatty acids are low, and rise progressively over the early hours of extrauterine life.[131] These elevations occur in the absence of a demonstrable fall in plasma insulin, but in the presence of increased glucagon, growth hormone, cortisol, presumably epinephrine secretion and increased sympathetic tone. Cold or relative cold exposure is associated with a marked reduction in adipose tissue stores and increased oxygen consumption in neonatal rabbits.[129] In humans, cold exposure results in a two- to threefold increase in circulating free fatty acids within 30 min.[132]

Free fatty acids can be directly utilized by heart, kidney, and muscle,[133] thus decreasing glucose utilization. A portion of free fatty acids undergo ketogenesis within the liver with the generation of ketone bodies (β-hydroxybutyrate, acetoacetate, and acetone). As pointed out above, this not only supplies the energy for hepatic gluconeogenesis but provides acetyl CoA to activate pyruvate carboxylase, and shares with gluconeogenesis the mutual production and utilization of oxidized pyridine nucleotide. There would appear to be no enzymatic limitation to hepatic ketogenesis since addition of fatty acids to fetal hepatic homogenates from both human and rat sources results in acetoacetate formation.[134,135] This would imply that the low concentrations of circulating ketone bodies in the fetus is a substrate-limited phenomenon.

At the time of delivery, cord β-hydroxybutyrate concentrations are often moderately elevated and fall rapidly in the first 60 to 120 min of life.[68] These ketone bodies represent transplacental transfer of maternal ketoacids. The rapid fall is most likely secondary to neonatal utilization. More recent studies in subhuman primate infants as well as fetal and neonatal human infants have demonstrated that as much as 50 percent of brain energy requirements are met by the oxidation of β-hydroxybutyrate and acetoacetate.[136–138] These alternative substrates may be of prime importance during the early hours of life by decreasing central nervous system glucose utilization at a time when hepatic glucose production may be compromised. Brain utilization of ketone bodies may further account for the absence of CNS symptoms during the transient period of "physiologic hypoglycemia" during the first few hours of life.

METABOLIC DERANGEMENTS OF FUEL HOMEOSTASIS IN THE NEONATE

General Considerations

Derangements of fuel metabolism in the neonate are manifested, as in the growing child or adult, by disturbances in blood glucose homeostasis. In contrast to the adult, where diabetes and hence hyperglycemia is the most prevalent disorder, hypoglycemia is very common in the neonate while hyperglycemic syndromes are rare.

Glucose is rapidly transported across the placenta so that the fetal plasma glucose level closely approximates the maternal concentrations. Consequently, the fetus during gestation is not dependent on its own hepatic gluconeogenesis. As described above, the gluconeogenic mechanisms in the fetus are not fully developed until near or soon after birth.

With regard to energy requirements, in highly developed countries the neonate upon delivery is placed in a position of being fully dependent upon his own resources, whereas in less sophisticated societies he is supported by being put immediately to the breast. The normal healthy newborn does have adequate stores of fat and glycogen to sustain a short period of caloric deprivation and appears capable of mobilizing these substrates as energy sources. For example, within a few hours after delivery, the plasma free fatty acids are elevated,[131] and glucagon evokes a glycemic response.[139,140] However, glycogen stores are limited and within a short period of time the neonate becomes dependent upon gluconeogenesis as the sole mechanism for meeting the obligate glucose requirements of the CNS and other glucose-dependent tissues. Despite these considerations it has been common practice to withhold feeding of normal neonates for 12 h, and even longer periods of caloric deprivation have been suggested in the past for low-birth-weight infants to avoid the problem of aspiration.[141]

DEFINITION, SIGNS, AND SYMPTOMS OF HYPOGLYCEMIA

Children and adults are usually symptomatic when the true blood glucose reaches a concentration of approximately 40 mg/100 ml. Symptoms are frequently unrecognized despite extremely low blood glucose levels in newborn infants.

Two factors which are frequently overlooked when interpreting the glucose concentrations are the analytic method used and whether blood or serum (plasma) is being examined. Since the water content of whole blood is approximately 15 percent less than serum, and glucose is not completely equilibrated between red cell water and serum, serum or plasma glucose levels will be approximately 15 percent higher than whole blood values. A large number of chemical and enzymatic methods are currently in use for the determination of glucose. The enzymatic methods using glucose oxidase or a combination of hexokinase and glucose-6-phosphate dehydrogenase specifically measure glucose. On the other hand, a variety of reducing methods are not as specific for glucose and, therefore, may occasionally give falsely elevated levels in the newborn infant.[142]

The clinical symptomatology associated with a rapid and acute fall in the blood glucose in the child and adult is usually easily interpreted. The signs and symptoms reflect primarily excessive epinephrine secretion (i.e., sweating, weakness, tachycardia, nervousness, and hunger). In the neonate, hypoglycemic symptoms are nonspecific, are less obvious, and may be completely overlooked or absent. Hypoglycemia should be suspected in any neonate with poor feeding, jitteriness, perioral cyanosis, lethargy, or seizures. Further, hypoglycemia should be anticipated in any infant known to be at high risk (e.g., infants of diabetic mothers, small-for-gestational-age infants, and neonatal asphyxia) (see below).

Since the normal fetus is exposed to an ambient plasma glucose level similar to the mother, there is no *a priori* reason to believe that, upon delivery, the glucose-dependent tissues of the neonate are more tolerant to a lower glucose supply than those of the adult. Indeed, the very opposite seems more likely, since many critical structures have yet to reach maturation. In this context it is difficult to accept current definitions of significant hypoglycemia—i.e., the presence of at least two sequential blood glucose values under 30 mg/100 ml during the first 72 h of life and 40 mg/100 ml thereafter in the full-sized infant born at term, and under 20 mg/100 ml in the infant of low birth weight.[66]

A great amount of effort has been spent in the investigation of neonatal hypoglycemia over the past 15 to 20 yr. Not unlike other areas of pediatrics, the practice of neonatology has undergone numerous changes, and the conditions under which many of these studies were performed in which "normal" blood glucose values were derived may no longer be applicable to presently accepted neonatal standards of care. Conditions of the studies that defined the normal range of blood glucose in full-term infants were for the most part uncontrolled regarding feeding-fasting regimens.[143–145]

The definition of hypoglycemia in the low-birth-weight neonate within the first 72 h of life is based on neonates (1) who had prolonged periods of caloric deprivation,[145–147] (2) who by definition are abnormal (premature or small for gestational age), and (3) who would appear to have a defect in gluconeogenesis (see below). Although the value of <20 mg/100 ml represents the lower limits of two standard deviations from the mean glucose concentration in the low-birth-weight infants studied, this value does not represent the "normal," much less the "ideal," blood glucose concentration since it was derived from an abnormal population. Evaluation of 53 premature infants breast fed immediately after birth demonstrated that the lowest mean plasma glucose value to be 54 mg/100 ml, which occurred at 36 h of life.[148]

Disorders in fuel homeostasis in the neonate can be divided into two general categories—those that are transient (e.g., hypo- and hyperglycemia associated with the small-for-gestational-age infant) and those that are chronic (e.g., hypoglycemia due to β-cell tumor or hepatic gluconeogenic enzyme defects). Table 141-3 lists the disorders that will be considered in more detail below.

Table 141-3. Disorders of Fuel Homeostasis in the Neonate

- Transient
  - SGA infant
    - Hypoglycemia
    - Hyperglycemia
  - Infant of the diabetic mother
  - Erythroblastosis
  - Miscellaneous—sepsis, hypoxemia, hypothermia
- Chronic
  - Sustained hyperinsulinemia
    - β-cell adenoma
    - β-cell hyperplasia
    - Nesidioblastosis
    - Functional β-cell secretory disorders
  - Endocrine deficiencies
    - Growth hormone
    - ACTH
    - Cortisol
  - Hepatic enzyme deficiencies
    - Glucose-6-phosphatase
    - Fructose-1,6-diphosphatase
    - Glycogen synthetase
    - Galactose-1-phosphate uridyl transferase
    - Fructose-1-phosphate aldolase

Although it is well documented that the nadir of blood glucose frequently occurs within 2 to 3 h following birth, we feel that this should not be construed as being either the normal or desirable concentrations for later hours of life. Until further studies relating to the effect of early feeding on the blood glucose concentrations have been performed, the authors follow the policy of trying to maintain the plasma glucose concentrations above 40 mg/100 ml in all neonates.

THERAPY

It is the author's current policy to monitor the blood glucose level of all high-risk infants (i.e., small-for-gestational-age infants, premature infants, infants of diabetic mothers, etc.) at 1-to-2-h intervals with Dextrostix (Ames). Since variable and inconsistent results are frequently observed with this method at low blood glucose concentrations, test results with Dextrostix are frequently compared with plasma glucose values determined by reliable laboratory methods. If the blood glucose level by Dextrostix is 45 mg/100 ml or less, a blood specimen is obtained for measurement of glucose by the glucose oxidase method, and the infant is started immediately on a feeding of 5-percent glucose followed subsequently at 2-to-3-h intervals with standard formula feedings. Throughout this time, the blood glucose level is monitored before each feeding; in the large majority of intances, adequate glucose concentrations are maintained by this practice. If, however, the plasma glucose value remains below 40 mg/100 ml by specific measurement, an intravenous infusion of 10- to 20-percent glucose is begun. Specific rates of glucose administration have been reported;[66] however, it is our opinion that the variability in requirements between patients is so great that the rate of administration needs to be individualized and the patient given an amount of glucose that will maintain his plasma glucose above 40 mg/100 ml. This approach to therapy requires frequent monitoring of the blood glucose and close observation of the volume of fluid being administered. On rare occasions, hypoglycemia persists despite this infusion, and then cortisone acetate is administered intramuscularly at 8-h intervals (total dosage is 5 mg/kg body wt/day). On this regimen, the blood glucose level has been readily stabilized in the vast majority of infants. Usually, the intravenous infusion of glucose can be tapered after 48 h and cortisone acetate therapy gradually eliminated during the subsequent 4 to 5 days. If hypoglycemia persists for more than 72 h on this regimen or is recurrent following cessation of therapy, causes for chronic hypoglycemia should be considered.

THE SMALL-FOR-GESTATIONAL-AGE INFANT

Infants whose weights are below the 10th percentile for gestational age[149] have been found to have an increased risk of both hypoglycemia and transient neonatal hyperglycemia. These infants have been termed intrauterine-growth-retarded or small-for-gestational-age (SGA) infants. The cause of the growth retardation is not clear but may be related to placental insufficiency; however, chromosomal defects and congenital viral syndromes have been implicated.[150]

HYPOGLYCEMIA IN THE SGA INFANT

Lubchenco and Bard[149] have shown that the risk for the development of blood sugar levels less than 30 mg/100 ml in the SGA infant was correlated best with the degree of maturation of

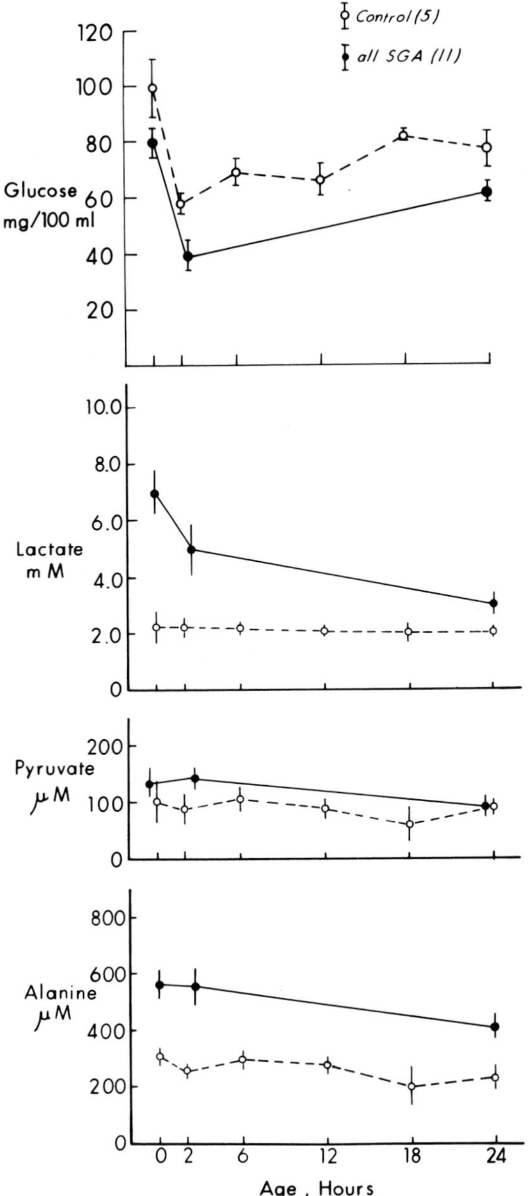

Fig. 141-9. Plasma glucose, blood lactate, blood pyruvate, and plasma alanine concentrations of the normal and SGA infants during the first 24 h of life (mean ± SEM). (From N. Engl. J. Med. *291*:322, 1974, with permission.)

the infant—i.e., the incidence of hypoglycemia was 67 percent in premature, 25 percent in term, and 18 percent in post-term SGA infants. The factors predisposing these infants to the development of hypoglycemia could theoretically be a defect in any one of the essential requirements for the maintenance of normal glucose homeostasis which includes the integrity of the hepatic gluconeogenic and glycogenolytic pathways, sufficient endogenous gluconeogenic substrate, and appropriate hormonal secretion to modulate the first two processes.

The information in the literature together with studies from the authors' laboratory have demonstrated elevated plasma concentrations of growth hormone and cortisol in low-birth-weight infants.[68] Therefore, it must be concluded that the pituitary gland and the pituitary adrenal axis are responding appropriately in the early hours of life. Insulin has been implicated in a variety of specific clinical and pathologic disorders in the newborn (see below), but hyperinsulinemia has not been found in these infants. It has recently been demonstrated that these infants have a hyperglucagonemic response to alanine infusion,[76] which mitigates against glucagon insufficiency as being the etiology of the hypoglycemia.

In regard to substrate availability, a few SGA infants have had free fatty acids, glycerol, and ketone bodies determined in the first 24 h of life,[68,151] but sufficient data are lacking for any general conclusions regarding formation or utilization of these important substrates.

Hyperlactatemia and hyperalaninemia are well-established findings in patients with defects in hepatic gluconeogenesis either congenital in origin (i.e, glucose-6-phosphatase or fructose 1,6-diphosphatase deficiencies)[152] or acquired defects (i.e., lactic acidosis).[153] Both hyperalaninemia and hypoglycemia have been observed within early hours of life in SGA infants of hypertensive mothers.[154] Lindblad *et al.*[155] also noted hyperalaninemia in a group of SGA infants of malnourished mothers, but no comment was made about the glucose concentrations of those infants. Studies from our laboratory have clearly demonstrated hyperlactatemia together with hyperaminoacidemia in the SGA infant.[68] Figure 141-9 compares the plasma glucose, alanine, blood lactate, and pyruvate in 5 full-term and 11 SGA infants from birth through the first 24 h of life, and Figure 141-10, the concentrations of the various gluconeogenic amino acids in cord blood and their respective potential entrance into the gluconeogenic pathway. The persistence of hyperlactatemia and hyperalaninemia is most compatible with a defect in gluconeogenesis, compromising the ability of the infant to utilize gluconeogenic substrates entering at or below pyruvate. With decreased hepatic gluconeogenesis, a larger proportion of hepatic glucose release must be derived from stored glycogen, which results in rapid depletion (Fig. 141-4) and would explain the poor glycemic responses observed in these infants upon challenge with glucagon.[139,140]

Since hypoglycemia develops in only 40 to 50 percent of SGA infants,[68,149] a spectrum of laboratory and clinical findings obviously exists. Significant inverse correlations of plasma glucose and lactate and of glucose and alanine support a causative relation

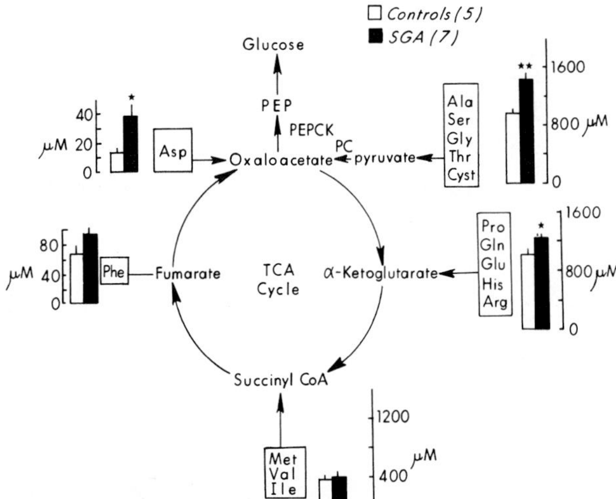

Fig. 141-10. Summed concentrations (mean ± SEM) of the individual amino acids in the cord plasma of the SGA and normal infants at their respective potential entrance into the gluconeogenic pathway. CoA: coenzyme A; PC: pyruvate carboxylase; PEP: phosphoenol pyruvate; PEPCK: phosphoenol pyruvate carboxykinase; TCA: tricarboxylic acid. $**p < 0.01$; $*p < 0.05$. (From N. Engl. J. Med. *291*:322, 1974, with permission.)

between gluconeogenic substrates and the plasma glucose concentration.[68] These observations, together with the pattern of other potential gluconeogenic amino acids, and the inability of the SGA infant to utilize administered alanine as a gluconeogenic substrate[76,156] during the first day of life as compared to normal infants, are strong evidence for a transient defect in hepatic gluconeogenesis.

HYPERGLYCEMIA IN THE SGA INFANT

Hyperglycemia and glycosuria during the first month of life are uncommon. An occasional case may represent the initial episode of true insulin-dependent diabetes mellitus while others have been associated with overwhelming infection and/or CNS disease ending in death. In 1926, Ramsey described the first well-documented case of a clinical entity simulating true diabetes mellitus,[157] which subsequently has been referred to as transient diabetes in the newborn, pseudodiabetes of the newborn, infantile glucosuria, and temporary neonatal hyperglycemia. Characteristically the disorder presents within the first 6 weeks of life with hyperglycemia, glycosuria, and dehydration, but ketonuria, if present, is minimal. This disorder most commonly affects the SGA infant, and recovery appears to be complete.

The etiology of this syndrome and its association with other forms of diabetes mellitus remains obscure. In approximately one-third there is a positive family history of diabetes mellitus.[158] In a few patients studied at autopsy, no characteristic abnormalities have been found in the pancreas.[159–163] A flat oral glucose tolerance test has been observed in the mothers of some of these infants. It has been suggested that the β cells of these infants are hypoplastic due to the lack of a normal glucose stimulus in utero,[164–167] which, in light of the data presented above on insulin secretion in the fetus, would make this postulate highly unlikely. Further, several mothers have given birth to infants with this syndrome[168–170] who have had normal or diabetic carbohydrate tolerance.

Few studies dealing with glucose-insulin relationships have been reported in these infants. Gentz and Cornblath[158] reported 2 patients, one of whom had plasma insulin concentrations of 6 and 17 μU/ml, when the blood glucose was 1280 and 2300 mg/100 ml, respectively. Following remission of the hyperglycemia in these infants, oral and intravenous glucose tolerance tests were normal.

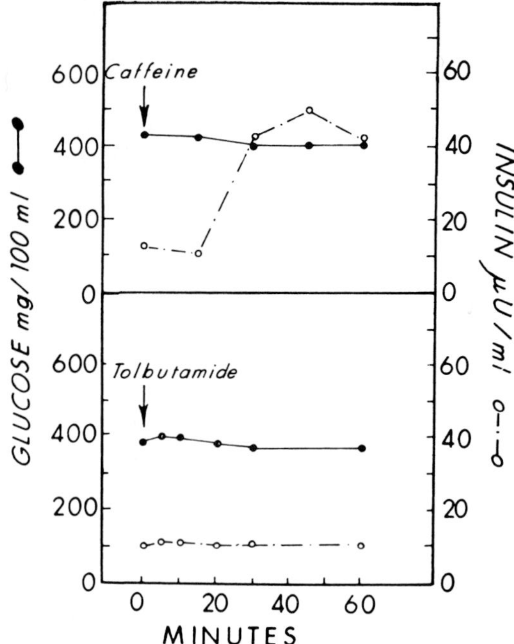

Fig. 141-11. Responses to intramuscular caffeine benzoate (4 mg/kg) at 9 days of age and intravenous sodium tolbutamide (20 mg/kg) at 18 days of age in an infant with transient neonatal diabetes. (From J. Pediatr. *81*:97, 1973, with permission.)

The authors have had the opportunity to study a patient with this syndrome.[171] Although insulin was detectable on all occasions, the concentrations during the diabetic phase were markedly reduced for the degree of hyperglycemia, suggesting that glucose-mediated insulin release was severely impaired. Intramuscular injection of caffeine, a potent nucleotide phosphodiesterase inhibitor, caused an increase in plasma insulin from 12 to 50 μU/ml with

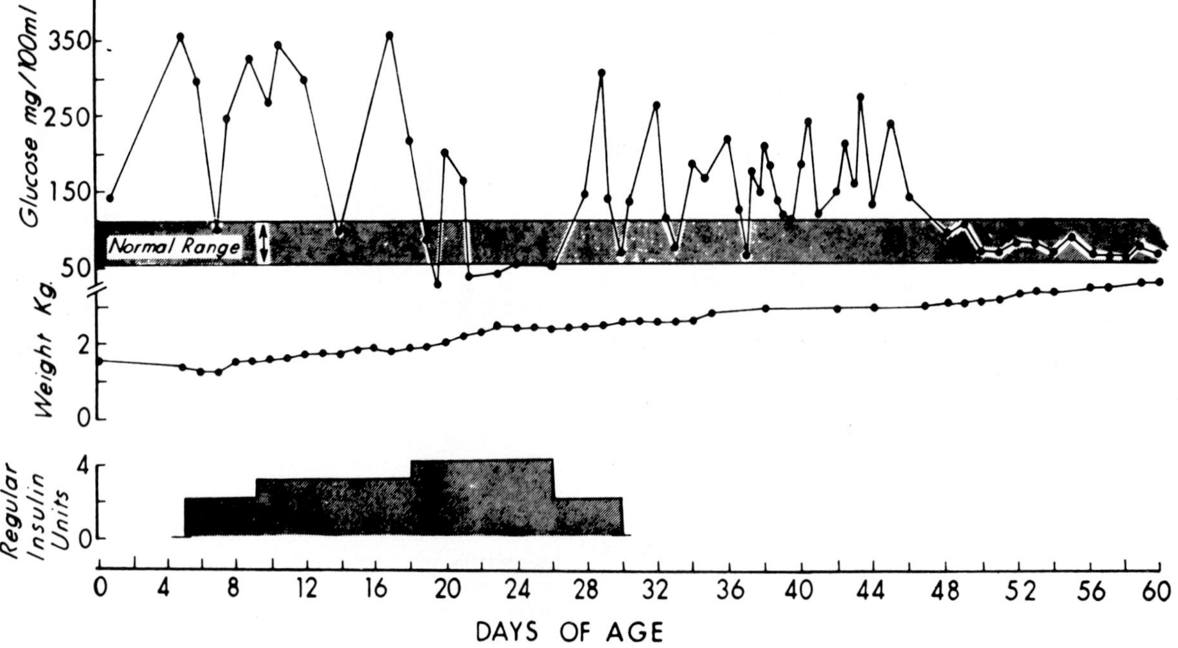

Fig. 141-12. Plasma glucose, body weight, and insulin therapy of an infant with transient neonatal diabetes. (From J. Pediatr. *81*:97, 1973, with permission.)

only a slight decrease in plasma glucose (Fig. 141-11). The failure of a fall in glucose may be related to a simultaneous increase in hepatic cyclic AMP concentrations resulting in increased glucose output by the liver.[172]

Tolbutamide administration during the hyperglycemic phase (Fig. 141-11), resulted in neither a detectable increase in circulating insulin nor a decrease in plasma glucose. These results are in accord with in vitro studies on human fetal pancreas,[57–59] and suggest that the pancreatic β cells of this patient were insensitive to tolbutamide- and glucose-mediated insulin release.

After 25 days of insulin therapy (Fig. 141-12), the child gradually developed normal glycemia, and all insulin was discontinued. Fourteen days following her last dose of insulin, fasting glucose ranged between 80 and 130 mg/100 ml and insulin 10 to 26 μU/ml. Repeat tolbutamide testing revealed a normal glucose response with plasma insulin increasing from a fasting concentration of 27 to 60 μU/ml within 2 min of injection (Fig. 141-13). When challenged with intravenous glucose, the infant demonstrated a normal glucose tolerance test. There was, however, a marked delay in insulin release, the peak insulin occurring at 30 min following the intravenous injection of glucose (Fig. 141-13).

These findings suggest that the defect in patients with transient neonatal diabetes may be an initial failure of the β cell to respond to glucose and tolbutamide at a time when insulin is present in the pancreas. As considered in detail above, normal neonates also demonstrate varying degrees of decreased sensitivity of insulin release to glucose. Thus, the defect seen in infants with transient neonatal diabetes may be quantitative in nature. Since caffeine, a phosphodiesterase inhibitor, is capable of releasing insulin during the transient diabetic phase, it is postulated that the defect may be related to delayed maturation of the adenyl cyclase-cyclic adenosine monophosphate system as a result of either a deficiency of β-cell adenyl cyclase or of an increased activity of the nucleotide phosphodiesterase. This hypothesis is consistent with the transient nature of the disorder.

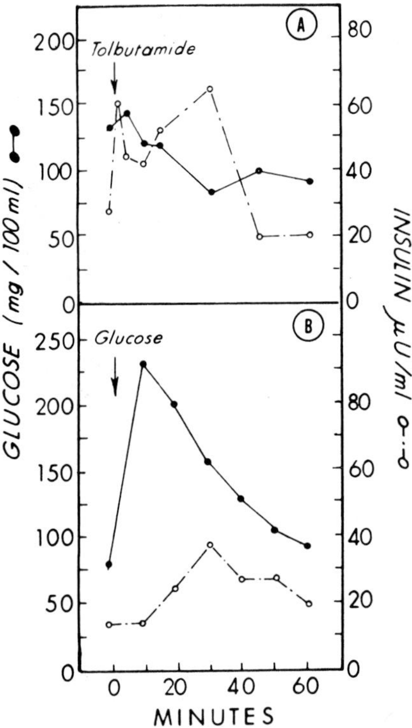

Fig. 141-13. A: response to intravenous sodium tolbutamide (20 mg/kg) at 52 days of age; B: response to intravenous glucose (0.75 g/kg) at 59 days of age in an infant with transient neonatal diabetes. (From J. Pediatr. *81*:97, 1973, with permission.)

INFANT OF THE DIABETIC MOTHER

While the ability to conceive does not apparently differ between diabetic and nondiabetic women, fetal wastage, neonatal mortality, and morbidity are significantly higher than in the normal population. These complications are directly related to vascular disease in the mother and not to the degree of insulin dependence, the age of onset, nor the duration of diabetes. White's classification[173] has subsequently been modified by Cornblath and Schwartz (Table 141-4).[66] Class A in this schema includes women with gestational diabetes and prediabetes. The gestational diabetic is defined as the woman who develops abnormal glucose tolerance during pregnancy, and postpartum reverts to a normal tolerance; the prediabetic includes pregnant women with a genetic predisposition to the disease including a strong family history of diabetes, a history of previously overweight infants (>4000 g), or unexplained stillbirth beyond 28 weeks' gestation.[66] By definition, the pregnant prediabetic has a normal glucose tolerance, and neither subclass is symptomatic or receiving insulin therapy during pregnancy.

Table 141-4. Modified White[66] Classification of Diabetes and Pregnancy

Class A:	High fetal survival, no insulin, minimal dietary regulation Gestational diabetes—abnormal glucose tolerance test during pregnancy which reverts to normal within a few weeks after delivery Prediabetes—normal glucose tolerance test, but family history of diabetes, previous large infants or unexplained stillbirths
Class B:	Onset of diabetes in adult life after age 20 yr, duration less than 10 yr, no vascular disease
Class C:	Diabetes of long duration (10–19 yr) with onset during adolescence (over 10 yr) with minimal vascular disease
Class D:	Diabetes of 20 yr or more duration, onset before age 10 yr, evidence of vascular disease (i.e., retinitis, albuminuria, hypertension)
Class E:	Patients with D, plus demonstrable calcification of pelvic vessels
Class F:	Patients with D, plus nephritis

In a retrospective study by Dekaban and Baird,[174] abortions, stillbirths, neonatal deaths, and abnormal survivors were significantly higher in overt and prediabetics as compared to controls (Table 141-5). When the diabetic mothers were classified according to the criteria given in Table 141-4, fetal loss was 14.5 percent for combined classes B and C, and 29 percent for combined classes D through F. Other factors that have been shown to affect the outcome of the pregnancy are toxemia and hydramnios.[66]

It is generally accepted that the neonates of overt insulin-

Table 141-5. Pregnancies of Diabetics

	Total No.	Abortions (%)	Stillbirths (%)	Neonatal Deaths (%)	Abnormal Survivors (%)
Diabetics	157	30.0	11.5	8.3	3.8
Prediabetics	78	20.5	5.1	1.3	2.6
Controls	249	12.4	1.2	3.0	0.4

Adapted from Dekaban and Baird: J. Pediatr. 55:563, 1959, with permission.

dependent diabetics (classes B–F) have increased survival if the pregnancy is interrupted between 35 and 37 weeks of gestation. Delivery prior to 35 weeks is associated with excessive neonatal mortality and delivery after 37 weeks with an increased incidence of stillbirths.

The infant of the diabetic mother is generally a "large-for-date" infant. However, despite their size these infants are physiologically immature. Diabetic mothers with severe vascular disease may give birth to SGA infants. The excessive weight is due to increased body fat and enlargement of certain viscera, primarily liver and heart.[175,176] They often exhibit several clinical problems associated with their prematurity including: respiratory distress due to hyaline membrane disease (the leading cause of death), nonhemolytic hyperbilirubinemia, hypocalcemic tetany, polycythemia, and rarely renal vein thrombosis.[176] Congenital anomalies are three times more frequent among these infants than normal controls.

CARBOHYDRATE HOMEOSTASIS

Pedersen *et al*[177] suggested that prolonged and excessive exposure of the fetus in a diabetic mother to hyperglycemia resulted in stimulation of the pancreatic β cell to synthesize and secrete excessive insulin. The high levels of glucose and insulin would thus result in increased synthesis and storage of fat, glycogen, and protein in utero.

Soon after birth severe symptomatic hypoglycemia occurs in 10 to 20 percent and asymptomatic hypoglycemia in up to 50 percent of these infants. The etiology of the hypoglycemia is felt to be secondary to hyperinsulinemia on the basis of (1) pathologic evidence of β-cell hyperplasia presumed to be secondary to in utero exposure to chronic hyperglycemia, (2) decreased circulating concentrations of free fatty acids and ketone bodies, and (3) more rapid disappearance of glucose whether administered by oral or intravenous routes.[175] Accurate estimations of plasma insulin by radioimmunoassay in these patients has been complicated by transplacental transfer of maternal antiinsulin IgG. In utero, the infant of the diabetic mother undoubtedly has high plasma insulin levels resulting from the sustained hyperglycemia; but postnatally there has been no solid evidence until recently that hyperinsulinemia persists following birth. β-cell function has been studied in the presence of antiinsulin antibodies by measurement of C-peptide, the connecting segment of the proinsulin molecule which is secreted in equimolar concentrations with insulin and does not cross-react in the insulin immunoassay. Preliminary data have shown significantly higher levels of C-peptide immunoreactivity in umbilical cord blood of infants of insulin-requiring diabetic mothers than in normal controls.[175]

Under the influence of a constant hyperglycemic stimulus and hyperinsulinemia in utero one might anticipate abnormalities in glucose homeostasis secondary to delayed induction of hepatic gluconeogenic and glycogenolytic enzymes resulting in compromised hepatic glucose production and release. This speculation is supported by a recent study in which alanine infusion was ineffective in producing a glycemic response at a time of hypoglycemia,[178] and this possible delay in enzyme induction may parallel the inhibitory effect of high glucose which inhibits PEPCK induction in the newborn rat.[122]

ERYTHROBLASTOSIS

Infants with erythroblastosis fetalis also have a high incidence of hypoglycemia which is secondary to hyperinsulinemia.[179] β-cell hyperplasia has been found at postmortem examination in these infants. No etiology is apparent that accounts for the β-cell hyperplasia and subsequent hyperinsulinemia observed in these patients.

BECKWITH-WIEDEMANN SYNDROME

β-cell hyperplasia has been observed in the Beckwith-Wiedemann syndrome.[180–182] This disorder is characterized by macroglossia, omphalocele, hyperplastic visceromegaly, and frequently hypoglycemia. Subsequent to the original descriptions of this syndrome, a large number of additional somatic abnormalities have been described; the interested reader is referred to several recent reviews.[181,182] The hypoglycemia, when it occurs in these neonates, is profound but spontaneously improves over the first few days of life. Hyperinsulinemia and elevated insulin-like activity have been documented in a number of these infants. Any newborn with macroglossia and/or exomphalos should be prospectively followed for the development of hypoglycemia so that prompt therapy can be instituted to minimize the CNS dysfunction so frequently observed with this disorder.

SEPSIS, HYPOXEMIA, HYPOTHERMIA

Neonatal bacterial sepsis is associated with hypoglycemia and accelerated rates of glucose disappearance to iv glucose administration.[183,184] Whether the hypoglycemia is secondary to poor antecedent caloric intake or the effects of circulating endotoxins on glucose homeostatic mechanisms has not been established. However, hypoglycemia has been observed in adults with gram-negative bacteremia.[185,186] In animal studies, gram-negative infection and exogenously administered endotoxins have been associated with hypoglycemia, hepatic glycogen depletion, and decreased rates of gluconeogenesis.[187,188]

Neonatal hypoxemia frequently is associated with hypoglycemia in the early hours of life.[189] In neonatal animal studies, it has been observed that tissue oxygenation is a prerequisite for the establishment of hepatic gluconeogenesis.[121] Therefore under the stress of hypoxemia, hepatic glycogen stores would be rapidly depleted, and with a superimposed functional defect in gluconeogenesis, hypoglycemia would ensue.

Hypoglycemia has also been associated with hypothermia in the newborn infant.[190] Cause and effect are not clear, since hypothermia is a common finding in adults with hypoglycemia. Hypoglycemia in the neonate in association with hypothermia may well be related to more rapid utilization of endogenous glycogen stores in the face of a decreased ability to perform gluconeogenesis.

SUSTAINED HYPERINSULINEMIA

Chronic hyperinsulinemia can result from a variety of different β-cell abnormalities: β-cell adenoma, diffuse β-cell hyperplasia, nesidioblastosis (i.e., neoformation of β cells from the ductal epithelium), and functional β-cell secretory disorders without detectable histologic abnormality. Any of these disorders of the β cell may present in the neonatal period as is illustrated in the following case report.

M. V. SLCH #75-1555. The patient was the 3020 gr product of a full-term pregnancy of a Gravida I, Para O, 16-yr-old woman. The infant was delivered by caeserean section due to cephalopelvic disproportion following a 12-h labor.

The infant did well until 3 days of age when he began vomiting and refused feedings. He soon developed generalized seizures. Laboratory data were all within normal limits except for a plasma glucose of 23 mg/100 ml. His plasma glucose remained low on glucose infusion together with frequent feedings and it was necessary to administer cortisone acetate intermuscularly at 8-h intervals to maintain his plasma glucose above 40 mg/100 ml (see Therapy section). After several days of steroid therapy, withdrawal of this drug resulted in the return of symptomatic hypoglycemia. Multiple determinations of plasma insulin were elevated relative to the plasma glucose. Diazoxide (15 mg/kg) failed to affect the hyperinsulinemia and hypoglycemia.

At laparotomy a 1×1-cm nodule was found in the head of the pancreas, the location of which necessitated a 90-percent resection. This nodule histologically consisted of many giant islets separated by thick bands of connective tissue. The islets contained α, β, and δ cells in the same relative numbers and distribution as in normal-sized islets. The edges of many of the enlarged islets contained ducts in continuity with islet cells. The size, number, and cellular composition of the islets in the tail of the pancreas were normal in appearance. Often individual islet cells or small groups were incorporated in otherwise normal acini.

Postoperatively the patient had transient hyperglycemia which returned to normal within 48 h. Reevaluation at 6 months of age demonstrated a normal 24-h fasting glucose-insulin profile and a mildly abnormal glucose tolerance test. There was no clinical or laboratory evidence of exocrine pancreatic insufficiency. Three years postsurgery the child continues to do well.

An islet cell adenoma of the pancreas is a rare finding in children; less than 50 cases have been reported.[191] A much more common pathologic finding in children with organic hyperinsulinism is β-cell hyperplasia. Recently, Brown and Young[192] and Yakovac and associates[193] reported that in 10 of 13 children who had had partial pancreatectomy for "idiopathic hypoglycemia," increased numbers of β cells were present in the exocrine portion of the pancreas. In these children nesidioblastosis would appear to be the persistence of elements of the fetal pancreas. Nesidioblastosis cannot be diagnosed by routine staining methods; rather, insulin-specific staining techniques (e.g., aldehyde-fuchsin and pinacyanole metachromasia) are required to establish this diagnosis. It has been suggested that this entity may account for many of the cases of hypoglycemia due to hyperinsulinemia, which on routine histologic examination have normal-appearing islets of Langerhans. However, there may be instances of organic hyperinsulinemia in children in which a functional defect in insulin secretion exists which cannot be identified even by sophisticated histologic examination. At the present time one cannot distinguish clinically, on the basis of plasma-insulin responses to fasting and provocative stimulatory agents (e.g., glucose, leucine, and tolbutamide) the entities of β-cell adenoma, β-cell hyperplasia, nesidioblastosis, and functional β-cell secretory disorders.

Medical management of hyperinsulinemia has included the long-term use of glucocorticoids and dietary manipulations. In general, the response to such treatment has been poor.[194] The hyperglycemic effect of diazoxide is due, at least in part, to suppression of pancreatic insulin secretion,[195–197] and this drug has been reported to be effective in treating many forms of childhood hypoglycemia.[195–199] There have been several infants with proven pancreatic adenomas in which diazoxide was ineffective in controlling hypoglycemia.[191,200,201] In a dosage range of 10 to 15 mg/kg body wt/day, the side-effects have consisted of hypertrichosis, advancement of bone age, mild hyperuricemia, and IgG deficiency.

There is no uniform agreement on the therapeutic effectiveness of pancreatic surgery in children with hyperinsulinism. Obviously, it is curative in β-cell adenoma. The variable results reported with this procedure reflect, at least in part, the heterogeneity of the underlying pathology (i.e., β-cell hyperplasia, nesidioblastosis, and functional β-cell secretory disorders) and the extent of the pancreatectomy.[152] Since subtotal pancreatectomy in a child performed by an experienced surgeon carries relatively little risk,[152,202] and the pathologic basis for hyperinsulinism cannot be defined by clinical testing, the authors feel that any infant with hypoglycemia and proven hyperinsulinemia persisting beyond the age of 2 weeks and not responding to standard medical measures is a candidate for pancreatic exploration. If an adenoma is not found after careful inspection and palpation, a subtotal pancreatectomy is indicated in which 75 to 85 percent of the pancreas is removed. Obviously, long-term follow-up of these patients is required before definitive conclusions on the efficacy of surgical therapy can be made. However, current results would indicate a significant number of children are benefited by this form of therapy.[152,202,202a]

ENDOCRINE DEFICIENCIES

Hypoglycemia is a frequent occurrence in neonates and children with primary and secondary adrenal insufficiency (i.e., Addison's disease,[203,204] congenital adrenal hyperplasia,[204] and isolated ACTH deficiency[205]). A 20-percent incidence has been noted in panhypopituitarism, monotrophic growth hormone, or various combinations of trophic hormonal deficiencies including growth hormone and ACTH.[206–208] The pathophysiology of the hypoglycemia in these endocrine disorders has generally been assumed to reflect decreased activity of gluconeogenic enzymes and accelerated rates of glucose utilization. We have studied 5 children with ACTH and growth-hormone deficiency.[209] Prior to replacement therapy, all of the subjects developed hypoglycemia, ketosis, and hypoalaninemia within 30 h of total caloric restriction. Hormone replacement (growth hormone 1 mg/day and cortisone acetate 25 mg/m^2/24 h) prevented hypoglycemia, increased circulating concentrations of amino acids, decreased ketosis, and decreased urinary nitrogen losses during a subsequent fast. Hepatic gluconeogenesis would appear to be intact in these patients since a normal glycemic response to alanine infusion was observed prior to and following replacement therapy in one of our patients. The improvement in glucose homeostasis and decreased excretion of urea nitrogen would imply decreased hepatic gluconeogenesis and glucose utilization perhaps by increasing peripheral utilization of fatty acids.

HEPATIC ENZYME DEFICIENCIES

GLUCOSE-6-PHOSPHATASE DEFICIENCY (GLYCOGEN STORAGE DISEASE TYPE I)

The glycogen storage diseases are inherited defects characterized by either a deficient or abnormally functioning enzyme involved in the degradation of glycogen. Glycogen storage diseases type II (deficient lysosomal α-1,4-glucosidase) and type IV (amylo-1,4 $\rightarrow$ 1,6-transglucosidase—brancher enzyme), as well as those due to specific muscle enzyme defects, are not considered in this chapter because they are not associated with hypoglycemia. In addition, deficiencies of amylo-1,6-glucoside and phosphorylase (glycogen storage diseases III and VI, respectively) rarely present with neonatal hypoglycemia and usually present with asymptomatic hepatomegaly at an older age. The interested reader is referred to recent reviews of these topics.[210,211]

The first case of hypoglycemia associated with hepatomegaly and ketonuria was reported by Snapper and van Creveld[212] in 1928. The following year, Von Gierke[213] demonstrated increased glycogen deposition in the liver and kidney of a similar patient, and 23-years later Cori and Cori[214] reported the absence of glucose-6-phosphatase in patients with the hepatic form of glycogen storage disease.

Since hydrolysis of glucose-6-phosphate is the final common enzymatic event in the release of glucose from either the gluconeogenic or glycogenolytic pathway, the absence of glucose-6-phosphatase typically results in severe hypoglycemia associated with marked ketosis and lactic acidosis. Hepatomegaly, growth retardation, hyperlipidemia, and hyperuricemia are also common clinical features of this disorder. Chronic hypoglycemia provokes the increased secretion of various hormones (i.e., catecholamines, glucagon, and cortisol) and suppresses insulin secretion, resulting in both increased glycogenolysis and amino acid flux to the liver. Consequently, lactic acidosis which develops is a result of increased formation and decreased utilization. Ketosis is a concomitant of exaggerated lipolysis and accelerated hepatic ketogenesis secondary to the chronic hypoinsulinemia.[215] Hyperuricemia reflects decreased renal clearance secondary to elevated blood lactate and ketone body concentrations, which compete for a common renal tubular secretory site,[215–217] as well as increased de novo uric acid production,[218–222] which may result in chronic gouty arthritis. Hypercholesterolemia and hypertriglyceridemia together with increased lipid stores in the liver appear related to increased lipogenesis.[215,219,223] Despite marked hepatomegaly due to excessive lipid and glycogen storage, there is generally little impairment of other hepatic functions.[210]

Glucose-6-phosphatase is also normally present in kidney and intestinal mucosa. Although the kidneys demonstrate excessive storage of glycogen, renal function is normal except for occasional glycosuria and aminoaciduria.[224] Recurrent diarrhea has been observed in some infants, but the relationship to absent glucose-6-phosphatase in the gastrointestinal tract is not apparent.[215,225] Clotting abnormalities have been observed in some patients,[210,226] but the relationship to the primary defect is not known.

Although occasional patients present with only mild clinical biochemic abnormalities (hypoglycemia after 15 to 20 h of fasting and subnormal but detectable glycemic responses to glucagon, fructose, and galactose administration[227], glucose-6-phosphatase activity cannot be demonstrated in liver biopsy specimens. Conversely, several well-studied cases, presenting with all of the clinical features of glucose-6-phosphatase deficiency and biopsy-proved hepatic glycogen storage, have been reported in which normal levels of this enzyme have been found.[227–231] These patients demonstrate the importance of defining the pathogenic basis of the disorder by both clinical studies (i.e., infusion tests, responses to fasting) and hepatic enzyme analyses. This suggests that other factor(s) may be involved in regulating the degradation of glycogen and hydrolysis of hepatic glucose-6-phosphate besides the currently identified enzymic systems.[227]

FRUCTOSE-1,6-DIPHOSPHATASE DEFICIENCY

Hepatic fructose-1,6-diphosphatase deficiency is a newly described gluconeogenic enzyme defect. The presenting signs and symptoms are indistinguishable from glycogen storage disease type I. However, excessive glycogen storage does not occur since the glycogenolytic pathway is intact. Hepatomegaly is secondary to lipid storage but liver function studies are generally normal. Lactic acidosis, ketoacidosis, hyperlipidemia, and hyperuricemia in this condition are presumed to have the same pathogenesis as in glucose-6-phosphatase deficiency.

The first report of this entity by Baker and Winegrad[232] was followed within a few months by the description of 4 additional cases.[233–237] The 5 children ranged in age from 5 months to 5.5 yr at the time of diagnosis. Several of these patients presented with hypoglycemia and acidosis in the neonatal period. One female infant died at 6 months of age, and the diagnosis was made by postmortem liver enzyme analysis.[236] Another died at 9 months of age with severe metabolic acidosis following extensive body burns.[237] The other 2 females and 2 male patients were living at the time of the respective reports. In 3 of the 5 families[232,235,236] there were 5 affected siblings who presented with hepatomegaly and died in the neonatal or early childhood period from unexplained metabolic acidosis. Postmortem histologic examination of the liver in 3 of the siblings revealed fatty infiltration similar to that found in the 5 index cases. Consanguinity was noted in 2 of the 5 families,[235,236] and on the basis of available data, this disorder appears to be inherited as an autosomal recessive trait.

Since the glycogenolytic system is intact, glucagon administration produces a hyperglycemic response in the immediate postprandial period but not after a short fast.[234,236] Glucose, galactose, maltose, and lactose are utilizable carbohydrates and can be stored as glycogen and metabolized. Since fructose, glycerol, and the gluconeogenic amino acids enter the gluconeogenic pathway at or below the level of fructose-1,6-diphosphatase (Fig. 141-6), these substances cannot be converted to glucose. Infusions of these substrates cause the accumulation of lactate and consequent lactic acidosis, and produce a rapid fall in the blood glucose level. The mechanism of this hypoglycemic effect has not been clarified, but one possibility is that the accumulation of triose phosphates below the level of fructose-1,6-diphosphatase may acutely inhibit glycogenolysis in a manner similar to that resulting from the accumulation of fructose-1-phosphate in patients with hereditary fructose intolerance.

DIAGNOSIS AND TREATMENT

Fasting hypoglycemia, hepatomegaly, and signs and symptoms of severe metabolic acidosis (i.e., episodic hyperventilation) are highly suggestive of either glucose-6-phosphatase or fructose-1,6-diphosphatase deficiency. Although each of these disorders has a similar clinical presentation including hypoglycemia, hyperlacticacidemia, ketosis, hyperlipidemia, and hyperuricemia, they can be readily distinguished by the responses to infusions of various gluconeogenic precursors. In both conditions, alanine, glycerol, and fructose infusions do not produce a glycemic response but result in a rapid rise in blood lactate and pyruvate. (Because of reported complications associated with glycerol infusion,[238] the authors avoid its use as a diagnostic tool.) The infusion of galactose provokes similar effects in patients with glucose-6-phosphatase deficiency, whereas in fructose 1,6-diphosphatase deficiency, a normal glycemic response without demonstrable change in blood lactate is observed. Glucagon further differentiates between these two disorders in that the hormone will produce a prompt glycemic response in the fed state in patients with fructose-1,6-diphosphatase deficiency but no significant response in those with glucose-6-phosphatase deficiency.

Definitive diagnosis of these two disorders is made by determining specific enzyme activities and glycogen content in liver biopsy specimens. In type I glycogen storage disease, glucose-6-phosphatase is totally absent and hepatic glycogen content is greater than 5 percent by weight. An occasional patient is seen with all the clinical stigmata of this disorder, including an elevated hepatic glycogen content, in whom the activities of glucose-6-phosphatase and other known glycogenolytic enzymes in the liver biopsy are normal. It has been suggested that in these rare patients, factors (as yet unidentified) are deficient that are required for normal in vivo glucose-6-phosphatase activity.[227] In fructose-1,6-diphosphatase deficiency, the enzyme is totally absent, and hepatic glycogen content may be normal or low depending upon the caloric intake immediately before the liver biopsy is obtained. In addition, fructose-1,6-diphosphatase activity has been observed in white blood cells, which may be a useful adjunct in the diagnosis of this enzyme deficiency.[237] Further experience will be necessary to determine if leukocyte enzyme deficiency is always concordant with the hepatic defect.

Since a depressed glucose-6-phosphatase activity precludes glucose output from either glycogenolytic or gluconeogenic sources, therapy in severely affected children is not satisfactory. Constant intravenous infusions of glucose can correct the secondary metabolic abnormalities.[239] Several drugs have been tried—including glucagon,[240,241] glucocorticoids,[242] thyroxine,[241] epinephrine,[242] and androgens[243]—with poor results. Diazoxide has been used in a few patients with apparently some benefit.[198,199] Since galactose and fructose cannot be converted to glucose, sucrose and lactose must be removed from the diet and carbohydrate should be given in the form of starch, maltose, and glucose. Total protein should be restricted to the minimal amount required for positive nitrogen balance (i.e., approximately 2g/kg body wt/day) since amounts in excess of this will predispose to lactic acidosis. The diet currently in use in our laboratory provides 60 percent of caloric requirements as carbohydrate, 15 percent as protein, and the remainder as fat; it is given in feedings at 3 to 4 hourly intervals around the clock. In those patients in whom lactic acidosis remains a persistent problem, sodium bicarbonate is given in an oral dose of 2 to 3 mEq/kg body wt/day.

Portacaval shunts or transpositions have been performed in 5 children with type I[239,244–246] and 1 patient with type III[247] glycogen storage diseases. The rationale for this operative approach is the observation that diversion of portal blood flow in dogs results in the delivery of glucose-rich blood directly into the systemic circulation and in a decrease in hepatic glycogen content.[248] One patient died in the postoperative period following portacaval transposition.[239] The others have had only limited improvement in their ability to maintain adequate blood sugar concentrations. Recent studies have demonstrated biochemical improvement and accelerated growth utilizing nocturnal nasogastric infusions of glucose or formula.[248a,248b]

Most severely affected children exhibit severe brain damage and growth retardation, and die early in life. A few patients have been followed into adult life,[218,249] but a question exists as to the exact nature of the types of glycogen storage diseases these patients have since hepatic enzyme studies were not carried out in all cases. Although it is frequently stated that the metabolic manifestations of this disorder improve with age, these observations are not well documented.

In our patient with fructose-1,6-diphosphatase deficiency, a diet containing 56 percent utilizable carbohydrate (glucose, maltose, and lactose), 12 percent protein, and 32 percent fat has been effective in controlling the chronic lactic acidosis and hypoglycemia. On this diet she has demonstrated normal growth and development for the past 7 yr.[234] However, during intercurrent infections associated with fever and vomiting, she continues to develop lactic acidosis, ketoacidosis, and plasma glucose concentrations of less than 3 mg/100 ml. Surprisingly, despite this profound hypoglycemia, the patient remains alert and without seizure activity—findings often observed in glucose-6-phosphatase deficiency. It must be presumed that other energy sources, such as ketone bodies, are being utilized for cerebral metabolism. These metabolic abnormalities are rapidly corrected with intravenous administration of glucose.

GLYCOGEN SYNTHETASE DEFICIENCY

Fasting hypoglycemia from birth has been reported in identical twins and their younger siblings, in whom liver biopsy studies in one twin demonstrated fatty metamorphosis, absence of glycogen, and a lack of glycogen synthetase activity.[250] Parr and associates[251] observed a 4-month-old infant with hypoglycemia in whom no glycogen was demonstrable in muscle, liver, kidney, and adrenal glands. The liver showed fatty infiltration, absent hepatic glycogen synthetase and phosphorylase, and markedly diminished glucose-6-phosphatase. Similar histologic findings were also observed in two siblings who had clinical hypoglycemia. Since all of these studies were carried out on postmortem tissue, the significance of these findings are open to question.

GALACTOSE-1-PHOSPHATE URIDYL TRANSFERASE DEFICIENCY (GALACTOSEMIA)

Infants with galactosemia are intolerant to products containing lactose and galactose, and present with hypoglycemia, diarrhea, and vomiting following meals and failure to thrive. The accumulation of galactose-1-phosphate in tissues reflects the inability to convert this substrate to glucose-1-phosphate (Fig. 141-6) and results in hepatosplenomegaly, jaundice, lenticular cataracts, mental retardation, and renal tubular abnormalities.[252] The occurrence of postprandial hypoglycemia in this disorder appears to be due to inhibition of phosphoglucomutase by galactose-1-phosphate, thereby resulting in acute inhibition of glycogenolysis.[253] Diagnosis is relatively easy and should be considered in all infants with failure to thrive together with any of the above physical manifestations or symptoms. Elimination of galactose from the diet early in life prevents further manifestations of the disease.

FRUCTOSE-1-PHOSPHATE ALDOLASE DEFICIENCY (HEREDITARY FRUCTOSE INTOLERANCE)

This disorder is dominated by symptoms of hypoglycemia and vomiting following ingestion of foods containing fructose. Fructosuria is present only after meals, and these patients frequently manifest hepatomegaly, jaundice, aminoaciduria, and failure to thrive. The hypoglycemia following fructose ingestion is a result of accumulation of fructose-1-phosphate which inhibits the phosphorylase system and gluconeogenesis at the level of fructose-1,6-diphosphate aldolase (Fig. 141-6).[254] Since most neonates are not exposed to fructose in the first weeks to month of life, this diagnosis can only be entertained in those special circumstances in which an infant is receiving sucrose-containing foods.

The diagnosis of galactosemia or hereditary fructose intolerance should be considered in infants presenting with hypoglycemia in the immediate postprandial period together with hepatomegaly and failure to thrive. In these disorders, nonglucose-reducing substances (i.e., galactose, fructose) will be present in the urine following meals. The definitive diagnosis of galactosemia is made by determining the galactose-1-phosphate uridyl transferase activity in red blood cells; a galactose infusion test is not required and is contraindicated. Hereditary fructose intolerance is diagnosed by the hypoglycemic and hypophosphatemic responses produced by the cautious intravenous infusion of fructose (0.25 g/kg body wt); the intravenous route of fructose administration obviates the distressful symptoms of nausea or vomiting associated with oral ingestion.[254]

REFERENCES

1. Longo, L. D.: Disorders of placental transfer. In Assali NS (ed): Pathophysiology of Gestation, vol II. New York, Academic, 1972, p 1.
2. Dancis, J., Olsen, G., Folkart, G.: Transfer of histidine and xylose across the placenta and into the red blood cell and amniotic fluids. *Am J Physiol 194:* 44, 1958.
3. Stephens, R. J.: The development and fine structure of the allantoic placental barrier in the bat *Tadarida brasiliensis cynocephala. J Ultrastruct Res 28:* 371, 1969.
4. Longo, L. D., Power, G. G., Forster, R. E.: Respiratory function of the placenta as determined with carbon monoxide in sheep and dogs. *J Clin Invest 46:* 812, 1967.
5. Meschia, G., Battaglia, F. G., Bruns, P. D.: Theoretical and experimental study of transplacental diffusion. *J Appl Physiol 22:* 1171, 1967.
6. Flexner, L. B., Cowie, D. B., Hellman, L. M. *et al:* The permeability of the human placenta to sodium in normal and abnormal pregnancies and the supply of sodium to the human fetus as determined with radioactive sodium. *Am J Obstet Gynecol 55:* 469, 1948.
7. Flexner, L. B., Roberts, R. B.: The measurement of placental permeability with radioactive sodium. *Am J Physiol 128:* 154, 1939.
8. Vosburgh, G. J., Flexner, L. B., Cowie, D. B., *et al:* The rate of renewal in woman of the water and sodium of the amniotic fluid as determined by tracer techniques. *Am J Obstet Gynecol 56:* 1156, 1948.
9. Comar, C. L.: Radiocalcium studies in pregnancy. *Ann NY Acad Sci 64:* 281, 1956.
10. Bothwell, T. H., Pribilla, W. F., Mebust, W., *et al:* Iron metabolism in the pregnant rabbit; iron transport across the placenta. *Am J Physiol 192:* 615, 1958.
11. Logothetopoulos, J., Scott, R. F.: Concentration of iodine-131 across the placenta of the guinea pig and the rabbit. *Nature (London) 175:* 775, 1955.
12. Dancis, J., Money, W. L., Springer, D.: Transport of amino acids by placenta. *Am J Obstet Gynecol 101:* 820, 1968.
13. Ghadimi H., Pecora, P.: Free amino acids of cord plasma as compared with maternal plasma during pregnancy. *Pediatrics 33:* 500, 1964.
14. Hill, P. M. M., Young, M.: Net placental transfer of free amino acids against varying concentrations. *J Physiol 235:* 409, 1973.
15. Christensen, H. N., Streicher, J. A.: Association between rapid growth and elevated cell concentration of amino acids: I. In fetal tissue. *J Biol Chem 175:* 95, 1948.
16. Dancis, J., Shafran, M.: The origin of plasma proteins in the guinea pig fetus. *J Clin Invest 37:* 1093, 1958.
17. Adam, P. A. J., Teramo, K., Raiha, N., *et al:* Human fetal insulin metabolism early in gestation response to acute elevation of the fetal glucose concentration and placental transfer of human insulin I-131. *Diabetes 18:* 409, 1969.
18. Adam, P. A. J., King, K. C., Schwartz, R.: Human placental barrier to ^{125}I-glucagon early in gestation. *J Clin Endocrinol Metab 34:* 772, 1972.
19. Robertson, A. F., Sprecher, H.: A review of human placental lipid metabolism and transport. *Acta Paediatr Scand 57, Suppl 183:* 1, 1968.
20. Kayden, H. J., Dancis, J., Money, W. L.: Transfer of lipids across the guinea pig placenta. *Am J Obstet Gynecol 104:* 564, 1969.
21. Portman, O. W., Behrman, R. E., Soltys, P.: Transfer of free fatty acids across the primate placenta. *Am J Physiol 216:* 143, 1969.
22. Gelfand, M. M., Strean, G. J., Pavilanis, V., *et al:* Studies in placental permeability. Transmission of poliomyelitis antibodies, lipoproteins, and cholesterol in single and twin newborn infants. *Am J Obstet Gynecol 79:* 117, 1960.
23. Goldwater, W. H., Stetten, D. W., Jr: Studies in fetal metabolism. *J Biol Chem 169:* 723, 1947.
24. Widdas, W. F.: Inability of diffusion to account for placental glucose transfer in the sheep and consideration of the kinetics of a possible carrier transfer. *J Physiol (London) 118:* 23, 1952.
25. Widdas, W. F.: Transport mechanisms in the foetus. *Br Med Bull 17:* 107, 1961.
26. Howard, J. M., Krantz, K. E.: Transfer and use of glucose in the human placenta during in vitro perfusion and the associated effects of oxytocin and papaverine. *Am J Obstet Gynecol 98:* 445, 1967.
27. Longo, L. D., Kleinzeller, A.: Transport of monosaccharides by placental cells. *Fed Proc, Fed Am Soc Exp Biol 29:* 802, 1970.
28. Schwartz, R.: Metabolic fuels in the foetus. *Proc R Soc Med 61:* 1231, 1968.
29. Villee, C. A.: Regulation of blood glucose in the human fetus. *J Appl Physiol 5:* 437, 1953.
30. Hagerman, D. D., Villee, C. A.: The transport of fructose by human placenta. *J Clin Invest 31:* 911, 1953.
31. Battaglia, F. C., Meschia, G.: Foetal metabolism and substrate utilization. In Conline, R. K. S., Cross, K. W., Dawes, J. S., Nathanielsz, P. W. (eds): Foetal and Neonatal Physiology. Sir Joseph Bancroft Centenary Symposium. Cambridge, Cambridge University Press, 1973.
32. Burd, L. I., Jones, M. D., Jr, Simmons, M. A., *et al:* The role of lactate as a major metabolic substrate in the ovine fetus. *Pediatr Res 9:* 348, 1975.
33. Cahill, G. F., Jr: The physiology of insulin in man. The Banting Memorial Lecture, 1971. *Diabetes 20:* 785, 1971.
34. Fain, J. N., Kovacev, V. P., Scow, R. O.: Antilipolytic effect of insulin in isolated fat cells of the rat. *Endocrinology 78:* 773, 1966.
35. Exton, J. H., Jefferson, L. S., Jr, Butcher, R. W., *et al:* Gluconeogenesis in the perfused liver: The effects of fasting, alloxan diabetes, glucagon, epinephrine, adenosine-3′,5′-monophosphate and insulin. *Am J Med 40:* 709, 1966.
36. Fajans, S. S., Floyd, J. C., Jr, Knopf, R. F., *et al:* Effect of amino acids and proteins on insulin secretion in man. *Recent Prog Horm Res 23:* 617, 1967.
37. Pagliara, A. S., Karl, I. E., DeVivo, P. C., *et al:* Hypoalaninemia: A concomitant of ketotic hypoglycemia. *J Clin Invest 51:* 1440, 1972.
38. Cahill, G. F., Jr, Herrera, M. G., Morgan, A. P., *et al:* Hormone fuel interrelationships during fasting. *J Clin Invest 45:* 1751, 1966.
39. Bondy, P. K.: Disorders of carbohydrate metabolism. In Bondy, P. K. (ed): Duncan's Diseases of Metabolism. Philadelphia, Saunders, 1969, p 199.
40. Weber, G., Singhal, R. L., Suvastava, S. K.: Action of glucocorticoid as inducer and insulin as suppressor of biosynthesis of hepatic gluconeogenic enzymes. *Adv Enzyme Regul 3:* 369, 1965.
41. Jost, A., Jacquot, R.: Recherches sur les facteurs endocriniens de la charge en glycogéne du foie factus chez le lapin. *Ann Endocrinol (Paris) 16:* 849, 1955.
42. Kaplan, S. A.: Hypopituitarism. In Gardner, L. I. (ed): Endocrine and Genetic Diseases of Childhood. Philadelphia, Saunders, 1969, p 98.
43. Liu, H. M., Potter, E. L.: Development of the human pancreas. *Arch Pathol 74:* 439, 1962.
44. Emery, J. L., Bary, H. P. R.: Involutionary changes in the islets of Langerhans. *Biol Neonate 6:* 15, 1964.
45. Robb, R.: The development of islets of Langerhans in man. *Arch Dis Child 36:* 229, 1961.
46. Hellman, B: The development of the mammalian endocrine pancreas. *Biol Neonate 9:* 263, 1966.
47. Milner, R. D. G.: The development of insulin secretion in man. In Jonxis, J. H. P., Visser, H. K. A., Troestra, J. A. (eds): Metabolic Processes in the Foetus and Newborn Infant. Baltimore, Williams & Wilkins, 1971, p 193.
48. Steinke, J., Driscoll, S.: The extractable insulin content of pancreas from fetuses and infants of diabetic and control mothers. *Diabetes 14:* 573, 1965.
49. Assan, R., Boillot, J.: Pancreatic glucagon and glucagon-like material in tissues and plasmas from human foetuses 6–26 weeks old. In Jonxis, J. H. P., Visser, H. K. A., Troestra, J. A. (eds): Metabolic Processes in Foetus and Newborn Infant. Baltimore, Williams & Wilkins, 1971, p 210.

50. Girard, J. R., Kervran, A., Soufflet, E., *et al:* Factors effecting secretion of insulin and glucagon by the rat fetus. *Diabetes 23:* 310, 1973.
51. Alexander, D. P., Britton, H. G., Cohen, N. M.: Plasma concentrations of insulin, glucose, free fatty acids and the response to a glucose load before and after birth. *Biol Neonate 14:* 178, 1969.
52. Basset, J. M., Thorburn, G. D.: The regulation of insulin secretion by the ovine foetus in utero. *J Endocrinol 50:* 59, 1971.
53. Milner, R. D. G., Hales, C. N.: Effect of intravenous glucose on concentrations of insulin in maternal and umbilical cord plasma. *Br Med J 1:* 284, 1965.
54. Obenshain, S. S., Adam, P. A. S., King, K. C., *et al:* Human fetal insulin responses to sustained maternal hyperglycemia. *N Engl J Med 283:* 566, 1970.
55. Mintz, D. H., Chez, R. A., Horger, E. O.: Fetal insulin and growth hormone metabolism in the subhuman primate. *J Clin Invest 48:* 176, 1969.
56. Willes, R. F, Boda, J. M., Manns, J. G.: Insulin secretion by the ovine fetus in utero. *Endocrinology 84:* 520, 1969.
57. Lambert, A. E., Juno, A., Stauffacher, W., *et al:* Organ culture of fetal rat pancreas. I. Insulin release induced by caffeine and by sugars and some derivatives. *Biochim Biophys Acta 184:* 529, 1969.
58. Esponosa, M. M. A., Driscoll, S. G., Steinke, J.: Insulin release from isolated human fetal pancreas. *Science 168:* 1111, 1970.
59. Milner, R. D. G., Ashworth, M. A., Barson, A. J.: Insulin release from human foetal pancreas in response to glucose, leucine and arginine. *J Endocrinol 52:* 497, 1972.
60. Chez, R. A., Mintz, D. H., Hutchinson, D. L.: Effect of theophylline on glucagon and glucose mediated plasma insulin responses in subhuman primate fetus and neonate. *Metabolism 20:* 805, 1971.
61. Grasso, S., Messina, A., Saporito, N.: Effect of theophylline, glucagon and theophylline plus glucagon on insulin secretion in the premature infant. *Diabetes 19:* 837, 1970.
62. Reitano, G., Grasso, S., Distefano, G., *et al.* The serum insulin and growth hormone response to arginine and to arginine with glucose in the premature infant. *J Clin Endocrinol 33:* 924, 1971.
63. Grasso, S., Messina, A., Distefano, G., *et al:* Insulin secretion in the premature infant, response to glucose and amino acids. *Diabetes 22:* 349, 1973.
64. Tobin, J. D., Roux, J. F., Soeldner, J. S.: Human fetal insulin response after acute maternal glucose administration during labor. *Pediatrics 44:* 668, 1969.
65. Milner, R. D. G., Hales, C. N.: Effect of intravenous glucose on concentration of insulin in maternal and umbilical-cord plasma. *Br Med J 1:* 284, 1965.
66. Cornblath, M., Schwartz, R.: Disorders of Carbohydrate Metabolism in Infancy. Philadelphia, Saunders, 1966.
67. Joassin, G., Parker, M. L., Pildes, R. S., *et al.:* Infants of diabetic mothers. *Diabetes 16:* 306, 1967.
68. Haymond, M. W., Karl I. E., Pagliara, A. S.: Increased gluconeogenic substrates in the small-for-gestational infant. *N Engl J Med 291:* 322, 1974.
69. Adam, P. A. J.: Control of glucose metabolism in the human fetus and newborn infant. *Adv Metab Disord 5:* 183, 1971.
70. Falorni, A., Fracassini, F., Masi-Benedetti, F., *et al:* Glucose metabolism and insulin secretion in the newborn infant. *Diabetes 23:* 1972, 1974.
71. Jarrousse, C., Rosselin, G.: Interaction of amino acids and cyclic AMP on the release of insulin and glucagon by newborn rat pancreas. *Endocrinology 96:* 168, 1975.
72. Fiser, R. H., Jr, Erenberg, A., Sperling, M. A., *et al:* Insulin-glucagon substrate interrelationships in the fetal sheep. *Pediatr Res 8:* 951, 1974.
73. Fiser, R. H., Williams, P. R., Sperling, M. A., *et al:* Glucagon secretory maturation in the neonatal sheep: Relationship to cyclic AMP. *Pediatr Res 9:* 350, 1975.
74. Sperling, M. A., Delamater, P. V., Phelps, D., *et al:* Spontaneous and amino acid stimulated glucagon secretion in the immediate postnatal period: Relation to glucose and insulin. *J Clin Invest 53:* 1159, 1974.
75. Lowry, M. F., Adams, P. A. J.: Lack of gluconeogenesis from alanine at birth. *Pediatr Res 9:* 353, 1975.
76. Williams, P. R., Fiser, R. H. Jr., Sperling, M. A., *et al:* Effects of oral alanine feeding on blood glucose, plasma glucagon and insulin concentrations in small for gestational age infants. *N Engl J Med 292:* 612, 1975.
77. Harris, R. J.: Plasma nonesterified fatty acids and blood glucose levels in healthy and hypoxemic newborn infants. *J Pediatr 84:* 578, 1974.
78. Alexander, G., Bell, A. W., Hales, J. R. S.: The effect of cold exposure on the plasma levels of glucose, lactate, free fatty acids and glycerol on the blood gases and acid-base status in young lambs. *Biol Neonate 20:* 9, 1972.
79. Greengard, O.: The developmental formation of enzymes in rat liver. In Litwack, G. (ed): Biochemical Actions of Hormones. London, Academic, 1970, p 53.
80. Cahill, G. F., Jr: Starvation in man. *New Engl J Med 282:* 668, 1970.
81. Nuttall, F. Q.: Mechanisms of insulin action on glycogen synthesis. In Greep, R. O., Astwood, B. (eds): Handbook of Physiology, vol 1, sec 7. Baltimore, American Physiological Society, Waverly Press, 1972, p 395.
82. Ballard, F. J., Oliver, I. T.: Glycogen metabolism in embryonic chick and neonatal rat liver. *Biochim Biophys Acta 71:* 578, 1963.
83. Shelley, H. J., Neligan, G. A.: Neonatal hypoglycemia. *Br Med Bull 22:* 34, 1966.
84. Shelley, H. J.: Carbohydrate reserves in the newborn infant. *Br Med J 1:* 273, 1964.
85. Barbehenn, E. K., Wales, R. G., Lowry, O. H.: The explanation for the blockade of glycolysis in early mouse embryos. *Proc Natl Acad Sci USA 71:* 1056, 1974.
86. Burch, H. B., Kulman, M., Skerjance, J., *et al:* Changes in patterns of enzymes of carbohydrate metabolism in the developing rat kidney. *Pediatrics 47:* 119, 1971.
87. Lea, M. A., Walker, D. G.: Glycogenesis in the guinea pig liver during development. *Dev Biol 15:* 51, 1967.
88. Jost, A., Hatley, J.: Influence de la decapitation sur la teneur en glycogene du foie du foetus de lapin. *CR Soc Biol 143:* 146, 1949.
89. Jacquot R., Kretchmer, N.: Effect of fetal decapitation on enzymes of glycogen metabolism. *J Biol Chem 239:* 1301, 1964.
90. Jacquot, R.: Recherches sur le controle endocrinien de l'accumulation de glycogene dans le foie chez 6 foetus de rat. *J Physiol (Paris) 51:* 655, 1959.
91. Margolis, F. L., Roffi, J., Jost, A.: Norepinephrine methylation in fetal rat adrenals. *Science 154:* 275, 1966.
92. Parker, L. N., Nobel, E. P.: Prenatal glucocorticoid administration and the development of the epinephrine-forming enzyme. *Proc Soc Exp Biol Med 126:* 734, 1967.
93. Snell, K., Walker, D. G.: Glucose metabolism in the newborn rat. Hormonal effects in vivo. *Biochem J 134:* 889, 1973.
94. Blazquez, E., Rubalcara, R., Montesano, R., *et al:* "Glucagon resistance" in fetal and neonatal rats. *Clin Res 23:* 315A, 1975.
95. Girard, J. R., Cuendet, G. S., Marliss, E. B., *et al:* Fuels, hormones, and liver metabolism at term and during the early postnatal period in the rat. *J Clin Invest 52:* 3190, 1973.
96. Exton, J. H., Mallette, L. E., Jefferson, L. S., *et al:* The hormonal control of hepatic gluconeogenesis. *Recent Prog Horm Res 26:* 411, 1970.
97. Ross, B. D., Hems, R., Krebs, H. A.: The rate of gluconeogenesis from various precursors in the perfused rat liver. *Biochem J 102:* 942, 1967.
98. Marliss, E. B., Aoki, R. R., Pozefsky, J., *et al:* Muscle and splanchnic glutamine and glutamate metabolism in post absorptive and starved man. *J Clin Invest 50:* 814, 1971.
99. Felig, P., Wahren, J., Karl, I. E., *et al:* Glutamine and glutamate metabolism in normal and diabetic subjects. *Diabetes 22:* 573, 1973.
100. Felig, P., Pozefsky, T., Marliss, E., *et al:* Alanine: Key role in gluconeogenesis. *Science 167:* 1003, 1970.
101. Garber, H. J., Karl, I. E., Kipnis, D. M.: Alanine and glutamine synthesis and release from skeletal muscle. II. The precursor role of amino acids in alanine and glutamine synthesis. *J Biol Chem 251:* 836, 1976.
102. Christensen, N. J.: Hypoadrenalinemia during insulin hypoglycemia in children with ketotic hypoglycemia. *J Clin Endocrinol Metab 38:* 107, 1974.
103. Garber, A. L., Karl, I. E., Kipnis, D. M.: Adrenergic control of alanine and glutamine formation in skeletal muscle. *Clin Res 22:* 468a, 1974.
104. Cahill, G. F. Jr, Aoki, T. T., Marliss, E. B: Insulin and muscle protein. In Steiner, D. F., Freinkel, N.(eds): Handbook of Physiology, sec 7, Endocrinology, Endocrine Pancreas, vol 1. Washington, Waverly Press, 1972.
105. Chaussain, J. L.: Glycemic responses to 24 hour fast in normal children and children with ketotic hypoglycemia. *J Pediatr 82:* 438, 1973.

106. Sherwin, R., Hendler, R., Felig, P.: Effect of ketone infusion on amino acid and nitrogen metabolism in man. *J Clin Invest 55:* 1382, 1975.
107. Ruderman, N. B., Houghton, C. R. S., Hems, R.: Evaluation of the isolated perfused rat hind quarter for the study of muscle metabolism. *Biochem J 124:* 639, 1971.
108. Helmrath, T. A., Bieber, L.: Development of gluconeogenesis in neonatal pig liver. *Am J Physiol 227:* 1306, 1974.
109. Coleman, J. E.: Metabolic interrelationships between carbohydrates, lipids, and protein. In Bondy, P. K. (ed): Diseases of Metabolism, ed 6. Philadelphia, Saunders, 1969, p 89.
110. Felig, P., Owen, O. E., Wahren, J., *et al:* Amino acid metabolism during prolonged starvation. *J Clin Invest 48:* 584, 1969.
111. Owen, O. E., Felig, P., Morgan, A. P., *et al:* Liver and kidney metabolism during prolonged starvation. *J Clin Invest 48:* 574, 1969.
112. Adibi, S. A.: Influence of dietary deprivations on plasma concentrations of free amino acids in man. *J Appl Physiol 25:* 53, 1968.
113. Haymond, M. W., Karl, I. E., Pagliara, A. S.: Ketotic hypoglycemia: An amino acid substrate limited disorder. *J Clin Endocrinol Metab 38:* 521, 1974.
114. Mersmann, H. J.: Glycolytic and gluconeogenic enzyme levels in pre- and postnatal pigs. *Am J Physiol 220:* 1297, 1971.
115. Yeung, D., Stanley, R. S., Oliver, I. T.: Development of gluconeogenesis in neonatal rat liver: Effect of triamcinolone. *Biochem J 105:* 1219, 1967.
116. Ballard, F. J., Hanson, R. W.: Phosphoenol pyruvate carboxykinase and pyruvate carboxylase in developing rat liver. *Biochem J 104:* 866, 1967.
117. Vernon, R. G., Walker, D. G.: Adaptive behavior of some enzymes involved in glucose utilization and formation in the rat liver during the weaning period: Changes in activity of some enzymes involved in glucose utilization and formation in developing rat liver. *Biochem J 106:* 321, 1968.
118. Ballard, F. J.: Carbohydrates. In Stave, V. (ed): Physiology of the Perinatal Period, vol. 1. New York, Appleton-Century-Crofts, 1970, p 417.
119. Philippidis, H., Ballard, F. J.: The development of gluconeogenesis in rat liver. Experiments in vivo. *Biochem J 113:* 651, 1969.
120. Yeung, D., Oliver, I. T.: Gluconeogenesis from amino acids in neonatal rat liver. *Biochem J 103:* 744, 1967.
121. Ballard, F. J.: The development of gluconeogenesis in rat liver: Controlling factors in the newborn. *Biochem J 124:* 265, 1971.
122. Yeung, D., Oliver, I. T.: Factors affecting the premature induction of phosphopyruvate carboxylase in neonatal rat liver. *Biochem J 108:* 325, 1968.
123. Yeung, D., Oliver, I. T.: Induction of phosphopyruvate carboxylase in neonatal rat liver by adenosine-3′,5′-cyclic monophosphate. *Biochemistry 7:* 3231, 1968.
124. Wicks, W. D.: Regulation of hepatic enzyme synthesis by cyclic AMP. *Ann NY Acad Sci 185:* 152, 1971.
125. Kirby, L., Hahn, P.: Enzyme induction in human fetal liver. *Pediatr Res 7:* 75, 1973.
126. Shimazu, T., Amakawa, A: Regulation of glycogen metabolism in liver by the autonomic nervous system. II. Neural control of glycogenolytic enzymes. *Biochim Biophys Acta 165:* 335, 1968.
127. Philippidis, H., Ballard, R. J.: The development of gluconeogenesis in rat liver: Effects of glucagon and ether. *Biochem J 120:* 385, 1970.
128. Windle, W. F.: Physiology of the Fetus. Springfield, Thomas, 1971, p 34.
129. Dawes, G. S.: Foetal and Neonatal Physiology. Chicago, Year Book Medical Publishers, 1968, p 247.
130. Schaffer, A. J., Avery, M. E.: Diseases of the Newborn, ed 3. Philadelphia, Saunders, 1971, p 21.
131. Melichar, V., Novak, M., Zoula, J., *et al:* Energy sources in the newborn. *Biol Neonate 9:* 298, 1965/66.
132. Pribylova, H., Rylander, E: Free fatty acids, glycerol, glucose and β-hydroxybutyrate in plasma of infants protected from cooling and exposured to cold at various times after birth. *Biol Neonate 20:* 425, 1972.
133. Lockwood, E. A., Bailey, E.: Some aspects of fatty acid oxidation and ketone body formation and utilization during development of the rat. *Enzyme 15:* 239, 1973.
134. Drahota, Z., Hahn, P., Kleinzeller, A., *et al:* Acetoacetate formation by liver slices from adult and infant rats. *Biochem J 93:* 61, 1964.
135. Hahn, P., Vavrouskova, E., Jirasek, J., *et al:* Acetoacetate formation by livers from human fetuses aged 8–17 weeks. *Biol Neonate 7:* 348, 1964.
136. Levitsky, L. L., Paton, J. B., Fisher, D. E.: Cerebral utilization of alternative substrates to glucose: An explanation for asymptomatic neonatal hypoglycemia. *Pediatr Res 7:* 418, 1973.
137. Kraus, H., Schlenker, S., Schivedesky, D: Developmental changes of cerebral ketone body utilization in human infants. *Hoppe-Seyler's Z Physiol Chem 355:* 164, 1974.
138. Adams, P. A. J., Raiha, N., Rahiala, F., *et al:* Oxidation of glucose and D-B-OH butyrate by the early human fetal brain. *Acta Paediatr Scand 64:* 17, 1975.
139. Cornblath, M., Ganzon, A. F., Nicholopoulos, D., *et al:* Studies of carbohydrate metabolism in the newborn infant. III. Some factors influencing the capillary blood sugar and the response to glucagon during the first hours of life. *Pediatrics 27:* 378, 1961.
140. Cornblath, M., Wybregt, S. H., Baens, G. S.: Studies of carbohydrate metabolism in the newborn infant. VII. Tests of carbohydrate tolerance in premature infants. *Pediatrics 32:* 1007, 1963.
141. Schaffer, A. S.: Diseases of the Newborn. Philadelphia, Saunders, 1966, p 951.
142. Hallman, N.: Studies on the blood sugar of newborn children and the children of diabetic mothers. *Mod Probl Pediatr 4:* 535, 1959.
143. Cornblath, M., Odell, G. B., Levin, E. Y.: Symptomatic neonatal hypoglycemia associated with toxemia of pregnancy. *J Pediatr 55:* 545, 1959.
144. Creery, R. D. G., Parkinson, T. J.: Blood glucose changes in the newborn. *Arch Dis Child 28:* 134, 1953.
145. Pagliara, A. S., Karl, I. E., Haymond, M., *et al:* Hypoglycemia in infancy and childhood. (Reply) *J Pediatr 83:* 694, 1973.
146. Ward. O. C.: Blood sugar studies on premature babies. *Arch Dis Child 28:* 194, 1953.
147. Baens, S. G., Lundeen, E., Cornblath, M.: Studies of carbohydrate metabolism in the newborn infant. *Pediatrics 31:* 580, 1963.
148. Ditchburn, R. K., Wilkinson, R. H., Davies, P. A., *et al.* Plasma glucose levels in infants 2,500 g and less fed immediately after birth with breast milk. *Biol Neonate 11:* 29, 1967.
149. Lubchenco, L. O., Bard, H.: Incidence of hypoglycemia in newborn infants classified by birthweight and gestational age. *Pediatrics 47:* 831, 1971.
150. Drillien, C. M.: The small-for-date infant:etiology and prognosis. *Pediatr Clin North Am 17:* 9, 1970.
151. Gertz, J. C., Warner, R., Persson, B. E., *et al:* Intravenous glucose tolerance, plasma insulin free fatty acids and beta-hydroxybutyrate in underweight newborn infants. *Acta Paediatr Scand 58:* 481, 1969.
152. Pagliara, A. S., Karl, I. E., Haymond, M., *et al:* Hypoglycemia in infancy and childhood. Part II. *J Pediatr 82:* 558, 1973.
153. Marliss, E. B., Aoki, T. T., Toews, C. H., *et al.* Amino acid metabolism in lactic acidosis. *Am J Med 52:* 474, 1972.
154. Lindblad, B. S.: The venous plasma free amino acid levels during the first hours of life. I. After normal and short gestation and gestation complicated by hypertension, with special reference to the "small for dates" syndrome. *Acta Pediatr Scand 59:* 13, 1970.
155. Lindblad, B. S., Rahimtoola, R. J., Kahn, N.: The venous plasma free amino acid levels during the first hours of life. II. In a lower socio-economic group of a refugee area in Karachi, West Pakistan, with special reference to the "small for dates" syndrome. *Acta Pediatr Scand 59:* 21, 1970.
156. Mastyan, J., Schultz, K., Horvath, M.: Comparative glycemic responses to alanine in normal term and small for gestational age infants. *J Pediatr 85:* 276, 1974.
157. Ramsey, W. R.: Glucosuria of the newborn treated with insulin. *Trans Am Pediatr Soc 38:* 100, 1926.
158. Gentz, J. C. H., Cornblath, M.: Transient diabetes of the newborn. *Adv Pediatr 16:* 345, 1969.
159. Devine, J.: A case of diabetes mellitus in a young infant, *Arch Dis Child 13:* 189, 1938.
160. Lewis, E., Eisenberg, H.: Diabetes mellitus neonatorium. *Am J Dis Child 49:* 408, 1955.
161. Hickish, G.: Neonatal diabetes. *Br Med J 1:* 95, 1956.
162. Tidd, J. T., Stanage, W. F.: Congenital diabetes mellitus. *South Dakota J Med 18:* 15, 1965.
163. Osborne, G. R.: Congenital diabetes. *Arch Dis Child 40:* 332, 1965.
164. Gerrard, J. W., Chin, W.: The syndrome of transient diabetes. *J Pediatr 61:* 89, 1962.
165. Ferguson, A. W., Mulner, R. D. G.: Transient neonatal diabetes mellitus in sibs. *Arch Dis Child 45:* 80, 1970.
166. Aziz, E. M., Lipsitz, P. J.: A case of transient hypoglycemia and hyperglycemia in a full-term neonate. *Clin Pediatr 12:* 363, 1973.
167. Dacon-Voutetakis, C., Anagnostakis, D., Xanthon, M.: Macroglos-

sia transient neonatal diabetes mellitus and intrauterine growth failure: A new distinct entity? *Pediatrics 55:* 127, 1975.
168. Coffey, J. D., Wormack, N. C.: Transient neonatal diabetes in half sisters. *Am J Dis Child 45:* 480, 1967.
169. Hager, H., Herbst, R.: Das transitorische diabetes mellitus syndrom des neuge borenen ein Krankbeutsbild sue generes. *Z Kinderheilk 95:* 324, 1966.
170. Pagliara, A. S.: Unpublished observations.
171. Pagliara, A. S., Karl, I. E., Kipnis, D. M.: Transient neonatal diabetes. Delayed maturation of the pancreatic beta cell. *J Pediatr 82:* 97, 1973.
172. Ensinck, J. W., Stole, R. W., Gale, C. C., *et al:* Effect of aminophylline on the secretion of insulin, glucagon, luteinizing hormone and growth hormone in humans. *J Clin Endocrinol 31:* 153, 1970.
173. White, P., Kosby, P., Duckers, J.: The management of pregnancy complicating diabetes and of children of diabetic mothers. *Med Clin North Am 37:* 1481, 1953.
174. Dekaban, A., Baird, R.: The outcome of pregnancy in diabetic women. 1. Fetal wastage, mortality and morbidity in the offspring of diabetic and normal control mothers. *J Pediatr 55:* 563, 1959.
175. Pildes, R. S.: Infants of diabetic mothers. *N Engl J Med 289:* 902, 1973.
176. Pedersen, J.: The Pregnant Diabetic and Her Newborn: Problems and Management. Baltimore, Williams & Wilkins, 1967.
177. Pedersen, J., Bojsen-Moller, B., Poulsen, H.: Blood sugar in newborn infants of diabetic mothers. *Acta Endocrinol (Copenhagen) 15:* 33, 1954.
178. Williams, P. R., Sperling, M. A., Racasa, Z.: Blunting of spontaneous, and amino acid stimulated glucagon secretion in infants of diabetic mothers (IDM). *Diabetes 24 (Suppl 2):* 411, 1975.
179. Barnett, C. T., Oliver, T. K. Jr.: Hypoglycemia and hyperinsulinisms in infants with erythroblastosis fetalis. *N Engl J Med 278:* 1260, 1968.
180. Combs, J. T., Grunt, J. A., Brandt, I. K.: New syndrome of neonatal hypoglycemia: Associated with viceromegaly, macroglossia, microcephaly and abnormal umbilicus. *N Engl J Med 275:* 236, 1966.
181. Filippi, G., McKensick, V. A.: The Beckwith-Wiedemann syndrome (the exomphalos-macroglossia-gigan-tisus syndrome): Report of two cases and review of the literature. *Medicine 49:* 279, 1970.
182. Cohen, M. D., Gorlin, R. J., Femgold, M., *et al:* The Beckwith-Wiedemann syndrome: Seven new cases. *Am J Dis Child 122:* 515, 1971.
183. Yeung, C. Y.: Hypoglycemia in neonatal sepsis. *J Pediatr 77:* 812, 1970.
184. Yeung, C. Y., Lee, V. W. Y., Yeung, M. B.: Glucose disappearance rate in neonatal infection. *J Pediatr 82:* 486, 1973.
185. McFadzean, A. J. S., Yeung, R. T. T.: Hypoglycemia in suppurative pancholangitis due to Clonorchis sinensis. *Trans R Soc Trop Med Hyg 59:* 179, 1965.
186. LaNone, K. F., Mason, A. D. Jr., Daniels, J. P.: The impairment of gluconeogenesis by gram-negative infection. *Metabolism 17:* 606, 1968.
187. Bergman, R. K., Munoz, J.: Hypoglycemia and its relationship to histamine sensitization in mice. *Proc Soc Exp Biol Med 131:* 42, 1969.
188. Shands, J. W. Jr., Miller, V., Martin, H.: The hypoglycemic activity of endotoxin I. Occurrence in animals hyper-reactive to endotoxin. *Proc Soc Exp Biol Med 130:* 413, 1969.
189. Harris, R. J.: Plasma non-esterified fatty acid and blood glucose levels in healthy and hypoxemic newborn infants. *J Pediatr 84:* 578, 1974.
190. Greenberg, R. E., Christiansen, O.: The critically ill child: Hypoglycemia. *Pediatrics 46:* 915, 1970.
191. Schwartz, J. F., Zwiren, G. T.: Islet cell adenomatosis and adenoma in an infant. *J Pediatr 79:* 232, 1971.
192. Brown, R. E., Young, R. B.: A possible role for the exocrine pancreas in the pathogenesis of neonatal leucine-sensitive hypoglycemia. *Am J Dig Dis 15:* 65, 1970.
193. Yakovac, W. C., Baker, L., Hummeler, K.: Beta cell nesidioblastosis in idiopathic hypoglycemia of infancy. *J Pediatr 79:* 226, 1971.
194. DiGeorge, A. M., Auerbach, V. H.: Leucine induced hypoglycemia: A review and speculations. *Am J Med Sci 240:* 792, 1960.
195. Mereu, T. R., Kassoff, A., Goodman, D.: Diazoxide in the treatment of infantile hypoglycemia. *N Engl J Med 275:* 1455, 1966.
196. Drash, A., Wolff, F.: Drug therapy in leucine-sensitive hypoglycemia. *Metabolism 13:* 487, 1964.
197. Tabachnik, I. I. A., Gulvenkian, A., Seidman, F.: The effect of a benzothiadiazine. *Diabetes 13:* 408, 1964.
198. Rennert, O. M., Mukhopadhyay, D.: Diazoxide in Von Gierke's disease. *Arch Dis Child 43:* 358, 1968.
199. Spergel, G., Bleicher, S. J.: Effects of diazoxide administration on plasma glucose, insulin and lipids in Von Gierke's disease. *Diabetes 15:* 406, 1966.
200. Buist, N. R. M., Campbell, J. R., Castro, A., *et al:* Congenital islet cell adenoma causing hypoglycemia in a newborn. *Pediatrics 47:* 605, 1971.
201. Salinas, E. D., Mangurten, H. H., Robert, S. S., *et al:* Functioning islet cell adenoma in the newborn. *Pediatrics 41:* 646, 1968.
202. Hamilton, J. P., Baker, L., Kaye, R., *et al:* Subtotal pancreatectomy in the management of severe persistent idiopathic hypoglycemia in children. *Pediatrics 39:* 49, 1967.
202a. Thomas, C. G., Underwood, L. E., Carney, C. N., *et al:* Neonatal and infantile hypoglycemia due to insulin excess: New aspects of diagnosis and surgical management. *Ann Surg 185:* 505, 1977.
203. McQuarrie, I.: Idiopathic spontaneously occuring hypoglycemia in infants: Clinical significance of problem and treatment. *Am J Dis Child 87:* 399, 1954.
204. Cahill, G. F. Jr.: Action of adrenal cortical steroids on carbohydrate metabolism. The human adrenal cortex. In Christy, N. P. (ed). New York, Harper & Row, 1971, p 205.
205. Martin, M. M., Martin, A. L. A.: Idiopathic hypoglycemia—A defect in hypothalamic ACTH-releasing factor secretion. *Pediatr Res 5:* 396, 1971.
206. Brasel, J. A., Wright, J. C., Wilkins, L., *et al:* An evaluation of 75 patients with hypopituitarism in childhood. *Am J Med 38:* 484, 1965.
207. Goodman, H. G., Grumbach, M. M., Kaplan, S. L.: Growth and growth hormone. II. A comparison of isolated growth hormone deficiency and multiple pituitary-hormone deficiencies in 35 patients with idiopathic dwarfism. *N Engl J Med 278:* 57, 1968.
208. Wilber, J. F., Odell, W. D.: Hypoglycemia and dwarfism associated with isolated deficiency of growth hormone. *Metabolism 14:* 590, 1965.
209. Haymond, M. W., Karl, I. E., Weldon, V. V., *et al:* The role of growth hormone and cortisone on glucose and gluconeogenic substrate regulation in fasted hypopituitary children. *J Clin Endocrinol 42:* 846, 1976.
210. Drash, A., Field, J.: The glycogen storage diseases, DM, October 1971.
211. Howell, R. R.: The glycogen storage diseases. In Stanbury, J. B., Wyngaarden, J. G., Fredrickson, D. A. (eds): The Metabolic Basis of Inherited Disease. New York, McGraw-Hill, 1972, p 149.
212. Snapper, I., van Creveld, S.: Un cas d'hypoglycemic acetonie chez un enfant. *Bull Soc Med Hop Paris 52:* 1315, 1928.
213. Von Gierke, E.: Hepato-nephromegalia glykogenica (Glykogenspeicherkrankheitden leber nieren). *Beitr Pathol Anat 82:* 497, 1929.
214. Cori, G. T., Cori, C. F.: Glucose-6-phosphatase in the liver in glycogen storage disease. *J Biol Chem 199:* 661, 1952.
215. Howell, R. R., Ashton, D. M., Wyngaarden, J. B.: Glucose-6-phosphatase deficiency glycogen storage disease. Studies on the interrelationships of carbohydrate, lipid and purine abnormalities. *Pediatrics 29:* 553, 1962.
216. Jeandet, J., Lestradet, H.: L'hyperlactacidémie, cause probable de l'hyperuricémie dans la glycogénose hépatique, *Rev Fr Etud Clin Biol 6:* 71, 1961.
217. Fine, R. N., Strauss, J., Donnell, G. N.: Hyperuricemia in glycogen storage disease type I. *Am J Dis Child 112:* 572, 1966.
218. Alepa, F. P., Howell, R. R., Klinenberg, J., *et al:* Relationships between glycogen storage disease and tophaceous gout. *Am J Med 42:* 58, 1967.
219. Jakovic, S., Sorensen, L. B.: Studies of uric acid metabolism in glycogen storage disease associated with gouty arthritis. *Arthritis Rheum 10:* 129, 1967.
220. Kelley, W. N., Rosenbloom, F. M., Seegmiller, J. E., *et al:* Excessive production of uric acid in type I glycogen storage disease. *J Pediatr 72:* 448, 1968.
221. Howell, R. R.: The interrelationship of glycogen storage disease and gout. *Arthritis Rheum 8:* 780, 1965.
222. Howell, R. R.: Hyperuricemia in childhood. *Fed Proc 27:* 1078, 1968.
223. Ockerman, P. A.: In vitro studies of adipose tissue metabolism of glucose, glycerol and free fatty acids in glycogen storage disease type I. *Clin Chem Acta 12:* 383, 1965.

224. Lampert, F., Mayer, H., Tocci, P. M., *et al:* Fanconi syndrome in glycogen storage disease. In Nyhan, W. (ed): Amino Acid Metabolism and Genetic Variation. New York, McGraw-Hill, 1967, p 353.
225. Sidbury, J. B. Jr., Heick, J. M. C.: Glycogen storage disease: A review with emphasis on gastrointestinal manifestations. *South Med J 61:* 915, 1968.
226. Lowe, C. V., Ambrus, J. L., Ambrus, C. M., *et al:* Bleeding diathesis in children with liver glycogen disease and in their parents. *J Clin Invest 29:* 1007, 1960.
227. Spencer-Peet J., Norman, M. E., Lake, B. D., *et al:* Hepatic glycogen storage disease, clinical and laboratory findings in 23 cases. *Q J Med 40:* 95, 1971.
228. Sokal, J. E., Lowe, C. V., Sarcione, E. J., *et al:* Studies of glycogen metabolism in liver glycogen disease (Von Gierke's disease): Six cases with similar metabolic abnormalities and responses to glucagon. *J Clin Invest 40:* 364, 1961.
229. Briggs, J. N., Haworth, J. C.: Liver glycogen disease. *Am J Med 36:* 443, 1964.
230. Francois, R., Hermier, M., Ruitton-Ugliengo: Un cas de glycogénose hépatique sans déficit enzymatique reconnu. Essai de tratement par le glucagon-retard associé à un régime riche en hydrates de carbone. *Pediatrie 20:* 37, 1965.
231. Senior, B., Loridan, L.: Functional differentiation of glycogenoses of the liver with respect to the use of glycerol. *N Engl J Med 279:* 965, 1968.
232. Baker, L., Winegrad, A. I.: Fasting hypoglycemia and metabolic acidosis associated with deficiency of hepatic fructose-1,6-diphosphatase activity. *Lancet 2:* 13, 1970.
233. Pagliara, A. S., Karl, I. E., Keating, J., *et al:* Hepatic fructose-1,6-diphosphatase deficiency: A cause of lactic acidosis and hypoglycemia in infancy. *Clin Res 19:* 481, 1971.
234. Pagliara, A. S., Karl, I. E., Keating, J., *et al:* Hepatic fructose-1,6-diphosphatase deficiency: A cause of lactic acidosis and hypoglycemia in infancy. *J Clin Invest 51:* 2115, 1972.
235. Baerlocher, K., Gitzelman, R., Nussli, R., *et al:* Infantile lactic acidosis due to hereditary fructose-1,6-diphosphatase deficiency. *Helv Paediatr Acta 26:* 489, 1971.
236. Hülsmann, W. C., Fernandes, J.: A child with lactacidemia and fructose diphosphatase deficiency in the liver. *Pediatr Res 5:* 633, 1971.
237. Melancon, S. B., Khachadurian, A. K., Nadler, H. L., *et al:* Metabolic and biochemical studies in fructose-1,6-diphosphatase deficiency. *J Pediatr 82:* 650, 1973.
238. Hagnevik, K., Gordon, E., Lins, L., *et al:* Glycerol-induced haemolysis with hemoglobinuria and acute renal failure. *Lancet 1:* 75, 1974.
239. Folkman, J., Philippart, A., Tze, J., *et al.* Portacaval shunt for glycogen storage disease: Value of prolonged intravenous hyperalimentation before surgery. *Surgery 72:* 306, 1972.
240. Lowe, C. V., Sokal, J. E., Doray, B. H., *et al:* Biochemical studies and specific therapy in hepatic glycogen storage disease. *J Clin Invest 38:* 1021, 1959.
241. Koulischen, N., Pickering, D. E.: Glycogen storage disease: A study on the effect of sodium 1-thyroxine and glucagon. *Am J Dis Child 91:* 103, 1956.
242. Field, R. A.: Glycogen deposition disease. In Stanbury, J. B., Wyngaarden, J. G., Frederickson, D. A. (eds): The Metabolic Basis of Inherited Disease. New York, McGraw-Hill, 1960, p 141.
243. Eberlein, W. R., Illingworth, B. A., Sidbury, J. B.: Heterogeneous glycogen storage disease in siblings and favorable response to synthetic androgen administration. *Am J Med 33:* 20, 1962.
244. Riddell, A. G., Davies, R. P., Clark, A. D.: Portacaval transposition in the treatment of glycogen storage disease. *Lancet 2:* 1146, 1966.
245. Hermann, R. E., Mercer, R. D.: Portacaval shunt in the treatment of glycogen storage: Report of a case. *Surgery 65:* 499, 1969.
246. Boley, S. J., Cohen, M. I., Gliedman, M. L.: Surgical therapy of glycogen storage disease. *Pediatrics 46:* 929, 1970.
247. Starzl, T. E., Marchioro, T. L., Sexton, A., *et al:* The effect of portacaval transposition on carbohydrate metabolism: Experimental and clinical observations. *Surgery 57:* 687, 1965.
248. Sexton, A. W., Marchioro, T. L., Waddell, W. R., *et al:* Liver deglycogenation after portacaval transposition. *Surg Forum 15:* 120, 1964.
248a. Greene, H. L., Slonim, A. E., O'Neil, J. A., *et al:* Continuous intragastric infusion of glucose in management of defective gluconeogenesis with hypoglycemia. *Am J Dis Child 132:* 241, 1978.
248b. Ehrlich, R. M., Robinson, B. H., Freedman, M. H., *et al:* Nocturnal intragastric infusion of glucose in management of defective gluconeogenesis with hypoglycemia. *Am J Dis Child 132:* 241, 1978.
249. van Creveld, S.: Clinical course of glycogen storage disease. *Chem Weekbl 57:* 445, 1961.
250. Lewis, G. M., Spencer-Peet, J., Stewart, K. M.: Infantile hypoglycemia due to inherited deficiency of glycogen synthetase in liver. *Arch Dis Child 38:* 40, 1963.
251. Parr, J., Teree, T. M., Larner, J: Symptomatic hypoglycemia, visceral fatty metamorphosis and aglycogenosis in an infant lacking glycogen synthetase and phosphorylase. *Pediatrics 35:* 770, 1965.
252. Segal, S.: Disorders of galactose metabolism. In Stanbury, J. B., Wyngaarden, J. B., Fredrickson, D. S. (eds): The Metabolic Basis of Inherited Disease. St Louis, McGraw-Hill, 1972, p 174.
253. Illingworth, B.: Enzymatic defects as causes of hypoglycemia. *Diabetes 14:* 333, 1965.
254. Froesch, E. R.: Essential fructosuria and hereditary fructose intolerance. In Stanbury, J. B., Wyngaarden, J. B., Fredrickson, D. S. (eds): The Metabolic Basis of Inherited Disease. St Louis, McGraw-Hill, 1972, p 131.

142

Somatic Growth and Maturation

Robert L. Rosenfield

Growth is an inherent property of life. The integrated function of many of the hormonal, metabolic, and other growth factors discussed in preceding chapters is necessary for normal somatic growth. This chapter will first briefly review the biologic and biochemic bases of growth. Secondly, it will deal in detail with the overall result of these processes—normal growth. Finally, the diagnosis and management of disorders of growth will be discussed.

THE CELLULAR METABOLIC BASIS OF GROWTH

The overall biologic basis of growth is becoming apparent, but knowledge of the exact nature and sequence of the underlying biochemic events is very sketchy. Cellular developmental processes may well be regulated to a great extent by the same mechanisms that determine physiologic responses in the mature cell.[1] There is considerable evidence that indicates that cyclic nucleotides (cAMP and cGMP) may be important regulators of growth. In vitro studies indicate cyclic nucleotides to be determinants of cell motility, adhesiveness, mitotic activity, differentiation, and morphogenesis.[1–3] In addition, the pattern of adenylate cyclase activity has been correlated with biochemical and structural development of several tissues in the rat.[4] The situation is complex because the effects of cAMP are known to vary with cell type and available substrates. For example, cAMP inhibits proliferation of many cell lines, but stimulates that of others. Furthermore, cAMP action may vary with cell maturation and the phase of the mitotic cycle. In some systems, cGMP effects are similar to those of cAMP. In other systems, cGMP is antagonistic to cAMP, and the ratio of intracellular cAMP to cGMP changes in phase with mitotic events. As a consequence of this information, it has been hypothesized that growth is initiated by signals at the cell surface which modify cyclic nucleotide production (Fig. 142-1).[1,5,6] Inducers suspected of acting in this fashion are peptide hormones, neurotransmitters (e.g., β-adrenergic catecholamines, serotonin, acetylcholine), prostaglandins, collagen, and lectins. Cell contacts may also signal through this mechanism via genetically determined specific surface antigens.[7] Altered cAMP-dependent protein kinase activity then mediates the cAMP effect. The mechanism whereby this chain of events initiates growth is unknown. There is evidence that cAMP enhances DNA transcription, promotes RNA and nucleoprotein synthesis, and affects the activity of certain cytoplasmic enzymes. Some growth stimulants appear to be relatively tissue-specific, such as nerve growth factor. Whether these act via cyclic nucleotides or via other mechanisms is unknown.

Following an appropriate stimulus, cell proliferation begins with increased DNA synthesis, a process requiring DNA-polymerase, deoxyribonucleotide, magnesium, and DNA template.[8] Subsequently, RNA synthesis increases and results in production of the multitude of new proteins necessary to bring about cell growth. Whether intercellular transmission of mRNA induces cell growth is a matter under investigation. Polyamine biosynthesis is closely coupled to RNA synthesis and growth.[9] The entire growth process requires an intact cell which is nourished by an optimal milieu (with respect to pH, trace minerals, and substrates for structural and energy purposes) and which contains the necessary specific genetic information.

Growth occurs by mitosis (increase in cell number: hyperplasia) and increase in cell size (hypertrophy).[10] The relative contribution of each of these parameters to growth has been assessed by chemical[10] and quantitative morphologic[11] means. The former technique is based on the principle that the DNA content of the cell nucleus is constant. Consequently, the ratio of protein (or, in the case of muscle, creatinine excretion) to DNA content is an indicator of cell size. The ratio, cell number: cell size, typically decreases with normal development of organs.[12,13]

DETERMINANTS AND PATTERNS OF NORMAL SOMATIC GROWTH

INTRAUTERINE GROWTH

Following fertilization, cell proliferation proceeds by mitotic division.[14] Cellular enlargement begins when cleavage of the fertilized egg is complete. The ratio of increments in cell number to cell size is probably higher during the period of differentiation than at any other normal period of life.[12,13] Differentiation (diversification of structure and function) takes place mainly throughout the first trimester of pregnancy and is grossly complete by 16 weeks' gestation in man. Thereafter, the general pace of cellular and biochemic differentiation slows, but continues to occur at tissue-

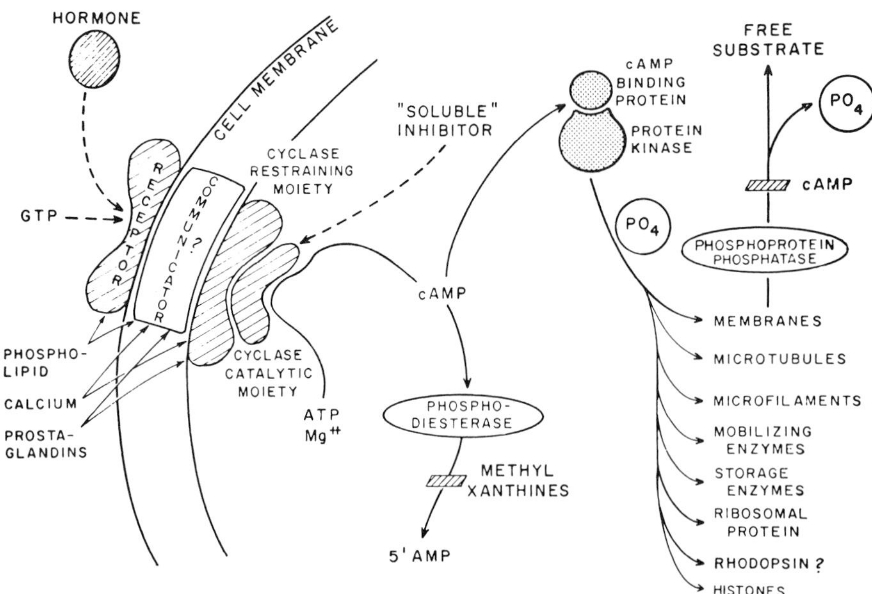

Fig. 142-1. A recently proposed model which depicts the role of cAMP in mediating the growth-promoting effects of hormones or other extracellular growth-inducing substances. Inhibition of phosphoprotein phosphatase by cAMP and of phosphodiesterase by methylxanthines is shown. Activation of phosphodiesterase by calcium is not depicted. [Reprinted from Bitensky, M. W., and Gorman, R. E.: Prog. Biophys. Mol. Biol. *26:* 411, 1973, with permission.]

and organ-specific rates. The biochemic basis for early skeletal differentiation has been characterized in considerable detail.[15] By 28 weeks' gestation the process of differentiation is often sufficiently complete to permit extrauterine life. By this time the pulmonary alveoli may be sufficiently mature to allow oxygen exchange. As with other organs and tissues, functional maturation lags behind anatomic maturation, and competence at sustaining ventilation improves with increasing production of pulmonary surfactant with age. Until potentially viable, the fetus is termed immature. Thereafter, the fetus born before 37 weeks' gestation is considered premature.

To a great extent normal fetal growth is dependent upon those factors necessary for normal postnatal growth (discussed in the following section—i.e., genetic endowment, an optimal biochemic milieu, and freedom from toxic factors). However, fetal requirements differ from those of the postnatal child in some significant respects. For example, the fetus is dependent upon placental, uterine, and maternal factors. On the other hand, growth in utero seems relatively free from some of the hormonal controls so important in extrauterine life.

Several major normal family and environmental variables have been identified which are related to birth weight independently of gestational age.[16–19]

1. Fetal sex. Male infants consistently average 150 g larger than females at term, the difference not being significant before about 38 weeks' gestation.
2. Sibling birth weight. The prediction of size at birth is about one-third more accurate when sibling weight is taken into account.
3. Maternal size. Both maternal height and weight correlate loosely with birth weight. There is dispute over which is the major factor. Each 10 kg by which a mother's mid-pregnancy weight differs from the average is associated with a 150-g increase in birth weight. Socioeconomic status does not seem to influence fetal growth independently of maternal size.
4. Maternal nutrition. A variety of observations strongly indicate that maternal undernutrition during the third trimester is a factor deleteriously affecting size at birth.[21,22] Most data suggest that a nutritious diet may provide an optimal upper input beyond which dietary supplementation plays relatively little role.
5. Maternal smoking. Birth weight is reduced in proportion to length of smoking history.[23,24] Nicotine and carbon monoxide have been incriminated.
6. Altitude. Infants born at an altitude of 10,000 ft have an average birth weight 270 g less than the U.S.A. average. This is probably related to the lower PO_2 of the mother.[25]

The following variables affect birth-weight, seemingly via utero-placental factors:

1. Parity. Later babies tend to be 100 g heavier than the first after 32 weeks' gestation, an effect that has been ascribed to more efficient uterine blood flow.
2. Multiparity. Growth is unaffected by the number of fetuses until about 30 weeks.[26,27] Subsequently, the rate of weight gain slows, such that twins, for example, each average about 700 g less than singletons at term. Compromise in fetal nutrition may underlie this discrepancy (see "Fetal Malnutrition"). Whether this is due to limitations in utero-placental blood flow or in placental mass is controversial.[26,28] Monozygous twins, especially monochorionic, are more discordant in size (and anomalies) than dizygotic.[29] This discrepancy may be related to unequal distribution of blood flow, placental arteriovenous anastomoses between monozygous twins being somewhat more frequent.
3. Placental weight. The extent to which the correlation between the size of the placenta and baby is due to nutritional factors and placental functional factors is unknown.[28,30]

Although thyroxine (T4) and growth hormone (GH) are essential for normal postnatal somatic growth, they may not play an important role in fetal somatic growth. This concept has arisen on the basis of several lines of clinical and experimental evidence. Neither hormone crosses the placenta well, so fetal levels are primarily of fetal origin.[31,32] The congenitally hypothyroid human is well known to be of normal size at birth.[33] The congenitally hyposomatotrophic human is often of normal size.[34,35] Fetal hypophysectomy by means of decapitation or thyroid ablation of the experimental animal do not necessarily prevent attainment of normal fetal size.[36] The conclusions reached on the basis of this information must be accepted with some qualification. Some T4 does cross the placenta, albeit inefficiently, and may contribute to growth. Furthermore, bone maturation of the congenitally hypothyroid fetus becomes impaired during the last trimester of pregnancy.[37] Body size and organ cellularity of anencephalics can be correlated with the amount of pituitary tissue, and organ size in experimental anencephaly does not necessarily reflect organ growth.[34] Furthermore, about 50 percent of congenitally GH-deficient or GH-resistant patients are short at birth.[38] It has been suggested that maternal GH may be trophic for placental growth and function, and thus influence growth of specific fetal tissues.[39]

Preliminary evidence indicates that somatomedin activity of umbilical cord serum rises during gestation in correlation with weight to become comparable to that of normal children.[40–41a] The possibility that somatomedin production might be independent of GH in the fetus must be considered. However, not only may fetal growth be independent of GH, but it may be independent of somatomedin as well. Fetal rat cartilage has been reported to be resistant to somatomedin.[42] (See Chapter 140).

Other hormones may be important to the growth of the fetoplacental unit. Placental lactogen (PL) and prolactin may be growth-promoting hormones. PL is weakly anabolic.[43] The placental concentration of the former hormone shows a small but strong correlation with birth size of twins as well as with placental size.[28] This effect of PL may be mediated via its effects on the placenta, fetal blood levels being relatively low (19 ng/ml).[44] PL levels are reportedly depressed in mothers of underweight newborns.[44a] Although prolactin probably has only about 5 percent the anabolic potency of GH,[45] it may contribute to nitrogen retention in the fetus, in whom levels appear to be quite high.[46] Insulin has been postulated to contribute to normal intrauterine growth.[47] Sex hormones may be important for somatic growth in utero, just as at puberty. It is noteworthy that sex steroid levels of the fetus are equal to or greater than those of the pubertal male with respect to the levels of free plasma testosterone, estradiol, and dehydroepiandrosterone.[48,49] The effects of sex hormones on fetoplacental growth are complex and poorly understood. For example, estrogen promotes fetal bone development,[50] yet, some evidence suggests that estrogen inhibits placental and fetal growth.[51]

The normal rate of third-trimester fetal somatic growth has been estimated from cross-sectional data regarding size attained by live-born babies of various gestational ages. The standards for birth size collected by Lubchenco and colleagues are shown in Figure 142-2.[16,52] These standards are the most widely used in the United States. They are not universally representative, and their major merits and drawbacks should be kept in mind. The data include multiple parameters and were collected from the charts of 5635 Caucasian infants born in Denver, Colorado, to a medically indigent, mixed ethnic population. They share the deficiencies common to most such studies—namely, that it is difficult to accurately estimate gestational age, that it is possible that prematurity may represent the consequences of an unidentified unphysiologic state, and that there is an arbitrary element in case selection. The median weight of Denver infants after 30 weeks' gestation is approximately 100 g below that in U.S. coastal areas.[53,54] The

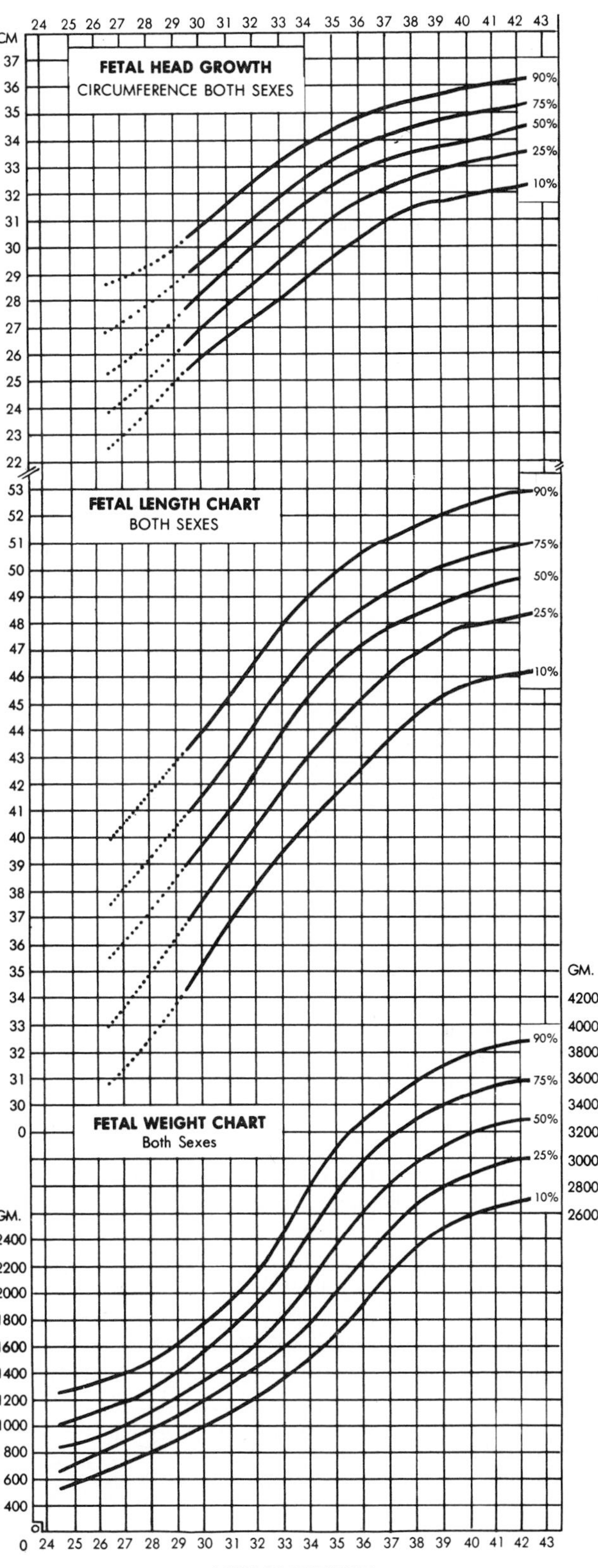

Fig. 142-2. Intrauterine growth chart. [Modified from Lubchenco, L. O., *et al.*: Pediatrics *32:* 793, 1963, *37:* 403, 1966.]

geographic difference seems independent of parental socioeconomic bracket. The 10th percentile of the Lubchenco standards with respect to weight corresponds closely with the 3rd to 5th percentile of babies born at lower altitudes.[17,53–56] The 10th percentile of the Lubchenco standards for length averages about 1.2 cm below the 3rd percentile for Montreal newborns. It is not clear whether there are any systematic differences between the intrauterine growth of Negroes and Caucasians.[56,57] The 90th percentile for birth weight of young premature infants reported by Lubchenco *et al.* is markedly lower than that reported from New York and Baltimore.[58] The overall pattern of fetal growth shown by all workers indicates that the rate of weight gain is fastest during the early portion of the 3rd trimester in parallel with growth of subcutaneous fat and muscle. Linear growth, on the other hand, is fastest during the 2nd trimester[59] and begins to slow at about 34 weeks. Head circumference reflects brain growth to a great extent (see "Concomitants of Normal Growth"). Secondary ossification centers appear radiographically in fetal enchondral bone in the order calcaneus, talus, distal femoral epiphysis, proximal tibial epiphysis, and cuboid, according to necropsy data.[60] The gestational age by which each of these centers appears in about 50 percent of the population is 24, 28, 36, 38, and 42 weeks, respectively.

Data regarding growth of premature infants (i.e., pre-term: born before 37 weeks' gestation) outside the uterus are beginning to appear. The data suggest that such infants grow in length at the same rate they would have grown in utero.[61–63] Consequently, small, but seemingly consistent, differences are apparent between the length of pre-term and full-term infants at 1 to 5 yr of age. Premature infants' weights tend to increase along the fetal growth percentile into which they fall in the first few days of life. Weight seems appropriate for height once these measurements can be plotted on the postnatal standards used for full-term infants.

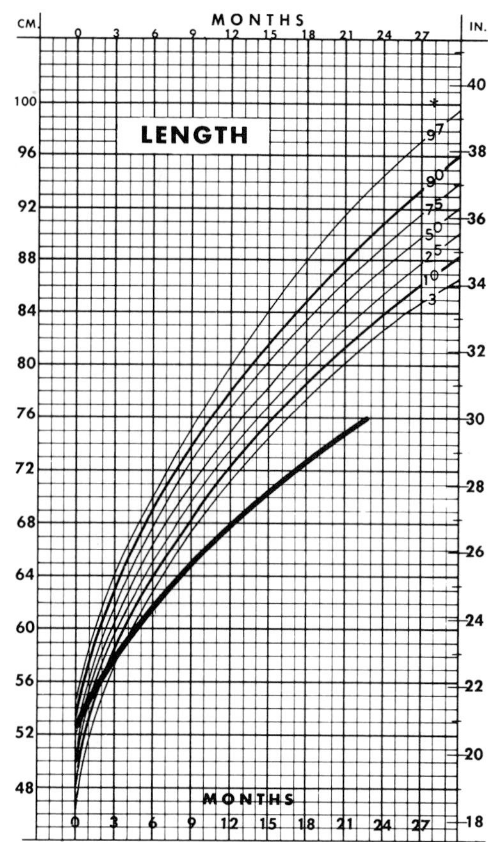

Fig. 142-3. Neonatal growth record of T. R., UC# 11462587, a child with congenital hyposomatotropism. He was born with cleft palate, bilaterally cleft lip, and a small penis. The diagnosis of growth hormone deficiency was first suspected when he was 3 yr of age and 32 inches tall. At that time a newborn sibling, who had a claft palate, cleft lip, and congenital heart disease, died; at autopsy no pituitary gland was found. T. R.'s growth velocity was 3.25 cm/yr by 5 to 9 yr of age. Standard is that of Stuart and Meredith.[126]

POSTNATAL GROWTH

Determinants and Patterns

Infancy. The factors regulating growth during the first 1 to 2 yr of life are not well understood. Linear growth velocity is most rapid in infancy and decreases geometrically during this period, unlike the situation thereafter.[64] Significant shifts in linear growth percentile rank occur in two-thirds of normal infants. A stable linear growth channel is almost always established by 2 yr of age.[65] Furthermore, the body segments of infants do not necessarily grow in proportion to one another as in the remainder of the prepubertal period.[66] The bases of the unique mode of bone growth of infants have not been studied. The author suspects that the growth pattern of infants is the resultant of an initial vector, which results from the factors uniquely affecting intrauterine growth (e.g., maternal size and fetoplacental function), superimposed upon a vector that represents the effects of the factors that determine subsequent postnatal growth (e.g., genetic, endocrine, and other factors discussed in the next section). Some such postulate seems necessary to explain why infants congenitally deficient in GH or thyroid hormone grow more rapidly in the neonatal period than in later childhood (Fig. 142-3).[66a] Birth size correlates loosely with subsequent early childhood growth.[66b]

Childhood. Linear growth through childhood (1 to 2 yr to puberty) normally proceeds at a rate that is predictable (see Growth Standards) and results from a predictable rate of bone growth. Linear growth occurs primarily by enchondral bone formation. The chondrocytes of the physis lay down an orderly cartilage template. The cartilage becomes calcified, chondrocyte degeneration occurs, and the cartilage cross-bands are lysed. This leaves longitudinal spicules extending in to the metaphysis. Mesenchymal cells then differentiate into osteoblasts which deposit osteoid onto this template. Calcification then occurs and remodeling of this primary spongiosa than progresses according to the demands of physical stress by progressive transformation of bone cells to osteoclasts. The cycle of bone cell differentiation for structural purposes is closely linked to the overall metabolic needs for calcium and phosphorus homeostasis by its responsiveness to hormones, especially parathormone and calcitonin.[67]

There is a strong tendency for an organism to grow at a rate that will permit it to reach a genetically predetermined target size. This "developmental canalization" of growth occurs in man as it does in lower organisms.[68] As a consequence, normal prepubertal children after 2 yr of age have a strong tendency to grow along a given height-attained percentile. This channel can be expressed mathematically as a single logistic function of time and growth velocity betwen 1 and 2 yr of age.[69] However, spontaneous, long-term shifts in the statural growth track may occur in normal children. On rare occasions, a gradual change of as much as 40 percentile positions in height-attained may occur over a period of several years.[66,70]

Deflections from an individual's growth channel are firmly resisted. Healthy children maintain their centile position with respect to height-attained by means of short-term fluctuations in growth velocity.[71,72] These oscillations may be marked, growth sometimes ranging down to nil over 3-month periods. It is unknown whether these changes are related to minor intercurrent illness.[73] The variations tend to be seasonal, a "blooming" trend most often occurring in the spring and summer. Even from year to year, normal children may shift in their centile position with respect to velocity-growth in order to maintain their centile position with respect to distance-growth. Changes in growth rate in compensation for chronic illness-induced alterations in growth seem to be related to the above oscillations. Such compensatory changes may completely preserve the child's height potential. "Catch-up" growth occurs upon relief from a chronic illness that has retarded growth. During the period of recovery, the growth-velocity deficit which has been incurred is matched by an equal velocity excess.[74] The rate of compensatory growth exceeds that expected for the age at which growth had been arrested. Catch-up growth has been documented following successful treatment of hypothyroidism (Fig. 142-4), renal acidosis, malnutrition, and Cushing's syndrome.[68,75] Compensatory deceleration of linear growth has been noted following adequate therapy of virilizing disease.[76] In the latter situation linear growth proceeds without advance of bone maturation. Complete compensation cannot occur in either growth-retarded or accelerated cases if the growth disorder is of many years' duration and extends too close to puberty. The mechanisms by which the developmental channel is maintained are unknown. The factors involved may be inherent, analogous to those determining cell density in tissue culture.[77] The possibility that subtle changes in hormone dynamics may mediate compensatory growth seems unlikely, but has not been thoroughly investigated. Data on GH levels during recovery from malnutrition in rats is conflicting[78,79] GH responsiveness to provocative stimuli does not correlate with the growth of hypothyroid patients before or after replacement therapy.[80]

An individual's growth channel has genetic origins. Parental height correlates with child height by 2 yr ($r = 0.5$).[65,81] Some of the determinants for bone-growth proportions reside on the sex chromosomes. On the basis of studies in men with two Y chromosomes, it seems as if this chromosome may enhance stature independently of sex hormone production.[82,83] This influence may be expressed antenatally.[84] Studies of prepubertal patients with Klinefelter's syndrome have led to the conclusion that their extra X chromosome is greatly responsible for their long-leggedness and

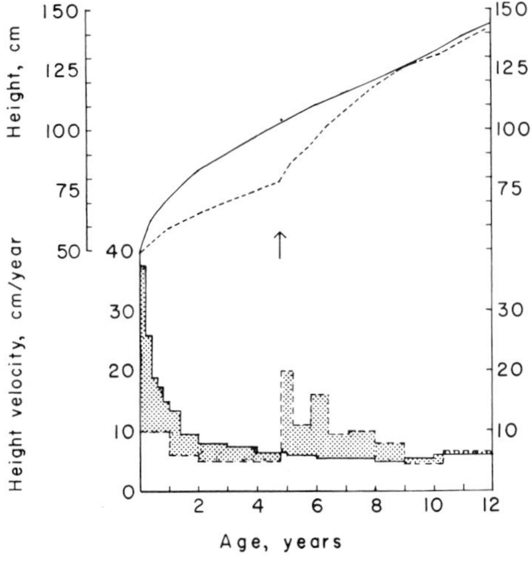

Figure 142-4. Height and height velocity for a girl with hypothyroidism. Solid line shows 25th percentile; dotted line shows the patient. Arrow indicates onset of treatment. Hatched areas show that the amount of growth velocity excess occurring during therapy equals the amount of growth velocity deficit accrued prior. [From Forbes, G. B.: Pediatr. Res. *8:* 929, 1974, with permission.]

eunuchoid proportions.[85] The short arm of the X chromosome also clearly carries genetic determinants for bone growth (see "Intrinsic Shortness"). A variety of evidence from pathologic states indicates that other genetic determinants of growth lie on the autosomes.

Adequate nutrition is essential for optimal somatic growth and maturation.[86–88] Multiple factors are involved. Energy sources, calories and oxygen, seem particularly critical for cell multiplication. Between about 2 and 13 percent of normal energy consumption goes into promoting growth.[89,90] Oxygen consumption and metabolic rate per kilogram body weight fall concomitantly with age.[91,92] This pattern of energy consumption through most of postnatal life is related to the relative size of the high-energy-requiring organs (brain, liver, heart, and kidney). At about the time of puberty, an increasing amount of energy is consumed by the expanding muscle mass. Protein intake seems relatively critical for normal growth in cellular size. Protein intake must be adequate with respect to both amount and provision of essential aminoacids or their ketoanalogues, else nitrogen accretion and growth cannot occur.[93–95] Essential fatty acids are necessary for normal growth in lower animals, but this may not hold true for primates.[96] Vitamins A and D are important growth factors.[97] Trace elements are important for normal growth.[98,98a] There is considerable current interest in the necessity of zinc for normal growth and sexual maturation.[99,100] These metals are probably essential because of their role as cofactors for enzyme function. In this regard, the pH must be maintained at that optimal for enzyme activity.[101]

Normal neuromuscular activity and blood circulation are well known to be necessary for limb growth, as discussed in a later section. It is quite possible that the general level of activity also promotes growth. Viteri has reported decreased efficiency of nitrogen accretion and decreased growth in inactive rats.[102]

Hormones are essential "catalysts" of growth. Yet as can be seen from the above discussion, they are not the only growth-promoting factors. Hormones bring about specific patterns of cell growth.[89] Growth hormone (GH) and thyroid hormone are especially important for cell multiplication, as determined in muscle. GH action on epiphyseal cartilage maturation is probably distinct from that on cartilage proliferation. Thyroid hormone has more noticeable effects on cell size than growth hormone. However, these effects of thyroid hormones are paradoxical, cell size being small in congenital hypothyroidism, large in acquired hypothyroidism. This may indicate a more important role of thyroxine in protein synthesis at earlier ages. Insulin seems primarily involved with increase in cell size. Androgens are capable of stimulating both hyperplasia and hypertrophy in target organs, to an extent which may be steroid-[103] and organ-specific. Trophic hormones (e.g., TSH) are well known to bring about hyperplasia of their target organs. Estrogens are thought to promote growth in muscle cell size, but inhibit cell multiplication in this tissue.[104]

Somatomedin probably mediates the growth-promoting effect of GH (see Chapter 10), but several lines of evidence suggest that somatomedin levels are also controlled by factors other than GH. Serum somatomedin activity increases with age, unlike GH levels.[105,105a] Somatomedin levels and growth may be normal with subnormal or absent serum GH in two conditions. The first of these is obesity.[105] It is doubtful whether this situation is entirely brought about by the accompanying hyperinsulinism, though insulin is a growth-promoting hormone.[106] The blood insulin level achieved in obese man is probably too low to mimic somatomedin.[107] The second occurs after the successful therapy of craniopharyngioma or similarly located tumors.[108,109] Most such patients are obese and are treated with vasopressin. The obesity has led to the postulate that hyperinsulinism in involved. If prolactin is responsible for somatomedin generation in such patients, the porcine prolactin which contaminates commercial vasopressin may be more important than endogenous prolactin, the levels of which are normal.[109–111] A negative-feedback link between cartilage growth and somatomedin generation is a possibility about which to cautiously speculate in view of the following information. Somatomedin activity of serum may be elevated in some patients with Turner syndrome and achondroplasia, and depressed in cerebral gigantism.[105,112] Rat cartilage explants become less responsive to somatomedin with age (vis-à-vis the above-noted rise in somatomedin levels with age).[42] A further factor influencing somatomedin activity is somatomedin inhibitory "factor" present in serum.[106]

Glucocorticoids in supraphysiologic doses are inhibitors of linear growth. This effect can be overcome to some extent by GH or testosterone administration.[113,114] Evidence is accumulating which suggests that this action of corticoids is mainly mediated by inhibition of somatomedin generation.[105–115] It is noteworthy that the dose of cortisone reported to inhibit somatomedin generation is that which is critical for growth-inhibition, 45 mg/m²/day.[116] Glucocorticoids have inconsistent effects on GH release in children[117] and on inhibition of somatomedin-promoted cartilage synthesis.[105,115] Pharmacologic doses of estrogen also inhibit growth, seemingly by interfering with somatomedin production.[115]

The possibility that sex hormones play a role in normal prepubertal growth is a subject worthy of further study. Boys have higher plasma testosterone levels and a slightly greater growth rate in early infancy than girls.[118] Otherwise, gonadal development and growth proceed faster in girls than boys.[119] Adrenocortical production of 17-ketosteroids begins to increase at about 6 yr of age.[120] It has been reported that dehydroepiandrosterone sulfate promotes calcification of cartilage,[121] and subandrogenic doses of androstenedione promote growth.[122] In support of the concept that sex hormones play a role in growth prepubertally is the observation that inexplicable growth arrest has been observed in a hypoadrenal, hypogonadal girl.[123]

Puberty. The timing of the onset of the adolescent growth spurt is clearly a determinant of mature height. Mathematical modelling of individual growth curves has led to the suggestions that (1) the adolescent growth component begins at an average age of 6 yr in girls and 9 yr in boys, (2) the amount of adolescent statural growth is very similar in both sexes, and (3) the greater ultimate height of boys compared to girls results mostly from their longer period of prepubertal growth.[69] This calculated pubertal component seems to begin 3 to 4 yr before the appearance of secondary sexual characteristics, as does the growth of lean body mass;[124] however, it does not clearly evidence the greater peak linear growth velocity of boys.[125]

Age influences the capacity for growth in response to pubertal stimuli. There is a tendency for older children to have a less intense growth spurt than early maturing children.[125] This tendency is also seen at comparable levels of bone maturation.[126]

Increased secretion of sex hormones clearly initiates the major pubertal growth spurt.[127,128] During the course of sexual maturation, the epiphyseal cartilage plates become progressively obliterated, with resultant fusion of the shafts and epiphyseal ossification centers, at which time linear growth ceases. The limited amount of data available indicate that the peak growth velocity of boys occurs when plasma testosterone levels are in the adult male range,[129] corresponding to a testosterone production rate of 100 to 150 mg/m²/month.[130] Physiologic levels of estrogen contribute to the pubertal growth spurt of girls.[123] Increased GH secretion may occur during puberty;[127,128] this tendency has been particularly noticeable when blood has been sampled frequently around the clock.

Normal Growth Standards

Normal measurements are depicted in Figures 142-5 to 142-8 and Table 142-1.[71,125,131,132] Linear growth occurs at a nearly constant rate through the prepubertal years. Growth averages 7.4 cm (2.9 in.) between 3 and 4 yr of age and 5.6 cm (2.2 in.) between 9 and 10 yr of age in boys, for example. The temporary growth acceleration of puberty is maximal after the onset of sexual maturation. The magnitude of this pubertal growth spurt is not apparent by inspection of height-attained standards because the pubertal spurts of individuals occur out of phase. In fact, the normal child may dip below the 3rd percentile of such graphs transiently if puberty occurs at a later-than-average age. In order to appreciate the normal pattern of growth during adolescence, one must turn to growth-velocity standards. The velocity standards, depicted as inserts in Figures 142-4 and 142-6, are centered upon the age at which peak height velocity occurs. These standards thus illustrate the normal pattern of growth with respect to years before and after the time of peak growth. For example, these standards show that the 3rd percentile for linear growth ranges from 3.45 cm/yr prepubertally, to 7.2 cm/yr at the time of peak pubertal growth in boys. The respective figures are 3.86 cm/yr and 6.26 cm/yr for girls. There is a tendency for early maturers to follow a higher centile than late maturers. Similar velocity curves result if growth increments are plotted according to years before and after menarche (Fig. 142-9).[133] In late puberty, deceleration of growth occurs. In girls, this slowing usually begins shortly prior to the onset of menses; hence, girls generally achieve only 7 cm further growth subsequent to menarche. Only about 1 cm of growth occurs after fusion is complete in the femur and tibia. Statural growth ceases at median ages of 17 yr in girls, 21 yr in boys.[134]

The growth standards given in Figures 142-4 to 142-7 are recent ones for British children as obtained by Tanner and his associates. The most widely used standards in the United States have been those of Stuart and Meredith, collected in 1930 to 1945, the 50th percentile of which is given in Table 142-1. Comparison of recent British and American data[135] reveals the following points. Yearly increments in growth are slightly (about 0.5 cm/yr), but significantly, greater in the American children. Consequently, somatic milestones are achieved about ½ yr later in the British children and centiles come to differ by a few centimeters in midchildhood. The 5th and 50th percentiles for height of American children correspond to about the 10th and 55th, respectively, for the British. The mean height of American 18-yr-olds in 1962 to 1975 exceeds that in 1930 to 1945 by about 2.3 cm.

Growth of non-Caucasian American children differs from that of Caucasians in some particulars. Black children from 5 to 12 yr are approximately 2 cm taller than white, matched for income. Puberty occurs about 0.28 yr earlier than in whites, and after 14 yr the size of Negroes and Caucasians is virtually identical.[81,136,137] Median heights of Oriental-American boys are less than those of Caucasians by about 5 cm during the prepubertal years, but they undergo a later growth spurt to catch up in height by 14 yr. However, the statural differences between Oriental and white girls are not resolved by 14 yr of age and seem to be inherent. The prepubertal growth rate of all these groups is similar.

Body proportions change in concert with growth. The limbs are relatively short in infancy. By about 9 yr of age adult proportions are reached (Table 142-1). Table 142-1 is based upon extrapolations from data published in 1932. Ranges are given because they

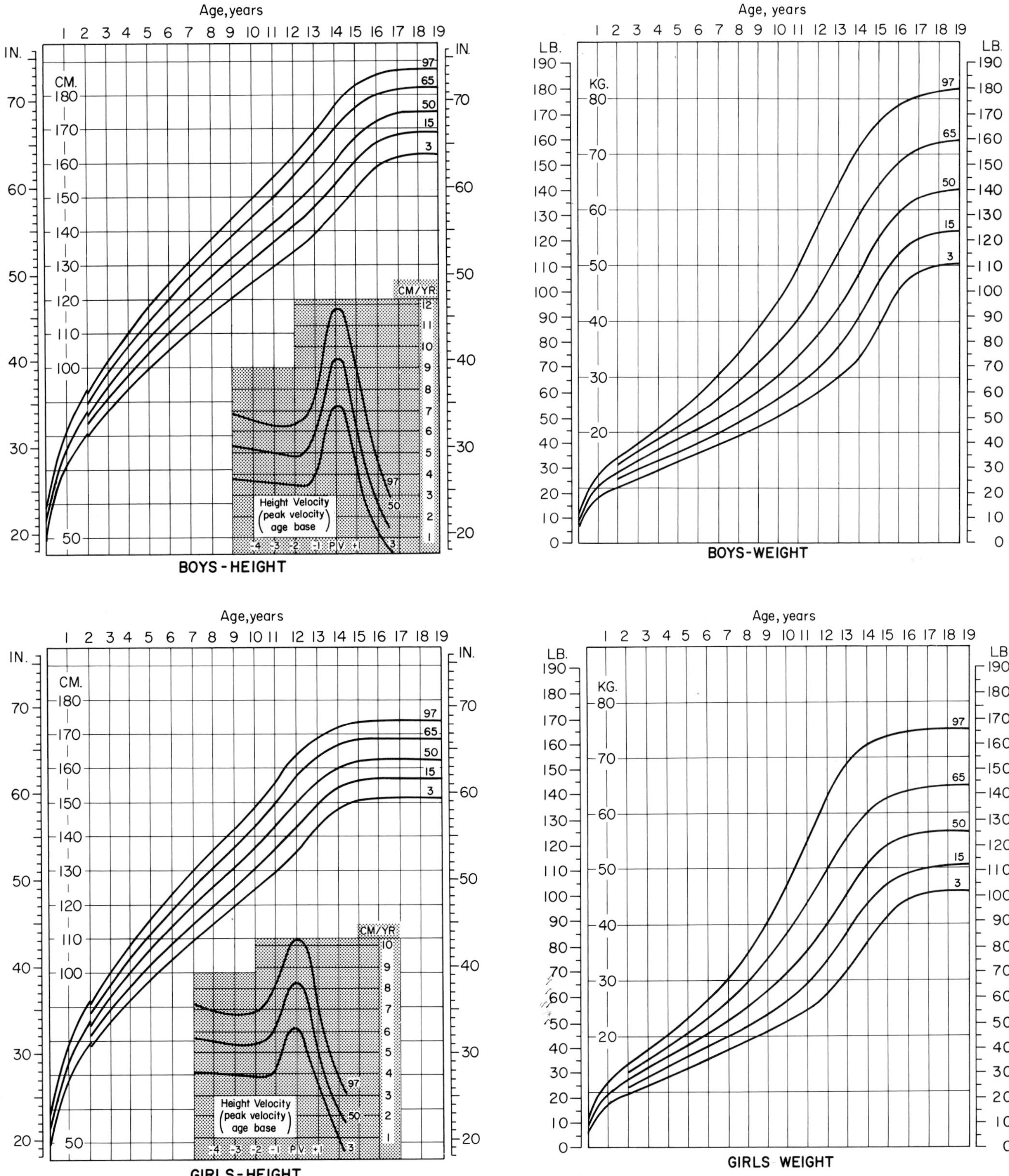

Figs. 142-5 to 142-8. Standards for height and weight of normal children. [redrawn from Tanner, J. M., *et al.*: Arch. Dis. Child. *41:* 454, 613, 1966]. Note that inserts for linear growth velocity are not based upon chronologic age, but rather upon years ± that at which peak growth velocity occurs.

are useful approximations; the author has seen normal, mature teenagers with body proportions outside the expected limits—e.g., upper/lower ratios of 0.81. Occasional marked variations in segmental proportions appear during puberty.[66] Facial configuration matures as well. The change in the nasal root can be documented by measurement of the intercanthal and interorbital distances (Table 142-2).[138–141] Head circumference increases most rapidly during the 1st yr (Figs. 142-10 and 142-11).[142] It is related to both skeletal and brain growth. Consequently, the relationship of head circumference to height is not a simple one and has been a subject of controversy.[143–145] It seems appropriate to plot the head circumference of GH-deficient children versus height age rather than

Table 142-1. Body Proportions (inches)

	Boys					Girls				
Age (yr.)	Height	Span: Avg. & Range	Upper Segment: Avg. & Range	Lower Segment: Avg. & Range	Ratio: U/L	Height	Span: Avg. & Range	Upper Segment: Avg. & Range	Lower Segment: Avg. & Range	Ratio: U/L
Birth	19.9	19.0 (19.1–21.0)	12.5 (11.9–12.9)	7.4 (6.8–7.8)	1.70	19.8	18.8 (18.0–19.8)	12.4 (12.0–13.0)	7.3 (6.8–7.8)	1.70
0.5	26.1	25.0 (23.9–26.1)	16.2 (15.6–16.7)	9.9 (9.5–10.6)	1.62	25.7	24.5 (23.5–25.5)	15.8 (15.3–16.3)	9.9 (9.4–10.4)	1.60
1	29.6	28.4 (27.3–29.5)	18.4 (17.8–19.0)	11.9 (11.3–12.5)	1.54	29.2	27.9 (26.8–29.0)	17.6 (17.4–18.6)	11.6 (11.0–12.2)	1.52
1.5	32.2	31.0 (30.1–32.5)	19.1 (18.8–20.0)	13.1 (12.3–13.5)	1.50	31.8	31.4 (29.4–31.6)	18.9 (18.3–19.5)	12.9 (12.3–13.4)	1.46
2	34.4	33.0 (32.4–34.9)	20.3 (17.6–18.8)	14.1 (11.3–12.4)	1.42	34.1	33.7 (32.6–34.8)	20.1 (19.5–20.9)	14.0 (13.3–14.7)	1.41
3	37.9	36.6 (35.4–38.2)	21.7 (21.0–22.6)	16.2 (15.5–17.1)	1.33	37.7	36.3 (34.7–37.5)	21.4 (20.5–22.1)	16.0 (15.1–16.7)	1.30
4	40.7	39.5 (37.8–40.9)	22.9 (21.8–23.6)	17.8 (16.9–18.5)	1.24	40.6	38.6 (37.1–39.9)	22.6 (21.8–23.4)	18.0 (17.1–18.7)	1.22
5	43.8	42.7 (41.2–44.3)	23.2 (22.2–24.2)	20.6 (16.6–21.6)	1.19	43.2	41.5 (40.0–43.2)	23.0 (21.9–23.9)	20.3 (19.2–21.2)	1.15
6	46.3	45.4 (43.6–47.0)	24.4 (23.4–25.4)	21.9 (20.8–22.8)	1.12	45.6	44.1 (42.3–45.5)	23.8 (22.8–24.8)	22.0 (21.2–23.2)	1.10
7	48.9	48.3 (46.2–49.8)	25.1 (23.9–26.1)	23.8 (22.6–24.8)	1.07	48.1	46.7 (45.1–48.5)	24.7 (23.6–25.8)	23.4 (22.4–24.6)	1.06
8	51.2	51.2 (49.1–52.9)	26.0 (24.9–27.1)	25.2 (23.9–26.3)	1.03	50.4	49.5 (47.8–51.4)	25.5 (24.4–26.6)	24.9 (23.9–26.1)	1.02
9	53.3	53.7 (51.5–55.5)	26.8 (25.6–28.0)	26.5 (25.1–27.5)	1.02	52.3	51.9 (50.0–53.8)	26.4 (25.2–27.6)	25.9 (24.7–27.1)	1.01
10	55.2	55.8 (53.5–57.7)	27.5 (26.1–28.8)	27.7 (26.3–28.9)	0.99	54.6	55.4 (52.6–56.6)	27.3 (26.1–28.7)	27.3 (26.1–28.7)	1.00
11	56.8	57.7 (55.5–59.7)	28.2 (26.9–29.6)	28.6 (27.2–29.8)	0.98	57.0	57.7 (55.4–59.6)	28.3 (27.0–29.6)	28.7 (27.3–29.9)	0.99
12	58.9	60.2 (58.1–62.7)	28.9 (27.5–30.3)	30.0 (28.5–31.3)	0.98	59.8	60.8 (58.2–62.6)	25.7 (28.3–31.1)	30.4 (28.5–31.4)	0.99
13	61.0	62.5 (60.2–64.9)	30.0 (28.6–31.6)	31.0 (29.5–32.5)	0.97	61.8	62.4 (60.1–64.7)	30.9 (29.6–32.4)	30.9 (29.6–32.4)	1.00
14	64.0	65.9 (63.2–68.2)	31.4 (29.9–32.9)	32.5 (31.1–34.1)	0.97	62.8	63.4 (61.1–65.7)	31.4 (30.2–33.0)	31.4 (30.0–32.8)	1.01
15	66.1	68.4 (65.8–71.0)	32.7 (31.2–34.2)	33.3 (31.8–34.8)	0.98					

Modified from Wilkins, L.: The Diagnosis and Treatment of Endocrine Disorders in Childhood and Adolescence, ed. 3. Springfield, Ill., Thomas, 1965, and Engelbach, W.: Endocrine Medicine. Springfield, Ill., Thomas, vol. 1, p. 261. Span and upper/lower measurements are those appropriate for modal heights according to the standards of Stuart, H. C., and Stevenson, S. S.: In Nelson, W. E. (ed.): Textbook of Pediatrics, ed. 7. Philadelphia, Saunders, 1959, p. 12.

chronologic age.[144,146] The head size of hypothyroid children is normal for age, however.[146a] The anterior fontanel normally closes by about 15 months of age; abnormal fontanel size for age may indicate disorders of somatic growth.[147]

Bone growth is normally accompanied by a predictable sequence and rate of bone maturation. Ossification centers first appear, then undergo modelling in shape, and, in the case of epiphyseal centers, finally go through fusion with the shaft. Several methods are available for assessing bone maturation.[148] The most widely used is the atlas method of Gruelich and Pyle, using an anterior-posterior roentgenogram of the left hand and wrist.[126] The Gruelich-Pyle standards are shown schematically in Figures 142-12 and 142-13. Skeletal maturity is expressed as "bone age" or "skeletal age." The bone age is the age at which the observed

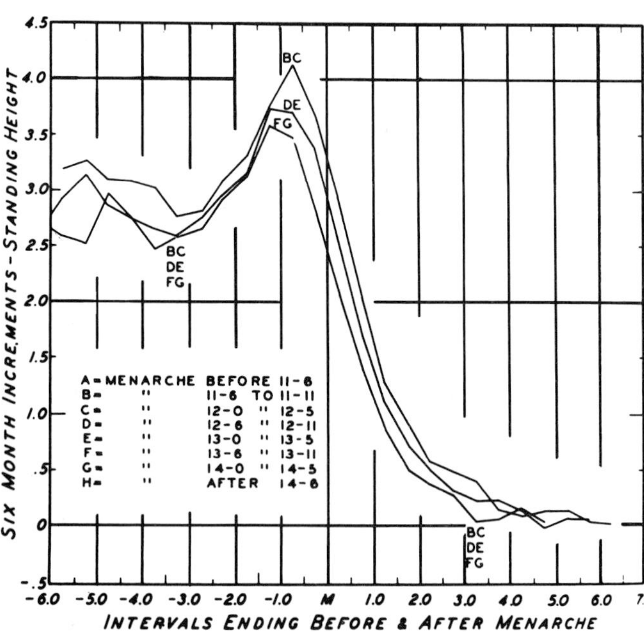

Fig. 142-9. Growth increments (cm) in years before and after menarche. Groups of cases menstruating at different ages arranged so that points corresponding to the advent of menarche are in the same vertical line. [Modified from Shuttleworth, F. K.: Monogr. Soc. Res. Child. Dev., Natl. Res. Counc. *2:* No. 5, 1937.]

Table 142-2. Normal Intercanthal Distance in Both Sexes

Age (yr)	Avg. and Range (cm)[a]
0	2.0 (1.3–2.6)
0.5	2.3 (1.6–2.7)
1.0	2.5 (2.1–3.1)
1.5	2.5 (2.1–3.1)
2.0	2.6 (2.1–3.1)
3.0	2.6 (2.2–3.2)
4.0	2.6 (2.2–3.2)
5.0	2.7 (2.2–3.4)
6.0	2.7 (2.2–3.4)
7.0	2.9 (2.4–3.4)
8.0	2.9 (2.4–3.5)
9.0	3.0 (2.4–3.5)
10.0	3.0 (2.4–3.5)
11.0	3.0 (2.4–3.5)
12.0	3.0 (2.4–3.6)
13.0	3.0 (2.4–3.7)
14.0	3.0 (2.4–3.7)
15.0	3.1 (2.5–3.6)
16.0	3.2 (2.7–3.8)
17.0	3.2 (2.7–3.8)
18.0	3.2 (2.9–3.8)

[a]Extrapolated and smoothed.[138,139] Non-Caucasian children's measurements average about 0.2 cm greater.[140] The variability may be reduced if head circumference is taken into account.[141]

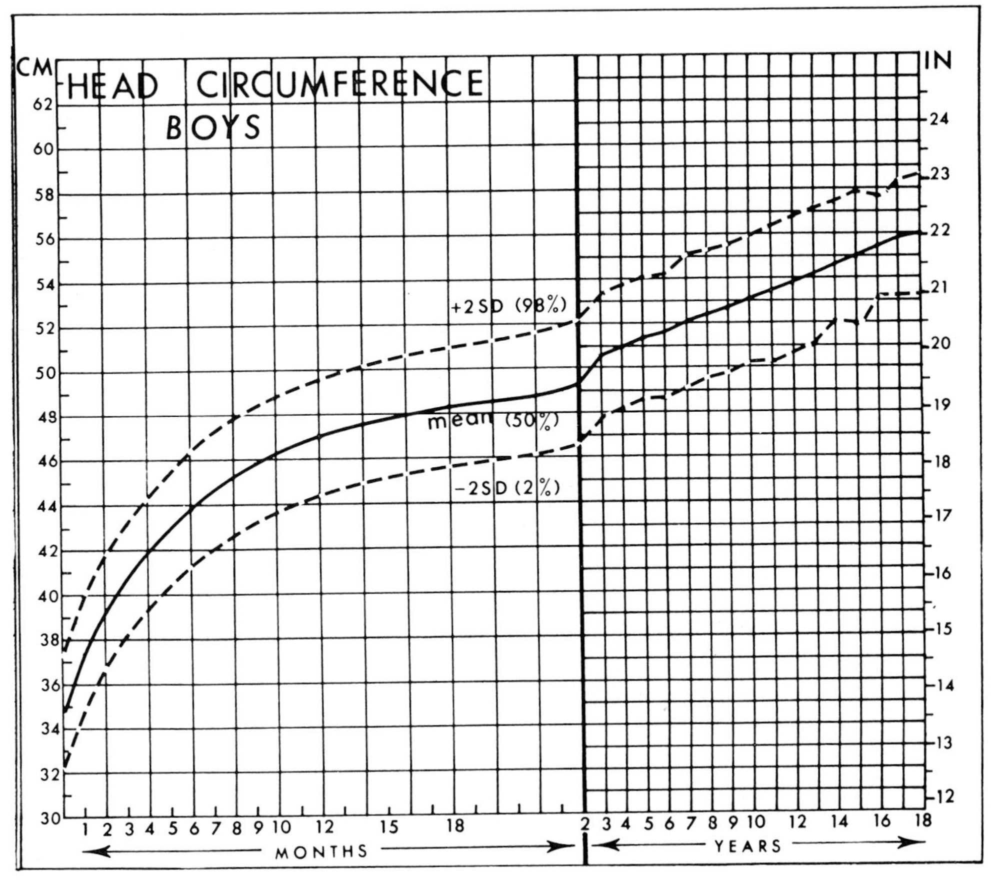

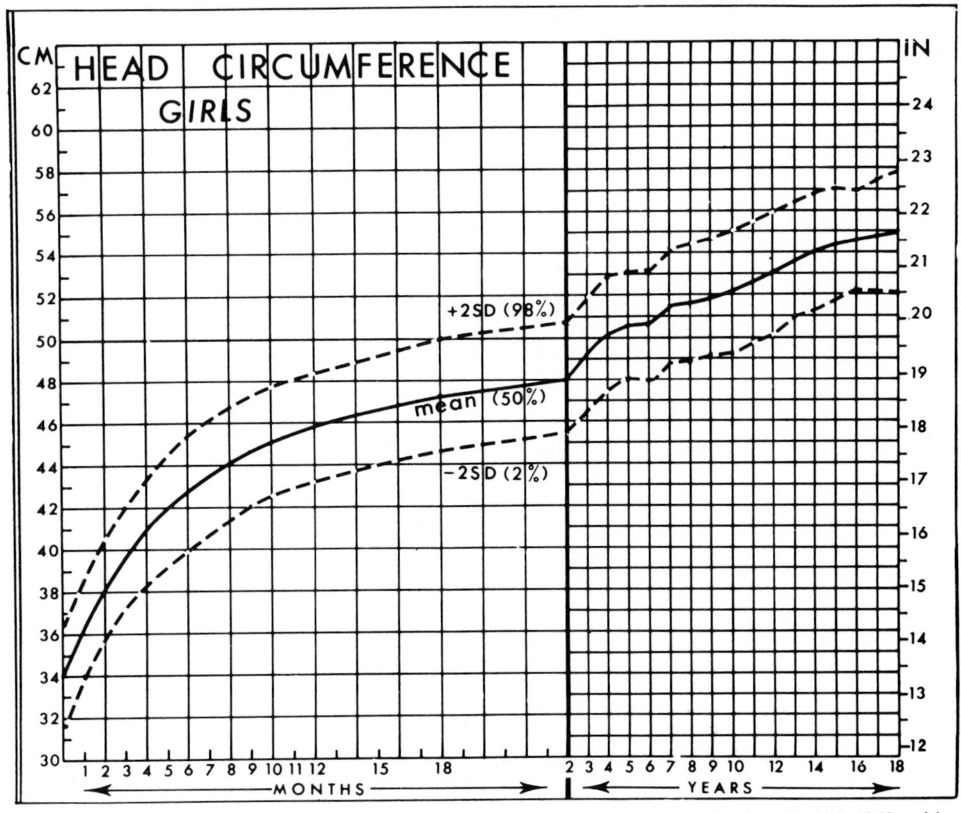

Figs. 142-10, 142-11. Interracial standards for head circumference. [From Nellhaus, G.: Pediatrics *41:* 106, 1968, with permission.]

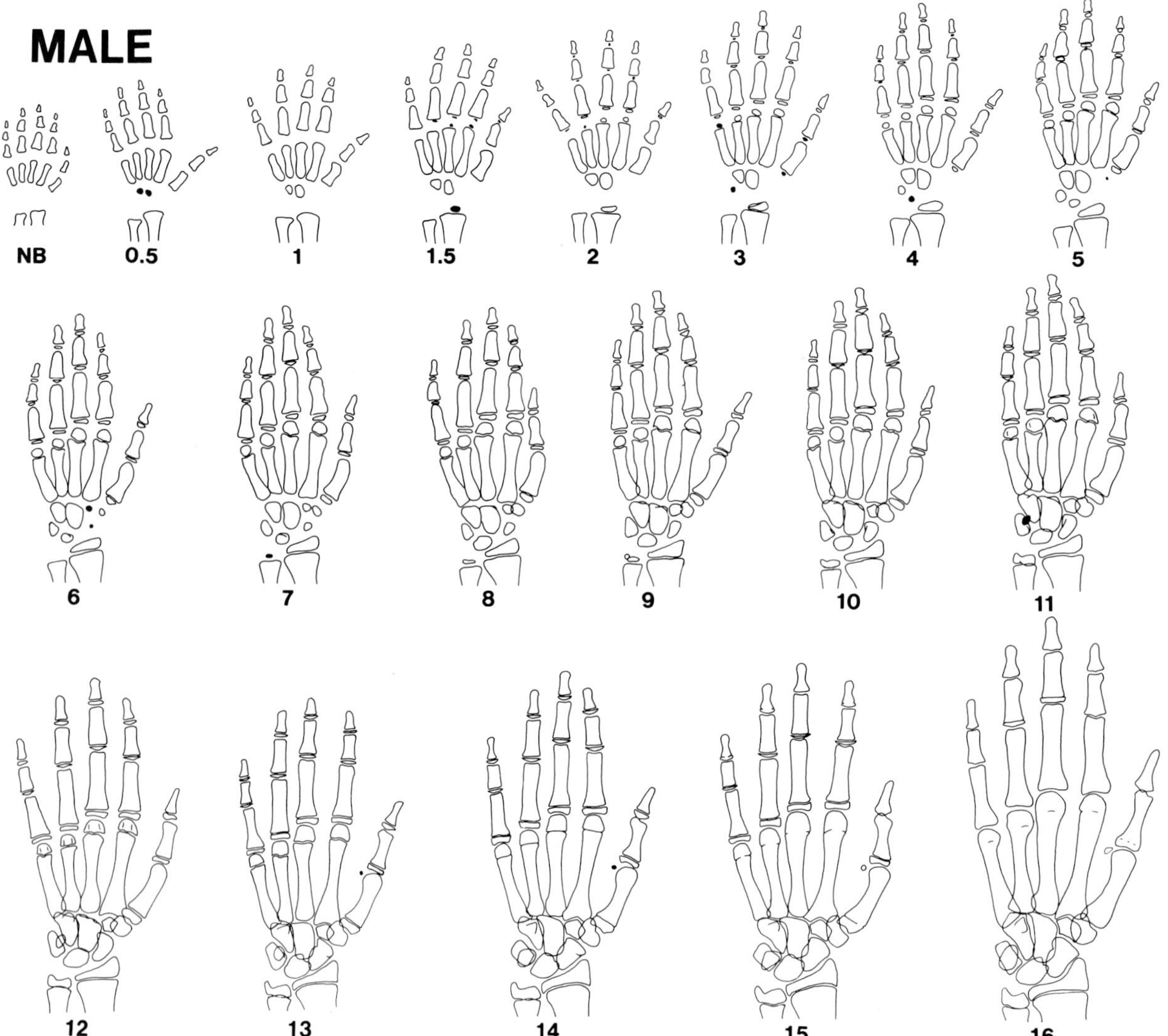

Figs. 142-12, 142-13. Progression of ossification of the hand and wrist. Tracings modified from standards of Gruelich and Pyle[126] according to manner of Wilkins.[33] Newly appeared ossification centers are shown in black. Late pre-fusion is depicted as a single line at the junction of epiphysis and shaft. Bony projections which appear as a double-contour within the outlines of a center are not illustrated after their appearance has matured.

degree of bone maturation would be typical. The evaluation is most reliable if a skeletal age is assigned to each bone of the hand film, and the average calculated.[149] The Gruelich-Pyle method's major drawbacks are the paucity of centers in early childhood and the subjective nature of the assessment of modelling. These difficulties contribute to the relatively wide coefficients of variation before puberty (Table 142-3). During puberty, as epiphyseal fusion commences, fewer indicators become available in the hand films from which to precisely assess the skeletal age. The asymmetries and variations in sequence of ossification observed in wrist X-rays in normal children are within the variability of the initiation of ossification.[150] Skeletal development of young Negro children is about 0.67 SD advanced over Caucasians of comparable economic status.[151]

Bone age correlates better with overall somatic maturation than chronologic age, height, or weight.[152] Peak height velocity

Table 142-3. Standard Deviations for Bone Age and Height Prediction According to Chronological Age[126]

	Chronological Age (yr)																
	1.0	2.0	3.0	4.0	5.0	6.0	7.0	8.0	9.0	10.0	11.0	12.0	13.0	14.0	15.0	16.0	17.0
Bone age (months)																	
Boys	2.1	4.0	6.0	7.0	8.4	9.3	10.1	10.8	11.0	11.4	10.5	10.4	11.1	12.0	14.2	15.1	15.4
Girls	2.7	4.0	5.6	7.2	8.6	9.0	8.3	8.8	9.3	10.8	12.3	14.0	14.6	12.6	11.2		
Height prediction (inches)[a]																	
Boys								1.47	1.27	1.33	1.14	1.09	1.21	1.21	0.88	0.49	0.41
Girls								1.73	1.46	1.37	1.15	1.06	0.62	0.42	0.38	0.26	0.20

[a]Validating sample

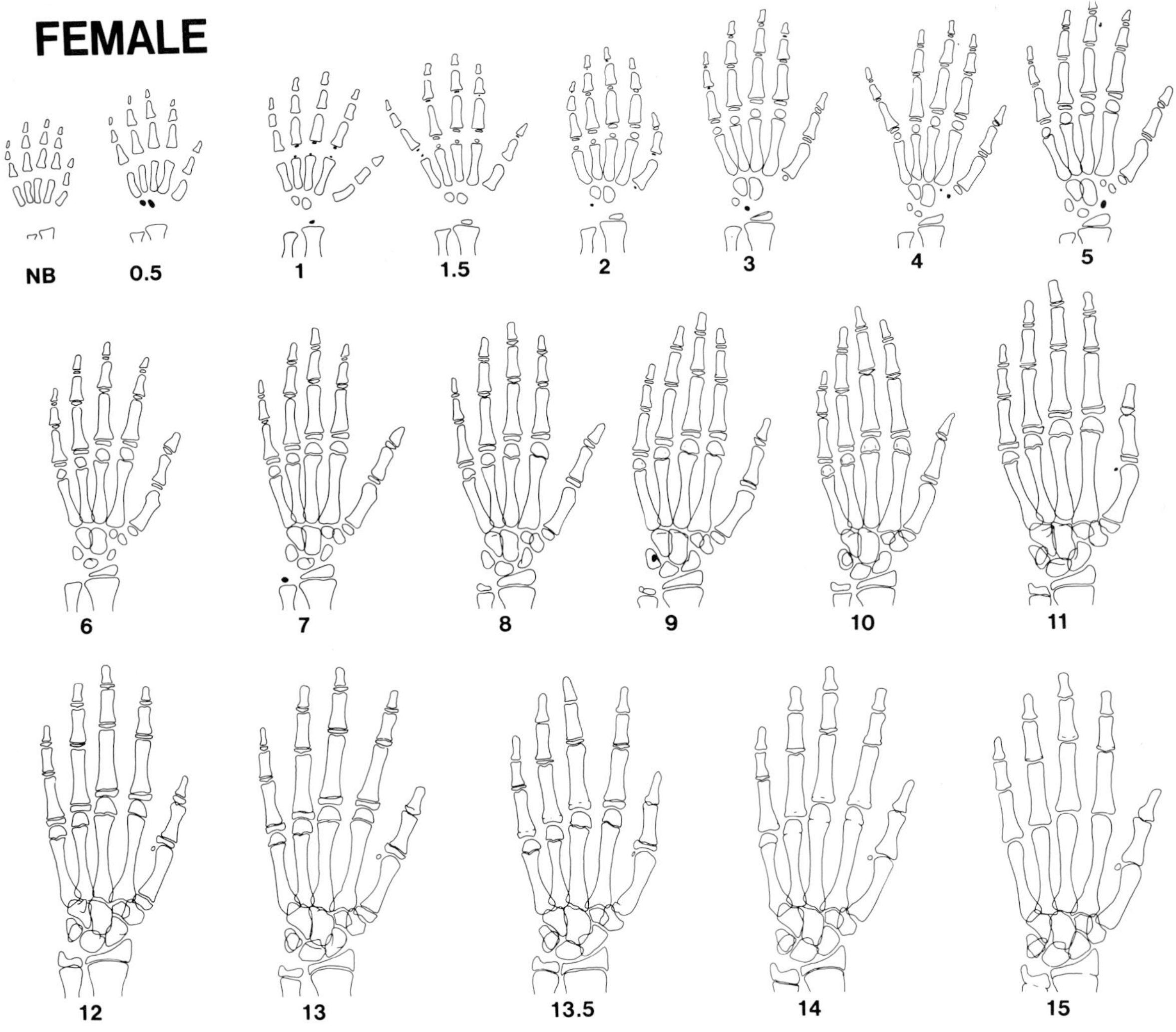

phase differences are 25 percent less when plotted against skeletal age instead of chronologic age.[71] Performance in sporting events is similarly related best to bone age.[153] The specifics of the relationship between sex hormones and bone age have not been well defined.

Weight is a labile parameter relative to height, being sensitive to acute illnesses and short-term changes in mode of living. Whether nutrition is appropriate is generally assessed by comparing a child's centile position for weight to that for height. Normal weight is more accurately described by using formulas that estimate normal weight for height according to body width[154] or percentile standards of fatness. Fat stores increase markedly during the first 9 months of life. Growth of adipose tissue then levels off, such that subcutaneous fat thickness decreases until about 7 yr of age.[73] There is then a preadolescent increase in net lipid.[124] During puberty, fat stores tend to increase slightly in girls and decrease in boys. Percentiles of fatness at menarche are shown in Figure 142-14.[155]

CONCOMITANTS OF SOMATIC GROWTH

Brain growth is probably nearly complete with respect to neuronal number by mid-pregnancy.[156] The major portion of the brain spurt in weight and cell number which commences in mid-pregnancy and continues postnatally is due to glial multiplication and myelination. It is during this time that dendritic branching and synapsing occur. Cerebellar development begins several weeks later than cerebral development, and ends earlier. The development of posture and reflexes is used widely to estimate gestational age.[157,158]

Normal fetal maturation has various endocrinologic and metabolic concomitants that have proven useful in estimating fetal well-being antenatally and gestational age. The feto-placental unit is responsible for the normal increase in mother's estrogen levels throughout pregnancy.[159] Placental lactogen production generally parallels the changes in estrone levels.[159] Amniotic fluid total cortisol and lecithin/sphingomyelin ratios increase sharply after 34 weeks' gestation.[160] Palpable breast tissue appears at 36 weeks. The testes are found in the inguinal canal in small premature infants and do not come to lie in the scrotum until about 36 weeks' postconception. It is of interest that the energy metabolism and RNA polymerase activity of maternal leukocytes are correlated with fetal growth.[161] Frank peripheral edema is present in the young premature and disappears by approximately 32 weeks' gestation. About 5 percent of the weight of the term newborn seems attributable to sodium and water retention and is lost in the first few days of extrauterine life.[162] Therefore, salt and water requirements in the first few days of life are 50 to 75 percent, respectively, of those thereafter.

Postnatal organ and tissue growth occur in characteristic pat-

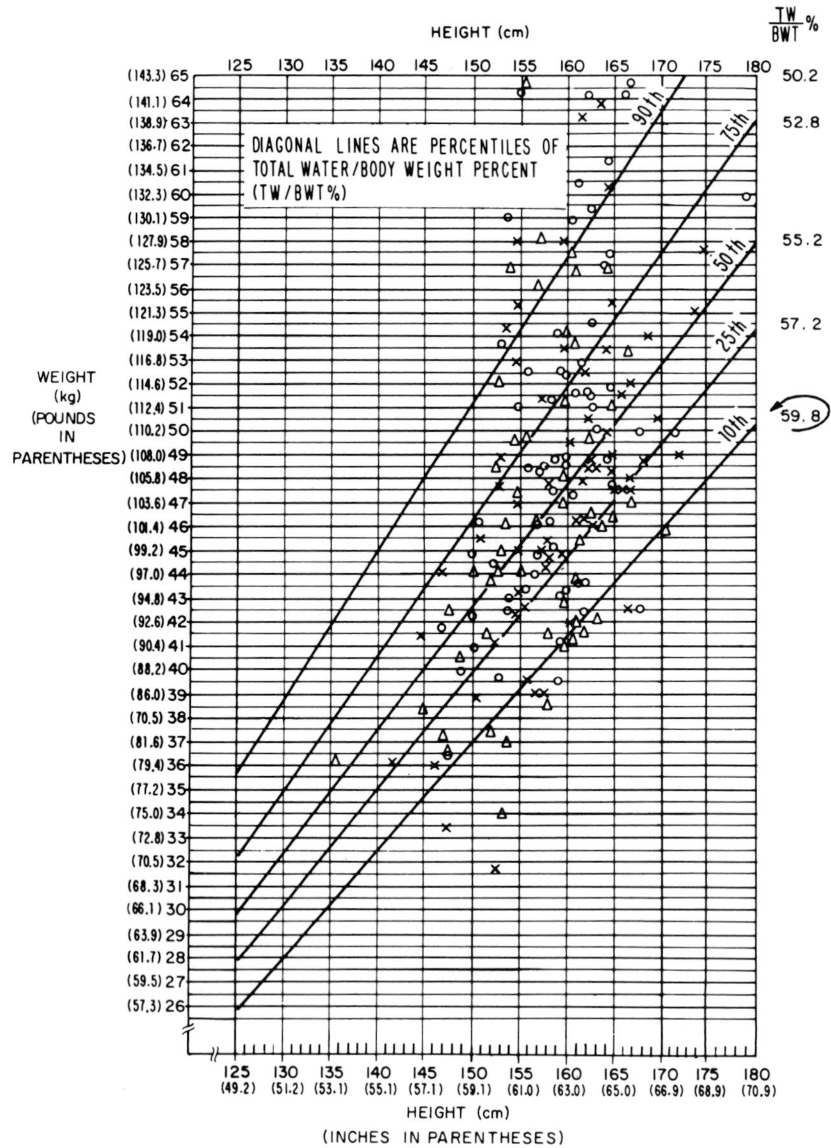

Fig. 142-14. Percentiles of total water as a percentage of body weight related to height and weight at menarche. These are percentiles of fatness for Caucasian girls at menarche. The height and weight of the menarchal individuals from whom the percentiles were calculated are depicted by the symbols. The minimal weight necessary at a particular height for the onset of menses is very close to the 10th percentile of fatness. This is indicated on the weight scale by the 10th percentile diagonal line of total water/body weight percent (59.8%) as it crosses the vertical height lines. [From Frisch, R. E., and McArthur, J. W.: Science *185:* 949, 1974, with permission.]

terns.[73,130,163] The growth of most organs follows the general somatic model (Figs. 142-5 to 142-8): respiratory and digestive organs, kidneys, cardiovascular system, spleen, liver, and musculature as a whole. Consequently, blood volume closely approximates 8 percent of body weight throughout life. The neuronal growth pattern differs: 50 percent of adult brain weight is achieved at 1 yr, nearly 100 percent by about 8 yr of age. Bursal lymphoid tissue mass grows to exceed adult levels between 8 and 18 yr of age, the peak occurring at 11 to 12 yr. Thymic size is two-thirds of maximum in infancy, is maximal in the preadolescent, then regresses during puberty. The growth of the reproductive organs is relatively slow until about a year before the appearance of secondary sexual characteristics.

Primary teeth begin to calcify before birth. The timing of calcification and eruption of the permanent teeth follows a consistent pattern (Table 142-4) and is dependent upon many of the nutritional and hormonal factors that determine somatic growth.[164] Nevertheless, the correlation between dental and bone maturation is not a good one.[131]

Body water undergoes important changes with age (Table 142-5). Calorie expenditure; salt, hormone, and drug dosage; and glomerular filtration rate change in proportion to water requirements. Two schemes for calculating average water, etc., needs are given in Table 142-5, one based on surface area and another empirically based on weight.[165,166] One hundred calories are required per 100 ml water. Normal sodium and potassium requirements are 3 and 2 mEq/100 ml water, respectively. The extracellular compartment is relatively larger in children than adults, falling from about 40 percent at 1 week to 30 percent at 3 to 6 months to 20 percent at maturity.

Commensurate with bone growth occur striking changes in the level of serum phosphorus and alkaline phosphatase.[167] The concentration of serum phosphorus falls steadily from a range of about 5 to 7.5 mg/100 ml in infancy to one of about 3 to 5 mg/100 ml

Table 142-4. Chronology of Human Dentition

Tooth		Calcification Begins	Crown Completed	Eruption	Root Completed	Root Resorption Begins
Primary	I	14 wk	4 months	6–8 months	1½–2 yr	5–6 yr
	II	16 wk	5 months	8–10 months	1½–2 yr	5–6 yr
	III	17 wk	9 months	16–20 months	2½–3 yr	6–7 yr
	IV	15½ wk	6 months	12–16 months	2–2½ yr	4–5 yr
	V	18–19 wk	10–12 months	20–30 months	3 yr	4–5 yr
Upper Permanent	1	3–4 months	4–5 yr	7–8 yr	10 yr	
	2	1 yr	4–5 yr	8–9 yr	11 yr	
	3	4–5 months	6–7 yr	11–12 yr	13–15 yr	
	4	1½–1¾ yr	5–6 yr	10–11 yr	12–13 yr	
	5	2–2½ yr	6–7 yr	10–12 yr	12–14 yr	
	6	8 months	2½–3 yr	6–7 yr	9–10 yr	
	7	2½–3 yr	7–8 yr	12–14 yr	14–16 yr	
	8	7–9 yr	12–16 yr	17–30 yr	18–25 yr	
Lower Permanent	1	3–4 months	4–5 yr	6–7 yr	9 yr	
	2	3–4 months	4–5 yr	7–8 yr	10 yr	
	3	4–5 months	6–7 yr	10–11 yr	12–14 yr	
	4	1¾–2 yr	5–6 yr	10–12 yr	12–13 yr	
	5	2¼–2½ yr	6–7 yr	11–12 yr	13–14 yr	
	6	8 months	2½–3 yr	6–7 yr	9–10 yr	
	7	2½–3 yr	7–8 yr	12–13 yr	14–15 yr	
	8	8–10 yr	12–16 yr	17–30 yr	18–25 yr	

From Rosenstein: In Barnett, H. (ed.): Pediatrics, ed. 15. New York, Appleton-Century-Crofts, 1972, with permission.

in the adult. Serum alkaline phosphatase falls from about 40 to 140 IU/liter in infancy to about 20 to 40 IU/liter in adults; the decline is interrupted by a secondary peak during the late preadolescent and adolescent years. The bone isozyme accounts for the difference in phosphatase levels between children and adults and presumably reflects osteoblastic activity. A downward trend is observed in serum calcium and parathormone levels with growth, but it is not prominent; and for practical purposes the plasma levels of these substances can be considered stable at adult levels.

Plasma hormone concentrations are, in general, similar in children and adults. In the case of some hormones—e.g., cortisol—this signifies that the secretion rate changes in proportion to surface area.[168] In the instance of other hormones—e.g., thyroxine—this is accomplished in spite of changes in hormone metabolism and secretion.[169] Examples of exceptions to the general rule about equivalency of hormone levels are free thyroxine (up to 20 percent higher during infancy),[31] renin and aldosterone (falling progressively throughout childhood),[170,171] and, of course, sex steroid, LH, and FSH levels.

Table 142-5. Changes in Average Water Requirements with Growth

Age[a]	Weight[a] (kg)	Surface Area (meters^2)	Predicted Daily Water Need (ml) by surface area[b]	by weight[c]
1 week	3.0	0.2	286	300
5 months	6.0	0.3	428	600
1.0 yr	10.0	0.45	642	1000
5.5 yr	20.0	0.80	1140	1500
9.0 yr	30.0	1.00	1430	1700
14.5 yr	50.0	1.50	2140	2100
Adult	70.0	1.75	2500	2500

[a]Data for males.
[b]Calculated on the assumption of 2500 ml total requirements in an adult whose surface area is 1.75 m^2.
[c]Calculated as 100 ml/kg up to 10 kg body weight; 1000 ml + 50 ml/kg from 10 to 20 kg; 1500 ml + 20 ml/kg over 20 kg.
Modified from Holliday, M. A.: In Maxwell, M. H., and Kleeman, C. R. (eds.): Clinical Disorders of Fluid and Electrolyte Metabolsm, ed. 1. New York, McGraw-Hill, 1962, p. 445; and Butler, A. M., and Richie, R. H.: *N. Engl. J. Med. 262:* 903, 1960. The water requirements given are approximately 50 percent above basal needs.

DIAGNOSTIC APPROACH TO GROWTH DISORDERS

Growth derangements can be classified according to the relationship between chronologic age (CA), height age (HA), weight age (WA), bone age (BA), and growth rate. The HA is the age for which a child's height would be average (i.e., at the 50th percentile). The WA and BA are similarly defined. For example, a subject with the height and bone development of an average 6-yr-old has a HA and BA of 6, regardless of his CA.

Growth disturbances are caused by a myriad of disorders. The physician is faced with an awesomely long differential diagnosis. In addition, he must keep in mind that about one-third of children whose size is outside the 95-percent confidence limits of normal have a growth pattern that is a variation of normal.[33] The most common of these variants are children who have a genetically limited growth potential or those who have an unexpectedly good growth potential on the basis of being "constitutionally" delayed in entering puberty. A two-step approach simplifies the diagnostic decisions. First, the disorder of growth is categorized as to whether it is a primary disturbance of height or weight by the relationship between HA and WA. A child with a primary disorder of linear growth has a weight that is appropriate for his length (WA $\simeq$ HA). A child with a primary nutritional disorder has a height that is considerably closer to the norm than the weight (e.g., WA<HA). Secondly, disturbances of linear growth may be understood on the basis of one general principle: *Normal linear growth proceeds at a predictable rate and is accompanied by a predictable rate of advance of bone age.* Two corollaries of this proposi-

Table 142-6. Percentage of Mature Height Achieved at a Given Bone Age

	Skeletal Age (yr)												
	6.0	6.5	7.0	7.5	8.0	8.5	9.0	9.5	10.0	10.5	11.0	11.5	12.0
PERCENTAGE OF MATURE HEIGHT													
Boys													
Average[a]			69.5	70.9	72.3	73.9	75.2	76.9	78.4	79.5	80.4	81.8	83.4
Accelerated[a]			67.0	68.3	69.6	70.9	72.0	73.4	74.7	75.8	76.7	78.6	80.9
Retarded[a]	68.0	70.0	71.8	73.8	75.6	77.3	78.6	80.0	81.2	81.9	82.3	83.2	84.5
Girls													
Average	72.0	73.8	75.7	77.2	79.0	81.0	82.7	84.4	86.2	88.4	90.6	91.4	92.2
Accelerated			71.2	73.2	75.0	77.1	79.0	80.9	82.8	85.6	88.3	89.1	90.1
Retarded	73.3	75.1	77.0	78.8	80.4	82.3	84.1	85.8	87.4	89.6	91.8	92.6	93.2

[a]With respect to whether the bone age is or is not within 1 yr of chronological age.

tion are (1) all correctable diseases that interfere with growth do so by interfering with the progression of bone growth, hence, bone age, and conversely, (2) if a child's bone age progresses normally, there is no correctable disease underlying his shortness. The only exception to these rules occurs in pituitary gigantism. Based upon these principles, disorders of intrauterine and postnatal growth can be approached in a discriminatory manner.

"Dwarfism" means marked shortness, and the term should be applied only if predicted adult height (see below) or the child's height is less than 4 SD from the mean. The expression carries implications of deformity to laymen. Actually, only some dwarfs are disproportionate ("imperfect"); many are proportionate ("perfect" or "ateliotic" dwarfs = midgets).

The proper evaluation of the growth rate and bone development is essential to the clinical assessment of patients with disturbances of linear growth. The most common error in the diagnosis of growth disorders is the physician's reliance on "routine" height measurements which have been taken inaccurately. Height can be measured reproducibly with less than 1 cm error if taken and rechecked in standard fashion: without shoes and with correct posture (standing "at attention": heels nearly together; heels, buttocks, shoulders, and occiput touching the vertical plane; abdominal muscles flat, and the lower margin of the orbit held in the horizontal plane which includes the external auditory meatus). Measurements should be made at approximately the same time of day, to avoid the effect of the diurnal variation that seems to result from postural changes and vertebral settling. This decrease in height between the early morning and late afternoon averages 1.54 cm.[172] The longitudinal growth rate cannot be accurately evaluated over periods of less than 6 to 12 months because of the short-term fluctuations which sometimes occur.

Bone development is assessed roentgenographically (see previous section). The film may reveal the unexpected presence of a bone dystrophy or ossification disturbance (Fig. 142-15). The radiogram then should be assigned a *precise* bone age; a statement that the bone age is "significantly retarded," "compatible with the chronologic age," etc., is useless in growth diagnosis. The limitations of the determination of skeletal age should be kept in mind, however. The limits of normal variations have been discussed above. Overall skeletal maturation does not correlate well with the rate of linear growth or growth potential in some bone dystrophies or dysostoses (Fig. 142-15).[173] The maturation of certain ossification centers, particularly among the carpals, may be specifically altered in certain bone dysplasias. The normal variations and asymmetries may be exaggerated in a variety of growth disorders, whether growth is altered generally (Fig. 142-16) or locally.[174] In cases where body proportions are altered, a skeletal survey is indicated, as the hand and wrist are not involved in some dysplasias.

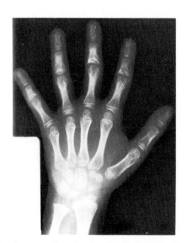

Fig. 142-15. Hand x-ray taken for the determination of bone age of a 9.75-yr-old girl whose height age was 4.75. Note the cone-shaped epiphyses and their ultimate premature fusion, characteristic of the rhinotricho-phalangeal syndrome. Consideration of only the overall retardation of bone age, without evaluation of the abnormal bone structure, would lead to an overestimation of this girl's mature height.

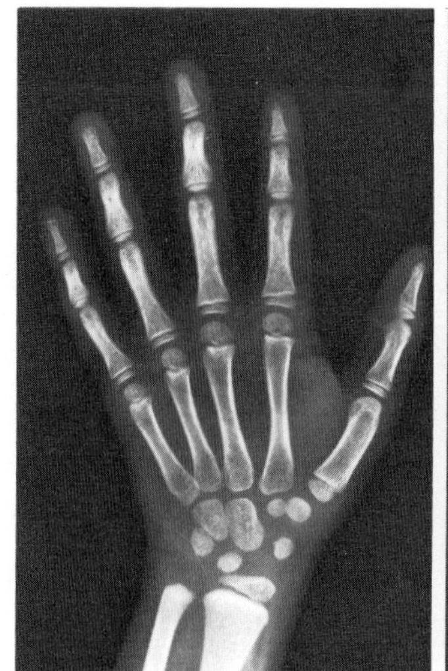
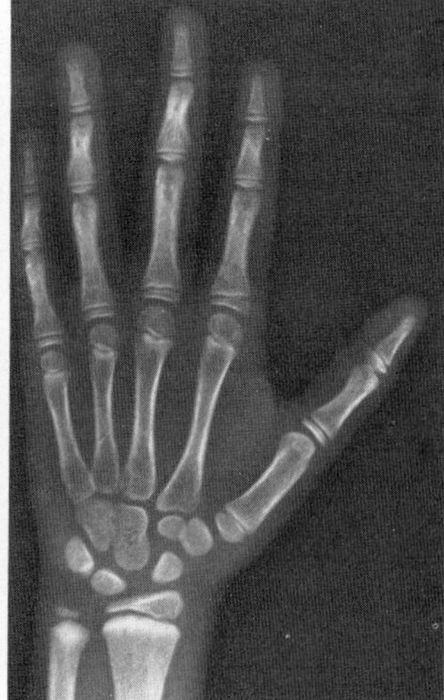

Fig. 142-16. Left: hand x-ray of a 4.75 yr-old girl (A.M., UC# 1143217-6) at the time of presentation for premature breast development. Bone age: 6 yr. Right: repeat x-ray three months later at time of diagnosis for feminizing tumor. Note rapid appearance advancement of BA, particularly with regard to the ossification of the pisiform, a 9-year center.

12.5	13.0	13.5	14.0	14.5	15.0	15.5	16.0	16.5	17.0	17.5	18.0	18.5
85.3	87.6	90.2	92.7	94.8	96.8	97.6	98.2	98.7	99.1	99.4	99.6	100.0
82.6	85.0	87.5	90.5	93.0	95.8	97.1	98.0	98.5	99.0			
86.0	88.0											
94.1	95.8	97.4	98.0	98.6	99.0	99.3	99.6	99.7	99.9	99.95	100.0	
92.4	94.5	96.3	97.2	98.0	98.6	99.0	99.3	99.5	99.8			
94.9	96.4	97.7	98.3	98.9	99.4	99.6	99.8	99.9	100.0			

PREDICTION OF ADULT HEIGHT AND AGE OF PUBERTY

The most widely used method of predicting the mature height of a normal child from his preadolescent height is that devised by Bayley and Pineau which involves the use of the bone age (Table 142-6). One can also predict the amount of growth remaining in body segments from the bone age (Table 142-7).[175] The principle is that the degree of bone maturation is inversely proportional to the amount of epiphyseal cartilage growth remaining. It follows that if a child's bone and height age are equal, he has the potential to reach an average adult height. The Bayley-Pineau tables show the percentage of mature height that has been achieved at skeletal ages of 6 yr or more; different figures apply if the skeletal age differs by over 1 yr from the average. The statistical error inherent in this method is given in Table 142-3. Spontaneous shifts by as much as 5 inches in predicted height may occur in 3 percent of the population for reasons that are unclear.[176] The error is not reduced by serial readings.[149]

In order to reduce the error in height prediction, elaborate tables have recently been devised that empirically take into consideration not only a child's bone age and height, but mid-parent stature (the average of the parents' heights) and weight.[177] Genetic influences can instead be roughly accounted for by adding to the prediction one-third the amount that mid-parent height differs from the average.[178]

Interestingly, the influence of weight upon ultimate height is a negative one in both sexes, which supports the Frisch-Revelle concept that greater weight is associated with earlier puberty, hence earlier cessation of growth. Frisch and associates have extensively explored statistically the relationship between weight and puberty. At peak growth velocity and menarche, the average height of early- and late-maturing girls differs, but not their average weight.[179] The same is true of boys with respect to peak growth velocity except for the very latest maturing boys. It has been hypothesized that the critical weight for these maturational events represents a critical body composition with respect to fatness. One can predict the age of menarche for prepubertal girls better by using percentiles of fatness than by using percentiles of height, weight, or weight for height or pubertal stage.[180] Percentiles of fatness at menarche for girls of various heights and weights are given in Figure 142-14.[155] Menstrual status, in turn, influences the prediction of ultimate height.[178,181]

Though there is considerable variation, skeletal age correlates better with age of menarche and peak height velocity than does chronologic age, weight, or height.[152] It seems as if bone and neuroendocrine maturation have common determinants. Though there is a statistical relationship between a critical weight and menarche (Fig. 142-14), this cannot be relied upon to predict the onset of menses in the individual child.[182] For example, fatness cannot be used to predict menarche in the prepubertal or early pubertal obese girl. Consequently, the bone age is in most circumstances the single best available predictor of pubertal events. In girls, menarche has been demonstrated to occur at a mean skeletal age of approximately 13 yr.[126,183] By extrapolation, one can expect breast development in girls, testicular enlargement in boys, and pubic hair appearance in boys to occur at average bone ages of 10.5, 11.5, and 12.75 yr, respectively.

DISORDERS OF INTRAUTERINE GROWTH

INTRAUTERINE GROWTH RETARDATION (IUGR)

Intrauterine growth retardation (IUGR) is defined as birth size inappropriately small for gestational age,[184] and is commonly equated with sizes below the 10th percentile on the Lubchenco standards. Although this working definition leaves something to be desired with respect to certain normal variables (see above), there is no doubt that it is of practical significance. Clinically, IUGR can be subdivided into disorders that primarily retard linear growth and those that primarily hinder fetal "nutrition." Several conditions falling into the former group are known to be characterized by a decrease in cell number in various organs—for example, congenital rubella, some congenital malformations of the heart, hypoxia,

Table 142-7. Percentage of Ultimate Length of Femur and Tibia Which Is Attained at a Given Skeletal Age

	Skeletal Age (yr)										
	8.0	9.0	10.0	11.0	12.0	13.0	14.0	15.0	16.0	17.0	18.0
PERCENTAGE OF FINAL LENGTH											
Boys	0.70	0.74	0.77	0.81	0.85	0.90	0.94	0.97	0.99	0.99	1.00
Girls	0.78	0.81	0.85	0.90	0.93	0.96	0.98	0.99	0.99	1.00	1.00

Calculated from data of Anderson, M. *et al.*: *J. Bone Joint Surg*. *45-A:* 1, 1963. Based on measurements of orthoroentgenograms which include both proximal and distal epiphyses. An average of 71 percent of femoral growth occurs at its lower end and 57 percent of tibial growth occurs at its upper end. Note correspondence of percentage of long-bone growth to percentage of whole-body growth at a given bone age. (Table 142-6).

and certain primordial dwarfs.[104,185] This suggests that bone, too, is endowed with a subnormal population of cells in these disorders. On the other hand, experimental data indicate that fetal malnutrition retards growth in both cell number and cell size. Cell number is particularly vulnerable to insult relatively early in the critical periods of organ development.[12] The extent to which subnormal endowment in cell number is related to the capacity for "catch-up" growth remains to be determined. It seems unlikely that deficits in cell population are necessarily lasting, in light of the knowledge that maturational increases in this parameter occur. As a group, IUGR infants are hypermetabolic,[92] a finding probably most closely related to the relatively greater size of the high-energy-consuming organs, such as brain, compared to somatic size.[91] A high neonatal mortality rate is found in infants with IUGR.[186–188] To some extent this is due to associated serious congenital anomalies. In addition, another factor may be hypoglycemia, for which fetal malnutrition is an important predisposing element.[189,190]

Primordial (Congenital) Dwarfs Presenting With IUGR

Disorders of fetal linear growth result from genetic, chromosomal, infectious, drug-induced, and unknown causes. They are sometimes associated with disproportionate body segments or multiple nonskeletal anomalies, which are, in turn, important clues to the presence of true dwarfism.[191–197a]

Abnormal skeletal proportions with IUGR usually indicate that one is dealing with bone dysplasia as the cause of an intrinsic growth disorder. These generalized disturbances of bone and cartilage growth results in permanent dwarfism. Several of the osteochondrodystrophies are manifest at birth. Achondroplasia is the most frequent of these disorders. It is characterized by short-limbed dwarfism, narrowing of the spinal canal characteristically appreciated on anterior-posterior roentgenograms, broad metacarpals and phalanges, and a prominent, bossed forehead. Achondrogenesis and thanatrophic dwarfism are lethal disorders. Other dystrophies recognizable at birth are chondrodysplasia punctata (congenital stippled epiphyses) of the autosomal recessive and coumadin-induced[198] types, metatrophic dwarfism (in which body proportions change with development), diastrophic dwarfism ("twisted," in reference to the multiple joint contractures), chondroectodermal dysplasia (Ellis-van Creveld syndrome), some other forms of mesomelic dwarfism, asphyxiating thoracic dysplasias (Jeune and Jarcho-Levin types[197b]), spondyloepiphyseal dysplasia, spondylometaphyseal dysplasia,[197c] cleidocranial dysplasia (formerly termed a dysostosis until it was recognized that generalized bone changes develop with time), camptomelic ("bent") dwarfism and "nonlethal achondrogenesis."[199] The reader is referred to the above-referenced reviews, atlases, and books for comprehensive discussions of these disorders. It should be kept in mind that the terminology underwent a change in 1970 and that previously unrecognized dystrophies are described often.[199a] Most of these disorders have a characteristic hereditary pattern, and families should be counselled appropriately. Metabolic bone disease, such as hypophosphatasia, may cause IUGR with deformities.

Proportionate IUGR may indicate an intrinsic generalized growth disorder. This is particularly likely if there are craniofacial abnormalities or multiple congenital anomalies, but may be the case with few if any obvious stigmata.

Facial disproportion in a small newborn may be the only evidence of a serious congenital defect in skeletal growth. A facies characterized by upturned nostrils and upper lip suggests the Cornelia-de Lange syndrome if associated with confluent eyebrows, and the elfin facies syndrome with its predisposition to hypercalcemia if associated with aortic stenosis.[200] Micrognathia with microcephaly suggests Virchow-Seckel (bird-headed) or Bloom[201] (see "Delayed Growth," below) dwarfism. IUGR with pseudohydrocephalus (relatively normal-sized head with small face) is termed Russell dwarfism or, if asymmetry is present in addition, Silver dwarfism.

Table 142-8 gives examples of multiple nonskeletal anomaly syndromes in which proportionate dwarfism presents as IUGR.[202–206] Multiple congenital anomalies may be due to chromosomal abnormalities, genetic disorders, congenital infection, or exposure to teratogenic drugs. The recent development of chromosomal-banding techniques has led to the documentation of the basis of previously unrecognized birth defect syndromes.[207] Many multiple congenital anomaly syndromes of unknown causes may be explained upon improvement in techniques for examining chromosomes in fine detail. "New" genetic disorders are being de-

Table 142-8. Examples of Multiple Congenital Birth Defect Syndromes Characterized by Proportionate IUGR and Subsequent Intrinsic Growth Failure

Etiology	Common Features	Reference
Autosomal Trisomy		
D	mental retardation, congenital heart disease, 3rd branchial arch syndrome, foot and hand deformities, bilateral cleft palate and lip, microphthalmia, colobomata	200
E	mental retardation, congenital heart disease, foot and hand deformities, 3rd branchial arch anomaly	
Genetic		
Leprechaunism	congenital lipodystrophy, small and wizened face	196
Meiten's syndrome	flexion contractures, corneal opacity, nystagmus, mental retardation	201
Camptodactyly	flexion contractures, camptodactyly, pulmonary hypoplasia, hypertelorism	202
Congenital Infection		
Rubella	hepatosplenomegaly, thrombocytopenia, anemia, patent ductus arteriosus, catarract, deafness	203
Drugs		
Aminopterin	skull anomalies, foot anomalies, low and malformed ears	192
Hydantoin	mental retardation, seizures, terminal digit hypoplasia, hypertelorism	204

scribed frequently. Congenital rubella often leads to permanent growth retardation; about 50 percent of cases are below the 10th percentile in adulthood.[208] The severity of the growth failure in congenital rubella seems to correlate with onset of infection in very early gestation and persistence of infection postnatally.[205] Two or more minor malformations are sometimes clues to an occult major malformation. Although 14 percent of newborns have a single minor anomaly, only 0.8 percent have two minor malformations, and the latter group has a fivefold increased incidence of a major defect.[196] Smith has illustrated the most important of the minor defects: (1) eyes: epicanthal folds, slanting palpebral fissures, hypertelorism; (2) ears: auricular malformation, low-set-slanted; (3) hands and feet: abnormal creases, dermatoglyphics, nail shape, digit formation; (4) skin, hair, teeth dysplasias; (5) mouth: frenulum, palatal arch abnormalities; and (6) genitalia: "saddle" scrotum, hypoplasia of labia majora. Hypertelorism (Table 142-3), dematoglyphics, and abnormal ear position are quantifiable. A single or absent umblical artery has also been claimed to be a clue to serious congenital anomalies.[209–211]

IUGR with few, if any, obvious external abnormalities may also be associated with limited growth potential. Bone dysplasia may present in this fashion—e.g., tubular stenosis (Kenny's syndrome).[196] Turner's syndrome is well known to sometimes present in this manner. Congenital infection with cytomegalovirus may stunt growth-cell proliferation. It has been suspected that growth potential is limited in the case of maternal addiction to ethanol or heroin.[209,210] Whether the shortness of stature persists through puberty is open to question, but permanent short stature might be suspected in the case of opiates on the basis of the finding of subnormal cell numbers in several organs. On the other hand, the isolated retardation of linear growth resulting from tetracycline exposure is temporary.[212,213]

The prognosis for postnatal growth depends upon the specific diagnosis. The various atlases referenced at the beginning of this section are invaluable in this regard. In the absence of clear-cut objective criteria, one should not prognosticate about future dwarfism and development until the patient is old enough to permit a fairly accurate assessment of potential for adult height and other areas of interest—e.g., intellectual development. The difficulty in making an exact diagnosis in infants with these problems is reminiscent of the mid-century dialectic with respect to the diagnosis of mongolism (Down's syndrome). There was considerable dispute as to which physical findings were the most reliable diagnostic signs: simian creases? epicanthal folds?, etc. These disputes were laid to rest with the discovery that chromosome "21" excess was consistent, and that the phenotypic expression of the trisomy varied. Similarly, many atypical malformation syndromes may prove to represent the partial expression of some single genetic defect.[214] However, until the chemical basis for each form of dwarfism is known and testable, one must not prognosticate on the basis of a diagnosis made from criteria which are not clear-cut. It is also important to remember that in some cases with multiple malformations, particularly when there are cerebral or craniofacial anomalies, postnatal growth failure may not be due to an intrinsic defect in skeletal growth, but mediated by GH deficiency.[215–220]

Management requires attention to the basic underlying disorder. Prophylaxis is possible with respect to certain of these disorders—e.g., interdiction of teratogenic drugs, active immunization to prevent congenital rubella, and amniocentesis in women at risk to permit abortion of fetuses afflicted with Down's syndrome or other congenital metabolic errors detectable prior to 20 weeks' gestation.[221] Treatment is often only expectant and supportive. Genetic counselling should not be overlooked. Guidance and advice with respect to handling congenital malformations or the mental retardation so frequently associated are important aspects of care.

Fetal "Malnutrition"

Fetal malnutrition results from fetal, placental, and maternal disturbances. Many cases in which the newborn appears to be undernourished have no obvious cause. Fetal factors include multiple fetuses and inherent metabolic disorders. Evidence for malnutrition of twins is most clear in those sets in which there is marked discrepancy of size. This situation arises because of placental arteriovenous anastomoses. The smaller (donor) twin of such a parabiotic set has organ abnormalities characteristic of malnutrition.[27,222] Placental insufficiency (infarcts, etc.) and postmaturity are associated with fetal undernutrition. Maternal disorders resulting in fetal malnutrition include vascular disease, undernutrition, drug addiction, and various chronic diseases, including neuropsychiatric disorders.[11,22,223,224] The rare syndrome of neonatal diabetes mellitus[47,225,226] is associated with proportionate retardation of intrauterine weight and length.

The pathogenesis of fetal undergrowth in these diverse situations may prove to be quite different. The poor uterine perfusion of toxemia[227] is often assumed to stunt the fetus by simply limiting the supply of protein and calories. Levitsky and co-workers, however, reported metabolic differences between rats whose intrauterine growth had been stunted by different mechanisms. Insulin levels were higher in hypoglycemic pups born after uterine vascular insufficiency than in those born to malnourished mothers.[228] The IUGR of heroin addicts' babies cannot always be attributed to coincident undernutrition.[211] Fetal hypoinsulinism has been postulated to contribute to the growth failure of infants presenting with diabetes neonatally.[47]

Infants with fetal malnutrition tend to be short for gestational age if the insult begins early and is of long duration.[229] Maturation of enchondral and membranous bone is retarded in most cases.[60,230,231]

The prognosis for these small-for-gestational-age (SGA) infants requires consideration of three major parameters.

Growth. Data regarding this area are meager.[19,61,62,229] The mean growth of these infants in length and weight is inclined to proceed appropriately for their gestational age. Bone growth velocity is usually normal, too.[232] Since IUGR infants have a low mean birth length for gestational age, they tend to grow in the 3rd to 10th percentile postnally. Consequently, their length is less than that of truly premature infants of comparable birth weight at 1 yr, a tendency that persists at 10 yr of age. Since bone maturation of IUGR babies is retarded somewhat, it seems as if they tend to follow a "delayed" growth pattern and have the potential to reach a relatively average adult height (see below). It is interesting that about 40 percent of the very small (< 3rd percentile) have a supranormal rate of linear growth within the first 6 months of life, and one cannot predict on the basis of size at birth which infants will "catch up" in this manner. It has been suggested that insulin is involved in the catch-up growth of IUGR.[229a] Neonatal diabetics may achieve a normal length by 1 yr of age.[223,233]

Hypoglycemia. The incidence of neonatal hypoglycemia is higher in underweight than in normal-sized infants of comparable gestational age.[188] The pathogenesis and management of the hypoglycemia is discussed in Chapter 89. The outlook for the infant depends upon prompt recognition and proper management of this complication.

Intellectual Development. There is considerable current interest in the possibility that fetal malnutrition may impair subsequent intellectual development irreparably. Studies in experimental animals indicate cerebral weight and DNA to be significantly depressed not only in first-, but also in second-generation offspring of protein-deficient mothers.[234]

Whether a comparable situation occurs in humans is open to question.[156] A 300-g discrepancy in birth weight of monozygotic twins reportedly leads to a significant 5-point disparity in IQ scores.[235] There is no doubt that placental insufficiency is associated with a high incidence of subsequent frank neurologic abnormalities in the affected infants.[236] The brain damage is not necessarily attributable to antenatal lack of foodstuffs; it may be partially due to neonatal hypoglycemia.

The treatment of fetal malnutrition is preventive with respect to maternal health care. This requires optimal nutritional provisions and attention to proper treatment of underlying maternal diseases. The infant born small for gestational age should likewise be provided an optimal diet. Early feeding may prevent neonatal hypoglycemia.[237] If hypoglycemia occurs, it must be treated promptly. It is important not to mislabel these infants as "dwarfs" because of an unusual facies or head size. About half of the IUGR infants who follow a delayed growth pattern postnatally respond to hGH therapy in replacement doses in spite of seemingly normal GH reserve.[238] There are no means of predicting which patients will benefit. The positive responses are not as great or sustained as those of hyposomatotrophic dwarfs. If the supply of hGH were not limited, this treatment would deserve further evaluation.

CONGENITAL OVERGROWTH

Hyperinsulinism is characteristic of most syndromes of fetal overgrowth. Infants of diabetic mothers become overweight unless there is placental insufficiency. This is because of increased adiposity and enlargement of certain organs, particularly the liver and heart, where cell hypertrophy predominates over hyperplasia. Length is increased to a lesser extent than weight. Brain growth is usually normal. Fetal hyperinsulinism seems to be the key factor in the overgrowth. There is also a correlation with maternal obesity.[239] Infants of prediabetic mothers are similarly affected, but usually less severely.[240–242] Treatment has been discussed in Chapter 86. Erythroblastosis fetalis infants are also hyperinsulinemic. It has been suggested that β cells become hyperplastic in response to inactivation of insulin by the placenta[243] or by products of hemolysis.[244] Hyperinsulinism and hypoglycemia correlate with severity of the anemia. However, the overweight of the erythroblastic fetuses seems mostly attributable to the development of edema.[245] Treatment is not only directed at the hypoglycemia, as for infants of diabetic mothers, but toward alleviating the perinatal hyperbilirubinemia and anemia. Infants with the Beckwith-Wiedemann syndrome resemble the overgrown infants of diabetic mothers in general appearance, but have several congenital anomalies.[246–250] Gigantism is not necessarily present at birth. The most consistent external features are macroglossia and umbilical abnormalities (ranging from hernia to omphalocele). Microcephaly occurs in at least 25 percent of cases. Occasionally there is hemihypertrophy. Most patients are probably hyperinsulinemic. Glucagon deficiency has been suspected on occasion.[251] However, hyperplasia of various visceral (kidney) and endocrine organs (pancreas, adrenal fetal cortex and medulla, pituitary amphophils, gonadal interstitial cells) is the rule, and there is a high incidence of postnatal intraabdominal tumor development. The disorder has occurred in sibships, so is thought to be hereditary (autosomal recessive). Growth during childhood is usually rapid, and accompanied by an accelerated bone age. In treating these patients, a major effort must be directed toward detection and vigorous treatment of hypoglycemia; the hypoglycemia tendency tends to regress within 4 months. Surgery may be required for the umbilical abnormality or macroglossia. Observation for tumors and supportive counselling are important thereafter. A lethal "variant" of the syndrome has been described in which there are no umbilical anomalies.[252]

The only other fetal overgrowth syndromes have been reported to have high plasma levels of branched-chain amino acids.[253,254] Cerebral gigantism (Soto's syndrome) is characterized by the presence of acromegalic features and cerebral dysfunction (usually mild mental retardation and dilated ventricular system), but normal GH levels and dynamics. Most are large at birth, all grow rapidly in early childhood though bone age is normal, yet only a few can be expected to achieve an excessive adult height. The disorder has been reported in concordant monozygotic twins.[255] Management is confined to supportive counselling. Weaver *et al.* reported 2 unrelated male infants with rapid linear growth, characteristic facies, and multiple contractures.[254] Their bone age was disproportionately advanced and long bone modelling seemed disturbed, with splaying of the distal femurs.

The neonatal mortality of babies inappropriately large for gestational age is quite high.[256] This problem seems to reflect the fact that this group includes infants of diabetic mothers and infants with severe hemolytic disease of the newborn. When these disorders are excluded from consideration, the risks to the overweight baby are increased only modestly.[186]

DISORDERS OF POSTNATAL GROWTH

PRIMARY DISTURBANCES OF GENERALIZED LINEAR GROWTH

Linear Growth Retardation

Classification. Primary disturbances of linear growth result from aberrations of inherent bone growth or of the extrinsic factors which affect the rate of bone development. The latter perturbations may be permanent, requiring treatment, or may have been temporary, the insult having regressed prior to the time medical consultation is sought. Hence, these growth-retarding disturbances fall into three categories, according to the relationship between chronologic age, height age, bone age, and growth rate (Table 142-9).[257,258] The table indicates that a 9-yr-old child with a height age of 6 and a bone age of 9 will be small as an adult. Since his bone age is normal, linear growth has almost certainly occurred at a normal rate. On the other hand, a 9-yr-old of the same size (HA = 6) with a bone age of 6 typically has a normal growth potential, but may or may not haye grown at a normal rate.

The nosology used here is somewhat different than that which is widely used. This has been done in an attempt to clarify and simplify the nomenclature because the author has found that the common terminology is confusing to students and many physicians. *Intrinsically small-boned* individuals have been frequently called "genetic" or "primordial" (congenital) dwarfs. These latter terms are misleading for two reasons. First, the genetic or familial basis may not be obvious, and other growth disorders may be familial. Secondly, not all are truly dwarfed. *Arrested growth* is the term applied to characterize individuals with a subnormal growth rate to emphasize their normal growth potential. A growth rate less than 50 percent of normal is due to endocrine, metabolic, or severe

Table 142-9. Classification of Causes of Short Stature

Diagnostic Category	BA[a]	Growth Rate	Abbreviated Differential Diagnosis
Intrinsic shortness	~CA	normal	chromosomal & genetic abnormalities, bone dysplasias, primordial dwarfs, familial
Arrested growth	~HA	subnormal	hyposomatotrophism, hypothyroidism, Cushing's syndrome, pH disturbance, hypoalbuminemia, severe malnutrition, severe systemic disease
Delayed growth	~HA	normal	variation of normal, undernutrition, hypoxia, hypophosphatemia, chronic illness, drugs

[a]BA: bone age; CA: chronologic age; HA: height age.

systemic disease until proven otherwise. *Delayed growth* is the term applied to the situation in which a child with a retarded bone age grows at a normal rate. This growth pattern commonly occurs as a variation of normal, often with a family precedent of similar development, a situation commonly termed "constitutional growth retardation." The author objects to this latter terminology because it conveys no clear meaning as to the situation. The overall maturation of individuals with this growth pattern seems to have been set back at a critical period in infancy or antenatally, but continues at a normal pace thereafter. These children's height-attained curves lay below but virtually parallel to the 3rd percentile, and their bone ages advance at a normal rate after about 2 yr of age. Our terminology has been chosen to emphasize that such a person's growth potential is normal and spontaneously achieved. Delay in the onset of puberty, the pubertal growth spurt, and the attainment of adult stature are inherent parts of this growth pattern.

Diagnosis and Therapy of Specific Disorders: Intrinsic Shortness. Intrinsic disorders of bone growth are usually congenital, though the patients may not display the disorder until after birth. Children with these problems usually grow below but parallel to the normal height-attained percentiles (Fig. 142-17). Most such patients simply have a short parent and are otherwise normal.

Examples of intrinsic dwarfism with associated defects are given in Table 142-10.[259–271] A chromosomal defect is found in less than 10 percent of patients with multiple congenital malformations; however, this estimate may change as karyotyping techniques improve. Growth retardation and cerebral dysfunction are the most characteristic features of autosomal aneuploidy. Thyroid autoimmunity has been reported to be a factor predisposing toward chromosomal nondisjunction, the event underlying these disorders.[272] Down's syndrome (trisomy 21 and variants thereof) is the most common multiple malformation syndrome in man. The growth impairment is slightly more pronounced in the lower extremities than in the trunk.[273]

The most characteristic features of Turner's syndrome are short stature and gonadal dysgenesis (Table 142-11).[274–287] Shortness is a more consistent finding in those patients who lack genetic material on the short arm of X that is gonadal failure.[275,288] Consequently, all girls with intrinsic short stature must be considered to have Turner's syndrome until proven otherwise; a normal buccal smear is not an adequate assurance of normalcy in this regard. Mild intrauterine growth retardation occurs sometimes. Growth arrest becomes apparent in the teenage years due to hypogonadism. Although a growth spurt can be induced by sex hormone therapy (see below), a final height of only about 58 inches can be expected.[123]

One of the most perplexing problems in the classification of syndromes of intrinsic short stature is that of the Noonan syndrome. This term has been used interchangeably with "male Turner syndrome" because only a small number (probably less than 20 percent) of males with the Turner phenotype have a sex chromosomal abnormality. At present the author feels it is best to apply the term "Noonan" to those patients of either sex with normal external genitalia who have a Turner-like phenotype but whose sex chromosomes are normal. The Noonan syndrome may be transmitted as an autosomal dominant disorder; partial deletion of a 6–12 autosome has been reported once.[281] "Turner's" syndrome is reserved for those individuals with abnormal sex chromosomes. Although the anomalies may be identical in many patients with their syndrome and though chromosomal mosaicism has not been thoroughly ruled out in most patients with the Noonan syndrome, the genetics and overall incidence of certain malformations (Table 142-11) are different. Consequently, the terminology proposed here is a practical one on which to prognosticate. Patients so classified as having Noonan's syndrome have a better prognosis for gonadal function and height than those with Turner's syndrome.

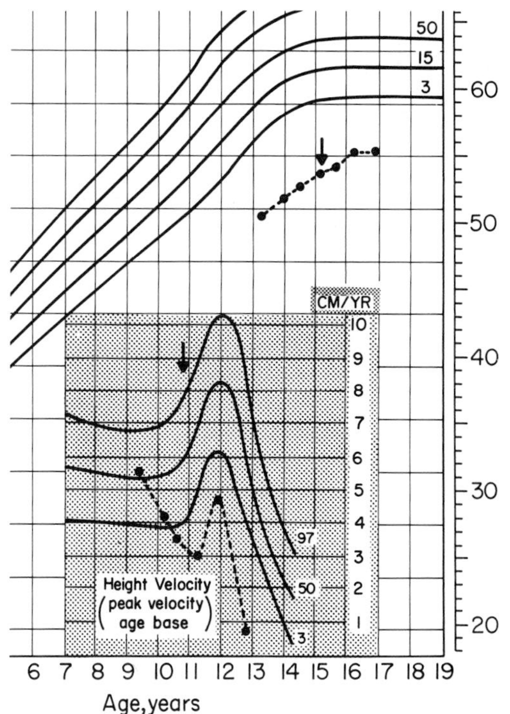

Fig. 142-17. Growth pattern of patient with Turner's syndrome. Note typically normal growth rate, below but parallel to third percentile for height attained in the early teenage years followed by deceleration and arrest of bone maturation in the mid-teens. Arrow indicates the start of estrogen treatment; this therapy is followed by a transient growth spurt.

Table 142-10. Examples of Congenital Multisystem Disorders Giving Rise to Intrinsic Dwarfism of Postnatal Onset

Syndromes	Common Associated Features	References
Chromosomal		
Trisomy 21 (Down)	characteristic facies, hypotonia, mental retardation	196
Turner	high palate, gonadal dysgenesis	259
Calcium-phosphorus disturbance		
pseudohypoparathyroidism (Albright dysostosis)	mental retardation, brachydactyly	196
Genital abnormalities		
Smith-Lemli-Opitz	male pseudohermaphroditism, microcephaly, characteristic facies, syndactyly	260, 261
Aarskog	scrotal anomalies, cryptorchidism, characteristic facies, hand webbing	262, 263
Mucopolysaccharidoses		264
Osteochondrodystrophies and dysostoses		191–197
Premature senility		
progeria (Hutchinson-Gilford)	onset in infancy, facies characteristic, arteriosclerosis, lipodystrophy (generalized), mental retardation	265
Cockayne	onset in early childhood, lipodystrophy (generalized), retinitis pigmentosa, photosensitivity, mental retardation, microcephaly	196
Werner	onset in late childhood, facies characteristic, atherosclerosis, catarract	266
Skin ± hair defects		
poikiloderma congenita (Rothmund-Thomson)	telangiectasia, skin dysplasia, catarract	267
Passwell	ichthyosis, poikiloderma, mental retardation	268
Sjögren-Larsson	ichthyosis, spasticity	269
Contractures		
Freeman-Sheldon	"whistling face", finger contractures, clubfeet	270
Winchester	"claw hands", osteolysis, catarracts	271
Moore-Federman	joint limitation, short limbs	196

Other endocrine disorders may be associated with intrinsic short stature. Restoration of calcium balance does not correct the short stature of patients with pseudohypoparathyroidism. Male genital abnormalities are accompanied by the development of short stature in the syndromes of Robinow, Smith-Lemli-Opitz, and Aarskog, and with aneuploidy of certain autosomes.[205] In the Robinow syndrome (mesomelia, penile hypoplasia, and hemivertebrae),[199a] the mesomelia is present at birth, yet overall length may be within normal limits. In the latter syndromes, the dwarfism is sometimes manifested as IUGR.

The mucopolysaccharide storage diseases are characterized by various combinations of skeletal and joint deformity, mental deterioration, corneal clouding, deafness, and hepatosplenomegaly. The osteochondrodystrophies are almost all associated with short stature. Such dystrophies are the major cause of obviously disproportionate dwarfism. However, some of these disorders have only subtle deformity (e.g., dyschondrosteosis), no deformities [e.g., tubular stenosis (see above)], or the skeletal abnormality or malformation makes its appearance only gradually (e.g., spondyloepiphyseal dysplasia tarda and rhinotrichophalangeal syndrome). The dysostoses (malformations of single bones, singly or in combination) are not usually accompanied by intrinsic short stature. There are exceptions to this generalization, as in the brachydactyly type E, Weill-Marchesani, and Rubenstein-Taybi syndromes. In some malformation syndromes, [289–291] insufficient data is available to deduce whether the short stature is intrinsic or has an endocrine basis—for example, GH deficiency as has been described in Fanconi anemia.[292] Abnormalities of cellular growth in vitro have been noted in some types of primordial dwarfs, particularly those characterized by a prematurely senile appearance. The decreased growth of isolated cells from patients with progeria[293] may be attributable to deficient repair of DNA chains of unknown cause.[294,295] A decreased rate of mitotic division of fibroblasts from patients with Werner's syndrome has also been noted (see Chapter 151).[266] Generalized, symmetric chromosomal instability has been found in Bloom's syndrome (see above); recent evidence suggests a defect in DNA chain growth.[295,296] The development of skin, hair, or joint abnormalities is common to several of the congenital syndromes of intrinsic growth failure in the absence of skeletal dysplasia. In addition, defects of these structures may occur in association with dystrophic disorders of bone (e.g., McKusick's metaphyseal chondrodysplasia, Epstein's syndrome).[297]

Arrest of linear growth by extensive bone irradiation is discussed below.

The proper management of these disorders requires specific diagnosis. The various atlases referenced above are invaluable in this regard. It has been estimated that in only about half the patients with multiple defects has a pattern or cause been discerned.[196] As is the case with IUGR, "new" disorders are being delineated regularly,[205,298–300] and further advances in this area can be expected, as discussed above. Genetic counselling is indicated for the hereditary aspects of these disorders. Guidance must be given in the management of associated abnormalities and psychosocial problems. Attention must be directed toward treatment of associated endocrine or metabolic disease. Frankness as to the prognosis for ultimate height is the best course to follow. Dwarfed

Table 142-11. Approximate Percentage Incidence of Selected Abnormalities in the Turner and Noonan Syndromes[a]

Abnormality	Turner's Syndrome[259,274–278]	Noonan's Syndrome[280–284]
1. Short stature (<10%)	100/80?[b]	90/90
2. Gonadal failure	99/85?	≦10/≦10[c]
3. Cryptorchidism	NA/33[d]	NA/50
4. Hypertelorism[e]	<25†	100
5. High palate	80	75
6. Neck webbed	50	10
7. Neck short	68	100
8. Cubitus valgus	68	30
9. Chest deformity[f]	50	50
10. Coarctation of aorta	20	<1
11. Pulmonic stenosis	10	50[g]
12. Mental retardation	10[h]	25
13. Pigmented moles, multiple	50	<10

[a]Defined on the basis of presence (Turner) or absence (Noonan) of sex-chromosome abnormality. The Turner syndrome in the female results from the deletion of genetic material on the short arm of the X-chromosome. Various sex chromosomal abnormalities have been reported in Turner syndrome in the male—e.g., XO, XXY, XO/XY, XO/XY/XYY, XX_i/XXY_r. Malignant hyperpyrexia has only been reported in the Noonan syndrome.[285]
[b]Female/male.
[c]The distinction between delayed puberty and hypogonadism has seldom been made.[286]
[d]Not applicable.
[e]Hypertelorism is not mentioned in four large series of cases of the Turner syndrome.[259,274–276] However, it has been reported in 25 percent of one large series in which it was mentioned[277] and in 33–44 percent of the chromatin-negative patients with congenital heart disease.[280]
[f]Chest deformity: pectus or apparent increase in internipple distance.[287]
[g]The high incidence of congenital heart disease in Noonan's syndrome may be due to ascertainment, Dr. Noonan being a cardiologist. A variety of other congenital heart defects have been reported in both syndromes.
[h]Males seem to have a greater incidence of mental retardation, though this may be a matter of ascertainment.

children tend to be treated as babies or mascots. These children need advice in means of projecting their age and maturity.[301]

There is no therapy that will clearly improve the ultimate height of children with intrinsic growth disorders. Treatment with low doses of androgens or androgen derivatives for 6-month periods has been recommended by some:[176,302–305] Δ^1-17 α-methyltestosterone (Dianabol®), 0.02 to 0.03 mg/kg/day; oxandrolone, 2-oxo-17 α-methyldihydrotestosterone (Anavar), 0.075 to 0.125 mg/kg/day; and 9 α-fluoro-11 β-hydroxy-17 α methyltestosterone (Halotestin), 2.5 mg/day, and methyltestosterone 5 mg/day have been most widely used. Virilization is unusual under these conditions. Some children so treated evidence an improvement in predicted height as great as the largest spontaneous shifts in untreated children; in others, predicted height falls. It would seem that generally these agents temporarily accelerate the growth rate such that the child reaches his ultimate height sooner. At least a 6-month period must elapse after each course of therapy before the effect of therapy on predicted height can be judged. The risk of deleteriously affecting adult height may be greater if treatment is begun before 9 yr. Human GH in pharmacologic doses (5 U/day im) increases the rate of growth in many nonhypopituitary dwarfs.[306,307] Growth is proportionate at this dose, but glucose intolerance may develop. If plentiful supplies of very pure GH, GH-releasing factor, or somatomedin become available, further trials of such therapy are warranted.

Arrested growth. This growth pattern can almost always be proven to result from endocrine, metabolic, or severe systemic disease. A sustained growth rate of less than 50 percent of the 3rd percentile is clearly abnormal. Intermediate rates of growth are abnormal if the child deviates further and further below the 3rd percentile on height-attained standards.

Deficiency of growth hormone (GH) production or action causes the most subtle presentation of any growth disorder because the child may be normal in every respect but growth. GH deficiency in "hypopituitarism" seems usually to arise from hypothalamic dysfunction rather than pituitary disease.[111] Most cases detected after referral for unexplained growth retardation are idiopathic and represent a monotropic GH deficit.[258] The second most common cause of GH deficiency is a tumor in the region of the hypothalamus and adenohypophysis and/or its treatment. GH deficiency may also arise congenitally. Congenital hyposomatotrophism may arise on a hereditary basis or in association with congenital anomalies (see previous section), particularly, but not exclusively those affecting the development of the brain or midline craniofacial structures. The significance of the abnormalities of GH release observed in patients with simple microcephaly or mental retardation and growth failure remains to be better defined.[218,219,308] GH deficiency may also be acquired on the basis of trauma, infection, neoplasm, irradiation, or cerebrovascular disease. Acquired hypopituitarism is sometimes functional. Functional hypopituitarism is potentially reversible with improvement in the psychosocial environment. This situation was originally described in severely disturbed children who had been emotionally deprived and who were from homes with abnormal parental interaction.[309] The author's experience suggests that children with this disorder may not be overtly disturbed. In most such patients GH secretion in response to many stimuli is subnormal promptly upon hospital admission, but may be normal subsequently.[310–312] Selective hypothalamic dysfunction or malnutrition may explain the growth failure in the latter group of patients. Defects in ACTH and TSH release are occasionally found. Deficient GH action on a genetic basis may account for rare cases of otherwise inexplicable growth failure (Table 142-12). Laron-dwarfs (type III) have characteristic craniofacial disproportion. These dwarfs are clearly resistant to both endogenous and exogenous GH.[313–315] On the basis of the

Table 142-12. Characteristics of Isolated GH-Deficient and GH-Resistant States

Characteristic	Type of Dwarfism[a] Deficiency (I)	Laron (III)	Pygmy (IV)
GH levels and responses	low	high[b]	normal
Somatomedin levels	low	low	?
Insulin sensitivity	present	present	present
Insulinopenia[c]	+	+	+
Glucose tolerance	poor	variable	normal
Response to hGH therapy			
early:			
somatomedin level	normal	unchanged	normal
insulinopenia	responsive	unchanged	unchanged
free fatty acids[d]	responsive	responsive	responsive
growth	yes	subnormal	?

[a]Roman numerals refer to the classification of Merrimee and co-workers.[304] Type II, which resembles type I except for the presence of adult-type chemical diabetes, has not been definitively delineated in children.
[b]GH levels are usually (60%–85%) high and usually poorly suppressible by glucose.
[c]In response to arginine or glucose administration.
[d]A large dose of hGH may be required to demonstrate this.

evidence to date, it is most likely that these dwarfs lack the GH receptors involved in somatomedin generation and direct GH actions with the possible exception of lipolysis. African pygmies have been postulated to have GH resistance on less certain grounds. The most appealing theory is that they have selective end-organ resistance to somatomedin. Other theories invoked to explain certain features of both type-III and -IV dwarfism are production of a functionally abnormal GH or heterogeneity of GH and somatomedin receptors. Considerable research remains to be done to define these syndromes and their pathogensis.

The diagnosis of GH deficiency is more difficult than one might imagine. The GH level and response of normal children must be characterized in each laboratory because of differences in standards and radioimmunoassay techniques. Less than half of normal fasting children manifest a serum GH level indicative of normal GH reserve. About 10 percent of normal children will not respond to any single, "definitive" provocative test.[316] On the other hand, some GH-deficient patients may achieve normal serum GH levels in response to certain pharmacologic stimuli. For these reasons, the author's practice is to screen subjects for eusomatotrophism by a "clinical bioassay," the accurate recording of growth velocity over a 6- to 12-month period. If the growth rate is clearly normal, it is extremely unlikely that a GH deficit exists that will require replacement therapy. If the growth rate is marginal, screening tests for GH status may be useful, particularly if the results are clearly normal. If the growth velocity is inexplicably 50 percent or less of normal, definitive testing of GH dynamics is surely indicated. When the assay of serum somatomedin levels becomes refined and generally available, this may be the best diagnostic parameter.

The best screening tests are the fasting GH response to estrogen (e.g. diethylstilbesterol 5 mg bid for 3 days) and to exercise (to the point of moderate fatigue and breathlessness). About 70 percent of normals will respond to each of these tests. The latter procedure, in particular, has not been well standardized with regard to stimulus-response characteristics relative to definitive testing, or for the incidence of falsely positive responses in hyposomatotrophic children.

The "definitive" tests for children's GH status which are the most widely used are: the insulin tolerance test (ITT), L-dopa test (LDT), arginine tolerance test (ATT), and the glucagon tolerance test. Sleep testing may prove to be of great value.

The ITT is performed by administering 0.1 to 0.15 U/kg of regular insulin as an iv push, preferably diluted in a protein-containing solution such as Plasmanate. If the patient has a history compatible with spontaneous hypoglycemia, half this dose of insulin should be used. The LDT is probably best performed by acclimating the patient to the drug in doses of 0.25 g/1.73 m^2 tid with meals for 2 days, then testing the fasting patient's response to 0.5g/1.73 m^2.[111] The ATT is performed by infusing 0.5 g/kg iv over a 30-min period. Ingestion of a British high-protein broth (Bovril) gives similar results. Glucagon is administered intramuscularly in a dose of 0.5 to 1.0 mg 2 h after β-adrenergic blockade with 20 to 40 mg propranolol orally. Blood samples are collected at 15- to 30-min intervals for 2 to 3 h after administration of each of these test substances. Blood sampling at artibrary times after the onset of sleep yields about 70 percent positive responses in normal children; it is quite likely that systematic, frequent sampling throughout sleep, especially if correlated with sleep stages, would be more definitive.

The author prefers to initiate testing with the LDT for safety's sake and use the ITT or ATT if confirmation of the GH-deficient state is required. The diagnosis of GH deficiency can be made with about 99 percent confidence if the GH response is subnormal to two "definitive" tests. Normalcy of response is customarily based on consideration of the peak GH concentration at any time during the test, including the control specimen.

The reproducibility of these tests has not been thoroughly investigated. The GH response to a test may be depressed by glucose, obesity, or hypothyroidism. Poor GH release during the ITT cannot be interpreted if the blood sugar falls less than 40 to 50 percent. Glucose administration blocks the response to insulin and to L-dopa.[317] Puberty and the administration of estrogens or androgens enhance GH-responsitivity to provocative tests. Glucocorticoids in pharmacologic doses have variable and inconsistent effects on GH dynamics in children. The diagnosis of GH deficiency need not be made on an "all-or-none" basis. Incomplete cases have been described which have intermediate levels of GH in response to provocative tests;[111,318] such patients respond to "replacement" doses of HGH. The ATT and glucagon tests have on rare occasions yielded normal results in GH-deficient patients.[111,316,319]

Human GH (hGH) is the mainstay of treatment of hyposomatotrophic dwarfs.[320–321] GH from other species does not promote growth in man. hGH is extracted from pituitary glands obtained postmortem, and the limited supply has been distributed in the United States by the National Pituitary Agency, 210 West Fayette Street, Baltimore, Maryland. Recently hGH has been made available commercially under special conditions by Calbiochem (U.S.A.) and Kabi (Sweden). GH replacement therapy is usually initiated with 2 IU (about 0.11 IU/kg) im three times a week. An improved rate of growth on hGH therapy confirms the diagnosis. Ninety percent of children so treated will grow at least 5.0 cm during the 1st yr of therapy, and the growth will be proportionate (Fig. 142-18). Linear growth seems related to the log-dose of gHG. A fivefold increase in dose tends to increase growth by 50 percent and give a more consistent response.[321,322] Younger patients and completely GH-deficient patients tend to accelerate more rapidly. The nonresponders cannot necessarily be predicted from short-term studies of nitrogen balance, serum urea nitrogen, phosphorus, cholesterol, free fatty acids, glucose tolerance, calciuria, or hydroxyprolinuria.[323–325] The growth rate of responders wanes with time. This may be less of a problem with intermittant therapy.[326] Replacement treatment with hGH can be expected to normalize carbohydrate and fat metabolism as well as growth. In teenagers, hGH therapy is associated with accelerated pubertal development.[327,328] Potential deleterious effects of hGH therapy are hypothyroidism,[329,330] slipped femoral capital epiphysis or Legg-Perthe disease,[331–333] and, questionably, enlargement of preexisting tumors.[331] An inadequate growth rate developing in the course of therapy may be attributable to several factors[331]:

1. The hGH dose per unit size becomes inadequate.
2. The somatomedin response to hGH may decrease.
3. Significant antibody titers may develop. About 40 percent of patients treated with hGH develop antibodies; in less than 40 percent of these is the growth rate poor.[334] A high hGH binding capacity and high antibody affinity are poor prognostic factors. Therapy should be interrupted and another preparation of hGH administered when the antibody titer falls.[335,336]
4. TSH deficiency may gradually develop.[330]
5. Glucocorticoid therapy may interfere. Hyposomatotrophic children are unusually sensitive to the growth-inhibiting effects of these steroids. Therefore, these hormones should be replaced only if there are clinical

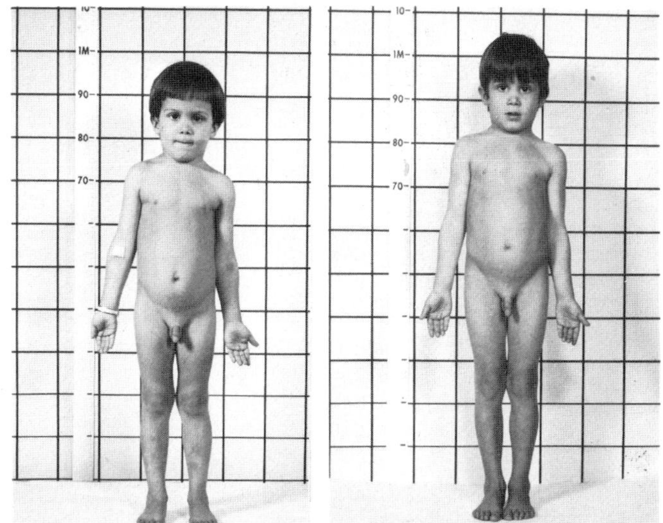

Fig. 142-18. Growth hormone-deficient patient before (left) and after (right) one year's treatment with hGH. Note that the growth spurt is accompanied by normal maturation of body proportions.

symptoms or signs of glucocorticoid deficiency, such as lethargy, cachexia, or hypoglycemia. If necessary, cortisol should be given in the lowest maintenance dose that will restore health, 5 to 20 mg/m²/day in 3 divided doses.[116,320,337]

6. Undernutrition.[338]
7. Improper administration of hGH, e.g., into a single injection site.

Ancillary treatment may be useful in enhancing the response to hGH. Thyroid hormone is necessary for growth, and its administration may promote growth even in the presence of normal free thyroxine levels.[329] Androgen derivatives in the "subandrogenic" doses discussed above may stimulate growth.[339,340] A preliminary report suggests that stimulation of appetite by cyproheptidine may promote growth.[341]

Retardation of bone maturation and linear growth is the most consistent feature of long-standing hypothyroidism. In only rare instances is the thyroid metabolic status not reflected in the free thyroxine (T_4) level.[31,329] The differential diagnosis and management of hypothyroidism are discussed in detail elsewhere (Chapter 33). Some comments about T4 dosage in children are in order here, however. The replacement dose of thyroid hormone in children is greater than one might expect on the basis of body size because fractional T4 turnover is greater in children than in adults.[169] Hence, the average replacement dose of L-thyroxine for infants is 10 μg/kg/day; this requirement gradually changes with growth to reach the adult level of 2.5 μg/kg/day.[341a–c] Dosage can be adjusted according to the serum level achieved. Quarter- or half-replacement is recommended for the initial therapy of long-standing hypothyroidism, where myxedema heart or latent adrenal insufficiency is suspected. The most frequent error in the treatment of childhood hypothyroidism is failure to adjust the dosage to a full replacement level prior to discharge from the hospital; infants lost to followup in the interim may sustain irreparable brain damage due to failure to increase T_4 dosage appropriately.

Glucocorticoid excess, whether due to spontaneous Cushing's syndrome or to therapeutic glucocorticoids, results in linear growth failure. Growth seems to be the most sensitive indicator of corticoid excess, for growth arrest may be the only clear clinical sign of Cushing's syndrome.[342] Diagnostic and therapeutic approaches to Cushing's syndrome are discussed in Chapter 95. Catch-up growth usually occurs after alleviation of the hypercortisolism.[68,343,344] The cause for failure of catch-up growth to occur in an occasional case is unclear. Mosier feels this is due to a subtle destructive effect of corticoids on the growth plate;[345] however, the failure of catch-up usually occurs in teen-agers. The extent to which age is the deciding factor is unknown. The potential for further growth and pubertal development if hypothalamo-pituitary function is preserved must be kept in mind when advising therapy for children with Cushing's syndrome. In cases due to adrenal hyperplasia, the author presently advises bilateral total adrenalectomy, unless there is evidence of a space-occupying mass in the region of the sella turcica. A transsphenoidal approach to pituitary tumors is preferred in the hope of best preserving function of uninvolved pituitary tissue. Too little is known about the effects of hypothalamo-pituitary irradiation on GH and gonadotropin regulation to warrant subjecting children to x-ray therapy unnecessarily. In cases in which growth failure accompanies glucocorticoid therapy of serious nonendocrine disease, it may be difficult to decide whether the growth problem is due to the disease or the steroid. Over 45 mg/m²/day of cortisone acetate usually inhibits growth.[116] The decision about steroid dose is particularly difficult since the relationship between steroid analog dose and the inhibitory effects of the steroid on growth, ACTH release, and inflammation do not seem to be proportionate. For example, prednisone seems to suppress growth in doses half as great as those required for suppression of ACTH[346] and inflammation.[347] Furthermore, there are individual differences in steroid metabolism which influence the degree of steroid side-effects.[339] If it is necessary to document the fact that the patient's steroid dose is excessive, it is the author's practice to determine the plasma dehydroepiandrosterone sulfate level and/or the response to metyrapone. Evidence of subnormal adrenocortical function is taken as evidence that the patient's therapeutic steroid dose is supraphysiologic.

In cases in which growth inhibition is attributable to glucocorticoid treatment of nonendocrine disease, there are three possible alternatives: (1) Use another form of therapy. (2) Lower the daily steroid dose if the underlying disease can be so controlled. (3) Switch the patient to alternate *morning* prednisone therapy.[349] "Alternate-day" administration of prednisone often results in preservation of the desired therapeutic effect while avoiding the unwanted cushingoid changes.

Several generalized metabolic disturbances retard growth. Any chronic disturbance of pH retards growth. Alkalosis arrests growth unless well controlled.[350] Acidosis, such as resulting from renal tubular disease, renal failure, disturbed aminoacid or lactate metabolism, and glycogen storage disease, causes growth retardation.[101,196,351,352] The situation in chronic renal failure is complex, with diminished somatomedin and vitamin D activity and undernutrition contributing to growth failure.[353–356] Hypoalbuminemia is a common thread in several diseases causing linear growth failure, such as regional enteritis (Fig. 142-19), liver disease, and nephrosis.[73,357,358] However, hypoalbuminemia may be only a marker because available data, admittedly meager, suggests that hereditary analbuminemia is not characterized by growth failure.[359] Poor control of diabetes mellitus may result in dwarfism with hepatomegaly (Mauriac's syndrome).[360]

Severe malnutrition as in kwashiorkor and marasmus or deficiency of an essential amino acid (as discussed above) clearly diminished growth velocity. The mechanism whereby growth failure comes about in starvation seems to be complex: somatomedin-GH homeostasis,[105,361] triiodothyronine production,[362,362a] vita-

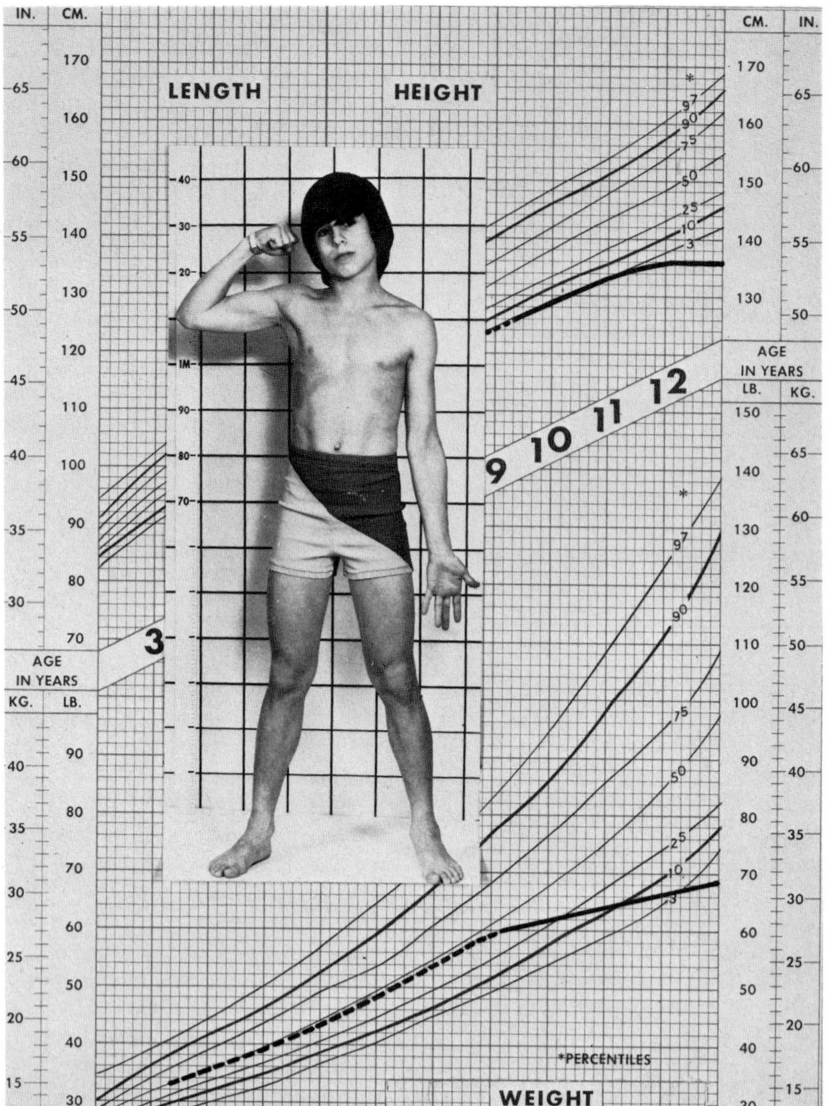

Fig. 142-19. D. T., UC# 779037-1. Picture at 13 yr of age at the time of referral for short stature and delayed puberty. Growth records show plateauing of weight commencing around 9 yr of age, of height 1 to 2 yr later. The data are plotted on the normal standards of Stuart and Meredith.[126] The history was unremarkable except for some vague abdominal cramps and loose stools. The photograph shows his seemingly good health, nutritional status, and excellent musculature, in keeping with his interest in competitive swimming. Examination revealed no clear-cut findings. Serum albumin was 3.05, globulin 3.65 g/dl. He was proved to have regional enteritis.

min[363] and mineral balance,[99,100] and probably insulin production may be disturbed. Congenital copper deficiency causes failure to thrive, mental deterioration, kinky hair, and bone changes.[364]

Severe chronic disease, such as juvenile rheumatoid arthritis, may halt growth through undetermined mechanisms.[365]

On some occasions, preadolescent growth deceleration may be the first indication of an intrinsic growth disorder, such as Turner's syndrome[366] or spondyloepiphyseal dysplasia tarda.[367] Determination of the bone age will permit recognition of the intrinsic nature of these problems; this criterion becomes more reliable in the second decade. On the other hand, growth arrest may result from disorders that usually manifest themselves as *delays* in growth, as in hypophosphatemia. Virtually complete growth failure will ensue in gonadal dysgenesis patients once the bone age reaches about 14 yr unless sex hormones are administered.[368]

With the exception of hyposomatotrophism, the nature of the disorder causing arrested growth will usually be obvious from a carefully taken medical history and thorough examination and/or determination of certain tests readily available from most routine laboratories: serum thyroxine, electrolytes, calcium, phosphorus, urea nitrogen, albumin, globulin, complete blood count, erythrocyte sedimentation rate, and urinalysis. Treatment must be directed toward the underlying disease. Acidosis should be treated with sodium bicarbonate and/or potassium citrate solutions; alkalosis with potassium chloride and possibly spironolactone or triampterine. Dihydrotachysterol in doses of about 0.25 to 0.75 mg is the agent of choice in the therapy of renal osteodystrophy. The prognosis depends on the basic disease and the degree of malnutrition.

Delayed Growth and Development. This growth pattern usually occurs as a variation of normal, but may result from ongoing health disturbances. Disease may be postulated to lead to this mode of growth in at least two different ways. First, an early and sustained 10-percent disturbance of linear growth rate can be calculated to lead to nearly 5 cm of growth retardation within the first 3 yr of life, but only about 2.5 cm of deviation from normal over the next 5 yr. Alternatively, undernutrition or unknown factors may prevent catch-up growth after alleviation of an insult to growth in early childhood.

A delayed growth pattern occurs far and away most commonly as a "constitutional" variation of normal. The typical child is perfectly healthy, and the course is one of normal birth size, deviation into a growth channel below the 3rd percentile on distance-standards beginning at about 1 to 2 yr of age (Fig. 142-20), height and bone age advancement below but parallel to the 3rd percentile from about 2 yr of age, and delayed puberty and pubertal growth spurt, culminating in an average adult height. This condition is unusual in girls. There is often a history of a parent or close relative with a similar growth pattern; this information is useful in the management of the child's psychological outlook but should not be relied upon diagnostically. The diagnosis of constitutionally delayed growth is made if careful medical history, examination, and screening tests (complete blood count, erythrocyte sedimentation rate, urinalysis, serum electrolytes, calcium, phosphorus, urea nitrogen, and proteins) are nonrevealing. One study indicates that such children may be insulinopenic;[369] however, the study was uncontrolled for ethnic background and nutritional status. From the bone age, prediction can be made regarding the potential for adult height and the approximate time of onset of puberty. After the skeletal age has reached 10 yr, gonadotropin levels should be checked to determine if the patient's delayed puberty is due to primary hypogonadism. There is at present no means of reliably differentiating organic hypogonadotropism from delayed puberty until the patient is 18 yr old. If the tests are

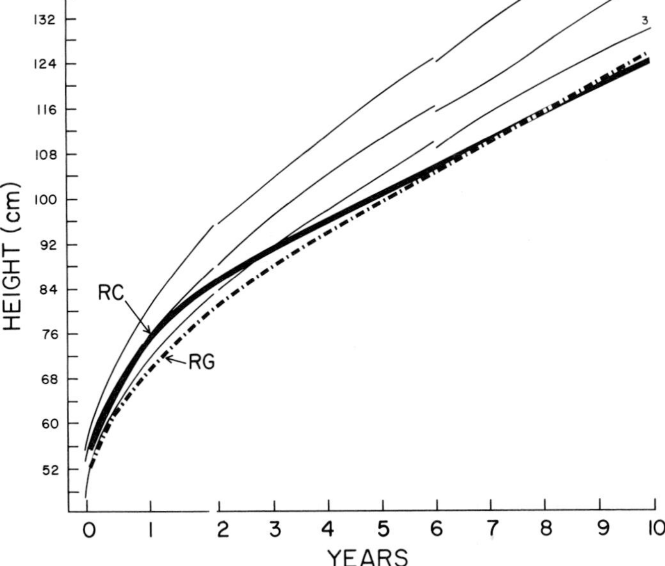

Fig. 142-20. Growth pattern in "constitutionally" delayed growth and development. Pediatrician's growth curves of 2 boys with constitutional delay of growth and development. Data are plotted in relation to the standards of Stuart and Meredith.[126] Note that diminished linear growth velocity began at about 1 to 2 yr of age. R. G., UC# 1206046, had a history of frequent upper respiratory tract infections from 7 to 15 months of age. R. C., UC# 1261844, had a concussion at 2 yr of age and occasional asthmatic attacks since; extensive testing revealed no evidence of endocrine, metabolic, or systemic disease. HIs father had a history of delayed puberty. Bone age of both boys was retarded 3.5 yr when first seen by the author at 9.5 to 10 yr of age.

normal, and the expectations for continued linear growth and pubertal development are not fulfilled, the child should be reevaluated.

The first step in managing a patient with delayed development is to reassure him as to his probable normalcy. He should also be assured that a pubertal growth spurt will surely occur, probably spontaneously. The wide normal variation in the pattern and timing of the pubertal spurt should be explained in detail, and he should be informed of his predicted ultimate height. Meanwhile, the psychologic state of the child should be considered. Amazingly, the majority of children with delayed puberty do not have overt psychologic symptoms. Obviously, complex compensations and sublimations occur. However, peer group pressures may make adjustment to shortness and sexual infantilism especially difficult for some by 13-or-so years.[370] A poor self-image may lead to social withdrawal and feelings of hopelessness in such children. Physical immaturity may prolong psychologic immaturity. A short course of sex hormone therapy may alleviate these anxieties. The treatment of short stature in preadolescents was already discussed. If puberty is delayed beyond 13 or 14 yr of age, the age at which 90 percent of girls and boys, respectively, have begun to mature, cautious sex hormone therapy may be considered. Before undertaking the induction of puberty, the child and his family must be warned of the possibility that adult-replacement doses of androgen and estrogen will cause a disproportionate advance of bone age relative to linear growth. Hence, they may lose as much as 2.5 cm in predicted height for each course of treatment. Those children who are more concerned with eventual height than immediate gains often choose to forego medical intervention at this point. In order to minimize the possibility of loss of growth potential, the author recommends that the initial course of therapy for the induction of sexual development consist of six monthly injections of 50 mg/m^2 repository testosterone in boys, 1 mg depot estradiol in girls. The patient's growth, development, and predicted height should be carefully reevaluated immediately upon completion of the therapeutic regimen and again 6 months later before undertaking a second course of therapy. Depot testosterone 100 to 150 mg/m^2/month and depot estradiol 1.5 to 2 mg/month closely approximate mid-pubertal sex hormone production in boys[130] and girls,[123] respectively. The author prefers to administer injections of repository forms of sex hormones to avoid the occasional side-effects of steroid analogs and to avoid the frequent injections necessary if chorionic gonadotropin is used for puberty induction. Thyroid hormone is a controversial, though relatively benign, mode of treatment of constitutionally delayed growth.[371] Hypothyroidism has been documented in the presence of normal free thyroxine and triiodothyronine levels.[329] If treatment is to be undertaken, the following precautions seem necessary to avoid prolonged unnecessary dependence on the hormone: (1) control observations for two consecutive 6-month periods, and (2) observation for the height acceleration and transient weight loss characteristic of the juvenile hypothyroidal patient's response to replacement therapy 3 and 6 months after treatment is begun.

Prolonged undernutrition is associated with a delayed growth pattern. In a cross-sectional survey of apparently healthy Denver children, most who were zinc-deficient were found to be short.[372] However, we have not found zinc deficiency in 12 children with constitutional delay in growth.[372a] A study of monozygotic twins discordant for diabetes mellitus has revealed a growth-retarding effect of this disease.[373]

Tissue hypoxia causes a delayed growth pattern. This is the case in chronic anemia[374] and congenital heart disease.[375,376] Whether poor tissue perfusion mediates the growth retardation of patients with left-to-right shunts is unknown; correction of the shunt before 8 yr of age results in catch-up growth if there are no complicating factors.[377] Other factors have also been implicated in the growth retardation of children with congenital heart disease: intrinsic intrauterine dwardism, malnutrition, and hypoinsulinism.[376,378]

Rickets causes a delayed growth pattern. Several lines of evidence indicate that the growth retardation is a consequence of the hypophosphatemia.[379–381] For example, vitamin D therapy may heal resistent rickets, but the growth rate will not improve unless phosphate supplementation is given as well.

Chronic illness of a variety of organ systems may cause growth retardation, particularly among whose who are socioeconomically disadvantaged.[73] The mechanisms of growth failure in these circumstances are not clear. Prolonged usage of stimulant drugs for the therapy of hyperactive children may be associated with reversible retardation of growth.[382] Dextroamphetamine reportedly causes a change of about 4 centiles yearly; methylphenidate (Ritalin) seems to affect growth only in doses over 20 mg daily. The extent to which the postulated effect of these drugs is mediated via their anorectic action or via depletion of hypothalamic neurotransmitters by displacement is unknown. The average size of mentally defective children is moderately less than normal.[273] The possibility is great that this is due to inclusion of patients with unrecognized chromosomal, endocrine, metabolic, and nutritional disorders.

Excessive Linear Growth

Classification. Supranormal height occurs either because of inherent endowment or a persistently excessive rate of bone growth. Growth-promoting disturbances fall into three categories (Table 142-13). Intrinsic tallness is characterized by a normal bone age. Intrinsically tall people are literally "large-boned." The height-attained plot of these individuals parallels the 97th percentile but is above it. Both pituitary gigantism and advanced growth patterns are characterized by supranormal growth velocity. In pituitary gigantism, the bone age is normal; hence adult height is predictably great. "Advanced growth" is the term applied here to the growth pattern in which the linear growth spurt is accompanied by an advanced skeletal age. Subjects with this latter growth pattern do not have an excessive predicted adult height, and puberty usually occurs at an early age. The initial diagnostic procedures used in approaching the case of a child with supranormal height are those used in approaching the problem of linear growth retardation. One can go a long way toward reaching a proper diagnosis by simply examining the relationship between CA, HA, BA, and growth rate (Table 142-13).

Diagnosis and Therapy of Specific Disorders. Intrinsic tallness. This growth pattern usually occurs as a "constitutional" variation

Table 142-13. Classification of Excessive Height

Diagnostic Category	BA	Growth Rate	Abbreviated Differential Diagnosis
intrinsic tallness	≅CA	normal	familial, marfanoid syndromes
pituitary gigantism	≅CA	supranormal	GH excess
advanced growth	≅HA	supranormal	variation of normal, sex precocity, hyperthyroidism, lipodystrophy, infant giants

of normal in families of above-average stature. An above-average height is often a social disadvantage for girls, but rarely one for boys. Consequently, females frequently present to endocrinologists seeking treatment for what they consider to be "excessive" height. The medical evaluation should include judgement of the patient's personality, psychosocial status, posture, outlook if nature is allowed to take its course, and expectations of therapy. In some cases, inordinate concerns about height may be but one aspect of a major adolescent adjustment reaction. From determination of skeletal age, one can get considerable diagnostic information and predict adult height. Many tall girls will not wish to undertake treatment when they find out their ultimate height will "only" be 6 feet. It is the author's policy to consider the possibility of therapy for girls whose predicted adult height is in the range of 6 feet or more. The essence of therapy is high-dose estrogen which produces premature epiphysial closure. The pros and cons of treatment are frankly discussed. Therapy induces rapid feminization and, sometimes, an early acceleration of growth. The therapeutic regimen outlined below is reported to reduce ultimate height by 3 to 6.5 inches if the girl's bone age is 11 yr.[383,384] Others report less height reduction in such patients;[385,386] whether this discrepancy is due to differences in estrogen dosage or differences in bone age interpretation is unknown. Later institution of treatment leads to less striking results. No significant effect is demonstrable once the skeletal age is over 13 yr. The risks are the inherent errors in predicting height (Table 142-3), the known exceptional complications of large doses of estrogen (thrombophlebitis, jaundice, etc.), and the unknown possible complications. Regarding the latter, it must be kept in mind that there are no large follow-up studies of the incidence of ovarian cysts, "post-pill amenorrhea," vaginal cancer, etc., in females so treated.[387] Treatment consists of high-dose estrogen (e.g., 10 to 15 mg of Premarin[R]) daily and continuously until epiphyseal fusion is complete. It is best to acclimate the patient to the estrogen by commencing with one-quarter to one-sixth of the full dose, and increasing this gradually over a 4- to 6-week period. A progestin is added cyclically to normalize the endometrial cycle; 10 mg medroxyprogesterone acetate for 5 days monthly brings about withdrawal bleeding in the face of continuous estrogen administration. Boys have been treated for "excessive" height with repository testosterone in doses of 200 mg or more every 2 weeks.[388]

The differenital diagnosis of inherent tallness includes the marfanoid syndromes (long extremities, tendency toward scoliosis): Marfan syndrome proper, homocystinuria, and the type-2 polyendocrine syndrome. The true Marfan syndrome is characterized by joint hypotonia, scoliosis, dislocation of lenses, aortic aneurysm, and mitral regurgitation in the full-blown state.[389] Fibroblasts from such patients are known to accumulate excessive amounts of hyaluronic acid in tissue culture.[390] Until the nature of the basic cellular defect is elucidated, there would seem to be no means of documenting this disorder in patients in whom it is incompletely expressed. Mental retardation, joint contractures, and a tendency to thromboembolism are clinical features unique to homocystinuria, permitting its differentiation from the Marfan syndrome.[389,391,392] Biochemical improvement of some cases has been reported to result from treatment with pyridoxine.[393] A marfanoid habitus may be a clue to Sipple's syndrome: familial medullary carcinoma of the thyroid, mucosal neuromas, pheochromocytoma, and parathyroid adenoma or hyperplasia.[394,395] Sex hormone therapy for overgrowth may be indicated in these disorders.

Pituitary Gigantism. Hypersecretion of GH is the cause of this growth pattern. In many cases, the children have some acromegalic features.[396–399] Paradoxically, excessive GH secretion does not advance the bone age, GH-deficiency being characterized by a delay in bone maturation. This seems to indicate that the GH effect on epiphyseal cartilage maturation is a "permissive" one and not essential to the GH effect in promoting linear growth. The diagnosis and therapy of acromegaly are discussed in Chapter 18.

Advanced Growth. Such a pattern occurs most often as a variation of normal. These children have a height and bone age in about the 95th percentile during the preadolescent years. They then enter puberty earlier than their peers and tower above them in height. Their predicted adult height is, of course, normal since they cease to grow earlier than their classmates. Explanation of the normalcy of this growth pattern usually is sufficient to allay any anxieties which the children might have. Sexual precocity advances bone age markedly out of proportion to height; the advance in bone age is not apparent within the first few months of onset, however (Fig. 142-16). The degree of disproportion depends upon the age of onset and the amount of sex hormone production. Unless the disorder is arrested, epiphyseal fusion will occur prematurely and growth will cease at an early age. The diagnosis and therapy of precocious puberty are discussed in Chapter 108. Hyperthyroidism tends to accelerate linear growth and bone maturation proportionately, and predicted ultimate height is not affected.[400] Craniostenosis is a common feature of thyrotoxicosis in young children.[401] Most infant giants follow this growth pattern; these syndromes are usually, but not necessarily, apparent at birth.

The diagnosis of congenital lipodystrophy as a cause of disturbed growth must be based upon clinical findings (see Chapter 88).[402,403] Poor fat stores are present at birth. Fatty liver, hyperlipemia, muscular hypertrophy, acromegaloid features, and a growth spurt tend to become apparent in infancy. About half the patients are mentally retarded. Acanthosis nigricans and adult-type diabetes mellitus tend to appear eventually, the latter not becoming manifest until about 12 yr of age. Linear growth acceleration is proportionate to bone-age advance during the first few years of life and then wanes in later childhood. Consequently, growth ceases early and adult height is normal. The age of onset of puberty is normal; hence, it occurs at a later-than-average skeletal age. Soft-tissue roentgenograms characteristically demonstrate the lack of fat-muscle interface. Hypermetabolism is frequently demonstrable. Variable disturbances of GH and ACTH release have been found. The etiology of the disorder is unclear. Many cases seem to have an autosomal recessive basis. The postulates as to the mechanism of lipodystrophy range from diencephalic overproduction of lipolytic hormones[404] to a primary deficit in fat tissue.[405] Pituitary irradiation and hypophysectomy have not proved to be successful forms of therapy.

PRIMARY DISTURBANCES OF NUTRITION

Pediatric Aspects of Malnutrition

Primary disturbances of nutrition characteristically retard weight gain more than linear growth. The linear growth pattern of moderately malnourished children is not strikingly abnormal, resembling that of normal children who have a "constitutional" delay in growth. When undernutrition is of a severe degree for a long time, the linear growth rate becomes clearly abnormal. Other than its effects on growth, malnutrition leads to widespread disturbance of metabolic and endocrine, immune, and psychomotor function.[406–411] Malnutrition is discussed in detail in Chapter 150.

Famine is the most common cause of starvation on a worldwide scale. Severe deficiency of both calories and protein during early infancy leads to marasmus; severe predominant deficiency of protein at weaning leads to kwashiorkor.[87] The former syndrome is characterized by wasting, the latter by hypoalbuminemia, edema, and hepatomegaly. Insufficient quantities of food are available to the most socioeconomically disadvantaged groups in the United States.[412] However, the major cause of childhood starvation in much of this country is deprivation on a psychosocial basis. This situation can be found in all socioeconomic groups and demands inquiry into the interpersonal relationships between the family, caretakers, and child. Anorexia may develop as a consequence of chronic disease of almost any organ, certain metabolic disturbances, and brain tumors. Idiopathic infantile hypercalcemia exemplifies a chronic metabolic disorder inhibiting growth. Infants with the severe form of this disease develop anorexia in infancy, then fail to gain weight, and eventually linear growth arrest occurs as the disorder persists.[413–415] The facial appearance of these patients is unusual; the extent to which this is due to inherent factors[207] and hypercalcemia[414] is unclear. Management is much the same as for vitamin D intoxication.[416] Brain tumors may cause emaciation while well-being is preserved. This has been termed the "diencephalic syndrome" because of its usual, though not invariable, association with tumors of the anterior hypothalamus or optic tract. Linear growth failure occasionally ensues secondarily. The mechanism whereby an especially profound absence of body fat comes about is unknown. Disturbances of the regulation of appetite or of the secretion of pituitary lipotrophic hormones, such as GH, have been postulated. Most of the tumors seem responsive to radiotherapy.[417–419]

Chronic emesis may be due to space-occupying intracranial masses or obstruction anywhere along the gastrointestinal tract. A psychologic basis may be present at any age, exemplified by rumination in infants and self-induced vomiting in older children. Partial compression of the duodenum by the superior mesenteric artery is a surgically curable disorder which in its early stage is difficult to distinguish from anorexia nervosa.[420] Malabsorption in children is most often due to cystic fibrosis of the pancreas, coeliac disease, bowel fistula, or immunologic deficiency disease. However, it may be associated with hypoparathyroidism. Tumors of the chromaffin or APUD (amine precursor uptake and decarboxylation) system are potential causes of chronic diarrhea via production of serotonin, prostaglandins, enteric hormones, and other substances.[421] Metabolic wastage may occur from loss of energy substrate, as in diabetes mellitus, or hypermetabolism, as in thyrotoxicosis and pheochromocytoma. Lack of adipose tissue gives the appearance of emaciation in lipodystrophy.

Treatment of undernutrition must be multifactorial.[422] In severe malnutrition, rapid protein and calorie replenishment are to be

Table 142-14. Role of Endocrine and Metabolic Disease in Malnutrition

Cause of Malnutrition	Endocrine-Metabolic Cause
inadequate intake of nutrients	
starvation	hypercalcemia,
anorexia	aminoacidopathies, diencephalic syndrome
loss of nutrients	
emesis	(see anorexia)
malabsorption	hypoparathyroidism, chromaffin or APUD tumors
metabolic wastage	
substrate loss	diabetes mellitus
hypermetabolism	hyperthyroidism, pheochromocytoma
lack of adipose tissue	lipodystrophy

avoided. Problems of mineral and water balance must be tended to. Attention must be directed toward complications such as intercurrent sepsis, vitamin deficiencies, and sugar intolerance. Weight gain cannot be expected to resume until calories are provided in amounts appropriate to the age of the child.[423] Once nutritional therapy is begun, one may see a lag of 1 week or longer before weight gain ensues.[424,425] Cyproheptidine (Periacten) has been recommended as an appetite stimulant.[426]

There is considerable concern about the possibility of there being permanent sequelae of malnutrition in childhood. The ultimate stature of severely affected patients is in doubt. Recent evidence suggests that those in whom linear growth has been retarded tend to catch up in height and then follow a delayed growth pattern if the malnutrition is reversed.[87,88,427] More worrisome is the possibility of transient malnutrition leading to subsequent intellectual impairment. Experimental evidence indicates that a finite period of malnutrition in early life permanently interferes with indices of brain development.[428,429] Whether the human brain is particularly and irreversibly vulnerable to malnutrition at the most critical developmental stages is unknown.[156] In fact, though brain growth is retarded in malnourished infants, there is evidence of rapid recovery with treatment.[430] Human malnutrition does not occur in isolation from other adverse influences of emotional, social, cultural, and physical sorts. Consequently, the clear correlation of malnutrition with subsequent intellectual impairment does not constitute proof of a cause-and-effect relationship.

Pediatric Aspects of Obesity

The problem of defining obesity in children is more difficult than in adults.[431–433] Two to 15 percent of children have been estimated to weigh 40 percent or more above average for height. Whether the borderline-obese child (weight around the 90th percentile for height) is at risk for anything other than adult obesity is not at all clear. The topic of obesity is discussed in detail in Chapter 148.

As in adults, the vast majority of obesity in children seems to have a functional basis, arising from excessive intake of calories relative to energy expenditure ("exogenous" or "regulatory" obesity). About one-third of obese children have " developmental" obesity: a history of weight gain since early infancy, a tendency toward an increase in lean body mass, and a modest increase of the linear growth rate which is proportionate to advancement of the skeletal age.[434,435] Other obese children have "reactive" obesity: a later onset of obesity, seemingly in response to emotional stresses (which are often not easily identified), and normal lean body mass and growth. Knittle and Hirsch and others have proposed that there is a sensitive period in man, lasting only until about 1 yr of age, during which the ultimate population of adipocytes is determined.[436,437] They postulate that the increased number of fat cells in developmental obesity predisposes to lifelong obesity. This concept has recently come under criticism because the techniques for quantitating fat cells do not record empty ones.[433]

The management of exogenous obesity in children is basically the same as that in adults. However, there are two special considerations. Stringent dietary restriction for the purpose of bringing about marked weight loss is to be avoided in the growing child. Nitrogen retention, essential for well-being and maturation, is relatively sensitive to caloric restriction during the period of rapid growth.[438] Secondly, psychologic immaturity prevents all young children and many teen-agers from complying with a long-term program for weight reduction. For these reasons, the first step in management of the obese child is to aim to modify psychologic factors and dietary activity with the aim of *maintaining* weight so that the child will "grow-into-it."

Organic diseases represent uncommon causes of obesity. The differential diagnosis of obesity consists of hypothalamic disorders, primary hyperinsulinism, Cushing's syndrome, and hypothyroidism. The diagnosis of a hypothalamic cause for an individual's obesity cannot be made unless there is evidence of a hypothalamic lesion (such as vasomotor instability), organic brain dysfunction (especially psychomotor seizures), or endocrine disturbance [e.g., hypogonadotropism (Froehlich syndrome), sexual precocity, diabetes insipidus, etc.]. Hypothalamic disease may be acquired (e.g., tumor) or congenital (e.g., Prader-Willi syndrome, Laurence-Moon-Biedl syndrome). The Prader-Willi syndrome is the most common of these. The most consistent features of this syndrome are benign hypotonia, mental retardation, small hands and feet, and hypogonadotropic hypogonadism (with cryptorchidism in males).[439–441] The Laurence-Moon-Biedl syndrome is characterized by mental retardation, retinitis pigmentosa, polydactyly, and hypogonadotropism.[441a] The expressivity of the syndrome is variable. The management of hypothalamic obesity is similar to that of exogenous obesity. Obesity is a common result of primary hyperinsulinism and is due to compensatory hyperphagia combined with the lipogenic effect of insulin. The clinical diagnosis of Cushing's syndrome and hypothyroidism are greatly simplified in children by the fact that linear growth arrest is the most consistent finding. Consequently, a normal linear growth rate effectively rules out these disorders; only when frank virilization coexists with glucocorticoid excess might there be an exception to this rule.[114]

Some of the complications seen in adult obesity are found in childhood obesity. Emotional disorders, adult-type diabetes mellitus, and pickwickian syndrome have all been observed in children.

LOCALIZED DISTURBANCES OF SOMATIC GROWTH

Growth of isolated structures may be abnormal in association with generalized abnormalities of growth; these disorders have been discussed above. Local growth may also be abnormal in an isolated or multifocal pattern without a disturbance of overall growth. Those aspects of localized growth disturbances that are of endocrinologic interest are noted here.

CONGENITAL

Hormone administration or hormonal disturbances at critical periods of development have been associated with localized somatic malformations: cortisone re cleft palate;[442] estrogen-progestin contraceptives re vascular-tracheoesophageal-limb-reduction anomalies (VATER association);[443] diabetes mellitus re sacral, palatal, and cardiac anomalies.[1,442,444–447] Whether the latter is an effect of hyperglycemia, hyperinsulinism, sulfonylurea, acetonemia, or insulin antagonism is unknown.

Congenital hemiasymmetry is linked with endocrine disorders and neoplasia. Wilms' tumor, adrenal carcinoma, and hepatic tumors occur more frequently in patients with congenital hemihypertrophy and their families than is expected by chance.[448–450] Wilms' tumor and congenital renal dysplasia also occur in association with pseudohermaphroditism.[451] It seems possible that a genetically determined error during a critical period of embryogenesis underlies these associations. Hemihypertrophy is also linked with endocrine dysfunction and neoplasia in von Recklinghausen's neurofibromatosis (adrenal carcinoma, thalamic tumors)[452] and the Beckwith-Wiedemann syndrome. Increased serum nerve-growth-stimulating activity has recently been reported in neurofibromatosis patients.[453]

The topic of congenital malformations of somatic, endocrine, and other organs is discussed more comprehensively in several treatises.[193,196,442,454]

ACQUIRED

The deleterious effects of a variety of disorders affecting limb growth may be mediated by alterations in blood circulation. The result of occlusion of the arterial flow to a limb is the most obvious instance. It has been shown that longitudinal growth of the arm is retarded out of proportion to bone maturation after sacrifice of the subclavian artery.[455] Growth of an entire limb is well known to be stunted in limbs of children paralyzed from any lesion, whether it be of the lower motor neuron as in poliomyelitis, or of the upper motor neuron, as in cerebral vascular accidents. It is unknown whether growth is affected because of a direct "trophic" effect of innervation or whether activity of the limb somehow promotes normal growth, possibly by promoting the circulation. Local inflammatory disease about a joint may accelerate epiphyseal maturation and lead to premature epiphyseal fusion and cessation of growth.[365] Trauma to the epiphyseal plate will result in growth arrest unless circulation is intact and the anatomy is restored.

Epiphyseal growth will also be arrested by x-irradiation in high, tumoricidal doses. The exact dose-response relationship between radiation dose and the rate of bone growth has not been established in man for either therapy with x-ray alone or in combination with such potentiating agents as actinomycin D, nor is there information about the relative sensitivity to x-ray of the various physeal centers. Vertebral growth may be affected by doses of around 4000 rads.[456] After extensive vertebral irradiation for treatment of malignant tumors, significant reductions in overall linear growth velocity can be expected in surviving patients.

REFERENCES

1. McMahon, D.: Chemical messengers in development: A hypothesis. *Science 185:* 1012, 1974.
2. Pastan, I., and Johnson, G. S.: Cyclic AMP and the transformation of fibroblasts. *Adv. Cancer Res 19:* 303, 1974.
3. Bitensky, M. W., and Gorman, R. E.: Cellular responses to cyclic AMP. *Prog. Biophys. Mol. Biol. 26:* 411, 1973.
4. Kohrman, A. F.: Patterns of development of adenyl cyclase activity and norepinephrine responsiveness in the rat. *Pediatr. Res. 7:* 575, 1973.
5. Burger, M. M., Bombik, B. M., Breckenridge, B. M., *et al.*: Growth control and cyclic alterations of cyclic AMP in the cell cycle. *Nature* [*New Biol.*] *239:* 161, 1972.
6. Ryan, W. L., and Heidrick, M. F.: Inhibition of cell growth in vitro by adenosine 3′,5′-monophosphates. *Science 162:* 1484, 1968.
7. Pious, D.: Cell surfaces, genetics, and congenital malformations. *J. Pediatr. 86:* 162, 1975.
8. Villee, C. A.: Biologic principles of growth. In Falkner, F. (ed.): *Human Development.* Philadelphia, Saunders, 1966, p. 1.
9. Russell, D. H. (ed.): Polyamines in Normal and Neoplastic Growth. New York, Raven, 1973.
10. Cheek, D. B., Graystone, J. E., and Read, M. S.: Cellular growth, nutrition, and development. *Pediatrics 45:* 315, 1970.
11. Naeye, R. L.: Malnutrition. Probable cause of fetal growth retardation. *Arch. Pathol. 79:* 284, 1965.
12. Winick, M., and Noble, A.: Quantitative changes in DNA, RNA, and protein during prenatal and postnatal growth in the rat. *Devel. Biol. 12:* 451, 1965.
13. Mukherjee, A. B., Hastings, C., and Cohen, M. M.: Nucleic acid synthesis in various organs of developing human fetuses. *Pediatr. Res. 7:* 696, 1973.
14. Arey, L. B.: Developmental Anatomy, [ed. 6]. Philadelphia, Saunders, 1954, pp. 11 and 62.
15. Levitt, D., Ho, P.-L. and Dorfman, A.: Differentiation of cartilage. In Moscona, A. A. (ed.): The Cell Surface in Development. New York, Wiley, 1974, p. 101.
16. Lubchenco, L. O., Hansman, C., Dressler, M., and Boyd, E: Intrauterine growth as estimated from liveborn birth-weight data at 24 to 42 weeks of gestation. *Pediatrics 32:* 793, 1963.
17. Thomson, A. M., Billewicz, W. Z., and Hytten, F. E.: The assessment of fetal growth. *J. Obstet. Gynacol.* Br. Commonw. *75:* 90, 1968.
18. Wingerd, V., and Schoen, E. J.: Factors influencing length at birth and height at five years. *Pediatrics 53:* 737, 1974.
19. Beck, G. J., and van der Berg, B. J.: The relationship of the rate of intrauterine growth of low-birth-weight infants to later growth. *J. Pediatr. 86:* 504, 1975.
20. Tanner, J. M., Lejahraga, H., and Turner, G.: Within-family standards for birth-weight. *Lancet 2:* 193, 1972.
21. Bergner, L., and Susser, M. W.: Low birth weight and prenatal nutrition: An interpretive review. *Pediatrics 46:* 946, 1970.
22. Stein, Z., and Susser, M.: The Dutch famine, 1944–1945, and the reproductive process. II. *Pediatr. Res. 9:* 76, 1975.
23. Hadden, W., Jr., Nesbitt, R. E. L., and Garcia, R.: Smoking and pregnancy: Carbon monoxide in blood during gestation and at term. *Obstet. Gynecol. 18:* 262, 1961.
24. Mosier, H. D., and Armstrong, M. K.: Effects of maternal intake of nicotine on fetal and newborn rats. *Proc. Soc. Exp. Biol. Med. 116:* 956, 1964.
25. Battaglia, F. C.: Placental clearance and fetal oxygenation. *Pediatrics 45:* 563, 1970.
26. Naeye, R. C.: The fetal and neonatal development of twins. *Pediatrics 33:* 546, 1964.
27. Naeye, R. L., Benirschke, K., Hagstrom, J. W. C., and Marcus, C. C.: Intrauterine growth of twins as estimated from liveborn birthweight data. *Pediatrics 37:* 409, 1966.
28. MacMillan, D. R., Brown, A. M., Matheny, A. P., Jr., and Wilson, R. S.: Relations between placental concentrations of chorionic somatomammotropin (placental lactogen) and growth: A study using the twin method. *Pediatr. Res. 7:* 719, 1973.
29. Fogel, B. J., Nitowsky, H. M., and Gruenwald, P.: Discordant anomalies in monozygotic twins. *J. Pediat. 66:* 64, 1965.
30. Winick, M.: Cellular growth of the human placenta. III. Intrauterine growth failure. *J. Pediatr. 71:* 390, 1967.
31. Rosenfield, R. L., Refetoff, S., Hoffer, P. B., *et al.:* Diagnosis of thyroid diseases in pediatrics. In James, A. E., Wagner, H. N., and Cooke, R. E. (eds.): *Pediatric Nuclear Medicine.* Philadelphia, Saunders, 1974. p. 376.
32. King, K. C., Adam, P. A. J., Schwartz, R., and Teramo, K.: Human placental transfer of human growth hormone. *Pediatrics 48:* 534, 1971.
33. Wilkins, L.: The Diagnosis and Treatment of Endocrine Disorders in Childhood and Adolescence, ed. 3. Springfield, Ill., Thomas, 1965.
34. Naeye, R. L., and Blanc, W. A.: Organ and body growth in anencephaly. *Arch. Pathol. 91:* 140, 1971.
35. Sadeghi-Nejad, A., and Senior, B.: A familial syndrome of isolated "aplasia" of the anterior pituitary. *J. Pediatr. 84:* 79, 1974.
36. Jost, A.: Hormonal factors in development of the fetus. Cold Spring Harbor Symp *19:* 167, 1954.
37. Smith, D. W., and Popick, G.: Large fontanels in congenital hypothyroidism: A potential clue toward earlier recognition. *J. Pediatr. 80:* 753, 1972.
38. Laron, Z., and Pertzelan, A.: Somatotropin in antenatal and perinatal growth and development. *Lancet 1:* 680, 1969.
39. Sara, V. R., Lazarus, L., Stuart, M. C., and King, T.: Fetal brain growth: Selective action by growth hormone. *Science 186:* 446, 1974.
40. Hinz, R. L., Seeds, J. M., and Johnsonbaugh, R. E.: Somatomedin and growth hormone in the newborn. *Pediatr. Res. 8:* 369/95, 1974 (Abstract).
41. Tato, L., Du Caju, M. V. L., Prévõt, C., and Rappaport, R.: Early variations of plasma somatomedin activity in the newborn. *J Clin. Endocrinol. Metab. 40:* 534, 1975.
41a. Gluckman, P. D., and Brinsmead, M. W.: Somatomedin in cord blood: Relationship to gestational age and birth size. *J. Clin. Endocrinol. Metab. 43:* 1378, 1976.
42. Heins, J. N., Garland, J. T., and Daughaday, W. H.: Incorporation of ^{35}S-sulfate into rat cartilage explants *in vitro:* Effects of aging on responsiveness to stimulation by sulfation factor. *Endocrinology 87:* 688, 1970.
43. Kaplan, S. L., and Grumbach, M. M.: Studies of a human and simian placental hormone with growth hormone-like and prolactin-like activities. *J. Clin. Endocrinol. Metab. 24:* 80, 1964.

44. Kaplan, S. L., and Grumbach, M. M.: Serum chorionic growth hormone-prolactin and serum pituitary growth hormone in mother and fetus at term. *J. Clin. Endocrinol. Metab. 25:* 1370, 1965.
44a. MacMillan, D. R., Hawkins, R., and Collier, R. N.: Chorionic somatomammotrophin as index of fetal growth. *Arch. Dis. Child. 51:* 120, 1976.
45. Blizzard, R. M., Drash, A. L., Jenkins, M. E., *et al.:* Comparative effects of animal prolactins and human growth hormone (HGH) in hypopituitary children. *J. Clin. Endocrinol. Metab. 26:* 852, 1966.
46. Guyda, H. J., and Friesen, H. G.: Serum prolactin levels in humans from birth to adult life. *Pediatr. Res. 7:* 534, 1973.
47. MacDonald, M. J.: Neonatal diabetes. *Lancet 1:* 737, 1974.
48. Forest, M. G., Ances, I. G., Tapper, A. J., and Migeon, C. J.: Percentage binding of testosterone, androstenedione and dehydroepiandrosterone in plasma at the time of delivery. *J. Clin. Endocrinol. Metab. 32:* 417, 1971.
49. Kenny, F. N., Angsusingha, K., Stinson, D., and Hotchkiss, J.: Unconjugated estrogens in the perinatal period. *Pediatr. Res. 7:* 826, 1973.
50. Abdul-Karim, R. W., and Marshall, C. D.: Influence of maternal oophorectomy on the collagen and calcium contents of fetal bone. *Obstet. Gynecol. 34:* 837, 1969.
51. Abdul-Karim, R. W., Nesbitt, R. E. L., Jr., Drucker, M. H., and Rizk, P. T.: The regulatory effect of estrogens on fetal growth. I. Placental and fetal body weights. *Am. J. Obstet. Gynecol. 109:* 656, 1971.
52. Lubchenco, L. O., Hansman, C., and Boyd, E.: Intrauterine growth in length and head circumference as estimated from live births at gestational ages from 26 to 42 weeks. *Pediatrics 37:* 403, 1966.
53. Babson, S. G., Behrman, R. E., and Lessel, R.: Fetal growth. *Pediatrics 45:* 937, 1970.
54. Gruenwald, P.: Growth of the human fetus. II. *Am. J. Obstet. Gynecol. 94:* 1120, 1966.
55. Usher, R., and McLean, F.: Intrauterine growth of live-born Caucasian infants at sea level. *J. Pediatr. 74:* 901, 1969.
56. Scott, R. B., Hiatt, H. H., Clark, B. G., *et al.:* Growth and development of Negro infants. IX. *Pediatrics 29:* 65, 1962.
57. Freeman, M. G., Graves, W. L., and Thompson, R. L.: Indigent Negro and Caucasian birth weight-gestational age tables. *Pediatrics 46:* 9, 1970.
58. Battaglia, R. C., Frazier, T. M., and Hellegers, A. E.: Birth weight, gestational age, and pregnancy outcome with special reference to high birth weight-low gestational age infant. *Pediatrics 37:* 417, 1966.
59. Watson, E. H., and Lowrey, G. H.: Growth and Development of Children, ed. 4. Chicago, Year Book Medical Publishers, 1962, p. 42.
60. Pryse-Davies, J., Smithan, J. H., and Napier, K. A.: Factors influencing development of secondary ossification centres in the fetus and newborn. *Arch. Dis. Child. 49:* 425, 1974.
61. Babson, S. G.: Growth of low-birth-weight infants. *J. Pediatr. 77:* 11, 1970.
62. Cruise, M. O.: A longitudinal study of the growth of low birth weight infants. I. *Pediatrics 51:* 620, 1973.
63. Wingerd, J., Schoen, E. J., and Solomon, I. L.: Growth standards in the first two years of life based on measurements of white and black children in a prepaid health care program. *Pediatrics 47:* 818, 1971.
64. Duncan, B., Lubchenco, L. O., and Hansman, C.: Growth charts for children 0 to 18 years of age. *Pediatrics 54:* 497, 1974.
65. Smith, D. W., Truog, W., Rogers, J. E., Greitzer, L. J., Skinner, A. L., McCann, J. J., and Harvey, M. A. S.: Shifting linear growth during infancy. *J. Pediatr. 89:* 225, 1976.
66. Maresh, M. M.: Linear growth of long bones of extremities from infancy through adolescence. *Am. J. Dis. Child. 89:* 725, 1955.
66a. Lovinger, R. D., Kaplan, S. L., and Grumbach, M. M.: Congenital hypopituitarism associated with neonatal hypoglycemia and microphallus: Four cases secondary to hypothalamic hormone deficiencies. *J. Pediatr. 87:* 1171, 1975.
66b. Garn, S. M., and Shaw, H. A.: Birth size and growth appraisal. *J. Pediatr. 90:* 1049, 1977.
67. Rasmussen, H., and Bordier, P.: The cellular basis of metabolic bone disease. *N. Engl. J. Med. 289:* 25, 1973.
68. Prader, A., Tanner, J. M., and von Harnack, G. A.: Catch-up growth following illness or starvation. *J. Pediatr. 62:* 646, 1963.
69. Bok, R. D., Wainer, H., Peterson, A.; *et al.:* A parameterization for individual human growth curves. *Hum. Biol. 45:* 63, 1973.
70. Reed, R. B., and Stuart, H. C.: Patterns of growth in height and weight from birth to eighteen years of age. *Pediatrics 24* (p. 2): 904, 1959.
71. Tanner, J. M., Whitehouse, R. H., and Takaishi, M.: Standards from birth to maturity for height, weight, height velocity, and weight velocity: British Children, 1965. Part II. *Arch. Dis. Child. 41:* 613, 1966.
72. Marshall, W. A.: Evaluation of growth rate in height over periods of less than one year. *Arch. Dis. Child. 46:* 414, 1971.
73. Tanner, J. M.: Growth at Adolescence. London, Blackwell, 1962, p. 130.
74. Forbes, G. B.: A note on the mathematics of "catchup" growth. *Pediatr. Res. 8:* 929, 1974.
75. Barr, D. G. D., Shmerling, D. H., and Prader, A.: Catch-up growth in malnutrition studied in celiac disease after institution of gluten-free diet. *Pediatr. Res. 6:* 521, 1972.
76. Bongiovanni, A. M., Moshang, T., Jr., and Parks, J. S.: Maturational deceleration after treatment of congenital adrenal hyperplasia. *Helv. Pediatr. Acta 28:* 127, 1973.
77. Glinos, A. D.: Density dependent regulation of growth and differentiated function in suspension cultures of mouse fibroblasts. In Kulonen, E., and Pikkarainen, J. (eds.): *Biology of Fibroblast,* New York, Academic, 1973, p. 155.
78. VanderLaan, W. P.: Growth hormone and nutrition. In Raiti, S. (ed.): *Advances in Human Growth Hormone Research.* Washington, D.C., U.S. Government, 1974, p. 853.
79. Mosier, H. D.: Discussion. In Raiti, S. (ed.): *Advances in Human Growth Hormone Research,* Washington, D.C., U.S. Government, 1974, p. 858.
80. MacGillivray, M. H., Aceto, T., Jr., and Frohman, L. A.: Plasma growth hormone responses and growth retardation in hypothyroidism. *Am. J. Dis. Child. 115:* 273, 1968.
81. Wingerd, J., Solomon, I. L., and Schoen, E. J.: Parent-specific height standards for preadolescent children of three racial groups, with method for rapid determination. *Pediatrics 52:* 555, 1973.
82. Leading article: The YY syndrome. *Lancet 1:* 583, 1966.
83. Santen, R. J., DeKretser, D. M., Paulsen, C. A., and Vorhees, J.: Gonadotrophins and testosterone in the XYY syndrome. *Lancet 2:* 371, 1970.
84. Ounsted, C., and Ounsted, M.: Effect of Y chromosone on fetal growth-rate. *Lancet 2:* 857, 1970.
85. Caldwell, P. D., and Smith, D. W.: The XXY (Klinefelter's) syndrome in childhood: Detection and treatment. *J. Pediatr. 80:* 250, 1972.
86. McCance, R. A., and Widdowson, E. M.: Nutrition and growth. *Proc. R. Soc. London 156:* 326, 1962.
87. Graham, G. G.: The later growth of malnourished infants; effects of age, severity, and subsequent diet. In McCance, R. A., and Widdowson, E. M. (eds.): *Calorie Deficiencies and Protein Deficiencies.* Boston, Little Brown, 1968, p. 301.
88. Dreizen, S., Spirakis, C. N., and Stone, R. E.: A comparison of skeletal growth and maturation in undernourished and well-nourished girls before and after menarche. *J. Pediatr. 70:* 256, 1967.
89. Cheek, D. B.: Cellular growth, hormones, nutrition, and time. *Pediatrics 41:* 30, 1968.
90. Hommes, F. A., Drost, Y. M., Geraets, W. X. M., and Reijenga, M. A. A.: The energy requirement for growth: An application of Atkinson's metabolic price system. *Pediatr. Res. 9:* 51, 1975.
91. Holliday, M. A.: Metabolic rate and organ size during growth from infancy to maturity and during late gestation and early infancy. *Pediatrics 47* (p. 2): 169, 1971.
92. Sinclair, J. C., and Silverman, W. A.: Intrauterine growth in active tissue mass of the human fetus, with particular reference to the undergrown baby. *Pediatrics 38:* 48, 1966.
93. Holt, L. E., Jr.: Some problems in dietary amino acid requirements. *Am. J. Clin. Nutr. 21:* 367, 1968.
94. Fisch, R. O., Gravem, H. J., and Feinberg, S. B.: Growth and bone characteristics of phenylketonurics. *Am. J. Dis. Child. 112:* 3, 1966.
95. Cahill, G. F., Jr.: Nitrogen versatility in bats, bears, and man. *N. Engl. J. Med. 290:* 686, 1974.
96. Holman, R. T.: Essential fatty acid deficiency. Prog. Chem. Fats Other Lipids *9* (p. 2): 275, 1968.
97. DeLuca, H. F.: Mechanism of action and metabolic effect of vitamin D. *Vitam. Horm. 25:* 315, 1968.

98. Clement, D. H., Fomon, S. J., Forbes, G. B., *et al.*: Trace elements in infant nutrition. *Pediatrics 26:* 715, 1960.

98a. Ulmer, D. D.: Trace elements. *New Engl. J. Med. 297:* 318, 1977.

99. Halsted, J. A., Ronagby, H. A., Abadi, P., *et al.*: Zinc deficiency in man. *Am. J. Med. 53:* 277, 1972.

100. Sandstead, H. H., Prasad, A. S., Schubert, A. R., *et al.*: Human zinc deficiency, endocrine manifestations, and response to treatment. *Am. J. Clin. Nutr. 20:* 422, 1967.

101. Cooke, R. E., Boyden, D. G., and Haller, E.: The relationship of acidosis and growth retardation. *J. Pediatr. 57:* 326, 1960.

102. Viteri, F. E.: (The effect of inactivity on the growth of rats fed diets adequate or restricted with respect to normal caloric intake), in (New Concepts about Old Aspects of Malnutrition), Mexico, Fondo Editorial Nestle de la Academia Mexicana de Pediatria, 1973 (Spanish).

103. Baulieu, E. E., Lasnitzki, I., and Robel, P.: Metabolism of testosterone and action of metabolites on prostate glands grown in organ culture. *Nature 219:* 1155, 1968.

104. Cheek, D. B. (ed.). *Human Growth.* Philadelphia, Lea and Febiger, 1968.

105. Van Den Brande, J. L., DeCaju, M. V. L.: Plasma somatomedin activity in children with growth disturbances. In Raiti, S. (ed.): *Advances in Human Growth Hormone Research.* Washington, D.C., U.S. Government, 1974, p. 98.

105a. D'Ercole, A. J., Underwood, L. E., and Van Wyk, J. J.: Serum somatomedin-C in hypopituitarism and in other disorders of growth. *J. Pediatr. 90:* 375, 1977.

106. Salter, J., and Best, E. H.: Insulin as a growth hormone. *Br. Med. J. 2:* 353, 1953.

107. Salmon, W. D., Jr.: Effects of somatomedin on cartilage metabolism: Further observations on an inhibitory serum factor. In Raiti, S. (ed.): *Advances in Human Growth Hormone Research.* Washington, U.S. Government, 1974, p. 76.

108. Finkelstein, J. W., Kream, J., Ladan, A., and Helmann, L.: Sulfation factor (somatomedin): An explanation for continued growth in the absence of immunoassayable growth hormone in patients with hypothalamic tumor. *J. Clin. Endocrinol Metabl. 35:* 13, 1972.

109. Kenny, F. M., Guyda, H. J., and Wright, J. C.: Prolactin and somatomedin in hypopituitary patients with "catch-up" growth following operations for craniopharyngioma. *J. Clin. Endocrinol. Metab. 36:* 378, 1973.

110. Costin, G., Kogut, M. D., Phillips, L. S., and Daughaday, W. H.: Craniopharyngioma: The role of insulin in promoting postoperative growth. *J. Clin. Endocrinol. Metabl. 42:* 370, 1976.

111. Porter, B. A., Rosenfield, R. L., and Lawrence, A. M.: The levodopa test of growth hormone reserve in children. *Am. J. Dis. Child. 126:* 590, 1973.

112. Daughaday, W. H., Laron, Z., Pertzelan, A., and Heins, J. N.: Defective sulfation factor generation: A possible etiologic link in dwarfism. *Trans. Assoc. Am. Phys. 82:* 129, 1969.

113. Root, A. W., Bongiovanni, A. M., and Eberlein, W. R.: Studies of the secretion and metabolic effects of human growth hormone in children with glucocorticoid-induced growth retardation. *J. Pediatr. 75:* 826, 1969.

114. Shahidi, N. T., and Crigler, J. F., Jr.: Evaluation of growth and of endocrine systems in testosterone-corticosteroid-treated patients with aplastic anemia. *J. Pediatr. 70:* 233, 1967.

115. Phillips, L. S., Herington, A. C., and Daughaday, W. H.: Hormone effects on somatomedin action and somatomedin generation. In Raiti, S. (ed.): *Advances in Human Growth Hormone Research.* Washington, U.S. Government, 1974, p. 50.

116. Blodgett, F. M., Burgin, L., Iezzoni, D., *et al.*: Effects of prolonged cortisone therapy on the statural growth, skeletal maturation and metabolic status of children. *N. Engl. J. Med. 254:* 636, 1956.

117. Root, A. W., Rosenfield, R. L., Bongiovanni, A. M., and Eberlein, W. R.: The plasma growth hormone response to insulin-induced hypoglycemia in children with retardation of growth. *Pediatrics 39:* 844, 1967.

118. Forest, M. G., Cathiard, A. M., and Bertrand, J. A.: Evidence of testicular activity in early infancy. *J. Clin. Endocrinol. Metab. 37:* 148, 1973.

119. Faiman, C., and Winter, J. S. D.: Sex difference in gonadotrophin concentrations in infancy. *Nature 232:* 130, 1971.

120. Migeon, C. J., Keller, A. R., Lawrence, B., and Shepard, T. H., III: Dehydroepiandrosterone and androsterone levels in human plasma. *J. Clin. Endocrinol. Metab. 17:* 1051, 1957.

121. Puche, R. C., and Romano, M. C.: Effect of dehydroepiandrosterone sulfate on the mineral accretion of chick embryo frontal bones cultivated *in vitro.* Calcif. Tissue Res. *4:* 39, 1969.

122. Skinner, J. D., Mann, T., and Rowson, L. E. A.: Androstenedione in relation to puberty and growth of the male calf. *J. Endocrinol. 40:* 261, 1968.

123. Rosenfield, R. L., and Fang, V. S.: The effects of prolonged physiologic estradiol therapy on the maturation of hypogonadal teen-agers. *J. Pediatr. 85:* 830, 1974.

124. Cheek, D. B., Mellits, D., and Elliott, D. A.: Body water, height and weight during growth in normal children. *Am. J. Dis. Child. 112:* 312, 1966.

125. Tanner, J. M., Whitehouse, R. H., and Takaishi, M.: Standards from birth to maturity for height, weight, height velocity, and weight velocity: British children, 1965. I. *Arch. Dis. Child. 41:* 454, 1966.

126. Gruelich, W. W., and Pyle, S. I.: Radiographic Atlas of Skeletal Development of the Hand and Wrist. Palo Alto, Stanford, 1959.

127. Finkelstein, J. W., Roffwarg, H. P., Boyar, R. M., *et al.*: Age-related change in the twenty-four-hour spontaneous secretion of growth hormone. *J. Clin. Endocrinol. Metab. 35:* 665, 1972.

128. Plotnick, L. P., Thompson, R. G., Kowarski, A., *et al.*: Circadian variation of integrated concentration of growth hormone in children and adults. *J. Clin. Endocrinol. Metab. 40:* 240, 1975.

129. Lee, P. A., Jaffe, R. B., and Midgley, A. R.: Serum gonadotropin, testosterone, and prolactin concentrations throughout puberty in boys. *J. Clin. Endocrinol. Metab. 39:* 664, 1974.

130. Zachmann, M., and Prader, A.: Anabolic and androgenic effect of testosterone in sexually immature boys and its dependency on growth hormone. *J. Clin. Endocrinol. Metab. 30:* 85, 1970.

131. Stuart, H. C., and Stevenson, S. S.: Physical growth and development. In Nelson, W. E. (ed.): Textbook of Pediatrics, ed. 7. Philadelphia, Saunders, 1959, p. 12.

132. Engelbach, W.: Endocrine Medicine. Springfield, Ill., Thomas, 1932, vol. 1, p. 261.

133. Shuttleworth, F. K.: Sexual maturation and physical growth of girls age six to nineteen. *Monogr. Soc. Res. Child. Dev., Natl. Res. Counc. 2:* No. 5, 1937.

134. Roche, A. F., and Davila, G. H.: Late adolescent growth in stature. *Pediatrics 50:* 874, 1972.

135. Hamill, P. V. V., Johnston, F. E., and Grams, W.: *Height and weight of children. Vital and Health Statistics,* Ser. 11, No. 104, Washington, U.S. Government, 1970.

136. Barr, G. D., Allen, C. M., and Shinefield, H. R.: Height and weight of 7500 children of three skin colors. *Am. J. Dis. Child. 124:* 866, 1972.

137. Garn, S. M., Clark, D. C., and Trowbridge, F. L.: Tendency toward greater stature in American black children. *Am. J. Dis. Child. 126:* 164, 1973.

138. Laestadius, N. D., Aase, J. M., and Smith, D. W.: Normal inner canthal and outer orbital dimensions. *J. Pediatr. 74:* 465, 1969.

139. Pryor, H. B.: Objective measurement of interpupillary distance. *Pediatrics 44:* 973, 1969.

140. Juberg, R. C., Sholte, F. G., and Touchstone, W. J.: Normal values for intercanthal distances of 5- to 11-year-old American blacks. *Pediatrics 55:* 431, 1975.

141. Mehes, K., and Kitzveger, E.: Inner canthal and intermammillary indices in the newborn infant. *J. Pediatr. 85:* 90, 1974.

142. Nellhaus, G.: Head circumference from birth to eighteen years. *Pediatrics 41:* 106, 1968.

143. O'Connell, E. J., Feldt, R. H., and Stickler, G. B.: Head circumference, mental retardation, and growth failure. *Pediatrics 36:* 62, 1965.

144. Krieger, I.: Head circumference, mental retardation and growth failure. *Pediatrics 37:* 384, 1966.

145. Illingworth, R. S., and Lutz, W.: Head circumference of infants related to body weight. *Arch. Dis. Child. 40:* 672, 1965.

146. Cloutier, M. D., and Stickler, G. B.: Head circumference in children with idiopathic hypopituitarism. *Pediatrics 42:* 209, 1968.

146a. Burt, L., and Kulin, H. E.: Head circumference in children with short stature secondary to primary hypothyroidism. *Pediatrics 59:* 628, 1977.

147. Popich, G. A., and Smith, D. W.: Fontanels: Range of normal size. *J. Pediatr. 80:* 749, 1972.

148. Graham, C. B.: Assessment of bone maturation—Methods and pitfalls. *Radiol. Clin. North Am. 10:* 185, 1972.

149. Roche, A. F., Eyman, S. L., and Davila, G. H.: Skeletal age prediction. *J. Pediatr. 78:* 997, 1971.
150. Baer, M. J., and Durkatz, J.: Bilateral asymmetry in skeletal maturation of the hand and wrist. *Am. J. Phys. Anthropol. 15:* 180, 1957.
151. Garn, S. M., Sandusky, S. T., Nagy, J. M., and McCann, M. B.: Advanced skeletal development in low-income Negro children. *J. Pediatr. 80:* 965, 1972.
152. Donovan, B. T., and Van der Werff ten Bosch, J. J.: *Physiology of Puberty.* London, Arnold, 1965.
153. Cumming, G. R., Garand, T., and Borysyk, L.: Correlation of performance in track and field events with bone age. *J. Pediatr. 80:* 970, 1972.
154. Pryor, H. B.: Charts of normal body measurements and revised width-weight tables in graphic form. *J. Pediatr. 68:* 615, 1966.
155. Frisch, R. E., and McArthur, J. W.: Menstrual cycles as a determinant of minimum weight for height necessary for their maintenance or onset. *Science 185:* 949, 1974.
156. Dobbing, J.: The later growth of the brain and its vulnerability. *Pediatrics 53:* 2, 1974.
157. Dubowitz, L. M. S., Dubowitz, V., and Goldberg, C.: Clinical assessment of gestational age in the newborn infant. *J. Pediatr. 77:* 1, 1970.
158. Finnstrom, O.: Studies on maturity in newborn infants. VI. *Acta. Paediatr. Scand. 61:* 33, 1972.
159. DeHertogh, R., Thomas, K., Bietlot, Y., *et al.:* Plasma levels of unconjugated estrone, estradiol, and estriol and of HCS throughout pregnancy in normal women. *J. Clin. Endocrinol. Metab. 40:* 93, 1975.
160. Fencl, M., and Tulchinsky, D.: Total cortisol in amniotic fluid and fetal lung maturation. *N. Engl. J. Med. 292:* 133, 1975.
161. Metcoff, J., Wikman-Coffelt, J., Yoshida, T., *et al.:* Energy metabolism and protein synthesis in human leukocytes during pregnancy and in placenta related to fetal growth. *Pediatrics 51:* 866, 1973.
162. Dancis, J., O'Connell, J. R., and Holt, L. E., Jr.: A grid for recording the weight of premature infants. *J. Pediatr. 33:* 570, 1948.
163. Ross Laboratories (ed.): Children are Different. Columbus, Ross Laboratories, 1970.
164. Rosenstein, S. N.: In Barnett, H. (ed.): *Pediatrics*, ed. 15. New York, Appleton-Century-Crofts, 1972.
165. Holliday, M. A.: Fluid and Electrolyte disturbances in pediatrics. In Maxwell, M. H., and Kleeman, C. R. (eds.): *Clinical Disorders of Fluid and Electrolyte Metabolism,* ed. 1. New York, McGraw-Hill, 1962, p. 445.
166. Butler, A. M., and Richie, R. H.: Simplification and improvement in estimating drug dosage and fluid and dietary allowances for patients of varying sizes. *N. Engl. J. Med. 262:* 903, 1960.
167. Arnaud, S. B., Goldsmith, R. S., Stickler, G. B., *et al.:* Serum parathyroid hormone and blood minerals: Interrelationships in normal children. *Pediatr. Res. 7:* 485, 1973.
168. Kenny, F. M., Preeyasombat, C., and Migeon, C. J.: Cortisol production rate. II. *Pediatrics 37:* 35, 1966.
169. Oddie, T. H., Meade, J. H., Jr., and Fisher, D. A.: An analysis of published data on thyroxine turnover in human subjects. *J. Clin. Endocrinol. Metab. 26:* 425, 1966.
170. Sassard, J., Sann, L., Vincent, M., Francois, R., and Cier, J. F.: Plasma renin activity in normal subjects from infancy to puberty. *J. Clin. Endocrinol. Metab. 40:* 524, 1975.
171. Beitins, I. Z., Graham, G. G., Kowarski, A., and Migeon, C. J.: Adrenal function in normal infants and in marasmus and kwashiorkor: Plasma aldosterone concentration and aldosterone secretion rate. *J. Pediatr. 84:* 444, 1974.
172. Strickland, A. L., and Shearin, R. B.: Diurnal height variation in children. *J. Pediatr. 80:* 1023, 1972.
173. Visveshwara, N., Rudolph, N., and Dragutsky, D.: Syndrome of accelerated skeletal maturation in infancy, peculiar facies, and multiple congenital anomalies. *J. Pediatr. 84:* 553, 1974.
174. Poznanski, A. K., Garn, S. M., Kuhns, L. R., and Sandusky, S. T.: Dysharmonic maturation of the hand in congenital malformation syndromes. *Am. J. Phys. Anthropol. 35:* 417, 1971.
175. Anderson, M., Green, W. T., and Messner, M. B.: Growth and predictions of growth in the lower extremities. J. Bone Joint Surg. *45-A:* 1, 1963.
176. Bayer, L. M., and Bayley, N.: Growth pattern shifts in healthy children: Spontaneous and induced. *J. Pediatr. 62:* 631, 1963.
177. Roche, A., Wainer, H., and Thissen, D.: The RWT method for the prediction of adult stature. *Pediatrics 56:* 1026, 1975.
178. Tanner, J. M., Whitehouse, R. H., Marshall, W. A., and Carter, B. S.: Prediction of adult height, bone age, and occurrence of menarche, at ages 4 to 16 with allowance for midparent height. *Arch. Dis. Child. 50:* 14, 1975.
179. Frisch, R. E.: Critical weight at menarche, initiation of the adolescent growth spurt, and control of puberty. In Grumbach, M. M., Grave, G. D., and Mayer, F. E. (eds.): Control of the Onset of Puberty. New York, Wiley, 1974, p. 403.
180. Fisch, R. E.: A method of prediction of age of menarche from height and weight at ages 9 through 13 years. *Pediatrics 53:* 384, 1974.
181. Frisch, R. E., and Nagel, J. S.: Prediction of adult height of girls from age of menarche and height at menarche. *J. Pediatr. 85:* 838, 1974.
182. Johnston, F. E., Roche, A. F., Schell, L. M., and Wettenhall, N. B.: Critical weight at menarche. A critique of a hypothesis. *Am. J. Dis. Child. 129:* 19, 1975.
183. Frisancho, A. R., Garn, S. M., and Rohmann, C. G.: Age at menarche: A new method of prediction and retrospective assessment based on hand x-rays. *Hum. Biol. 41:* 42, 1969.
184. Warkany, J., Monroe, B. B., and Sutherland, B. S.: Intrauterine growth retardation. *Am. J. Dis. Child. 102:* 127, 1961.
185. Medovy, H.: New parameters in neonatal growth—cell number and cell size. *J. Pediatr. 71:* 459, 1967.
186. Lubchenco, L. O., Searls, D. T., and Brazie, J. V.: Neonatal mortality rate: Relationship to birth weight and gestational age. *J. Pediatr. 81:* 814, 1972.
187. Miller, H. C.: Fetal growth and neonatal mortality. *Pediatrics 49:* 392, 1972.
188. North, A. F.: Small-for-dates neonates. I. *Pediatrics 38:* 1013, 1966.
189. Lubchenco, L., and Bard, H.: Incidence of hypoglycemia in newborn infants classified by birth weight and gestational age. *Pediatrics 47:* 831, 1971.
190. Pildes, R. S., Forbes, A. E., and Cornblath, M.: Studies of carbohydrate metabolism in the newborn infant. IX. Blood glucose levels and hypoglycemia in twins. *Pediatrics 40:* 69, 1967.
191. Bergsma, D. (ed.): *First Conference on the Clinical Delineation of Birth Defects. IV. Skeletal Dysplasias.* Birth Defects: Original Article Series, vol. 5, 1969.
192. Bergsma, D. (ed.): *Birth Defects Atlas and Compendium.* Baltimore, National Foundation, 1973.
193. McKusick, V. A.: *Mendelian Inheritance in Man.* ed. 2. Baltimore, Johns Hopkins, 1968.
194. Cremin, B. J., and Beighton, P.: Dwarfism in the newborn; the nomenclature, radiological features and genetic significance. *Br. J. Radiol. 47:* 77, 1974.
195. Rubin, P.: *Dynamic Classification of Bone Dysplasias.* Chicago, Year Book, 1964.
196. Smith, D. W.: *Recognizable Patterns of Human Malformation.* Philadelphia, Saunders, 1970.
197. Scott, C. I.: The genetics of short stature. *Prog. Med. Genet. 8:* 243, 1972.
197a. Langer, L. O., Jr.: Check list of conditions associated with retarded longitudinal growth. *Clin. Pediatr. 8:* 142, 1969.
197b. Pérez-Comas, A., and García-Castro, J. M.: Occipito-facial-cervicothoracic-abdomino-digital dysplasia; Jarcho-Levin syndrome of vertebral anomalies. *J. Pediatr. 85:* 388, 1974.
197c. Bailey, J. A.: Forms of dwarfism recognizable at birth. *Clin. Orthop. 76:* 157, 1971.
198. Warkany, J.: A warfarin embryopathy? *Am. J. Dis. Child. 129:* 287, 1975.
199. Romeo, G., Zonana, J., Rimoin, D. L., et al.: Heterogeneity of nonlethal severe short-limed dwarfism. *J. Pediat. 91:* 918, 1977.
199a. Wadlington, W. B., Tucker, V. L., and Schimke, R. N.: Mesomelic dwarfism with hemivertebrae and small genitalia (the Robinow syndrome). *Am. J. Dis. Child. 126:* 202, 1973.
200. Jones, K. L., and Smith, D. W.: The Williams elfin facies syndrome. *J. Pediatr. 86:* 718, 1975.
201. Bloom, D.: The syndrome of congenital telangiectatic erythema and stunted growth. *J. Pediatr. 68:* 103, 1966.
202. Rosenfield, R. L., Breibart, S., Isacs, H., Jr., *et al.:* Trisomy of chromosomes 13–15 and 17–18: Its association with infantile arteriosclerosis. *Am. J. Med. Sci. 244:* 763, 1962.
203. Mietens, C., and Weber, H.: A syndrome characterized by corneal opacity, nystagmus, flexion contracture of the elbows, growth failure, and mental retardation. *J. Pediatr. 69:* 624, 1966.

204. Pena, S. D. J., and Shokeir, M. H. K.: Syndrome of camptodactyly, multiple ankyloses, facial anomalies, and pulmonary hypoplasia. A lethal condition. *J. Pediatr. 85:* 373, 1974.
205. Michaels, R. H., and Kenny, F. M.: Postnatal growth retardation in congenital rubella. *Pediatrics 43:* 251, 1969.
206. Hanson, J. W., and Smith, D. W.: The fetal hydantoin syndrome. *J. Pediatr. 87:* 285, 1975.
207. Lewandowski, R. C., and Yunis, J. J.: New chromosomal syndromes. *Am. J. Dis. Child. 129:* 515, 1975.
208. Menser, M. A., Dods, L., and Harley, J. D.: A twenty-five-year follow-up of congenital rubella. *Lancet 2:* 1347, 1967.
209. Palmer, R. H., Ouelette, E. M., Warner, L., and Leichtman, S. R.: Congenital malformations in offspring of a chronic alcoholic mother. *Pediatrics 53:* 490, 1974.
210. Kandall, S. R., Albin, S., Lowinson, J., Berle, B., Eidelman, A. I., and Gartner, L. M.: Differential effects of maternal heroin and methadone use on birthweight. *Pediatrics 58:* 681, 1976.
211. Feingold, M., Fine, R. N., and Ingall, D.: Intravenous pyelography in infants with single umbilical artery. *N. Engl. J. Med. 270:* 1178, 1964.
212. Cohlan, S. Q., Bevelander, G., and Tiamsic, T.: Growth inhibition of prematures receiving tetracycline: Clinical and laboratory investigation of tetracycline-induced bone fluorescence. *Am. J. Dis. Child. 105:* 453, 1963.
213. Demers, P., Fraser, D., Goldbloom, R. B., *et al.:* Effects of tetracyclines on skeletal growth and dentition. *Canad. Med. Assoc. J. 99:* 849, 1968.
214. Pinsky, L., and Fraser, F. C.: Atypical malformation syndromes. *J. Pediatr. 80:* 141, 1972.
215. Sadehi-Nejad, A., and Senior, B.: Autosomal dominant transmission of isolated growth hormone deficiency in iris-dental dysplasia (Rieger's syndrome). *J. Pediatr. 85:* 644, 1974.
216. Hoyt, W. F., Kaplan, S. L., Grumbach, M. M., and Glaser, J. S.: Septo-optic dysplasia and pituitary dwarfism. *Lancet 1:* 893, 1970.
217. Pochedly, C., Collipp, P. J., Wolman, S. R., *et al.:* Fanconi's anemia with growth hormone deficiency. *J. Pediatr. 79:* 93, 1971.
218. Dacou-Voutetakis, C., Karpathios, T., Logothetis, N., *et al.:* Defective growth hormone secretion in primary microcephaly. *J. Pediatr. 85:* 498, 1974.
219. Castells, S., Voeller, K. K., Vinas, C., and Lu, C.: Cerebral dwarfism: Association of brain dysfunction with growth retardation. *J. Pediatr. 85:* 36, 1974.
220. Cantu, J. M., Hernandez, A., Larracilla, J., *et al.:* A new x-linked recessive disorder with dwarfism, cerebral atrophy, and generalized keratosis follicularis. *Pediatrics 84:* 564, 1974.
221. Dorfman, A. (ed.): *Antenatal Diagnosis.* Chicago, University of Chicago, 1972.
222. Naeye, R.: Organ abnormalities in a human parabiotic syndrome. *Am. J. Pathol. 46:* 299, 1965.
223. Schiff, D., Colle, E., and Stern, L.: Metabolic and growth patterns in transient neonatal diabetes. *N. Engl. J. Med. 287:* 119, 1972.
224. Pagliara, A. S., Karl, I. E., and Kipnis, D. B.: Transient neonatal diabetes: Delayed maturation of the pancreatic beta cell. *J. Pediatr. 82:* 97, 1973.
225. Miller, H. C., and Hassanein, K.: Fetal malnutrition in white newborn infants: Maternal factors. *Pediatrics 52:* 504, 1973.
226. Naeye, R., Blanc, W., and Paul, C.: Effects of maternal nutrition on the human fetus. *Pediatrics 52:* 494, 1973.
227. Morris, N., Osborn, S. B., and Wright, H. P.: Effective circulation of the uterine wall in late pregnancy. *Lancet 1:* 323, 1955.
228. Levitsky, L., Speck, S., and Shulman, S.: Response to fasting in intrauterine growth retardation: A comparison of experimental models. *J. Pediatr. 86:* 972, 1975.
229. Fitzhardinge, P. M., and Steven, E. M.: The small-for-date infant. I. Later growth patterns. *Pediatrics 49:* 671, 1972.
229a. Colle, E., Schill, D., Andrew, G., Bauer, C. B., and Fitzhardinge, P.: Insulin responses during catch-up growth of infants who were small for gestational age. *Pediatrics 57:* 363, 1976.
230. Philip, A. G. S.: Fontanel size and epiphyseal ossification in neonates with intrauterine growth retardation. *J. Pediatr. 84:* 204, 1974.
231. Scott, K. E., and Usher, R.: Epiphyseal development in fetal malnutrition syndrome. *N. Engl. J. Med. 270:* 822, 1964.
232. Wilson, M. G., Meyers, H. I., and Peters, A. H.: Postnatal bone growth of infants with fetal growth retardation. *Pediatrics 40:* 213, 1967.
233. Dacou-Voutetakis, C., Anagnostakis, D., and Xanthous, M.: Macroglossia, transient neonatal diabetes mellitus and intrauterine growth failure: A new distinct entity? *Pediatrics 55:* 127, 1975.
234. Zamenhof, S., van Marthens, E., and Grauel, L.: DNA (cell number) in neonatal brain: Second generation (F_2) alteration by maternal (F_0) dietary protein restriction. *Science 172:* 850, 1971.
235. Babson, S. G., and Phillips, D. S.: Growth and development of twins dissimilar in size at birth. *N. Engl. J. Med. 289:* 937, 1973.
236. Wallace, S. J., and Michie, E. A.: A follow-up study of infants born to mothers with low estriol excretion during pregnancy. *Lancet 2:* 560, 1966.
237. Rabor, I. F., Oh, W., Wu, P. Y. K., *et al.:* The effects of early and late feeding of intrauterine fetally malnourished infants. *Pediatrics 42:* 261, 1968.
238. Foley, T. P., Jr., Thompson, R. G., Shaw, M., *et al.:* Growth responses to human growth hormone in patients with intrauterine growth retardation. *J. Pediatr. 84:* 635, 1974.
239. Verdy, M., Gagnon, M.-A., and Caron, D.: Birth weight and adult obesity in children of diabetic mothers. *N. Engl. J. Med. 290:* 376, 1974.
240. Block, M. B., Pildes, R. S., Mossabhoy, N. A., *et al.:* C-peptide immunoreactivity: A new method for studying infants of insulin-treated diabetic mothers. *Pediatrics 53:* 923, 1974.
241. Naeye, R. L.: Infants of diabetic mothers: A quantitative morphologic study. *Pediatrics 35:* 980, 1965.
242. Pildes, R. S.: Infants of diabetic mothers. *N. Engl. J. Med. 289:* 902, 1973.
243. Schiff, D., and Lowy, C.: Hypoglycemia and excretion of insulin in urine in hemolytic disease of the new-born. *Pediatr. Res. 4:* 280, 1970.
244. Gries, F. A., and Driscoll, S. G.: *In vitro* studies of insulin inactivation with reference to erythroblastosis fetalis. *Blood 30:* 359, 1967.
245. Gruenwald, P.: Growth of the human fetus. I. *Am. J. Obstet. Gynecol. 94:* 1112, 1966.
246. Beckwith, J. B.: Macroglossia, omphalocele, adrenal cytomegaly, gigantism, and hyperplastic visceromegaly. In Bergsma, D. (ed.): *Birth Defects: Original Article Series 2:* 188, 1969.
247. Cohen, M. M., Jr., Gorlin, R. J., Feingold, M, and ten Bensel, R. W.: The Wiedemann syndrome. *Am. J. Dis. Child. 122:* 515, 1971.
248. Filippi, G., and McKusick, V. A.: The Beckwith-Weidemann syndrome. *Medicine 49:* 279, 1970.
249. Roe, T. F., Kershnar, A. K., Weitzmann, J. J., and Madrigal, L. S.: Beckwith's syndrome with extreme organ hyperplasia. *Pediatrics 52:* 372, 1973.
250. Schiff, D., Colle, E., Wells, D., and Stern, L.: Metabolic aspects of the Beckwith-Wiedemann syndrome. *J. Pediatr. 82:* 258, 1973.
251. Gotlin, R. W., and Silver, H. K.: Neonatal hypoglycemia, hyperinsulinism, and absence of pancreatic alpha-cells. *Lancet 1:* 1346, 1970.
252. Perlman, M., Goldberg, G. M., Bar-Ziv, J., and Danovitch, G.: Renal hamartomas and nephroblastomatosis with fetal gigantism: A familial syndrome. *J. Pediatr. 83:* 414, 1973.
253. Bejar, R. L., Smith, G. F., Park, S., *et al.:* Cerebral gigantism: Concentrations of amino acids in plasma and muscle. *J. Pediatr. 76:* 105, 1970.
254. Weaver, D. D., Graham, C. B., Thomas, I. T., and Smith, D. W.: A new overgrowth syndrome with accelerated skeletal maturation, unusual facies, and camptodactyly. *J. Pediatr. 84:* 547, 1974.
255. Hook, E. B., and Reynolds, J. W.: Cerebral gigantism: Endocrinological and clinical observations of six patients including a congenital giant, concordant monozygotic twins, and a child who achieved adult gigantic size. *J. Pediatr. 70:* 900, 1967.
256. Battaglia, F. C., Frazier, T. M., and Hellegers, A. E.: Birth weight, gestational age, and pregnancy outcome with special reference to high birth weight-low gestational age infant. *Pediatrics 37:* 417, 1966.
257. Mellman, W. J., Bongiovanni, A. M., and Hope, J. W.: The diagnostic usefulness of skeletal maturation in an endocrine clinic. *Pediatrics 23:* 530, 1959.
258. Root, A. W., Bongiovanni, A. M., and Eberlein, W. R.: Diagnosis and management of growth retardation with special reference to the problem of hypopituitarism. *J. Pediatr. 78:* 737, 1971.
259. Lemli, L., and Smith, D. W.: The XO syndrome: A study of the differentiated phenotype in 25 patients. *J. Pediatr. 63:* 577, 1963.
260. Smith, D. W., Lemli, L., and Opitz, J. M.: A newly recognized syndrome of multiple congenital anomalies. *J. Pediatr. 64:* 210, 1964.
261. Pinsky, L., and DiGeorge, A. M.: A familial syndrome of facial and

skeletal anomalies associated with genital abnormality in the male and normal genitals in the female. *J. Pediatr. 66:* 1049, 1965.
262. Aarskog, D.: A familial syndrome of short stature associated with facial dysplasia and genital anomalies. *J. Pediatr. 77:* 856, 1970.
263. Sugarman, G. I., Rimoin, D. L., and Lachman, R. S.: The facial-digital-genital (Aarskog) syndrome. *Am. J. Dis. Child. 126:* 248, 1973.
264. Dorfman, A., and Matalon, R.: The mucopolysaccharidoses. In Stanbury, J. B., Wyngaarden, J. B., and Frederickson, D. S. (eds.): *The Metabolic Basis of Inherited Disease,* New York, McGraw-Hill, 1972, p. 1218.
265. DeBusk, F. L.: The Hutchinson-Gilford progeria syndrome. *J. Pediatr. 80* (pt. 2): 697, 1972.
266. Epstein, C. J., Martin, G. M., Schultz, A. L., and Motulsky, A. G.: Werner's syndrome. *Medicine 45:* 177, 1966.
267. Silver, H. K.: Rothmund-Thomson syndrome: An oculocutaneous disorder. *Am. J. Dis. Child. 111:* 182, 1966.
268. Passwell, J., Zipperkowski, L., Katznelson, D., *et al.:* A syndrome characterized by congenital ichthyosis with atrophy, mental retardation, dwarfism, and generalized aminoaciduria. *J. Pediatr. 82:* 466, 1973.
269. Selmanowitz, V. J., and Porter, M. J.: The Sjogren-Larsen syndrome. *Am. J. Med. 42:* 412, 1967.
270. Weinstein, S., and Gorlin, R. J.: Cranio-carpo-tarsal dysplasia or the whistling face syndrome. *Am. J. Dis. Child. 117:* 427, 1969.
271. Hollister, D. W., Rimoin, D. L., Lachman, R. S., *et al.:* The Winchester syndrome: A nonlysosomal connective tissue disease. *J. Pediatr. 84:* 701, 1974.
272. Fialkow, P. J.: Autoimmunity and chromosomal aberrations, *Am. J. Hum. Genet. 18:* 93, 1966.
273. Mosier, H. D., Grossman, H. J., and Dingman, H. F.: Physical growth in mental defectives. *Pediatrics 36* (suppl.): 465, 1965.
274. Haddad, H. M., and Wilkins, L.: Congenital anomalies associated with gonadal aplasia. *Pediatrics 23:* 885, 1959.
275. Ferguson-Smith, M. A., Alexander, D. S., Bowen, P., *et al.:* Clinical and cytogenetical studies in female gonadal dysgenesis and their bearing on the cause of Turner's syndrome. *Cytogenetics 3:* 355, 1964.
276. Engel, E., and Forbes, A. P.: Cytogenetic and clinical findings in 48 patients with congenitally defective or absent ovaries. *Medicine 44:* 135, 1965.
277. Goldberg, M. B., Scully, A. L., Solomon, I. L., and Steinbach, H. L.: Gonadal dysgenesis in phenotypic female subjects. *Am. J. Med. 45:* 529, 1968.
278. Carballo, E. C.: Turner's syndrome and Noonan's syndrome. *J. Pediatr. 75:* 729, 1969.
279. Curts, F. L., Pucci, E., Scappaticci, S., *et al.:* XO and male phenotype. *Am. J. Dis. Child. 128:* 90, 1974.
280. Rainier-Pope, C. R., Cunningham, R. D., Nadas, A. S., and Crigler, J. F., Jr.: Cardiovascular malformations in Turner's syndrome. *Pediatrics 33:* 919, 1964.
281. Heller, R. H.: The Turner phenotype in the male. *J. Pediatr. 66:* 48, 1965.
282. Noonan, J. A.: Hypertelorism with Turner phenotype. *Am. J. Dis. Child. 116:* 373, 1968.
283. Collins, E., and Turner, G.: The Noonan syndrome—A review of the clinical and genetic features of 27 cases. *J. Pediatr. 83:* 941, 1973.
284. Nora, J. J., Nora, A. H., Sinha, A. K., *et al.:* The Ullrich-Noonan syndrome (Turner phenotype). *Am. J. Dis. Child. 127:* 48, 1974.
285. Pinsky, L., and Levy, E. P.: Malignant hyperpyreia or the XX-XY Turner phenotype. *J. Pediatr. 83:* 896, 1973.
286. Saez, J. M., Morera, A. M., and Bertrand, J.: Testicular endocrine function in males with Noonan's syndrome. *Lancet 2:* 1078, 1969.
287. Wilson, J. G.: Comment on internipple distance. *J. Pediatr. 85:* 148, 1974.
288. Razdan, A. K., Rosenfield, R. L., and Kim, M. H.: Endocrinologic characteristics of partial ovarian failure. *J. Clin. Endocrinol. Metab. 43:* 449, 1976.
289. Armendares, S., Antillon, F., Del Castillo, V., and Jiminez, M.: A newly recognized inherited syndrome of dwarfism, craniostenosis, retinitis pigmentosa, and multiple congenital malformations. *J. Pediatr. 85:* 872, 1974.
290. Hoefnagel, D., and Benirschke, K.: Dyscephalia mandibulo oculofacialis (Hallerman-Streiff syndrome). *Arch. Dis. Child. 40:* 57, 1965.
291. Tay, C. H.: Ichthyosiform erythroderma, hair shaft abnormalities and mental and growth retardation. *Arch. Derm. 104:* 4, 1971.
292. Zachmann, M., Illig, R., and Prader, A.: Fanconi's anemia with isolated growth hormone deficiency. *J. Pediatr. 80:* 159, 1972.
293. Danes, B. S.: Progeria: A cell culture study on aging. *J. Clin. Invest. 50:* 2000, 1971.
294. Epstein, J., Williams, J. R., and Little, J. B.: Deficient DNA repair in human progeroid cells. *Proc. Natl. Acad. Sci. 70:* 977, 1973.
295. Regan, J. D., and Setlow, R. B.: DNA repair in human progeroid cells. *Biochem. Biophys. Res. Commun. 59:* 858, 1974.
296. Hand, R., and German, J.: Delayed DNA chain growth in Bloom's syndrome. *J. Clin. Invest. 53:* 31a, 1974.
297. Epstein, C. J., Graham, C. B., Hodgkin, W. E., *et al.:* Hereditary dysplasia of bone with kyphoscoliosis, contractures and abnormally shaped ears. *J. Pediatr. 73:* 379, 1968.
298. Rimoin, D. L., Fletcher, B. D., and McKusick, V. A.: Spondylocostal dysplasia. *Am. J. Med. 45:* 948, 1968.
299. Ruvalcaba, R. H. A., Reichert, A., and Smith, D. W.: A new familial syndrome with osseous dysplasia and mental deficiency. *J. Pediatr. 79:* 450, 1971.
300. Rüdiger, R. A., Schmidt, W., Loose, D. A., and Passarge, E.: Severe developmental failure with coarse facial features, distal limb hypoplasia, thickened palmar creases, bifid uvula, and ureteral stenosis: A previously unidentified familial disorder with lethal outcome. *J. Pediatr. 79:* 977, 1971.
301. Money, J.: Dwarfism. Questions and answers in counseling. *Rehabil. Lit. 28:* 134, 1967.
302. Bettman, H. K., Goldman, H. S., Abramowicz, M., and Sobel, E. H.: Oxandrolone treatment of short stature: Effect on predicted mature height. *J. Pediatr. 79:* 1018, 1971.
303. Johanson, A. J., Brasel, J. A., and Blizzard, R. M.: Growth in patients with gonadal dysgenesis receiving fluoxymesterone. *J. Pediatr. 75:* 1015, 1969.
304. Sobel, E. H., Raymond, C. S., Quinn, K. V., and Talbot, N. B.: The use of methyltestosterone to stimulate growth: Relative influence on skeletal maturation and linear growth. *J. Clin. Endocrinol. Metab. 16:* 241, 1956.
305. Yaffe, S. J., Bierman, C. W., Cann, H. M., *et al.:* Counseling and synthetic steroids in short stature without organic disease. *Pediatrics 53:* 285, 1974.
306. Crawford, J. D., Bode, H. H., and Botstein, P. M.: Human growth hormone and nonhypopituitary disorders. In Raiti, S. (ed.): *Advances in Human Growth Hormone Research,* Washington, D.C., U.S. Government, 1974, p. 757.
307. Escamilla, R. F.: Non-hypopituitary dwarfs and human growth hormone therapy. In Raiti, S. (ed.): *Advances in Human Growth Hormone Research.* Washington, D.C., U.S. Government, 1974, p. 765.
308. Frasier, S. D., Hilburn, J. M., and Smith, F. G., Jr.: Dwarfism and mental retardation: The serum growth hormone response to hypoglycemia. *J. Pediatr. 77:* 136, 1970.
309. Powell, G. F., Brasel, J. A., and Blizzard, R. M.: Emotional deprivation and growth retardation simulating idiopathic hypopituitarism. *N. Engl. J. Med. 276:* 1271, 1967.
310. Silver, H. K., and Finkelstein, M.: Deprivation dwarfism. *J. Pediatr. 70:* 317, 1967.
311. Krieger, I., and Millinger, R. C.: Pituitary function in the deprivation syndrome. *J. Pediatr. 79:* 216, 1971.
312. Powell, G. F., Hopwood, N. J., and Barratt, E. S.: Growth hormone studies before and during catch-up growth in a child with emotional deprivation and short stature. *J. Clin. Endocrinol. Metab. 37:* 674, 1973.
313. Rabinowitz, D., and Merimee, T. J.: Isolated human growth hormone deficiency and related disorders. *Isr. J. Med. Sci. 9:* 1599, 1973.
314. Laron, Z., Pertzelan, A., Karp, M., *et al.:* Administration of growth hormone to patients with familial dwarfism with high plasma immunoreactive growth hormone. *J. Clin. Endocrinol. Metab. 33:* 332, 1971.
314a. Daughaday, W. H., Laron, Z., Pertzelan, A., and Heins, J. N.: Defective sulfation factor generation: A possible etiological link in dwarfism. *Trans. Assoc. Am. Phys. 82:* 129, 1969.
315. Elders, M. J., Garland, J. T., Daughaday, W. A., *et al.:* Laron's dwarfism: Studies on the nature of the defect. *J. Pediatr. 83:* 253, 1973.
316. Frasier, S. D.: A review of growth hormone stimulation tests in children. *Pediatrics 53:* 929, 1974.
317. Mims, R. B., Scott, C. L., Modebe, O. M., and Bethune, J. E.: Prevention of L-dopa-induced growth hormone stimulation by hyperglycemia. *J. Clin. Endocrinol. Metab. 37:* 660, 1973.

318. Joss, E. E., and Zuppinger, K. A.: The significance of intermediate plasma growth hormone levels in growth-retarded children. *J. Pediatr. 81:* 1092, 1972.
319. Parker, M. L., and Daughaday, W. H.: Growth retardation: Correlation of plasma growth hormone responses to insulin and arginine with subsequent metabolic and skeletal responses to GH treatment. In Pecile, A., and Muller, E. E. (eds.): *Growth Hormone*. Amsterdam, Excerpta Medica, 1968, p. 398.
320. Aceto, T., Jr., Frasier, S. D., Hayles, A. B., *et al.*: Collaborative study of the effects of humam growth hormone in growth hormone deficiency. I. First year of therapy. *J. Clin. Endocrinol. Metab. 35:* 483, 1972.
321. Aceto, T., Jr., Frasier, S. D., Hayles, A. B., *et al.*: Collaborative study of the effects of human growth hormone in growth hormone deficiency. III. First eighteen months of therapy. In Raiti, S. (ed.): *Advances in Human Growth Hormone Research,* Washington, D.C., U.S. Government, 1974, p. 695.
322. Frasier, S. D.: Personal communication, 1974.
323. Wright, J. C., Brasel, J. A., Aceto, T., Jr., *et al.*: Studies with human growth hormone (HGH), *Am. J. Med. 38:* 499, 1965.
324. Hubble, D.: Studies with human growth hormone. *Arch. Dis. Child. 41:* 17, 1966.
325. Clayton, B. E., Tanner, J. M., and Vince, F. P.: Diagnostic and prognostic value of short-term metabolic response to human growth hormone in short stature. *Arch. Dis. Child. 46:* 405, 1971.
326. Kirkland, R. T., Kirkland, J. L., Librik, L., and Clayton, G. W.: Results of intermittant human growth hormone (HGH) therapy in hypopituitary dwarfism. *J. Clin. Endocrinol. Metab. 37:* 204, 1973.
327. Goodman, H. G., Grumbach, M. M., and Kaplan, S. L.: Growth and growth hormone. II. *N. Engl. J. Med. 278:* 57, 1968.
328. Sheikolislam, B. M., and Stempfel, R. S., Jr.: Hereditary isolated somatotrophin deficiency: Effects of human growth hormone administration. *Pediatrics 49:* 362, 1972.
329. Porter, B. A., Refetoff, S., Rosenfield, R. L., *et al.*: Abnormal thyroxine metabolism in hyposomatotrophic dwarfism and inhibition of responsiveness to TRH during GH therapy. *Pediatrics 51:* 668, 1973.
330. Lippe, B. M., Van Herle, A. J., La Franchi, S. H., *et al.*: Reversible hypothyroidism in growth hormone-deficient children treated with human growth hormone. *J. Clin. Endocrinol, Metab. 40:* 612, 1975.
331. Kaplan, S. L., Savage, D. C. L., Suter, S., *et al.*: Antibodies to human growth hormone arising in patients treated with human growth hormone: Incidence, characteristics, and effects on growth. In Raiti, S. (ed.): *Advances in Human Growth Hormone Research,* Washington, D.C., U.S. Government, 1974, p. 725.
332. Ridler, M. W., and Brook, C. G. D.: Slipped upper femoral epiphypsis following treatment with human growth hormone. *J. Bone Joint Surg. 56-A:* 1719, 1974.
333. Rennie, W., and Mitchell, H N.: Slipped femoral capital epiphysis occurring during growth hormone therapy. *J. Bone Joint Surg. 56-B:* 703, 1974.
334. Frasier, S. D., Aceto, T., Jr., Hayles, A. B.; *et al.*: Collaborative study of the effects of human growth hormone in growth hormone deficiency. II. Development and significance of antibodies to human growth hormone during the first year of therapy. *J. Clin. Endocrinol. Metab. 38:* 14, 1974.
335. Underwood, L. E., Voina, S. J., and Van Wyck, J. J.: Restoration of growth by human growth hormone (Roos) in hypopituitary dwarfs immunized by other human growth hormone preparations. *J. Clin. Endocrinol. Metab. 38:* 288, 1974.
336. Raiti, S.: Letter to the editor. *J. Clin. Endocrinol. Metab. 39:* 964, 1974.
337. Van den Brande, J. L., Van Wyk, J. J., French, F. S., *et al.*: Advancement of skeletal age of hypopituitary children treated with thyroid hormone plus cortisone. *J. Pediatr. 82:* 22, 1973.
338. Frasier, S. D., and Rallison, M. L.: Growth retardation and emotional deprivation: Relative resistance to treatment with human growth hormone. *J. Pediatr. 80:* 603, 1972.
339. Raiti, S., Trias, E., Levitsky, L., and Grossman, M. S.: Oxandrolone and human growth hormone. *Am. J. Dis. Child. 126:* 597, 1973.
340. MacGillivray, M. H., Kolotkin, M., and Munschauer, R. W.: Enhanced linear growth responses in hypopituitary dwarfs treated with growth hormone plus androgen *versus* growth hormone alone. *Pediatr. Res. 8:* 103, 1974.
341. Agustin, A. V., deLevie, M., Radfar, N., *et al.*: Enhanced linear growth rate, weight gain, and insulin release in hypopituitarism by cyproheptadine (CP) plus human growth hormone (HGH) versus HGH alone. *Pediatr. Res. 9:* 287, 1975.
341a. Rezvani, I., and DiGeorge, A. M.: Reassessment of the daily dose of oral thyroxine for replacement therapy in hypothyroid children. *J. Pediatr. 90:* 291, 1977.
341b. Abbassi, V., and Aldige, C.: Evaluation of sodium L-thyroxine (T_4) requirement in replacement therapy of hypothyroidism *J. Pediatr. 90:* 298, 1977.
341c. Sato, T., Suzuki, Y., Taketani, T., Ishiguor, K., and Nakajima, H.: Age related change in pituitary threshold for TSH release during thyroxine replacement therapy for cretinism. *J. Clin. Endocrinol. Metab. 44:* 553, 1977.
342. Lee, P. A., Weldon, V. V., and Migeon, C. V.: Short stature as the only clinical sign of Cushing's syndrome. *J. Pediatr. 86:* 89, 1975.
343. Loridan, L., and Senior, B.: Cushing's syndrome in infancy. *J. Pediatr. 75:* 349, 1969.
344. Strickland, A. L., Underwood, L. E., Voina, S. J., *et al.*: Growth retardation in Cushing's syndrome. *Am. J. Dis. Child. 123:* 207, 1972.
345. Mosier, H. D., Smith, F. G., Jr., and Schultz, M. A.: Failure of catch-up growth after Cushing's syndrome in childhood. *Am. J. Dis. Child. 124:* 251, 1972.
346. Migeon, C. J.: Updating the treatment of congenital adrenal hyperplasia. *J. Pediatr. 73:* 805, 1968.
347. Van Metre, T. E., Niermann, W. A., and Rosen, L. T.: A comparison of the growth suppressive effect of cortisone, prednisone, and other adrenal cortical hormones. *J. Allergy 31:* 531, 1960.
348. Kozower, M., Veatch, L., and Kaplan, M. M.: Decreased clearance of prednisolone, a factor in the development of corticosteroid side effects. *J. Clin. Endocrinol. Metab. 38:* 407, 1974.
349. Soyka, L. F.: Alternate-day corticosteroid therapy. *Adv. Pediatr. 19:* 47, 1972.
350. Simopoulos, A. P., and Bartter, F. C.: Growth characteristics and factors influencing growth in Bartter's syndrome. *J. Pediatr. 81:* 56, 1972.
351. Nash, M. A., Torrado, A. D., Greifer, I., *et al.*: Renal tubular acidosis in infants and children. *J. Pediatr. 80:* 738, 1972.
352. Moses, S. W., and Gutman, A.: Inborn errors of glycogen metabolism. *Adv. Pediatr. 19:* 95, 1972.
353. Simmons, J. M., Wilson, C. J., Potter, D. E., and Holliday, M. A.: Relation of calorie deficiency to growth failure in children on hemodialysis and the growth response to calorie supplementation. *N. Engl. J. Med. 285:* 642, 1974.
354. Saenger, P., Wiedemann, E., Schwartz, E., *et al.*: Somatomedin and growth after renal transplantation. *Pediatr. Res. 8:* 163, 1974.
355. Stickler, G. B., and Bergen, B. J.: A review: Short stature in renal disease. *Pediatr. Res. 7:* 978, 1973.
356. Broyer, M., Kleinknecht, C., Loirat, C., *et al.*: Growth in children treated with long-term hemodialysis. *J. Pediatr. 84:* 642, 1974.
357. Beeken, W. L.: Absorptive defects in young people with regional enteritis. *Pediatrics 52:* 69, 1973.
358. Teng, C. T., Daeschner, C. W., Jr., Singleton, E. B., *et al.*: Liver disease and osteoporosis in children. *I. J. Pediatr. 59:* 684, 1961.
359. Waldmann, T. A., Gordon, R. S., Jr., and Rosse, W.: Studies on the metabolism of the serum proteins and lipids in a patient with analbuminemia. *Am. J. Med. 37:* 960, 1964.
360. Editorial: The Mauriac syndrome. *Diabetes 2:* 415, 1953.
361. Raghuramulu, N., and Rao, K. S. J.: Growth hormone secretion in protein-calorie malnutrition. *J. Clin. Endocrinol. Metab. 38:* 176, 1974.
362. Portnay, G. I., O'Brian, J. T., Bush, J., *et al.*: The effect of starvation on the concentration and binding of thyroxine and triiodothyronine in serum and on the response to TRH. *J. Clin. Endocrinol. Metab. 39:* 199, 1974.
362a. Chopra, I. J., Chopra, U., Smith, S. R., Reza, M., and Solomon, D. H.: Reciprocal changes in serum concentrations of 3, 3′,5′-triiodothyronine (reverse T_3) and 3, 3'5-triiodothyronine (T_3) in systemic illnesses. *J. Clin. Endocrinol. Metab. 41:* 1043, 1975.
363. Ellis, R. W. B.: Growth and health of Belgian children during and before the German occupation (1940-1944). *Arch. Dis. Child. 20:* 97, 1945.
364. Danks, D. M., Stevens, B. J., Campbell, P. E., *et al.*: Menkes' kinky-hair syndrome. *Lancet 1:* 1100, 1972.
365. Ansell, B. M., and Bywaters, E. G. L.: Growth in Stills' disease. *Ann. Rheum. Dis. 15:* 295, 1956.
366. Hsu, L. Y. F., and Hirschhom, K.: Unusual Turner mosaicism (45, X/47, XXX; 45, X/46, XX_{qi}; 45, X/46, XX_r): detection through

deceleration from normal linear growth or secondary amenorrhea. *J. Pediatr. 79:* 276, 1971.

367. Bannerman, R. M.: X-linked spondyloepiphyseal dysplasia tarda (SDT). In Bergsma, D. (ed.): *Birth Defects Orig. Article Ser. 5:* 48, 1969.
368. Acheson, R. M.: Maturation of the skeleton. In Falkner, F. (ed.): *Human Development.* Philadelphia, Saunders, 1966, p. 465.
369. Karp, M., Laron, Z., and Doron, M.: Insulin secretion in children with constitutional familial short stature. *J. Pediatr. 83:* 241, 1973.
370. Rothchild, E., and Owens, R. P.: Adolescent girls who lack functioning ovaries. *J. Am. Acad. Child. Psych. 11:* 88, 1972.
371. Hermosa, B. D., and Sobel, E. H.: Thyroid in the treatment of short stature. *J. Pediatr. 80:* 988, 1972.
372. Hambidge, K. M., Hambidge, C., Jacobs, M., and Baun, J. D.: Low levels of zinc in hair, anorexia, poor growth, and hypogeusia in children. *Pediatr. Res. 6:* 868, 1972.
372a. Solomons, N. W., Rosenfield, R. L., Jacob, R. A., and Sandstead, H. H.: Growth retardation and zinc nutrition. *Pediatr. Res. 10:* 923, 1976.
373. Tattersall, R. B., and Pyke, D. A.: Growth in diabetic children. *Lancet 2:* 1105, 1973.
374. Ashcroft, M. T., Sarjeant, G. R., and Desai, P.: Heights, weights, and skeletal age of Jamaican adolescents with sickle cell anemia. *Arch. Dis. Child. 47:* 519, 1972.
375. Linde, L. M., Dunn, O. J., Schireson, R., and Rasof, B.: Growth in children with congenital heart disease. *J. Pediatr. 70:* 413, 1967.
376. Naeye, R. L.: Anatomic features of growth failure in congenital heart disease. *Pediatrics 39:* 433, 1967.
377. Umansky, R., and Hauck, A. J.: Factors in the growth of children with patent ductus arteriosis. *Pediatrics 30:* 540, 1962.
378. Hait, G., Gruskin, A. B., and Paulsen, E. P.: Insulin suppression in children with congestive heart failure. *Pediatrics 50:* 451, 1972.
379. Harrison, H. E., Harrison, H. C., Lifshitz, F., and Johnson, A. D.: Growth disturbance in hereditary hypophosphatemia. *Am. J. Dis. Child. 112:* 290, 1966.
380. Glorieux, F. H., Scriver, C. R., Reade, T. M., *et al.:* Use of phosphate and vitamin D to prevent dwarfism and rickets in X-linked hypophosphatemia. *N. Engl. J. Med. 287:* 481, 1972.
381. McEnery, P. T., Silverman, F. N., and West, C. D.: Acceleration of growth with combined vitamin D-phosphate therapy of hypophosphatemic resistant rickets. *J. Pediatr. 80:* 763, 1972.
382. Safer, D. J., and Allen, R. P.: Factors influencing the suppressant effects of two stimulant drugs on the growth of hyperactive children. *Pediatrics 51:* 660, 1973.
383. Greenblatt, R. B., McDonough, P. G., and Mahesh, V. B.: Estrogen therapy in inhibition of growth. *J. Clin. Endocrinol. Metab. 26:* 1185, 1966.
384. Greenblatt, R. B., McDonough, P. G., and Mahesh, V. B.: Projection of growth. *J. Clin. Endocrinol. Metab. 27:* 1761, 1967.
385. Schoen, E. J., Solomon, I. L., Warner, O., and Wingird, J.: Estrogen treatment of tall girls. *Am. J. Dis. Child. 125:* 71, 1973.
386. Wettenhall, H. N. B., Cahill, C., and Roche, A. F.: Tall girls: A survey of 15 years of management and treatment. *J. Pediatr. 86:* 602, 1975.
387. Gardner, L. I.: The child with "excessive" height prediction. *Am. J. Dis. Child. 129:* 17, 1975.
388. Zachmann, M., Ferrandez, A., Mürset, G., Vnehm, H. E., and Prader, A.: Testosterone treatment of excessively tall boys. *J. Pediatr. 88:* 116, 1975.
389. McKusick, V. A.: *Heritable Disorders of Connective Tissues,* 4th ed. St. Louis, Mosby, 1972.
390. Lamberg, S. I., and Dorfman, A.: Synthesis and degradation of hyaluronic acid in cultured fibroblasts of Marfan's disease. *J. Clin. Invest. 52:* 2428, 1973.
391. Carey, M. C., Donovan, D. E., FitzGerald, O., and McAuley, F. D.: Hemocystinuria. I. *Am. J. Med. 45:* 7, 1968.
392. Bianchine, J. W.: The Marfan syndrome revisited. *J. Pediatr. 79:* 717, 1971.
393. Barber, G. W., and Spaeth, G. L.: The successful treatment of homocystinuria with pyridoxine. *J. Pediatr. 75:* 463, 1969.
394. Schimke, R. N.: Phenotype of malignancy: The mucosal neuroma syndrome. *Pediatrics 52:* 283, 1973.
395. Kaplan, E. L., and Peskin, G. W.: Physiologic implications of medullary carcinoma of the thyroid gland. *Surg. Clin. North Am. 51:* 125, 1971.
396. Costin, G., Fefferman, R. A., and Kogut, M. D.: Hypothalamic gigantism. *J. Pediatr. 83:* 419, 1973.
397. AvRuskin, T. W., Sau, K., Tang, S., and Juan, C.: Childhood acromegaly: Successful therapy with conventional radiation and effects of chlorpromazine on growth hormone and prolactin secretions. *J. Clin. Endocrinol, Metab. 37:* 380, 1973.
398. Frasier, S. D., and Kogut, M. D.: Adolescent acromegaly. Studies of growth-hormone and insulin metabolism. *J. Pediatr. 71:* 832, 1967.
399. Saxena, K. M., and Crawford, J. D.: Acromegalic gigantism in an adolescent girl. *J. Pediatr. 62:* 660, 1963.
400. Schlesinger, S., MacGillivray, M. H., and Manschauer, R. W.: Acceleration of growth and bone maturation in childhood thyrotoxicosis. *J. Pediatr. 83:* 233, 1973.
401. Wilroy, R. S., Jr., and Etteldorf, J. N.: Familial hyperthyroidism including two siblings with neonatal Graves' disease. *J. Pediatr. 78:* 625, 1971.
402. Seip, M.: Generalized lipodystrophy. Ergeb. Inn. Med. Kinderheilkd. *31:* 65, 1971.
403. Mabry, C. C., and Hollingsworth, D. R.: Failure of hypophysectomy in generalized lipodystrophy. *J. Pediatr. 81:* 990, 1972.
404. Mabry, C. C., Hollingsworth, D. R., Upton, C. V., and Corbin, A.: Pituitary-hypothalamic dysfunction in generalized lipodystrophy. *J. Pediatr. 82:* 625, 1973.
405. Senior, B., and Loridan, L.: Fat cell function and insulin in a patient with generalized lipodystrophy. *J. Pediatr. 74:* 972, 1969.
406. Beitins, I. Z., Kowarski, A., Migeon, C. J., and Graham, G. G.: Adrenal function in normal infants and in marasmus and kwashiorkor. *J. Pediatr. 86:* 302, 1975.
407. Caddell, J. L.: Studies in protein-calorie malnutrition. II. *N. Engl. J. Med. 276:* 535, 1967.
408. Ferguson, A. C., Lawlor, G. J., Jr., Neumann, C. G., *et al.:* Decreased rosette-forming lymphocytes in malnutrition and intrauterine growth retardation. *J. Pediatr. 85:* 717, 1974.
409. McAnulty, P. A., and Dickerson, J. W. T.: The cellular response of the weanling rat thymus gland to undernutrition and rehabilitation. *Pediatr. Res. 9:* 778, 1973.
410. McFarlane, H., Ogbeide, M. I., Reddy, S., *et al.:* Biochemical assessment of protein-calorie malnutrition. *Lancet 1:* 392, 1969.
411. Waterlow, J. C.: Observations on the mechanisms of adaptation to low protein intakes. *Lancet 2:* 1091, 1968.
412. Owen, G. M., Kram, K. M., Garry, P. J., *et al.:* A study of nutritional status of preschool children in the United States, 1968–1970. *Pediatrics 53:* (pt. 2): 598, 1974.
413. Bongiovanni, A. M., Eberlein, W. R., and Jones, I. T.: Idiopathic hypercalcemia of infancy, with failure to thrive. *N. Engl. J. Med. 257:* 951, 1957.
414. Friedman, W. F., and Mills, L. F.: The relationship between vitamin D and the craniofacial and dental anomalies of the supravalvular aortic stenosis syndrome. *Pediatrics 43:* 12, 1969.
415. Seelig, M. S.: Vitamin D and cardiovascular, renal, and brain damage in infancy and childhood. *Ann. N.Y. Acad. Sci. 147:* 537, 1969.
416. Fraser, D., Kidd, B. S. L., Kooh, S. W., and Paunier, L.: A new look at infantile hypercalcemia. *Pediatr. Clin. North Am. 13:* 503, 1966.
417. Addy, D. P., and Hudson, F. P.: Diencephalic syndrome of infantile emaciation. *Arch. Dis. Child. 47:* 338, 1972.
418. Fishman, M. A., and Peake, G. T.: Paradoxical growth in a patient with the diencephalic syndrome. *Pediatrics 45:* 973, 1970.
419. Pimstone, B. L., Sobel, J., Meyer, E., and Eale, D.: Secretion of growth hormone in the diecephalic syndrome of childhood. *J. Pediatr. 76:* 886, 1970.
420. Wayne, E. R., and Burrington, J. D.: Extrinsic duodenal obstruction in children. *Surg. Gynecol. Obstet. 136:* 87, 1973.
421. Soergel, K. H.: Hormonally mediated diarrhea. *N. Engl. J. Med. 292:* 970, 1975.
422. Wharton, B. A., Jelliffe, D. B., and Stanfield, J. P.: Do we know how to treat kwashiorkor? *J. Pediatr. 72:* 721, 1968.
423. Krieger, I., and Chen, Y. C.: Calorie requirements for weight gain in infants with growth failure due to maternal deprivation, undernutrition, and congenital heart disease. *Pediatrics 44:* 647, 1969.
424. de Oliveira, J. E. D., Seatera, L., de Oliveira Netto, N., and Duarte, G. G.: The nutritive value of soya milk and cow's milk in malnourished children: A comparative study. *J. Pediatr. 69:* 670, 1966.
425. Keating, J. P., and Ternberg, J. L.: Amino acid-hypertonic glucose treatment for intractable diarrhea in infants. *Am. J. Dis. Child. 122:* 226, 1971.

426. Van Metre, T. E., Jr.: Factors affecting the rate of linear growth and weight gain of asthmatic children. *South. Med. J. 55:* 1305, 1962.
427. Hansen, J. D. L., Freesemann, C., Moodie, A. D., and Evans, D. E.: What does nutritional growth retardation imply? *Pediatrics 47:* (pt. 2): 299, 1971.
428. Winick, M., and Noble, A.: Cellular response in rats during malnutrition at various ages. *J. Nutr. 89:* 300, 1966.
429. Winick, M.: Malnutrition and brain development. *J. Pediatr. 74:* 667, 1969.
430. De Levie, M., and Nogrady, M. B.: Rapid brain growth upon restoration of adequate nutrution causing false radiologic evidence of increased intracranial pressure. *J. Pediatr. 76:* 523, 1970.
431. Bray, G. A.: Obesity: A serious symptom. *Ann. Int. Med. 77:* 797, 1972.
432. Knittle, J. L.: Obesity in childhood: A problem in adipose tissue cellular development. *J. Pediatr. 81:* 1048, 1972.
433. Mann, G. V.: The influence of obesity on health. *N. Engl. J. Med. 291:* 178, *291:* 226, 1974.
434. Forbes, G. B.: Lean body mass and fat in obese children. *Pediatrics 34:* 308, 1964.
435. Cheek, D. B., Schultz, R. B., Parra, A., and Reba, R. C.: Overgrowth of lean and adipose tissue in adolescent obesity. *Pediatr. Res. 4:* 268, 1970.
436. Knittle, J. L., and Hirsch, J.: Effect of early nutrition on the development of rat epididymal fat pads: Cellularity and metabolism. *J. Clin. Invest. 47:* 2091, 1968.
437. Brook, C. G. D.: Evidence for a sensitive period in adipose-cell replication in man. *Lancet 2:* 624, 1972.
438. Heald, F. P., and Hunt, S. M.: Caloric dependency in obese adolescents as affected by degree of maturation. *J. Pediatr. 66:* 1035, 1965.
439. Hall, B. D., and Smith, D. W.: Prader-Willi syndrome. *J. Pediatr. 81:* 286, 1972.
440. Parra, A., Cervantes, C., and Schultz, R. B.: Immunoreactive insulin and growth hormone responses in patients with Prader-Willi syndrome. *J. Pediatr. 83:* 587, 1973.
441. Tolis, G., Lewis, W., Verdy, M., *et al.:* Anterior pituitary function in the Prader-Labhart-Willi (PLW) syndrome. *J. Clin. Endocrinol. Metab. 39:* 1061, 1974.
441a. Klein, D., and Ammann, F.: The syndrome of Laurence-Moon-Bardet-Biedl and allied diseases in Switzerland. *J. Neurol. Sci. 9:* 479, 1969.
442. Warkany, J., and Kalter, H.: Congenital malformations. *N. Engl. J. Med. 265:* 993, 1961.
443. Nora, J. J., and Nora, A. H.: Can the pill cause birth defects? *N. Engl. J. Med. 291:* 731, 1974.
444. Reid, R. A.: Diabetes and congenital anomalies. *Lancet 1:* 1030, 1970.
445. Rowland, T. W., Hubbell, J. P., Jr., and Nadas, A. S.: Congenital heart disease in infants of diabetic mothers. *J. Pediatr. 83:* 815, 1973.
446. Kucera, J.: Exposure to fat solvents: A possible cause of sacral agenesis in man. *J. Pediatr. 72:* 857, 1968.
447. Vallance-Owen, J., Braithwaite, F., Wilson, J. S. P., *et al.:* Cleft lip and palate deformities and insulin antagonism. *Lancet 2:* 912, 1967.
448. Miller, R. W.: Relation between cancer and congenital defects in man. *N. Engl. J. Med. 275:* 87, 1966.
449. Parker, D. A. and Skalko, R. G.: Congenital asymmetry report of 10 cases with associated developmental abnormalities. *Pediatrics 44:* 584, 1969.
450. Meadows, A. T., Lichtenfeld, J. L., and Koop, C. E.: Wilms' tumor in three children of a woman with congenital hemihypertrophy. *N. Engl. J. Med. 291:* 23, 1974.
451. Barakat, A. Y., Papadopoulou, Z. L., Chandra, R. S.: *et al.:* Psudohermaphroditism, nephron disorder, and Wilms' tumor: A unifying concept. *Pediatrics 54:* 366, 1974.
452. Fienman, N. L., and Yakovac, W. C.: Neurofibromatosis in childhood. *J. Pediatr. 76:* 339, 1970.
453. Schenkein, I., Bueker, E. D., Helson, L., *et al.:* Increased nerve-growth-stimulating activity in disseminated neurofibromatosis. *N. Engl. J. Med. 290:* 613, 1974.
454. Holmes, L. B.: Inborn errors of morphogenesis. *N. Engl. J. Med. 291:* 763, 1974.
455. Currarino, G., and Engle, M. A.: The effects of ligation of the subclavian artery on the bones and soft tissues of the arms. *J. Pediatr. 67:* 808, 1965.
456. Young, R. C., De Vita, V. T., and Johnson, R. E.: Hodgkin's disease in childhood. *Blood 42:* 163, 1973.

ACKNOWLEDGMENTS

This chapter was written while the author was under the tenure of USPHS Research Career Development Award HD-70152. Portions of this work were supported by USPHS grants HD-06308 and HD-07110.

143

Metabolic Effects of Insulin, Glucagon, and Glucose in Man: Clinical Applications

Thomas T. Aoki
George F. Cahill, Jr.

INTRODUCTION

In 1912, Benedict and Joslin[1] performed metabolic balance studies on diabetics in whom blood sugar control was attempted by the only therapeutic modality then available, i.e., severe dietary restriction, especially of carbohydrates. They showed that these patients excreted large quantities of urea, glucose, and ketoacids in their urine each day (suggesting that both endogenous and exogenous protein were being converted into glucose by the liver, with excess glucose appearing in the urine.)

In 1921, Banting and Best[2] administered acid–alcohol extracts of fetal calf and dog pancreas to diabetic dogs and effected a reversal of their diabetes. The following year similar extracts of beef pancreas were used clinically, and physicians noted marked increases in both total body weight and lean body mass following treatment. In 1924, Wiechmann,[3,4] a German physician, reported that the administration of glucose to normal subjects and insulin to diabetic subjects resulted in a lowering of circulating α-amino nitrogen levels, and, in particular, in a narrowing of the negative arteriovenous α-amino nitrogen difference across the forearm. Other investigators[5,6] subsequently confirmed these observations not only in man but in rats and rabbits as well. In 1938, Mirsky[7] showed that the administration of insulin to nephrectomized dogs resulted in a marked reduction in the rate of formation of nonprotein nitrogen, and hence, indirectly, of endogenous protein catabolism. The mechanism by which the reduction of catabolism was accomplished was suggested by the further observation that the levels of amino acids in muscle were significantly reduced. Based on these experiments, however, it was not possible to differentiate enhanced protein synthesis from decreased muscle proteolysis.

Supported in part by UPHS Grants AM-05077 and AM-15191. Dr. Aoki is an Investigator, Howard Hughes Medical Institute.

In 1955, Russell[8] noted that insulin prevented the rise in α-amino nitrogen levels in eviscerated rats and subsequently postulated that insulin directly enhances muscle amino acid uptake. With the availability of nonmetabolizable amino acids such as α-amino isobutyric acid, it was quickly determined by a number of investigators that insulin directly enhances uptake of this substance into certain tissues such as muscle and liver. It was soon discovered, somewhat disconcertingly, that a number of amino acids are present in extraordinarily high concentrations within muscle cells—an observation that made kinetic studies somewhat difficult. Nevertheless, Manchester[9] has compiled a list of amino acids whose intracellular concentrations in muscle are enhanced by insulin (Table 143-1). It is important to note that it is possible to separate protein synthesis from amino acid transport in studies by the appropriate protein synthesis inhibitor (i.e., puromycin, cycloheximide) and to clearly establish that one may take place without the other. Indeed, the initiation of protein synthesis in muscle is not dependent on glucose availability, glucose transport, or RNA synthesis.[10,11]

Our understanding of the mechanisms involved in the initiation, execution, and termination of both protein synthesis and

Table 143-1. Intracellular Accumulation of Amino Acids: Effects of Insulin

Accumulation Enhanced by Insulin	
Alanine	α-Aminoisobutyric acid
Glycine	Cycloleucine
Histidine	Ethionine
Methionine	Isovaline
Proline	Sarcosine
Serine	
Threonine	
Accumulation Not Enhanced by Insulin	
Alanine	β-Alanine
Arginine	γ-Aminobutyric acid
Aspartic acid	Canavanine
Cystine	α,γ-Diaminobutyric acid
Glutamic acid	ρ-Fluorophenylalanine
Histidine	α-Methyltyrosine
Isoleucine	Norleucine
Leucine	Ornithine
Lysine	α-Aminobicyclo 2,2,1 heptene-2-carboxylic acid
Phenylalanine	
Threonine	
Tryptophan	

degradation in mammalian cells remains largely incomplete. The limited picture that is now available (drawn mainly from stu bacteria, to a lesser extent from studies in rats, and to a very small degree from studies directly in man) is rich in possibilities, not only in regard to the variety of proteins to be produced and removed but also with respect to the regulation of the processes themselves.

Insulin-stimulated protein synthesis apparently requires that the insulin molecule attach to the appropriate receptor on the cell membrane. The work of Cuatrecasas[12] established that insulin need not enter the adipocyte in order to increase glucose transport or glucose oxidation by isolated rat adipose tissue cells. In addition, this investigator showed that lipogenesis was stimulated while lipolysis was inhibited under the same conditions. With the attachment of insulin to its receptor on the cell membrane, a second messenger, as yet uncharacterized, is synthesized, and, as shown by Wool et al.,[13] one of its effects requires the synthesis of a protein (e.g., enzyme or cofactor). A very rapid effect is the phosphorylation of an already present protein with a weight of 130,000 daltons.[14] At any rate, a signal is eventually transmitted to loci inside the cell, including the nucleus, to activate certain processes and to initiate protein synthesis.

As can be seen from this very brief description, intervention or regulation is possible at a wide number of sites. For example, does the initiating signal for protein synthesis or inhibition of degradation need to be a hormone (e.g., insulin)? The answer to this question is apparently "no," since muscle hypertrophy does occur in exercised diabetic rats. How and by what means does insulin, or more correctly, its second message, initiate peptide chain synthesis as well as decrease proteolysis? How does it initiate de novo formation of new protein-synthesizing units, the polysomes, and synthesis of RNA, which is involved in both transcription of the nuclear code (mRNA) and delivery of amino acids to the polysomes (tRNA)? The questions are almost endless and the years of research that lie ahead will be both exciting and challenging.

PROTEIN TURNOVER

Since a normal 70-kg individual has only approximately 6 kg of metabolically mobilizable protein (Fig. 143-1) mainly in the form of muscle (but also as enzymes, albumin, etc.), a loss of more than 2 kg will result in or be accompanied by such marked muscle weakness that the affected individual will have difficulty with such simple tasks as breathing or coughing. Therefore, the rate at which

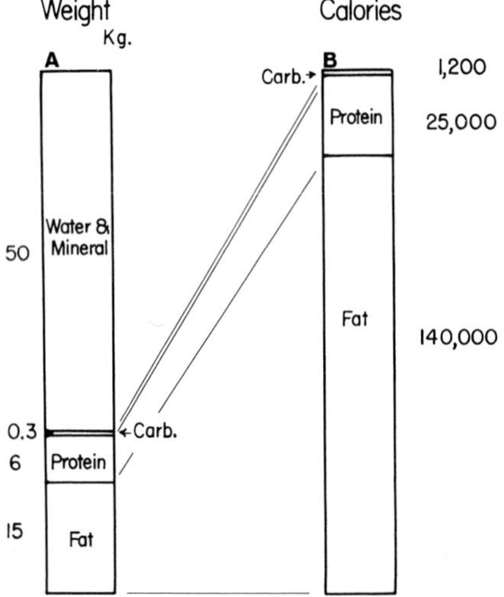

Fig. 143-1. Mobilizable fuel reserves in a normal 70-kg individual on a weight (A) and caloric (B) basis.

man can synthesize and degrade protein is of more than academic interest. Waterlow[15,16] used ^{14}C-lysine infusions to show that total body protein is in a continuous state of flux, with total protein turnover in normal man being on the order of 1.5–3.0 g/kg/day. Since body protein is primarily in the form of muscle, it is probable that this tissue is relatively labile and thereby represents a modest but significant alternative fuel depot upon which various tissues, especially brain, can draw (muscle degradation → hepatic gluconeogenesis → glucose) when the small stores of carbohydrate (hepatic glycogen, extracellular glucose) have been rapidly depleted, as after a 12-h fast. Repletion of any protein debt, as in fasting man, is predictably swift. In view of the foregoing, it appears to be advantageous that both synthesis and degradation of protein are differentially regulated.

PROTEIN CATABOLISM

Amino acid efflux from the forearm muscle bed of postabsorptive normal man has been measured by a number of investigators.[17–21] It has been calculated that 0.5–1.0 g/kg/day of amino acids is released.[19] Assuming that intracellular amino acid concentrations do not change, this quantity of substrate must be derived from proteolysis of muscle protein. Parenthetically, since hydrolysis of any peptide bond is essentially an irreversible step, initial hydrolysis of a single peptide bond of any protein will be followed by the eventual hydrolysis of the entire protein molecule. The mechanism(s) by which this process is initiated and terminated is not known. Of importance to the researcher, approximately one histidine molecule per molecule of actin[22,23] or myosin[23,24] is methylated in the 3 position. Since this amino acid (3-methylhistidine) cannot be reincorporated into protein nor metabolized,[25] it must be excreted in the urine.[26] It would thus appear to be a superb marker of net proteolysis.

As alluded to previously, there appears to be separate regulation of the synthesis and degradation of protein. The importance of this distinction is suggested by the work of Schimke.[27,28] and others,[29,30] who have reported that some rat liver enzymes are maintained or changed primarily by variable and highly characteristic proteolytic rather than synthetic rates. In addition, when rats are fed a diet deficient in one more essential amino acid,[31] proteolysis is augmented, resulting in a greater nitrogen loss than that incurred by starvation alone. The administration of cortisone to rats[32] can preferentially increase proteolysis and result in a greater loss of lean body tissue than can be attributed to a reduction or inhibition of protein synthesis alone. Similarly, the accelerated muscle atrophy observed after denervation is probably due to a preferential increase in proteolysis. The manner in which intracellular proteolysis is regulated and keyed to the metabolic needs of the entire organism has been attributed by some not only to insulin but (based upon isolated perfused rat liver studies[33] and studies on various muscle preparations[34]) to circulating amino acid levels as well. Of interest, Woolfolk and Stadtman[35] have reported that amino acids in bacterial systems may function as cofactors by direct allosteric alteration of enzymes in both synthetic and catabolic reactions.

INSULIN AND PROTEIN CATABOLISM

As mentioned previously, amino acid efflux from human muscle amounts to approximately 0.5–1.0 g/kg/day.[19,20] When a high but physiologic quantity of insulin is infused into human forearm muscle, amino acid efflux is markedly reduced; the major changes are manifested by the branched-chain amino acids. Similarly, when 20 U of regular insulin is infused into individuals who are undergoing therapeutic fasts and whose brains are primarily using ketoacids for fuel,[36] there is a modest but significant reduction in urinary urea nitrogen excretion coincident with marked decreases in circulating amino acid levels. Finally, Hinton et al.,[37] in an attempt to minimize nitrogen loss in severely burned patients, infused massive quantities of both insulin and glucose and were able to effect a striking reduction in urinary urea excretion. Determination of plasma arteriovenous amino acid differences across the forearm of patients in diabetic ketoacidosis showed a marked reduction in both glutamine and alanine release following insulin therapy.[38] In summary, insulin clearly plays a preeminent role in the regulation of overall proteolysis in man.

PROTEIN ANABOLISM: EFFECT OF INNERVATION AND ACTIVITY

Recent studies have been published that suggest that other nonhormonal mechanisms, in particular neuromuscular mechanisms, may be at least as important in the regulation of mammalian protein metabolism as those involving hormones (i.e., insulin). Perhaps the strongest evidence supporting this view comes from the work of Goldberg.[39–41] He divided the gastrocnemius muscle (therby forcing the ipsilateral soleus to become weight bearing) of both starved diabetic and nondiabetic rats and showed that hypertrophy of the soleus muscle occurred despite (1) the lack of provisioning of amino acids from exogenous sources and (2) the absence of insulin. He concluded that "compensatory hypertrophy clearly takes precedence over hormonal growth and even over endocrine signals for muscle depletion." As might be expected, the metabolic similarity between insulin's metabolic effects and that of muscle activity extends to both amino acid transport[42] and stimulation of protein synthesis; this finding, in turn, suggests that they may both operate through some common step in the initiation of protein synthesis (possibly the same second messenger).

The biochemical and structural character of a given muscle is to a great extent determined by the type of work or exercise it performs and the nature of its innervation. For example, red muscle is associated with repetitive or continuous contractions, is characterized by an active protein synthetic rate that is highly responsive to insulin, has a rich capillary blood supply, contains oxidative enzymes, and is innervated mainly by slow conducting axons (e.g., soleus). In contrast, white muscle (gastrocnemeius, flexor digitorum longus) is associated with fast contractions (i.e., fight or flight situations), has a relatively sparse blood supply, contains glycogen and glycolytic enzymes, and is innervated with fast conducting axons. When the nerve supplying a red muscle is divided and rerouted to a white muscle, and vice versa, the muscle initially biochemically dedifferentiates and then assumes the biochemical character, complete with the characteristic capillary blood supply, of the muscle to which the nerve originally ran. Thus, "the energy metabolism of the muscle fibers is determined by the nerve supply."[43] In the final analysis, it is mainly exercise, and to a much less extent food or insulin, that can increase muscle mass, presumably due to the ability of exercise to change the "set" of muscle to any given level of insulin and substrate.

METABOLIC EFFECTS OF GLUCOSE ON NITROGEN METABOLISM

Attempts to characterize the metabolic effects of glucose on nitrogen metabolism extend back at least to the work of Cathcart in 1909. After fasting for 40 h, he placed himself on a pure carbohydrate diet (40 Cal/kg) and noted a marked decrease in nitrogen excretion.[44] As noted elsewhere in this section, Weichmann reported that the administration of glucose to normal subjects resulted in a lowering of circulating α-amino nitrogen levels.[3,4] In 1946, Gamble[45] reported that maximal nitrogen conservation in normal subjects was achieved by the daily ingestion of approximately 100–200 g glucose. More recently, Crofford et al.[46] infused glucose (25 g over 5 min) and glucose and insulin (0.1 U/kg) into normal subjects and reported a decline in the levels of six essential amino acids (valine, leucine, isoleucine, threonine, phenylalanine, and tyrosine). Since the decline in levels of these amino acids was accentuated by the addition of the insulin, it appeared that it was the insulin elicited by the glucose infusion that was primarily responsible for the observed changes.

From the above studies it is not possible to definitively determine what role glucose and insulin each played in the amino acid–lowering effect seen following glucose administration. However, using the forearm technique described by Andres et al.,[47] Pozefsky et al.[19] infused physiologic quantities of insulin into the forearm of normal subjects and were able to significantly diminish the resting efflux of virtually all 20 amino acids; in so doing, they showed that insulin rather than glucose was responsible for the amino acid–lowering effect noted previously.

From the foregoing, it is apparent that a very close relationship obtains between carbohydrate and protein metabolism and that insulin plays a key mediating role. However, equal in importance to the role of insulin in this relationship is that of transaminases in general, and of glutamic–pyruvic transaminase in particular. These enzymes establish the common ground—namely the relationship between the amino acids and their ketoacid derivatives (e.g., alanine⟷pyruvic, leucine⟷α-ketoisocaproic acid)—between the two areas of metabolism. Their action emphasizes how tightly carbohydrate and amino acid metabolism are intertwined: an increase or decrease in given substrate couple (e.g., alanine or leucine) is closely associated with commensurate increase or decrease in its deaminated equivalent (e.g., pyruvate[48] or α-ketoisocaproate, respectively).

The importance of this relationship from a metabolic standpoint is underscored by the discovery that the amino acids released from muscle (the individual quantities of which appear to be only slightly related to free intracellular amino acid concentrations[49]) are almost stoichiometrically removed by the splanchnic bed, with alanine and glutamine being preeminent.[20] Alanine in particular is preferentially removed by the liver and converted into glucose (hepatic gluconeogenesis); the glucose is transported back to peripheral tissues, including muscle, where it is glycolyzed to lactate and pyruvate. At this point, amino groups from amino acids being oxidized in muscle (the branched-chain amino acids, leucine, valine, and isoleucine in particular) are transferred to pyruvate, which is then transformed into alanine. This energy–ammonia shuttle has been aptly labeled the *alanine cycle*. Initially, a similar role had been ascribed to glutamine, an amino acid released from muscle in even greater quantities than alanine.[20] However, subsequent studies have revealed[50] that much of this amino acid is removed by the gastrointestinal tract rather than by the liver; its metabolic fate, other than its use in ammonia formation by the kidney, is as yet unknown.

With the identification of insulin as a primary agent in the regulation of nitrogen metabolism in man, it remains to be determined when and under what conditions certain tissues, especially muscle and adipose tissue, are sensitive to insulin. As most inpatients, for one reason or another, are temporarily on hypocaloric diets, the study of tissue response(s) to glucose and insulin in fasting man seems particularly appropriate.

METABOLIC EFFECTS OF GLUCOSE AND INSULIN IN FASTING MAN

When relatively small quantities of glucose (100–200 g/day) are ingested by normal man, nitrogen conservation is observed.[45] When overweight but otherwise normal subjects ingest similar hypocaloric glucose meals (37.5 g every 6 h for 7 days), nitrogen conservation, as evidenced by diminished urinary urea nitrogen excretion[51] and inhibition of renal ammoniagenesis, is also seen (Fig. 143-2). Despite this marked effect on nitrogen metabolism, a gradual but significant elevation in blood β-hydroxybutyrate, acetoacetate, and plasma free fatty acid levels occurs. In addition, despite the repetitive stimulation of the pancreas at 6 h intervals, blood glucose and serum insulin levels decline significantly. Thus, a gradual adaptation to the fasting metabolic state[52] develops along with maximal nitrogen conservation when hypocaloric quantities of glucose are ingested by these subjects. Interestingly, levels of amino acids, except for a slight decline in alanine and slight increases in glycine and threonine, show little change.

After 3 weeks of total fasting, when the subjects have adapted to the fasting state (see Chapter 51 by Felig), the small glucose meals of 37.5 g taken every 6 h are again resumed and several important responses and one important lack of response are seen (Fig. 143-3). First, plasma amino acids (especially the glucogenic amino acids), which had declined dramatically during the fast, now return to near normal levels, while the elevated levels of glycine

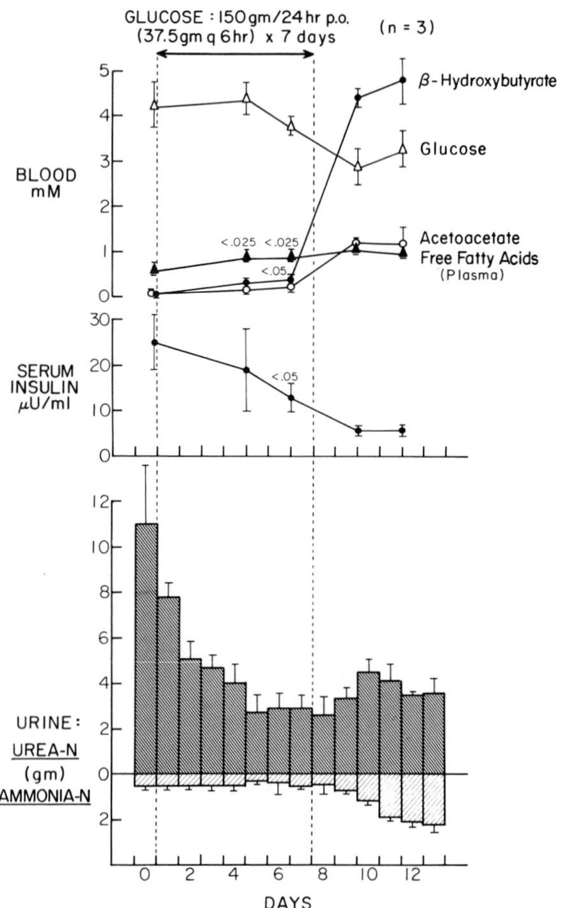

Fig. 143-2. Blood and urine changes in 3 subjects placed on a diet of 150 g glucose/24 h (37.5 g every 6h) for 7 days. Insulin declines while plasma free fatty acids and the ketoacids increase significantly. At the end of the glucose administration, the subjects were totally fasted for 21 days.

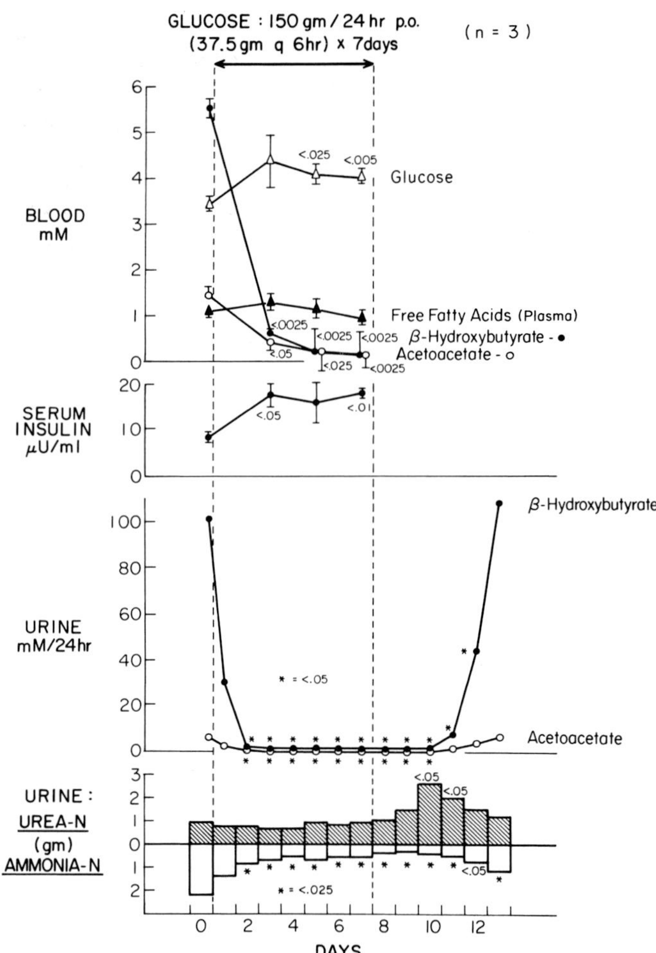

Fig. 143-3. Blood and urine changes in 3 subjects who, after fasting for 3 weeks, ingested 150 g glucose/24 h (37.5 g every 6 h) for 7 days, and then resumed their fasts again. Note the prompt decline in the blood ketoacid levels concomitant with an equally striking diminution in both urinary ketoacid and ammonia nitrogen excretion. In contrast, plasma free fatty acid levels remained elevated.

and threonine decline to the prefast values. Blood β-hydroxybutyrate and acetoacetate and urinary ketoacid levels rapidly decline to postabsorptive levels within 48 h. Nitrogen conservation is once again accomplished, as evidence by inhibition of renal ammoniagenesis and a slight diminution of urinary urea nitrogen excretion. Perhaps most importantly, plasma free fatty acid levels fail to decline during the entire week of glucose, suggesting that adipose tissue, unlike muscle, continues to be relatively insulin resistant. Thus, in a rather striking way, it is clear that body tissues may exhibit differential sensitivities to insulin and, most likely, other hormones as well, probably as a function of the nutritional status of the subject at hand as well as the duration of the altered nutrition itself.

If 150 g glucose are infused over a 24 h period into subjects that have fasted for 4–6 weeks, plasma glucose and serum insulin levels promptly increase while blood and urine β-hydroxybutyrate and acetoacetate levels decline (Fig. 143-4). Marked diminutions in virtually all circulating amino acid levels are seen (Fig. 143-5). Urinary urea and ammonia nitrogen levels inexplicably decline the day following rather than the day of the glucose infusion. Plasma free fatty acid levels remain elevated during and following the study period.

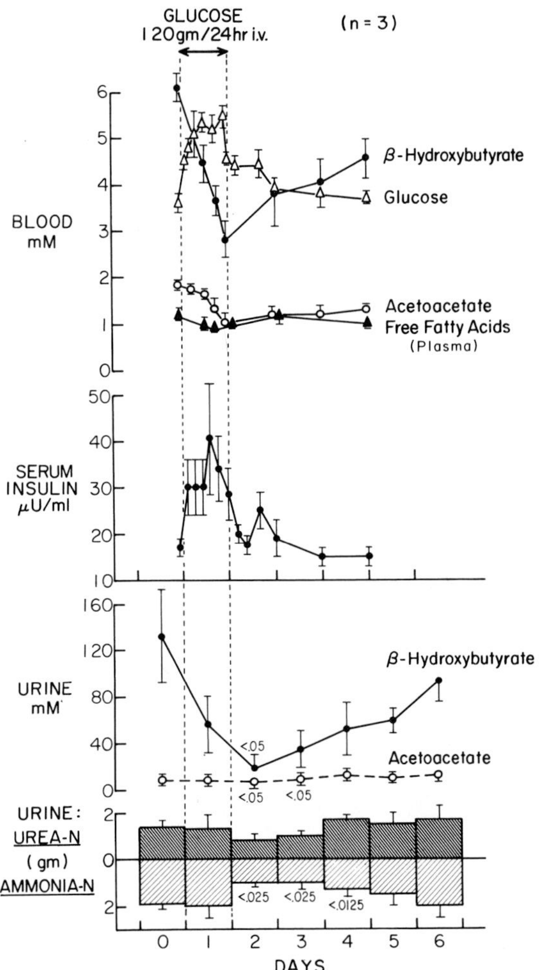

Fig. 143-4. Blood and urine changes in 3 fasting subjects who received 120 g glucose intravenously over a 24-h period. Note the decline of the ketoacids in both blood and urine while serum insulin and blood glucose levels rose. A reduction in both urea and ammonia nitrogen was seen on the days following the glucose infusion. Again, plasma free fatty acid levels did not change significantly.

When 20 U of crystalline zinc insulin are infused into fasted subjects over a 24-h period, blood glucose (Fig. 143-6) and circulating amino acid levels (Fig. 143-7) fall precipitously while serum insulin concentrations double. Blood ketoacid levels drop slightly but rapidly return to preinfusion levels. Urinary urea nitrogen excretion declines modestly but significantly during the study period. Again, despite a doubling of insulin levels, plasma free fatty acid levels do not change and remain elevated during the study and even after.

Thus, it appears that when postabsorptive or fasted man is placed on a low-glucose diet (50–150 g/day), maximal nitrogen conservation takes place while fat mobilization (the most abundant fuel) is permitted. That fat mobilization is a most important and singular event is suggested by the inability of oral or parenteral glucose administration and even intravenous insulin to inhibit it. However, these manuevers are capable of affecting ketogenesis. Thus, the body has made a strong commitment to maximally utilize fat for fuel, with obviously logical teleologic benefit.

In summary, since many hospitalized patients, for one reason or another, are on hypocaloric diets (by mouth or vein), clinicians should be aware of what can be achieved by the simple administration of glucose and/or insulin with respect to nitrogen conservation. Finally, it should be emphasized that the metabolic consequences described here are characteristic of subjects or patients (1) whose insulin-secreting capability is normal and (2) whose tissues are capable of responding appropriately to insulin.

METABOLIC ROLE OF GLUCAGON

Glucagon is a small (3485 daltons) straight-chain polypeptide that is made up of 29 l-amino acids[53] and is synthesized in the α cells of the pancreas. It is relatively insoluble in water but is soluble in both acidic and basic solutions. Although its usual configuration is that of random coil,[54] it can also assume a β structure (acidic gels) or α-helix (crystal state).[55]

With the development of a reliable radioimmunoassay for glucagon,[56] investigators began the difficult task of cataloguing the metabolic effects of this hormone. Early and even current studies assessing endogenous production have been made difficult due to a number of substances that possess immunoreactivity characteristics that are quite similar to pancreatic glucagon.[58] Nevertheless, an impressive array of information has been published concerning this hormone, and some of it will be mentioned here.

With the attachment of a glucagon molecule to a specific glucagon receptor (noncovalent bond) on the hepatocyte,[58] protein kinase activity is increased via cAMP, and glycogenolysis is thereby accelerated. In addition, the activities of enzymes involved in hepatic amino acid trapping,[59] gluconeogenesis, and ureogenesis are increased.[60–62] Of interest, amino acid incorporation into both muscle[63] and liver protein[64] is inhibited by pharmacologic quantities of glucagon.

Pancreatic glucagon output in normal man appears to vary inversely with blood glucose concentration.[65] Thus, glucagon secretion can be inhibited by a glucose infusion in normal subjects or animals; however, it is poorly inhibited in diabetic subjects with impaired insulin-secretory mechanisms, and this inhibition is apparently increased but not completely corrected by good control of the blood glucose level.[66] Thus, it appears that both insulin and glucose availability play important roles in the regulation of glucagon secretion.

Single amino acids,[67] especially asparagine and alanine, and protein meals[68,69] have been shown to elicit glucagon secretion. Indeed, Unger et al.[70] have proposed that glucagon secretion is necessary to offset the hypothetical hypoglycemia that would be induced by the hyperinsulinemia occasioned by the ingestion of a protein meal. These investigators consider this bihormonal mechanism for glucose homeostasis essential for man's well-being.

More recently investigators have begun to appreciate the important role of the sympathetic nervous system in regulating glucagon secretion. Direct stimulation of the ventromedial nucleus of the hypothalamus[71] of the rat and the autonomic nerves supplying the canine pancreas[72] result in the secretion of glucagon. Indeed, exercise has been shown to be associated with increased glucagon production in both man[73] and dogs.[74]

Glucagon, in pharmacologic dosage, also exerts inotropic and chronotropic effects on the heart.[75] It also increases glomerular filtration rate and renal plasma flow[76] and is associated with increased urinary excretion of sodium, potassium, chloride, and inorganic phosphorous.[77]

It might be anticipated, in view of the foregoing, that the assignment to this hormone of a metabolic role in fuel regulation might be somewhat difficult. In part, this uncertainty is due to somewhat controversial properties attributed to it. For example, it

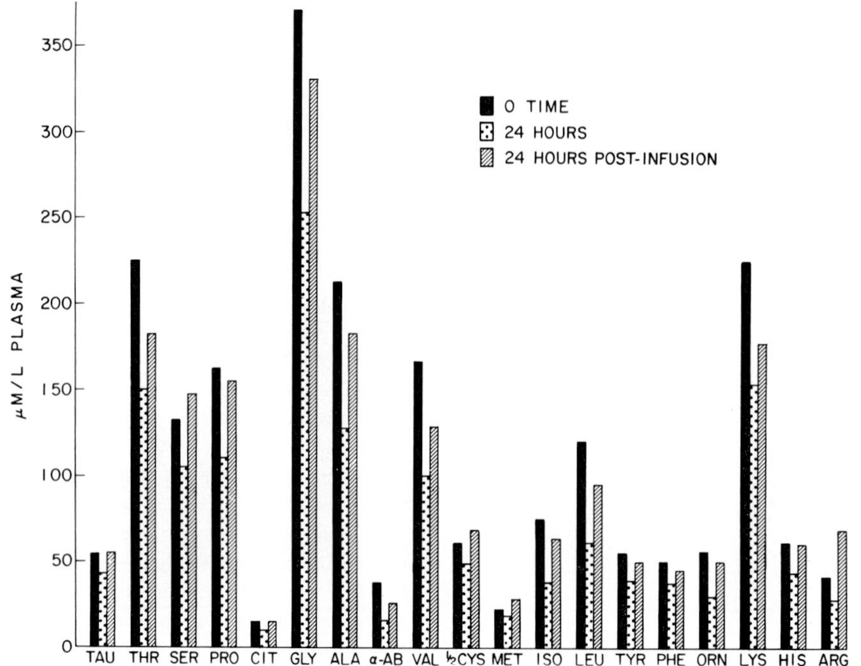

Fig. 143-5. Plasma amino acid levels prior to, during, and following the completion of the glucose infusion. Levels of virtually all amino acids declined during the study. Note the prompt trend toward pre-infusion levels following cessation of the glucose infusion.

was initially considered to be a hormone that initiated protein catabolism. This claim was based on studies in which increased urea nitrogen excretion was observed after pharmacologic quantities of glucagon were infused into normal subjects[78,79] or animals.[80,81] Indeed, this hormone is markedly elevated in hypercatabolic patients, such as those in diabetic ketoacidosis,[38,82,83] and patients suffering from major trauma,[84] either accidental or surgical. In addition, it is known to be elevated during the first 3–5 days of a fast,[85] a time associated with increased muscle breakdown.[86] Further substantiation of this hypothesis was provided by studies in which large quantities of glucagon (10 mg/24 h for 2 days or 1 mg/24 h for 2 days) were infused into subjects undergoing therapeutic fasts. Urinary urea nitrogen excretion promptly and significantly increased during the infusion and declined subsequent to the cessation of the study.[87] However, calculation of the increased nitrogen lost in the urine revealed that the nitrogen had come primarily, if not entirely,from the extracellular compartment and not from body tissues.

More recently, Fitzpatrick et al.[88] administered glucose (720 g/day) into normal man for 8 days, thereby maximally conserving nitrogen . On days 7 and 8 of the glucose infusion, glucagon (1 mg/24 h for 2 days) was also infused. They were able to show that urinary urea nitrogen excretion did increase but was not associated with a concomitant increase in 3-methyl-histidine excretion. Thus, the increased nitrogen loss was not at the expense of muscle but probably of liver. In addition, a patient with a glucagonoma in whom plasma glucagon levels of 2000–3000 pg/ml were common has had daily 3-methyl-histidine excretion rates[89] within normal limits.[26] Furthermore, when physiologic quantities of glucagon are infused systemically into subjects undergoing therapeutic fasts, urea nitrogen excretion diminishes.[87,90] Finally, Pozefsky et al. infused glucagon into the forearm muscle bed of normal subjects and failed to document any change in the resting output of amino acids from muscle.[91] Thus, it would appear that glucagon is not a primary "catabolic" hormone with respect to muscle; instead, it probably facilitates the uptake and metabolism of amino acids

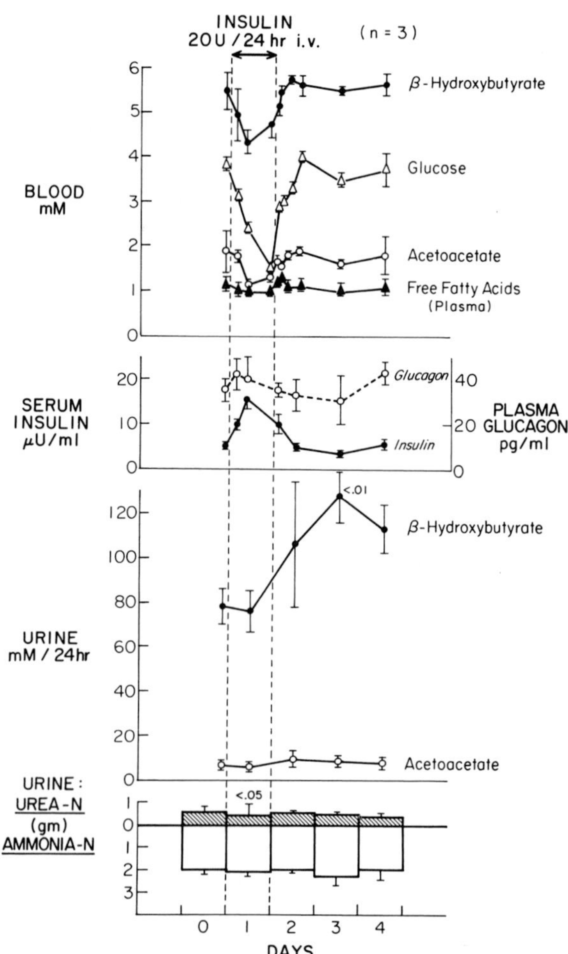

Fig. 143-6. Blood and urine changes in 3 totally fasted (3–4 weeks) individuals prior to, during, and following the infusion of 20 U of crystalline zinc insulin over a 24-h period. Note the prompt decline in blood glucose. Again, plasma free fatty acids did not decline during the infusion.

already in the extracellular fluid and directly facilitates proteolysis in liver.

A similar analysis of the role played by glucagon in the pathogenesis of diabetes is currently underway. While postabsorptive values of this hormone in diabetics are the same as in control subjects, hyperglucagonemia usually occurs only in diabetic patients in response to α cell challenges such as arginine[83] or protein meals.[92] The finding that somatostatin preferentially diminishes α cell activity[93] has been a great boon to the clinical investigator attempting to determine the role of glucagon in fuel homeostasis. However, the recent report that hepatic blood flow was reduced by 35 percent during the infusion period has been somewhat sobering.[94] In summary, the relative importance of the role played by glucagon in overall fuel regulation remains to be established.

MUSCLE MASS, PROTEIN MEALS, BRANCHED-CHAIN AMINO ACIDS, HORMONES, AND REDOX STATE

It is within the setting of the nutritional state and activity level of the individual that insulin and, apparently to a much lesser extent, glucagon play their roles in maintaining the nitrogen mass at an optimal level for survival. Mention has been made elsewhere of the exquisite sensitivity of muscle proteolysis to insulin in fasting man, and to the relative insensitivity of ketogenesis and lipolysis to these changes in insulin level. The work of Pozefsky et al.[19] suggests that in normal postabsorptive man a similar sensitivity to insulin exists in muscle. This sensitivity of muscle to small changes in insulin level is of paramount importance, for it indicates that at relatively low levels of insulin (about 10 μU/ml) muscle anabolism is stimulated, while at lower levels muscle proteolysis occurs (in the absence of physical activity). In this situation, if nitrogen levels are already optimized for a given individual, excess calories (carbohydrate, protein, or fat) are diverted to fat deposition.

Following the ingestion of a protein meal by a normal postabsorptive individual, constituent amino acids pass from the gut via the portal vein to the liver, where virtually all the glucogenic amino acids are removed. In contrast, the branched-chain amino acids appear to pass through the splanchnic bed.[68] This amino acid pattern is very similar to that seen when rat livers are perfused with glucagon.[59] It is therefore presumed that since glucagon is released in large quantities following the ingestion of a protein meal, glucagon is largely responsible for the appearance of the branched-chain amino acids in the systemic circulation, while the low levels of insulin permit the removal of the glucogenic amino acids by the liver. It is therefore most fortunate that the branched-chain amino acids are the only amino acids that do not stimulate glucagon secretion in dogs[67] and, presumably, man. Since the branched-chain amino acids appear to be the preferred amino acid fuel in peripheral tissues (muscle and fat), this pattern seems to be most appropriate. Parenthetically, the ingestion of a protein meal by a nitrogen-depleted individual is followed by both high insulin and high glucagon levels, which should favor the delivery of virtually all of the essential and nonessential amino acids to peripheral tissues.[69] In an individual whose nitrogen stores are optimal, following the ingestion of a protein meal only small quantities of insulin appear peripherally, along with large amounts of glucagon, thereby favoring the peripheral delivery of only the branched-chain amino acids. It should be remembered, however, that for reasons that are not well understood, preferential accretion or synthesis of protein by exercised muscle may occur[40] despite the relative or absolute absence of insulin or exogenous sources of amino acids. It should also be apparent that the very lability and responsiveness of muscles to insulin permits it to play a central metabolic role whether man is fasting, eating, or exercising (see Chapter 146).

It is well known that in at least one situation of protein wasting, namely diabetic ketoacidosis, levels of branched-chain amino acids are elevated while only alanine and glutamine are being released in large quantities.[38] Since the branched-chain amino acids are not being released from or taken up by muscle

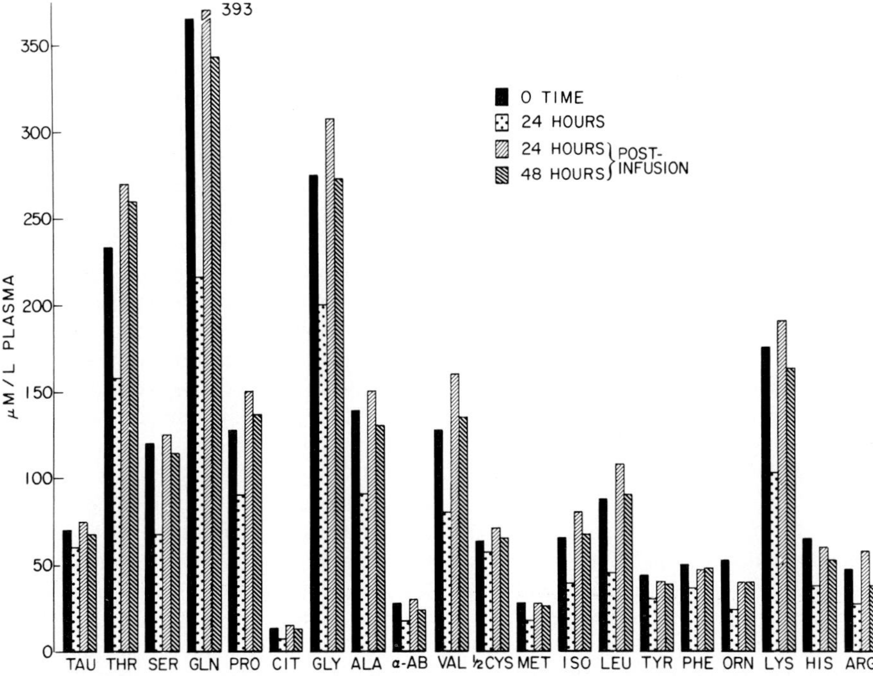

Fig. 143-7. Plasma amino acid levels prior to, during, and 24 h and 48 h following the cessation of the insulin infusion. Note the generalized hypoaminoacidemia that ensued during the infusion and the prompt return toward pre-infusion levels following the end of the study.

(with the possible exception of valine), the most likely source of the increased circulating levels of the branched-chain amino acids is the liver.[95] It therefore follows that since the proposed major stimulus to branched-chain amino acid release from liver is glucagon, this hormone is elevated.[38,82,83] However, in most other situations in which a normal insulin-secreting mechanism and tissue(s) capable of responding appropriately to this hormone are present, levels of the branched-chain amino acids appear to vary directly with on-going protein synthesis or inhibition of muscle proteolysis. Thus, in prolonged fasted man, in whom nitrogen conservation is clearly evidenced, branched-chain amino acids are low. When normal man is infused with large quantities of glucose (about 700g/day) and clearly reaches the floor of urinary nitrogen excretion,[96] branched-chain amino acids are also very low. In addition, as would be predicted, patients who have glucagonomas, but have apparently normal tissue responsiveness to insulin and insulinsecreting capability, branched-chain amino acid levels are low. Presumably the mild hyperglycemia present in many of these subjects stimulates insulin secretion, which in turn decreases both muscle and liver proteolysis.[97]

From the foregoing, it appears that muscle protein synthesis and/or proteolysis may be keyed to both insulin and circulating branched-chain amino acid levels. Thus moderately high insulin levels in combination with high branched-chain amino acid levels, as after a protein meal, would result in increased amino acid uptake by muscle, leading eventually to protein synthesis. Very low or no insulin in combination with elevated levels of branched-chain amino acid would not be associated with branched-chain amino acid removal by muscle from the circulation. Insulin levels of approximately 10 μU/ml might be associated with inhibition of proteolysis and normal or low levels of branched-chain amino acids. The precise mechanisms operative in normal postabsorptive man remain to be clarified.

More recently, a mechanism by which nitrogen conservation could be effected in fasting man has been proposed.[98] The proposed central role played by the branched-chain amino acids pivots around the irreversible oxidative decarboxylation step, which requires the cofactor nicotinamide adenine dinucleotide (NAD^+). In fasting man, muscle appears to be the most reduced tissue, as reflected by determination of redox pairs such as lactate/pyruvate and β-hydroxybutyrate/acetoacetate in both cytosol and mitochondria, respectively. Thus, lack of NAD^+ would inhibit the oxidative decarboxylation of the branched-chain amino acids, and this block may increase intracellular concentrations of these amino acids, which may in turn signal the termination of proteolysis. Since the branched-chain amino acids are "amino fats," and since fasting man rapidly substitutes free fatty acids and ketoacids to meet virtually all of his fuel requirements, it seems reasonable to predict that decreased concentration of NAD^+ would be associated with decreased branched-chain amino acid oxidation.

CLINICAL APPLICATIONS

The concepts developed in the preceding sections are applicable to virtually every patient admitted to a hospital for more than a few days. Thus, it is not sufficient to merely calculate and then meet the theoretical caloric requirements of patients based on their height and weight; rather, such factors as physical activity and, perhaps more importantly, the patient's metabolic readiness, in terms of hormone secretion and tissue responsiveness to these hormones, to embrace the various therapeutic modalities that might be offered must be considered. In addition, these hypotheses must undergo continual reevaluation in order to ensure that therapeutic support and the changing clinical status of the patient are appropriately meshed. One illustrative situation is the type of nutritional support that should be provided to patients who, for one reason or another, are unable to ingest their meals.

In 1946, Gamble reported[45] that 100 g of glucose by mouth was able to almost maximally conserve nitrogen, and this protein-sparing effect of glucose has been confirmed by others using both small and large quantities of glucose either ingested or infused.[51,96,99,100] Common to these investigations, however, were subjects whose insulin-secreting mechanisms were intact and whose tissues were capable of responding appropriately to this hormone.

Recently, a number of investigators have begun to evaluate the potential role of fat emulsions and, in particular, to examine their effect on nitrogen metabolism in man. Of interest, Brennan et al. showed that the nitrogen conservation observed in normal subjects receiving soybean oil infusions as their sole caloric source was primarily attributable to the glycerol added to each bottle of fat emulsion for osmotic purposes.[101] Thus, the 16–20 g of glycerol arising from hydrolysis of endogenous triglycerides may be in part responsible for the nitrogen conservation seen in fasting man. Finally, some studies have indicated that significant quantities of the infused fat accumulate in hepatic reticuloendothelial cells.[102]

Most recently, however, attention has been directed toward the use of solutions of essential and nonessential amino acids. A number of investigators have attempted to determine whether or not the provisioning of amino acid solutions of various types might diminish or mitigate patients' nitrogen losses. Indeed, some investigators[103–105] have even suggested that isotonic amino acid rather than 5 percent glucose in water solution be given routinely. Their hypothesis was as follows:[105] The infusion of glucose (100–150 g/day) elicits a pronounced increase in circulating insulin levels (note the necessity for the presence of a normal insulin-secreting mechanism). These elevated insulin levels inhibit lipolysis and ketogenesis (note the requirement for the same sensitivity to insulin of both hepatic and adipose tissue, as in postabsorptive rather than prolonged fasted man). Thus, the total caloric or energy deficit must apparently be met by increased mobilization of muscle protein (for hepatic gluconeogenic purposes). Hence, indirectly, the infusion of some glucose, followed by increased insulin levels, was considered to be theoretically catabolic. In contrast, these investigators maintained that the use of amino acid solutions, presumably less potent insulin secretagogues, permit lipolysis and ketogenesis to continue. Ketogenesis was held to be pivotol since the brain, the major consumer of glucose in man, could use the ketoacids, β-hydroxybutyrate and acetoacetate, in lieu of glucose for fuel. Furthermore, these investigators reported that supplying 70–90 g of amino acids to patients in the postabsorptive state could, within a 24-h period, bring the patients into zero or positive balance.[103]

At first glance, this hypothesis appears to be quite attractive. Unfortunately, it does not withstand a more critical assessment. First, insulin levels alone impart relatively little information. The knowledge usually desired is the responsiveness of various tissues (e.g., muscle, fat, liver) to relatively low or high levels of this hormone in particular. For example, basal insulin levels in overweight individuals are usually quite elevated when compared to normal controls.[106,107] In addition, the adipose tissue of these subjects is usually markedly resistant to insulin,[108–111] again underscoring the fact that it is not insulin levels per se but rather the metabolic reaction of tissues to prevailing levels of this hormone that is important. In addition, despite having somewhat higher insulin levels, fasting obese subjects usually have higher basal free fatty acid levels than do normal weight controls. Second, during fasting (as noted previously) adipose tissue becomes quite resistant to the effects of insulin with respect to lipolysis and remains so despite the fact that these subjects may be quite physically active, thereby suggesting a non–activity-related metabolic adaptation. Thus, increased insulin levels need not be associated with inhibition of lipolysis or ketogenesis. Indeed, a very modest but significant reduction in urinary urea nitrogen excretion can be seen while both adipose and hepatic tissue responses are virtually nonexistent following a systemic infusion of insulin into fasting subjects (Fig. 143-6).

Third, when glucose meals are fed to obese subjects prior to their initiation of a therapeutic fast, urea nitrogen excretion is clearly diminished while urinary ammonia nitrogen excretion remains negligible due to inhibition of ketogenesis. A small, gradual, and significant increase in plasma free fatty acid and blood β-hydroxybutyrate and acetoacetate levels is seen during the course of the study (Fig. 143-2). Following the completion of 3 weeks of total fast, when the glucose meals are reintroduced, blood β-hydroxybutyrate and acetoacetate levels rapidly decline, as does urinary ammonia nitrogen levels (Fig. 143-3). Importantly, there is no increased nitrogen mobilization despite the fact that a hypocaloric glucose meal is being administered. Clearly, the body is using free fatty acids and glucose. Thus ketogenesis is neither needed (since glucose is being provided) nor desirable since an obligatory loss of nitrogen (as NH_3^+) would thereby be necessitated. In addition, free fatty acid levels remain elevated during the entire period, underscoring the lack of effect of elevated insulin levels on lipolysis. Bear in mind that these subjects are nitrogen depleted and yet (1) they conserve nitrogen and (2) free fatty acid levels remain unchanged during the study period, despite increased insulin levels. Note particularily that ketosis necessitates an obligatory additional 2–2.5 g of ammoniagenesis by the kidney (representing a loss of 12–15 g protein/day).

In view of the foregoing discussion, the ultimate disposition of an amino acid load appears to be a function of (1) prevailing insulin levels, (2) tissue (adipose, muscle, liver) responsiveness to insulin and, to a lesser extent, glucagon, (3) the nutritional status of the subject, and (4) the physical activity of the individual. High insulin levels maintained by a normal insulin-secreting mechanism favor the peripheral uptake of amino acids by muscle and diminish their breakdown, while low levels favor or permit amino acid removal, primarily by the liver. These actions are based on the presence of appropriate tissue response(s), for if there is any diminution in muscle response to insulin, as in trauma,[37,84] there may be increased breakdown and release of amino acids by these tissues. If there is no nitrogen deficit, then only the "wear and tear" quantities of protein need be replenished. Finally, if physical activity is increased, necessitating increased muscle mass, increased quantities of administered nitrogen, primarily in the form of protein and amino acids, are retained in the form of lean body mass.

Thus, it would be predicted that a prolonged fasted (i.e., nitrogen-depleted) individual would respond with relatively high insulin levels and would retain amino acids peripherally in order that muscle mass could be quickly restored to optimal levels.[69] It would also be expected that a traumatized individual (one who is excreting more than 20 g of urinary urea nitrogen/day in the absence of exogenous sources of nitrogen and is incapable of elevating peripheral levels of insulin communsurate with the degree of glycemia) would not be able to incorporate administered nitrogen as muscle protein. However, it is conceivable that such an individual could retain some nitrogen, but as liver proteins, some of which have a $t_{1/2}$ measurable in hours[28–30] rather than days. Support for this concept can be found in those investigations in which normal subjects ingested 200 g of meat[68] or other proteins.[112] In all such studies only branched-chain amino acids escaped from the splanchnic bed to peripheral tissues, and the vast bulk of the essential and nonessential amino acids presumably were captured and retained in the form of glycogen, protein, and, to a lesser extent, amino acids.

The administration of glucose (about 150 g/day) should and does conserve nitrogen in normal postabsorptive subjects. However, if these individuals should then suffer significant trauma and subsequently develop some degree of insulin resistance, neither ingested nor intravenously administered glucose would be capable of eliciting adequate release of insulin and nitrogen would not be conserved.

If isotonic amino acids are administered to normal individuals, nitrogen balance remains negative.[113] The provisioning of both glucose and amino acids might be expected to result in less loss or greater conservation of nitrogen, primarily due to inhibition of ammonia nitrogen production (secondary to a decrease or inhibition of ketogenesis).[114] However, the administration of glucose and amino acids to traumatized individuals with some degree of peripheral insulin resistance and/or inappropriately low insulin levels relative to prevailing (elevated) levels of glucose probably will not be followed by removal of amino acids by peripheral tissues.

The key to nitrogen retention is thus the metabolic readiness of muscle to respond to insulin mainly by extracting circulating amino acids. The process is slow, under the most extreme circumstances, since the $t_{1/2}$ of muscle turnover is on the order of days.[41]

In contrast, when amino acids or amino acids plus glucose are administered to subjects whose nitrogen stores are optimal or nearly so, muscle is probably not involved in removing amino acids. Rather, the liver appears to remove amino acids acutely, as after a protein meal, and then rapidly unload them as urea and/or glucose. An extreme example of this hepatic capability can be seen in the vampire bat,[115] who can ingest one-half its body weight (30 g) in blood at one sitting. The bat is then land bound for the next 30 min, during which time its liver is busily converting the ingested proteins into urea and glucose. At the end of the 30-min period, the bat has urinated enough water and urea so that it can once again fly.

CONCLUSION

The complex interrelationships that exist between protein, carbohydrate, and lipid metabolism in both normal and abnormal man appear to be primarily under the influence of the following:

1. Prevailing insulin levels
2. Tissue (muscle, adipose, liver) responsiveness to insulin and, to a lesser extent, glucagon
3. Nutritional status of the individual
4. Physical activity status of the individual

Changes in any one of these variables will necessitate adjustments in the other three; the results will be dependent on the nature, both qualitative and quantitative, of these adjustments.

ACKNOWLEDGMENT

We wish to express our deep appreciation of the contributions made by Dzidra Rumba, Patricia Hatch, Velta Ramolins, Adacie Allen, and Michael Arcangeli in the investigations reported in this paper.

REFERENCES

1. Benedict, F. G., Joslin, E. P.: A study of metabolism in severe diabetes. Washington, D.C., Carnegie Institute, Publ 176, 1912.
2. Best, C. H.: Epochs in the history of diabetes. In R. W. Williams (ed): Diabetes, New York, Hoeber, 1960, pp 1–13.
3. Wiechmann, E.: Über den einfluxx des insulins auf den aminosäurengehalt von blut und harn beim diabetikor. *Z Ges Exp Med 44:* 158, 1924.
4. Wiechmann, E.: Zur-permeabilitäts theorie des diabetes mellitus. *Dtsch Arch Klin Med 150:* 186, 1926.
5. Luck, J. M., Morrison, G., Wilbur, L. F.: The effect of insulin on the amino acid content of blood. *J Biol Chem 77:* 151, 1928.
6. Luck, J. M., Morse, S. W.: The effects of insulin and adrenalin on the amino acid content of blood. *Biochem J 27:* 1648, 1933.
7. Mirsky, I. A.: The influence of insulin on the protein metabolism of nephrectomized dogs. *Am J Physiol 124:* 569, 1938.
8. Russell, J. A.: Hormonal control of amino acid metabolism. *Fed Proc 14:* 696, 1955.
9. Manchester, K. L.: The control by insulin of amino acid accumulation in muscle. *Biochem J 117:* 457, 1970.
10. Manchester, K. L.: Insulin and protein synthesis. In: Biochemical Actions of Hormones, vol 1. New York, Academic, 1970, pp 267–320.
11. Wool, I. G., Castles, J. J., Leader, D. P., Fox, A.: Insulin and the function of muscle ribosomes. In Steiner, D. F., Freinkel, N. (eds): Handbook of Physiology, sect 7, Endocrinology, vol 1, Endocrine Pancreas. Baltimore, Williams and Wilkins, 1972, ch 24, pp 385–394.
12. Cuatrecasas, P.: Interaction of insulin with the cell membrane, the primary action of insulin. *Proc Natl Acad Sci U.S.A. 63:* 450, 1969.
13. Wool, I. G., Stirewalt, W. S., Kurihara, K., et al: Mode of action of insulin in the regulation of protein biosynthesis in muscle. *Recent Prog Horm Res 24:* 139, 1968.
14. Avruch, J., Leone, G. R., Martin, D. B.: Effects of epinephrine and insulin on phosphopeptide metabolism in adipocytes. *J Biol Chem 251:* 1511, 1976.
15. Waterlow, J. C.: Lysine turnover in man measured by intravenous infusion of 1-(U-^{14}C) lysine. *Clin Sci 33:* 507, 1967.
16. Waterlow, J. C.: The assessment of protein nutrition and metabolism in the whole animal, with special reference to man. In Munroe, H. N. (ed): Mammalian Protein Metabolism, vol 30, New York Academic, 1969, pp 326–390.
17. London, D. R., Foley, T. H., Webb, C. G.: Evidence for the release of individual amino acids from resting human forearm. *Nature 208:* 588, 1965.
18. London, D. R., Prenton, M. A.: Beta-adrenergic receptors and the plasma amino acid response to insulin in man. *Clin Sci 35:* 55, 1968.
19. Pozefsky, T., Felig, P., Tobin, J. D., Soeldner, J. S., Cahill, G. F., Jr.: Amino acid balance across tissues of the forearm in postabsorptive man. Effects of insulin at two dose levels. *J Clin Invest 48:* 2273, 1969.
20. Marliss, E. B., Aoki, T. T., Pozefsky, T., Most, A. S., Cahill, G. F., Jr.: Muscle and splanchnic glutamine and glutamate metabolism in postabsorptive and starved man. *J Clin Invest 50:* 814, 1971.
21. Aoki, T. T., Brennan, M. F., Müller, W. A., Soeldner, J. S., Cahill, G. F., Jr.: Amino acid levels across normal forearm muscle: whole blood vs plasma. *Adv Enzyme Regul 12:* 3, 1974.
22. Asatoor, A. M., Armstrong, M. D.: 3-Methylhistidine, a component of actin. *Biochem Biophys Res Commun 26:* 168, 1967.
23. Johnson, P., Perry, S. V.: Biological activity and the 3-methylhistidine content of actin and myosin. *Biochem J 119:* 293, 1970.
24. Trayer, I. P., Harris, C. I., Perry, S. V.: 3-Methylhistidine and foetal forms of skeletal muscle myosin. *Nature 217:* 452, 1968.
25. Long, C. L., Haverberg, L. N., Young, V. R., et al: Metabolism of 3-methylhistidine in man. *Metabolism 24:* 929, 1975.
26. Young, V. R., Haverberg, L. N., Bilmazes, C., Munro, H. N.: Potential use of 3-methylhistidine excretion as an index of progressive reduction in muscle protein catabolism during starvation. *Metabolism 22:* 1429, 1973.
27. Schimke, R. T.: The importance of both synthesis and degradation in the control of arginase levels in rat liver. *J Biol Chem 239:* 3808, 1964.
28. Schimke, R. T.: Regulation of protein degradation in mammalian tissues. In Monro, H. N. (ed): Mammalian Protein Metabolism, vol 4. New York: Academic, 1970, pp 177–228.
29. Kuehl, L., Sumsion, E. N.: Turnover of several glycolytic enzymes in rat liver. *J Biol Chem 245:* 6616, 1970.
30. Segal, H. L., Matsuzawa, T., Halder, M., Abraham, G. J.: What determines the half-life of proteins in vivo? Some experiences with alanine aminotransferase of rat tissue. *Biochem Biophys Res Commun 36:* 764, 1969.
31. Sidransky, H., Verney, E.: Skeletal muscle protein metabolism changes in rate force-fed a diet inducing an experimental kwashiorkor-like model. *J Clin Nutr 23:* 1154, 1970.
32. Goldberg, A. L.: Protein turnover in skeletal muscle. II. Effect of denervation and cortisone on protein catabolism in skeletal muscle. *J Biol Chem 244:* 3223, 1969.
33. Schimassek, H., Gerok, W.: Control of the levels of free amino acids in plasma by the liver. *Biochemistry 342:* 407, 1965.
34. Goldberg, A. L., St John, A. C.: Intracellular protein degradation in mammalian and bacterial cells: Part 2. *Ann. Rev. Biochem. 45:* 747, 1976.
35. Woolfolk, C. A., Stadtman, E. R.: Regulation of glutamine synthetase. III. Cumulative feedback inhibition of glutamine synthetase from Escherichia coli. *Arch Biochem Biophys 118:* 736, 1967.
36. Owen, O. E., Morgan, A. P., Kemp, H. G., et al: Brain metabolism during fasting. *J Clin Invest 46:* 1589, 1967.
37. Hinton, P., Allison, S. P., Littlejohn, S., Lloyd, J.: Insulin and glucose to reduce catabolic response to injury in burned patients. *Lancet 1:* 767, 1971.
38. Aoki, T. T., Assal, J. P., Manzano, F., Kozak, G. P., Cahill, G. F., Jr.: Plasma and cerebrospinal fluid amino acid levels in diabetic ketoacidosis before and after corrective therapy. *Diabetes 24:* 463, 1975.
39. Goldberg, A. L.: Role of insulin in work-induced growth of skeletal muscle. *Endocrinology 83:* 1071, 1968.
40. Goldberg, A. L.: Protein synthesis during work-induced growth of skeletal muscle. *J Cell Biol 36:* 653, 1968.
41. Goldberg, A. L.: Mechanisms of growth and atrophy of skeletal muscle. In: Progress in Muscle Biology. New York: Dekker, 1972, ch 5, pp 89–118.
42. Goldberg, A. L., Goodman, H. M.: Amino acid transport during work-induced growth of skeletal muscle. *Am J Physiol 216:* 1111, 1969.
43. Romanul, F. C. A.: Reversal of enzymatic profiles and capillary supply of muscle fibers in fast and slow muscles after cross innervation. In Pernow, B., Saltin, B., (eds): Muscle Metabolism During Exercise. New York, Plenum, 1971.
44. Cathcart, E. P.: The influence of carbohydrate and fats on protein metabolism. *J Physiol 39:* 311, 1909.
45. Gamble, J. L.: Physiological information gained from studies on the life raft ration. *Harvey Lect 42:* 247, 1946–1947.
46. Crofford, D. B., Fels, P. W., Lacy, W. W.: Effect of glucose infusion on the individual plasma amino acids in man. *Proc Soc Exp Biol Med 117:* 11, 1964.
47. Andres, R., Zierler, K. L., Anderson, H. M., et al: Measurement of blood flow and volume in the forearm of man; with notes on the theory of indicator-dilution and on production of turbulence, hemolysis, and vasodilitation by intra-vascular injection. *J Clin Invest 33:* 482, 1954.
48. Rossini, A. A., Aoki, T. T., Ganda, O. P., Soeldner, J. S., Cahill, G. F., Jr.: Alanine-induced amino acid interrelationships. *Metabolism 24:* 1185, 1975.
49. Cahill, G. F., Jr., Aoki, T. T., Marliss, E. B.: Insulin and muscle protein. In Steiner, D. F., Freinkel, N. (eds): Handbook of Physiology, sect 7, Endocrinology, vol 1, Endocrine Pancreas. Baltimore, Williams and Wilkins, 1972, pp 563–577.
50. Felig, P., Wahren, J., Raf, L.: Evidence of inter-organ amino acid transport by blood cells in humans. *Proc Natl Acad Sci U.S.A. 70:* 1775, 1973.
51. Aoki, T. T., Müller, W. A., Brennan, M. F., Cahill, G. F., Jr.: Metabolic effects of glucose in brief and prolonged fasted man. *Am J Clin Nutr 28:* 507, 1975.
52. Cahill, G. F., Jr., Herrera, M. G., Morgan, A. P., et al: Hormone-fuel interrelationships during fasting. *J. Clin Invest 45:* 1751, 1966.
53. Bromer, W. W., Sinn, L. G., Staub, A., et al: The amino acid sequence of glucagon. 1. Amino acid composition and terminal amino analyses. *J Am Chem Soc 79:* 2794, 1957.
54. Bromer, W. W.: Chemistry of glucagon and gastrin. In Steiner, D. F., Freinkel, N. (eds): Handbook of Physiology, section 7, Endocrinology, vol 1, Endocrine Pancreas. Baltimore, Williams and Wilkins, 1972, pp 133–138.

55. Gratzer, W. B., Bailery, E., Beaven, G. H.: Conformational states of glucagon. *Biochem Biophys Res Commun 28:* 914, 1967.
56. Unger, R. H., Eisentraut, A. M., McCall, M. S. et al: Glucagon antibodies and their use for immunoassay for glucagon. *Proc Soc Exp Biol Med 102:* 621, 1959.
57. Eisentraut, A. M., Ohneda, A., Aguilar-Parada, E., Unger, R. H.: Immunologic discrimination between pancreatic glucagon and enteric glucagon-like immunoreactivity (GLI) in tissues and plasma. *Diabetes 17* [*Suppl 1*]*:* 321, 1968.
58. Rodbell, M., Birnbaumer, L., Pohl, S. L., Sundby, F.: The reaction of glucagon with its receptor: evidence for discrete regions of activity and binding in the glucagon molecule. *Proc Natl Acad Sci U.S.A. 68:* 909, 1971.
59. Mallette, L. E., Exton, J. H., Park, C. R.: Control of gluconeogenesis from amino acids in the perfused rat liver. *J Biol Chem 244:* 5713, 1969.
60. Weber, G., Lea, M. A., Hird Convery, H. J., Stamm, N. B.: Regulation of gluconeogenesis and glycolysis; studies of mechanisms controlling enzyme activity. In Weber, G. (ed): Advances in Enzyme Regulation, vol 15. London, Pergamon, 1967, pp 257–298.
61. Weber, G., Singhal, R. L., Stamm, N. B., Srivastava, S. K.: Hormonal induction and suppression of liver enzyme biosynthesis. *Fed Proc 24:* 745, 1965.
62. McLean, P., Novello, F.: Influence of pancreatic hormones on enzymes concerned with urea synthesis in rat liver. *Biochem J 94:* 410, 1965.
63. Beatty, C. H., Peterson, R. D., Bocek, R. M., Craig, N. C., Welebar, R.: Effect of glucagon on incorporation of glycine-C-14 into protein of voluntary skeletal muscle. *Endocrinology 73:* 721, 1963.
64. Pryor, J., Berthet, J.: The action of adenosine 3′,5′-monophosphate on the incorporation of leucine into liver protein. *Biochem Biophys Acta 43:* 556, 1960.
65. Ohneda, A., Aguilar-Parada, E., Eisentraut, A. M., Unger, R. H.: Control of pancreatic glucagon secretion by glucose. *Diabetes 18:* 1, 1969.
66. Unger, R. H.: Diabetes and the alpha cell. The Banting Memorial Lecture 1975. *Diabetes 25:* 136, 1976.
67. Rocha, D. M., Faloona, G. R., Unger, R. H.: Glucagon-stimulating activity of 2o amino acids in dogs. *J Clin Invest 51:* 2346, 1972.
68. Aoki, T. T., Brennan, M. F., Müller, W. A., et al: Amino acid levels across normal forearm muscle and splanchnic bed after a protein meal. *Am J Clin Nutr 29:* 340, 1976.
69. Aoki, T. T., Muller, W. A., Brennan, M. F., Cahill, G. F., Jr.: Blood cell and plasma amino acid levels across forearm muscle during a protein meal. *Diabetes 22:* 768, 1973.
70. Unger, R. H., Ohneda, A., Aguilar-Parada, E., Eisentraut, A. M.: The role of aminogenic glucagon secretion in blood glucose homeostasis. *J Clin Invest 48:* 810, 1969.
71. Frohman, L. A., Bernardis, L. L.: Effect of hypothalamic stimulation on plasma glucose, insulin and glucagon levels. *Am J Physiol 221:* 1596, 1971.
72. Marliss, E. B., Girardier, L., Seydoux, J., et al: Glucagon release induced by pancreatic nerve stimulation in the dog. *J Clin Invest 52:* 1246, 1973.
73. Felig, P., Wahren, J., Hendler, R., Ahlborg, G.: Plasma glucagon levels in exercising man. *N Engl J Med 287:* 184, 1972.
74. Böttger, I., Schlein, E. M., Faloona, G. R., Knochel, J. P., Unger, R. H.: The effect of exercise on glucagon secretion. *J Clin Endocrinol Metab 35:* 117, 1972.
75. Parmley, W. W., Glick, G., Sonnenblick, E. H.: Cardiovascular effects of glucagon in man. *N Engl J Med 279:* 12, 1968.
76. Serratto, M., Earle, D. P.: Effect of glucagon on renal functions in the dog. *Proc Soc Exp Biol Med 102:* 701, 1959.
77. Avioli, L. V.: The effect of glucagon on mineral and electrolyte metabolism. In Lefebvre, P. J., Unger, R. H. (eds): Glucagon Molecular Physiology, Clinical and Therapeutic Implications. London, Pergamon, 1972, pp 181–186.
78. Kibler, R. F., Taylor, W. J., Myers, J. D.: The effect of glucagon on net splanchnic balances of glucose, amino acid nitrogen, urea, ketones, and oxygen in man. *J Clin Invest 43:* 904, 1964.
79. Landau, R. L., Lugibihl, K.: Effect of glucagon on concentration of several free amino acids in plasma. *Metab Clin Exp 18:* 265, 1969.
80. Woodside, K. H., Mortimore, G. E.: Control of proteolysis in the perfused rat liver: influence of amino acids, insulin and glucagon. *Fed Proc 29:* 379, 1970 (abstract).
81. Guder, W., Hepp, K. D., Wieland, O.: The catabolic action of glucagon in rat liver. *Biochem Biophys Acta 222:* 593, 1970.
82. Assan, R., Hautecouverture, G., Guillemant, S.: Evolution de paramétres hormonaux (glucagon, cortisol, hormone somatotrope) et énergétiques (glucose, acides gras, glycérol libre) dans dix acidocétoses diabétiques graves traitées. *Pathol Biol 17:* 1095, 1969.
83. Unger, R. H., Aguilar-Parada, E., Muller, W. A. Eisentraut, A. M.: Studies of pancreatic alpha cell function in normal and diabetic subjects. *J Clin Invest 49:* 837, 1970.
84. Meguid, M. M., Brennan, M. F., Aoki, T. T. et al: Hormone–substrate interrelationships following trauma. *Arch Surg 109:* 776, 1974.
85. Aguilar-Parada, E., Eisentraut, A. M., Unger, R. H.: Effects of starvation on plasma pancreatic glucagon in normal man. *Diabetes 18:* 717, 1969.
86. Pozefsky, T., Tancredi, R. G., Moxley, R. T., Dupre, J., Tobin, J. D.: Effects of brief starvation on muscle amino acid metabolism in nonobese man. *J Clin Invest 57:* 444, 1976.
87. Marliss, E. B., Aoki, T. T., Unger, R. H., Soeldner, J. S., Cahill, G. F., Jr.: Glucagon levels and metabolic effects in fasting man. *J Clin Invest 49:* 2256, 1970.
88. Fitzpatrick, G., Meguid, M. M., Gitlitz, P. H., Brennan, M. F.: Glucagon infusion in normal man: effects on 3-methylhistidine excretion and plasma amino acids. *Metabolism 26:* 477, 1977.
89. Horton, E. S., Aoki, T. T., Weir, G. C.: Personal communication.
90. Aoki, T. T., Müller, W. A., Brennan, M. F., Cahill, G. F., Jr.: Effect of glucagon on amino acid and nitrogen metabolism in fasting man. *Metabolism 23:* 805, 1974.
91. Pozefsky, T., Tancredi, R. G., Moxley, R. T., Dupre, J., Tobin, J. D.: Metabolism of forearm tissues in man. Studies with glucagon. *Diabetes 25:* 128, 1976.
92. Müller, W. A., Faloona, G. R., Aguilar-Parada, E., Unger, R. H.: Abnormal alpha cell function in diabetes: response to carbohydrate and protein ingestion. *N Engl J Med 283:* 109, 1970.
93. Gerich, J. E., Lorenzi, M., Karam, J. H., Schneider, V., Forsham, P. H.: Abnormal pancreatic glucagon secretion and postprandial hyperglycemia in diabetes mellitus. *J.A.M.A. 234:* 159, 1975.
94. Wahren, J., Felig, P.: Somatostatin (SRIF) and glucagon in diabetes: failure of glucagon suppression to improve I.V. glucose tolerance and evidence of an effect of SRIF on glucose absorption. *Clin Res 24:* 416A, 1976.
95. Mallette, L. E., Exton, J. H., Park, C. R.: Effects of glucagon on amino acid transport and utilization in the perfused rat liver. *J Biol Chem 244:* 5724, 1969.
96. O'Connell, R. C., Morgan, A. P., Aoki, T. T., Ball, M. R., Moore, F. D.: Nitrogen conservation in starvation graded responses to intravenous glucose. *J Clin Endocrinol Metab 39:* 555, 1974.
97. Mallinson, C. N., Bloom, S. R., Warin, A. P., Salmon, P. R., Cox, B.: A glucagonoma syndrome. *Lancet 2:* 1, 1974.
98. Aoki, T. T., Toews, C. J., Rossini, A. A., Ruderman, N. B., Cahill, G. F., Jr.: Glucogenic substrate levels in fasting man. *Adv Enzyme Regul 13:* 329, 1975.
99. Fitzpatrick, G. F., Meguid, M. M., O'Connell, R. C. et al: Nitrogen sparing by carbohydrate in man: intermittent to continuous enteral compared with continuous parenteral glucose. *Surgery 78:* 105, 1975.
100. Young, V. R., Scrimshaw, N. S.: Endogenous nitrogen metabolism and plasma free amino acids in young adults given a "protein free" diet. *Br J Nutr 22:* 9, 1968.
101. Brennan, M. F., Fitzpatrick, G. F., Cohen, K. H., Moore, F. D.: Glycerol: major contributor to the short term protein sparing effect of fat emulsions in normal man. *Ann Surg 182:* 386, 1975.
102. Scow, R. O.: Transport of triglyceride: its removal from blood circulation and uptake by tissues. In Meng, H. C., Law, D. H. (eds): Parenteral Nutrition. Proceedings of International Symposium, Vanderbilt University School of Medicine, Nashville, Tenn. Springfield, Ill. Thomas, 1970, ch 24, pp 294–338.
103. Blackburn, G. L., Flatt, J. P., Clowes, G. H. A., O'Donnell, T. E.: Peripheral intravenous feeding with isotonic amino acid solutions. *Am J Surg 125:* 447, 1973.
104. Blackburn, G. L., Flatt, J. P., Clowes, G. H. A., Jr., O'Donnell, T. F., Hensle, T. E.: Protein sparing therapy during periods of starvation with sepsis or trauma. *Ann Surg 177:* 588, 1973.
105. Flatt, J. P., Blackburn, G. L.: The metabolic fuel regulatory system: implications for protein-sparing therapies during caloric deprivation and disease. *Am J Clin Nutr 27:* 175, 1974.
106. Bagdade, J. D., Bierman, E. L., Porte, D., Jr.: The significance of basal insulin levels in the evaluation of the insulin response to

glucose in diabetic and non-diabetic subjects. *J Clin Invest 46:* 1549, 1967.

107. Felig, P., Marliss, E. B., Cahill, G. F., Jr.: Plasma amino acid levels and insulin secretion in obesity. *N Engl J Med 281:* 811, 1969.

108. Rabinowitz, D., Zierler, K. L.: Forearm metabolism in obesity and its response to intra-arterial insulin. Characterization of insulin resistance, i.e. evidence for adaptive hyperinsulinism. *J Clin Invest 41:* 2173, 1962.

109. Chlouverakis, C., White, P. A.: Obesity and insulin resistance in the obese hyperglycemic mouse (obob). *Metabolism 18:* 998, 1969.

110. Stauffacher, W., Crofford, O. B., Jeanrenaud, B., Renold, A. E.: Comparitive studies of muscle and adipose tissue metabolism in lean and obese mice. *Ann N.Y. Acad Sci 131:* 528, 1965.

111. Stauffacher, W., Lambert, A. E., Vecchio, D., Renold, A. E.: Measurement of insulin activities in pancreas and serum of mice with spontaneous ("obese" and "New Zealand obese") and induced (GTG) obesity and hyperglycemia and considerations on the pathogenesis of the spontaneous syndrome. *Diabetologia 3:* 230, 1967.

112. Frame, E. G.: The levels of individual free amino acids in the plasma of normal man at various intervals after a high-protein meal. *J Clin Invest 37:* 1710, 1958.

113. Tweedle, D., Brennan, M. F., Ftizpatrick, G., Ball, M. R., Moore, F. D.: Protein conservation with peripheral isotonic amino acid solutions. *Surg Forum 26:* 32, 1975.

114. Wolfe, B. M., Culebras, J. M., Tweedle, D., Moore, F. D.: Effect of glucose on the nitrogen-sparing effect of amino acids given intravenously. *Surg Forum 27:* 39, 1976.

115. Wimsatt, W. A., Guerriere, A.: Observations on the feeding capacities and excretory function of captive vampire bats. *J Mammal 43:* 17, 1962.

144

Hormonal Control of Lipoprotein Metabolism

Gustav Schonfeld

INTRODUCTION

The heterogeneous group of complex molecules known as lipids form important structural elements and perform essential metabolic functions in animals. Lipids and lipoproteins are also involved in a number of human diseases, the most prevalent of which is atherosclerosis.

Atherosclerotic cardiovascular disease is the leading cause of death in the Western world. The disease process can involve all of the major arteries of the body, producing lesions in the walls of blood vessels that may result in partial or complete occlusions of the lumens of the involved vessel. Weakening of arterial walls may also occur, leading to aneurysmal dilatations. The overall effect is interference with the flow of arterial blood to vital organs and the production of symptoms of ischemia involving most of the major organ systems of the body, including the central nervous system, the heart, the intestines, the kidneys, and the extremities. Although the initiating causes and the factors that lead to the progression of the atherosclerotic process have not been completely delineated, it is clear that certain human populations have a greater propensity for developing clinical atherosclerosis than do others. Some of the factors that put people at higher than usual risk include high blood pressure, cigarette smoking, and hypercholesterolemia (and other kinds of hyperlipoproteinemia). The strong connection between hyperlipoproteinemia and atherosclerosis, and the hope that atherosclerosis may be prevented by the treatment of hyperlipoproteinemia, represent some practical motivation for research into the causes of hyperlipoproteinemia in man.

Lipids enter the body as food, and many are also synthesized de novo. Triglycerides (triacylglycerols) comprise 40 percent of the total caloric intake of Americans, and more than 90 percent of the mass of adipose tissue (which in turn comprises 10–35 percent of body weight). Cholesterol, which is the metabolic precursor of steroid hormones and bile acids and is an important constituent of plasma membranes, is ingested and synthesized in approximately equal amounts (0.4–0.8 g/ day). About 1–2 g of phospholipids are ingested daily. The total body synthesis of these substances, which serve primarily as structural elements of various cell and organelle membranes and of the plasma lipoproteins, has not been accurately estimated.

Although virtually all tissues synthesize some lipids, more than 95 percent of cholesterol and a large proportion of the triacylglycerols are synthesized by two tissues: the absorptive cells of the gastrointestinal tract and the parenchymal cells of the liver. Triacylglycerols are also synthesized in large amounts in adipose tissue. Rates of synthesis and turnover of these substances are regulated, in part, by the quantity and composition of the diet and by endogenous diurnal cycles. Various hormones are also important.

Lipids are transported from one tissue to another through plasma by lipoproteins—water-soluble complexes that contain several moieties of lipids and apoproteins. The lipoproteins containing dietary lipids are assembled in and secreted from the absorptive cells of the gut, whence they find their way into the blood stream and transport lipids to "peripheral" tissues. Endogenously assembled triacylglycerols are exported from liver by very low density lipoproteins (VLDL).

Transport of lipids from gut and liver to "peripheral" tissues is essential in the nutrition of the organism. Some transport in the opposite direction also occurs. This may be important in the turnover of lipids in cell membranes and in preventing the accumulation of lipids within tissues (e.g., in the arterial wall). Cholesterol arriving to the liver in lipoproteins may be excreted unchanged directly into bile, or it may be converted to bile salts prior to secretion. Thus, the "reverse transport" of lipids in plasma lipoproteins may play a role in the excretion of cholesterol and in bile acid synthesis.

Levels of lipoproteins in plasma are determined by the rates of two processes: (1) *input,* which is influenced by genetic, metabolic, and hormonal factors operating at the level of the liver and/ or gut; and (2) *catabolism,* which is regulated by genetic, metabolic, and hormonal factors operating on "peripheral" tissues such as the heart, skeletal muscle, adipose tissue, and plasma itself.

An acquaintance with lipid and lipoprotein metabolism is

---

*It should be noted that apolipoproteins are known by two different nomenclatures. The one used in this text is based on the ABC system of Alaupovic: apolipoproteins are named alphabetically in the chronologic order of their discoveries. The alternative nomenclature is based on the carboxyl terminal amino acids of the apolipoproteins.

important in clinical medicine because the hyperlipoproteinemias are among the most frequently encountered clinical disorders in man. These aberrations may be "primary," or "secondary" to hormonal or other diseases. There are particularly strong associations between hyperlipoproteinemia and diabetes mellitus. People with hyperlipoproteinemia are peculiarly susceptible to atherosclerosis, a susceptibility that is greatly enhanced in patients who have both hyperlipoproteinemia and diabetes mellitus.

FAT DIGESTION AND ABSORPTION

The typical 2500-cal American diet contains 110 g (1000 cal) of fat. More than 95 percent of this fat is in the form of triacylglycerol. Intakes of cholesterol and phospholipids are approximately 800 mg and 2000 mg/day, respectively.[1]

Dietary lipids undergo a progressive emulsification after they enter the small intestine (Fig. 144-1), which reduces the relatively large pieces of fat into progressively smaller droplets of oil. Conjugated bile salts are essential in this process.[2] Specific lipases, which act at the interfaces of the oil and aqueous phases, hydrolyze the fatty ester bonds of the dietary triacylglycerols, cholesterol esters, and phosphoacylglycerols, producing fatty acids, mono- and diacylglycerols, glycerol, free cholesterol, and lysophosphatidylcholine.[3]

Glycerol and lysophosphatidylcholine are water soluble and readily enter the aqueous phase of chyme. However, the other lipid moieties are hydrophobic and need to be rendered soluble as mixed micelles. These molecular aggregates, which have Stokes radii ranging from 23 to 35 nm and form optically clear solutions, are composed primarily of monoacylglycerols, fatty acids, lysophosphatidylcholine, and bile salts, but small amounts of cholesterol are also incorporated into them and are thereby solubilized.[4] Any unsolubilized cholesterol probably passes out unabsorbed through the intestine. Bile acids must be present in the small

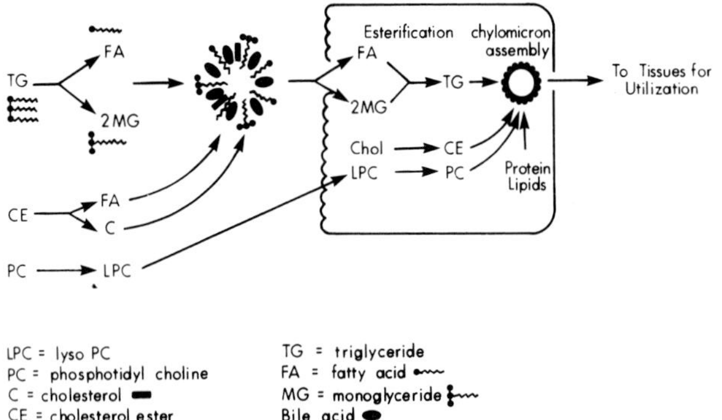

Fig. 144-1. Digestion and absorption of fat in the duodenum and jejunum. The various lipid moieties are hydrolyzed by pancreatic lipases and the resulting fatty acids, monoacylglycerol, and small amounts of cholesterol combine with bile acids to form mixed micelles. These structures move across the unstirred water layer up to the brush border cell membrane of the intestinal absorptive cell. Lipids penetrate the cell membrane. Within the cell, triacylglycerol, cholesterol esters, and phospholipids are reconstituted by esterification. Lipids and apoproteins synthesized in the gut cell are assembled into chylomicrons, which are secreted into the intestinal lymph. Chylomicrons enter the venous system via the thoracic duct. Chylomicron-triacylglycerols in the vascular compartment are hydrolyzed to fatty acids and glycerol by lipoprotein lipase. Both glycerol and fatty acids readily enter peripheral tissues.

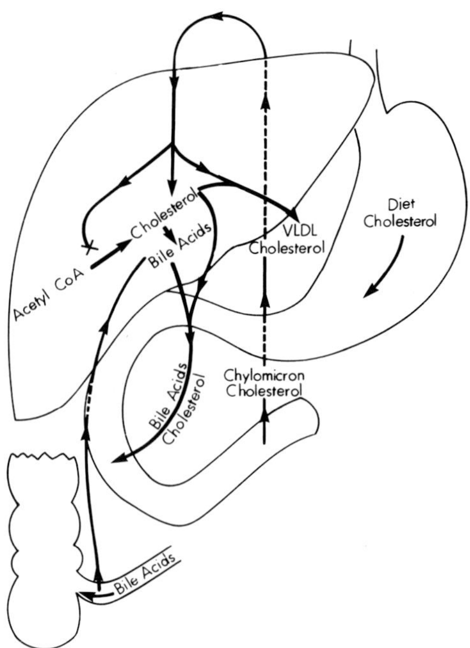

Fig. 144-2. Interrelations of cholesterol and bile acid metabolism. Dietary cholesterol enters the liver from partially catabolized chylomicrons, the "remnants." In liver, cholesterol inhibits (×) further cholesterol synthesis from acetyl CoA. Cholesterol is secreted from liver as part of the VLDL particle. In addition, both dietary and newly synthesized cholesterol serve as precursors for bile acid synthesis (although the latter may be the preferred substrate). Bile acids are secreted into the duodenum, where they aid in the emulsification, digestion, and absorption of fats, including cholesterol. In the terminal ileum 95 percent of secreted bile acids are reabsorbed into the blood stream and enter the liver. In the liver, bile acids control further synthesis of bile acids (↓). They may also be resecreted into the bile, forming the enterohepatic circulation of bile salts.

intestine at or above their critical micellar concentrations for micelles to be formed.

Micelles in the aqueous phase move across the unstirred water layer[5] that surrounds the microvilli, up to the cell membrane of the absorptive cell, where long-chain fatty acids, monoacylglycerols, and cholesterol penetrate the cell membrane. Bile salts remain in the lumen to be absorbed farther "downstream" in the terminal ileum.[6] Most fat absorption occurs in the duodenum and proximal jejunum.[7]

Absorbed lipids are reesterified (Fig. 144-1) on the intracellular side of the brush border (to triacylglycerol, cholesterol ester, and phosphotidylcholine), and along with apoproteins they are assembled into chylomicrons (see below). These particles are extruded from the basal or the lateral surfaces of the absorptive cells into the lacteals. The chylomicron-containing intestinal lymph is collected into the major lymphatic ducts and emptied into the venous system via the thoracic duct[7–9] (Fig. 144-2).

Using the complex processes just outlined, the human intestine absorbs only about 40 percent of the dietary cholesterol daily (300 mg). This limitation, which represents a "line of defense" against hypercholesterolemia in man, may be related to the incomplete micellar solubilization of cholesterol and to the relatively slow rates of transport of cholesterol across the brush border membrane. By contrast, the ability of the intestine to absorb fatty acids is virtually unlimited. More than 95 percent of normal intakes (which are 100-fold greater than those of cholesterol) are absorbed, and even very large (e.g., 2-fold) increases in dietary intakes of fat do not result in steatorrhea.[7–10]

METABOLISM OF LIPIDS

CHOLESTEROL AND BILE ACIDS

Cholesterol Biosynthesis

Synthesis[11,12] (Fig. 144-3) begins in the cytoplasm with acetyl coenzyme A (CoA). Acetyl CoA is produced in mitochondria and is not transported across the mitochondrial membrane. Instead, citrate is synthesized from mitochondrial acetyl CoA and oxaloacetate by citrate synthase, and citrate is transported into the cytosol. In the cytosol, citrate is converted back to acetyl CoA by the citrate cleavage enzyme.[13]

In the first sequence of reactions, two cytosolic enzymes—acetoacetyl CoA thiolase and HMG-CoA synthase—convert acetyl CoA to HMG-CoA,[14,15] and HMG-CoA is reduced to mevalonate by means of HMG-CoA reductase, an enzyme loosely bound to the microsomal fraction of the cell.[16–19] A parallel pathway for the production of HMG-CoA exists in the mitochondria. However, the mitochondria do not possess HMG-CoA reductase; instead they contain HMG-CoA lyase, which catalyzes the production of acetoacetate.[20,21] Thus ketogenesis and cholesterol synthesis are compartmentalized beginning with acetyl CoA.

The next major sequence is the conversion of mevalonate to squalene, by means of several enzymatic reactions. The final group of reactions consists of the conversion of squalene to cholesterol via lanosterol and several other steroid intermediates. These intermediates are hydrophobic, but they are solubilized and made available to the microsomal enzymes, which catalyze these final conversions by means of a sterol carrier protein.[22,23]

Control of Cholesterol Synthesis

The overall rate of synthesis of cholesterol (measured by the incorporation of two carbon precursors to sterols) is at its maximum at night and reaches minimum levels during the daylight hours (Table 144-1).[24–26,28] This diurnal variation has been particularly well documented in the rat. High-cholesterol diets, biliary obstruction, and starvation inhibit cholesterol synthesis. Diets low in cholesterol and interference with the intestinal reabsorption of bile acids with resins or by surgical diversion of biliary flow increase rates of cholesterol synthesis.[29–33] Insulin and thyroid hormone increase cholesterol synthesis, whereas glucagon and glucocorticoids[34–37] are inhibitory.

The regulatory effects of diets on hepatic cholesterol synthesis are probably mediated by dietary cholesterol (not bile acids), which reaches the liver via lipoproteins produced in the intestine (Fig. 144-2).[28,38,39] Experiments have shown that hepatic cholesterogenesis in the rat is inhibited in vivo by the infusion of lipoproteins, the magnitude of inhibition being directly related to the cellular uptake of cholesterol from any given class of lipoproteins (Table 144-2). Thus, when the same degree of hypercholesterolemia is produced by the intravenous infusion of lipoproteins, the largest amount of hepatic uptake and the greatest inhibition of synthesis are obtained with chylomicrons. These results indicate that chylomicron-cholesterol is the most effective regulator of hepatic cholesterol synthesis, albeit the other lipoproteins are not without effect.

Table 144-1. Control of Cholesterol Synthesis in Rats

Group	Midnight*	9:00 a.m.	Noon	9:00 p.m.
Control	100	33	17	92
Cholesterol fed	7	—	7	—
Cholestyramine	—	—	173	360
Fasting	—	14	—	20

Adapted from Bortz et al.: Biochim. Biophys. Acta *316:* 366, 1973.[27]

Cholesterol (400 mg) or cholestyramine (400 mg) were given by gastric tube as a single dose. Hepatic cholesterol synthesis from ^{14}C-acetate was measured 12–24 h later, at the times indicated. In control animals, peak synthetic rates (100 percent) at midnight were 6-fold greater than minimum rates (17 percent) at noon. A single oral dose of cholesterol depressed cholesterol synthesis to 7 percent. Bile sequestration by cholestyramine increased synthesis 10-fold at noon (173 versus 17 percent). Fasting for 24 h was inhibiting.

*Rates are expressed relative to controls at midnight, which have been set to 100 percent.

Table 144-2. Control of Hepatic Synthesis of Cholesterol by Intestinal and Hepatic Lipoproteins

	Cholesterol Input	
	Δ Cholesterol Esters*	Cholesterol Synthesis
Chylomicrons	0.108 ± 0.011	6.5
Serum lipoproteins	0.002 ± 0.003	19.7

Various fractions of intestinal lipoproteins (chylomicrons) or hepatic (serum) lipoproteins were injected intravenously into rats. Analyses were performed 12 h later. The amounts of cholesterol injected were matched for the two types of lipoproteins. Clearly, more cholesterol enters the liver from chylomicrons than from serum lipoproteins (0.108 vs 0.002). Cholesterol synthesis was inhibited more by chylomicrons than by serum lipoproteins.

*Increases of hepatic cholesterol contents (over baseline) produced per unit mass of cholesterol injected.

Adapted from Nervi and Dietschy: J. Biol. Chem. *250:* 8704, 1975.[39]

Brown et al.[40,41] have demonstrated in human fibroblasts that the physiologic inhibition of cellular cholesterol synthesis involves several steps: (1) the binding of lipoproteins to specific receptor sites on cell membranes; (2) the interiorization of the lipoproteins by phagocytosis; (3) their "disassembly" in phagolysosomes, including the hydrolysis of cholesterol esters and of apoproteins; and (4) the movement of cholesterol out of the phagolysosome, presumably to the sites where HMG-CoA is inhibited. None of the intracellular events, including the regulation of cholesterol synthesis, occurs in the absence of cellular receptor sites.[41–43] The situation described for the skin fibroblast also appears to hold for arterial smooth muscle cells[44–46] and leukocytes.[47,48] Lipoprotein-arterial smooth muscle cell interactions, in addition to regulating intracellular cholesterol metabolism, may also be important in regulating the proliferation of the smooth muscle cells.[49,50]

Receptor sites for chylomicron remnants have recently been identified on liver cell membranes. This finding and the efficiency of chylomicrons (or chylomicron "remnants") in moving cholesterol into the liver cell, and in "turning off" cholesterol synthesis suggests that lipoprotein—cell membrane interactions and the interiorization of cholesterol are important in regulating cholesterol synthesis in the liver as well.

Intestinal cholesterogenesis in gut wall is probably regulated by the cholesterol absorbed into the absorptive cell from the gut lumen, although bile acids are also important because they determine rates of cholesterol penetration into the cell. Thus, both hepatic and intestinal cholesterol synthesis are under dietary regulation.

The HMG-CoA reductase reaction is an important regulatory site in cholesterogenesis.[43] Rates of cholesterol synthesis and activities of HMG-CoA reductase parallel each other closely during the diurnal cycle and following a variety of metabolic perturbations.

Variations in the *activity* of HMG-CoA reductase are fre-

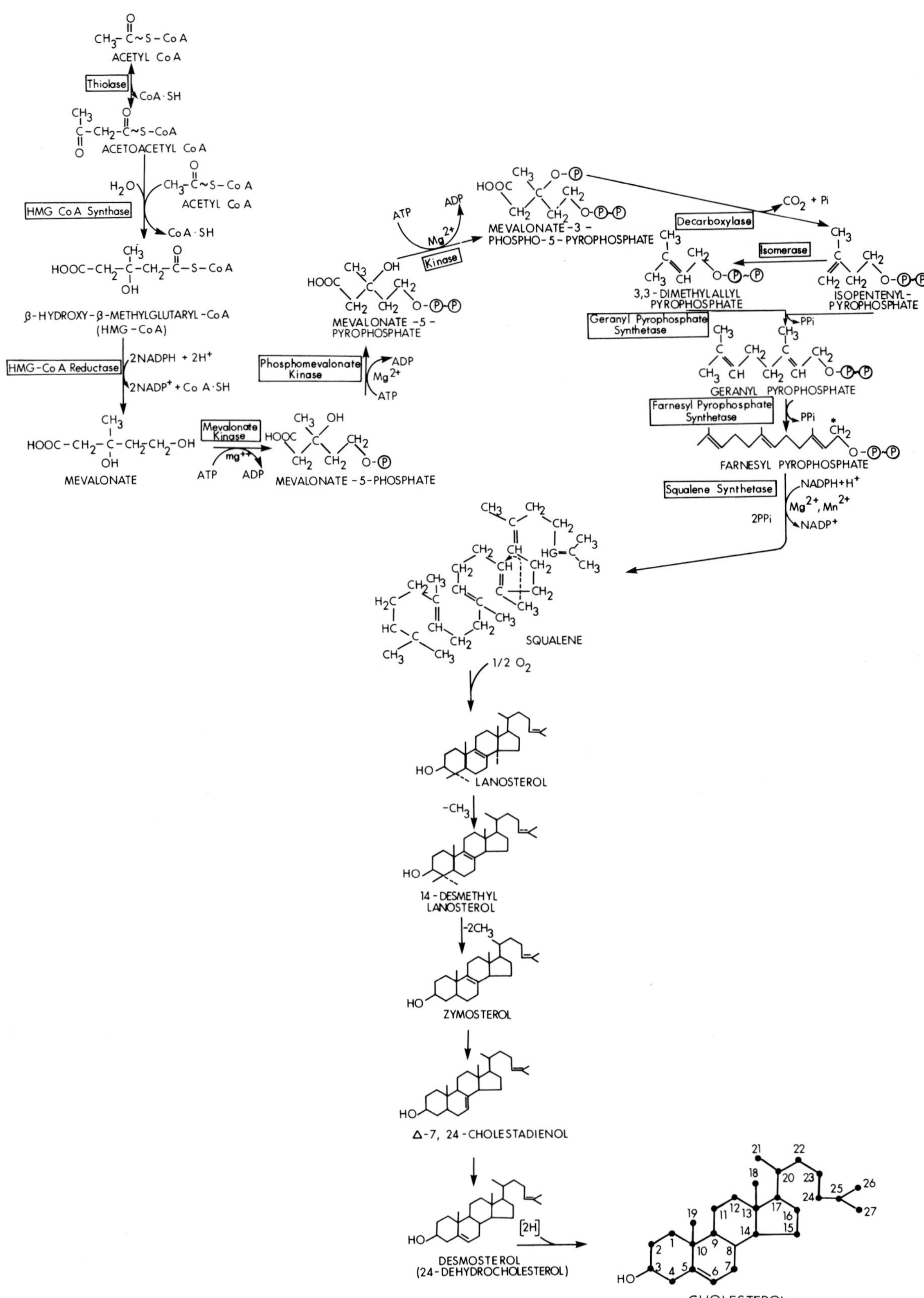

Fig. 144-3. Biosynthesis of cholesterol. The three major subdivisions of the biosynthetic scheme are as follows: A. Acetyl CoA → HMG-CoA; this sequence occurs in the cytosol. B. HMG-CoA → squalene. The major rate-limiting step, HMG-CoA reductase, occurs in this sequence; the enzymes of this sequence are located in the microsomes. C. Squalene → cholesterol; most of the sterol intermediates are water insoluble in isolated form, and thus the sterol carrier protein (SCP) is important in solubilizing the sterols (SCP–sterol complex) and in making the interactions with the microsomal enzymes of this sequence possible.

quently accompanied by changes in the rates of synthesis of *enzyme protein,*[51] some of which may be prevented by inhibition of the production of messenger RNA, suggesting that the activity of the enzyme may be regulated at the translational step of its synthesis.[52] However, recent work suggests that changes in activity and enzyme synthesis (or catabolism) are not invariably coupled, i.e., that "allosteric" effects may also be operative[53] in the case of some "cholesterologenic" enzymes.

It was originally thought that the HMG-CoA reductase reaction was the *only* one affected during variations in cholesterol synthetic rates. However, other enzymatic activities may also be affected, albeit to a lesser extent. For example, feeding of high-cholesterol diets affects the activities of acetoacetyl CoA thiolase, HMG-CoA synthase, and of some of the enzymes involved in the conversion of mevalonate to squalene.[14,15] The sterol carrier protein is another potential site of regulation.[11,22,23]

Catabolism of Cholesterol and Production of Bile Acids

Cholesterol leaves the body primarily through the biliary secretions, which are excreted in the stool either as neutral sterols (i.e., unchanged cholesterol, or cholesterol partially metabolized by gut bacteria, e.g., cholestanol or coprosterol) or as bile salts (acidic sterols). The cyclopentanophenanthrene ring is not degraded in mammalian cells, but some neutral sterols are degraded by intestinal bacteria; 10 percent or less is excreted via the skin.

Bile acid synthesis[54,55] (Fig. 144-4) occurs in the microsomal fraction of the liver. Some of the hydroxylation steps resemble those performed by the "detoxifying" mixed microsomal oxydases and require cytochrome P_{450}. Isotopic equilibrium experiments indicate that there are at least two pools of cholesterol in the liver cell.[56] The pool containing edogenously synthesized cholesterol may be the preferred but is not the sole substrate for bile acid synthesis.

The initial reaction of the synthetic sequence results in the introduction of an α-hydroxyl group at the 7 position of cholesterol by the 7-α-hydroxylase enzyme. The oxidation of the hydroxyl group at the 3 position, and the shifting of the double bond from the Δ^5 to the Δ^4 position, results in the production of 7-hydroxy-4-cholestene-3-one, which serves as the common precursor for the two primary bile acids, cholic acid and chenodeoxycholic acid. The divergent pathways to cholic and chenodeoxycholic acids begin with the 12-α-hydroxylase and the 5-β-reductase reactions, respectively.

Bile acids differ from cholesterol in that (1) the Δ^5 double bond is fully saturated, (2) there are α-hydroxyl groups at the 3, 7, and 12 positions, (3) the side chain is diminished by three carbon atoms, and (4) a carboxyl group is introduced at the terminal C-24 position. Before they are secreted into the bile canaliculi, bile acids are conjugated either with taurine or glycine at C-24. Thus, the products secreted from liver are conjugated bile salts.

A major site of regulation of the overall synthesis of the bile acids is the 7-α-hydroxylase step.[57,58] Other potential sites of regulation are at the branch point between cholic and chenodeoxycholic acids.

Following their secretion into the bile and entry into the duodenum, bile salts participate in the digestion of fat as previously described (Figs. 144-1 and 144-2). Bacteria in the gut deconjugate bile acids and convert primary to secondary bile acids. Cholic acid is converted to deoxycholic acid, and chenodeoxycholic acid to lithocholic acid. Secondary bile acids are absorbed in the terminal ileum along with the primary bile acids and become parts of the total circulating bile acid pool. Bacteria also catabolize the steroid nucleus.

Approximately 95 percent of the bile acids secreted during a 24-h period are reabsorbed (Fig. 144-2). The 5 percent lost is regained by dietary intake and by de novo synthesis of cholesterol and bile acids. Thus, the total body content of sterols is thought to be held at a relatively constant steady-state level, albeit the tendency is toward increases in tissue cholesterol content with age.[59-61]

Bile, in addition to containing primary and secondary bile acids, also contains cholesterol and phospholipids. The relative proportions in which these three constituents are secreted determines the degree of saturation of bile with respect to cholesterol, and this in turn is related to the lithogenicity of the bile[62] (i.e., its propensity to form cholesterol crystals and eventually cholesterol gallstones).

Controls of Bile Acid Synthesis

The rate of synthesis of the bile acids parallels the rate of synthesis of cholesterol in most instances. Thus, bile acid synthesis is at its maximum during the dark phase of the diurnal cycle, and at its minimum during the light phase. Diversion of bile flow, or the binding of bile acids with resins, which results in interference with their reabsorption in the ileum, increases the synthesis of cholesterol and bile acids simultaneously. Similarly, obstruction of bile flow inhibits the production of both molecules.[63,64] The intake of high-calorie and high-carbohydrate diets stimulates the synthesis of both cholesterol and bile acids.[65,66]

By contrast, high-fat and high-cholesterol diets inhibit cholesterogenesis, but they stimulate cholesterol and bile acid secretion. Thus, several mechanisms exist for limiting the accumulation of cholesterol: (1) limited absorption from the gastrointestinal tract; (2) the reciprocal relationship between dietary absorption and the rate of endogenous synthesis of cholesterol; and (3) the variable excretion of sterols in bile as cholesterol or as bile acids, or both (Fig. 144-2).

These "mechanisms of defense" operate at various levels of efficiency in different species of animals. For example, in the rabbit, most of the cholesterol is absorbed, the "feedback inhibition" of hepatic cholesterogenesis is inefficient, and reexcretion of cholesterol (either unchanged or as bile acids) is incomplete. Therefore, rabbits are rendered very hypercholesterolemic by high-cholesterol diets (plasma cholesterols rise from less than 30 to more than 1000 mg/dl in a few days). Rats, on the other hand, although they absorb large amounts of cholesterol, possess very efficient machinery for regulation of cholesterol and bile acid synthesis. Consequently, it is very difficult to render rats hypercholesterolemic by diet alone. Man is variable but he tends to fall between these two extremes.[67,68]

Cholesterol in Blood

The cholesterol in plasma may be derived from a variety of sources, including (1) the diet (chylomicrons and chylomicron degradation products), (2) cholesterol synthesized by liver on its way to the periphery (VLDL, LDL), or (3) cholesterol synthesized by a variety of tissues on its way in the opposite direction (high-density lipoproteins, HDL).

Approximately 70 percent of plasma cholesterol is esterified with long-chain fatty acids. Most of the esterification is thought to occur in plasma, catalyzed by the enzyme lecithin:cholesterol acyltransferase (LCAT; see below).

In normolipemic man on an "American" diet, 60–70 percent of the cholesterol in plasma is carried by LDL and approximately

75 percent of the cholesterol arises from sources other than diet.[30,59] However, the distribution of cholesterol among the lipoproteins and the relative contribution of the various sources to the cholesterol of plasma is determined by the metabolic and hormonal state of the individual. For example, 3–4 h after a meal, a greater portion of plasma cholesterol comes from the diet and is carried by chylomicrons than after a 12–24 h fast. On the other hand, the hypercholesterolemia which accompanies several days or more of starvation cannot be due to diet, and the de novo synthesis of cholesterol virtually ceases.[25,26,69,70] Therefore, the hypercholesterolemia must be due to the mobilization of tissue cholesterol (probably from the adipose tissue, a large reservoir of cholesterol) and the transport of this cholesterol in lipoproteins. Hepatic synthesis and secretion of bile acids during starvation are greatly slowed. The latter may also contribute to the hypercholesterolemia by delaying the clearance of cholesterol from plasma.

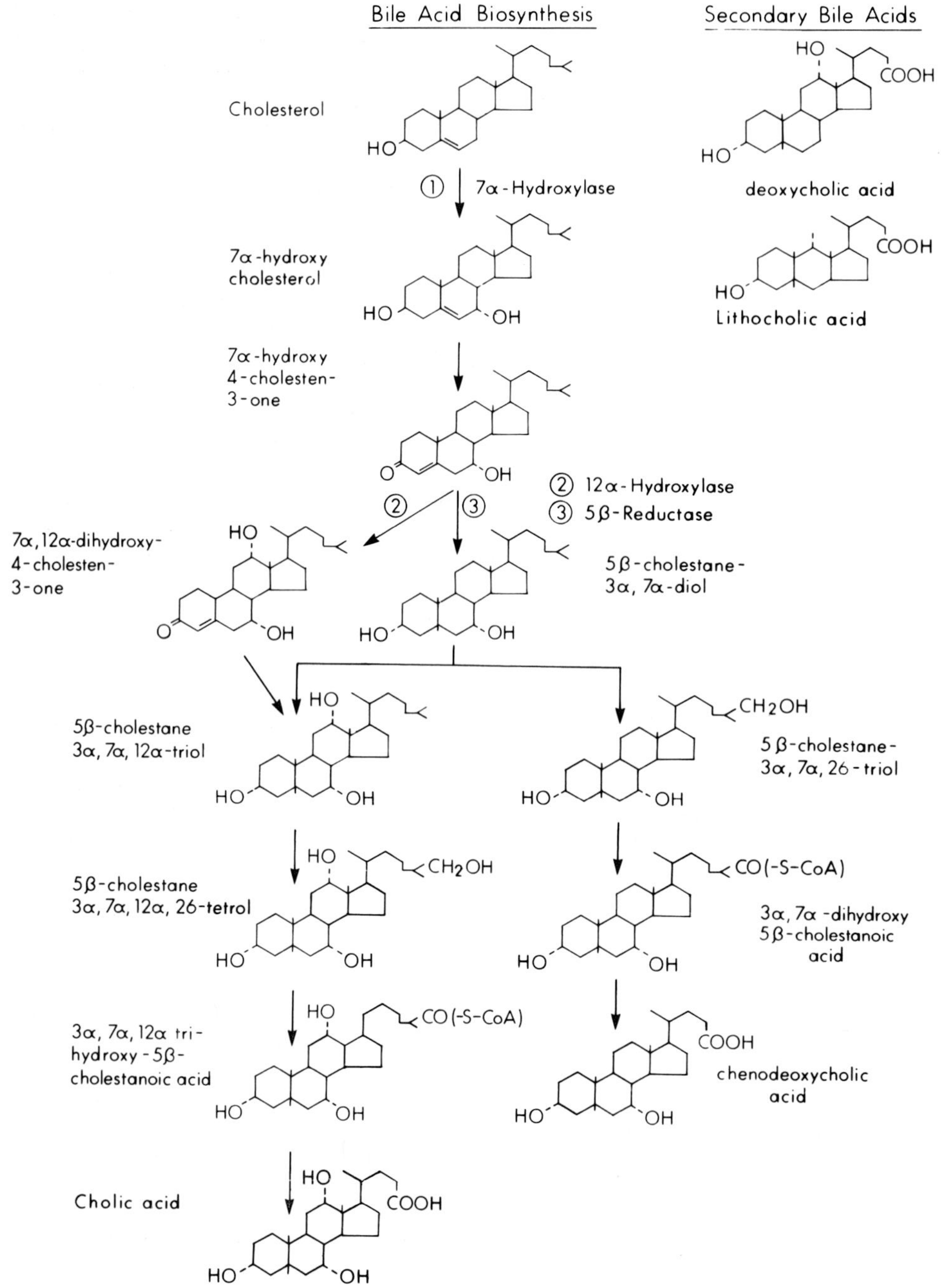

Bile Acid Biosynthesis

Secondary Bile Acids

Cholesterol

① 7α-Hydroxylase

deoxycholic acid

7α-hydroxy cholesterol

Lithocholic acid

7α-hydroxy 4-cholesten-3-one

② 12α-Hydroxylase

③ 5β-Reductase

7α,12α-dihydroxy-4-cholesten-3-one

5β-cholestane-3α, 7α-diol

5β-cholestane 3α, 7α, 12α-triol

5β-cholestane-3α, 7α, 26-triol

5β-cholestane 3α, 7α, 12α, 26-tetrol

3α, 7α-dihydroxy 5β-cholestanoic acid

3α, 7α, 12α tri-hydroxy-5β-cholestanoic acid

chenodeoxycholic acid

Cholic acid

Fig. 144-4. Biosynthesis of bile acids. The hydroxylase enzymes that catalyze these reactions resemble the microsomal mixed function oxydases of the liver cell in their localization and in their requirements for cytochrome P_{450}. Other enzymes appear to be localized to the cytosol. The hepatic cholesterol that serves as precursor appears to be distributed into more than one intracellular kinetic "pool." Cholesterol synthesized de novo may be the preferred substrate. The major overall rate-limiting step is at 7-α-hydroxylase (1). Activities of 12-α-hydroxylase (2) and 5-β-reductase (3) may determine the relative amounts of cholic and deoxycholic acid synthesized.

Secondary bile acids are produced by intestinal bacteria. These acids too are reabsorbed in the terminal ileum and become part of the circulating (enterohepatic) bile acid pool.

TRIACYLGLYCEROL

Triacylglycerol Biosynthesis and Degradation

Two pathways, both located in the endoplasmic reticulum of the cell, are available for the formation of triacylglycerols[12] (Fig. 144-5). The "glycerolphosphate" pathway predominates in liver and adipose tissue, the "monoglyceride" pathway in gut mucosa.[9,10]

Long-chain fatty acyl CoA and sn-glycerol-3-phosphate are the required starting materials for the glycerolphosphate pathway.[71,72] The former are contributed by endogenous de novo synthesis, or by exogenous fatty acids that arrive at the cell unesterified complexed to albumin, or esterified in lipoproteins.[73] Following their entry into the cytosol, fatty acids are converted to fatty acyl CoA before they enter the synthetic pathway:[71]

$$\text{Fatty acid} + \text{ATP} + \text{CoA} \xrightarrow[\text{(thiokinase)}]{\text{fatty acyl CoA ligase}} \text{Fatty acyl CoA} + \text{AMP} + \text{PP}_i. \quad (1)$$

sn-Glycerol-3-phosphate is contributed by glycolysis, specifically by the reduction of dihydroxyacetonephosphate.[74] In liver

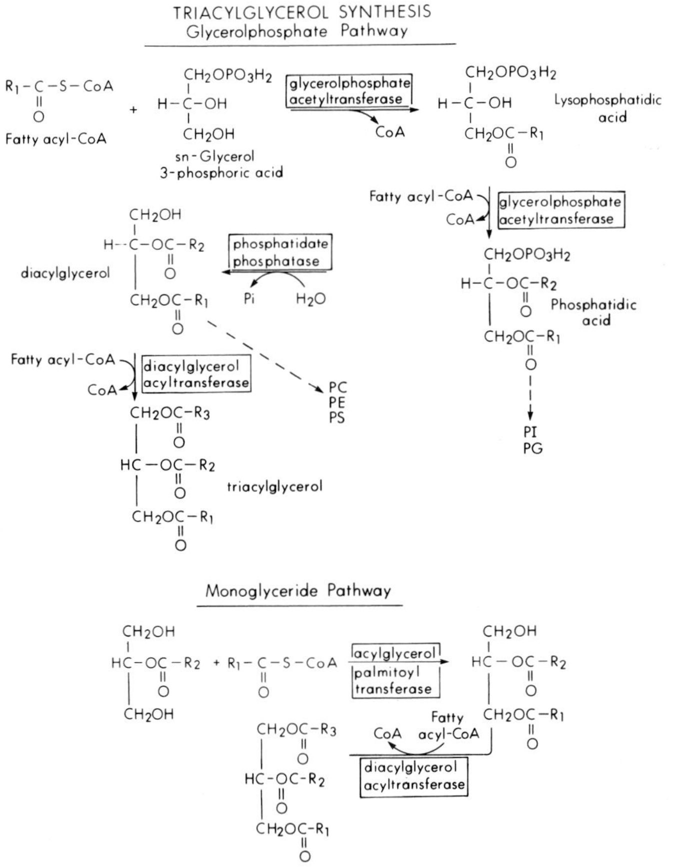

TRIACYLGLYCEROL SYNTHESIS
Glycerolphosphate Pathway

$R_1-C(=O)-S-CoA$ (Fatty acyl-CoA) + $CH_2OPO_3H_2$ / $H-C-OH$ / CH_2OH (sn-Glycerol 3-phosphoric acid) —[glycerolphosphate acetyltransferase]→ CoA + $CH_2OPO_3H_2$ / $H-C-OH$ / $CH_2OC(=O)-R_1$ (Lysophosphatidic acid)

Fatty acyl-CoA → CoA [glycerolphosphate acetyltransferase] → $CH_2OPO_3H_2$ / $H-C-OC(=O)-R_2$ / $CH_2OC(=O)-R_1$ (Phosphatidic acid) → PI, PG

[phosphatidate phosphatase] (H_2O → Pi) → CH_2OH / $H-C-OC(=O)-R_2$ / $CH_2OC(=O)-R_1$ (diacylglycerol) → PC, PE, PS

Fatty acyl-CoA → CoA [diacylglycerol acyltransferase] → $CH_2OC(=O)-R_3$ / $HC-OC(=O)-R_2$ / $CH_2OC(=O)-R_1$ (triacylglycerol)

Monoglyceride Pathway

CH_2OH / $HC-OC(=O)-R_2$ / CH_2OH + $R_1-C(=O)-S-CoA$ —[acylglycerol palmitoyl transferase]→ CH_2OH / $HC-OC(=O)-R_2$ / $CH_2OC(=O)-R_1$

Fatty acyl-CoA → CoA [diacylglycerol acyltransferase] → $CH_2OC(=O)-R_3$ / $HC-OC(=O)-R_2$ / $CH_2OC(=O)-R_1$

Fig. 144-5. Biosynthesis of triacylglycerol. Two pathways are depicted. The "glycerophosphate" pathway is predominant in most tissues; the "monoglyceride" pathway predominates in the intestinal absorptive cell. The acyltransferase enzymes are located in microsomes. Phosphatidate phosphatase activity is found primarily in the cytosol (90 percent soluble, 10 percent microsomal). This enzyme is rate limiting for the glycerolphosphate pathway. Other important sites of control include the two branch points at phosphatidic acid and at diacylglycerol.

(but not in adipose tissue) glycerolphosphate can also be produced by the phosphorylation of glycerol:

$$\text{Glycerol} + \text{ATP} \xrightarrow[\text{Mg}^{++}]{\text{glycerokinase}} \text{sn-Glycerol-3-phosphate} + \text{ADP}. \quad (2)$$

The assembly of triacylglycerols from these precursors is catalyzed by three microsomal acyltransferases and phosphatidate phosphatase[75,76] (Fig. 144-5); 10 percent of the latter activity is in the microsomal fraction and 90 percent is in the cytosol.

The first step in synthesis is the transfer of an acyl CoA group onto the C-1 position of sn-glycerol-3-phosphate[77] (Fig. 144-5). This reaction is catalyzed by glycerolphosphate acyltransferase. Next is the esterification of the C-2 position, resulting in the production of phosphatidic acid, a key intermediate in the pathway because it is located at a branch point. One branch leads to triacylglycerol, phosphatidylcholine, and phosphatidylethanolamine, and the other to phosphatidylglycerol and phosphatidylinositol. This point in the pathway is also important because phosphatidic acid phosphatase, the enzyme that removes phosphate and converts phosphatidate to diacylglycerol, is rate limiting.[78]

Diacylglycerol is also a branch point—one branch leads to triacylglycerol, and the other to phosphatidyl choline, phosphatidylethanolamine, and phosphatidylserine.[77–79]

The glycerol "monophosphate" pathway of triacylglycerol synthesis (Fig. 144-5) in the gut serves to reassemble the monoacylglycerol and fatty acids produced during the intraluminal hydrolysis of triacylglycerols.[9,10] During the course of intraluminal hydrolysis and cellular reesterification, there is some randomization of molecules. As a result, the triacylglycerol compositions of diet and chylomicrons, although very similar, are not identical.

The triacylglycerols formed in gut mucosa and in liver are not catabolized within those tissues, nor are they stored to any great extent; rather they are "exported" to plasma via lipoproteins (see below). By contrast, the triacylglycerols of adipose tissue are stored for variable periods of time and mobilization occurs as needed. This is effected by lipolysis via the hormone-sensitive lipase.[73,80] The resulting glycerol and free fatty acids are liberated into plasma. Glycerol is soluble in plasma water, but free fatty acids are not; they are transported complexed with albumin.

Control of Triacylglycerol Synthesis

The regulation of triacylglycerol synthesis is a complex process, a point well illustrated by the changes that occur in liver following the feeding of diets high in carbohydrates[77–79,81] (Table 144-3). Rates of glycolysis increase, thereby providing increased amounts of sn-glycerol-3-phosphate. Levels and activities of acetyl CoA carboxylase and fatty acid synthetase also rise,[82–87] yielding larger amounts of fatty acids, and activities of phosphatidate phosphorylase, the rate-limiting enzyme, go up severalfold.[79]

The increased availability of precursors (sn-glycerol-3-phosphate and fatty acids) and the higher activity of the rate-limiting enzyme increase the rate of flow through the synthetic pathway. This would tend to increase the synthesis of both triacylglycerol and phospholipids; however, the activity of diacylglycerol acyltransferase is increased, while the activities of the enzymes that catalyze the production of phospholipids from phosphatidic acid and from diacylglycerol are diminished or kept constant. Thus, with high-carbohydrate diets the formation of triacylglycerol is favored at the expense of phospholipids.

Similar detailed knowledge of the changes that accompany the

Table 144-3. Stimulation of Hepatic Triacylglycerol (TG) Synthesis by Carbohydrate

Diet	TG Content (mg/g liver)	1,3-^{14}C-Glycerol Incorporation into TG (cpm × 10^3/g liver)
Rat chow (7)*	5.6	3.5
	±0.5	±0.7
75% Fructose (7)	25.3†	15.1†
	±2.8	±1.6
75% Glucose (7)	14.0†	10.5†
	±1.4	±1.0

Rats were given chow or the diets indicated ad lib for 4 days. Results are means ± 1 SEM. Clearly, both diets were followed by increases in hepatic triacylglycerol contents and synthesis.
*Number of rats.
†Means significantly different from chow group at $p < 0.001$.
Adapted from Waddell and Fallon: J. Clin. Invest. *52:* 2725, 1973.[81]

other metabolic and/or hormonal perturbations that alter lipid synthesis are not available. However, overall rates of glycerol lipid synthesis have been demonstrably altered in connection with a variety of metabolic and hormonal factors. In general, the "fed state" promotes triacylglycerol synthesis in both liver and adipose tissue while the "starvd state" promotes ketogenesis and lipolysis.[88] In this respect, insulin[86,89] and glucagon (or insulin lack)[90–92] mimic the fed and starved states, respectively. Thyroid hormone has divergent effects on liver and adipose tissue, increasing the synthesis of triacylglycerol in the former and decreasing it in the latter.[93] The sex steroids enhance hepatic triacylglycerol synthesis.[94]

Triacylglycerol in Blood

The triacylglycercols circulating in plasma are associated exclusively with lipoproteins. In plasmas of normal fasting (12–14 h) subjects, the majority of the triacylglycerol is carried in the VLDL fraction; 3–6 h after a fatty meal, a large proportion of plasma triacylglycerol is in the chylomicrons.

Most of the fatty acids in acylglycerols of fasting normal subjects originate from the free fatty acids of plasma. Fatty acids are taken up by liver, reesterified, and secreted as VLDL-triacylglycerols. Since in the fasting state most plasma free fatty acids arise from adipose tissue, the VLDL-acylglycerol fatty acids represent adipose tissue fatty acids that had been "recycled" through the liver.[73,95]

VLDL-acylglycerol fatty acids can also arise from other sources, depending upon the nutritional, metabolic, and hormonal state of the individual. For example, in obese or alcoholic men the liver synthesizes and stores larger than normal amounts of triacylglycerols. These "endogenous" lipids are also secreted with VLDL.[96,97] As a result, the VLDL-acylglycerols of obese or alcoholic subjects contain a mixture of hepatic and adipose tissue fatty acids even after 12–14 h of fasting; 3–6 h after a fatty meal, most of the plasma triacylglycerol fatty acids come from the diet and are carried in chylomicrons (S_f >400) or chylomicron "remnants" (that are isolated with VLDL).[98]

PHOSPHOLIPIDS

Phospholipid Metabolism

The glycerolphospholipids are synthesized by microsomal enzymes as indicated in Figures 144-6 and 144-7.[12,99,100] The choline-, serine- and ethanolamine-containing lipids are derived from diacylglycerol (Fig. 144-6), while the inositol- and glycerol-containing ones originate from phosphatidic acid via cytidine diphosphate–diacylglycerol (Fig. 144-7). In addition to the above "de novo" pathways, phosphatidylcholine can also be produced from phosphatidylethanolamine by reaction (3) (below).

Phosphatidylserine can be produced by interchange of ethanolamine for serine:

$$\text{Phosphotidylethanolamine} + \text{Serine} \rightarrow \text{Phosphatidylserine} + \text{Ethanolamine.} \quad (4)$$

In addition to alterations in the "head groups," acyl groups can also turn over independently of the rest of the molecule. Phospholipases A_1 and A_2 deacylate at the C-1 or C-2 positions of glycerol, respectively, producing lysophosphatidyl residues. The latter are reacylated as shown in (5) (below).

Thus, individual glycerolphospholipids are synthesized directly de novo (Figs. 144-6 and 144-7) or they may be produced from similar molecules by "base interchange" (reaction 4), by chemical alteration of the base group (reaction 3), or by deacylation–reacylation (reaction 5).

It has been well established that phospholipids are essential for membrane function.[101–103] Obviously, versatility in the production of glycerophospholipids enables the cell to alter the composition of its membrane phospholipids rapidly at very specific points. Indeed such alterations accompany variations in the availability of substrate; the functional consequences for membrane function have not been completely elucidated. However, rapid alterations in phosphatidylinositol compositions do accompany certain membrane functions.[101]

Irreversible catabolism of glycerophosphatides is catalyzed by lysophospholipase(s) (phospholipase B) that attack(s) the lysophosphatides:

$$\text{Lysophophosphatidylcholine} + H_2O \xrightarrow{\text{phospholipase B}} \text{Phosphorylcholine} + \text{Fatty acid} \quad (6)$$

The metabolism of the sphingomyelins will not be reviewed here.[11,100]

Phospholipids in Blood

Virtually all of the phospholipids in plasma are carried in lipoproteins, except for the lyso compounds, which are water soluble and are found in the nonlipoprotein fraction of plasma (d >1.21).[102,103] Most phospholipids are transported by the HDL. Approximately 70 percent of the plasma phospholipid mass consists of phosphatidylcholine and 20 percent of sphingomyelin. The serine-, ethanolamine-, and inositol-containing phospholipids, and phosphatidic acid, each make up less than 3 percent.

Phospholipids enter the plasma with chylomicrons, VLDL, and presumably HDL. Some phospholipids may be acquired by

$$\text{Phosphatidylethanolamine (PE)} + \text{3, 5-Adenosylmethionine} \xrightarrow{\text{PE methyltransferase}} \text{Phosphatidylcholine} + \text{3, 5-Adenosylhomocysteine.}$$

$$\text{Lysophosphatidylcholine} + \text{Acyl CoA} \xrightarrow{\text{acyl CoA: phospholipid acyltransferase}} \text{Phosphatidylcholine} \pm \text{CoASH.} \quad (5)$$

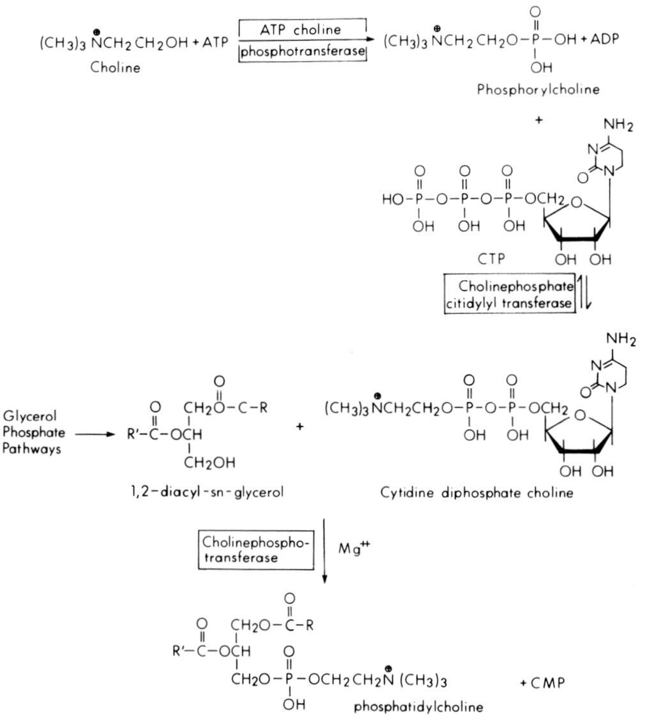

Fig. 144-6. Biosynthesis of phosphatidylcholine. First, choline is phosphorylated; phosphorylcholine is then converted to cytidine diphosphocholine. The latter reacts with diacylglycerol to form phosphatidylcholine. Note that the diacylglycerol moiety is furnished by the glycerolphosphate pathway. Phosphatidylcholine may also be synthesized from other phospholipids (see text).

HDL from cell membranes, including the membrane of the red cell (see function of HDL in section on Cholesterol "Reverse Transport"). There is also an active interchange of phospholipids between lipoproteins. Thus each phospholipid class, in each of the lipoproteins, probably arises from several sources. Virtually nothing is known about the regulation of entry into or exit of phospholipids from plasma.

One well characterized and very important function of plasma phosphatidylcholine is its role as an acyl donor in the esterification of cholesterol in plasma via the LCAT enzyme:[104]

$$\text{Cholesterol} + \text{Phosphatidylcholine} \xrightarrow{\text{LCAT}} \text{Cholesterol ester} + \text{2-lysophosphatidylcholine.} \qquad (7)$$

Deficiency of this enzyme results in gross disturbances in the metabolism and structure of lipoproteins, red cells, corneas, and kidneys. [104]

PHYSIOLOGY OF LIPOPROTEINS

In previous sections, the digestion and absorption of fat were briefly outlined, and the synthetic and catabolic pathways of the major lipids and their modes of regulation were reviewed. In this section we shall discuss the structure and the metabolism of lipoproteins.

Liproproteins have been characterized in man to a greater extent than in other species because of the importance of lipoproteins in human disease and the relative ease with which samples of sufficient size are obtainable for study. Hence, the classification of the lipoproteins in all species is derived from the system devised for man. Two sets of operational nomenclatures have been developed: one is based on the behavior of lipoproteins in the analytic ultracentrifuge (densities, or flotation rates, S_f;)[105] the other is based on their electrophoretic mobilities (Table 144-4).[106,107] Chylomicrons (S_f >400), VLDL (S_f 20–400), LDL (S_f 0–20), and HDL (F 0–20), (ultracentrifugal nomenclature), have the electrophoretic mobilities of gamma, pre-β (α_2), β, and α (α_1) globulins, respectively. There is also a minor class of lipoproteins in human plasma known as *sinking preβ*, or *Lp(a)* lipoprotein. The densities at which the various classes of lipoproteins are isolated from plasma by preparative ultracentrifugation are given in Table 144-4.

A correspondence between the ultracentrifugal and electrophoretic nomenclatures has been established in man[107] and in other species, but the agreement is not absolute. In man, most VLDL isolated by ultracentrifugation migrates as prebeta-lipoprotein; however, a VLDL of β mobility is present in type III hyperlipoproteinemia.[107] Most HDL migrates as α-lipoprotein, but Lp(a), a lipoprotein of high density present in variable amounts in all subjects,[108] migrates as preβ-lipoprotein.

A conceptual (rather than operational) classification for lipoproteins has been proposed by Alaupovic,[109] According to this theory, there are a number of lipoprotein "families" identified by their apolipoproteins (Table 144-4). The various density classes are

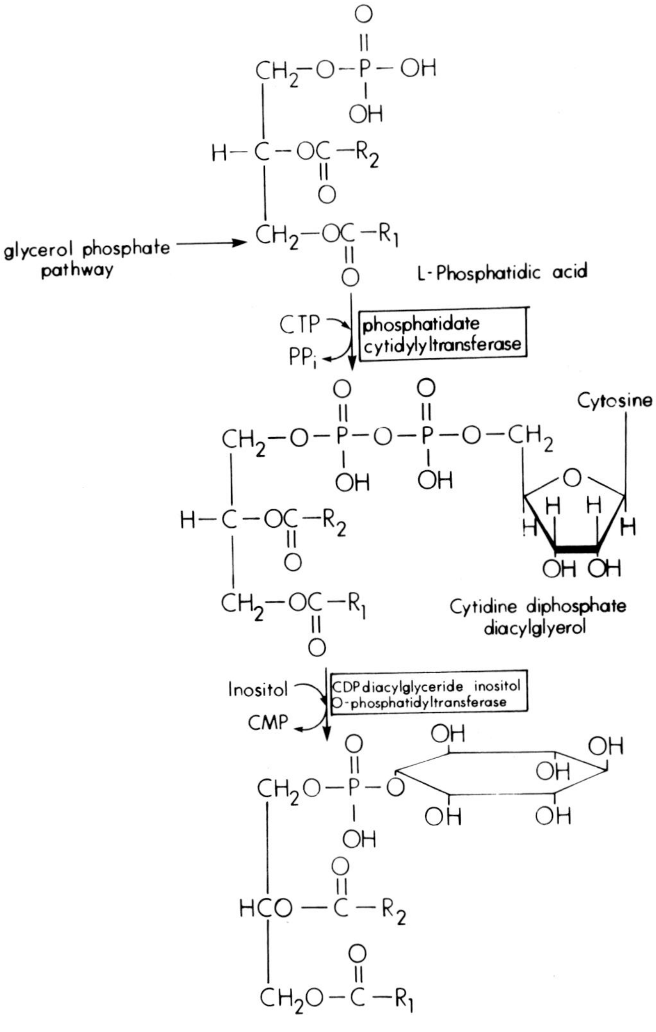

Fig. 144-7. Biosynthesis of phosphatidylinositol. Phosphatidic acid furnished by the glycerolphosphate pathway serves as an essential intermediate in this synthesis.

Table 144-4. Lipoproteins of Human Plasma

Density Class*	Density Range (g/ml)	Floatation Range (S_f)	Electrophoretic Mobility	Lipoprotein Family	Particles Found in Density Class
Chylomicrons	0.95–0.97	>400	Origin	LpA LpB LpC	Exogenous particles from gut; large endogenous particles from liver
VLDL	0.95–1.006	20–400*	α_2 globulin	LpB LpC LpE	Endogenous particles from liver; small exogenous particles from gut; chylomicron remnants; type III β-VLDL
LDL	1.006–1.063	0–20	β globulin	LpB LpC LpD	Degradation products of VLDL; abnormal LDL in type IV: LCAT deficiency; Tangier disease, obstructive jaundice; Lp(a)
Lp(a)	1.060–1.090	0–4	α_2 globulin	LpB Lp(a) Albumin	HDL_1; Lp(a)
HDL	1.063–1.21	F 1–10†	α_1 globulin	LpC LpA LpD	Lp(a); HDL of LCAT deficiency and abetalipoproteinemia; HDL_{1-3}
VHDL	>1.21				Phosphoprotein

Data from references 105, 107, and 109.

The density and electrophoretic nomenclatures are based on "operational" considerations, whereas the "lipoprotein family" is a conceptual classification that holds that each lipoprotein family is defined by its characteristic apolipoprotein (e.g., lipoprotein A (LpA) is the family containing apolipoprotein A (ApoA), LpB is the family containing ApoB, etc.). According to this theory, each density or electrophoretic class may contain one or more of the lipoprotein families free or complexed to each other. (See also Table 144-13.)

*VLDL may be divided into density subclasses, e.g., S_f 20–50, 50–100, 100–400. Subclasses differ from each other in the lipid and apoprotein compositions (see also Table 144-5).

†HDL may be divided into HDL_2 (1.063–1.125) and HDL_3 (1.125–1.21). The two HDL subclasses are differentially affected by some metabolic perturbations. HDL, contains Lp(a) and a lipoprotein which accumulates on very high cholesterol diets.

made up of complexes of these lipoprotein families. For example, lipoprotein A (LpA) and lipoprotein B (LpB) families consist of various lipids bound to apolipoprotein A (ApoA) and apolipoprotein B (ApoB). VLDL, according to this concept, consist of a complex of at least two lipoprotein families, LpB and LpC.

The current clinical lipoprotein phenotyping methods are based on lipoprotein electrophoretic techniques (and determinations of lipids in plasma); consequently, the electrophoretic nomenclature is the most popular in clinical practice. However, since we will be describing the chemistry and metabolism of lipoproteins isolated from plasma by ultracentrifugation, we will follow the ultracentrifugal terminology throughout this presentation.

COMPOSITION

Before data on the composition of the various classes of lipoproteins are presented, it should be pointed out that lipoproteins arise in at least two tissues. Furthermore, as a result of the interactions of lipoproteins with each other and with lipoprotein catabolic enzymes in plasma (see below), each lipoprotein class isolated by ultracentrifugation may contain particles of diverse metabolic origin (Table 144-4). Thus partially degraded chylomicrons and VLDL known as "remnants" both float as intermediate-density lipoproteins (IDL or LDL_1, d 1.006–1.019); in addition, for a few hours following a fat-containing meal, the VLDL density class contains VLDL of hepatic origin as well as chylomicron remnants.[110–114] Finally, abnormal lipoproteins may be present under some circumstances.[104,115,116] This potential for the metabolic heterogeneity of lipoproteins isolated by ultracentrifugation necessitates careful selection and close metablic control of the subjects who donate their lipoproteins for metabolic and structural studies.

Isolated lipoproteins contain a variety of lipids and apolipoproteins in various proportions[117,118] (Table 144-5). Chylomicrons, the least dense, contain approximately 90 percent triglycerides and 1–2 percent protein. Conversely, HDL, the most dense, contain 3 percent triglycerides, and 50 percent protein. VLDL and LDL fall between these extremes. Clearly, the densities of lipoproteins are related to their relative content of protein and lipid.

Lipoproteins also differ with respect to their apoprotein compositions. Chylomicrons contain 5–10 percent ApoB, 60–70 percent ApoC, and small amounts of other apoproteins[119] (Table 144-6), whereas VLDL contain a larger proportion of ApoB.[120–122] LDL-protein consists of 80–90 percent ApoB.[123,124] HDL contains

Table 144-5. Composition of Human Lipoproteins

Density Class	Diameter (Å)	TG	Chol.	Chol. Esters	Phospholipids	Protein
Chylomicrons	750–6000	86	1	5	7	2
VLDL	250–750	50	7	13	20	10
LDL	170–260	8	10	30	30	22
HDL	70–120	8	4	12	24	52

Courtesy of Wiley.

Abbreviations: TG, triacylglycerol; chol., cholesterol.

Compositions are given as percent of dry weight.

Adapted from Skipski, in Nelson (ed.): Blood Lipids and Lipoproteins, 1972.

Table 144-6. Apoprotein Contents of Human Lipoproteins

	ApoA			ApoC					
Density Class	A-I (R-gln I)	A-II (R-gln II)	ApoB* (R-ser)	C-I (R-ser)	C-II (R-glu)	C-III (R-ala)	Lp(a)	ApoD (ApoA-III)	Arginine Rich (ApoE)
Chylomicrons	Trace	Trace	5–10		60–70				+†
VLDL‡	<1	Trace	37 (20–60)	3	6	40		ND§	12 (7–15)
LDL	ND	ND	>80		<10			+	Trace
Lp(a)‖	ND	ND	65		ND		20	—	—
HDL	65–70	20–25	ND		5–10			1–2	ND

Values represent percent of total apoprotein mass.
*ApoB is not completely defined; it may represent two or more proteins.
†+: Identified by disc gel electrophoresis or immunologically, no quantitative estimates available.
‡VLDL subclasses vary in apoprotein composition. The S_f 100–400 subfraction contains 20 percent ApoB, 7 percent arginine-rich apoprotein, and 70 percent ApoC. S_f 20–50 contains 60 percent ApoB, 15 percent arginine-rich apoprotein, and 25 percent ApoC. S_f 50–100 has an intermediate apoprotein composition.
§ND: none detected.
‖Lp(a) contains albumin (~15 percent) in addition to ApoB and the specific Lp(a) apoprotein.
Data from references 117–129.

virtually no ApoB; 90 percent of the protein of HDL consists of ApoA-I and ApoA-II.[125–127] The "arginine-rich" protein[126,128] and ApoD are minor apoproteins.[129] Some of the biochemical characteristics and physiologic functions of apoproteins are listed in Tables 144-7 and 144-8. ApoF and ApoG have just been described; their functions are unknown (Table 144-7).

STRUCTURE

The interactions of lipids with proteins determine the structures and many of the functions of plasma lipoproteins and cell membranes. Thus, the chemistry of these interactions is an important biologic problem. Studies of lipoprotein structure have added much cogent information to this area of biology.

HDL have been studied in greatest detail because they are relatively abundant and easy to handle (e.g., HDL apoproteins are readily soluble in aqueous solvents); most of the studies summarized below apply to HDL. It is generally agreed upon from electron microscopic[135] and small-angle x-ray scattering studies[136,137] that most lipoproteins isolated from normal plasmas are spheres (Fig. 144-8). The sizes of lipoproteins have been assessed from electron micrographs, x-ray scattergrams, or homodyne spectroscopy[138]. Analytical ultracentrifugation has yielded data on densities and molecular weights.[105,139] The latter has also been determined by column chromatography[140]. Lipoproteins vary in diameter from 70 to 5000 αA (HDL and chylomicrons, respectively) (Table 144-5). Molecular weights range from 150,000 for HDL to several hundred millions for the chylomicrons.

Lipoprotein structures are divided into outer "surface" areas and inner "core" regions. Phospholipids and apoproteins are thought to be located on or near the surfaces of lipoproteins because they are water soluble. Acylglycerols and cholesterol esters are in the core and cholesterol is in the "interfacial" region between core and surface. These theoretical constructs are supported by several experimental observations: Apoproteins in intact lipoproteins are subject to enzymatic[141] and chemical[142] modifications. Apoproteins also react with antisera; however, it is clear that not all regions on the apoprotein are equally reactive, suggesting that parts of apoproteins may be "masked" by lipid–protein or protein–protein interactions.[143,144] Phospholipids are also subject to digestion by specific phospholipases[145] and the ^{31}P moiety of phospholipids is easily accessible to the chelation by Eu^{+++}.[146] Triacylglycerol is in the core, yet it is attacked by lipoprotein lipase. How this is accomplished is not known.

Small-angle x-ray studies have revealed electron-dense regions representing the outer surface of HDL and electron-poor areas in the center of HDL.[136] The former are said to represent the hydrophilic proteins and phospholipids, while the latter represent hydrophobic lipids. These results support the enzymatic, chemical, and immunologic studies cited above.

Information about the configurations and interactions of the various chemical moieties has been obtained by spectroscopic

Table 144-7. Some Characteristics of Human Apolipoproteins

	ApoA			ApoC					
	A-I*	A-II*	ApoB	C-I*	C-II	C-III*	ApoD (ApoA-III)	Arginine Rich (ApoE)	Lp(a)
Molecular wt.	28,311	17,380	36,000–38,000 26,000 250,000–260,000	6,631	10,000	8,751	20,000	33,000	
No. of AA	245	77		57	Glu	79		Ala	
C-terminal AA	Gln	Gln	Ser	Ser		Ala	Ser		
N-terminal AA	Asp	PCA†	Glu	Thr	Thr	Ser		Lys	
Missing AA	Ileu	His		Cys	Cys	Ileu			
	Cys	Arg		His	His	Cys	Cys	Cys	
		Tryp		Tyr					
Sialic acid (mole/mole)	0	0				0–2			66 μg/mole

*The amino acid sequences are known.
†PCA: pyrrolidone carboxylic acid.
Data from references 117, 120, 123, 126, 128–134. ApoF and ApoG have been just described (refs 263, 264).

Table 144-8. Physiologic Functions of Apoproteins

Apoprotein	Physiologic Function	Pathophysiologic Role
A-I	Activation of LCAT[231,232]	Reduced to 1%–2% of normal levels in hypoalphalipoproteinemia (Tangier disease); A-I deficiency may lead to decreased "reverse transport" of cholesterol, and the deposition of cholesteryl esters in the tissues of Tangier disease patients[156,224]
A-II	Binds lipids avidly, structural role in HDL	Reduced to 10%–15% of normal in Tangier disease
B	Essential in transporting lipids from gut and liver in chylomicrons and VLDL	Reduced to <<0.1% of normal levels in abetalipoproteinemia; these patients have extremely low levels of blood lipids,[156] probably due to lack of secretion of VLDL and chylomicrons
C-I	Activation of LCAT, activation of lipoprotein lipase (LPL_{C-I})[209]	Unknown
C-II	Activation of lipoprotein lipase[207–209]	C-II and C-III together modulate lipoprotein lipase activity in vitro; absence of C-II[262] and disturbed C-II/C-III ratios[248] have been noted in some cases of hyperprebetalipoproteinemia and hyperchylomicronemia
C-III	Inhibition of C-II activation of lipoprotein lipase[207]	
D (thin-line peptide)	Unknown[129]	Unknown
E-I, II, III (arginine rich)	Unknown, may serve as a recognition marker between lipoproteins and cells[126,128]	E-I and E-II increased and E-III absent or decreased in the VLDL of patients with dysbetalipoproteinemia[247] (type III); ApoE increased in the lipoproteins of animals fed a high-cholesterol diet
Lp(a)	Unknown[108]	Unknown

techniques [e.g., circular dichroism, intrinsic fluorescence, fluorescent probes, nuclear magnetic resonance, and electron spin resonance]. Some of these techniques yield information about the tertiary structures of proteins; others probe the microenvironments that surround "reporter" molecules and are thus capable of determining the identity and location of some of the chemical groups involved in lipid–protein or protein–protein interactions.

These techniques have revealed that a large proportion of the apoproteins in situ in intact lipoproteins have helical conformations (e.g., 60–70 percent in HDL) and that binding of lipids increases the helicity and stabilizes the tertiary structures of the apoproteins. These studies, and others utilizing apoprotein fragments, strongly suggest that binding of lipids to proteins is greatest in the helical regions of apoproteins. Segrest et al. have proposed [147,148] that the helical regions of apoproteins present two surfaces—one polar and the other apolar—for lipid–protein interactions. The hydrophobic lipids interact with the apolar surface of the protein helix while the charged phospholipids and other proteins interact with the polar side. Thus, the surface components of lipoproteins appear to be arranged in an orderly fashion. By contrast, the core lipids (triacylglycerol and cholesterol esters) have much more freedom on the inside of the molecule.

Several models for HDL structure are available (Fig. 144-8). The Assmann and Brewer model[149] depicts HDL as a sphere in which apoproteins in *globular* configurations float as "icebergs in a sea of lipids." In this structure ApoA-I and ApoA-II are held together by protein–protein interactions, phospholipids interact with ApoA-II, and the other lipids interact with the hydrophobic fatty acid "tails" of phospholipids. A similar model has been proposed by Stoffel et al.[150] In the model of Verdery and Nichols, apoproteins are *stretched out* on the surfaces of HDL[151]. This model suggests a location for each of the molecular moieties of HDL. Our reasons for stressing these structural features become obvious when one considers that lipoprotein catabolism in plasma requires interactions between the lipoproteins themselves, between lipoproteins and specific enzymes, and between lipoproteins and tissues. The regulation of cellular cholesterol synthesis also depends on the last interaction. Each of these interactions is likely to be influenced by the structures of the lipoproteins.

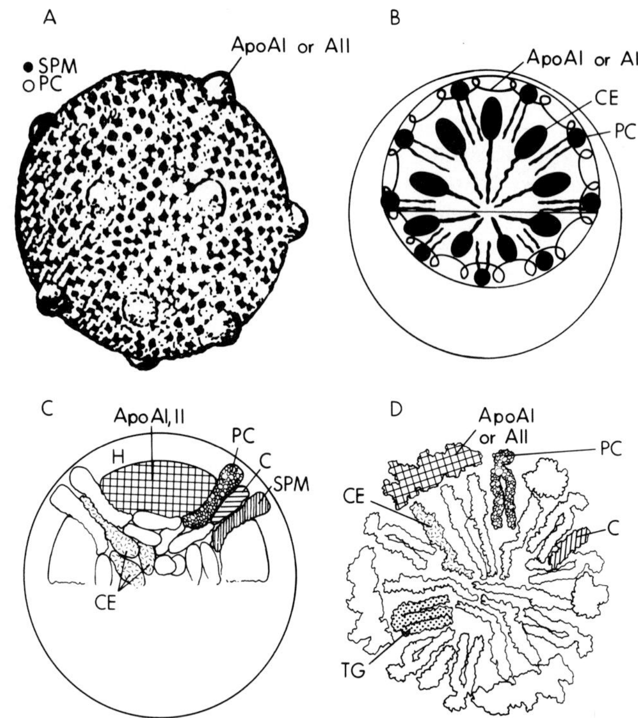

Fig. 144-8. Models of HDL structure. PC, phosphatidylcholine; SPM, sphingomyelin; C, cholesterol; CE, cholesterol ester; TG, triacylglycerol; H, hydrated shell. Each model depicts a spherical structure with apoproteins and "heads" of phospholipids on or close to the surface. Fatty acid "tails" of phospholipids and neutral lipids are directed inward toward the core. A. Assman and Brewer[149] propose that apoproteins are *globular* and are partially buried within the lipids "as icebergs in a sea of lipids." B. Segrest et al.[147] favor a fibrillar configuration for apoproteins on the surface of HDL. C. According to Stoffel et al.[150] apoproteins form depressions between the "heads" of the phospholipids. D. Verdery and Nichols[151] place the apoproteins protruding from the surface.

PRODUCTION

Processes

Of the lipoproteins circulating in plasma, all of the chylomicrons (by definition), some VLDL, and perhaps some HDL are produced in the absorptive cell of the gut mucosa. Most VLDL and HDL are also assembled in the liver. LDL is probably not synthesized as such in man, but is assumed to be a product of the intravascular "processing" of VLDL. Some HDL may also arise from surface components of chylomicrons and VLDL which are "shed" during the catabolism of these triglyceride-rich particles. Thus, LDL may be a "core" remnant and some HDL "surface" remnants. The site of synthesis of Lp(a) is not known.

The production of lipoproteins probably involves several steps analogous to those of other secretory proteins:[152,153] (1) synthesis of several lipid and protein components, (2) coordination of synthesis, (3) transport of endogenous and exogenous lipids and proteins to sites of assembly, (4) assembly of lipids and proteins, (5) storage, and (6) discharge from the cell (Fig. 144-9).

Lipoprotein production has been studied by biochemical and electron microscopic techniques[154] in a number of systems of varying complexity, i.e., isolated subcellular fractions of gut mucosa and hepatic cells, intact dispersed liver cells, liver slices, perfused loops of bowel, the perfused isolated liver, and the liver in situ in man and dog.

Apoproteins, in common with other proteins, are synthesized on membrane-bound polyribosomes,[155] whence they are presumably released into the cysternae of the endoplasmic reticulum. It is not known whether each of the hepatic parenchymal or intestinal absorptive cells is capable of synthesizing all apoproteins or whether there is "specialization" among cells; nor is it known whether, within cells, the various apoproteins are synthesized in proximity to each other in "clusters" of polyribosomes, or whether there are specific, spatially separated sites of synthesis for each apoprotein. Similarly, although it is clear that the synthesis of apoproteins must be coordinated, the releveant molecular mechanisms have not been identified. However, it is clear that the active synthesis of ApoB in both gut and liver is an absolute prerequisite for lipoprotein production in those tissues. [156] In abetalipoproteinemia, in which ApoB is apparently not synthesized, fat is absorbed into the cells of the gut and esterification of long-chain dietary fatty acids proceeds, but chylomicron assembly is halted. Therefore dietary fats do not enter the lacteals and blood stream; instead they accumulate in the intestinal cell. Secretion of hepatic VLDL is also virtually absent.

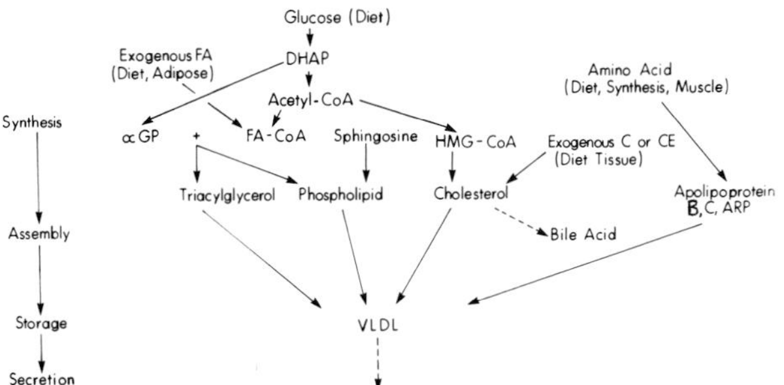

Fig. 144-9. Production of VLDL. The major stages in production are synthesis, assembly, storage, and secretion. The major steps in lipid and apoprotein synthesis are indicated. All of the terminal synthetic steps are located on microsomes. Assembly probably begins in the endoplasmic reticulum and is completed in the Golgi apparatus, where lipoproteins are recognizable by electron microscopy. VLDL and chylomicrons are stored in the cysternae of the Golgi apparatus. Secretion occurs by means of the tubulin–actin apparatus of the cell and resembles the secretion of insulin and other secretory proteins.

Lipids are synthesized in microsomes presumably close to the sites of apoprotein synthesis and in coordination with protein synthesis.

For assembly, the various component moieties must be brought into proximity with each other. Lipids absorbed from gut lumen or taken up from portal blood and incorporated into intestinal and hepatic lipoproteins must also find their way to the sites of assembly. For free fatty acids[8] and cholesterol[22,23] this intracellular movement may involve two different transport proteins. Assembly probably begins somewhere in the endoplasmic reticulum. However, lipoprotein structures are first recognizable by electron microscopy only in the cysternae of the Golgi apparatus.[8,154] Here, too, the sugar moieties are added to ApoC-III.[157] Assembly itself has not been studied in vivo, but lipids and apoproteins form complexes when they are incubated together in vitro, suggesting that noncovalent binding of lipids to proteins may occur in the absence of exogenous energy,[158] i.e., when components are in close proximity in proper proportions and conformations.

VLDL particles isolated from the Golgi apparatus of rat liver,[159] and VLDL similarly isolated from gut mucosa, greatly resemble their counterparts in blood and intestinal lymph, respectively, with respect to size, shape, and composition, although there is some question as to whether these particles acquire ApoC before or after secretion. On the other hand, HDL is secreted from liver and gut as a relatively simple structure that acquires considerably more complexity following its entry into plasma.[160] Thus, the ApoA- and ApoB-containing lipoproteins seem to follow different and unique pathways of production.

VLDL and chylomicrons seem to be secreted by microtubular mechanisms that resemble the secretion of other secretory proteins (e.g., insulin) in that the process is inhibited by colchicine and vincristine.[161] The roles of the microtubules in HDL secretion have not been examined.

Control

A process as complex and interrelated as the one involved in the production of lipoproteins is potentially controllable at many points. Even if the individual steps of production were known in detail, it would be difficult to identify the physiologically important regulatory sites. Such detailed information is in fact not available. Therefore, much of the experimental work has concentrated on evaluating the effects of hormonal and/or metabolic perturbations on overall production.

Among the factors known to increase hepatic VLDL production are obesity and hypercaloric diets,[162,163] isocaloric high-carbohydrate diets[164], ethanol[165], female sex,[166] pregnancy,[167] and hormones such as insulin,[168] thyroxine,[169] and estrogens.[94,170] Some patients with diabetes mellitus[171] and some patients with "primary" hyperlipoproteinemia[172,173] may also overproduce VLDL. Where studied, VLDL-apoprotein and lipid production are increased simultaneously. Factors that decrease production are fasting, glucagon, cAMP,[92] and hypothyroidism.[169] Some diabetics also produce too little VLDL[171] Patients with abetalipoproteinemia[156] secrete virtually no VLDL or chylomicrons. Patients with Tangier disease[156] have very little HDL in their plasmas. This is due to greatly increased catabolism of HDL.

A number of chemical agents, such as inhibitors of RNA translation and transcription,[174] orotic acid, ethionine,[175] and agents that aggregate contractile proteins,[161] have the net effect of reducing VLDL output.

Variations in VLDL output are accompanied by parallel variations in hepatic synthesis of the component moieties. For example, increased availability of fatty acids or high-carbohydrate diets, in addition to increasing triacylglycerol synthesis, also increase cholesterol[64] and VLDL-protein synthesis,[178] with the greatest increase being in the VLDL–non-ApoB. Phospholipid synthetic rates appear to be affected to a lesser extent. Decreased VLDL production is accompanied by inhibited triacylglycerol cholesterol and fatty acid synthesis. Furthermore, fatty acids that reach the liver in increased quantities during inhibited VLDL production are shunted to ketogenesis, while triacylglycerol synthesis is decreased.[92] Since the synthetic rates of several component moieties are altered in parallel with overall VLDL production and secretion, it is difficult to identify a single site of "primary" stimulation or inhibition, if indeed such a primary site exists.

Although alterations in triacylglycerol synthesis are closely correlated with VLDL secretion, rates of triacylglycerol synthesis do not, by themselves, determine rates of secretion of VLDL. When increasing amounts of fatty acids are made available to the liver, increasing amounts are taken up and esterified to triacylglycerol and to phospholipids. Under these circumstances, VLDL secretory rates parallel the esterification of lipids initially, but at some point secretory rates plateau in spite of continuing increases in rates of esterification. At this point larger than usual numbers of lipoproteins are indentifiable in the Golgi apparatus.

This dissociation of lipid synthesis from VLDL secretion suggests that the rate-limiting step to overall VLDL production lies somewhere beyond lipid synthesis. The accumulation of VLDL particles in the Golgi system may indicate that *secretion* is that rate-limiting step. However, limitations of apoprotein synthesis and lipoprotein assembly have not been ruled out.

As rates of VLDL secretion increase, both the numbers of particles and their sizes increase.[176] Particles become relatively enriched with triacylglycerol and the composition of the apoproteins is altered.[177,178] These changes imply that although the synthesis and assembly of the various moieties are coordinated, they are not tightly "coupled."

Eaton and Schade have suggested that the activities of all the factors that affect VLDL production by the liver are mediated by two hormones—insulin and glucagon.[179] Factors that enhance production are said to increase the activity of insulin relative to glucagon and inhibitory factors have the opposite effect.

Chylomicron production is known to be controlled in part by the amounts and chemical characteristics of the fatty acids being absorbed.[9,10,180] In analogy with the liver, the process can be disrupted by protein synthesis inhibitors and by colchicine.[181] Effects of hormones have not been studied.

It should be remembered that increased lipoprotein production is not always accompanied by hyperlipoproteinemia, because in some cases catabolic rates may also be enhanced. This results in an increased flux of lipids through the plasma compartment with relatively minor changes in plasma levels. The same reasoning may be applied to decreased VLDL production and hypolipoproteinemia. In fact, various combinations of production and catabolism may be imagined, resulting in either high or low levels of plasma lipoproteins. For this reason, it may be difficult to foretell what effects any given metabolic or hormonal stimulus, administered for the first time, will have on plasma levels.

CATABOLISM

The catabolism of lipoproteins involves three body compartments: (1) the plasma; (2) the interstitial space, and (3) the intracellular space. Following their entry into plasma the triacylglycerols of chylomicrons and VLDL are hydrolyzed by lipoprotein lipase,[182] to free fatty acids and glycerol. They are then available for uptake and utilization by "peripheral" tissues. It is by this means that dietary or hepatic triacylglycerols become available to peripheral tissues.[183] Most chylomicron- or VLDL-cholesterol esters are taken up by the liver.[184–186]

As they lose their triacylglycerols, chylomicrons and VLDL become progressively smaller in size (IDL, or "remnants").[111,112] These products differ from the originals in that they are relatively enriched in cholesterol esters and apoproteins. They are depleted of triacylglycerols and phospholipids. The composition of the apoproteins is also altered; i.e., remnants have relatively more ApoB and arginine-rich protein and less ApoC than do larger lipoproteins.[121,122] A proportion of the remnants are taken up by liver; the rest are converted to LDL and reenter the blood stream.[111–113,187–189] LDL leave the vascular compartment to enter the interstitial space; then uptake by liver and other tissues serves the dual purpose of lipoprotein catabolism and regulation of cholesterol synthesis. Those LDL that escape uptake by tissues presumably reenter the plasma with the lymphatic fluid.[190]

Lipoprotein Lipase–ApoC

The transformations of lipoproteins in plasma involve a number of interactions between the lipoproteins themselves, and between lipoproteins and enzymes (Fig. 144-10). The first interaction after the entry of chylomicrons and VLDL into plasma involves the ApoC of HDL. These apoproteins exchange readily between HDL and chylomicrons or VLDL.[191,192] Two to four hours after a fatty meal, ApoC levels rise in the plasma chylomicron fraction and fall in the HDL fraction, suggesting that ApoC have moved from HDL to chylomicrons. Later, during fat absorption (at 8–12 h), ApoC appear to move back to HDL. Similarly, when rates of VLDL secretion into plasma are increased by high-carbohydrate diets, plasma VLDL-ApoC levels rise[178] and ApoC-II increase relative to ApoC-III. The potential importance of these changes in ApoC lies in the fact that these apoproteins modulate the activity of lipoprotein lipase (see below).

The next interaction is between lipoproteins and lipoprotein lipase. The enzyme, which has been identified in several organs (including the aorta, heart, skeletal muscle, adipose tissue, mammary gland, lung, and kidney[193]) is secreted from cells[194] in an "activated" form by a colchicine-inhibitable mechanism[195,196] and finds its way to the luminal surfaces of local vascular endothelial cells.[194] Enzyme activities in plasmas of untreated subjects are very low, but activities are greatly increased within a few minutes of the intravenous injection of heparin,[197] suggesting that the enzyme is loosely bound to endothelial cells and is "extracted" into plasma by heparin.[198] A hepatic triacylglycerol lipase, a phospholipase, and monoacylglycerol lipase activities are also released into plasma by heparin,[199–202] the roles of the latter two activities in lipoprotein metabolism is not clear. "Hepatic lipase" will be discussed below.

Lipoprotein lipase has been purified from heart, adipose tissue, and postheparin plasma of several species,[203–206] but its molecular mechanism of action is not yet known. It is clear, however, that the enzyme is virtually inactive against protein-free lipid emulsions, whereas it is quite active when ApoC-II is included in the emulsions (Table 144-8).[207–209] ApoC-III appears to inhibit the activation by ApoC-II. This protein requirement is a unique feature of lipoprotein lipase. Other characteristics of the enzyme that distinguish it from other lipases are its inhibitability by 1 M NaC1 and by protamine.

There are two proposals for the interactions between lipoprotein lipase and lipoproteins. One holds that lipoprotein lipase functions as a solid-phase enzyme.[194,210] Lipoproteins in blood become attached to the arterial wall via the enzyme, hydrolysis of triacylglycerols occurs, and remnants reenter the moving blood stream. The other theory[211] proposes that, as a result of the interaction of lipoproteins with the cell wall (Fig. 144-10), the enzyme is detached from the endothelium and circulates with the lipoproteins. Hydrolysis occurs within the moving blood stream rather than at the vessel wall. According to the secondary theory, the enzyme on the lipoproteins also fulfills another important function, that of serving as a recognition marker on remnants for recognition sites on the liver cell membrane (see below).

Enzymatic contents of specific capillary beds correlate well with uptakes of fatty acids by tissues, suggesting that lipoprotein lipase is important in determining the amount of hydrolysis products, generated from lipoproteins, that become available to the local tissues.[212,213] Indeed, the levels of lipoprotein lipase in tissue vary depending upon the metabolic and hormonal state of the animal. For example, during starvation or exercise, lipoprotein lipase activity in heart muscle increases, while activity in adipose tissue falls.[214] Insulin,[215,216] glucagon,[217] estrogens,[218,219] and oxandrolone[220] each affect lipase activity. Insulin and oxandrolone increase, the others decrease activity.

Interesting changes in lipase activity have been demonstrated in the mammary gland during lactation. Levels begin to rise shortly before parturition and reach levels many-fold higher during lactation. Similar alterations are produced by treatment with prolactin.[221] This change places the mammary gland in an advantageous position to utilize lipoprotein triacylglycerols for milk lipid production. Thus, local alterations in enzyme levels appear to be important in determining how the hydrolysis products will be distributed among competing tissues.

The sums of the activities in all tissues, i.e., total "effective" body levels of enzyme (along with production rates of lipoproteins). are assumed to determine plasma levels and rates of flux of triacylglycerol through plasma. Total effective levels of enzyme are impossible to determine directly in vivo, but indirect measurements have been made that correlate well with kinetic assessments of VLDL catabolism.[222] The importance of this enzyme in lipoprotein metabolism is made dramatically evident by the gross abnormalities of lipoprotein metabolism in subjects with familial type I hyperlipoproteinemia (hyperchylomicronemia), in whom enzyme activity is virtually absent.[223,224]

LCAT-ApoA-I

Another set of interactions that appear to be important in the intravascular metabolism of chylomicrons and VLDL is their transformation by LCAT (Fig. 144-10). This enzyme is secreted into the blood stream from the liver.[225] It has been purified from the blood of man.[226,227] Norum et al. showed some time ago[104] that LCAT is responsible for the production of most of the cholesterol esters in plasma by means of reaction 7 (page 1863). According to them, HDL serves as the natural "substrate" for the LCAT reaction, i.e., the phosphatidylcholine in HDL serves as acyl donor, and the cholesterol in HDL serves as acyl recipient. Cholesterol esters exchange readily between lipoproteins (e.g., be-

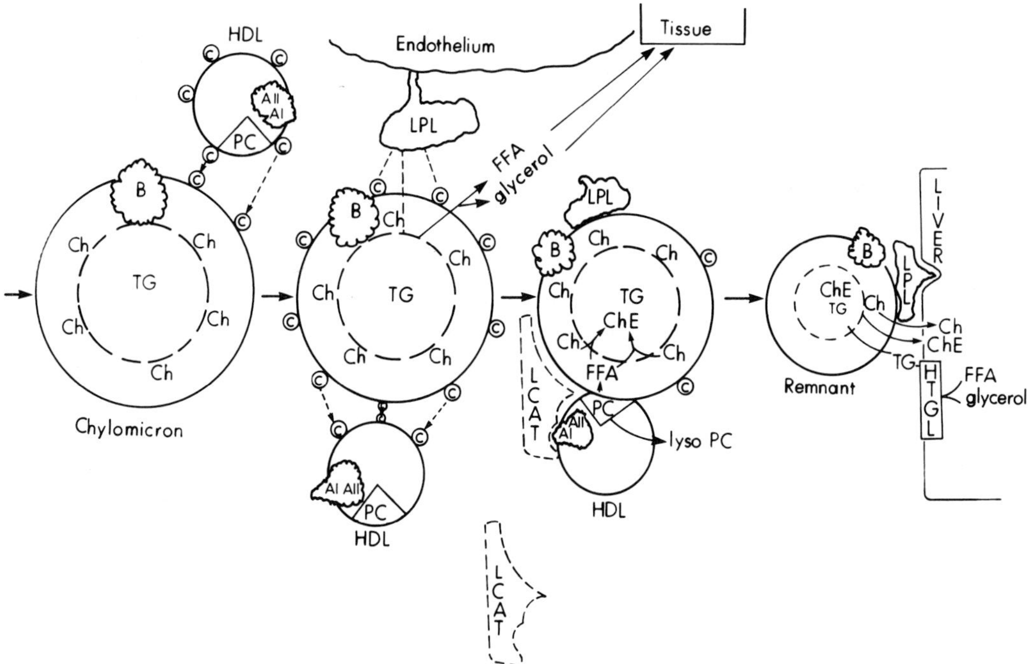

Fig. 144-10. Intravascular catabolism of lipoproteins. Following their entry into plasma, chylomicrons acquire ApoC from HDL. Lipoprotein lipase (LPL) catalyzes the hydrolysis of chylomicron- (and VLDL-) triacylglycerols (TG). The resulting free fatty acids (FFA) and glycerol are available for uptake by "peripheral" tissues. The activity of LPL is modulated by ApoC. As triacylglycerol hydrolysis proceeds, chylomicrons lose volume and become progressively smaller "remnants." ApoC return to HDL. Cholesterol esterification (ChE) in plasma is catalyzed by LCAT. Acyl groups (FFA) are transferred from phosphatidylcholine (PC) to cholesterol (Ch). In the process PC is converted to lyso PC, which is water soluble and enters the acqueous phase. The ChE, formed either in HDL or in chylomicrons, enters the core region of chylomicrons and remnants. The LCAT reaction is accelerated by ApoA-I and ApoC-I. Thus ChE formation requires interaction between remnants, HDL, and LCAT. According to Felts et al.,[211] LPL is removed from endothelium by lipoproteins and becomes part of a lipoprotein-LPL complex. LPL serves as a recognition marker for the hepatic uptake and eventual intracellular "disassembly" of remnants. Hepatic triacylglycerol lipase (HTGL) may aid in further hydrolysis of remnant-TG. Those remnants not entering hepatocytes may be converted to LDL. Therefore the partition of remnants between hepatic uptake or conversion of LDL may determine plasma LDL levels, at least in part.

tween HDL and VLDL.[228] This led to the postulate that the cholesterol esters of lipoproteins originate from the action of LCAT on HDL. Originally it was thought that HDL is the sole substrate for LCAT; however, recent evidence shows that LCAT also esterifies VLDL-cholesterol directly.[229]

In either case, cholesterol esters make an important contribution to VLDL and chylomicron catabolism by providing neutral lipids to replace the glycerides lost from the "core" of VLDL through the action of the lipases; this is important in maintaining the sphericity of particles. The activity of LCAT is increased in vivo by ApoA-I and ApoC-I;[230,231] i.e., both LCAT "substrates" contain apoproteins that could modulate LCAT activity in vivo.

The physiologic importance of both LCAT and HDL are well illustrated by two inherited deficiency diseases, LCAT deficiency[104,232] and hypoalphalipoproteinemia (Tangier disease).[156] Both conditions are associated with gross disturbances of lipid and lipoprotein metabolism (Tables 144-12 and 144-13).

Cellular Catabolism

The last step in the intravascular "processing" of VLDL and chylomicrons is their exit from blood vessels into the interstitial compartment as partially catabolyzed lipoproteins. Exit may occur by pinocytic uptake of lipoproteins into the endothelial cell and vesicular transport through the cell, or lipoproteins may penetrate into the interstitial space between endothelial cells. In either case, the final steps in lipoprotein catabolism occur inside parenchymal cells of tissues.

Some of the chylomicron or VLDL remnants generated by the action of lipoprotein lipase are taken up by liver. According to Felts et al. [211] lipoprotein lipase serves as a recognition marker on the surface of the remnants. Details of the lipoprotein–cell interactions and intracellular catabolism are not available, but presumably the pinocytic uptake and lysosomal "disassembly" described for LDL and the fibroblast[43,233–235] are also operative here. Thus, it appears that some proportion of the circulating chylomicrons and VLDL, having donated their loads of triacylglycerols to the periphery, return to the liver for disassembly. The apoprotein moieties here may be "recycled" into freshly secreted VLDL, or, more likely, they are degraded to amino acids. The cholesterol esters are hydrolyzed and the cholesterol is used for bile acid synthesis, for storage, or for resecretion with VLDL. This cholesterol also regulates hepatic cholesterol synthesis.

Remnants are also taken up by other tissues.[47,236–238] The quantitative importance of this for overall lipoprotein catabolism is not known, but uptake by arterial smooth muscle cells is thought to be important in the genesis and delayed resolution of atherosclerotic lesions.[49,50,239] Indeed, it is this concept and the hope that lowering of plasma lipoprotein levels will prevent or delay coronary artery disease that underlie the therapy of most of the hyperlipoproteinemias.

Finally, some remnants are converted to LDL. This is thought to occur at the liver cell membrane, perhaps through the activity of hepatic triacylglycerol lipase,[114,185,211] a molecule closely related to lipoprotein lipase. Hepatic lipase has been isolated from liver cell membranes.[240] It is not activated by ApoC-II, nor inhibited by 1 M NaCl.[199,200] Since LDL differs from remnants both with respect to lipids and apoproteins (Tables 144-5 and 144-6), the conversion must include losses not only of triacylglycerol (perhaps via hepatic lipase), but also loss of surface components. How the latter occurs is not known.

The liver may also add some stabilizing factor to LDL, since hepatectomy results in enhanced clearance of LDL from the circulation.[241] If it is true that LDL production occurs from remnants at the liver cell surface, the partitioning of remnants between hepatic uptake and LDL production could be an important control point for determining plasma LDL levels and the propensity for atherogenesis. The other determinant of LDL levels is peripheral catabolism initiated via the cell membrane receptor. As noted previously, cellular catabolism of LDL involves recognition, uptake, and disassembly.[43] LDL disassembly by fibroblasts has already been discussed; other tissues seem to follow similar patterns of behavior.[46,47]

CHOLESTEROL "REVERSE TRANSPORT"

HDL, in addition to participating in the metabolism of VLDL and chylomicrons in plasma as a donor of ApoC and cholesterol esters, may also participate in the metabolism of cholesterol by peripheral tissues. Cholesterol is readily removed from cells by HDL or HDL apoproteins.[242] Should this occur in vivo, the cholesterol of peripheral tissues could enter the plasma via HDL and become esterified by means of the LCAT reaction. Since cholesterol esters cannot exchange with cell membranes, cholesterol would be "trapped" in plasma HDL. However, the cholesterol esters of lipoproteins do exchange freely with liver. Thus, it is possible to envision a transport of cholesterol from "periphery" to liver by means of HDL.

Table 144-9. Hyperlipoproteinemia According to NIH Criteria

Lipoprotein Phenotype	Abnormality		Causes of Secondary Hyperlipoproteinemia
	Ultracentrifugal Nomenclature	Electrophoretic Nomenclature	
I	Hyperchylomicronemia	Chylomicron band	Uncontrolled diabetes, dysglobulinemias (especially systemic lupus erythematosus), hypothyroidism
IIA	LDL increased	Increased βeta band	Porphyria, hypothyroidism, biliary obstruction, nephrosis, dysglobulinemias (especially myeloma), pregnancy
IIB	LDL plus VLDL increased	Increased βeta and pre-β bands	Same as for IIA
III	Accumulation of "remnants" or IDL (degradation products of chylomicrons and/or VLDL)	"Floating β," "broad β"	Hypothyroidism, alcoholism, dysglobulinemias, uncontrolled diabetes
IV	VLDL increased	Increased pre-β	Lipodystrophy, diabetes, alcohol intake, glucocorticoids, chronic renal disease, estrogens, pregnancy, glycogen storage disease
V	VLDL and chylomicrons increased	Increased pre-β and chylomicron bands	Alcoholism, pancreatitis, dysglobulinemias, uncontrolled diabetes

Hyperlipoproteinemias are defined by the elevations of individual classes of lipoproteins. The elevations may be primary, or secondary to other diseases.[223,224]

Table 144-10. Plasma Cholesterol and Triglyceride Levels

		Males		Females	
	Age	Mean	95th Percentile	Mean	95th Percentile
Cholesterol	10–14	165	205	165	205
	15–19	150	200	165	220
	20–29	180	235	180	235
	30–39	205	270	190	250
	40–49	215	280	210	285
	50–59	215	280	220	210
Triglycerides	10–14	65	145	75	150
	15–19	80	160	75	150
	20–29	105	250	90	210
	30–39	130	300	100	225
	40–49	140	380	110	240
	50–59	140	330	120	260

Values are expressed in mg/dl. Data are based on analysis of 1000 subjects. Each cell had more than 50 subjects. Values were obtained by the Auto-Analyzer II procedure on extracted plasma. Less specific methods, using unextracted serum such as the SMA-12 procedure may give values 15–25 percent higher. We consider cholesterol values above the 95th percentile to represent hypercholesterolemia, but arbitrarily consider triglyceride values above 200 mg/dl to represent hypertriglyceridemia (see text).
Data from Schonfeld, Weidman, and Witztum, unpublished observations.

DISORDERS OF LIPOPROTEIN METABOLISM IN MAN

DEFINITIONS

The hyperlipoproteinemias comprise a large group of heterogeneous disorders the classification of which is presently in a state of flux. The classification currently in widest use is a descriptive one that uses abnormalities in the levels of plasma lipoproteins (Table 144-9) as the basis for classification. The marked advances of the past few years in the field of lipid transport and in the genetics of hyperlipoproteinemia have started a trend toward the classification of lipoprotein disorders on the basis of their pathophysiology (see below and table 144-13).

In clinical practice, hyperlipidemia (elevations of plasma triglycerides, cholesterol, or both) is recognized first. Hyperlipidemia is then converted to hyperlipoproteinemia to make a specific diagnosis.

Hyperlipidemia is diagnosed when plasma levels of cholesterol, triglycerides, or both are elevated under well-defined conditions. Since the time of the last meal greatly influences lipid and lipoprotein levels, normal lipid values have been defined in the fasting state. Therefore, samples of blood must be drawn after 12–14 h of fasting. Diet and drugs also affect lipoproteins; therefore, the subject should not be eating an atypical diet nor be taking any medication known to alter lipoprotein levels. Because acute illnesses may also change lipid levels, diagnosis of lipoprotein disorders should be delayed until any acute illness has abated. Finally, it is useful to draw more than one baseline blood sample (e.g., three samples 2–4 weeks apart) to assess the degree of spontaneous fluctuation in any individual before any therapy is begun.

It is clear from Table 144-10 that the levels of both cholesterol and triglycerides are strongly related to age and to sex. Hypercholesterolemia can be defined as any value above the 95th percentile for the appropriate age and sex of the patient. However, it is worth distinguishing "normal" values derived by statistical calculations from "ideal" values derived by risk factor analysis. In the case of cholesterol, "ideal" values would probably be closer to 200 mg/dl than to the 95th percentile values. The same 95th percentile criteria are applied in the case of hypertriglyceridemia in subjects below the age of 20. However, on the basis of risk factor analysis most workers in the field consider triglyceride levels above 200 mg/dl to be undesirably high. This criterion is therefore arbitrarily applied to the age groups above 20 years. If hyperlipidemia is present, one needs to distinguish between primary and secondary causes (Table 144-9). The latter consist of a variety of disorders that are accompanied by disturbances in lipid or lipoprotein metabolism. In these cases, the lipoprotein abnormalities usually regress with the treatment of the primary disorder.

Having diagnosed hyperlipidemia it is useful to know which lipoproteins are responsible for the elevations of the lipids because, as stated above, the currently most widely accepted classification of lipid disorders (primary and secondary) is based on elevations of specific classes of lipoproteins in plasma (Table 144-9). For this classification it is necessary to quantify the lipoproteins levels in plasma. Several methods are available. The most accurate one measures the lipid contents of individual lipoprotein fractions by a combination of chemical, ultracentrifugal, and precipitation techniques. More simplified schemes have been devised for estimating the lipoprotein classes in plasma for clinical practice (e.g., lipoprotein electrophoresis). From a knowledge of the plasma

Table 144-11. Practical Approach to Phenotyping

Lipids	Plasma	Type
Chol. high, TG normal	Clear	IIA
Chol. high, TG > 200–400 mg/dl	Chylomicrons absent, plasma clear to turbid	LDL-chol. < 190: IV LDL-chol. > 190: IIB (suspect III)
Chol. high, TG 400–1000 mg/dl	Chylomicrons absent, plasma turbid	IV
	Chylomicrons present, plasma turbid	V (suspect III)
Chol. high, TG > 1000 mg/dl	Chylomicrons present, plasma turbid	V
	Chylomicrons present, plasma clear	I
Chol. normal, TG high	Chylomicrons absent, plasma turbid	IV

Abbreviations: chol., cholesterol; TG, triglycerides.
When plasma triglycerides are less than 400 mg/dl, LDL-cholesterol (in mg/dl) may be estimated from the following formula: LDL-cholesterol = total cholesterol − [(TG/5) + 45], where (TG/5) is an estimate of VLDL-cholesterol.

cholesterol and triglyceride levels and the lipoprotein electrophoresis one can estimate which lipoproteins are increased and whether lipoproteins of abnormal mobility are present. It is also possible to identify chylomicrons or the presence of abnormal amounts of VLDL by the inspection of plasma that has been kept at 4°C for 16–24 h. Using these bits of information, the diagnosis of over 80 percent of the patients as to phenotype (according to the NIH criteria) can be made (Table 144-11). However, disorders of lipid transport, especially hyperalphalipoproteinemia and the type I and type III hyperlipoproteinemias can be diagnosed with *certainty* only by the use of special techniques. In addition to the lipoprotein abnormalities, the hyperlipoproteinemias are associated with signs and symptoms involving many organ systems; they may be useful aids in making a diagnosis and are listed for the familial disorders in Table 144-12.

The value of the phenotypic classification of primary hyperlipoproteinemia has recently been questioned on several grounds:[243–245] (1) the apparent phenotype of any individual may change with diet, therapy, intercurrent illness, etc., confusing both patient and doctor; (2) not all of the phenotypes correspond to genetic entities (e.g. types IIb, IV, and V); (3) some of the phenotypes are heterogeneous with respect to symptomatology and prognosis; and (4) therapy is not yet specific enough to warrant the many subdividions. The objections are valid but the phenotyping system remains useful, provided it is remembered that the classification is but a shorthand method for describing the hyperlipoproteinemia and phenotyping must be done under the strict conditions specified above. The results of therapy are followed by estimating triglyceride and cholesterol levels. Phenotyping of treated patients is unnecessary and may be misleading.

Other classifications of the hyperlipidemias are being attempted based on current understanding of the pathophysiology and genetics of hyperlipoproteinemias (one example is shown in Table 144-13). The primary hyperlipoproteinemias for which the pathophysiology has been worked out reasonably well include:

1. Lipoprotein lipase deficiency (type I)[223]
2. Defective LDL hypercholesterolemia (type II)[246]
3. LDL-receptor–deficient or–defective monogenic hypercholesterolemia (type II)[41,42]
4. Broad beta disease (type III), a disorder of apolipoprotein E[247]
5. ApoC-II-deficient hypertriglyceridemia (type V)[248,262]

Perhaps 10 percent or less of patients with hyperlipoproteinemia fall into these well-defined categories. There remain large populations of patients with the following:

6. Primary hypertriglyceridemia (type IV)
7. Primary hypercholesterolemia (type IIa)
8. Primary elevations of both lipids (types IIb, IV, and V)

In some instances the hypertriglyceridemia (type IV and V) is due to overproduction of VLDL; in other cases, it is due to the poor clearance of lipoproteins from plasma. The molecular bases of these kinetic defects are not known. Patients with primary hypertriglyceridemia (6, 7) may come from families with "familial hypertriglyceridemia" or from families with "combined or multiple phenotype hyperlipidemia" (these families contain individuals with types II, IV, and V hyperlipoproteinemia). The large groups of patients with isolated hypercholesterolemia (7), or "mixed" hyperlipidemia (8), also comprise heterogeneous populations in terms of metabolism and/or genetics; e.g., in addition to monogenic (e.g., LDL-receptor netative) hypercholesterolemia, there are patients with "sporadic" and "polygenic" hypercholesterolemia, and also "familial combined hyperlipidemia."[249]

Although the descriptive and pathophysiologic classifications serve to increase our understanding of the primary hyperlipoproteinemias, they provide us with more information than we need for therapy at the present time. As will be seen, for a practical approach it is sufficient to know whether the disorder consists primarily of elevations of triglycerides, cholesterol, or both and whether or not chylomicrons are present.

Table 144-12. Presenting Complaints in Primary Dyslipoproteinemia

Organ or System	Symptom	Disorder
Skin	Eruptive xanthoma	Types I and V
	Palmar xanthoma	Type III
	Xanthelasma	Types II and III
	Tuberous and tendinous xanthoma	Types II and II, cerebrotendinous xanthomatosis, β-sitosterolemia
Eye	Arcus corneae	All
	Cataract	LCAT deficiency
Ear, nose, throat	Large orange tonsils	Tangier disease
	Yellow plaques on buccal mucosa	Type II
Pulmonary	None described	
Heart	Coronary artery disease	Types II–V, particularly type II
	Aortic valvular disease	Homozygous type II
Gastrointestinal	Abdominal pain	Types I and V
	Hepatosplenomegaly	Types I and V, LCAT deficiency
	Malabsorption, steatorrhea	Abetalipoproteinemia
Renal	Glomerular disease	LCAT deficiency
	Renovascular disease	Types II and III
Neuromuscular	Gait disturbance	Abetalipoproteinemia
	Peripheral neuropathy	Tangier disease
Hematologic	Normocytic anemia	LCAT deficiency
	Acanthocytosis	Abetalipoproteinemia
Rheumatologic	Fibrositis–arthritis involving particularly ankles and Achilles tendon	

Data from references 156, 223, 224.

DIET THERAPY

Two issues must be addressed with regard to therapy directed at lowering plasma lipid levels. First, who should be treated? There is no debate about the necessity of treating symptomatic hyperlipidemia (e.g., pancreatitis and/or eruptive xanthoma), and most would agree that clear-cut familial (type II or III) hyperlipidemia should be treated even though there is no definitive evidence that this would reverse the high coronary risk of these individuals. Beyond this, there is controversy because some studies show that coronary prevention by diets or drugs is possible, while others show no benefit.[250–254] Most experts would tend to treat all those with diagnosed hyperlipidemia. The most controversial question is whether steps should be taken to lower the lipid levels of whole Western populations. The second general question is what modalities of therapy ought to be employed—diets, drugs, surgery, or combinations?[223,255–258]

If the goal is to achieve "ideal" lipid values in large populations (e.g., cholesterol and triglyceride values each of 200 mg/ dl or less in adults), then dietary manipulation seems at the moment the only practical way of achieving this goal, given that 20–40 percent of adult Americans are estimated to have values above these "ideals."[259] For the subjects with distinct hyperlipoproteinemia, combined diet and drug therapy is feasible. Surgery is still experimental and will not be discussed here.

Diets for Lowering Plasma Cholesterol

Dietary cholesterol makes significant contributions to the plasma cholesterol levels of many patients with hypercholesterolemia. Therefore, significant decreases in their plasma cholesterols could be achieved by drastically decreasing the cholesterol contents of prevailing diets. However, it is unlikely that many patients could or would follow extremely restrictive diets. However, changes in the polyunsaturated/saturated fat (P/S) ratio also affect plasma cholesterol levels and increases of this ratio represent another effective and reasonably convenient way to achieve modest cholesterol lowering. Therefore, most workers favor diets that combine moderate restriction of dietary cholesterol (from ~800 down to <300 mg/day) with increases in the P/S ratio (from ~0.3 up to >2.0). Such diets cause as much as 25 percent reductions of serum cholesterol in healthy young adults under controlled conditions and 7–16 percent reductions when applied to a variety of free living or semiconfined populations of adults with and without hypercholesterolemia. The effect of total caloric intake is of relatively minor importance in determining plasma cholesterol (in contrast to its major importance in hypertriglyceridemia). However, subjects who are obese and have associated hypertriglyceridemia (e.g., type IIb) may experience significant drops in cholesterol with caloric restrictions. Although questions have been raised as to the potential carcinogenicity or gallstone-producing properties of "polyunsaturated diets," the available evidence is against these possibilities. Indeed, diets with P/S ratios of 4.0–5.0 and lower contents of cholesterol can be used for subjects with severe hypercholesterolemia.

A variety of approaches are available to individuals for the construction of cholesterol-lowering diets. The aim is to reduce intakes of animal fats, organ foods, milk products, and shrimp and to increase the intake of vegetable oils, fish, and fowl. Even children can be taught to adhere to low-cholesterol diets in order to achieve some lowering of plasma lipids (Fig. 144-11). For those not wishing to give up beef and veal, a "soft-fat" meat containing large amounts of unsaturated fats has been developed. However, at this time, soft-fat beef is available only to experimenters. Diet literature and professional help are readily available through most affiliates of the American Heart Association.

Diets to Reduce Triglyceride Levels

Chylomicrons are normally cleared from the plasma 8–12 h after a meal; their presence in fasting plasma (type I and V) indicates a deficient clearing mechanism for dietary triglycerides. For such individuals, diet therapy is aimed at reducing the exogenous fat load so that the circulating chylomicron levels will be reduced. "Medium-chain triglycerides," which are not absorbed with chylomicrons, may be used as fat supplements in individuals with severe fat intolerance.

In most cases, plasma triglyceride elevations are due to excess VLDL. In contrast to the relatively simple relationship between chylomicrons and dietary fat, many factors affect VLDL levels, including obesity, caloric excess, high-carbohydrate diets, and alcohol consumption.[260] The relative potency of each of these factors is debated, but clearly all of them lead to higher VLDL levels in some patients. Therefore, triglyceride elevations not due to chylomicrons (type IIb, III, and IV) can be treated by various combinations of reduction toward ideal body weight, reduced carbohydrate intake, and avoidance of simple sugars and alcohol. Therapy is tailored to the individual patient. It is common experience that in the vast majority of patients with hypertriglyceridemia dietary therapy *alone* will reduce triglyceride levels toward normal values, in many cases dramatically (Fig. 144-12).

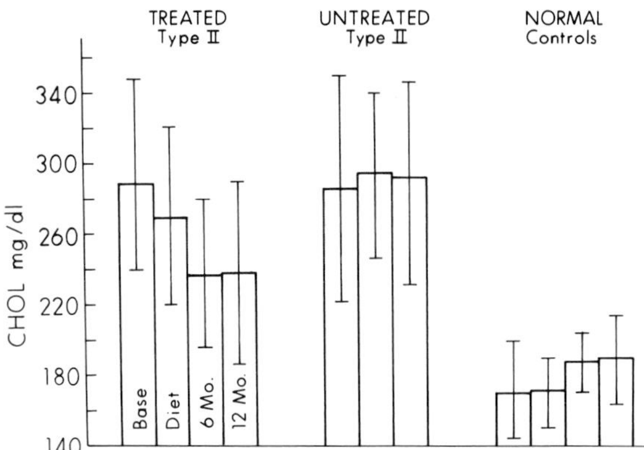

Fig. 144-11. Effects of diet and colestipol resin therapy in children (ages 5–15) with familial type II hyperlipoproteinemia. The children were divided into three groups: "Treated" ($N = 7$) children were judged to have good adherence by independent observers (parents, physicians, and dietitians). After baseline period, an NIH type IIA diet (cholesterol restricted to 300 mg/day, P/S ratio ~2) was prescribed. After 3 months, colestipol-HCL (20 g/day) was begun. "Untreated" ($N = 7$) children were judged to have minimal adherence to diet or medication regimen and exhibited poor clinic attendance as well. "Normal" ($N = 7$) children were normolipemic siblings of the treated and untreated groups. They received no diet or medication. Three lipid determinations were made on all subjects at monthly intervals for the baseline and dietary periods, and three observations at bimonthly intervals on drug therapy. The three lipid analyses of each period were used for calculations. Each bar and bracket represents the group mean ± SD. Cholesterol values remained unchanged in the untreated and control groups. Modest reductions with diet and drug therapy were achieved. Even in the "treated" group adherence to both diet and drug was suboptimal. (Data from Schwarz, Alpers, and Schonfeld, unpublished observations.)

Table 144-13. Pathogenetic Classification of Primary and Secondary Dyslipoproteinemias

Condition	Putative Mechanisms and Metabolic Consequences	Associated Clinical Condition
	Abnormal Rates of Production	
Secondary hyperlipoproteinemias		
Type II	Overproduction of VLDL and increased VLDL conversion to LDL	Nephrosis
Type IV	VLDL overproduction, alcohol stimulation of lipid synthesis	Alcoholism
	VLDL overproduction, part of general response of liver to urinary losses or protein	Nephrosis
	Mixed picture, some patients overproduce VLDL, others have slow clearance	Diabetes mellitus
	Hepatic overproduction of VLDL, decreased fat cell LPL	Corticosteroid therapy
	Shunting of glucose-6-phosphate toward glycolysis and fatty acid synthesis results in increased hepatic VLDL production	Glycogenosis, type I (von Gierke)
Hyperlipoproteinemia of pregnancy	Levels of all lipoproteins increase, hepatic triacylglycerol synthesis and VLDL output are increased	Pregnanacy and estrogen therapy
Hyperlipoproteinemia of obesity	Enhanced secretion of VLDL	Mild (105% ideal body weight) to severe obesity
Abetalipoproteinemia (acanthocytosis)	Presumed deficient synthesis of ApoB; vanishing small levels of VLDL, LDL, and chylomicrons	Fat malabsorption, abnormal red cells, nervous system disorder
	Defective Lipoproteins	
Hyperbetalipoproteinemia* (type II)	Defection LDL not "recognized" by cells leading to deficient LDL catabolism and accumulation of LDL in plasma	Familial accelerated atherosclerosis
Primary dysbetalipoproteinemia* (type III)	Deficiency of ApoE-III and increased ApoE-I and ApoE-II in VLDL; abnormal catabolism of remnants, accumulation of abnormal B migrating VLDL	Familial; accelerated atherosclerosis
Hyperchylomicronemia–hyperprebetalipoproteinemia* (primary type V)	Decreased ApoC-I and ApoC-II activatable lipoprotein lipase; decreased ratios of ApoC-II/ApoC-III; chylomicrons not hydrolyzed by normal postheparin lipase; low lipase activity and/or abnormal activation of lipase, deficient VLDL and chylomicron catabolism, accumulation of VLDL and chylomicrons	Possible familial; glucose intolerance, pancreatitis, eruptive xanthoma
Hyperlipoproteinemia of liver disease (Lp-X)	Production and release of abnormal LDL, called Lp-X, by liver	Obstructive jaundice
Hyperlipoproteinemia of paraproteinemia (secondary type V)	Formation of abnormal lipoprotein substrates in plasma because of complexing of paraprotein with lipoproteins, results in high VLDL and chylomicron levels	Consequences of hyperchylomicronemia, e.g., pancreatitis, eruptive xanthoma
	Abnormal Catabolism	
Primary hyperchylomicronemia* (type I)	Lipoprotein lipase deficiency; absent ApoC-I activatable lipase and decreased ApoC-II activated lipase; deficient chylomicron catabolism, accumulation of chylomicrons	Hepatosplenomegaly, abdominal pain, eruptive xanthoma, pancreatitis
Primary hyperbetalipoproteinemia* (type II)	Deficient or defective cellular receptors for LDL, leading to deficient catabolism of LDL, disturbed regulation of cholesterol synthesis, accumulation of LDL	Severe atherosclerosis in early life, familial
Secondary type IV or type V hyperlipoproteinemia of renal disease	Lipoprotein lipase deficiency or inhibition, delayed clearance of VLDL in plasma	Uremic syndrome, accelerated athersclerosis
Hypoalphalipoproteinemia (Tangier disease)	Greatly accelerated turnover of HDL-proteins, low levels of abnormal HDL	Storage of cholesterol esters in tonsils, spleen, marrow; peripheral neuropathy

Table 144-13. *(Continued)*

Condition	Putative Mechanisms and Metabolic Consequences	Associated Clinical Condition
	Abnormal Catabolism	
Hyperlipoproteinemia of lupus erythematosus (secondary type I or type V)	Circulating antiheparin, interference with lipoprotein lipase release or with lipase–lipoprotein interaction	Syndrome of clinical lupus erythematosus
Hyperlipoproteinemia of hypothyroidism (secondary Type II or Type III)	Diminished lipid synthesis in liver, lower activities and rates of synthesis of lipoprotein lipase in adipose tissue leading to slowed clearance and accumulation of LDL in plasma	Syndrome of hypothyroidism
Diabetic lipemia (secondary type V)	Deficient tissue synthesis and/or activation of lipoprotein lipase, deficient catabolism of VLDL and chylomicrons	Clinical complications of diabetes mellitus including atherosclerosis
	Unknown and Mixed Etiologies	
Primary hyperprebetalipoproteinemia* (type IV)	Overproduction of VLDL and/or deficient catabolism, accumulation of VLDL; mixed etiology, none well defined	Glucose intolerance, obesity, hyperuricemia, hypertension
Hyperlipoproteinemia of porphyria (secondary type II)	Excess accumulation of LDL, etiology unknown	Syndrome of porphyria
Hyperalphalipoproteinemia	High HDL-cholesterol levels	Longevity, decreased prevalence of atherosclerosis
Hypobetalipoproteinemia	Low LDL-cholesterol levels	Longevity

*Primary hyperlipoproteinemia.

Summary

Intelligent use of either the cholesterol- or triglyceride-lowering diets or combinations of them can lead to correction of the hyperlipoproteinemia in over 50 percent of patients. However, the diets must be adequately explained and follow-up of patients is essential. Trained nutritionists are very helpful in this area of therapy.

With respect to lowering of lipids of Western populations there is still controversy. However, based on considerations of safety, cholesterol-lowering efficacy, and potential for coronary prevention, it is the recommendation of the Nutrition Committee of the American Heart Association that moderate cholesterol-lowering diets (cholesterol 300 mg/day, P/S ratio ~2.0) can and should be followed by most adult Americans. Indeed, most experts feel that if prevention of atherosclerosis by dietary modification is to be maximally effective, dietary changes should be instituted at an early age, especially in those children at high risk.

DRUG THERAPY

Drug therapy in hyperlipoproteinemia is reserved for those patients whose dietary response is deemed suboptimal and in whom lowering of lipoprotein levels is thought to be important. The latter group consists of patients who are symptomatic from their hyperlipoproteinemia or are at particularly high risk for the development of vascular disease by virtue of family history or due to the presence of other coronary risk factors. Diet therapy is continued as drugs are added because the effects of the two modalities are frequently additive.

Drugs may be divided into those that are effective in (1) the hypercholesterolemias, (2) the hypertriglyceridemias, or (3) both. Several excellent reviews have recently been published.[255–258]

Cholesterol (LDL)-Lowering Drugs

Cholestyramine and Colestipol-HCL. The current drugs of choice for treatment of hypercholesterolemia (type II) are cationic polymeric resins that bind bile acids in the intestine. With usual

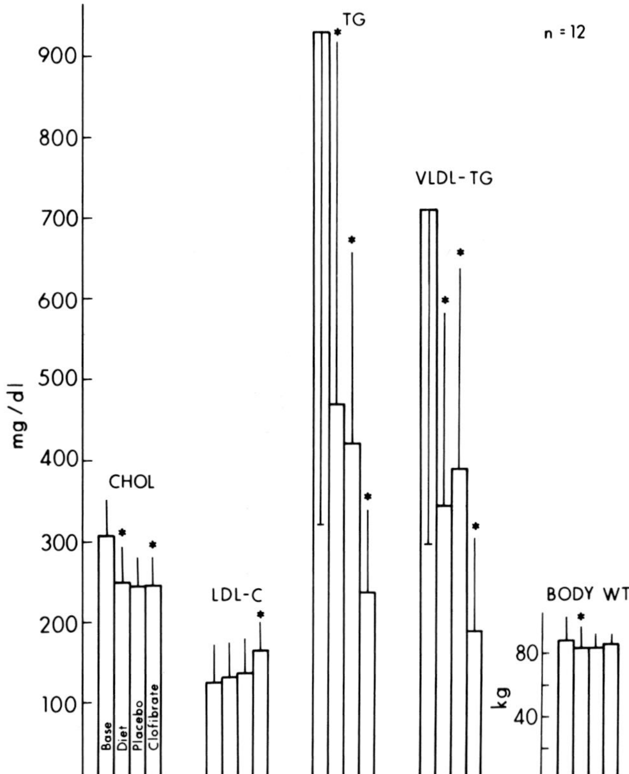

Fig. 144-12. Results of diet and clofibrate therapy in type IV hyperlipoproteinemia. All patients were adults with primary type IV. NIH type IV diet was prescribed (carbohydrates restricted to 35 percent of calories with restriction of simple sugars and alcohol). Significant reductions in total triglycerides as well as VLDL-triglyceride were observed on diet alone. Clofibrate given in this double-blind placebo versus active drug study produced a further lowering of triglycerides LDL-cholesterol rose. *, Means versus baseline period significantly different by paired t test ($p \leq 0.01$). (Data from Schonfeld and Witztum, unpublished observations.)

therapeutic doses the net excretion of bile acids in stool is increased several-fold. This is followed by enhanced hepatic cholesterol and bile acid synthesis. The greater movement of sterols from liver to bile and out of the body is associated with higher rates of production of VLDL and greater fractional rates of catabolism of plasma LDL. Thus there is an increased flux of VLDL and LDL through the plasma. The biochemical mechanisms that underlie the associations between hepatic cholesterol–bile acid synthesis and VLDL–LDL metabolism are not clear, but the results of therapy are a variable elevation of VLDL-cholesterol and -triglyceride levels and a persistent 25–35 percent lowering of plasma LDL-cholesterol levels in children and in adults (Fig. 144-11, Table 144-14).

The major advantages of the bile acid–binding resins for clinical practice are their effectiveness in lowering plasma cholesterol and the fact that they are "nonsystemic," i.e., they are not absorbed from the gut. The latter attribute greatly limits their potential for producing allergic or toxic reactions. In fact, side effects are limited to local effects produced by the bulkiness of the drugs, e.g., bloating and constipation. No serious side effects have been reported. Cholestyramine and colestipol may interfere with the absorption of certain drugs (e.g., digoxin, thyroxine) or nutrients (e.g., fat-soluble vitamins, iron). Problems may be avoided by taking other medications 1–2 h before the resins are ingested.

β-Sitosterol. β-Sitosterol, a plant sterol preparation that also contains small amounts of campesterol and stigmasterol lowers plasma cholesterol an average of about 10 percent without appreciably affecting triglycerides. It probably acts by competitively inhibiting the absorption of cholesterol from the gut lumen without more than 1–2 percent of the dietary β-sitosterol itself being absorbed. The major disadvantage of β-sitosterol is its relatively low efficacy. In addition, some infants and rare adults do absorb large amounts (20–30 percent) of dietary plant sterols and appreciable amounts of plant sterols are found in plasmas of these subjects. In the rare adults with β-sitosterolemia, xanthomas containing plant sterols have been found. The drug is not widely used at the present time.

Table 144-14. Effect of Long-Term Treatment with Colestipol on Lipoprotein Lipids

	Before* (mg/dl)	After† (mg/dl)	p‡
Total cholesterol (chol.)	345 ± 66	258 ± 63	<0.001
Total triglyceride (TG)	121 ± 37	133 ± 39	NS
VLDL-chol.	13.5 ± 6.3	15.8 ± 7.9	NS
VLDL-TG	65.4 ± 30.8	83.2 ± 35.2	NS
VLDL-TG/VLDL-Chol.	5.41 ± 2.45	5.46 ± 0.84	NS
LDL-Chol	277 ± 67	188 ± 53	<0.001
LDL-TG	38.1 ± 9.9	32.6 ± 8.7	<0.01
LDL-TG/LDL-Chol.	0.14 ± 0.03	0.18 ± 0.06	<0.005
HDL-Chol.	50.6 ± 13.7	51.2 ± 16.3	NS
HDL-TG	9.7 ± 3.7	10.6 ± 4.7	NS
HDL-TG/HDL-Chol.	0.20 ± 0.07	0.21 ± 0.06	NS

The mean of three observations for each period for each of 12 patients was used to calculate the mean ± SD for the value of each lipoprotein and for the TG/chol. ratio of each lipoprotein.

*Mean of three determinations, made at monthly intervals before therapy, on each of 12 subjects.

†Mean of three consecutive determinations done after the longest period of therapy for that patient (3–12 months).

‡Paired Student's t test. NS: not significant.

Data from reference 261.

D-Thyroxine. D-Thyroxine, the dextroisomer of the natural thyroid hormone is an effective LDL-cholesterol–lowering agent that probably acts by increasing the catabolism of LDL. Effects on plasma triglycerides are small and variable. Its use is limited to young subjects with type IIa hypercholesterolemia who have no heart disease and whose progress can be adequately monitored by medical personnel. It is contraindicated for anyone with known heart disease.

Cholestyramine, β-sitosterol, and D-thyroxine have been approved by the Food and Drug Administration (FDA) for use in the treatment of hypercholesterolemia. Colestipol is not yet approved. Two other drugs that have been used for other medical indications have been used experimentally in the treatment of hypercholesterolemia: para-aminosalicylic acid (PAS-C) and neomycin. The FDA has not approved these drugs in the treatment of hypercholesterolemia; they are to be considered experimental drugs with respect to hypercholesterolemia.

Triglyceride (VLDL)-Lowering Drugs

Clofibrate. Clofibrate is probably the most widely used medication for the treatment of hyperlipoproteinemia. In contrast with the resins, which are bulky powders, clofibrate is a capsule, which is easy and convenient for the patient to take. It is modestly effective in type II, moderately effective in type IV, and very effective in type III hyperlipoproteinemia (Fig. 144-9 to 144-11, Tables 144-12 and 144-13). Clofibrate primarily lowers VLDL levels and works best when used in conjunction with diet therapy. In fact, poor adherence to diet can result in large elevations of VLDL even when adherence to drug therapy is adequate. One undesired affect of clofibrate is a rise of LDL levels as VLDL levels fall. This happens most often in patients with type IV hyperlipoproteinemia and may require an adjustment of diet or the addition of an anticholesterol drug (Fig. 144-11).

In animal and in vitro experiments clofibrate decreases lipolysis in adipose tissue, diminishes fatty acid and triglyceride synthesis in liver, and reduces hepatic secretion of VLDL. These data suggest that at least in animals (primarily the rat) clofibrate lowers plasma lipids by decreasing VLDL input into plasma. However, experiments in man have not demonstrated inhibition of VLDL secretion. Instead, in man clofibrate therapy is followed by increased activity of lipoprotein lipase and increased fecal excretion of bile acids. These results are more compatible with enhanced rates of lipoprotein catabolism. The molecular bases underlying these effects in man are not known.

Clofibrate is a systemic drug and several side effects have been reported. The most frequent is a mild elevation of hepatic enzymes in blood that seems to have no deleterious effects. Other side effects include cardiac arrhythmias and a myopathic syndrome that occurs primarily in persons with chronic renal disease. Drug interactions, particularly with anticoagulants, and the reduced dosage requirements in subjects with renal disease are well known.

Nicotinic Acid. Nicotinic acid and its derivatives are potent depressants of plasma triglyceride (VLDL and chylomicron) levels particularly in type III and type V hyperlipoproteinemias in which decreases in plasma triglycerides of 50–90 percent have been obtained. Nicotinic acid has also been used in type IIb and type IV hyperlipoproteinemia with a decrease of approximately 25 percent in triglycerides; in type IIa hyperlipoproteinemia triglyceride and cholesterol levels fell by approximately 10 percent each.

The mode of action of nicotinic acid is unknown. In the rat it is a powerful inhibitor of lipolysis in adipose tissue and it also decreases hepatic cholesterol and triglyceride synthesis. Its mode of action in man is controversial. Some workers feel that its primary effect, like that in the rat, is inhibition of VLDL secretion by liver; others feel that its major effect is an increase in the catabolism of VLDL and chylomicrons.

The considerations that keep this group of medications from being "first line" drugs relate to the fact that they are systemic and have unpleasant and potentially serious side effects. The former include flushing, itching, dry skin, acanthosis nigricans, nausea, and diarrhea, and the latter, hyperglycemia, hyperuricemia, and hepatic toxicity. It should be noted that the serious side effects are unusual and reversible, and the mild ones can be avoided or overcome by the administration of the drugs at slowly increasing increments until therapeutic doses are reached.

Progestational and Anabolic Steroids. Progestational and anabolic steroids have been used only experimentally in the treatment of hypertriglyceridemia, particularly type V disease, in a limited number of cases. In these subjects 30–50 percent decreases in triglycerides have been obtained and the therapeutic effect has been accompanied by increased activities in postheparin lipoprotein lipase. No deleterious effects have been recorded. This approach to the therapy of hypertriglyceridemia deserves further experimental exploration.

ACKNOWLEDGMENTS

The invaluable aid of Bonnie Larson, Dr. Joseph Witztum, and Lillie Beal is appreciated. The work of the author is supported by NIH Contract NO1-HU-2-2916-L, NIH Grants HL 15427 and HL 15308, and by grants from the Upjohn Company and Ayerst Laboratories.

REFERENCES

1. The National Diet–Heart Study Final Report. *Circulation 37* [Suppl 1]: 125, 1968.
2. Hofmann, A. F.: Gastroenterology: physical events in lipid digestion and absorption. *Fed Proc 29:* 1317, 1970.
3. Brockerhoff, H., Jensen, R. G.: Lipolytic Enzymes. New York, Academic, 1974.
4. Mansbach, C. M. II, Cohen, R. S., Leff, P. B.: Isolation and properties of the mixed lipid micelles present in intestinal content during fat digestion in man. *J Clin Invest 56:* 781, 1975.
5. Westergaard, H., Dietschy, J. M.: The mechanism whereby bile acid micelles increase the rate of fatty acid and cholesterol uptake into the intestinal mucosal cell. *J Clin Invest 58:* 97, 1976.
6. Tyor, M. P., Garbutt, J. T., Lack, L.: Metabolism and transport of bile acids in the intestine. *Am J Med 51:* 614, 1971.
7. Borgstom, B.: Fat digestion and absorption. In Smyth, D. H. (ed): Biomembranes, Intestinal Absorption, vol 4B. New York, Plenum, 1974, p 555.
8. Ockner, R. K., Manning, J. M.: Fatty acid binding protein (FABP) in small intestine: identification, isolation and evidence for its role in cellular fatty acid transport. *J Clin Invest 54:* 326, 1974.
9. Gangl, A., Ockner, R. K.: Intestinal metabolism of lipids and lipoproteins. *Gastrenterology 68:* 167, 1975.
10. Brindley, D. N.: The intracellular phase of fat absorption. In Smyth, D. H. (ed): Biomembranes, Intestinal Absorption, vol 4B. New York, Plenum, 1974, p 621.
11. Dempsey, M. E.: Regulation of steroid biosynthesis. *Annu Rev Biochem 43:* 967, 1974.
12. Lehninger, A. L.: Biochemistry: Molecular Basis of Cell Structure and Function, ed 2, New York, Worth, 1975.
13. Lowenstein, J. M.: The pyruvate dehydrogenase complex & the citric acid cycle. In Florkin, M., Storz, E. H. (eds): Comprehensive Biochemistry, vol 18S, suppl: Pyruvate and Fatty Acid Metabolism. Amsterdam, Elsevier, 1971.
14. Clinkenbeard, K. D., Sugiyama, T., Moss, J., Reed, W. D., Lane, M. D.: Molecular and catalytic properties of cytosolic acetoacetyl coenzyme A thiolase from avian liver. *J Biol Chem 248:* 2275, 1973.
15. Clinkenbeard, K. D., Sugiyama, T., Reed, W. D., Lane, M. D.: Cytoplasmic 3-hydroxy-3-methylglutaryl coenzyme A synthase from liver. *J Biol Chem 250:* 3124, 1975.
16. White, L. W., Rudney, H.: Biosynthesis of 3-hydroxy-3-methylglutarate and mevalonate by rat liver homogenates *in vitro*. *Biochemistry 9:* 2713, 1970.
17. Brown, M. S., Dana, S. E., Siperstein, M. D.: Properties of 3-hydroxy-3-methylglutaryl coenzyme A reductase solubilized from rat liver and hepatoma. *J Biol Chem 249:* 6585, 1974.
18. Tormanen, C. D., Redd, W. L., Srikantaiah, M. V., Scallen, T. J.: Purification of 3-hydroxy-3-methylglutaryl coenzyme A reductase. *Biochem Biophys Res Commun 68:* 754, 1976.
19. Clinkenbeard, K. D., Reed, W. D., Mooney, R. A., Lane, M. D.: Intracellular localization of the 3-hydroxy-3-methylglutaryl coenzyme A cycle enzymes in liver. *J Biol Chem 250:* 3108, 1975.
20. Decker, K., Barth, C.: Compartmentation of the early steps of cholesterol biosynthesis in mammalian liver. *Mol Cell Biochem 2:* 179, 1973.
21. Chapman, M. J., Miller, L. R., Antko, J. A.: Localization of the enzymes of ketogenesis in rat liver mitochondria. *J Cell Biol 58:* 284, 1973.
22. Scallen, T. J., Schuster, M. W., Dhar, A. K.: Evidence for a noncatalytic carrier protein in cholesterol biosynthesis. *J Biol Chem 246:* 224, 1971.
23. Ritter, M. C., Dempsey, M. E.: Squalene and sterol carrier protein: structural properties, lipid-binding, and function in cholesterol biosynthesis. *Proc Natl Acad Sci USA 70:* 265, 1973.
24. Shapiro, D. J., Rodwell, V. W.: Diurnal variation and cholesterol regulation of hepatic HMG-CoA reductase activity. *Biochem Biophys Res Commun 37:* 867, 1969.
25. Slakey, L. L., Craig, M. C., Beytia, E., et al: The effects of fasting and refeeding and time of day on the levels of enzymes effecting the conversion of β-hydroxy-β-methylglutaryl coenzyme A to squalene. *J Biol Chem 247:* 3014, 1972.
26. Bortz, W. M.: On the control of cholesterol synthesis. *Metabolism 22:* 1507, 1973.
27. Bortz, W. M., Steele, L., Arkens, L., et al: Structure of the alteration of hepatic cholesterol synthesis in the rat. *Biochim Biophys Acta 316:* 366, 1973.
28. Weis, H. J., Dietschy, J. M.: The interaction of various control mechanisms in determining the rate of hepatic cholesterogenesis in the rat. *Biochim Biophys Acta 398:* 315, 1975.
29. Goodman, D. S., Nobile, R. P., Dell, R. B.: The effects of colestipol resin and of colestipol plus clofibrate on the turnover of plasma cholesterol in man. *J Clin Invest 52:* 2646, 1973.
30. Wilson, J. D., Lindsey, C. A., Jr.: Studies on the influence of dietary cholesterol on cholesterol metabolism in the isotopic steady state in man. *J Clin Invest 44:* 1805, 1965.
31. Quintao, E., Grundy, S. M., Ahrens, E. H., Jr.: Effects of dietary cholesterol on the regulation of total body cholesterol in man. *J Lipid Res 12:* 233, 1971.
32. Miller, N. E., Clifton-Bligh, P., Nestel, P. J.: Effects of colestipol, a new bile-acid-sequestering resin, on cholesterol metabolism in man. *J Lab Clin Med 82:* 876, 1973.
33. Moutafis, C. D., Myant, N. B.: Cholesterol metabolism in a patient with familial hyperbetalipoproteinaemia during periods of high and low cholesterol intake. *Atherosclerosis 14:* 305, 1973.
34. Nepokroeff, C. M., Lakshmanan, M. R., Ness, G. C., Dugan, R. E., Porter, J. W.: Regulation of the diurnal rhythm of rat liver β-hydroxyβ-methylglutaryl coenzyme A reductase activity by insulin, glucagon, cyclic amp and hydrocortisone. *Arch Biochem Biophys 160:* 387, 1974.
35. Ness, G. C., Dugan, R. E., Lakshmanan, M. R., Nepokroeff, C. M., Porter, J. W.: Stimulation of hepatic β-hydroxy-β-methylglutaryl coenzyme A reductase activity in hypophysectomized rats by L-triiodothyronine. *Proc Natl Acad Sci USA 70:* 3839, 1973.
36. James, M. J., Sabine, J. R.: Adrenal hormones and the control of hepatic cholesterol. *Proc Aust Biochem Soc 6:* 42, 1973.
37. Bhathena, S. J., Avigan, J., Schreiner, M. A.: Effect of insulin on sterol and fatty acid synthesis and hydroxymethylglutaryl CoA reductase activity in mammalian cells grown in culture. *Proc Natl Acad Sci USA 71:* 2174, 1974.
38. Weis, H. J., Dietschy, J. M.: Failure of bile acids to control hepatic cholesterogenesis: evidence for endogenous cholesterol feedback. *J Clin Invest 48:* 2398, 1969.

39. Nervi, F. O., Dietschy, J. M.: Ability of six different lipoprotein fractions to regulate the rate of hepatic cholesterogenesis in vivo. *J Biol Chem 250:* 8704, 1975.
40. Brown, M. S., Faust, J. R., Goldstein, J. L.: Role of the low density lipoprotein receptor in regulating the content of free and esterified cholesterol in human fibroblasts. *J Clin Invest 55:* 783, 1975.
41. Brown, M. S., Goldstein, J. L.: Expression of the familial hypercholesterolemia gene in heterozygotes: mechanism for a dominant disorder in man. *Science 185:* 61, 1974.
42. Khachadurian, A. K., Kawahara, F. S.: Cholesterol synthesis by cultured fibroblasts: decreased feedback inhibition in familial hypercholesterolemia. *J Lab Clin Med 83:* 7, 1974.
43. Brown, M. S., Goldstein, J. L.: Receptor-mediated control of cholesterol metabolism. *Science 191:* 150, 1976.
44. Assmann, G., Brown, B. G., Mahley, R. W.: Regulation of 3-hydroxy-3-methylglutaryl coenzyme A reductase activity in cultured swine aortic smooth muscle cells by plasma lipoproteins. *Biochemistry 14:* 3996, 1975.
45. Weinstein, D. B., Carew, T. E., Steinberg, D.: Uptake and degradation of low density lipoprotein by swine arterial smooth muscle cells with inhibition of cholesterol biosynthesis. *Biochim Biophys Acta 424:* 404, 1976.
46. Bierman, E. L., Stein, O., Stein, Y.: Lipoprotein uptake and metabolism by rat aortic smooth muscle cell in tissue culture. *Circ Res 35:* 136, 1974.
47. Kayden, H. J., Hatam, L., Beratis, N. G.: Regulation of 3-hydroxy-3-methylglutaryl coenzyme A reductase activity and the esterification of cholesterol in human long term lymphoid cell lines. *Biochemistry 15:* 521, 1976.
48. Fogelman, A. M., Edmond, J., Seager, J., et al: Abnormal induction of 3-hydroxy-3-methylglutaryl coenzyme A reductase in leukocytes from subjects with heterozygous familial hypercholesterolemia. *J Biol Chem 250:* 2045, 1975.
49. Ross, R., Glomset, J. A.: Atherosclerosis and the arterial smooth muscle cell. *Science 180:* 1332, 1973.
50. Fisher-Dzoga, K., Chen, R., Wissler, R. W.: Effects of serum lipoproteins on the morphology, growth, and metabolism of arterial smooth muscle cells. *Adv Exp Med Biol 43:* 299, 1974.
51. Higgins, M. J. P., Brady, D., Rudney, H.: Rat liver 3-hydroxy-3-methylglutaryl coenzyme A reductase: a comparison and immunological study of purified solubilized preparations, and alteration of enzyme levels by choylestyramine feeding. *Arch Biochem Biophys 163:* 271, 1974.
52. Erickson, S. K., Davison, A. M., Gould, R. G.: Correlation of rat liver chromatin-bound free and esterified cholesterol with the circadian rhythm of cholesterol biosynthesis in the rat. *Biochim Biophys Acta 409:* 59, 1975.
53. Sugiyama, T., Clinkenbeard, K., Moss, J., et al: Multiple cytosolic forms of hepatic beta-hydroxy-beta-methylglutaryl CoA synthase: possible regulatory role in cholesterol synthesis. *Biochem Biophys Res Commun 48:* 255, 1972.
54. Danielsson, H.: Mechanisms of bile acid synthesis. In Nair, P. P., Kritchevsky, D. (eds): The Bile Acids: Chemistry, Physiology and Metabolism, vol 2. New York, Plenum, 1973, p 1.
55. Danielsson, H., Sjovall, J.: Bile acid metabolism. *Annu Rev Biochem 44:* 233, 1975.
56. Mitropoulos, K. A., Myant, N. B., Gibbons, G. F., et al: Cholesterol precursor pools for the synthesis of cholic and chenodeoxycholic acids in rats. *J Biol Chem 249:* 6052, 1974.
57. Einarsson, K., Hellstrom, K., Kallner, M.: Feedback regulation of bile acid formation in man. *Metabolism 22:* 1477, 1973.
58. Mitropoulos, K. A., Balasubramaniam, S., Myant, N. B.: The effect of interruption of the enterohepatic circulation of bile acids and of cholesterol feeding on cholesterol 7α-hyroxylase in relation to the diurnal rhythm in its activity. *Biochim Biophys Acta 326:* 428, 1973.
59. Grundy, S. M., Ahrens, E. H. Jr.: Measurement of cholesterol turnover, synthesis, and absorption in man, carried out by isotope kinetic and sterol balance methods. *J Lipid Res 10:* 91, 1969.
60. Goodman, D. S., Nobel, R. P.: Turnover of plasma cholesterol in man. *J Clin Invest 47:* 231, 1968.
61. Crouse, J. R., Grundy, S. M., Ahrens, E. H. J. R.: Cholesterol distribution in the bulk tissues of man: variation with age. *J Clin Invest 59:* 1292, 1972.
62. Redinger, R. N., Small, D. M.: Bile composition, bile salt metabolism and gall stones. *Arch Intern Med 130:* 618, 1972.
63. Garbutt, J. T., Kenney, T. J.: Effect of cholestyramine on bile acid metabolism in normal man. *J Clin Invest 57:* 2781, 1972.
64. Bortz, W. M., Steele, L. A.: Synchronization of hepatic cholesterol synthesis, cholesterol and bile acid content, fatty acid synthesis and plasma free fatty acid levels in the fed and fasted rat. *Biochim Biophys Acta 306:* 85, 1973.
65. Whyte, H. M., Nestel, P. J., Pryke, E. S.: Bile acid and cholesterol excretion with carbohydrate rich diets. *J Lab Clin Med 81:* 818, 1971.
66. Nestel, P. J., Schreibman, P. H., Ahrens, E. H. Jr.: Cholesterol metabolism in human obesity. *J Clin Invest 52:* 2389, 1973.
67. Spritz, N., Ahrens, E. H., Jr., Grundy, S.: Sterol balance in man as plasma cholesterol concentrations are altered by exchanges of dietary fats. *J Clin Invest 44:* 1482, 1965.
68. Nestel, P. J., Poyser, A.: Changes in cholesterol synthesis and excretion when cholesterol intake is increased. *Ann Intern Med 25:* 1591, 1976.
69. Nestel, P. J.: Cholesterol metabolism in anorexia nervosa and hypercholesterolemia. *J Clin Endocrinol Metab 38:* 325, 1974.
70. Swaner, J. C., Connor, W. E.: Hypercholesterolemia of total starvation: its mechanism via tissue mobilization of cholesterol. *Am J Physiol 229:* 365, 1975.
71. Kornberg, A., Pricer, W. E., Jr.: Enzymatic synthesis of the coenzyme A derivatives of long chain fatty acids. *J Biol Chem 204:* 329, 1953.
72. Kornberg, A., Pricer, W. E., Jr.: Enzymatic esterification of α-glycerophosphate by long chain fatty acids. *J Biol Chem 204:* 345, 1953.
73. Steinberg, D.: Fatty acid mobilization—mechanisms of regulation and metabolic consequences. *Biochem Soc Symp 24:* 111, 1963.
74. Pollock, R. J., Hajra, A. K., Agranoff, B. W.: The relative utilization of acyl dihydroxyacetonephosphate and glycerolphosphate pathways for synthesis of glycerolipids in various tumors and normal tissues. *Biochim Biophys Acta 380:* 421, 1975.
75. Hubscher, N. G., Smith, E., Sedgwick, B.: Stimulation of biosynthesis of glyceride. *Nature 216:* 449, 1967.
76. Young, D. L., Lynen, F.: Enzymatic regulation of 3-sn-phosphatidylcholine and triacylglycerol synthesis in states of altered lipid metabolism. *J Biol Chem 244:* 377, 1969.
77. Lamb, R. G., Fallon, H. J.: The formation of monoacylglycerophosphate from sn-glycerol-3-phosphate by a rat liver particulate preparation. *J Biol Chem 245:* 3075, 1970.
78. Lamb, R. G., Fallon, H. J.: An enzymatic explanation for dietary induced alterations in hepatic glycerolipid metabolism. *Biochim Biophys Acta 348:* 179, 1974.
79. Fallon, H. J., Barwick, J., Lamb, R. G., et al: Studies of rat liver microsomal diglyceride acyltransferase and cholinephosphotransferase using microsomal-bound substrate: effects of high fructose intake. *J Lipid Res 16:* 107, 1975.
80. Burns, T. W., Mohs, J. M., Langley, P. E., et al: Regulation of human lipolysis. In vivo observations on the role of adrenergic receptors. *J Clin Invest 53:* 338, 1974.
81. Waddell, M., Fallon, H. J.: The effect of high-carbohydrate diets on liver triglyceride formation in the rat. *J Clin Invest 52:* 2725, 1973.
82. Majerus, P. W., Kilburn, E.: Acetyl coenzyme A carboxylase. The roles of synthesis and degradation in regulation of enzyme levels in rat liver. *J Biol Chem 244:* 6254, 1969.
83. Strauss, A. W., Alberts, A. W., Hennessy, S., et al: Regulation of synthesis of hepatic fatty acid synthetase: polysomal translation in a cell-free system. *Proc Natl Acad Sci USA 72:* 4366, 1975.
84. Strawser, L. D., Larrabee, A. R.: Studies on the synthesis of rat liver fatty acid synthetase. *J Biol Chem 254:* 720, 1976.
85. Nakanishi, S., Numa, S.: Purification of rat liver acetyl coenzyme A carboxylase and immunochemical studies on its synthesis and degradation. *Eur J Biochem 16:* 161, 1970.
86. Volpe, J. J., Vagelos, P. R.: Regulation of mammalian fatty-acid synthetase. The roles of carbohydrate and insulin (liver/adipose tissue/brain/fructose/diabetes). *Proc Natl Acad Sci USA 71:* 889, 1974.
87. Craig, M. C., Porter, J. W.: Synthesis of fatty acid synthetase by isolated liver cells obtained from rats in different nutritional or hormonal states. *Arch Biochem Biophys 159:* 606, 1973.
88. Nikkila, E. A.: Control of plasma and liver triglyceride kinetics by carbohydrate metabolism and insulin. *Adv Lipid Res 7:* 63, 1969.
89. Alcindor, L. G., Infante, R., Soler-Argilaga, C., et al: Effect of a single insulin administration on the hepatic release of triglycerides into the plasma. *Biochim Biophys Acta 306:* 347, 1973.
90. Corder, C. N., Kalkhoff, R. K.: Hepatic lipid metabolism in alloxan-diabetic rats. *J Lab Clin Med 73:* 551, 1969.

91. Woodside, W. F., Heimberg, M.: The effects of anti-insulin serum, insulin, and glucose on output of triglycerides and on ketogenesis by the perfused rat liver. *J Biol Chem 251:* 13, 1976.
92. Heimberg, M., Weinstein, I., Kohout, M.: The effects of glucagon, dibutyryl-3′, 5′-adenosine monophosphate, and concentration of free fatty acid on hepatic lipid metabolism. *J Biol Chem 244:* 5131, 1969.
93. Roncari, D. A., Murthy, V. K.: Effects of thyroid hormones on enzymes involved in fatty acid and glycerolipid synthesis. *J Biol Chem 250:* 4134, 1975.
94. Kekki, M., Nikkila, E. A.: Plasma triglyceride turnover during use of oral contraceptives. *Metabolism 20:* 878, 1971.
95. Havel, R. J., Kane, J. P., Balasse, E. O., et al: Splanchnic metabolism of free fatty acids and production of triglycerides of very low density lipoproteins in normotriglyceridemic and hypertriglyceridemic humans. *J Clin Invest 49:* 2017, 1970.
96. Barter, P. J., Nestel, P. J., Carroll, K. F.: Precursors of plasma triglyceride fatty acid in humans. Effects of glucose consumption, clofibrate administration, and alcoholic fatty liver. *Metabolism 21:* 117, 1972.
97. Barter, P. J., Nestel, P. J.: Precursors of plasma-triglyceride fatty acids in obesity. *Metabolism 22:* 779, 1973.
98. Edelin, Y. H., Kinsell, L. W., Michaels, G. D., et al: Relation between dietary fat and fatty acid composition of endogenous and exogenous very low density lipoprotein triglycerides ($d < 1.006$). *Metabolism 17:* 544, 1968.
99. Vanden Bosch, H.: Phosphoglyceride metabolism. *Annu Rev Biochem 43:* 243, 1974.
100. Thompson, G. A., Jr.: Phospholipid metabolism in animal tissues. In Ansell, G. B., Dawson, R. M. C., Hawthorne, J. N. (eds): Form and Function of Phospholipids. Amsterdam, Elsevier, 1973, p 67.
101. Hawthrone, J. N.: Phospholipid metabolism and transport of materials across the cell membrane. In Ansell, G. B., Dawson, R. M. C., Hawthrone, J. N. (eds): Form and Function of Phospholipids. Amsterdam, Elsevier, 1973, p 423.
102. Jackson, R. L., Gotto, A. M., Jr.: Phospholipids in biology and medicine. *N Engl J Med 290:* 24, 1974.
103. Jackson, R. L., Gotto, A. M., Jr.: Phospholipids in biology and medicine. *N Engl J Med 290:* 87, 1974.
104. Norum, K. R., Glomset, J. A., Gjone, E.: Familial lecithin: cholesterol acyl transferase deficiency. In Stanbury, J. B., Wyngaarden, J. B., Fredrickson, D. S. (eds): Metabolic Basis of Inherited Diseases, ed 3. New York, McGraw-Hill, 1972, p 531.
105. Lindgren, F. T., Jensen, L. C.: The isolation and quantitative analysis of serum lipoproteins. In Nelson, G. J. (ed): Blood Lipids and Lipoproteins: Quantitation, Composition and Metabolism. New York, Wiley, 1972, p 181.
106. Fredrickson, D. S., Lees, R. S.: A system for phenotyping hyperlipoproteinemia. *Circulation 31:* 321, 1965.
107. Fredrickson, D. S., Levy, R. I., Lindgren, F. T.: A comparison of heritable abnormal lipoprotein patterns as defined by two different techniques. *J Clin Invest 47:* 2446, 1968.
108. Albers, J. J., Hazzard, W. R.: Immunochemical quantification of human plasma Lp(a) lipoprotein. *Lipids 9:* 15, 1974.
109. Alaupovic, P.: Studies on the composition and structure of plasma lipoproteins. Distribution of lipoprotein families in major density classes of normal human plasma lipoproteins. *Biochim Biophys Acta 260:* 689, 1972.
110. Ockner, R. K., Hughes, F. B., Isselbacher, K. J.: Very low density lipoproteins in intestinal lymph: origin, composition and role in lipid transport in the fasting state. *J Clin Invest 48:* 2079, 1969.
111. Redgrave, T. G.: Formation of cholesteryl-ester-rich particulate lipid during metabolism of chylomicrons. *J Clin Invest 49:* 465, 1970.
112. Mjos, O. D., Faergeman, O., Hamilton, R. L., et al: Characterization of remnants produced during the metabolism of triglyceride-rich lipoproteins of blood plasma and intestinal lymph in the rat. *J Clin Invest 56:* 603, 1975.
113. Eisenberg, S., Bilheimer, D. W., Levy, R. I., et al: On the metabolic conversion of human plasma very low density lipoprotein to low density lipoprotein. *Biochim Biophys Acta 326:* 361, 1973.
114. Faergeman, O., Sata, T., Kane, J. P., et al: Metabolism of apoprotein B of plasma very low density lipoproteins in the rat. *J Clin Invest 54:* 1396, 1975.
115. Seidel, D., Alaupovic, P., Furman, R. H.: A lipoprotein characterizing obstructive jaundice. I. Method for quantitative separation and identification of lipoproteins in jaundiced subjects. *J Clin Invest 48:* 1211, 1969.
116. Hazzard, W. R., Porte, D., Jr., Bierman, E. L.: Abnormal lipid composition of very low density lipoproteins in diagnosis of broad-beta disease (type III hyperlipoproteinemia). *Metabolism 21:* 1009, 1972.
117. Fredrickson, D. S., Lux, S. E., Herbert, P. N.: The apolipoproteins. *Adv Exp Med Biol 26:* 25, 1972.
118. Morrisett, J. D., Jackson, R. L., Gotto, A. M.: Lipoproteins: structure and function. *Annu Rev Biochem 44:* 183, 1975.
119. Kostner, G., Holasek, A.: Characterization and quantitation of the apolipoproteins from human chyle chylomicrons. *Biochemistry 11:* 1217, 1972.
120. Brown, W. V., Levy, R. I., Fredrickson, D. S.: Further characterization of apolipoproteins from the human plasma very low density lipoproteins. *J Biol Chem 245:* 6588, 1970.
121. Eisenberg, S., Bilheimer, D., Lindgren, F., et al: On the apoprotein composition of human plasma very low density lipoprotein subfractions. *Biochim Biophys Acta 260:* 329, 1972.
122. Kane, J. P., Sata, T., Hamilton, R. L., et al: Apoprotein composition of very low density lipoproteins of human serum. *J Clin Invest 56:* 1622, 1975.
123. Kane, J. P., Richards, E. G., Havel, R. J.: Subunit heterogeneity in human serum beta lipoprotein. *Proc Natl Acad Sci USA 66:* 1075, 1970.
124. Smith, R., Dawson, J. R., Tanford, C.: The size and number of polypeptide chains in human serum low density lipoproteins. *J Biol Chem 247:* 3376, 1972.
125. Kostner, G., Alaupovic, P.: Studies of the composition and structure of plasma lipoproteins. Separation and quantification of the lipoprotein families occurring in the high density lipoproteins of human plasma. *Biochemistry 11:* 3419, 1972.
126. Shore, V. G., Shore, B.: The apolipoproteins: their structure and functional roles in human-serum lipoproteins. In Nelson, G. J. (ed): Blood Lipids and Lipoproteins: Quantitation, Composition and Metabolism. New York, Wiley, 1972, p 789.
127. Scanu, A. M., Edelstein, C., Keim, P.: Serum lipoproteins. In Putnam, F. W. (ed): The Plasma Proteins, ed 2, vol 1. New York, Academic, 1975, p 317.
128. Utermann, G.: Isolation and partial characterization of an arganine-rich apolipoprotein from human plasma very low density lipoproteins: apolipoprotein E. *Hoppe Seylers Z Physiol Chem 356:* 1113, 1975.
129. McConathy, W. J., Alaupovic, P.: Studies on the isolation and partial characterization of apolipoprotein D and lipoprotein D of human plasma. *Biochemistry 15:* 515, 1976.
130. Brewer, H. B., Jr., Lux, S. E., Ronan, R., et al: Amino acid sequence of human Apolip-Gln-II (ApoA-II), an apolipoprotein islated from the high-density lipoprotein complex. *Proc Natl Acad Sci USA 69:* 1304, 1972.
131. Jackson, R. L., Sparrow, J. T., Baker, H. N., et al: The primary structure of apolipoprotein-serine. *J Biol Chem 249:* 5308, 1974.
132. Brewer, H. B., Jr., Shulman, R., Herbert, P., et al: The complete amino acid sequence of alanine apolipoprotein (ApoC-III), an apolipoprotein from human plasma very low density lipoproteins. *J Biol Chem 249:* 4975, 1974.
133. Sparrow, J. T., Gotto, A. M., Morrisett, J. D.: Chemical synthesis and biochemical properties of peptide fragments of apolipoprotein-alanine. *Proc Natl Acad Sci USA 70:* 2124, 1973.
134. Shulman, R. S., Herbert, P. N., Wehrly, K., et al: The complete amino acid sequence of C-I (ApoLp-Ser), and apolipoprotein from human very low density lipoproteins. *J Biol Chem 250:* 182, 1975.
135. Forte, T., Nichols, A. V.: Application of electron microscopy to the study of plasma lipoprotein structure. *Adv Lipid Res 10:* 1, 1972.
136. Laggner, P., Muller, K., Kratky, O., et al: Studies on the structure of lipoprotein A of human high density lipoprotein HDL_3: The spherically averaged electron density distribution. *FEBS Lett 33:* 77, 1973.
137. Tardieu, A., Mateu, L., Sardet, C., et al: Structure of human serum lipoproteins in solution. II. Small-angle x-ray scattering study of HDL_3 and LDL. *J Mol Biol 101:* 129, 1976.
138. DeBlois, R. W., Uzgiris, E. E., Devi, S. K., et al: Application of laser self-beat spectroscopic technique to the study of solutions of human plasma low-density lipoproteins. *Biochemistry 12:* 2645, 1973.
139. Adams, G. H., Schumaker, V. N.: Equilibrium banding of low-density lipoproteins. III. Studies of normal individuals and the effects of diet and heparin-induced lipase. *Biochim Biophys Acta 210:* 462, 1970.
140. Sata, T., Havel, R. J., Jones, A. L.: Characterization of subfractions

of triglyceride-rich lipoproteins separated by gel chromatography from blood plasma of normolipemic and hyperlipemic humans. *J Lipid Res 13:* 757, 1972.

141. Camejo, G.: The structure of human density lipoprotein: a study of the effect of phospholipase A and trypsin on its components and of the behavior of the lipid and protein moieties at the air–water interphase. *Biochim Biophys Acta 175:* 290, 1969.

142. Gotto, A. M., Levy, R. I., Lux, S. E., et al: A comparative study of the effects of chemical modification on the immunochemical and optical properties of human plasma low-density lipoprotein(s) and apoproteins. *Biochem J 133:* 369, 1973.

143. Schonfeld, G., Pfleger, B.: The structure of human high density lipoprotein and the levels of apolipoprotein A-I in plasma as determined by radioimmunoassay. *J Clin Invest 54:* 236, 1974.

144. Schonfeld, G., Pfleger, B., Roy, R.: Structure of human high density lipoprotein reassembled in vitro. *J Biol Chem 250:* 7943, 1975.

145. Pattnaik, N. H., Kezdy, F. J., Scanu, A. M.: Kinetic study of the action of snake venom phospholipase A_2 on human serum high density lipoprotein 3. *J Biol Chem 251:* 1984, 1976.

146. Assmann, G., Sokoloski, E. A., Brewer, H. B., Jr.: ^{31}P Nuclear magnetic resonance spectroscopy of native and recombined lipoproteins. *Proc Natl Acad Sci USA 71:* 549, 1974.

147. Segrest, J. P., Jackson, R. L., Morrisett, J. D., et al: A molecular theory of lipid–protein interactions in the plasma lipoproteins. *FEBS Lett 38:* 247, 1974.

148. Jackson, R. L., Morrisett, J. D., Gotto, A. M., Jr., et al: The mechanism of lipid binding by plasma lipoproteins. *Mol Cel Biochem 6:* 43, 1975.

149. Assmann, G., Brewer, H. B., Jr.: A molecular model of high density lipoproteins. *Proc Natl Acad Sci USA 71:* 1534, 1974.

150. Stoffel, W., Zierenberg, O., Tunggal, B. D., et al: ^{13}C Nuclear magnetic resonance spectroscopic studies on lipid–protein interactions in human high-density lipoprotein (HDL): a model of the HDL particle. *Hoppe Seylers Z Physiol Chem 355:* 1381, 1974.

151. Verdery, R. G. III, Nichols, A. V.: Arrangement of lipid and protein in human serum high density lipoproteins: a proposed model. *Chem Phys Lipids 14:* 123, 1975.

152. Margolis, S., Capuzzi, D.: Serum-lipoprotein synthesis and metabolism. In Nelson, G. J. (ed): Blood Lipids and Lipoproteins: Quantitation, Composition and Metabolism. New York, Wiley, 1972 p 825.

153. Palade, G.: Intracellular aspects of the process of protein synthesis. *Science 189:* 347, 1975.

154. Hamilton, R. L., Regen, D. M., Gray, M. E., et al: Lipid transport in liver. I. Electron microscopic identification of VLDL in perfused rat liver. *Lab Invest 16:* 305, 1967.

155. Kessler, J. I., Stein, J., Dannacker, D., et al: Biosynthesis of low density lipoprotein by cell-free preparations of rat intestinal mucosa. *J Biol Chem 245:* 5281, 1970.

156. Fredrickson, D. S., Gotto, A. M., Levy, R. I.: Familial lipoprotein deficiencies. In Stanbury, J. B., Wyngaarden, J. B., Fredrickson, D. S. (eds): Metabolic Basis of Inherited Diseases. New York, McGraw-Hill, 1972, p 493.

157. Lo, C. H., Marsh, J. B.: Biosynthesis of plasma lipoproteins. Incorporation of ^{14}C-glucosamine by cells and subcellular fractions of rat liver. *J Biol Chem 245:* 5001, 1970.

158. Morrisett, J. D., Sparrow, J. T., Hoff, H. E., et al: Methods for studying lipid–protein interactions. *Baylor Univ Cardiovasc Res Center Bull 12:* 39, 1973.

159. Mahley, R. W., Bersot, T. P., LeQuire, V. S., et al: Identity of very low density lipoprotein apoproteins of plasma and liver Golgi apparatus. *Science 168:* 380, 1970.

160. Marsh, J. B.: Apoproteins of the lipoproteins in a non-recirculating perfusate of rat liver. *J Lipid Res 17:* 85, 1976.

161. Marchand, Y. L., Singh, A., Assimacopoulos-Jeannet, F., et al: A role for the microtubular system in the release of very low density lipoproteins by perfused mouse livers. *J Biol Chem 248:* 6862, 1973.

162. Schonfeld, G., Pfleger, B.: Overproduction of very low-density lipoproteins by livers of genetically obese rats. *Am J Physiol 220:* 1178, 1971.

163. Robertson, R. P., Gavareski, D. J., Henderson, J. D., et al: Accelerated triglyceride secretion, a metabolic consequence of obesity. *J Clin Invest 52:* 1620, 1973.

164. Quarfordt, S. H., Frank, A., Shames, D. M., et al: Very low density lipoprotein triglyceride transport in type IV hyperlipoproteinemia and the effects of carbohydrate-rich diets. *J Clin Invest 49:* 2281, 1970.

165. Kudzma, D. J., Schonfeld, G.: Alcoholic hyperlipidemia: induction by alcohol but not by carbohydrate. *J Lab Clin Med 77:* 384, 1971.

166. Olefsky, J., Farguhar, J. W., Reaven, G. M.: Sex differences in the kinetics of triglyceride metabolism in normal and hypertriglyceridaemic human subjects. *Eur J Clin Invest 4:* 121, 1974.

167. Hillman, L., Schonfeld, G., Miller, J. P., et al: Apolipoproteins in human pregnancy. *Metabolism 24:* 943, 1975.

168. Nikkila, E. A.: Control of plasma and liver triglyceride kinetics by carbohydrate metabolism and insulin. *Adv Lipid Res 7:* 63, 1969.

169. Nikkila, E. A., Kekki, M.: Plasma triglyceride metabolism in thyroid disease. *J Clin Invest 51:* 2103, 1972.

170. Glueck, C. J., Fallat, R. W., Scheel, D.: Effects of estrogenic compounds on triglyceride kinetics. *Metabolism 24:* 537, 1975.

171. Nikkila, E. A., Kekki, M.: Plasma triglyceride transport kinetics in diabetes mellitus. *Metabolism 22:* 1, 1973.

172. Havel, R. J.: Pathogenesis, differentiation and management of hypertriglyceridemia. *Adv Intern Med 15:* 117, 1969.

173. Nikkila, E. A., Kekki, M.: Measurement of plasma triglyceride turnover in the study of hypertriglyceridemia. *Scand J Clin Lab Invest 27:* 97, 1971.

174. Bar-On, H., Kook, A. I., Stein, O., et al: Assembly and secretion of very low density lipoproteins by rat liver following inhibition of protein synthesis with cycloheximide. *Biochim Biophys Acta 306:* 106, 1973.

175. Pottenger, L. A., Frazier, L. E., DuGien, L. H., et al: Carbohydrate composition of lipoprotein apoproteins isolated from rat plasma and from the livers of rats fed orotic acid. *Biochem Biophys Res Commun 54:* 770, 1973.

176. Ruderman, N. B., Jones, A. L., Krauss, R. M., et al: A biochemical and morphologic study of very low density lipoproteins in carbohydrate-induced hypertriglyceridemia. *J Clin Invest 50:* 1355, 1971.

177. Schonfeld, G.: Changes in the composition of very low density lipoprotein during carbohydrate induction in man. *J Lab Clin Med 75:* 206, 1970.

178. Schonfeld, G., Weidman, S. W., Witztum, J. L., et al: Alterations in levels and interrelations of plasma apolipoproteins induced by diet. *Metabolism 25:* 261, 1976.

179. Eaton, R. P., Schade, D. S.: Glucagon resistance as a hormonal basis for endogenous hyperlipaemia. *The Lancet 1:* 937, 1973.

180. Fraser, R., Cliff, W. J., Courtice, F. C.: The effect of dietary fat load on the size and composition of chylomicrons in thoracic duct lymph. *Q J Exp Physiol 53:* 390, 1968.

181. Glickman, R. M., Perotto, J. L., Kirsch, K.: Intestinal lipoprotein formation: effect of colchicine. *Gastroenterology 70:* 347, 1976.

182. Korn, E. D.: Clearing factor, a heparin-activated lipoprotein lipase. II. Substrate specificity and activation of coconut oil. *J Biol Chem 215:* 15, 1955.

183. Robinson, D. S.: The clearing factor lipase and its action in the transport of fatty acids between blood and tissues. *Adv Lipid Res 3:* 133, 1963.

184. Olivecrona, T.: Metabolism of chylomicrons labeled with C^{14}-glycerol-H^3-palmitic acid in the rat. *J Lipid Res 3:* 439, 1962.

185. Faergman, O., Havel, J. R.: Metabolism of cholesteryl esters of rat very low density lipoproteins. *J Clin Invest 55:* 1210, 1975.

186. Stein, O., Stein, Y., Goodman, D. S., et al: The metabolism of chylomicron cholesteryl ester in rat liver. A combined radio autographic–electron microscopic and biochemical study. *J Cell Biol 43:* 410, 1969.

187. Blanchette-Mackie, E. J., Scow, R. O.: Effects of lipoprotein lipase on the structure of chylomicrons. *J Cell Biol 58:* 689, 1973.

188. Barter, P. J., Nestel, P. J.: Precursor product relationship between pools of very low density lipoprotein triglyceride. *J Clin Invest 51:* 174, 1972.

189. Sigurdsson, G., Nicoll, A., Lewis, B.: Conversion of very low density lipoprotein to low density lipoprotein. *J Clin Invest 56:* 1481, 1975.

190. Reichl, D., Simons, L. A., Myant, N. B., et al: The lipids and lipoproteins of human peripheral lymph, with observations on the transport of cholesterol from plasma and tissues into lymph. *Clin Sci Mol Med 45:* 313, 1973.

191. Havel, R. J., Kane, J. P., Kaseyap, M. L.: Interchange of apolipoproteins between chylomicrons and high density lipoproteins during alimentary lipemia in man. *J Clin Invest 52:* 32, 1973.

192. Schonfeld, G., Gulbrandsen, C. L., Wilson, R. B., et al: Catabolism of human very low density lipoproteins in monkeys. *Biochim Biophys Acta 270:* 426, 1972.

193. Yasuoka, S., Setsuro, F.: Relationship between clearing factor lipase and lipases in tissues. *J Biochem 70:* 749, 1971.
194. Schotz, M. C., Stewart, J. E., Garfinkel, A. S., et al: Isolated fat cells: morphology and possible role of released lipoprotein lipase in deposition of lipoprotein fatty acid. *Adv Exp Med Biol 4:* 161, 1969.
195. Chajek, T., Stein, O., Stein, Y.: Colchicine-induced inhibition of plasma lipoprotein lipase release in the intact rat. *Biochim Biophys Acta 380:* 127, 1975.
196. Borensztajn, J., Rone, M. S., Sandros, T.: Effects of colchicine and cycloheximide on the functional and non-functional lipoprotein lipase fractions of rat heart. *Biochim Biophys Acta 398:* 394, 1975.
197. Fredrickson, D. S., Ono, K., Davis, L. L.: Lipolytic activity of post heparin plasma in hyperglyceridemia. *J Lipid Res 4:* 24, 1963.
198. Stewart, J. E., Schotz, M. C.: Release of lipoprotein lipase activity from isolated fat cells. II. Effect of heparin. *J Biol Chem 249:* 904, 1974.
199. Ehnholm, C., Greten, H., Brown, W. V.: A comparative study of post-heaprin lipolytic activity and a purified human plasma triacylglycerol lipase. *Biochim Biophys Acta 360:* 68, 1974.
200. Krauss, R. M., Levy, R. I., Fredrickson, D. S.: Selective measurement of two lipase activities in postheparin plasma from normal subjects and patients with hyperlipoproteinemia. *J Clin Invest 54:* 1107, 1974.
201. Ehnholm, C., Shaw, W., Greten, H., et al: Purification from human plasma of a heparin-released lipase with activity against triglyceride and phospholipids. *J Biol Chem 250:* 6756, 1975.
202. Noma, A., Okabe, H., Sakurada, T., et al: Determination and properties of monoglyceride hydrolase in human post-heparin plasma. *Clin Chem Acta 54:* 177, 1974.
203. Garfinkel, A. S., Schotz, M. C.: Separation of molecular species of lipoprotein lipase from adipose tissue. *J Lipid Res 13:* 63, 1972.
204. Greten, H., Walter, B., Brown, W. V.: Purification of a human post heparin plasma triglyceride lipase. *FEBS Lett 27:* 306, 1972.
205. Bensadoun, A., Ehnholm, C., Steinberg, D., et al: Purification and characterization of lipoprotein lipase from pig adipose tissue. *J Biol Chem 249:* 2220, 1974.
206. Ehnholm, C., Kinnunen, P. K. J., Huttunen, J. K., et al: Purification and characterization of lipoprotein lipase from pig myocardium. *Biochem J 149:* 649, 1975.
207. Brown, V. W., Baginsky, M. L.: Inhibition of lipoprotein lipase by an apoprotein of human very low density lipoprotein. *Biochem Biophys Res Commun 46:* 375, 1972.
208. Havel, R. J., Fielding, C. J., Olivecrona, T., et al: Cofactor activity of protein components of human very low density lipoprotein in the hydrolysis of triglycerides by lipoprotein lipase from different sources. *Biochemistry 12:* 1828, 1973.
209. Ganesan, D., Bass, H. B.: Isolation of C-I and C-II activated lipoprotein lipases and protamine insensitive triglyceride lipase by heparin–Sepharose affinity chromatography. *FEBS Lett 53:* 1, 1975.
210. Fielding, C. J.: Lipoprotein lipase: evidence for high and low-affinity binding sites. *Biochemistry 15:* 879, 1976.
211. Felts, J. M., Itakura, H., Crane, R. T.: The mechanism of assimilation of constituents of chylomicrons, very low density lipoproteins and remnants—a new theory. *Biochem Biophys Res Commun 66:* 1467, 1975.
212. Garfinkel, A. S., Baker, N., Schotz, M. C.: Relationship of lipoprotein lipase activity to triglyceride uptake in adipose tissue. *J Lipid Res 8:* 274, 1967.
213. Huttunen, J. K., Ehnholm, C., Kekki, M., et al: Post-heparin plasma lipoprotein lipase and hepatic lipase in normal subjects and in patients with hypertriglyceridaemia: correlations to sex, age and various parameters of triglyceride metabolism. *Clin Sci Mol Med 50:* 249, 1976.
214. Huttunen, J. K., Ehnholm, C., Nikkila, E. A., et al: Effect of fasting on two postheparin plasma triglyceride lipases and triglyceride removal in obese subjects. *Eur J Clin Invest 5:* 435, 1975.
215. Garfinkel, A. S., Nilsson-Ehle, P., Schotz, M. C.: Regulation of lipoprotein lipase induction by insulin. *Biochim Biophys Acta 424:* 264, 1976.
216. Pykalisto, O. J., Smith, P. H., Brunzell, J. D.: Determinants of human adipose tissue lipoprotein lipase. Effect of diabetes and obesity on basal and diet-induced activity. *J Clin Invest 56:* 1108, 1975.
217. Borensztajn, J., Keig, P., Rubenstein, A. H.: The role of glucagon in the regulation of myocardial lipoprotein lipase activity. *Biochem Biophys Res Commun 53:* 603, 1973.
218. Ence, T. J., Wilson, D. E., Flowers, C. M., et al: Heparin metabolism and heparin-released lipase activity during long-term estrogen–progestin treatment. *Metabolism 25:* 139, 1976.
219. Hamosh, M., Hamosh, P.: The effect of estrogen on the lipoprotein lipase activity of rat adipose tissue. *J Clin Invest 55:* 1132, 1975.
220. Ehnholm, C., Huttunen, J. K., Kinnunen, P. J., et al: Effect of oxandrolone treatment on the activity of lipoprotein lipase, hepatic lipase and phospholipase A_1 of human postheparin plasma. *N Engl J Med 292:* 1314, 1975.
221. Zinder, O., Hamosh, M., Fleck, T. R. C., et al: Effect of prolactin on lipoprotein lipase in mammary gland and adipose tissue of rats. *Am J Physiol 226:* 744, 1974.
222. Porte, D., Jr., Bierman, E. L.: The effect of heparin infusion on plasma triglyceride in vivo and in vitro with a method for calculating triglyceride turnover. *J Lab Clin Med 73:* 631, 1969.
223. Fredrickson, D. S., Levy, R. I.: Familial hyperlipoproteinemia. In Stanbury, J. B., Wyngaarden, J. B., Fredrickson, D. S. (eds): Metabolic Basis of Inherited Diseases, ed 3. New York, McGraw-Hill, 1972, p 545.
224. Lees, R. S., Wilson, D. E., Schonfeld, G., et al: The familial dyslipoproteinemia. *Prog Med Genet 9:* 237, 1973.
225. Osuga, T., Portman, O. W.: Origin and disappearance of plasma lecithin: cholesterol acyltransferase. *Am J Physiol 220:* 735, 1971.
226. Fielding, C. J., Fielding, P. E.: Purification and substrate specificity of lecithin–cholesterol acyl transferase from human plasma. *FEBS Lett 15:* 355, 1974.
227. Albers, J. J., Cabana, V. G., Barden Stahl, Y. D.: Purification and characterization of human plasma lecithin: cholesterol acyltransferase. *Biochemistry 15:* 1083, 1976.
228. Nichols, A. V., Smith, L.: Effect of very low-density lipoproteins on lipid transfer in incubated serum. *J Lipid Res 6:* 206, 1965.
229. Marcel, Y. L., Vezina, C.: Lecithin:cholesterol acyltransferase of human plasma: role of chylomicrons, very low, and high density lipoproteins in the reaction. *J Biol Chem 248:* 8254, 1973.
230. Fielding, C. J., Shore, V. G., Fielding, P. E.: A protein cofactor of lecithin:cholesterol acyltransferase. *Biochem Biophys Res Commun 46:* 1493, 1972.
231. Soutar, A. K., Garner, C. W., Baker, H. N., et al: Effect of the human plasma apolipoproteins and phosphatidylcholine acyl donor on the activity of lecithin: cholesterol acyltransferase. *Biochemistry 14:* 3057, 1975.
232. Gjone, E.: Familial LCAT deficiency. *Acta Med Scand 194:* 353, 1973.
233. Goldstein, J. L., Brown, M. S.: Binding and degradation of low density lipoproteins by cultured human fibroblasts. *J Biol Chem 249:* 5153, 1974.
234. Goldstein, J. L., Brunschede, B. Y., Brown, M. S.: Inhibition of the proteolytic degradation of low density lipoprotein in human fibroblasts by chloroquine, concanavalin A and triton WR 1339. *J Biol Chem 250:* 7854, 1975.
235. Goldstein, J. L., Dana, S. E., Faust, J. R., et al: Role of lysosomal acid lipase in the metabolism of plasma low density lipoprotein. *J Biol Chem 250:* 8487, 1975.
236. Bierman, E. L., Eisenberg, S., Stein, O., et al: Very low density lipoprotein "remnant" particles: uptake by aortic smooth muscle cells in culture. *Biochim Biophys Acta 329:* 163, 1973.
237. Reichl, D., Postiglione, A., Myant, N. B.: Uptake and catabolism of low density lipoproteins by human lymphocytes. *Nature 260:* 634, 1976.
238. Onitiri, A. C., Lewis, B., Bentall, H., et al: Lipoprotein concentrations in serum and in biopsy samples of arterial intima. *Atherosclerosis 23:* 513, 1976.
239. Zilversmit, D. B.: A proposal linking atherogenesis to the interaction of endothelial lipoprotein lipase with triglyceride-rich lipoproteins. *Circ Res 33:* 633, 1973.
240. Ledford, J. H., Alaupovic, P.: Subcellular fractionation, partial purification and characterization of neutral triacylglycerol lipase from pig liver. *Biochim Biophys Acta 398:* 132, 1975.
241. Sniderman, A. D., Carew, T. E., Chandler, J. G., et al: Paradoxical increase in rate of catabolism of low-density lipoproteins after hepatectomy. *Science 183:* 526, 1973.
242. Jackson, R. L., Gotto, A. M., Stein, O., et al: A comparative study on the removal of cellular lipids from Landschutz ascites cells by human plasma apolipoproteins. *J Biol Chem 250:* 7204, 1975.
243. Lees, R. S.: A progress report on lipoprotein phenotyping. *J Lab Clin Med 82:* 529, 1973 (editorial).

244. Fredrickson, D. S.: It's time to be practical. *Circulation 51:* 209, 1975.
245. Levy, R. I.: The meaning of lipid profiles. *Postgrad Med 57:* 34, 1975.
246. Higgins, M. J. P., Lecamwasam, D. S., Galton, D. J.: A new type of familial hypercholesterolaemia. *Lancet 2:* 737, 1975.
247. Utermann, G., Jaeschke, M., Menzel, J.: Familial hyperlipoproteinemia type III: deficiency of a specific apolipoprotein (apo E-III) in the very low density lipoproteins. *FEBS Lett 56:* 352, 1975.
248. Carlson, L. A., Ballantyne, D.: Changing relative proportions of apolipoproteins C-II and C-III of very low density lipoproteins in hypertriglyceridemia. *Atherosclerosis 23:* 563, 1976.
249. Goldstein, J. L., Schrott, H. G., Hazzard, W. R., et al: Hyperlipidemia in coronary heart disease, II. Genetic analysis of lipid levels in 176 families and delineation of a new inherited disorder, combined hyperlipidemia. *J Clin Invest 52:* 4544, 1973.
250. Stamler, J.: Preventive Cardiology. New York, Grune & Stratton, 1967.
251. Artheriosclerosis: Report by National Heart and Lung Institute Task Force on Arteriosclerosis, vol 2. DHEW Publ No. (NIH), 1971, pp 72–219.
252. Spaet, T. H.: Optimism in the control of atherosclerosis. *N Engl J Med 291:* 576, 1974.
253. Wissler, R. W.: Atherosclerosis—its pathogenesis in perspective. Comparative pathology of the heart. *Adv Cardiol 13:* 10, 1974.
254. Dayton, S., Pearce, M. L.: Prevention of coronary heart disease and other complications of atherosclerosis by modified diet. *Am J Med 46:* 751, 1969.
255. Levy, R. I., Fredrickson, D. S. Schulman, R., et al: Dietary and drug treatment of primary hyperlipoproteinemia. *Ann Intern Med 77:* 267, 1972.
256. Lees, R. S., Wilson, D. E.: The treatment of hyperlipidemia. *N Engl J Med 284:* 186, 1971.
257. Yeshurun, D., Gotto, A. M., Jr.: Drug treatment of hyperlipidemia. *Am J Med 60:* 379, 1976.
258. Levy, R. I.: Drug therapy of hyperlipoproteinemia. *JAMA 21:* 2334, 1976.
259. Wood, P. D. S., Stern, M. P., Silvers, A., et al: Prevalence of plasma lipoprotein abnormalities in a free-living population of the Central Valley, California. *Circulation 45:* 114, 1972.
260. Schonfeld, G., Kudzma, D. J.: Type IV hyperlipoproteinemia—a critical appraisal. *Arch Intern Med 132:* 55, 1973.
261. Witztum, J. L., Schonfeld, G., Weidman, S. W.: The effects of colestipol on the metabolism of very-low-density lipoproteins in man. *J Lab Clin Med 88:* 1008, 1976.
262. Breckenridge, W. C., Little, J. A., Steiner, G., et al.: Hypertriglyceridemia associated with deficiency of apolipoprotein C-II. *N Engl J Med 298:* 1265, 1978.
263. Olofsson, S.-O., McConathy, W. J., Alaupovic, P.: Isolation and partial characterization of a new acidic apolipoprotein (apolipoprotein F) from high density lipoproteins of human plasma. *Biochemistry 17:* 1032, 1978.
264. Ayrault-Jarrier, M., Alix, J.-F., Polonovski, J.: Une nouvelle proteine des lipoproteines du serum humain: isolement et caracterisation partielle d'une apolipoproteine G. *Biochimie 60:* 65, 1978.

145

Adrenocortical Regulation of Salt and Water Metabolism: Physiology, Pathophysiology, and Clinical Syndromes

Edward N. Ehrlich

In normal man the volume, distribution, and concentration of body fluids remain remarkably constant despite wide variations in quantity and relative proportions of ingested water and solutes. Such constancy of the internal environment requires close coordination between independent regulatory systems that govern sodium and water metabolism. These systems are extremely complex, but essentially each consists of an afferent limb, which is capable of detecting changes in body fluid status, and an efferent limb, which transmits neural and endocrine signals to the major effector organ, the kidney, that lead to appropriate adjustments in renal excretion of sodium and water.

This chapter is mainly concerned with the role of the adrenal cortex in the regulation of fluid and electrolyte metabolism and the pathophysiology of disorders that result from abnormal secretion of adrenocortical hormones. Aldosterone and other mineralocorticoids secreted by the adrenal have significant effects upon renal handling of sodium and potassium, and glucocorticoids, such as cortisol, facilitate water excretion. Adrenocortical hormones, however, are only a few of many factors involved in fluid and electrolyte homeostasis. Indeed, factors other than aldosterone play a major role in determining excretion of sodium, and water balance is controlled mainly by antidiuretic hormone. Although well-defined fluid and electrolyte disorders can be related to specific disturbances of adrenocortical function, there are important clinical features that cannot be attributed directly to the effects of the abnormally secreted corticoid(s). Some of the associated metabolic abnormalities reflect secondary renal responses that are independent of adrenocortical regulation; others are not completely understood.

The pathophysiology of the clinical disorders of fluid and electrolyte metabolism that result from abnormal secretion of adrenocortical hormones is complex. The precise role of individual corticoids in the pathogenesis of these disorders can be appreciated only when viewed against the overall process of fluid and electrolyte metabolism. Accordingly, the physiology of body fluid regulation and renal mechanisms that govern water and electrolyte excretion will be reviewed before considering the clinical derangements that have been associated with disturbances of adrenocortical function.

NORMAL PHYSIOLOGY

EXTRACELLULAR FLUID HOMEOSTASIS

Osmolarity of body fluids is mainly dependent upon mechanisms that regulate water metabolism, specifically hypothalamic centers that control the release of antidiuretic hormone and modulate the sensation of thirst. These mechanisms have been discussed in Chapter 19. Most cell membranes are freely permeable to water. Therefore, osmolarity of intracellular and extracellular fluid compartments tends to be identical due to physical forces of osmosis and diffusion, and, as a corollary, the distribution of body water is dependent upon the quantity of solute each compartment contains. Sodium is the principal extracellular cation. In contrast the sodium content of intracellular fluid is extremely low due to active outward extrusion of sodium ions by cell membranes. Since extracellular

Supported in part by the Madison General Hospital Endocrine Research Fund.

solute consists mainly of sodium salts, the volume of the extracellular compartment is determined by its sodium content.[1,2]

Loss of body sodium initially results in decreased extracellular osmolarity. This results in movement of extracellular water down the osmotic gradient into cells, and at the same time suppresses release of antidiuretic hormone, leading to increased renal excretion of water. Both effects produce contraction of extracellular fluid volume. Conversely, increased sodium intake tends to raise osmolarity of extracellular fluids, cellular water moves into the extracellular space to maintain osmotic equilibrium, and antidiuresis occurs due to stimulation of antidiuretic hormone. These effects result in expansion of the extracellular volume. Since renal mechanisms controlling sodium excretion are responsive to fluctuations in extracellular fluid volume, loss or gain of body sodium ultimately leads to corresponding changes in sodium excretion.[3,4] However, extracellular fluid volume is not restored to normal by these alterations in sodium excretion alone. This requires a final adjustment in extracellular water content, mediated by an appropriate change in antidiuretic hormone. Thus, extracellular fluid volume, although determined by sodium content, is regulated by mechanisms that govern both sodium and water balance.

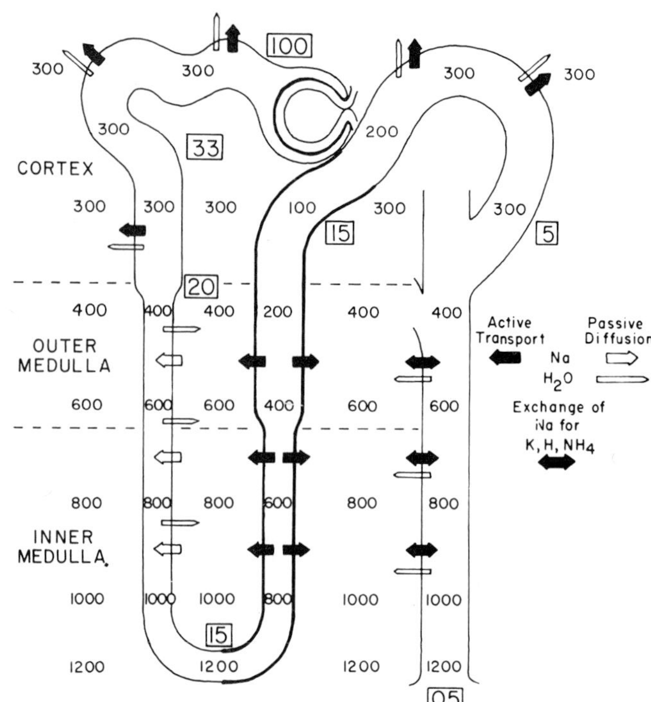

Fig. 145-1. Summary of reabsorption and excretion of ions and water in the nephron.[11] Concentrations are given in m/sm/liter. Boxed numerals are estimated percentages of filtrate remaining within the tubule. Recent evidence indicates that chloride is actively reabsorbed by the ascending limb of Henle's loop.[16,17] (From Windhager, E. E.: Mechanisms of reabsorption and excretion of ions and water. In Pitts, R. F. (ed): Physiology of the Kidney and Body Fluids. Chicago, Year Book Medical Publishers, 1974, p. 134).

RENAL SODIUM EXCRETION

The amount of sodium excreted in the urine represents the net difference between glomerular filtration and tubular reabsorption of sodium. In a normal adult the kidney filters approximately 20,000 meq of sodium daily, an enormous amount compared to the 100–200 meq excreted daily in the urine with normal sodium intake.[5,6] Even if sodium intake were increased far beyond the usual range, the quantity of sodium excreted in order to maintain balance still would be an extremely small fraction of the filtered load. Thus, because of the high filtration rate, tubular reabsorption of sodium must be sustained at an almost equivalent rate in order to prevent sodium depletion. Very small fluctuations in either rate of filtration or tubular reabsorption of sodium theoretically could result in substantial changes in sodium excretion. It has not always been clear which of these variables determines the quantity of sodium excreted.

The glomerular filtration rate is remarkably stable in man and does not respond appreciably to usual variations in sodium intake.[7] Furthermore, experimentally induced fluctuations in filtration rate are accompanied by corresponding, proportionate changes in tubular sodium reabsorption that tend to minimize the resultant change in sodium excretion.[8] This adjustment in sodium reabsorption in response to changes in filtration, so-called *glomerulotubular balance,* seems to take place in the proximal tubule.[9,10]

Reabsorption and excretion of filtrate by the nephron is summarized in Figure 145-1. Approximately 70 percent of filtered sodium is reabsorbed in the proximal tubule. Sodium concentration remains constant throughout this segment of the nephron, indicating that reabsorption of sodium and water is isotonic.[11,12] Sodium is reabsorbed in the proximal tubule by an active transport process, and it was assumed that this generates an osmotic gradient that results in passive reabsorption of water.[11–14] However, when measured directly, the osmotic gradient between tubular lumen and peritubular fluid in the proximal tubule was found insufficient to account for the quantity of filtrate reabsorbed. Recent evidence supports the hypothesis that coupled transfer of water and sodium in the proximal tubule occurs through intercellular channels as well as transcellularly.[11,12,14,15] Fluid entering the loop of Henle is still isoosmotic. Its quantity depends upon the filtered sodium load and the amount of sodium reabsorbed by the proximal tubule. The descending limb of the loop of Henle and probably also the thin ascending limb do not actively transport sodium, but they are freely permeable to water. On the other hand, the thick ascending limb is capable of reabsorbing sodium chloride but is relatively impermeable to water. The transport process in the ascending limb is unique in that chloride is actively transported and sodium moves passively along the electrical potential gradient generated by the active transport of chloride ions.[16,17] Reabsorption of sodium chloride in the thick ascending limb contributes not only to overall tubular sodium reabsorption, but also has a special significance in providing the single effect for the countercurrent multiplier system that establishes the large osmotic gradient in the medullary interstitium for reabsorption of water from the medullary collecting duct.[11,1]

The distal nephron reabsorbs only a small fraction of filtrate only 10–20 percent of the total.[11] However, in contrast to the proximal tubule, where filtrate is reabsorbed isoosmotically, sodium and water reabsorption are not tightly coupled in the distal nephron, and each may vary independently.[11–14] Thus, bulk reabsorption of filtrate occurs in the proximal tubule, but the distal nephron has the special capability of adjusting the composition of the filtrate in accordance with differing proportions of salt and water usually ingested. Sodium reabsorption in the distal convoluted tubule involves an active transport mechanism capable of effecting net inward movement of sodium ions against a high electrochemical gradient.[11–14] This transport mechanism is specifically stimulated by aldosterone and other steroids possessing mineralocorticoid activity.[19,20] Active sodium reabsorption also occurs in the collecting duct and this, too, may be responsive to mineralocorticoids. Although only a very small fraction of overall sodium reabsorption takes place in the collecting duct, extremely low sodium concentrations, as low as 1–2 meq/liter are achieved in this segment during salt deprivation.[21] In contrast, with very large amounts of dietary sodium and limited water intake the concentration of sodium in urine may be fourfold greater than in plasma.

Water reabsorption in the distal nephron, as previously noted, is passive and is governed by permeability changes induced by antidiuretic hormone. The osmolarity of filtrate entering the distal nephron is approximately 100 mosmol/kg. This degree of hypoosmolarity achieved in the ascending limb of the loop of Henle is unchanged by extremes in water intake. However, in the distal nephron marked changes in concentration of tubular fluid are induced. During water diuresis there is further dilution of the hypotonic fluid leaving the loop of Henle, since the distal nephron is relatively impermeable to water and active reabsorption of ions continues. On the other hand, during water deprivation urine osmolality may exceed 1200 mosmol/kg as fluid in collecting duct is free to equilibrate with the hypertonic medullary interstitium.

REGULATION OF TUBULAR SODIUM REABSORPTION

As previously stated, the amount of sodium excreted in the urine represents the very small net difference between the much larger quantities of sodium that are filtered and reabsorbed by the kidney. Since changes in filtration have a minimal influence upon sodium excretion, factors controlling reabsorption must be the major determinant.

The adrenal cortex plays an important role in regulating sodium excretion by secreting mineralocorticoids, which increase renal sodium reabsorption. Aldosterone is the major mineralocorticoid produced by the adrenal, and its rate of secretion fluctuates in a manner consistent with its presumed function as a regulator of sodium balance, i.e., it varies inversely with changes in sodium intake.[22] Aldosterone and other mineralocorticoids act mainly upon the distal tubule, where they stimulate reabsorption of sodium and stimulate secretion of potassium, hydrogen, ammonium, and magnesium ions.[19,23] Mineralocorticoids probably also stimulate sodium reabsorption in the collecting duct,[21] but whether they have such action on the proximal tubule or the ascending limb of the loop of Henle is controversial.[20,23]

Mineralocorticoids increase active sodium transport in a variety of epithelial tissues in various species, including sweat and salivary glands, intestinal epithelium, and renal tubules in man.[23] The subcellular action of mineralocorticoids is similar to that of other steroid hormones. It involves initial binding of the steroid to a cytosol receptor in the target tissue and transfer of the steroid–receptor complex to the cell nucleus, where it interacts with chromatin. This in turn leads to induction of proteins that mediate the physiologic effects of the steroid.[24] The nature and intracellular site of action of the mineralocorticoid-induced protein has not been defined, but several hypotheses have been proposed. These hypotheses are summarized in Figure 145-2, which schematically depicts the active sodium transport process in a mineralocorticoid-responsive cell. It is noteworthy that there is a 1-h latent period before biologic effects of mineralocorticoids become apparent in in vitro preparations[25] or before there is an appreciable decline in urinary sodium excretion in vivo.[26] This latent period, which is independent of the concentration of mineralocorticoid, presumably is required for synthesis of the induced protein. Aldosterone inhibitors, such as spironolactone and progesterone, presumably act by competing with the active corticoid for cytosol-binding sites.[27]

Endocrinologists have tended to emphasize the role of adrenocortical hormones in regulation of sodium reabsorption. However, during the past decade it has become evident that factors other than aldosterone also play an important, perhaps predominant, role in regulating sodium reabsorption. In 1961 deWardener and his co-workers showed that saline infusions resulted in overall

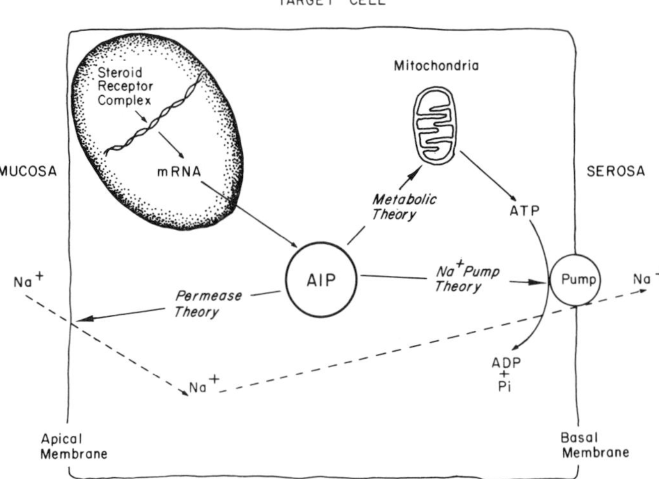

Fig. 145-2. Active sodium transport in a mineralocorticoid-responsive cell and postulated sites of action of aldosterone-induced protein (AIP). Na^+ enters the apical cell membrane along its electrochemical gradient and is extruded by an Na^+,K^+-activated ATPase ("pump") located in the basal membrane. AIP has been postulated to act at three possible sites: (1) at apical entry step (permease theory); (2) directly on NaK-ATPase (pump theory); (3) on oxidative pathways generating high-energy intermediates to fuel the pump (metabolic theory). (From Feldman et al: *Am. J. Med. 53:* 545, 1972.)

depression of tubular sodium reabsorption independent of any change in mineralocorticoid activity and that the resultant natriuresis persisted even when the glomerular filtration rate was reduced by obstructing the aorta.[28] Their experiments not only demonstrated that changes in tubular reabsorption could be a major determinant of sodium excretion, but also stimulated a widespread search for nonaldosterone factors that might influence tubular sodium reabsorption. Subsequently, it was shown by micropuncture techniques that the depression of sodium reabsorption during saline loading occurs in the proximal tubule.[29] Since then, numerous experiments have been performed to study proximal sodium reabsorption, and several possible mechanisms have been proposed to explain the depression that occurs in response to volume hyperexpansion.[2,5,30,31] However, this complex process is still incompletely understood.

One possible explanation is that filtrate is redistributed among nephrons having different reabsorptive capacities. The nephron population of the kidney is not homogenous. Cortical nephrons possessing short loops of Henle have limited sodium-reabsorbing capacity compared to juxtamedullary nephrons possessing longer loops. A redistribution of filtrate to cortical nephrons would favor sodium excretion, whereas redistribution to juxtamedullary nephrons would favor sodium retention.[32] Furthermore, there is experimental evidence suggesting that variations in salt intake result in the appropriate redistribution of filtrate required to adjust sodium excretion.[33]

Other theories emphasize the role of physical factors, i.e., hydrostatic and oncotic pressures in peritubular capillaries, with modulation of proximal tubular sodium reabsorption.[5,30,33] These hypotheses are based on experimental evidence showing that passive uptake of reabsorbate in the proximal tubule is indirectly related to hydrostatic pressure and directly related to plasma protein oncotic pressure in the peritubular capillaries.[34,35] Furthermore, the natriuresis induced by saline infusions was shown to be associated with decreased renal vascular resistance and reduced filtration fraction.[5,36] This leads to increased hydrostatic pressure and decreased oncotic pressure in peritubular capillaries, thereby retarding isotonic reabsorption by the proximal tubule. More recently, Brenner and his associates have presented data supporting the role of changes in peritubular oncotic pressure in the natriuresis induced by volume expansion.[37,38] Other recent studies indicate that increased membrane permeability may be required for expression of the physical forces that lead to decreased reabsorption.[30,39]

Lee and DeWardener suggest that a humoral agent may be responsible for the depression of proximal sodium absorption that occurs in response to saline loading.[40] Evidence for the existence of such a natriuretic hormone is based on results of cross-circulation experiments in animals in which volume hyperexpansion induced in donor animals resulted in natriuresis in recipients.[40,41] Factors have been extracted from blood and urine of saline-loaded animals or man which depress sodium transport in vitro and increase sodium excretion in vivo.[42,43] There is evidence suggesting that the hypothalamus or neurohypophysis may be the source of a natriuretic hormone.[40] A potent natriuretic factor, seemingly distinct from vasopressin or oxytocin has been isolated from the posterior pituitary that may participate in the tubular response to volume hyperexpansion.[44] Others have proposed that a natriuretic hormone may be secreted by the kidney, possibly from the juxtaglomerular apparatus.[31]

It has been postulated that sodium reabsorption in the distal convoluted tubule and the collecting ducts also may be influenced by nonaldosterone effects.[45,46] Regardless of the precise site of action of the various factors that influence tubular sodium reabsorption, it seems each may have a somewhat special, but complementary role in regulating renal sodium excretion. Changes in aldosterone cannot be responsible for moment-to-moment adjustments in sodium excretion in view of the prolonged latent period and duration of action of this steroid. However, because of these very qualities, aldosterone would tend to stabilize the extracellular fluid volume, particularly the blood volume as it relates to renal hemodynamics, within a range in which more immediate-acting modulating factors can be optimally effective. Sodium balance may eventually be restored spontaneously in the face of deficient or excessive aldosterone secretion, presumably reflecting long-term effects of nonaldosterone factors, but extracellular fluid volume in such circumstances will remain contracted or expanded unless drastic, appropriate changes are made in salt intake.

VOLUME REGULATION AND RENAL SODIUM EXCRETION

It is apparent that the various factors, aldosterone and nonaldosterone, that regulate renal sodium excretion are responsive to changes in extracellular fluid volume. This is not surprising, since extracellular fluid volume is determined by its sodium content. However, it is not clear how deviations in extracellular volume are detected, or how such information is integrated and transmitted to effector organs in response to these deviations. Current opinion holds that sodium excretion responds to changes in the "effective blood volume" rather than to the actual volume of extracellular fluid per se.[47] According to this hypothesis, sensors located at strategic sites within the cardiovascular tree detect local changes in transmural pressure or the degree of stretching of the vascular wall.[47,48] These sensors include baroreceptors located in the aorta and carotid sinus, stretch receptors in the cardiac atria and great veins, and baroreceptors in the afferent glomerular arterioles that modulate secretion of renin by juxtaglomerular cells. Multiple stimuli arising from these sites would have to be integrated and interpreted somewhere in the central nervous system, probably the hypothalamus. Efferent signals then would be transmitted via neural and humoral pathways to various end organs that determine the effective blood volume, i.e., the heart, kidneys, and peripheral vessels.

The role of the kidney in volume homeostasis is multifaceted. In addition to being an effector organ with respect to regulating sodium excretion, it has receptors that can detect fluctuations in effective blood volume or sodium balance,[49] and it also has effector mechanisms that can directly or indirectly initiate appropriate changes in sodium reabsorption. Thus, the kidney not only responds to aldosterone, but it also regulates aldosterone secretion. The juxtaglomerular apparatus of the kidney secretes renin, a proteolytic enzyme, that cleaves its substrate, a circulating α_2-globulin synthesized by the liver, to produce the decapeptide, angiotensin I. Converting enzyme found mainly in the lung removes two terminal amino acids from angiotensin I, forming angiotensin II, an octapeptide. Angiotensin II stimulates aldosterone secretion by glomerulosa cells of the adrenal cortex, and it is also a potent vasoconstrictor.[50]

As shown in Figure 145-3, the juxtaglomerular apparatus is comprised of juxtaglomerular cells surrounding the afferent glomerular arteriole and the macula densa, consisting of specialized cells at the origin of the distal tubule. Renin release from juxtaglomerular cells is inversely related to pressure changes in the afferent glomerular arteriole, and in the macula densa there appears to be a direct relationship between distal tubular sodium delivery and renin release.[49,50] Renin secretion is also influenced by the sympathetic nervous system. Renal sympathectomy or β-adrenergic blockade decreases baseline plasma renin activity and the renin response to hypovolemic stimuli. Furthermore, either renal nerve stimulation or increased circulating catecholamine may directly result in enhanced renin release independent of changes in renal perfusion pressure or sodium delivery to the distal tubule.

Nonaldosterone effects upon sodium reabsorption also are probably mediated by changes in volume perceived within the kidney itself, since subtle changes in intrarenal vascular tone

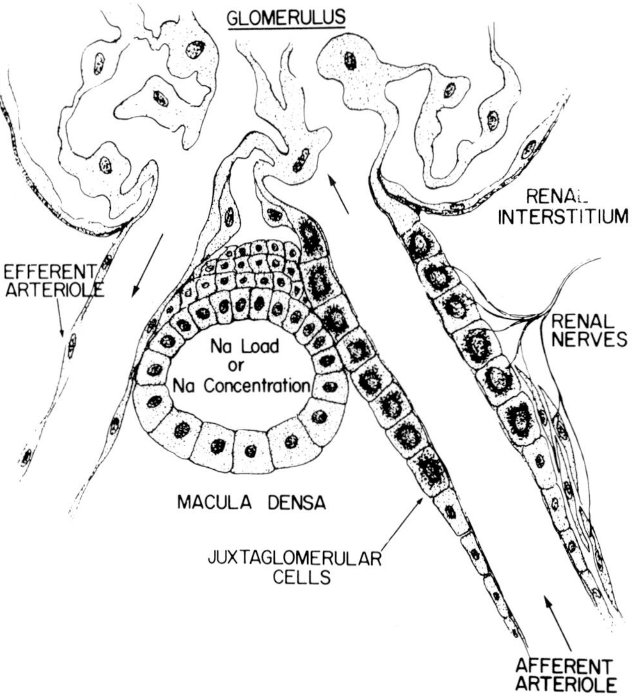

Fig. 145-3. Juxtaglomerular apparatus. (From Davis: *Circ. Res. 28:* 301, 1971.)

would be the primary determinant of hemodynamic influences upon sodium excretion.[5,31] As noted above, some workers have suggested that the kidney also regulates the release of a natriuretic hormone. According to this hypothesis the juxtaglomerular apparatus produces a natriuretic hormone in addition to renin. Thus, the juxtaglomerular cells would not only respond to increased pressure by releasing a natriuretic hormone that acts upon the proximal tubule, but also by suppressing renin release.

POTASSIUM EXCRETION

Potassium excreted in the urine is not the result of the net difference between glomerular filtration and tubular reabsorption, as is the case with sodium excretion.[23,51] Most of the filtered potassium is reabsorbed proximally.[52] Only 5–10 percent of the filtered load reaches the distal tubule regardless of the dietary intake of potassium.[53] Thus, most of the potassium excreted in the urine is due to tubular secretion in the distal nephron. Although potassium secretion is dependent upon distal sodium reabsorption, microperfusion and micropuncture studies indicate that it is not stoichiometrically coupled to active inward transport by a carrier-mediated ion-exchange process.[53,54] Rather, it seems that potassium moves passively into the lumen along an electrical potential gradient generated by active sodium transport.[55]

The kaliuretic effect of mineralocorticoids is poorly understood. Secretion of potassium in the late distal tubule is impaired by adrenalectomy, but the transtubular potential difference remains normal.[56] This is difficult to reconcile with the assumption that mineralocorticoids facilitate potassium secretion by increasing the potential gradient generated by sodium reabsorption. Other studies also suggest that the effect of aldosterone upon potassium secretion may be unrelated to its effect upon sodium transport. Inhibition of new protein synthesis by actinomycin D blocks the sodium-retaining effect of aldosterone in adrenalectomized rats, but not the kaliuretic effect.[57]

Potassium secretion by the kidney is also affected by acid–base status.[51,58] Alkalosis is usually associated with increased potassium excretion and acidosis is accompanied by a decrease in urinary potassium. Observations of this reciprocal relationship between potassium and hydrogen ion excretion have led to the assumption that these two cations compete for the same transport site. However, recent studies do not support this concept; they suggest that acid–base changes modify factors that govern potassium uptake across the peritubular membrane of cells of the distal convoluted tubule.[58]

Thus, tubular secretion of potassium in the distal nephron is influenced by three factors: distal sodium delivery, acid–base status, and the level of mineralocorticoid activity. Aldosterone may also affect the disposition of potassium in cells outside the kidney. There is evidence suggesting that mineralocorticoids facilitate the entry of potassium into muscle cells during potassium loading.[59]

FACTORS REGULATING ALDOSTERONE SECRETION

The adrenal cortex consists of two functionally independent, anatomically distinct secretory components. The inner cortical zones, the fasiculata and reticularis, comprise a single functional unit that secretes 15–20 mg/day of cortisol, a glucocorticoid. Cortisol secretion normally follows a diurnal pattern.[60] It reaches a peak early in the day and declines to negligible quantities toward midnight. Recently, it has been shown that this diurnal pattern actually results from a series of discontinuous bursts of secretory activity during the early part of the day with virtual cessation of secretion for several hours just before and after midnight. Overall cortisol secretion is increased by physical and emotional stress. Such stress-related stimuli override the baseline regulatory mechanism, and resultant increments are superimposed upon the usual nycto-hemeral pattern. Both the stress response and the baseline cortisol secretory pattern are dependent upon ACTH released by the anterior pituitary under the influence of hypothalamic corticotropin-releasing factor.

The other adrenocortical component, consisting of an irregular outer zone of glomerulosa cells, normally secretes 50–150 μg/day of aldosterone, a potent mineralocorticoid.[23] Aldosterone secretion varies inversely with changes in dietary sodium intake or the effective blood volume,[22,61] and these variations are closely accompanied by parallel changes in plasma renin activity[22,62] (Fig. 145-4). Moreover, aldosterone secretion in man is stimulated by infused angiotensin and the resultant increments are sustained during prolonged stimulation.[63] These observations support the assumption that aldosterone responses to changes in salt balance or volume status are regulated by the renin–angiotensin system.

The possible role of ACTH in regulation of aldosterone secretion has been a subject of renewed interest. Early studies indicated that aldosterone secretion is unresponsive to a small dose of ACTH.[64] Aldosterone secretion is stimulated by pharmacologically large doses of exogenous ACTH, but the response is transient and subsides after the first 24 h despite continued ACTH administration.[22,65] Thus, it seemed unlikely that the much lower quantities of ACTH normally secreted by the pituitary could have a significant influence upon aldosterone secretion. However, recent studies indicate that aldosterone secretion is as responsive as cortisol to infusions of physiologic concentrations of ACTH.[66] Aldosterone secretion also displays a diurnal pattern that is roughly synchronous with cortisol,[67] and its secretory activity is episodic like that of cortisol.[68] Peak plasma aldosterone levels coincide more often with cortisol than with plasma renin activity,[68] as shown in Figure 145-5. Although these correlations suggest that diurnal variations and spontaneous fluctuations in aldosterone secretion are influenced by ACTH, this is not borne out by the observation that the pattern is not disrupted by suppression of ACTH with dexamethasone.[68]

The concentration of plasma potassium may play a significant role in regulation of aldosterone secretion, particularly in mediating responses observed in the anephric state.[69] Aldosterone secretion increases sharply in response to barely perceptible increments in plasma potassium concentration, and it decreases with potassium depletion. Stimulation of aldosterone secretion by potassium presumably is due to a direct effect of this ion upon glomerulosa cells, and plasma renin activity is thereby depressed[70] (Fig. 145-6).

CLINICAL DISORDERS DUE TO MINERALOCORTICOID EXCESS

PATHOPHYSIOLOGY

Metabolic Effects of Excess Mineralocorticoid Activity

The renal effects of mineralocorticoids have been described above. They act mainly upon the distal nephron to induce increased sodium reabsorption and promote potassium secretion. Accordingly, it might be anticipated that exposure to excessive mineralocorticoid activity would result in unremitting sodium retention manifested by edema and congestive heart failure, as well

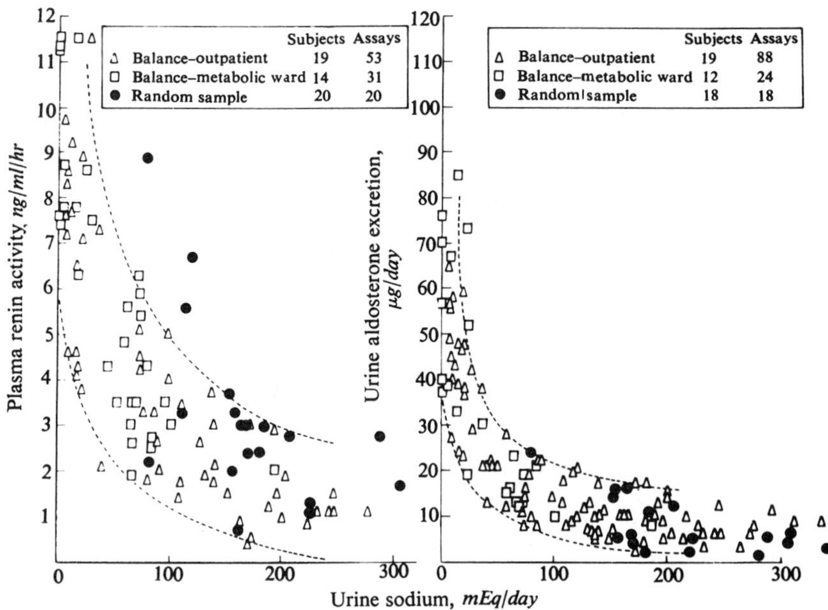

Fig. 145-4. Relationship of plasma renin activity and aldosterone excretion to urinary sodium in normal subjects. (From Laragh et al: *Am. J. Med. 52:* 633, 1972.)

as hypertension. However, the clinical syndrome of mineralocorticoid excess is characterized by hypokalemia and hypertension, and overt evidence of sodium retention is minimal or absent. Other features include metabolic alkalosis and manifestations of mild impairment of renal concentrating ability. Clinical features of the syndrome of mineralocorticoid excess are listed in Table 145-1.

Table 145-1. Clinical Features of the Syndrome of Mineralocorticoid Excess

Limited sodium retention; no overt edema
Hypertension
Hypokalemia
Metabolic alkalosis
Polyuria; slightly increased plasma osmolality

Sodium and Potassium Balance. When large amounts of a potent mineralocorticoid are administered to normal subjects, the resulting sodium retention subsides within a short period, usually 4–7 days, and sodium balance resumes despite continued treatment.[71,72] After resumption of balance, larger doses of mineralocorticoid do not induce further sodium retention. The restoration of sodium balance and apparent refractoriness to the sodium-retaining action of mineralocorticoids has been termed the *escape phenomenon*. The renal response to excess mineralocorticoid is depicted schematically in Figure 145-7.

Escape has been related to depression of proximal tubular sodium reabsorption in response to volume expansion resulting from stimulation of distal sodium transport.[73] Presumably, inhibition of proximal reabsorption during chronic and acute expansion involves similar mechanisms. Escape occurs as proximal sodium

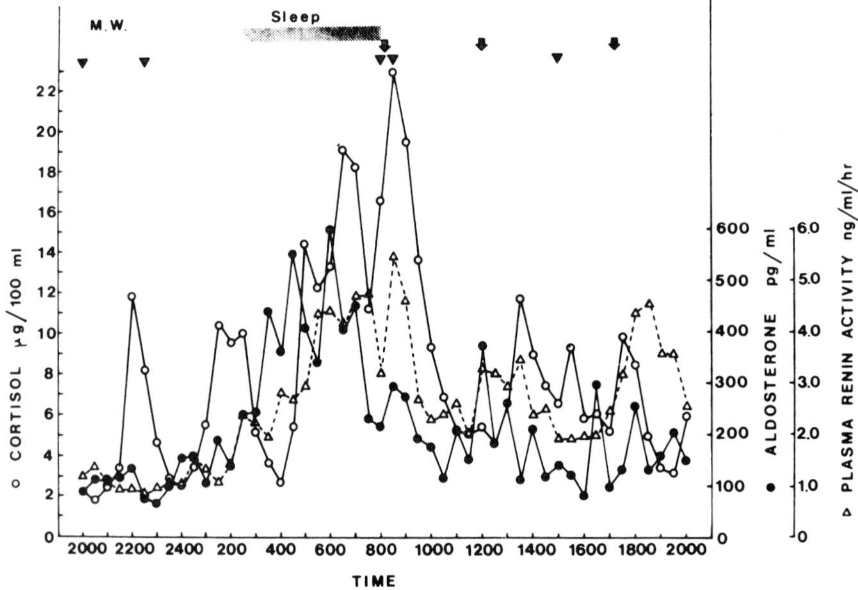

Fig. 145-5. Twenty-four–hour rhythm of plasma aldosterone, cortisol, and renin activity in a normal man. (From Katz et al: *J. Clin. Endocrinol. Metab. 40:* 125, 1975.)

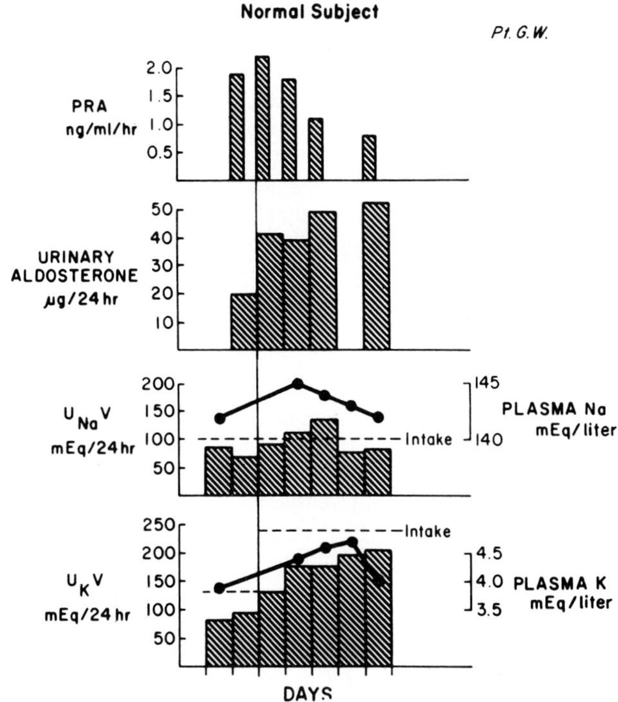

Fig. 145-6. Effect of potassium loading on plasma renin activity (PRA), aldosterone excretion, and sodium balance in a normal man. (From Brunner et al: *J. Clin. Invest. 49:* 2128, 1970.)

rejection overcomes enhanced distal reabsorption. Thus, escape is not a response to mineralocoriticoids per se, but rather to the volume expansion they induce. Overt edema does not occur because cumulative sodium retention usually is limited by the onset of escape to no more than 200–300 meq. Sodium retention is accompanied from the outset by kaliuresis, which may be reinforced as escape occurs since more sodium is delivered to the distal tubule. Thus, the limited accumulation of body sodium and urinary potassium wasting characteristic of the clinical syndrome of mineralocorticoid excess can be reproduced experimentally in man. However, the severity of hypokalemia in many clinical cases of mineralocorticoid excess is much greater than can be produced by prolonged administration of comparable doses of mineralocorticoid to normals.[71,72] This observation has raised the possibility that other factors may contribute to the pathogenesis of hypokalemia in the clinical disorders.[74]

Blood Pressure. Hypertension is a characteristic feature of clinical syndromes of mineralocorticoid excess. However, exogenous mineralocorticoids have a variable effect upon blood pressure in man. Mild elevations may occur in some individuals during prolonged treatment when salt intake is liberal;[71,72] it can be prevented by restricting dietary salt.[75] Thus, mineralocorticoids do not appear to have an immediate, direct pressor effect. Rather, the development of hypertension seems to be related to altered sodium metabolism, not only in response to the increased extracellular fluid volume,[75] but also to changes in the water and electrolyte content of arteriolar walls.[76]

Acid–Base Balance.[77] Mineralocorticoids increase secretion of potassium and hydrogen ions into the distal tubular lumen by an exchange process that is dependent upon the rate of sodium reabsorption. Therefore, hydrogen ion secretion is enhanced by mineralocorticoids only if an ample supply of sodium is delivered to the distal tubule. This condition usually is ensured because proximal sodium reabsorption is reduced by volume hyperexpansion unless sodium intake is severely restricted. Potassium secretion is accelerated preferentially when distal sodium reabsorption is stimulated, but hydrogen ion secretion increases progressively as potassium depletion develops. Accordingly, a loss of hydrogen ions will not occur if potassium depletion is prevented by potassium chloride supplementation.[78] Thus, generation of metabolic alkalosis in the syndrome of mineralocorticoid excess is due to the loss of acid in the urine resulting from stimulation of distal sodium transport, but it may be markedly influenced by intake of sodium and potassium.

The alkalosis generated by the action of mineralocorticoids upon the distal nephron is maintained by the increased proximal resorptive capacity that results from potassium depletion.[79] Proximal reabsorption of bicarbonate is also influenced by changes in extracellular fluid volume.[80] Volume expansion, such as occurs in mineralocorticoid excess, tends to depress proximal bicarbonate reabsorption, thereby partially offsetting the effect of potassium depletion. The increased bicarbonate load cannot be completely reabsorbed by the distal nephron and some leaks into the urine. Thus, the metabolic alkalosis in the syndrome of mineralocorticoid excess is associated with a more alkaline urine and tends to be less severe than in states of metabolic alkalosis induced by diuretics or protracted vomiting, in which proximal bicarbonate reabsorption is enhanced by volume contraction.

Although metabolic alkalosis in the syndrome of mineralocorticoid excess seems to be explained by known renal mechanisms, it has not been possible to reproduce a similar degree of alkalosis by administering mineralocorticoids to normal subjects for 3 months.[81] Plasma bicarbonate increased by no more than 3 meq/liter and plasma potassium did not fall below 3.1 meq/liter. The slight rise in bicarbonate induced by exogenous aldosterone, as

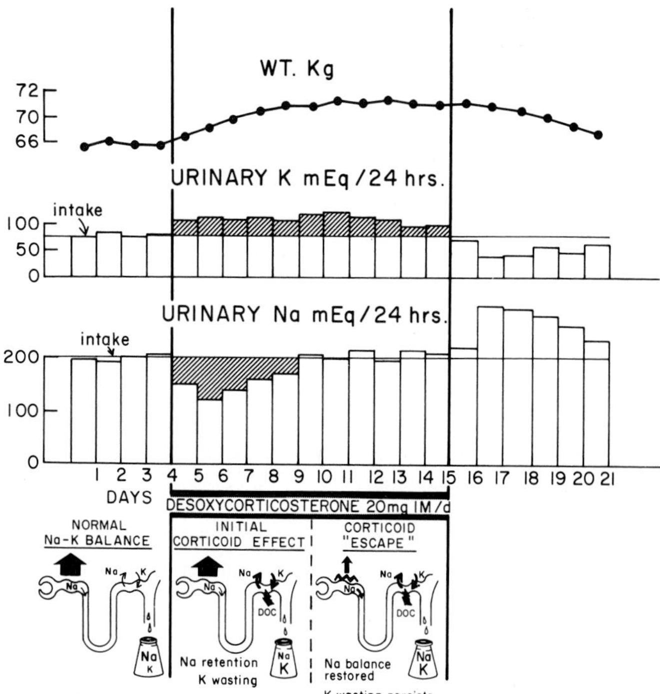

Fig. 145-7. Renal response to prolonged treatment with desoxycorticosterone acetate in normal man, showing renal adjustments involved in mineralocorticoid "escape."

well as the much higher level noted in reported cases of primary aldosteronism, correlated inversely with potassium concentration.[81] These observations suggested that severity of alkalosis induced by aldosterone is determined by the degree of potassium deficiency. Again, the failure of exogenous aldosterone to produce as severe a degree of potassium depletion as in primary aldosteronism is unexplained.

Renal Concentrating Ability. The syndrome of mineralocorticoid excess is associated with impaired ability to concentrate the urine. This defect may be manifested by mild hypernatremia, slightly elevated plasma osmolality, and polyuria. Polyuria is most prominent at night, i.e., nocturia, which may be due to the reversal of the normal diurnal pattern of water and electrolyte excretion that has been observed in primary aldosteronism.[82]

Impairment of urinary concentrating ability in the syndrome of mineralocorticoid excess is presumably due to potassium depletion.[83] The degree of impairment has been related to the severity and duration of potassium deficiency, and the resulting defect may persist for many years after potassium repletion. Decreased urinary concentration also may be at least partly due to suppression of antidiuretic hormone by chronic volume hyperexpansion.

Mineralocorticoids Secreted by the Adrenal

The syndrome of mineralocorticoid excess can result from exposure to excessive amounts of any corticoid or other agent possessing mineralocorticoid activity. Almost all naturally occurring and synthetically derived corticoids have both mineralo- and glucocorticoid activity, but they are designated as one or the other on the basis of their predominant activity. Desoxycorticosterone has only mineralocorticoid activity and its potency is modest compared to aldosterone. Aldosterone reportedly has approximately one-third the glucocorticoid activity of cortisone,[84] but this would be negligible with quantities of aldosterone secreted in clinical circumstances. Cortisol, a glucocorticoid, has modest mineralocorticoid activity that may contribute to manifestations of mineralocorticoid excess observed in some cases of Cushing's syndrome. Corticosterone has moderate glucocorticoid and mineralocorticoid activity in man and will produce manifestations of mineralocorticoid excess when present in amounts sufficient to satisfy glucocorticoid requirements. Relative mineralocorticoid and glucocorticoid activities of these corticoids are summarized in Table 145-2.

Desoxycorticosterone and corticosterone are direct precursors in aldosterone biosynthesis, but they also are by-products of cortisol production (Fig. 145-8). The magnitude of steroidogenic processes involved in cortisol biosynthesis is so much greater than that of those engaged in aldosterone production that almost all desoxycorticosterone and corticosterone secreted by the adrenal is related to cortisol production and is ACTH dependent. Sodium retention and kaliuresis that occur in response to administered ACTH probably are related to increased secretion of these ACTH-dependent mineralocorticoids rather than to mineralocorticoid activity of cortisol.[65] Recently considerable attention has been directed toward 18-hydroxydesoxycorticosterone as a possible pathogenic factor in some cases of low-renin hypertension.[85,86] This corticoid, normally secreted in small amounts by the human adrenal cortex, is also ACTH dependent. It seems to have sodium-retaining and antidiuretic but no kaliuretic action in rats.[87] Its metabolic effects have not been extensively evaluated in man.

Table 145-2. Relative Potencies of Corticosteroids

Corticosteroid	Glucocorticoid Activity	Mineralocorticoid Activity
Cortisol	1	1
Cortisone	0.8	0.8
Corticosterone (compound B)	0.35	0.2
11-Desoxycortisol (compound S)	0	0
11-Desoxycorticosterone	0	20
Aldosterone	0.3	400
9α-Fluorocortisol	10.0	400

CLINICAL SYNDROMES

Exposure to excessive amounts of any of the various agents possessing mineralocorticoid activity should result in similar manifestations, i.e., the syndrome of mineralocorticoid excess. However, the various clinical disorders that result in excessive secretion of mineralocorticoid may be distinguished by special features that accompany or are superimposed upon the syndrome of mineralocorticoid excess. These distinguishing features are dependent upon the nature of the underlying pathologic process, the relative glucocorticoid potency of the causative mineralocorticoid, or the biologic activity of by-products associated with secretion of the mineralocorticoid. The various disorders are described below.

Aldosteronism

The term *aldosteronism* should be restricted to the state of mineralocorticoid excess that results from exposure to *excessive* amounts of aldosterone. The occurrence of a very high rate of aldosterone secretion does not in itself justify the assumption that it represents *hypersecretion* or that a state of *aldosteronism* exists. Aldosterone secretion normally varies considerably in response to changes in dietary sodium intake or the effective blood volume.[22,61,62] With extreme sodium deprivation aldosterone secretion rates are markedly elevated, reaching levels as high or even higher than in some cases of aldosteronism (Fig. 145-4). However, this is a normal compensatory response to threatened sodium depletion. Accordingly, even the most striking elevations induced by extreme sodium depletion or reductions in the effective blood volume would not be excessive and should not be so regarded, since aldosterone secretion in this circumstance is not augmented to a higher level than required to restore sodium balance or the effective blood volume. Norms for aldosterone secretion can be defined only in relation to the state of sodium balance or the effective blood volume.

Primary Aldosteronism.

Conn's Syndrome: This name refers to the pathologic state that results from hypersecretion of aldosterone from a solitary, functionally autonomous adrenocortical adenoma. The first case, reported by Conn in 1954, presented primarily with overt neuromuscular difficulties: tetany, periodic weakness, and "paralyses."[88] Although hypertension apparently had been present for many years it was of moderate severity and uncomplicated. Severe hypokalemia was present, accounting for muscle weakness. Tetany presumably was related to hypomagnesemia. Surgical exploration revealed a single, large (4-cm diameter) benign cortical adenoma in the right adrenal. Following excision of the adenoma the abnormal findings promptly disappeared. Subsequently, early

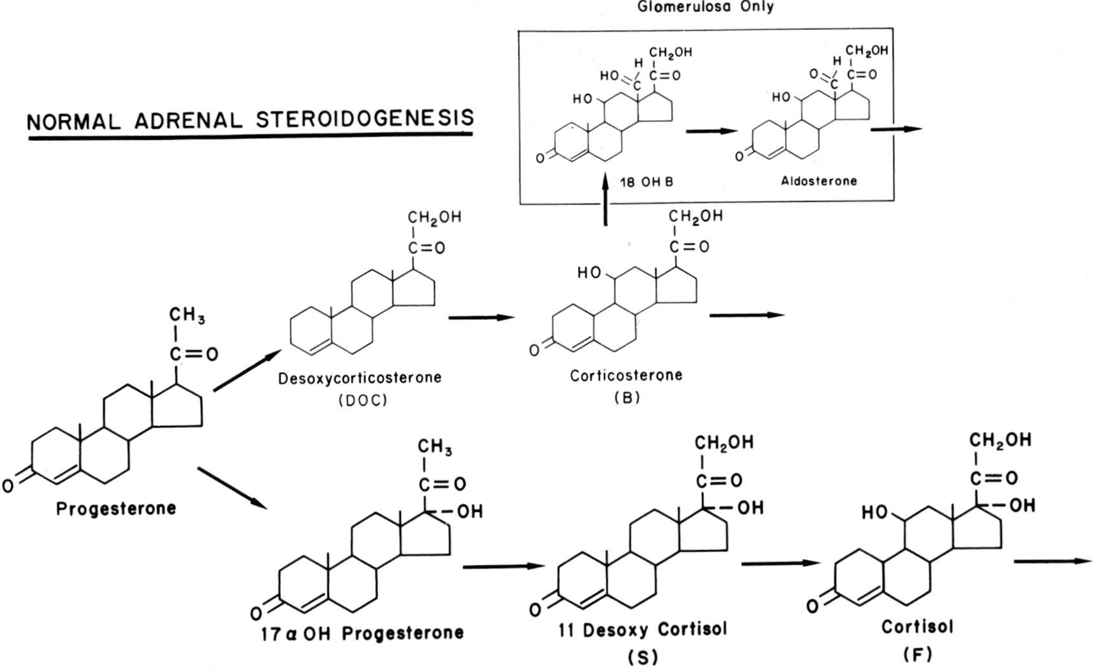

Fig. 145-8. Final pathways of aldosterone and cortisol biosynthesis.

case finding efforts were directed toward hypertensive patients with hypokalemia. The presumptive diagnosis of primary aldosteronism was made in such individuals by finding increased urinary excretion of aldosterone or an elevated aldosterone secretion rate. With recognition of primary aldosteronism depending mainly upon these criteria, its reported incidence, according to Conn et al., up to July 1962 was only 145 cases.[89]

Unfortunately, early criteria were not always a reliable guide to diagnosis of primary aldosteronism. Hypertensive patients with overt hypokalemia and aldosterone hypersecretion clearly unrelated to prior diuretic therapy were found at operation to have no apparent adrenal abnormality or bilateral nodular adrenocortical hyperplasia, and their hypertension was not relieved by total adrenalectomy. A possible cause for such misdiagnosis soon became apparent with the recognition that aldosterone secretion is abnormally elevated in advanced stages of essential hypertension[90] or in cases of renovascular hypertension,[91] because of renal ischemia. Resultant activation of the renin-angiotensin system stimulates aldosterone secretion, causing secondary aldosteronism and adrenal hyperplasia. The development of practical methods for assaying plasma renin activity seemed to offer a reasonable means of differentiating primary and secondary aldosteronism. Secondary aldosteronism was supposedly distinguished by high levels of plasma renin activity;[92] finding suppressed renin activity in patients with evidence of increased aldosterone secretion was assumed to be uniquely diagnostic of an autonomous adosterone-producing adenoma.[93]

Idiopathic Aldosteronism (pseudoprimary aldosteronism): Even when the preoperative diagnosis of primary aldosteronism is based upon finding hypertension with hypokalemia, evidence of aldosterone hypersecretion, and subnormal renin, not all patients are found to have solitary adrenal adenomas at surgery. Many patients with all the above features of primary aldosteronism have bilateral nodular hyperplasia or grossly normal-appearing adrenals, and their hypertension is not ameliorated by bilateral adrenalectomy.[94] These cases have been designated as "idiopathic" or pseudoprimary aldosteronism.[94,95] Aldosterone secretion in some patients with idiopathic aldosteronism is readily suppressed by administration of mineralocorticoids, which affords a means of distinguishing these preoperatively from surgically curable cases of primary aldosteronism due to solitary adenoma.[94]

Measurements of plasma aldosterone concentration may afford another means of identifying patients with aldosterone-producing adenomas. Biglieri et al reported that the plasma aldosterone concentration after overnight recumbency was greater than 19.5 ng/100 ml in patients with surgically-proven adenomas, whereas it was less than 19.5 ng/100 ml in patients with idiopathic aldosteronism. Furthermore, after 4 hours of upright posture, plasma aldosterone concentration *fell* in 19 of 25 patients with aldosterone-producing adenomas; in patients with idiopathic aldosteronism the plasma aldosterone concentration increased briskly in response to upright posture.[94b] Until the reliability of such measurements of the plasma aldosterone concentration is established, preoperative differentiation between bilateral hyperplasia and a solitary adenoma may require selective adrenal vein catheterization, which permits venographic examination and measurements of aldosterone concentration in adrenal vein blood, as discussed in Chapter 98.

The pathogenesis of adrenal nodular hyperplasia with aldosterone hypersecretion and suppressed renin is unclear. These findings suggest that aldosterone-producing cells are stimulated by an agent other than angiotensin. Another possibility is that suppressed renin reflects a later stage in the evolution of secondary aldosteronism in which chronic hyperstimulation by angiotensin eventually leads to autonomous function of hyperplastic cells. Cases in which aldosterone secretion is suppressed by administered mineralocorticoids may represent an intermediate stage in which there is only partial autonomy. The observation of somewhat higher renin levels in cases of bilateral hyperplasia with suppressible aldosterone is consistent with the proposition that renin becomes suppressed as adrenal cells undergo a transition from angiotensin-dependent hyperplasia to autonomous function.[94]

The significance of plasma renin measurements in diagnosing

primary aldosteronism has changed considerably during the past decade. In the mid-1960s great reliance was placed upon this determination as a means of screening normokalemic hypertensive patients for primary aldosteronism. The combined findings of aldosterone hypersecretion and suppressed plasma renin activity were assumed to be uniquely diagnostic of primary aldosteronism due to a solitary adenoma.[93] Based on their initial experience in applying these criteria, Conn et al. proposed that the incidence of normokalemic primary aldosteronism in the essential hypertensive population may be as high as 20 percent.[96] More recent estimates seem to indicate an incidence of less than 3 percent, and normokalemic cases are a distinct rarity.[97]

Current diagnostic features include hypertension, hypokalemia, aldosterone hypersecretion resistant to suppressive procedures, and suppressed plasma renin activity. Although plasma renin measurements are helpful in interpreting elevated aldosterone values, the finding of suppressed renin activity is not as specific as previously assumed; subnormal renin values are found in a large number of patients with essential hypertension,[98] and they cannot aid in differentiating surgically curable primary aldosteronism due to an adenoma from idiopathic aldosteronism, which is not ameliorated by adrenalectomy. Such differentiation is absolutely essential for proper surgical management, and presently it may be achieved only by employing adrenal venography or scintillation scanning or by sampling adrenal vein blood for aldosterone measurements.[99,100] These procedures have been discussed in Chapter 98.

Glucocorticoid-Suppressible Aldosteronism: Sutherland et al. described a father and son with clinical findings identical to primary aldosteronism, i.e., benign hypertension, potassium deficiency, increased aldosterone secretion rate, raised plasma volume, and suppressed plasma renin activity.[101] The father underwent adrenal exploration and no adenoma was found. The left adrenal was excised and showed nodular hyperplasia; hypertension persisted postoperatively. All abnormalities in father and son were relieved by dexamethasone, 2 mg daily.

Subsequently, other cases of glucocorticoid-suppressible aldosteronism have been reported.[102–104] The condition appears to be familial, but the mode of inheritance is unclear. Biochemical studies seemed to rule out steroidogenic defects such as 21-hydroxylase, 11 β-hydroxylase, or 17-hydroxylase deficiency. In several cases, urinary 17-hydroxycorticoids or 17-ketogenic steroids were slightly elevated,[101,104] whereas in others these urinary metabolites were depressed.[102,103] In one report several weeks of glucocorticoid treatment were required for a complete response.[104] This suggested that prolonged trials with dexamethasone might be advisable in patients with evidence of primary aldosteronism to rule out any glucocorticoid-suppressible cases, particularly if diagnostic procedures fail to identify an adenoma.

Secondary Aldosteronism

This label refers to the pathologic state that results from overproduction of aldosterone due to hyperstimulation of the adrenals by the renin-angiotensin system. The term should not be applied without qualification to clinical situations in which aldosterone secretion increases in response to sodium depletion or to a reduced effective blood volume, which is a normal compensatory response mediated by the renin-angiotensin system. Although aldosterone secretion and plasma renin activity are increased in either circumstance, secondary aldosteronism is characterized by hypertension and metabolic features of mineralocorticoid excess, such as hypokalemia and alkalosis, whereas compensatory responses result in markedly diminished sodium excretion but do not raise blood pressure above normal. Causes of secondary aldosteronism and the various conditions that result in compensatory increases in aldosterone secretion are listed in Table 145-3.

Accelerated and Renovascular Hypertension: Secondary aldosteronism most commonly is caused by disorders that compromise renal perfusion, i.e., accelerated malignant essential hypertension or renal artery stenosis.[91,92,105] Reduced mean pressure in the afferent glomerular arteriole activates the renin–angiotensin system, which in turn stimulates aldosterone production and leads to manifestations of mineralocorticoid excess. Thus, hypokalemia is a common occurrence in advanced stages of essential hypertension and severe forms of renal artery stenosis.[91,92,106] Total adrenalectomy usually relieves the hypokalemia but does not effectively lower the blood pressure. Thus, it is doubtful that aldosterone hypersecretion is a major factor in the pathogenesis of hypertension in secondary aldosteronism.

It has been proposed that in malignant hypertension and lesser degrees of essential hypertension associated with high renin values blood pressure elevations are sustained or reinforced mainly by the vasoconstrictor and vasculotoxic effects of the excessively high angiotensin levels, and the associated aldosterone hypersecretion contributes a volume-dependent component to the hypertensive process only when sodium excretion is impeded by renal damage.[105,107] Several clinical observations tend to support the proposition that hypertension in these hyperreninemic states may be due to direct vascular effects of angiotensin. Hypertension in such cases is not effectively controlled by therapeutic measures that produce volume depletion,[107] but it is dramatically relieved by propranolol, which inhibits renin release; lowering of blood pressure is commensurate with the depression of renin activity produced by propranolol.[108] Malignant hypertension, which often cannot be controlled, and even may be aggravated by removal of excess fluid and salt during hemodialysis, is dramatically improved by nephrectomy.[109]

On the other hand, there is no clear relationship between plasma renin levels and the occurrence of hypertension in renal artery stenosis. Although peripheral plasma renin activity frequently is elevated in renovascular hypertension, in many cases it is normal or low.[110] Functionally significant renovascular lesions are distinguished by finding substantially higher renal vein renin levels on the affected side than on the contralateral side, even when peripheral plasma renin activity is not elevated, and differences between the two sides are amplified by upright posture or

Table 145-3. Causes of Secondary Aldosteronism

I. Pathologic: excessive stimulation of aldosterone secretion
   A. Renovascular hypertension
      1. Accelerated essential hypertension
      2. Renal artery stenosis
   B. Juxtaglomerular cell tumors
II. Physiologic: compensatory response to volume depletion
   A. Sodium depletion
   B. Normal pregnancy
   C. Cirrhosis
   D. Nephrotic syndrome
   E. Idiopathic edema
   F. Diuretic therapy*
   G. Bartter's Syndrome†

*Aldosterone hypersecretion contributes to hypokalemia.
†Relationship of aldosterone to pathogenesis of hypokalemia is uncertain.

sodium depletion.[111] The differing levels of peripheral plasma renin activity noted in patients with renovascular hypertension have their counterparts in experimental animal models.[92,105] When one renal artery is clipped and the other kidney is left untouched, hypertension results which is characterized by increased plasma renin activity, volume contraction, and natriuresis from the normal kidney. In this model striking reductions in blood pressure occur following administration of angiotensin antibodies or peptide angiotensin antagonists. When one renal artery is clipped and the other kidney is removed, the ensuing hypertension is characterized by low or normal renin, because of impaired sodium excretion. Since manifestations of excessive renin secretion may be related to direct effects of components of the renin-angiotensin system as well as to aldosterone, perhaps it would be more appropriate to designate the resultant syndrome as secondary "hyperrenism" rather than "aldosteronism."

Differentiation of secondary from primary aldosteronism usually is not difficult. Malignant hypertension is associated with evidence of impaired renal function and high renin values. Rarely, malignant hypertension may result from primary aldosteronism,[112] but diagnosis of such cases may be of academic interest, since removal of the offending aldosteronoma would not effect a cure once renal damage had occurred. Secondary aldosteronism due to renal artery occlusion may simulate primary aldosteronism, since renal function may not be severely impaired.[106] However, peripheral renin values would not be suppressed, although they are not elevated in all cases of renovascular hypertension.

Renin-Secreting Tumors (primary reninism): Renin-secreting tumors are a rare cause of a hypertensive syndrome characterized by markedly increased plasma renin activity, aldosterone hypersecretion, and hypokalemia.[113] Almost all of these tumors have been of renal origin and usually are comprised of cellular elements of the juxtaglomerular apparatus. Histopathologically, juxtaglomerular cell tumors resemble hemangiopericytomas, but some also contain cells similar to paraganglionomas or carotid body tumors, as well as tubular components.[114] Excessive renin production has also been attributed to Wilm's tumors and to a clear cell carcinoma of the kidney.[115,116] Ectopic renin production from an oat cell carcinoma has also been suspected in one reported case.[117]

Failure to recognize the cause of aldosteronism in several cases has led to adrenalectomy, which did not relieve hypertension. Removal of the tumor by unilateral nephrectomy results in a prompt decline in plasma renin activity to subnormal levels and cure of hypertension. Thus, hypertension in this syndrome also seems to be maintained mainly by a component of the renin–angiotensin system, presumably angiotensin II, rather than by aldosterone. Evidence that these tumors are capable of secreting renin is found in studies showing that tumor tissue has a very high concentration of renin; this is shown by identifying renin in tumor cells with immunofluorescent staining techniques and by demonstrating renin production in tumor cell incubates.[118]

Renin secretion in patients with these tumors does not respond to maneuvers that affect sodium balance. However, normal circadian variations and responses of plasma renin activity to postural stimuli have been observed, indicating that renin production by the tumor is not completely autonomous.[118] Thus, responsiveness to changes in salt balance seems to depend upon the normal anatomic relationship of juxtaglomerular cells to the nephron; but dislocated cells presumably retain the capacity to respond to systemically transmitted humoral agents such as sympathomimetic amines.

Diagnosis of renin-secreting tumors could be difficult. Demonstration of markedly elevated plasma renin activity in hypertensive patients with hypokalemia would distinguish this syndrome from primary aldosteronism but not from renovascular hypertension with secondary aldosteronism. Renal vein renin measurements would not in themselves be diagnostic, since unilateral overproduction of renin would be found with either renal artery stenosis or a renin-secreting tumor. Selective renal arteriography may reveal a tumor, but if none is visualized, the failure to identify a renovascular lesion in a patient with unilaterally elevated renin secretion should make one highly suspicious of a renin-secreting tumor. Most patients with this syndrome have been young, and hypertension has not always been associated with hypokalemia. Although only a small number of cases have been reported, the actual incidence is unknown. The diagnosis of a renin-secreting tumor should be considered in young hypertensives with elevated plasma renin activity whether or not there is hypokalemia.

Compensatory Responses to Volume Depletion:

Dietary sodium deprivation: Sodium depletion and other conditions that reduce the effective blood volume stimulate renin release, which leads to increased aldosterone secretion. This is a normal compensatory response, and, accordingly, renin and aldosterone secretion do not increase more than required to restore the effective blood volume. Nonetheless, aldosterone and renin may rise to very high levels during extreme sodium deprivation,[62,119] higher than in many cases of secondary aldosteronism, but hypertension and hypokalemia do not occur. On the contrary, as shown in Figure 145-9, potassium balance actually becomes positive despite increased aldosterone secretion. Presumably, the lack of kaliuresis is related to decreased distal tubular sodium delivery

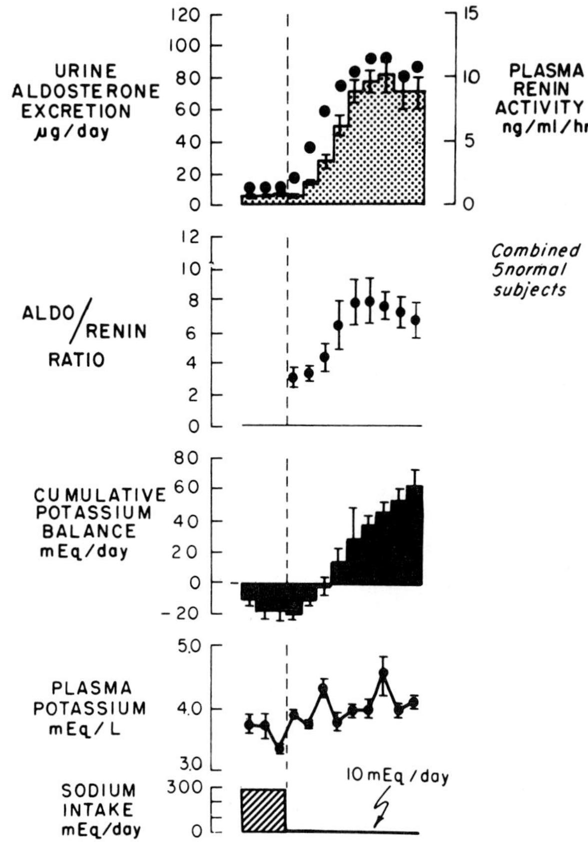

Fig. 145-9. Effect of sodium depletion on aldosterone excretion and potassium balance. (From Laragh et al: *Am. J. Med. 53:* 649, 1972.)

because proximal sodium reabsorption is enhanced by the hypovolemia associated with sodium depletion. Thus, when aldosterone increases in response to sodium deprivation, it causes sodium retention unaccompanied by potassium wasting; the threat of volume depletion is successfully countered by an appropriate reduction in sodium excretion, and the effective blood volume is restored to normal without pathologic consequences.

Pregnancy: Normal pregnancy is associated with markedly increased levels of aldosterone, desoxycorticosterone, as well as estrogens, which possess sodium-retaining activity in humans.[120–122] Nonetheless, pregnant women do not exhibit metabolic manifestations of mineralocorticoid excess, and blood pressure actually falls below prepregnancy values during the first trimester. Indeed, there is considerable evidence that normal pregnancy results in a tendency toward sodium depletion despite the salt-retaining action of the aforementioned steroids.[123]

Aldosterone secretion is regulated by normal mechanisms during pregnancy.[124] Increased aldosterone is associated with elevated plasma renin activity and both are as responsive to changes in salt intake or posture as in nongravidas. The very high rate of aldosterone excretion in pregnancy is readily suppressed by administered mineralocorticoids, and diuretic-induced salt loss results in further increments in aldosterone excretion. Thus, since renin activity and aldosterone secretion can respond normally to variations in salt intake or in the effective blood volume, it is reasonable to assume that the activity of the renin–angiotensin–aldosterone system is increased during normal pregnancy only to the extent required to maintain salt and/or volume homeostasis.

More direct evidence that aldosterone secretion must be augmented to prevent sodium depletion is provided by studies in which aldosterone secretion in third trimester women was experimentally decreased by administering the heparinoid, RO 1-8307.[125] Heparin and several related heparinoids selectively impair aldosterone production by means of an undefined mechanism.[126] As shown in Figure 145-10, when the increased secretion of aldosterone in normal gravidas was reduced by prolonged treatment with the heparinoid, substantial sodium losses ensued. One subject developed clinical evidence of sodium depletion. It is particularly noteworthy that sodium losses occurred during treatment even though aldosterone excretion did not fall below normal nongravid levels. After stopping treatment reversal of natriuresis did not occur until aldosterone excretion had risen to previous high control rates. The occurrence of substantial sodium losses in the face of higher than normal aldosterone excretion rates indicates that augmented aldosterone secretion is required to maintain sodium balance. It also strongly supports the proposition that potent factors oppose the sodium-retaining effects of aldosterone during pregnancy.

Several known factors in pregnancy promote sodium loss. The glomerular filtration rate is increased by 50 percent.[127] Consequently, there must be a commensurate increment in tubular reabsorption of sodium if salt-wasting is to be avoided. Another factor promoting sodium excretion is increased progesterone production. Progesterone is natriuretic by virture of its capacity to inhibit the action of mineralocorticoids.[128] Thus, the convergent effects of at least these two factors result in a sodium-losing tendency that is offset by increased aldosterone secretion. The need to retain additional sodium for the developing conceptus and for physiologic expansion of the maternal extracellular fluid spaces imposes a further stimulus for increased aldosterone production.[129] In addition, there is relaxation of vascular smooth muscle during pregnancy, perhaps due to progesterone[130a] or to vasodepressor effects of prostaglandins which are increased in pregnancy.[130b] These not

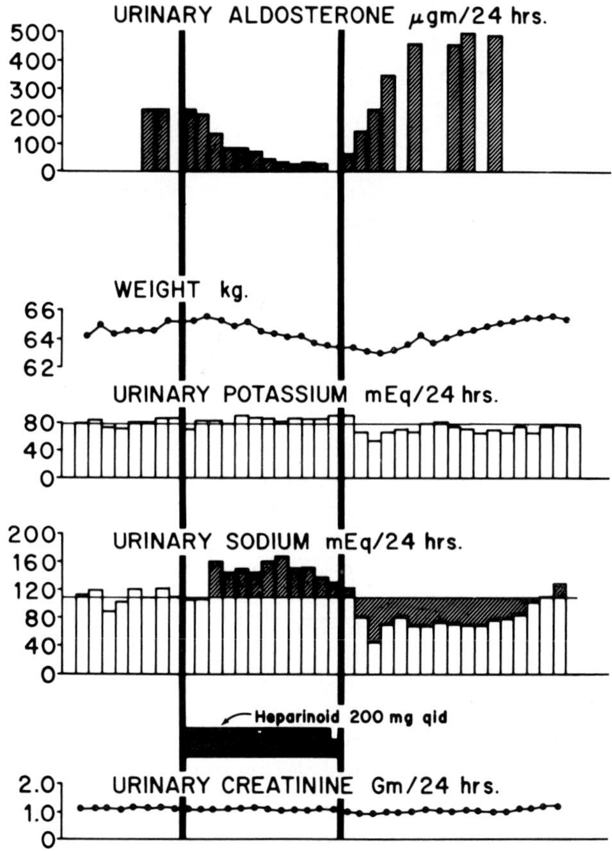

Fig. 145-10. Effect of intramuscular administration of the heparinoid RO1-8307 to a normal 21-year-old third trimester primigravida. (From Ehrlich: *Am. J. Obstet. Gynecol. 109:* 963, 1971.)

only may account for the lowering of blood pressure observed in early midpregnancy, but also would tend to accentuate the reduction in effective blood volume that occurs upon assuming the upright posture. This may explain the remarkable influence that slight changes in posture have upon plasma renin activity and renal sodium handling in normal pregnant women.[131] Merely changing from a lateral recumbent to a supine position results in a substantial rise in plasma renin activity and sharply reduced sodium excretion.

The compensatory increase in aldosterone secretion during pregnancy does not produce potassium wasting, probably because the tendency toward sodium depletion results in diminished distal tubular sodium delivery, just as in sodium deprivation in nongravidas. However, a remarkable finding in pregnancy is that renal potassium excretion is not increased by mineralocorticoid administration and high salt intake, even after escape occurs.[132] There is evidence that the absence of kaliuresis in this circumstance may be due to progesterone.

The cause of excessive sodium retention in preeclampsia is obscure. Aldosterone secretion and plasma renin concentration are lower in preeclampsia than in normal pregnancy and in severe cases may be reduced to normal nongravid levels.[133–135] Thus, increased aldosterone does not seem to play a role in maintaining the preeclamptic state, and presumably is not involved in its pathogenesis. Since the high rate of aldosterone secretion in normal pregnancy is suppressed by high salt intake or administered mineralocorticoids, the progressive decline in aldosterone secretion with increasing severity of preeclampsia probably is due to excessive sodium retention caused by factors other than aldosterone. Preeclampsia is also characterized by spasm of vascular smooth muscle, and this might tend to increase the *effective* blood volume and contribute to the suppressive influence of the retained sodium.

As previously noted, desoxycorticosterone is secreted in large amounts during normal pregnancy.[121,124] If desoxycorticosterone secretion were unresponsive to volume hyperexpansion, as in nonpregnant individuals, it would present a substantial nonsuppressible level of mineralocorticoid activity. During maternal complications such as preeclampsia, in which aldosterone secretion may be appropriately suppressed, persistently high desoxycorticosterone levels, although reported to be no higher than in normotensive pregnancies, might be excessive relative to the existing degree of sodium retention and contribute to the pathogenesis of hypertension.

Hypoalbuminemic states (nephrotic syndrome and hepatic cirrhosis): In nephrotic syndrome more albumin is lost in the urine than can be replaced by hepatic synthesis, because of altered glomerular permability; in hepatic cirrhosis there is reduced synthesis of albumin by the liver. In either situation hypoalbuminemia results, and the effective blood volume is reduced because of the decreased intravascular oncotic pressure. Activation of the renin–angiotensin system leads to increased aldosterone production and urinary sodium excretion is markedly diminished. This is identical to the compensatory response induced by sodium deprivation in normal individuals. However, in contrast to chronic sodium deprivation, in which a normal effective blood volume is reestablished promptly and maintained by an appropriate reduction in sodium excretion, the decreased effective blood volume in hypoalbuminemic states cannot be restored to normal even by the most avid retention of sodium. Because of the decreased intravascular oncotic pressure, retained sodium and associated water transudes into the interstitial space and hypovolemia is not repaired. Sodium retention is unremitting and gross edema develops. In cirrhosis, increased hydrostatic pressure in the portal circulation is an additional local factor that favors transudation of fluid into the peritoneal cavity and ascites forms. Thus, the compensatory response in these conditions is excessive in the sense that it produces pathologic consequences; perhaps for this reason the term *secondary aldosteronism* may be appropriate.

Hypokalemia is not a prominent feature of these hypoalbuminemic states. In cirrhosis hypokalemia may frequently result from gastrointestinal losses coupled with poor nutrition or prior diuretic therapy, and avid retention of sodium may not only be unassociated with renal potassium wasting but at times may occur with a positive potassium balance.[136,137] The lack of kaluresis in this circumstance may not be entirely explained on the basis of decreased distal tubular sodium delivery since hypoalbuminemia reduces peritubular oncotic pressure, which would be expected to oppose the increase in proximal tubular reabsorption that occurs with hypovolemia. Nonetheless, fractional proximal sodium reabsorption is increased in patients with cirrhosis who retain sodium.[78] Recent evidence suggests that proximal sodium reabsorption may not be increased in nephrotic syndrome, so that excessive sodium retention must be due to greatly increased distal reabsorption.[138] The effectiveness of aldosterone inhibitors such as spironolactone in promoting natriuresis in these edematous patients is consistent with the proposition that there is substantial distal sodium reabsorption, which is dependent upon increased mineralocorticoid activity, presumably from aldosterone.

Diuretic therapy: Diuretics induce renal loss of body fluids by interfering with tubular reabsorption of sodium at various nephron sites. Thiazides, ethacrynic acid, and furosemide inhibit sodium reabsorption in the ascending limb of Henle's loop.[139–141] This action of thiazides is limited to the cortical segment; ethacrynic acid and furosemide act upon the entire ascending limb and are more potent natriuretic agents than thiazides. Any of these diuretics is capable of producing a brisk natriuretic response associated with kaliuresis. Spironolactone, triamterene, and amiloride inhibit distal tubular sodium reabsorption.[140,142,143] These diuretics do not induce very substantial sodium losses, but they decrease potassium excretion. They are often referred to as *potassium-sparing diuretics*.

Administration of diuretics may result in volume depletion, which activates the renin–angiotensin–aldosterone system. Although this compensatory response limits the sodium loss, it also contributes to development of electrolyte disturbances during prolonged treatment with diuretics that act upon the loop of Henle. Inhibition of sodium reabsorption at this site results in increased sodium delivery to the distal nephron even though sodium reabsorption in the proximal convoluted tubule is increased by volume contraction. Thus, conditions in the distal nephron are more similar to those in primary aldosteronism than to those in sodium deprivation, and as in primary aldosteronism they result in hypokalemia and metabolic alkalosis. However, in contrast to primary aldosteronism, in which the extracellular fluid volume is hyperexpanded, diuretics result in volume contraction, which increases proximal bicarbonate reabsorption. This tends to reinforce the alkalosis generated by enhanced distal hydrogen ion secretion and may account for the urine pH being lower than in primary aldosteronism. Hypokalemic alkalosis is a well-recognized side effect of long-term therapy with potent diuretics, and its occurrence ordinarily does not present a diagnostic problem. However, occasionally hypokalemic alkalosis may be due to surreptitious self-administration of diuretics, in which case the diagnosis may be suspected only by results of careful metabolic studies and can be confirmed by analyzing urine for excreted diuretics.[144]

Potassium-sparing diuretics rarely produce sufficient sodium loss to cause appreciable volume depletion. However, they may result in life-threatening hyperkalemia if administered to patients with impaired potassium excretion due to renal disease.[145] These diuretics may be especially useful when used in conjunction with more potent non–potassium-sparing diuretics, since they counter the effects of the compensatory rise in aldosterone, reinforcing the natriuresis while minimizing the loss of potassium and hydrogen ions.[140]

Bartter's syndrome: In 1962 Bartter and co-workers described two patients who were normotensive but exhibited features of secondary aldosteronism, i.e., hypokalemic alkalosis, increased aldosterone secretion, and markedly elevated serum angiotensin concentrations.[146] Blood pressure was remarkably insensitive to infused angiotensin. Renal biopsies revealed hyperplasia and hypertrophy of the juxtaglomerular apparatus. An example of juxtaglomerular hyperplasia is shown in Figure 145-11. An adrenal gland excised from one patient was grossly normal but histologic examination showed hypertrophy of the zona glomerulosa.

One of the patients was dwarfed and the other was of normal stature but had grown slowly; both were mentally retarded. Glomerular abnormalities were noted in both patients. In one, approximately 40 percent of glomeruli were atrophic, the abnormal glomeruli always being associated with a greatly enlarged juxtaglomerular apparatus. The glomerular filtration rate was decreased in this patient. In the other, glomeruli were about twice the size of normal. Urinary concentrating ability was impaired and was not improved by administration of antidiuretic hormone. Renal hydrogen ion excretion was normal, as evidenced by the response to ammonium chloride administration.

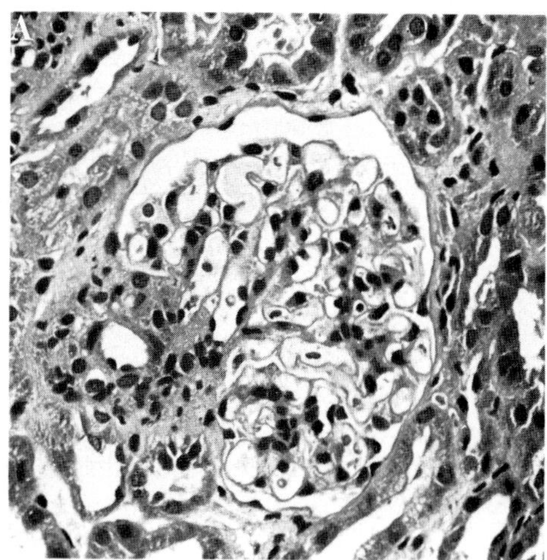

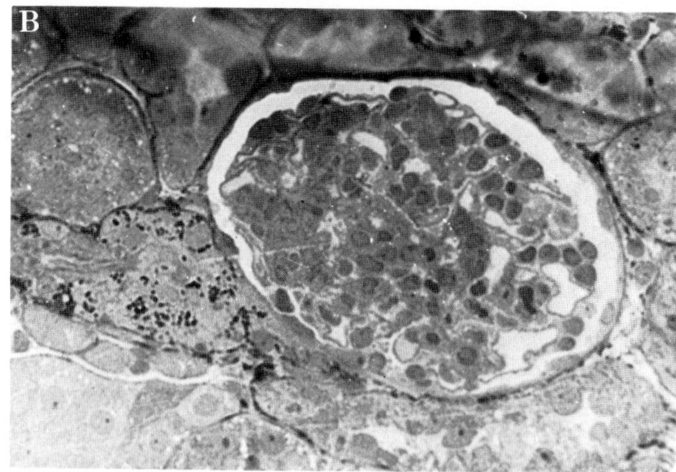

Fig. 145-11. Light micrographs of glomeruli from a patient with Bartter's syndrome. A. Markedly enlarged juxtaglomerular apparatus completely surrounding the afferent arteriole. H&E. B. Epon-embedded section showing multiple granules in the enlarged juxtaglomerular apparatus. Toluidine blue. (From Trygstad et al: *Pediatrics 44:* 235, 1969.

Aldosterone secretion was not suppressed by oral salt loading or infused albumin. During sodium deprivation one patient conserved sodium normally, whereas urinary sodium loss continued to exceed intake in the other. However, sodium excretion in the latter patient fell to zero during the infusion of albumin, indicating that the kidney was capable of conserving sodium. Serum potassium concentration was not restored fully to normal by sodium deprivation even when potassium intake was raised to 170–250 meq/day. Administration of spironolactone produced potassium retention and a rise in serum potassium concentration, associated with increased sodium excretion and negative sodium balance. Bartter and co-workers postulated that the primary defect was impaired vascular responsiveness to the pressor effect of angiotensin, requiring a compensatory increase in renin secretion to maintain a normal blood pressure and effective blood volume. Increased renin would not elevate the blood pressure to hypertensive levels, but would lead to aldosterone hypersecretion and metabolic manifestations of aldosterone excess.

Another hypothesis is that the syndrome results from a defect in proximal sodium reabsorption. Pathophysiologic consequences of such an abnormality would resemble those induced by diuretic therapy. Activation of the renin–angiotensin system stimulates a compensatory rise in aldosterone secretion, which prevents excessive sodium loss; but, because of increased distal sodium delivery, it also causes severe hypokalemia and alkalosis. This hypothesis is supported by the observation of persistent urinary sodium wasting during dietary sodium deprivation in some patients with the syndrome.[147,148] Although most conserve sodium normally in response to this challenge, this might be achieved in the face of defective proximal reabsorption by an adaptive increase in distal sodium reabsorption sustained by high levels of aldosterone.

In one reported case increased aldosterone secretion was depressed by administration of albumin, aminoglutethimide, and dexamethasone.[149] Surprisingly, the reduction in aldosterone was not accompanied by an appreciable rise in sodium excretion and urinary potassium wasting did not subside. In another case, subtotal adrenalectomy did not correct hypokalemia even though aldosterone secretion was decreased substantially,[150] and persistent hypokalemia has been noted following total adrenalectomy.[148] These observations suggest that there must be a primary defect in tubular potassium transport as well as impaired sodium reabsorption. Accordingly, based on recent advances in our knowledge of sodium chloride reabsorption by the kidney, Kurtzman and Gutierrez presented a hypothesis involving a single tubular defect to explain Bartter's syndrome.[150a] Since sodium and potassium are reabsorbed passively in the thick ascending limb of the loop of Henle along the gradient established by active *chloride* transport,[16,17,51] a defect in the chloride transport mechanism would result in urinary losses of both sodium chloride and potassium chloride. Resultant volume contraction would activate the renin-angiotensin system leading to increased aldosterone secretion, thereby reinforcing the hypokalemia, but potassium wasting would persist even in the absence of aldosterone because of the primary tubular defect.

Another intriguing observation is that elevated plasma renin activity and aldosterone secretion in a patient with Bartter's syndrome were promptly lowered by propranolol.[151] However, despite the fall in aldosterone, sodium excretion *decreased,* and the serum potassium level failed to rise. The authors of this report proposed that elevated renin was the cause of volume depletion rather than the result of it. They cited the observation that large doses of angiotensin may have a natriuretic effect and demonstrated a slight rise in fractional sodium and potassium excretion during infusion of a small, subpressor dose of angiotensin to their patient while endogenous renin was depressed by propranolol. However, their hypothesis is difficult to reconcile with the findings in renin-secreting tumors, in which increased renin secretion leads to secondary aldosteronism with hypertension.

Glomerular lesions such as those described by Bartter and co-workers have been noted in other case reports.[147,152] Examination of serial sections of glomeruli by light and electron microscopy reveals defects that could result in glomerulodistal tubular shunts, perhaps due to early glomerulitis.[152] Such a lesion could result in increased delivery of proximal fluid directly into the distal convoluted tubule. Another interesting observation is that erythrocyte sodium transport is abnormal in patients with Bartter's syndrome and their relatives.[153] If this alteration could be related to the pathophysiology of Bartter's syndrome it would lend support to the assumption that there is a genetically determined defect of membrane ion transport. Recent observations indicate that urinary prostaglandins E_2 and $F_{2\alpha}$ are increased in patients with Bartter's syndrome. Treatment with prostaglandin synthetase inhibitors, indomethacin or ibuprofen, in sufficient doses to depress prostglandin excretion resulted in partial or complete reversal of hyperreninemia and hyperaldosteronism, but did not produce sustained amelioration of hypokalemia.[153a] Although these findings provide additional evidence that prostaglandins play an important role in the release of renin, very recent studies in hypokalemic dogs seem to indicate that the increased production of prostaglandins in Bartter's syndrome is secondary to potassium depletion.[153b]

Treatment of Bartter's syndrome generally is unsatisfactory. Lowering aldosterone secretion by means of adrenalectomy or opposing its action by administering spironolactone or triamterene usually produces only a transient rise in the serum potassium level and may result in excessive urinary sodium loss. Potassium supplements usually do not restore the serum potassium concentration to normal, but the growth rate has increased following partial correction of potassium depletion.[147] Perhaps propranolol will prove useful in the treatment of Bartter's syndrome when used in combination with other drugs such as spironolactone. The variant features in some cases, such as suppressibility of aldosterone, lack of clearly elevated aldosterone secretion, decreased renal function, and impaired hydrogen ion secretion, as well as differences observed in the ability to conserve sodium and in familial incidence may indicate that there is more than one etiology for the syndrome. Juxtaglomerular hyperplasia and refractoriness to the pressor effects of infused angiotensin are not distinctive findings. Presumably, any abnormality that causes sodium depletion or hypovolemia could result in increased renin secretion and decreased sensitivity to exogenous angiotensin. Indeed, juxtaglomerular hyperplasia has been described in a patient with volume depletion due to gastrointestinal loss of fluid and electrolyte.[154]

Idiopathic edema: Idiopathic edema is a clinical condition that occurs almost exclusively in women of childbearing age; it is characterized by intermittent, generalized swelling without apparent cardiac, renal, or hepatic disease. Typically, affected women complain vociferously of periodic bouts of facial puffiness, swelling of the extremities, abdominal distention, and fullness of the breasts, which worsen with physical activity. Other common complaints include lassitude and postural weakness, which may be accentuated by hypokalemia and volume depletion secondary to excessive use of potent diuretics. Women presenting with this syndrome are often emotionally unstable and seem irritable or depressed. Objective evidence of swelling, such as pitting edema, may not be apparent to the examining physician, but patients describe swelling of such proportions that larger than usual size clothing must be worn, and they are able to document marked fluid retention by recording weight gains exceeding 10 lb from morning to night. Episodes of swelling usually are unrelated temporally to the menstrual cycle, but may be superimposed upon premenstrual tension, which also is associated with varying degrees of sodium retention and altered emotional states.

Postural factors are important in the pathophysiology of idiopathic edema.[155–158] Women with the syndrome retain sodium avidly when they are upright and excrete sodium normally during recumbency. The excessive sodium retention that occurs when women with idiopathic edema assume the upright posture is associated with a greater rise in plasma renin activity and rate of aldosterone excretion than in normal women.[156] These findings could indicate either that the renin–angiotensin–aldosterone system is hyperresponsive to postural stimuli in idiopathic edema or that the effective blood volume is diminished to a greater degree than normal by upright posture. The observation that patients with idiopathic edema have a more pronounced fall in systolic blood pressure and a greater increase in leg volume than normal women when they stand up is consistent with the latter possibility.[156] Furthermore, the exaggerated responses of renin, aldosterone, and sodium exretion to upright posture in patients with idiopathic edema are reduced toward normal by leg bandaging, which presumably limits the drop in effective blood volume.[156]

The reason for the impaired ability of patients with this syndrome to maintain a normal effective blood volume in the standing position is not clear. Findings in various case studies suggest that the effective blood volume may be compromised by several mechanisms. Venous dilatation, possibly due to effects of ovarian hormones, with dependent pooling of blood may be a common pathogenic factor.[157] Venomotor tone is reduced by pregnancy or administration of oral contraceptives.[130] Other mechanisms suggested in individual case reports include abnormal albumin metabolism,[159] increased capillary permeability,[155] and abnormal hemodynamic responses to upright posture due to occult cardiomyopathy.[160] Careful hemodynamic studies in 11 women with idiopathic edema supported hypotheses that upright posture results in excessive pooling of fluid in dependent parts of the body, but only 1 woman had evidence of abnormal cardiac function.[161]

Diagnosis of idiopathic edema can be made on the basis of a characteristic history and evidence of marked weight fluctuations induced by changes in posture. Any patient in whom the diagnosis is suspected should be asked to keep a careful record of morning and evening weights for at least 1 week. Patients with idiopathic edema are very difficult to manage. They seem unwilling to tolerate even the mildest manifestations of the syndrome and any subjective sensation of swelling brings forth an unrelenting demand for complete relief. Potent diuretics should be avoided. They aggravate the tendency toward volume depletion, causing orthostatic symptoms, and may also produce hypokalemia. Mild diuretics, particularly aldosterone antagonists, may be useful, but remain effective only if used intermittently. Sympathomimetics, such as ephedrine, often diminish sodium retention and alleviate orthostatic symptoms. The occasional case due to underlying cardiomyopathy is dramatically benefited by digitalization[161].

Syndromes Not Caused by Aldosterone

Desoxycorticosterone and Corticosterone.

Cushing's Syndrome: Hypokalemic alkalosis occurs occasionally in Cushing's syndrome. It is relatively uncommon in bilateral adrenal hyperplasia due to Cushing's disease,[162] more frequent in adrenocortical carcinoma,[163] and a predominant feature of the ectopic ACTH syndrome.[164] Indeed, when severe hypokalemia does occur in Cushing's syndrome it raises strong suspicion of a malignant etiology—either primary adrenal carcinoma or a nonadrenal neoplasm that secretes ACTH.[163,165] Hypokalemic alkalosis in Cushing's disease (bilateral adrenal hyperplasia) usually is not a manifestation of aldosterone excess, since aldosterone secretion is either low or normal.[162,166] Although the presence and severity of hypokalemia seems to be directly related to the degree of cortisol hypersecretion,[162] development of the metabolic abnormality most likely is due to increased secretion of ACTH-dependent mineralocorticoids, such as desoxycorticosterone and corticosterone, rather than to the relatively weak mineralocorticoid activity of cortisol itself.[165,166] The ectopic ACTH syndrome, which is often associated with higher plasma ACTH levels than found in Cushing's disease,[167] is also associated with correspondingly greater increases in secretion of desoxycorticosterone and corticosterone.[165,166] Therefore, it is not surprising that hypokalemic alkalosis is such a prominent finding in the ectopic ACTH syndrome, although it is difficult to understand the minimal evidence of hypercortisolism that characterizes this syndrome.

Hypokalemia also has been attributed to desoxycorticosterone and corticosterone in Cushing's syndrome due to adrenocortical neoplasms. Increased desoxycorticosterone secretion in some cases of adrenocortical carcinoma may be due to an 11β-hydroxylation block. Evidence for this is provided by studies demonstrating increased excretion of tetrahydrodesoxycortisol (THS) in patients with adrenal cancer.[168,169] Lipsett and co-workers reported that THS excretion was increased in every one of 13 patients with adrenal tumors who had increased urinary corticoid excretion.[168] Thus, urinary 17-hydroxycorticoids measured in cases of adrenal cancer may be comprised mainly of metabolites of 11-desoxycortisol, a biologically inactive corticoid. This would explain the minimal evidence of cortisol excess in some patients with markedly elevated urinary corticoid excretion. The alterations in corticoid biosynthesis resulting from this acquired 11β-hydroxylation defect are similar to those induced by metyrapone or those observed in the hypertensive type of congenital adrenal hyperplasia (Fig. 145-12, see below).

Congenital Adrenal Hyperplasia: Desoxycorticosterone secretion is increased in the hypertensive type of congenital adrenal hyperplasia due to 11β-hydroxylase deficiency.[170–172] Abnormal corticoid biosynthesis resulting from this defect is shown in Figure 145-12. Although hypertension in this disorder is ascribed to mineralocorticoid activity from increased desoxycorticosterone, it is difficult to explain the absence of hypokalemia in most reported cases. This disorder may be associated with variable degrees of virilization and onset of manifestations may be delayed until adulthood.[172] Thus, it occurred to some investigators that mild variants of this type of congenital adrenal hyperplasia might be a cause of hypertension in some adults, either alone, particularly in men, or in association with slight evidence of androgen excess in women, such as in the Stein-Leventhal syndrome. Since the hallmark of 11β-hydroxylase deficiency is the finding of substantial quantities of 11-desoxycortisol metabolites in the urine, urinary THS measurements were performed in 88 hypertensive patients; but they did not reveal a case with evidence of this syndrome.[173]

Corticosterone and desoxycorticosterone secretion are increased in congenital adrenal hyperplasia due to 17α-hydroxylase deficiency.[174,175] Abnormal corticoid biosynthesis resulting from this defect is shown in Figure 145-13. This syndrome is characterized by hypertension, hypokalemic alkalosis, and sexual immaturity in females or male pseudohermaphroditism in genetic males. The sexual abnormalities are due to defective 17-hydroxylation activity in the gonads resulting in the absence of sex steroid production. The diagnosis can be suspected in postpubertal individuals with the above sexual abnormalities, low urinary excretion of 17-ketosteroids and 17-hydroxycorticoids, and low aldosterone and sex steroid measurements. In prepuberty, the syndrome would be less obvious in females than in males, and in either case, low urinary 17-ketosteroids and plasma sex steroid concentrations would not distinguish them from normal prepubertal individuals whose values are also low.

18-Hydroxydesoxycorticosterone (18(OH)DOC) Excess. Some considered the finding of suppressed plasma renin activity in patients with essential hypertension to be presumptive evidence of mineralocorticoid excess, and they suspected that an unknown mineralocorticoid might be involved in the pathogenesis of the hypertension, particularly in cases with low aldosterone.[176] 18(OH)DOC, an ACTH-dependent steroid, is normally secreted by human adrenal in amounts comparable to aldosterone.[86] Although it seems to have less sodium-retaining activity than desoxycorticosterone, it has a hypertensive action when administered to rats.[87]

Excess 18(OH)DOC secretion was found in 10 of 30 cases of essential hypertension with suppressed plasma renin activity.[86] The mean urinary 18(OH)DOC excretion was significantly higher in hypertensive patients with suppressed plasma renin activity than in hypertensives with normal renin responsiveness. Suppression of 18(OH)DOC secretion with dexamethasone treatment was associated with a decline in blood pressure. Four of five patients became normotensive when treated with large doses of spironolactone. Surgical exploration in five patients revealed adrenal abnormalities ranging from hyperplasia to adenomas, but only two of these patients became normotensive following adrenalectomy. It has been suggested that 10–20 percent of patients with low renin hypertension have elevated 18(OH)DOC excretion in urine.[85]

Studies in rats suggest that 18(OH)DOC has sodium-retaining and antidiuretic effects but is not kaluretic.[87] This might explain the

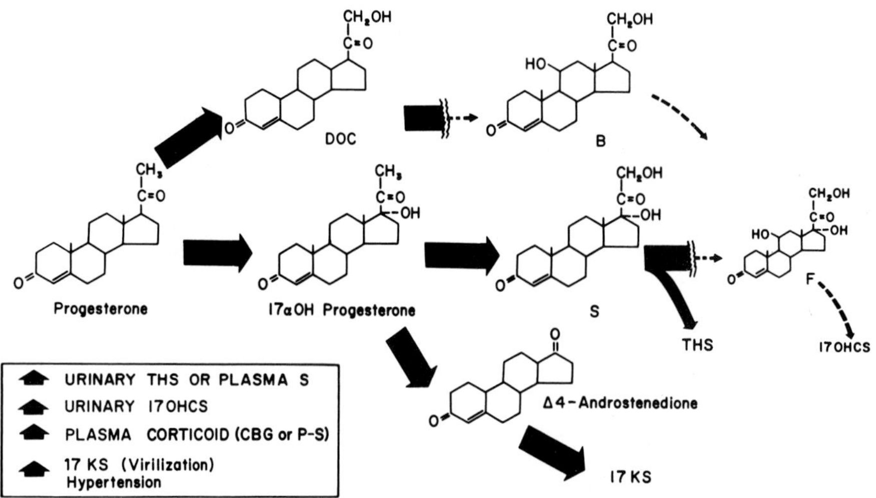

Fig. 145-12. Steroidogenic abnormalities in 11β-hydroxylase deficiency.

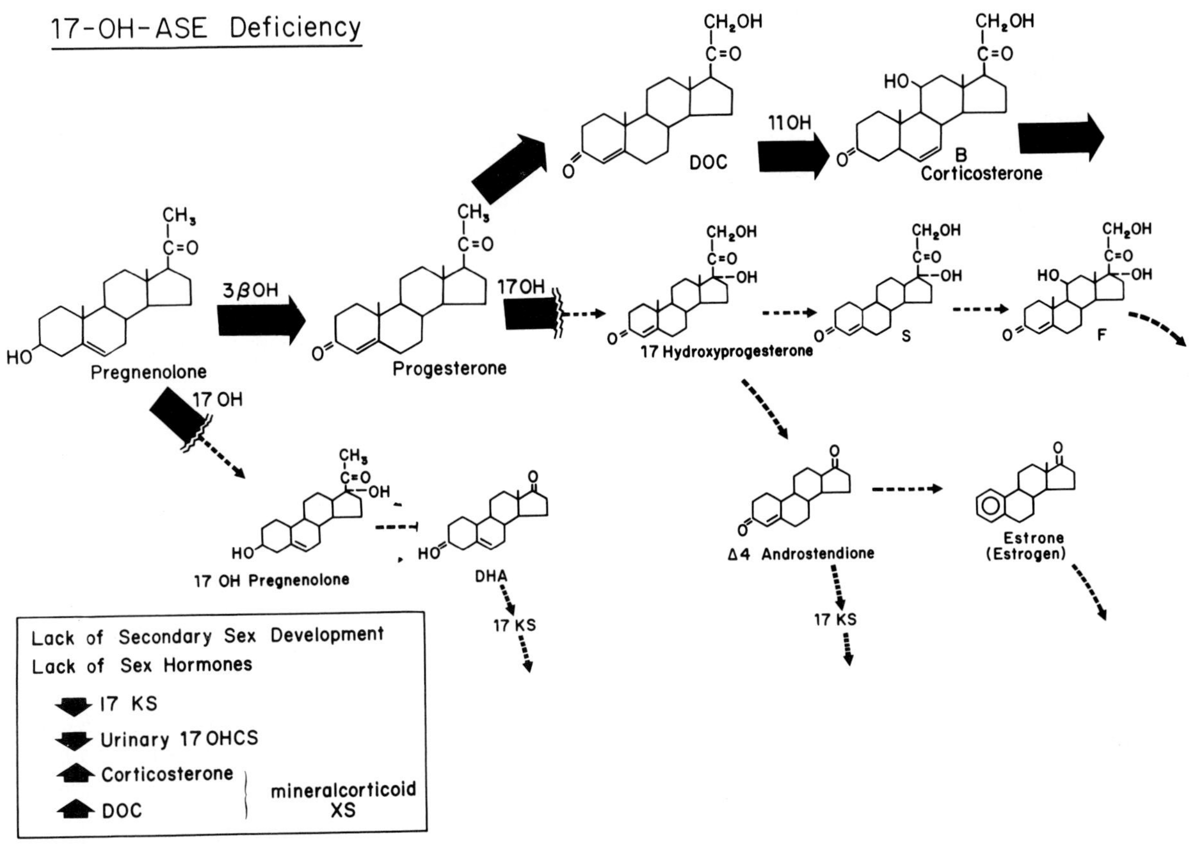

Fig. 145-13. Steroidogenic abnormalities in 17α-hydroxylase deficiency (Biglieri's syndrome).

lack of hypokalemia in cases of low renin hypertension with increased 18(OH)DOC secretion. However, the sodium-retaining effect of 18(OH)DOC is relatively weak, and it is difficult to understand how blood pressure elevations could result from the increments in secretion noted in the hypertensive patients. Recently, it has been proposed that 18(OH)DOC might be a precursor of a more potent corticoid of higher biologic potency.[177] Incubations of adrenal tissue from a patient with low renin hypertension showed a disproportionate conversion of 18(OH)DOC to dihydroxy DOC. This conversion product did not stimulate sodium transport in toad bladders and did not have significant mineralocorticoid activity in the rat, but it seemed to enhance the effect of aldosterone, perhaps due to a positive allosteric effect. Obviously, further studies are required to define the role of 18(OH)DOC and its derivatives in hypertensive disorders in man.

Licorice-Induced Syndrome of Mineralocorticoid Excess. Glycyrrhizinic acid, a constituent of licorice obtained from the root of the plant *Glycyrrhiza glabra,* has significant mineralocorticoid-like activity.[178] When ingested in licorice candy or in medications containing licorice extract, it can produce a clinical disorder that is characterized by hypertension and hypokalemia and resembles primary aldosteronism or other syndromes of mineralocorticoid excess.[179,180] Hypokalemia induced by licorice intoxication may be severe enough to cause myopathy with myoglobulinuria.[181] Hypokalemia and hypertension subside when licorice intake is discontinued.

Glycyrrhizinic acid was purified from crude licorice extract as the ammonium salt by Louis and Conn.[182] Administration of 2–5 g of the pure ammoniated compound to normal subjects results in marked sodium retention and kaliuresis as well as suppression of plasma renin activity and aldosterone secretion. The mineralocorticoidlike effects of glycyrrhizinic acid presumably are due to a direct renal action that is antagonized by the mineralocorticoid inhibitor, spironolactone.[183] Structurally, glycyrrhizinic acid resembles a cyclopentanophenanthrene steroid (Fig. 145-14).

Confectioner's licorice extract, which is the material used by all major licorice candy manufacturers in the United States, contains approximately 25 percent ammoniated glycyrrhizin. The average amount of this extract used by candy manufacturers is 2–3 percent by weight of the finished product.[184] Intoxication has resulted from chronic ingestion of two to three 36-g licorice candy bars daily, providing only about 0.5 g of active principle.[182]

The possibility of excessive licorice ingestion should be considered in any patient presenting with the syndrome of mineralocorticoid excess, especially if plasma renin activity and aldosterone secretion are suppressed. Patients often may reveal that licorice was ingested instead of regular meals as a self-styled weight reduction program. In past years intoxication was more often related to medications containing licorice extract. Patients frequently developed hypertension when licorice was used in treatment of peptic ulcers,[185] and fatal hypokalemia was observed in tuberculous patients treated with para-aminosalicylic acid flavored with licorice extract.[186]

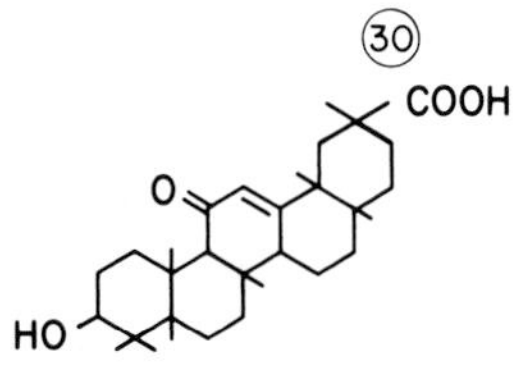

(30) COOH
O
HO

Fig. 145-14. Structural configuration of glycyrrhizinic acid.

Renal Disorders Simulating the Syndrome of Mineralocorticoid Excess

Liddle's Syndrome. Clinical disorders have been described with features of the syndrome of mineralocorticoid excess that cannot be related to the effects of any known mineralocorticoid; they have been attributed to intrinsic renal defects. Liddle's syndrome is characterized by hypertension and hypokalemic alkalosis with negligible aldosterone secretion.[187] It is familial and affects individuals of both sexes. Manifestations presumably result from increased distal tubular sodium reabsorption and potassium secretion independent of the effect of any known mineralocorticoid. Spironolactone, a mineralocorticoid inhibitor, does not improve abnormal electrolyte excretion in these patients. However, administration of triamterene, which interferes with distal tubular ion transport by means of an action that does not involve mineralocorticoid inhibition,[140,142] results in natriuresis and deceased potassium excretion. Blood pressure and serum electrolytes are restored to normal by treatment with triamterene in combination with low-salt diet, and they remain normal with long-term treatment with this regimen. Increased sodium transport has been observed in erythrocytes of patients with Liddle's syndrome, whereas sodium transport in erythrocytes from patients with primary aldosteronism did not differ from normal.[188] Demonstration of this abnormality in nonrenal tissue suggests that there might be a generalized, inherited abnormality of sodium transport in Liddle's syndrome.

Other Renal Disorders. Childhood occurrence of hypokalemia and renal potassium wasting, without hypertension, has also been ascribed to renal disorders. In familial juvenile nephronophthisis there is a chronic renal disorder manifested by persistent hypokalemia, polyuria, polydipsia, and growth retardation.[189] Aldosterone excretion is not elevated and can be suppressed by high salt intake. These children have obvious renal pathology consisting of progressive interstitial nephritis and glomerular damage, which eventually results in terminal renal failure. A striking feature of the disease is the absence of protein and formed elements in the urine despite extensive parenchymal damage. Hypokalemia and impaired ability to concentrate the urine may be the earliest indications of this disorder.

A nonhypertensive familial disorder characterized by hypokalemia and hypomagnesemia was described by Gitelman and co-workers.[190] These patients had high-normal aldosterone secretion rates and clearly elevated plasma renin activity. Spironolactone administration resulted in reversal of potassium wasting and natriuresis excretion, suggesting that abnormal electrolyte excretion was at least partly due to increased mineralocorticoid activity. Renal function was not impaired in these patients, and renal biopsies were not performed. Except for aldosterone values, which were high-normal rather than clearly elevated, clinical findings in these cases are the same as in Bartter's syndrome.

HYPOALDOSTERONISM

PATHOPHYSIOLOGY

Renal sodium wasting associated with impaired ability to excrete potassium are fundamental disturbances in electrolyte metabolism in Addison's disease that lead to hyponatremia, decreased extracellular fluid and blood volumes, hypotension, reduced glomerular filtration, nitrogen retention, and hyperkalemia. If untreated, there is progressive volume depletion, ultimately resulting in cardiovascular collapse complicated by severe hyperkalemia, and death ensues. Administration of replacement doses of a mineralocorticoid reverses these abnormalities and restores electrolyte balance to normal without affecting metabolic derangements due to glucocorticoid deficiency. Based on these observations, it has been assumed that the electrolyte disturbances characteristic of Addison's disease are manifestations of mineralocorticoid deficiency, and, accordingly it would be expected that the syndrome resulting from selective aldosterone deficiency would be characterized mainly by evidence(s) of sodium depletion associated with hyperkalemia.

However, although sodium wasting and hyponatremia are prominent features of congenital aldosterone deficiency in children, most adult cases of hypoaldosteronism have been characterized mainly by hyperkalemia. Indeed, it has even been argued that uncomplicated selective analdosteronism is essentially asymptomatic, and that some degree of renal insufficiency must be present in order for hyperkalemia to occur.[191,192] This argument is supported by observations that totally adrenalectomized patients seemingly remain asymptomatic without mineralocorticoid replacement therapy, while taking only a glucocorticoid, i.e., cortisone acetate 50 mg/day, and most adult cases of hypoaldosteronism with severe hyperkalemia have been associated with some evidence of intrinsic renal disease.

On the other hand, it has been clearly demonstrated that totally adrenalectomized patients maintained on cortisone alone are incapable of withstanding sodium deprivation.[193] Substantial negative sodium balances occur in these patients when dietary sodium intake is restricted. During the initial phase of sodium depletion, there is isotonic contraction of extracellular fluid and plasma volume, which is reasonably well tolerated, particularly if sodium loss is gradual. As sodium depletion approaches 50 percent of total exchangeable sodium, small additional losses rapidly lead to severe, symptomatic hyponatremia, associated with a rise in blood urea nitrogen and serum creatinine concentration. The relative water retention that must occur as hyponatremia develops probably is related to volume contraction, which limits the quantity of filtrate reaching diluting sites in the ascending limb of Henle's loop, and also stimulates release of antidiuretic hormone. Potassium retention occurs in these adrenalectomized subjects during sodium deprivation, but hyperkalemia is mild to moderate. Upon resuming high salt intake, prompt symptomatic improvement occurs even before there is an appreciable rise in the serum sodium concentration.

In an earlier study, performed prior to the availability of cortisone or other active glucocorticoid preparations, Thorn and co-workers observed the effects of withdrawing desoxycorticosterone acetate from patients with Addison's disease whose usual maintenance therapy consisted only of this mineralocorticoid.[194] Sudden withdrawal of therapy resulted in renal sodium loss and precipitated a crisis without necessarily causing a fall in serum sodium concentration.

Clinical observations that adrenalectomized or Addison's disease patients treated with cortisone alone seem to get along reasonably well do not justify the conclusion that a potent mineralocorticoid is not needed to maintain normal volume homeostasis or that uncomplicated selective analdosteronism is asymptomatic. The absence of overt manifestations in these patients is dependent upon several factors. The ability to tolerate mineralocorticoid deficiency is directly related to the sodium intake; with extremely high sodium intake aldosterone secretion normally is suppressed to a negligible rate. Therefore, providing salt supplements to patients with adrenal insufficiency is not merely a symptomatic treatment, but produces a physiologic state in which there is a reduced mineralocorticoid requirement. Moreover, sodium deprivation does not result in unremitting sodium loss in the absence of a mineralocorticoid. Nonaldosterone factors come into play and renal sodium excretion decreases as volume depletion progresses.[193,195] The presence and severity of symptoms is dependent upon the extent of hypovolemia that must develop before sodium balance is restored, and this in turn is related to the degree of sodium deprivation. Therefore, although sodium balance can be maintained in the absence of a mineralocorticoid, the plasma volume is extremely susceptible to changes in sodium intake. Moderate degrees of hypovolemia may be well tolerated, but any small additional sodium losses or further reductions in dietary sodium intake would result in rapid development of symptomatic hypovolemia with hyponatremia and hyperkalemia, as observed in metabolic studies of the effects of sodium deprivation in adrenalectomized patients treated with cortisome alone.[193]

Thus, impaired ability to conserve sodium is a characteristic feature of uncomplicated selective aldosterone deficiency. However, the development and severity of symptoms is dependent upon the extent of sodium depletion that develops. Substantial sodium depletion ultimately leads to hyponatremia with mild to moderate hyperkalemia. Disproportionately severe hyperkalemia does not occur unless renal function is diminished by intrinsic renal disease.

CLINICAL SYNDROMES

Patients with hypoaldosteronism have presented diverse findings and few cases have been characterized by typical features of aldosterone deficiency. The most common manifestation has been severe hyperkalemia, often resulting in cardiac arrhythmias or neuromuscular disturbances.[191,196,197] Indeed, at first glance, reported cases seem to present a confusing array of findings, with aldosterone deficiency being the only common feature. However, when considered on the basis of pathophysiologic mechanisms, as is customary with other endocrine-deficiency states, a more consistent relationship becomes apparent between the clinical findings and the various causes of hypoaldosteronism. Aldosterone deficiency may result from an intrinsic adrenal defect, i.e., primary aldosterone deficiency, or from lack of stimulation of aldosterone secretion because of defective regulatory mechanisms, i.e., secondary aldosterone deficiency (hyporeninemic hypoaldosteronism). Manifestations of aldosterone deficiency may also be due to an inability of the kidney to respond to aldosterone, i.e., pseudohypoaldosteronism. The pathogenesis and clinical features of these various types of hypoaldosteronism are discussed in the following sections. The various possible causes of hypoaldosteronism are summarized in Figure 145-15.

Primary Aldosterone Deficiency

Primary hypoaldosteronism is the clinical state that results from selective impairment of aldosterone secretion due to an intrinsic adrenal abnormality, either functional or anatomic. The diagnosis of primary hypoaldosteronism is based upon demonstrating the following: a subnormal rate of aldosterone secretion that is not increased by sodium deprivation and fails to respond to stimulation by administered angiotensin or ACTH; increased activity of the renin–angiotensin system; and preservation of normal cortisol secretion.

Congenital or Acquired Adrenal Defects. Aldosterone secretion may be selectively impaired by enzymatic defects in aldosterone biosynthesis. Cases of congenital hypoaldosteronism have been attributed to either 18-dehydrogenase or 18-hydroxylase deficiency.[198–200] These disorders most often occur in families and usually present as sodium-wasting syndromes in infancy. Clinical manifestations include growth retardation and failure to thrive associated with hyponatremia and hyperkalemia. Electrolyte abnormalities are restored to normal and growth rate is improved by administration of replacement doses of a potent mineralocorticoid and dietary salt supplements. Enzyme deficiencies in these cases have been deduced by measuring secretion of aldosterone precursors and their urinary metabolites. Defective 18-dehydrogenation has been postulated in cases with evidence of markedly increased production of 18-hydroxycorticosterone, the immediate precursor of aldosterone.[198,200] The steroidogenic abnormality is shown in Figure 145-16. Recognition of this steroidogenic defect may be facilitated by the fact that the major urinary metabolite of 18-

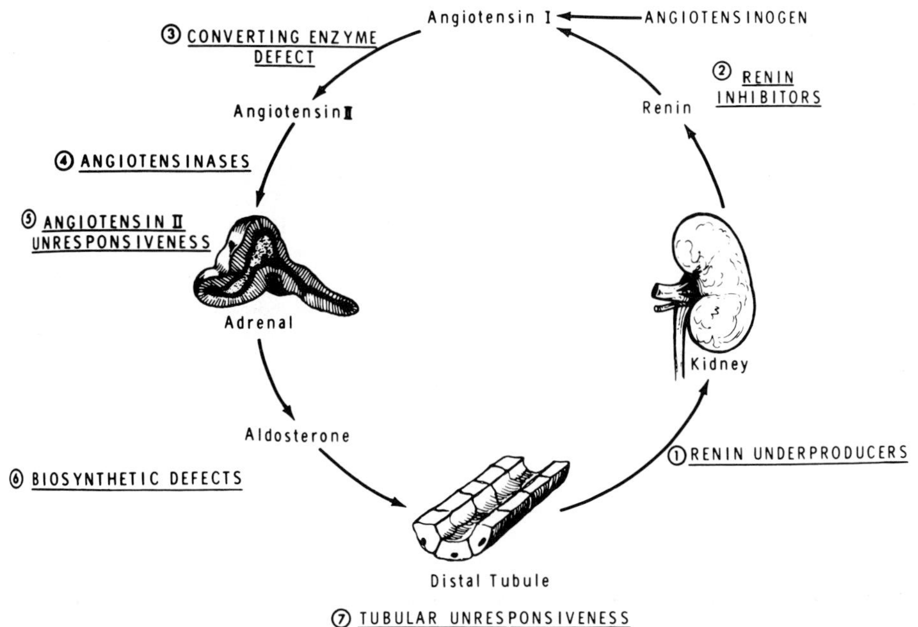

Fig. 145-15. Possible causes of aldosterone deficiency. (From Perez et al: *Ann. Intern. Med. 76:* 757, 1972.)

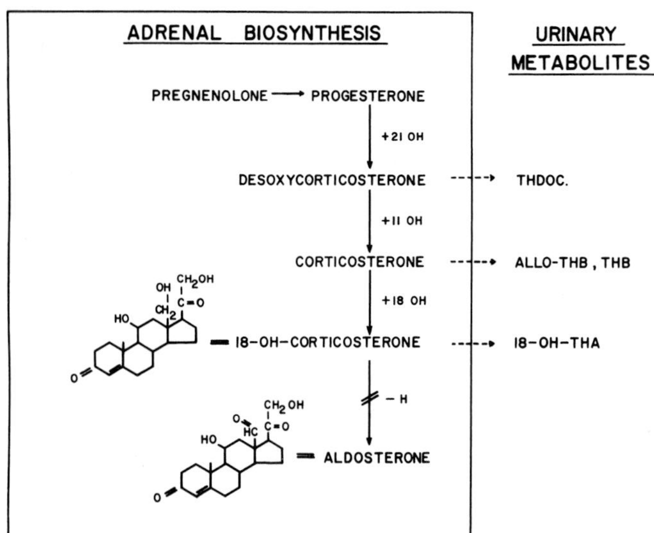

Fig. 145-16. Aldosterone biosynthetic pathways and urinary metabolites of major aldosterone precursors; an 18-dehydrogenase defect is shown. (From David et al: *Pediatrics 41:* 403, 1968.)

hydroxycorticosterone, 18-hydroxytetrahydro-compound A is Porter-Silber positive. Therefore, urinary corticoids may be elevated by the excessive excretion of 18-hydroxytetrahydro-compound A and this increment can be suppressed by administration of desoxycorticosterone and salt, but not by dexamethasone.[200]

Deficient 18-hydroxylase may be suspected in aldosterone deficiency when there is evidence of increased corticosterone and subnormal 18-hydroxycorticosterone production. By these criteria an acquired defect in 18-hydroxylation was proposed as a possible cause of selective aldosterone deficiency in older patients.[191,201] However, it cannot be assumed that the corticosterone measured in these cases necessarily is related to a defect in aldosterone biosynthesis, since corticosterone normally is secreted proponderantly from ACTH-dependent pathways. Thus, a destructive lesion involving only the zona glomerulosa would result in findings very similar to those in defective 18-hydroxylation. Secretion of aldosterone and its steroidogenic precursors, such as 18-hydrocorticosterone, would be markedly decreased, but corticosterone would not be appreciably reduced. These findings in a case of isolated hypoaldosteronism associated with idiopathic hypoparathyroidism most likely reflected selective atrophy of aldosterone-producing cells due to an autoimmune process, although an acquired 18-hydroxylation defect could not be excluded.[201] Aldosterone deficiency in this patient resulted in severe hyponatremia and only moderate hyperkalemia.

An unusual adrenocortical disorder has been described, characterized mainly by the development of manifestations of aldosterone deficiency late in adult life. Findings suggested the presence of abnormally high 20α-hydroxysteroid dehydrogenase activity, possibly resulting in diversion of adrenal steroidogenesis toward production of inactive 20α-hydroxylated derivatives rather than normal end products.[202] Adrenals obtained at autopsy had a remarkable appearance. Grossly, they were hypoplastic; microscopically, normal adrenal tissue was almost completely replaced by atypical large cells. The morphologic picture was identified as cytomegalic type of congenital adrenal hypoplasia. This patient rapidly developed severe hyponatremia and hyperkalemia when mineralocorticoid replacement therapy was withdrawn. A case with similar clinical features was reported by Molnar and coworkers, but neither plasma 20α-hydroxyprogesterone nor urinary pregnanediol was measured.[203]

Drug-Induced Aldosterone Deficiency. Aldosterone secretion can be selectively inhibited by heparin or related synthetic congeners, such as the heparinoid RO1-8307.[126,204–207] Treatment with these agents in doses ranging upward from 200 mg/day results in a distinct natruresis and modest potassium retention commencing within 2–3 days, coinciding with the depression of aldosterone secretion. The aldosterone-lowering effect does not seem to involve inhibition of any component of the renin–angiotensin system, since plasma renin activity increases and renin substrate is unchanged during treatment with heparinoid. Furthermore, aldosterone secretion is diminished by administration of heparin or RO1-8307 in patients with primary aldosteronism in whom renin is suppressed.[206] Heparinoid administration has been reported to reduce the width of the zona glomerulosa in rats,[208] and long-term treatment with heparin caused irreversible atrophy of the glomerulosa in a man.[209]

Several chemical agents, including metyrapone and aminoglutethimide, impair the synthesis of aldosterone as well as cortisol.[210,211] Aldosterone secretion may be inhibited by large doses of op′-DDD, but hypercortisolism in Cushing's syndrome may be successfully treated by administering smaller doses that do not affect aldosterone production.[212] Another agent, SU-9055, may inhibit 18-oxidation of corticosterone.[213] These drugs are generally recognized as inhibitors of adrenal steroidogenesis and their therapeutic application is restricted mainly to patients with malignant adrenocortical disorders, and occasionally to cases of adrenal hyperfunction of benign etiology. On the other hand, heparin is commonly administered as an anticoagulant, and its capacity to inhibit aldosterone secretion is not widely appreciated. Usual anticoagulant doses of heparin are sufficient to impair aldosterone secretion. Therefore, it would seem reasonable to monitor serum electrolytes during heparin therapy, particularly in patients with cardiovascular or renal disease who might tend to develop hyperkalemia as the result of aldosterone deficiency.

Secondary Aldosterone Deficiency

Secondary aldosterone deficiency is the condition that results from impaired function of aldosterone regulatory mechanisms. Clinically, it has been related almost exclusively to malfunction of the renin–angiotensin system, but long-standing hypopituitarism may occasionally lead to deficient aldosterone secretion, perhaps reflecting severe, generalized adrenal atrophy due to lack of ACTH.[214,215] Since aldosterone secretion may be dependent upon more than one regulatory factor, the term *hyporeninemic hypoaldosteronism* specifically defines aldosterone deficiency that is secondary to reduced function of the renin-angiotensin system. The diagnosis of hyporeninemic hypoaldosteronism should be based upon the following findings: abnormally low aldosterone secretion that is not responsive to sodium deprivation, but responds to stimulation by administered angiotensin or ACTH; subnormal plasma levels of angiotensin or renin activity that fail to respond to volume-depleting maneuvers; and preservation of normal cortisol secretion. Possible causes of impaired function of the renin-angiotensin system are discussed below.

Chronic Suppression of Renin Secretion. Aldosterone secretion and plasma renin activity may remain low and fail to respond to appropriate stimuli for a prolonged period following chronic suppression by volume hyperexpansion.[96,216,217] Thus, aldosterone deficiency often occurs following surgical excision of an aldosterone-producing adenoma; consequently, sodium wasting, potassium retention, and postural hypotension may be apparent during the first postoperative month. The prolonged suppression of aldosterone excretion after surgical treatment of primary aldosteronism is shown in Figure 145-17. Restoration of normal responsiveness of the renin–angiotensin–aldosterone system is gradual, although somewhat more rapid than recovery of the corticotropin–cortisol axis following long-term glucocorticoid suppression. Recovery of normal function is initiated by a rise in renin secretion that may reach supranormal levels within the first 2 weeks, but several more weeks may be required before aldosterone secretion is capable of responding to direct or indirect stimuli, and baseline aldosterone secretion may remain low for several months.[93,216] Persistent suppression of aldosterone secretion also has been observed in patients who chronically ingest massive quantities of baking soda.[217,217a] These patients develop transient hypoaldosteronism characterized by orthostatic hypotension and hyperkalemia after the self-medication is discontinued. Presumably, chronic volume hyperexpansion induced by the continuously high intake of sodium bicarbonate results in profound suppression of the renin-angiotensin-aldosterone system.

These consequences of prolonged suppression of aldosterone secretion have important implications that must be considered in any situation in which there is aldosterone deficiency. First, the association of aldosterone hyposecretion with subnormal plasma renin activity, as in hyporeninemic hypoaldosteronism, may not be due to an intrinsic defect in the renin–angiotensin system, but could reflect lack of recovery from the suppressive influence of chronic volume hyperexpansion. Second, aldosterone secretion that fails to respond to angiotensin or ACTH, even if associated with increased renin activity, is not necessarily indicative of an intrinsic adrenal abnormality, but could represent an intermediate stage in recovery from chronic suppression. Therefore, conclusions regarding pathophysiology of aldosterone deficiency may not be valid if based upon measurements of the various components of the renin–angiotensin–aldosterone system at a single point in time; they must be based upon serial observations over a protracted period.

Autonomic Insufficiency. Aldosterone secretion and plasma renin activity are frequently reduced in patients with autonomic insufficiency.[218,219] During prolonged sodium deprivation, in this disorder aldosterone secretion eventually increases and becomes responsive to infused angiotensin or ACTH, suggesting that aldosterone deficiency is secondary to chronic lack of stimulation rather than an adrenal defect. Presumably, impaired function of the renin–angiotensin–aldosterone system is due to disruption of sympathetic pathways, which, as previously noted, play an important role in regulating renin release.[50] This assumption is supported by the observation that responsiveness of renin activity and aldosterone secretion to sodium deprivation and to upright posture is restored by intravenous infusions of catecholamines.[220]

Autonomic insufficiency is characterized by severe orthostatic hypotension, which often is dramatically improved by treatment with mineralocorticoids and dietary salt supplements. Sodium conservation is impaired in some patients with autonomic insufficiency.[218,221,222] This observation, coupled with the finding of aldosterone deficiency in many patients with autonomic insufficiency, has led to the suggestion that mineralocorticoid administration provides specific replacement therapy rather than a pharmacologic effect. However, there is no correlation between the occurrence of renal salt wasting and aldosterone deficiency in this syndrome.[222] Furthermore, favorable responses to treatment with mineralocorticoids do not correlate with the occurrence of impaired sodium conservation or reduced aldosterone secretion, but improvement of orthostatic hypotension does not occur unless substantial sodium retention is induced by therapy. These observations are consistent with the proposition that orthostatic hypotension in this syndrome probably is related directly to loss of sympathetic vasomotor tone, rather than salt wasting. However, even though administered mineralocorticoids are not needed as replacement therapy to correct a defect in sodium conservation, the induced sodium retention tends to restore the effective blood volume to normal, mimicking the effect of the compensatory rise in aldosterone secretion that occurs in hypoalbuminemic states or idiopathic edema.

Hyporeninemic Hypoaldosteronism. This term has been used to describe a syndrome observed in older patients with selective aldosterone deficiency and low plasma renin levels.[223–227] It is characterized clinically by severe hyperkalemia, which develops particularly when sodium intake is low and may be accompanied by hyperchloremic acidosis.[225] These patients have mild to moderate renal insufficiency and often are hypertensive.[226] During sodium deprivation aldosterone secretion and plasma renin activity

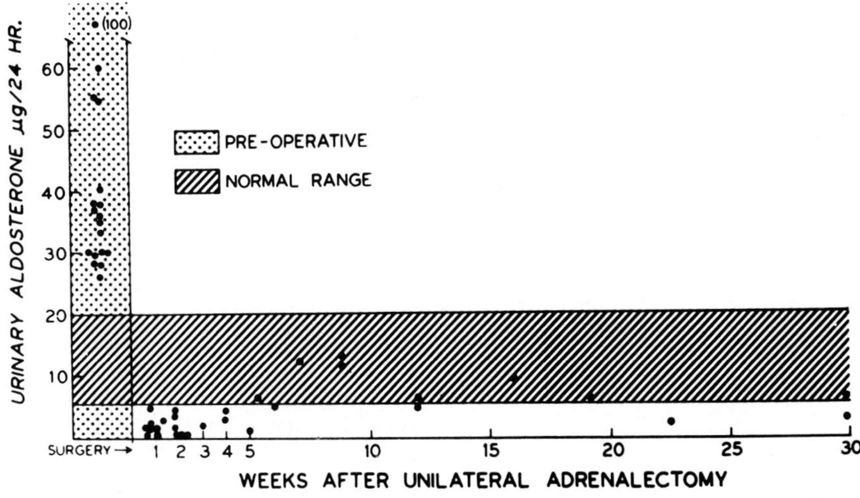

Fig. 145-17. Composite pre- and postoperative levels of urinary aldosterone in 18 patients with primary aldosteronism. (From Biglieri et al: *J. Clin. Endocrinol. Metab. 26:* 553, 1966.)

remain low, and sodium wasting occurs. Accordingly, it has been assumed that aldosterone deficiency is secondary to diminished renin secretion. This assumption is supported by finding subnormal plasma renin concentrations and normal or slightly elevated renin substrate.[223] However, the presence of renin inhibitors has not been specifically excluded. Although aldosterone secretion often is unresponsive to direct stimulation by ACTH or angiotensin, this has been assumed to be due to chronic lack of stimulation rather than an intrinsic defect of aldosterone-secreting cells.

Decreased renin secretion could be due to acquired impairment of renin synthesis or release. Hyporeninemic hypoaldosteronism often is associated with diseases, such as pyelonephritis, diabetes, nephrosclerosis, hyperparathyroidism, or gout, that could damage the juxtaglomerular apparatus along with other interstitial structures of the kidney.[223] Diabetes may also play a more direct role, since studies indicate that function of the renin–angiotensin system is reduced in alloxan-treated diabetic rats, and the degree of hypofunction is inversely related to the severity of hyperglycemia.[228] Additional factors that contribute to the frequent occurrence of hypoaldosteronism in diabetic patients are discussed in a separate section below.

However, renin deficiency in hyporeninemic hypoaldosteronism could also be due to chronic suppression of the renin–angiotensin system. Indeed, a patient with chronic volume hyperexpansion induced by a unique renal lesion presented the same clinical features as hyporeninemic hypoaldosteronism.[229] In this case hypertension and severe hyperkalemia associated with suppression of renin and aldosterone secretion presumably were due to a tubular defect that resulted in enhanced proximal sodium reabsorption. Prolonged dietary sodium restriction corrected all clinical manifestations, and there was an associated rise of renin and aldosterone to normal levels. Similarly, extracellular fluid volume and total exchangeable sodium were found to be increased in patients with hyporeninemic hypoaldosteronism, and a gradual increase in plasma renin activity and plasma aldosterone was observed when sustained reductions in extracellular volume were induced by prolonged treatment with furosemide.[227] The mechanism of volume expansion in patients with hyporeninemic hypoaldosteronism is unclear, but the underlying renal disease may result in impaired ability to excrete sodium. Suppression of the renin–angiotensin system may also be related to hypertension that frequently occurs in this syndrome.[227] Patients with low renin hypertension also may have subnormal aldosterone responses during sodium deprivation[230,231] and may fail to conserve sodium normally.[231,232] Abnormal adrenal responsiveness to angiotensin has been postulated in a few hypertensives in whom aldosterone secretion remained low during sodium restriction despite very high plasma levels of angiotensin.[233] As suggested above, these findings may represent a later stage in recovery from suppression, since restoration of normal aldosterone responsiveness is preceded by supranormal levels of plasma renin activity. Incidentally, these hypertensive patients developed hyperkalemia during the period of low intake. Thus, hyporeninemic hypoaldosteronism and low renin hypertension have many features in common. Severe hyperkalemia would be very apt to occur in patients with low renin hypertension if they developed even a mild degree of renal insufficiency, in which case the clinical picture would be indistinguishable from hyporeninemic hypoaldosteronism with hypertension.

Pseudohypoaldosteronism

Manifestations of aldosterone deficiency may be due to failure of the kidneys to respond to mineralocorticoids. This could result from defective renal tubules or from factors that inhibit the action of mineralocorticoids. Patients with excessive urinary losses of sodium, chloride, and water due to chronic renal disease rather than adrenal insufficiency were first described three decades ago by Thorn and co-workers, who suggested the term *salt-losing nephritis*.[234] Severe hyperkalemia, which occurs infrequently in nonoliguric chronic renal insufficiency, is a prominent feature of salt-losing nephropathy.[235] Salt wasting and hyperkalemia are potent stimuli for increased aldosterone secretion, and hypersecretion of aldosterone may be observed in patients with salt-losing nephropathy.[236] However, sodium depletion and hyperkalemia will persist in the face of markedly increased aldosterone secretion if impairment of tubular function is severe enough to make them refractory to the action of mineralocorticoids. In such cases the kidneys fail to respond to further increments in aldosterone secretion during sodium deprivation or to large doses of administered mineralocorticoids.[236] Severe hyperkalemia may also occur during treatment with aldosterone inhibitors, such as spironolactone or triamterene, especially if renal function is impaired, even though these agents normally induce a compensatory increase in aldosterone secretion.[145]

In some patients with sodium-losing nephropathy, aldosterone secretion does not rise and may even fall below normal because the juxtaglomerular apparatus is damaged by the same pathologic process that causes tubular injury.[237] Sodium depletion and hyperkalemia in these patients may be corrected by administration of larger than usual replacement doses of mineralocorticoid. Similarly, severe hyperkalemia developed in an adrenalectomized woman with chronic pyelonephritis despite treatment with usual replacement doses or cortisone acetate and fluorocortisol acetate, and was corrected by massive doses of fluorocortisol acetate.[238] The enhanced mineralocorticoid requirement in this case was postulated to be due to renal tubular damage. Hyperkalemia and hyperchloremic acidosis without evidence of sodium wasting have been described in chronic pyelonephritis with only moderate degrees of azotemia.[239,240] An acquired tubular defect resulting in impaired secretion of potassium and hydrogen ions was assumed, although aldosterone deficiency was not ruled out by aldosterone measurements, and no attempt was made to correct the metabolic abnormalities with mineralocorticoid therapy.

Because the kidney harbors the regulatory system and the target cells for aldosterone, it is apparent that both could be affected by any process that damages the kidney. Therefore, it frequently may be very difficult to make a clear distinction between pseudo- and secondary hypoaldosteronism. Even if aldosterone secretion increases substantially in response to tubular refractoriness, the rise may be limited by some degree of impairment of renin release, and the increment may be subnormal for the circumstance. Furthermore, it may not be possible to assess accurately different degrees of tubular damage by observing renal responsiveness to exogenous mineralocorticoids.

Diabetes Mellitus and Hypoaldosteronism

Diabetes mellitus is common in adult patients with hypoaldosteronism. According to one survey, 19 of 67 patients with selective hypoaldosteronism also had diabetes.[241] Such frequent association of these two conditions is not surprising when one considers the various abnormalities in diabetes that result in decreased aldosterone secretion or blunted renal responsiveness to mineralocorticoids. As noted above, diabetic nephropathy may lead to hyporeninemic hypoaldosteronism, not only because of interstitial damage due to pyelonephritis,[223] but also because diabetic glomerulosclerosis can result in hyalinization of juxtaglomerular cells.[228] Renin release also can be impaired by autonomic neuropathy in diabetic patients.[218,219] Studies in alloxan-treated rats suggest that renin secretion may be reduced by hyperglycemia per se,[228] and the recently reported finding of "big renin" in plasma of diabetic patients suggested that hypoaldosteronism may result from defective conversion of a biologically inactive precursor to active renin.[241] The latter report also presented evidence suggesting that hypoaldosteronism in diabetics may result from specific defects in aldosterone biosynthesis.[241] Furthermore, a synergistic effect between insulin and aldosterone upon potassium metabolism has been observed in diabetic patients with aldosterone deficiency.[242] In these patients a paradoxical rise in serum potassium levels in response to glucose was blunted by aldosterone, but was abolished by prior administration of insulin.[242] Thus, hypoaldosteronism is a frequent occurrence in diabetics and carries the added risk of severe, life-threatening hyperkalemia due to associated renal insufficiency or due to the paradoxical rise in potassium that may be induced by hyperglycemia when both insulin and aldosterone are deficient. Indeed, the advisability of administering 10–50 gm of glucose intravenously to comatose diabetic patients as a "therapeutic test" has been questioned because of the risk of glucose-induced hyperkalemia.[243]

REFERENCES

1. Pitts, R. F.: Physiology of the Kidney and Body Fluids, ed 3. Chicago, Year Book, 1974, p 11.
2. Klahr, S., Slatapolsky, E.: Renal regulation of sodium excretion. *Arch Intern Med 131:* 780, 1973.
3. Strauss, M. B., Davis, R. K., Rosenbaum, J. D., et al: Production of increased renal sodium excretion by the hypertonic expansion of extracellular fluid volume in recumbent subjects. *J Clin Invest 31:* 80, 1952.
4. Epstein, F. H.: Renal excretion of sodium and the concept of a volume receptor. *Yale J Biol Med 29:* 282, 1956.
5. Earley, L. E., Daugharty, T. M.: Sodium metabolism. *N Engl J Med 281:* 72, 1969.
6. Renkin, E. M., Robinson, R. R.: Glomerular filtration. *N Engl J Med 290:* 785, 1974.
7. Berliner, R. W.: Outline of Renal Physiology. In Strauss, M. B., Welt, L. G. (eds): *Diseases of the Kidney,* ed 2. Boston, Little, Brown, 1971, p 37.
8. Wesson, L. G., Jr., Anslow, W. P., Smith, H. W.: The excretion of strong electrolytes. *Bull NY Acad Med 24:* 586, 1948.
9. Dirks, J. H., Cirksena, W. J., Berliner, R. W.: Effects of saline infusion on sodium reabsorption by proximal tubule of dog. *J Clin Invest 44:* 1160, 1965.
10. Rector, F. C., Jr., Brunner, F. P., Seldin, D. W.: Mechanism of glomerulotubular balance. I. Effect of aortic constriction and elevated ureteropelvic pressure on glomerular filtration rate, proximal reabsorption, transit time and tubular size in proximal tubule of rat. *J Clin Invest 45:* 590, 1966.
11. Windhager, E. E.: Mechanisms of reabsorption and excretion of ions and water. In Pitts, R. F. (ed): *Physiology of the Kidney and Body Fluids,* ed 3. Chicago, Year Book, 1974, p 99.
12. Giebisch, G.: Coupled ion and fluid transport in the kidney. *N Engl J Med 287:* 913, 1972.
13. Giebisch, G., Windhager, E. E.: Renal tubular transfer of sodium, chloride and potassium. *Am J Med 36:* 643, 1964.
14. Giebisch, G.: Functional organization of proximal and distal tubular electrolyte transport. *Nephron 6:* 260, 1969.
15. Diamond, J. M., Bossert, W. H.: Standing gradient osmotic flow. A mechanism for coupling of water and solute transport in epithelia. *J Gen Physiol 50:* 2061, 1967.
16. Burg, M. B., Green, N.: Function of the thick ascending limb of Henle's loop. *Am J Physiol 224:* 659, 1973.
17. Kokko, J. P.: Membrane characteristics governing salt and water in the loop of Henle. *Fed Proc 33:* 25, 1974.
18. Marsh, D. J.: Osmotic concentration and dilution of urine. In Rouiller, C., Muller, A. F. (eds): *The Kidney: Morphology, Biochemistry, Physiology,* vol 3. New York, Academic, 1971, p 71.
19. Vander, A. J., Wilde, W. S., Malvin, R. L.: Stop-flow analysis of aldosterone and steroidal antagonist SC-8109 on renal tubular sodium kinetics. *Proc Soc Exp Biol Med 103:* 525, 1960.
20. Hierholzer, K., Stolte, H.: The proximal and distal tubular action of adrenal steroids on Na reabsorption. *Nephron 6:* 188, 1969.
21. Stein, J. H.: The role of the collecting duct in the regulation of excretion of sodium and other electrolytes. *Kidney Int 6:* 1, 1974.
22. Bartter, F. C., Mills, I. H., Biglieri, E. G., et al: Studies on the control and physiologic action of aldosterone. *Recent Prog Horm Res 15:* 311, 1959.
23. Mulrow, P. J., Forman, B. H.: The tissue effects of mineralocorticoids. *Am J Med 53:* 561, 1972.
24. Feldman, D., Funder, J. W., Edelman, I. S.: Subcellular mechanisms in the action of adrenal steroids. *Am J Med 53:* 545, 1972.
25. Crabbe, J.: Stimulation of active sodium transport by the isolated toad bladder with aldosterone *in vitro*. *J Clin Invest 40:* 2103, 1961.
26. Barger, A. C., Berlin, R. D., Tulenko, J. F.: Infusion of aldosterone, 9-α-fluorohydrocortisone, and antidiuretic hormone into renal artery of normal and adrenalectomized unanesthetized dogs: effect on electrolyte and water excretion. *Endocrinology 62:* 804, 1958.
27. Sharp, G. W. G., Leaf, A.: Mechanism of action of aldosterone. *Phys Rev 46:* 593, 1966.
28. DeWardener, H. E., Mills, I. H., Clapham, W. F., et al: Studies on the efferent mechanism of the sodium diuresis which follows the administration of intravenous saline in the dog. *Clin Sci 21:* 249, 1961.
29. Dirks, J. H., Cirksena, W. J., Berliner, R. W.: Effects of saline infusion on sodium reabsorption by proximal tubule of dog. *J Clin Invest 44:* 1160, 1965.
30. Knox, F. G., Davis, B. B.: Role of physical and neuroendocrine factors in proximal electrolyte reabsorption. *Metabolism 23:* 793, 1974.
31. Mills, I. H.: Renal regulation of sodium excretion. *Ann Rev Med 21:* 75, 1970.
32. Barger, A. C.: Renal hemodynamic factors in congestive heart failure. *Ann NY Acad Sci 139:* 276, 1966.
33. Thurau, K., Horster, M.: Micropuncture studies on the filtration rate of single superficial and juxtamedullary glomeruli in the rat kidney. *Arch Ges Physiol 301:* 1159, 1963.
34. Earley, L. E., Martino, J. A., Friedler, R. M.: Factors affecting sodium reabsorption by proximal tubule as determined during blockade of distal sodium reabsorption. *J Clin Invest 45:* 1668, 1966.
35. Daugherty, T. M., Belleau, L. J., Martino, J. A., et al: Interrelationship of physical factors affecting sodium reabsorption in dog. *Am J Physiol 215:* 1442, 1968.
36. Earley, L. E., Friedler, R. M.: Changes in renal blood flow and possibly intrarenal distribution of blood during natriuresis accompanying saline loading in dog. *J Clin Invest 44:* 929, 1965.
37. Brenner, B. M., Troy, J. L., Daugharty, T. M.: On the mechanism of inhibition in fluid reabsorption by the renal proximal tubule of the volume-expanded rat. *J Clin Invest 50:* 1596, 1971.
38. Daugharty, T. M., Ueki, I. F., Nicholas, D. P., et al: Comparative renal effects of isooncotic and colloid-free volume expansion in the rat. *Am J Physiol 222:* 225, 1972.
39. Bank, N., Yarger, W. E., Aynedjian, H. S.: A microperfusion study of sucrose movement across the rat proximal tubule during renal vein constriction. *J Clin Invest 50:* 294, 1971.
40. Lee, J., DeWardener, H. E.: Neurosecretion and sodium excretion. *Kidney Int 6:* 323, 1974.
41. Sonnenberg, H., Veress, A. T., Pearce, J. W.: A humoral component of the natriuretic mechanism in sustained blood volume expansion. *J Clin Invest 51:* 2631, 1972.
42. Buckalew, V. M., Jr., Lancaster, C. D., Jr.: The association of a humoral sodium transport inhibitory activity with renal escape from chronic mineralocorticoid administration in the dog. *Clin Sci 42:* 69, 1972.
43. Sealey, J. E., Laragh, J. H.: Further studies of a natriuretic substance occurring in human urine and plasma. *Circ Res 28[Suppl 2]:* 32, 1971.
44. Gitelman, H. J., Blythe, W. B.: Isolation of a natriuretic factor from the posterior pituitary. *Clin Res 20:* 594, 1972.
45. Bennett, C. M.: Effect of extracellular expansion upon sodium reabosrption in the distal nephron of dogs. *J Clin Invest 52:* 2548, 1973.

46. Sonnenberg, H.: Renal response to blood volume expansion: distal tubular function and kidney excretion. *Am J Physiol 223:* 916, 1972.
47. Smith, H. W.: Salt and water volume receptors. *Am J Med 23:* 623, 1957.
48. Pitts, R. F.: Regulation of volume and osmolar concentration of extracellular fluid volume, in Pitts, R. F. (ed): *Physiology of the Kidney and Body Fluids,* ed 3. Chicago, Year Book, 1974, p 242.
49. Davis, J. O.: The control of renin release. *Am J Med 55:* 333, 1973.
50. Oparil, S., Haber, E.: The renin–angiotensin system. *N Engl J Med 291:* 389, 1974.
51. Schultze, R. G.: Recent advances in the physiology and pathophysiology of potassium excretion. *Arch Intern Med 131:* 885, 1973.
52. Berliner, R. W.: Renal mechanism for potassium excretion. *Harvey Lect 55:* 141, 1961.
53. Malnic, G., Klose, R. M., Giebisch, G.: Micropuncture study of distal tubular potassium and sodium transport in rat nephron. *Am J Physiol 211:* 529, 1966.
54. Malnic, G., Klose, R. M., Giebisch, G.: Microperfusion study of distal tubular potassium and sodium transfer in rat kidney. *Am J Physiol 211:* 548, 1966.
55. Giebisch, G.: Renal potassium excretion, in Rouiller, C., Muller, A. F. (eds): *The Kidney,* vol 3. New York, Academic, 1971, p 329.
56. Hierholzer, K., et al: Micropuncture study of renal transtubular concentration gradients in adrenalectomized rats. *Pfluegers Arch 285:* 193, 1965.
57. Figmonari, G. M., Fanestil, D. D., Edelman, I. S.: Induction of RNA and protein synthesis in the action of aldosterone in the rat. *Am J Physiol 213:* 954, 1967.
58. Malnic, G., de Mello-Aires, M., Giebisch, G.: Potassium transport across renal distal tubules during acid–base disturbances. *Am J Physiol 221:* 1192, 1971.
59. Adler, S.: An extrarenal action of aldosterone on mammalian skeletal muscle. *Am J Physiol 218:* 616, 1970.
60. Nelson, D. H.: Regulation of glucocorticoid release. *Am J Med 53:* 590, 1972.
61. Ulick, S., Laragh, J. H., Lieberman, S.: The isolation of a urinary metabolite of aldosterone and its use to measure the rate of secretion of aldosterone by the adrenal cortex in man. *Trans Assoc Am Phys 71:* 225, 1958.
62. Laragh, J. H., Sealey, J., Brunner, H. R.: The control of aldosterone secretion in normal and hypertensive man: abnormal renin–aldosterone patterns in low renin hypertension. *Am J Med 53:* 649, 1972.
63. Ames, R. P., Borkowski, H. J., Sicinski, A. M., et al: Prolonged infusions of angiotensin II and norepinephrine and blood pressure, electrolyte balance, aldosterone and cortisol secretion in normal man and in cirrhosis with ascites. *J Clin Invest 44:* 1171, 1965.
64. Bledsoe, T., Island, D. P., Liddle, G. W.: Studies of the mechanism through which sodium depletion increases aldosterone biosynthesis in man. *J Clin Invest 45:* 524, 1966.
65. Biglieri, E. G., Shambelan, M., Slaton, P. E., Jr.: Effect of adrenocorticotropin on desoxycorticosterone, corticosterone and aldosterone excretion. *J Clin Endocrinol 28:* 1090, 1968.
66. Kem, D. C., Sanchez-Gomez, C., Kramer, N. J., et al: Plasma aldosterone and renin activity response to ACTH infusion in dexamethasone-suppressed normal and sodium-depleted man. *J Clin Endocrinol 40:* 116, 1975.
67. Williams, G. H., Cain, J. P., Dluhy, R. G., et al: Studies of the control of plasma aldosterone concentration in normal man: I. Response to posture, acute and chronic volume depletion, and sodium loading. *J Clin Invest 51:* 1731, 1972.
68. Katz, F. H., Romfh, P., Smith, J. A.: Diurnal variation of plasma aldosterone, cortisol and renin activities in supine man. *J Clin Endocrinol 40:* 125, 1975.
69. Davis, J. O.: Are there unidentified factors in the control of aldosterone secretion? *N Engl J Med 286:* 100, 1972.
70. Brunner, H. R., Baer, L., Sealey, J., et al: The influence of potassium administration and potassium deprivation on plasma renin in normal and hypertensive subjects. *J Clin Invest 49:* 2128, 1970.
71. Relman, A. S., Schwartz, W. B.: The effect of DOCA on electrolyte balance in normal man and its relation to sodium chloride intake. *Yale J Biol Med 24:* 540, 1952.
72. August, J. T., Nelson, D. H., Thorn, G. W.: Response of normal subjects to large amounts of aldosterone. *J Clin Invest 37:* 1549, 1958.
73. Martino, J. A., Earley, L. E.: The profile of tubular sodium reabsorption in normal man before and after escape from a mineralocorticoid and in patients with pathologic sodium retention. *J Clin Invest 47:* 1472, 1968 (abstract).
74. Leutscher, J. A., Jr.: The syndrome of mineralocorticoid excess. *Ann Intern Med 48:* 1424, 1958.
75. Tobian, L.: Interrelationship of electrolytes, juxtaglomerular cells and hypertension. *Physiol Rev 40:* 280, 1960.
76. Mendlowitz, M.: Vascular reactivity in essential and renal hypertension in man. *Am Heart J 73:* 121, 1967.
77. Seldin, D. W., Rector, F. C., Jr.: The generation and maintenance of metabolic alkalosis. *Kidney Int 1:* 306, 1972.
78. Seldin, D. W., Welt, L. G., Cort, J. H.: The role of sodium salts and adrenal steroids in the production of hypokalemic alkalosis. *Yale J Biol Med 29:* 229, 1956.
79. Kunau, R. T., Jr., Frick, A., Rector, F. C., Jr., et al: Micropuncture study of the proximal tubular factors responsible for maintenance of alkalosis during potassium deficiency in the rat. *Clin Sci 38:* 223, 1968.
80. Kurtzman, N. A.: Regulation of renal bicarbonate reabsorption by extracellular volume. *J Clin Invest 49:* 586, 1970.
81. Kassirer, J. P., London, A. M., Goldman, D. M., et al: On the pathogenesis of metabolic alkalosis in hyperaldosteronism. *Am J Med 49:* 306, 1970.
82. Lennon, E. J., Reutz, P. P., Engstrom, W. W.: Reversal of diurnal rhythm in excretion of water and salt in primary hyperaldosteronism. *Am J Med 30:* 475, 1961.
83. Hollander, W., Jr., Blythe, W. B.: Nephropathy of potassium depletion. In Strauss, M. B., Welt, L. G. (eds): *Diseases of the Kidney.* Boston, Little, Brown, 1971, p 952.
84. Gaunt, R., Renzi, A. A., Chart, J. J.: Aldosterone—a review. *J Clin Endocrinol 15:* 621, 1955.
85. Melby, J. C., Dale, S. L., Wilson, T. E.: 18-Hydroxy-11-deoxycorticosterone in human hypertension. *Circ Res 28[Suppl 2]:* 11, 1971.
86. Melby, J. C., Dale, S. L., Grekin, R. J., et al: 18-Hydroxy-11-desoxycorticosterone (18-OH DOC) secretion in experimental and human hypertension. *Rec Prog Horm Res 28:* 287, 1972.
87. Birmingham, M. K., MacDonald, M., Rochefort, J. G.: Adrenal function in normal rats and in rats bearing regenerated adrenal glands. In McKerns, K. W. (ed): Functions of the Adrenal Cortex. New York, Appleton-Century-Crofts, 1968, p 647.
88. Conn, J. W.: Presidential address, part II. Primary aldosteronism, a new clinical syndrome. *J Lab Clin Med 45:* 6, 1955.
89. Conn, J. W., Knopf, R. F., Nesbit, R. M.: Clinical characteristics of primary aldosteronism from an analysis of 145 cases. *Am J Surg 107:* 159, 1964.
90. Laragh, J. H., Ulick, S., Januszewicz, V., et al: Electrolyte metabolsim and aldosterone secretion in benign and malignant hypertension. *Ann Intern Med 53:* 259, 1960.
91. Laragh, J. H., Sealey, J. E., Sommers, S. C.: Patterns of adrenal secretion and urinary excretion of aldosterone and plasma renin activity in normal and hypertensive subjects. *Circ Res 19[Suppl 1]:* 158, 1966.
92. Masson, G. M. C.: The renin–angiotensin–aldosterone system. In Page, I. H., McCubbin, J. W. (eds): Renal Hypertension. Chicago, Year Book, 1968, p 239.
93. Conn, J. W., Cohen, E. L., Rovner, D. R.: Suppression of plasma renin activity in primary aldosteronism. *JAMA 190:* 213, 1964.
94. Biglieri, E. G., Stockigt, J. R., Schambelan, M.: Adrenal mineralocorticoids causing hypertension. *Am J Med 52:* 623, 1972.
94a. Biglieri, E. G., Schambelan, M., Brust, N., et al: Plasma aldosterone concentration. Further characterization of aldosterone-producing adenomas. *Circ Res 34–35(Suppl 1):* 183, 1974.
95. Baer, L., Sommers, S. C., Krakoff, L. R., et al: Pseudoprimary aldosteronism: an entity distinct from true primary aldosteronism. *Circ Res 26–27[Suppl 1]:* 1, 1970.
96. Conn, J. W., Cohen, E. L., Rovner, O. R., et al: Normokalemic primary aldosteronism: detectable cause of curable "essential" hypertension. *JAMA 193:* 200, 1965.
97. Crane, M. G., Harris, J. J., Varner, J. J., Jr.: Hyporeninemic hypertension. *Am J Med 52:* 457, 1972.
98. Spark, R. F.: Low renin hypertension and the adrenal cortex. *N Engl J Med 287:* 343, 1972.
99. Melby, J. C.: Identifying the adrenal lesion in primary aldosteronism. *Ann Intern Med 76:* 1039, 1972.
100. Conn, J. W., Morita, R., Cohen, E. L., et al: Primary aldosteronism. Photoscanning of tumors after administration of ^{131}I-19-iodocholesterol. *Arch Intern Med 129:* 417, 1972.

101. Sutherland, D. J. A., Ruse, J. L., Laidlaw, J. C.: Hypertension, increased aldosterone secretion and low plasma renin activity relieved by dexamethasone. *Can Med Assoc J 95:* 1109, 1966.
102. New, M. I., Peterson, R. E.: A new form of congenital adrenal hyperplasia. *J Clin Endocrinol 27:* 300, 1967.
103. Miura, K., Yoshinaga, K., Goto, K., et al: A case of glucocorticoid-responsive hyperaldosteronism. *J Clin Endocrinol 28:* 1807, 1968.
104. Giebink, G. S., Gotlin, R. W., Biglieri, E. G., et al: A kindred with familal glucocorticoid-suppressible aldosteronism. *J Clin Endocrinol 36:* 715, 1973.
105. Laragh, J. H.: Vasoconstrictor-volume analysis for understanding and treating hypertension. The use of renin and aldosterone profiles. *Am J Med 55:* 261, 1973.
106. Laidlaw, J. C., Yendt, E. R., Gornell, A. G.: Hypertension caused by renal artery occlusion simulating primary aldosteronism. *Metabolism 9:* 612, 1960.
107. Kurtzman, N. A., Pillay, V. K. G., Rogers, P. W., et al: Renal vascular hypertension and low plasma renin activity. Interrelationship of volume and renin in the pathogenesis of hypertension. *Arch Intern Med 133:* 195, 1974.
108. Buhler, F. R., Laragh, J. H., Baer, L., et al: Propranolol inhibition of renin secretion. A specific approach to diagnosis and treatment of renin-dependent hypertensive diseases. *N Engl J Med 287:* 1209, 1972.
109. Vertes, V., Cangiano, J. L., Berman, L. B., et al: Hypertension in end-stage renal disease. *N Engl J Med 280:* 978, 1969.
110. Laragh, J. H., Baer, L., Brunner, H. L., et al: Renin, angiotensin and aldosterone system in pathogenesis and management of hypertensive vascular disease. *Am J Med 52:* 633, 1972.
111. Hunt, J. C., Sheps, S. G., Harrison, E. G., Jr., et al: Renal and renovascular hypertension. A reasoned approach to diagnosis and management. *Arch Intern Med 133:* 988, 1974.
112. Kaplan, N. M.: Primary aldosteronism with malignant hypertension. *N Engl J Med 269:* 1282, 1963.
113. Robertson, P. W., Klidjian, A., Harding, L. K., et al: Hypertension due to a renin-secreting tumour. *Am J Med 43:* 963, 1967.
114. Schambelan, M., Howes, E. L., Jr., Stockigt, J. R., et al: Role of renin and aldosterone in hypertension due to a renin-secreting tumor. *Am J Med 55:* 86, 1973.
115. Mitchell, J. D., Baxter, T. J., Blair-West, J. R., et al: Renin levels in nephroblastoma (Wilms' tumour). Report of a renin-secreting tumor. *Arch Dis Child 45:* 376, 1970.
116. Hollifield, J. W., Page, D. L., Smith, C., et al: Renin-secreting clear cell carcinoma of the kidney. *Arch Intern Med 135:* 859, 1975.
117. Hauger-Klevene, J. H.: High plasma renin activity in an oat cell carcinoma: a renin-secreting carcinoma? *Cancer 26:* 1112, 1970.
118. Conn, J. W., Cohen, E. L., Lucas, C. P.: Primary reninism. Hypertension, hyperreninemia, and secondary aldosteronism due to renin-producing juxtaglomerular cell tumors. *Arch Intern Med 130:* 682, 1972.
119. Ford, H. C., Pieters, H. P., Bailey, R. E.: Aldosterone and sodium conservation: the effect of acute dietary sodium deprivation on the plasma concentration, the metabolic clearance and the secretion and excretion rates of aldosterone in normal subjects. *J Clin Endocrinol 28:* 451, 1968.
120. Watanabe, M., Meeker, C. I., Gray, M. J., et al: Secretion rate of aldosterone in normal pregnancy. *J Clin Invest 42:* 1619, 1963.
121. Brown, R. D., Strott, C. A., Liddle, G. W.: Plasma deoxycorticosterone in normal and abnormal human pregnancy. *J Clin Endocrinol 35:* 736, 1972.
122. Christy, N. P., Shaver, J. C.: Estrogens and the kidney. *Kidney Int 6:* 366, 1974.
123. Ehrlich, E. N., Lindheimer, M. D.: Sodium metabolism, aldosterone, and the hypertensive disorders of pregnancy. *J Reprod Med 3:* 106, 1972.
124. Ehrlich, E. N., Oparil, S., Lindheimer, M. D.: Role of the augmented aldosterone secretion in regulation of volume homeostasis in pregnancy. In Fregly, M. J., Fregly, M. S. (eds): Oral Contraceptives and High Blood Pressure. Gainesville, Dolphin, 1974, p 274.
125. Ehrlich, E. N.: Heparinoid-induced inhibition of aldosterone secretion in pregnant women. The role of augmented aldosterone secretion in sodium conservation during normal pregnancy. *Am J Obstet Gynecol 109:* 1963, 1971.
126. Schlatmann, R. J. A. F. M., Prenen, H., Jansen, A. P., et al: The natriuretic action of heparin and some related substances. *Lancet 1:* 314, 1960.
127. Sims, E. A. H.: The kidney in pregnancy. In Strauss, M. B., Welt, L. G. (eds): *Diseases of the Kidney,* ed 2. Boston, Little, Brown, 1971, p. 1155.
128. Landau, R. L., Lugibihl, K.: Inhibition of the sodium-retaining influence of aldosterone by progesterone. *J Clin Endocrinol 18:* 1237, 1958.
129. Chesley, L. C.: Disorders of the kidney, fluids, electrolytes, In Assali, N. (ed): *Pathophysiology of Gestational Disorders,* vol 1. New York, Academic, 1972, p 355.
130. Goodrich, S. M., Wood. J. E.: Peripheral venous distensibility and velocity of venous flow during pregnancy or during oral contraceptive therapy. *Am J Obstet Gynecol 90:* 740, 1964.
130a. Bay, W. H., Farris, T. F.: Studies of circulation during pregnancy. *Clin Res 23:* 468A, 1975 (Abstr).
131. Lindheimer, M. D., del Greco, F., Ehrlich, E. N.: Postural effects on Na and steroid excretion, and serum renin activity during pregnancy. *J Applied Physiol 35:* 343, 1973.
132. Ehrlich, E. N., Lindheimer, M. D.: Effect of administered mineralocorticoids or ACTH in pregnant women. Attenuation of kaliuretic influence of mineralocorticoids during pregnancy. *J Clin Invest 51:* 1301, 1972.
133. Vande Wiele, R. L., Gurpide, E., Kelly, W. G., et al: The secretory rate of progesterone and aldosterone in normal and late pregnancy. *Acta Endocrinol 35*[*Suppl 51*]: 159, 1960.
134. Watanabe, M., Meeker, C. I., Gray, M. J., et al: Aldosterone secretion rates in abnormal pregnancy. *J Clin Endocrinol 25:* 1665, 1965.
135. Weinberger, M. H., Kramer, N. J., Petersen, L. P., et al: Sequential changes in the renin-angiotensin-aldosterone systems and plasma progesterone concentration in normal and abnormal human pregnancy. In Lindheimer, M. D., Katz, A. I., Zuspan, F. P. (eds): Hypertension in Pregnancy. New York, Wiley, 1976, pp. 263–269.
136. Ricketts, W. E., Eichelberger, L., Kirsner, J. B.: Observations on the alterations in electrolytes and fluid balance in patients with cirrhosis of the liver with and without ascites. *J Clin Invest 30:* 1157, 1951.
137. Rivera, A., Pena, J. C., Barcena, C., et al: Renal excretion of water, sodium and potassium in cirrhosis of the liver. *Metabolism 10:* 1, 1961.
138. Grausz, H., Lieberman, R., Earley, L. E.: Effect of plasma albumin on sodium reabsorption in patients with nephrotic syndrome. *Kidney Int 1:* 47, 1972.
139. Earley, L. E., Orloff, J.: Thiazide diuretics. *Ann Rev Med 15:* 149, 1964.
140. Frazier, H. S., Yager, H.: Drug therapy. The clinical use of diuretics. *N Engl J Med 288:* 246, 1973.
141. Cannon, P. J., Kilcoyne, M. M.: Ethacrynic acid and furosemide: renal pharmacology and clinical use. *Prog Cardiovasc Dis 12:* 99, 1969.
142. Liddle, G. W.: Aldosterone antagonists and triamterene. *Ann NY Acad Sci 139:* 466, 1966.
143. Bull, M. B., Laragh, J. H.: Amiloride, a potassium-sparing natriuretic agent. *Circulation 37:* 45, 1968.
144. Katz, F. H., Eckert, R. C., Gebott, M. D.: Hypokalemia caused by surreptitious self-administration of diuretics. *Ann Intern Med 76:* 85, 1972.
145. Greenblatt, D. J., Koch-Weser, J.: Adverse reactions to spironolactones. A report from the Boston collaborative drug surveillance program. *JAMA 225:* 40, 1973.
146. Bartter, F. C., Pronove, P., Gill, J. R., Jr., et al: Hyperplasia of the juxtaglomerular complex with hyperaldosteronism and hypokalemic alkalosis. A new syndrome. *Am J Med 33:* 311, 1962.
147. Cannon, P. J., Leeming, J. M., Sommers, S. C., et al: Juxtaglomerular cell hyperplasia and secondary hyperaldosteronism (Bartter's syndrome): a reevaluation of the pathophysiology. *Medicine 47:* 107, 1968.
148. Trygstad, C. W., Mangos, J. A., Bloodworth, J. M. B., Jr., et al: A sibship with Bartter's syndrome: failure of total adrenalectomy to correct the potassium wasting. *Pediatrics 44:* 234, 1969.
149. Goodman, A. D., Vagnucci, A. H., Hartroft, P. M.: Pathogenesis of Bartter's syndrome. *N Engl J Med 281:* 1435, 1969.
150. Bryan, G. T., MacCardle, R. C., Bartter, F. C.: Hyperaldosteronism, hyperplasia of the juxtaglomerular complex, normal blood pressure, and dwarfism: report of a case. *Pediatrics 27:* 43, 1966.
150a. Kurtzman, N. A., Gutierrez, L. F.: Hypothesis. The pathophysiology of Bartter syndrome. *JAMA 234:* 758, 1975.

151. Modlinger, R. S., Nocolis, G. L., Krakoff, L. R., et al: Some observations on the pathogenesis of Bartter's syndrome. *N Engl J Med 9:* 1023, 1973.
152. Biava, C., Desjardins, R., Bravo, E., et al: Glomerular changes with glomerulo-distotubular shunts in patients with Bartter's syndrome. *Lab Invest 20:* 575, 1969.
153. Gardner, J. D., Simopoulos, A. P., Lapey, A., et al: Altered membrane sodium transport on Bartter's syndrome. *J Clin Invest 51:* 1565, 1972.
153a. Gill, J. R., Jr., Frolich, J. C., Bowden, R. E., Taylor, A. A., et al: Bartter's syndrome: a disorder characterized by high urinary prostaglandins and a dependence of hyperreninemia on prostaglandin synthesis. *Am J Med 61:* 43, 1976.
153b. Galvez, O. G., Roberts, B. W., Bay, W. H., Ferris, T. F.: Hemodynamic changes with hypokalemia. *Clin Res 24:* 559A, 1976.
154. Pasternack, A., Perheentupa, J., Launiala, K., et al: Kidney biopsy findings in familial chloride diarrhea. *Acta Endocrinol 55:* 1, 1967.
155. Streeten, D. H. P., Louis, L. H., Conn, J. W.: Secondary aldosteronism in "idiopathic edema." *Trans Assoc Am Physicians 73:* 227, 1960.
156. Kuchel, O., Horky, K., Gregarova, I., et al: Inappropriate response to upright posture: a precipitating factor in the pathogenesis of idiopathic edema. *Ann Intern Med 73:* 245, 1970.
157. Fisher, D. A., Morris, M. D.: Idiopathic edema and hyperaldosteronuria: postural venous plasma pooling. *Pediatrics 35:* 413, 1965.
158. Hill, S. R., Jr., Hood, W. G., Jr., Farmer, T. A., Jr., et al: Idiopathic edema. Report of a case with orthostatic edema and hyperaldosteronism. *N Engl J Med 263:* 1342, 1960.
159. Gill, J. R., Jr., Cox, J., Delea, C. S., et al: Idiopathic edema II. Pathogenesis of edema in patients with hypoalbuminemia. *Am J Med 52:* 452, 1972.
160. Gill, J. R., Jr., Mason, D. T., Bartter, F. C.: "Idiopathic" edema resulting from occult cardiomyopathy. *Am J Med 38:* 475, 1965.
161. Obeid, A. I., Streeten, D. H. P., Eich, R. H.: Cardiac function in idiopathic edema. *Arch Intern Med 134:* 253, 1974.
162. Christy, N. P., Laragh, J. H.: Pathogenesis of hypokalemic alkalosis in Cushing's syndrome. *N Engl J Med 265:* 1083, 1961.
163. Bagshawe, K. D.: Hypokalemia, carcinoma, and Cushing's syndrome. *Lancet 2:* 284, 1960.
164. Meador, C. K., Liddle, G. W., Island, D. P., et al: Cause of Cushing's syndrome in patients with tumors arising from "nonendocrine tissue." *J Clin Endocrinol 22:* 693, 1962.
165. Crane, M. G., Harris, J. J.: Desoxycorticosterone secretion rates in hyperadrenocorticism. *J Clin Endocrinol 26:* 1135, 1966.
166. Schambelan, M., Slaton, P. E., Jr., Biglieri, E. G.: Mineralocorticoid production in hyperadrenocorticism. *Am J Med 51:* 299, 1971.
167. Liddle, G. W., Island, D. P., Meador, C. K.: Normal and abnormal regulation of corticotropin in man. *Rec Prog Horm Res 18:* 125, 1962.
168. Lipsett, M. B., Hertz, R., Ross, G. T.: Clinical and pathophysiologic aspects of adrenocortical cancer. *Am J Med 35:* 374, 1963.
169. Touchstone, J. C., Bulachenko, H., Richardson, E. M., et al: The excretion of pregnane-3α,17α,21-triol-20-one (tetrahydro S) in normal and pathologic urine. *J Clin Endocrinol 17:* 250, 1957.
170. Eberlein, W. R., Bongiovanni, A. M.: Congenital adrenal hyperplasia with hypertension: unusual steroid pattern in blood and urine. *J Clin Endocrinol 15:* 1531, 1955.
171. Bongiovanni, A. M., Root, A. W.: The adrenogenital syndrome. *N Engl J Med 268:* 1283, 1963.
172. Gabrilove, J. L., Sharma, D. C., Dorfman, R. I.: Adrenocortical 11β-hydroxylase deficiency and virilism first manifest in the adult woman. *N Engl J Med 272:* 1189, 1965.
173. Green, O. C., Migeon, C. J., Wilkins, L.: Urinary steroids in hypertensive form of congenital adrenal hyperplasia. *J Clin Endocrinol 20:* 929, 1960.
174. Biglieri, E. G., Herron, M. A., Brust, N.: 17-Hydroxylation deficiency in man. *J Clin Invest 45:* 1946, 1966.
175. New, M. I., Suvannakul, L.: Male pseudohermaphrodism due to 17α-hydroxylase deficiency. *J Clin Invest 49:* 1930, 1970.
176. Spark, R. F., Melby, J. C.: Hypertension and low plasma renin activity: presumptive evidence for mineralocorticoid excess. *Ann Intern Med 75:* 831, 1971.
177. Dale, S. L., Melby, J. C.: Altered adrenal steroidogenesis in "low renin" essential hypertension. *Trans Assoc Am Physicians 87:* 248, 1974.
178. Molhuysen, J. A., Gerbrandy, J., deVries, L. A., et al: A licorice extract with deoxycortone-like action. *Lancet 2:* 381, 1950.
179. Conn, J. W., Rovner, D. R., Cohen, E. L.: Licorice-induced pseudoaldosteronism. *JAMA 205:* 492, 1968.
180. Holmes, A. M., Marrott, P. K., Young, J., et al: Pseudohyperaldosteronism induced by habitual ingesting of licorice. *Postgrad Med J 46:* 625, 1970.
181. Gross, E. G., Dexter, J. D., Roth, R. G.: Hypokalemic myopathy with myoglobinuria associated with licorice ingestion. *N Engl J Med 274:* 602, 1966.
182. Louis, L. H., Conn, J. W.: Preparation of glycyrrhizinic acid, the electrolyte-active principle of licorice. Its effects upon metabolism and upon pituitary adrenal function in man. *J Lab Clin Med 47:* 20, 1956.
183. Salassa, R. M., Mattox, V. R., Rosevear, J. W.: Inhibition of the "mineralocorticoid" activity of licorice by spironolactone. *J Clin Endocrinol 22:* 1156, 1962.
184. Personal communication, Whitman, R. H., Sales Manager, MacAndrews and Forbes Co (MAFCO).
185. Revers, F. E.: Licorice juice in therapy of ventricular and duodenal ulcers. *Ned Tijdschr Geneeskd 92:* 2968, 1948.
186. Roussak, N. J.: Fatal hypokalemic alkalosis with tetany during liquorice and P.A.S. therapy. *Br Med J 1:* 360, 1952.
187. Liddle, G. W., Bledsoe, T., Coppage, W. S., Jr.: A familial renal disorder simulating primary aldosteronism but with negligible aldosterone secretion. *Trans Assoc Am Physicians 76:* 199, 1963.
188. Gardner, J. D., Lapey, A., Simopoulos, A. P., et al: Abnormal membrane sodium transportation in Liddle's syndrome. *J Clin Invest 50:* 2253, 1971.
189. Mangos, J. A., Opitz, J. M., Lobeck, C. C., et al: Familial juvenile nephronophthisis. An unrecognized renal disease in the United States. *Pediatrics 34:* 337, 1964.
190. Gitelman, H. J., Graham, J. B., Welt, L. G.: A new familial disorder characterized by hypokalemia and hypomagnesemia. *Trans Assoc Am Physicians 79:* 221, 1966.
191. Vagnucci, A. H.: Selective aldosterone deficiency. *J Clin Endocrinol 29:* 279, 1969.
192. Hills, A. G.: Pathogenesis of hyperkalemia in hypoaldosteronism. *J Clin Endocrinol 29:* 988, 1969.
193. Lipsett, M. B., Pearson, O. H.: Sodium depletion in adrenalectomized humans. *J Clin Invest 37:* 1394, 1958.
194. Thorn, G. W., Dorrance, S. S., Day, E.: Addison's disease: Evaluation of synthetic desoxycorticosterone acetate therapy in 158 patients. *Ann Intern Med 16:* 1053, 1942.
195. Rosenbaum, J. D., Papper, S., Ashley, M. M.: Variations in renal excretion of sodium independent of change in adrenocortical hormone dosage in patients with Addison's disease. *J Clin Endocrinol 15:* 1459, 1955.
196. Hudson, J. B., Chobanian, A. V., Relman, A. S.: Hypoaldosteronism: a clinical study of a patient with an isolated adrenal mineralocorticoid deficiency resulting in hyperkalemia and Stokes-Adams attacks. *N Engl J Med 257:* 529, 1957.
197. Lambrew, C. T., Carver, S. T., Peterson, R. E.: Hypoaldosteronism as a cause of hyperkalemia and syncopal attacks in a patient with complete heart block. *Am J Med 31:* 81, 1961.
198. Ulick, S., Gautier, E., Vetter, K. K., et al: An aldosterone biosynthetic defect in a salt-losing disorder. *J Clin Endocrinol 24:* 669, 1964.
199. Visser, H. K. A., Cost, W. S.: A new hereditary defect in the biosynthesis of aldosterone: urinary C21-corticosteroid pattern in three related patients with a salt-losing syndrome suggesting an 18-oxidation defect. *Acta Endocrinol 47:* 589, 1964.
200. David, R., Golan, S., Drucker, W.: Familial aldosterone deficiency: enzyme defect, diagnosis, clinical course, *Pediatrics 41:* 403, 1968.
201. Marieb, N. J., Melby, J. C., Lyall, S. S.: Isolated hypoaldosteronism associated with idiopathic hypoparathyroidism. *Arch Intern Med 134:* 424, 1974.
202. Ehrlich, E. N., Straus, F. H., II, Hunter, R. L., et al: Cytomegalic adrenocortical hypoplasia and increased plasma 20α-hydroxypregn-4-en-3-one in a man's exhibiting the features of selective mineralocorticoid deficiency. *J Clin Endocrinol 29:* 523, 1969.
203. Molnar, G. D., Mattox, V. R., Mason, H. L., et al: Chronic adrenocortical dysfunction including aldosterone deficiency: studies of steroid and electrolyte metabolism. *J Clin Endocrinol 19:* 1023, 1959.
204. Schlatmann, R., Jansen, A., Prenen, H., et al: The natriuretic and

aldosterone suppressive action of heparin and some related polysulfated polysaccharides. *J Clin Endocrinol 24:* 35, 1964.

205. Bailey, R. E., Ford, H. C.: The effect of heparin on sodium conservation and on the plasma concentration, the metabolic clearance and the secretion and excretion rates of aldosterone in normal subjects. *Acta Endocrinol 60:* 249, 1969.

206. Conn, J. W., Rovner, D. R., Cohen, E. L., et al: Inhibition by heparinoid of aldosterone biosynthesis in man. *J Clin Endocrinol 26:* 527, 1966.

207. Abbott, E. C., Gornall, A. G., Sutherland, D. J. A., et al: The influence of a heparin-like compound on hypertension, electrolytes and aldosterone in man. *Can Med Assoc J 94:* 1155, 1966.

208. Abbott, E. C., Monkhouse, F. C., Steiner, J. W., et al: Effect of a sulfated mucopolysaccharide (RO1-8307) on the zona glomerulosa of the rat adrenal. *Endocrinology 78:* 651, 1966.

209. Wilson, I. D., Goetz, F. C.: Selective hypoaldosteronism after prolonged heparin administration. *Am J Med 36:* 635, 1964.

210. Coppage, W. S., Island, D., Smith, M.: Inhibition of aldosterone secretion and modification of electrolyte excretion in man by a chemical inhibitor of 11β-hydroxylation. *J Clin Invest 38:* 2101, 1959.

211. Fishman, L. M., Liddle, G. W., Island, D. P., et al: Effects of amino-glutethimide on adrenal function in man. *J Clin Endocrinol 27:* 481, 1967.

212. Temple, T. E., Jr., Jones, D. J., Jr., Liddle, G. W., et al: Treatment of Cushing's disease. Correction of hypercortisolism by o,p′-DDD without induction of aldosterone deficiency. *N Engl J Med 281:* 801, 1969.

213. Bledsoe, T., Island, D. P., Riondel, A. M., et al: Modification of aldosterone secretion and electrolyte excretion in man by a chemical inhibitor of 18-oxidation. *J Clin Endocrinol 24:* 740, 1964.

214. Ross, E. J., Van't Hoff, W., Crabbe, J., et al: Aldosterone secretion in hypopituitarism and after hypophysectomy in man. *Am J Med 28:* 229, 1960.

215. Williams, G. H., Rose, L. I., Dluhy, R. G., et al: Aldosterone response to sodium restriction and ACTH stimulation in panhypopituitarism. *J Clin Endocrinol 32:* 27, 1971.

216. Biglieri, E. G., Slaton, P. E., J. R., Silen, W. S., et al: Postoperative studies of adrenal function in primary aldosteronism. *J Clin Endocrinol 26:* 553, 1966.

217. Lowder, S. C., Brown, R. D.: Hypertension corrected by discontinuing chronic sodium bicarbonate ingestion. Subsequent transient hypoaldosteronism. *Am J Med 58:* 272, 1975.

217a. Oster, J. R., Periz, G. O., Rosen, M. S.: Hyporeninemic hypoaldosteronism after chronic sodium bicarbonate abuse. *Arch Intern Med 136:* 1179, 1976.

218. Slaton, P. E., Jr., Biglieri, E. G.: Reduced aldosterone excretion in patients with autonomic insufficiency. *J Clin Endocrinol 27:* 37, 1967.

219. Boticelli, J. T., Lange, R. L., Kelly, O. A.: Postural hypotension with decreased central blood volume and impaired aldosterone response. *Am J Med 37:* 147, 1964.

220. Gordon, R. D., Kuchel, O., Liddle, G. W., et al: Role of the sympathetic nervous system in regulating renin and aldosterone production in man. *J Clin Invest 46:* 599, 1967.

221. Shear, L.: Renal function and sodium metabolism in idiopathic orthostatic hypotension. *N Engl J Med 268:* 347, 1963.

222. Shear, L.: Orthostatic hypotension. *Arch Intern Med 122:* 467, 1968.

223. Schambelan, M., Stockigt, J. R., Biglieri, E. G.: Isolated hypoaldosteronism in adults. A renin deficiency syndrome. *N Engl J Med 287:* 573, 1972.

224. Weidman, P., Reinhart, R., Maxwell, M. H., et al: Syndrome of hyporeninemic hypoaldosteronism and hyperkalemia in renal disease. *J Clin Endocrinol 36:* 965, 1973.

225. Perez, G., Siegel, L., Schreiner, G. E.: Selective hypoaldosteronism with hyperkalemia. *Ann Intern Med 76:* 757, 1972.

226. Gossain, V. V., Ferrara, E. V., Werk, E. E.: Impaired renin responsiveness with secondary hypoaldosteronism. *Arch Intern Med 132:* 885, 1973.

227. Oh, M. S., Carroll, H. J.: Clemmons, J. E., et al: A mechanism for hyporeninemic hypoaldosteronism in chronic renal disease. *Metabolism 23:* 1157, 1974.

228. Christlieb, A. R.: Diabetes and hypertensive vascular disease. *Am J Cardiol 32:* 593, 1973.

229. Gordon, R. D., Geddes, R. A., Pawsey, C. G. K., et al: Hypertension and severe hyperkalemia associated with suppression of renin and aldosterone and completely reversed by dietary sodium restriction. *Aust Ann Med 4:* 287, 1970.

230. Weinberger, M. H., Dowdy, A. I., Nokes, G. W., et al: Plasma renin activity and aldosterone secretion in hypertensive patients during high and low sodium intake and administration of diuretic. *J Clin Endocrinol 28:* 359, 1968.

231. Jose, A., Crout, J. R., Kaplan, N. M.: Suppressed plasma renin activity in essential hypertension: roles of plasma volume, blood pressure, and sympathetic nervous system. *Ann Intern Med 72:* 9, 1970.

232. Jose, A., Kaplan, N. M.: Plasma renin activity in the diagnosis of primary aldosteronism: failure to distinguish primary aldosteronism from essential hypertension. *Arch Intern Med 123:* 141, 1969.

233. Christlieb, A. R., Hickler, R. B., Lauler, D. P., et al: Hypertension with inappropriate aldosterone stimulation. *N Engl J Med 281:* 128, 1969.

234. Thorn, G. W., Koepf, G. F., Clinton, M., Jr.: Renal failure simulating adrenocortical insufficiency. *N Engl J Med 231:* 76, 1944.

235. Nussbaum, H. E., Bernhard, W. G., Mattia, V. D., Jr.: Chronic pyelonephritis simulating adrenocortical insufficiency. *N Engl J Med 246:* 289, 1952.

236. Popovtzer, M. M., Katz, F. H., Pinggera, W. F., et al: Hyperkalemia in salt-wasting nephropathy. Study of the mechanism. *Arch Intern Med 132:* 203, 1973.

237. Gerstein, A. R., Kleeman, C. R., Gold, F. M., et al: Aldosterone deficiency in chronic renal failure. *Nephron 5:* 90, 1968.

238. Daughaday, W. H., Rendleman, D.: Severe symptomatic hyperkalemia in an adrenalectomized woman due to enhanced mineralocorticoid requirement. *Ann Intern Med 66:* 1197, 1967.

239. Lathem, W.: Hyperchloremic acidosis in chronic pyelonephritis. *N Engl J Med 258:* 1031, 1958.

240. Carroll, H. J., Farber, S. J.: Hyperkalemia and hyperchloremic acidosis in chronic pyelonephritis. *Metabolism 13:* 808, 1964.

241. de Leiva, A., Christlieb, A. R., Melby, J. C., et al: Big renin and biosynthetic defect of aldosterone in diabetes mellitus. *N Engl J Med 295:* 639, 1976.

242. Goldfarb, S., Cox, M., Singer, I., et al: Acute hyperkalemia induced by hyperglycemia: hormonal mechanisms. *Ann Intern Med 84:* 426, 1976.

243. Viberti, G. C.: Glucose-induced hyperkalemia: A hazard for diabetics? *Lancet 1:* 690, 1978.

146

Metabolic Adaptation to Physical Exercise in Man

John Wahren

INTRODUCTION

The metabolic processes of muscle tissue serve to transform chemical energy into mechanical energy. This is achieved primarily by the oxidation of carbohydrate and lipid substrates to provide the ATP necessary for the contractile process. Although of fundamental importance for man's ability to carry out exercise, the mechanisms and conditions regulating the supply and utilization of different fuels by contracting muscle remained relatively unexplored until fairly recently. Until the early 1950s our understanding of substrate utilization by human skeletal muscle was based primarily on animal experiments, in vitro analyses of muscle tissue, and studies of pulmonary oxygen uptake and carbon dioxide release in man. The development since then of new investigative procedures and analytical methods has greatly increased the possibilities of studying the metabolic and hormonal adaptation that occurs in response to physical exertion in man.

To study the metabolic exchange of an intact organ or tissue, one needs to collect both arterial and venous blood. It was therefore a great step forward when procedures for the percutaneous catheterization of arteries and veins became available[1] and radiologic techniques made it possible to direct catheters to the body's major vessels, thereby making it possible to determine the regional arteriovenous (AV) concentration differences for oxygen, carbon dioxide, and blood substrates. However, in order to obtain a quantitative estimate of regional substrate exchange, data on AV differences must be supplemented with determinations of blood flow. Several techniques—based on indicator dilution, isotope clearance, or thermodilution—have been developed for this and it is now possible to measure blood flow to the limbs[2–4] or to the liver[5,6] during exercise. The product of blood flow and AV difference for a substrate provides an estimate of the net exchange per unit time for that region, thereby allowing quantitative calculations of the contribution to metabolism made by blood-borne substrates. In addition, the use of radioactive isotopes, primarily ^{14}C, for labeling substrates and metabolites has facilitated specific, quantitative estimation of the systemic or regional turnover of substrates during exercise.

In order to evaluate the metabolic events inside muscle tissue and the utilization of fuels stored within the muscle cell, it is necessary to obtain muscle specimens for analysis. Such studies used to be limited to animal experiments. In 1962 a needle biopsy technique was presented by Bergström[7] with which muscle specimens could be obtained safely and repeatedly from the quadriceps muscle or other muscle groups during exercise in man.

It is the purpose of this chapter to present some of the major recent findings regarding the metabolic adaptation to exercise, with the emphasis on quantitative human data. Unless otherwise stated, the findings refer to the postabsorptive state after 12–14 h of fasting. It should be recognized that as man proceeds from the fed to the adapted fasting state, important biochemical and hormonal changes occur through which a continuous supply of fuel is maintained to meet the metabolic expenditures. Inasmuch as the human body continues to adapt to fasting for several days, exercise studies undertaken after 12–14 h of fasting reflect two superimposed states—the transition from the fed to the fasted state and the metabolic response to exercise. This fact should be borne in mind when interpreting results from prolonged periods of exercise.

SUBSTRATE DEPOTS OF THE BODY

CARBOHYDRATE STORES

The depots of carbohydrate substrates in body fluids and tissues of normal man are presented in Table 146-1. The body contains approximately 20 g of free glucose, distributed in extracellular water and the intracellular compartment of the liver cells. Although small, the blood pool has the important task of maintain-

Table 146-1. Substrate Stores in Normal Man

Fuel	Weight (kg)	Energy (kcal)
Circulating fuels		
Glucose (extracellular water)	0.020	80
Free fatty acids (plasma)	0.0004	4
Triglycerides (plasma)	0.004	40
Total		124
Tissue stores		
Fat		
Adipose tissue triglycerides	15	140,000
Intramuscular triglycerides	0.3	2,800
Protein (mainly muscle)	10	41,000
Glycogen		
Liver	0.085	350
Muscle	0.350	1,450
Total		185,600

ing a continuous supply of glucose to the glucose-dependent tissues. In the basal state the dominant glucose-consuming tissue is the brain. Replenishment of the blood glucose pool occurs continuously from the liver; no other organ produces significant amounts of glucose in the basal state. The hepatic glucose output derives from glycogenolysis (70–75 percent) as well as from de novo synthesis of glucose (gluconeogenesis) from glucose precursors such as lactate, amino acids, glycerol, and pyruvate (25–30 percent)[8,9] taken up by the liver.

The hepatic glycogen concentration in subjects ingesting a mixed diet is approximately 50 g/kg wet tissue.[10] Assuming a liver weight of 1500–1800 g, the total glycogen store in the liver may be estimated at 75–90 g. This substrate depot has an important function in the body's adjustment to varying energy requirements. After 10–12 h of fasting, mobilization of liver glycogen proceeds at a rate of approximately 50 mg/min/kg liver[11]—thereby contributing to maintain the blood glucose level. As discussed below, this rate accelerates substantially during physical exertion. Although we do not know just how large a part of the liver glycogen is available for mobilization during exercise, the fact that the liver is almost entirely depleted after 1 week on a carbohydrate-free diet[11] suggests that the major part can be utilized during exercise, too. The liver depot of glycogen refills relatively slowly; 12–36 h (depending on diet and physical activity) are required for full restitution after a period of severe exercise. When a carbohydrate-rich diet is ingested after exercise, the liver glycogen content recovers to levels above the control value.[11]

In addition to the liver depot, an important store of glycogen is contained in muscle tissue. Here the concentration is approximately 9–16 g/kg wet muscle, the values being lowest in arm and shoulder muscles and highest in samples from the lower extremities.[12] The muscle glycogen concentration does not seem to vary with either age or sex. Assuming that the total muscle mass accounts for approximately 40 percent of body weight, the glycogen depot in skeletal muscle can be estimated at 300–400 g, making this the largest carbohydrate store of the body. This estimate agrees quite well with indirect evaluations based on the respiratory quotient (RQ) and prolonged exhaustive exercise.[13]

The muscle glycogen content does not vary under resting basal conditions and decreases slowly during prolonged fasting.[14] It is during physical exercise that muscle glycogen is primarily utilized physiologically, as discussed below. As muscle tissue lacks glucose-6-phosphatase and there is no hydrolysis of phosphorylated glycolytic intermediary metabolites, the amounts of glucose that leave muscle either at rest or during exercise are quantitatively insignificant. Consequently, only the local glycogen store of the exercising muscle can be utilized as fuel; the glycogen content of a resting muscle does not change, even when other muscle groups are exercised to exhaustion.[15]

Recent studies have emphasized the profound differences in muscle glycogen restitution after exercise in subjects ingesting different diets. A diet rich in carbohydrate greatly enhances glycogen resynthesis after exercise; the muscle glycogen content recovers to a peak that is higher than the preexercise level, an overshoot that is confined to the glycogen-depleted muscle.[16] With a diet consisting mainly of protein and fat, on the other hand, the resynthesis of glycogen after rigorous exercise is greatly delayed.[17]

The key enzyme in the regulation of glycogen synthesis is glycogen synthetase, of which there are two forms; one (D form) is dependent and the other (I form) is independent of glucose-6-phosphate for its activity.[18,19] It is widely accepted that most physiologic alterations involving accelerated glycogen synthesis can be explained by increased activity of the I form synthetase. However, this does not seem to apply either to the increase in glycogen synthesis following a period of exercise or to the overshoot in muscle glycogen content observed on a carbohydrate-rich diet.[14,15] Although glycogen resynthesis clearly depends on substrate availability as well as on the I form synthetase, the mechanisms behind the intriguing overshoot phenomenon are still obscure.

Studies in subjects in whom the muscle glycogen concentration has been varied by dietary manipulation have illustrated that the size of the carbohydrate stores influences the capacity to perform heavy work. The physiologic importance of the muscle glycogen depot is underscored by the direct correlation between the initial glycogen content of muscle and an individual's ability to tolerate prolonged heavy bicycle exercise,[20,21] suggesting that the glycogen concentration may become a limiting factor in this context.

The blood glucose pool and the glycogen stored in the liver and in muscle tissue are thus the quantitatively important depots of carbohydrate. Their relative importance as sources of fuel during exercise depends on the type and duration of the exercise performed. Muscle glycogen is of use in meeting the energy requirements of those muscle fibers in which it is contained but not as a reservoir for repletion of blood glucose. In contrast, liver glycogen represents a readily mobilizable source of blood glucose that may be gradually depleted during periods of fasting or rapidly mobilized in response to exercise.

ADIPOSE TISSUE

It has been known for more than a century that fat is the body's principal form of stored energy. Early studies by Benedict on prolonged fasting[22] demonstrated that fat-derived substrates provide the major part of the calories utilized during food deprivation. However, only during the last 15 years has greater insight been gained into the physiologic mechanisms behind the deposition, mobilization, and utilization of lipid substrates.

Man's ability to tolerate marked extremes in caloric intake and fuel consumption is in part a consequence of his ability to store energy in an economical form. While fuel may be accumulated in the body as carbohydrate, protein, or fat, the last of these has by far the highest calorie:weight ratio; because of its anhydrous nature, adipose tissue is on this basis approximately eight times more economical as a depot than glycogen and protein. Moreover, the white fat of the body is readily expended without adverse effects and can meet the substrate requirements of many different body tissues.

The average 70-kg man has approximately 15 kg of fat in the form of adipose tissue triglycerides, representing about 140,000 kcal (Table 146-1). In addition, intramuscular triglycerides can be estimated at 300 g,[23] corresponding to an additional 2800 kcal. The energy stored in the body's triglyceride depots is enough to permit survival during 2 to 3 months of total food deprivation. By comparison, liver and muscle carbohydrate stores and circulating fuels, in the form of glucose, free fatty acids (FFA), or triglycerides, are quantitatively insignificant. Protein, mainly in the form of muscle tissue, has a large caloric potential—approximately 24,000 kcal (Table 146-1)—but only a minor part is available under normal circumstances since (unlike adipose tissue triglyceride and glycogen in muscle and liver) protein in both muscle and other tissues primarily serves purposes other than caloric storage.

Hydrolysis of the adipose tissue triglycerides (lipolysis) leads to the release of FFA and glycerol to the blood stream. The regulation of adipose tissue lipopolysis during exercise involves the sympathetic nervous system.[24] Norepinephrine, liberated at sympathetic nerve endings, potently stimulates fat mobilization. Like epinephrine, it activates the adenyl cyclase system to form increased amounts of cAMP. This substance, in turn, activates a lipolytic system in the adipose tissue cell which catalyzes the hydrolysis of the stored triglycerides. Plasma levels of epinephrine as well as of norepinephrine increase during exercise.[25,26] Increased plasma concentrations of catecholamines are not as effective in eliciting lipolysis as augmented activity in sympathetic nerves to adipose tissue,[27] suggesting that sympathetic outflow is more important than circulating catecholamines for FFA mobilization during exercise. While it is the sympathetic nervous activity to adipose tissue that permits the rapid acceleration of lipolysis during exercise, changes in the hormonal milieu are probably of importance too. In particular, the fall in concentration of insulin[26,28] and the rise in glucagon[26,28,29] and growth hormone[30] concentrations with exercise are likely to contribute to a sustained release of FFA from adipose tissue, particularly during prolonged exercise.

It is not known just which adipose tissues are responsible for the augmented FFA mobilization during physical exertion, though regional differences have been described in the sympathetic innervation of adipose tissue.[31] The contribution from subcutaneous tissue of the arms and legs is trivial during exercise[32,33] and the splanchnic area shows a net FFA uptake,[34] suggesting that the bulk of FFA must derive from adipose tissue of the trunk.

MUSCLE GLYCOGEN UTILIZATION

MUSCLE FIBER COMPOSITION AND RECRUITMENT PATTERNS

In normal human skeletal muscle two major types of muscle fibers can be identified on the basis of different histochemical characteristics.[35] The red fibers (type I, slow-twitch fibers) are rich in capillaries, oxidative enzymes, and lipids, while the white fibers (type II, fast-twitch fibers) show high concentrations of glycolytic enzymes but lower capillary and mitochondrial densities.[36] Thus, the red fibers show a high oxidative capacity while the white fibers are engaged primarily in glycolytic metabolism. The glycogen content is approximately the same in the two fiber types.[35] Most muscle groups contain 40–50 percent red fibers; fiber composition varies greatly between individuals but only slightly between two muscles from the same subject.

Muscle fibers within the same motor unit are structurally homogeneous, i.e., each motor unit comprises only one type of muscle fiber.[37] The size of the motor neuron appears to be of functional significance. Red fiber motor neurons are small and show low spinal thresholds and a tonic discharge pattern, while the motor neurons activating white fibers are large, show high thresholds, and discharge phasically. The intensity and duration of the neurogenic stimulus thus tend to determine the type of fiber that is activated. For work of light intensity and rhythmic type, such as bicycling or walking, it appears that the low-threshold motor neurons and hence the red muscle fibers are recruited, the white fibers being activated only very transiently at the onset of exercise.[38,39] In contrast, exercise of higher intensity or work involving rapid, sudden movements as well as strong isometric contractions is accompanied by recruitment of the high-threshold motor neurons activating the white fibers.[39,40] It is thus conceivable, as discussed below, that the activation pattern for enzymatically and metabolically different muscle fibers may provide a background to the changing pattern of substrate utilization by skeletal muscle.

GLYCOGEN UTILIZATION

The occurrence of glycogen in muscle tissue was first described by Claude Bernard in 1859.[41] The utilization of this glycogen during exercise has been recognized for a long time but until recently it was thought that this was mainly for anaerobic metabolism and the production of lactate. While it is true that the lactate released by muscle at the onset of exercise, as well as that formed during very strenuous exertion, is derived from glycogen, the primary metabolic fate of muscle glycogen is terminal oxidation. The important role of glycogen in aerobic muscle metabolism was identified by Hultman and co-workers,[14,42,43] and much subsequent work has been devoted to characterizing the utilization of muscle glycogen under a variety of physiologic conditions.

There are two major factors that influence the consumption of muscle glycogen during work: the duration and the intensity* of the exercise performed. During prolonged, submaximal exercise the glycogen concentration decreases in a curvilinear manner[14,42] (Fig. 146-1). A rapid decline in concentration at the onset of work is accompanied by a sharp increase in blood lactate levels. After the initial phase of exercise, glycogen utilization slows down,

*The intensity of exercise may be graded in absolute terms (watts or kilogram-meters/minute; 1 watt = 6.135 kg-m/min) or in terms of relative work capacity (percent of maximal aerobic capacity). In this chapter "mild" exercise refers to an intensity of approximately 400 kg-m/min (65 W), or 25–30 percent of maximal capacity; "moderate" exercise refers to approximately 800 kg-m/min (130 W), or 40–50 percent of maximal capacity; and "severe" or "heavy" exercise refers to a work intensity of approximately 1200 kg-m/min (200 W) or 70–80 percent of maximal capacity.

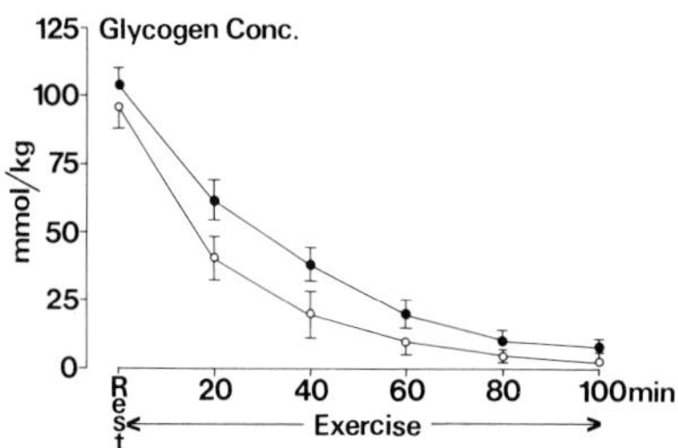

Fig. 146-1. Glycogen content of quadriceps muscle at rest and during submaximal exercise in trained (●) and untrained (○) subjects (mean ± SE). Glycogen concentration is given in millimoles glucosyl units per kilogram muscle. (Data courtesy of Dr. B. Saltin.)

possibly because the circulatory adaptation to exercise makes other substrates available to the contracting muscle. As exercise proceeds beyond 60–80 min the rate of glycogen utilization drops still further; there is now a relative lack of muscle glycogen and the utilization of blood-borne substrates gradually increases.

The influence of work intensity on the rate of muscle glycogenolysis has been demonstrated indirectly[44] as well as by direct measurements of muscle glycogen consumption. The rate of muscle glycogen utilization during the first 5–10 min of exercise shows a curvilinear relationship to work load for dynamic work[43] (Fig. 146-2) as well as for static contractions.[45] The rise in the rate of utilization is more pronounced at the heavier work intensities. The most rapid muscle glycogenolysis is seen in connection with short-term, heavy isometric contractions, when the rate may be 10 times greater than during heavy dynamic work.

The utilization of glycogen in response to exercise differs between the two types of muscle fiber. During light to moderately heavy exercise, demanding less than 60 percent of the maximal pulmonary oxygen uptake, glycogen depletion seems to be confined to the red fibers,[39] as illustrated in Figure 146-3. Only when the glycogen content of these fibers decreases during prolonged work, do the white fibers gradually become activated and their glycogen utilized. During exercise of higher intensity, close to or above the maximal aerobic power, depletion of glycogen occurs chiefly in the white fibers and only to a smaller extent in the red. Isometric contractions are accompanied by glycogen utilization primarily in the white fibers; utilization is in fact confined to these fibers if the contraction tension is at least 20 percent of the maximal.[40] Glycogen utilization therefore seems to occur preferentially in one of the two types of muscle fiber, depending on the exercise conditions. This may help to explain why subjects become exhausted even though the muscle tissue still contains significant amounts of glycogen—the muscle fibers containing this glycogen may not be activated under the given conditions of exercise.

These studies were performed in the postabsorptive, basal state. As some form of nutrition, usually rich in carbohydrate, is often taken in connection with heavy exercise or athletics, it would be of interest to know whether less muscle glycogen is used during exercise when extra glucose is supplied. The data available suggest that this is not the case with prolonged heavy exercise.[14] At a lower work load (less than 50 percent of maximal oxygen uptake), however, the administration of glucose significantly reduces glycogen consumption.[46] Similarly, the infusion of nicotinic acid, which inhibits the mobilization of FFA from adipose tissue, is associated with an augmented utilization of muscle glycogen during work, particularly during prolonged exercise.[47] Thus it can be concluded that, although glycogen utilization plays an important and at times a dominant role in aerobic muscle metabolism, its rate of consumption is modified by alterations in the supply of blood-borne fuels.

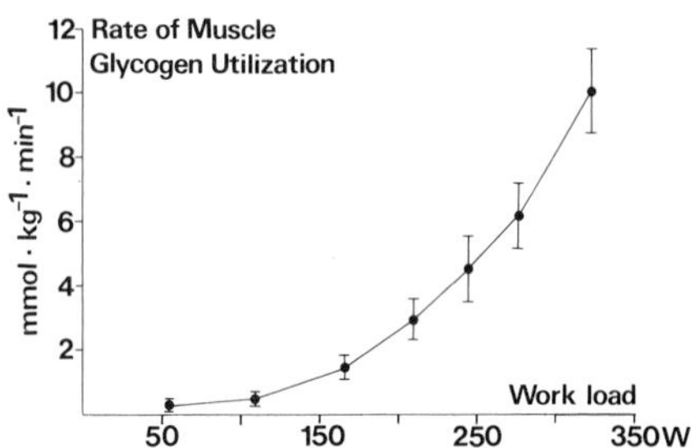

Fig. 146-2. Estimated rate of leg muscle glycogen utilization during the first 5–10 min of exercise at different work loads (mean ± SE). (Data courtesy of Dr. B. Saltin.)

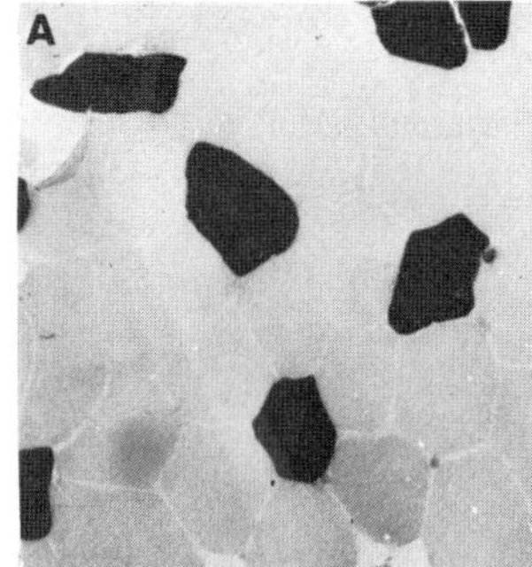

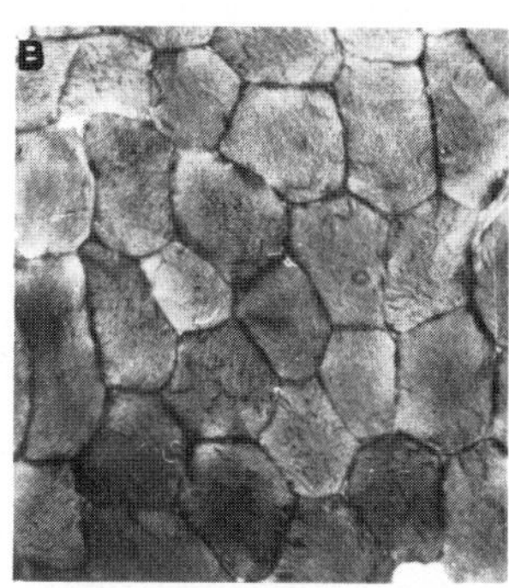

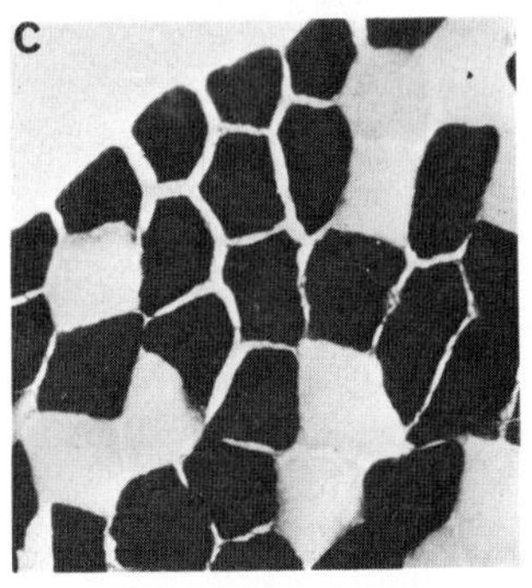

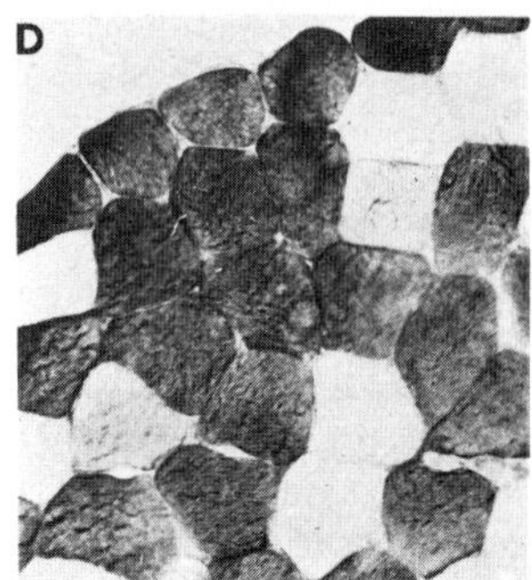

Fig. 146-3. Serial sections of quadriceps muscle samples. A, B. At rest. C, D. After exercise for 3 h at a work load corresponding to 30 percent of maximal oxygen uptake. Sections A and C were stained for myofibrillar ATPase and show red fibers (light) and white fibers (dark). Sections B and D were stained for glycogen using the PAS reaction. Serial sections A and B, representing the resting state, demonstrate an even distribution of glycogen in the two fiber types. Serial sections C and D illustrate selective depletion of glycogen in the red fibers following prolonged mild exercise. (Data courtesy of Dr. B. Saltin.)

BLOOD GLUCOSE TURNOVER

GLUCOSE UPTAKE BY MUSCLE

Uptake of blood glucose by contracting skeletal muscle has been recognized for almost 90 years.[48] However, following the discovery of the important role of the plasma FFA as energy-yielding substrates (see below), glucose was generally relegated to a minor role with respect to energy metabolism in muscle. In recent years studies have been made in man of the quantitative contributions of blood glucose to the energy needs engendered by exercise, and it is now clear that the role of blood glucose is determined by the duration and intensity of the exercise performed.

In the resting state, there is a small positive AV difference for glucose across the forearm tissues, indicating glucose uptake.[49] At the onset of moderately heavy rhythmic forearm exercise this difference becomes smaller, and after 1–2 min it is reversed, indicating a net release of glucose from the forearm.[50,51] Since glucose-6-phosphatase is not present in muscle tissue, the mechanism behind this finding probably does not involve hydrolysis of glucose-6-phosphate. Some clues may be provided by the breakdown pattern of glycogen, in which most of the glycosyl units are converted to glucose-6-phosphate by the action of myophosphorylase. In the degradation process, debranching of the glycogen molecules (catalyzed by amylo-1,6-glucosidase and oligo-1.4-1.6-glucantransferase) involves the formation of free glucose corresponding to 8–10 percent of the glycogen.[52] During conditions of low to moderate rates of glycogenolysis, this glucose is probably phosphorylated rapidly in the hexokinase reaction, whereas during heavy exercise with rapid glycogen degradation, increased amounts of intracellular glucose will be formed. At this time the hexokinase reaction may be operating slowly or not at all, due in part to inhibition by accumulating glucose-6-phosphate and in part to substrate deficiency as a consequence of lowered levels of ATP. Under such circumstances it is conceivable that the transport of glucose across the cell membrane into the cell is reversed. This transient release of glucose from muscle to blood is quantitatively insignificant, but the observation may help explain the divergent results reported for glucose uptake by muscle during exercise in man.

After the initial 1–2 min of exercise the forearm muscles show a small net uptake of glucose and a considerable release of lactate. As work continues, glucose uptake increases progressively and the release of lactate gradually subsides (Fig. 146-4).[51] Quantitative calculations show that net glucose uptake by forearm muscle may be 15 times the basal value after 10 min of exercise and as much as 35 times after 60 min.[51] The contribution of glucose to the carbohydrate oxidation as well as to the total oxidative metabolism of forearm muscles can be estimated from the local RQ and the AV differences for oxygen, glucose, and lactate. Such calculations show that under resting conditions carbohydrate oxidation plays a minor role,[49,51] and FFA are the dominant fuel. After 10 min of exercise this situation has altered: the RQ indicates that the major part of the oxygen uptake is now being used for carbohydrate oxidation; lactate is released in excess of the simultaneous glucose uptake, suggesting that muscle glycogen is the dominant source of carbohydrate substrate in this situation. However, at the end of a prolonged period of exercise (40–60 min) the situation has changed again: the RQ value indicates that about half of the oxidative metabolism is carbohydrate oxidation, nearly all of which can be accounted for by glucose uptake from the blood.[51]

During the early phase of exercise, lactate output from contracting muscle is at its peak (Fig. 146-4), lower rates of release being seen with increasing duration of work at submaximal work loads. It used to be believed that lactate output is a sign of muscle hypoxia even during mild exercise. However, recent measurements of the steady-state oxidation–reduction level of mitochondrial NAD of contracting skeletal muscle have demonstrated adequate oxygenation even during lactate production.[53] This indicates that lactate production is not necessarily a result of hypoxic stimulation of anaerobic glucolysis. Instead, at mild to moderate levels of work it may reflect an imbalance between the rate of glycolysis and the rate of pyruvate utilization in the citric acid cycle. However, although lactate release does not necessarily imply muscle hypoxia, it does not rule out the possibility of hypoxia during the initial phase of exercise or during very heavy work.

Owing to the small muscle volume involved, glucose utilization during prolonged forearm exercise does not substantially challenge blood glucose homeostasis. However, the pattern of blood glucose utilization is similar during exercise with large muscle groups. When healthy individuals exercised on a bicycle ergometer at mild to strenuous work loads (65, 130, and 200 W), the arterial levels of glucose either did not change or increased during a 40-min exercise period.[8] The AV difference for glucose and the leg blood flow both increased at all levels of work intensity. Net glucose uptake by the leg increased 7-fold above the resting value after 40 min of light exercise, and 10- and 20-fold at the heavier work intensities. Leg glucose uptake rose gradually during the exercise, in keeping with the observations from forearm exercise. For leg exercise, blood glucose oxidation accounts for a growing fraction of both the total and the carbohydrate oxidation of the leg during progressive exercise at all levels of work intensity (Fig. 146-5), thereby helping to make up for the gradually diminishing stores of carbohydrate in the exercising muscle. Thus, although muscle glycogen is likely to be the dominant carbohydrate substrate during the initial phase of exercise, the utilization of blood glucose rises steadily with time. After 40 min of exercise, blood glucose can (assuming that the glucose taken up by the leg muscles is completely oxidized) sustain as much as 75–90 percent of the carbohydrate metabolism and 30–35 percent of the total oxidative metabolism of the leg (Fig. 146-5).

As mild exercise is continued beyond 40 min the rate of glucose utilization increases further, reaching a peak at 90–180 min, at which time glucose uptake may account for 35–40 percent of total metabolism.[28] Mild hypoglycemia may subsequently develop and leg uptake of glucose decline slightly. From these observations it can be concluded that during exercise with the large muscle groups of the leg, as well as during rhythmic work with the forearm flexors, blood glucose is a quantitatively important substrate for oxidation by working muscle.

Turning to the mechanism behind the rise in glucose uptake by muscle during exercise, it is noteworthy that exercise induces a significant fall in the plasma insulin concentration (Fig. 146-6).[8,28,54]

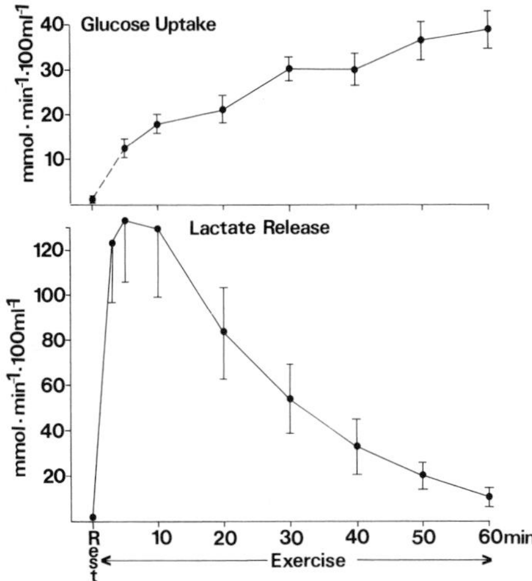

Fig. 146-4. Glucose uptake and release of lactate by the forearm tissues at rest and during prolonged rhythmic forearm exercise using a hand ergometer (work load 1.5 W) (mean ± SE). (Data from Jorfeldt and Wahren.[51])

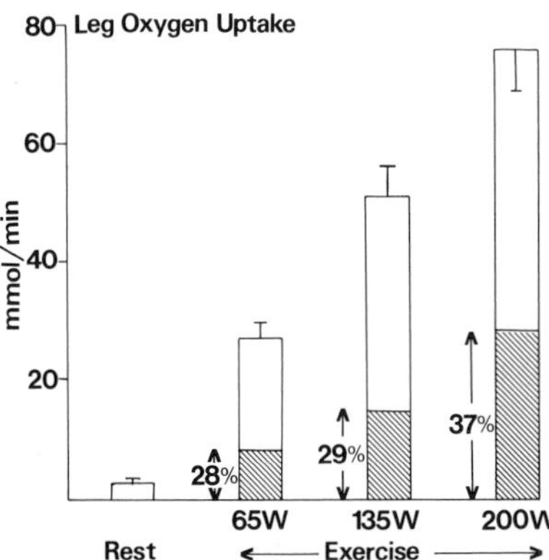

Fig. 146-5. Leg oxygen uptake at rest and after 40 min of bicycle exercise at work loads of 65, 130, and 200 W. Hatched area indicates the proportion of the oxygen uptake that may be accounted for by glucose oxidation. (Data from Wahren et al.[8])

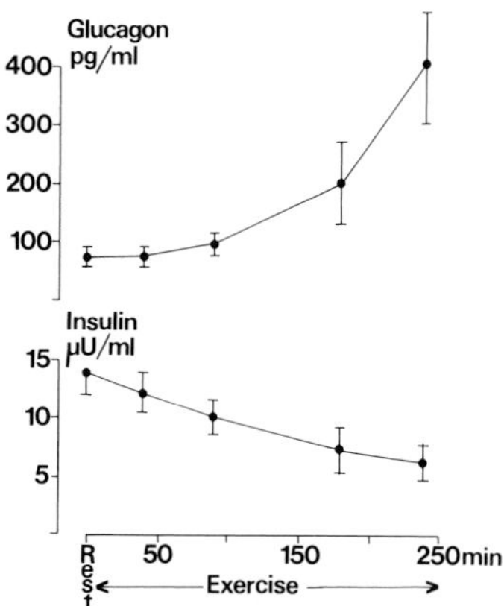

Fig. 146-6. Arterial concentrations of insulin and glucagon during prolonged mild exercise (mean ± SE). (Data from Ahlborg et al.[28])

The divergent responses of circulating glucose and insulin, particularly during strenuous exercise, suggest that insulin secretion is in fact inhibited during physical work, probably as a consequence of increased liberation of catecholamines.[25,26] It has been postulated that exercise-induced hypoinsulinemia serves to limit blood glucose uptake by muscle, thereby increasing its availability to the brain. However, this does not appear to be the case since glucose uptake increases during exercise in the face of falling concentrations of insulin. Furthermore, insulin-dependent patients with juvenile diabetes who have been without insulin for 24 h also show a marked rise in muscle glucose utilization during physical exertion.[55] One can therefore conclude that glucose uptake during exercise does not depend on the ability to secrete increased quantities of insulin. It is still conceivable, however, that the presence of low concentrations of insulin exerts a permissive effect on glucose uptake by contracting muscle, and it should be noted that the augmented blood flow and enlarged capillary surface area during exercise augment the total delivery of insulin to the working muscle. It has also been suggested that the contractile process results in the release by muscle of a humoral substance ("muscle activity factor") that stimulates glucose utilization by exercising muscle.[56] However, studies involving perfused muscle have failed to support the existence of such a humoral factor.[57,58]

Direct examination of the glucose exchange across the cerebral circulation reveals that glucose remains the sole substrate oxidized during exercise and that its rate of utilization is unchanged from the resting state.[59] Moreover, during one-leg exercise, the glucose uptake by the nonexercising leg is unchanged or slightly increased above the basal level.[60] These observations refute the previously advanced hypothesis that part of the increased uptake of blood glucose to the exercising muscles is provided for by a reduced uptake by inactive muscle or the brain.

HEPATIC GLUCOSE OUTPUT

The magnitude of the glucose utilization by exercising muscle clearly indicates that during exercise with large muscle groups the turnover of the blood glucose pool must accelerate considerably. Since the arterial glucose concentration is maintained or even increased during heavy exercise, one can conclude that the augmented peripheral utilization is accompanied by continuous replenishment of the pool. The kidney has the capacity to synthesize significant amounts of glucose, particularly in the prolonged fasted state,[61] but direct measurements in the overnight fasted state indicate that there is no net renal glucose production at rest or during exercise.[8] Since the liver is the only other organ capable of significant gluconeogenesis and since muscle glycogenolysis, in the absence of glucose-6-phosphatase in muscle, is unlikely to contribute significantly to the blood glucose level, it can be concluded that the liver is the dominant and probably the sole source of the increased amounts of glucose utilized during exercise.

The output of glucose from the liver in the basal state, documented in numerous studies involving hepatic venous catheterization, is of the order of 100–200 mg/min. Judging from the splanchnic uptake of glucose percursors (lactate, glucogenic amino acids, glycerol, and pyruvate), approximately 20–25 percent of the basal glucose release derives from gluconeogenesis.[8,9] The remainder is a result of hepatic glycogenolysis, as indicated by direct measurements of hepatic glycogen degradation rates of postabsorptive man.[11]

The output of glucose from the liver rises in response to exercise;[62] maximal increments 4–5-fold above the basal level have been observed during strenuous exertion (Fig. 146-7).[8] The intensity and duration of exercise are the major factors determining the absolute rate of glucose release as well as the relative contributions of glycogenolysis and gluconeogenesis. During exercise of mild intensity (65 W) and short duration (10–30 min), total glucose output rises progressively, by 25–100 percent and the contribution from gluconeogenesis remains comparable to that observed in the basal state.[8] During moderate to severe exercise (130–200 W), glucose release rises 2–5 times the basal value and the contribution from gluconeogenesis decreases to 6–11 percent.[8] This relative decrease in gluconeogenesis does not represent a fall in the absolute uptake of gluconeogenic precursors below basal resting levels, but it does indicate that precursor uptake fails to keep pace with the overall increase in hepatic glucose output. Although both splanchnic fractional extraction (the fraction of the arterial concentration taken up by the splanchnic tissues) and arterial concentrations of lactate, pyruvate, glycerol, and alanine increase during exercise, the fall in splanchnic blood flow induced by moderate to severe exercise is such as to preclude an increment in glucose precursor uptake. Thus the major source of hepatic glucose output during short-term exercise, particularly at heavy work loads, is hepatic glycogenolysis. The extent of hepatic glycogen depletion during 40 min of severe exercise is approximately 18–20 g.[8]

The importance of hepatic glucose production for blood glucose homeostasis during physical work and as a substrate for exercising muscle is underscored by the close agreement between estimated rates of glucose uptake by leg muscle and splanchnic glucose release (Fig. 146-8). Splanchnic glucose output exceeds leg uptake in the resting state, since it is the brain that accounts for the

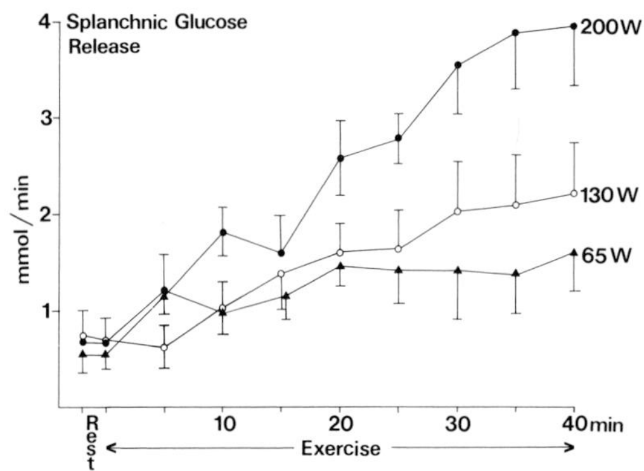

Fig. 146-7. Splanchnic glucose output at rest and during bicycle exercise at work loads of 65, 130, and 200 W (mean ± SE). (Data from Wahren et al.[8])

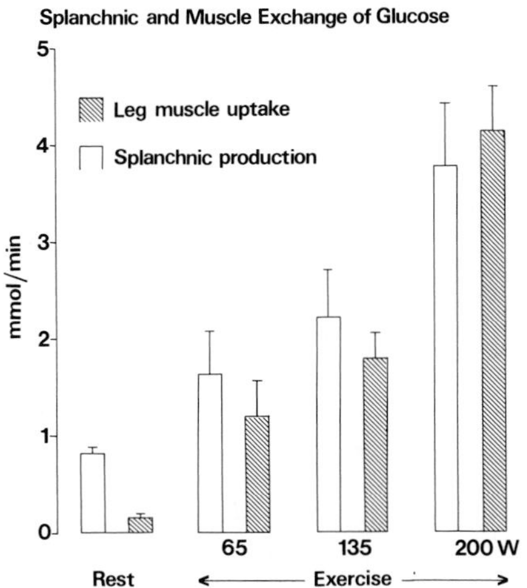

Fig. 146-8. Comparison of estimated glucose exchange of the legs and the splanchnic area in the basal state and after 40 min of exercise at different work loads (mean ± SE). (Data from Wahren et al.[8])

major part of total glucose utilization in the basal postabsorptive state. With increasing physical activity the brain's share of total glucose turnover diminishes and splanchnic output corresponds more and more closely to leg glucose uptake.

Exercise lasting several hours can be maintained only at low work intensities, corresponding to 25–35 percent or less of maximal oxygen uptake. In response to work of this intensity, glucose output rises by 80–100 percent and remains at this level throughout a 4-h exercise period.[28] Total glucose release during this time amounts to approximately 75 g. This large output derives in part from hepatic glycogenolysis, but the rate of gluconeogenesis also accelerates (Fig. 146-9). Prolonged exercise elicits an increased splanchnic fractional extraction as well as augmented arterial levels of alanine, lactate, and glycerol, causing the splanchnic uptake of these glucose precursors to rise 2–10-fold above basal levels. Of the 75 g of glucose released from the liver during 4 h of exercise, approximately 15–20 g may stem from gluconeogenesis and the

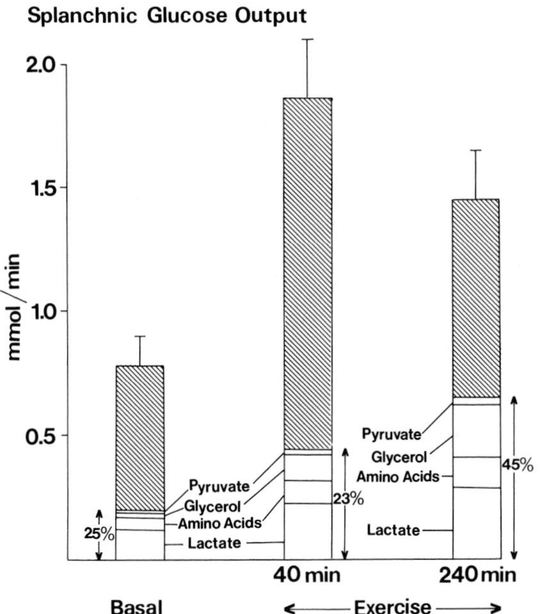

Fig. 146-9. Splanchnic glucose output and uptake of glucogenic precursor substrates in the basal state and during prolonged exercise (mean ± SE). (Data from Ahlborg et al.[28])

other 55–60 g from glycogenolysis, indicating that three-fourths of the hepatic glycogen store is dissipated during this form of exercise.[28] Accordingly, prolonged, mild exercise differs from short-term work in that the contribution from gluconeogenesis increases instead of falling. When exercise is extended over 8 h or more, virtually the entire hepatic glucose output is attributable to gluconeogenesis.[63]

As to the factors responsible for the augmented hepatic glucose output during exercise, it is noteworthy that serum insulin decreases in short-term[8] as well as in prolonged exercise.[28] As the liver is highly sensitive to small changes in insulin,[9] one could expect such a decrease to result in stimulation of hepatic glycogenolysis and gluconeogenesis. At heavy work intensities[26,29] and during prolonged exercise involving mild hypoglycemia,[28] increases in plasma glucagon may also contribute to hepatic glucose production (Fig. 146-6). In addition, increments in growth hormone[30] and catecholamines may be of importance in this context.

Recent studies suggest that changes in the circulating levels of insulin, glucagon, and glucose are not the sole (or primary) determinants of hepatic glucose production in exercise. When the concentrations of insulin, glucagon, and glucose in plasma are maintained at basal levels during exercise by means of an intravenous glucose infusion, the normal 2–3-fold increase in hepatic glucose production is not affected.[64] Furthermore, infusion of insulin and maintenance of hyperinsulinemia in excess of 100 μU/ml does not inhibit exercise-induced stimulation of hepatic glucose output.[64] Thus, factors other than the prevailing concentrations of insulin and glucagon contribute to the regulation of hepatic glucose output in exercise. Sympathetic adrenergic activity and release of catecholamines are both augmented in exercise and may be of importance for this regulation.

LIPID METABOLISM

FFA

The fact that fat is utilized as a fuel by exercising human muscle was demonstrated by Christensen and Hansen in 1939.[13] The finding was deduced from the RQ and no evidence was obtained about the form in which the fat was utilized. Methods for the direct measurement of fat metabolism by exercising muscle did not become available until 1956, at which time three independent groups[65–67] identified the important role of FFA in the transport of fuel from adipose tissue stores to other organs, where FFA are taken up and utilized in energy metabolism. FFA are "free" only in the sense that they are not esterified but possess a free carboxyl group. In plasma, FFA are bound to albumin, which serves as a transport protein for the water-insoluble FFA molecules. The plasma FFA fraction is a mixture of several fatty acids of different chain lengths and numbers of double bonds; palmitic, stearic, oleic, and linoleic acids make up approximately 85 percent of the total plasma FFA. In healthy postabsorptive individuals the plasma FFA constitute only a small part of the total blood lipids, the plasma level of FFA being approximately 400–700 μmol/liter.[68]

ARTERIAL CONCENTRATION AND TURNOVER OF FFA

Although the plasma FFA concentration is low, the FFA pool is essential for the supply of fuel to body tissues. In the basal state FFA turnover is approximately 600 μmol/min and the half-life of the plasma pool is of the order of 3 min. With the exception of the brain, most tissues have the capacity to metabolize FFA; muscle and liver are the major sites of FFA removal under basal conditions. However, not all the FFA taken up by the peripheral tissues are oxidized—some recirculate in the form of lipoprotein-bound triglycerides. This explains why the FFA turnover expressed in kilocalories exceeds the body's basal energy requirement. The turnover of FFA in the basal state is directly correlated to the plasma FFA concentration. Consequently, the magnitude of the FFA turnover is regulated primarily by the rate of adipose tissue lipolysis.

At the onset of work involving large muscle groups, such as bicycle exercise, the arterial FFA concentration drops transiently for the first 10–20 min,[69] as increased removal of FFA by muscle outstrips FFA mobilization. There is then a gradual rise in the arterial FFA level to and above the basal level, concurrently with augmented rates of FFA mobilization from adipose tissue. When exercise continues for 10–12 h, arterial FFA reaches plateau values 4–5 times those at rest.[70] During exercise with small muscle groups or of low work intensity, the balance between removal and mobilization of FFA can be maintained during the initial phase and the transient fall in arterial FFA is not seen.[32] As in the resting state, during exercise there is a direct linear correlation between FFA turnover and arterial concentration, although the turnover is then greater for a given arterial level of FFA.[71]

The individual FFA differ markedly in their arterial concentrations during exercise (Fig. 146-10). The increments during prolonged exercise are most pronounced for oleic acid and palmitic acid, whereas the linoleic acid concentration rises only slightly and stearic and arachidonic acids do not rise at all.[71] This is probably because palmitic and oleic acids predominate in the exercise-induced increase in FFA mobilization from adipose tissue triglycerides. Arachidonic acid occupies an exceptional position among the plasma FFA: its concentration is independent of the total FFA level, it is not influenced by the administration of nicotinic acid (a potent inhibitor of adipose tissue lipolysis), and there is no uptake of this acid to either muscle or liver.[72] The regulation of the plasma arachidonic acid concentration would thus seem to differ completely from that of the other FFA.

MUSCLE METABOLISM OF FFA

The study of FFA metabolism in skeletal muscle in man is complicated by the simultaneous uptake and release of FFA that occurs both at rest and during exercise (Fig. 146-11).[32,33,73] The

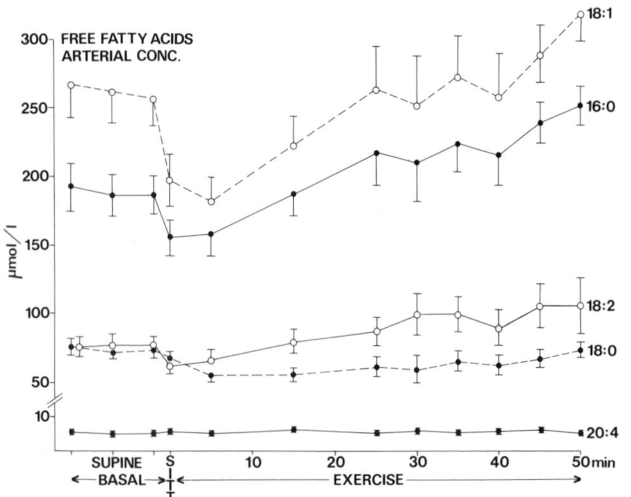

Fig. 146-10. Arterial concentrations of palmitic (16:0), stearic (18:0), oleic (18:1), linoleic (18:2) and arachidonic (20:4) acids at rest in the supine and sitting positions and during upright exercise at a work load of 65 W (mean ± SE). (Data from Hagenfeldt et al.[71])

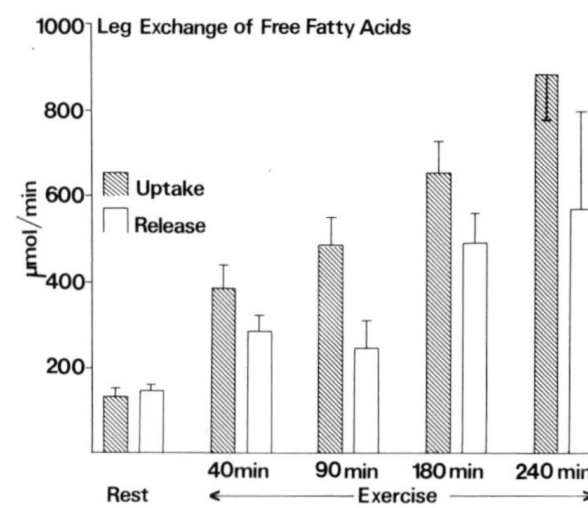

Fig. 146-11. Leg uptake and release of FFA at rest and during prolonged submaximal bicycle exercise. Uptake and release of FFA were calculated from ^{14}C-oleic acid data (mean ± SE). (Data from Ahlborg et al.[28])

FFA released from muscle may derive from lipolysis in adipose tissue interspersed between the muscle fibers or from hydrolysis of intracellular triglycerides in the muscle tissue itself. This phenomenon necessitates the use of isotopic techniques for the measurement of both regional FFA exchange and oxidation. Oleic or palmitic acid is generally used as a tracer of the entire FFA fraction since these are the individual FFA with the highest concentrations and their fractional uptake in both muscle and liver is very similar to that of total FFA.[32,72]

At rest about 50 percent of the FFA entering the forearm or the leg are removed during each circulation.[71,73] As approximately the same amount or slightly less is released into the circulation, there is only a small or no net AV difference for FFA. Most of the FFA taken up are stored for several hours; only a small fraction are oxidized rapidly. In the postabsorptive state the local RQ for muscle is close to 0.7, indicating that fat substrates almost exclusively are being oxidized.

The uptake of FFA by exercising limb muscles during bicycle exercise or forearm work rises in direct proportion to the arterial FFA inflow, expressed as the product of arterial concentration and plasma flow. The same has been found to hold during prolonged starvation with greatly elevated arterial levels of FFA.[74] These findings demonstrate that the FFA transport mechanism does not reach a saturation point even under the extreme metabolic conditions associated with prolonged starvation. It would thus seem that the magnitude of FFA uptake in muscle is regulated not by the muscle itself, but primarily by outside factors, such as the rate of FFA mobilization from adipose tissue.

The uptake of FFA during moderately heavy exercise is not sufficient to account for the muscle's entire oxidation of fat, as evaluated from the local RQ, indicating that this oxidation may include fatty acids other than those taken up from plasma, as discussed below. During prolonged fasting, when the FFA uptake is larger (as a consequence of the higher FFA levels), the rate of fat oxidation during exercise is largely unchanged. Thus, in this situation the exercising muscle seems to be capable of increasing the fraction of its fat metabolism that involves the immediate oxidation of plasma FFA.[74]

The oxidation of FFA by exercising muscle may be studied by measuring the $^{14}CO_2$ output after administering a ^{14}C-labeled tracer. It appears that during work of light intensity, all of the FFA taken up are oxidized immediately.[75] For moderately heavy or strenuous work, on the other hand, no more than 50–60 percent of the FFA may be oxidized immediately.[32,75] The remaining radioactivity–not released as $^{14}CO_2$—can be recovered, not in the muscle tissue, but as water-soluble metabolites in a perchloric acid extract of blood. Labeled 3-hydroxybutyrate has been identified among these metabolites, but 20–60 percent of the radioactivity appears to be present in the form of acetate.[71,75]

These findings may indicate that during work of high intensity the production of acetyl coenzyme A (CoA) exceeds the simultaneous capacity for its oxidation in the citric acid cycle. Such a metabolic situation is likely to develop in skeletal muscle in view of its high capacity for glycolysis and its relative scarcity of mitochondria. Furthermore, the high rate of ATP consumption for muscle contraction may reduce the energy charge of the adenine nucleotides, thereby reducing its inhibitory influence on the breakdown of substrates to acetyl CoA. The resulting enhanced glycolysis is (because of the cytoplasmic redox state) diverted into production of lactate, while the intramitochondrial overproduction of acetyl CoA may either result in deacylation, yielding acetate, or be channeled into synthesis of 3-hydroxybutyrate. The above metabolic situation is probably a consequence of insufficient mitochondrial oxidative capacity of the muscle in relation to the work load applied. Support for this is obtained from the finding that physical training is associated with an augmented ability of muscle to oxidize fatty acids.[76] A diminished capacity of the leg muscles to oxidize FFA during even mild exercise has been demonstrated in patients with occlusions of the leg arteries.[71] In these subjects the oxygen extraction from blood was close to maximal, suggesting that tissue hypoxia may have contributed to the diminished capacity for FFA oxidation.

KETONE BODIES

In the resting state there is a net uptake of both acetoacetate and 3-hydroxybutyrate by human skeletal muscle that is directly proportional to the arterial concentrations.[77] For both substances the fractional uptake across the forearm muscle is as high as 50 percent; but, because of their relatively low arterial concentrations in the postabsorptive state, the contribution to total substrate exchange is only about 3–5 percent, assuming complete oxidation.

During a period of exercise the positive AV difference across an exercising limb gradually diminishes and is presently replaced by a small net release of acetoacetate.[77] Failure of the exercising muscle to utilize available ketone bodies may be a consequence of elevated intracellular levels of acetoacetate and 3-hydroxybutyrate, secondary to incomplete FFA oxidation, as discussed above. The contributions made by acetoacetate and 3-hydroxybutyrate to the total substrate supply of exercising muscle are accordingly negligible in the postabsorptive state.

Ketone body utilization is of particular interest during prolonged fasting, inasmuch as these substances then accumulate in the extracellular fluid, reaching concentrations 10–20-fold above basal. Following a prolonged period of starvation, resting skeletal muscle shows a small uptake of acetoacetate and a simultaneous release of 3-hydroxybutyrate;[78,79] for the two combined there is no significant net uptake or release. Furthermore, dynamic exercise elicits no significant net exchange for either substrate in spite of their markedly elevated arterial levels.[78]

The background to the failure of skeletal muscle to utilize ketone bodies in prolonged fasting is unclear. Although FFA and ketone bodies compete as fuels in muscle metabolism, the preference for one over the other probably depends mainly on their relative concentrations. During prolonged fasting, blood levels of ketone bodies exceed the level of FFA, but the intracellular FFA level is higher in muscle than in plasma.[80] Consequently, it is conceivable that the concentrations of the competitive substrates at the intracellular sites of metabolism are not adequately reflected by their plasma levels and that the intracellular FFA concentration during prolonged fasting may in fact be higher than that of either acetoacetate or 3-hydroxybutyrate. This is in keeping with results for brain metabolism during starvation, indicating that nearly all of the 3-hydroxybutyrate and acetoacetate formed (except that excreted in the urine) is utilized as fuel for the central nervous system.[61,81]

INTRAMUSCULAR LIPIDS

Several studies in exercising man have emphasized the failure of FFA metabolism to account for the entire fat oxidation as evaluated from the RQ. In healthy subjects exercising at a low work intensity, only 30–50 percent of the exhaled CO_2 could be attributed to the oxidation of plasma FFA, whereas the RQ indicated an almost exclusive utilization of fat substrates.[82] Likewise, direct studies of FFA metabolism of forearm and leg muscle during exercise have demonstrated that FFA uptake and oxidation may account for approximately 50 percent of the total fat oxidation.[32,33] The combined findings on FFA oxidation by muscle and the local RQ values thus strongly suggest that during exercise skeletal muscle obtains fatty acids from sources other than circulating FFA. It has therefore been suggested that triglyceride stores in muscle tissue contribute fatty acids for oxidation.

It has long been known that droplets of neutral fat occur in skeletal muscle; they are found in close proximity to the mitochondria and are abundant in human muscle, particularly in the red fibers.[83] The concentration of triglyceride in human quadriceps muscle is approximately 10 mg/kg muscle[23] and the total pool of intramuscular triglyceride can be estimated at a maximum of 300 g (Table 146-1). Direct measurements of changes in the local lipid stores in connection with exercise in animal studies have yielded contradictory but largely negative results. However, the relevance of these findings to intact man is uncertain, and it seems difficult to conceive a function other than supply of fuel for the lipid droplets stored in the red muscle fibers. Recent results in healthy volunteers exercising to exhaustion on a bicycle ergometer support this view.[23] Muscle biopsy samples were obtained from the lateral portion of the quadriceps muscle before and after prolonged exhaustive exercise. A 25 percent reduction in triglyceride content was observed after exercise, with no change in phospholipid content. Intramuscular triglyceride stores were estimated to contribute two-thirds of the fatty acids for total fat oxidation during this form of exercise, indicating a quantitatively important role for intramuscular lipids in the supply of substrate to human muscle during heavy exercise.

AMINO ACID METABOLISM

BASAL STATE

In the resting, basal state muscle is in negative nitrogen balance, as indicated by a consistent net output of most amino acids from muscle tissue (Fig. 146-12).[84–86] The pattern of this release is quite distinctive in that the combined output of alanine and glutamine exceeds that of all other amino acids, accounting for more than 50 percent of total α-amino nitrogen release.[87,88] The negative balance of amino acids for muscle tissue is complemented by a consistent uptake of a number of amino acids by the splanchnic tissues.[85,89,90] As in the case of peripheral output, alanine and glutamine dominate this uptake (Fig. 146-13).

Data on the relative contributions of hepatic and extrahepatic tissues to net splanchnic balances in man indicate that the gut rather than the liver is responsible for the uptake of glutamine by the splanchnic area.[86,91] In contrast, the gut releases alanine and, to a lesser extent, other amino acids to portal venous blood.[85,86]

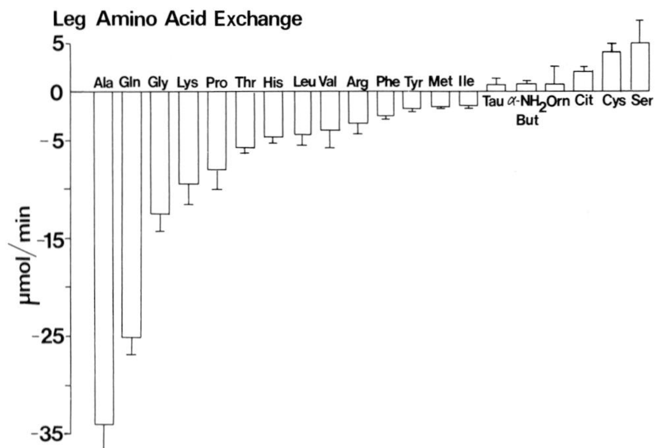

Fig. 146-12. Net exchange of individual amino acids across the legs in the basal state (mean ± SE). (Data from Felig et al.[85,86])

Determinations of the splanchnic uptake of alanine from arterial hepatic venous differences will therefore be lower than the true hepatic uptake, possibly by as much as 50 percent. Of the amino acids taken up by the liver, alanine in particular is readily converted to glucose, as illustrated by studies involving the incorporation of ^{14}C-alanine into blood glucose in human subjects.[92] Thus with regard to output from muscle, uptake by liver, and efficiency in conversion to glucose, alanine is preeminent among amino acids as a glucose precursor. Inasmuch as the extrahepatic splanchnic tissues do not contribute to glucose production, it seems that glutamine is not an important glucose precursor in man.

The primacy of alanine output from muscle is unexpected inasmuch as alanine comprises only 5–8 percent of the amino acid residues in muscle protein.[93] This discrepancy led to the suggestion that alanine is synthesized de novo in muscle tissue by transamination of pyruvate.[85,94] Moreover, on the basis of the evidence that alanine is a glucose precursor, a glucose–alanine cycle has been proposed in which alanine is synthetized in muscle by transamination of glucose-derived pyruvate and is transported to the liver, where its carbon skeleton is reconverted to glucose.[85,94,95]

EXERCISE

During exercise several important alterations in amino acid metabolism are elicited. Mild bicycle exercise causes arterial alanine levels to rise by 20–25 percent while more intense exertion is accompanied by a rise of 60–100 percent.[85,96] In contrast, the concentrations of all other amino acids are unchanged with light exercise, while strenuous exertion elicits increases of 8–35 percent in the levels of isoleucine, leucine, methionine, tyrosine, and phenylalanine. The augmented arterial concentration of alanine during work is primarily caused by an increased release from exercising muscle, alanine being the only amino acid for which a consistent net output is demonstrable during exercise. The net alanine release rises in proportion to the work intensity. A rise of 50 percent has been observed with light work and increments of 100–500 percent are reported for heavier exercise.[85] During work as well as in the resting state there is a direct linear correlation between arterial alanine and pyruvate levels.

Contrasting with the response of alanine metabolism to exercise in normal subjects are the changes observed in patients with McArdle's syndrome, a disorder characterized by a lack of muscle phosphorylase. In this condition, exercise-induced muscle glycolysis and pyruvate formation are markedly decreased.[97] In these patients, exercise causes arterial levels and muscle concentrations of pyruvate to fall. In a like manner, arterial alanine decreases, and instead of an increased peripheral output, alanine together with other amino acids is taken up by muscle, where they serve as an auxiliary fuel during exercise.[97] Moreover, studies of amino acid metabolism have also been undertaken in patients with a familial myopathy characterized by myoglobinuria, hyperpyruvicemia, and hyperlactatemia.[98] In these patients, who show a markedly accelerated muscle glycolysis during exercise, the increased pyruvate availability is accompanied by an augmented formation of alanine.[99] The above observations in healthy individuals and in patients with myopathies all support the hypothesis that alanine formation in muscle is related to glucose utilization and the availability of pyruvate.

With respect to the source of the amino groups for alanine synthesis, it is noteworthy that the branched-chain amino acids (valine, leucine, and isoleucine) are preferentially catabolized in muscle.[100,101] During exercise the oxidation of these amino acids in muscle tissue is stimulated,[100] as is the conversion of aspartate to oxaloacetate.[102] Exercise is also known to increase the production of ammonia by muscle.[103] Recent studies have indicated that ammonia formation in muscle occurs by virtue of a cyclic interconversion of the purine nucleotides, adenosine monophosphate and inosine monophosphate.[104] The ammonia thus liberated may be used for the synthesis of glutamate (via reductive amination of α-ketoglutarate), which subsequently undergoes transamination with pyruvate to form alanine. The functional significance of augmented alanine production by exercising muscle with respect to body nitrogen metabolism may thus derive from the fact that it provides a nontoxic alternative to ammonia in the transport of amino groups from muscle to the liver. In addition, alanine synthesis by muscle may be useful with respect to ATP production.[105] Conversion of glucose to alanine provides 6 mol ATP, compared to the 2 mol provided by conversion to lactate. Furthermore, to the extent that alanine formation facilitates the oxidation of the branched-chain amino acids, an additional 32–42 mol of ATP will be generated per mole of amino acid oxidized.[95] In prolonged exercise, selective uptake of the branched-chain amino acids by the exercising limb has been demonstrated,[28] suggesting that these amino acids may in fact contribute to the fuel supply of exercising muscle.

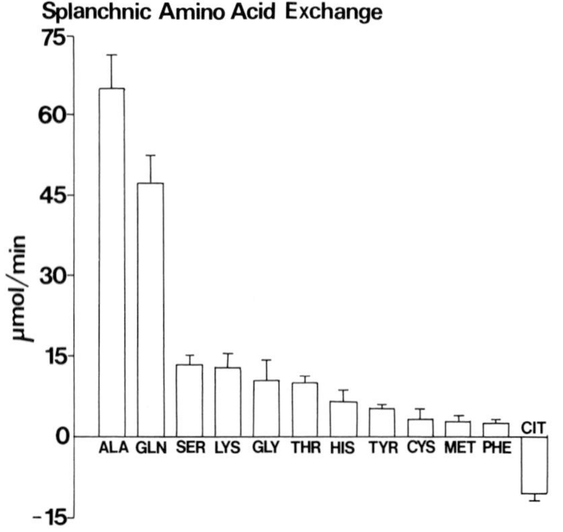

Fig. 146-13. Net exchange of individual amino acids across the splanchnic vascular bed in the basal state (mean ± SE). (Date from Felig et al.[85,86])

Brief exercise does not substantially modify the basal splanchnic amino acid uptake, but prolonged periods of exercise are accompanied by marked alterations in splanchnic amino acid metabolism.[28] As exercise continues beyond the first hour, the output of alanine from exercising muscle remains above the basal level. At this time the splanchnic uptake of alanine, as well as other amino acids, rises even more rapidly, with the result that their arterial concentration falls; the increase in the splanchnic uptake primarily reflects an augmented fractional extraction. After 4 h of exercise, amino acid uptake has risen 140 percent above the basal value and total glucose precursor uptake can then account for as much as 45 percent of splanchnic glucose output.[28] Thus, increased splanchnic amino acid uptake, particularly of alanine, makes an important contribution to the augmented rate of hepatic gluconeogenesis during prolonged exercise.

The findings regarding muscle and liver exchange of alanine support the existence of a glucose–alanine cycle in man (Fig. 146-14).[85,94,95] Accordingly, alanine may be synthesized in muscle from pyruvate and released to the blood. Circulating alanine is then extracted by the liver, where its carbon skeleton is reconverted to glucose. The influence of exercise on this cyclic interconversion differs between brief and prolonged work. Brief exercise seems to increase the rate of alanine formation in muscle in excess of its net uptake by the liver; as a consequence the alanine concentration of arterial plasma rises. Prolonged exercise, on the other hand, causes the rate of alanine uptake by the liver to rise above its rate of formation by exercising muscle, with the result that the arterial alanine level falls.

INTEGRATED ASPECTS OF SUPPLY AND USE OF FUELS

CHOICE OF FUELS IN THE RESTING STATE

After an overnight fast the local RQ of muscle is close to 0.7,[32,49] suggesting that fatty acids are the major energy-yielding substrate. Accordingly, FFA uptake by resting muscle is about 50 percent of the arterial concentration and, if oxidized, is sufficient to account for approximately 90 percent of the oxygen consumption.[73] However, only a small fraction of the FFA taken up is oxidized immediately to CO_2; the remainder presumably enters intracellular triglyceride pools.[33] Available data suggest a continuous breakdown and resynthesis of stored triglyceride, so that FFA and endogenous fatty acid together provide the bulk of fuel for oxidation. There is a quantitatively minor uptake of acetoacetate and 3-hydroxybutyrate which, if oxidized, may account for 5–8 percent of the oxygen uptake.[77] In addition, there is a small uptake

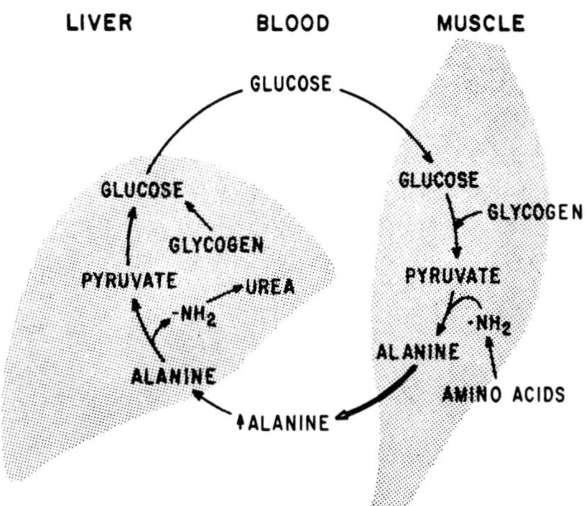

Fig. 146-14. Glucose–alanine cycle. Alanine is synthesized in muscle by transamination of glucose-derived pyruvate; it is subsequently taken up by the liver, where its carbon skeletons are utilized in gluconeogenesis and the amino groups are incorporated into urea. Glucose is released to the blood and then taken up by muscle. (From Felig and Wahren: *J. Clin. Invest. 50:* 2703, 1971.)

of glucose by resting muscle.[8,49] However, there is also a net release of lactate as a result of glycolysis in muscle and probably also in erythrocytes. The fraction of glucose oxidized after being taken up to muscle is probably very small; alternatively, glucose may participate in glycogen synthesis or it may leave the muscle as lactate or alanine after transamination of glucose-derived pyruvate.[85]

SUPPLY AND USE OF FUELS DURING EXERCISE

During the initial phase of exercise, before blood flow and the mobilization of oxygen and blood-borne substrates have increased, the contracting muscle has to rely on intramuscular stores for energy production. The immediate fuels include the phosphagens ATP and creatine phosphate, of which muscle contains a limited store.[106] At the onset of muscular contraction primarily the white fibers are activated, and resynthesis of ATP and creatine phosphate may be accomplished through degradation of glycogen to lactate. Shortly after the onset of work, the red fibers are recruited in parallel with ceasing white fiber activity, and oxidative metabolism accelerates. The major part of the rise in blood flow to working muscle occurs within the first 1–2 min, thereby increasing the oxygen, FFA, and glucose available for extraction.

Glycogen degradation, as evidenced by lactate production, occurs even at the onset of exercise at a low work load.[107] The production of lactate gradually diminishes and may cease after the first minutes. During further light exercise, which raises the basal oxygen consumption only 2–3-fold, the uptake of blood-borne substrates (predominantly FFA) may suffice to meet the energy requirement,[108] but with heavier exercise the degradation of glycogen continues. As the availability of oxygen increases, more and more of the glycogen undergoes terminal oxidation and lactate production gradually diminishes.

The importance of glycogen as an intramuscular fuel depot is underscored by the finding of a reduced exercise tolerance in patients with McArdle's syndrome.[109,110] These individuals lack myophosphorylase, the enzyme responsible for muscle glycogen degradation. At the onset of even light work they experience intense muscular fatigue, stiffness, and swelling of the contracting muscles, as well as marked tachycardia and hyperventilation. After a few minutes the symptoms may subside and the patient can continue exercising for an unlimited period (second-wind phenomenon); but if the work load is raised the symptoms reappear.[109] In accordance with these patients' inability to degrade glycogen, lactate does not accumulate in blood during exercise. Subjects with this syndrome can have their ability to exercise improved by the intravenous administration of glucose or emulsified fat or by having the arterial level of FFA and the local blood flow increased by the administration of isoproterenol.[109,110] Their subjective symptoms appear at the time during exercise when the muscle depends to a great extent on glycogen utilization for the resynthesis of energy-rich phosphagens. The ability of these patients to achieve a "second wind" is related to the inflow of blood-borne substrates, inasmuch as an augmentation of local blood flow and/or arterial substrate concentrations, notably FFA, enhances their capacity to continue exercise.[109] These patients' dependence on fuel supply from the blood is further underscored by the finding that they are unable to reach a second wind or to continue exercise if adipose tissue lipolysis is blocked by infusion of nicotinic acid, thereby substantially reducing the availability of plasma FFA.[109]

The glycogen content of muscle gradually falls during prolonged exercise; the rate of utilization is related to the severity of the work. The first hour of exercise is accompanied by an increased mobilization of FFA from adipose tissue and of glucose from the liver. The relative importance of these substrates increases with continued exercise. The uptake of FFA from the blood after 1–4 h of moderately heavy bicycle exercise accounts for 40–60 percent of the oxygen uptake, almost all FFA taken up by the working muscles being oxidized immediately. The concurrent uptake of glucose may account for 30–40 percent of total oxidative metabolism and the entire estimated carbohydrate oxidation. Together glucose and FFA may account for more than 90 percent of the total metabolism after 4 h of exercise.[28]

The overall pattern of fuel utilization during mild to moderate exercise for prolonged periods may thus be characterized as a triphasic sequence in which intramuscular substrates, notably glycogen, blood glucose, and FFA successively predominate as the major energy-yielding substrate. During exercise at a high work intensity there is a more persistent dependence on local fuel depots. The muscle glycogen content falls gradually and exhaustion generally coincides with depletion of glycogen stores. Blocking FFA release from adipose tissue by the administration of nicotinic acid during this type of exercise results in an accelerated rate of glycogen utilization and probably also of blood glucose uptake by muscle.[47] The local RQ indicates that fat oxidation continues in spite of low FFA levels, and direct measurements of the intramuscular lipids of exercising quadriceps muscle suggest that intramuscular triglycerides contribute fuel in this situation.[23] However, this source of substrate apparently cannot be utilized to an extent sufficient to obviate the need for glycogen or plasma FFA during exercise.

POSTEXERCISE RECOVERY

At the termination of work there is a redistribution of blood flow in that blood flow to the previously exercising limbs decreases and perfusion of the splanchnic bed rises to its basal level. The overall effect of the recovery phase on glucose metabolism is initiation of repletion of glycogen stores in muscle as well as liver. Glucose uptake by muscle remains 3–4-fold above basal levels for at least 40 min after exercise is stopped.[111] In the absence of augmented lactate release or oxygen consumption[111] these findings suggest a resynthesis of muscle glycogen. Repletion of liver glycogen is facilitated by a rapid decline in splanchnic glucose output after exercise, basal levels being reached by 40 min after exercise. Simultaneously there is an augmented splanchnic uptake of gluconeogenic substrates. This is particularly prominent in the case of lactate and pyruvate.[111] Splanchnic uptake of these glucose precursors during recovery exceeds the rates observed during exercise and is 3–4-fold greater than in the basal state. Smaller increments are observed for splanchnic alanine uptake. This augmentation in precursor utilization is a consequence of a rise in splanchnic blood flow, elevations in arterial levels, and increased fractional extraction. The net effect is a doubling of the proportion of glucose output attributable to gluconeogenesis as compared to the resting state.[111] Arterial levels of FFA reach a peak of approximately twice the exercise value during the early recovery phase,[112] thereby increasing the availability of FFA to the liver and presumably facilitating hepatic gluconeogenesis. Repletion of liver glucogen thus appears to begin even in the absence of glucose ingestion by means of augmented recycling to glucose of glucose-derived carbon skeletons.

The hormonal changes during the recovery period are characterized by a rapid increase in insulin levels within the first 2–10 min of the recovery phase.[111] Of particular interest is the greater rise in insulin concentration that occurs in hepatic venous as compared to arterial blood. Coupled with the increment in splanchnic blood flow, these observations suggest a true increase in insulin delivery during recovery (perhaps mediated via a cessation of inhibitory adrenergic signals) irrespective of alterations in peripheral insulin catabolism. In view of the marked sensitivity of hepatic glycogenolysis to insulin,[9] the rise in insulin may be a major factor responsible for the decline in hepatic glucose output to basal levels. In contrast to the rapid changes in circulating insulin, glucagon concentrations remain elevated in the recovery period[29] and may thereby contribute to the augmented hepatic uptake of gluconeogenic precursors.

PROTEIN CATABOLISM AND ANABOLISM

Prolonged exercise as well as the recovery period after brief exercise are associated with an increased uptake of alanine by the liver for gluconeogenesis. In addition, increased utilization of branched-chain amino acids by muscle, presumably for oxidation as energy-yielding substrates, is seen in prolonged exercise.[28] To the extent that there is a net flow of branched-chain amino acids from liver to muscle, this catabolic effect occurs at the expense of liver rather than muscle protein.[28] Regardless of the site of proteolysis, exercise would thus be expected to result in a negative nitrogen balance. Early studies, however, did not demonstrate an increase in urinary nitrogen loss during exercise.[113,114] However, more recent data reveal a 60 percent increase in urea production and in blood urea nitrogen concentration during prolonged, severe exercise in well-trained subjects (cross-country skiers).[115] The failure to observe similar evidence of protein catabolism in earlier studies may relate to the sensitivity of the techniques employed. In addition, intermittent exercise of mild intensity during which blood urea concentrations remain unaltered[63,70] may differ from more severe, sustained exercise with respect to its influence on protein catabolism.

In contrast to the transient catabolic effects of continuous, prolonged exercise and the early postexercise recovery period, repeated bouts of exercise are accompanied by protein anabolism manifested by muscle hypertrophy as a long-term effect. This hypertrophic effect is demonstrable even in the face of starvation.[116] The anabolic effects of repeated contraction have been shown to occur in resting muscle and to involve an inhibition in protein catabolism as well as stimulation of protein synthesis.[117] The alternation between a catabolic process during contraction and an augmented anabolic response in the postcontraction resting state is not unique to protein metabolism, but is also demonstrable for glycogen synthesis, as discussed above.

EFFECTS OF PHYSICAL TRAINING

A program of endurance training, besides eliciting alterations in the capacity of the cardiovascular system to transport and distribute oxygen during exercise, induces both structural and functional changes in the exercising muscle; the muscle mass and the size of the muscle cells increase, as does the number of capillaries per muscle fiber.[118,119] Recent studies have emphasized the marked biochemical adaptations in muscle that occur in response to physical training. Skeletal muscle develops an increased capacity for aerobic metabolism as a consequence of adaptive changes in the muscle mitochondria.[120] There is electron-microscopic evidence that this adaptation involves an increase in both the size and the number of muscle mitochondria.[121,122] A substantial rise in the total mitochondrial protein fraction has been reported[120] concomitant with augmented activity by the mitochondrial respiratory-chain enzymes, linking the oxidation of NADH and succinate to oxygen.[120] Moreover, the activities of mitochondrial ATPase,[123] citric-acid cycle enzymes,[124] and the rate-limiting enzymes involved in the activation, transport, and catabolism of long-chain fatty acids[76] are markedly enhanced by physical training. The enzymes involved in ketone body utilization likewise increase in activity following endurance training.[125] The mitochondria obtained from trained muscle exhibit tightly coupled oxidative phosphorylation, indicating that the increment to mitochondrial oxidative capacity is associated with a parallel rise in aerobic ATP generation.

Unlike the mitochondrial oxidative enzymes, the enzymes involved in glycolysis and glycogenolysis of muscle do not respond significantly to physical training.[126,127] Hexokinase is the only exception; its activity is increased in untrained animals by just a few light bouts of exercise. However, this is probably not a training effect in the same sense as the rise in activity of the oxidative enzymes. The lack of a training effect on the glycolytic enzymes may have to do with the fact that at submaximal steady-state exercise the conversion of glycogen and glucose to pyruvate and lactate is determined not so much by the concentrations of the rate-limiting enzymes as by the operation of a number of feedback control mechanisms.

The activity of alanine transaminase is reported to rise in response to physical training.[128] As a result of this adaptation, a greater proportion of the pyruvate formed in muscle during exercise may be converted into alanine and less into lactate as alanine transaminase becomes increasingly effective in competing with lactate dehydrogenase for pyruvate.

The intracellular stores of glycogen and fat are also influenced by endurance training. Increased glycogen synthetase and glycogen concentration have been observed following physical training.[129] There is likewise an increased incorporation of palmitic acid into intracellular fatty acid stores, and probably augmented levels of intramuscular triglycerides.[130] Exercise training also raises the muscle myoglobin content,[131] thereby probably facilitating oxygen utilization in muscle by increasing its rate of diffusion through the cytoplasm to the mitochondria. Red and white muscle fibers do not appear to be affected differently by training; training in fact appears to magnify the normal differences between them.[132] Thus, studies reporting an increased proportion of red fibers in subjects engaged in endurance training and an augmented fraction of white fibers in weight-lifters and sprinters[35] probably reflect a natural selection rather than a training effect.

Considering the increased activity of mitochondrial oxidative enzymes following physical training, it is understandable that the pattern of substrate utilization by muscle also changes. Thus, during exercise at the same intensity, a greater percentage of the total oxidative metabolism derives from fatty acid oxidation in trained individuals, compared to untrained.[43,44,133] This difference is referable in part to the adaptive increase in the capacity of muscle to oxidize fatty acids. Furthermore, training appears to be associated with a greater rate of release of fatty acids from adipose tissue.[134,135] This results in elevated levels of FFA in plasma, thereby increasing the availability of FFA to muscle. The muscle's enhanced capacity to oxidize fatty acids, coupled with the increased rate of FFA mobilization, accounts for the greater utilization of fat-derived substrates for muscle oxidation in physically trained individuals. This is also reflected in a lower RQ and a slower depletion of muscle glycogen stores in trained as compared to untrained individuals at submaximal work intensities (Fig. 146-1).[43]

Depletion of muscle glycogen and hypoglycemia have been cited as factors responsible for the development of fatigue during prolonged heavy exercise, obliging the individual to discontinue work or reduce his pace.[17,21] The shift that physical training induces in the source of carbon for muscle oxidation—toward a greater fatty acid utilization—contributes to a glycogen-saving effect, thus postponing the depletion of glycogen stores and probably the occurrence of fatigue.

DIABETES MELLITUS

It has been known for a long time that in diabetic patients physical activity reduces the insulin requirements, improves glucose tolerance, and occasionally precipitates periods of hypoglycemia. The interaction of exercise and diabetes is, however, more complex, inasmuch as the relative contributions of carbohydrate and fat substrates to total oxidative metabolism are influenced as well as the rates of gluconeogenesis and ketogenesis. In general, the effect of exercise on glucose metabolism is dependent on the interval since insulin administration and the level of blood substrates at the time exercise is started.

In patients with juvenile diabetes performing moderately heavy short-term exercise 24 h after insulin withdrawal, glucose uptake by the exercising leg is similar to that of healthy controls.[55,136] As noted above, these observations support the conclusion that increased glucose uptake in exercise is not dependent on increased availability of insulin.[8] In spite of the similarity to healthy individuals with regard to glucose uptake from the blood, the contribution of fatty acids to total oxygen consumption by the exercising limb is increased by almost 50 percent in diabetes.[55] This greater dependence on blood-borne fatty acids is probably a consequence of the higher plasma levels of FFA as well as the decreased availability of muscle glycogen in hyperglycemic diabetic patients.[137]

Diabetic patients resemble controls in their total rate of hepatic glucose release in response to exercise but differ with regard to the effect of exercise on gluconeogenesis (Fig. 146-15). In the normal group the absolute rate of gluconeogenic precursor utilization during exercise does not change from the resting state, resulting in a decrease of 50 percent or more in the relative contribution from gluconeogenesis.[8] In diabetics, who already show an augmented rate of precursor uptake in the resting basal state,[138] gluconeogenesis rises during exercise to 2–3 times the resting rate.[55] This increase in gluconeogenic precursor uptake during short-term exercise is a consequence of an increased splanchnic

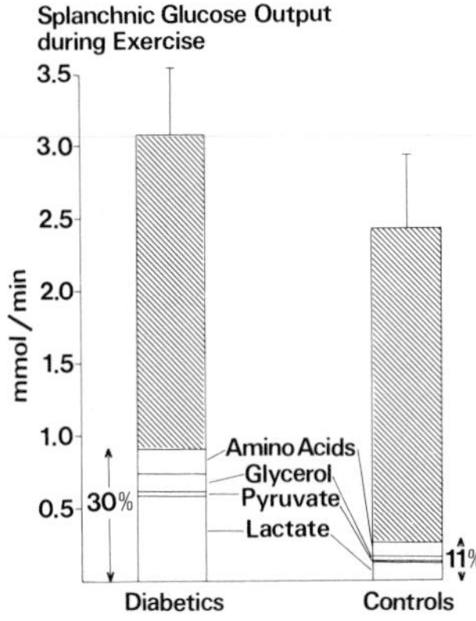

Fig. 146-15. Splanchnic glucose output and uptake of glucogenic precursor substrates in diabetic patients and controls after 40 min of bicycle exercise at work loads corresponding to 55 percent of maximal capacity. (Data from Hunter and Sukkar.[54])

fractional extraction as well as elevated arterial levels of precursor substrates. The stimulative effect of short-term exercise on gluconeogenesis in diabetes is thus comparable to that observed with long-term exercise (4 h or more) in healthy subjects, in whom the gluconeogenic component rises.[28] The similarity to prolonged exercise in normal subjects extends to muscle amino acid metabolism as well. Diabetic subjects demonstrate a consistent uptake of branched-chain amino acids by the exercising leg after 40 min,[55] while in normal subjects a comparable response is observed after 4 h.[28] These findings thus suggest that, as compared to the normal state, diabetes exerts an accelerating influence on the metabolic adaptation to exercise.

With regard to the influence of exercise on "diabetic control," the degree of insulin deficiency at the time of exercise, as reflected in the blood glucose and ketone concentrations, is of importance in determining the overall response. In nonketotic diabetic patients with blood glucose levels of 200–300 mg/100 ml or less, moderately heavy exercise performed 24 h after insulin withdrawal results in a fall in blood glucose.[55] In such patients, ketone production by the liver is not stimulated by exercise.[55] In contrast, in patients with more severe hyperglycemia (blood glucose above 350 mg/100 ml) and mild ketonemia (blood ketones 2–3 mmol/liter), brief exercise results in a 50–100 mg/100 ml rise in blood glucose. Furthermore, ketone production in such patients is increased 2–3-fold above basal, resting levels.[55] This tendency of exercise to intensify the diabetic state in certain circumstances may reflect the need for permissive concentrations of insulin[58] and the increase in insulin-antagonizing hormones such as glucagon,[26,29] catecholamines,[26] and growth hormone.[30]

REFERENCES

1. Berneus, B., Carlsten, A., Holmgren, A., and Seldinger, S.: Percutaneous catheterization of peripheral arteries as a method for blood sampling. *Scand. J. Clin. Lab. Invest. 6:* 217, 1954.
2. Wahren, J.: Quantitative aspects of blood flow and oxygen uptake in the human forearm during rhythmic exercise. *Acta Physiol. Scand. 67* [Suppl. 269]: 1, 1966.
3. Ganz, V., Hlavová, A., Froněk, A., Linhart, J., and Přerovský, J.: Measurement of blood flow in the femoral artery in man at rest and during exercise by local thermodilution. *Circulation 30:* 86, 1964.
4. Jorfeldt, L., and Wahren, J.: Leg blood flow during exercise in man. *Clin. Sci. 41:* 459, 1971.
5. Bradley, S. E.: Measurements of hepatic blood flow. In Potter, V. R. (ed): Methods in Medical Research, vol. 1. Chicago, Year Book, 1948, p. 199.
6. Rowell, L. B., Kraning, K. B., II, Evans, T. O., et al: Splanchnic removal of lactate and pyruvate during prolonged exercise in man. *J. Appl. Physiol 21:* 1773, 1966.
7. Bergström, J.: Muscle electrolytes in man. Determined by neutron activation analysis on needle biopsy specimens. A study on normal subjects, kidney patients, and patients with chronic diarrhea. *Scand. J. Clin. Lab. Invest. 14* [*Suppl. 68*]*:* 1, 1962.
8. Wahren, J., Felig, P., Ahlborg, G., and Jorfeldt, L.: Glucose metabolism during leg exercise in man. *J. Clin. Invest. 50:* 2715, 1971.
9. Felig, P., and Wahren, J.: Influence of endogenous insulin secretion on splanchnic glucose and amino acid metabolism in man. *J. Clin. Invest. 50:* 1702, 1971.
10. Nilsson, L. H:son: Liver glycogen content in man in the postabsorptive state. *Scand. J. Clin. Lab. Invest. 32:* 317, 1973.
11. Nilsson, L. H:son, and Hultman, E.: Liver glycogen in man—the effect of total starvation or a carbohydrate-poor diet followed by carbohydrate refeeding. *Scand. J. Clin. Lab. Invest. 32:* 325, 1973.
12. Hultman, E.: Muscle glycogen in man determined in needle biopsy specimens. Method and normal values. *Scand. J. Clin. Lab. Invest. 19:* 209, 1967.
13. Christensen, E. H., and Hansen, O.: Untersuchungen über die Verbrennungsvorgänge bei langdauernder, schwerer Muskelarbeit. *Skand. Arch. Physiol. 81:* 152, 1939.
14. Hultman, E.: Studies on muscle metabolism of glycogen and active phosphate in man with special reference to exercise and diet. *Scand. J. Clin. Lab. Invest. 19,* Suppl 94: 1, 1967.
15. Bergström, J., and Hultman, E.: A study of the glycogen metabolism during exercise in man. *Scand. J. Clin. Lab. Invest. 19:* 218, 1967.
16. Hultman, E., and Bergström, J.: Muscle glycogen synthesis in relation to diet studied in normal subjects. *Acta Med. Scand. 182:* 109, 1967.
17. Bergström, J., Hermansen, L., Hultman, E., and Saltin, B.: Diet, muscle glycogen and physical performance. *Acta Physiol. Scand. 71:* 140, 1967.
18. Danforth, W. H.: Glycogen synthetase activity in skeletal muscle. *J. Biol. Chem. 240:* 588, 1965.
19. Villar-Palasi, C., and Larner, J.: Feedback control of glycogen metabolism in muscle. *Fed. Proc. 25:* 583, 1966.
20. Karlsson, J., and Saltin, B.: Diet, muscle glycogen, and endurance performance, *J. Appl. Physiol. 31:* 203, 1971.
21. Pernow, B., and Saltin, B.: Availability of substrates and capacity for prolonged heavy exercise in man. *J. Appl. Physiol. 31:* 416, 1971.
22. Benedict, F. G.: A study of prolonged fasting. Washington DC, Carnegie Institute, Publ. No. 203, 1915.
23. Carlson, L. A., Ekelund, L.-G., and Fröberg, S. O.: Concentration of triglycerides, phospholipids and glycogen in skeletal muscle and of free fatty acids and β-hydroxybutyric acid in blood in man in response to exercise. *Eur. J. Clin. Invest. 1:* 248, 1971.
24. Havel, R. J.: Autonomic nervous system and adipose tissue. In Renold, A. E., and Cahill, G. F., Jr., (eds): Handbook of Physiology, section 5. Washington, DC, American Physiological Society, 1965, p. 575.
25. Häggendal, J., Hartley, H., and Saltin, B.: Arterial noradrenaline concentration during exercise in relation to the relative work levels. *Scand. J. Clin. Lab. Invest. 3:* 337, 1970.
26. Galbo, H., Holst, J. J., and Christensen, N. J.: Glucagon and plasma catecholamine responses to graded and prolonged exercise in man. *J. Appl. Physiol. 38:* 70, 1975.
27. Ballard, K., Cobb, C. A., and Rosell, S.: Vascular and lipolytic responses in canine subcutaneous adipose tissue following infusion of catecholamines. *Acta Physiol. Scand. 81:* 246, 1971.
28. Ahlborg, G., Felig, P., Hagenfeldt, L., Hendler, R., and Wahren, J.: Substrate turnover during prolonged exercise in man: splanchnic and leg metabolism of glucose, free fatty acids and amino acids. *J. Clin. Invest. 53:* 1080, 1974.
29. Felig, P., Wahren, J., Hendler, R., and Ahlborg, G.: Plasma glucagon levels in exercising man. *N. Engl. J. Med. 287:* 184, 1972.
30. Hunter, W. M., Fonseka, C. C., and Passmore, R.: The role of growth hormone in the mobilization of fuel for muscular exercise. *Q. J. Exp. Physiol. 50:* 406, 1965.
31. Ballard, K., and Rosell, S.: The unresponsiveness of lipid metabolism in canine mesenteric adipose tissue to biogenic amines and to sympathetic nerve stimulation. *Acta Physiol. Scand. 77:* 442, 1969.
32. Hagenfeldt, L., and Wahren, J.: Human forearm muscle metabolism during exercise. II. Uptake, release and oxidation of individual FFA and glycerol. *Scand. J. Clin. Lab. Invest. 21:* 263, 1968.
33. Havel, R. J., Pernow, B., and Jones, N. I.: Uptake and release of free fatty acids and other metabolites in the legs of exercising men. *J. Appl. Physiol. 23:* 90, 1967.
34. Hagenfeldt, L., and Wahren, J.: Effect of exercise on splanchnic exchange of free fatty acids. *Metabolism 22:* 815, 1973.
35. Gollnick, P. D., Armstrong, R. B., Saubert, C. W., IV, Piehl, K., and Saltin, B.: Enzyme activity and fiber composition in skeletal muscle of untrained and trained men. *J. Appl. Physiol. 33:* 312, 1972.
36. Essén, B., Jansson, E., Henriksson, J., Taylor, A. W., and Saltin, B.: Metabolic characteristics of fiber types in human skeletal muscle. *Acta Physiol. Scand. 94:* 153, 1975.
37. Edström, L., and Kugelberg, E.: Histochemical composition of distribution of fibres and fatigability of single motor units. *J. Neurol. Neurosurg. Psychiatry 31:* 424, 1968.
38. Grimby, L., and Hannertz, J.: Recruitment order of motor units on voluntary contraction: changes induced by proprioceptive afferent activity. *J. Neurol. Neurosurg. Psychiatry 31:* 565, 1968.
39. Gollnick, P. D., Piehl, K., and Saltin, B.: Selective glycogen depletion pattern in human muscle fibres after exercise of varying intensity and at varying pedalling rates. *J. Physiol. 241:* 45, 1974.
40. Gollnick, P. D., Karlsson, J., Piehl, K., and Saltin, B.: Selective

glycogen depletion in skeletal muscle fibres of man following sustained contractions. *J. Physiol. 241:* 59, 1974.
41. Bernard, C.: De la matière glycogène considerée comme condition de developpement de certains tissus, chez le foetus, avant l'apparition de la fonction glycogénique du foie. *C. R. Acad. Sci. 48:* 673, 1859.
42. Saltin, B., and Karlsson, J.: Muscle glycogen utilization during work of different intensities. In Pernow, B., and Saltin, B. (eds): Muscle Metabolism During Exercise. New York, Plenum, 1971, p. 289.
43. Hermansen, L., Hultman, E., and Saltin, B.: Muscle glycogen during prolonged severe exercise. *Acta Physiol. Scand. 71:* 129, 1967.
44. Christensen, E. H., and Hansen, O.: Respiratorischer Quotient und O_2-Aufnahme. *Skand. Arch. Physiol. 81:* 180, 1939.
45. Ahlborg, B., Bergström, J., Ekelund, L.-G., et al.: Muscle metabolism during isometric exercise performed at constant force. *J. Appl. Physiol. 33:* 224, 1972.
46. Hultman, E.: Muscle glycogen stores and prolonged exercise. In Shephard, R. J. (ed): Frontiers of Fitness. Springfield, Ill., Thomas, 1971, p. 37.
47. Bergström, J., Hultman, E., Jorfeldt, L., Pernow, B., and Wahren, J.: The effect of nicotinic acid on physical working capacity and metabolism of muscle glycogen in man. *J. Appl. Physiol. 26:* 170, 1969.
48. Chauveau, M. A., and Kaufmann, M.: Expériences pour la détermination du coefficient de l'activité nutritive et respiratoire des muscles en repos et en travail. *C. R. Acad. Sci. 104:* 1126, 1887.
49. Andres, R., Cader, G., and Zierler, K. L.: The quantitatively minor role of carbohydrate in oxidative metabolism by skeletal muscle in intact man in the basal state. Measurements of oxygen and glucose uptake and carbon dioxide and lactate production in the forearm. *J. Clin. Invest. 35:* 67, 1956.
50. Wahren, J.: Human forearm muscle metabolism during exercise. IV. Glucose uptake at different work intensities. *Scand. J. Clin. Lab. Invest. 25:* 129, 1970.
51. Jorfeldt, L., and Wahren, J.: Human forearm muscle metabolism during exercise. V. Quantitative aspects of glucose uptake and lactate production during prolonged exercise. *Scand. J. Clin. Lab. Invest. 26:* 73, 1970.
52. Field, R. A.: Glycogen deposition diseases. In Stanbury, J. B., Wyngaarden, J. B., and Fredrickson, D. S. (eds): The Metabolic Basis of Inherited Disease. New York, McGraw-Hill, 1966, p. 141.
53. Jöbsis, F. F., and Stainsby, W. N.: Oxidation of NADH during contractions of circulated mammalian skeletal muscle. *Resp. Physiol. 4:* 292, 1968.
54. Hunter, W. M., and Sukkar, M. Y.: Changes in plasma insulin levels during muscular exercise. *J. Physiol. 196:* 110, 1968.
55. Wahren, J., Hagenfeldt, L., and Felig, P.: Splanchnic and leg exchange of glucose, amino acids and free fatty acids during exercise in diabetes mellitus. *J. Clin. Invest. 55:* 1303, 1975.
56. Goldstein, M. S.: Humoral nature of hypoglycemia in muscular exercise. *Am. J. Physiol. 200:* 67, 1961.
57. Szabo, A. J., Mahler, R. J., and Szabo, O.: Influence of exercise upon serum factors and its secondary effect on glucose utilization by the resting muscle. *Horm. Metab. Res. 4:* 139, 172.
58. Berger, M., Hagg, S., and Ruderman, N. B.: Glucose metabolism in perfused skeletal muscle. Interaction of insulin and exercise on glucose uptake. *Biochem. J. 146:* 231, 1975.
59. Ahlborg, G., and Wahren, J.: Brain substrate utilization during prolonged exercise. *Scand. J. Clin. Lab. Invest. 29:* 397, 1972.
60. Ahlborg, G., Hagenfeldt, L., and Wahren, J.: Substrate utilization by the inactive leg during one-leg or arm exercise. *J. Appl. Physiol. 39:* 718, 1975.
61. Owen, O. E., Felig, P., Morgan, A. P., Wahren, J., and Cahill, G. F., Jr.,: Liver and kidney metabolism during prolonged starvation. *J. Clin. Invest. 48:* 574, 1969.
62. Rowell, L. B., Masoro, E. J., and Spencer, M. J.: Splanchnic metabolism in exercising man. *J. Appl. Physiol. 20:* 1032, 1965.
63. Young, D. R., Pelligra, R., Shapira, J., Adachi, R. R., and Skrettingland, K.: Glucose oxidation and replacement during prolonged exercise in man. *J. Appl. Physiol. 23:* 734, 1967.
64. Felig. P., and Wahren, J.: Role of insulin and glucagon in the regulation of hepatic glucose production during exercise. *Diabetes 28,* 1978 (in press).
65. Dole, V. P.: A relation between non-esterified fatty acids in plasma and the metabolism of glucose. *J. Clin. Invest. 35:* 150, 1956.
66. Gordon, R. S., Jr., and Cherkes, A.: Unesterified fatty acids in human blood plasma. *J. Clin. Invest. 35:* 206, 1956.
67. Laurell, S.: Plasma free fatty acids in diabetic acidosis and starvation. *Scand. J. Clin. Lab. Invest. 8:* 81, 1956.
68. Hagenfeldt, L.: The concentrations of individual free fatty acids in human plasma and their interrelationships. *Ark Kemi 29:* 57, 1968.
69. Carlson, L. A., and Pernow, B.: Studies on blood lipids during exercise. I. Arterial and venous plasma concentrations of unesterified fatty acids. *J. Lab. Clin. Med. 53:* 833, 1959.
70. Young, D. R., Pelligra, R., and Adachi, R.: Serum glucose and free fatty acids in man during prolonged exercise. *J. Appl. Physiol. 21:* 1047, 1966.
71. Hagenfeldt, L., Wahren, J., Pernow, B., Cronestrand, R., and Ekeström, S.: Free fatty acid metabolism of the leg muscles during exercise in patients with obliterative iliac and femoral artery disease before and after reconstructive surgery. *J. Clin. Invest. 51:* 3061, 1972.
72. Hagenfeldt, L., Wahren, J., Pernow, B., and Räf, L.: Uptake of individual free fatty acids by skeletal muscle and liver in man. *J. Clin. Invest. 51:* 2324, 1972.
73. Rabinowitz, D., and Zierler, K. L.: Role of free fatty acids in forearm metabolism in man quantitated by use of insulin. *J. Clin. Invest. 41:* 2191, 1962.
74. Hagenfeldt, L., and Wahren, J.: Metabolism of free fatty acids and ketone bodies in skeletal muscle. In Pernow, B., and Saltin, B. (eds): Muscle Metabolism During Exercise. New York, Plenum, 1971, p. 153.
75. Hagenfeldt, L., and Wahren, J.: Human forearm muscle metabolism during exercise. VII. FFA uptake and oxidation at different work intensities. *Scand. J. Clin. Lab. Invest. 30:* 429, 1972.
76. Mole, P. A., Oscai, L. B., and Holloszy, J. O.: Increase in levels of palmilyl CoA synthetase, carnitine palmityltransferase, and palmityl CoA dehydrogenase, and in the capacity to oxidize fatty acids. *J. Clin. Invest. 50:* 2323, 1971.
77. Hagenfeldt, L., and Wahren, J.: Human forearm muscle metabolism during exercise. III. Uptake, release and oxidation of β-hydroxybutyrate and observations on the β-hydroxybutyrate/acetoacetate ratio. *Scand. J. Clin. Lab. Invest. 21:* 314, 1968.
78. Hagenfeldt, L., and Wahren, J.: Human forearm muscle metabolism during exercise. VI. Substrate utilization in prolonged fasting. *Scand. J. Clin. Invest. 27:* 299, 1971.
79. Owen, O. E., and Reichard, G. A., Jr.: Human forearm metabolism during progressive starvation. *J. Clin. Invest. 50:* 1536, 1971.
80. Schonfeld, G., and Kipnis, D. M.: Glucose–fatty acid interactions in the rat diaphragm in vivo. *Diabetes 17:* 422, 1968.
81. Owen, O. E., Morgan, A. P., Kemp, H. G., et al.: Brain metabolism during fasting. *J. Clin. Invest. 46:* 1589, 1967.
82. Havel, R. J., Naimark, A., and Borchgrevink, C. F.: Turnover rate and oxidation of free fatty acids of blood plasma in man during exercise: studies during continuous infusion of palmitate-1-C^{14}. *J. Clin. Invest. 42:* 1054, 1963.
83. Gauthier, G. F., and Padykula, H. A.: Cytological studies of fiber types in skeletal muscle. A comparative study of the mammalian diaphragm. *J. Cell. Biol. 28:* 333, 1966.
84. London, D. R., Foley, T. H., and Webb, C. G.: Evidence for the release of individual amino acids from resting human forearm. *Nature 208:* 588, 1965.
85. Felig, P., and Wahren, J.: Amino acid metabolism in exercising man. *J. Clin. Invest. 50:* 2703, 1971.
86. Felig, P., Wahren, J., and Räf, L.: Evidence of inter-organ amino acid transport by blood cells in humans. *Proc. Natl. Acad. Sci. U.S.A. 70:* 1775, 1973.
87. Pozefsky, T., Felig, P., Tobin, J. D., Soeldner, J. S., and Cahill, G. F., Jr.: Amino acid balance across tissues of the forearm in postabsorptive man. Effects of insulin at two dose levels. *J. Clin. Invest. 48:* 2773, 1969.
88. Marliss, E. B., Aoki, T. T., Pozefsky, T., Most, A. S., and Cahill, G. F., Jr.: Muscle and splanchnic glutamine and glutamate metabolism in postabsorptive and starved man. *J. Clin. Invest. 50:* 814, 1971.
89. Carlsten, A., Hallgren, B., Jagenburg, R., Svanborg, A., and Werkö, L.: Arterio-hepatic venous differences of free fatty acids and amino acids. Studies in patients with diabetes or essential hypercholesterolemia, and in healthy individuals. *Acta Med. Scand. 181:* 199, 1967.
90. Felig, P., Owen, O. E., Wahren, J., and Cahill, Jr., G. F.: Amino acid metabolism during prolonged starvation. *J. Clin. Invest. 48:* 584, 1969.

91. Felig, P., Wahren, J., Karl, I., et al: Glutamine and glutamate metabolism in normal and diabetic subjects. *Diabetes 22:* 573, 1973.
92. Felig, P., Marliss, E., Pozefsky, T., and Cahill, G. F., Jr.: Amino acid metabolism in the regulation of gluconeogenesis in man. *Am. J. Clin. Nutr. 23:* 986, 1970.
93. Kominz, D. R., Hough, A., Symonds, P., and Laki, K.: The amino acid composition of actin, myosin, tropomyosin and the meromysins. *Arch. Biochem. Biophys. 50:* 148, 1954.
94. Felig, P., Pozefsky, T., Marliss, E., and Cahill, G. F., Jr.: Alanine: key role in gluconeogenesis. *Science 167:* 1003, 1970.
95. Mallette, L. E., Exton, J. H., and Park, C. R.: Control of gluconeogenesis from amino acids in the perfused rat liver. *J. Biol. Chem. 244:* 1003, 1970.
96. Carlsten, A., Hallgren, B., Jagenburg, R., Svanborg, A., and Werkö, L.: Arterial concentrations of fatty acids and free amino acids in healthy human individuals at rest and at different work loads. *Scand. J. Clin. Lab. Invest. 14:* 185, 1962.
97. Wahren, J., Felig, P., Havel, R. J., et al: Amino acid metabolism in McArdle's syndrome. *N. Engl. J. Med. 288:* 774, 1973.
98. Larsson, L.-E., Linderholm, H., Müller, R., Ringqvist, T., and Sörnäs, R.: Hereditary metabolic myopathy with paroxysmal myoglobinuria due to abnormal glycolysis. *J. Neurol. Neurosurg. Psychiatry 27:* 361, 1964.
99. Wahren, J., Felig, P., and Linderholm, H.: Amino acid metabolism in patients with a hereditary myopathy with paroxysmal myoglobinuria. *Acta Medica Scand.,* 1978, in press.
100. Turner, L. V., and Manchester, K. L.: Influence of denervation on the free amino acids of rat diaphragm. *Biochem. Biophys. Acta 320:* 352, 1973.
101. Miller, L. L.: The role of the liver and the non-hepatic tissues in the regulation of free amino acid levels in the blood. In Holden, J. T. (ed): Amino Acid Pools. *Proceedings of the Symposium on Free Amino Acids,* City of Hope Medical Center. Amsterdam, Elsevier, 1962, p. 708.
102. Randle, P. J., England, P. J., and Denton, R. M.: Control of the tricarboxylate cycle and its interactions with glycolysis during acetate utilization in rat heart. *Biochem. J. 117:* 677, 1970.
103. Parnas, J. K.: Ammonia formation in muscle and its source. *Am. J. Physiol. 90:* 467, 1929.
104. Lowenstein, J., and Tornheim, K.: Ammonia production in muscle: the purine nucleotide cycle. *Science 171:* 397, 1971.
105. Odessey, R., Khairallah, E. A., and Goldberg, A. L.: Origin and possible significance of alanine production by skeletal muscle. *J. Biol. Chem. 249:* 7623, 1974.
106. Hultman, E., Bergström, J., and McLennan Andersson, N.: Breakdown and resynthesis of phosphorylcreatine and adenosine triphosphate in connection with muscular work in man. *Scand. J. Clin. Lab. Invest. 19:* 56, 1967.
107. Pernow, B., and Wahren, J.: Lactate and pyruvate formation and oxygen utilization in the human forearm muscles during work of high intensity and varying duration. *Acta Physiol. Scand. 56:* 267, 1962.
108. Klassen, G. A., Andrew, G. M., and Becklake, M. R.: Effect of training on total and regional blood flow and metabolism in paddlers. *J. Appl. Physiol. 28:* 397, 1970.
109. Pernow, B., Havel, R., and Jennings, D. B.: The second wind phenomenon in McArdle's syndrome. *Acta Med. Scand.* [*Suppl.*] *472:* 294, 1967.
110. Porte, D., Jr., Crawford, D. W., Jennings, D. B., Aber, C., and McIlroy, M. B.: Cardiovascular and metabolic responses to exercise in a patient with McArdle's syndrome. *N. Engl. J. Med. 275:* 406, 1966.
111. Wahren, J., Felig, P., Hendler, R., and Ahlborg, G.: Glucose and amino acid metabolism during recovery after exercise. *J. Appl. Physiol. 34:* 838, 1973.
112. Hagenfeldt, L., and Wahren, J.: Turnover of free fatty acids during the recovery after exercise. *J. Appl. Physiol. 39:* 247, 1975.
113. Wilson, B. W., Long, W. L., and Thompson, H. C.: Changes in the composition of urine after muscular exercise. *J. Biol. Chem. 65:* 755, 1925.
114. Thomas, K.: Über das physiologische Stickstoffminimum. *Arch. Anat. Physiol.* [*Suppl.*] p. 249, 1910.
115. Refsum, H. E., and Strömme, S. B.: Urea and creatinine production and excretion in urine during and after prolonged heavy exercise. *Scand. J. Clin. Lab. Invest. 33:* 247, 1974.
116. Goldberg, A. L.: Relationship between hormones and muscular work in determining muscle size. In Alfred, N. (ed): Cardiac Hypertrophy. New York, Academic, 1971, p. 39.
117. Goldberg, A. L., Howell, E. M., and Li, J. B.: Physiological significance of protein degradation in animal and bacterial cells. *Fed. Proc. 33:* 112, 1974.
118. Hermansen, L., and Wachtlova, M.: Capillary density of skeletal muscle in well-trained and untrained men. *J. Appl. Physiol. 30:* 860, 1971.
119. Petren, T., Sjöstrand, T., and Sylvén, B.: Der Einfluss der trainings auf die Heufigkeit der Capillaren in Herz- und Skelettmuskulatur, *Arbeitsphysiol. 9:* 376, 1936.
120. Holloszy, J. O.: Biochemical adaptations in muscle. Effects of exercise on mitochondrial oxygen uptake and respiratory enzyme activity in skeletal muscle. *J. Biol. Chem. 242:* 2278, 1967.
121. Gollnick, P. D., and King, D. W.: Effect of exercise and training on mitochondria of rat skeletal muscle. *Am. J. Physiol. 216:* 1502, 1969.
122. Kiessling, K.-H., Piehl, K., and Lundquist, C.-G.: Effect of physical training on ultrastructural features in human skeletal muscle. In Pernow, B., and Saltin, B. (eds): Muscle Metabolism During Exercise. New York, Plenum, 1971, p. 97.
123. Oscai, L. B., Holloszy, J. O.: Biochemical adaptations in muscle II. Response of mitochondrial adenosine triphosphatase, creatine phosphokinase, and adenylate kinase activities in skeletal muscle to exercise. *J. Biol. Chem. 246:* 6968, 1971.
124. Holloszy, J. O., Oscai, L. B., Don, I. J., and Molé, P. A.: Mitochondrial citric acid cycle and related enzymes: adaptive response to exercise. *Biochem. Biophys. Res. Commun. 40:* 1368, 1970.
125. Winder, W. W., Baldwin, K. M., and Holloszy, J. O.: Enzymes involved in ketone utilization in different types of muscle: adaptation to exercise. *Eur. J. Biochem. 47:* 461, 1974.
126. Baldwin, K. M., Winder, W. W., Terjung, R. L., and Holloszy, J. O.: Glycolytic enzymes in different types of skeletal muscle: adaptation to exercise. *Am. J. Physiol. 225:* 962, 1973.
127. Lamb, D. R., Peter, J. B., Jeffress, R. N., and Wallace, H. A.: Glycogen, hexokinase, and glycogen synthetase adaptations to exercise. *Am. J. Physiol. 217:* 1628, 1969.
128. Molé, P. A., Baldwin, K. M., Terjung, R. L., and Holloszy, J. O.: Enzymatic pathways of pyruvate metabolism in skeletal muscle: adaptations to exercise. *Am. J. Physiol. 224:* 50, 1973.
129. Morgan, T. E., Cobb, L. A., Short, F. A., Ross, R., and Gunn, D. R.: Effects of long-term exercise on human muscle mitochondria. In Pernow, B., and Saltin, B. (eds): Muscle Metabolism During Exercise. New York, Plenum, 1971, p. 87.
130. Morgan, T. E., Short, F. A., and Cobb, L. A.: Effect of long-term exercise on skeletal muscle lipid composition. *Am. J. Physiol. 216:* 82, 1969.
131. Pattengale, P. K., and Holloszy, J. O.: Augmentation of skeletal muscle myoglobin by a program of treadmill running. *Am. J. Physiol. 213:* 783, 1967.
132. Short, F. A., Cobb, L. A., Kawabori, J., and Goodner, C. J.: Influence of exercise training on red and white rat skeletal muscle. *Am. J. Physiol. 217:* 327, 1969.
133. Issekutz, B., Miller, H. I., and Rodahl, K.: Lipid and carbohydrate metabolism during exercise. *Fed. Proc. 25:* 1415, 1966.
134. Havel, R. J., Carlson, L. A., Ekelund, L.-G., and Holmgren, A.: Turnover rate and oxidation of different free fatty acids in man during exercise. *J. Appl. Physiol. 19:* 613, 1964.
135. Issekutz, B., Jr., Miller, H. I., Paul, P., and Rodahl, K.: Aerobic work capacity and plasma FFA turnover. *J. Appl. Physiol. 20:* 293, 1965.
136. Sanders, C. A., Levinson, G. E., Abelmann, W. H., and Freinkel, N.: Effect of exercise on the peripheral utilization of glucose in man. *N. Engl. J. Med. 271:* 220, 1964.
137. Roch-Norlund, A. E., Bergström, J., Castenfors, H., and Hultman, E.: Muscle glycogen in patients with diabetes mellitus. Glycogen content before treatment and the effect of insulin. *Acta Med. Scand. 187:* 445, 1970.
138. Wahren, J., Felig, P., Cerasi, E., and Luft, R.: Splanchnic and peripheral glucose and amino acid metabolism in diabetes mellitus. *J. Clin. Invest. 51:* 1870, 1972.

147

Starvation

Philip Felig

INTRODUCTION

The endocrine and metabolic response to starvation represents an integrated fuel–hormone interplay designed to maintain euglycemia while meeting the substrate requirements of specific tissues, notably the brain, and at the same time minimizing losses of body protein.[1] The adaptive nature of the response takes into account the composition and expendability of body fuel stores as well as the fuel requirements of individual tissues. Although prolonged starvation is rarely encountered as a medical problem in Western civilization today, shorter periods of food deprivation may result in the development of symptomatic hypoglycemia in a variety of disease states (see Chapter 90). The normal physiologic response to fasting thus provides a basis for evaluating the pathophysiology of hypoglycemia. Furthermore, in various disease states characterized by debilitation (metastatic cancer, uremia, severe inflammatory bowel disease), starvation is often an important contributory cause of death. In such patients the following sequence of events is often encountered: decreased food intake → protein wasting → weakness of respiratory muscles → atelectasis → pneumonia → death. The inability to conserve body protein stores in such patients reflects a failure of the normal homeostatic mechanisms present in healthy subjects undergoing prolonged periods of food deprivation. In the discussion that follows, the normal response to starvation will be viewed as a continuum that can be divided into three phases: the postabsorptive state (6–12 h after food intake); short-term starvation (lasting 3–7 days); and prolonged starvation (2 weeks or longer).

BODY FUEL STORES

The calories consumed in the typical American or Western European diet consist of 40–45 percent carbohydrate, 40 percent fat, and 15–20 percent protein. The composition of the fuels stored in the human body, however, is far different from that ingested in the diet.[2] Carbohydrate represents a calorically insignificant fuel store. The combined caloric value of liver glycogen (70 g), muscle glycogen (200 g), and circulating blood glucose (20 g) amounts to approximately 1100 Calories, well below the total caloric expenditure of a single day, even under basal conditions. Nevertheless, liver glycogen represents an important source of carbohydrate to meet the ongoing needs of the brain, particularly in the interval between the evening meal and breakfast and during bursts of augmented glucose utilization accompanying exercise.[3] However, liver glycogen is rapidly depleted as starvation extends beyond 18–24 h.[4] The teleologic basis of the limitation in stored carbohydrate derives not only from its decreased caloric density (4 kcal/g as compared to 9 kcal/g in fat), but also from the large amount of tissue water obligated in the storage of glycogen (4 ml/g). Thus, to store an equivalent number of calories as carbohydrate requires more than eight times the mass (weight) necessary for storage as fat.

By far the largest reservoir of body fuel is in the form of fat, stored as triglyceride. In a nonobese person, body fat amounts to 20 percent of total body weight and has a caloric value of 130,000–140,000 Calories, accounting for 80 percent of total body fuel storage. This amount of calories could meet basal caloric requirements for approximately 2 months. In obese subjects, fat tissue may provide for the storage of over 500,000 Calories. Regardless of the degree of adiposity, fat clearly represents the most expendable as well as the most plentiful fuel available to man.

The fuel whose depletion limits survival in starvation, however, is neither fat nor carbohydrate, but protein. The major reservoir of body protein is in muscle tissue, amounting to 10 kg (exclusive of tissue water), or 40,000 Calories. Because of protein's importance in body structure, in muscle function, and as a catalytic agent (enzymes), depletion of body protein by 30–50 percent is incompatible with survival, despite residual, mobilizable fat tissue.[5] Death in starvation results not from hypoglycemia, but, as noted above, from loss of respiratory muscle function leading to terminal pneumonia.

Of particular importance in the homeostatic response to starvation is the interchangeability of fuels. Body protein (by virtue of its constituent amino acids, other than leucine) is readily converted to glucose (gluconeogenesis). Carbohydrate availability for obligate, glucose-dependent tissues (e.g., brain) thus does not cease with depletion of liver glycogen. On the other hand, fatty acids containing an even number of carbon atoms (comprising over 95 percent of the total fatty acids stored as triglyceride) cannot be converted to glucose; mammalian tissue lacks the enzymatic steps necessary for net gluconeogenesis from acetyl CoA. Thus, to the extent that blood glucose is terminally oxidized in starvation and replenished by gluconeogenesis, there will be an obligate dissolution of body protein stores.

POSTABSORPTIVE STATE

The changeover from the fed to the fasted condition can best be examined in the context of the postabsorptive state—the condition that exists 6–12 h after food ingestion. While this interval represents a nonsteady state, it is nevertheless a readily identifiable reference point. In the postabsorptive condition, adipose tissue releases free fatty acids (FFA) to meet the fuel requirements of muscle and heart as well as parenchymal tissues (liver, kidney). The respiratory quotient of resting muscle is thus close to 0.7.[6] Carbohydrate utilization in this circumstance occurs primarily in the brain, which terminally oxidizes glucose at a rate of 125 g/day.[7] Smaller amounts of glucose are utilized by resting muscle[6] and by obligate anaerobic tissues such as the formed elements of the blood and the renal medulla (Fig. 147-1). While several tissues thus contribute to glucose utilization, production of glucose is limited to the liver. Maintenance of euglycemia depends on release of glucose from the liver at a rate equal to the combined utilization in

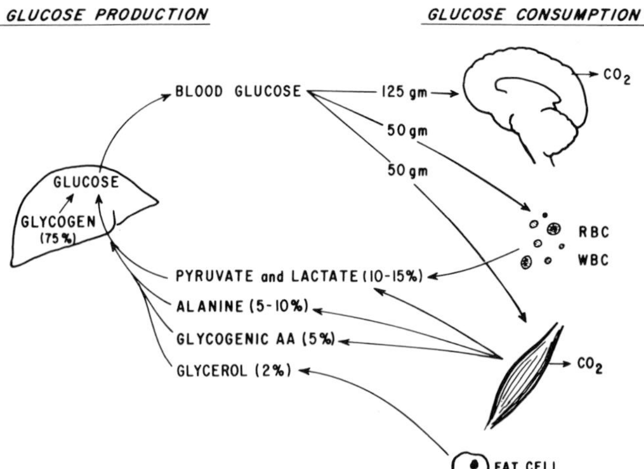

Fig. 147-1. Glucose production and utilization in postabsorptive man. The values for glucose uptake represent the amounts consumed per day; in the case of muscle this refers to the resting state. Glucose output from the liver derives from glycogenolysis (25 percent). As starvation extends beyond 12 h, glycogen stores are depleted and the contribution from gluconeogenesis increases.

brain and peripheral tissues (150–250 g/day; 2–3 mg/kg body weight/min; 6–10 g/hr). In the absence of such glucose production, the blood glucose level would be halved in 40–60 min. Approximately 75 percent of the glucose released after an overnight fast is derived from glycogen, the remainder being formed by gluconeogenesis.[7] Thus after no more than a 6–12- h period of food abstinence the metabolic "set" has already been converted from feeding to fasting, as evidenced by lipolysis (fat mobilization), glycogenolysis, and gluconeogenesis. Since, as noted above, liver glycogen stores (70 g) can sustain cerebral glucose requirements for less than 24 h, as fasting extends beyond the postabsorptive state greater reliance is placed on gluconeogenesis.

GLUCONEOGENESIS

Gluconeogenesis refers to the processes whereby glucose is formed from noncarbohydrate sources. The principal precursor substrates from which glucose may be derived are amino acids, pyruvate, lactate, and glycerol. The latter three substrates represent glycolytic intermediates, inasmuch as they are formed from glucose in the Embden-Myerhoff pathway. Consequently, glucose formation from these precursors represents a recycling of substrates (the Cori cycle in the case of lactate) rather than de novo glucose synthesis. In fact, it is by means of this recycling process that muscle glycogen can contribute to blood glucose homeostasis. Since muscle lacks the enzyme glucose-6-phosphatase, its glycogen cannot be released into the blood stream as glucose. However, lactate and pyruvate formed from muscle glycogen are released to the liver, where they are converted to glucose.

With respect to gluconeogenesis from amino acids, all amino acids other than leucine are potentially glycogenic. However, the pattern of interorgan amino acid exchange is such that alanine is the major amino acid available for hepatic gluconeogenesis.[7,8] After an overnight fast, muscle is in negative nitrogen balance, releasing all amino acids other than serine. However, the output of alanine and glutamine exceeds that of all other amino acids. While glutamine is taken up mainly by the gut and kidney (where it is converted to ammonia), alanine is extracted by the liver for conversion to glucose[7,8] (Fig. 147-2A). The predominance of alanine in the outflow of amino nitrogen from muscle has been explained on the basis of its synthesis in situ by transamination of glucose-derived pyruvate.[8] In circumstances of increased pyruvate formation, such as muscular exercise, alanine formation is markedly accelerated.[9] Recent studies indicate that the branched-chain amino acids (valine, leucine, and isoleucine) that are selectively catabolized in muscle provide the amino groups for alanine synthesis.[10–12] Isotopic studies[11] as well as balance data[7] indicate that 60–70 percent of the alanine carbon skeletons are glucose derived. Thus gluconeogenesis from this amino acid represents, in part, a recycling of carbon substrate (the glucose–alanine cycle) analogous to the Cori cycle for lactate.[7]

The intermediary steps in the synthesis of glucose involve mainly a reversal of the glycolytic pathway. However, at several points, pathways and enzymes unique to the gluconeogenic process are employed (Fig. 147-2B). Since the final step in glycolysis, the conversion of phosphoenolpyruvate to pyruvate, is thermodynamically irreversible, the "upward" flow of pyruvate to glucose is achieved by initially converting pyruvate to oxaloacetate (by pyruvate carboxylase) and subsequent formation of phosphoenol pyruvate (catalyzed by phosphoenolypyruvate carboxykinase). The steps involved in the conversion of pyruvate to phosphoenolpyruvate represent a major site of hormonal control, par-

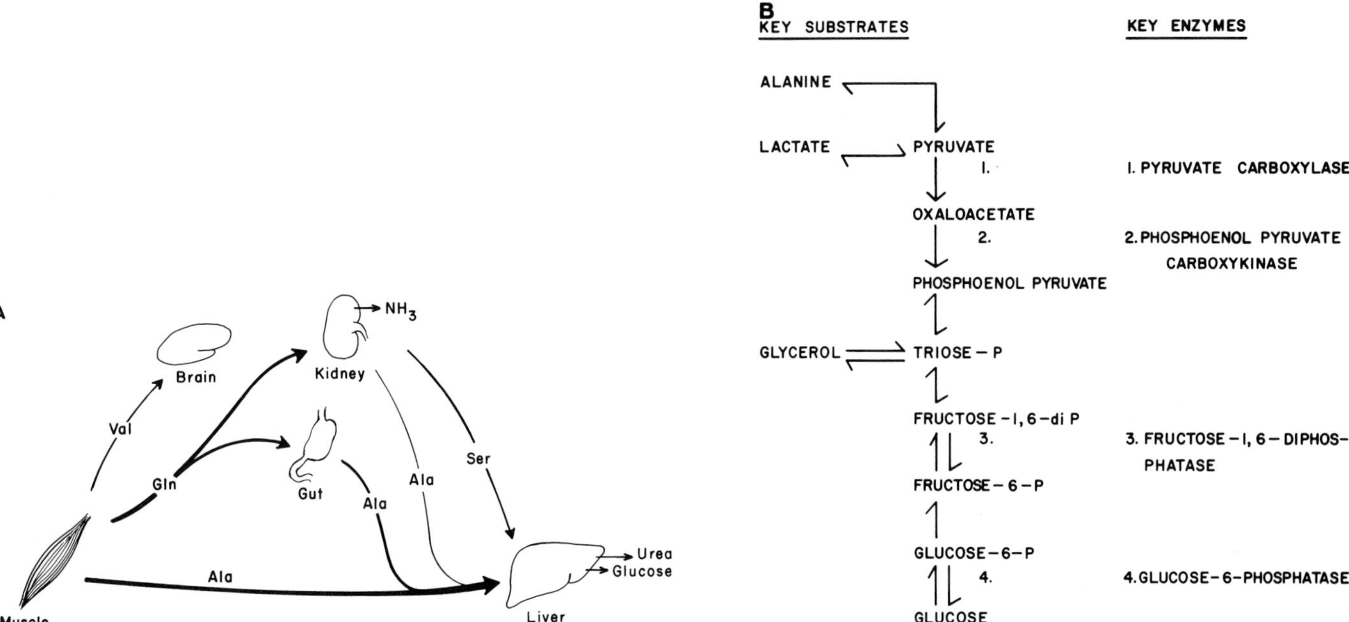

Fig. 147-2. A. Interorgan amino acid exchange in normal postabsorptive man. The key role of alanine in amino acid output from muscle and gut tissue and uptake by the liver is shown. B. Gluconeogenic pathway. The quantitatively important substrates are alanine and lactate; glycerol and pyruvate contribute to a lesser extent. The key rate-limiting enzymatic steps are also shown.

ticularly the stimulatory action of glucagon.[13] Furthermore, pyruvate carboxylase is allosterically activated by acetyl CoA. In this manner augmented oxidation of fatty acids in the liver serves to enhance gluconeogenesis. Other enzymes unique to the gluconeogenic pathway are fructose-1-6-diphosphatase, which catalyzes the formation of fructose-6-phosphate from fructose-1-6-diphosphate, and glucose-6-phosphatase, which permits dephosphorylation of glucose and liberation of this hexose into the blood stream.

The overall regulation of gluconeogenesis depends on substrate availability, the hormonal milieu, and enzyme activity. In the postabsorptive state, 30–40 percent of the alanine and lactate delivered to the liver is extracted by hepatic cells. An augmentation in gluconeogenesis can thus be achieved as a result of increased hepatic extraction of gluconeogenic precursors or, alternatively, by increasing precursor supply. Contrariwise, inhibition of gluconeogenesis may be achieved by diminishing precursor availability or altering hepatic uptake and/or disposal of available precursors. The data suggest that the physiologic regulation of gluconeogenesis in starvation involves all of these mechanisms. Early in starvation (see below) gluconeogenesis is increased by means of augmented hepatic extraction of available precursors. In prolonged starvation gluconeogenesis progressively declines as a result of decreased precursor availability (see below). In contrast, the diminution in gluconeogenesis associated with glucose-mediated insulin secretion involves an inhibition of hepatic gluconeogenic processes despite on-going precursor availability.[14,15]

Returning to the postabsorptive state, gluconeogenesis accounts for 25–30 percent of total hepatic glucose production (Fig. 147-1). Lactate is the major gluconeogenic precursor (15 percent), followed by alanine (5–10 percent) and, to a much lesser extent, glycerol (1 percent) and pyruvate (1 percent). The quantitative considerations are such that gluconeogenic mechanisms become crucial to the maintenance of euglycemia in circumstances in which glycogen stores have been depleted (fasting extending beyond 12–18 h) or in which glycogen is mobilized at an accelerated rate (prolonged exercise, pregnancy).

FAT MOBILIZATION AND KETOGENESIS

Utilization of body fat as an energy-yielding fuel is initiated by the breakdown of stored triglyceride in adipose tissue, resulting in the liberation of FFA and glycerol (lipolysis). This hormone-sensitive step (see below) is actively proceeding in the postabsorptive state, as evidenced by the net flow of fatty acids from adipose tissue to muscle, liver, heart, and kidney. The concentration of FFA in the postabsorptive state (500–800 μeq/liter) is twofold greater than that observed 2 h after meal ingestion.[16]

Concomitant with the uptake and oxidation of FFA in muscle, FFA are oxidized by the liver, where they form ketone acids: β-hydroxybutyric acid and acetoacetic acid. These ketone acids are interconvertible via a reversible oxidoreductive step analogous to the interconversion of lactate and pyruvate. They circulate in a ratio of 3:1 (favoring β-hydroxybutyrate), which reflects the intramitochondrial redox state, mainly of muscle. The formation of ketone acids within the liver involves the enzymatic transfer of fatty acyl CoA across the mitochondrial membrane (catalyzed by acylcarnitine transferase), followed by β-oxidation, giving rise to acetyl CoA. Condensation of two molecules of acetyl CoA yields acetoacetyl CoA, which is converted to acetoacetic acid.

The rate of ketogenesis is determined by the availability of precursor FFA as well as the nutritionally determined hormonal milieu. When FFA are elevated in the *fed state* by ingestion of a fat meal (and administration of heparin), ketogenesis is minimally enhanced, presumably because insulin levels are not sufficiently reduced in such fed subjects.[17] Conversely, it can be demonstrated in the isolated liver that in the fasted state, ketogenesis is enhanced at any given level of FFA availability.[18] The factors altering the metabolic set in the fed or fasted state are believed to be insulin and glucagon[19] (see below). The data suggest that the hormone-sensitive step in hepatic ketogenesis that is accelerated in starvation involves the acylcarnitine transferase reaction.[20]

The importance of ketone acids in starvation derives from their effects on acid–base homeostasis and fluid balance, and, perhaps most importantly, on their utilization as oxidizable substrates. The pK of β-hydroxybutyrate as well as acetoacetate is such as to result in complete dissociation in body water, thereby causing a metabolic acidosis. The loss of these anions in the urine, while calorically negligible (<100 Cal/day), obligates a loss of cations in the form of sodium (resulting in a diuresis) or ammonia (resulting in protein depletion). On the other hand, in prolonged fasting the availability of ketones as an energy-yielding fuel permits a decrease in glucose utilization and gluconeogenesis, thereby sparing body protein stores.

Besides ketogenesis, an alternative fate of FFA uptake by the liver is reesterification with α-glycerophosphate to form triglyceride. It has been suggested that the rate of fatty acid oxidation (and ketone formation) is determined by the efficiency of triglyceride synthesis, which in turn is influenced by the availability of α-glycerophosphate. However, a decrease in hepatic α-glycerophosphate has not been observed in starvation.[8] The available evidence thus suggests that triglyceride-synthesizing pathways are intact in starvation. Fatty acids, however, are shunted into the oxidative pathway because of activation of the key step in this sequence, the acylcarnitine transferase reaction.[20]

In the postabsorptive state, the rate of lipolysis is such as to result in the mobilization of approximately 7 g of fatty acids per hour. FFA are taken up by the liver at a rate of 3 g/hr, where disposal occurs in fairly equal proportions along each of three pathways: terminal oxidation to CO_2, formation of ketone acids, and synthesis of triglycerides.[21] The net result is that ketone acids circulate in the postabsorptive condition in concentrations no greater than 0.5 mM. Such levels pose no threat to acid–base equilibrium nor to protein conservation (in obligating urinary ammonia excretion). Nevertheless, ketogenesis is clearly demonstrable within a 6–12 h interval after meal ingestion and thus should not be viewed as a toxic process limited to disease states.

GLUCOREGULATORY HORMONES

From the foregoing discussion it should be readily apparent that the key processes characterizing the response to starvation (glycogenolysis, gluconeogenesis, lipolysis, ketogenesis) become operative within brief periods of food abstinence. The cardinal factors governing these processes are the glucoregulatory hormones, insulin and glucagon. The response to starvation is characterized by a fall in plasma insulin from the levels present in the fed state, and by a rise in plasma glucagon.

Insulin

The secretion of insulin is stimulated by virtually all ingested substrates, particularly glucose. Following meal ingestion, circulating insulin (in nonobese subjects) falls from peak levels of 50–150 μU/ml (1 h postprandially) to concentrations of 15–20 μU/ml in the postabsorptive state. In the latter circumstance insulin does not disappear from the circulation nor does its secretion cease. It is estimated that insulin is released into the systemic circulation in postabsorptive subjects in rates of 0.5–1.0 U/hr. (22)

The sensitivity of the processes involved in regulating insulin secretion are such that changes in blood glucose (induced by iv glucose infusion) of no more than 10–15 mg/100 ml are sufficient to cause a 50 percent or more change in insulin levels and marked alterations in glycogenolysis. (14) Similar changes in insulin will alter lipolysis. The decline in secretion of insulin (initiated by the postprandial drop in blood sugar) is thus the key signal that sets in motion the matabolic response to starvation.

The overall physiologic effect of insulin may be characterized as stimulation of a variety of processes designed to enhance fuel storage (glycogen synthesis, fat synthesis and storage, protein synthesis). A fall in insulin results in the reverse effect on each of these processes. As noted above, lipolysis is exquisitly sensitive to insulin (by virtue of a hormone-sensitive lipase in the fat cell), so that fatty acid mobilization and utilization is accelerated as serum insulin falls. Simultaneously, intrahepatic β-oxidative pathways are accelerated (by virtue of activation of the acylcarnitine transferase reaction). Glycogenolytic and gluconeogenic mechanisms in the liver are also stimulated. Finally, amino acid mobilization from muscle is enhanced as protein synthetic processes decline while catabolic reactions increase in activity.

Because of the all important role of gluconeogenesis in fasting, the mechanism whereby insulin influences gluconeogenesis deserves special emphasis. The increases in insulin secretion observed with a carbohydrate meal result in the conversion of the liver from an organ of glucose production to one of glucose utilization.[15] This involves not only stimulation of glycogen synthesis but also inhibition of gluconeogenesis. The site of action of insulin in regulating gluconeogenesis is primarily in the liver rather than by virtue of a primary effect on precursor availability. This is evidenced by the fact that circulating levels of the quantitatively important gluconeogenic substrates alanine and lactate may increase (or remain stable) after a carbohydrate meal, yet their extraction by the liver falls by 50–100 percent.[14,15] The fall in insulin to basal postabsorptive levels is accompanied by an increase in hepatic uptake and utilization of gluconeogenic precursors. It should be noted that larger increments in insulin are required to inhibit gluconeogenesis as compared to glycogenolysis.[14,23]

While the locus of insulin's action is the liver in regulating gluconeogenesis, clear-cut effects of insulin in regulating amino acid mobilization are readily demonstrable. A fall in circulating amino acids involving primarily the branched-chain amino acids (valine, leucine, and isoleucine) accompanies a rise in insulin secretion,[8] while the reverse (elevated levels of branched-chain amino acids) is observed with insulin deficiency.[24] The selectivity of the action of insulin on branched-chain amino acid levels may derive from their role as a fuel for muscle[10] as well as their importance in regulating protein synthesis in muscle.[11]

Glucagon

In recent years, primarily as a consequence of the work of Unger, it has become apparent that food intake or deprivation influences circulating levels of glucagon as well as insulin. The basal postabsorptive level of glucagon (50–100 pg/ml) represents an increment from the suppressed concentrations observed after ingestion of a carbohydrate meal.[25] The overall importance of these basal concentrations to glucose homeostasis in the postabsorptive state is demonstrable from experiments with somatostatin, a tetradecapeptide that inhibits glucagon as well as insulin secretion.[26] Administration of somatostatin to healthy subjects results in a decline in postabsorptive blood glucose of approximately 40 mg/100 ml over a 1-h period.[26,27] This hypoglycemic effect is entirely a consequence of inhibition of hepatic glucose output.[28] Thus, despite a fall in insulin to extremely low levels, maintenance of hepatic glycogenolysis is dependent on basal levels of circulating glucagon. This action of glucagon on glycogenolysis is mediated via changes in hepatic adenyl cyclase activity. Glucagon also functions in starvation as a stimulus to gluconeogenesis. For example, in 3-day fasted, glycogen-depleted subjects, somatostatin-induced hypoglucagonemia results in a marked fall in hepatic glucose production, indicating inhibition of gluconeogenesis.[28] On the other hand, the lipolytic effects of glucagon probably represent a pharmacologic rather than a physiologic effect.

It should be noted that increased secretion of glucagon contributes to glucose homeostasis not only in the postabsorptive state but in the protein-fed individual as well.[25,29] In such subjects, an increment in serum insulin sufficient to inhibit glycogenolysis occurs in the absence of carbohydrate intake. A fall in hepatic glucose output and in blood glucose would thus be expected after a protein meal. The maintenance of euglycemia in this circumstance depends on the protein-induced increment in glucagon which serves to counteract the glycogen-sparing effects of insulin.[25,29]

SHORT-TERM STARVATION

The integrated fuel–hormone response to relatively brief starvation (3–7 days) represents an acceleration of gluconeogenic, lipolytic, and ketogenic processes that are already functioning at a less rapid rate in the postabsorptive condition. Stimulation of gluconeogenesis is necessitated by the rapid depletion of glycogen stores and the need to provide glucose for consumption by the brain. Lipolysis allows for the mobilization of the most abundant fuel supply available to the fasted individual, body fat. Ketogenesis may be viewed as a mechanism whose usefulness becomes apparent in prolonged starvation, at which point ketones function as fuel for the brain and as a signal for protein conservation in muscle.[30]

The chief factors mediating the enhancement in gluconeogenesis and ketogenesis as fasting extends from 12 h to 3 days or 1 week are a drop in plasma insulin and a rise in glucagon (Fig. 147-3). As noted above, the sensitivity of the pancreatic β cells is such that decrements in blood glucose of 5–10 mg/100 ml/day that occur during each day of a 3-day fast are sufficient to result in a measurable decline in circulating insulin levels.[31] A simultaneous rise in glucagon is observed which reaches its peak (50–100 percent above postabsorptive levels) at 3 days.[32] Interestingly, the rise in glucagon that occurs early in human starvation has recently been shown to be largely a consequence of decreased hormonal catabolism rather than a result of hypersecretion.[33]

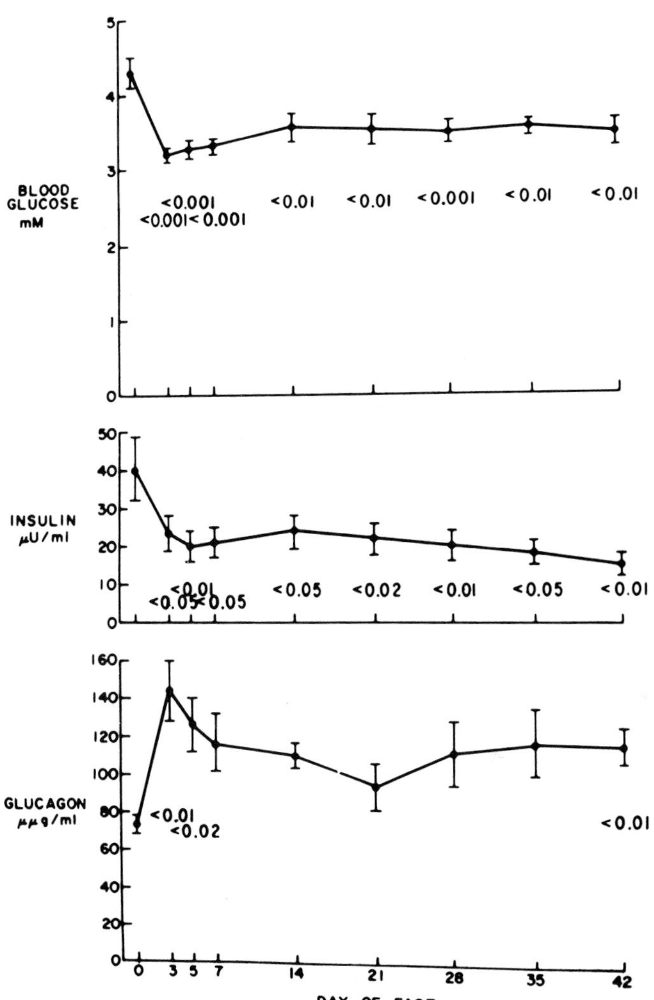

Fig. 147-3. Blood glucose, serum insulin, and plasma glucagon response to prolonged starvation. (From Marliss et al.: *J. Clin. Invest. 49:* 2256, 1970.)

The altered levels of insulin and glucagon accelerate gluconeogenic and ketogenic processes by virtue of their effects on hepatic and, in the case of insulin, peripheral tissues. The prime locus of the increase in gluconeogenesis is an augmentation in hepatic extraction of alanine despite a fall in plasma alanine levels.[34] The augmented rate of alanine extraction in brief starvation is comparable to that observed in other insulinopenic states such as diabetes[35] and prolonged exercise.[9] The overall rate of gluconeogenesis increases 2–3-fold above postabsorptive levels and, in view of the depletion in liver glycogen, accounts for virtually the entire output of glucose from the liver.[7,34] An increase in proteolysis and amino acid mobilization from muscle (to supply glucose precursors) accompanies the rise in hepatic gluconeogenesis.[36] This is reflected in negative nitrogen balance at the rate of 10–12 g/day, indicating breakdown of 75–100 g protein/day. A progressive rise in the blood levels of the insulin-sensitive branched-chain amino acids (valine, leucine, and isoleucine) is also observed, providing further similarity to the diabetic state.[34]

At the same time the increase in gluconeogenesis takes place, ketone production by the liver is enhanced. The fall in insulin stimulates lipolysis, thereby increasing the delivery of FFA. In addition, changes in the β-oxidative pathway within the liver induced by the change in insulin and glucagon favor ketone formation at the expense of alternative pathways of FFA disposal. The result is that the liver, after a 3-day fast, utilizes FFA at twice the rate observed in postabsorptive man and produces ketones at a rate of 75–100 g/day.[21] The lipolytic and ketogenic activity also serves to enhance gluconeogenesis by (1) providing FFA to meet hepatic energy requirements, (2) furnishing acetyl CoA, which stimulates pyruvate carboxylase (a rate-limiting enzyme in gluconeogenesis; see above), and (3) altering the hepatic redox state to favor glucose synthesis.

The overall sequence of events characterizing early starvation is shown in Figure 147-4 and may be summarized as follows. Ongoing glucose utilization by the brain results in depletion of liver glycogen and a small decline in blood glucose (5–10 mg/100 ml). As

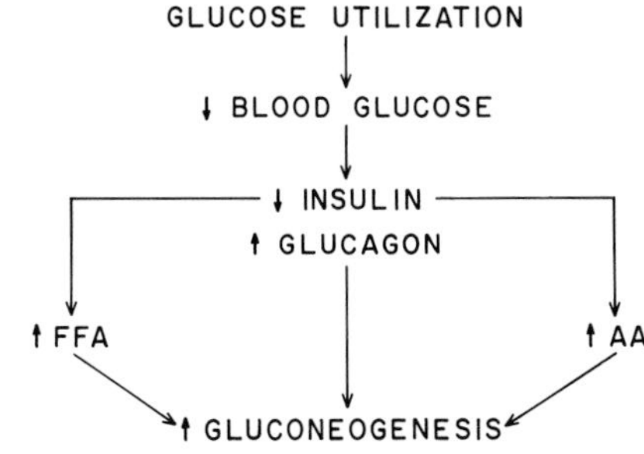

Fig. 147-4. Metabolic adaptation during the early or gluconeogenic phase of starvation.

a result, β cell secretion is reduced and insulin levels decline. An accompanying rise in glucagon is observed, which may be mediated primarily by diminished hormonal catabolism rather than hypersecretion. The bihormonal changes influence intrahepatic events (augmented alanine uptake and conversion to glucose, increased acylcarnitine transferase activity) so as to accelerate gluconeogenesis as well as ketogenesis. Contributing to these effects are peripheral actions of hypoinsulinemia, which enchance the mobilization of FFA and amino acids from adipose tissue and muscle, respectively.

PROLONGED STARVATION

Continuation of the events described in early starvation would facilitate the maintenance of euglycemia as well as dissipation of fat stores, but at the expense of body protein. As noted above, fatty acids cannot be converted to glucose; net gluconeogenesis occurs only from protein-derived precursors. Persistence of gluconeogenesis and proteolysis at rates observed early in starvation would result in dissipation of 30–50 percent of body protein (a life-threatening situation) within 4–6 weeks, well before body fat stores have been fully mobilized. Studies in obese subjects (whose body protein mass is comparable to nonobese subjects) reveal that fasts lasting 6 weeks to 6 months (in a hospital setting) can be tolerated without ill effect. The adaptive mechanism permitting for such extended periods of starvation involves a progressive decrease in protein breakdown. As shown originally in the classical studies of Benedict[37] and repeatedly confirmed by others,[38] the rate of urinary nitrogen loss in prolonged fasting falls progressively, reaching levels as low as 3 g/day, indicating dissolution of no more than 20 g of body protein (Fig. 147-5). The nature of the nitrogenous end products also changes, from predominantly urea in early starvation, to primarily ammonia after 10 days of fasting (Fig. 147-5).

GLUCONEOGENESIS

A decline in protein breakdown necessitates a simultaneous reduction in gluconeogenesis. Direct measurements of glucose production in prolonged fasted subjects (3–6 weeks) reveal that hepatic glucose production falls from postabsorptive rates of 150–250 g/day to approximately 50 g/day.[34,38] An additional 40 g of glucose is produced by the kidney, which in prolonged starvation contributes to gluconeogenesis in amounts equal to the liver.[38] Theoretically, the marked decline in hepatic glucose production could be ascribed to inhibition of hepatic processes involved in the uptake and utilization of gluconeogenic substrates, diminished precursor (alanine) release from the periphery (i.e., muscle), or a combination of these processes. In fact, the rate-limiting step is in the periphery, where a marked diminution in muscle release of alanine as well as other amino acids is observed[34a] (Fig. 147-6). Prolonged fasting thus clearly differs from early starvation (3-day fast), in which there is a rise in muscle alanine output.[36] Accompanying this fall in alanine output is a progressive decline in circulating alanine levels (Fig. 147-6) that exceeds the fall observed in all other amino acids.[34] Underscoring the role of alanine availability in regulating gluconeogenesis are observations on hepatic alanine uptake. The fractional extraction of alanine by the liver in prolonged starvation is no less than that observed in the overnight fasted state.[34] Furthermore, administration of exogenous alanine to prolonged fasted subjects results in a prompt rise in blood glucose, indicating unimpaired intrahepatic gluconeogenic pathways.[39,40]

In contrast to the fall in glucose output from the liver, the kidney subserves an important role as a site of glucose formation in prolonged fasting.[38] This contrasts with the situation in postabsorptive man or in physiologic circumstances of augmented glucose production such as exercise,[3] or even in pathologic situations such as the hyperglycemic diabetic;[41] in none of these conditions is net addition of glucose from the kidney to the blood stream observed. Based on in vitro studies linking renal gluconeogenesis and ammoniagenesis,[42] it has been suggested that the enhanced ammonia excretion dictated by the ketonuria of starvation (Fig. 147-5) serves as a stimulus of renal glucose production.

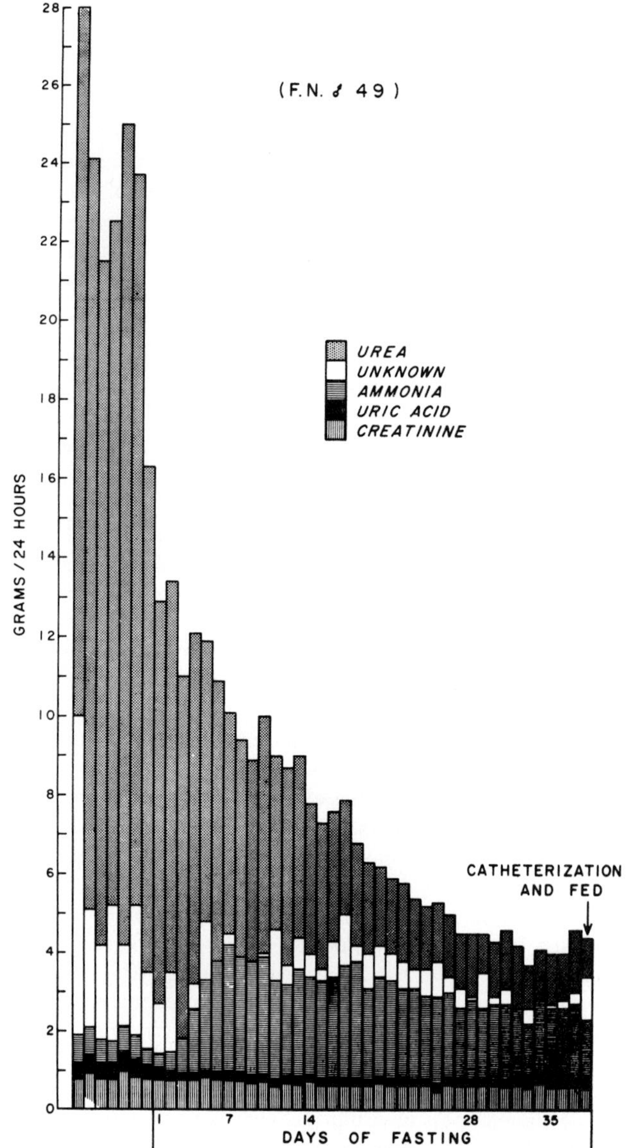

Fig. 147-5. Urinary nitrogen excretion during prolonged starvation. Nitrogen losses decline markedly as starvation extends beyond 1 week. (From Owen et al.: *J. Clin. Invest. 48:* 574, 1969.)

KETONE METABOLISM

Despite the contribution of the kidney to gluconeogenesis, total glucose production in prolonged fasting (90 g/day) is one-half or less of that observed in postabsorptive man.[38] In the absence of adaptive changes in glucose consumption, severe hypoglycemia and attendant derangement in brain function would rapidly ensue. As shown in Figure 147-3, blood glucose levels reach a plateau of 50–70 mg/100 ml within 3 days of fasting and subsequently stabi-

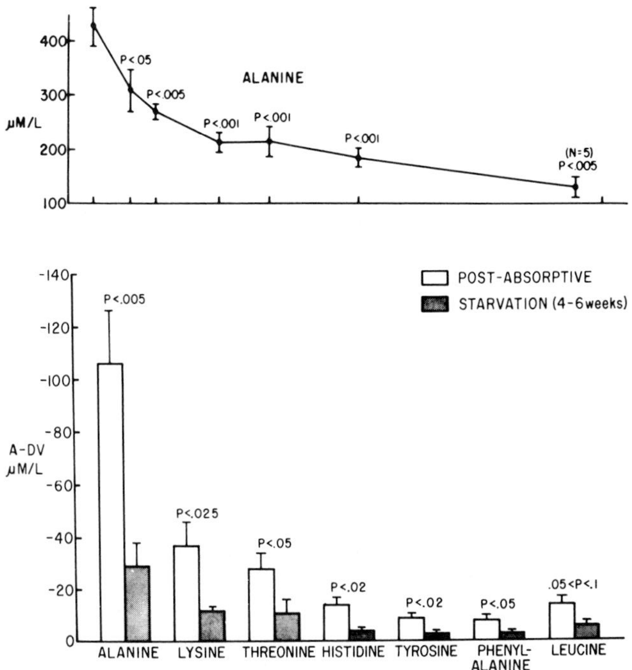

Fig. 147-6. A. Changes in plasma alanine during prolonged starvation. B. Changes in muscle release of amino acids during prolonged starvation. The decrease in alanine output from muscle is the factor responsible for hypoalaninemia and the decrease in hepatic gluconeogenesis in the late phase of starvation. (Data from Felig et al.[34,34a])

lize. Even more striking is the fact that prolonged fasted subjects have no problem in maintaining cerebral function in the face of a marked reduction in glucose availability. This seeming paradox is resolved by the observation that ketone acids become a major fuel for the brain in prolonged fasting.[43] The uptake of ketone acids by the brain is sufficient to account for 50 percent or more of its fuel requirements. A corresponding decline in brain uptake of glucose permits euglycemia in the face of diminished glucose production. As a corollary of this shift in fuels by the brain, prolonged fasted subjects are resistant to the symptomatic effects of insulin hypoglycemia.[44] In experimental animals this dependence on ketones serves to protect animals from insulin-induced seizures despite unchanged responsiveness to other central nervous system irritants.[45]

The mechanism responsible for ketone utilization by the brain in prolonged starvation is primarily substrate availability. Studies in experimental animals and man reveal that ketone-oxidizing enzymes are already active in the brain after an overnight fast.[46,47] The progressive increase in brain ketone utilization is thus a reflection of a rising arterial ketone concentration.[38] It is of interest in this regard that blood ketone levels (particularly β-hydroxybutyrate) continue to rise for 3–4 weeks of starvation,[4] while FFA levels as well as hepatic ketone production rates reach peak levels within 3–10 days.[38,48] The events of prolonged starvation thus appear to be directed at raising the arterial concentration of ketone acids so as to augment their availability to the brain without necessitating an increase in ketogenesis. This adaptation is achieved by a progressive decrease and/or saturation of extracerebral pathways of ketone utilization as starvation continues beyond 3 days.[49] For example, muscle uptake of ketones in prolonged starvation falls by 75 percent as compared to the early fasting period.[50,51] Finally, a rapid rise in the net rate of ketone reabsorption by the renal tubule between 3 and 10 days of starvation serves to diminish urinary ketone losses and thereby accentuate ketone accumulation in blood.[52]

REGULATORY MECHANISMS

A major question in prolonged starvation is the nature of the signal(s) responsible for the adaptive changes described. Specifically, what factor(s) is (are) responsible for decreased muscle protein catabolism and lessened alanine availability for gluconeogenesis in prolonged fasting? The key roles demonstrated for insulin and glucagon in early starvation immediately raise the possibility of a similar function in prolonged fasting. However, insulin levels that reach their nadir in 7–10 days remain at low levels throughout prolonged fasting (Fig. 147-3). The hypoinsulinemia responsible for accelerated gluconeogenesis and proteolysis in early starvation thus cannot be invoked as an explanation of diminished gluconeogenesis and protein conservation in prolonged starvation. In the case of glucagon, a return to basal, postabsorptive levels occurs as starvation continues beyond 3 days (Fig. 147-3) as a result of a progressive diminution in secretion as well as turnover.[33] Furthermore, a role for glucagon in regulating muscle proteolysis or alanine availability has not been established.

Recently it has been suggested that hyperketonemia may of itself provide the protein-sparing signal to muscle tissue. In prolonged fasted subjects a rise in blood ketone acid levels induced by infusion of exogenous β-hydroxybutyrate has been accompanied by a reduction in urinary nitrogen losses and a fall in circulating alanine levels.[53] Furthermore, a selective effect of ketones of reducing alanine formation and release from muscle and of inhibiting proteolysis and amino acid catabolism has been observed.[53] These observations suggest that ketones act not only as substrate for the brain but as the "signal" to muscle tissue limiting proteolysis and secondarily reducing availability to the liver of precursor (alanine) for gluconeogenesis.[30,53]

The overall metabolic response to prolonged starvation is summarized in Figure 147-7. Ongoing hepatic ketogenesis accompanied by a diminution in extracerebral ketone utilization results in a progressive rise in blood ketones. Increased availability of ketones leads to their uptake by the brain and a concomitant reduction in cerebral glucose utilization. Simultaneously, the hyperketonemia provides a signal to muscle that results in diminished proteolysis, lessened muscle output of alanine, and, consequently, a reduction in hepatic gluconeogenesis. In this manner the twin goals of euglycemia and protein conservation are achieved in prolonged fasting.

OTHER HORMONAL CHANGES

The preceding discussion has emphasized the role of insulin and glucagon in the metabolic response to fasting, particularly in early starvation. A variety of other hormonal changes, however, have also been demonstrated. An increase in circulating growth hormone,[54] a diminished secretion of cortisol,[55] a fall in serum

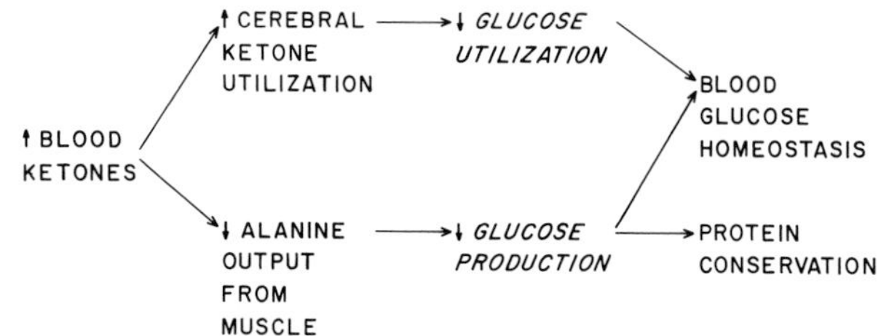

Fig. 147-7. Metabolic adaptation to prolonged starvation. Ketones play a central role, replacing glucose as substrate for the brain and signaling a reduction in protein calabolism and alanine output from muscle. In this manner, protein conservation is achieved and glucose homeostasis is maintained.

triiodothyronine,[56] and increased levels of catecholamines[57] have all been noted in starvation. In contrast to the changes in insulin (and probably glucagon), hormones such as growth hormone and cortisol exert primarily a permissive rather than a regulatory role in starvation (i.e., normal glucose homeostasis requires their presence but is not dependent on changes in secretion).

GROWTH HORMONE

An increase in growth hormone levels has been repeatedly documented in briefly fasted individuals.[54] However, the timing and magnitude of the increase in growth hormone is quite variable. In most instances growth hormone levels have returned to baseline by 5–10 days despite a progressive increase in lipolysis.[31,38] Furthermore, in growth hormone–deficient dwarfs the lipolysis and ketosis are at least as great as in healthy subjects.[58] In addition, administration of exogenous growth hormone to prolonged fasted subjects fails to augment protein conservation. Thus growth hormone does not play an essential role in either the lipolytic effects of early starvation or the protein conservation of late starvation. On the other hand, growth hormone–deficient dwarfs have a greater decline in blood glucose than is observed in healthy subjects.[58] Accompanying this hypoglycemic response is an exaggerated fall in serum insulin.[58] Thus the normal glucose–insulin relationship of starvation is not dependent on growth hormone, but the setting of the blood glucose concentration at which this relationship takes place is reduced in growth hormone–deficient subjects.

GLUCOCORTICOIDS

Fasting hypoglycemia is also observed in patients with Addison's disease or selective deficiency of ACTH. Measurements of urinary free cortisol indicate a progressive decline in secretion during early starvation.[55] This has been attributed to a decline in turnover acting to raise circulating cortisol levels and thereby inhibiting ACTH secretion.[55] An excess of cortisol in spontaneous Cushing's disease or in subjects treated with exogenous cortisone acetate fails to increase protein wasting in starvation.[60] Thus, neither the brisk proteolytic and gluconeogenic response of early starvation nor the protein conservation of late starvation can be attributed to changes in cortisol secretion. As in the case of growth hormone, cortisol acts primarily to influence the "glucostat"—the blood glucose setting at which normal interrelationships with insulin are observed: with cortisol deficiency fasting hypoglycemia and hypoinsulinemia are observed; with cortisol excess a rise in fasting glucose and fasting hyperinsulinemia is noted.[60]

CATECHOLAMINES

Catecholamines can influence glucose homeostasis in a variety of ways: inhibition of insulin secretion (via α-adrenergic receptors); stimulation of glycogenolysis, lipolysis, and glucagon secretion; and antagonism to the action of insulin in promoting glucose uptake by fat and muscle tissue. In starvation an increase in plasma and urinary nonepinephrine and unchanged plasma epinephrine have been observed.[57,61] Although the glycogenolytic effect of norepinephrine is only one-fifth that of epinephrine, in vivo studies suggest that norepinephrine released at sympathetic nerve endings in the liver is the more important mediator of glycogenolysis in glucopenic states.[62,63] On the other hand, neither the lipolytic nor the hyperglucagonemic response to fasting is altered by β-adrenergic blockade.[64,65] Thus, while there is little doubt that sympathoadrenal mechanisms contribute importantly to the acute counterregulatory response engendered by an abrupt fall in blood glucose as manifested by glycogenolysis, this system is less important in the more gradual homeostatic response to fasting.

THYROID

Until recently, starvation was felt to have little effect on thyroid physiology. Serum thyroxin (T_4) was noted to be unchanged or only slightly reduced. A small reduction in the intensity of T_4 binding in serum was also observed, so that the free T_4 concentration remained within normal limits. More recent studies have shown a profound decline (50 percent) in free triiodothyrorine (3,5,3′-triiodothyronine, free T_3) in fasted subjects.[56] This reduction in free T_3 occurs in patients in whom endogenous thyroid hormone secretion has been suppressed by administration of replacement doses of exogenous hormone, suggesting an alteration in peripheral conversion of T_4 to T_3 rather than suppression of endogenous thyroid secretion of T_3.[56] This conclusion is supported by the demonstration of increased levels of reverse T_3 (3,3′,5′-triiodothyronine) in fasted subjects.[66] Thus starvation results in a shift in the peripheral conversion of T_4 from the metabolically active T_3 to the calorigenically inactive form, reverse T_3. This effect of starvation on T_3 levels appears to be related to the carbohydrate content of the diet;[67] it is demonstrable in anorexia nervosa as well.[68] The physiologic significance of the fall in serum free T_3 is that it provides an explanation for the well-recognized reduction in basal metabolic rate (oxygen consumption) that accompanies prolonged fasting (see the section on Weight Loss: Energy Expenditure).

GONADOTROPINS AND SEX STEROIDS

Anovulation and hypomenorrhea or amenorrhea are well-recognized complications of caloric deprivation. Reductions in plasma follicle-stimulating hormone have been observed in starvation along with a loss of the midcycle luteinizing hormone surge. A progressive decline in urinary androgen excretion is also noted in fasted subjects.[55]

EFFECT OF AGE AND SEX

The decline in blood glucose engendered by a 24–72 h fast is more marked in children than in adults,[69] and more severe in women than in men.[70] In a large number of healthy children subjected to a fast, hypoglycemia was frequently noted.[71] These children exhibited an appropriate reduction in serum insulin. Similarly, in healthy premenopausal nonpregnant women, the decline in plasma glucose during a 72-h fast was 15–25 mg/100 ml lower than in healthy men, reaching mean values of 40 mg/100 ml at 75 h.[71] Despite the seemingly hypoglycemic response, no symptoms of hypoglycemia were encountered.

The basis of these effects of age and sex remains to be established. In the child, as in the premature infant, the relatively large size of the brain as compared to the liver may result in an imbalance between cerebral glucose requirements and hepatic glucose production (glycogenolysis and gluconeogenesis). An alternative explanation is decreased availability of gluconeogenic precursors, particularly alanine, in normal children and women.[69] A role for hypoalaninemia in the exaggerated hypoglycemia of starvation observed in normal pregnancy (see below) and in children with the syndrome of ketotic hypoglycemia has been demonstrated.[72,73]

ACCELERATED STARVATION

A number of physiologic and pathologic conditions exist in which the normal response to starvation, particularly with respect to the fall in blood glucose and insulin and the rise in blood ketones, is accelerated and exaggerated. The effect of age and sex in augmenting the hypoglycemia and hypoinsulinemia of starvation has been noted above. More striking changes in blood glucose and ketones are observed in normal pregnancy and in patients with alcoholic ketoacidosis. In addition, the response to prolonged exercise (4 h or more) in many respects resembles accelerated starvation. It should be noted that the various abnormal fasting hypoglycemic states (e.g., islet cell tumor, adrenal insufficiency, acute hepatic necrosis) cannot be construed as an acceleration of normal processes, but rather represent a failure of normal homeostatic mechanisms, (e.g., failure of insulin to decline, failure of glycogenolytic and/or gluconeogenic processes, etc.).

PREGNANCY

In pregnancy, the fuel requirements of the developing fetus are met primarily by the consumption of glucose, inasmuch as little if any transfer of FFA occurs across the placenta. The rate of glucose utilization by the fetus at term is estimated at 6 mg/kg/min, well in excess of adult utilization rates of 2 mg/kg/min.[74] In addition to glucose transfer taking place, amino acids are actively transported across the placenta for fetal protein synthesis and possibly for oxidative processes as well. The ongoing siphoning of glucose and amino acids persists during periods of maternal fasting as well as feeding. As a consequence, the maternal response to starvation is characterized by an accelerated and exaggerated fall in blood glucose. Maternal hypoglycemia results in hypoinsulinemia and a concomitant exaggeration of starvation ketosis.[75] In addition, the fall in plasma alanine is also accentuated in pregnancy as a result of ongoing transfer of alanine to the fetus.[72] That maternal gluconeogenic mechanisms remain intact is indicated by the prompt rise in blood glucose after exogenous alanine is administered.[72] Thus the maternal hypoglycemia of pregnancy is initiated by fetal siphoning of glucose and perpetuated by the transfer to the fetus of gluconeogenic precursors.[72]

The starvation ketosis of pregnancy is of particular interest in view of the possible adverse consequences of hyperketonemia to the fetus. On the basis of indirect data in humans,[76] it is likely that maternal ketones are transferred to the fetus, and the enzymes necessary for ketone oxidation have been identified in fetal brain tissue.[46] In contrast to the seemingly inoccuous effects of ketone uptake by the brain of the fasting adult (see above), maternal ketonemia in pregnancy has been associated with a significant reduction in the I.Q. of offspring tested at age 4.[77] Thus the psychoneurologic development of the fetal brain may be impaired by the transfer of ketones from the maternal to the fetal circulation. These observations underscore the importance of avoiding periods of fasting or fad diets involving severe carbohydrate restriction during pregnancy.[78]

ALCOHOLIC KETOACIDOSIS

In normal subjects, peak rates of ketone production and utilization observed in prolonged fasting are associated with blood ketone levels that remain below 8mM, while serum bicarbonate generally remains above 14 meq/liter.[38] Briefer periods of fasting (1–3 days) are accompanied by ketone levels of less than 3–4 mM. In contrast, in alcoholics a period of binge drinking accompanied by protracted vomiting and poor food intake may result in an exaggerated starvation ketosis in which ketone acids accumulate to levels of 8–12 mM and a metabolic acidosis is observed.[79] The clinical picture in such patients varies from deep coma to an alert state in which deep, rapid respiration (Kussmaul breathing) is noted. Arterial pH is often reduced to less than 7.2 and the anion gap is increased from normal levels of 15 meq/liter to greater than 25 meq/liter. In about 25 percent of cases the blood glucose level is less than 50 mg/100 ml. The nature of the metabolic acidosis is often not recognized or is mistakenly attributed to lactate, since the semiquantitative nitroprusside reaction for ketones (Acetest, Ketostix, Ames Co.) is often only faintly positive. This is due to the high ratio of β-hydroxybutyrate (which is not detected in the nitroprusside test) to acetoacetate.

A variety of mechanisms may be responsible for the accelerated ketosis observed in alcoholics. Alcohol may exaggerate ketogenesis via (1) a direct lipolytic effect, (2) altered intramitochondrial redox potential resulting in conversion of oxaloacetate to malate and consequently decreased Krebs cycle activity, and (3) stimulation of intramitochondrial mechanisms involved in the transfer and oxidation of fatty acids. In most instances a prompt clinical response follows the administration of glucose-containing fluids. Treatment with insulin is generally not required; in patients with accompanying hypoglycemia insulin treatment is contraindicated.

EXERCISE

The metabolic and hormonal effects of exercise are described in detail in Chapter 146. In a variety of respects the response to prolonged (4 h or more) submaximal exercise is quite comparable to a 3-day fast. Blood glucose levels decline by 20–25 mg/100 ml, serum insulin falls, and glucagon rises.[80] Concomitantly, there is an increase in the splanchnic fractional extraction of alanine and an elevation in the plasma levels of the branched-chain amino acids. The similarity between metabolic changes in prolonged exercise and at 3 days of starvation may reflect a common homeostatic mechanism directed at minimizing the fall in blood glucose associated with depletion of liver glycogen stores in the face of normal to increased rates of glucose utilization.[80]

WEIGHT LOSS

The rate of weight loss observed during fasting varies with the duration of starvation. During the initial 3–5 days of fasting, weight loss occurs at a rate of 1–2 kg/day. Thereafter, the rate of weight loss declines, reaching rates of 0.3 kg/day after 3 weeks or more. The variable rates of weight loss in starvation can be attributed to a transient, early diuretic effect, changes in energy expenditure, and alterations in the composition of the tissues catabolized.

DIURESIS

The early studies of Benedict,[37] conducted over 50 years ago, and the subsequent work of Gamble[81] demonstrated that weight loss early in starvation was well in excess of that attributable to the tissue metabolism necessary to meet caloric requirements. The accelerated rate of weight loss is a consequence of a diuretic effect of fasting due to increased losses of urinary sodium. The natriuresis is not dependent on sodium deprivation per se, inasmuch as it persists in fasting subjects given sodium supplements.[82] On the other hand, the key role of caloric deprivation in the development of the diuresis is reflected by the prompt reduction in sodium excretion observed in normal subjects given a sodium-restricted but calorically adequate diet.

Urinary sodium losses in starvation reach a peak of 100–150 meq/day at 3–4 days and return to baseline by 7–8 days (Fig. 147-8). The cumulative loss of sodium amounts to 250–350 meq and is accompanied by much smaller losses of chloride (40–100 meq).[82,83] Although a transient increase in glomerular filtration rate may occur in starvation, the peak losses of sodium cannot be explained

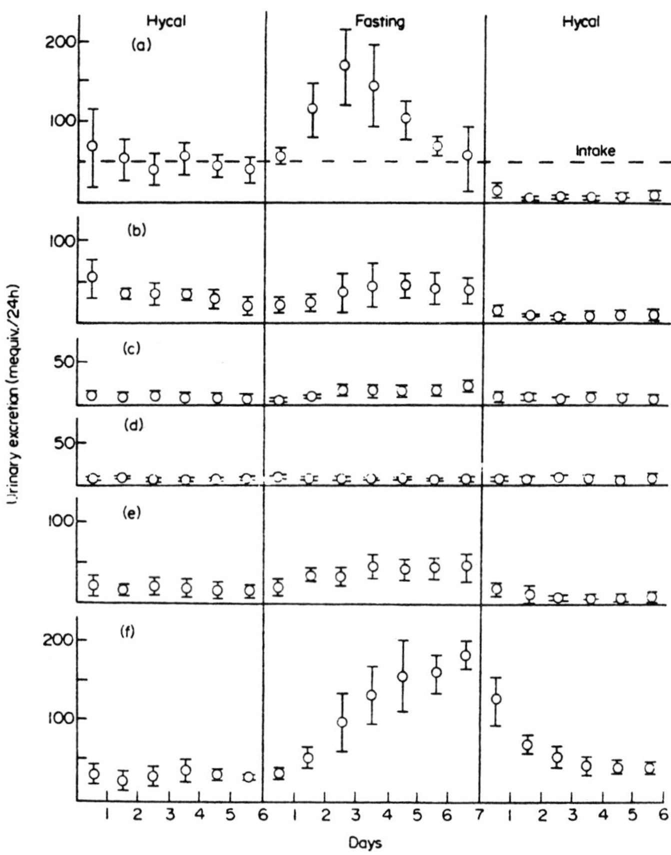

Fig. 147-8. Daily urinary excretion of (a) sodium, (b) potassium, (c) calcium, (d) magnesium, (e) titratable acid, and (f) ammonium in subjects ingesting a constant amount of sodium chloride (50 mEq/day) in the fed state ("Hycal") and during fasting. (From North et al.[82])

on this basis. Neither can altered mineralocorticoid excretion be invoked as an explanation of the natriuresis. Urinary aldosterone excretion increases during the first week of starvation, the exact opposite of the changes expected if this hormone were responsible for the loss of sodium.[84] Furthermore, the diuresis of starvation cannot be blunted by exogenous mineralocorticoid administration.[84] Recent studies suggest that the natriuresis of starvation is largely a consequence of obligatory cation loss to cover the excretion of metabolically generated anions, particularly the ketone acids β-hydroxybutyrate and acetoacetate.[82,83] During the first week of fasting urinary ammonia excretion lags behind the increase in ketone acid excretion and is insufficient to cover the organic acid anions. It is during this period of imbalance between ammonia excretion and ketonuria that maximum rates of sodium excretion are observed.[82,83] Furthermore, in fasting a direct linear correlation is observed between the changes in urinary cations and in organic acid anion excretion. The failure to observe an ongoing sodium diuresis as starvation continues beyond 7 days is explained by the increase in urinary ammonia excretion that ultimately reaches levels sufficient to cover anion losses.

The fact that some obligatory coverage of metabolically generated anions is not the sole explanation of the natriuresis of starvation is suggested by the increase in urinary chloride that is also observed during fasting.[82,83] Since the filtered load of ketone acids reaches levels of 500 mmol/min, the nonreabsorbable portion of ketone acids may act as an osmotic diuretic, thereby increasing the excretion of sodium and chloride.[52,83] In addition physiologic increments in glucagon induced by infusion of exogenous hormone have been observed to induce a natriuresis that is not reversed by mineralocorticoids.[85,86] Inasmuch as the changes in plasma glucagon (Fig. 147-3) correspond to the changes in sodium loss (peak levels at 3–4 days with a subsequent return to baseline; Fig 147-8), the transient hyperglucagonemia of starvation may be a contributory factor in the natriuresis.[84,86]

ENERGY EXPENDITURE

The decline in the rate of weight loss as fasting continues reflects not only changes in fluid balance but changes in energy expenditure as well. The basal metabolic rate is observed to decline by 20 percent over a 3-week period of starvation.[87] In addition, the caloric expenditure accompanying activities such as walking may decrease by as much as 30 percent.[88] In obese subjects, in whom total caloric expenditure in the fed state even in a hospital setting may amount to 3500 Cal/day (because of their large surface area and the work required to move their large mass), the reduction in energy expenditure observed after 3 weeks of fasting may amount to 1000 Cal/day. Such a decline in energy expenditure would be expected to result in a saving of at least 150 g of body weight per day (100 g fat, 10 g protein, and 40 g water that would accompany the protein losses). As to the mechanism of this decline in metabolic rate, the recent demonstration that plasma free T_3 falls by 50 percent in starvation may be of particular interest.[56] The accompanying increase in plasma levels of reverse T_3 (see above) would not be expected to counteract the reduction in T_3 inasmuch as reverse T_3 is metabolically inactive.[56] Thus the changes in peripheral de-iodination of T_4 to T_3 observed in starvation may reflect a mechanism designed to conserve endogenous fuel stores by limiting caloric expenditure.

BODY COMPOSITION

The effects of starvation or hypocaloric diets on body composition have been the subject of intensive inquiry in recent years. Unfortunately, the techniques available (densitometry, potassium balances) are not sufficiently sensitive or accurate to provide conclusive data regarding the extent of losses of lean body mass as compared to fat tissue.[89] Conclusions based on measurements of body composition have frequently been marred by marked discrepancies between the caloric equivalent of the estimated losses of fat and lean tissue and the actual energy expenditure of the fasted subjects.[89] A more accurate assessment can be achieved by examining losses of urinary nitrogen and measurements of respiratory quotient. In the subject fasted for 3 weeks, approximately 180 g of adipose tissue are dissipated per day.[38] An additional 150 g of lean tissue is lost, representing 30 g of protein and 120 g of water. Total weight loss amounts to about 300 g/day. Earlier in starvation, when the mechanisms involved in protein conservation have not as yet come into play, lean tissue is dissipated at the rate of approximately 400 g (75–80 g protein) per day and fat dissipation is less marked. The greater reliance on calorically dense fat tissue (9 Cal/g) as compared to lean body mass (1 Cal/g including tissue water) as starvation progresses provides an additional explanation for the decline in the rate of weight loss.

REFEEDING

The hormonal and metabolic changes that characterize the fasting state are rapidly reversed by refeeding. Of particular interest has been the effect of specific and limited quantities of nutrients in altering the response to starvation. The classic studies of Gamble demonstrated that provision of as little as 100 g carbohydrate/day reduced nitrogen losses during the first week of starvation from 12 g/day to 5–6 g/day.[81] More recent studies have shown that this protein-sparing effect is related to decreased urea production, suggesting an accompanying inhibition in hepatic gluconeogenesis.[90] An even greater reduction in body protein breakdown is observed when the carbohydrate intake is increased to 700 g/day.[90] In more prolonged fasting (3–6 weeks), at which time nitrogen losses are already reduced to 5–6 g/day, the protein-sparing effect of carbohydrate is equally effective.[90,91] In prolonged starvation, glucose feeding causes a rise in insulin, a fall in blood and urinary ketones, and a reduction in nitrogen losses involving primarily ammonia. Urinary urea losses are only minimally reduced, suggesting unchanged rates of hepatic gluconeogenesis. The prompt reduction in ammonia is probably a consequence of an inhibition of ketogenesis. Interestingly, blood ketones fall despite unchanged FFA levels, suggesting that in starvation intrahepatic processes involved in ketogenesis are more sensitive to small increases in insulin than is peripheral lipolysis.[90]

Nitrogen losses in starvation may also be reduced by providing nutrients other than carbohydrate. Administration of exogenous ketones causes a significant reduction in nitrogen losses as well as a further fall in plasma alanine.[53] It has been suggested that this effect of ketones is mediated by inhibition of branched-chain amino acid catabolism in muscle.[53,12] Infusion of an amino acid mixture (100 g) may also result in a reduction of net nitrogen losses to zero.[92] In contrast, the combined infusion of carbohydrate and amino acids is less effective in restoring nitrogen balance.[92] The greater effectiveness of the pure amino acid mixture remains unexplained, although the accompanying ketosis has been suggested as the factor that may limit protein breakdown.[92]

Evidence that refeeding may permit the reutilization of urea formed in starvation has recently been presented. Administration of the α-keto analogues of the branched-chain amino acids to prolonged fasted subjects results in decreased losses of urea.[93] This effect occurs in the absence of changes in insulin or glucagon. It has been postulated that the urea that would otherwise have been irreversibly lost in the urine is utilized for the synthesis of branched-chain amino acids from their α-keto analogues.[93] Since the branched-chain amino acids have been shown to have a unique effect in stimulating protein synthesis and inhibiting protein catabolism in muscle,[11] the overall effect is a net reduction in protein catabolism.

In addition to influencing nitrogen losses and ketogenesis, refeeding has a profound effect on sodium and water balance. When fasting subjects are refed a pure carbohydrate diet, there is a marked retention of sodium and often the development of "refeeding edema." Refeeding with protein causes less sodium retention, whereas pure fat administration results in an ongoing natriuresis.[94] As in the case of the natriuresis of starvation, changes in mineralocorticoid secretion cannot account for the sodium retention of the refed state.[84] A lag in the decline of urinary ammonia excretion as compared to ketone excretion may account for the positive sodium balance that develops during the initial period of carbohydrate refeeding.[82,83] Since the administration of a pure fat diet is accompanied by ongoing ketosis, a dissociation between ketonuria and ammonia excretion is not observed and sodium retention would not be expected.

STARVATION AS THERAPY OF OBESITY

The increasing incidence of obesity, the growing awareness of its adverse effects on metabolism and overall morbidity, and the high failure rate of most diet programs have led to the search for more effective means of achieving weight loss. Interest in starvation as a therapeutic modality for the extremely obese patient was stimulated by the report by Bloom that nine obese subjects lost 9–22 lb during a 4–9 day fast.[95] Particularly encouraging was the lack of undesirable symptoms and the continuing weight loss in five of the subjects who successfully followed a hypocaloric diet after completion of the fast. Subsequent studies have confirmed the general lack of symptoms and the fact that all patients lose weight during the fast, although at varying rates. In obese patients, weight loss during the first week may be as rapid as 3–4 lb/day. Subsequently the rate of weight loss slows to ½–1 lb/day (see above, the section on Weight Loss). Severely obese patients have been treated in this manner for periods of 3 months to over 1 year, in some instances losing 100–150 lb.[96] Despite the reports of success in achieving weight reduction during fasting, the safety as well as effectiveness of starvation in achieving long-term weight reduction must be examined before considering its use as a therapeutic measure. On both accounts, (safety as well as efficacy), it is clear that fasting has only limited usefulness in the management of obesity.

COMPLICATIONS

Most disturbing have been the isolated reports of sudden death in patients on a starvation regimen.[97–99] In some of the cases, the patients had severe heart failure, cardiac arrhythimias, and evidence of digitalis toxicity,[97] circumstances in which starvation with its attendant electrolyte losses (particularly potassium) should be considered contraindicated. Death was also reported during refeeding of a young girl who had been reduced to less than ideal weight.[100] Although fragmentation of myocardial fibrils was the suggested cause of death,[100] the validity of those findings has been questioned.[101,102]

Perhaps the most disabling symptom observed during very prolonged fasts is orthostatic hypotension. In subjects fasted more than 3 weeks, the incidence of symptomatic orthostatic hypotension is more than 50 percent.[103] In hypertensive patients, blood pressure may fall to normal levels. As to the mechanism of the hypotension, the early natriuretic response may be an important factor. However, the hypotension is most marked late in fasting, while urinary sodium and fluid loss occurs primarily early in starvation. In fact, unless forced to drink water, prolonged fasted patients may become oliguric with urine volumes less than 300 ml/day. Other factors that may be contributory are decreased activity of the sympathetic nervous system or altered responsiveness to catecholamines. Of interest with respect to the latter possibility is the reduction in circulating free T_3 in starvation (see above); it is well recognized that thyroid hormones may alter the responsiveness to catecholamines.

While the sodium loss occurring in early fasting gradually falls to less than 10 meq/day, ongoing losses of potassium in the order of 15 meq/day are usually observed throughout starvation. Although the serum potassium may remain in the low-normal range, the deficit in total body potassium may amount to 10–25 percent (300–800 meq). Symptomatically, the potassium losses are manifest as generalized muscle weakness. Metabolic alkalosis and tetany are not observed because of the accompanying hyperketonemia.

Hyperuricemia develops during starvation in virtually all patients.[103] Serum uric acid levels may reach 17–20 mg/100 ml in female as well as male patients. However, acute gouty arthritis is only occasionally observed, generally in patients with a prior history of acute gout.[104,105] The mechanism of the hyperuricemia probably involves diminished urinary excretion secondary to a competitive action of ketones on the tubular secretion of uric acid.[106] Treatment with allopurinol effectively prevents the hyperuricemia of starvation. In patients with a history of gout or prior elevations in uric acid, treatment with allopurinol should be instituted at the time fasting is initiated.

Other untoward side effects observed in fasting include a mild, normochromic and normocytic anemia and evidence of vitamin deficiencies in the form of glossitis, gingival bleeding, and dry skin. These can readily be prevented by administering a multivitamin supplement during the fast.

Despite the above complications, most noteworthy has been the general lack of complaints in fasting patients. Frequently the hunger observed in the first 2 days is replaced by a feeling of anorexia. The latter has been attributed to the progressive rise in ketones. Headaches are commonly observed but are not persistent or severe.

LONG-TERM RESULTS

The success in achieving weight loss during the fast has been followed by a disappointingly high failure rate in maintaining the weight loss on a long-term basis. Follow-up of patients fasted for prolonged periods reveals that only 15–30 percent continue to follow a diet and lose additional weight or even maintain the weight loss achieved during the fast.[105,107,108] The magnitude of weight loss achieved during the fast and the attainment of ideal weight are of no prognostic significance with regard to long-term success. A positive correlation has been observed between follow-up attendance as an outpatient and on-going weight loss. This relationship, however, may reflect the greater motivation of the patient rather than the efficacy of the outpatient regimen.

ADVANTAGES AND INDICATIONS

The advantages of starvation remain those emphasized initially by Bloom:[95] the patient is impressed that he *can* lose weight and that he has the will power to forget food. The fast may give added motivation for subsequent dieting since considerable progress in weight reduction has already been made. In addition, a hypocaloric diet may be more tolerable after prolonged fasting. Finally, the fast provides an opportunity for patient education: the patient should receive intensive dietary instruction so that the effects of the fast can be sustained by subsequent dieting.

Despite these advantages, the side effects and infrequency of long-term success severely limit the usefulness of prolonged starvation as therapy for obesity. Treatment should consequently be restricted to patients with marked or severe obesity (60 percent or more above ideal weight) in whom dietary regimens have repeatedly failed. Starvation is contraindicated in patients with evidence of severe congestive heart failure, cardiac arrhythmias, electrolyte imbalance, or cerebral ischemia. In all instances, prolonged fasting requires inpatient hospitalization. Vitamin and potassium supplements and allopurinol (where indicated) should be administered, as noted above. Throughout the fast patients should be encouraged to drink water so as to prevent oliguria. Recently a high success rate was reported in patients treated with relatively brief fasting (5–7 days) as outpatients followed by an intensive educational and dietary program.[109]

COMPARATIVE PHYSIOLOGY OF STARVATION

In man, the adaptation to fasting, as described in detail above, consists of an initial gluconeogenic phase followed by selective utilization of fat and ketones that allows for protein sparing. In various animal species, depending in part on the availability of fat stores, a wide spectrum of responses is observed. In the mouse and rat, in whom fat stores are quite limited, starvation results in death in 3–8 days.[110] At the time of death, there is no visible adipose tissue. Although the hormonal changes (hypoinsulinemia and hyperglucagonemia) are similar to those observed in man, the fuel response is quite different. The findings in the mouse and rat suggest the rapid exhaustion of very limited fuel reserves stored as triglyceride followed by protein depletion and death. In mutant strains of mice with large fat stores (the *obob* mouse), lipolysis, ketogenesis, and protein conservation, mimicking the response in man, are observed.[110]

At the opposite end of the spectrum from the mouse in its response to starvation is the black bear. During winter sleep (a period of reduced physical activity but near normal body temperature), the bear is able to go without food for periods of 3 months.[111] During this time, there is no net loss of urea nor any decrease in lean body mass.[111] In these animals caloric requirements are entirely met by the mobilization and oxidation of body fat. This ability to inhibit net production of urea while metabolizing only fat as the source of energy is unique to the winter sleep period as it cannot be duplicated when such animals are starved in the summer.[112] With regard to the mechanism by which lean body mass is conserved, it does not involve an inhibition of protein catabolism. Protein breakdown and urea formation continue during winter sleep. However, urea is absorbed across the urinary bladder and its nitrogen is reutilized for amino acid synthesis and incorporation into protein.[112]

REFERENCES

1. Cahill, G. F., Jr. Starvation in man. *N. Engl. J. Med. 282:* 668, 1970.
2. Felig, P. Nutritional maintenance and diet therapy in acute and chronic disease. In Beeson, P., and McDermott, W. (eds.): Cecil-Loeb Textbook of Medicine, ed. 14. Philadelphia, Saunders, 1975, p. 1389.
3. Felig, P., and Wahren, J. Fuel homeostasis in exercise. *N. Engl. J. Med. 293:* 1078, 1975.
4. Hultman, E., and Nilsson, L. H. Liver glycogen in man. Effect of different diets and muscular exercise. *Adv. Exp. Med. Biol. 11:* 143, 1971.
5. Garrow, J. S., Fletcher, K., and Halliday, D. Body composition in severe infantile malnutrition. *J. Clin. Invest. 44:* 417, 1965.
6. Andres, R., Cader, G., and Zierler, K. L. The quantitatively minor role of carbohydrate in oxidative metabolism by skeletal muscle in intact man in the basal state. *J. Clin. Invest. 35:* 671, 1956.
7. Felig, P. The glucose–alanine cycle. *Metabolism 22:* 179, 1973.
8. Felig, P. Amino acid metabolism in man. *Ann. Rev. Biochem. 44:* 933, 1975.
9. Felig, P., and Wahren, J. Amino acid metabolism in exercising man. *J. Clin. Invest. 50:* 2703, 1971.
10. Buse, M. G., Biggers, J. F., Frederici, K. H., and Buse, J. F. Oxidation of branched chain amino acids by isolated hearts and diaphragms of the rat. *J. Biol. Chem. 247:* 8085, 1972.
11. Odessey, R., Khairallah, A., and Goldberg, A. L. Origin and possible significance of alanine production by skeletal muscle. *J. Biol. Chem. 249:* 7623, 1974.
12. Palaiologos, G., and Felig, P. Effects of ketone bodies on amino acid metabolism in isolated rat diaphragms. *Biochem. J. 154:* 709, 1976.
13. Exton, J. H. Progress in endocrinology and metabolism, gluconeogenesis. *Metabolism 21:* 945, 1972.
14. Felig, P., and Wahren, J. Influence of endogenous insulin secretion on splanchnic glucose and amino acid metabolism. *J. Clin. Invest. 50:* 1702, 1971.
15. Felig, P., Wahren, J., and Hendler, R. Influence of oral glucose ingestion on splanchnic glucose and gluconeogenic substrate metabolism. *Diabetes 24:* 468, 1975.
16. Dole, V. P. A relation between nonesterified fatty acids in plasma and the metabolism of glucose. *J. Clin. Invest. 35:* 150, 1956.

17. Grey, N. J., Karl, I., and Kipnis, D. M. Physiologic mechanisms in the development of starvation ketosis in man. *Diabetes 24:* 10, 1975.
18. McGarry, J. D., Meier, J. M., and D. W. Foster. The effects of starvation and refeeding on carbohydrate and lipid metabolism in vivo in the perfused rat liver. *J. Biol. Chem. 248:* 270, 1973.
19. Schade, D. S., and Eaton, R. P. Glucagon regulation of plasma ketone body concentration in human diabetes. *J. Clin. Invest. 56:* 1340, 1975.
20. McGarry, S. J., and Foster, D. W. Acute reversal of experimental diabetic ketoacidosis in the rat with (+)-decanoylcarnitine. *J. Clin. Invest. 52:* 877, 1973.
21. Havel, R. J. Caloric homeostasis and disorders of fuel transport. *N. Engl. J. Med. 287:* 1186, 1972.
22. Turner, R. C., Grayburn, J. A., Newman, G. B., et al. Measurement of the insulin delivery rate in man. *J. Clin. Endocrinol. Metab. 33:* 279, 1971.
23. Liljenquist, J. E., Chiasson, J. L., Finger, F. E., et al. Differential effect of insulin on glycogenolysis and gluconeogenesis. *Diabetes 23* [*Suppl. 1*]: 349, 1974.
24. Felig, P., Marliss, E., Ohman, J., et al. Plasma amino acid levels in diabetic ketoacidosis. *Diabetes 19:* 727, 1970.
25. Unger, R. H. Apha- and beta-cell interrelationships in health and disease. *Metabolism 23:* 581, 1974.
26. Gerich, J. F., Lorenzi, M., Schneider, V., et al. Effects of somatostatin on plasma glucose and glucagon levels in human diabetes. *N. Engl. J. Med. 291:* 544, 1974.
27. Alford, F. G., Bloom, S. R., Nabarro, J. D. N. et al. Glucagon control of fasting glucose in man. *Lancet 2:* 974, 1974.
28. Felig. P., Wahren, J., Sherwin, R., et al. Insulin and glucagon in normal physiology and diabetes. *Diabetes 25:* 1091, 1976.
29. Wahren, J., Felig, P., and Hagenfeldt, L. Effect of protein ingestion on splanchnic and leg metabolism in normal man and patients with diabetes mellitus. *J. Clin. Invest. 57:* 987, 1976.
30. Felig, P. The metabolic events of starvation. *Am. J. Med. 60:* 119, 1976.
31. Cahill, G. F., Herrera, M. G., Morgan, A. P., et al. Hormone–fuel interrelationships during fasting. *J. Clin. Invest. 45:* 1751, 1966.
32. Marliss, E. B., Aoki, T. T., Unger, R. H., Soeldner, J. S., and Cahill, G. F., Jr. Glucagon levels and metabolic effects in fasting. *J. Clin. Invest. 49:* 2256, 1970.
33. Fisher, M., Sherwin, R., Hendler, R., et al. The kinetics of glucagon in man: effects of starvation. *Proc. Natl. Acad. Sci. U.S.A.*, 1976 (in press).
34. Felig, P., Owen, O. E., Wahren, J., and Cahill, G. F., Jr. Amino acid metabolism in prolonged starvation. *J. Clin. Invest. 48:* 584, 1969.
34a. Felig, P., Pozefsky, T., Marliss, E., and Cahill, G. F., Jr. Alanine: key role in gluconeogenesis. *Science 167:* 1003, 1970.
35. Wahren, J., Felig, P., Cerasi, E., et al. Splanchnic and peripheral glucose and amino acid metabolism in diabetes mellitus. *J. Clin. Invest. 51:* 1870, 1972.
36. Pozefsky, T., Tancredi, R. G., Moxley, R. T., et al. Effects of brief starvation on muscle amino acid metabolism in nonobese man. *J. Clin. Invest. 57:* 444, 1976.
37. Benedict, F. G. A study of prolonged fasting. Washington, D.C., Carnegie Institute Publ. No. 203, 1915.
38. Owen, O. E., Felig, P., Morgan, A. P., Wahren, J., and Cahill, G. F., Jr. Liver and kidney metabolism during prolonged starvation. *J. Clin. Invest. 48:* 574, 1969.
39. Felig, P., Marliss, E., Owen, O. E., and Cahill, G. F., Jr. Role of substrate in the regulation of hepatic gluconeogenesis in man. *Adv. Enzyme Regul. 7:* 41, 1969.
40. Felig, P. Interaction of insulin and amino acids in the regulation of gluconeogenesis. *Isr. J. Med. Sci. 8:* 262, 1972.
41. Wahren, J., and Felig, P. Renal substate exchange in human diabetes mellitus. *Diabetes 24:* 730, 1975.
42. Goodman, A. D., Fuisz, R. E., and Cahill, G. F., Jr. Renal gluconeogenesis in acidosis, alkalosis and potassium deficiency: its possible role in the regulation of renal ammonia production. *J. Clin. Invest. 45:* 612, 1966.
43. Owen, O. E., Morgan, A. P., Kemp, H. G., et al. Brain metabolism during fasting. *J. Clin. Invest. 46:* 1589, 1967.
44. Drenick, E. J., Alvarez, L. C., Tamasi, G. C., et al. Resistance to symptomatic insulin reactions after fasting. *J. Clin. Invest. 51:* 2757, 1972.
45. Tamasi, G. C., and Drenick, E. J. Resistance to insulin convulsions in fasted mice. *Endocrinology 92:* 1277, 1973.
46. Page, M. A., and Williamson, D. H. Enzymes of ketone body utilization in human brain. *Lancet 2:* 66, 1971.
47. Hawkins, R. A., Williamson, D. H., and Krebs, H. A. Ketone body utilization by adult and suckling rat brain in vivo. *Biochem. J. 122:* 13, 1971.
48. Garber, A. J., Menzel, P. H., Boden, G., and Owen, O. E. Hepatic ketogenesis and gluconeogenesis in humans. *J. Clin. Invest. 54:* 981, 1974.
49. Owen, O. E., Reichard, G. A., Jr., Markus, H., et al. Rapid intravenous sodium acetoacetate infusion in man. *J. Clin. Invest. 52:* 2606, 1973.
50. Owen, O. E., and Reichard, G.: Human forearm metabolism during progressive starvation. *J. Clin. Invest. 50:* 1536, 1971.
51. Reichard, G. A., Jr., Owen, O. E., Haff, A. C., et al. Ketone body production and oxidation in fasting humans. *J. Clin. Invest. 53:* 508, 1974.
52. Sapir, D. G., and Owen, O. E. Renal conservation of ketone bodies during starvation. *Metabolism 24:* 23, 1975.
53. Sherwin, R. S., Hendler, R. G., and Felig, P. Effect of ketone infusion on amino acid and nitrogen metabolism in man. *J. Clin. Invest. 55:* 1382, 1975.
54. Merimee, T., and Fineberg, S. E. Growth hormone secretion in starvation: a reassessment. *J. Clin. Endocrinol. Metab. 39:* 385, 1974.
55. Hendrikx, A. Aspects of Steroid Metabolism in Obese Subjects under Various Nutritional Conditions. Brussels, Arscia Vitgaven, 1968.
56. Portnay, G. I., O'Brian, J. T., Bush, J., et al. The effect of starvation on the concentration and binding of thyroxine and triiodothyronine in serum and on the response to TRH. *J. Clin. Endocrinol. Metab. 39:* 199, 1974.
57. Januszewicz, W., Sznajderman-Ciswicka, M., and Wocial, B. Urinary excretion of catecholamines in fasting obese subjects. *J. Clin. Endocrinol. Metab. 271:* 130, 1967.
58. Merimee, T., Felig, P., Marliss, E., et al. Glucose and lipid homeostasis in the absence of human growth hormone. *J. Clin. Invest. 50:* 574, 1971.
59. Felig, P., Marliss, E. B., and Cahill, G. F., Jr. Metabolic response to human growth hormone during prolonged starvation. *J. Clin. Invest. 50:* 411, 1971.
60. Owen, O. E., and Cahill, G. F., Jr. Metabolic effects of exogenous glucocorticoids in fasted man. *J. Clin. Invest. 52:* 2596, 1973.
61. Christensen, N. J. Plasma norepinephrine and epinephrine in untreated diabetics during fasting and after insulin administration. *Diabetes 32:* 1, 1974.
62. Brodows, R. G., Pi-Sunyer, F. X., and Campbell, R. G. Neural control of counterregulatory events during glucopenia in man. *J. Clin. Invest. 52:* 1841, 1973.
63. Brodows, R. G., Pi-Sunyer, F. X., and Campbell, R. G. Sympathetic control of hepatic glycogenolysis during glucopenia in man. *Metabolism 24:* 617, 1975.
64. Pinter, E. J., and Pattee, C. J. Some data on the metabolic function of the adrenergic nervous system in the obese during starvation. *J. Clin. Endocrinol. Metab. 28:* 106, 1968.
65. Walter, R. M., Dudl, R. J., Palmer, J. P., et al. The effect of adrenergic blockade on the glucagon responses to starvation and hypoglycemia in man. *J. Clin. Invest. 54:* 1214, 1974.
66. Vegenakis, A. G., Burger, A. Portnay, G. I., et al. Diversion of peripheral thyroxine metabolism from activating to inactivating pathways during complete fasting. *J. Clin. Endocrinol. Metab. 41:* 191, 1975.
67. Spaulding, S. W., Chopra, I. J., Sherwin, R. S., et al. Effect of caloric restriction and dietary composition on serum T_3 and reverse T_3 in man. *J. Clin. Endocrinol. 42:* 197, 1976.
68. Moshang, T., Jr., Parks, J. S., Baker, L., et al. Low serum triiodothyronine in patients with anorexia nervosa. *J. Clin. Endocrinol. Metab. 40:* 470, 1975.
69. Santiago, J., Haymond, M., Karl, I., et al. Comparative substrate and hormone responses to fasting in normal adults and children. Program, 56th Annual Meeting, Endocrine Society, Atlanta, June 1974.
70. Merimee, T. J., and Tyson, J. E. Stabilization of plasma glucose during fasting. Normal variations in two separate studies. *N. Engl. J. Med. 291:* 1275, 1974.
71. Chaussain, J. L. Glycemic response to 24 hour fast in normal

children and children with ketotic hypoglycemia. *J. Pediatr. 82:* 438, 1973.
72. Felig, P., Kini, Y. J., Lynch, V., et al. Amino acid metabolism during starvation in human pregnancy. *J. Clin. Invest. 51:* 1195, 1972.
73. Pagliara, A. S., Karl, I. E., DeVivo, D. C., et al. Hypoalaninemia: a concomitant of ketotic hypoglycemia. *J. Clin. Invest. 51:* 1440, 1972.
74. Page, E. W. Human fetal nutrition and growth. *Am. J. Obstet. Gynecol. 104:* 378, 1969.
75. Felig, P., and Lynch, V. Starvation in human pregnancy: hypoglycemia, hypoinsulinemia, and hyperketonemia. *Science 170:* 990, 1970.
76. Kim, Y. J., and Felig, P. Maternal and amniotic fluid substrate levels during caloric deprivation in human pregnancy. *Metabolism 21:* 507, 1972.
77. Churchill, J. A., and Berendes, H. W. Intelligence of children whose mothers had acetonuria during pregnancy. In: Perinatal Factors Affecting Human Development. Washington, D.C., Pan American Health Organization, Scientific Publ. No. 185, 1969.
78. Felig, P. Maternal and fetal fuel homeostasis in human pregnancy. *Am. J. Clin. Nutr. 26:* 988, 1973.
79. Levy, L. J., Duga, J., Girgis, M., et al. Ketoacidosis associated with alcoholism in nondiabetic subjects. *Ann. Intern. Med. 78:* 213, 1973.
80. Alborg, G., Felig, P., Hagenfeldt, L., et al. Substrate turnover during prolonged exercise in man: splanchnic and leg metabolism of glucose, free fatty acids, and amino acids. *J. Clin. Invest. 53:* 108, 1974.
81. Gamble, J. L. Physiological information from studies on the life raft ration. *Harvey Lect. 42:* 247, 1946–1947.
82. North, K. A. K., Lascelles, D., and Coates, P. The mechanisms by which sodium excretion is increased during a fast but reduced on subsequent carbohydrate refeeding. *Clin. Sci. Mol. Med. 46:* 423, 1974.
83. Sigler, M. H. The mechanism of the natriuresis of fasting. *J. Clin. Invest. 55:* 377, 1975.
84. Spark, R. F., Arky, R. A., Boulter, P. R., et al. Renin, aldosterone and glucagon in the natriuresis of fasting. *N. Engl. J. Med. 292:* 1335, 1975.
85. Boulter, P. R., Spark, R. F., and Arky, R. A. Dissociation of the renin–aldosterone system and refractoriness to the sodium-retaining action of mineralocorticoid during starvation in man. *J. Clin. Endocrinol. Metab. 38:* 248, 1974.
86. Saudek, C. D., Boulter, P. R., and Arky, R. A. The natriuretic effect of glucagon and its role in starvation. *J. Clin. Endocrinol. Metab. 36:* 761, 1973.
87. Bray, G. A. Effect of diet and triiodothyronine on the activity of glycerol phosphate dehydrogenase and on the metabolism of glucose and pyruvate by adipose tissue of obese patients. *J. Clin. Invest. 48:* 1413, 1969.
88. Drenick, E. J., and Dennin, H. F. Energy expenditure in fasting obese men. *J. Lab. Clin. Med. 81:* 421, 1973.
89. Grande, F. Energy balance and body composition changes: a critical study of three recent publications *Ann. Intern. Med. 68:* 467, 1968.
90. Aoki, T. T., Muller, W. A., Brennan, M. F., et al. Metabolic effects of glucose in brief and prolonged fasted man. *Am. J. Clin. Nutr. 28:* 507, 1975.
91. O'Connell, R. C., Morgan, A. P., Aoki, T. T., et al. Nitrogen conservation in starvation: graded responses to intravenous glucose. *J. Clin. Endocrinol. Metab. 39:* 555, 1974.
92. Blackburn, G. L., Flatt, J. P., Clowes, G. H. A., Jr., et al. Protein-sparing therapy during periods of starvation with sepsis or trauma. *Ann. Surg. 177:* 588, 1973.
93. Sapir, D. G., Owen, O. E., Pozefsky, T., et al. Nitrogen sparing induced by a mixture of essential amino acids given chiefly as their ketoanalogues during prolonged starvation in obese subjects. *J. Clin. Invest. 54:* 974, 1974.
94. Veverbrants, E., and Arky, R. A. Effects of fasting and refeeding. I. Studies on sodium, potassium, and water excretion on a constant electrolyte and fluid intake. *J. Clin. Endocrinol. Metab. 29:* 55, 1969.
95. Bloom, W. L. Fasting as an introduction to the treatment of obesity. *Metabolism 8:* 214, 1959.
96. Kollar, E. J., Aitkinson, R. M., and Alfin, D. L. The effectiveness of fasting in the treatment of superobesity. *Psychosomatics 10:* 125, 1968.
97. Hermann, L. S., and Iversen, M. Death during therapeutic starvation. *Lancet 2:* 217, 1968.
98. Kahan, A. Death during therapeutic starvation. *Lancet 1:* 1378, 1968.
99. Cubberley, P. J., Poster, A. S., and Schulman, C. L. Lactic acidosis and death after the treatment of obesity by fasting. *N. Engl. J. Med. 272:* 628, 1965.
100. Garnett, E. S., Barnard, D. L., Ford, J., et al. Gross fragmentation of cardiac myofibrils after therapeutic starvation for obesity. *Lancet 1:* 914, 1969.
101. Macadam, R. F., and Jackson, A. M. Fragmentation of cardiac myofibrils after therapeutic starvation. *Lancet 1:* 1050, 1969.
102. Lawlor, T. Fragmentation of cardiac myofibrils after therapeutic starvation for obesity. *Lancet 1:* 105, 1969.
103. Drenick, E. J., Swendseid, M. E., Bland, W. H., et al. Prolonged starvation as treatment for severe obesity. *J.A.M.A. 187:* 14, 1964.
104. Drenick, E. J. Hyperuricemia, acute gout, renal insufficiency, and urate nephrolithiasis due to starvation. *Arthritis Rheum. 8:* 988, 1965.
105. Munro, J. F., and Duncan, L. J. P. Fasting in the treatment of obesity. *Practioner 208:* 493, 1972.
106. Goldfinger, S., Klinenberg, J. R., and Seegmiller, J. E. Renal retention of uric acid induced by infusion of beta-hydroxybutyrate and acetoacetate. *N. Engl. J. Med. 272:* 351, 1965.
107. Ashley, B. C. E. Drastic dietary reduction of obesity. *Med. J. Aust. 1:* 593, 1964.
108. Innes, J. A., Campbell, I. W., Campbell, C. J., et al. Long-term follow-up of therapeutic starvation. *Br. Med. J. 2:* 356, 1974.
109. Davidson, J. K. Controlling diabetes mellitus with diet therapy. *Postgrad. Med. 59:* 114, 1976.
110. Cuendet, G. S., Loten, E. G., Cameron, D. P., et al. Hormone-substrate responses to total fasting in lean and obese mice. *Am. J. Physiol. 228:* 276, 1975.
111. Nelson, R. A., Wahner, H. W., Jones, J. D., et al. Metabolism of bears before, during, and after winter sleep. *Am. J. Physiol. 224:* 491, 1973.
112. Nelson, R. A., Jones, J. D., Wahner, H. W., et al. Nitrogen metabolism in bears; urea metabolism in summer starvation and in winter sleep and role of urinary bladder in water and nitrogen conservation. *Mayo Clin. Proc. 50:* 141, 1975.

148

Syndromes of Obesity

Ethan A. H. Sims

INTRODUCTION

The study of management of obesity over recent decades has been a sad, dull story. What other clinical disorder, so clearly comprising a variety of syndromes, has been treated as an undifferentiated single entity when the attempt is made to correlate investigative data? In what other disorder has the physician so regularly resorted to blaming the patient for "noncompliance" when therapeutic efforts are frustrated?

Recently, however, the rising incidence of obesity in Western society has led to research that is developing new concepts regarding the importance of cellular hyperplasia, energy balance, thermogenesis, endocrine disorders, and mechanisms of appetite. New emphasis is being placed on genetic predisposition, and a series of syndromes of obesity in animals are being clarified, each of which may have its human counterpart. There is greater interest in the value of increased physical activity along with caloric restriction in promoting general health and maintaining weight reduction. More rational methods have been developed for treating the overweight patient with the potentially reversible form of diabetes and what may prove to be the equally reversible associated hypertension. Thus, there begins to be hope of providing both therapy and preventive measures.*

DEFINITION AND MEASUREMENT OF OBESITY

DEFINITION

The derivation of the word *obese* implies a single etiology of overeating, since it incorporates the Latin prefex *ob-*, or over, with *edere,* to eat. In reality, many obese people eat less than their peers but expend relatively less energy.[9] A simple medical or social definition is "the state of having an excess accumulation of body fat." The problem remains of defining "an excess."

The tables of the Metropolitan Insurance Company are the traditional reference for obesity, although many authors have pointed out their limitations.[10] In particular, they do not distinguish between obesity and overweight, and different body types have differing degrees of fit with a supposed ideal.[11] A person may fall within the normal range in weight but have an abnormal body fat content and a correspondingly reduced lean body mass. As discussed later in this chapter, such a person may also have a greater degree of metabolic abnormality than a well-trained person with increased adipose mass. A second consideration that is overlooked in indices of obesity is whether an increase in body fat represents hyperplasia of adipose tissue cells or hypertrophy, in which cells are enlarged but normal in number (the two anatomic classes defined by Hirsch et al.[12]). Conversely, a person built along the lines of a football lineman may be overweight according to the tables but may have a normal percentage of body fat and be in excellent physical shape. The distribution of body fat may also be an index of endocrine dysfunction and may be evaluated by regional measurements.[13] Finally, in evaluating obesity, the hyperplasia of other tissues should not be neglected. Naeye and Roode[14] have found that in some young obese accident victims there was hyperplasia of the cells of the liver, spleen, and heart, as well as an

---

*A number of general references are available: Garrow[1] has recently written a critical and thoroughly readable book on energy balance in man. In 1973, a comprehensive international conference on obesity was sponsored by the Fogarty International Center.[2] A second conference was held in 1977. The Medical Research Council of the British Department of Health and Social Security has sponsored a valuable report on obesity.[2a] The proceedings of several recent European conferences on obesity and energy balance are available[3–6] as well as other recent books and reviews.[7,8,111]

increase in the cytoplasmic mass per cell. Thus, obesity should not only be regarded as a disorder of fat storage.

MEASUREMENT OF BODY FAT

A variety of techniques are available for estimation of body fat, but none have a high degree of accuracy. The recent critique of Grande[15] evaluates the many assumptions and sources of error. Durnin and Womersley[16] have developed normal standards for the sum of four skinfold measurements that take into consideration the increase in thickness with age. These standards, however, are based on a limited population in the United Kingdom and may be merely defining as normal the physical deterioration of an affluent and underexercised society. Possibly, a single standard, as proposed by Seltzer and Mayer,[17] is preferable for screening. An independent, accurate, but somewhat cumbersome technique based on the uptake of cyclopropane or ^{85}Kr has been introduced by Lesser and co-workers.[18] Irsigler et al. have recently described a method for simultaneously measuring specific gravity by combined submersion under water and a pneumatic method to measure residual volume of the lung and intestinal gases.[19] Tables for evaluation of skinfold measurements and of several other indices of body fat are included in Part 1 of the Fogarty International Center volume.[2]

EPIDEMIOLOGY AND COMPLICATIONS OF OBESITY

The incidence of obesity is apparently increasing in our Western society. Military induction data from the United States show an increase in incidence in draftees from 1918 to 1943 and again to 1955.[20] The recent extensive United States Public Health Survey[21] indicates that the incidence is high in men, but higher in women, particularly black women in the 45–74-year-old age group (33 percent). It is higher in white than in black men (16 percent in white men and 10.6 percent in black men ages 20–44). Women with lower incomes, regardless of race, are more obese. In the younger age group, higher income in men is associated with higher prevalence of obesity.

The key question is the degree to which obesity contributes to disease. The relation to diabetes is well known and is discussed in later sections. The increased incidence of gall bladder disease may be related to the excessive hepatic excretion of cholesterol and supersaturation of the bile with respect to this lipid. Caloric restriction does not decrease this effect, but achievement of a more ideal weight does.[22] The exact relation of obesity to various types of cardiovascular disease has been a matter of controversy.[23] One of the largest prospective studies of the development of vascular disease is the Framingham Study of 5209 persons, originally 30–62 years of age at entry. After 18 years of follow-up,[24] the findings differ from those most frequently quoted, which were based on the 12th year of follow-up. On the basis of multivariate analysis, weight gain was found to be associated with a rise in serum lipids, increase in blood pressure, impairment of glucose tolerance, and a slight rise in plasma uric acid concentrations. Weight loss was associated with a reduction in these risk factors. Particularly in women, overweight was associated at postmortem with increased left ventricular weight and thickness, suggesting increased cardiac workload. The average annual overall mortality was not greater in the obese, but coronary mortality and sudden death rates were higher in the obese, consistent with life insurance data. Morbidity was also increased for all forms of cardiovascular disease, except peripheral arterial disease. Relative to the lean, obese women had a higher incidence of congestive failure and cerebral infarction than men. The positive correlation of obesity with coronary heart disease persisted when allowance was made for other risk factors by multivariate analysis. Intermittent claudication showed a negative correlation with obesity. In women, the net effect of obesity was present but small for cerebral infarction and for cardiovascular event, with the exception of congestive failure. In men, all vascular manifestations were related to obesity, but only in the case of angina and coronary attacks was the relationship significant with the numbers available. In women only, the coronary insufficiency syndrome was related to relative weight taking the associated risk factors into account.

The authors conclude that obesity predisposes to development of hyperlipidemia, impaired glucose tolerance, hypertension, and hyperuricemia, and that by increasing these atherogenic factors obesity is an important contributor to cardiovascular mortality. This presupposes a direct cause and effect relationship between "obesity" and the metabolic abnormalities, a question to be discussed later in this chapter. Seltzer,[25] Mann,[23] and others have emphasized that excess weight is associated with increased mortality only when in excess of 25–30 percent above ideal weight, but in the Framingham Study, to date at least, the risk of major cardiovascular events rises linearly in proportion to the degree of overweight without any critical threshold. The Framingham investigators emphasize that when the atherogenic factors are present, the addition of obesity does not enhance the prediction of cardiovascular disease. Thus they agree with the conclusion of Keys,[10] based on the findings of the seven-country study and on reanalysis of other data, that obesity is not a major independent predictive factor, but they disagree with the conclusion that obesity as a contributing factor is not important. In a recent study by Weinsier et al.[10a] of 1483 male U.S. Air Force crew members reviewed for various medical defects, percent body fat was estimated by dilution of tritiated water. There was a low order of correlation between body fat and blood pressure, serum cholesterol, and triglycerides. The means of those with coronary disease and control subjects did not differ. The findings in this low-risk group of subjects, however, cannot be extrapolated to the general population.

There are somewhat antique data from insurance statistics to suggest that weight reduction may reduce cardiovascular mortality.[26] Only limited conclusions can be drawn from this information, however, since bias must have influenced selection of the particular 2300 people who managed to reduce their weight. Prospective studies are needed in which the obese subjects are classified into the types of obesity, so that meaningful conclusions can be drawn. It is quite likely that patients with certain types of obesity may be harmed by misguided attempts to return to them a weight supposedly normal for them. At present we cannot answer the question whether by diet, increased physical activity, and refraining from smoking an obese patient in a good state of training could maintain a normal risk for cardiovascular disease while still remaining obese. After all, such a person, in transporting his extra ballast, would be following the advice of preventive cardiologists in increasing his physical activity. This could provide a welcome alternative to many.

One problem common to large prospective studies and other investigative work is that all fat people are grouped together under a common heading, when in reality there may be important etiologic subgroups. This disregard may confound the results. We know that there are well-defined different types of obesity in animals,[27] and no editorial board would accept a report of a study based on a mixed assortment. We also know, for instance, that in certain strains of animals diabetes is not a "risk factor" developing as a late sequel to obesity, but is an integral part of the syndrome. In man, obese patients with diabetes or hyperlipidemia in their familial background may have a prognosis and response to treatment quite different from that of those with uncomplicated obesity. This points to the critical need for an agreed-upon classification and data base in the field of obesity.

CLASSIFICATION OF THE SYNDROMES OF OBESITY

The many attempts at classification of obesity have been reviewed elsewhere.[28] In both investigative and clinical fields there is a need for a uniform, comprehensive data base and for a diagnostic classification of the syndromes of obesity. When gross endocrine disorder has been excluded, it has been the usual practice in clinical work to use von Noorden's designation of "exogenous obesity." Since all obesity is exogenous with respect to energy balance, this pseudodiagnosis merely serves to deaden further thought. In addition, the designation "exogenous" has come to imply that the patient is at fault for allowing such a state to develop, and this in turn relieves the physician of the need to pursue prime causes, and possible points of attack on the problem may therefore be overlooked.

It is now possible to classify patients anatomically into one or other of the broad classifications, delineated by Bjurulf[29] and clarified by Hirsch and Knittle,[30] of hyperplastic–hypertrophic or hypertrophic obesity. Early onset favors the former and adult-onset the latter (see section on control of Adipose Tissue Cellularity). A further anatomic or etiologic description can often be made. Unfortunately, to estimate adipocyte number with any certainty requires cumbersome techniques, as described below. However, if the adipose mass is increased threefold or to more than 170 percent of ideal weight, it can be assumed that hyperplasia exists since the human fat cell, unlike that of the rat, apparently has limits of maximum size.[31]

One or more factors in the patient's background may be significant in perpetuating the obesity, and it is often as important to recognize these as it is to make a specific diagnosis. Thus, the first step in the approach to a patient who is overweight should be to assemble, by means of interview and perhaps questionnaire, all information relevant to the problem, including the objective findings of physical examination and laboratory work. This may be facilitated by the use of an algorithm as a guide to the minimal work-up of patients with obesity.[32] On this basis an etiologic diagnosis is made when possible. In the case of endocrine disorder it may be indicated at which functional level (satellite gland, pituitary, or hypothalamus) there is malfunction. Finally, other relevant problems, both present and potential, should be listed and carried as active problems until resolved.

In Table 148-1 a detailed anatomic and etiologic classification is outlined, with a listing of contributory factors. This classification is based on that developed at the University of Vermont and was adopted by the Advisory and Editorial Board for Obesity of the Fogarty International Center.[2] It is hoped that after appropriate modification some such classification and data base can be generally adopted both for clinical and investigative work.

Table 148-1. Classification and Problem-Oriented Approach to Obesity

I. Recommended data base of factors relevent to obesity in man
  - A. Familial background (genetic and/or environmental)
    1. Obesity with juvenile onset
    2. Obesity with adult onset
    3. Diabetes mellitus
       a. Overt
       b. Suspected (history of large birth weights)
    4. Hyperlipidemias, types III and IV
    5. Accelerated cardiovascular disease
    6. Specific endocrine disorders associated with obesity As listed under III-B and -C
  - B. Functional profile
    1. Details of gestation
    2. Age of onset of obesity
    3. Rate of progression during main stages of life
       a. Weight
       b. Rate of gain or loss of weight
    4. Age of onset of puberty
  - C. Socioeconomic factors
    1. Social pressures
    2. Occupational pressures
    3. Forced inactivity
    4. Reliance on labor-saving devices
  - D. Nutritional factors
    1. Composition of diet
    2. Gorging pattern of eating
    3. Intake of alcohol
  - E. Psychologic factors
    1. Attitude of patient, family, and friends toward his or her obesity and its probable causes
    2. Psychologic disturbances (primary or secondary to the Obesity)
  - F. FactorsAffecting Energy Balance
    1. Physical Activity
       a. Type and pattern
       b. Degree
    2. Endocrine
       a. Oral contraceptives
       b. Glucocorticoid excess
       c. Inappropriate insulin treatment
    3. Drugs
       a. Oral hypoglycemic agents
       b. Phenothiazine tranquilizers
       c. Cyproheptadine
       d. Amphetamines and anorectic agents
  - G. Addictions
    1. Smoking, pack years
    2. Alcohol
  - H. Physical examination
    1. Distribution of excess adipose tissue and body measurements
    2. Hair distribution (android, gynecoid, and excess)
  - I. Laboratory measurements*

II. Anatomic classification
  - A. Hypercellular–hypertrophic, usually associated with early onset and universal distribution of obesity
  - B. Hypertrophic, usually of late onset

III. Etiologic classification
  - A. Primary endocrine
    1. Hyperinsulimenia: insulinoma
    2. Glucocorticoid excess: adrenocortical tumor
    3. Associated with other endocrine disorder
       a. Diabetes mellitus, non–insulin-dependent
       b. Polycycstic ovarian syndrome (Stein-Leventhal)
       c. Primary hypogonadism
       d. Primary hypothyroidism
  - B. Pituitary–hypothalamic
    1. Cushing's disease due to pituitary dysfunction

Table 148-1. *(Continued)*

2. Hypothalamic and/or pituitary tumors
   a. Solid tumors
   b. Leukemic infiltration
   c. Histiocytosis-X
3. Hypothalamic or hypopituitary hypogonadism
4. Inflammatory lesions of the hypothalamus
5. Trauma or surgical injury
6. Pseudotumor cerebri
7. Empty sella syndrome

C. Genetic syndromes associated with obesity
1. Laurence-Moon-Bardet-Biedl syndrome
2. Hyperostosis frontalis interna
3. Alstrom's syndrome
4. Prader-Willi syndrome
5. Pseudo hypoparathyroidism

D. Possibly genetic in origin
1. Down's syndrome
2. Familial obesity
   a. Massive obesity with familial incidence
   b. Associated with diabetes
   c. Associated with familial hyperlipidemia

E. In lieu of specific etiologic diagnosis: relevant problems and contributory factors assembled from the data base (I).

*For laboratory data base and diagnostic algorithm, see Bray, Jordan, and Sims.[32]

CONTROL OF ADIPOSE TISSUE CELLULARITY

It has become widely accepted that an increase in the number of fat cells occurs only during the early years and adolescent period and that any changes in the size of the adipose tissue depot are accomplished by change in cell lipid content. The corollary is that persons with obesity of early onset are saddled with increased number of cells, which inevitably perpetuate the obesity. In its broad outlines there is impressive evidence to support this concept. It has been useful in focusing attention on the early years and possible factors controlling hyperplasia. However, in cases of established obesity of early onset it has increased the general pessimism of physician and patient regarding any hope of successful treatment. Some authors have questioned the universality of this doctrine as applied to the individual patient.[1,23,33] It is thus pertinent to examine the techniques for estimating cell number and the factors that affect proliferation of these cells.

ESTIMATION OF HYPERPLASIA AND HYPERTROPHY OF ADIPOSE TISSUE

As emphasized above, the hyperplasia and hypertrophy of adipose tissue is shared by other tissues in some, but not all, young obese patients. There may or may not be a proportional increase in lean body mass.[14,34] Ideally, to characterize a patient completely, measurement would be made of both protein:DNA of muscle and of cell size or lipid content of adipocytes.

There are several techniques for estimating cell size and number. Hirsch and Gallian made their classic studies by estimating cell size and number by electronically counting the osmium-fixed globules from adipocytes and independently measuring lipid content per cell.[35] The latter, divided into total body fat, gives an estimate of cell number. Other techniques estimate cell size by micrometer measurement after separation with collagenase[36] or by measurement after partial fixation.[37] The observations of Van et al.[38] and of Poznanski et al.[39] suggest that adipocytes depleted of lipid do not revert to cells identical with fibroblasts. However, neither the Hirsch technique nor any other so far devised can count either lipid-depleted adipocytes or cells destined to become adipocytes prior to lipid accumulation. In experimental animals it is possible to identify preadipocytes by prior administration of a pulse of radioactive thymidine.[31] A second problem is that the variation of accessible cells from site to site is so great that the estimated cell number may vary by as much as 85 percent depending on the site selected; thus several sites should be averaged.[40] A third problem is that the available sites may not be representative of the body as a whole. Lemonnier and Alexiu[41] have even shown that in mice cells of the perirenal depots may respond to change in nutrition in the opposite direction to those in other storage areas.

FACTORS AFFECTING ADIPOSE TISSUE MORPHOLOGY

In Animals

Diet. Diet has been the subject of much experimentation.[30] Severe manipulation of litter size in rats can decrease adipocyte number as a part of general runting of other body tissues. However, Lemonnier and Alexiu[41] have shown in mice made obese by a high-fat diet that even adults can achieve an increase in cell number. If dams are fed a suitable high-fat diet during gestation, offspring develop hypertrophy of fat cells, but not hyperplasia. Zucker obese rats respond to preweaning overfeeding with an increase in cell numbers. Early underfeeding reduces cell number in the control, but not in the affected rats.[42]

Endocrine. It has not been possible to increase adipocyte number in rats by administering insulin from an early age.[43] In hypophysectomized and in normal rats growth hormone stimulated incorporation of tracer into DNA of stromal cells, but not of primitive fat cells.[44]

Cold. Therriault and Mellin[45] have reported that young rats weighing 50–75 g, when maintained at 5 C, develop a progressive increase in the number of epididymal adipose tissue cells that is linear over the range observed (to 500 g). Recent studies in our laboratory have not confirmed this.[46]

Exercise. Oscai et al.[47] have shown that rats trained like Olympic swimmers, working out for 6h/day, 6 days/week develop fewer and smaller epidymal fat cells than their sedentary controls, even though they have free access to food. One would like to know whether during their later years they are as, or more, subject as their peers to development of a middle-aged spread.

Hypothalamic Injury. Lesions of the ventromedial hypothalamus in rats have produced hypertrophy of adipose tissue without hyperplasia,[30] even though such lesions produce a variety of secondary endocrine derangements.

Inactivity with Free Access to Food. It is well known that confinement of an animal leads to an increase in weight and body fat. Data on the effect of this situation on adipose cell number were not available until Young[48] demonstrated that woodchucks kept in captivity from an early age are not only fatter, but have an increase in adipocyte number of approximately 40 percent in comparison with those freshly brought from the wild. The increase in cell number can also occur after weaning.[49] It is not yet established whether inactivity, change in composition of the diet, or boredom is most important in producing the hyperplasia.

In Man

Experimental Obesity in Normal Man. The normal volunteer subjects studied in Vermont[50] gained 20–25 percent above their basal weight by overeating a mixed diet. The change in adipose cell size was proportional to the increase in body fat. Later measurements by Salans et al.,[51] based on aspiration biopsies of three sites and counted by the Hirsch and Gallian technique,[35] showed no increase in cell number. The possibility that newly generated preadipocytes were missed or that more prolonged gain in weight would have given a different result is not excluded.

Spontaneous Obesity. The classic study of Hirsch et al.[12] demonstrated that massively obese patients may have as many as four times the normal number of adipocytes, and that the number is not affected by reduction in weight. Brook et al., in England,[52] concluded that there are two periods in development when adipocyte hyperplasia is most apt to take place: during the first year of life and again during early puberty. However, it is difficult to exclude prenatal factors. In a study of cell number in a selected group of patients coming to bypass surgery, Salans et al.[40] found that an increase in cell number was almost exclusively limited to those with early-onset obesity. We have come to assume that such a history indicates cellular hyperplasia and may take a pessimistic attitude regarding the patient for that reason. However, recent evidence suggests that such an assumption may not be entirely valid. First, the technical difficulties of obtaining representative estimates has been mentioned. Second, another study has produced results in contrast to those of Salans et al., perhaps due to a different selection of subjects. Hirsch and Batchelor[31] have reviewed 106 patients of all ages and types of obesity who were studied with multiple fat biopsies at Rockefeller Hospital. There was still an order of inverse correlation between age of onset and adipose cell number, but there was considerable crossover in that some patients with onset in childhood showed only hypertrophy, and others with onset in the adult years had definite cellular hyperplasia. Possibly further studies correlating such factors as family history of obesity or diabetes, gestational and perinatal history, endocrine status, and other possible contributing factors may yield a less confusing pattern.

Cheek et al.[34] conducted a detailed study of the body composition of a group of 23 children with varying family histories of obesity and of diabetes. Among the girls they found two groups with respect to advanced maturation and increased ratio of nuclei and protein to DNA of muscle. They suggested that excess growth hormone could account for the differences. Adipocyte number was not estimated. Again, there is a need to correlate such measurements with other data.

DOES ADIPOCYTE NUMBER PREDETERMINE SUBSEQUENT DEVELOPMENT OF OBESITY?

To date there are only suggestive data, and a final answer must await the results of prospective studies. Some animal data bear on this point. Widdowson and Shaw[33] underfed piglets from 10 days of age, so that at 1 year there were minimal countable adipocytes. When refed, however, their genetic predisposition toward obesity overcame this handicap. Adipocytes were restored and they tended to become obese. Johnson et al.[42] obtained essentially similar results from over- and underfeeding Zucker fatty rats. Prospective data are not yet available relative to later obesity in animals in which hypercellularity has been produced by confinement.

A related question is whether, in time, cell number may regress if weight is lost. Serial follow-up of the studies of Salans et al.[40] of patients undergoing bypass surgery should give an answer to this question in patients with the hyperplasia type of obesity.

GENERAL ASPECTS OF OBESITY

We have been through an era when psychologists and psychiatrists have credited various psychological disorders with being primary causes of obesity, and this has often added a burden of guilt to those already handicapped. More recently, psychologic factors associated with being obese and prejudices against obese people are being emphasized.[53] There is incontrovertible evidence in animals that a number of types of obesity may be inherited.[27] Mayer[9] and Seltzer[54] have revived the question of the relative contribution of environmental and social factors versus genetic factors in producing obesity in man. The studies by Newman et al.[55] and others of twins raised together or apart indicate that genetic factors are highly significant, but that environmental factors also play a role. The observations of Withers[56] of adopted children are often cited as evidence of the predominant influence of heredity in determining obesity, since the children physically resembled their true rather than their foster parents. However, adoption did not take place until a mean age of 14.5 months, with a range of 10 days to 8 years, so that perinatal and early childhood influences could not be entirely excluded.[57] It is also likely that the various types of obesity may have different patterns of inheritance.

Obesity and adult-onset diabetes are commonly associated. It is the common assumption that obesity, with its associated insulin resistance, may eventually produce diabetes in a susceptible individual; but there is much to suggest that, as in experimental animals, the diabetes and the obesity may be manifestations of the same basic disorder.[54] In fact, in many species of animals and in man with adult-onset diabetes, the two are often so closely interrelated that the term "diabesity" could be used for the syndrome. Hypertension is also frequently a concomitant of obesity, diabetes, and hyperlipidemia, and is usually at least temporarily reversible by caloric restriction or weight loss. When reversible, perhaps this could be called "obetension"!

ENDOCRINE CHANGES AND INSULIN RESISTANCE

The endocrine changes in spontaneous obesity are outlined in Table 148-2. Of these, the most important clinically is the increase in plasma insulin, which at times may represent an increase in insulin secretion of well over 100–200 percent.[58] This represents a change in releasable insulin, rather than in the threshold to glucose stimulation.[59,60] The paradox of increased insulin secretion in obesity associated with diabetes is clarified by the demonstration of Perley and Kipnis[61] that in the face of the insulin resistance of obesity there is still a relative insulin deficiency. Given a comparable stimulus of hyperglycemia, the nondiabetic obese secrete more insulin than the normal. If the normal is given a stimulus of hyperglycemia comparable to that of a diabetic obese person, the response of the normal will be less than that of the diabetic, but the response of the obese diabetic will be less than that of a nondiabetic obese person given a comparable stimulus. In other words, the diabetic is unable to surmount the insulin resistance of obesity.

The nature of the islet hyperplasia and insulin resistance in obesity has been a matter of intense investigation and considerable

Table 148-2. Endocrine and Metabolic Changes in Spontaneous and Experimental Obesity

	Spontaneous Obesity	Experimental Obesity*	
		I	II
Adipose tissue			
Cell size	↑	↑	
Cell number	↑	Unchanged	
Caloric balance			
Calories required to maintain obese state (kcal/m²)	1300	2700	1800
Return to starting weight	Rapid	Rapid	
Spontaneous physical activity	↓	↓	
Appetite late in the day	↑	↑	↓
Fasting concentrations in blood			
Cholesterol	↑	↑	
Triglycerides	↑	↑	↑
Free fatty acids	↑	Unchanged or ↓	
Amino acids	↑	↑	
Glucose	N† or ↑	↑	N
Insulin	↑	↑	↑
Glucose tolerance			
Oral	↓	↓	↓
Intravenous	↓	↓	
Insulin release			
To oral glucose	↑	↑	↑
To iv glucose	↑	↑	
To iv arginine	↑	↑	↑
Evidence of insulin resistance			
Insulin: glucose ratio	↑	↑	↑
Adipose tissue metabolism sensitivity to insulin in vitro	↓	↓	
Forearm muscle metabolism			
Insulin-stimulated glucose uptake	↓	↓	↓
Insulin inhibition of release of branched-chain amino acids		↓	
Hormones possible affecting insulin resistance			
Glucocorticoids			
Plasma cortisol	N or ↓	Unchanged	
Cortisol production rate	↑	↑	
Urinary 17-hydroxycorticoids	↑ ‡	↑ ‡	
Growth hormone			
Response to glucose	↓	↓	N
Response to arginine	↓	↓	N
Nocturnal rise		↓	

From Ref.[111].
*I, from excess of a mixed diet; II, from adding fat to the diet.
†N: normal.
‡Normal range per kilogram body weight.

controversy,[62] and it has recently been reviewed by Mahler.[63] It is a matter of great clinical importance, since the increased demand on the pancreas presumably must hasten the emergence of overt diabetes in those who have diabetes in their background.

It is clear that resistance to insulin occurs in adipose tissue cells,[8,40] and most attention has been given to this tissue. However, adipose tissue accounts for only a small percentage of glucose uptake, and any explanation for insulin resistance must take into account the demonstrated resistance of other tissues. In spontaneous obesity, as originally shown by the pioneer studies of Rabinowitz and Zierler,[64] the muscle of the forearm is resistant to stimulation of glucose uptake by insulin. Horton et al.[65] found the same to be true in our subjects with experimental obesity; in addition, there was a decrease in the ability of insulin to inhibit the release of branched-chain amino acids from muscle.[70] Felig et al.[66] have shown by human catheterization experiments that an important site of resistance to insulin in obesity is the liver. They found that splanchnic glucose production was not increased, but, exactly as found in non–insulin-dependent diabetics, the hepatic uptake of alanine, lactate, glycerol, and free fatty acids was greater in obese subjects than in normal. The normal inhibition of splanchnic glucose output from insulin infusion was reduced in the obese, and comparable infusions of glucose gave a greater insulin response. Consistent with this evidence of resistance, Soll et al.[67] have reported an apparent reduction of receptor sites for insulin in hepatic cellular membranes of ob/ob mice, and the same has been shown in lymphocytes.

IS INSULIN RESISTANCE PRIMARY OR IS IT SECONDARY TO WEIGHT GAIN AND OVERFEEDING?

Experimental Weight Loss and Weight Gain

Weight loss by obese subjects restores insulin response and sensitivity toward normal.[68] At the University of Vermont we have studied the reverse situation, namely, the response of volunteers who have no family history of diabetes or of obesity to prolonged overfeeding with various types of diets.[50] The findings are summarized in Table 148-2. Essentially, all of the endocrine changes seen in spontaneous obesity could be reproduced in direction, if not necessarily in magnitude, by overeating a diet of mixed composition. All the changes were within the normal range. These findings are frequently cited as indicating that changes such as the hyperinsulinemia must necessarily be secondary to the obesity, and not causal; however, they simply indicate that these changes may be secondary and do not exclude other mechanisms in some of the syndromes of obesity.[69]

Controlled studies employing various diets have indicated the following: Under comparable conditions of diet there was a decrease in tolerance to oral and intravenous glucose and an increase in the response of insulin following gain in weight. On the other hand, an increase in the ratio of carbohydrate to fat in the diet was associated with improved oral and intravenous tolerance to glucose at basal weight, and at both initial and peak weight with increase in plasma insulin. In vitro, the responses of adipose tissue to insulin were diminished in association with gain in weight, but they were enhanced by a higher rate of carbohydrate to fat in the diet. Weight gain brought about by taking a supplement of fat, as opposed to carbohydrate, in the diet produced a comparable hyperinsulinemia and impairment of glucose tolerance. As noted in the preceding section, there is also a reversible increased resistance of muscle to the action of insulin.[65,70]

Relation of Endocrine Changes to Insulin Resistance

Growth hormone response to a variety of stimuli is reduced in spontaneous obesity. This is also true in experimental obesity in man when excess carbohydrate in a mixed diet is given, but not when excess fat is added to the diet.[50] Thus, it is unlikely that growth hormone produces the insulin resistance, which occurs with both types of overfeeding.

Cortisol. Production rates of cortisol are increased in spontaneous obesity, and O'Connell et al.[71] have found the same in experimental obesity. In relation to body size or surface area, however, there is no increase. Serum cortisol is not increased in either type of obesity, so it is an unlikely candidate to add to the insulin resistance.

Glucagon. The evidence for an increased concentration of glucagon in obesity is conflicting. Gossain et al.[72] found normal plasma values in obese subjects before and after weight reduction. There was normal suppression by glucose, but an increased response to intravenous arginine. In contrast, Wise et al.[73] found a diminished response to infusion of alanine and to starvation. The relative number of α cells is decreased in the pancreatic islets of mice with inherited obesity (ob/ob), but in view of the islet hypertrophy, there is an increase in the total mass. More work is needed before a role of glucagon can be ruled out in any of the syndromes of obesity.

Prolactin. This hormone may have an important role in human obesity, particularly in view of its suspected major role as a liporegulatory hormone in birds and lower animals.[74] There is also indirect evidence that it may play a similar role in the hamster in modulating fat deposition and reproductive function.[75] Its physiologic action in this respect is dependent upon entrainment by antecedent secretion of steriod hormones. Ovine prolactin increases lipogenic enzymes in pigeon liver in vivo,[76] and, depending on the environment of steroidal hormone action, affects the activity of lipoprotein lipase in various tissues of the rat.[77] Studies directed toward clarifying its role will have to take into consideration the profiles of secretion of the hormones that are synergistic to its action. Copinschi et al.[78] found basal concentrations of prolactin to be lower in four obese males than in controls; but the prolactin response after insulin-induced hypoglycemia was not impaired, in contrast to that of growth hormone.

Thyroid Hormone. The role of thyroid hormone in obesity and overfeeding is discussed below in relation to energy balance.

Insulin. Finally, there is the possibility that insulin itself may produce its own resistance, as discussed below.

Cellular Mechanisms of Insulin Resistance

Much attention has been given to the fat cell as a source of insulin resistance, even though it can account for only a relatively small proportion of the uptake of ingested glucose. It has been known for some time that the enlarged fat cell is less sensitive to the antilipolytic and lipogenic action of insulin.[79] This may be a partial explanation for the fact that in man the upper limit of fat storage per cell is approximately 1.2 μg. The effect of increased size, however, must be dissociated from effects of change in diet. Salans and Dougherty[80] showed in rats given controlled diets that increased size was associated with increased basal incorporation of 1-^{14}C-glucose into triglyceride–glycerol, but there was a decreased effect of insulin in stimulating glucose incorporation into triglyceride–glycerol and oxidation to CO_2. The same pattern of response was seen in adipose tissue from obese patients undergoing a reducing regimen[81] and in subjects with experimental obesity.[50] The effect of variation in intake of carbohydrate from 100 to 300 g/m^2, given as isocaloric diets with constant protein, was compared in volunteers and patients in both the lean and fattened states. While taking comparable diets, the enlarged cells from the obese patients and volunteers had a diminished response to insulin; but the effect of increased dietary carbohydrate was overriding to such a degree that the enlarged cells from subjects taking a high-carbohydrate diet had a greater response to insulin than those from the ‹me subject when studied in the lean state.[119]

Other important variables are the state of growth of an animal and whether there is active weight gain or loss at the time of study.[80] During active gain, basal glucose metabolism and the response to insulin of large cells may be greater than that of smaller cells taken from nonobese subjects at stable weight or from obese subjects losing weight. While actively losing weight, the response may be much less than normal.[81]

Finally, Curtis-Pryor[82] has speculated that prostaglandins may normally inhibit lipolysis through a negative-feedback mechanism and that in certain types of obesity there may be a biochemical error leading to overproduction of prostaglandins.

Cellular Site of Insulin Resistance in Obesity

The binding of insulin to its receptor is described elsewhere in this volume (Chapter 153). Changes in the number of receptor sites have been described that at first appeared to explain the resistance to the action of insulin of adipose tissue and other cells, but exceptions and findings contradictory to any single explanation became apparent, and metabolic changes distal to the receptor site have been sought. It now appears that the data must be interpreted in the light of the type of obesity and the particular circumstances of study in both man and animals.

In animals a series of studies form Roth's laboratory[67] have shown that in the ob/ob obese mouse the number of insulin receptor sites of hepatocytes, adipocytes, and thymic lymphocytes was reduced. The same was found to be true of the ob/db diabetic obese mouse and of the mouse treated with gold–thioglucose or with an excess of glucocorticoids. Fasting restored the sensitivity and number of active receptor sites. It was suggested that sustained increase in the concentration of insulin was a major factor in reducing its own receptor sites, a phenomenon termed *negative cooperativity*. There is conflicting evidence as to whether simple enlargement of adipocytes, as in the aging rat, leads to reduction of receptor sites, as both decreased and unchanged numbers have been found.

In man there has been conflicting data regarding the relationship between insulin resistance and insulin binding. Archer et al.[83] found a reduction in insulin binding of isolated monocytes in obesity. However, in 9 severely obese patients, all with hyperinsulinemia and adipocyte enlargement, Amatruda et al.[84] found no reduction of insulin-binding receptors, and attributed the insulin resistance to dilution of sites on the surface of the membrane or to a metabolic change within the cell. Olefsky[85] has shown that the conflicting findings may be reconciled if the subjects are characterized with respect to age of onset of obesity and type of obesity. In his study of 14 male subjects, 9 had hyperinsulinemia and averaged 50 years of age; these 9 had decreased insulin binding to both adipocytes and monocytes. Five patients without hyperinsulinemia were younger, averaging 33 years of age; 4 of these 5 had normal binding to adipocytes and monocytes. These 4 may well have represented the subjects with early onset of obesity. Since the patients in the study of Amatruda et al.[84] all had morbid obesity and presumably early onset, they, too, probably represented the hyperplastic type of obesity.

This analysis suggests that there may be differences in the mechanism of insulin resistance between those early-onset hyperplastic obesity and the late-onset hypertrophic obese, but there are questions to be resolved. The young patients in Olefsky's study[85] who had normal insulin binding had enlarged fat cells, but no hyperinsulinemia; those in the study by Armatruda et al.[84] also had enlarged fat cells and normal binding, but in addition had hyperinsulinemia. The difference may be due to the conditions of study since, as discussed above, the antecedent diet, the level of physical activity, and the course of the weight gain may all affect insulin resistance and could do so at a point distal to the binding of insulin to the receptor. The circumstances surrounding biopsy and the technique used may also be important. Clearly, there is a need for studies both of human subjects well characterized for the type of their obesity and of animals with the various syndromes of obesity that are well controlled for all these variables.

The studies of Cushman and Salans[86] have shown that diet may affect insulin resistance, and that insulin resistance may vary independently of receptor-site binding. They measured equilibrium insulin binding and the response to stimulation by insulin of glucose metabolism in adipocytes of rats raised from weaning on isocaloric diets containing either a high or a low ratio of carbohydrate to fat. With a high intake of carbohydrate, the binding per cell and antilipolytic effect of insulin in the presence of epinephrine was unaffected, but the stimulatory effect of insulin on glucose oxidation and lipogenesis was markedly increased. Alteration of cell size by hypercaloric diets also dissociated equilibrium insulin binding from the effect of insulin on glucose metabolism. This finding further emphasizes the need for control of diet in any studies of insulin resistance.

Rate of Insulin Release in Relation to Insulin Resistance

The work of Albisser et al.[87,88] has shown that the rate of secretion of insulin in response to a glucose load is critical in determining its effect. They used a computer-controlled device to infuse insulin in pancreatectomized dogs challenged with a glucose infusion. Direct control of insulin release that related insulin dosage to the concentration of circulating blood sugar only slowly corrected hyperglycemia and called for excessive insulin production. On the other hand, control based on the incremental rise of glucose and the predicted need for insulin, a response similar to the normal rapid delivery of the readily releasable pool of insulin in vivo, minimized rise of glucose and accomplished this with approximately one-fifth the amount of insulin. Thus, delayed delivery of insulin alone may lead to a state of insulin resistance or, at least, raised insulin to glucose ratios. In addition, reactive hypoglycemia from secretion of too much insulin too late, as seen in early diabetes, can provoke endocrine responses to inhibit glucose utilization. As delayed insulin response is one of the earliest signs of diabetes,[89] this delay may be an important contributor to insulin resistance.

Role of Total Adipose Tissue Mass in Insulin Resistance

Flatt[90] has suggested that the increased adipose mass in obesity may explain the hyperinsulinemia and insulin resistance by providing an increased total release of circulating fatty acids. Insulin determines the rate of entry of glucose into the cell, but, according to the Hales-Randle hypothesis of the glucose-fatty acid cycle,[91] the rate of oxidation is influenced by the concentration of free fatty acids. In an analysis of the data of Björntorp et al.[92] from a study of insulin concentration and free fatty acid turnover in obesity, Flatt has pointed out that the actual rate of free fatty acid release per kilogram of adipose tissue decreases as adiposity increases, and that the increment in insulin concentrations in obesity is therefore only partially negated by insulin resistance. The antilipolytic effect of insulin is thus stronger in obese than in normal subjects. The net result is a functional hyperinsulinism that favors further accumulation of fat stores.[93] Nestel and Whyte[94] have shown that the turnover rate of fatty acids is proportional to body weight, and Gomez et al.[95] have shown that infusion of fatty acids in man can increase the concentration of insulin without change in serum glucose, all of which is consistent with Flatt's hypothesis.

Effect of Exercise on Insulin Resistance

The role of increased physical activity is a most important, but unitl recently, neglected aspect of carbohydrate metabolism in obesity. Just as in the case of variation in the intake of carbohydrate, variation in physical activity can bring about dissociation between adipocyte size and adipose tissue mass and insulin sensitivity. Björntorp[96] has shown that a course of physical training for middle-aged, severely obese men strikingly reduced the plasma insulin concentration, even though the total body fat was not reduced. At first the effect of such training is in the opposite direction, but thereafter the reduction of plasma insulin and improved glucose tolerance persists for several days. This improvement is more marked in the obese than in the lean, and it is not explained by a change in cortisol, growth hormone, or epi- and norepinephrine response (Björntrop, personal communication). As a result of physical training, normal subjects with free access to food reduce their body fat, but this is not true of those with lifelong obesity.

The improvement in insulin sensitivity without change in adipose tissue mass may seem inconsistent with the concept proposed by Flatt, but we do not know what effect training may have on the rate of lipolysis.

Clinical Implications of Insulin Resistance

Insulin resistance is an important concomitant of obesity, and may be partially overcome by weight loss. It may also be overcome by an increase in physical activity, even though the adipose tissue mass is not reduced. A parallel reduction in serum lipids may be expected and may perhaps lead to a reduction in the incidence of cardiovascular disease, although we do not have prospective studies to support this statement. In those people genetically predisposed to diabetes, it is reasonable to assume that the development of overt diabetes may be forestalled or prevented and that overt non–insulin-dependent diabetes may frequently be put in remission. There may also be an improvement in an unmeasureable but important parameter—a sense of well-being.

LIPID METABOLISM IN OBESITY

Obesity, hyperinsulinemia (with or without glucose tolerance), and hyperlipidemia are frequently associated. Obesity occurs in 90 percent of patients with primary or endogenous hyperlipidemia (type IV of Frederickson).[97] When hypertriglyceridemia occurs in association with diabetes, it is difficult to know whether it is the result of a primary hyperlipidemia or it is secondary to the diabetes. Brunzell et al.[98] have found that when such patients present with serum triglyceride concentrations above 500 mg/dl, there is a high incidence of nondiabetic relatives with type IV hypertriglyceridemia; thus it is likely that they suffer from the familial disorder. Obese diabetic patients with lesser degrees of hypertriglyceridemia lack this relationship, and thus the disorder is probably secondary. There have been conflicting opinions as to which of the possible factors plays a primary role in the hypertriglyceridemia often associated with obesity. The contradictory results of various studies may be the result of lack of control of the antecedent diet or of the level of physical activity. As noted above, Björntorp[96] has shown that in middle-aged men physical training can reduce serum triglycerides, as well as insulin, even though there is no change in body fat.

MECHANISMS PRODUCING HYPERTRIGLYCERIDEMIA IN OBESITY

Some investigators have suggested that the increased serum insulin plays a primary role. The group at Stanford[99] suggests that the primary factor is the cellular resistance to insulin associated with obesity. Mild elevation of glucose then causes hyperinsulinemia, which in turn contributes to glyceride production by the liver. There is much evidence to support this scheme. Bagdade et al.[100] have shown that basal insulin correlates closely with degree of obesity. In a study carefully controlled for weight and age, however, Bagdade et al.[101] found no increase in basal insulin concentrations in patients with primary type IV hyperlipidemia and no direct relationship between insulin response and the hypertriglyceridemia. They concluded that, through its associated abnormalities, obesity could contribute to, but did not cause, the lipid disorder.

Much of the fatty acid of triglyceride associated with prebetalipoprotein has its origin in peripheral adipocytes.[97] The increased release from the enlarged adipose tissue depot[90] and the increased turnover of fatty acids may well contribute to hepatic glyceride formation.

The type and distribution of obesity has an important bearing on lipid disturbances. In their well-known study of factory workers, Albrink and Meigs[102] found that those who had gained over 4.5 kg of weight in adult years were more hyperlipidemic and that skinfold measurements indicating central deposition of fat were also more often associated with hyperlipidemia. We now know that most such individuals represent hypertrophic obesity with predominantly cellular enlargement and with increased basal lipolysis, hyperinsulinemia, and insulin resistance.

There is general agreement that in both primary and secondary type IV hyperlipidemia weight reduction is highly effective in lowering the serum triglycerides.[97] In view of Björntorp's finding[96] that physical training will lower plasma lipids, even though body fat is not reduced, it seems logical to combine the two treatments. Both should be rigorously pursued before pharmacologic treatment is considered.

CHOLESTEROL METABOLISM IN OBESITY

Hypercholesterolemia and Obesity

Hypercholesterolemia and obesity are not highly correlated. In a cooperative study of renovascular hypertension when age was taken into consideration, no correlation of obesity with serum cholesterol was found. This includes the assumption, however, that just because serum cholesterol increases with age in our population, this is a normal phenomenon of aging, which may not be the case. Nestel et al.[103] have shown an increase in production rate of cholesterol in obesity, and the balance studies of Miettinen[104] indicate that this may represent almost a doubling of the rate. Farkas et al.[105] have shown that the adipose tissue represents a large storage pool for cholesterol and provides a small amount of de novo synthesis, which may be significant when there is obesity.

Gallstone Formation in Obesity

The increase of cholesterol turnover in obesity has another important consequence. Bennion and Grundy[22] have found in a comprehensive study that the bile is consistently supersaturated with respect to cholesterol in obese subjects as opposed to matched controls, and that this was due to increased secretion into bile rather than to a decreased output of bile acids and phospholipids. This quite probably accounts for the increased incidence of cholelithiasis in the obese. During acute caloric restriction, as in starvation or protein-sparing modified fasts, mobilization of cholesterol and decrease of the solubilizing factors may actually increase the supersaturation, but once loss is achieved, the saturation is less.

CLINICAL IMPLICATIONS

There are thus several ways in which obesity may contribute to disturbance of both lipid and carbohydrate metabolism. These can often be reversed by weight loss, a diet low in calories and carbohydrate, and increased physical activity. As Björntorp recently stated:[96] "Physical training seems to be associated with a rejuvenation of carbohydrate and lipid metabolism in the non-obese subject," and he might have added in the obese as well. These options should be thoroughly tried in both varieties of type IV hyperlipidemia and usually should be the only ones considered for management of the secondary form.

ESTROGEN METABOLISM IN OBESITY

Changes in body weight are associated with variations in the time of onset of puberty and in ovulation, and recently a correlation between increased body weight and the incidence of breast and endometrial carcinoma has been established. This may be explained in part by the finding of Fishman et al.[106] that the metabolites of estradiol are altered in such a way that overall estrogenic effect is increased. The percentage of glucuronides as estradiol and estriol (which has also now been shown to be a potent estrogen) is increased, while that of 2-hydroxyestrone, which may block the cytosol receptor, is decreased. In anorexia nervosa the reciprocal changes are found.

ENERGY BALANCE AND THYROID FUNCTION IN NORMALS AND IN THE OBESE*

Every physician encounters patients who insist that they eat very little and still cannot lose weight, while some of their peers appear to eat without limit and do not gain. We usually attribute the former to unreliable reporting and treat the patient condescendingly or blame him for not following our advice. We conclude that the latter, those overeating with impunity, must simply be very active. Knowing that the caloric equivalents of protein, carbohydrate, and fat in vivo are 4, 4, and 9 kcal/g, respectively, we assume that excess calories must lead to a proportionate gain in weight.

RESPONSE OF NORMALS TO OVERFEEDING

In the early studies of experimental obesity at the University of Vermont[50] it soon became apparent that many of the subjects could ingest impressive amounts of food, up to 10,000 kcal of a mixed diet per day in some cases, and not gain at the anticipated rate; there were also marked differences between individuals in ability to gain. It was also noted in the first 19 subjects that the calories required to hold the weight gain exceeded those necessary to maintain basal weight by an amount that could not readily be accounted for by the increase in body size. This observation suggested the phenomenon described by the German writers at the turn of the century and referred to as *Luxuskonsumption,* i.e., an increase in heat production to produce a stable body weight in the face of increased intake.

The term *Luxuskonsumption* was used by Neumann,[107] who found over a period of 2 years that he could vary his intake by as much as 800 kcal/day while maintaining stable, if not necessarily the same, body weight. It seems likely that he was influenced by Rubner,[108] who had completed his series of meticulous studies of energy balance in dogs. Rubner's summary statement is consistent with present evidence respecting energy balance in both over- and undernutrition:

> We must distinguish between the period of undernutrition, the period of nutritional equilibrium, the period of pure weight gain, and the period of heat increase. The stream of food increases, but it does not determine the size of consumption. Apparently the organism does. At first the organism builds reserves, then it deposits additional substance, and finally, with increasing heat production, it gets rid of the ample food intake, at least in part.

Neumann's concept had only a few supporters, particularly Gulick,[109] who in 1922, also carried out careful studies on himself and noted the same phenomenon in a malnourished subject during refeeding. These early studies have been summarized by Graefe.[110] Many subsequent workers could not find such an ability of normals to adapt to excess intake.[111] However, N. Ashworth et al.[112] gave substantial supplements of food by liquid formula to volunteers by gavage at bedtime, and found that the calories could not be completely accounted for in terms of subsequent weight gain or reduction of intake. In more recent years, the possibility of adaptation to excess intake was revived by the report of Miller et al.[113] that, following overfeeding of 2000 kcal for several weeks, the energy cost of physical exercise and what has come to be called the *thermic effect of feeding* were increased, although they found resting metabolic rate unaltered.

Studies involving the fourth group of volunteers of the Vermont Study of Experimental Obesity[50] were closely monitored in a totally supervised institutional prison environment. They verified that maintenance requirements following weight gain from excess of a mixed diet were significantly greater than those in the baseline period. An estimated 2700 kcal/m^2 (37 kcal/kg) did not completely maintain the increased weight, while 1800 kcal/m^2 (27 kcal/kg) was adequate in the baseline period. Both these values are in contrast to the 1300–1700 kcal/m^2 that is usually adequate to maintain body weight after weight reduction in spontaneously obese subjects. It should be noted that this was a selected group of subjects not entirely representative of the general population, and also that the intake of coffee and smoking were not controlled.

In collaboration with Goldman and his associates[114] at the U.S. Army Research Institute of Environmental Medicine, thermogenesis studies were conducted with volunteers undergoing overfeeding in the Vermont Study. Measurements of heat production while basal, during various forms of exercise and at rest, and before and following standard meals were made while the volunteers were living in a chamber with constant environment. Unfortunately, the thermogenesis studies were not carried out in the initial groups of volunteers who gained 20–25 percent in weight during prolonged overeating of a mixed diet. One study of long-term overfeeding of fat was carried out in a group of volunteers in a clinical research center. They were given 1100 cal/day of relatively unsaturated fat as a supplement to a closely controlled basal diet. They gained weight over a 3-month period with surprising efficiency,[50] but had to overcome complete loss of appetite. Measurements at the end of the period of weight gain gave no evidence of an adaptive increase in thermogenesis in association with meals, exercise, or resting metabolic rate. In concurrent studies at the University of Vermont, Hanson,[115] likewise, found no change in the efficiency of graded muscular work. More efficient gain in weight from adding fat to the diet has long been recognized in animal husbandry.[116]

To date five collaborative short-term studies involving short-term overfeeding of carbohydrate, fat,[115a] or protein[115b] for periods of 3 weeks have been carried out. Resting metabolic rate was increased after increased intake of each of the three elements of the diet, but the thermic response to meals beyond the resting rate was unchanged. The resting rate was decreased, but not to basal rates, after withdrawal of the caloric supplement. In contrast to the findings of Miller et al.[113] and of Apfelbaum et al.[117] but consistent with that of Whipp et al.[118] in a similar study, no change was detected in the efficiency of muscular exercise. The changes in the metabolism of thyroid hormone during these studies of short-term overfeeding are discussed below.

A number of different mechanisms could account for the increased caloric requirements in normal subjects of over 1500 kcal/day to maintain the weight gained by long-term increase in intake of a mixed diet: (1) replacement of tissue of low caloric density or excess water and electrolyte initially retained with calorically dense but lighter fat during the period of apparent equilibrium; (2) an increased caloric requirement associated with weight gain, which in active subjects is not adequately corrected

*Much of the material in this section is reprinted with permission from Clin. Endocrinol. Metab., 1976.

for by simply relating caloric intake to surface area; (3) increased fecal loss; or (4) an adaptive increase in thermogenesis. Evidence suggesting that the first three of these possibilities acting alone or in combination are inadequate to account for the increased caloric requirements is discussed elsewhere.[111,114] However, evidence for an adaptive increase in thermogenesis has been increasing.

POSSIBLE MECHANISMS OF DIET-INDUCED THERMOGENESIS

There are numerous biochemical reactions by which animals and plants can generate excess heat in a variety of biologic adaptations; these are reviewed in a wide-ranging and intriguing paper by Hochachka[120] and in a recent review of cellular thermogenesis by Himms-Hagen.[121] For example, the philodendron can uncouple respiration and raise its temperature in the tissues concerned with the dissemination of its scent by as much as 10 C above the ambient temperature; also, as shown by Clarke et al.,[122] before take-off on a cold morning the bumble bee uses the futile cycle of fructose-6-phosphate to fructose-1,6-diphosphate to warm its wing muscles.

There are a number of metabolic pathways whose use could result in an adaptive increase in thermogenesis in animals. These have recently been reviewed by Hegsted,[123] Stirling and Stock,[124] and Garrow,[1] and only the bare outlines will be suggested here. There have also been a number of symposia concerned with this subject.[6,125,125a,126] Such pathways are known to be activated in adaptation to cold.[127] In an extensive review, Meerson[128] has discussed the mechanisms whereby new protein may be synthesized and mitochondria replicated as a part of adaptation to cold and anoxia. There is an intriguing possibility that some of the differences in thermogenic response in man may be a reflection of differences or changes in mitochondrial density.

Ever since Lavoisier demonstrated animal respiration, there has been a tendency to assume that animals constantly burn their substrates with the same even flame and with the same efficiency, generally estimated as 39–40 percent for carbohydrate and fat and 32–34 percent for protein. However, as Hegsted[123] points out, there is no reason to believe that this maximum is achieved or is constant in different individuals and under different conditions. Some of the mechanisms that can produce less efficient utilization of substrates for synthesis of tissue or mechanical work are discussed below.

Cost of Storage and Later Utilization of Fuels

On the basis of data on oxygen consumption by adipose tissue during lipogenesis, Ball[129] has estimated that 11 percent of the energy present in glucose is lost in the conversion of glucose to fat, an energy loss twice that incurred during the conversion of glucose into glycogen. Flatt[93] has reevaluated the cost of glucose conversion to fat, including in his estimate the caloric value of the high-energy bonds formed by substrate phosphorylation; according to this estimate, 20 percent of the caloric value of the glucose channeled into the lipogenic pathways is expended to produce the ATP required for synthesis of fatty acid.

After a meal, a significant portion of the amino acids ingested is thought to be converted to muscle protein. Flatt[93] estimates the metabolic cost for this storage (which is provided by oxidation of carbohydrate and fat,) at 20 percent of the caloric content of the protein synthesized. When this protein is mobilized during the postabsorptive phase and the amino acids are used for energy production, additional metabolic energy is required to convert the gluconeogenic amino acids to glucose and to incorporate the nitrogen into urea. This again requires an energy expenditure equal to some 30 percent of the protein calories originally ingested. Thus, an amount of metabolic fuel equal in amount to 50 percent of the calories supplied by dietary protein could be expended for ATP generation in order to allow for the temporary storage of the amino acids through protein synthesis, followed by the obligatory ATP expenditure for gluconeogenesis and ureagenesis during the catabolism of the ingested amino acids.

Inefficient Generation of ATP

In place of the usual coupling of oxidation to ATP generation with a P:O ratio of 3, there are cytochromes that yield a ratio of 1 or even of 0; flavin-linked oxidations, as in the oxidation of succinate, yields a P:O ratio of only 2. This is also the case in the oxidation of α-glycerophosphate via the mitochondrial dehydrogenase (EC 1.1.2.1). This enzyme is increased by thyroid hormone[130] and during the increase in thermogenesis in response to cold. In rats that had been given a diet inadequate in protein and were overeating, apparently to obtain adequate protein, Stirling and Stock[131] found the efficiency of weight gain to be low. In fact, the calories that could not be accounted for ultimately equaled the entire final energy content of the carcass. The mitochondrial α-glycerophosphate dehydrogenase of the liver was increased 20-fold over that of the control animals. A similar inefficiency of weight gain has been found by Tulp et al.[132] in rats given, from birth, a diet containing only 8 percent casein. The stunted rats eat more than the controls in proportion to their body size, but gain less per unit of food ingested. Their thyroid response is discussed below.

Uncoupling of Oxidative Phosphorylation

The medical profession's first ill-conceived attempt to solve the problem of obesity by means of a pill[133] involved the use of dinitrophenol, an agent that uncouples mitochondrial respiration. Uncoupling also accounts for the generation of heat by brown fat; in this process the fatty acids from hydrolysis of triglycerides themselves act as uncoupling agents, and heat, but little ATP, is generated.[120] However, there has been no demonstration of brown fat in adult men.

Inefficient Utilization of ATP and Futile Cycles

As already noted, intermittent eating, with temporary storage of energy as fat or glycogen, is inefficient with respect to energy balance. There are also a number of steps in metabolic pathways in which the direction of flow is controlled by separate enzymes and in which recycling will waste the energy derived from synthesis of ATP.[124] Examples of these steps are (1) glucose to glucose-6-phosphate, (2) fructose-6-phosphate to fructose-1,6-diphosphate, and (3) phosphoenolpyruvate to pyruvate. Williamson et al.[134] have suggested that such cycling may be involved in the control of the rate of gluconeogenesis in the liver. In adipose tissue, energy-wasting recycling may occur in a fatty acid synthesis–oxidation cycle and in a triglyceride hydrolysis–reesterification cycle.[124]

Variation in "Specific Dynamic Action" and the Hypermetabolism of Refeeding

Specific dynamic action has been the term for the increase in metabolic rate that occurs after ingestion of protein and it has been regarded as a fixed increment. Krebs[135] has attributed the extra heat production to the energy requirements for urea synthesis and the wasting of some of the energy of amino acid degradation in the formation of ATP. In other words, the effect is attributed entirely to catabolism of amino acids. However, Garrow and Hawes[136] have continuously monitored oxygen uptake in studying the effect of meals that either increase or decrease the rate of urea production. They found a similar increase in metabolic rate for a given energy content of test meal, regardless of the nutrient content. These findings are consistent with those of A. Ashworth[137] in studies of infants with protein-calorie malnutrition. She found that during refeeding the resting metabolic rate was not increased and was not affected by variations in the composition of the diet. She attributed the increased metabolic rate in response to meals to the energy cost of growth during growth spurts occurring in association with meals. Fleagle et al.[138] have also noted an inefficiency of weight gain with respect to caloric intake on refeeding squirrel monkeys that have been malnourished with respect to protein. If the increase in metabolic rate in these situations reflects increased protein synthesis, it is quite a different phenomenon from the adaptive increase in metabolic rate which may serve to dispose of excess calories in a nongrowing subject. Certainly there is enough evidence to indicate that *specific dynamic action* is neither specific for protein, nor a fixed entity, and the term had best be discarded in favor of the more general term *diet-induced thermogenesis*.

Effect of Mental State

Miller[139] has made the interesting suggestion that the thermic response to overfeeding may vary in a given individual depending on his general state of anxiety or relaxation. In the Vermont Study[50] the most inefficient use of calories for weight gain was noted in subjects under stress of imprisonment.

Ionic Pump Activity

It has been suggested that a high proportion of the resting energy utilization of the body is devoted to keeping the primordial sea water out of our cells, i.e., in operation of a "sodium pump." It is estimated that 35 percent of the resting metabolism of liver is devoted to maintaining the cellular gradient of sodium and of potassium, while in brain this may require 50 percent, in kidney 40 percent, and in muscle, bulk lean body mass, 19 percent.[126] It is possible that variations in the efficiency of this process might explain some of the variation in energy requirements between individuals. The rate of ionic pumping can be varied in particular organs by the action of three hormones. Insulin may increase the turnover of potassium ion 1.5-fold in muscle, and norepinephrine can increase the permeability of brown fat cells to sodium 8-fold. Ismail-Beigi and Edelman[140] have shown that thyroxine (T_4) albeit in pharmacologic doses, increases the activity of the ATP-dependent sodium pump, and suggest that this accounts for the calorigenic action. In the presence of an ion leak, energy could be dissipated without producing any change in intra- or extracellular concentrations.

Changes in Thyroid Function

An abnormality in thyroid function has long been sought to explain the ease of weight gain in the obese.

In our subjects with increased diet-induced thermogenesis following overfeeding with a mixed diet or with carbohydrate, Danforth et al.[141] have found significant increases in serum triiodothyronine (T_3) with no change in T_4. There was also a significant decrease in serum 3,3′5′-triiodothyronine, "reverse T_3" (rT_3), an isomer of T_3 with minimal physiologic activity. This compound, as well as most of the serum T_3, is believed to be generated in the periphery, probably in the liver,[142] by monodeiodination of T_4, either in the outer (beta) ring, forming T_3 or in the inner (alpha) ring, forming rT_3. It should also be emphasized that all of these changes following overfeeding have been within the conventional limits of normal for both T_3 (137 ± 4 to 169 ± 9 ng/100 ml) and rT_3 (33 ± 4 to 21 ± 4 ng/100 ml). It is not yet established whether there is a direct causal relationship between the changes in thyroid hormone and the changes in thermogenesis. That there may be such a direct relationship, however, is suggested by the additional finding that there was no change in the formation of either hormone in the subjects who gained efficiently from the addition of excess fat to their diet and gave no evidence of increased oxygen uptake (heat production) not explained by increase in body size.[114]

The importance of the composition of the diet became further apparent when it was found by Danforth et al.[141,141a] that volunteers fed isocaloric diets low in carbohydrate, or containing no carbohydrate, developed changes in T_3 and rT_3 opposite to those from feeding excess carbohydrate. Serum T_3 was reduced and rT_3 increased when carbohydrate was restricted in the diet, again without changes in serum T_4. These results are consistent with the observations of Portnay et al.[143] in starvation. It seems likely, therefore, that diet-induced alterations of the metabolism of thyroid hormone are associated in some manner with the carbohydrate content of the diet, and probably also with the relative state of nutrition.

Kinetic studies of thyroid function have been carried out by Danforth[143a] in subjects of the Vermont Study, described above, who were given excess carbohydrate, fat, or protein for periods of approximately 3 weeks. Serum concentration of T_3 increased in all groups, and rT_3 was decreased 30 percent. There was no change in T_4 or in T_3 serum binding, and T_4 kinetics were unaffected by overeating. However, T_3 metabolic clearance rate increased in each group. Thus, the production of T_3 is increased during short-term overfeeding of each component of the diet, thyroidal secretion of T_4 is of minor importance, and the origin of the increased production of T_3 is from altered peripheral conversion of T_4 to T_3.

Recent studies have indicated that T_3 directly affects the number of β-adrenergic receptors in the myocardium.[143b] One might speculate that the increased sensitivity to catecholamines may be important in explaining the increase in thermogenesis. One may also speculate that a similar mechanism may explain, in part, the hypertension frequently associated with spontaneous obesity and overfeeding.

An adaptation in which resting metabolic rate were increased in the face of an excess of food of poor quality would have obvious survival value, since it could permit an animal to eat to obtain enough of a scarce nutrient, protein or minerals, and yet have less chance of paying the penalty of becoming obese. An adaptation by which resting metabolism were reduced in the face of deprivation of food would also be advantageous. That such is the case has been demonstrated in the classic study by Benedict of his fasting subject[144] and of Keys et al. in the Minnesota study of malnutrition.[145a] More recently, Bray[146] and Apfelbaum et al.[117] have also shown a reduction in metabolic rate during caloric deprivation. There is, however, no convincing evidence that the energy cost of physical work is altered under these conditions.

The critical questions remain, however, whether there is a difference in resting metabolic rate in any of the varieties of obesity, whether the thermic response to food is impaired, and whether any change in the metabolism of thyroid hormone can explain ease of weight gain.

ENERGY BALANCE AND THYROID FUNCTION IN THE OBESE

Garrow[1] has reviewed the discordant studies of resting metabolic rate in the obese and has concluded that an adequate comparison with lean controls cannot be made using available methods. Intraindividual comparisons can be made, however.

Miller and Parsonage[147] have studied a group of 29 women selected as difficult weight losers from a large national slimming club in England. They were kept reasonably active in a country house and were closely monitored with a tightly controlled intake of 1500 kcal for 3 weeks. Twenty lost weight as might be expected, but nine were able to maintain their weight. Metabolic rates were significantly lower in the latter group, and metabolic rate correlated better than any other parameter with ability to lose. Since these patients with low metabolic rates represented only one-third of a highly selected group, the finding of reduced metabolic rates of this degree must be rare.[147a]

It is apparent that individuals vary widely in their resting metabolic rates.[145] In fact, as has been pointed out by Thomas,[148] we are not entirely individuals, but rather symbiotic colonies that include the myriad of mitochondria, which, as he states "are probably primitive bacteria that swam into ancestral precursors of our cells and stayed there." We are dependent upon them for almost all of our energy. They respond to cues that we do not understand and they are capable of replicating themselves under conditions of muscular exercise, hyperthyroidism, hypoxia, and cold exposure.[128] Perhaps, when we understand more of these mechanisms, we may be able to treat certain varieties of obesity by regimes that more directly affect the resting metabolic rate.

In continuation of the Vermont Study, Danforth et al.[148a] have evaluated thyroid function in 4 moderately overweight young men who ate approximately 1800 kcal carbohydrate/day in excess of requirements for maintenance. The mean serum T_3 increased (127 $\pm$ 3 versus 157 $\pm$ 10 ng/100 ml) and rT_3 decreased (47 $\pm$ 4 versus 39 $\pm$ 5 ng/100 ml) for the group. However, the changes in T_3 and rT_3 were not significant in 2 of the subjects. The 2 subjects who showed the expected changes also showed an increase in thermogenesis similar to that of their lean counterparts. Further studies will be required to determine whether there may be subpopulations of obese subjects who do not show the same response to overfeeding with carbohydrate as normals.

Thyroid hormone increases the activity of the flavin-dependent mitochondrial α-glycerophosphate dehydrogenase in adipose tissue. Galton and Bray[130] found this to be reduced in adipose tissue of obese patients. They point out that this reduction could result in more glycerol becoming available for triglyceride formation. Conversely, Stirling and Stock[131] have emphasized that an increase in the mitochondrial enzyme also results in a lower P:O ratio of oxidative phosphorylation and thus could contribute to diet-induced thermogenesis.

EFFECT OF SMOKING ON APPETITE AND LACK OF EFFECT ON THERMOGENESIS

Many persons continue smoking cigarettes because they have noted that they gain excessive weight on stopping. This phenomenon might be explained by the report of Glauser et al.[149] that laboratory workers had higher mean resting metabolic rate and protein-bound iodine when smoking an average of 1.6 packs of cigarettes per day than after stopping, although statistical significance was marginal. In a recent study in our laboratory employing an on–off–on design with 3-week periods of identical food intake, no change in weight, resting metabolic rate, thermic response to exercise or meals, or weighted body temperatures were noted. There was also no change in serum T_3 or T_4 or in their response to thyrotropin-releasing hormone (TRH).[150] There was, however, a significant increase in appetite ratings during the nonsmoking period, and, at least in moderate smokers, this appears to be the main explanation for the tendency of reformed smokers to gain weight. Along with the change in appetite, the thyrotropin (TSH) response to TRH was increased, while the prolactin response to TRH was not. The young subjects of this study smoked only 1 pack of cigarettes per day and abstained for only 3 weeks; it is possible that a more prolonged study of more hardened addicts might reveal more definite metabolic changes.

CLINICAL AND OTHER IMPLICATIONS OF VARIATIONS IN THERMOGENESIS

Individual Variation in Weight Gain

Indivduals vary both in their ease of gaining weight and in their ability to lose weight in response to variation of intake. Weight gain from overeating carbohydrate or a mixed diet can, it appears, be modified to a limited extent by an adaptive increase in thermogenesis. We do not yet know whether this response may be impaired in some patients with spontaneous obesity and, if so, the extent to which this may contribute to the obesity. At most, perhaps 10–20 percent of excess calories can be expended in this manner.

Response of Metabolic Rate to Caloric or Carbohydrate Restriction

When intake is below maintenance and when carbohydrate is restricted, as in a reducing program, there is an adaptive decrease in resting metabolic rate that decreases the net deficit of calories. When a patient fails to gain or lose weight according to our expectations, allowance should be made for these adaptive changes, and the patient should be considered innocent until proven guilty of distorting his or her account of intake.

Response of T_3 to Restriction of Caloric Intake

A reduction of serum T_3 and an increase in conversion of T_4 to the inert rT_3 is part of the adaptation to restricted intake. This survival mechanism does not appear to be useful in the present context. However, present knowledge does not permit us to say whether giving thyroid hormone to counter the decrease in thermogenesis is indicated. Protein catabolism is also accelerated, and one must weigh the advantages against the disadvantages. Increasing physical activity, which increases and conditions lean body mass, is a preferable alternative means of restoring caloric expenditure.

Concept of Adaptive Thermogenesis and Its Implications

The concept of adaptive thermogenesis has broader implications. Four English nutritionists recently stated:[151]

> We believe that the energy requirements of man and his balance of intake and expenditure are not known . . . It is possible that the 30 percent of the world's population who have an "adequate" intake are really eating too much and that an unknown proportion of the rest are not undernourished.

The results of the studies of energy balance of individuals described in this section are consistent with this concept.

REGULATION OF APPETITE AND SATIETY

It seems clear that the body is not so unwise as to entrust the regulation of such an important matter as the intake of food to any simple or single mechanism. This complex subject has been discussed at two recent symposia[2,152] and in recent reviews[1,153] and cannot be considered in detail here. There are, however, new models and approaches to the question of regulation that will be alluded to briefly.

To dissociate short-term satiety factors possibly released from the proximal gut, Koopmans[154] has developed a model in which the intestines of parabiotic rats are spliced in such a manner that one rat borrows 30 cm of intestine from the other of the pair.

Several ingenious models alter the pattern of substrates that an animal "sees" during energy deprivation. Van Itallie's group[153] have enriched the diet of rats with odd-chain fatty acids that yield 1 mol glucose on catabolism. This dividend of carbohydrate is sensed by the organism when deprived. Sullivan et al.[155,156] have blocked the endogenous production of fatty acids by giving the nontoxic, nonmetabolizable isomer of citrate (–)-hydroxycitrate, to rats; they found through pair-feeding experiments that the resulting reduction of weight and body fat is brought about by inhibition of appetite.

There are intimations that the seat of the soul with respect to appetite may have to be moved to the liver, as this organ appears to be capable of responding directly with afferent signals to glucose infusion or changes in hepatic stores of carbohydrate.[157] Some years ago Brobeck[158] suggested that animals eat to keep warm. Now we have a suggestion that they eat to keep the fires burning in their liver and can sense the temperature. It has been reported that if rats are equipped with implanted heaters over their livers, eating may be inhibited by raising the temperature a few degrees.[159]

The concept that an animal with a ventromedial hypothalamic lesion becomes obese as a result of simple hyperphagia must be modified by evidence in animals and in man that such lesions may produce a primary hyperinsulinemia.[160,161] Signals transmitted via the vagus nerve are apparently essential for perpetuation of the obesity, gastric hyperacidity, and hyperinsulinemia in the lesioned rat, since vagotomy at the level of the diaphragm reverses these abnormalities.[162] On the other hand, vagotomy does nothing for the insatiable appetite of the Zucker rat,[163] which appears to have an obligatory trapping of glyceride in its adipose tissue, perhaps analogous to the kindred described by Galton et al., in whom a primary enzymatic abnormality of adipose tissue is suspected.[164] In the fatty rats, Zucker showed in one of her last studies that caloric deprivation does not proportionally reduce fat stores, and the deprived animals develop an appetite so insatiable that they may consume their own tails. To my knowledge no one has suggested a psychologic basis for this overeating.

An intricate story has been elucidated as to how tryptophane, the precursor of serotonin, crosses the central nervous system barrier. Active transport is required, and there is direct competition by the branched-chain amino acids, the release of which is inhibited by insulin.[165] Thus, availability of carbohydrate and secretion of insulin may modulate serotonin production and, in turn, behavior.

Finally, in this potpourri of models, the provocative suggestion may be mentioned that a peptide hormone from the upper intestine, cholecystokinin–pancreozymin may specifically inhibit feeding behavior in rats[166] when given in large doses. Several investigators have found, however, that intake of water is inhibited along with appetite. In man the infusion of this hormone, or its analogue, caerulein, does not inhibit appetite.[167]

TREATMENT OF THE SYNDROMES OF OBESITY

Since obesity is not a single entity, but rather a number of syndromes with obesity as a common expression, no single therapeutic maneuver or stereotyped method can be expected to meet the needs of all patients. It is essential to characterize the individual patient as fully as possible, as suggested at the beginning of this chapter, and to establish the various factors that may contribute toward his obesity.

The statistics for success of treatment of run-of-the-mill obesity are discouraging.[168] However, these are based on the options of treatment formerly available, and no study has been made to date to consider the prognosis for weight loss in relation to types of obesity. In addition, it is quite possible that the approach to cooperating with the patient in management of his disorder has not been an appropriate or effective one.

WHO SHOULD BE TREATED?

The factors affecting prognosis have already been discussed. A person with hypertrophic obesity is more apt to have metabolic derangements,[169] but at the same time may be more responsive to treatment, since the desired end result is to have cells with a normal content of lipid. It is clear that the maturity-onset diabetic, the hyperlipidemic patient, types III–V, those with osteoarthritis, and those with hypertension or cardiovascular problems all stand to benefit from weight reduction as well as those with milder degrees of obesity who, 10 or 20 years hence, will probably be in the same plight. Perhaps when we look at percent body fat or percent overweight, we are looking at the wrong parameter. Heavy people with a generous muscle mass show none of the metabolic changes of the usual spontaneously obese.[170] Just to whittle away a portion of stored fat may accomplish little with respect to later degenerative disease. On the other hand, much harm may be done through inappropriate efforts to mold all to a preconceived "ideal" weight.[53,171] This may be particularly true if it means attempting to maintain a reduced patient, initially hyperplastic, in a state in which each cell is relatively depleted. Björntorp et al.[170a] found that obese women undergoing a program of weight reduction reached a plateau of weight loss, and that this occurred when the adipocyte cell size fell within the normal range, and not when any particular percent of body fat was reached.

METHOD OF TREATMENT

Dietary Restriction and Increased Activity.

Conventional Balanced Diet. The major problem in treating the various forms of obesity is maintaining the weight loss that is achieved. Hence various regimens must be judged by their long-term as well as their immediate success. The spontaneous obese, like those with experimental obesity, gravitate toward their original weight. It is quite possible that inducing futile oscillations in weight may be more harmful than remaining overweight. If gradual weight loss can be achieved by a balanced diet and program of increased activity that could be maintained indefinitely, the loss should be more permanent. There are certainly many people with a tendency toward obesity who maintain a normal weight by this means, while attracting no attention to themselves or their routines. Preliminary reports from the large outpatient department at Grady Memorial Hospital suggest that with a positive approach weight loss can be achieved by conventional means rigorously applied. As a part of withdrawing treatment with sulfonylurea from several thousand obese diabetic patients, Davidson[172] has employed a program of perfected dietary instruction, home supervision, exercise, and 25 h of instruction per patient and achieved enough loss to control the diabetes. It is clear that simply handing a diet to a patient is inadequate. A negative attitude toward achieving retraining proves self-fulfilling. In the patient severely handicapped by the more serious forms of obesity an attitude of blame merely adds to the patient's burden. The ideal for this lifelong problem is for the professional to develop a relationship with the patient more as cooperating client than passive recipient of advice or blame.[173]

There are definite metabolic effects from a gorging pattern of eating rather than a nibbling pattern,[174] but there is no evidence that weight loss is accelerated by one or the other pattern of eating. However, young male volunteers, taking a single daily meal, produced higher serum cholesterol values and slightly impaired glucose tolerance.[175]

Details of dietary prescription are given by Mayer.[176] A pictorial dietary guide has been developed by the Diabetic Clinic of the Grady Memorial Hospital.[172]

Experimental Unbalanced Regimens. Teleologically, the tendency toward obesity has been perpetuated because it represents preparation for possible famine. It is not surprising, therefore, that starvation should have had many medical proponents as a means of treating obesity. As described in the preceding chapter, man is superbly adapted to withstanding starvation. From the studies of Cahill's laboratory (Chapter 147) it is known that the central nervous system can utilize ketones effectively as a source of energy. There have been many advocates of diets sufficiently low in carbohydrate to produce ketosis to obtain some of the benefits of starvation. These have been reviewed by Van Itallie et al.,[153] who conclude: "Apart from the bargain basement philosophy that underlies so many proposed methods of weight reduction . . . the bargains are often illusory." Hood[177] found that the rate of weight loss from diets of 1000 kcal producing mild ketosis did not differ from those with more liberal carbohydrate, and there was no difference in appetite.

Interest in an essentially carbohydrate-free diet was rekindled by Apfelbaum et at.[117,178] in France. They have extensively studied the effect of giving only approximately 55 g of casein, suitably supplemented. Net nitrogen balance was restored after approximately 2 weeks. Blackburn et al.[179] in the United States have emphasized this advantage and have attributed the nitrogen-sparing effect to reduction of the antilipolytic effect of insulin, permitting fatty acids and ketones to be used maximally as a substitute for glucose derived from protein as fuel. The β-hydroxybutyric acid inhibits release from muscle of the gluconeogenic amino acid, alanine, and the small amount of dietary protein supplies the branched-chain amino acids essential to minimize protein catabolism. Needless to say, such a regimen requires supplements of vitamins and electrolytes, and trace element depletion may present problems from long-term use. On the positive side, many patients report abatement of appetite and others an elevation of mood, which in certain cases may outweigh potential hazards of the diet. These hazards have been summarized recently[153,180] and are very real for a patient with renal insufficiency or gout, although the net effect of a ketogenic regimen may be less in obese patients, who are notoriously resistant to ketosis. Long-term hazards are calcium depletion secondary to the acidosis, leading to osteoporosis, and menstrual disturbance in young women.

A portion of the enthusiasm for the ketogenic diets may be due to the rapid weight loss that a ketogenic diet produces. In a study in which changes in body composition were carefully assessed, Yang and Van Itallie[181] compared the effects over 10-day periods of 800-calorie formulas either carbohydrate-free or containing carbohydrate adequate to prevent ketosis. Weight loss was most marked with the former diet, but this was entirely in the form of water and electrolyte, since the decrease in energy content of the body was the same, and at the end of this short period nitrogen loss was comparable. Equally careful long-term studies of the nitrogen balance are needed. Greenberg et al.[182] have tested, again in short-term experiments, the premise of Flatt and Blackburn. In assessing nitrogen balance following operations they could detect no difference in nitrogen balance when comparing the effect of intravenous amino acids versus the same with added glucose. Infusion of lipids, which should further spare nitrogen, was also without effect. In both situations nitrogen balance was the same. In this situation, however, catabolic stresses other than dietary deprivation were operating, and again, long-term studies are needed. The fatalities associated with use of the so-called liquid protein diets, consisting of a variety of commercially available protein hydrolysates, as opposed to biologically complete proteins, have been described in a recent publication.[182a]

It is naive to believe that any one solution exists for the complicated problem of obesity. There is a need for controlled studies in which the obesity is classified as to type and stage as well as possible, so that more can be learned about which type of management is suitable under various conditions. Controlled studies are also necessary to sort out the degree to which the enthusiasm and bias of the physician or professional contributes to acceptance of success of a given regimen.

Initial studies[183] and much anecdotal experience suggests that a protein-sparing regimen may be of value as a temporary measure for obese patients with maturity-onset diabetes and a high degree of insulin resistance, as described in a later section. Such a regimen may provide more effective and comprehensive treatment of hypertension in overweight patients than that provided by drugs.

Exercise in the Management of Obesity. Particularly when the physical strength and level of physical activity of the patient are low, and when dietary restriction has, as we have seen, lowered the resting metabolic rate, the patient has a hard row to hoe in attempting to reduce by diet alone. However, increasing physical activity is a valuable and logical adjunct that may permit weight loss even with a more liberal diet. Contrary to general belief, moderate exercise is not inevitably followed by an increase in appetite. Time spent exercising is time lost to eating on two counts: it is not possible to do both at the same time, and the interest and stimulation derived from physical activity reduces the boredom which is the shortest route to snacking. Many take out their slide rules and calculate that since so little time can be spent in vigorous exercise, this is an unrewarding way to attempt to lose weight, but they neglect to consider other important benefits of increased activity: (1) a sense of well-being; (2) the possibility that the insulin resistance of obesity may be reversed;[96] (3) glucose tolerance is improved; (4) there is to some degree, protection against cardiovascular accidents. For the young and well-motivated patient an aerobic form of exercise is recommended,[184] and for the busy adult perhaps less demanding programs that can be adapted to the daily routine.[185]

It is instructive both for the patient and his physician to keep a daily log of physical activity along with a record of food intake. Convenient charts for this purpose that also give the caloric value of physical activity are available.[2] At best, what is considered as "exercise" can make up but a small portion of the day's total caloric expenditure; modifying the day's routine to include more standing, walking, bending, and stair-climbing may accomplish more. What is really involved is a change in life style. The techniques of behavioral self-modification are useful in helping patients to assume responsibility for the daily management of their own problems.

Behavioral Self-Modification

The underlying assumption of behavioral self-modification is that, whatever the prime cause, there are learned patterns of eating and of activity and inactivity that can be pinpointed and systematically corrected. Both eating habits and physical activity are given attention. For details the reader is referred to summaries by Stuart,[186] who originated the approach. As he states: "Unfortunately the effective limits of this approach are unknown at present. We do not know whether it will meet the needs of the grossly obese, for example." Again, this points up the need to characterize and classify as well as possible the patient entering into such studies before this question can be answered.

Endocrine and Drug Therapy

The possible role of thyroid hormone in the management of obesity has been discussed above under Energy Balance.

The use of chorionic gonadotrophin, a Phoenix-like treatment that refuses to die, has been critically reviewed by Albrink.[187] A prospective randomized study showed an apparent efficacy, but on further statistical analysis of the data the highest statistical correlation is found between the number of injections of either placebo or test substance and the weight lost.[188]

Asher[189] has summarized the various direct and indirect benefits of the use of anorectic agents in the logistics of treating obesity. The statistical evaluations of the various agents and the difficulties of meaningfully conducting such clinical trials have been critically reviewed by Garrow,[1] who concludes: "These trials demonstrate that it is possible to promote significant weight loss by anorectic drugs, but that the effect is not lasting." All of the amphetamine derivatives have been placed in classes II and III by the Federal Drug Agency and the Drug Enforcement Administration, with the exception of fenfluramine, which is in class IV. While amphetamines and derivatives present problems as "uppers," modifications of the molecule have produced in fenfluramine a "downer" with a high incidence of serious depression, particularly following withdrawal. Development of the latter drug has shown that it is possible to dissociate the stimulatory action of this group of drugs from the appetite suppressing, and it is hoped that in the future even more specific appetite suppressants may be developed. However, like the use of oral hypoglycemic agents in diabetes or of drugs for treatment of hypertension in the overweight, they carry the hazard that they may be used as substitutes for other options of treatment that are more effective on a long-term basis. In view of the lack of proven long-term efficacy, risk of addiction, and considerable side reactions and expense, their cost–benefit ratio must be carefully evaluated for each patient.

Jejunal Bypass

Intestinal bypass surgery for the severe, refractory forms of obesity is a potentially and sometimes dramatically helpful measure that is currently being evaluated. It is of interest that in successful cases, although diarrhea does not appear to be the inhibiting factor, appetite may be in abeyance in the presence of relative weight loss and relative starvation.[190] Discussion of the pros and potentially serious cons of this procedure are beyond the scope of this chapter; the reader is referred to other sources.[191]

MANAGEMENT OF OBESITY COMPLICATED BY DIABETES OR HYPERTENSION

Obesity and Diabetes

One of the most serious problems in relation to obesity is its association with diabetes, either as an integral part of the syndrome or as a precipitating factor in those who are genetically predisposed. The management of the non-insulin-dependent, nonketosis-prone obese diabetic, whether the diabetes is of juvenile or adult onset, is quite different from that of the insulin dependent.

Over 90 percent of adult onset diabetics are obese, and perhaps 50 percent are seriously obese. As we have seen, obesity is associated with insulin resistance, which may either precipitate or aggravate existing diabetes, and presumably may increase the likelihood of its progressing to an insulin-dependent stage. There is also evidence, cited above, that obesity may be a risk factor for cardiovascular disease, either directly or indirectly. Yet the majority of treatment programs elected for the group of patients with obesity and diabetes have served mainly to make them fatter. This is not surprising, since a major role of insulin is that of a storage hormone.

Consideration of the optimal treatment has recently been dominated by the controversy arising from the University Group Diabetes Project (UGDP) of the U.S. National Institutes of Health regarding the effects of various treatments for adult-onset diabetes.[192] Controversy has centered around the finding of increased cardiovascular mortality in those who took a sulfonylurea drug. This increase only amounts to approximately a 1 percent increase in mortality. Meanwhile, other results of the study that may be much more important in the long run have been overlooked. These results include the following:

Sulfonylurea Drugs. Sulfonylurea drugs may act mainly through increasing the release of insulin. They add to the hyperinsulinemia of spontaneous obesity, and insulin has been shown to reduce its own receptors through negative cooperativity, as described above. This may explain why, after the initial drop in weight shared by all treatment groups, those taking tolbutamide increased their weight by approximately 8 percent.[192]

Phenformin. Since phenformin does not increase insulin secretion, it was hoped that it might favor weight loss. However, the phenformin group fared no better than the placebo group in this respect.[193] There was an increase in both total and cardiovascular mortality.

Insulin. Many have mistakenly interpreted the lesson to be learned from the UGDP study as follows: "If diet alone fails, turn to insulin." However, insulin is contraindicated for the obese diabetic except in those cases in which pancreatic reserve has become irretrievably exhausted or in which every attempt at weight reduction has failed. In the UGDP study, both fixed and variable doses of insulin were associated with a gain in weight above the initial value; this in turn presumably led to a higher degree of insulin resistance.

The five treatment options selected initially by the UGDP investigators represented the prevailing options of symptomatic treatment in 1960. They did not include the newer options for treatment such as behavioral self-modification programs, in which patterns of both eating and exercising are altered, and the use of modified fasts. The critical point is that these newer options, vigorously applied, have the capability of reversing the overt diabetic state. The chief health hazard of the oral agents may be not the increased risk of cardiovascular death, but the fact that their availability draws attention away from the measures that can bring about long-lasting improvement in the quality of the patient's life. It is estimated that, at the time of writing, 1,500,000 diabetics, of whom some 1,300,000 are probably overweight, are being given an oral agent. Increasing numbers of clinics and individuals are finding that diabetes combined with obesity can best be treated without oral agents. The largest public clinic for diabetics in the

United States, at the Grady Memorial Hospital in Atlanta, has had over 3 years of experience with alternative treatment.[172] Sixty percent of patients being given oral agents had no increase in blood sugar when these agents were discontinued. With an intensified program of education, including 25 h of individual and group instruction, it was possible to discontinue insulin therapy as well for essentially all patients who were above ideal body weight. Admittedly, by the time they come to see us, patients with non–insulin–dependent diabetes usually have advanced obesity and diminished capacity for physical activity. Ideally, rehabilitative efforts for those at risk should be started much earlier in life.

Obesity and Hypertension

Obesity in general is quite frequently associated with hypertension,[7] but whether it is an important determinant of hypertension is a matter of debate.[10a,23,24] Essentially no attention has been given to the study of the relationship between the various types of obesity and hypertension. It is an unsubstantiated clinical impression that adult-onset obesity of the "cushingoid" variety, with more central deposition of fat, is more commonly associated with hypertension and is in turn commonly associated with the risk factors of hyperlipidemia and diabetes.

A reasonable goal of treatment would be to reduce the associated risk factors at the time the blood pressure is brought down. However, it is quite common to see patients whose hypertension is "well controlled" through use of diuretics or more potent antihypertensive agents who are still hyperlipidemic or insulin resistant. It is well known that an aggressive effort to achieve weight loss, whether by a diet of rice, as one extreme, or the currently popular protein-sparing fasts as the other, may often restore blood pressure to normal. Starvation or semistarvation may exert its antihypertensive effect by a number of mechanisms. These include limitation of sodium intake and reduced sensitivity to mineralocorticoids. Another possible mechanism may involve diminished production of T_3 from T_4, which occurs in starvation[143] or during reduced intake of carbohydrate.[141a] As noted above, T_3 has been shown to modulate the number of β-adrenergic receptors[143b] and hence could affect blood pressure through altering sensitivity to catecholamines. If an aggressive regimen of protein-sparing starvation is used as an adjunct in the management of the obese hypertensive or diabetic obese hypertensive patient, it is possible to discontinue diuretics at the start, and very often to discontinue other antihypertensive agents later.[183a]

The priorities for research in this important area of public health have recently been assessed by the Hypertension Task Force of the National Institutes of Health.[183b] There is a close parallel between the options available for the treatment of diabetes and those available for management of hypertension in the overweight patient. Just as the use of sulfonylurea drugs or insulin may be inappropriate and counterproductive for treatment of the overweight diabetic, the pharmaceutical approach to management of hypertension in the overweight may be equally inappropriate. If a total program of physical rehabilitation through revision of diet and weight loss can reverse the hypertension, it is inappropriate to use diuretics and antihypertensives, particularly if they merely lower the blood pressure and do not correct the other risk factors for cardiovascular disease.

PREVENTION OF OBESITY

Obesity is a family problem in several ways. It occurs in families with a history of obesity and has a strong genetic component. The family unit also reflects the culture of the times in its habits of eating, physical activity, work, and recreation, and provides the environmental influences that may promote obesity. Treatment, to be effective, usually involves changes in life style both for the obese individual and the surrounding family. Unfortunately, it is a fact of life that our present system of health care does not foster the care of entire families, or reward attention to preventive measures. It seems as if there is no way to make the time available for outreach, and no method of prepayment that includes the cost of patient education. However, in the case of obesity, the methods and approaches for treatment and prevention go hand in hand.

The physician treating an obese person must look at family history along with other factors in order to classify the type of obesity he is dealing with. He has a corresponding opportunity to involve the patient's family in revising habits of nutrition and physical activity. It is quite possible that physicians who use their opportunities for preventive education effectively can do a great deal to reduce the incidence of obesity, particularly that of the hypertrophic type. The dental profession has waged a successful war against dental caries in the last decade by emphasizing simple daily routines of hygiene and nutrition for all members of families under their care.

In regard to the culture of our times, we have been subjected to a successful involuntary program of behavior modification for the last 30 years by the availability and advertising of activity-sparing technology and the continual access to food. We have been eating more than we need to and moving our bodies less than we were designed to do. The media do all they can to promote overeating of carbohydrate-rich foods and to maintain the sedentary habits of their clientele. However, recently the physician has had some unexpected allies in the public's renewed interest in food of good quality and reasonable cost and in physical fitness. Even Madison Avenue has taken note of this trend and now couples its promotion of soft drinks with pictures of people energetically engaged in sports. Schools have increased their emphasis on sports that can be continued throughout life, such as cross-country skiing, swimming, tennis and hiking, instead of competitive team sports that cater to the athletically endowed adolescents who need them least.

The two major common types of obesity are best considered separately with respect to possible prevention, although many of the same principles apply to both.

HYPERPLASTIC–HYPERTROPHIC OBESITY

The hyperplastic–hypertrophic obesity, predominantly of juvenile onset, is often of massive proportions and resistant to permanent correction. To be in any way effective, preventive measures must be directed early in their lives to those at risk. Close attention to a family history of obesity and development of overweight in childhood aids in identifying this population.

In our present state of knowledge, we cannot say whether the course of obesity in childhood can be effectively moderated by restricting infant nutrition. Laboratory experience with such an attempt in the Zucker rat, subject to hyperplastic obesity, suggest that it is limited to effect.[42] However, a retrospective study of the incidence of obesity in later years in those who survived a period of famine in Holland during the Second World War indicated that those who were restricted in calories between birth and 6 months of age were significantly affected, but older age groups were not.[183c] Another consideration is that a serious attempt to apply a nutritional strait jacket to the very young could affect other development adversely. Grinker et al.[194] have described the adverse psychologic reactions that may result from such an attempt.

Nevertheless, at least the gross overfeeding typical of our culture can be avoided. A fat baby is not necessarily a healthy baby. Hirsch has suggested that mothers can learn to be better signal detectors. Does a baby's crying and restlessness indicate true hunger calling for feeding or other forms of distress?

For the child who develops early obesity, the last major opportunity to intervene effectively may be in the preadolescent period. In order to be effective, such intervention probably must be far-reaching enough to affect the total family way of life in such a way as to increase the general level of daily activity while modifying eating habits. Dwyer and Mayer[195] have found on follow-up that an intervention program designed to increase physical activity of obese schoolgirls had minimal long-term effect. Decreased physical activity in such girls has been well documented, but this may not be the basic problem. Bradfield et al.[196] found that obese schoolgirls in California spent 70 percent of their time at minimal activity, but he also found that their friends were equally inactive.

During young adult years, the contraceptive pill should not be given to those with a tendency toward obesity unless there is a clear understanding of the consequences and acceptance of a program designed to compensate. Similarly, use of those tranquilizers that promote weight gain, such as the phenthiazine derivatives, should be avoided, particularly in combination with the contraceptive pill.

Pregnancy is normally followed by weight gain, and in the obese a succession of pregnancies may lead to increases in weight by giant steps. Again, such consequences can be mitigated by effective education, delineating goals and responsibilities. Since some pregnant women are subject to reactive hypoglycemia and intense hunger, attention should be given to providing frequent feedings with a relative reduction in carbohydrate to minimize this effect.

HYPERTROPHIC ADULT-ONSET OBESITY

It is in this type of obesity that the greatest impact can be made through preventive and corrective measures. In theory, we should be able to prevent almost all of it. This disorder is more potentially reversible than the preceding one and there is a greater association with secondary metabolic disorder. There is predominantly adipocyte enlargement; thus to achieve weight reduction it may only be necessary to achieve normality of cell size. There is predominantly central deposition of fat; this is associated with a greater incidence of disorders of carbohydrate and lipid metabolism.[96] By attacking the obesity, an important impact can be made upon the major and increasing public health problem of diabetes.

It is certain that genetically predisposed individuals will have to reckon with their tendency to gain weight throughout the course of their lives.

As outlined above, prevention consists mainly of helping a patient to understand and accept a lifelong limitation. To live successfully with it requires changes in habits and responsibility on the part of the patient to monitor continuously one of the most personal aspects of daily life. It is important that therapeutic programs be tailored to meet the individual patient's needs and that patients be made aware of the options open to them and be encouraged to take part in choosing a way to live with susceptibility to weight gain. If they share as much as possible in developing their life plan, they will feel rewarded when it works for them. In a relationship of this sort, there will be no place for accusing the patient of cheating when things go wrong.

Obviously, an additional requirement for effective preventive measures is good habits of communication between pediatricians, internists, obstetricians, and mental health personnel. Hopefully, it will become easier to exchange professional knowledge and information about specific patients as we learn to apply modern communications technology to improve records. Hopefully, it also will not be long before health insurance will cover the costs of patient education.

REFERENCES

1. Garrow, J. S.: Energy Balance and Obesity in Man. New York, American Elsevier, (ed): 1974.
2. Bray, G. A. (ed): Obesity in Perspective, Fogarty International Series on Preventive Medicine, Vol 2, Parts 1 and 2. Washington, DC, US Government Printing Office, 1975.

2a. James, W. P. T. (Scientific Secretary of the Working Group): Report on Obesity. London, Her Majesty's Stationary Office.

3. Burland, W. L., Samuel, P. D., Yudkin, J.: Obesity Symposium: Proceedings of the Servier Research Institute Symposium. Edinburgh, Churchill Livingstone, 1974.
4. Vague, J., Boyer, J., Addison, G. M.: The Regulation of the Adipose Tissue Mass. Proceedings of the IV International Meeting of Endocrinology, Marseille, July 10–12, 1973. Amsterdam, Excerpta Medica, 1974.
5. Howard, A. (ed): Recent Advances in Obesity Research: Proceedings of the 1st International Congress on Obesity, Royal College of Physicians. London, Newman, 1975.
6. Jequier, E. (ed): Regulation of Energy Balance in Man: 2nd Congress, Lausanne, March 14–16, 1974. Geneva, Editions Médecine et Hygiènes, 1975.
7. Bray, G. A.: The Obese Patient, Vol. IX. In Smith, L. H., Jr. (ed): Major Problems in Internal Medicine. Philadelphia, W. B. Saunders, 1976.
8. Jeanrenaud, B., Hepp, D. (eds): Adipose Tissue: Regulation and Metabolic Functions. New York, Academic Press, 1970.
9. Mayer, J.: Inactivity as a Major Factor in Adolescent Obesity. *J Ann Acad Sci 131:* 502, 1965.
10. Keys, A.: Overweight and the Risk of Heart Attack and Sudden Death. In Bray, G. A. (ed): Obesity in Perspective, Fogarty International Series on Preventive Medicine, vol 2, part 2. Washington, DC, US Government Printing Office, 1975, p 215.

10a. Weinsier, R. L., Fuchs, R. J., Kay, T. D., Triebwasser, J. H., Lancaster, M. C.: Body Fat: Its Relationship to Coronary Heart Disease, Blood Pressure, Lipids and Other Risk Factors Measured in a Large Male Population. *Am J Med 61:* 815, 1976.

11. Seltzer, C. C.: Limitation of Height–Weight Standards (Insurance Company Tables). *N Engl J Med 272:* 1132, 1965.
12. Hirsch, J., Knittle, L. J., Salans, L. B.: Cell Lipid Content and Cell Number in Obese and Non-Obese Human Adipose Tissue. *J Clin Invest 45:* 1023, 1966.
13. Vague, J., Boyer, J., Jubelin, J., et al: Adipomuscular Ratio in Human Subjects. In Vague J (ed): Proceedings of the 3rd International Meeting of Endocrinologists, Marseille, 1968. *Amsterdam, Excerpta Medica,* 1969, p 363.
14. Naeye, R. L., Roode, P.: The Sizes and Numbers of Cells in Visceral Organs in Human Obesity. *Am J Clin Pathol 54:* 251, 1970.
15. Grande, F.: The Assessment of Body Fat in Man. In Bray, G. A. (ed): Obesity in Perspective, Fogarty International Center Series on Preventive Medicine, vol 2, part 2. Washington, DC, US Government Printing Office, 1975, p 189.
16. Durnin, J. V. G. A., Womersley, J.: Body Fat Assessed from Total Body Density and Its Estimation from Skinfold Thickness: Measurement on 481 Men and Women Aged from 16 to 72 Years. *Br J Nutr 32:* 77, 1974.
17. Seltzer, C. C., Mayer, J.: A Simple Criterion of Obesity. *Postgrad Med 38:* A-101, 1965.
18. Lesser, G. T., Deutsch, S., Markofsky, J.: Use of Independent Measurement of Body Fat to Evaluate Overweight and Underweight. *Metabolism 20:* 792, 1971.
19. Irsigler, K., Heitkamp, J., Schlick, W., Schmid, P.: Diet and Energy-Balance in Obesity. (A Methodological Approach). In Jequier, E. (ed): Regulation du Bilan d'Energie chez l'Homme. Geneva, Editions Medecine et Hygiene, 1975, p 72.
20. Karpinos, B. D.: Current Weight–Height Relationships of Youths of Military Age. *J Am Statis Assoc 57:* 895, 1962.

21. Preliminary Findings of the First Health and Nutrition Examination Survey, United States, 1971–1972: Dietary Intake and Biochemical Findings. Rockville, Md, US Public Health Service, Health Resources Administration, National Center for Health Statistics, Publ. No. HRA 74-1219-1, 1974.
22. Bennion, L. J., Grundy, S. M.: Effects of Obesity and Caloric Intake on Biliary Lipid Metabolism in Man. *J Clin Invest 56:* 996, 1975.
23. Mann, G. V.: The Influence of Obesity on Health. *N Engl J Med 291:* 178, 226, 1974.
24. Kannel, W. B., Gordon, R.: Obesity and Cardiovascular Disease. The Framingham Study. In Burland, W. L., Samuel, P. D., Judkin, J. (eds): Obesity Symposium, Proceedings of a Servier Research Institute Symposium held in December 1973. Edinburgh, Churchill Livingstone, 1974, p 24.
25. Seltzer, C. C.: Some Re-evaluations of the Build and Blood Pressure Study, 1959 as Related to Ponderal Index, Somatotype and Mortality. *N Engl J Med 274:* 254, 1966.
26. Dublin, L. I.: Relation of Obesity to Longevity. *N Engl J Med 248:* 971, 1953.
27. Bray, G. A., York, D. A.: Genetically Transmitted Obesity in Rodents, *Physiol Rev 51:* 598, 1971.
28. A Classification of the Obesities. In Bray, G. A. (ed): Fogarty International Center Series on Preventive Medicine, vol 2, part 1. Washington, DC US Government Printing Office, 1975, p 13.
29. Bjurulf, P.: Atherosclerosis and Body Build with Special Reference to Size and Number of Subcutaneous Fat Cells. *Acta Med Scand* [*Supp*] *349:* 1, 1959.
30. Hirsch, J., Knittle, J. L.: Cellularity of Obese and Nonobese Human Adipose Tissue. *Fed Proc 29:* 1516, 1970.
31. Hirsch, J., Batchelor, B.: Adipose Tissue Cellularity in Human Obesity. *Clin Endocrinol Metab 5:* 299, 1976.
32. Bray, G. A., Jordan, H. A., Sims, E. A. H.: Evaluation of the Obese Patient. I. An Algoritm. *JAMA 235:* 1487, 1976.
33. Widdowson, E. M., Shaw, W. T.: Full and Empty Fat Cells. *Lancet 2:* 905, 1973.
34. Cheek, D. B., Schultz, R. B., Parra, A., Rebay, R. T. C.: Overgrowth of Lean and Adipose Tissues in Adolescent Obesity. *Pediatr Res 4:* 268, 1970.
35. Hirsch, J., Gallian, E.: Methods for the Determination of Adipose Tissue Cell Size in Man and Animals. *J Lipid Res 9:* 110, 1968.
36. Bray, G. A.: Measurement of Subcutaneous Fat Cells from Obese Patients. *Ann Intern Med 73:* 565, 1970.
37. Sjöstrom, L., Smith, U., Krotkiewski, M., Björntrop, P.: Cellularity in Different Regions of Adipose Tissue in Young Men and Women. *Metabolism 21:* 1143, 1972.
38. Van, R. R. L., Bayliss, C. E., Roncari, D. A. K.: Cytological and Enzymological Characterization of an Adipocyte Precursor Pool Found in Adult Man. *Clin Res 23:* 334A, 1975.
39. Poznanski, W. J., Rushton, J., Waheed, I.: The Origin and Metamorphosis of the Human Fat Cell. In Vague, J., Boyer, J., Addison, G. M. (eds): The Regulation of the Adipose Tissue Mass, Proceedings of the 4th International Meeting of Endocrinology, Marseille, 1973. *Amsterdam, Excerpta Medica,* 1974, p 145.
40. Salans, L. B., Cushman, S. W., Weisman, R. E.: Studies of Human Adipose Tissue. Adipose Cell Size and Number in Nonobese and Obese Patients. *J Clin Invest 52:* 929, 1973.
41. Lemonnier, D., Alexiu, A.: Nutritional, Genetic and Hormonal Aspects of Adipose Tissue Cellularity. In Vague, J., Boyer, J., Addison, G. M. (eds): The Regulation of the Adipose Tissue Mass, Proceedings of the 4th International Meeting of Endocrinology, Marseille, 1973. Amsterdam, Excerpta Medica, 1974, p 159.
42. Johnson, P. R., Stern, J. S., Greenwood, M. R. C., Zucker, L. M., and Hirsch, J.: Effect of Early Nutrition on Adipose Cellularity and Pancreatic Insulin Release in the Zucker Rat. *J Nutr 103:* 738, 1973.
43. Salans, L. B., Zarnowski, M. J., Segal, R.: Effect of Insulin upon the Cellular Character of Adipose Tissue. *J Lipid Res 13:* 616, 1972.
44. Hollenberg, C. H., Vost, A.: Nutritional and Hormonal Regulation of DNA Synthesis in Rat Adipose Tissue. In Jeanrenaud, B., Hepp, D. (eds): Adipose Tissue: Regulation and Metabolic Functions. New York, Academic Press, 1970, p 125.
45. Therriault, D. G., Mellin, D. B.: Cellularity of Adipose Tissue in Cold-Exposed Rats and the Calorigenic Effect of Norepinephrine. *Lipids 6:* 486, 1971.
46. Rathbun, L., Tulp, O. L., and Sims, E. A. H.: Growth and Adipose Tissue Development in Cold-Adapted Rats. *Clin Res,* 1978, in press.
47. Oscai, L. G., Babirak, S. P., McGarr, J. A., Spirakis, C. N.: Effect of Exercise on Adipose Tissue Cellularity. *Fed Proc 33:* 1956, 1974.
48. Young, R. A.: The Woodchuck, *Marmota Monax,* as a Biomedical Model for the Study of Obesity. Ph.D. Dissertation, University of Vermont, May, 1975.
49. Young, R. A.: Unpublished Observations.
50. Sims, E. A. H., Danforth, E. Jr., Horton, E. S., Bray, G. A., Glennon, J. A., Salans, L. B.: Endocrine and Metabolic Effects of Experimental Obesity in Man. Recent *Prog Horm Res 29:* 457, 1973.
51. Salans, L. B., Horton, E. S., Sims, E. A. H.: Experimental Obesity in Man: Cellular Character of the Adipose Tissue. *J Clin Invest 50:* 1005, 1971.
52. Brook, C. G. D., Lloyd, J. K., Wolf, O. H.: Relation Between Age of Onset of Obesity and Size and Number of Adipose Cells. *Br Med J 2:* 25, 1972.
53. Allon, N.: The Stigma of Overweight in Everyday Life. In Bray, G. A. (ed): Obesity in Perspective, Fogarty International Series on Preventive Medicine, vol 2, part 2. Washington, DC, US Government Printing Office, 1975, p 83.
54. Seltzer, C. C.: Genetics and Obesity. In Vague, J. (ed): Pathophysiology of Adipose Tissue, Proceedings of the Third International Meeting of Endocrinology, Marseille, 1968. *Amsterdam, Excerpta Medica,* 1974, p 325.
55. Newman, H. H., Freeman, F. N., Holzinger, K. J.: Twins: Study of Heredity and Environment. Chicago, University of Chicago Press, 1937, p 72.
56. Withers, R. F. J.: Problems in the Genetics of Human Obesity. *Eugen Rev 56:* 81, 1964.
57. Withers, R. F. J.: Personal Communication.
58. Genuth, S. M., Przybylski, R. J., Rosenberg, D. M.: Insulin Resistance in Genetically Obese, Hyperglycemic Mice. *Endocrinology 88:* 1230, 1971.
59. Pelkonen, R., Taskinen, M. R., Nikkilä, E. A.: Early Response to Plasma Insulin to Small Doses of Intravenous Glucose: Effect of Obesity. *J Clin Endocrinol Metab 39:* 418, 1974.
60. Karam, J. H., Grodsky, G. M., Ching, K. N., Schmid, F. T., Burvill, K. T., Forsham, P. H.: "Staircase" Glucose Stimulation of Insulin Secretion in Obesity. *Diabetes 23:* 763, 1974.
61. Perley, M. J., Kipnis, D. M.: Plasma Insulin Response to Oral and Intravenous Glucose: Studies in Normal and Diabetic Subjects. *J Clin Invest 46:* 1954, 1967.
62. Rabinowitz, D.: Some Endocrine and Metabolic Aspects of Obesity. *Annu Rev Med 21:* 241, 1970.
63. Mahler, R. J.: The Pathogenesis of Pancreatic Islet Cell Hyperplasia and Insulin Insensitivity in Obesity. *Adv Metab Disord 7:* 213, 1974.
64. Rabinowitz, D., Zierler, K. L.: Forearm Metabolism in Obesity and Its Response to Intra-arterial Insulin. Characterization of Insulin Resistance and Evidence for Adaptive Hyperinsulinism. *J Clin Invest 41:* 2173, 1962.
65. Horton, E. S., Runge, C. F., Sims, E. A. H.: Forearm Metabolism in Human Experimental Obesity. *J Clin Invest 49:* 45a, 1970 (abstract).
66. Felig, P., Wahren, J., Hendler, R., Brundin, T.: Splanchnic Glucose and Amino Acid Metabolism in Obesity. *J Clin Invest 53:* 582, 1974.
67. Soll, A. H., Kahn, C. R., Neville, D. M. Jr., Roth, J.: Insulin Receptor Deficiency in Genetic and Acquired Obesity. *J Clin Invest 56:* 769, 1975.
68. Kalkhoff, R. K., Kimm, H. J., Cerletty, J., Ferrou, C. A.: Metabolic Effects of Weight Loss in Obese Subjects. Changes in Plasma Substrate Levels, Insulin and Growth Hormone Responses. *Diabetes 20:* 83, 1971.
69. Sims, E. A. H., Danforth, E. Jr.: The Role of Insulin in Obesity. *Isr J Med Sci 10:* 1222, 1974.
70. Felig, P., Horton, E. S., Runge, C. F., Sims, E. A. H.: Experimental Obesity in Man: Hyperaminoacidemia and Diminished Effectiveness of Insulin in Regulating Peripheral Amino Acid Release. Program of the 53rd Meeting, Endocrine Society, June, 1971 (abstract 29).
71. O'Connell, M., Danforth, E. Jr., Horton, E. S., Salans, L. B., Sims, E. A. H.: Experimental Obesity in Man. III. Adrenocortical Function. *J Clin Endocrinol Metab 36:* 323, 1973.
72. Gossain, V. V., Matute, M. L., Kalkhoff, R. K.: Relative Influence of Obesity and Diabetes on Plasma Alpha-Cell Glucagon. *J Clin Endocrinol Metab 38:* 238, 1974.

73. Wise, J. K., Hendler, R., Felig, P.: Evaluation of Alpha-Cell Function by Infusion of Alanine in Normal, Diabetic and Obese Subjects. *N Engl J Med 288:* 487, 1973.
74. Meier, A. H.: Prolactin, the Liporegulatory Hormone. In Dellmann, H. D., Johnson, J. A., and Klachko, D. M. (eds): Comparative Endocrinology of Prolactin. New York, Plenum Press, 1977.
75. Joseph, M. M., Meier, A. H.: Circadian Component in the Fattening and Reproductive Responses to Prolactin in the Hamster. *Proc Soc Exp Biol Med 146:* 1150, 1974.
76. Goodridge, A. G., Ball, E. G.: The Effect of Prolaction on Lipogenesis in the Pigeon. *In Vivo* Studies. *Biochemistry 6:* 1676, 1682, 1967.
77. Zinder, O., Bray, G. A.: Lipoprotein Lipase Activity in Human Adipose Tissue in Obesity. In Bray, G. A. (ed): Obesity in Perspective, Fogarty International Center Series on Preventive Medicine, vol 2, part 2. Washington, DC, US Government Printing Office, 1975, p 263.
78. Copinschi, G., L'Hermite, M., Leclercq, R., Virasoro, E., Robyn, C.: Prolactin Release After Insulin-Induced Hypoglycemia in Obese Subjects. In Vague, J., Boyer, J., Addison, G. M. (eds): The Regulation of the Adipose Tissue Mass, Proceedings of the 4th International Meeting of Endocrinology, Marseille, 1973. Amsterdam, Excerpta Medica, 1974, p 288.
79. Goldrick, R. B., McLoughlin, G. M.: Lipolysis and Lipogenesis from Glucose in Human Fat Cells of Different Sizes. Effects of Insulin, Epinephrine, and Theophylline. *J Clin Invest 49:* 1213, 1970.
80. Salans, L. B., Dougherty, J. W.: The Effect of Insulin upon Glucose Metabolism by Adipose Cells of Different Size. Influence of Cell Lipid and Protein Content, Age, and Nutritional State. *J Clin Invest 50:* 1399, 1971.
81. Salans, L. B., Cushman, S. W., Horton, E. S., Danforth, E. Jr., Sims, E. A. H.: Hormones and the Adipocyte: Factors Influencing the Metabolic Effects of Insulin and Adrenaline. In Bray, G. A. (ed): Obesity in Perspective, Fogarty International Series on Preventive Medicine, vol 2, part 2. Washington, DC, US Government Printing Office, 1975, p 204
82. Curtis-Prior, P. B.: Prostaglandins and Obesity. *Lancet 1:* 897, 1975.
83. Archer, J. A., Gorden, P., Roth, J.: Defect in Insulin Binding to Receptors in Obese Man. Amelioration with Caloric Restriction. *J Clin Invest 55:* 166, 1975.
84. Amatruda, J. M., Livingston, J. N., Lockwood, D. H.: Insulin Receptor: Role in the Resistance of Human Obesity to Insulin. *Science 188:* 264, 1975.
85. Olefsky, J. M.: Decreased Insulin Binding to Adipocytes and Circulating Monocytes from Obese Subjects. *J Clin Invest 47:* 1165, 1976.
86. Cushman, S. W., Salans, L. B.: Effects of Adipose Cell Size on Modulation of Epinephrine Response by Extracellular Fatty Acid Accumulation. *Fed Proc 34:* 939, 1975 (abstract).
87. Albisser, A. M., Leibel, B. S., Ewart, T. G., Davidovac, Z., Botz, C. K., Zingg, W.: An Artifical Endocrine Pancreas. *Diabetes 23:* 389, 1974.
88. Albisser, A. M., Leibel, B. S., Ewart, T. G., Davidovac, Z., Botz, C. K., Zingg, W., Schipper, H., Ginder, R.: Clinical Control of Diabetes by the Artificial Pancreas. *Diabetes 23:* 397, 1974.
89. Cerasi, E., Luft, R.: Followup of Non-Diabetic Subjects with Normal and Decreased Insulin Response to Glucose Infusion (First Report). *Horm Metab Res* [*Suppl 5*]*:* 113, 1974.
90. Flatt, J. P.: Role of the Increased Adipose Tissue Mass in the Apparent Insulin Insensitivity of Obesity. *Am J Clin Nutr 25:* 1189, 1972.
91. Randle, P. J., Garland, P. B., Hales, C. N., Newsholme, E. A.: The Glucose–Fatty-Acid Cycle. Its Role in Insulin Sensitivity and the Metabolic Disturbances of Diabetes Mellitus. *Lancet 1:* 785, 1963.
92. Björntorp, P., Bergman, H., Varnauskas, E., Lindholm, B.: Lipid Mobilization in Relation to Body Composition in Man. *Metabolism 18:* 840, 1969.
93. Flatt, J. P.: Personal communication.
94. Nestel, P. J., Whyte, H. M.: Plasma Free Fatty Acid and Triglyceride Turnover in Obesity. *Metabolism 17:* 1122, 1968.
95. Gomez, F., Jéquier, E., Chabot, V., Büber, V., Felber, J. P.: Carbohydrate and Lipid Oxidation in Normal Human Subjects: Its Influence on Glucose Tolerance and Insulin Response to Glucose. *Metabolism 21:* 381, 1972.
96. Björntorp, P.: The Effects of Exercise in Human Obesity. In Burland, W. L., Samuel, P. D., Judkin, J. (eds): Obesity Symposium, Proceedings of the Servier Research Institute Symposium, December 1973. Edinburgh, Churchill Livingstone, 1974, p 171.
97. Fredrickson, D. S., Levy, R. I., Lees, R. S.: Fat Transport in Lipoproteins—An Integrated Approach to Mechanisms and Disorders. *N Engl J Med 276:* 34, 94, 148, 215, 273, 1967.
98. Brunzell, J. D., Hazzard, W. R., Motulsky, A. G., Bierman, E. L.: Evidence for Diabetes Mellitus and Genetic Forms of Hypertriglyceridemia as Independent Entities. *Metabolism 24:* 1115, 1975.
99. Farquhar, J. W., Olefsky, J., Stern, M., Reaven, G. M.: Obesity, Insulin, and Triglycerides. In Bray, G. A. (ed): Obesity in Perspective, Fogarty International Center Series on Preventive Medicine, vol 2, part 2. Washington, DC, US Government Printing Office, 1975, p 313.
100. Bagdade, J. D., Porte, D. Jr., Brunzell, J. D.: Basal and Stimulated Hyperinsulinism: Reversible Metabolic Sequelae of Obesity. *J Lab Clin Med 83:* 563, 1974.
101. Bagdade, J. D., Bierman, E. L., Porte, D. Jr.: Influence of Obesity on the Relationship Between Insulin and Triglyceride Levels in Endogenous Hypertriglyceridemia. *Diabetes 20:* 664, 1971.
102. Albrink, M. J., Meigs, J. W.: The Relationship Between Serum Triglycerides and Skinfold Thickness in Obese Subjects. *Ann NY Acad Sci 131:* 673, 1965.
103. Nestel, P. J., Schreibman, P. H., Ahrens, E. H. Jr.: Cholesterol Metabolism in Human Obesity. *J Clin Invest 52:* 2389, 1973.
104. Miettinen, T. A.: Cholesterol Production in Obesity. *Circulation 44:* 842, 1971.
105. Farkas, J., Angel, A., Avigan, M. I.: Studies on the Compartmentation of Lipid in Adipose Cells. II. Cholesterol Accumulation and Distribution in Adipose Tissue Components. *J Lipid Res 14:* 344, 1973.
106. Fishman, J., Boyar, R. M., Hellman, L.: Influence of Body Weight on Estradiol Metabolism in Young Women. *J Clin Endocrinol Metab 41:* 989, 1975.
107. Neumann, R. O.: Experimentelle Beigrage zur Lehre von dem täglichen Nahrungsbedarf des Menschen unter besonderer Berücksichtigung der Notwendigen Eiweissmenge. *Arch Hyg 45:* 1, 1902.
108. Rubner, M.: Die Gesetze des Energieverbrachs bei der Ernahrung Franz Deuticke Lipzig and Vienna: Markoff, A., Sandri-White, A., (transl), Joy, J. T. (ed). Natick, Mass, U.S. Army Research Institute of Environmental Medicine, 1968.
109. Gulick, A.: A Study of Weight Regulation in Adult Human Body During Overnutrition. *Am J Physiol 60:* 371, 1922.
110. Graefe, E.: Metabolic Diseases and Their Treatment. New York, Lea & Febiger, 1933, p 551.
111. Sims, E. A. H.: Experimental Obesity, Dietary Induced Thermogenesis and Their Clinical Implications in Obesity. *Clin Endocrinol Metab 5:* 377, 1976.
112. Ashworth, N., Hunt, J. N., Creedy, Makon, S., Newland, P.: Effect of Nightly Food Supplements on Food Intake in Man. *Lancet 2:* 685, 1962.
113. Miller, D. S., Mumford, P., Stock, M. J.: Gluttony. 2. Thermogenesis in Overeating Man. *Am J Clin Nutr 20:* 1223, 1967.
114. Goldman, R. F., Haisman, M. F., Bynum, G., Horton, E. S., Sims, E. A. H.: Experimental Obesity in Man: Metabolic Rate in Relation to Dietary Intake. In Bray, G. A. (ed): Obesity in Perspective, Fogarty International Center Series on Preventive Medicine, vol 2, part 2. Washington, DC, US Government Printing Office, 1975, p 165.
115. Hanson, J.: Exercise Responses Following Production of Experimental Obesity. *J Appl Physiol 35:* 587, 1973.
115a. Burse, R. L., Goldman, R. F., Danforth, E. Jr., Horton, E. S., Sims, E. A. H.: Effect of Excess Carbohydrate and Fat Intake on Resting Metabolism. *Fed Proc 36:* 1456, 1977.
115b. Burse, R. L., Goldman, R. F., Danforth, E. Jr., Robbins, D. C., Horton, E. S., Sims, E. A. H.: Effect of excess protein intake on metabolism *The Physiol 20:* 100, 1977.
116. Blaxter, K. L.: Energy Utilization and Obesity in Domesticated Animals. In Bray, G. A. (ed): Obesity in Perspective, Fogarty International Center Series on Preventive Medicine, vol 2, part 2. Washington, DC, US Government Printing Office, 1975, p 127.
117. Apfelbaum, M., Bostsarron, J., Lacatis, D.: Effect of Caloric Restriction and Excessive Caloric Intake on Energy Expenditure. *Am J Clin Nutr 24:* 1404, 1971.
118. Whipp, B. J., Bray, G. A., Koyal, S. N.: Exercise Energetics in

Normal Man Following Acute Weight Gain. *Am J Clin Nutr 26:* 1284, 1973.

119. Horton, E. S., Danforth, E. Jr., Sims, E. A. H., Salans, L. B.: Endocrine and Metabolic Alterations in Spontaneous and Experimental Obesity. In Bray, G. A. (ed): Obesity in Perspective, Fogarty International Center Series on Preventive Medicine, vol 2, part 5. Washington, DC, US Government Printing Office, 1976, p 323.
120. Hochachka, P. W.: Regulation of Heat Production at the Cellular Level. *Fed Proc 33:* 2162, 1974.
121. Himms-Hagen, J.: Cellular Thermogenesis. *Annu Rev Physiol 38:* 315, 1976.
122. Clarke, M. G., Bloxham, D. P., Holland, P. C., Lardy, H. A.: Estimation of the Fructose–Diphosphatase–Phosphofructokinase Substrate Cycle in the Flight Muscle of *Bombus affinis. Biochem J 134:* 589, 1973.
123. Hegsted, D. M.: Energy Needs and Energy Utilization. *Nutr Rev 32:* 33, 1974.
124. Stirling, J. L., Stock, M. J.: Non-conservative Mechanisms of Energy Metabolism in Thermogenesis. In Apfelbaum, M. (ed): Energy Balance in Man. Paris, Masson, 1973, p 219.
125. Hill, F. W. (ed): Energy Costs of Intermediary Metabolism in the Intact Animal. *Fed Proc 30:* 1434, 1971.
125a. Kinney, J. M. (ed): Assessment of Energy Metabolism in Health and Disease, 1st Ross Conf on Medical Research, June 25–28, 1978 (in press).
126. Apfelbaum, M. (ed): Energy Balance in Man. Paris, Masson, 1973.
127. Smith, R. E., Hoijer, D. J.: Metabolism and Cellular Function in Cold Acclimation. *Physiol Rev 42:* 60, 1962.
128. Meerson, F. Z.: Role of Synthesis of Nucleic Acids and Protein in Adaptation to the External Environment. *Physiol Rev 55:* 79, 1975.
129. Ball, E. G.: Some Energy Relationships in Adipose Tissue Metabolism and Obesity. *Ann NY Acad Sci 131:* 225, 1965.
130. Galton, D. J., Bray, G. A.: Metabolism of α-Glycerol Phosphate in Human Adipose Tissue in Obesity. *J Clin Endocrinol 27:* 1573, 1967.
131. Stirling, J. L., Stock, M. J.: Metabolic Origins of Thermogenesis Induced by Diet. *Nature 220:* 801, 1968.
132. Tulp, O.L., Desilets, E. J., Danforth, E. Jr., Horton, E. S.: Increased Plasma Triiodothyronine (T3) Concentrations in Experimental Protein Malnutrition. *Clin Res 23:* 594A, 1975 (abstract).
133. Tainter, M. L., Stockton, A. B., Cutting, W. C.: Use of Nitrophenol in Obesity and Related Conditions. A Progress Report. *JAMA 101:* 1472, 1933.
134. Williamson, J. R., Jakob, A., Scholz, R. Energy Cost of Gluconeogenesis in Rat Liver. *Metabolism 20:* 13, 1971.
135. Krebs, H. A.: The Metabolic Fate of Amino Acids. In Munro, H. N., Allison, J. B. (eds): Mammalian Protein Metabolism, vol 1. New York, Academic, 1964, p 125.
136. Garrow, J. S., Hawes, S. F.: The Role of Amino Acid Oxidation in Causing "Specific Dynamic Action" in Man. *J Nutr 27:* 211, 1972.
137. Ashworth, A.: Metabolic Rates During Recovery from Protein-Calorie Malnutrition: The Need for a New Concept of Specific Dynamic Action. *Nature 223:* 407, 1969.
138. Fleagle, J. G., Samonds, K. W., Hegsted, D. M.: Physcial Growth of Cebus Monkeys, *Cebus albifrons,* During Protein and Calorie Deficiency. *Am J Clin Nut 28:* 246, 1975.
139. Miller, D. S.: Thermogenesis in Everyday Life. XXVI International Congress of Physiological Sciences, New Delhi, 1974 (abstract).
140. Ismail-Beigi, F., Edelman, I. S.: The Mechanism of the Calorigenic Action of Thyroid Hormone. Stimulation of Na^+—K^+-Activated Adenosinetriphosphatase Activity. *J Gen Physiol 57:* 710, 1971.
141. Danforth, E. Jr., Desilets, E. J., Horton, E. S., Sims, E. A. H., Burger, A. G., Braverman, L. E., Vagenakis, A. G., Ingbar, S. H.: Reciprocal Serum Triiodothyronine (T_3) and Reverse (rT_3) Induced by Altering the Carbohydrate Content of the Diet. *Clin Res 23:* 573A, 1975 (abstract).
141a. Danforth, E. Jr.: Hormonal Interrelationships in Response to Carbohydrate-Free Isocaloric Diets in Normal Man. *Diabetes 20:* 343, 1971.
142. Chopra, I. J.: Study of Extrathyroidal Conversion of T4 to T3 in Vitro: Evidence that Reverse T_3 is a Potent Inhibitor of T_3 Production. *Clin Res 24:* 142A, 1976 (abstract).
143. Portnay, G. I., O'Brian, J. T., Bush, J., Vagenskis, A. G., Azizi, F., Arky, R., Ingbar, S. H., Braverman, L. E.: Effects of Prolonged Starvation on Serum TSH, T4 and T3 Concentration in Man. *Clin Res 21:* 958, 1973.
143a. Danforth, E. Jr.: Increased Triiodothyronine (T_3) Metabolic Clearance Rate During Overnutrition. XIth Acta Endocrinologica Congress, Lausanne, June 19–23, 1977 (abstract).
143b. Williams, L. T., Leftkowitz, R. J., Watanabe, A. M., Hathaway, D. R., Besch, H. R. Jr.: Thyroid Hormone Regulation of Myocardial Beta-Adrenergic Receptor Number. *Clin Res 25:* 458, 1977.
144. Benedict, F. G.: A Study of Prolonged Fasting. Washington, DC, Carnegie Institution of Washington, Publ No 203, 1915.
145. Keys, A., Taylor, H. L., Grande, F.: Basal Metabolism and Age of Adult Man. *Metabolism 22:* 579, 1973.
145a. Keys, A., Brozek, J., Henschel, A., Mickelson, O., Taylor, H. L.: The Biology of Human Starvation. Minneapolis, University of Minnesota Press, 1950, p 1385.
146. Bray, G. A.: Effect of Caloric Restriction on Energy Expenditure in Obese Patients. *Lancet 2:* 397, 1969.
147. Miller, D. S., Parsonage, S.: Resistance to Slimming. Adaptation or Illusion. *Lancet 1:* 773, 1975.
147a. Kleiber, M.: The Fire of Life. New York, Krieger, 1975, pp 453.
148. Thomas, L.: The Lives of a Cell. New York, Viking, 1974.
148a. Danforth, E. Jr., Horton, E. S., and Sims, E. A. H.: Thyroid Hormone Metabolism and Thermogenesis in Spontaneous Obesity. 5th Internat Congress of Endocrin. Hamborg, Fed Rep of Germany, 1976.
149. Glauser, S. C., Glauser, E. M., Reidenberg, M. M., Rusy, B. F., Tallarida, R. T.: Metabolic Changes Associated with the Cessation of Cigarette Smoking. *Arch Environ Health 20:* 377, 1970.
150. Burse, R. L., Bynum, G. D., Pandolf, K. B., Goldman, R. F., Sims, E. A. H., Danforth, E. Jr.: Increased Appetite and Unchanged Metabolism upon Cessation of Smoking with Diet Held Constant. *Physiologist 18:* 157, 1975.(abstract).
151. Durnin, J. V. G. A., Edholm, O. G., Miller, D. S., Waterlou, J. C.: How Much Food Does Mean Require? *Nature, 242:* 418, 1973.
152. Novin, D., Wyrwicka, W., Bray, G. A. (eds): Hunger: Basic Mechanisms and Clinical Implications. New York, Raven. 1975.
153. Van Itallie, T. B., Smith, N. S., Quartermain, D.: Short-Term and Long-Term Components in the Regulation of Food Intake: Evidence for a Modulatory Role of Carbohydrate Status. *Am J Clin Nutr 30(5):* 742, 1977.
154. Koopmans, H. S.: Regulation of Food Intake During Long-Term Loss of Food From the Intestine of the Rat. *Proc Soc Expt Biol 157:* 480, 1978.
155. Sullivan, A. C., Triscari, J., Hamilton, J. G., Miller, U. N., Wheatley, V. R.: Effect of (−)-Hydroxycitrate upon the Accumulation of Lipid in the Rat. I. Lipogenesis. II. Appetite. *Lipids 9:* 121, 129, 1974.
156. Sullivan, A. C., Triscari, J.: Possible Interrelationship Between Metabolic Flux and Appetite. In Novin, D., Wyrwicka, W., Bray, G. A. (eds): Hunger: Basic Mechanisms and Clinical Implications. New York, Raven, 1975, p 115.
157. Niijima, A.: Afferent Impulse Discharges from Glucoreceptors in the Liver of the Guinea Pig. *Ann NY Acad Sci 157:* 690, 1969.
158. Brobeck, J. R.: Nature of Satiety Signals. *Am J Clin Nutr 28:* 806, 1975.
159. XXVI International Congress of Physiological Sciences on Physiology of Food and Fluid Intake. Jerusalem, October, 1974.
160. York, D. A., Bray, G. A.: Dependence of Hypothalamic Obesity on Insulin, the Pituitary, and the Adrenal Gland. *Endocrinology 90:* 885, 1972.
161. Bray, G. A. Gallagher, T. F. Jr.: Manifestations of Hypothalamic Obesity in Man: A Comprehensive Investigation of Eight Patients and a Review of the Literature. *Medicine 54:* 301, 1975.
162. Powley, T. L., Opsahl, C. A.: Ventromedial Hypothalamic Obesity Abolished by Subdiaphragmatic Vagotomy. *Am J Physiol 226:* 25, 1974.
163. Opsahl, C. A., Powley, T. L.: Failure of Vagotomy to Reverse Obesity in the Genetically Obese Zucker Rat. *Am J Physiol 226:* 34, 1974.
164. Galton, D. J., Gilbert, C., Reckless, J. F. D., Kaye, J.: Triglyceride Storage Disease: A Group of Inborn Errors of Triglyceride Metabolism. *Q J Med 43:* 63, 1974.
165. Wurtman, R. J., Fernstrom, J. D.: Effects of the Diet on Brain Neurotransmitters. *Nutr Rev 32:* 193, 1974.
166. Gibbs, J., Young, R. C., Smith, G. P.: Cholecystokinin Decreases Food Intake in Rats. *J Comp Physiol Psychol 84:* 488, 1973.

167. Goetz, H., Sturdevant, R.: Effect of Cholecystokinin on Food Intake in Man. *Clin Res 23:* 98A, 1975 (abstract).

168. Feinstein, A. R.: The Treatment of Obesity: An Analysis of Methods, Results and Factors Which Influence Success. *J Chronic Dis 11:* 349, 1960.

169. Björntorp, P., Bengtsson, C., Blohme, G., Jonsson, A., Sjöstrom, L., Tibblin, E., Tibblin, G., Wilhelmsen, L.: Adipose Tissue Fat Cell Size and Number in Relation to Metabolism in Randomly Selected Middle-aged Men and Women. *Metabolism 20:* 927, 1971.

170. Kalkhoff, R., Ferrou, C.: Metabolic Differences Between Obese Overweight and Muscular Overweight Men. *N Engl J Med 284:* 1236, 1971.

170a. Björntorp, P., Calgren, G., Isaksson, B., Krotkiewski, M., Larsson, B., and Sjöström, L.: Effect of an Energy-reduced Dietary Regimen in Relation to Adipose Tissue Cellularity in Obese Women. *Am J Clin Nut 28:* 45, 1975.

171. Bruch, H.: The Psychological Handicaps of the Obese. In Bray, G. A. (ed): Obesity in Perspective, Fogarty International Center Series on Preventive Medicine, vol 2, part 2. Washington, DC, US Government Printing Office, 1975, p 111.

172. Davidson, J. K.: Educating Diabetic Patients About Diet Therapy. *Int Diabetes Fed Bull 20:* 3, 1975.

173. Sims, D. F.: Cooperating Clients or Passive Recipients: The Suggestions of a Patient. In Steiner, G., Lawrence, P. (eds): The Education of the Diabetic (in press).

174. Bray, G. A.: Lipogenesis in Human Adipose Tissue: Some Effects of Nibbling and Gorging. *J Clin Invest 51:* 537, 1972.

175. Young, C. M., Hutter, L. F., Scanlan, S. S., Rand, C. E., Lutevak, L., Simko, V.: Metabolic Effects of Meal Frequency on Normal Young Men. *J Am Diet Assoc 61:* 391, 1972.

176. Mayer, J.: Overweight: Causes, Costs and Control. Englewood Cliffs, NJ, Prentice-Hall, 1968.

177. Hood, C. E. A., Goodhart, J. M., Fletcher, R. F., Gloster, J., Bertrand, P. V., Crooke, A. C.: Observations on Obese Patients Eating Isocaloric Reducing Diets with Varying Proportions of Carbohydrate. *Br J Nutr 24:* 39, 1970.

178. Apfelbaum, M., Bost-Sarron, J., Brigant, L., Dapen, H.: La Composition du Poids au Cours de la Diète Hydrique: Effets de la Supplèmentation Protidique. *Gastroenterologia 108:* 121, 1967.

179. Blackburn, G. L., Bistrian, B., Flatt, J. P.: Role of Protein-Sparing Starvation in Obesity. In Howard, A. (ed): Recent Advances in Obesity Research, Proceedings of the First International Congress on Obesity, 1974. London, Newman, 1975, p 279.

180. American Medical Association Council on Foods and Nutrition: A Critique of Low-Carbohydrate Ketogenic Weight-Reducing Regimens. *JAMA 224:* 1415, 1973.

181. Yang, M.-U., Van Itallie, T. B.: Composition of Weight Lost During Short-Term Weight Reduction. Metabolic Responses of Obese Subjects to Starvation and Low-Caloric Ketogenic and Non-Ketogenic Diets. *J Clin Invest 58:* 722, 1976.

182. Greenberg, G. R., Marliss, E. G., Anderson, G. H., Langer, B., Spence, W., Tovee, E. B., Jeegeebhoy, N. K.: Protein-Sparing Therapy: Effects of Added Hypocaloric Glucose or Lipid. *N Engl J Med 294:* 1411, 1976.

183. Bistrian, B. R., Blackburn, G. L., Flatt, J. P., Sizer, J., Scrimsaw, N. S., Sherman, M.: Nitrogen Metabolism and Insulin Requirements in Obese Diabetic Adults on a Protein-Sparing Modified Fast. *Diabetes 25:* 494, 1976.

183a. Lindner, P. G., Blackburn, G. L.: Multidisciplinary Approach to Obesity Utilizing Fasting Modified by Protein Sparing Therapy. *Obesity/Bariatric Med 5:* 198, 1976.

183b. Hypertension Task Force of the National Institutes of Health, National Heart, Lung and Blood Institute. Report. Section on Obesity. (in press).

183c. Ravelli, G. -P.: Obesity in Young Men After Famine Exposure In Utero and Early Infancy. *N Engl J Med 295:* 349, 1976.

184. Cooper, K. H.: The New Aerobics. New York, Bantam, 1970.

184a. Cooper, M., and Cooper, K. H.: Aerobics for Women. New York, Bantam, 1977.

185. Morehouse, L. E., Gross, L.: Total Fitness in 30 Minutes a Week. New York, Pocket Books, 1976.

186. Stuart, R. B.: Behavioral Control of Eating: A Report. In Bray, G. A. (ed): Obesity in Perspective, Fogarty International Center Series on Preventive Medicine, vol 2, part 2. Washington, DC, US Government Printing Office, 1975, p 367.

187. Albrink, M. J.: Chorionic Gonadotropin and Obesity. *Am J Clin Nutr 22:* 681, 1969.

188. Asher, W. L., Harper, H. W.: Effect of Human Chorionic Gonadotrophin on Weight Loss, Hunger, and Feeling of Well-being. *Am J Clin Nutr 26:* 211, 1973.

189. Asher, W. L.: The Clinical Assessment of Anorectic Drugs. In Bray, G. A. (ed): Obesity in Perspective, Fogarty International Center Series on Preventive Medicine, vol 2, part 2. Washington, DC, US Government Printing Office, 1975, p 445.

190. Mills, M. J., Stunkard, A. J.: Behavioral Changes Following Surgery for Obesity. American Psychologic Society, 128th Annual Meeting, Anaheim, Calif, May 5–9, 1975.

191. Scott, H. W., Dean, R. H., Shull, H. J., Gluck, F. W.: Metabolic Complications of Jejunoileal Bypass Operations for Morbid Obesity. *Annu Rev Med 27:* 397, 1976.

192. Report of the Committee for the Assessment of Biometric Aspects of Controlled Trials of Hypoglycemic Agents. *JAMA 231:* 583, 1975.

193. Knatterud, G. L., Klimt, C. R., Osborne, R. K., Meinert, C. L., Martin, D. B., Hawkins, B. S.: The University Group Diabetes Program: A Study of the Effects of Hypoglycemic Agents on Vascular Complications in Patients with Adult-Onset Diabetes. V. Evaluation of Phenformin Therapy. *Diabetes 24 [Suppl 1]:* 65, 1975.

194. Grinker, J., Hirsch, J., Levin, B.: The Affective Responses of Obese Patients to Weight Reduction: A Differentiation Based on Age at Onset of Obesity. *Psychosom Med 35:* 57, 1973.

195. Dwyer, J. T., Mayer, J.: A Preventive Programme for Obesity Control. In Burland, W. L., Samuel, P. D., Yudkin, J. (eds): Obesity Symposium, Proceedings of a Servier Research Institute Symposium, December 1973. Edinburgh, Churchill Livingstone, 1974, p 253.

196. Bradfield, R. B., Paulos, J., Grossman, L.: Energy Expenditure and Heart Rate of Obese High School Girls. *Am J Clin Nutr 24:* 1482, 1971.

149

The Metabolic Response to Injury and Infection

John M. Kinney
Philip Felig

When the body is injured it responds both locally and generally. The local response is described as a form of "inflammation," while the word "shock" has been used in a similar way to describe the early general response to injury. The intensity of the general response depends on the severity of the injury. The pioneering observations of Cuthbertson[1] established the metabolic response to physical injury over 40 years ago. The initial observations in humans and subsequent work in the rat led this investigator to separate the metabolic response into an early "ebb" or shock phase, with depressed vitality, followed by a "flow" or catabolic phase, with a resurgence of vitality having certain similarities to inflammation.[2] The idea that injury can occur with or without shock is misleading. There must always be some general response to an injury, and certain metabolic responses are overlooked if one's focus is only on the shock that occurs when the response reaches a certain magnitude.

This discussion is limited to the changes associated with organic metabolism that occur in the ebb and flow phases of convalescence after injury or infection. Cuthbertson introduced the concept of the ebb phase as being the early response to physical injury, which may or may not be of sufficient magnitude to be considered "shock" from hemorrhage or trauma. In this chapter the metabolic response to infection has also been divided into an ebb or septic shock phase and a flow phase for similar reasons of convenience. Obviously, certain differences must be kept in mind when extending the concept of ebb and flow phases to the response to infection. The metabolic changes that occur after the infective exposure but before the onset of fever are considered part of the ebb phase. The flow phase may be considered to occur when the circulatory responses to the febrile state have stabilized at the new level. The transition from the ebb to the flow phase of infection is poorly defined from a metabolic viewpoint but presumably occurs sometime during the early part of the febrile response.

It is now apparent that the metabolic response to starvation differs in important respects from that of injury and even more from that of infection. Thus the metabolic response of any given hospital patient is the net effect of the responses to many factors, particularly varying degrees of starvation, injury, and infection. Since partial starvation is a common element of convalescence associated with injury and infection, the present understanding of the metabolic response to starvation should be considered (as discussed in Chapter 147) in understanding the response to injury and infection.

THE METABOLIC RESPONSE TO HEMORRHAGE AND INJURY

EBB PHASE

Body Weight

There has been little attention to changes in body weight in either the experimental animal or in the surgical patient during the ebb phase following injury. This is because the ebb phase is fairly brief in duration and also because the clinical emphasis at this time is on support of ventilation, circulation, and vital organ function. However, this lack of attention to changes in body weight during resuscitation from acute injury is often associated with subsequent confusion regarding changes in body weight during the flow phase that follows. A clinical axiom is that a patient should not gain weight acutely unless this is necessary to support the circulation. However, the relationship between fluid loads and acute increases in body weight are seldom appreciated.[3] This is, in part, because a gain in body weight is not the result of merely the fluid administered but rather the balance between the fluid administered and the various routes of loss during that time. The increases in body weight during resuscitation should never be a guide to the amount and type of resuscitation. The therapy obviously should be determined by the response to hemodynamic variables and vital organ function. The extent of acute increase in body weight should be noted, however, because this then constitutes the extent of acute water load that should be excreted during the ensuing few days. It is commonly assumed that this excretion will take place promptly, and thus it is seldom monitored by following serial body weights.

The availability of accurate bed scales for intensive care reveals that many patients who enter the hospital with acute fluid loading during the ebb phase do not excrete their fluid loads promptly during the flow phase. A study by Gump and co-workers[4] revealed that in a group of 15 such patients, approximately one-third excreted their fluid load promptly, another third did not excrete their fluid load until after 1 week, while the other third still had significant fluid retention after 2 weeks. In general, the more serious the problem and the more there are continuing complications following the initial cause for shock, the more prolonged is the fluid retention. Posttraumatic pulmonary failure, or "shock lung," is characterized by the appearance of interstitial pulmonary edema, a serious complication that seems to occur more readily in the background of unsuspected fluid retention following initial fluid loading. The delayed appearance of pulmonary deterioration in the injured and infected patient is often dealt with in terms of local infection and the clearance of pulmonary secretions. Important as these factors are, the combined aspects of the metabolic response to injury may also play an important role. This includes the insidious appearance of interstitial pulmonary edema as part of a retained fluid load following initial treatment and also the progressive muscle protein breakdown that may produce some compromise of the muscles of breathing.

Energy Metabolism

There is widespread agreement that during the ebb phase, both oxygen and body temperature tend to be reduced, with a corresponding decrease in production. The ebb phase after major hemorrhage is accompanied by a metabolic acidosis, an increase in plasma catecholamine levels, and the development of an oxygen debt. Manger and co-workers[5] demonstrated in canine hemorrhagic shock that control of pH alone or increased delivery of oxygen alone did not alter the survival rate, while an improved survival resulted when both pH and oxygen delivery were treated following hemorrhage. Crowell and Smith[6] demonstrated a reproducible correlation between the cumulative oxygen deficit and survival after hemorrhage in the dog. Oxygen deficits of 100 mg/kg or less were not lethal, while deficits of 120 ml/kg produced a LD_{50}, and deficits of 140 ml/kg or greater were invariably fatal. Jones and co-workers[7] went on to show that the time of irreversibility (when blood began to be taken up from the reservoir) was correlated with the time the animal took to reach an oxygen deficit of 120 ml/kg and that the oxygen deficit was reached sooner than the time of reversal of blood flow. Vladeck and co-workers[8] studied the differences between rapid (under 4 hours) and slow hemorrhage in man. They found that oxygen transport in rapid bleeding was limited by reduced oxygen content and low cardiac output, but in slow bleeding, oxygen transport was primarily limited by reduced arterial oxygen content. The rapid bleeding seemed to be associated with a partially compensated metabolic acidosis, reflecting poor tissue perfusion and anaerobic carbohydrate metabolism. The patients with slow bleeding were commonly alkalotic from hyperventilation in the face of adequate oxygen delivery to tissues.

Halmagyi and co-workers[9] presented data in canine shock that femoral oxygen usage was related to femoral arterial blood flow and then subsequently found a linear relationship between systemic arterial resistance and O_2 consumption in both normovolemic and hypovolemic animals, suggesting an important role for precapillary sphincters in determining O_2 consumption in shock. Thus these investigators concluded that the mechanism of maintaining total body O_2 consumption in low flow states is similar to that described for regional circuits and that reduced O_2 uptake in shock has no specific predictive value.

Wilson and co-workers[10] studied the oxygen consumption of 100 critically ill patients who had undergone major trauma or operation. Of 20 patients with a reduced oxygen consumption, 80 percent died, while only 30 percent died if a normal or increased oxygen consumption was present. The finding of a refractory decrease in oxygen consumption is obviously a grave sign, but lethality is difficult to relate to the extent of decreased energy metabolism except in extreme cases. Patients in shock usually have no control values available for their resting oxygen uptake. Also, shock studies usually involve general anesthesia in a way that produces a uniform and stable baseline, which is not the case in patients being treated in an intensive care unit. In addition, patients who are found to be in shock have had the condition for a variable period of time and have presumably been accumulating an unknown oxygen deficit before they are first seen. Furthermore, it appears that oxygen store (approximately 2 liters in the average adult human body) can be shifting during the course of measuring external oxygen consumption during the acute phases of treatment. Thus the external measurements may provide the sum of both the actual tissue utilization of oxygen and the changes in body gas stores which are difficult to separate.

Hind Limb Ischemia

The experimental study of injury requires a well-defined and reproducible form of injury, most commonly involving hemorrhage, long bone fracture, endotoxin injection, or a thermal burn. Stoner and colleagues[11] have perfected the technique of bilateral hind limb ischemia in the rat. The extent of the injury can be varied by altering the amount of the muscle damaged, the duration of ischemia, and the environmental conditions. Stoner[12] summarized the findings with this form of injury in 1960, emphasizing that "shock" is primarily a state of decreased energy output. The period of 4 to 6 hours after release of the hind limb tourniquet was characterized by falling oxygen consumption, decreased muscular activity, and falling body temperature. The survival period after hind limb ischemia could be divided into two parts: in the first part, the tissues have an adequate oxygen supply, while in the second, there is a failure of oxygen transport. The first phase lasts about 4 hours. The amount of glucose entering tissue metabolism is reduced, and there is even a greater reduction in glucose and pyruvate oxidation. Stoner proposed that shock might be a defense mechanism to husband vital energy needs, and he noted that the greater the metabolic stores at the time of the injury, the better was the prognosis for the rat.

Carbohydrate Metabolism

Carbohydrate metabolism during the ebb phase began with the observations of Claude Bernard a century ago, when he found that the blood sugar in a dog subjected to experimental hemorrhage rose to twice normal levels. This early observation has since been confirmed by numerous investigators, and in humans the hyperglycemic response seems to have a rough correlation with the degree of the injury. The blood sugar generally remains high as shock progresses until the late stages, when hypoglycemia supervenes in the untreated animal or patient, particularly if the environmental temperature is high. Early in the ebb phase, increased glycogenolysis has been reported in skeletal muscle[11] and in liver[13] for animals subjected to hind limb ischemia. Cardiac muscle glycogen and brain glycogen both decreased terminally after being maintained near normal levels. Bloom and Ward[14] emphasized that anoxia produced much less acute depletion of liver glycogen than did blood loss, indicating that blood loss produced a more complex reaction than that of simple decrease in oxygen availability. In contrast to the increased glycogenolysis, the rate of oxidation of carbohydrate is decreased soon after injury.[15] This is consistent with the abnormal glucose tolerance test observed following injury.[16]

Gluconeogenesis, the synthesis of glucose from noncarbohydrate precursors such as lactate, glycerol, and amino acids, may be modified during the ebb phase. Shoemaker and co-workers[17] demonstrated increased hepatic output of glucose during the hypovolemic period after injury. Ashby and co-workers[18] concluded from studies with labeled glucose that there was little change in gluconeogenesis but a block in pyruvate oxidation. Kovach[19] concluded that gluconeogenesis in the liver was inhibited.

It is well known that increased circulating lactate and pyruvate are often present in various shock states. It is generally considered to be the result of anaerobic glycolysis, which is assumed to be the result of inadequate perfusion of muscle. However, lactate accumulation may be potentiated by the relative functional failure of liver and other tissues that remove lactate from the blood under normal conditions. Elevation of blood lactate provides a rough index of the severity of the metabolic response to hemorrhage or injury. Broder and Weil[20] first emphasized that the blood lactate that remained elevated despite all efforts at treatment had a significant correlation with reduced survival of the patient. Schumer[19] and Drucker[22] have reported impairment in the oxidation of pyruvate following experimental hemorrhagic shock. The nature of the injury may influence the production or uptake of lactate during the ebb phase, where lactate levels may be increased more after hemorrhage than after endotoxin shock. Spitzer and co-workers[23] have suggested that elevated lactate levels following severe hemorrhage in the dog may be associated with increased utilization of FFA for lipid synthesis rather than oxidation.

The early phase of hypovolemia in the conscious dog was found by Weiner and Spitzer[24] to be characterized by an enhanced concentration, turnover, and oxidation of lactate to the point where lactate became the major metabolic substrate. Lactate metabolism in hemorrhagic shock was studied in the dog by Halmagyi and co-workers.[25] Changes in femoral and mesenteric lactate production failed to account for rising arterial lactate levels. These workers suggested that no single organ or tissue, such as muscle, played a predominant role in the lactate production of hemorrhagic shock.

Fritz and co-workers[26] found that adding hypertonic glucose to the resuscitation of hemorrhagic shock in the sheep produced a significant increase in survival.

McCoy and Drucker[27] have summarized the changes in carbohydrate metabolism in hypovolemic shock as being depletion of hepatic glycogen stores while gluconeogenesis is inadequate to sustain the initial hyperglycemic response to hemorrhage. As a consequence, the initial hyperglycemia is followed by a falling blood sugar. Infusion of glucose at this time restores, at least briefly, the mechanisms that support the circulation in the presence of a greatly depleted circulatory volume. But this particular role of glucose in supporting the failing circulation remains uncertain. The deterioration during hypovolemic shock appears to be hastened by prior starvation or anything that will have reduced hepatic glycogen levels.[28] Russell and co-workers[29] indicated a continued uptake of glucose by peripheral tissues in late experimental shock, and Randle[30] has demonstrated an increased cellular uptake of glucose under hypoxic conditions. Thus the late falling level of blood sugar reflects a combination of depleted hepatic glycogen stores, insufficient gluconeogenesis, and a continuing movement of glucose into peripheral tissues.

Gradual depletion of liver and muscle glycogen and reduced gluconeogenesis account for the late hypoglycemia in advanced shock. Cerebral glycogen levels are maintained, although liver and muscle glycogen levels are markedly reduced. In rats and mice starved prior to shock produced by hemorrhage or tourniquet, a more rapid decline in blood sugar and in liver and muscle glycogen is observed. These animals survive for briefer periods than did controls that had been adequately fed. When the blood sugar was maintained at normal levels, however, the fatal course of hemorrhagic shock in dogs was not changed. This is somewhat at variance with the findings of Drucker,[31] who reported that the prior nutrition of rats subjected to hypovolemic shock influenced their response. There was a greatly reduced tolerance to hemorrhagic shock when the body weight was maintained on a low-protein, high-carbohydrate diet, which was associated with continued hyperglycemia. Thus glucose available in the blood appeared to be inhibited from tissue utilization by unknown mechanisms. Fundamental changes in carbohydrate metabolism, which take place at the cellular and subcellular levels independently of blood sugar, may be decisive in determining recovery.

Protein Metabolism

Most studies of the effect of injury on protein metabolism have been made on patients or experimental animals in the flow or catabolic phase after recovery from the ebb or shock phase. Little is known concerning the role of protein or of protein breakdown in the ebb phase. Plasma protein concentration may change in shock owing to shifts in water and electrolytes and to shifts and losses of plasma proteins themselves. Frank and co-workers[32] reported a delay in the synthesis of albumin, prothrombin, and fibrinogen by the liver of the dog in shock. The early response of the serum proteins to injury is complex because the synthesis rates of some proteins are increased, while that of others appears to be decreased. Owen[33] has reviewed the literature describing plasma protein changes associated with injury. The work of many investigators seems to indicate that various forms of injury result in a decrease in serum albumin and an increase in an alpha globulin. The level of fibrinogen is very variable, although high levels are noted in the presence of any inflammation, and a deficit can be restored in a few hours. Getzen and co-workers[34] found that serum protein levels in canine hemorrhagic shock fell faster than the hematocrit changes, with the early drop of albumin being faster than the globulins. These findings were interpreted as showing a leakage of protein into the interstitial space, particularly the albumin, which is of smaller size than the globulins.

Observations by Schumer and others[35] have shown that during shock there is a relative increase in the $alpha_2$ globulin concentration of plasma, while albumin falls and fibrinogen tends to increase. Gordon[36] reported that in the rat the synthesis of $alpha_1$ globulin was increased within 5 hours after injury. Wannemacher[37] reported that liver protein synthesis was incresed within 5 hours after injury. Cuthbertson and Tilstone[38] conclude that the acute effects of injury on plasma protein turnover are best explained in terms of an increase in metabolic turnover of the protein concerned and the appearance of an abnormal $alpha_2$ globulin. All the proteins acutely affected are synthesized in the liver, which is stimulated to increase protein synthesis through the action of some unknown mediator generated by the injury. The proteins that rise in concentration, such as haptoglobin and fibrinogen, are assumed to reflect an increased synthesis that temporarily is greater than catabolism. In the case of proteins where the plasma concentrations fall, such as albumin and transferrin, increased catabolism must exceed whatever the synthesis rate is. Net transfer of protein from the intravascular to the extravascular compartment may contribute to the fall in plasma concentrations, although this effect is probably minor. In burn injury the surface loss of protein can represent a serious and continuing loss of newly synthesized protein such as albumin.

Engle[39] demonstrated that hemorrhagic shock in the rat is characterized by rising blood levels of amino nitrogen, mainly because of an increase in breakdown of proteins in peripheral tissue associated with a decreased ability of the anoxic liver to metabolize amino acids. Rosen and Levenson[40] observed in rats, 12 hours after a severe burn, that plasma values for taurine were strikingly elevated; values for asparagine, isoleucine, leucine, tyrosine, phenylalanine, and methionine were mildly elevated; while values for proline and valine were decreased. These workers studied the amino acids from soldiers with battle injuries and shock and found increases in phenylalanine, tyrosine, lysine, taurine, and alanine, while isoleucine, proline, and glycine tended to be decreased.[41] There was no consistent rise in total free amino acids during or after shock in this study. There was a rise in a plasma amino conjugate fraction observed earlier in burned rats, however, which seemed to rise in parallel with plasma urea. The precise composition of the amino conjugates seemed to vary, and their metabolic significance remained unclear. In the goat, Gillette and co-workers[42] demonstrated that massive trauma raises the plasma NPN, urea, creatinine, creatine, and magnesium levels markedly. These increases were well beyond those to be expected from decreased renal function. The source of the increased amino acids in experimental injury according to Cuthbertson[43] is not the "reserve protein," since hyperaminoacidemia following injury was also found in animals that had been fed for a considerable period on a very low protein diet. The increase in blood amino acids also occurred in adrenalectomized rats subjected to trauma, while the posttraumatic hyperglycemia was not observed in such animals.

Elwyn and co-workers[44] recently studied the interorgan transport of amino acids in the dog with chronic catheter implantations subjected to hemorrhage. These workers found an increased splanchnic and decreased peripheral blood flow and oxygen consumption. Blood concentrations of most amino acids showed little change during hemorrhage but increased markedly after retransfusion. Most amino acids showed peripheral tissue output and hepatic uptake during the control period, and both declined progressively during shock. After retransfusion there appeared to be a net transport of some compounds from the periphery to the liver, while others had a net movement from liver to peripheral tissues. Hepatic protein catabolism accompanied by decreased hepatic uptake of amino acids and net peripheral amino acid release appeared to be the main cause of increased blood amino acid concentrations. While changes in pH, Po_2, and blood flow were of physiological and metabolic significance early in hemorrhage, changes in amino acid concentrations in blood and their movements between tissues remained nearly normal until late in shock and appeared to have little immediate significance for the metabolic fate of the animal.

Fat Metabolism

Shoemaker and co-workers[17] examined the changes in circulating lipids during successive stages of hypovolemic shock. In the early stage, there was a net increase in the release of triglycerides from the liver and an increased uptake of free fatty acids. This effect was brief and returned to control levels as shock progressed. In the late stage, free fatty acids and phospholipids were released into the circulation. The nonhepatic splanchnic tissues seem to respond to hemorrhage with an increased output of FFA, triglycerides, and phospholipids, which decrease in the late terminal stages of hypovolemia. Studies of the response to hemorrhage in the dog by Kovach[45] showed increased arterial glycerol concentrations when arterial FFA levels did not rise. This observation was attributed to a reduction in blood flow in the subcutaneous adipose tissue.

A nonlinear relationship between the plasma FFA levels and the concentration of free plasma tryptophane was found in rats with different nutritional states, although factors other than FFA exist. This relationship was destroyed by limb ischemia in the rat.[46] A fall in the total tryptophan in plasma with certain drugs was assumed to be the result of altered distribution in the interstititial space rather than altered metabolism. In uninjured rats the irreversible disposal rate of plasma tryptophan was not affected by the level of free plasma tryptophan. In the injured rat the rate was not altered during limb ischemia but was decreased after removal of the tourniquets. Increased competition for tissue entry by other neutral amino acids and the decrease in body temperature could be factors in this fall.

Barton[47] studied the metabolism of labeled β-hydroxybutyrate and acetoacetate in the rat following tourniquet shock. Here it appeared that the contribution of ketones to whole body oxygen consumption rose from 7 to 15 percent in the early phase after this injury. Total ketone bodies in the blood did change after injury in postabsorptive rats but did fall after injury in starved rats, while the β-hydroxybutyrate/acetoacetate ratio fell after injury in both postabsorptive and starved rats.[48] This ratio in the liver did not change in either group until terminal stages, indicating adequate hepatic oxygenation in the early response to injury. In control postabsorptive and starved rats the level of liver total ketones was correlated with plasma FFA. After injury in postabsorptive rats the liver ketones rose and remained higher than would be predicted from controls, suggesting increased ketogenesis compatible with inhibition of complete oxidation of FFA after injury. In contrast, the liver total ketones did not change after injury in starved rats.

The "diabetes of injury" is characterized by hyperglycemia independent of the appearance of ketosis. The occurrence of very high levels of ketones in the injured patient, uncomplicated by starvation, is not common. Smith and co-workers[49] found some of their acutely injured patients to have normal blood lactate levels but ketones that were elevated up to seven times the normal value, together with a tendency to increased free fatty acids. By comparison, a diabetic injured patient may have blood ketone levels up to 80 times the normal value.

Cell Fractions

At the end of World War II, McShan and colleagues[50] published studies on rats subjected to drum shock or tourniquet shock. These studies emphasized the belief of these workers that shock was a depletion of body energy stores due to overwhelming stimulation or an interference with the processes of energy mobilization. Lepage[51] performed tissue analyses on the above animals and demonstrated depletion of glycogen, ATP, phosphocreatine, and suggested late failure of processes of gluconeogenesis, thus depriving the animal of further substrate for glycolysis after glycogen stores were exhausted. Bell and co-workers[52] found that canine hemorrhagic shock was associated with lysosomal disruption, with rising plasma enzyme levels, and with loss of reticuloendothelial system function.

There has been a growing interest in mitochondria and oxidative phosphorylation during the ebb phase of experimental injury. Stoner and Threlfall[53] reported that during shock following removal of hind leg tourniquets in the rat, brain phosphocreatine levels remained unchanged and liver ATP only decreased shortly before death. This was in contrast to muscle, where both phosphocreatine and ATP levels declined shortly before death. In muscle, they found that both glucose-6-phosphate and fructose-1,6-diphosphate were increased, while in the liver, only the latter was increased in shock. More recently, Rush[54] has referred to the depressed levels of cell ATP in hemorrhagic shock and to the well-known increase in circulating levels of lactate associated with an increased output of lactate by the myocardium. Mela and co-workers[55] have studied *Escherichia coli* endotoxemia and hemorrhage in the rat, where they found liver lysosomal acid phosphatase activity to decrease in association with mitochondrial impairment. These changes were not reproduced by pure tissue hypoxia. Somogyi and co-workers[56] have suggested that the increased respiration capacity of rat brain mitochondria after injury might be related to the release of free fatty acids. Baue and Sayeed,[57] along with Mela and co-workers[58] have shown that, structurally, the mitochondria first swell, then broken membranes are demonstrable, and in the final stages of shock there is complete disappearance of the inner mitochondrial structure. These changes, with concomitant functional impairment, have been shown to occur in the rat liver mitochondria after endotoxin, hemorrhage, and ischemia. Similar changes have also been seen in human liver, skeletal muscle, and kidney.

Markley and Smallman[59] reported protection from burn shock in mice given intraperitoneal injections of various purine compounds. Chaudry and co-workers[60] have reported that hemorrhagic shock in the rat uniformly reduces the levels of ATP in both liver and kidney and that these levels remain low after resuscitation with blood plus electrolyte solution. An intravenous preparation of ATP-magnesium chloride was added to blood and restored ATP levels in both liver and kidney to normal.

FLOW PHASE

Weight Loss

There is general agreement that the extent of weight loss parallels the severity of the injury. Cuthbertson[61] reported that following long bone fracture in a healthy, young adult male, there was a parallel rise and return to normal of temperature, pulse, oxygen consumption, and nitrogen excretion during the first 12 days following injury. It was also noted that there were parallel changes in sulfur, phosphorus, and nitrogen excretion, suggesting breakdown of intracellular materials. Various observers have reported that the rate and extent of nitrogen loss roughly parallel the loss of body weight. Since these patients commonly do not receive a normal nitrogen intake, the resulting negative nitrogen balance is composed of both a postinjury increase in nitrogen excretion and an element of starvation. Weight loss in the early postoperative period will often be in the range of 200–400 g/day after an initial tendency to water retention. More severe injury may have sustained losses of 400–800 g/day.

Energy Metabolism

The rapid weight loss with fatigue and weakness in acute surgical catabolism led to the suggestion that perhaps the injury had caused a large resting energy demand and that body protein was being degraded for fuel purposes. Serial measurements of gas exchange and nitrogen excretion have been employed by Kinney and co-workers,[62] using the principles of indirect calorimetry, to construct a daily resting calorie balance along with the nitrogen balance. Such studies have revealed that uncomplicated postoperative convalescence has a resting metabolic expenditure (RME) within ±10 percent of the preoperative values. Multiple fractures commonly caused increases of 10 to 25 percent in RME for periods of 2 to 3 weeks. Major infections such as peritonitis cause variable increases from 15 to 50 percent of normal values. Major third-degree burns caused sustained hypermetabolism, which is commonly between 40 and 100 percent above normal values. This severe hypermetabolism appears within the first week after the burn and remains high until the burn surface is excised and grafted.

The increased nitrogen loss in surgical catabolism is largely expressed as an increase in synthesis and excretion of urea. Loss of body weight over a few days may be predominantly loss of water. Sustained weight loss over 2 weeks or more can be assumed to be made up of protein, fat, and water. Recent studies of cumulative calorie and nitrogen balance in patients with major injury and infection have shown that the protein contribution to the weight loss over a 3-week period following injury amounted to 10 to 14 percent of the weight loss, while the loss of body fat was in the range of 18 to 25 percent. The rate of weight loss in one subject over 3 weeks of total starvation was studied by Benedict. The weight loss was similar to that seen following major injury and infection despite the latter patients receiving 40 to 60 percent of their daily estimated calorie and nitrogen requirements. Analysis of the tissue composition of weight loss during 3 weeks of total starvation revealed 12 percent of the weight loss was body protein and approximately 26 percent was body fat.[63] This information suggests that body protein represents a surprisingly reproducible proportion of weight loss and is similar regardless of whether the weight loss is due to starvation alone.

Bergström and co-workers[64] have reported preliminary studies of energy-rich phosphate materials in muscle biopsies taken from 18 patients in an intensive care unit. Each patient had a stable circulation and urine output but required mechanical ventilation for adequate arterial oxygenation. Eight of the patients were biopsied within the first 5 days following admission for acute circulatory or ventilatory failure. The second group was biopsied between 6 days and 6 weeks while receiving total parenteral nutrition. The early biopsies showed an increase in muscle lactate and a decrease in phosphocreatine stores and ATP. The patients with prolonged disease despite a seemingly stable circulation had more pronounced decreases in ATP content, reaching only 50 percent of normal despite a normal lactate content. This low ATP level was thought by these workers to be primarily the result of increased formation and deamination of adenosine monophosphate in combination with a decreased rate of purine synthesis in the liver and/or decreased capacity for purine "salvage" in the muscle. These workers also noted that prolonged immobilization without metabolic disturbances did not change the total adenine content of muscle, while short-lasting severe metabolic acidosis was associated with significant decreases in total adenine content. Preliminary experience with this technique suggests that it may be an important means of monitoring the metabolic course of critically ill patients, since blood and urine measurements are not clearly indicative of intracellular changes.

Protein Metabolism

The best known feature of the metabolic response to injury, first observed by Cuthbertson, was the increase in nitrogen loss. This investigator and subsequently many others have shown that many different types of injury result in the breakdown of body protein. This is associated with a rise in urinary nitrogen, sulfur, phosphorus, potassium, magnesium, and creatine along with some increase in the resting oxygen consumption. These catabolic changes of the "flow" phase reach a maximum during 4 to 8 days after an injury such as a long bone fracture. The changes after an uncomplicated surgical operation are usually of lesser magnitude and may last for a shorter duration. The patient with multiple fractures and secondary infection, or a major thermal burn, can be expected to demonstrate a more prolonged catabolic response, with the cumulative nitrogen loss reaching 300 g or more in extreme cases. The rise in urinary nitrogen excretion is mainly as urea, the sulfur as sulfate, and the phosphorus as phosphate. Comparable disturbances of nitrogen metabolism following injury have been found in animals as divergent as man, sheep, earthworms and crabs.[65]

The source of the nitrogen and other intracellular constituents lost following injury has never been completely defined. However, the nitrogen/sulfur and nitrogen/potassium ratios of the urinary losses suggest that the nitrogen loss is mainly from muscle. The influence of previous nutrition on this response is discussed later in this section.

Moore and Ball[66] presented detailed balance studies of different forms of surgical injury, emphasizing the magnitude of the losses of both nitrogen and potassium that could occur. Moore and co-workers[67] perfected a multiple isotope dilution technique for studying the changes in body composition of surgical patients. These changes emphasized that the catabolic process involved shrinkage of the body cell mass with an absolute or relative expansion of extracellular or supporting volume and its constituents.

Whole Body Protein Turnover

Nitrogen balance techniques give information about net exchanges of nitrogen with the environment, but isotopic tracers or regional catheterization studies are needed to examine the dynamics of nitrogen within the body. A great deal of effort has been devoted to the kinetics of plasma protein turnover in man, but there is much less knowledge of rates of total protein synthesis. Sprinson and Rittenberg[68] used ^{15}N-glycine for this purpose and calculated that the rate of protein synthesis in adult man was approximately 300 g/day. Waterlow[69] developed a different approach, utilizing a continuous infusion of labeled amino acid. O'Keefe and co-workers[70] studied 5 postoperative patients using an infusion of ^{14}C-leucine. They reported a small decrease in synthesis with no increase in breakdown. The study is difficult to interpret, however, since the patients received a normal diet preoperatively and were given only water and electrolytes in the postoperative period. Crane and co-workers[71] studied protein turnover in 11 patients before and after elective orthopedic operation by giving labeled glycine orally every 4 hours for 32 hours. A constant protein intake was maintained throughout the study. The rate of protein synthesis fell from 3.83 g/kg/day to 2.94 after operation, with no change in the calculated rate of protein breakdown. These workers postulate a block in muscle protein synthesis as being responsible for the catabolic loss of nitrogen after injury. Studies by Long and co-workers,[72] utilizing ^{15}N-alanine in acutely ill septic surgical patients, have indicated that a negative nitrogen balance can be the result of an increased protein synthesis rate with an even greater increase in protein breakdown.

Plasma Proteins

The fall in albumin concentration and an increase in certain globulin fractions after injury was reported by Cuthbertson and Tompsett in 1935.[73] Since then,.a variety of new techniques has allowed the study of plasma proteins with increasing sophistication.[33,74–76]

All investigators agree that after trauma, albumin concentration decreases to reach a minimum by the third to the sixth day and gradually returns to normal over days to weeks, depending upon the severity of the injury. Fibrinogen concentration increases up to twice normal values following skeletal injury and burns. Alpha$_1$ antitrypsin and alpha$_1$ acid glycoprotein both increase up to 50 percent after injury, although the alpha$_1$ lipoprotein decreases by approximately 50 percent. The net effect is an increase in the alpha$_1$ proteins. Alpha$_2$ globulins, including ceruloplasmin and haptoglobin, are increased up to 100 percent after injury. The beta globulins, such as transferrin and beta lipoprotein, consistently show a decrease of 25 to 50 percent after injury. The immunoglobulins IgG, IgA, and IgM seem not to change significantly after injury unless there is a source of infections, as in burns, when the increases may be considerable. The C-reactive protein migrates in the gamma$_1$ region on electrophoresis. It is scarcely detectable in the serum of normal individuals but appears consistently after injury or inflammation. Crockson and co-workers[77] have suggested that it may be the best screening test for determining whether an "acute phase reaction" is present. The acute phase reactants have been described by Koj[78] as the plasma proteins that show an increase in concentration in the acute phase of inflammation.

There has been increasing effort over the past decade to examine the rates of synthesis and catabolism of individual plasma proteins after injury. Ballantyne and Fleck[79] found no increase in the absolute catabolic rate of albumin after injury but did observe an increase in the fractional catabolic rate. In contrast, Davies and Liljedahl[80] have reported an increased catabolism of albumin, fibrinogen, and IgG after major burns. The increased catabolism of albumin and IgG in burned patients appeared to be proportional to the degree of increase in resting metabolic expenditure. The distribution of albumin in the body, expressed as the extravascular/intravascular ratio, is markedly increased after injury, with the most severe changes found in the burn injury. Davies[81] studied the synthesis rate of albumin following burns utilizing ^{131}I-labeled proteins. He found that albumin synthesis appeared to be increased in the first few days and then decreased to below normal after about 5 days. The synthesis rate of IgG rose rapidly after injury. Davies and co-workers[82] also reported that fibrinogen synthesis was increased after injury. Ballantyne and co-workers[83] used the ^{14}C-carbonate method to study albumin synthesis in rabbits following femoral fracture. They observed that synthesis was significantly decreased on the third day after fracture, and this change could account for the decreased plasma concentrations of albumin found at that time. This is in contrast to Koj and McFarlane,[84] who found that the administration of endotoxin to rabbits led to an increased synthesis of both albumin (up 60 percent) and fibrinogen (up 400 percent) at 48 hours.

Many investigators have found that albumin synthesis in the liver is rapidly reduced in protein deprivation.[85–87] The catabolic rate of albumin apparently does not decrease immediately after the onset of protein deprivation but does so only after the concentration of plasma albumin has decreased significantly. When protein repletion is begun the synthesis rate of albumin responds with a very rapid increase. The catabolic rate increases very gradually as the plasma albumin concentration rises.

The prolonged increase in catabolic rate in the presence of a reduced total pool and low intravascular level of albumin in severely burned patients is in notable contrast to the reduced catabolism in the primary malnourished individual. Presumably, this difference is related to the different endocrine settings of the injured versus the malnourished patient. Fleck[75] observed no clear single gross trend in liver protein synthesis in injury. Polysome patterns in rat liver after injury and RNA synthesis studies are compatible with a general increase in protein synthesis up to 12 hours.[88]

Amino Acid Metabolism

E.B. Man found that plasma amino acid nitrogen usually fell during the 24 hours after operation in patients who had been in relatively good health and normal nutrition prior to operation.[89] The amino acid nitrogen remained low in the plasma throughout the early acute stage and slowly returned to normal as convalescence progressed. It was noted that if the patients were ill or malnourished before operation, the plasma amino acid nitrogen was commonly low preoperatively and was often not affected by operation. Thus the prompt fall in amino acid nitrogen was considered to be a normal part of the reaction to injury. No correlation was found with the levels of NPN or the nitrogen balance. Everson and Fritschel,[90] using a microbiologic assay, reported a significant decrease in the total plasma concentration of essential amino acids following operation. Nardi[91] observed increased amino acid excretion in burned patients. While the urinary amino acid loss was a small proportion of the total urinary nitrogen excretion, it consisted of the nonessential amino acids normally found in the urine plus certain essential amino acids such as threonine, leucine, isoleucine, lysine, and methionine. Traces of creatine were noted, indicating that the catabolic state was perhaps due to muscle tissue breakdown beyond that found with muscle disuse. Schønheyder and colleagues,[92] using ion exchange chromatography, found postoperative changes in both essential and nonessential amino acids of the plasma, which they interpreted as being due primarily to postoperative malnutrition.

The levels of individual plasma amino acids were studied in the postoperative patient by Dale and co-workers.[93] Immediately after an abdominal operation of moderate (vagotomy and pyloroplasty) or extensive (aortic aneurysm excision) nature, most plasma amino acids decreased promptly. The nonessential amino acids continued to fall for the first 2 days or more, while the essential amino acids returned to a higher concentration than immediately after operation. There appeared to be no correlation between these changes and the length of anesthesia or the severity of the operation. Increasing the postoperative intake of glucose caused only some increase in plasma alanine and a lower methionine level. These authors suggest that cystine and tyrosine may temporarily become essential amino acids after injury and that an associated rise in phenylalanine and methionine was perhaps due to transient liver dysfunction.

Woolf and co-workers[94] studied the changes in arterial amino acid concentrations associated with the catabolism of abdominal operation, major fractures, and postoperative sepsis. The pattern of changes found did not resemble that previously observed by these workers after glucocorticoid administration. In the patients with fractures, the concentrations of ornithine, taurine, and aspartic acid were lower than those of control values. The septic patients showed phenylalanine concentrations greater than normal on the first and third days. Four of these septic patients with increased phenylalanine levels also had elevated arterial methionine concentrations, suggesting impaired liver function.

Wedge and co-workers[95] studied the relationship between the branched-chain amino acids of plasma, nitrogen excretion, and circulating ketone bodies in a group of 16 male patients following bony and soft tissue injury and compared them with 4 adults undergoing elective skin grafts. It was found that the concentrations of the branched-chain amino acids rose significantly within 24 hours after injury and reached twice normal values by 4 days, in contrast to values for circulating alanine, glycine, and glutamate, which were slightly depressed. Patients undergoing skin grafting showed no significant change in their amino acids. The injured patients were divided into those with normal ketone levels and those who showed an initial hyperketonemia, defined as more than 0.2 mM/liter. In those injured patients with initial hyperketonemia, the increase in concentration of branched-chain amino acids at the fourth and seventh day after injury was significantly less than those with normal ketone levels and was accompanied by lower urinary nitrogen excretion throughout the entire period. These workers suggest that changes in the concentration of branched-chain amino acids after injury indicate a decreased uptake by muscle or an excessive release due to an imbalance between protein synthesis and protein catabolism in muscle tissue. The relationship between circulating ketone levels and nitrogen excretion is not clear; however, the studies of Sherwin and co-workers[96] are of interest in this regard. These investigators infused 3-hydroxybutyrate into starving subjects and showed that this caused a decrease in circulating blood alanine and in urinary nitrogen excretion without a detectable change in either circulating insulin or glucose.

Muscle Free Amino Acids

The supply of free amino acids to the tissues is of primary importance in protein metabolism. Herbert[97] studied the total free amino acid pool in different tissues of the rat and showed that the concentration of most of the amino acids was considerably higher in the tissues than in the plasma. He also found that the size of the pools of individual free amino acids differed widely. About 80 percent of free amino acids in the total body was found in skeletal muscle. A technique of percutaneous needle biopsy of skeletal muscle in man was introduced by Bergstrøm[98,99] and permits repeated sampling of muscle tissue. Vinnars and co-workers[100] reported changes in the free amino acids of muscle tissue following uncomplicated elective abdominal operation and in patients following more severe injury and septic postoperative complications. The first groups received only 1500 Kcal of carbohydrate daily after operation, while the latter group received 2,200 kcal and 9.5 g of nitrogen daily. The postoperative group, with a moderate degree of surgical catabolism, showed a definite increase in extracellular water content of muscle, while the intracellular water content was only slightly decreased. No significant change was seen in the total plasma free amino acid levels. In muscle, essential amino acids were unchanged, while the nonessential amino acids were decreased at 3 days following operation. The plasma pattern was changed, with an increase in phenylalanine and tyrosine and a decrease in isoleucine and histidine levels. The concentrations of serine and proline showed a more moderate decrease, while the level of leucine increased slightly. In the muscle there was a large decrease in glutamine, arginine, and lysine and significant falls in proline and glutamic acid levels. Major increases occurred in taurine, valine, and phenylalanine concentrations in muscle, with smaller increases in serine, glycine, alanine, and leucine. The transmembrane gradient showed marked increases for glycine, valine, serine, isoleucine, and leucine.

In severe surgical catabolism,[101] total muscle water content was increased more than after moderate injury. The increase is related both to the elevated extracellular water content and to the severity of the catabolic state. In contrast to the postoperative groups, the size of essential free amino acid pool was reduced in both the plasma and the muscle. The total nonessential amino acids was further decreased in plasma but was about the same as the postoperative group in muscle. Consequently the total amino acid pools were reduced in both plasma and muscle. In plasma, all the essential amino acids were markedly decreased except for phenylalanine, which was increased. In muscle, phenylalanine was increased and lysine decreased. The phenylalanine/tyrosine ratio in muscle was markedly increased in both plasma and muscle.

Munro[102] suggested that an abnormal plasma amino acid pattern might be a sign of protein catabolism. It is reasonable to expect that changes in the free amino acid pattern of muscle might also reflect protein catabolism. However, the work of Vinnars and colleagues[101] appears to indicate that there is no common pattern for the catabolism seen in uremia, diabetes, and starvation, but rather distinctive patterns are present for each condition. Likewise there may be a distinctive pattern for the response to injury and infection. While the above changes in plasma and muscle free amino acids require much further work for adequate interpretation, it appears definite that the changes following moderate and severe injury are distinctly different from those of starvation. Phenylalanine was found in low concentration in muscle after starvation, while it was elevated in injury. The injured patients had consistent falls in muscle lysine and glutamine. The decrease of muscle lysine in starvation may be considered as a sign of general muscle catabolism. The decrease in glutamine observed in the injured patients seems to be unique to surgical catabolism. This technique may offer an important method of separating the influence of trauma from that of starvation and of guiding the nutritional therapy of future patients in a more specific and rational manner.

Carbohydrate Metabolism

In 1877, Claude Bernard[103] documented an increase in the blood sugar as a feature of the response to injury. Studies from Cannon[104] onward have repeatedly confirmed this finding and shown that in burns, military casualties, and obstetric hemorrhage the response is roughly proportional to the degree of injury sustained. Howard[105] found in a study of battle casualties that the response to an oral glucose load was similar to that observed in diabetes mellitus, in that tolerance was less and the glucose lowering effect of intravenously injected insulin was reduced, a state termed "insulin resistance." Evans and Butterfield[106] used the term "pseudo-diabetes" (progressive hyperglycemia without ketosis) to describe similar but more severe changes in burned patients. The latter condition has since been recognized in various clinical settings as "nonketotic hyperosmolar coma."

The injured or infected patient often shows a mild to moderate hyperglycemia, which has been termed the "diabetes of injury." Even when this hyperglycemia is scarcely noticed, there will be an abnormal response to a glucose tolerance test, which has generally been interpreted to mean that glucose entry into cells is impaired. Giddings [107] studied the insulin response to glucose infusions during and after operation and documented the postoperative hyperglycemia and hyperinsulinemia found by others. The change in postoperative glucose dynamics is due to an increase in gluconeogenesis, however, and not to decreased peripheral glucose utilization.[108–109] Giddings and co-workers [109] noted that the basal glucose level remains slightly elevated for 5 days after elective abdominal operation. These investigators believe that raised plasma glucose values do not necessarily indicate reduced rates of peripheral glucose uptake, but rather that the concentration of glucose required to maintain normal rates of uptake has been increased.

Early suggestions that glucose intolerance might be due to the inability of the injured patient to oxidize glucose were disproved by the studies of Long and co-workers.[110] Their use of ^{14}C-glucose with a mathematical model of human glucose metabolism indicated that the injured patient oxidized glucose at normal or even increased rates in the presence of a stable circulation. An additional finding was that glucose turnover rate was increased above normal along with the associated hypermetabolism. Regional catheterization of surgical patients by Gump and co-workers[111] revealed an increased hepatic glucose output despite the presence of hyperglycemia. In addition, studies on the forearm with catheterization of the artery and deep vein revealed a normal curve of glucose uptake with rising levels of blood glucose, except that in the presence of surgical injury the curve was displaced to a high level of blood sugar consistent with "insulin resistance."

Preliminary studies by Aoki and co-workers[112] have shown that plasma amino acid levels in severely traumatized patients were depressed but that arterial venous differences for plasma amino acids across the forearm muscle were similar to control values. The half-life of labeled alanine was found to be decreased by one-half, a measure of hepatic gluconeogenesis. Long and co-workers[110] demonstrated that there was an increase in glucose production and in glucose oxidation after injury. Thus it seems clear that amino acids are released from muscle at an accelerated rate to be converted into glucose by the liver. Aoki and co-workers[112] suggest that since reparative tissues use only glucose for substrate, it is reasonable to assume that trauma initiates muscle hypercatabolism to provide fuel for reparative processes. Not only did the primordial response to injury not include the possibility of intravenously administered carbohydrate, but the ebb phase includes adrenergic suppression of insulin release and the flow phase is characterized by peripheral insulin resistance, tending to reduce the utilization of exogenously administered glucose. Furthermore, these mechanisms fail to suppress the increased production of endogenously synthesized glucose, despite the existence of hyperglycemia.

Long and associates[110] demonstrated an increased flow of glucose through the extracellular fluid compartment in acutely ill patients, and hepatic catheterization studies by Gump and co-workers[111] suggest that insulin inhibition of hepatic gluconeogenesis is reduced following injury. The kinetics of glucose movement have been studied in detail by Wilmore and co-workers[113] using the method of Hlad and Elrich.[114] During the initial period of burn shock, total body glucose was elevated, but the mass flow of glucose through the expanded glucose space was near normal. Following resuscitation, the rate of glucose disappearance was enhanced, while the proportionality constant for glucose disappearance was similar to that of normal individuals. The glucose "flow" was significantly elevated as a consequence of increased hepatic production, not altered peripheral glucose disappearance. Glucose flow was related to the extent of the injury and fell with time following the injury to return to normal levels with closure of the burn wound. The insulin response to glucose in the burn patients was dampened only during the ebb phase but was comparable to normal individuals during the height of the hypermetabolic flow phase. The increased glucose flow correlated well with the increased resting oxygen consumption, despite the fact that the respiratory quotient (R.Q.) of these patients was uniformly low, reflecting the oxidation of fat as the primary fuel. The increased flow of glucose from the liver to the periphery during the flow phase of the burn injury is associated with the increase in flow of three carbon intermediates (pyruvate, lactate, and alanine) back to the liver for resynthesis of new glucose. Wilmore[115] has suggested that ADP generated by the increased cycling of glucose closely controls the rate of fuel oxidation, which may be in part related to demands for increased heat production.

Fat Metabolism

Investigation of the changes in fat metabolism associated with injury has been limited. Moore[116] has emphasized the large loss of adipose tissue that can occur after injury. In a study of surgical patients not receiving TPN, indirect calorimetry indicated that 75 to 90 percent of the calorie expenditure was from body fat, while protein provided the remainder.[117] It is important to emphasize that fatty acids are an excellent source of calories as "two-carbon fragments" to be oxidized in the tricarboxylic cycle. However, the breakdown of fatty acids cannot yield a net gain of glycogen, glucose, or carbohydrate intermediates for the synthesis of the nonessential amino acids.

Fat macroglobules formed by aggregation of lipid particles have been demonstrated in the blood after both injury and elective operation. According to Sevitt,[118] these changes reflect the general metabolic changes associated with injury. Lepistö[119] reported a detailed study of the blood lipid changes following 43 patients who sustained fractures of the leg or pelvis. The serum triglycerides increased over 4 days, while a mild decrease in cholesterol and phospholipid levels were noted in 8 of the patients who were diagnosed as having the fat embolism syndrome. Lipoprotein fractionation showed no significant changes from normal.

Carlson and Hallberg[120] noted that the product for intravenous fat administration, known as Intralipid, was a convenient tracer for chylomicra because of similar behavior. Carlson and Rossner[121] developed an intravenous fat tolerance test utilizing this material. They observed a positive relationship between the decay slope and the fractional turnover rate of endogenous triglycerides. Further studies suggested that approximately half of the infused lipid solution was removed by skeletal muscle.

The mobilization and utilization of lipid after injury was summarized by Carlson.[122] He emphasized that in patients with major burns, there was a marked early rise in the plasma free fatty acids and that the increase appeared to be proportional to the size of the burn. At the same time, the plasma triglycerides were relatively unchanged from normal values. Upon infusion of the Intralipid, these burn patients showed only a slight increase in the plasma triglycerides, and the free fatty acid level actually decreased. These workers also noted that the clearance of the Intralipid was more rapid from the bloodstream in the presence of the hypermetabolic burn injury. Wilmore and co-workers[123] confirmed the more rapid clearance in burn patients. Wilmore also noted that 5 burn patients receiving long-term fat-free TPN had developed an essential fatty acid deficiency of the red cell membrane which responded promptly to intravenous fat administration.

Carlson and co-workers[124] studied the possibility of "excessive" mobilization of free fatty acids in the injured animal or patient. They infused norepinephrine for 24 hours into dogs, so that the free fatty acid level was 4 to 5 times the normal level. This resulted in fat droplets appearing in the myocardium, skeletal muscle, kidney, lungs and liver. The animals showed fever, tachypnea, increased oxygen consumption, and evidence of intravascular coagulation.

THE METABOLIC RESPONSE TO INFECTION

EBB PHASE

Any discussion of the ebb or shock phase after infection is more difficult than that for the ebb phase following hemorrhage or injury. A variety of pathogenic (and nonpathogenic) agents may be involved, and a variable amount of the clinical picture may be due to toxic factors that act independently of the presence of living organisms. The causative agents may be normally endogenous or acquired from the environment, particularly during hospitalization. Although the infective agent is important, the capacity of the host to respond effectively to the invasion is often of decisive importance. An invasion of microorganisms causes the body to initiate a variety of reactions which include those of obvious importance to host defense and other reactions that remain poorly understood but are assumed to relate somehow to mechanisms of host defense. Mobilization of phagocytes, the development of local inflammation, and the activation of immune mechanisms have distinct, identifiable roles in host defense. The large molecular size of endotoxins prevent their entering the cell; however, they activate various systems that pose widespread threats to homeostasis. A heat-labile plasma component, complement, is apparently needed for the activation of vasoactive substances that may be followed by disseminated intravascular coagulation. Platelets and white cells become aggregated and disrupted.

Beisel[125] has pointed out that certain patterns of metabolic response are highly consistent. These responses begin promptly following the initiation of the infectious process and are geared in their timing and magnitude to the clinical stages and severity of the illness. Many host biochemical events begin within hours of the invasion of the microorganism, well before the onset of any clinical sign or symptom of illness. Some subsequent metabolic responses coincide with the onset of fever, and still others accompany the onset of convalescence. A fulminating onset with chills, fever, and hypotension is usually assumed to be the result of endotoxemia in addition to the presence of microorganisms. The following discussion relates to selected metabolic events that have been reported to occur in septic shock or when an organ or tissue is subjected to the presence of live organisms or endotoxin.

Spink and co-workers[126] were instrumental in the recognition of shock associated with infection and the possible role of endotoxin. These workers noted an abrupt increase in temperature, hypotension, and tachycardia in half of a group of patients with brucellosis who were receiving an initial dose of tetracycline. This was postulated to be the result of destroying viable bacilli and liberating antigenic material into patients with acquired hypersensitivity. Subsequent studies showed that the shock response could be prevented by administering a lower dose of the antibiotic or by giving corticosteroid therapy. A large number of investigations have followed, with controversy still remaining in regard to: (1) Whether the shock syndrome seen with sudden bacteremia is similar to or different from the syndrome associated with endotoxemia, and (2) Whether the metabolic events in septic shock are different from those seen with other forms of shock of the same severity.

Liver damage is known to occur in many types of experimental injury and infection. White and co-workers[127] studied the hepatic ultrastructure of rats in endotoxemia, hemorrhage, and hypoxia, with special emphasis on mitochondrial changes. These workers demonstrated a heterogenous mixture of hepatic mitochondrial changes in both lethal hemorrhage and lethal endotoxemia but found that hypoxia and hypotension alone were apparently not responsible for generating the swollen mitochondrial matrices common to both endotoxemia and hemorrhage. This was of particular interest, since reports from this laboratory by Mela and co-workers[128] had shown that both hemorrhage and endotoxemia causes a severe depression of mitochondrial respiratory control ratio by both increasing state 4 rates and depressing state 3 rates, indicating a marked uncoupling effect.

The observation that hemorrhagic and endotoxic shock had certain similarities has led to the idea that perhaps toxic agents may enter the bloodstream during hemorrhagic shock. Herman and co-workers[129] have studied this hypothesis in the monkey and concluded that endogenous endotoxemia is not a common feature of hemorrhagic shock in baboons nor is it related to the duration or severity of hemorrhagic shock in this species.

Energy Metabolism

Duff and co-workers[130] studied 22 patients in shock with major sepsis and compared their clinical findings with two studies on dogs in which the animals received intravenous endotoxin or developed peritonitis from cecal ligation. The patients with septic shock had a falling oxygen consumption that could have been due to either arteriovenous shunting or to cellular damage and failure to take up oxygen. In the dogs receiving endotoxin, the failure of O_2 uptake was clearly due to inadequate capillary perfusion. In the dogs with peritonitis, half developed an increased cardiac output, which correlated with an increased blood flow in muscle. The animals with a hyperdynamic circulation were thought to have an intracellular defect causing a decreased O_2 uptake despite adequate oxygen delivery. Thus patients in septic shock may show a high or a low cardiac output, with intracellular damage to tissues, which starts early in the process as a result of circulating toxic factors or appear later as the result of a low flow state and resultant hypoxic damage. Reports in the literature are about evenly divided between those that report changes that can be attributed to toxic materials and those which result from inadequate perfusion.

Elevations of lactic acid are only moderate in the plasma of endotoxin shock dogs despite the presence of a large oxygen deficit in the tissue. The failure of lactic acid to rise proportionally to the degree of hypoxia was studied by Rush and Hsieh[54] by exposing canine liver slices to endotoxin. Endotoxin had no effect when added in vitro, but if first infected into dogs, it was followed by a prompt depression in oxygen consumption and liver water content within 10 minutes. These findings were interpreted to be effects of intermediate products that endotoxin causes to be released in vivo.

E. coli septicemia in the baboon was found by Cryer and co-workers[131] to depress plasma insulin and raise plasma glucose, a finding interpreted as a decreased insulin output. Berk and co-workers[132] noted that dogs receiving intravenous endotoxin could be divided into roughly equal numbers which showed an early rise and then a fall in blood glucose or an immediate and steady decline in blood sugar. These workers found that maintaining the blood glucose significantly increased survival in the animal after small doses of endotoxin but was no longer protective when large doses were given.

A comparison of acute hemorrhagic and endotoxic shock was conducted by Printen and co-workers[133] in dogs with comparable degrees of hypotension. FFA rose with endotoxemia but not with hemorrhage, while blood glucose was elevated more in hemorrhage than in sepsis. Thus the metabolic control of these substrates are mediated through pathways other than a simple response to hypotension.

The overall rate of glucogenesis in liver slices of the rat was shown by LaNoue and co-workers[134] to be impaired by *Pseudomonas* infection and *E coli.* endotoxin. The liver activity of glucose-6-phosphatase was significantly lower in the infected and endotoxic animals than in controls. These findings were thought to represent an explanation for the observation that rats dying of *Pseudomonas* infection had low blood sugars and a depletion of liver glycogen.

Levels of circulating glucose and triglyceride, together with plasma hormone levels, were followed for 12 hours by Griffiths and co-workers[135] after a single injection of *E coli.* in the dog. Dogs who succumbed in the first few hours showed elevations of triglyceride and norepinephrine which were greater than dogs surviving for 12 hours, while glucose, insulin, epinephrine, and cortisol were not significantly different. After 12 hours of bacteremia, dogs with increased serum triglyceride levels had higher norepinephrine and lower insulin levels than did dogs with an unchanged triglyceride value, suggesting increased fat mobilization. The low insulin in the hypoglycemic dogs with hypertriglyceridemia was thought to be the result of increased plasma norepinephrine. Fiser and co-workers[136] showed in monkeys that endotoxemia causes a marked increase in plasma triglycerides, which was partially prevented by carbohydrate administration. Endotoxin causes a decrease in plasma FFA and phospholipid but no change in cholesterol. Endotoxemic monkeys showed a delayed clearance of glucose and higher serum insulin levels than did control animals. However, none of these measurements provided an indicator of severity of the host response or of lethality.

The presence of hypertriglyceridemia has been observed during sepsis due to gram-negative bacteria in both human and animal studies, whereas plasma triglyceride concentrations have usually been normal or slightly elevated during gram-positive sepsis. Several investigators have suggested that endotoxin from gram-negative bacteria may be responsible for the elevation of serum triglycerides. Kaufmann and co-workers[137] sought to explore the mechanism of the hypertriglyceridemia by examining the effect of endotoxin on lipid disposal using both intravenous lipid-loading tests and studies of total plasma lipolytic activity after administration of heparin. The possible interference of endotoxin with lipid-clearing enzymes was explored by the in vitro addition of endotoxin to heparin-activated plasma of monkeys. Small doses of endotoxin produced increases in FFA without increased triglycerides for 2 to 6 hours after administration. Within 4 hours after larger doses of endotoxin, however, serum triglycerides were elevated with an impaired disposal of lipids. Once lipid-clearing enzymes were activated, endotoxin did not reduce the lipolytic activity in vitro. Thus endotoxin causes a hypertriglyceridemia in association with impaired lipid disposal by interfering with the activation of the lipid-clearing enzymes.

The importance of liver metabolism and energy production has been emphasized by Smith and Mukherjee[138] in studying septic shock in the mouse. The mice died when a critical number of bacteria had accumulated at any site in the carcass. A falling blood glucose was associated with defective oxygen transport at a time of increased oxygen demand. Liver mitochondria showed uncoupling of oxidative phosphorylation at a time of increase in blood FFA. Uncoupling of oxidative phosphorylation could be induced by suspending the mitochondria in various ratios of saturated and unsaturated fatty acids or in naturally occurring infected mouse serum. Mitochondria from the livers of infected mice could not be further uncoupled by such maneuvers.

Peroxisomes from evaginations of smooth endoplasmic reticulum may not exist as single entities but remain normally in continuity with the smooth endoplasmic reticulum. Canonico and co-workers[139] observed a reduction of two marker enzymes for peroxisomes, hepatic catalase, and urate oxidase activity in rats infected with pneumococci. These findings may be correlated with the observation that animals infected with *Diplococcus pneumoniae* have increases in hepatic cholesterol and triglycerides. It is suggested that during some bacterial infections, hepatic synthesis of acute phase serum proteins occurs at the expense of peroxisomal protein synthesis and results in a reduction of the peroxisomal protein pool and number of peroxisomes.

The metabolic effects of intravenous administration of live *Pseudomonas* organisms to dogs over 5 hours has been studied by Postel and Schloerb.[140] Acute lethality was associated with hypoglycemia and hypothermia, along with low insulin and high catecholamine levels in the plasma. Mortality could be reduced significantly by glucose administration.

FLOW PHASE

This discussion relates to the flow phase following the onset of infection, that is, the postresuscitation period when metabolic responses lasting days to weeks are evident. Although many organisms produce specific effects, much of what happens in bacterial infection reflects the standard responses of the body to the types of cellular damage produced. Stoner[141] has pointed out that the target tissue of a given infecting organism may be more pathognomonic than the reaction that it produces. The effects of pathogenic bacteria could perhaps be reproduced by chemical and physical injuries if they could be applied to the correct point in the metabolic pathways of the right cells. Bacterial infection is distinguished from other types of injury by the ability of the infecting agent to deliver the injury to specific and often localized sites in the body. As with other forms of injury, the host response to infection can be divided into the local response at the site of injury and the general or systemic response of the entire body.

The metabolic response to infection involves a number of underlying generalized metabolic responses of the host that presumably are related to aiding host defense in ways that are not well-defined. Recent studies indicate that catabolic responses during a febrile infection evolve in a sequence that is repetitive, predictable, and in certain ways analogous to the catabolic responses seen after injury. Fever appears to be the major stimulus for initiating catabolic losses during acute infection. Widespread catabolism of body tissues is not seen until the fever has become evident, leading early investigators to believe that the metabolic response to infection was primarily a response to fever. A febrile response requires excessive expenditure of body energy, even though the fever is generally accompanied by a diminished intake of food and other nutrients. Such changes lead inevitably to negative balances for many substances.

It has been taught that the increase in resting metabolism of the body can be predicted from the degree of elevation in the body temperature. DuBois[142] studied a variety of medical conditions and found an approximate increase of 13 percent for each degree Celsius rise in body temperature (7 percent for each degree Fahrenheit). He expressed the opinion that the effects of fever on the metabolic rate corresponded to the principle of van't Hoff: the velocity of chemical reactions is proportional to the temperature at which they occur. Therefore, at a temperature of 40.5° C (105°F) the average human body would have an increase of approximately 50 percent in its resting metabolic expenditure. Comparison of the resting metabolic expenditure in postoperative patients revealed that the 13 percent relationship of DuBois provided an approximate correlation for brief periods of low-grade fever.[143] This was in contrast to cases of major peritonitis and burns in which the energy expenditure was increased well beyond the value predicted from the extent of fever.[144] A study of the medical conditions from which DuBois drew his correlation between body temperature and resting metabolism reveals an interesting separation in different cases. Cases with chronic pulmonary tuberculosis tended to show a significant fever with minimal increase in the energy expenditure. These cases were in contrast to the severe cases of typhoid fever in which the same elevation in temperature was accompanied by a greater than average increase in energy expenditure. Coleman and other associates of DuBois[145] noticed that the pulmonary tuberculosis patients tended to excrete relatively small amounts of urinary nitrogen, while the typhoid patients had large urinary nitrogen losses and were extremely difficult to put into positive nitrogen balance by any form of supplemental oral intake. It seems probable that these two types of medical fever correspond to surgical patients in whom with late depletion there may be a fever and relatively small increase in energy expenditure, in contrast to early diffuse peritonitis in which the energy expenditure, as in the typhoid patients, is considerably in excess of that predicted from the fever.

Splanchnic Metabolism and Fever

The increase in resting heat production associated with fever has never been clearly identified as to the tissues involved or the chemical reactions that are responsible. Studies on nonshivering thermogenesis in small animals emphasize increased peripheral utilization of fatty acids. Yet the hypermetabolism of clinical fever may not be equivalent to nonshivering thermogenesis induced by environmental changes.

The old observation of increased net heat production following protein ingestion (specific dynamic action) has been linked to the deamination of certain amino acids. Cairnie and co-workers[146] have suggested that the increased heat production after skeletal injury in the rat might be due to an "endogenous specific dynamic action" that was underlying the increased nitrogen excretion. Since urea synthesis is increased in protein feeding, injury, and a variety of febrile conditions, and since the liver is the sole organ to synthesize urea, is the hypermetabolism of clinical fever limited to the liver?

The gastrointestinal blood supply under normal resting conditions could conceivably determine hepatic function through its domination of the substrate supply. But, in fact, the hepatic blood supply appears to be adjusted to the metabolic requirements of the body as a whole. Hepatic blood flow increases after a protein meal in proportion to the rise in cardiac output and blood flow to the entire body that occurs at the same time. Similar changes in systemic and hepatic circulation have been detected in man during febrile reactions to pyrogenic agents that increase total oxygen consumption. Liver temperature rises after protein feeding and during fever, presumably as a result of augmented hepatocellular metabolism. Myers[147] has confirmed that the relationship between cardiac output and arteriovenous oxygen differences for the whole body has a similar pattern to that which exists for the liver. Rapid intravenous injection of amino acids caused a prompt rise in the splanchnic oxygen consumption as a result of widening the arteriovenous oxygen difference without increasing hepatic blood flow. This pattern differs from that following the administration of an intravenous pyrogen to normal man, in which the arteriovenous oxygen difference remains essentially normal while hepatic blood flow is promptly increased.

The extent of increase in splanchnic blood flow and oxygen consumption was studied by Gump and co-workers in 15 patients who were febrile as a result of intraperitoneal infection.[148] Whole body and splanchnic blood flow were measured together with whole body and splanchnic oxygen consumption. One-third of the patients had no increase in oxygen consumption despite fever. Such patients had small increases in cardiac output with no significant change in the proportion of blood flow or oxygen consumption across the splanchnic bed. The patients with an increase in resting oxygen consumption always had an increased splanchnic blood flow. The increase in blood flow and oxygen consumption across the splanchnic viscera accounted for only 40 to 50 percent of the total increase, establishing that the hypermetabolism of this form of surgical fever involved tissues other than the liver and chemical reactions other than deamination and urea synthesis. It is of interest that 3 burn patients studied in a similar fashion revealed much larger increases in resting oxygen consumption; however, the resting blood flow to the liver was of the same order of magnitude as that seen with intra-abdominal infection.[149] This is consistent with the fact that the fever and the increase in nitrogen excretion of burn patients are of the same order of magnitude as those seen in cases of major peritoneal infection.

Protein Metabolism and Fever

At normal body temperature the rate of destruction of cell proteins occurs so slowly that the normal concentration of a specific type of protein is readily maintained by synthesis. As the body temperature rises, both the synthetic repair process and the destruction of the protein increase, although at widely different rates, until a temperature level is reached at which the rate of destruction equals the rate of repair. Any further increment in temperature leads to a rate of protein destruction that rapidly exceeds that for repair because of the great disparity in the temperature coefficients of the opposing processes. Metabolic activity begins to fail unless the system is cooled, and the cell dies at a temperature only a few degrees above the temperature of balance between production and breakdown. The temperature at which death occurs for indefinitely long exposure is called the thermal death point. For skin, the temperature corresponds to the threshold temperature for burn injury.

There appear to be qualitative changes in intermediary metabolism in febrile conditions of certain types. It has long been recognized that patients with a variety of acute infections "use protein extravagantly."[150] This toxic destruction of protein cannot be overcome except by the administration of supranormal amounts of protein and calories. The phenomenon is not a specific reaction to infection; it also occurs following severe injury or major surgical operation. The nitrogen loss cannot be attributed merely to accelerated energy expenditure, since protein can be conserved in both exercise and hyperthyroidism if caloric balance is maintained. The tendency to waste protein appears to be a reaction to injury that is most characteristic of previously healthy, well-nourished patients. Late in the convalescence after major infections, the nitrogen excretion is usually decreased below normal, and will show only minimal, if any, elevation with the onset of fever.

Beisel and co-workers[151] reported metabolic balance studies in 61 healthy male soldiers who underwent exposure to specific infective agents. Illness associated with three different kinds of infection was accompanied by a remarkably stereotyped pattern of catabolic response, the magnitude of metabolic change being related to the severity of the illness. Cumulative losses of the major intracellular elements—nitrogen, potassium, magnesium, and phosphorus—began shortly after the onset of illness and reached a maximum value after convalescence had begun. Although catabolic changes predominate, in certain patients the initiation of infection was accompanied by anabolic changes. Plasma amino acid levels decreased after exposure for several days prior to the onset of fever. Nitrogen balance became negative despite the fact that both anabolic and catabolic processes were occurring simultaneously during the febrile period of the infection. The investigators felt that the catabolism of muscle protein was serving to redistribute amino acids required for the synthesis of protein in other locations, as well as responding to increased requirements for gluconeogenesis.

Wannemacher and co-workers[152] demonstrated an endogenous mediator substance that is elaborated from polymorphonuclear leukocytes in the presence of various infective agents. This substance is not endotoxin.[153] The assay for this material is based on more rapid uptake of amino acids and zinc from the circulating bloodstream into the liver cells. It has been demonstrated that this amino acid uptake is not for gluconeogenesis but rather for protein synthesis, apparently for the synthesis of acute phase proteins as part of the metabolic response to infection. This is noteworthy because the organ that is responsible for the majority of new glucose formation during catabolic states is also the organ that is involved in acute phase protein synthesis, since all the acute phase proteins are glycoproteins. Stimulation of this process requires muscle protein breakdown in addition to the amount of breakdown that would be predicted by urea excretion. Therefore, this may help to explain the observation that the most rapid and extreme muscle wasting in clinical conditions is observed in the well-muscled young adult male who is febrile as a result of visceral injuries and secondary infection.

The contribution of alanine to the synthesis of glucose and the oxidation of alanine was evaluated by Long and co-workers[154] in normal and septic patients using ^{14}C-alanine. A significant increase was found in the conversion of alanine to glucose in the presence of sepsis. This occurred despite glucose administration, which would have markedly reduced this conversion in normal, postabsorptive man. It was of special interest that the percentage of alanine oxidized to CO_2 in 3 hours was the same in the septic patients as in normal man, suggesting that pyruvate oxidation was not depressed by this degree of sepsis.

Fat Metabolism

Gallin and co-workers[155] described an increase in the plasma concentration of several lipid moieties including triglyceride and FFA during gram-negative infections. Such increases were not observed in infections due to influenza or gram-positive cocci. These findings suggested the possibility that each different class of infecting microorganism might lead to a characteristic response of lipid metabolism within the host. However, this theory was not substantiated when tested by the same workers using the rabbit as an experimental animal.[156]

Fiser and co-workers[157] followed the serial changes in plasma lipids and lipoproteins of monkeys after infection with pneumoniae and salmonella. The pneumococci infection resulted in increased levels of plasma triglycerides, and prebeta lipoproteins. The salmonella group showed increased levels of triglycerides and prebeta and alpha lipoproteins together with decreases in phospholipids, cholesterol, and beta lipoproteins in plasma. The free fatty acid response in both groups was variable. In contrast to the many hormonal and metabolic responses that are relatively stereotyped during different infections, lipid responses appear to vary according to the nature of the invading organism as well as to the stage, severity, and duration of the illness.

Lees and co-workers[158] studied the influence of an experimental viral infection (sandfly fever) on plasma lipids and lipoprotein metabolism in healthy young men. Plasma triglycerides were seen to fall initially and then rise above control levels, suggesting an increased use of lipid for tissue fuel in the early febrile period. These workers noted that the mechanisms that mediated the metabolic responses to such a mild, self-limited virus infection took precedence over some of the ordinary demands of energy balance.

Kaufmann and co-workers[159] studied lipid disposal in monkeys following administration of *Salmonella typhimurium*. Salmonella infection was associated with reduced clearance of orally and intravenously administered lipid and markedly reduced postheparin lipolytic activity. Pneumoniae infection showed some impairment of oral but no impairment of intravenous lipid clearance, and postheparin lipolytic activity was only slightly reduced. An impairment of lipid disposal may contribute to hypertriglyceridemia during infection, particularly with gram-negative organisms.

When humans and experimental animals are fed an adequate diet, the concentration of ketone bodies in the liver and blood is very low. With prolonged fasting, large quantities of ketones are produced in the liver and transported to various tissues as a source of energy. Based on the increased nitrogen losses that are associated with most infectious processes, Wannemacher[160] has suggested that the infected host may not be able to evoke the physiological mechanisms normally utilized to conserve body protein. Neufeld and co-workers[161] conducted studies in the effect of several bacterial infections on the gluconeogenic and ketogenic activity of rat liver. During an infection the concentration of ketone bodies in the liver and blood is markedly depressed, and this depression is accompanied by a concomitant decrease in the concentration of circulating free fatty acids in the serum. These workers postulate decreased lipolysis in the infected host to account for these changes. They note the data of Ryan and co-workers[162] and of Zenser and associates,[163] which show that infection causes hyperinsulinemia. This hyperinsulinemia may be correlated with a reduction in fatty acid mobilization and perhaps the reduction in ketosis during sepsis. However, the decreased concentration of ketones and FFA in the plasma could be associated with increased utilization by peripheral tissue.

Fuel Interrelationships

The liver plays a unique role in regulating the metabolism of foodstuffs, particularly in relation to amino acids and glucose. This role is related to many factors, such as its anatomic position, its central importance in amino acid catabolism and gluconeogenesis, its rapid gain or loss of protein, and the fact that hormones that influence amino acid metabolism often have opposite effects on muscle and on the liver. The liver modulates the large fluctuations in amino acids of the portal vein during feeding and fasting to preserve a surprisingly uniform level and pattern of circulating amino acids. How does the liver discriminate in its output of amino acids according to the needs of peripheral tissues such as muscle? The liver does not catabolize the branched-chain amino acids. Do the peripheral tissues have some feedback signal to the liver for degrading essential amino acids other than the branched-chain amino acids? Further information is needed to answer these questions in regard to both normal food intake and starvation and to allow examination of how such fuel interrelationships are disturbed as a result of major injury or severe infection.

Abnormal energy metabolism and protein breakdown in injury and infection has been studied by Clowes and co-workers.[164] They present data that are interpreted to indicate a muscle fuel deficit in such conditions, causing muscle tissue to increase the oxidation of branched-chain amino acids with a corresponding increase in the output of alanine for hepatic gluconeogenesis. Border and co-workers[165] suggest that during injury and infection, the lack of a normal amino acid mixture coming to the liver from muscle results in potential restriction of hepatic synthesis of a variety of proteins, including those for export such as albumin. Skillman and colleagues[166] have shown improved albumin synthesis in postoperative patients when given 3.5 percent amino acids rather than a 5 percent glucose solution for intravenous nutrition.

ENDOCRINE RESPONSE TO INJURY AND INFECTION

As discussed in the previous section the metabolic response to injury and infection may be divided into an initial ebb or shock phase and a secondary flow phase. The responses in both phases depend in part on the nature of the precipitating event (trauma, sepsis, hemorrhage) as well as its severity. Nevertheless, certain aspects are fairly constant and permit a general description.

EBB PHASE OR SHOCK

The metabolic response to traumatic or septic shock is characterized by hypometabolism (decreased oxygen consumption and body temperature) in a setting of hyperglycemia and increased gluconeogenesis. The endocrine changes in this phase consist of hypoinsulinemia, increased glucocorticoid secretion, and augmented adrenal medullary activity.

Despite an elevation in blood glucose in the ebb phase, plasma insulin levels are reduced.[167,168] Hypoinsulinemia has been observed acutely after experimental bacteremia,[140] during the intraoperative period in patients undergoing abdominal surgery,[169] following acute blood loss,[170,171] and in association with extensive body burns.[168] In the last circumstance, the hypoinsulinemia was most marked in the patients with the most extensive thermal injury.[2]

Since the hypoinsulinemia of the shock phase occurs in the face of hyperglycemia, inhibition of pancreatic beta cell secretion is clearly evident. Of the physiological factors (other than hypoglycemia) capable of inhibiting beta-cell function, epinephrine and norepinephrine, by virtue of their alpha-adrenergic effects, are of particular importance.[172] Although the importance of the sympathetic nervous system in the response to stress has been recognized since the classical studies of Cannon, the role of circulating catecholamines has been more difficult to substantiate, primarily because of difficulties in the development of sensitive, reproducible assays. Nevertheless, a variety of studies implicate the adrenal medulla in the hypoinsulinemia of shock. Thus administration of ganglionic blockers or adrenalectomy abolishes both the hypoinsulinemic and hyperglycemic response.[173,174] In addition, elevations in urinary catecholamines have been observed early in the response to thermal[175] or hemorrhagic shock.[176]

The combined setting of decreased insulin secretion and elevations in catecholamines can account for the alterations in glucose metabolism observed in the ebb phase. Hypoinsulinemia favors an acceleration of glycogenolysis and gluconeogenesis. In addition to inhibiting insulin secretion, epinephrine stimulates glycogenolysis and gluconeogenesis and interferes with insulin-mediated uptake of glucose by peripheral tissues.[177] Consequently, hepatic glucose production and the utilization of gluconeogenic substrates is increased in traumatic or septic shock while glucose utilization is normal or reduced, resulting in hyperglycemia.[178] The decrease in glucose utilization is due not only to hypoinsulinemia but also to a diminished tissue responsiveness to whatever insulin is available.[179]

In contrast to the changes in insulin and catecholamines, it should be noted that glucagon levels are unchanged during the initial 24 to 48 hours after extensive body burns[168] or during the course of intra-abdominal surgery.[169] Consequently, hyperglucagonemia does not appear to be a contributory factor in the acute hyperglycemia of traumatic or septic shock.

Plasma cortisol levels have been noted to be elevated in proportion to the severity of the trauma during the first 24 hours after thermal injury.[168] However, inasmuch as the ebb phase is not characterized by major changes in amino acid or nitrogen metabolism (see above), the metabolic effects of these acute changes in adrenocortical secretion have not been clearly delineated.

FLOW PHASE

As discussed above, the flow phase following trauma or sepsis is characterized by hyperglycemia, hypermetabolism (increased oxygen consumption and fever), and markedly negative nitrogen balance, resulting in a decrease in body protein stores.

Insulin

In contrast to the hypoinsulinemia of the ebb or shock phase, hyperinsulinemia and insulin resistance are characteristic findings in the flow phase. Thus, in patients studied 24 to 48 hours after abdominal surgery, insulin levels are increased,[169,180] but glucose disappearance is reduced.[180,181] Impaired glucose tolerance is most marked after severe sepsis or trauma but is demonstrable even after mild viral illnesses.[182]

The coexistence of hyperinsulinemia and hyperglycemia indicates the presence of insulin resistance. After infection or trauma, as well as after hemorrhage, a decrease in insulin-stimulated uptake of glucose by muscle and fat tissue has been demonstrated.[162,183] The resistance to insulin may also contribute to alterations in muscle amino acid metabolism. An acceleration in muscle catabolism of branched-chain amino acids (leucine, isoleucine, and valine) has been demonstrated after trauma and sepsis.[184] These changes are analogous to those observed in muscles of rats with experimental diabetes.[185] Furthermore, the markedly negative nitrogen balance after trauma is reversible only by the administration of massive amounts of insulin and glucose.[186] Thus insulin resistance is a major factor in the development of the glucose intolerance and glucose overproduction and contributes, at least in part, to protein wasting and negative nitrogen balance in the flow phase. It should, however, be noted that in patients with very extensive body burns, the hypoinsulinemia observed in shock persists throughout the flow phase as well.[168]

Catecholamines

Since hyperglycemia is relatively mild, while nitrogen wasting is extensive following injury or infection, it is clear that factors other than insulin resistance or insulin lack must contribute to the metabolic disturbance. The role of catecholamines has received considerable attention in recent years.[115,175] Increased urinary levels of epinephrine and norepinephrine are evident after thermal injury or bacteremia.[140,168,175] A calorigenic effect of catecholamines has long been recognized. In addition, alpha- and beta-adrenergic blockade reduces the hypermetabolic response to burn injury.[175] These findings have led to the conclusion that catecholamines are major determinants of the insulin resistance and hypermetabolism of stress.[115,175]

Although there is little doubt that catecholamines contribute to the metabolic response to injury and infection, whether these hormones are the primary regulators of this response has not been established. Virtually all the available data have involved measurements of urinary rather than plasma catecholamine levels. What are needed are studies in which catecholamines are infused in doses that simulate the levels observed after trauma or infection. Until such data are available, it is unclear, for example, whether calorigenesis as observed after trauma is due to catecholamines.

Cortisol

Hypersecretion of cortisol is another characteristic response following trauma or sepsis.[168] The increase in cortisol is proportional to the severity of the trauma.[168] Furthermore, plasma cortisol is strongly correlated with increments in gluconeogenic substrates and plasma urea.[168] These observations thus support a role for hypercorticism in the protein dissolution as well as the glucose overproduction of the flow phase. However, the classical studies by Ingle[187] involving adrenalectomized animals given replacement doses of glucocorticoid clearly demonstrated a permissive rather than a regulatory role for the adrenal cortex in the nitrogen wasting that follows trauma.

Glucagon

A rise in plasma glucagon is observed 24 hours after intra-abdominal surgery[169] and 48 to 72 hours after therma injury.[168,188] Infection is also characterized by hyperglucagonemia.[189] In each of these conditions the magnitude of hyperglucagonemia is proportional to the severity of the injury or infection.[168,189] Inasmuch as administration of exogenous glucagon has been known to cause hyperglycemia and stimulate gluconeogenesis, hyperglucagonemia or a fall in the insulin/glucagon ratio (relative hyperglucagonemia) has been implicated as the mediator of stress-induced catabolism.[190] A variety of studies suggest that glucagon is of relatively minor importance, however.

Despite the elevations in glucagon, plasma levels of this hormone fail to correlate with hyperglycemia or changes in gluconeogenic substrates in either postoperative or burned patients.[168,169] Furthermore, infusions of glucagon causing plasma elevations in this hormone comparable to those observed with severe burns fail to induce hyperglycemia, glucose intolerance, or negative nitrogen balance.[191,192] In the absence of an absolute decline in insulin or a change in tissue responsiveness to insulin, glucagon (in physiological amounts) is not diabetogenic.[193] Accordingly, hyperglucagonemia is likely to contribute to hyperglycemia in the setting of tissue resistance to insulin which characterizes the flow phase; however, it is not the primary determinant of the catabolic response.

Summary

The flow phase following trauma, infection, or hemorrhage is characterized by insulin resistance and increased secretion of catecholamines, cortisol, and glucagon. No single hormonal change has been established as the primary or essential modulator of the metabolic alterations (hyperglycemia, hypermetabolism, and nitrogen wasting). Possibly it is the synergistic interaction of the individual components in this multihormonal response that determines the metabolic status of the patient.

ENVIRONMENTAL TEMPERATURE AND THE METABOLIC RESPONSE

EXPERIMENTAL INJURY

Environmental factors exert a profound effect on the response to injury in the rat and other small mammals. Qualitatively similar changes can be expected to occur in larger mammals such as man, although the exploration of this area is just beginning. The growing interest in the relation of environmental conditions to convalescence after various forms of trauma in man justifies a brief review of current knowledge from small animal studies.

Various investigators have shown that the rat has an increased mortality and shortened survival time following various forms of injury, when the ambient temperature is raised significantly above control values anywhere in the range of 10° to 37°C. Increasing the temperature of the damaged part increases the severity of the tissue damage and consequent loss of fluid into the area. At a later stage, both burns and surgical wounds of the skin have been shown to heal faster at 30°C than at 20°C, perhaps because of better circulation in the area of the wound.[194]

When rats are injured at an ordinary room temperature of about 20°C, the injury is rapidly followed by a fall in deep body or core temperature. Except in major hemorrhage, this is not due, in the early stages, to a failure of oxygen transport to the heat-producing organs. This is in contrast to the later stages leading to death, in which the picture is dominated by a failure of oxygen transport. An optimal temperature for survival after various forms of injury has been reported from many laboratories for various species. This optimal temperature is always below the thermoneutral zone and is associated with a temporary decrease in core temperature. Stoner[195] has observed that "from a teleological standpoint the optimum environmental temperature is one which allows the body temperature to fall at an optimum rate to a level which is not so low that unaided recovery is impossible yet which confers advantages by limiting the injury and husbanding the body's metabolic resources."

THE SPECIAL PROBLEM OF THE BURN PATIENT

No injury results in greater changes in the host for a longer period of time than a thermal burn. Twenty-five years ago, burn cachexia was frequently observed but poorly understood. Patients with large burns lost weight progressively, and weeks after injury, they became hypoalbuminemic and anemic. Skin grafts frequently failed to take, and the death rate was high. Cope et al.[196] in 1953 reported that burned patients demonstrated a chronic increase in metabolic rate without any change in the circulating levels of thyroid hormone. This report also noted that the hypermetabolism persisted until wound closure. Lieberman and Lansche[197] demonstrated an increase in evaporative heat loss and metabolic rate in burned rats and suggested that there was a causal relationship. They observed that both the evaporative heat loss and rate of heat production returned toward normal when such burn wounds were covered with a material impermeable to water. Caldwell et al.[198] demonstrated that thyroid function was not necessary for the hypermetabolism in burned rats and that increasing the ambient temperature for such animals resulted in a return to near normal of the metabolic rate without affecting the increased evaporative heat loss. With partitional calorimetry it was demonstrated that the decrease in metabolism effected by a warm ambient temperature was due to a decrease in heat loss by radiation, conduction, and convection.[199]

Caldwell et al.[200] showed that burned rats housed at 30°C, with their total caloric intake fixed at preburned levels, were able to maintain positive nitrogen balance and gain body weight, whereas similarly burned and nourished animals housed at 20°C lost weight rapidly and sustained a negative nitrogen balance for more than 40 days following the injury. Thus the reduction of dry heat loss for burned rats through the medium of increased ambient temperature above thermal neutrality resulted in a great nutritional advantage.

Goodall et al.[201] first recorded large increases in the rate of excretion of catacholamines in patient with large burns. These authors noted that the major portion of the increase was noradrenalin and that the amount of increase roughly paralleled the size of the burn.

Harrison and co-workers[202] showed a positive correlation between the metabolic rate and rate of catecholamine excretion for burned patients and postulated that an increased catecholamine excretion is responsible for the elevated metabolic rate seen in burned patients.

Zawacki et al.[203] studied 12 burned patients before and after their burn wounds had been covered for 12 hours with an impermeable material. In these 12 patients (average burn size, 40 percent BSA; average day of study, 14th PBD) with medium-size burns studied in the early postburn period, increased body temperature was, on average, 0.5°F. If there was no associated decrease in the rate of heat production, covering the burn wound should have resulted in a rise in body temperature of 1 degree per hour in some of these patients. From these observations, Zawacki challenged the idea that in man increased evaporative heat loss occurring through the burn wound was the primary drive for the hypermetabolism following thermal trauma.

In contrast to Zawacki, Neely et al.[204] found a prompt decrease in the metabolic rate of all but 1 of 6 burned patients after burn wounds were covered, but 5 of the 6 patients were febrile.

Birke and associates[205] studied burned patients at environmental temperatures of 22°C and 32°C. These investigators found a decrease in the rate of heat production and catecholamine excretion at 32°C as compared with 22°C without a change in the rate of evaporative heat loss. Similarly, Davis et al.[206] showed that housing burned patients in a warm (32°C), dry environment resulted in less loss of body weight, less excretion of urinary nitrogen, and a lower metabolic rate than did keeping them at an ambient temperature of 22°C.

Wilmore et al.[207] confirmed the findings of Birke and demonstrated further that the febrile patients showed increased tissue conduction and loss via radiation. This study also showed a lack of correlation between the rate of catecholamine excretion and metabolic rate when the metabolic rate was very high. Combined alpha and beta blockade of these patients produced a fall in metabolic rate, but 64 percent of the original increase persisted. Wilmore suggested that alterations in "hypothalamic function" due to injury resulting in increased catacholamine elaboration would explain the metabolic response to thermal injury. This explanation seems incomplete in view of (1) the persistent hypermetabolic state of Wilmore's patients following alpha and beta blockade, and (2) the inability of even adrenalin to produce more than a 30 to 35 percent increase in metabolic rate in man, while noradrenalin (which accounts for 90 percent of the late increase in catecholamine in burned patients) can produce only a 21 ± 8 percent increase in the metabolic rate in man.[208] Furthermore, burned rats with no adrenal medullary function are still hypermetabolic at ambient temperature of 20°C and 28°C, although they demonstrate chronic whole body hypothermia when housed at 20°C.[209]

In summary, burned humans demonstrate an increased metabolic rate that correlates very well with an increased evaporative heat loss. There is, in addition, a chronic febrile state with increased tissue conduction and dry heat loss as a result. Catecholamine turnover, principally of noradrenalin, is increased.

Elevating the ambient temperature for such patients results in a lowering of the metabolic rate, a decrease in the rate of excretion of catecholamines, a probable decrease in dry heat loss, and little or no change in the evaporative heat loss. Patients treated in this manner lose less body weight and excrete less urinary nitrogen.

These data indicate that the zone of thermal neutrality for the burned patient is increased. Wilmore states that the burned patient behaves as though he is internally warm rather than externally cold. The overall evidence suggests that he is both internally warm and externally cold. The burned patient acts as though the regulatory set point for body temperature had been shifted upward. Efforts to explain the hypermetabolic state following thermal trauma must include the metabolic effects of fever. Special consideration of the effects of fever should be given in the burned patient, for the fever persists for so long that the cumulative effect becomes more important than in many febrile states.

What, then, is the primary drive and/or drives for the hypermetabolic state following thermal trauma? One interpretation of the data supports the idea that increased evaporative heat loss and a chronic elevation of body temperature are the primary etiological factors producing an increased metabolic rate. The possibility of interaction between these two factors is very real, for an increase in metabolic rate may produce fever, and fever definitely increases the metabolic rate following the van't Hoff law as if the whole body had a Q_{10} of 2.3 to 2.5. Most of the data from both man and animals fit this idea. The metabolic effect of fever is subtle and has not been adequately studied. Even the basic cause of fever in burned patients is not understood. Increases in the excretion rates for catecholamines, principally noradrenalin, respond as if they are secondary to the chronic stress of hypermetabolism; increased release and turnover of catecholamines is a nonspecific response seen to some degree after all trauma and may not be a very effective way to increase heat production. Most investigators agree that the burned patient should be cared for in a warm, ambient environment.

HEAT METABOLISM AND THE SURGICAL PATIENT

A reduction in posttraumatic nitrogen loss and a more normal plasma protein metabolism have recently been shown in the rat and in man following fracture of a long bone if convalescence was in an environment of 28° to 30°C (82.4° to 86.0°F) rather than 20° to 21°C (68.0° to 69.8°F).[199] The mechanisms for this improvement is not clear and is the subject of active study. An ambient temperature below the thermoneutral zone in the patient area may cause an increased nitrogen loss as a result of a greater food requirement or of some unidentified neuroendocrine stimulus.

Burn patients are febrile before there is significant bacterial colonization of burn wounds. The fever appears in 2 to 4 days and later becomes obscured by fever from secondary bacterial pyrogens originating in the burn wound. Although evidence is lacking, one possible explanation of the early fever seen with thermal injury is the absorption of heat-modified protein fragments from the burn wound that have the capacity to act as pyrogens at a hypothalamic level. The neurosurgical patient with damage to the brain stem may demonstrate no thermoregulatory responses to a positive or negative thermal load. In such cases, the patient may actually require treatment as if he were poikilothermic.

Recent advances in construction of buildings have included high-rise elevators, decreased window space, artificial lighting, and so forth: all of which contribute to a separation of man from his natural environment. None of these architectural features have more physiological significance than modern ventilation and air conditioning. The ease of manipulating temperature, humidity, and air flow in modern hospitals has outdistanced our knowledge of physiological requirements and how they are altered in the critically ill patient. Too often, the ventilation and air conditioning are regulated for the comfort of the professional staff rather than for the physiological needs of the patients.

One suggestion has been that the thermoneutral zone (28° to 30°C) for seminude man should be the guide for the ambient temperature of hospital wards and particularly intensive care units. Perhaps in the hospital, graduated patient care from areas such as the recovery room and the intensive care unit to areas of intermediate care and limited care for late convalescence should be accompanied by changes in ambient temperature, from 25°C (77°F) for an area of intermediate care to conventional indoor temperature—21° to 22°C (70° to 72°F)—for late convalescence. Thus the transition in graduated medical care could have a parallel stepwise return toward the mild environmental stress associated with conditions of ordinary indoor living.

NUTRITIONAL CONSIDERATIONS DURING INJURY AND INFECTION

THE INFLUENCE OF NUTRITIONAL DEPLETION

The role of nutritional depletion in the metabolic response to injury and infection has been an area of confusion in the surgical literature. Abbott and Albertson[210] studied the nitrogen balance of surgical patients and concluded that the postoperative metabolic response was essentially that of the reduced voluntary food intake that usually follows major injury. Such conclusions make it important to differentiate between the metabolic response of starvation and that of injury. Such differences can provide perspective for considering the influence of *prior* nutritional depletion on the metabolic response to injury and infection.

Studies in partial and total starvation were summarized early in this chapter. Resting energy expenditure, nitrogen excretion, and blood sugar levels have been observed to decrease in somewhat parallel fashion with starvation. The resting energy expenditure, nitrogen excretion, and blood sugar levels all tend to increase with major injury and infection; thus the metabolic response in these conditions cannot simply be ascribed to partial starvation. The patients studied by Abbott and Albertson were mostly adult female patients undergoing cholecystectomy, which produces only a limited degree of operative injury. Hence the major metabolic features of injury were scarcely evident, and the authors concluded that the postoperative response was mainly that of partial starvation.

As described in the preceding sections, it is now reasonably clear that the source of most of the additional nitrogen, sulfur, and phosphorus lost in the urine in the flow phase after injury and infection is mainly from the labile protein of skeletal muscle, rather than from viscera such as liver. This labile protein is nutritionally dependent and readily mobilizable in the well-nourished patient. Associated with this increased breakdown of protein are accompanying increments in the urinary excretion of substances that also are notable constituents of muscle, namely phosphate, creatine, potassium, zinc, and to a lesser extent, magnesium.

The importance of a dietary-dependent, endogenous protein pool was demonstrated by Munro and Cuthbertson[211] and by

Munro and Chalmers,[212] who found no increase in urinary nitrogen following fracture of the femur in the rat if the animals had been fed a protein-free but calorie-adequate diet for some time before the injury. They also showed that the proportion of protein in the preinjury diet, but not the postinjury diet, quantitatively affected the response to trauma, as judged by nitrogen excretion of patients following two forms of gastrointestinal operations. Gastric operations on patients who had satisfactory nutrition prior to the operation were associated with a significant increase in nitrogen loss, while nitrogen excretion following operation was not increased in patients undergoing colon resection for chronic inflammatory disease whose nutrition was poor.[213] Thus the level of the previous nutrition will strongly influence the nitrogen excretion following injury and presumably following infection. It is of interest that the depleted patient with minimal increase in nitrogen loss following injury is also the one who shows the least increase in resting metabolic expenditure. The depleted patients who show this blunted response to injury would be expected to show the greatest improvement in nitrogen balance from any given level of parenteral nutrition.

EVOLUTION OF SURGICAL NUTRITION

The attitude of physicians and surgeons toward the role of nutrition in the management of the acutely injured or infected patient has been heavily conditioned by a blend of experimental studies, untested assumptions, and the availability of nutritional products that were sufficiently safe and inexpensive to become a part of patient management. It is only now that there is a growing recognition that every hospitalized patient demonstrates a metabolic response that is some particular blend of starvation, injury, and infection conditioned by age, sex, body size, and previous nutrition. During the decades just before and after World War I, pioneering studies were conducted on the metabolic response to starvation, injury, and infection. Benedict[214] conducted a remarkably detailed study of starvation in the normal adult male. Cuthbertson[215] correlated urinary excretion patterns of injured man with pulse, temperature, and basal oxygen consumption. DuBois[216] established the relationship of fever to increased energy metabolism in various types of clinical infection. Investigation of the fields of starvation, injury, and infection have proceeded along largely independent lines since that time.

During the 1930s the provision of intravenous fluids was largely limited to intravenous saline and occasionally glucose solutions, but with a significant incidence of febrile reactions. Isotonic glucose solutions represented the routine intraoperative and postoperative nutrition during the 1940s and 1950s. This was done for two reasons: The daily provision of 100 g of glucose would prevent starvation ketosis and provide nitrogen sparing. In addition the concept of "postoperative salt intolerance"[217] meant that solutions of glucose rather than sodium were the preferred way of giving 2–3 liters of fluid per day to the acute postoperative patient.

During the 1940s and 1950s, there was tremendous interest in the role of the adrenal cortex. The metabolic response to injury was assumed to be an obligatory neuroendocrine process in which the adrenal cortex played a central role. Attempts to treat the acutely injured patient by providing nitrogen as protein hydrolysate or crystalline amino acid solutions were generally thought to be inappropriate for two reasons: (1) the metabolic response to injury would ensure that the amino acids were "burned for energy," and (2) the inability to provide adequate calories intravenously would also ensure that the amino acids were burned for energy, since nitrogen equilibrium could not be obtained without caloric equilibrium. This reluctance to give parenteral sources of nitrogen was prevalent, despite the pioneering work of Robert Elman,[218] who demonstrated the clinical use of intravenous amino acids.

Efforts to devlop a safe and reliable intravenous fat preparation in the United States were terminated after initial promising results.[219] During the period of 1960 to 1966, Wretlind, Schuberth, and Hallberg[220] developed and utilized a new intravenous fat emulsion, with an unusually low incidence of undesirable side reactions.

The practice of monitoring surgical patients with an inlying catheter for serial measurements of central venous pressure became an acceptable clinical practice in the mid 1960s. Dr. Johnathan Rhodes and his associate, Dr. Stanley Dudrick,[221] recognized the potential of this practice for providing hypertonic intravenous nutrition to acutely ill and injured patients. Thus the combined experience from both sides of the Atlantic Ocean began to emphasize the importance of more adequate nutritional support in the acutely ill and injured patient. Several of the myths and fables of previous decades were demolished. One such myth held that it was impossible to achieve a positive nitrogen balance when intake was entirely limited to intravenous rather than oral routes. Wilmore and Dudrick[222] provided a dramatic demonstration that an infant could not only survive but also have a normal growth rate while receiving nothing but total parenteral nutrition, even without intravenous fat being commercially available in the United States. More recently, the concept that caloric equilibrium is necessary before nitrogen equilibrium can be established has been challenged by Blackburn and Flatt[223] with their studies of intravenous nutritional support providing amino acids alone. Some of the recent approaches to parenteral nutrition are discussed in more detail in the following section.

TOTAL PARENTERAL NUTRITION

Total parenteral nutrition (TPN) or hyperalimentation is a technique involving the infusion of a hypertonic glucose-amino acid mixture providing approximately 1000 Calories plus 30–50g of amino acids per liter of infusate.[224] In this manner the caloric as well as the nitrogen requirements are met during the hypermetabolic flow phase following trauma or sepsis. Because of the hyperosmolarity (600–800 milliosmol/liter) of the solutions (engendered by the low caloric density of carbohydrate), administration is via a catheter placed in a central vein (e.g., the superior vena cava). Rapid dilution of the infusion mixture by high blood flow in such vessels prevents the phlebitis and thrombosis that would occur if a peripheral vein were employed.

The studies of Dudrick and colleagues have clearly documented the effectiveness of TPN in patients with extensive body burns or multiple gastrointestinal fistulas complicated by sepsis.[225] Positive nitrogen balance and healing of wounds are more rapidly achieved than with conventional intravenous infusions even when supplemented by oral feedings.[225] The long-held notion that negative nitrogen balance cannot be circumvented in the flow phase of sepsis or trauma is no longer tenable. The key to reversal of the catabolic process in this circumstance is the provision of adequate calories (equivalent to the hypermetabolic expenditure) as well as amino acids in a dose of at least 1.5 g/kg of body weight. The importance of amino acids in the infusate is indicated by the fact that even in the absence of trauma or infection (i.e., in the fasted patient), intravenous glucose of itself will diminish but not entirely eliminate net protein catabolism.[226]

Total parenteral nutrition is not without risk to the patient.

Complications include sepsis (for which the catheter is most commonly the source), severe hyperglycemia, hypophosphatemia, hyperchloremic acidosis, and essential fatty acid deficiencies.[227,228] Strict attention to detail such as meticulous care of the puncture site, use of an on-line membrane filter, monitoring of blood glucose and electrolytes, and addition of phosphate to the infusate can eliminate most of these problems.[224,225]

ISOTONIC AMINO ACID MIXTURES

Because of the small but definite hazards associated with hypertonic infusates (TPN), an alternate approach involving the use of isotonic amino acids without glucose has been developed by Blackburn and colleagues.[229] These investigators have shown that negative nitrogen balance in the postoperative state can be reversed by administering a 100-g mixture of amino acids. The advantage of this technique is that a central venous catheter is not required.

In their original observations, Blackburn et al. emphasized the importance of avoiding glucose in the infusate.[229,230] Their reasoning was that glucose-induced hyperinsulinemia would prevent lipolysis and fat utilization and would thereby necessitate protein breakdown.[230] Subsequent studies have shown that isotonic amino acids are no less effective in improving nitrogen balance when combined with glucose.[231] Thus the underlying principle is not the maintenance of hypoinsulinemia but rather the availability of an exogenous source of amino acids.

While isotonic amino acids are an effective form of parenteral feeding in some postoperative patients, the precise indications for this form of therapy have not as yet been established. In patients with severe burns or extensive sepsis, isotonic amino acids have not been demonstrated to bring about the anabolism observed with TPN. On the other hand, in circumstances of more limited injury or trauma (including the postoperative state), it has not been established that improvement in nitrogen balance has sufficient clinical benefit (e.g., in accelerating wound healing or preventing sepsis) to warrant the added expense of isotonic amino acids as compared to dextrose-electrolyte solutions.

THE ROLE OF LIPID IN PARENTERAL NUTRITION

The availability of a parenteral fat emulsion providing approximately 1000 kcal/liter and capable of being given safely for prolonged periods obviously could assist greatly in meeting caloric needs of the injured or infected patient by eliminating the need for large fluid volumes and high glucose loads as well as perhaps the need for a central venous catheter. While certain preparations are widely used in Europe, FDA-approved intravenous fat only became available in the United States in 1976. Although the European experience is very encouraging, further information is required to define properly the guidelines for the use of intravenous fat.

Extensive work by Japanese and American investigators during the 1930s and 1940s has been reviewed by Thompson.[232] One of the most common side effects was the tendency toward chills, fever, and back pain. Schuberth and Wretlind[233] presented extensive experimental and clinical data on different fats and concluded that an emulsion of soybean oil and egg yolk phosphatides could be given as an intravenous infusion in man without any of the serious side effects associated with previous lipid preparations. There is general agreement that an intravenous fat emulsion, such as that developed by Wretlind and co-workers[234] and marketed under the name Intralipid, provides a material that can be promptly oxidized as a source of calories.

Carlson and Hallberg[235] reported that Intralipid was a convenient tracer for chylomicrons because of its similar metabolic behavior. After a single injection of either chylomicra or Intralipid, the disappearance from the bloodstream could be characterized as having a linear phase and a logarithmic phase. Thus it was possible to determine two rate constants for these phases. The rate constant K_1 of the linear phase was thought to reflect the total available enzyme activity responsible for eliminating chylomicra from the bloodstream. The rate constant K_2 was thought to represent the first-order reaction from the disappearance of chylomicra, probably reflecting, among other things, the distribution of the flow of substrate passing the enzyme site. These two rate constants are apparently altered following injury. After a surgical operation, there is a considerable increase in both K_1 and K_2. These effects appear to be specific for injury and are not seen after starvation alone.These findings reassured the investigators that it would be safe to administer intravenous fat emulsions to injured patients. since there appeared to be an increased capacity to remove the exogenous lipid from the bloodstream, despite the fact that levels of circulating lipids were already increased.

Hallberg and co-workers[236]presented a series of studies on fat emulsion for complete intravenous nutrition. These workers indicated that fat particles were eliminated from the bloodstream at a rate that differed depending upon whether a "critical concentration" was exceeded. Below the critical concentration, the elimination depended upon the triglyceride concentration. Above the critical concentration, there seemed to be a maximal elimination capacity. These workers reported on the clinical administration of Intralipid in 2781 infusions with a complication rate that was extremely low. Similar favorable results have been reported for introductory use of this material in the United States.[237]

In a series of papers published between 1971 and 1974, Carlson and Rossner[237] presented a method for an intravenous fat tolerance test using the fat emulsion Intralipid. When 1 ml of 10% Intralipid per kilogram of body weight was given, first-order kinetics for the removal of fat emulsion were generally found, and linear curves were obtained in a semilogarithmic plot. The K_2 value for the intravenous fat tolerance test was highly reproducible and repeated in the same subjects up to 6 months. There is a statistically significant positive relationship between the K_2 value and the fractional turnover rate of endogenous triglycerides. The arteriovenous concentration differences of Intralipid during a constant infusion were studied in several different animal tissue, and the following results were obtained: the myocardium appeared to remove approximately 14 percent; the splanchnic viscera, 25 percent; skeletal muscle, 47 percent; and subcutaneous adipose tissue, 13 percent of the infused Intralipid. No net removal was observed in the liver.

It is generally accepted that the intravenous fat solution Intralipid is a readily available source for oxidation. It also provides a rapid and effective treatment of the fatty acid deficiency that occurs with prolonged TPN using only carbohydrate and amino acids.[238] However, its use for nitrogen sparing requires further study. Long and co-workers[239] have reported that patients with major burns show progressive nitrogen retention with increasing carbohydrate intake, while equivalent increases in calories as fat are not associated with nitrogen retention. How much of these findings are the result of brief study periods and how much relate to intrinsic differences in the nitrogen-sparing properties of carbohydrate versus fat remain to be answered.

REFERENCES

1. Cuthbertson, D. P.: Observations on the disturbance of metabolism produced by injury to the limbs. *Q J Med 1:* 233–246, 1932.
2. Cuthbertson, D. P.: Post-shock metabolic response. *Lancet 1:* 433–437, 1942.
3. Gump, F. E., Kinney, J. M., Long, C. L., Gelber, R.: Measurement of water balance—a guide to surgical care. *Surgery 64:* 154–164, 1968.
4. Gump, F. E., Kinney, J. M., Iles, M., Long, C. L.: Duration and significance of large fluid loads administered for circulatory support. *J Trauma 10:* 431–439, 1970.
5. Manger, W. M., Nahas, G. G., Hassam, D., Habif, D. V., Papper, E. M.: Effect of pH control and increased O_2 delivery on the course of hemorrhagic shock. *Ann Surg 156:* 503–510, 1962.
6. Crowell, J. W., Smith, E. E.: Oxygen deficit and irreversible hemorrhagic shock. *Am J Physiol 206:* 313–316, 1964.
7. Jones, C. E., Crowell, J. W., Smith, E. E.: A cause-effect relationship between oxygen deficit and irreversible hemorrhagic shock. *Surg Gynecol Obstet 127:* 93–96, 1968.
8. Vladeck, B. C., Bassin, R., Kark, A. E., Shoemaker, W. C.: Rapid and slow hemorrhage in man. II. Sequential acid base and oxygen transport responses. *Ann Surg 173:* 331–336, 1971.
9. Halmagyi, D. F. G., Goodman, A. H., Neering, J. R.: Hindlimb blood flow and oxygen usage in hemorrhagic shock. *J Appl Physiol 27:* 508–513, 1969.
10. Wilson, R. F., Christensen, C., LeBlanc, L. P.: Oxygen consumption in critically ill surgical patients. *Ann Surg 176:* 801–804, 1972.
11. Stoner, H. B.: Studies on the mechanism of shock: The quantitative aspects of glycogen metabolism after limb ischaemia in the rat. *Br J Exp Pathol 39:* 635–651, 1958.
12. Stoner, H. B., Threlfall, C. J.: The effect of limb ischaemia on carbohydrate distribution and energy transformation, in Stoner HB, Threlfall CJ (ed): The Biochemical Response to Injury, Proceedings from Symposium, Council for International Organizations of Medical Sciences. Oxford, Blackwell, 1960.
13. Heath, D. F.: Liver metabolism after injury. *Adv Exp Med Biol 33:* 271–276, 1971.
14. Bloom, W. L., Ward, J. A.: Changes in carbohydrate metabolism during blood loss, shock and anoxia. *Metabolism 10:* 379–385, 1961.
15. Heath, D. F., Corney, P. L.: The effects of starvation, environmental temperature and injury on the rate of disposal of glucose by the rat. *Biochem J 136:* 519–530, 1973.
16. Stoner, H. B., Heath, D. F.: The effects of trauma on carbohydrate metabolism. *Br J Anaesthesiol 45:* 244–251, 1973.
17. Shoemaker, W. C., Stahr, L. J., Kim, S. I., Elwyn, D. H.: Sequential circulatory and metabolic changes in the liver and whole body during hemorrhagic shock, in Kovach AGB, Stoner HB, Spitzer JJ (ed): Neurohumoral and Metabolic Aspects of Injury. New York, Plenum Press, 1973, p 292.
18. Ashby, M. M., Heath, D. F., Stoner, H. B.: A quantitative study of carbohydrate metabolism in the normal and injured rat. *J Physiol 179:* 193–237, 1965.
19. Kovach, A. G. B., Sandor, P.: Effect of hemorrhagic shock on gluconeogenesis, oxygen consumption and redox state of perfused rat liver, in Kovach AGB, Stoner, HB, Spitzer JJ (ed): Neurohumoral and Metabolic Aspects of Injury. New York, Plenum Press, 1973, p 243.
20. Broder, G., Weil, M. H.: Excess lactate: An index of reversibility of shock in human patients. *Science 143:* 1457–1459, 1964.
21. Schumer, W.: Localization of the energy pathway block in shock. *Surgery 64:* 55–59, 1968.
22. Drucker, W. R., Kaye, M., Kendrick, R., Hoffman, N., Kingsbury, B.: Metabolic aspects of hemorrhagic shock. I. Changes in intermediary metabolism during hemorrhage and repletion of blood. *Surg Forum 9:* 49–54, 1958.
23. Spitzer, J. J., Wiener, R., Wolf, E. H.: Non-esterified fatty acid (FFA) metabolism following severe hemorrhage in the conscious dog, in Kovach AGB, Stoner HB, Spitzer JJ (ed): Neurohumoral and Metabolic Aspects of Injury. New York, Plenum Press, 1973, p 221.
24. Wiener, R., Spitzer, J. J.: Lactate metabolism following severe hemorrhage in the conscious dog. *Am J Physiol 227:* 58–62, 1974
25. Halmagyi, D. F. J., Goodman, A. H., Little, M. J., Varga, D.: Mesenteric and skeletal muscular lactate production in hemorrhagic shock (in press).
26. Fritz, S. D., Fitts, C. T., Lurie, D.: The effect of hypertonic glucose upon survival in hemorrhagic shock utilizing a re-stress model in sheep. *J Trauma 16:* 284–289, 1976.
27. McCoy, S., Drucker, W. R.: Carbohydrate metabolism, in Ballinger WF, Collins JA, Drucker WR, Dudrick SJ, Zeppa R (ed): Manual of Surgical Nutrition. Philadelphia, WB Saunders, 1975, p 13.
28. Strawitz, J. G., Hift, H., Ehrhardt, A., Cline, D. W.: Irreversible hemorrhagic shock in rats: Changes in blood glucose and liver glycogen. *Am J Physiol 200:* 261–263, 1961.
29. Russell, J. A., Long, C. N. H., Engel, F. L.: Biochemical studies on shock. II. The role of the peripheral tissues in the metabolism of protein and carbohydrate during hemorrhagic shock in the rat. *J Exp Med 79:* 1–7, 1944.
30. Randle, P. J., Smith, G. H.: Regulation of glucose uptake by muscle. I. The effect of insulin, anaerobiasis and cell poisons on the uptake of glucose and release of potassium by isolated rat diaphragm. *Biochem J 70:* 490–500, 1958.
31. Drucker, W. R., Howard, P. L., McCoy, S.: Influence of diet on response to hemorrhagic shock. *Ann Surg 181:* 698–704, 1975.
32. Frank, E. D., Frank, H. A., Fine, J.: Traumatic shock. XVIII. Plasma fibrinogen in hemorrhagic shock in the dog. *Am J Physiol 162:* 619–631, 1950.
33. Owen, J. A.: Effect of injury on plasma proteins, in Sobotka H, Stewart CP (ed): Advances in Clinical Chemistry, vol. 9. New York, Academic Press, 1967, p 1.
34. Getzen, L. C., Pollak, E. W., Wolfman, E. F. Jr.: Serum concentration during hemorrhagic shock. *Surg Gynecol Obstet 144:* 42–44, 1977.
35. Schumer, W., Kukral, J. C.: Metabolism of shock. *Surgery 63:* 630–636, 1968.
36. Gordon, A. H.: The effects of trauma and partial hepatectomy on the rates of synthesis of plasma protein by the liver, in Rothchild MA, Waldmann T (ed): Plasma Protein Metabolism. New York, Academic Press, 1970, p 351.
37. Wannemacher, R. W. Jr.: Ribosomal RNA synthesis and function as influenced by amino acid supply and stress. *Proc Nutr Soc 31:* 281–290, 1972.
38. Cuthbertson, D. P., Tilstone, W. J.: Metabolism during the post-injury period, in Sobotka H, Stewart CP (ed): Advances in Clinical Chemistry, vol. 12. New York, Academic Press, 1969, p 1.
39. Engel, F. L.: The significance of the metabolic changes during shock. *Ann NY Acad Sci 55:* 381–393, 1952.
40. Rosen, H., Levenson, S. M.: Nonprotein changes in serum and plasma of rats following thermal injury. *Proc Soc Exp Biol Med 83:* 91–97, 1953.
41. Levenson, S. M., Howard, J. M., Rosen, H.: Studies of the plasma amino acids and amino conjugates in patients with severe battle wounds. *Surg Gynecol Obstet 101:* 35–47, 1955.
42. Gilletee, R. W., Mansberger, A. R., Johnson, C. E., Kookootsedes, G. J.: A new preparation for the study of experimental shock from massive wounds. V. Changes in some serum electrolytes and nitrogenous fraction valves. *Surgery 43:* 740–746, 1958.
43. Cuthbertson, D. P.: Further observations on disturbance of metabolism caused by injury with particular reference to the dietary requirements of fracture cases. *Br J Surg 23:* 505–520, 1936.
44. Elwyn, D. H., Hamendra, C. P., Stahr, L.J., Kim, S. I., Shoemaker, W. C.: Interorgan transport of amino acids in hemorrhagic shock. *Am J Physiol 231:* 377–386, 1976.
45. Kovach, A. G. B.: Metabolic changes in haemorrhagic shock. *Adv Exp Med Biol 23:* 275–278, 1972.
46. Stoner, H. B., Cunningham, V. J., Elson, P. M., Hunt, A.: The effects of diet, lipolysis and limb ischaemia on the distribution of plasma tryptophan in the rat. *Biochem J 146:* 659–666, 1975.
47. Barton, R. N.: Ketone metabolism after trauma, in Porter R, Knight, J (ed): Energy Metabolism in Trauma. London, Churchill, 1970, p 173.
48. Barton, R. N.: Ketone-body concentrations in liver and blood after limb ischaemia in the rat. *Clin Sci 40:* 463–477, 1971.
49. Smith, R., Fuller, D. J., Wedge, J. H., Williamson, D. H., Alberti, G. G. M.: Initial effect of injury on ketone bodies and other blood metabolites. *Lancet 1:* 1–3, 1975.
50. McShan, W. H., Van Potter, R., Goldman, A., Shipley, E. A., Meyer, R. K.: Biological energy transformations during shock as shown by blood chemistry. *Am J Physiol 145:* 93–106, 1945.

51. LePage, G. A.: Biological energy transformations during shock as shown by tissue analyses. *Am J Physiol 146:* 267–281, 1946.
52. Bell, M. L., Herman, A. H., Smith, E. E., Egdahl, R. H., Rutenberg, A. M.: Role of lysosomal instability in the development of refractory shock. *Surgery 70:* 341–347, 1971.
53. Stoner, H. B., Threlfall, C. J.: The effect of limb ischaemia on carbohydrate distribution and energy transformation, in Stoner HB, Threlfall CJ (ed): The Biochemical Response to Injury. Oxford, Blackwell, 1960, p 105.
54. Rush, B. F., Hsieh, H.: In vivo and vitro effects of endotoxin on tissue metabolism. *Surgery 63:* 298–300, 1968.
55. Mela, L., Miller, L. D., Bacalzo, L. V., Jr., Olofsson, K., White, R. R., IV.: Role of intracellular variations of lysosomal enzyme activity and oxygen tension in mitochondrial impairment in endotoxemia and hemorrhage in the rat. *Ann Surg 178:* 727–735, 1973.
56. Somogyi, J., Cremer, J. E., Ikrényi, K. I.: Characterization of rat brain mitochondria, the effect of injury. *Adv Exp Med Biol 33:* 345–352, 1972.
57. Baue, A. E., Sayeed, M. M.: Alterations in the functional capacity of mitochondria in hemorrhagic shock. *Surgery 68:* 40–47, 1970.
58. Mela, L., Bacalzo, L. V., Miller, L. D.: Defective oxidative metabolism of rat liver mitochondria in hemorrhagic and endotoxin shock. *Am J Physiol 220:* 571–577, 1971.
59. Markley, K., Smallman, E.: Protection against burn, tourniquet and endotoxin shock by purine compounds. *J Trauma 10:* 508–607, 1970.
60. Chaudry, J. H., Mohammed, M. S., Baue, A. E.: Depletion and restoration of tissue ATP in hemorrhagic shock. *Arch Surg 108:* 208–211, 1974.
61. Cuthbertson, D. P.: Observations on the disturbance of metabolism produced by injury in the limbs. *Q J Med 1:* 233–246, 1932.
62. Kinney, J. M., Duke, J. H., Jr., Long, C. L., Gump, F. E.: Tissue fuel and weight loss after injury. Proceedings from Symposium on the Pathology of Trauma. *J Clin Pathol 4:* 65–72, 1970.
63. Kinney, J. M.: Surgical diagnosis, patterns of energy, weight and tissue change, in Wilkinson, A. W., Cuthbertson, D. P. (eds): Metabolism and the Response to Injury. Kent, Pitman Medical, 1976, p 121.
64. Bergström, J., Boström, H., Fürst, P., Hultman, E., Vinnars, E.: Preliminary studies of energy-rich phosphagens in muscle from severely ill patients. *Crit Care Med 4:* 197–204, 1976.
65. Needham, A. E.: The pattern of nitrogen excretion during regeneration in Oligochaetes. *J Exp Zool 3:* 189, 1955.
66. Moore, F. D.: The Metabolic Response to Surgery (ed 2). Springfield, Charles C Thomas; Oxford, Blackwell Scientific, 1952.
67. Moore, F. D.: The Body Cell Mass and Its Supporting Environment (ed 6). Philadelphia-London, WB Saunders, 1963.
68. Sprinson, D. B., Rittenberg, D.: The rate of interaction of the amino acids of the diet with the tissue proteins. *J Biol Chem 180:* 715–726, 1949.
69. Waterlow, J. C., Stephen, J. M. L.: The measurement of total lysine turnover in the rat by intravenous infusion of L-(U-^{14}C) lysine. *Clin Sci 33:* 489–506, 1967.
70. O'Keefe, J. D., Sender, P. M., James, W. P. T.: "Catabolic" loss of body nitrogen in response to injury. *Lancet 2:* 1035–1037, 1974.
71. Crane, C. W., Picou, D., Smith, R., Waterlow, J. C.: Protein turnover in patients before and after elective orthpaedic operations. *Br J Surg 64:* 129–133, 1977.
72. Long, C. L., Jeevanandam, B., Kim, B. M., Kinney, J. M.: Whole body protein synthesis and catabolism in septic man. *Am J Clin Nutr 30:* 1340–1344, 1977.
73. Cuthbertson, D. P., Tompsett, S. L.: Note on the effect of injury on the level of the plasma proteins. *Br J Exp Pathol 16:* 471–475, 1935.
74. Werner, M., Cohnen, G.: Changes in serum proteins in the immediate postoperative period. *Clin Sci 36:* 173–184, 1969.
75. Fleck, A.: Injury and plasma proteins, in Wilkinson AW, Cuthbertson DP (ed): Metabolism and the Response to Injury. London, Pitman Medical, 1976, p 229.
76. Davies, J. W. L.: Albumin turnover in burns and trauma, in Bianchi R, Mariani G, McFarlane AS (ed): Plasma Protein Turnover. London-Basingtoke, Macmillan Press, 1976, p 404.
77. Crockson, R. A., Payne, C. J., Ratcliff, A. P., Soothill, J. F.: Time sequence of acute phase reactive proteins following surgical trauma. *Clin Chim Acta 14:* 435–441, 1966.
78. Koj, A.: Synthesis and turnover of acute-phase reactants, in Porter R, Knight J (ed): Energy Metabolism in Trauma, Proceedings of a Ciba Foundation Symposium. London, Churchill, 1970.
79. Ballantyne, F. C., Fleck, A.: The effect of environmental temperature (20° and 30°) after injury on the concentration of serum proteins in man. *Clin Chim Acta 44:* 341–347, 1973.
80. Davies, J. W. L., Liljedahl, S-O.: Protein catabolism and energy utilization in burned patients treated at different environmental temperatures, in Porter R, Knight J (ed): Energy Metabolism in Trauma. Proceedings of a Ciba Foundation Symposium. London, Churchill, 1970.
81. Davies, J. W. L.: Protein metabolism following injury. *J Clin Pathol 4:* 56–64, 1970.
82. Davies, J. W. L., Liljedahl, S-O., Reizenstein, P.: Fibrinogen metabolism following injury and its surgical treatment. *Injury 1:* 178–185, 1970.
83. Ballantyne, F. C., Tilstone, W. J., Fleck, A.: Effect of injury on albumin synthesis in the rabbit. *Br J Exp Pathol 54:* 409–415, 1973.
84. Koj, A., McFarlane, A. S.: Effect of endotoxin on plasma albumin and fibrinogen synthesis rates in rabbits, as measured by the (^{14}C) carbonate method. *Biochem J 108:* 137–146, 1968.
85. Rothschild, M. A., Schreiber, S. S., Oratz, M., McGee, H. L.: The effect of adrenocortical hormones on albumin metabolism studied with albumin I^{131}. *J Clin Invest 37:* 1229–1235, 1958.
86. Hoffenberg, R.: Control of albumin degradation in vivo and in the perfused liver, in Rothschild MA, Waldmann T (ed): Plasma Protein Metabolism Regulation of Synthesis, Distribution and Degradation. London, Academic Press, 1970, p 239.
87. Jeejeebhoy, K. N., Bruce-Robertson, A., Ho, J., Sodtke, U.: The comparative effects of nutritional and hormonal factors on the synthesis of albumin, fibrinogen and transferrin, in McFarlane AS (chairman): Protein Turnover. Proceedings of a Ciba Foundation Symposium. Amsterdam, Associated Scientific, 1973.
88. Khan, S. N., Tilstone, W. J., Fleck, A., Broom, I.: Protein synthesis in the rat liver after fracture of the femur. *Proc Nutr Soc 33:* 93A–94A, 1974.
89. Peters, J. P., Van Slyke, D. D.: Amino acids, in Peters JP, Van Slyke DD (ed): Quantitative Clinical Chemistry: Interpretations, vol. 1. Baltimore, Williams & Wilkins, 1946, p 808.
90. Everson, T. C., Fritschel, M. J.: The effect of surgery on the plasma levels of individual essential amino acids. *Surgery 31:* 226–232, 1952.
91. Nardi, G. L.: Essential and nonessential amino acids in the urine of severely burned patients. *J Clin Invest 33:* 847–854, 1954.
92. Schønheyder, F., Bone, J., Skjoldborg, H.: Variations in plasma amino acid concentrations after abdominal surgical procedures. *Acta Chir Scand 140:* 271–275, 1974.
93. Dale, G., Young, F., Latner, A. L., Goode, A., Tweedle, D., Johnston, I. D. A.: The effect of surgical operation on venous plasma free amino acids. *Surgery 81:* 295–301, 1977.
94. Woolf, L. I., Groves, A. C., Moore, J. P., Duff, J. H., Finley, R. J., Loomer, R. L.: Arterial plasma amino acids in patients with serious postoperative infection and in patients with major fractures. *Surgery 79:* 283–292, 1976.
95. Wedge, J. H., De Campos, R., Kerr, A., Smith, R., Farrell, R., Ilie, V., Williamson, D. H.: Branched-chain amino acids, nitrogen excretion and injury in man. *Clin Sci Mol Med 50:* 393–399, 1976.
96. Sherwin, R. S., Hendler, R. G., Felig, P.: Effect of ketone infusion on amino acid and nitrogen metabolism in man. *J Clin Invest 55:* 1382–1390, 1975.
97. Herbert, J. D., Coulson, R. A., Hernandez, T.: Free amino acids in the canine and rat. *Comp Biochem Physiol 17:* 583–598, 1966.
98. Bergström, J.: Muscle electrolytes in man, determined by neutron activation analysis on needle biopsy specimens: A study on normal subjects, kidney patients and patients with chronic diarrhea. *Scand J Clin Lab Invest 14:* 1–110, 1962.
99. Bergström, J., Fürst, P., Norée, L-O., Vinnars, E.: Intracellular free amino acid concentration in human muscle tissue. *J Appl Physiol 36:* 693–697, 1974.
100. Vinnars, E., Bergström, J., Fürst, P.: Influence of the postoperative state on the intracellular free amino acids in human muscle tissue. *Ann Surg 182:* 665–671, 1965.
101. Vinnars, E., Fürst, P., Bergström, J., von Francken, I.: Intracellular free amino acids in muscle tissue in normal man and in different clinical conditions, in Wilkinson, AW, Cuthbertson DP (ed): Metabolism and the Response to Injury. London, Pitman Medical, 1976, p. 336.
102. Munro, H. N.: Free amino acid pools and their role in regulation, in Munro HN (ed): Mammalian Protein Metabolism, vol. 4. New York, Academic Press, 1970, p 299.

103. Bernard C. Leçons sur le Diabete. Paris, Librairie J.B. Baillere, 1877, p 408.
104. Cannon, W. B.: Traumatic Shock (ed 3). New York, Appleton, 1923, p 85.
105. Howard, J. M.: Studies of the absorption and metabolism of glucose following injury. *Ann Surg 141:* 321–326, 1955.
106. Evans, E. I., Butterfield, W. J. H.: The stress response in the severely burned. *Ann Surg 134:* 588–613, 1951.
107. Giddings, A. E. B.: The control of plasma glucose in the surgical patient. *Br J Surg 61:* 787–792, 1974.
108. Hayes, M. A., Brandt, R. L.: Carbohydrate metabolism in the immediate postoperative period. *Surgery 32:* 819–827, 1952.
109. Giddings, A. E. B., Rowlands, B. J., Mangnall, D., and Clark, R. G.: Plasma insulin and surgery II: Later changes and the effect of intravenous carbohydrates. *Ann Surg 186:* 687–693, 1977.
110. Long, C. L., Spencer, J. L., Kinney, J. M., Geiger, J. W.: Carbohydrate metabolism in normal man and effect of glucose infusion. *J Appl Physiol 31:* 102–109, 1971.
111. Gump, F. E., Long, C. L., Killian, P., Kinney, J. M.: Studies of glucose intolerance in septic injured patients. *J Trauma 14:* 378–388, 1974.
112. Aoki, T. T., Brennan, M. F., Muller, W. A., Cahill,G. F., Jr.: Nitrogen balance insulin and amino acid metabolism, in Brown H (ed): Protein Nutrition. Springfield, Charles C Thomas, 1974, p 180.
113. Wilmore, D. W., Mason, A. D., Jr., Pruitt, B. A., Jr.: Insulin response to glucose in hypermetabolic burn patients. *Ann Surg 183:* 314–320, 1976.
114. Hlad, C. J., Jr., Elrick, H., Witten, T. A.: Studies on the kinetics of glucose utilization. *J Clin Invest 35:* 1139–1149, 1956.
115. Wilmore, D. W.: Hormonal responses and their effect on metabolism. *Surg Clin North Am 56:* 999–1018, 1976.
116. Moore, F. D.: Metabolic Care of the Surgical Patient. Philadelphia, WB Saunders, 1959, p 15.
117. Duke, J. H., Jørgensen, S. B., Broell, J. R., Long, C. L., Kinney, J. M.: Contribution of protein to caloric expenditure following injury. *Surgery 68:* 168–174, 1970.
118. Sevitt, S.: The boundaries between physiology, pathology and after injury. *Lancet 12:* 1204–1210, 1966.
119. Lepistö, P. V.: Post-traumatic blood lipid changes and fat embolism. *J Trauma 16:* 52–57, 1976.
120. Carlson, L. A., Hallberg, D.: Studies on the elimination of exogenous lipids from the blood stream: The kinetics of the elimination of a fat emulsion and of chylomicrons in the dog after single injection. *Acta Physiol Scand 59:* 52–61, 1963.
121. Carlson, L. A., Rossner, S.: A methodological study of an intravenous fat tolerance test with Intralipid® emulsion. *Scand J Clin Lab Invest 29:* 271–280, 1972.
122. Carlson, L. A.: Mobilization and utilization of lipids after trauma: Relation to caloric homeostasis, in Porter R, Knight J (ed): Energy Metabolism in Trauma. Proceedings from a Ciba Foundation Symposium. London, Churchill, 1970.
123. Wilmore, D. W., Moylan, J. A., Helmkamp, G. M., Pruitt, B. A.: Clinical evaluation of a 10% intravenous fat emulsion for parenteral nutrition in thermally injured patients. *Ann Surg 178:* 503–513, 1973.
124. Carlson, L. A., Liljedahl, S-O., Wirsen, C.: Blood and tissue changes in the dog during and after excessive free fatty acid mobilization: A biochemical and morphological study. *Acta Med Scand 178:* 81–102, 1965.
125. Beisel, W. R.: Metabolic response to infection, in Creger WP, Coggins CH, Hancock EW (ed): Annual Review of Medicine: Selected Topics in the Clinical Sciences, vol. 26. Palo Alto, Annual Review, 1975, p 9.
126. Spink, W. W.: The ecology of human septic shock, in Hershey SG, Del Guercio LRM, McConn R (ed): Septic Shock in Man. Boston, Little, Brown, 1971, p 3.
127. White, R. R., Mela, L, Bacalzo L. V., Jr., Olofsson, K., Miller, L. D.: Hepatic ultrastructure in endotoxemia, hemorrhage, and hypoxia: Emphasis on mitochondrial changes. *Surgery 73:* 525–534, 1973.
128. Mela, L., Miller, L. D., Diaco, J. F., Sugarman, H. J.: Effect of *E. coli* endotoxin on mitochondrial energy-linked functions. *Surgery 68:* 541–549, 1970.
129. Herman, C. M., Kraft, A. R., Smith, K. R., Artnak, E. J., Chisholm, F. C., Dickson, L. G., McKee, A. E., Jr., Homer, L. D., Levin, J.: Relationship of circulating endogenous endotoxin to hemorrhagic shock in the baboon. *Ann Surg 179:* 910–916, 1974.
130. Duff, J. H., Wright, C. J., McLean, A. P. H., MacLean, L. D.: Oxygen consumption in septic shock, in Forscher BK, Lillehei RC, Stubbs SS (ed): Shock in Low- and High-Flow States. Amsterdam, Excerpta Medica, 1972.
131. Cryer, P. E., Herman, C. M., Sode, J.: Carbohydrate metabolism in the baboon subjected to gram-negative *(E. coli)* septicemia: I. Hyperglycemia with depressed plasma insulin concentrations. *Ann Surg 174:* 91–100, 1971.
132. Berk, J. L., Hagen, J. F., Beyer, W. H., Gerber, M. J.: Hypoglycemia of shock. *Ann Surg 171:* 400–408, 1970.
133. Printon, K. J., Keefe, W. E., Foster, E., Brown, W.: Fluxes in serum glucose and free fatty acid in early endotoxemia and hemorrhage. *Surg Gynecol Obstet 138:* 686–688, 1974.
134. LaNoue, K. F., Mason, A. D., Daniels, J. P.: The impairment of gluconeogenesis by gram-negative infection. *Metabolism 17:* 606–611, 1968.
135. Griffiths, J., Groves, A. C., Leung, F. Y.: Hypertriglyceridemia in gram-negative sepsis in the dog. *Surg Gynecol Obstet 136:* 897–903, 1973.
136. Fiser, R. H., Denniston, J. C., Beisel, W. R.: Endotoxemia in the rhesus monkey: Alterations in host lipid and carbohydrate metabolism. *Pediatr Res 8:* 13–17, 1974.
137. Kaufman, R. L., Matson, C. F., Beisel, W. R.: Hypertriglyceridemia produced by endotoxin: Role of impaired triglyceride disposal mechanisms. *J Infect Dis 133:* 548–555, 1976.
138. Smith, I. M., Mukherjee, K. L.: Liver metabolism and energy production in *Staphylococcus aureus* septic shock in mice, in Hinshaw LB, Cox BG (ed): The Fundamental Mechanisms of Shock. Proceedings of Symposium held in Oklahoma City. New York, Plenum Press, 1972.
139. Canonico, P. G., White, J. D., Powanda, M. C.: Peroxisome depletion in rat liver during pneumococcal sepsis. *Lab Invest 33:* 147–150, 1975.
140. Postel, J., Schloerb, P. R.: Metabolic effects of experimental bacteremia. *Ann Surg 185:* 475–480, 1977.
141. Stoner, H. B.: Specific and non-specific effects of bacterial infection on the host. Symposia of the Society for General Microbiology. XXII. Microbial Pathogenecity in Man and Animals, 1972. Printed in Great Britain.
142. DuBois, E. F.: Fever, in DuBois EF (ed): Basal Metabolism in Health and Disease. Philadelphia, Lea & Febiger, 1924, p 311.
143. Kinney, J. M., Roe, C. F.: Caloric equivalent of fever. I. Patterns of postoperative response. *Ann Surg 156:* 610–622, 1962.
144. Roe, C. F., Kinney, J. M.: The caloric equivalent of fever. II. Influence of major trauma. *Ann Surg 161:* 140–147, 1965.
145. Coleman, W., DuBois, E. F.: The influence of the high-calorie diet on the respiratory exchanges in typhoid fever. *Arch Intern Med 14:* 168–209, 1914.
146. Cairnie, A. B., Campbell, R. M., Pullar, J. D., Cuthbertson, D. P.: The heat production consequent on injury. *Br J Exp Pathol 38:* 504–511, 1957.
147. Myers, J. D.: The circulation in the splanchnic area, in Green HD (ed): Shock and Circulatory Homeostasis. New York, Josiah Macy Jr. Foundation, 1955, p 121.
148. Gump, F. E., Price, J. B., Jr., Kinney, J. M.: Whole body and splanchnic blood flow and oxygen consumption measurements in patients with intraperitoneal infection. *Ann Surg 171:* 321–328, 1970.
149. Gump, F. E., Price, J. B., Jr., Kinney, J. M.: Blood flow and oxygen consumption in patients with severe burns. *Surg Gynecol Obstet 130:* 23–28, 1970.
150. Peters, J. P., Van Slyke, D. D.: The net metabolism of protein, in Peters JP, Van Slyke DD (ed): Quantitative Clinical Chemistry Interpretations, vol. I. Baltimore, Williams & Wilkins, 1946, p 631.
151. Beisel, W. R., Sawyer, W. D., Ryll, W. D.: Metabolic effects of intracellular infections in man. *Ann Intern Med 67:* 744–779, 1972.
152. Wannemacher, R. W., Jr., DuPont, H. I., Pekarek, R. S., Powanda, M. C., Schwartz, A., Hornick, R. B., Beisel, W. R.: An exogenous mediator of depression of amino acids and trace metals in serum, during typhoid fever. *J Infect Dis 126:* 77–86, 1972.
153. Kampschmidt, R. F.: Effects of leukocytic endogenous mediator on metabolism and infection. *Ann Okla Acad Sci 4:* 62–68, 1974.
154. Long, C. L., Kinney, J. M., Geiger, J. W.: Nonsuppressability of gluconeogenesis by glucose in septic patients. *Metabolism 25:* 193–201, 1976.
155. Gallin, J. I., Kaye, D., O'Leary, W. M.: Serum lipids in infection. *N Engl J Med 281:* 1081–1086, 1969.

156. Gallin, J. I., O'Leary, W. M., Kaye, D.: Serum concentrations of lipids in rabbits infected with *Escherichia coli* and *Staphylococcus aureus*. *Proc Soc Exp Biol Med 133:* 309–313, 1970.
157. Fiser, R. H., Denniston, J. C., Beisel, W. R.: Infection with *Diplococcus pneumoniae* and *Salmonella typhimurium* in monkeys: Changes in plasma lipids and lipoproteins. *J Infect Dis 125:* 54–60, 1972.
158. Lees, R. S., Fiser, R. H., Beisel, W. R.: Effects of an experimental viral infection on plasma lipid and lipoprotein metabolism. *Metabolism 21:* 825–833, 1972.
159. Kaufmann, R. L., Matson, C. F., Rowberg, A. H., Beisel, W. R.: Defective lipid disposal mechanisms during bacterial infection in rhesus monkeys. *Metabolism 25:* 615–624, 1976.
160. Wannemacher, R. W., Jr.: Protein metabolism, in Ghadimi H (ed): Total Parenteral Nutrition: Premises and Promises. New York, John Wiley, 1975, p 85.
161. Neufeld, H. A., Pace, J. A., White, F. E.: The effect of bacterial infections on ketone concentrations in rat liver and blood and on free fatty acid concentrations in rat blood. *Metabolism 25:* 877–884, 1976.
162. Ryan, N. T., Blackburn, G. L., Clowes, G. H. A.: Differential tissue sensitivity to elevated endogenous insulin levels during experimental peritonitis in rats. *Metabolism 23:* 1081–1089, 1974.
163. Zenser, T. V., DeRubertis, F. R., George, D. T., Rayfield, E. J.: Infection-induced hyperglucagonemia and altered hepatic response to glucagon in the rat. *Am J Physiol 227:* 1299–1305, 1974.
164. Clowes, G. H. A., Jr., O'Donnell, T. F., Blackburn, G. L., Maki, T. N.: Energy metabolism and proteolysis in traumatized and septic man. *Surg Clin North Am 56:* 1169–1184, 1976.
165. Border, J. R., Chenier, R., McMenamy, R. H., Seibel, R., Birkhahn, R, Yu, L.: Multiple systems organ failure: Muscle fuel deficit with visceral protein malnutrition. *Surg Clin North Am 56:* 1147–1167, 1976.
166. Skillman, J. J., Rosenoer, V. M., Smith, P. C., Fang, M. S.: Improved albumin synthesis in postoperative patients by amino acid infusion. *N Engl J Med 295:* 1037–1040, 1976.
167. Ryan, N. T.: Metabolic adaptation for energy production during trauma and sepsis. *Surg Clin North Am 56:* 1073–1090, 1976.
168. Batstone, G. F., Alberti, K. G. M. M., Hinks, L., et al. Metabolic studies in subjects following thermal injury. Intermediary metabolites, hormones, and tissue oxygenation. *Burns 2:* 207–225, 1976.
169. Giddings, A. E. B., O'Connor, K. J., Rowlands, B. J., Mangnall, D., Clark, R. G.: The relationship of plasma glucagon to the hyperglycemia and hyperinsulinemia of surgical operation. *Br J Surg 63:* 612–616, 1976.
170. Carey, L. C., Lowery, B. D., Cloutier, C. T.: Blood sugar and insulin response of humans in shock. *Ann Surg 172:* 342–350, 1970.
171. Moss, G. S., Cerchio, G. M., Siegel, D. C., et al: Serum insulin response in hemorrhagic shock in baboons. *Surgery 68:* 34–39, 1970.
172. Lerner, R. L., Porte, D., Jr.: Epinephrine: Selective inhibition of the acute insulin response to glucose. *J Clin Invest 50:* 2453–2457, 1971.
173. Halmagyi, D. G. J., Gillett, D. J., Lazarus, L., Young, J. D.: Blood glucose and serum insulin in reversible and irreversible post hemorrhagic shock. *J Trauma 6:* 623–669, 1966.
174. Hiebert, J. M., Celik, Z., Soeldner, J. S., Egdahl, R. H.: Insulin response to hemorrhagic shock in the intact and adrenalectomized primate. *Am J Surg 12:* 501–507, 1973.
175. Wilmore, D. W., Long, J. M., Mason, A. D., Skreen, R. W., Pruitt, B. A., Jr.: Catecholamines: Mediator of the hypermetabolic response to thermal injury. *Ann Surg 180:* 653–669, 1974.
176. Skillman, J. J., Hedley-Whyte, J., Pallotta, J. A.: Cardio-respiratory, metabolic and endocrine changes after hemorrhage in man. *Ann Surg 174:* 911, 1971.
177. Shikama, H., Ui, M.: Adrenergic receptor and epinephrine-induced hyperglycemia and glucose intolerance. *Am J Physiol 229:* 962–970, 1976.
178. Wolfe, R. R., Miller, H. I., Spitzer, J. J.: Glucose and lactate kinetics in burn shock. *Am J Physiol 1:* E415–E418, 1977.
179. Chaudry, I. H., Sayeed, M. M., Baue, A. E.: Insulin resistance in experimental shock. *Arch Surg 109: 412–415, 1974.*
180. Ross, H., Johnston, I. D. A., Welborn, T. A., Wright, A. D.: Effect of abdominal operation on glucose tolerance and serum levels of insulin, growth hormone and hydrocortisone. *Lancet 2:* 563–566, 1966.
181. Howard, J. M.: Studies of the absorption of glucose following injury. *Ann Surg 1441:* 321–326, 1955.
182. Rayfield, E. J., Curnow, R. T., George, D. T., Beisel, W. R.: Impaired carbohydrate metabolism during a mild viral illness. *N Engl J Med 289:* 618–621, 1973.
183. Ryan, N. T., George, B. C., Egdahl, D. H., Egdahl, R. H.: Chronic tissue insulin resistance following hemorrhagic shock. *Ann Surg 180:* 402–407, 1974.
184. Ryan, N. T., George, B. C., Odessey, R., Egdahl, R. H.: The effect of hemorrhagic shock, fasting, and glucocorticoid administration on leucine oxidation and incorporation into protein by skeletal muscle. *Metabolism 23:* 901–903, 1974.
185. Buse, M. G., Herlong, H. G., Weigond, D. A.: The effect of diabetes, insulin and the redox potential on leucine metabolism by isolated rat diaphragm. *Endocrinology 98:* 1166, 1976.
186. Hinton, P., Allison, S. P., Littlejohn, S., Lloyd, J.: Insulin and glucose to reduce catabolic response to injury in burned patients. *Lancet 1:* 767–769, 1971.
187. Ingle, D. J., Ward, E. O., Kuizenga, M. H.: The relationship of the adrenal glands to changes in urinary non-protein nitrogen following multiple fractures in force-fed rat. *Am J Physiol 149:* 510, 1947.
188. Wilmore, D. W., Lindsey, C. A., Moylan, J. A., Faloona, G. A., Pruitt, B. A., Unger, R. H.: Hyperglucagonemia after burns. *Lancet 1:* 73–75, 1974.
189. Rocha, D. M., Santensamo, F., Faloona, G. R., Unger, R. H.: Abnormal pancreatic alpha cell function in bacterial infections. *N Engl J Med 288:* 700–703, 1973.
190. Unger, R. H.: Glucagon and the insulin:glucagon ratio in diabetes and other catabolic states. *Diabetes 20:* 834–838, 1971.
191. Sherwin, R. S., Fisher, M., Hendler, R., Felig, P.: Hyperglucagonemia and blood glucose regulation in normal, obese, and diabetic patients. *N Engl J Med 294:* 455–561, 1976.
192. Sherwin, R. S., Hendler, R., Felig, P.: Influence of hyperglucagonemia on urinary glucose, nitrogen and electrolyte excretion in diabetes. *Metabolism 26:* 53–57, 1977.
193. Felig, P.: Insulin, glucagon, and somatostatin in normal physiology and diabetes mellitus. *Diabetes 25:* 1091–1099, 1976.
194. Cuthbertson, D. P., Tilstone, W. J.: Metabolism during the postinjury period, in Sobotka H, Steward TP (eds): Advances in Clinical Chemistry, vol. 12. New York, Academic Press, 1969, p 1.
195. Stoner, H. B.: The effect of environment on the response to injury in the rat. *Postgrad Med J 45:* 555–558, 1969.
196. Cope, O., Nardi, G. L., Quijano, M., Rovit, R. L., Stanbury, J. B., Wight, A.: Metabolic rate and thyroid function following acute thermal trauma in man. *Ann Surg 137:* 165–174, 1953.
197. Lieberman, Z. H., Lansche, J. M.: Effects of thermal injury on metabolic rate on insensible water loss in the rat. *Surg Forum 7:* 83–88, 1957.
198. Caldwell, F. T., Osterholm, J. L., Sower, N. D., Moyer, C. A.: Metabolic response to thermal trauma of normal and thyroprivic rats at three environmental temperatures. *Ann Surg 150:* 976–988, 1959.
199. Caldwell, F. T., Hammel, H. D., Dolan, F.: A calorimeter for simultaneous determination of heat production and heat loss in the rat. *J Appl Physiol 21:* 1655–1671, 1966.
200. Caldwell, F. T.: Metabolic response to thermal trauma: II. Nutritional studies with rats at two environmental temperatures. *Ann Surg 155:* 119–126, 1962.
201. Goodall, McC., Stone, C., Haynes, B. W., Jr.: Urinary output of adrenaline and noradrenaline in severe thermal burns. *Ann Surg 145:* 479–487, 1957.
202. Harrison, T. S., Seaton, J. F., Feller, I.: Relationship of increased oxygen consumption to catecholamine excretion in thermal burns. *Ann Surg 165:* 169–172, 1967.
203. Zawacki, B. E., Spitzer, K. W., Mason, A. D., Johns, L. A.: Does increased evaporative water loss cause hypermetabolism in burned patients? *Ann Surg 171:* 236–240, 1970.
204. Neely, W. A., Petro, A. B., Holloman, G. H., Jr., Rushton, F. W., Turner, M. D., Hardy, J. D.: Researches on the cause of burn hypermetabolism. *Ann Surg 179:* 291–294, 1974.
205. Birke, G., Carlson, L. A., von Euler, U. S., Liljedahl, S-O., Plantin, L-O.: Studies on burns. XII. Lipid metabolism, catecholamine excretion, basal metabolic rate and water loss during treatment of burns with warm dry air. *Acta Chir Scand 138:* 321–333, 1972.
206. Davies, J. W. L., Liljedahl, S-O., Birke, G.: Protein metabolism in burned patients treated in a warm (32°C) or cool (22°C) environment. *Injury 1:* 43, 1969.
207. Wilmore, D. W., Long, J. M., Mason, A. D., Jr., Skreen, R. W.,

Pruitt, B. A.: Catecholamines: Mediator of the hypermetabolic response to thermal injury. *Ann Surg 180:* 653–669, 1974.

208. Steinberg, D., Nestel, P. J., Buskirk, E. R., Thompson, R. H.: Calorigenic effect of norepinephrine correlated with plasma free fatty acid turnover and oxidation. *J Clin Invest 43:* 167–176, 1964.
209. Caldwell, F. T.: Energy metabolism following thermal burns. *Arch Surg 111:* 181–185, 1976.
210. Abbott, W. E., Albertsen, K.: The effect of starvation, infection and injury on the metabolic processes and body composition. *Ann NY Acad Sci 110:* 941–964, 1963.
211. Munro, H. N., Cuthbertson, D. P.: Response of protein metabolism to injury. *Biochem J 37:* XII, 1943.
212. Munro, H. N., Chalmers, M. I.: Fracture metabolism at different levels of protein intake. *Br J Exp Pathol 26:* 396–404, 1945.
213. Johnston, I. D. A.: The endocrine response to trauma. *Sci Basis Med Ann Rev* p 224–241, 1968.
214. Benedict, F. G.: A study of prolonged fasting. Carnegie Institution of Washington, publication 203, 1915.
215. Cuthbertson, D. P.: Observations on the disturbance of metabolism produced by injury in the limbs. *Q J Med 1:* 233–246, 1973.
216. DuBois, E. F.: The basal metabolism in fever. *JAMA 77:* 352–357, 1921.
217. Coller, F. A., Campbell, K. N., Vaughan, H. H., Iob, V., Moyer, C. A.: Postoperative salt intolerance. *Ann Surg 119:* 533–542, 1944.
218. Elman, R. E.: Parenteral Nutrition in Surgery. New York, Paul B Hoeber, 1947.
219. Thompson, S. W.: The Pathology of Parenteral Nutrition with Lipids. Springfield, Charles C Thomas, 1974, p 111.
220. Hallberg, D., Schuberth, O., Wretlind, A.: Experimental and clinical studies with fat emulsion for intravenous nutrition. *Nutr Diet 8:* 245–281, 1966.
221. Dudrick, S. J., Steiger, E., Long, J. M., Rhoads, J. E.: Role of parenteral hyperalimentation in management of multiple catastrophic complications. *Surg Clin North Am 50:* 1031–1038, 1970.
222. Wilmore, D. W., Dudrick, S. J.: Growth and development of an infant receiving all nutrients exclusively by vein. *JAMA 203:* 860–864, 1968.
223. Blackburn, G. L., Flatt, J. P., Clowes, G. H. A., Jr., O'Donnell, T. F., Hensle, T. E.: Protein sparing during periods of starvation with sepsis or trauma. *Ann Surg 177:* 588–594, 1973.
224. Fischer, J.: Total Parenteral Nutrition. Boston, Little, Brown, 1975.
225. Dudrick, S. J., Macfadyen, B. V., Jr., Van Buren, C. T., Ruberg, R. L., Maynard, A. T.: Parenteral hyperalimentation. Metabolic problems and solutions. *Ann Surg 176:* 259, 1972.
226. O'Connell, R. C., Morgan, H. P., Aoki, T. T., Ball, M. A., Moore, F. D.: Nitrogen conservation in starvation:graded responses to intravenous glucose. *J Clin Endocrinol Metab 39:* 555–563, 1974.
227. Felig, P.: Nutritional maintenance and diet therapy in acute and chronic disease, in Beeson PB, McDermott W (ed): Textbook of Medicine (ed 14). Philadelphia, WB Saunders, 1975, p 1389.
228. Caldwell, M. D., Johnson, H. T., Othersen, H. B. Jr.: Essential fatty acid deficiency in an infant receiving prolonged parenteral alimentation. *J Pediatr 81:* 894–899, 1972.
229. Blackburn, G. L., Flatt, J. P., Clowes, G. H. A., O'Donnel, T. F.: Peripheral intravenous feeding with isotonic amino acid solutions. *Am J Surg 125:* 447, 1973.
230. Flatt, J. P., Blackburn, G. L.: The metabolic fuel regulatory system: Implications for protein sparing therapies during caloric deprivation and disease. *Am J Clin Nutr 27:* 175–187, 1974.
231. Greenberg, G. R., Marliss, E. B., Anderson, G. H., Langer, B., Spence, W., Tovee, B., Jeejeebhoy, K. N.: Protein-sparing therapy in postoperative patients. *N Engl J Med 294:* 1411–1416, 1976.
232. Thompson, S. W. : The Pathology of Parenteral Nutrition with Lipids. Springfield, Charles C Thomas, 1974.
233. Schuberth, O., Wretlind, A.: Intravenous infusions of fat emulsions, phosphatides and emulsifying agents. *Acta Chir Scand 278 (suppl):* 1–21, 1961.
234. Wretlind, A.: Metabolism of fat emulsion for intravenous nutrition, in Wilsinson AW, Cuthbertson DP (ed): Metabolism and the Response to Injury. Kent, Pitman Medical, 1976, p 69.
235. Carlson, L. A., Hallberg, D.: Studies on the elimination of exogenous lipids from the bloodstream: The kinetics of the elimination of a fat emulsion and of chylomicrons in the dog after a single injection. *Acta Physiol Scand 59:* 52–61, 1963.
236. Hallberg, D., Holm, I., Obel, A. L., Schuberth, O., Wretlind, A.: Fat emulsion for complete intravenous nutrition. II. Clinical studies. *Postgrad Med J 43:* 307–316, 1967.
237. Hansen, L. M., Hardie, W. R., Hidalgo, J.: Fat emulsion for intravenous administration: Clinical experience with Intralipid® 10%. *Ann Surg 184:* 80–88, 1976.
238. Carlson, L. A., Rossner, S.: A methodological study of an intravenous fat tolerance test with Intralipid® emulsion. *Scand J Clin Lab Invest 29:* 271–280, 1972.
239. Holman, R. T.: Essential fatty acid deficiency in humans, in Callic C, Jacini G, Pecile A (ed): Dietary Lipids and Postnatal Development. New York, Raven Press, 1973, p 127.
240. Long, J. M., Wilmore, D. W., Mason, A. D. Jr., Pruitt, B. A.: Effect of carbohydrate and fat intake on nitrogen excretion during total intravenous feeding. *Ann Surg 185:* 417–422, 1977.

150

Protein-Energy Malnutrition and Endocrine Function

Marilyn C. Crim
Hamish N. Munro

This chapter deals with the effects of protein and energy deprivation on endocrine function. In this field, much of the evidence and emphasis has been on the study of protein-energy malnutrition (PEM) during infancy and early childhood of humans and during the growth period of experimental animals. In consequence, we shall largely restrict our survey to responses during this developmental period. The topics of starvation and obesity, both of which are forms of malnutrition related particularly to abnormalities of energy intake, are dealt with elsewhere in this volume (Chapters 147 and 148). A considerable amount of original clinical evidence of hormonal changes in malnutrition has been conveniently assembled in the Kroc Foundation's recently published symposium on "Endocrine Aspects of Malnutrition."[1]

It would be satisfying to present a picture of animal experimentation showing how nutritional and endocrine factors interact and to use this evidence to interpret the hormonal studies that have been made in human cases of PEM. Unfortunately, little systematic experimental study has been made on animals of the mechanisms by which dietary components affect endocrine function. We shall therefore have to content ourselves with a prospective look at the type of information that should be collected from animal studies, together with a description of the findings in human malnutrition. First, however, it is necessary to describe the clinical picture of protein–energy malnutrition as it occurs in some of the world's less favored children in order to emphasize the complex etiology and features of this syndrome and to determine the validity of animal models of the condition.

Dr. M. C. Crim was the recipient of a Post-doctoral Fellowship from the National Institute of Arthritis and Metabolic Diseases, U.S. Public Health Service.

MALNUTRITION IN MAN AND ANIMALS

PROTEIN–ENERGY MALNUTRITION IN MAN

The clinical picture of malnutrition in infancy and childhood has been classically defined in terms of two syndromes, *kwashiorkor,* associated primarily with deficiency of protein in the diet, and *marasmus,* which is an overall deficit of food intake, especially of energy. In practice, however, PEM is a complex condition of multiple etiology that commonly presents as a spectrum between these two extremes. While primarily a result of less than adequate intake of protein and/or calories, the onset of PEM is influenced by many other factors such as stage of development, infections, child-rearing and food habits, and other cultural factors. Although most often seen in the developing countries in Asia, Africa, and Latin America, PEM has been occasionally reported in the slums of Europe and North America.[2–5]

Kwashiorkor occurs classically between the ages of 1 and 3 years in children whose diet is grossly deficient in protein, usually as a result of being transferred from breast milk to a starchy diet such as cassava, plantain, or cereal. The child with kwashiorkor shows growth failure, mental apathy, irritability, muscle wasting, and edema. There is usually palpable hepatomegaly associated with fatty infiltration and liver damage; diarrhea and anemia are also common features. In addition, changes in the color and texture of the hair, with depigmentation of the skin and dermatosis, are often evident. The most striking biochemical abnormality is the reduced level of plasma albumin, but the fall in serum transferrin content has recently proved to be a more sensitive index of severity.[6]

In contrast to kwashiorkor, marasmus occurs most commonly but not exclusively in children under 1 year of age. It is basically due to insufficient intake of food. A common cause is early cessation of breast-feeding, coupled with an inadequate supply of alternative food, which frequently is also a source of infectious disease, and this then exacerbates the dietary inadequacy. It can also be secondary to conditions such as celiac disease, in which malabsorption restricts utilization of the diet.[7] The main clinical features include marked growth failure, the child often being less than 60 percent of normal weight for age and having a reduced body length. The severe muscle wasting, loss of subcutaneous fat, and wizened facial features contrast with the characteristic protuberant abdomen. As in kwashiorkor, diarrhea and anemia are common, but there is no edema, and serum protein levels are nearly normal, suggesting better liver function.

Figure 150-1 shows children exhibiting the classical syn-

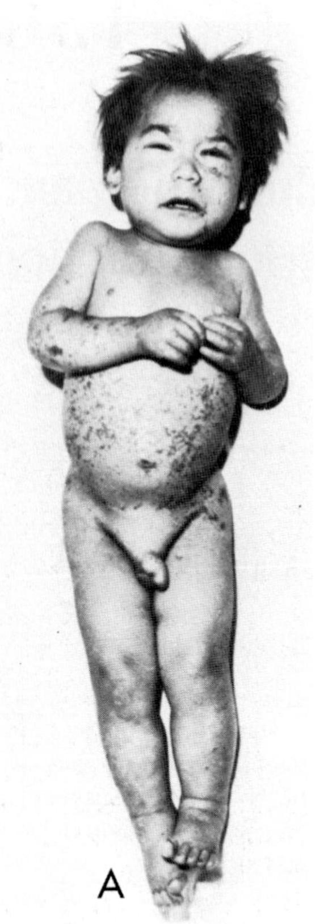

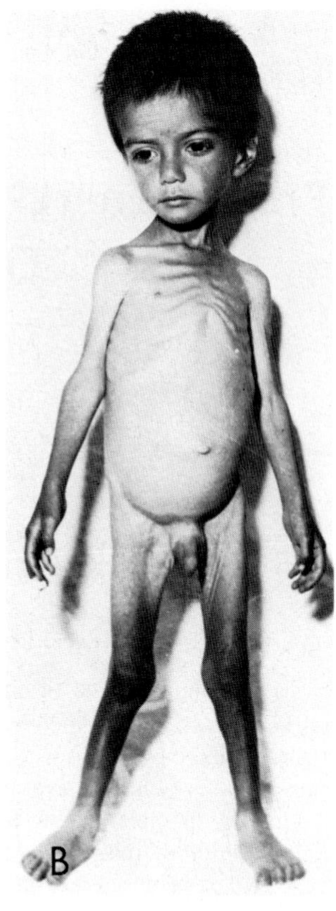

Fig. 150-1. Typical cases of kwashiorkor and marasmus. *Left,* child 1 year and 11 months old with kwashiorkor. Note the edema, the changes in skin and hair, and the evidence of mental distress. *Right,* child 4 years and 5 months old with typical marasmus, showing muscular wasting and lack of subcutaneous fat, but a protuberant abdomen. (Reproduced with permission from N. S. Scrimshaw and M. Behar, *Science 133:* 2039–2047, 1961. Copyright 1961 by the American Association for the Advancement of Science.)

dromes of kwashiorkor and marasmus.[2] In practice, many intermediate forms of PEM are seen, and these are by far the most common types of case encountered. A second difficulty in clinical classification is defining the degree of severity of PEM. Table 150-1 lists some typical biochemical findings in different types of PEM.[8] With the possible exception of serum transferrin levels, however, such biochemical measurements lack adequate precision for classifying severity. Most human nutritionists generally agree that anthropometric measurements provide the best criteria for diagnosing the degree of malnutrition. Height and weight are the most frequently used measurements, but skinfold thickness, head and chest circumference, and other physical measurements are also commonly employed.[9] Such measurements have been systematized in attempts to grade the type and degree of malnutrition. For example, the Gomez classification, which is widely used, is based on the deviation of the child's weight from a standard weight for his or her age.[10] On the other hand, Seoane and Latham have combined age, weight, and height in an attempt to distinguish children with acute malnutrition from those with chronic malnutrition or those who have been stunted as a consequence of past malnutrition.[11]

ANIMAL MODELS OF PROTEIN–ENERGY MALNUTRITION

Animal models have been used extensively in the experimental study of PEM. There has, however, been some controversy regarding the relevance of these models to the human syndromes of PEM and the validity of extrapolating data obtained from animals to man.[12] As discussed above, human PEM is the product of a complex situation with environmental factors such as infections as well as dietary components. For example, environmental factors have been implicated in the impairment of adrenocortical function identified by some investigators in PEM.[13] In addition, PEM expresses itself as several syndromes (kwashiorkor, marasmus, and marasmic kwashiorkor) according to whether the emphasis is on protein deficiency or on energy as well as protein deficiency, and animal models have to distinguish these differences in order to be valid. Nevertheless, some recent animal models closely resemble the human syndromes of PEM. For example, Anthony and Edozien[14] have induced a syndrome in the rat in which they have reproduced the edema of kwashiorkor. On the other hand, it is difficult to accept the claim[15] that force-feeding a diet deficient in one essential amino acid for several days produces experimental kwashiorkor.

If such animal models are used with discretion under appropriate conditions, it should be possible to identify individual factors in the etiology of PEM that are responsible for the observed changes in endocrine function. In addition, sites of dietary action on the control of hormonal levels can be determined on animal models using procedures that would be unacceptable in human experimentation. The choice of the animal model may be determined by a variety of factors, such as the size, cost, and biological

Table 150-1. Biochemical Findings in Children with Protein–Energy Malnutrition

Blood or Plasma Constituent		Marasmus (N = 72)	Marasmic Kwashiorkor (N = 72)	Kwashiorkor (N = 61)	Controls[a] (N = 50)
Hemoglobin	(g/100 ml)	10.1 ± 0.3	9.8 ± 0.3	9.7 ± 0.3	11.7 ± 0.1
Albumin	(g/100 ml)	2.80 ± 0.09	1.90 ± 0.05	1.51 ± 0.05	3.70 ± 0.07
IgG	(g/100 ml)	1.29 ± 0.21	1.28 ± 0.21	1.21 ± 0.08	0.90 ± 0.28
IgM	(mg/100 ml)	168 ± 10	265 ± 70	205 ± 22	61 ± 19
Transferrin	(μg/100 ml)	239 ± 15	138 ± 7	111 ± 8	357 ± 7
Iron	(μg/100 ml)	71 ± 10	54 ± 4	71 ± 6	69 ± 4
Cholesterol	(mg/100 ml)	109 ± 6	82 ± 5	77 ± 6	129 ± 5
Folic acid	(ng/ml)	9.4 ± 1.2	7.5 ± 0.9	5.1 ± 0.6	25 ± 1
Vitamin B_{12}	(pg/ml)	711 ± 82	1306 ± 294	906 ± 203	443 ± 60
Vitamin E	(mg/100 ml)	0.29 ± 0.02	0.26 ± 0.03	0.22 ± 0.02	0.42 ± 0.02
Vitamin A	(μg/100 ml)	37.6 ± 4.5	21.2 ± 2.0	23.6 ± 4.0	54 ± 5
Retinol-binding protein	(μg/ml)	23.3 ± 2.6	21.5 ±3.0	19.7 ± 5.7	30.0 ± 1.6

Reproduced with permission from R. E. Olson, *American Journal of Clinical Nutrition 28:* 626–637, 1975.
[a]Healthy villagers of same age.

relevance of the particular species. The clinical features of PEM have been reproduced successfully by various workers using the monkey and other nonhuman primates,[16–22] the pig,[23,24] the guinea pig,[25] the dog,[23] and the rat.[14,26–28] These various studies provide much detailed evidence regarding changes produced by malnutrition, notably protein deficiency (kwashiorkor). Since marasmic kwashiorkor is much more common than pure kwashiorkor, such models should be interpreted with care regarding their significance for PEM. In this connection, Platt et al.[23] discuss in some detail the relevance of their extensive studies of malnutrition in pigs and dogs to human PEM. With this in mind, changes in endocrine status of animal models of PEM will be presented in the appropriate sections to amplify endocrine changes observed in human PEM.

In using animal models, we should also recognize the influence of mammalian body size on metabolism and endocrine function, which should caution us in applying quantitative data obtained on small rodents to the much larger human species of mammal. Mammals vary in adult body size from the shrew (7 g) to the sperm whale (60,000 kg), and even within the range of species normally used experimentally there is a 2800-fold difference between the body weights of a mouse (25 g) and of a man (70 kg). It has long been known that energy metabolism diminishes in intensity with increasing size of the mammal, basal energy metabolism being about 108 kcal/kg/day for the mouse and 23 kcal/kg/day for the adult man, a fivefold difference. Various parameters of the intensity of protein metabolism also change in parallel with energy metabolism over the same range of species;[29] Table 150-2 represents some of these data for two commonly studied species, the rat and man. It shows that organs involved in metabolism form a smaller proportion of body weight in the larger mammals. Thus the liver of the rat is 4.1 percent of its body weight, but only 1.9 percent of the body weight of a man, which is a twofold decrease. The pituitary and adrenal glands are even more severely affected by body weight of the species; their sizes relative to body weight decline almost as much as does energy metabolism. The turnover of thyroxine also decreases from rat to man in parallel with the reduction in intensity of energy metabolism, but paradoxically the weight of the thyroid gland accounts for about the same proportion of the body over the range of mammals. Measurements of thyroid cell population showed that the number of thyroid cells relative to body size does, in fact, diminish twofold between the rat and man, and each cell had less RNA in the larger species.[30] The near-constancy of thyroid gland weight per kilogram of body weight is due to the amount of extracellular protein (colloid) in the gland which is proportional to plasma volume and thus forms a constant proportion of body weight. Thus, with a diminishing cell population but a constant amount of colloid, the thyroid glands of large mammals have bigger colloid vesicles than are found in the glands of small mammals.[29]

Table 150-2. The Influence of Body Size on Metabolic and Endocrine Parameters in Mammals

Measurement	Calculated Amount of Metabolic or Body Component per Kilogram of Body Weight: At 200 g (rat)	At 70 kg (man)	Ratio rat/man
Basal energy metabolism (kcal/day)	108	23	4.7
Liver weight (g)	41	19	2.1
Skeletal muscle weight (g)	450	450	1.0
Pituitary weight (mg)	360	80	4.5
Adrenal weight (mg)	380	120	3.2
Thyroid weight (mg)	150	90	1.7
Thyroid protein (mg)	13	18	0.7
Thyroid DNA (mg)	0.38	0.21	1.9
Thyroid RNA (mg)	0.43	0.15	2.9
Plasma thyroxine turnover (days^{-1})	—	—	4.6

Adapted from H. N. Munro, in *Mammalian Protein Metabolism* vol. 3, Academic Press, New York, 1969.

MECHANISMS INVOLVED IN ENDOCRINE ADAPTATIONS TO MALNUTRITION

SITES OF ENDOCRINE CHANGE IN MALNUTRITION

Many of the studies of the effects of experimental protein malnutrition on the endocrine systems of animals were carried out more than a decade ago (see Munro, ref. 31, for review), before the control of anterior pituitary function by the hypothalamus had been recognized and before modern techniques for hormone assay became available. In the light of this new information, a better understanding of the effects of malnutrition on endocrine function demands a detailed reexamination of the consequences of malnutrition at each step in the regulation of endocrine secretion. For example, Figure 150-2 illustrates the well-known sequence of events regulating formation and removal of plasma corticosteroids. At each step, nutritional status could influence (1) the functional capacity of the organ to make and secrete an endocrine product (CRF, ACTH, or corticosteroid), (2) the responsiveness of each organ to feedback or other control, and (3) the rate of degradation of the product secreted. Thus, a reduction of CRF formation by the hypothalamus, or of ACTH by the anterior pituitary gland, of the malnourished animal or human subject would tend to lower plasma levels of corticosteroids. On the other hand, reduced concentrations of liver enzymes degrading corticosteroids as a result of malnutrition would tend to elevate the plasma concentrations, and this would be followed by feedback inhibition of synthesis at the hypothalamic level. The final concentration of corticosteroid in the plasma would thus be a balance between the relative effects on liver degradation rate and on feedback inhibition. Finally, malnu-

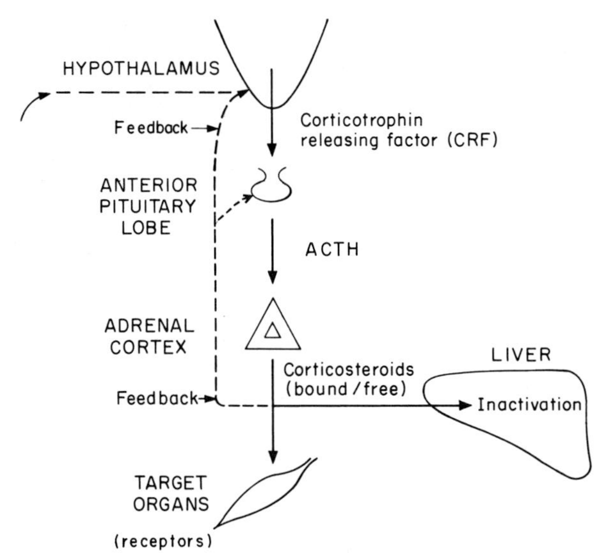

Fig. 150-2. The regulation of corticosteroid hormone production and removal.

trition could affect tissue responses to corticosteroids by altering the amount of corticosteroid-binding protein in the plasma (and thus the amount free in the plasma) and by changing the capacity of the tissue to respond to corticosteroids in malnourished animals (receptors, etc.).

The role of the liver in the regulation of plasma levels of hormones deserves detailed consideration, since (1) a considerable number of hormones (e.g., insulin, growth hormone, corticosteroids, estrogens, testosterone) are inactivated or otherwise metabolized by the liver, (2) the liver is sensitive to malnutrition, and (3) a nutrition-related change in liver function could thus be a causal factor in elevating or lowering plasma hormone levels. For example, half of the insulin secreted into the portal vein by the islets is normally extracted during its first passage through the liver.[32,33] This implies that a reduction in the capacity of the liver to inactivate insulin could result in abnormally large amounts of insulin appearing in the peripheral blood. We have employed this to explain some aspects of amino acid metabolism in cases of hepatic cirrhosis.[34]

There is rapid and extensive loss of protein and RNA from the livers of rats fed on diets providing inadequate quantities of protein and/or energy.[35,36] With this loss of liver protein goes reduction in the total amounts of many liver enzymes, including the complete disappearance of xanthine oxidase[37] and impaired liver function, as shown by a diminished capacity to clear sulfobromophthalein from the blood.[38] Some of these changes have been confirmed in human cases of PEM, but their clinical significance is uncertain.[39] Since the liver is the site of inactivation of a number of hormones, it would be important to know whether clinical or experimental PEM affects the capacity of the liver to perform these functions. Unfortunately, this question has *not* been pursued vigorously and would demand measurement of degradation of hormones in animals on deficient diets or perfusion of labeled hormones through the isolated livers of malnourished animals. However, there is enough evidence in the clinical and experimental literature to indicate that PEM can alter the metabolism of hormones inactivated by the liver. For example, Biskind[40] describes an experiment in which small amounts of estrone were implanted in the spleens of castrated female rats. The amount of estrone entering the portal vein was insufficient to bring on estrus when the rats received a normal diet but caused estrus when a low-protein cirrhosis-producing diet was fed. The impaired capacity of the liver of the protein-depleted rat to inactivate estrogens has been confirmed by others.[41] Similarly, the liver appears to be a major site of somatomedin production, and the capacity to produce somatomedin in response to growth hormone stimulation is reported to be impaired in clinical PEM.[42]

LONG-TERM EFFECTS OF MALNUTRITION ON ENDOCRINE FUNCTION

The role of individual hormones varies at different stages of growth and development,[43] and thus the effects of alterations in nutrient supply are likely to cause dissimilar changes at various stages of development. Even the age difference in the usual time of onset of kwashiorkor (1 to 3 years) and of marasmus (under 1 year) could result in different endocrine responses to similar deficiencies.

Of particular interest are animals studies showing how prenatal malnutrition can influence subsequent endocrine function after birth. In confirmation and extension of earlier work by Stephan et al.,[44] Zeman[45] malnourished rat dams during pregnancy and observed that the offspring with access to a normal diet nevertheless grew less rapidly and had a reduced capacity for growth hormone biosynthesis in vitro; the growth depression could be corrected by exogenous growth hormone administration. It has also been shown that rats malnourished in utero and during weaning[46,47] and then allowed access to an unrestricted diet have increased plasma corticosteroid levels later in life, especially in response to stress. It is not known how far the low growth hormone production or elevated corticosteroid formation contribute to the later poor growth performance of rats malnourished in early life.

Another long-term change in endocrine function is also reported by Zamenhof et al.,[48] who malnourished rat dams and found that when the female offspring were then allowed to grow on an adequate diet and were mated, their progeny were smaller at birth and suffered from diminished brain development. This is probably attributable to suboptimal endocrine performance during the pregnancy of the second-generation rats. Permanent endocrine underfunction following early malnutrition has also been suggested as occurring in human cases of PEM and was named "nutritional hypophysectomy."[49] However, the response of the malnourished child to nutritional rehabilitation shows that there is no permanent effect of early malnutrition on the capacity to grow,[50] and the Dutch famine study[51] indicates no effect of maternal malnutrition on physical growth or mental function of the offspring at 20 years of age. It will nevertheless be interesting to know whether the girls in this Dutch cohort, whose mothers were malnourished during pregnancy, do in fact produce infants of normal weight.

ENDOCRINE CHANGES OBSERVED IN PROTEIN–ENERGY MALNUTRITION

EVALUATION OF ENDOCRINE STATUS IN HUMAN MALNUTRITION

Identifying the primary site of action of malnutrition on endocrine status of man is difficult. In practice, plasma hormone levels are most commonly used to assess endocrine function in human subjects. The rates of secretion and of degradation of a hormone and even changes in plasma volume[52] all contribute to determining the hormone concentration in the plasma. It is important to assess which variable is responsible for any change in hormone level so that the nature of the change can be identified. As techniques for detecting hormones have become increasingly sophisticated, it will ultimately be desirable to document in man the responses of each element in the systems of endocrine control to variations in nutrient intake. In man, one usually has access only to blood and urine levels of endocrine secretions, often measured in isolation from the other components in the sequence. Certain hormones exist in the plasma in both a metabolically active free form and an inactive form bound to a plasma protein. The level of the latter can be sensitive to nutritional status (e.g., low albumin in kwashiorkor). Assessment of the biological activity of circulating hormones is particularly important. The peripheral effects of the hormones may also vary with nutritional status, that is, their capacity to bind to tissues and activate messenger systems. In addition, the time course of the changes in hormone levels resulting from PEM are seldom completely documented, including short-term diurnal changes.

The information about blood levels in malnourished subjects has sometimes been supplemented by provocative tests of the capacity of an endocrine organ. They are designed to determine the functional capacity of the organ to secrete hormone. Thus the function of the adrenal cortex is tested by its ability to release cortisol following administration of ACTH. Growth hormone secretion is evoked by giving arginine or lysine[53] or glucagon[54] and by hypoglycemia, but it is suppressed by hyperglycemia.[54] The physiological relevance of such tests is uncertain at this time.[55] Finally, in man, responses of tissues to hormone levels may serve as an indication of hormonal status, such as the number of circulating eosinophils, which are lowered following administration of corticosteroids.[56]

GROWTH HORMONE (HGH)

The studies of Hansen and his colleagues[50,57–59] demonstrated that HGH was elevated in both kwashiorkor and marasmus cases seen in South Africa (Fig. 150-3). In addition, the normal reduction in plasma HGH level caused by glucose loading was retarded. The HGH level diminished within 3 days of feeding with protein and reached control values within 3 weeks, whereas the HGH level was not restored when patients were fed a protein-free diet. In addition to the ameliorating effects of dietary protein, Hansen's studies have shown that plasma amino acid levels, notably alanine, may be relevant to the regulation of HGH levels.

In contrast, the Chilean studies of Mönckeberg[60–62] showed subnormal levels of HGH in marasmus but high levels in kwashiorkor. Furthermore, stimulation with arginine[60] evoked no release of HGH in Chilean cases of marasmus or kwashiorkor. Hansen[50] comments that the discrepancy with his data may be attributable to several factors, the most significant being that the Chilean marasmic children were tested 10 days after admission, whereas a reduction in HGH level was observed by Hansen's group within 3 days of initiating protein feeding. This criticism can also be leveled against the normal HGH levels observed by Godard[63] in marasmus cases in Bolivia. Nevertheless, Rao and Raghuramulu[64,65] obtained the same picture as Mönckeberg's group even though their kwashiorkor and marasmus cases were studied on admission. Parra et al.[66] in Mexico observed only a slight elevation of HGH in marasmic children soon after admission, with a distinct response to arginine administration, whereas these same authors recorded very high HGH levels in kwashiorkor, which resisted change following administration of arginine. In contrast, Suskind et al.[67] observed (like Hansen) a gross elevation of HGH in both marasmus and kwashiorkor, and especially in the former. Finally, Samuel and Deshpande[68] found elevation of HGH in a series of 54 marasmic infants in India.

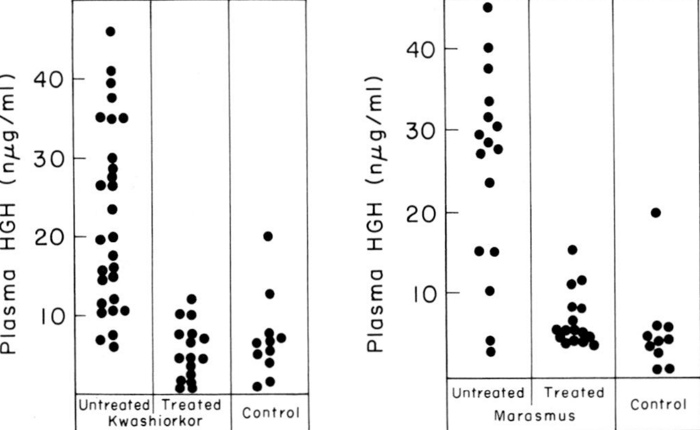

Fig. 150-3. Plasma growth hormone levels in cases of kwashiorkor (left panel) and marasmus (right panel) before and after treatment, compared with the levels in control infants. (Reproduced with permission from J. D. L. Hansen, in R. E. Olson (ed.), *Protein-Calorie Malnutrition*, Academic Press, New York, 1975, pp. 229–241.)

From these various studies on infants, it may be concluded that HGH levels have been uniformly found to be raised in kwashiorkor[50,60,63–67] but can be depressed,[60,63–65] unchanged,[66] or sometimes elevated[50,67,68] in marasmus. As regards adults, high HGH levels have also been noted in gross general malnutrition in Indians[69] and in malnourished hospital patients.[70] These elevations were also observed in normal adults undergoing total starvation[71,72] but not routinely in starving obese subjects,[72,73] thereby suggesting that body fat stores may determine the response of HGH to inadequate energy intake.

Recent evidence shows that at least some of the actions of HGH are dependent on formation of somatomedin. According to van Wyk,[74] the liver is the probable major site of synthesis of somatomedin. Synthesis rate is determined by HGH level in the plasma, and HGH may even be a precursor of somatomedin. In fact, somatomedin levels are depressed in PEM.[40] This may implicate the decreased liver function of PEM as the cause both of the elevated HGH and the lower somatomedin. Either the HGH is not being transformed adequately by the impaired liver or the low somatomedin level is stimulating excessive output of HGH through insufficient feedback repression. Since liver function is often less severely affected in marasmus, this may explain why HGH elevation has been more consistently observed in kwashiorkor than in marasmus. It might thus be more significant to measure somatomedin levels as indexes of endocrine functional status in kwashiorkor and marasmus. See Chapter 140 for further information concerning somatomedin.

Experimental studies on animals receiving diets deficient in protein (kwashiorkor type) have added some detail to the human picture. Srebnik and Nelson[75] fed rats on protein-free diets for 5 weeks and observed depletion of ICSH, FSH, and GH in the anterior pituitary gland without a reduction in TSH content. This picture was accompanied by histological evidence of exhaustion of the gland, which was also observed by Platt et al.[23] in their protein-depleted pigs and dogs. Despite this suggestion of pituitary hypofunction in experimental protein deficiency, the elevated plasma levels of growth hormone seen in human PEM were reproduced by Turner et al.[76] in protein-depleted rabbits. These elevated growth hormone levels in the depleted rabbits were unaffected by arginine or glucose administration, in agreement with the observations of Mönckeberg[60] and Hansen,[50] respectively, in human cases of PEM. It is thus obvious that a comprehensive study should be made on animals of the response of the hypothalamic-pituitary system, plasma growth hormone levels, and somatomedin production in malnutrition of both kwashiorkor and marasmic types. Finally, Turner et al.[77] have made the interesting observation on their protein-deficient rabbits that growth hormone causes a subnormal stimulation of protein synthesis when added in vitro to muscle from the depleted animals. This observation suggests that the target organs may be less responsive to the high levels of HGH observed in PEM, particularly in kwashiorkor. This thesis is compatible with the clinical observation of Hadden and Rutishauser[78] that growth hormone administration to children with PEM failed to evoke a metabolic response. On the other hand, Beas and Muzzo[62] found low levels of HGH in infantile marasmus and were able to stimulate the growth of these children by administering growth hormone.

INSULIN AND GLUCAGON

Whereas plasma HGH levels are often elevated in cases of PEM, insulin levels are frequently lowered. For example, Table 150-3 records the fasting levels of glucose, free fatty acids (FFA),

Table 150-3. Fasting Plasma Levels of Certain Metabolites in Infantile Malnutrition

Measurement	Malnourished[a] Children	Recovered[a] Children
Glucose (mg/100 ml)	67 ± 4	73 ± 3
FFA (μM)	707 ± 91	238 ± 39[b]
α-Amino nitrogen (mM)	2.6 ± 0.2	3.2 ± 0.2
Insulin (μU/ml)	7.3 ± 0.9	11.9 ± 1.2[b]
Growth hormone (ng/ml)	24.5 ± 4.6	8.7 ± 1.2[b]

Reproduced with permission from R. D. G. Milner, *Memoirs of Society for Endocrinology 18:* 191–210, 1970.
[a]Measurements made on 15 infants 1 to 6 days after admission (malnourished) and again at 6 to 12 weeks later (recovered). The data are the means ± standard errors.
[b]Difference significant ($P < 0.01$ by t test).

insulin, and growth hormone obtained by Milner[79] in Jamaican children with PEM at admission and following rehabilitation. Although the glucose level was not affected, the FFA and growth hormone levels were high on admission and fell on recovery, whereas the insulin level was initially low and rose after recovery. As in the case of HGH, there is lack of uniformity among investigators regarding the relative effects of kwashiorkor and marasmus on carbohydrate metabolism and the capacity to secrete insulin. Several authors[50,80,82] have observed a reduced capacity of kwashiorkor cases to remove intravenously administered glucose, whereas in marasmus the rate of glucose removal was often normal. However, Oxman[83] noted a decreased glucose tolerance in marasmics. In Hansen's cases,[50] oral administration of glucose failed to raise the plasma insulin level adequately in children with kwashiorkor, whereas in marasmus the defect in secretion was sometimes less severe. In earlier studies, Baig and Edozien[84] had observed low fasting insulin levels in kwashiorkor cases, whereas Hadden[81] found the insulin level to be normal in such children, but low in marasmic children. In normal subjects, both HGH and insulin levels respond to protein or amino acid administration. However, oral administration of a mixture of 10 essential amino acids to patients with PEM caused a normal rise in plasma-free amino acid levels and reduced the high HGH level but failed to raise plasma insulin concentration.[85]

Hansen[50] has considered the reasons for the failure of cases of PEM to secrete adequate amounts of insulin in response to carbohydrate administration. Dissection of the insulin secretory mechanism suggests that (1) islet-stimulating factors from the gut mucosa may be reduced as a result of mucosal atrophy in PEM,[86] a thesis that is supported by the larger secretion of insulin obtained by giving glucose intravenously rather than orally;[50] (2) release of insulin rather than synthesis of this peptide hormone may be the site of impairment, since Hansen[50] has observed that glucagon administration to cases of PEM can induce a normal elevation of insulin, although this response was not observed by Milner;[87] and (3) antagonism or resistance to insulin may occur in cases of PEM, as suggested by the failure of administered insulin to improve glucose tolerance.[80] Finally, the impairment in carbohydrate metabolism persists long after rehabilitation has been under way,[86,88,89] and this requires explanation.

In animal experiments, impaired glucose tolerance has been produced in pigs[23] and dogs[23,90] receiving inadequate intakes of protein. Rats on a low-protein diet were found to have low fasting insulin levels.[91] In rabbits on a diet low in protein, release of insulin in response to glucose[76] or to glucagon[92] was virtually absent. In addition, muscle from the rabbits on the low-protein diet had a reduced in vitro capacity to take up amino acids in response to insulin.[93] This may correlate with the observation of Heard and Turner[90] that dogs receiving a diet low in protein develop resistance to exogenous insulin, as has also been observed in human cases of PEM.[80] Thus the picture of changes in insulin levels and function in humans can be reproduced in considerable detail in animals.

There is no evidence regarding glucagon levels in human PEM. In rats, however, Anthony and Faloona[91] found that experimental protein deficiency caused no change in plasma glucagon levels, although the reduction in plasma insulin levels characteristic of PEM in humans and animal models was obtained.

ADRENOCORTICAL HORMONES

Castellanos and Arroyave[94] studied urinary excretion of adrenal steroid metabolites and observed an increased output in marasmus but not in kwashiorkor. This finding is compatible with increased adrenocortical activity in marasmus, but final interpretation depends on whether there were changes in renal function caused by malnutrition. A careful study of plasma cortisol levels and metabolism has been made by Alleyne and Young,[95] who compared unclassified cases of PEM before and after treatment. As shown in Table 150-4, the levels of cortisol in the plasma were elevated but still responded to ACTH stimulation and were also depressed by dexamethasone, indicating some preservation of control through the pituitary-adrenal axis. Measurement of the half-life of plasma cortisol showed a reduction in catabolism (Table 150-4), which could be due to diet-induced impairment of liver function. Since cortisol production rates expressed in relation to body weight were similar on admission and after recovery, it can be concluded that the raised plasma levels resulted solely from the diminished rate of degradation. If the production rates are expressed in absolute terms, there was a rise in output following recovery, which makes the reduction in the degradation rate an even more important factor in the elevation of the plasma level.

Alleyne and Young did not separate their cases of PEM into kwashiorkor and marasmus. However, many subsequent studies on cortisol metabolism do so. Some of these later investigators have concluded that the increase in plasma cortisol occurs mainly in marasmic children and less in kwashiorkor cases. Thus Prinsloo et al.[96] found no consistent increase in the plasma cortisol levels of children with kwashiorkor, nor did Brun,[97] who did, however, find an increment in untreated cases of marasmus. Similarly, Rao et al.[98] found that plasma cortisol was elevated in both marasmus and kwashiorkor but more so in the former. On the other hand, Schonland et al.[99] observed high plasma cortisol levels in kwashiorkor cases, which fell after treatment, and Abassy et al.[100] observed equal elevation of plasma cortisol in both conditions, without any

Table 150-4. Plasma Cortisol Levels and Rates of Cortisol Production and Degradation in Malnourished and Recovered Children

Measurement	Malnourished Children	Recovered Children
Plasma cortisol at midnight (μg/100 ml)	20.8	4.9
Plasma cortisol in morning (μg/100 ml)	28.2	11.5
Plasma cortisol 1 hr after ACTH[a] (μg/100 ml)	58.4	44.6
Plasma cortisol 2 days after dexamethasome (μg/100 ml)	10.5	—
Half-life of plasma cortisol (min)	180	80
Cortisol production rate (mg/kg/day)	0.41	0.34

Assembled from data of G. A. O. Alleyne and V. H. Young, *Clinical Science 33:* 189–200, 1967.
[a]Given as synacthen.

increase after administration of ACTH. Paisey et al.[101] also found similar elevations of cortisol in untreated cases of marasmus and kwashiorkor. Thus, cases of marasmus have been generally associated with raised plasma cortisol levels,[96–98,100,101] whereas kwashiorkor cases showed no change[96,97] or moderate[98] to extensive[99–101] elevations.

In any discussion of plasma cortisol levels, attention has to be paid to the amount of hormone free in the plasma and the amount bound to serum albumin and to transcortin. The free fraction, representing 10 percent of the total, is the physiologically active form. Both albumin and transcortin are made in the liver and can undergo a reduction as a consequence of malnutrition. It is therefore not surprising that there is an increase in the proportion of cortisol free in the plasma of untreated PEM cases and that this returns to normal proportions when the plasma protein concentrations are restored following treatment.[50,99,102,103] This leads to the conclusion that corticosteroid overactivity in PEM is greater than the total plasma values would suggest, and indeed there is some evidence of hypercorticism in PEM that may be a cause of the depressed cell-mediated immunity.[99]

Aldosterone secretion has been studied in PEM in Peru.[104,105] In marasmus, aldosterone levels were similar to those of age or height/weight-matched controls, whereas in kwashiorkor, elevated levels of aldosterone were observed. However, the rate of aldosterone secretion was increased in marasmus but not in kwashiorkor. The normal plasma level of the marasmic patient means that aldosterone is turning over more rapidly. The elevated plasma level of kwashiorkor, in spite of a normal production rate, implies that breakdown is retarded, presumably because of the greater liver damage in kwashiorkor than in marasmus. Like cortisol, aldosterone circulates loosely bound to serum albumin, and Leonard and McWilliam[106] have shown that the proportion of bound aldosterone decreases in kwashiorkor. However, the increased amount of unbound aldosterone may have less significance than in the case of cortisol, since aldosterone binding is normally rather loose.[105]

Many studies of the effects of malnutrition on the adrenocortical function of animals have been undertaken. Almost all of them describe observations on animals depleted of protein but not of calories. The earlier literature deals mainly with changes in adrenal gland weight and has been reviewed elsewhere.[31] Several investigators[23,107–109] have reported that prolonged ad libitum feeding of protein-deficient diets to animals failed to diminish the weight of the adrenal glands relative to *final* body weight, although the glands were small relative to *age* controls. Since prolonged malnutrition results in animals that differ markedly in size from their controls, Munro et al.[110] analyzed the adrenal glands of mature rats after only 11 days on a protein-free diet that did not cause serious weight loss and observed a loss of adrenal cell population (measured as DNA) and also a reduction in the protein, RNA, and phospholipid content per cell. However, in agreement with earlier investigators,[111–114] the adrenal glands of the protein-deficient animals responded normally to ACTH, suggesting that the hypofunction of the adrenal cortex was due to reduced secretion of ACTH. This conclusion is in agreement with the general loss of trophic hormones from the pituitary glands of protein-depleted animals[75] and is supported by a careful study of PEM in monkeys on restricted intakes of energy as well as protein.[22] In the latter study, plasma corticosteroid levels were considerably elevated, whereas the adrenal cortex showed marked atrophic changes. This picture also corresponds with studies of adrenal histology made on children dying of PEM. Despite the normal or elevated levels of cortisol in the plasma, fatal cases of PEM usually display a picture of atrophy at autopsy.[79,115] It has been suggested[116] that at first there is adrenal hyperfunction in response to malnutrition but that this is followed by adrenal exhaustion, which accounts for the terminal picture of atrophy. The proposal of a hypertrophic phase seems unnecessary if we accept that the elevated plasma cortisol levels in marasmus are due to a diminished rate of its degradation.

The study by Alleyne and Young[95] indicates that reduced degradation of cortisol plays a causal role in raising plasma levels of the hormone. In this connection, the most challenging relationship between nutritional status, liver function, and hormone action is that of the corticosteroids, since these are not only degraded in the liver by dehydrogenation followed by conjugation with glucuronic acid[117] but they also promote RNA and protein synthesis in the liver. In this context, Goodlad and Munro[118] examined the effect of diet on the anabolic response of the liver to administered corticosteroid. They fed groups of rats at three levels of dietary protein, at each of which two levels of energy intake were given, and administered cortisone over a 4-day period to some of the animals in each dietary group. As shown in Table 150-5, cortisone administration caused nitrogen balance on all six diets to become less favorable than in control animals fed at the same protein and energy level, but the magnitude of this response was unaffected by the type of diet. On the other hand, the deposition of protein and RNA in the liver caused by cortisone administration was significantly influenced by intake of energy but not by intake of protein. It is thus possible that plasma corticosteroids may be less able to induce their own inactivating liver enzymes in cases of marasmus (energy deficit), and thus the plasma concentrations of the hormone may be more elevated than in kwashiorkor (protein deficit), as had been claimed in some of the studies summarized above. It would therefore be instructive if the dietary studies of Goodlad and Munro could be extended to include turnover rates of administered corticosteroid under each nutritional condition. These experiments suggest that corticosteroid degradation rate *may* be affected by dietary energy level.

Table 150-5. Interaction of Dietary Protein and Energy Levels with the Response of Mature Female Rats to Cortisone Administration

Diet		N Balance (mg/4 days)			Liver Protein (mg N/100 g initial body weight)			Liver RNA (mg P/100 g initial body weight)		
Protein (g/day)	Energy (kcal/day)	Control	Cort.	Diff.	Control	Cort.	Diff.	Control	Cort.	Diff.
0	21	−95	−118	−23	52.3	62.1	+9.7	2.26	2.44	+0.18
	45	−65	−85	−20	49.9	67.0	+17.1	2.43	2.75	+0.32
1.2	21	−62	−82	−20	57.8	58.7	+0.9	2.32	2.33	+0.01
	45	+15	−35	−50	63.7	75.7	+12.0	2.65	3.10	+0.45
2.4	21	−15	−60	−45	64.2	73.7	+9.5	2.59	2.82	+0.23
	45	+38	−5	−43	71.3	84.3	+13.0	2.75	3.37	+0.62

Adapted from G. A. J. Goodlad and H. N. Munro, *Biochemical Journal 73:* 343–348, 1959.

Finally, the impact of nutrients on the control of adrenocortical function is also illustrated by studies made some years ago on RNA and protein metabolism in the livers of rats consuming different protein meals. Synthesis of RNA in the liver is stimulated within a few hours of feeding casein to rats, and this was attributed to the effects of a complete supply of all essential amino acids.[119] However, the giving of zein, which is deficient in tryptophan and lysine, also led to the same response.[120] The action of zein was traced to the large amount of leucine in zein. When leucine was given alone to rats, there was an increased uptake of precursors into liver RNA, accompanied by an increase in the protein content of the liver. These changes were then found to be associated with a rise in plasma corticosteroid levels[121] and could be eliminated by adrenalectomy.[122] The site of action of excess dietary leucine has not been established, but data from another laboratory[123] show that administered leucine causes depletion of the adrenal ascorbic acid content of normal rats but not of hypophysectomized rats. This finding suggests that hypothalamic-pituitary control of ACTH release is likely to be the location at which excessive levels of this amino acid exercises its effects on adrenocortical secretion and thus on liver metabolism. It is apparent that the exact site of action can be determined using newer techniques for exploring hypothalamic control of CRF release[124,125] and that the effects of other nutritional factors on endocrine function could be similarly evaluated. This type of study thus points the way to a more satisfying dissection of the control mechanisms by which nutritional changes affect endocrine function.

THYROID HORMONES

Classically, thyroid function has been assessed by basal metabolic rate determinations. The early measurements gave varied results in malnourished infants.[126,127] However, as Milner[79] points out, interpretations of BMR measurements are complicated by variations in body composition.[128–130] As an illustration of the difficulty of interpreting BMR, Montgomery[128] found in malnourished cases that BMR could be subnormal in relation to body weight but not necessarily in terms of body solids. Generally, it is agreed that an untreated malnourished child has a diminished oxygen consumption per unit of lean body mass.[131,132] In order to avoid the problem of body composition, Mönckeberg[60] has related oxygen consumption to height. In this way, he distinguishes a reduction in oxygen uptake in marasmus from none in kwashiorkor and postulates that this is due to the more adequate caloric intake of the latter group.

A more direct approach to the study of the impact of malnutrition on thyroid function is provided by modern methodology for measuring (1) uptake of radioactive iodine by the thyroid gland, (2) plasma levels of plasma protein-bound and butanol-extractable iodine, (3) triiodothyronine, (4) thyroxine, (5) free thyroxine, (6) thyroxine-binding globulin, (7) thyroxine-binding prealbumin capacity, (8) thyroid-stimulating hormone (TSH), (9) thyrotropin-releasing hormone (TRF), and (10) responses of various parameters of thyroid function to administered TSH and TRF.

Early investigations on marasmic infants of the uptake of radioactive iodine by the thyroid gland showed reduced capacity to capture iodine[133,134] and increased urinary excretion of iodine,[135] which correlates with evidence that protein-bound iodine[136,137] and butanol-extractable iodine[138,139] are low in the plasma of marasmic children. However, Hansen[50] considers that such tests tend to be unreliable indexes of thyroid function because of variations in iodine intake in the diet.

With the advent of immunoassays and other new procedures, more convincing evidence of changes in thyroid function in PEM has emerged. The most extensive studies are those of Graham and Blizzard,[140] who compared cases of kwashiorkor and cases of marasmic kwashiorkor in Peru with age-matched controls, an important consideration because the normal infant shows considerable age-related changes in plasma levels of TSH during growth. In the kwashiorkor series, there was extensive reduction in plasma thyroxine level, which could be correlated with reduced thyroxine-binding globulin in the plasma. This resulted in a greater proportion of thyroxine occurring in the unbound state, while the level of TSH remained within the normal range. In contrast, the marasmic infants showed only a small reduction in plasma thyroxine level, presumably because the concentration of thyroxine-binding globulin was normal, and thus there was no change in the proportion of unbound thyroxine; on the other hand, the level of TSH in the plasma of marasmic children was reduced to below detectable values. This picture receives support from other, less comprehensive surveys. Using a bioassay, Varga and Mess[141] found TSH to be undetectable in marasmus and normal or only moderately reduced in kwashiorkor. Similarly, Godard[142,143] had found in Bolivia that cases of kwashiorkor had normal TSH levels, whereas marasmic infants had decreased levels; in cases of PEM with gross hypoalbuminemia (kwashiorkor) in South Africa, Pimstone et al.[144] found plasma TSH values to be normal or raised. In mixed PEM cases in Uganda, Harland and Parkin[145] observed low TSH levels, and this was also noted in adults with malnutrition due to anorexia nervosa,[146] although not in a group of malnourished Indian adults.[147]

The responsiveness of the thyroid gland to TSH has been explored in marasmic as compared with control infants.[129] Administration of TSH increased ^{131}I uptake and plasma butanol-extractable iodine in both groups, and in addition the marasmic infants responded with an increase in BMR. However, by none of these parameters did TSH administration cause the marasmic infants to attain the normal range of values, and the authors conclude that the hypofunction of the thyroid gland in marasmus is due not only to a reduced level of TSH but also to decreased responsiveness of the gland to TSH. Finally, with the availability of thyrotropin-releasing factor (TRF), two groups have reported that normal or excessive responses to injection of this factor were obtained in cases of infantile kwashiorkor[144] and of adult malnutrition.[147] In both series, the level of TSH in the plasma was within the normal range before TRF injection; it would be interesting to know whether TRF is also fully effective in marasmic infants with depressed resting levels of TSH.

The impact of malnutrition on the function of the thyroid gland can be summarized as follows. In kwashiorkor, the main effect appears to be a reduction in the circulating level of total thyroxine as a result of the diminished amount of carrier protein in the plasma. Since there is no corresponding reduction in the levels of free thyroxine or TSH, it can be concluded that the thyroid gland in children with kwashiorkor is being stimulated at a normal level and is secreting adequate amounts of thyroxine. In contrast, cases of marasmus show a profound reduction in TSH level in the plasma, which must result in hypoactivity of the thyroid gland and diminished secretion of thyroxine. Nevertheless, in cases of marasmus the level of thyroxine in the plasma is normal[140] or even elevated,[130] and it must be concluded that removal of thyroxine is severely depressed. Recent evidence shows that conversion of thyroxine to triiodothyronine in the liver and elsewhere is impaired in malnutrition. Cases of PEM studied in Senegal[148] showed a much greater fall in plasma levels of triiodothyronine than of thyroxine. Similarly, obese subjects undergoing starvation had normal plasma levels of total thyroxine and slightly elevated free thyroxine, whereas total and free triiodothyronine levels were markedly decreased.[149] In starvation, it appears that thyroxine is deiodinated to an inactive form of triiodothyronine (3,3′,5′ triiodothyronine, "reverse T3").[150] The lower levels of biologically active triiodothyronine in the plasma of starving people may account for their reduced oxygen consumption and for the fall in urinary nitrogen output characteristic of starvation; the latter becomes elevated when triiodothyronine is administered during starvation.[151]

This distinction between thyroid function in the two types of PEM seems to be reflected in the findings of experimental studies of thyroid histology. Monkeys fed ad libitum on a protein-deficient (kwashiorkor-type) diet[16] showed no changes in thyroid structure, which is compatible with the observation of normal levels of TSH in the anterior pituitary glands of rats fed ad libitum on a protein-free diet[75] and with the normal plasma levels of TSH in clinical cases of kwashiorkor. In contrast, the experimental picture in marasmus is compatible with a diminished output of TSH when the diet is deficient in calories as well protein. In animals, Enwonwu[22,152] observed a flattened, atrophic thyroid gland structure in monkeys subjected to caloric as well as protein restriction, and Platt and his colleagues[23] also observed thyroid atrophy in young pigs receiving a diet low in protein and in calories; however, Platt et al. also observed thyroid atrophy when the extra calories were added to the low-protein diet. Differences in caloric intake of human cases of PEM may account for the contradictory findings in fatal cases of PEM with normal thyroid histology in Jamaica[153] and atrophy in Uganda.[115] The atrophic state of the thyroid gland in PEM must be readily reversible, since malnourished children respond promptly to dietary treatment by displaying catch-up growth[154] and restoration of normal metabolic rate.[155]

CATECHOLAMINES AND OTHER NEUROHORMONES

The catecholamine neurotransmitters and hormones (dopamine, norepinephrine, and epinephrine) are formed from tyrosine by specific neurones in the brain (dopamine and norepinephrine) and by the postganglionic sympathetic nerve terminals (norepinephrine) and are secreted from the adrenal medulla (norepinephrine and epinephrine). Interpretation of the amounts of these hormones and their metabolites excreted in the urine is thus complicated by the number of contributing tissues, of which the sympathetic nerves are the major source. In addition, some of the urinary dopamine and its metabolites are accounted for by dopamine of dietary origin.[156] The major metabolites found in the urine vary according to the catecholamine. Dopamine (dihydroxyphenylethylamine) is metabolized to dihydroxyphenylacetic acid and then oxidized to homovanillic acid, both of which appear in the urine. Norepinephrine and epinephrine undergo 0-methylation to form normetanephrine and metanephrine respectively, and both of these intermediate degradation products are further oxidized to vanillylmandelic acid.

Although the data are thus difficult to interpret, measurements have nevertheless been made of catecholamine metabolites in the urine of children with PEM. Bourgeois et al.[157] measured the combined urinary output of metanephrine and normetanephrine in undesignated cases of malnutrition in Brazil. The outputs of both metabolites relative to surface area were significantly below normal in untreated PEM cases, and there was a delayed response to hypoglycemic stress, indicating underfunctioning of the adrenal medulla. These deviations from normal values disappeared following nutritional rehabilitation. Other studies have been made of catecholamine metabolites. In kwashiorkor cases in Mexico, Parra et al.[158] observed a reduced output of dopamine per square meter of body surface area but no significant reduction in the urinary levels of norepinephrine, epinephrine, and vanillylmandelic acid. Cases of PEM studied in Guatemala[159] had an increased output of epinephrine (which the authors suggested might be due to infection), no change in norepinephrine excretion, a reduction in urinary dopamine level (attributed to a lower dietary intake of dopamine), and also a fall in vanillylmandelic acid output, which may have reflected diminished metabolism of norepinephrine. Finally, studies on malnourished infant rats[160] have demonstrated loss of catecholamines from the adrenal glands and epinephrine from the brain; on rehabilitation, the tissue levels of these catecholamines were restored to normal. Thus, malnutrition-related changes in catecholamine metabolism have been found without identification in man of the relative effects of malnutrition on the various organs producing catecholamines.

Serotonin is another neurotransmitter substance synthesized from an amino acid (tryptophan). Like the catecholamines, the first step in synthesis is decarboxylation by aromatic amino acid decarboxylase of a precursor to yield the corresponding amine. Again like the catecholamines, serotonin is made by specific brain cells and also by other tissues in the body. In recent studies on human subjects,[161] we found that the daily excretion of metabolites of serotonin and dopamine diminished when protein was removed from their diet. This was confirmed in rats, in which it was also observed that the stimulant effect of adding protein to the diet could be abolished by pretreating the animals with an inhibitor specific for aromatic amino acid decarboxylase in tissues other than the brain. Consequently, the observed changes in the urinary metabolites at different levels of protein intake did not include alterations in brain serotonin metabolism. However, there are many studies to show that availability of tryptophan to the brain regulates serotonin metabolism in that organ.[162] These include a long-term experiment with weanling rats consuming a diet in which corn (deficient in tryptophan) was the source of protein; the corn-fed animals showed reduced brain levels of serotonin.[163]

Since tryptophan is rate-limiting for serotonin synthesis, factors affecting entry of tryptophan into the brain have been explored by a number of investigators with contradictory conclusions. Among plasma amino acids, tryptophan is unique in being transported mainly bound to serum albumin, from which it can be displaced by free fatty acids competing preferentially for the albumin-binding sites.[164] It has therefore been postulated that the entry of tryptophan into the brain will depend on the concentration of free (non-albumin-bound) tryptophan[165] and that high levels of free fatty acids in the plasma will consequently raise brain tryptophan levels by displacing tryptophan from albumin and making more free tryptophan available.[166] This is contradicted by our studies on rats[167] in which carbohydrate feeding depressed the levels of plasma-free fatty acids, with consequent *reduction* in free plasma tryptophan, but this was accompanied by an *elevation* of brain tryptophan levels. Instead, the increased entry of tryptophan into the brain after a meal of carbohydrate can be correlated with a sharp reduction in the plasma levels of neutral amino acids competing for entry, notably the branched-chain amino acids.[162] This is relevant to the very considerable changes in the plasma levels of branched-chain and some other neutral amino acids observed in cases of PEM.[168] In cirrhosis of the liver, the plasma levels of branched-chain amino acids are depressed, whereas tryptophan concentration is often raised, and in such cases we have postulated that the freer access of tryptophan to the brain will increase serotonin formation and contribute to hepatic coma.[34]

By analogy to serotonin, formation of the hypothalamic releasing-factor peptides may turn out to be rate-limited by the entry of several amino acids into the brain and may therefore show even more complex competitive effects of changes in plasma amino acid levels. An understanding of the effects of PEM on the regulation of endocrine function may not be possible until the impact of plasma amino acid concentrations on hypothalamic function is unraveled.

ANTIDIURETIC HORMONE

The levels of antidiuretic hormone in the plasma and urine of children are elevated in kwashiorkor but are unchanged in marasmus.[169] Lack of information on rates of synthesis and removal of this hormone makes it impossible to deduce the cause of the elevated levels in kwashiorkor or to speculate whether they are related to the fluid retention of that condition.

CONCLUSIONS

Two general questions are worth pursuing further before closing. First, from the available clinical and animal data, can we begin to identify control points of hormone production and utilization that may be sensitive to protein and energy deficit and thus pave the way for definitive identification? Second, can we predict the metabolic consequences of the hormonal changes observed in PEM?

With regard to the first of these objectives, cases of kwashiorkor in different parts of the world show a surprisingly uniform picture of (1) elevation of plasma HGH levels with reduced somatomedin production, (2) a reduced level of insulin (both in the fasting state and in response to carbohydrate), (3) usually little or no rise in blood cortisol level, and (4) no change in plasma TSH levels but a fall in total thyroxine concentration consistent with the reduction in thyroxine bound to carrier protein but not associated with reduced free thyroxine. While the first of these observations (high HGH) suggests that there is overproduction of this hormone by the anterior hypophyseal lobe, the studies of Srebnik and Nelson[75] on rats receiving a protein-free diet without energy deficit (kwashiorkor model) showed reduced pituitary levels of HGH. The high plasma level of HGH may thus be due to even more extensively reduced removal of HGH. The lowered insulin production in kwashiorkor presumably represents a direct failure of insulin synthesis and/or release.

In marasmus the hormonal picture is somewhat different, although more variable in different clinical experiences than for kwashiorkor. Thus (1) the plasma level of HGH is *not* always raised, (2) insulin levels are usually normal, (3) plasma cortisol levels are more often elevated than in kwashiorkor, and (4) there is no reduction or even an elevation in plasma thyroxine level, but all investigators note a severe reduction in circulating TSH, and in caloric insufficiency the level of triiodothyronine is grossly reduced. The studies of Alleyne and Young[95] on children with PEM show reduced degradation of cortisol as the major reason for elevation of this hormone in PEM, and this is consistent with the observations of Goodlad and Munro[118] that energy intake can alter the response of the liver to corticosterone administered to rats. Degradation of thyroxine is probably also reduced in marasmic cases, since normal or elevated plasma levels are maintained despite evidence suggesting hypoactivity of the thyroid gland. The latter is shown by the reduced TSH levels of clinical cases of marasmus and by the finding of an atrophic thyroid gland in experimental marasmus in monkeys.[152] Since these phenomena occur in the presence of normal plasma thyroxine levels, we must assume a malnutrition-related loss of sensitivity of the hypothalamic-pituitary mechanism to plasma thyroxine content.

It is apparent from this summary of studies on clinical cases and experimental animals that insufficient evidence is presently available to indicate what points in hormone production and degradation are most susceptible to nutritional control. This will not materially improve until carefully designed experiments on animal models of kwashiorkor and marasmus are performed in which each step in hormone synthesis and breakdown is tested. In addition, there is now enough evidence to show that hormone receptors can probably be affected by nutritional status. Thus, Leathem[170] states that protein deficiency prevents the sexual organs of the rat from responding to androgens and gonadotropins, and evidence has been presented earlier in this review that the actions of administered insulin on carbohydrate utilization[81] and of growth hormone on muscle protein synthesis[77] can be impaired by malnutrition. In view of the considerable changes in plasma amino acid levels found in PEM,[168] it would seem important to assess the role of amino acid supply to the tissues on formation of releasing factors by the hypothalamus, on endocrine organ secretory function, and on the capacity of the target organs to respond.

An area in which more research effort would also be rewarding is the role of the liver in controlling degradation of hormones and thus influencing their plasma levels. It was pointed out earlier that several hormones (e.g., insulin, corticosteroids, sex hormones, and probably growth hormone) are metabolized in the liver and that this organ is susceptible to rapid changes in enzyme content in response to alterations in dietary protein and/or energy intake. The data of Goodlad and Munro[118] illustrate how the anabolic action of corticosteroids can be affected by each of these dietary factors. It would therefore be very informative to have direct studies on degradation of hormones by the livers of animals receiving kwashiorkor-type or marasmus-type diets. This could be combined with a study of the capacity of the liver of the malnourished animal to form hormone transport proteins so that the overall contribution of liver impairment in malnutrition to the hormonal picture of PEM could be evaluated.

Finally, attempts have been made[8] to interpret the metabolic changes observed in cases of PEM in terms of the known effects of hormones on biochemical processes. Cases of malnutrition with increased plasma cortisol and lowered plasma insulin levels would be expected to exhibit mobilization of amino acids from muscle, and the resulting flow of amino acids to the liver should promote gluconeogenesis. Increased plasma levels of growth hormone and depressed levels of insulin should result in mobilization of body fat. Thus, it would be predicted that the hormonal imbalances of PEM should lead to dissipation of muscle protein and fat stores. In marasmic cases, this may be offset to some extent by the reduced metabolic rate, which will conserve energy. This type of metabolic analysis may be premature because of possible reductions in the sensitivity of the target organs to hormone levels in PEM. Analysis of the metabolic consequences of the hormonal changes in PEM must therefore await a better understanding of the effects on the target organs.

REFERENCES

1. Gardner, L. I., Amacher, P. (eds). *Endocrine Aspects of Malnutrition*. The Kroc Foundation, Santa Ynez, Calif., 1973.
2. Scrimshaw, N. S. and Béhar, M. Protein malnutrition in young children. *Science 133:* 2039–2047, 1961.
3. Latham, M. C. Protein-calorie malnutrition in children and its rela-

tion to psychological development and behavior. *Physiol. Rev. 54:* 541–565, 1974.

4. Anonymous. Malnutrition and physical and mental development *Nutr. Rev. 28:* 176–177, 1970.
5. Viteri, F., Béhar, M., Arroyave, G., and Scrimshaw, N. S. Clinical aspects of protein malnutrition *in Mammalian Protein Metabolism* (ed. H. N. Munro and J. B. Allison), vol. 2. Academic Press, New York, 1964, pp. 523–568.
6. McFarlane, H. et al. Immunity, transferrin and survival in kwashiorkor. *Br. Med. J. 4:* 268–270, 1970.
7. Lloyd-Still, J. D., Wolff, P. H., Harwitz, I., and Schwachman, H. Studies on intellectual development after severe malnutrition in infancy in cystic fibrosis and other intestinal lesions. Cited by Latham, M. C. *in Physiol. Rev. 54:* 541–565, 1974.
8. Olson, R. E. Introductory remarks: Nutrient, hormone, enzyme interactions. *Am. J. Clin. Nutr. 28:* 626–637, 1975.
9. Jelliffe, D. B. *In The Assessment of the Nutritional Status of the Community.* World Health Organization Monogr. Ser. No. 33, Geneva, 1966.
10. Gomez, F. et al. Malnutrition in infancy and childhood with special reference to kwashiorkor. *Adv. Pediatr. 7:* 131–169, 1954.
11. Seoane, N. and Latham, M. C. Nutritional anthropometry in the identification of malnutrition in childhood. *J. Trop. Pediatr. 17:* 198–204, 1971.
12. Kirsch, R. E., Saunders, S. J. and Brock, J. F. Animal models and human protein-calorie malnutrition. *Am. J. Clin. Nutr. 21:* 1225–1228, 1968.
13. Paisey, R. B., Angers, M., and Frenk, S. Plasma cortisol levels in malnourished children with and without superimposed acute stress. *Arch. Dis. Child. 48:* 714–720, 1973.
14. Anthony, L. E. and Edozien, J. C. Experimental protein and energy deficiencies in the rat. *J. Nutr. 105:* 631–648, 1975.
15. Sidransky, H. and Verney, E. Chemical pathology of acute amino acid deficiencies. VII. *Arch. Pathol. 78:* 134–144, 1964.
16. Deo, M. G., Sood, S. K., and Ramalingaswami, V. Experimental protein deficiency: pathological features in the rhesus monkey. *Arch. Pathol. 80:* 14–23, 1965.
17. Follis, R. H. A kwashiorkor-like syndrome observed in monkeys fed maize. *Proc. Soc. Exp. Biol. Med. 96:* 523–528, 1957.
18. Coward, D. G. and Whitehead, R. G. Experimental protein-energy malnutrition in baby baboons. Attempts to reproduce the pathological features of kwashiorkor as seen in Uganda. *Br. J. Nutr. 28:* 223–237, 1972.
19. Kumar, V., Chase, H. P., Hammond, K., and O'Brien, D. Alterations in blood biochemical tests in progressive protein malnutrition. *Pediatrics 49:* 736, 1972.
20. Kerr, G. R., Allen, J. R., Scheffler, G., and Waisman, H. A. Malnutrition studies in the rhesus monkey. I. Effect on physical growth. *Am. J. Clin. Nutr. 23:* 739–748, 1970.
21. Ordy, J. M., Samorajski, T., Zimmerman, R. R., and Rady, P. M. Effects of post-natal protein deficiency on weight gain, serum proteins, enzymes, cholesterol, and liver ultrastructure in a subhuman primate *(macaca mulatta) Am. J. Pathol. 48:* 769–791, 1966.
22. Enwonwu, C. O., Stambaugh, R. V., and Jacobson, K. L. Protein-energy deficiency in non-human primates: biochemical and morphological alterations. *Am. J. Clin. Nutr. 26:* 1287–1302, 1973.
23. Platt, B. S., Heard, C. R. C., and Stewart, R. J. C. *In* Mammalian Protein Metabolism (ed. H. N. Munro and J. B. Allison), vol. 2. Academic Press, New York, 1964, pp. 445–521.
24. Grimble, R. F. and Whitehead, R. G. The relationship between an elevated serum amino acid ratio and the development of other biological abnormalities in the experimentally malnourished pig. *Br. J. Nutr. 23:* 791–804, 1969.
25. Enwonwu, C. O. Experimental protein-calorie malnutrition in the guineapig and evaluation of the role of ascorbic acid status. *Lab. Invest. 29:* 17–26, 1973.
26. Kirsch, R. E., Brock, J. F., and Saunders, S. J. Experimental protein-calorie malnutrition. *Am. J. Clin. Nutr. 21:* 820–826, 1968.
27. Grimble, R. F., Sawyer, M. B., and Whitehead, R. G. Time relationships between elevation of the serum amino acid ratio and the changes in liver composition in malnourished rats. *Br. J. Nutr. 23:* 879–888, 1969.
28. Enwonwu, C. O. and Sreebny, L. M. Experimental protein-calorie malnutrition in rats. Biochemical and ultrastructural studies. *Exp. Mol. Pathol. 12:* 332–353, 1970.
29. Munro, H. N. Evolution of protein metabolism in mammals, *in Mammalian Protein Metabolism* (ed. H. N. Munro), vol. 3. Academic Press, New York, 1969, pp. 133–182.
30. Begg, D., McGirr, E. M., and Munro, H. N. The protein and nucleic acid content of the thyroid glands of different mammals. *Endocrinology 76:* 171–177, 1965.
31. Munro, H. N. General aspects of the regulation of protein metabolism by diet and by hormones, *in Mammalian Protein Metabolism* (ed. H. N. Munro and J. B. Allison) vol. 1. Academic Press, New York, 1964, pp. 381–481.
32. Kraas, E., Bittner, R., Meves, M., and Beger, H. G. Insulinkonzentrationen im Pfortaderblut des Menschen nach Glucose-Infusion. *Klin. Wschr. 52:* 404–406, 1974.
33. Kaden, M., Harding, P., and Field, J. B. Effect of intraduodenal glucose administration on hepatic extraction of insulin in the anesthetized dog. *J. Clin. Invest. 52:* 2016–2028, 1973.
34. Munro, H. N., Fernstrom, J. D. and Wurtman, R. J. Insulin, plasma amino acid imbalance, and hepatic coma. *Lancet, 1:* 722–724, 1975.
35. Munro, H. N. and Naismith, D. J. The influence of energy intake on protein metabolism. *Biochem. J. 54:* 191–197, 1953.
36. Munro, H. N., Naismith, D. J., and Wikramanayake, T. W. The influence of energy intake on ribonucleic acid metabolism. *Biochem. J. 54:* 198–205, 1953.
37. Meikleham, V., Wells, I.C., Richert, D.A., and Westerfeld, W. W. Liver esterase and xanthine oxidase during protein depletion. *J. Biol. Chem. 192:* 651–661, 1951.
38. Wang, C. F. et al. Progressive changes in liver composition, function, body fluids and liver cytology during protein depletion in the rat and the effect of choline on these changes. *J. Lab. Clin. Med. 34:* 953–964, 1949.
39. Waterlow, J. C. The assessment of protein nutrition and metabolism in the whole animal with reference to man, in *Mammalian Protein Metabolism* (ed. H. N. Munro), vol. 3. Academic Press, New York, 1969, pp. 325–390.
40. Biskind, M. S. Nutritional therapy of endocrine disturbances. *Vitam. Horm. 5:* 147–185, 1946.
41. Vasington, F. E., Parker, A., Headley, W., and Vanderlinde, R. E. Relationship of low protein diet and ascorbic acid in estrogen inactivation by liver. *Endocrinology 62:* 557–564, 1958.
42. Grant, D. B. et al. Reduced sulphation factor in undernourished children. *Arch. Dis. Child. 48:* 596–600, 1973.
43. Miller, S. A. Protein metabolism during growth and development, in *Mammalian Protein Metabolism* (ed. H. N. Munro), vol. 3. Academic Press, New York, 1969, pp. 183–233.
44. Stephen, J. K. et al. Relationship of growth hormone to the growth retardation associated with maternal dietary restriction. *J. Nutr. 101:* 1453–1458, 1971.
45. Zeman, F. J., Shrader, R. E., and Allen, L. H. Persistent effects of maternal protein deficiency in post-natal rats. *Nutr. Rep. Int. 7:* 421–436, 1973.
46. Adlard, B. P. F. and Smart, J. L. Adrenocortical function in rats subjected to nutritional deprivation in early life. *J. Endocrinol. 54:* 99–105, 1972.
47. Tigner, J. C. and Barnes, R. H. Effect of postnatal malnutrition on plasma corticosteroid levels in male albino rats. *Proc. Soc. Exp. Biol. Med. 149:* 80–82, 1975.
48. Zamenhof, S., van Marthens, E., and Grauel, L. Prenatal nutritional factors affecting brain development. *Nutr. Rep. Int. 7:* 371–382, 1973.
49. Mulinos, M. G. and Pomeranz, L. Pseudohypophysectomy: A condition resembling hypophysectomy produced by malnutrition. *J. Nutr. 19:* 493–501, 1940.
50. Hansen, J. D. L. Endocrines and malnutrition, in *Protein-Calorie Malnutrition* (ed. R. E. Olson). Academic Press, New York, 1975, pp. 229–241.
51. Stein, Z., Susser, M., Saenger, G., and Marolla, F. Conclusions, *in Famine and Human Development.* Oxford University Press, London, 1975, pp. 229–236.
52. Srebnik, H. H. FSH and ICSH in pituitary and plasma of castrate protein-deficient rats. *Biol. Reprod. 3:* 96–104, 1970.
53. Turner, M. R. Dietary effects on the secretion and actions of growth hormone. *Proc. Nutr. Soc. 31:* 205–212, 1972.
54. Milner, R. D. G. and Wright, A. D. Plasma glucose, non-esterified fatty acid, insulin and growth hormone response to glucagon in the newborn. *Clin. Sci. 32:* 249–259, 1967.
55. Pimstone, B. Concluding remarks, *in Endocrine Aspects of Malnutrition,* Kroc Foundation Symposia Number 1 (ed. L. I. Gardner and

P. Amacher). The Kroc Foundation, Santa Ynez, Calif., 1973, pp. 487–492.

56. Góth, A., Lengyel, L., Bencze, E., Sávely, C., and Majsay, A. The role of amino acids in inducing hormone secretion. *Experientia 11:* 27–29, 1955.

57. Pimstone, B. L. et al. Growth hormone and protein-calorie malnutrition. Impaired suppression during induced hyperglycaemia. *Lancet 2:* 1333–1334, 1967.

58. Pimstone, B. L. et al. Studies on growth hormone secretion in protein-calorie malnutrition. *Am. J. Clin. Nutr. 21:* 482–487, 1968.

59. Pimstone et al., Growth hormone and kwashiorkor. *Lancet 2:* 779–780, 1966.

60. Mönckeberg, F. Adaptation to calorie and protein restriction in infants, *in Calorie Deficiencies and Protein Deficiencies* (ed. R. A. McCance and E. M. Widdowson). Churchill, London, 1968, pp. 91–106.

61. Mönckeberg, F. et al. Human growth hormone in infant malnutrition. *Pediatrics 31:* 58–64, 1963.

62. Beas, F., Muzzo, S. Growth hormone and malnutrition: the Chilean experience, *in Endocrine Aspects of Malnutrition* (ed. L. I. Gardner and P. Amacher). Kroc Foundation, Santa Ynez, Calif. 1973, pp. 1–18.

63. Godard, C. Plasma growth hormone levels in severe infantile malnutrition in Bolivia, *in Endocrine Aspects of Malnutrition.* (ed. L. I. Gardner and P. Amacher). Kroc Foundation, Santa Ynez, Calif., 1973, pp. 19–30.

64. Raghuramulu, N. and Rao, K. S. J. Growth hormone secretion in protein-calorie malnutrition. *J. Clin. Endocrinol. Metab. 38:* 176–180, 1974.

65. Rao, K. S. J. and Raghuramulu, N. Growth hormone and insulin secretion in protein-calorie malnutrition, as seen in India, *in Endocrine Aspects of Malnutrition* (ed. L. I. Gardner and P. Amacher). Kroc Foundation, Santa Ynez, Calif., 1973, pp. 91–98.

66. Parra, A. et al. Insulin-growth hormone adaptations in marasmus and kwashiorkor as seen in Mexico, *in Endocrine Aspects of Malnutrition* (ed. L. E. Gardner and P. Amacher). Kroc Foundation, Santa Ynez, Calif., 1973, pp. 31–43.

67. Suskind, R. et al. Interrelationships between growth hormone and amino acid metabolism in protein-calorie malnutrition, *in Endocrine Aspects of Malnutrition* (ed. L. I. Gardner and P. Amacher). Kroc Foundation, Santa Ynez, Calif., 1973, pp. 99–113.

68. Samuel, A. M. and Deshpande, U. R. Growth hormone levels in protein-calorie malnutrition. *J. Clin. Endocrinol. Metab. 35:* 863–867, 1972.

69. Smith, S. R., Edgar, P. J., Pozefsky, T., Chhetro, M. K., and Prout, T. E. Growth hormone in adults with protein-calorie malnutrition. *J. Clin. Endocrinol. Metab. 39:* 53–62, 1974.

70. Alvarez, L. C., Dimas, C. O., Castro, A., Rossman, L. G., Varderlaan, E. F., and Vanderlaan, W. P. Growth hormone in malnutrition. *J. Clin. Endocrinol. Metab. 34:* 400–409, 1972.

71. Marks, V., Howorth, N., Greenwood, F. Plasma growth-hormone levels in chronic starvation in man. *Nature 208:* 686–687, 1965.

72. Schwarz, F., van Riet, H. G., and Schopman, W. Serum growth hormone and energy supply in fasting obese patients. *Metabolism 15:* 194–205, 1966.

73. Beck, J. et al. Studies of insulin and growth hormone secretion in human obesity. *J. Lab. Clin. Med. 64:* 654–663, 1964.

74. Van Wyk, J. J. et al. The somatomedins: A family of insulin-like hormones under growth hormone control. *Recent Prog. Horm. Res. 30:* 259–295, 1974.

75. Srebnik, H. H. and Nelson, M. M. Anterior pituitary function in male rats deprived of dietary protein. *Endocrinology 70:* 723–730, 1962.

76. Turner, M. R., Allen, K. A., and Munday, K. A. Effects of age and diet on the secretion of insulin and growth hormone in rabbits. *Proc. Nutr. Soc. (Engl. Scot.) 33:* 56A, 1974.

77. Turner, M. R., Reeds, P., Munday, K. A. Action of growth hormone on protein synthesis in vitro in muscle from nonhypophysectomized rabbits fed protein-deficient diets. *Br. J. Nutr.* (in press).

78. Hadden, D. R. and Rutishauser, I. H. E. Effect of human growth hormone in kwashiorkor and marasmus. *Arch. Dis. Child. 42:* 29–39, 1967.

79. Milner, R. D. G. Malnutrition and the endocrine system in man. *Mem. Soc. Endocrinol. 18:* 191–210, 1970.

80. Bowie, M. D. Intravenous glucose tolerance in kwashiorkor and marasmus. *S. Afr. Med. J. 38:* 328–329, 1964.

81. Hadden, D. R. Glucose, free fatty acid, and insulin interrelations in kwashiorkor and marasmus. *Lancet 2:* 589–593, 1967.

82. Prinsloo, J. G., deBruin, J. P., and Kruger, H. Comparison on intravenous glucose tolerance tests and serum insulin levels in kwashiorkor and pellagra. *Arch. Dis. Child. 46:* 795–805, 1971.

83. Oxman, S., et al. Disturbances of carbohydrate metabolism in infantile marasmus. *Am. J. Clin. Nutr. 21:* 1285–1290, 1968.

84. Baig, H. A. and Edozien, J. C. Carbohydrate metabolism in kwashiorkor. *Lancet 2:* 662–665, 1965.

85. Milner, R. D. G. Metabolic and hormonal responses to oral amino acids in infantile malnutrition. *Arch. Dis. Child. 46:* 301–305, 1971.

86. Becker, D. J. et al. Insulin secretion in protein-calorie malnutrition. *Diabetes 20:* 542–551, 1971.

87. Milner, R. D. G. Metabolic and hormonal responses to glucose and glucagon in patients with infantile malnutrition. *Pediatr. Res. 5:* 33–39, 1971.

88. Milner, R. D. G. Endocrine adaptation to malnutrition. *Nutr. Rev. 30:* 103–106, 1972.

89. James, W. P. T. and Coores, H. G. Persistent impairment of insulin secretion and glucose tolerance after malnutrition. *Am. J. Clin. Nutr. 23:* 386–389, 1970.

90. Heard, C. R. C. and Turner, M. R. Glucose tolerance and related factors in dogs fed diets of suboptimal protein value. *Diabetes 16:* 96–107, 1967.

91. Anthony, L. E. and Faloona, G. R. Plasma insulin and glucagon levels in protein-malnourished rats. *Metabolism 23:* 303–306, 1974.

92. Munday, K. A. and Turner, M. R. Effect of protein deficiency on glucagon-stimulated insulin secretion, and on glycogen storage and release in rabbits. *Proc. Nutr. Soc 34:* 96A, 1975.

93. Allen, K. A., Munday, K. A. and Turner, M. R. Effects of age and postnatal diet on the protein synthetic actions of insulin and growth hormone. *Proc. Nutr. Soc. 33:* 113A, 1974.

94. Castellanos, H. and Arroyave, G. Role of the adrenocortical system in the response of children to severe protein malnutrition. *Am. J. Clin. Nutr. 9:* 186–195, 1961.

95. Alleyne, G. A. O. and Young, V. H. Adrenocortical function in children with severe protein-calorie malnutrition. *Clin. Sci. 33:* 189–200, 1967.

96. Prinsloo, J. G. et al. Integrity of the hypothalamo-pituitary-adrenal axis in kwashiorkor as tested with piromen. *S. Afr. Med. J. 48:* 2303–2305, 1974.

97. Brun, T. A. Hormonal disturbances and liver dysfunction in infantile malnutrition. Ph.D. thesis, University of California, Berkeley.

98. Rao, K. S. J., Sikantia, S. G. and Gopalan, C. Plasma cortisol levels in protein-calorie malnutrition. *Arch Dis. Child. 43:* 365–367, 1968.

99. Schonland, M. M., Shanley, B. C., Loening, W. E. K., Parent, M. A., and Coovadia, H. M. Plasma-cortisol and immunosuppression in protein-calorie malnutrition. *Lancet 2:* 435–436, 1972.

100. Abassy, A. S., Mikhail, M., Zeitoun, M. H., and Ragab, M. The suprarenal cortical function as measured by the plasma 17-hydroxycorticosteroid level in malnourished children. *J. Trop. Pediatr. 13:* 87–90 and 155–163, 1967.

101. Paisey, R. B., Angers, M., and Frenk, S. Plasma cortisol level in malnourished children with and without superimposed stress. *Arch. Dis. Child. 48:* 714–724, 1973.

102. Leonard, P. J. and MacWilliam, K. M. Cortisol binding in the serum in kwashiorkor. *J. Endocrinol. 29:* 273–276, 1964.

103. Leonard, P. J. Cortisol-binding in serum in kwashiorkor: East African studies, *in Endocrine Aspects of Malnutrition* (ed. L. I. Gardner and P. Amacher). Kroc Foundations, Santa Ynez, Calif., 1973, pp. 1–18.

104. Migeon, C. J. et al. Plasma aldosterone concentration and aldosterone secretion rate in Peruvian infants with marasmus and kwashiorkor, *in Endocrine Aspects of Malnutrition* (ed. L. I. Gardner and P. Amacher). Kroc Foundation, Santa Ynez, Calif., 1973, pp. 399–424.

105. Beitens, I. Z. et al. Adrenal function in normal infants and in marasmus and kwashiorkor: Plasma aldosterone concentration and aldosterone secretion rate. *J. Pediatr. 84:* 444–451, 1974.

106. Leonard, P. J. and MacWilliam, K. M. The binding of aldosterone in the serum in kwashiorkor. *Am. J. Clin. Nutr. 16:* 360–362, 1965.

107. Limson, M. and Jackson, C. M. Changes in the weights of various organs and systems of young rats maintained on a low-protein diet. *J. Nutr., 5:* 163–174, 1932.

108. Guggenheim, K. and Hegsted, D. M. Effect of desoxycorticosterone and posterior pituitary hormone on water and electrolyte metabolism in protein deficiency. *Am. J. Physiol. 172:* 23–28, 1953.

109. Leathem, J. H. Hormones in growth and development. *Recent Prog. Horm. Res. 14:* 141–176, 1958.
110. Munro, H. N., Hutchison, W. C., Ramaiah, T. R., and Neilson, F. J. The influence of diet on the weight and chemical constituents of the rat adrenal gland. *Br. J. Nutr. 16:* 387–395, 1962.
111. Ingle, D. W., Prestrud, M. C., Li, C. H., and Evans, H. M. The relationship of diet to the effect of adrenocorticotrophic hormone upon urinary nitrogen, glucose and electrolytes. *Endocrinology 41:* 170–176, 1947.
112. Moya, F., Prado, J. L., Rodriquez, R., Savard, K., and Selye, H. Effect of the dietary protein concentration upon the secretion of adrenocorticotrophin. *Endocrinology 42:* 223–229, 1948.
113. Handler, P. and Bernheim, F. Physiological basis for effects of low-protein diets on blood pressure of subtotally nephrectomized rats. *Am. J. Physiol. 162:* 368–374, 1950.
114. Selye, H. *The Physiological Pathology of Exposure to Stress.* Acta Inc., Montreal, 1950, p. 324.
115. Trowell, H. C., Davies, J. N. P., and Dean, R. F. A. *Kwashiorkor.* Arnold, London, 1954.
116. Gillman, J. & Gillman, T. *Perspectives in Human Malnutrition.* Grune & Stratton, New York, 1951, p. 584.
117. McCann, V. J. and Fulton, T. T. Cortisol metabolism in chronic liver disease. *J. Clin. Endocrinol. Metab. 40:* 1038–1044, 1975.
118. Goodlad, G. A. J. and Munro, H. N. Diet and the action of cortisone on protein metabolism. *Biochem. J. 73:* 343–348, 1959.
119. Clark, C. M., Naismith, D. J., and Munro, H. N. The influence of dietary protein on the incorporation of ^{14}C-glycine and ^{32}P into the ribonucleic acid of rat liver. *Biochim. Biophys. Acta 23:* 587–596, 1957.
120. Munro, H. N. and Mukerji, D. Ribonucleic acid metabolism in the liver after administration of individual amino acids. *Biochem. J. 69:* 321–326, 1958.
121. Munro, H. N., Steele, M. H. and Hutchison, W. C. Blood corticosterone-levels in the rat after administration of amino acids. *Nature 199:* 1182–1183, 1963.
122. Munro, H. N. and Mukerji, D. The mechanism by which administration of individual amino acids causes changes in the ribonucleic acid metabolism of the liver. *Biochem. J. 82:* 520–522, 1962.
123. Góth, A., Nadásdi, N., and Stadler, E. The effect of amino acids on pituitary-adrenal activity. *Vitam. Horm. Fermentforsch. 9:* 184–195, 1958.
124. Edwardson, J. A., Bennett, G. W., and Bradford, H. F. Release of amino acids and neurosecretory substances after stimulation of nerve-endings (synaptosomes) isolated from the hypothalamus. *Nature 240:* 554–556, 1972.
125. Edwardson, J. A. and Bennett, G. W. Modulation of corticotrophin-releasing factor from hypothalamic synaptosomes. *Nature 251:* 425–427, 1974.
126. Benedict, F. G. and Talbot, F. B. The gaseous metabolism of infants with special reference to its relationship to pulse rate and muscular activity. Publs. Carnegie Inst., No. 201, 1914.
127. Benedict, F. G. and Talbot, F. B. The physiology of the new-born infant. Character and amount of the catabolism, Publs. Carnegie Inst., No. 233, 1915.
128. Montgomery, R. D. Changes in the basal metabolic rate of the malnourished infant and their relation to body composition. *J. Clin. Invest. 41:* 1653–1663, 1962.
129. Beas, F., Mönckeberg, F., and Horwitz, I. The response of the thyroid gland to thyroid-stimulating hormone (TSH) in infants with malnutrition. *Pediatrics 38:* 1003–1008, 1966.
130. Parra, A. et al. Thyroid hormones and energy metabolism in marasmus and kwashiorkor as seen in Mexico, *in Endocrine Aspects of Malnutrition,* vol. 1. (ed. L. I. Gardner, and P. Amacher). Kroc Foundation, Santa Ynez, Calif., 1973, pp. 229–242.
131. Mönckeberg, F., Beas, F., Horwitz, I., Dabancens, A., and Gonzalez, M. Oxygen consumption in infant malnurition. *Pediatrics 33:* 554–561, 1964.
132. Varga, F. The respective effects of starvation and changed body composition on energy metabolism in malnourished infants. *Pediatrics 23:* 1085–1090, 1959.
133. Zubiran, S. and Gomez, F. Endocrine disturbances in chronic human malnutrition. *Vitam. Horm. 11:* 97–132, 1953.
134. Mönckeberg, F. et al. Captación de yodo radioactivo por el tiroides en el lactante desnutrido. *Rev. Chil. Pediatr. 28:* 173–175, 1957.
135. Szerdahelyi, F., Kertesz, L., and Peter, F. Untersuchungen über den Jod-Stoffwechsel atrophischer Säuglinge. *Mschr. Kinderheilk. 111:* 12–14, 1963.
136. Gomez, F., Ramos-Galvan, R., and Cravioto, G. Determinición de yodo unido a la proteina en niños desnutridos y durante su recuperación. *Rev. Mex. Pediatr. 24:* 94–99, 1955.
137. Valledor, Y. et al. Thyroid function disturbances in malnourished infants and small children. *Rev. Cuba Pediatr. 31:* 533–540, 1959.
138. Lifshitz, F., et al. Yodo hormonal en la desnutrición avanzada del niño. *Bol. Hosp. Inf. Mex. 19:* 319–326, 1962.
139. Beas, F., Mönckeberg, F., and Horwitz, I. The response of the thyroid gland to thyroid-stimulating hormone (TSH) in infants with malnutrition. *Pediatrics 38:* 1003–1008, 1966.
140. Graham, G. G. and Blizzard, R. M. Thyroid hormonal studies in severely malnourished Peruvian infants and small children, *in Endocrine Aspects of Malnutrition,* vol. 1 (ed. L. I. Gardner and P. Amacher) Kroc Foundation, Santa, Ynez, Calif., 1973, pp. 205–219.
141. Varga, F., Mess, B. Serum thyrotrophin in semistarvation. *Acta Paediatr. Hungar. 9:* 197–203, 1968.
142. Godard, C. Plasma growth hormone levels in severe infantile malnutrition in Bolivia, *in Endocrine Aspects of Malnutrition,* vol. 1 (ed. L. I. Gardner and P. Amacher). Kroc Foundation, Santa Ynez, Calif., 1973, pp. 19–30.
143. Godard, C. and Lemarchand-Beraud. Plasma thyrotropin levels in severe infantile malnutrition. *Horm. Res. 4:* 43–52, 1973.
144. Pimstone, B. L., Becker, D. J., and Hendricks, S. TSH response to synthetic thyrotropin releasing hormone in human PCM. *J. Clin. Endocrinol. Metab. 36:* 779–783, 1973.
145. Harland, P. S. E. G. and Parkin, J. M. TSH levels in severe malnutrition. *Lancet 2:* 1145, 1972.
146. Lundberg, P. O. et al. Effects of thyrotrophin-releasing hormone on plasma levels of TSH, FSH, LH and GH in anorexia nervosa. *Eur. J. Clin. Invest. 2:* 150–153, 1972.
147. Rastogi, G. K., Sawhney, R. C., Panda, N. C., and Tripathy, B. B. Thyroid hormone levels in adult protein calorie malnutrition (PCM). *Horm. Metab. Res. 6:* 528–529, 1974.
148. Ingenbleek, Y. and Beckers, C. Triiodothyronine and thyroid-stimulating hormone in protein-calorie malnutrition in infants. *Lancet 2:* 845–848, 1975.
149. Portnay, G. I., O'Brian, J. T., Bush, J., Vagenakis, A. G., Azizi, F., Arky, R. A., Ingbar, S. H., and Braverman, L. E. The effect of starvation on the concentration and binding of thyroxine and triiodothyrine in serum and on the response to TRH. *J. Clin. Endocrinol. Metab. 39:* 191–194, 1974.
150. Vagenakis, A. G., Burger, A., Portnay, G. I., Rudolph, M., O'Brian, J. T., Azizi, F., Arky, R. A., Nicod, P., Ingbar, S. H., and Braverman, L. E. Diversion of peripheral thyroxine metabolism from activating to inactivating pathways during complete fasting. *J. Clin. Endocrinol. Metab. 41:* 191–193, 1975.
151. Carter, W. J., Shakir, K. M., Hodges, S., Faas, F. H., and Wynn, J. O. Effect of thyroid hormone on metabolic adaptation to fasting. *Metabolism 24:* 1177–1183, 1975.
152. Worthington, B. S. and Enwonwu, C. O. Functional variations in the ultrastructure of the thyroid gland in malnourished infant monkeys. *Am. J. Clin. Nutr. 28:* 66–78, 1975.
153. Stirling, G. A. The thyroid in malnutrition. *Arch. Dis. Child. 37:* 99–102, 1962.
154. Hansen, J. D. L. et al. What does nutritional growth retardation imply? *Pediatrics 47:* 299–313, 1971.
155. Alvarada, G. Cited by Milner (88).
156. Moskowitz, M. A. and Wurtman, R. J. Catecholamines and neurologic diseases. *N. Engl. J. Med. 293:* 274–280, 1975.
157. Bourgeois, B., Schmidt, B. J., and Bourgeois, R. Some aspects of catecholamines in undernutrition, *in Endocrine Aspects of Malnutrition,* vol. 1 (ed. L. I. Gardner and P. Amacher). Kroc Foundation, Santa Ynez, Calif., 1973, pp. 163–173.
158. Parra, A. et al. Studies of daily urinary catecholamine excretion in kwashiorkor as observed in Mexico, *in Endocrine Aspects of Malnutrition,* vol. 1 (ed. L. I. Gardner and P. Amacher). Kroc Foundation, Santa Ynez, Calif., 1973, pp. 181–190.
159. Hoeldtke, R. D. and Wurtman, R. J. Excretion of catecholamines and catecholamine metabolites in kwashiorkor. *Am. J. Clin. Nutr. 26:* 205–210, 1973.
160. Shoemaker, W. J. and Wurtman, R. J. Perinatal undernutrition: accumulation of catecholamines in rat brain. *Science 171:* 1017–1019, 1971.
161. Nomura, M. et al. Excretion of 5-HIAA and HVA by humans and

rats in response to changes in dietary protein. *Proc. Soc. Neuroendocrinol.* (in press)

162. Fernstrom, J. D., Madras, B. K., Munro, H. N., and Wurtman, R. J. Nutritional control of the synthesis of 5-hydroxytryptamine in the brain, *in Aromatic Amino Acids in the Brain.* Ciba Foundation Symposium 22, Elsevier, New York, 1974, pp. 153–173.
163. Lytle, L. D., Messing, R. B., Fisher, L., and Phebus, L. Effects of chronic corn consumption on brain serotonin and the response to electric shock. *Science 140:* 692–694, 1975.
164. Lipsett, D., Madras, B. K., Wurtman, R. J., and Munro, H. N. Serum tryptophan level after carbohydrate ingestion: Selective decline in non-albumin-bound tryptophan coincident with reduction in serum free fatty acids. *Life Sci. 12* (part II): 57–64, 1973.
165. Knott, P. J. and Curzon, G. The relationship between plasma free tryptophan and brain tryptophan metabolism. *Nature 239:* 452–453, 1972.
166. Curzon, G. and Knott, P. J. Fatty acids and the disposition of tryptophan, *in Aromatic Amino Acids in the Brain.* Ciba Foundation Symposium 22, Elsevier, Amsterdam, 1974, pp. 217–229.
167. Madras, B. K., Cohen, E. L., Messing, R., Munro, H. N., and Wurtman, R. J. Relevance of free tryptophan in serum to tissue tryptophan concentrations. *Metabolism 23:* 1107–1116, 1974.
168. Holt, L. E. and Snyderman, S. E. Anomalies of amino acid metabolism, *in Mammalian Protein Metabolism,* vol. 2 (ed. H. N. Munro and J. B. Allison). Academic Press, New York, 1964, pp. 321–372.
169. Srikantia, S. G. and Mohanram, M. Antidiuretic hormone values in plasma and urine of malnourished children. *J. Clin. Endocrinol. Metab. 31:* 312, 1970.
170. Leathem, J. H. Some aspects of hormone and protein metabolic interrelationships, in *Mammalian Protein Metabolism,* vol. 1 (ed. H. N. Munro and J. B. Allison). Academic Press, New York, 1964, pp. 343–380.

151

Senescence

Samuel Goldstein

HORMONES AND AGING

The idea that endocrine failure causes aging is logical on *a priori* grounds because of the pervasive influence of hormones on homeostatic adaptation. In reality, this concept has long been entertained but repeated claims of rejuvenation following spurious maneuvers such as gonadal transplantation served to impede the progress of both aging and endocrinology as legitimate sciences. At this juncture, it is safe to say that no definite evidence exists to prove causality. What clearly emerges though, is a changing profile of each hormone system along an uneven front.

Certain conceptual nuances must be appreciated at the outset. In the usual approach, hormonal responses are followed over minutes, hours, and weeks. Although in exploring senescent changes we are also concerned with the short range, greater emphasis is placed on trends over the years. Additionally, serious pitfalls may be encountered in measurement. The level of a hormone in bodily fluids and the consequences of its stimulus represent the summation of several physiologic processes. Each may change throughout life within limits determined by intrinsic genetic mechanisms on the one hand and environmental perturbations on the other. Therefore, great individual variation may occur. Moreover, body composition changes throughout life, not only in the relative proportions of total water and fractional spaces of extra- and intracellular water,[1] but also with respect to the mass of secretory organs, proportion of hormone-producing cells, rates of secretion, hormone distribution space, circulating binding proteins, tissue receptors, and hormone degradation and excretion. It must also be appreciated that illness, so common in the elderly, can affect many of these parameters. In short, there may be a multiplicity of factors altering the effective delivery of hormone to target tissue, so that it is often difficult to judge whether differences between young and elderly individuals are apparent or real (Fig. 151-1).

It must also be appreciated that new discoveries will require revision of our body knowledge. The radioimmunoassay is generally supplanting the bioassay by providing more specificity and accuracy in measurement. Other explosive advances are now occurring that increasingly link the central nervous system to more classically conceived endocrine organs. Eminent examples are connections that exist between "transducer" neurons and the hypothalamic releasing factors[2] so that electrical stimulation of discrete parts of the hypothalamus can increase the activity of specific releasing factors in pituitary-portal blood.[3] We can also implicate substances such as dopamine, present in hypothalamic neurons, in the release of various factors such as leuteinizing hormone releasing factor (LRF) and follicle stimulating hormone releasing factor (FRF); indeed, we have learned that LRF and FRF are probably the same molecule.[4] To develop a clear picture of neuroendocrine relationships over the human life span, it would be desirable to know the concentrations of releasing factors in both the hypothalamus and pituitary-portal blood. For obvious reasons, such data are currently unobtainable during life. Even procuring sufficient amounts of fresh postmortem material is difficult, quite apart from problems of cleanly dissecting each region of the hypothalamus. However, indirect information is now available by measuring responses following the administration of exogenous releasing factors. This situation, in total, makes tentative any current review on the relationship between neuroendocrine physiology and the aging process.

In the present analysis, human findings will receive paramount emphasis. When information is lacking, animal experiments will be introduced in full recognition of the potential pitfalls that exist in extrapolation to man. Each integrated hormone axis will be dealt with individually, insofar as current knowledge allows, in an attempt to encompass all levels of function from the central nervous system to the hypothalmus, the pituitary, the trophic organ, and down to the peripheral target cell(s). Other reviews have appeared covering general hormonal changes over the life span, primarily in experimental systems.[5,6] A similar review of human aging has recently been published.[7]

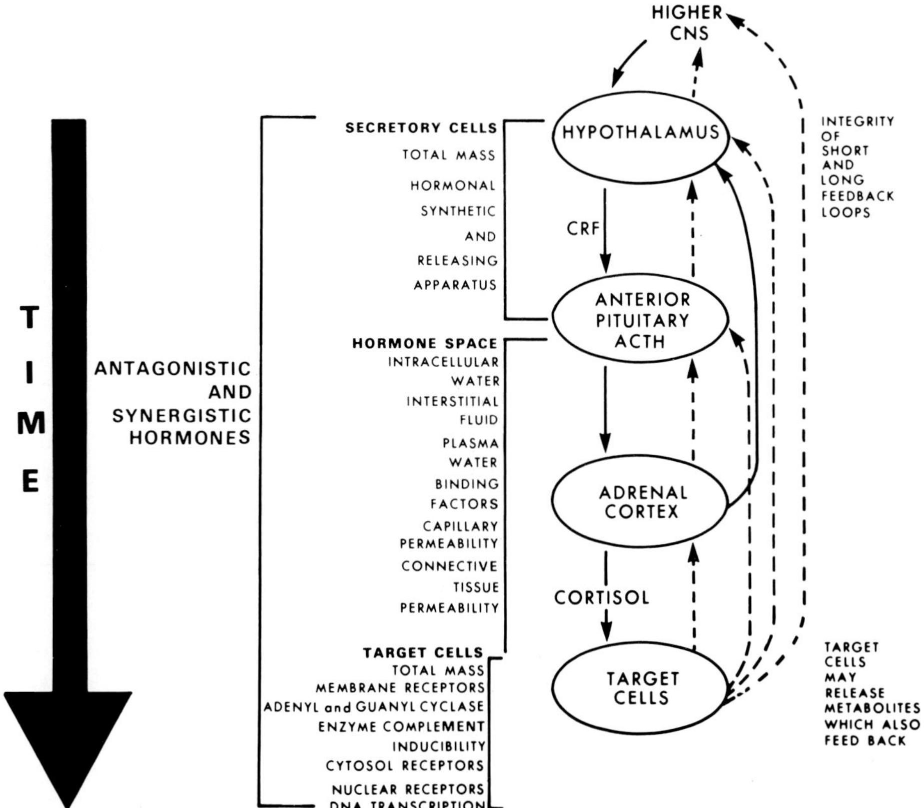

Fig. 151-1. Hierarchy between the nervous system and hormone-secreting glands, their feedback loops, and various physiologic, biochemical, and time-dependent factors that influence them, using the adrenal system as an example. ----, Possible feedback loops.

GONADAL AXIS

Females

Estrogen and Progesterone. The menopause represents the most discrete example of endocrine senescence.[8,9] Until recently, virtually all studies have been cross-sectional rather than the preferred but more difficult longitudinal surveys that follow the performance of given individuals during life. Nevertheless, they clearly demonstrate that the ovary is the primary site of failure. Both peripheral venous levels and urinary excretion of estrogen show a relatively precipitous decline around the menopause,[8,10] but after this time there is a further, more gradual drop in estrogen output due to continued ovarian failure.[11] Urinary excretion of pregnanediol, derived mainly from progesterone, also decreases markedly at the same time.[12] After age 60, excretion of biologically active estrogens remains about 20 percent of that prior to the menopause, which indicates that steroid precursors are converted peripherally to estrogenic substances. In fact, extraovarian estrone production via adrenal androstenedione increases progressively, so that elderly females, compared to young adults, show a 2–4-fold increase in this capability.[13]

Gonadotropins and Releasing Factors. With the menopausal decline in estrogen levels, negative feedback on the hypothalamic–pituitary axis is relaxed. This leads to marked increases of urinary gonadatropin output, which are maximal 15–19 years postmenopausally.[14] Early work was based on bioassays that measured the specific property of growth induction in gonads of immature or hypophysectemized rats. Utilizing this assay it appears that the pituitary content of follicle-stimulating hormone (FSH) and leuteinizing hormone (LH) remains constant well beyond the menopause.[14] Radioimmunoassays have now confirmed these earlier results and clearly demonstrate increased serum levels of FSH and LH in postmenopausal females.[15] Both hormones usually rise in parallel, although in some perimenopausal females with short cycles and lower estradiol levels, dissociation can occur, with FSH rising first.[16] More recent longitudinal studies[17] have found elevated FSH and LH levels 5–10 years before the menopause in the face of normal levels of estrogen, which indicates a gradual and progressive rather than a precipitous ovarian follicular failure. With the total number of follicles decreased, it follows that the number of receptors, and perhaps their affinity for gonadotropins, also fall well in advance of the clinically overt menopause. Thus, more FSH is needed to stimulate fewer follicles and produce a normal estrogen output.

Paradoxically, levels of LRF in postmenopausal females show a negative correlation with those of LH,[18] possibly due to short-loop feedback control of LRF secretion via plasma LH. Alternatively, LRF secretion may be independent of LH levels, but peaks of LH secretion could be a consequence of bursts of LRF secretion with the two peaks out of phase. A final possibility is that individual women may vary in pituitary sensitivity to LRF, the most sensitive having higher LH and lower LRF levels that, in turn, are related to varying degrees of estrogen deficiency.

Males

Testosterone. In aging males, classical studies demonstrate a decline both in plasma levels and urinary excretion of total urinary 17-ketosteroids.[9,19] When these findings are linked to the decreased testosterone levels found in spermatic vein blood[20] and are considered in conjunction with many reports of decreased free testosterone levels in peripheral plasma,[21,22] it seems clear that the age-dependent loss of testicular steroid output is predominantly due to gradual Leydig cell failure. The decreased plasma levels of free testosterone are partly determined by an increased binding capacity of the specific plasma-binding protein[23] that occurs despite a fall in the metabolic clearance rate for testosterone. In any case, the decreasing free testosterone fraction makes extrahepatic metabolism of this hormone less important.

Gonadotropins and Releasing Factors. Elevated gonadotropin levels are found in males over 45 years of age, but elevations are of a smaller magnitude and show a larger statistical variance than in menopausal females[14,21,22] (Fig. 151-2). Additionally, FSH and LH levels rise higher in the serum of elderly, compared to younger males following stimulation by intravenously administered LRF; this indicates that the reserve of the aging pituitary is in fact augmented.[21] However, there are also increased estrogen levels in aging men that, as in females, are due primarily to increasing conversion of androstenedione to estrone.[13] This may account for the fact that male gonadotropin levels increase to a lesser degree than expected from the decreasing testosterone levels; estrogens are more potent suppressors of pituitary gonadotropin secretion than testosterone.[24] Rising estrogen levels may also account for the increased amount of testosterone binding globulin in the elderly male.

In rats, the pituitary responsiveness to LRF is maximal in early life, in part related to the glandular content of LH and FSH.[25] Serum levels of these gonodotropins run parallel to pituitary content and, although no decline is seen after maturity, the larger variance in mean LH concentration observed in older animals after administration of LRF indicates individual differences in sensitivity. However, in vitro studies on LRF stimulation of rat pituitaries indicate that glandular content of LH is not the only factor that determines the quantity of hormone released.[26] Different patterns of release are observed around the time of puberty for female compared to male pituitaries even though no sex differences are found in hormone content of the gland. Thus, it appears that regulation occurs more distally, at the receptor or the coupled enzymatic machinery. This may help to explain the different mechanisms that determine the onset of puberty in the two sexes, as well as sex differences occurring during adulthood and senescence. However, other factors are undoubtedly involved. Atherosclerosis, so common in and beyond the fifth decade in both sexes, may play a role in some individuals by decreasing the gonadal blood supply. Nevertheless, it seems unlikely that ischemia is a universal cause, at least with respect to ovarian failure, for this is the most discrete of all endocrine involutionary processes. Furthermore, the absence of an abrupt climacteric in males in the face of actuarial evidence that females live longer than males, points to the further unlikelihood that failure of gonadal secretion causes aging of the whole organism.

THYROID AXIS

Some of the difficulty in interpreting thyroid physiology relates to our incomplete understanding of the exact role of thyroxine (T_4) and triiodothyronine (T_3). Basal levels of circulating T_3 decrease by almost one-half in healthy elderly persons,[27–29] although T_4 levels do not change, whether measured as protein-bound iodine or directly as free or protein-bound T_4.[27,28,30] The rate of T_4 turnover decreases by about one-half during adulthood, probably related to a gradual slowing in cellular degradation.[31] Concomitantly, the thyroid gland shows a progressive cellular infiltration and fibrotic replacement as well as decreased follicular size and a corresponding loss of stainable colloid.[32] Functionally, the gland has a decreased radioiodide uptake, but the variance increases significantly, probably due to frequently impaired renal function in the elderly, which slows the rate of iodide excretion. On the average, circulating thyroid-binding globulins rise slightly[33] despite the drop found in some subjects. There is clearly an age-associated fall in serum albumin. Although albumin may not be a significant vehicle for T_4 relative to the specific binding globulin, the decrease in both kinds of serum protein suggests that hepatic synthesis is impaired.[34]

Baseline levels of thyrotropin (TSH) do not change with age in either sex.[27,28,30] Following intramuscular injection of thyrotropin releasing hormone (TRH), elderly women achieve the same elevations of serum TSH as young women, although in contrast, males have an age-dependent reduction in peak values.[30] In one series, when elderly males were carefully matched with young subjects for height, weight, serum T_4, and free T_4 index,[27,28] peak TSH levels following injection of TRH declined from a mean of 14.3 to 6.1 μU/ml (Fig. 151-3). It is of interest that peak increments in serum T_4 following TRH administration show no sex or age dependency at a time when peak T_3 is significantly reduced with age in both sexes.[30] In total, these results suggest that aging, particularly in males, blunts the response at multiple sites in the chain of events from the pituitary receptor for TRH to the turnover of T_3. However, if hypofunction of the thyroid occurs with aging, one might expect to find elevations of TSH in analogy with the gonadal axis. There is little support for this view apart from one study[35] which

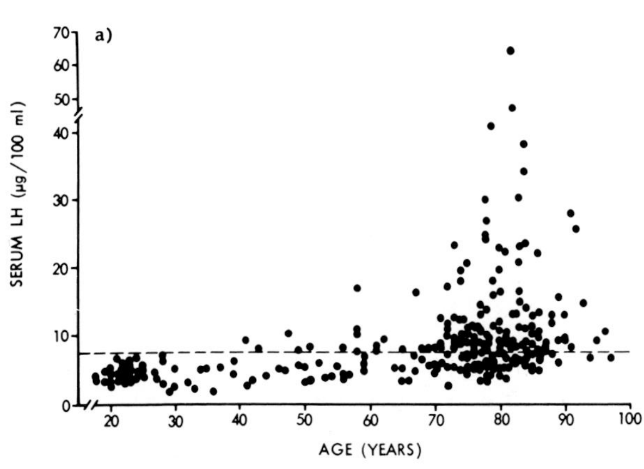

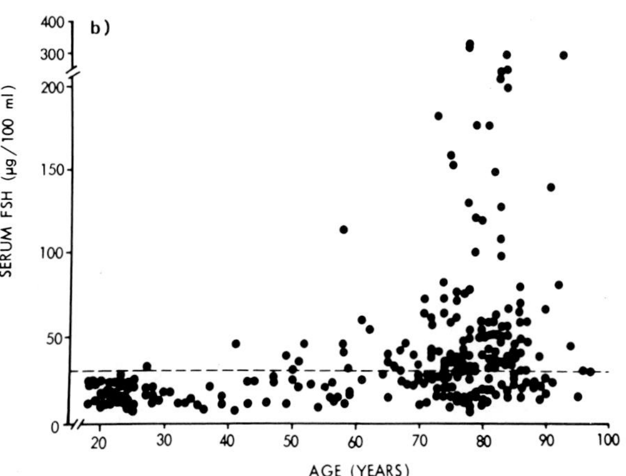

Fig. 151-2. Serum gonadotropin levels in men 18–97 years of age. a. LH. b. FSH.---, Upper limit of normal for men less than 45 years of age. (From Stearns et al.: Am. J. Med. *57:* 761, 1974.)

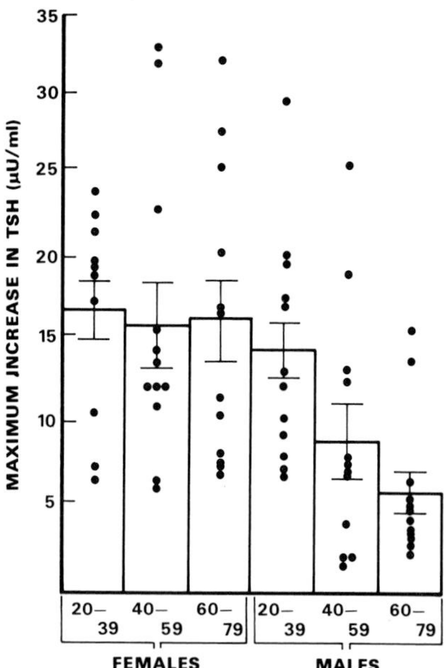

Fig. 151-3. Peak TSH levels as a function of age in males and females following iv administration of TRH. Vertical bars and brackets are the mean ± SEM. (Adapted from Snyder and Utiger: J. Clin. Endocrinol. *34:* 380, 1096, 1972.)

found that basal values of TSH defined a parabolic distribution, being highest in the early and later decades of life. In any event, it appears that TSH secretory capacity, like that of the gonadotropins is fully preserved in man and lower forms into advanced old age.[36]

Any consideration of thyroid function must include the basal metabolic rate (BMR) and oxygen consumption because of the close linkage between these parameters. It has been asserted that BMR decreases with age, but this decline may not be as dramatic as once believed. First, the apparent decline virtually disappears when expressed on the basis of remaining body water or creatinine excretion (Fig. 151-4). This is due to the progressive replacement of muscle mass with adipose tissue even in elderly persons who maintain ideal body weight; adipose tissue has a low water content and, compared to muscle, is relatively inert metabolically.[37] Second, recent more informative longitudinal surveys have found that reduction in BMR is much less marked even before provision is made for the adipose weight gain, being about 1–2 percent per decade of age in men 20–75 years old.[38]

Still to be elucidated vis-à-vis thyroid function and aging is the role of peripheral tissues and their component parts. For example, it was recently shown in isolated hepatic nuclei of hypothyroid rats (and in contrast to steroid hormones[39]) that T_3 acts directly in the nucleus independent of a specific cytosol protein.[40] Since liver is the major site of T_3 and T_4 turnover, studies are needed to clarify the total number of binding sites and their relative affinity to each hormone during aging. Furthermore, a significant proportion of circulating T_3 emanates from T_4 rather than from direct thyroidal secretion. Thus, it is likely that the decline in T_3 levels in the elderly is primarily a consequence of decreased peripheral conversion of T_4. However, the apparent diminished requirement for T_4 replacement therapy that occurs in aging man,[37] and the findings of increased sensitivity to T_4 in aging female cats,[41] suggest that T_4 exerts a significant direct effect on target tissues independent of conversion to T_3. Nevertheless, on the basis of preliminary evidence, T_3 seems to be more important than T_4 in the modulation of TSH secretion, probably related to the higher affinity of specific pituitary receptors for T_3.[42]

ADRENOCORTICAL AXIS

Glucocorticoids

Total output of cortisol and its metabolites is clearly reduced during human aging, but when expressed as a function of creatinine clearance, quantitative differences between young and old disappear.[9,43] Additionally, the proportions of individual metabolites in relation to the total output may change somewhat during aging, so that elderly men excrete a larger proportion of 11-hydroxylated derivatives. Despite this overall decline in glucocorticoid output, plasma levels of cortisol remain unchanged into advanced old age,[12,44] although its half-life in the circulation changes significantly (Fig. 151-5). Removal of administered hormone is 50 percent slower for a group of subjects over 65 years of age compared to adults 21–55 years old. From this information, and the early morning resting levels of cortisol, it can be calculated that only 23.5 μg cortisol/kg/h are needed to maintain plasma levels in elderly individuals, in comparison to 43 μg/kg/h in the young. This demonstrates that the adrenals of elderly individuals are faced with decreased demand in maintaining the same circulating levels of cortisol, perhaps in part because older people have a cortisol

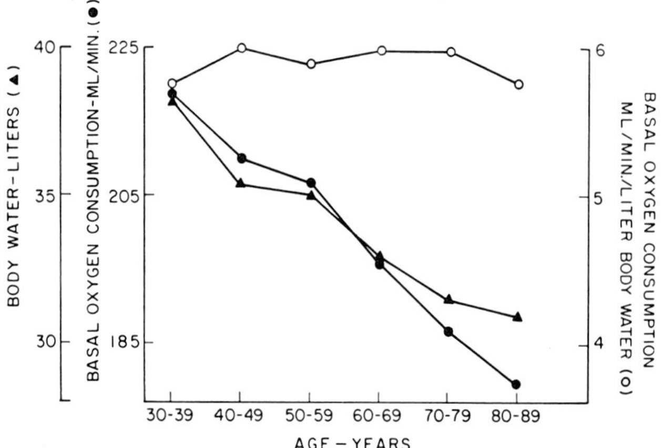

Fig. 151-4. Relationship of age to total body water (antipyrine space), basal oxygen consumption, and basal oxygen consumption per unit of body water. (From Gregerman, in Gitman (ed): Endocrines and Aging, 1967. Courtesy of Charles C. Thomas, Publishers.)

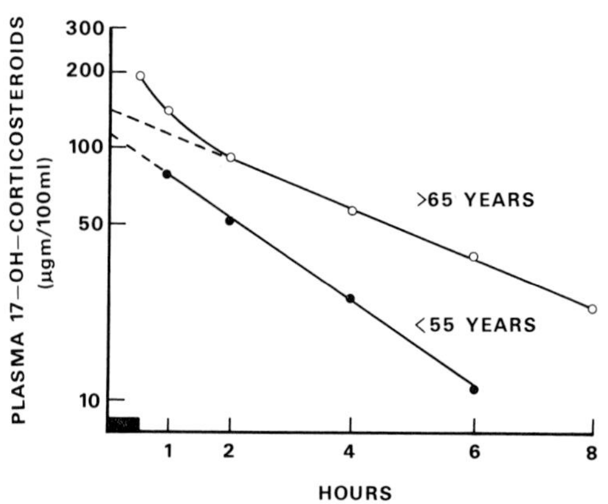

Fig. 151-5. Rate of disappearance of cortisol from the circulation after the infusion of 1 mg/kg body weight over a period of 30 min (■). ○, Normal subjects over 65 years old; •, normal subjects 21–55 years old. (Adapted from Samuels, in England, Pincus (eds): Hormones and the Aging Process, 1956. Courtesy of Academic Press.)

distribution volume that is 60 percent of the total mass, compared to 90 percent in young people. In addition, the infused cortisol takes about 90 min to equilibrate in tissues of the elderly, versus 30 min in younger subjects (Fig. 151-5). Taken together, the findings suggest that there is an increased amount and density of connective tissue and ground substance, a decreased functional mass of cells, and possibly diminished concentrations and affinities of steroid receptors.

Little information is available on changes in the levels of transcortin with age. Just as occurs with testosterone and thyroid-binding proteins, age-dependent changes in transcortin could influence the turnover of cortisol. We must also remember that each hormone may exert effects on other binding proteins, e.g., estrogen on thyroid- and testosterone-binding globulins.

Androgens

Urinary excretion of androgens decreases with advancing age in both males and females.[19] The major 17-ketosteroids in young adults, dehydroepiandrosterone and androsterone, drop about 50 percent, the former somewhat more severely.[12,19] However, the exact biologic significance of 17-ketosteroids is unknown, as is the precise contribution of the testes and ovaries to plasma levels and urinary output. Due to their profound influence on nitrogen metabolism, androgenic steroids could be critical determinants of bone, muscle, and organ mass generally, and, in turn, of glucocorticoid production. Whatever their role, it seems clear that adrenal androgens are more severely affected by age than are glucocorticoids.

ACTH

There is a tendency for the levels of serum ACTH to decrease in the elderly even though the metyrapone test indicates that no major limitation develops in hypothalamic–pituitary reserve.[46] Controversy exists regarding the glucocorticoid response to exogenous ACTH. In some studies,[45] but not in others,[44] elderly subjects have a decreased response, as reflected in plasma glucocorticoid levels. The apparent solution may be to correct for creatinine excretion, after which there appears to be little residual effect of age on ACTH-augmented plasma glucocorticoids or their total urinary excretion.[12] However, it has been suggested that this correction may not always be justified because of the poor correlation between the excretion of creatinine and glucocorticoids.[47] Moreover, since liver rather than muscle is the major site of steroid catabolism,[48] it is unlikely that a smaller muscle mass is the sole explanation for the fall in total glucocorticoid output during aging.

Following injection of ACTH, androgen responses are greatly suppressed in the elderly, compared to younger subjects. Although, in contrast to glucocorticoids, androgen output falls in parallel with creatinine excretion, it remains significantly decreased in the elderly even after correction.[47]

Formidable species differences also appear. At the extreme is the spawning Pacific salmon, in whom a huge outpouring of ACTH produces massive hypertrophy and exhaustion of the adrenal cortex, followed invariably by death.[49] In cattle,[50] the response to ACTH infusion is decreased, as it is in goats,[51] while an undiminished reserve potential is maintained in dogs.[52] If old rats are exposed to prolonged periods of adrenocortical stimulation, exhaustion cannot be produced.[53] In fact, when animals so treated are given an extra insult of ether-induced stress, the elderly animals respond better. This indicates that hypothalamic–pituitary mechanisms that respond to elevated blood corticoids following prolonged adrenocortical stimulation are set at a higher level with age.

RENIN–ANGIOTENSIN–ALDOSTERONE AXIS

Both baseline and stimulated renin levels decrease with each decade of adult life. Basal values at age 70 are 35 percent lower than at age 20,[54] and they are accompanied by a parallel drop in the plasma concentration, secretion rate, and metabolic clearance of aldosterone.[55] Decreased aldosterone output does not appear to be a consequence of altered sodium balance since in one series the dietary intake and the urinary excretion of sodium were at or below normal.[55] Moreover, the elderly group was as active physically as young subjects, making it unlikely that posture or activity were major factors. Nevertheless, it is possible that hormone secretion is decreased consequent to lowered sodium secretion, and hence, is secondary to reduced renal blood flow. Similarly, reduced aldosterone clearance could relate to impaired splanchnic circulation leading to reduced hormone extraction.

The age-dependent fall in renin activity and aldosterone excretion also occurs in patients with essential hypertension. However, in some cases[54] hypertension is nonexistent in the "low-renin" group, and, additionally, the low-renin group is older. Other studies give opposite results.[56] Thus, in normotensives, renin response does not decline with age, while some hypertensive subjects seem to have a normal or hyperresponsive renin system at the onset of the disease, followed later by a state of decreased renin responsiveness.

Many variables may contribute to this apparent controversy, especially patient selection and genetics. Thus, in certain rats that are predisposed to hypertension because of a genetically high output of mineralocorticoids, a correlation is found between steroid levels, an enlarged zona glomerulosa, and a low juxtaglomerular granularity, i.e., low renin output.[57] The same strain of rats can be bred to produce offspring with a low mineralocorticoid activity, a high juxtaglomerular index, and normotension. Still another genetic strain has been found with peculiar renal sodium and potassium handling in response to aldosterone that is related to poor hormone binding in the nucleus of renal tubular cells.[58] In sharp contrast, normal rats that are unselected genetically undergo a substantial reduction in the width of the zona glomerulosa with age. Moreover, this finding correlates with decreased juxtaglomerular cell granularity in the kidney as well as a diminution of neurosecretory material in the posterior pituitary.[59]

Although this situation points to complex heterogeneity in rats, by and large, the effects of inheritance and aging appear to be separable. Familial clustering of human hypertension is also well known, but in most cases specific molecular lesions have not yet been pinpointed. The same lack applies to human aging, in which information is still needed even relating plasma levels of hormones to morphology of the zona glomerulosa and juxtaglomerular apparatus. Furthermore, the exact role of excessive angiotensin generation (i.e., increased plasma renin activity) in various forms of renal and essential hypertension has still not been realized.[60] Two pressor mechanisms have now been invoked: vasoconstrictor hypertension associated with excess angiotensin in the face of high or normal renin; and volume (sodium) hypertension with low renin. The normal renin group may be a combination of high and low renin groups wherein arterial volume is inappropriate for vascular capacity.[60].

Scant information exists in elderly subjects regarding the pressor effect of angiotensin (as opposed to its stimulation of aldosterone secretion). One recent report clearly demonstrates that the peptide constricts the renal vasculature of old individuals just as well as that of the young, although a decreased vasodilator response to acetylcholine and a sodium load is demonstrable.[61]

More data are clearly needed in this important area. Since the problems of hypertension mainly become evident in middle age and beyond, standard values of plasma renin, angiotensin, and aldosterone will need to be carefully age controlled. As our general understanding of hypertension improves, we should be able to distinguish certain subgroups that are predisposed primarily through inheritance from others at risk mainly on the basis of age.

GROWTH HORMONE (GH)

Males

Basal GH levels do not change with advancing age in males, although there are diminished responses following arginine and insulin stimulation.[62] This is best explained by a concomitant increase in adiposity associated with age, and, in turn, with rising levels of fasting plasma glucose and the possibility of insulin resistance.[63] In fact, normal GH responses are seen in elderly persons during insulin-induced hypoglycemia if they are selected to have fasting euglycemia and a hypoglycemic response that is adequate to evoke GH secretion.[64,65] However, the peak of GH usually seen during sleep fails to appear in a majority of individuals over 50 years of age.[66] Under some circumstances, therefore, aging of human males is associated with a subtle rather than a generalized hyporesponsiveness of GH.

Females

Elderly females maintain higher basal levels of GH than males, just as occurs during youth. Unexpectedly, little difference is seen in mean GH values for pre- and postmenopausal women, although the mean serum phosphorus concentration is significantly higher after the menopause.[67] Since estrogens antagonize the end-organ response to GH it would be anticipated that GH levels would fall postmenopausally. Therefore, postmenopausal hyperphosphatemia may be due to a relative GH excess over estrogen. This analysis would apply only if the same end-organ responsiveness were preserved, but there is sketchy evidence that target sensitivity to GH may decrease in the elderly.[68]

Hypothalamic GH Factors

No age-related studies have yet been reported on hypothalamic releasing and inhibition factors for GH in man.[3,4] In senescent rats, the hypothalamus loses GH-releasing factor (GHRF) activity,[69] while their aging pituitaries respond poorly to hypothalamic extracts that possess potent GHRF activity in young animals. Regarding a causal relationship between GH and aging, some strains of dwarfed GH-deficient mice develop premature aging, but they apparently lack other pituitary factors as well.[70] Indeed, the life span of these mice can be extended about 50 percent by giving them daily injections of GH and T_4. It is probable that these hormones are only two factors among others that may be linked simultaneously to other defects, which, in total, produce premature aging.[71]

PARATHYROID HORMONE (PTH): INTERACTIONS WITH ESTROGEN

Serum PTH levels decrease with advancing age and, unexpectedly, no sex differences appear.[72] However, females with severe postmenopausal osteoporosis with compression fractures have mean PTH levels that are more than twofold higher than those of normal subjects of corresponding age. These studies clearly indicate that increased serum PTH levels are not a physiologic age-dependent process. They also suggest that rather than being a consequence of natural skeletal aging, osteoporosis affects a limited subgroup as a primary disturbance of calcium metabolism accompanied by increased serum PTH. Such information in conjuction with the knowledge that ovariectomy increases bone sensitivity to PTH,[73] provides ample reason for the debilitating osteoporosis in predisposed females. It must be emphasized that age-dependent skeletal changes are not simply the result of an altered balance between PTH and estrogen. Estrogen replacement therapy beginning at the time of menopause helps to improve bone density for 5–10 years, in comparison to no treatment, but the differences gradually diminish after 15 years and are no longer discernible by 20 years.[74]

THYROCALCITONIN (TCT)

Although the peripheral effect of TCT is greatly reduced during maturation of rats,[75] no TCT data are available in man, either for plasma levels or peripheral response. Aging humans seem to respond nicely to exogenous TCT, but the utility of the exogenous hormone in the treatment of osteoporosis is of dubious value.[76]

SYMPATHOADRENAL SYSTEM

It is still not possible to distinguish between catecholamines released from the adrenal medulla or from extramedullary sources, e.g., during neurotransmission; age changes could clearly have differential effects at each site. Total urinary excretion of epinephrine and norepinephrine appears to drop very slightly during human aging.[77] Following various challenges, there is a diminished catecholamine output in the elderly, perhaps reflecting a relative hypothalamic refractoriness.[78–80] However, recent work, using sensitive radioimmunoassays, indicates that there is an age-dependent increase in circulating norepinephrine that is particularly accentuated in the presence of hypothyroidism.[81]

Monoamine oxidase activity increases markedly with age in human brain, plasma, and circulating platelets.[82] Simultaneously, in the hindbrain 5-hydroxyindole acetic acid increases, while norepinephrine decreases in negative correlation with the levels of monoamine oxidase. In lower forms, similar age-related changes occur not only in catecholamine metabolism but also in the cholinergic system.[83,84] Depletion or imbalance of these substances with age may impair neurotransmission and psychomotor function and also blunt the neural connections with the endocrine system via transducer cells. Perhaps some instances of age-dependent depression and parkinsonism also relate to these findings.

THYMUS

The thymus gland has often been implicated in the altered immune response of aging individuals, but until now studies have been carried out almost entirely in mice. Recent purification of the thymic hormone, thymosin, a low molecular weight polypeptide, holds promise in elucidating certain age-dependent immune disorders of man. Serum levels of thymosin, whether measured by radioimmunoassay or bioassay, show a significant inverse correlation with age.[85] Furthermore, thymosin activity is considerably lower in the blood of patients with immunodeficiency disorders. Another recently characterized thymic hormone, thymopoietin,[86] may exert trophic influences not only on lymphoid tissue also on several other cells throughout the body in the development of cell-mediated and humoral immunity.

Although attempts at therapeutic intervention are only now

beginning,[87] the implications for staving off age-dependent diseases seem clear. Maintaining normal levels of thymic hormones may retard senescence of the immune system and delay onset of age-dependent diseases. Further developments in this exciting area are awaited expectantly.

PINEAL GLAND

Calcification of the human pineal is so common during adult life that this phenomenon has long been exploited as an intracranial radiologic marker. Despite the progressive calcium deposition, which in females particularly is accompanied by substantial fibrosis, parenchymal cells do not seem to atrophy significantly during aging.[88] Moreover, monoamine oxidase and other critical enzymes continue to be demonstrable histochemically, indicating that the capacity to inactivate histamine and serotonin and to synthesize melatonin persist with age. However, the exact functional significance of the pineal is still shrouded in mystery.[2] Its role in initiating pubescence by governing gonadotropin secretion seems increasingly important, as is its influence on complex circadian rhythms. It may turn out to be a critical organ in terms of senescence but further knowledge must be forthcoming.

POSTERIOR PITUITARY

Little information is available on the content of oxytocin or vasopressin (antidiuretic hormone, ADH) in the posterior pituitary, or the secretion capacity of the gland during mammalian aging. In aging rats, the capacity to put out ADH diminishes,[89] correlating nicely with the reduced content of neurosecretory material in the posterior pituitary.[59] There is a concomitant loss in the ability to excrete concentrated urine and a reciprocal rise in muscle sodium, but both can be reversed by the administration of ADH. In contrast, aging humans have a decreased response to exogenous ADH, measured as the loss of urinary concentrating capacity which appears to be a primary consequence of diminished glomerular filtration.[90] It is noteworthy that selected aging diabetics treated with chlorpropramide show an aberration in ADH secretion which manifests as inappropriate ADH activity. Chlorpropramide probably potentiates the peripheral effects of ADH rather than its secretion, so that these individuals apparently fail to reduce their ADH output in response to hypoosmolar volume expansion.[91] This provides further evidence for a generalized blunting of feedback control, in this case between posterior pituitary secretion, its renally mediated osmotic consequences, and the supraoptic and paraventricular nuclei of the hypothalamus.

PANCREATIC HORMONES

Insulin

Regardless of which diagnostic test is employed, there is a progressive deterioration of glucose tolerance decade by decade of life.[92] Still to be clarified is the precise relationship between the first and second phases of insulin release, although, in general, aging appears to be associated with blunting of both phases, and, frequently, an exaggerated length of the second phase.[92] Part of the cause of age-dependent decline in glucose tolerance may reside in the greater proportion of proinsulin that elderly subjects secrete, since this prohormone is considerably less potent than insulin in stimulating glucose uptake.[93] Elderly subjects who are carefully matched for weight with a group of younger individuals produce about 50 percent more proinsulin as a fraction of the total immunoreactivity after a glucose challenge.[93]

Few studies have addressed themselves directly to quantifying the number of islets during normal aging, their content of β cells, and the amount of extractable insulin. It appears, however, that these parameters are all reduced in the elderly, even when normal glucose tolerance persists.[94,95] Additionally, aging of overt diabetics, whether the diabetes is of juvenile or adult onset, is clearly associated with a further decline in an already depleted β cell mass[95] and secretory capacity, measured by the urinary output of C-reactive peptide.[96] In fact, the age-related decline of insulin output in the face of rising levels of blood sugar indicates a progressive β cell insensitivity to a glucose stimulus.[97]

Although the metabolic clearance and basal secretory rates of insulin appear unchanged in elderly people with normal glucose tolerance,[98] the status of insulin secretion and the sensitivity of peripheral tissues is in doubt. Some report that certain elderly normals have no change in either parameter,[98] but in another subgroup of elderly individuals who maintain euglycemia as well as young normals, this feat is accomplished only by having the capacity to sustain elevated levels of circulating insulin.[99] Perhaps the discrepancies can be ascribed to the fact that many tests have been performed on subjects who were not strictly comparable with regard to body weight or glucose tolerance. Thus, a more recent report on individuals who were carefully matched for both parameters indicates that young people maintain glucose homeostasis after a challenge with much lower plasma insulin levels than do their older counterparts.[100] Therefore, by avoiding some of the assumptions inherent in the use of the insulin/glucose ratio, it appears that old subjects are more resistant to endogenous insulin than are young subjects. Certainly, there is little debate regarding the relative insensitivity of peripheral tissues in adult-onset diabetics to insulin, whether exogenous or endogenous.[101,102]

Nonetheless, the relationships between insulin production and peripheral responsiveness is not always clear in a given individual. Even when ideal body weight is maintained in the elderly, it must be appreciated that adipose tissue has still replaced lean muscle mass. Intermediate influences may also be important, such as hemodynamic factors, circulating antagonists, capillary and interstitial permeability, or, in total, the effective delivery of insulin to target tissues. At the opposite pole of the feedback loop, the role of the glucostat in the ventral medial hypothalamus may also be critical in regulating glucose levels through appetite and autonomic neural control of insulin secretion.[103] Indeed, young people have a greater caloric flux than the elderly, and for this reason alone would produce more insulin. This multifactorial concept of aberrant glucose homeostasis during human aging is substantiated by observations in aging rats. There is a 60 percent reduction of insulin levels in portal venous blood following intragastric glucose feeding, as well as decreased insulin-binding capacity to hepatic plasma membranes.[104]

Decreased receptor concentrations may also play a role in human diabetes, at least in nonobese individuals with the adult-onset, insulin-dependent form. Thus, peripheral mononuclear leukocytes of such individuals appear to have half as many insulin-binding sites as normal controls, with the added possibility of a reduced affinity of each receptor.[105] However, again, it is critical to control for adiposity because this condition, even in the absence of diabetes, is associated with decreased receptor concentrations that can be reversed by caloric restriction. Moreover, there is controversy in this area, apparently related to the cell type examined, so that the monocyte accounts for most of the insulin binding.[106] While mononuclear cells of obese individuals have a decreased concentration of receptors, the monocyte fraction (expressed as a percentage of the total mononuclear leukocytes) apparently remains normal.[107] In contrast, adipocytes of obese nondiabetic subjects do not show receptor changes,[108] but in this situation it appears that either the density of receptors is decreased on the enlarged "obese" adipocytes or the distal enzymatic machinery is aberrant. Most important, however, and as yet unknown, are the effects of aging per se on the concentration and affinity of insulin receptors in adipocytes, liver, and muscle, the tissues accounting for most of the augmented glucose uptake following insulin stimulation.

Glucagon

Despite the limited information available, it seems that α cell content of glucagon and glucagon release following arginine challenge undergo no measurable change during aging.[109] Recently, it has become recognized that glucagon [and/or related enteroglucagon(s)] not only stimulates insulin secretion but also has profound effects on glucose tolerance in its own right.[110,111] Future studies of glucagon secretory dynamics, therefore, may reveal an important role of this hormone in the age-dependent rise of glucose intolerance.

GENERAL TISSUE RESPONSIVENESS

Although the picture is far from uniform or complete, there appears to be an overall decrease in tissue responsiveness during aging. Moreover, it seems likely that this is due to both a quantitative reduction in cell mass and a qualitative derangement within surviving cells. The best examples again are the menopausal ovary and the senescent testis, but other tissues are probably involved in a similar manner, even though they are often not detectable above the clinical horizon.

Neurohypophyseal Interactions: Dual Role as Effectors and Targets

It must be emphasized that many cells, particularly those in the neurohypophyseal axis, perform a dual role as both effectors and targets; each responds to the "end" hormone whose sequence of production it initiated. Moreover, many observations of altered neuroendocrine function cannot be thoroughly evaluated until the relative concentrations of glia and neurons (or, generally, connective tissue versus parenchyma) are known since each undoubtedly has a specific response to a given neurotransmitter or hormone. Nevertheless, gross differences are found in the chemical composition of the human brain during aging, and these are specific for each anatomic region.[112] Brain-specific proteins also change over the life span of the mouse.[113] In rats, administration of 17-β estradiol increases acetylcholinesterase activity in the cerebral hemispheres and cerebellum of immature adult animals but not in the elderly.[114] The most likely basis is a diminished concentration of estradiol receptors in the brain. Indeed, there is evidence in other systems that the decreased responsiveness of rat brain[115] and chicken brain[83] to norepinephrine and dopamine is mediated via loss of a receptor specifically linked to the regulatory rather than the catalytic subunit of adenyl cyclase. However, changes also occur at other sites. Androgenic sex steroids need to be converted enzymatically in peripheral tissues, particularly the accessory sex organs, to an active form, which is then bound to a specific cystosol receptor. Thus, age-dependent decrements appear at the level of peripheral enzymatic conversion.[116–118]

A selected subgroup of senescent female rats who are in constant estrous have continously elevated prolactin levels both in serum and the anterior pituitary; although ovarian follicles mature, ovulation does not occur and corpora lutea do not develop.[119] The anovulatory state is probably due to a relative deficiency of neurotransmitter catecholamines responsible for stimulating neurons that release LRF. This may have important implications for the high incidence of breast carcinoma in human females during perimenopause.[120] More generally, this and previous examples illustrate a breakdown of feedback circles whereby neurotransmitters and hormones normally influence the output of hypothalamic releasing factors.[79,80]

Hormone-Mediated Enzyme Induction

Age-dependent changes also appear in hormone-mediated enzyme induction. There is a prolongation in the time needed to induce two hepatic enzymes: glucokinase following glucose feeding, and tyrosine aminotransferase following intraperitoneal injection of ACTH.[104] However, these stimuli are indirect and exert their effects via the secretion of insulin and glucocorticoids, respectively. When the inducing hormone is given directly, the prolonged lag period reverts to normal, suggesting that extrahepatic factors are responsible. In fact, multiple sites from enteric absorption to hormone release and delivery are involved in this chain of events. Thus, insulin concentrations in portal venous blood following intragastric glucose feeding are reduced by 60 percent in elderly rats.[104] Additionally, aged liver membranes have a reduced concentration and affinity of receptors to bind insulin, although the analysis is complicated by increased liver cell ploidy and cell size. However, similar decrements in glucocorticoid binding have also been found in fat, prostate, skeletal muscle, and the cytosol of brain cerebral hemispheres.[121]

Hormone Receptors and Adenyl Cyclase

Hormone receptors seem to be critically important during aging, particularly in fat cells. For example, a selective decline occurs in the number of glucagon receptors relative to those for epinephrine and ACTH.[122] This is further borne out by the finding in rat adipocytes that norepinephrine stimulation of lipolysis decreases with age concomitant with a fall in adenyl cyclase activity and a rise in phosphodiesterase activity.[123] Adipose cells are unique because their size, which is partly related to age and partly to nutritional status, shows an inverse relationship to the concentration of hormone receptor.[124] Moreover, this situation appears to be similar in man.[125]

Age- and sex-dependent changes also occur in the adenyl cyclase of rat liver.[126] Basal activity is constant from weaning through senescence in male and female rats. During aging, the cyclase response to glucagon and epinephrine diminishes, with the decline in epinephrine response being particularly pronounced in males. The independent variation in levels of glucagon- and epinephrine-responsive adenyl cyclase suggest that genetically distinct cyclase systems exist for each hormone. Another possibility is that there is a single adenyl cyclase loosely affiliated with independently varying hormone receptors.

Vascular tissue responsiveness following stimulation with contractile agonists such as epinephrine and cyclic nucleotides also decreases with age in the rat.[127] This finding is also consistent with alterations in receptor–cyclic nucleotide systems, but, alternatively, in this case could relate to increased rigidity of arterial wall collagen.

POSSIBLE PITUITARY PACEMAKER OF AGING IN RATS

Recently, a pituitary factor has been described in rats that decreases peripheral tissue responsiveness to thyroid hormone.[71,128] Although it appears to be specific for thyroid function its effect is independent of TSH. Using a new measure called *minimal O_2 consumption,* the factor is first detectable at puberty, after which its effects begin to increase. Like BMR, minimal O_2

consumption decreases with age, but it apparently shows more specificity for the pituitary factor. Moreover, interfering with its output by hypophysectomy or otherwise delaying maturity prolongs the life span of the mouse. It has been proposed, therefore, that this factor may serve as a primary pacemaker of aging. However, its precise significance in the rat as well as its implications for man are still obscure. One would predict that levels of all hormones in the thyroid axis should rise with age in an attempt to overcome the inhibitory effects of this factor, but this is clearly not so.

INCREASED HORMONAL SENSITIVITY DURING AGING

Examples of increased hormonal sensitivity are uncommon. The supersensitivity to catecholamines that is seen after denervation may also appear during aging, particularly in the human cardiovascular system.[129] These observations are difficult to reconcile with what currently seems to be a generalized decline in functional competence of receptors and distal enzymatic machinery for cyclic nucleotides, at least when measured in vitro.[130] In vivo, there could be alterations in the balance between antagonistic hormones that are not revealed under in vitro conditions. However, the finding of an enhanced epinephrine effect in aging human fibroblasts is consistent with a cellular rather than a neurohumoral basis (see next section).

CONCLUSIONS

Aging is clearly accompanied by altered endocrine function, but attempts to assign causality may be overly simplistic and even futile. The severity of involvement varies considerably from system to system (Table 151-1), so that changes can often be demonstrated at various sites in the complex cycle of events from production of a hormone, to its delivery to the peripheral cell, to its later feedback effects. It is obvious, therefore, that aging can have selective effects on specific gene products. While the immediate molecular alteration is not always apparent, current techniques should soon enable us to define a precise basis in each case. In homeostatic terms, it is exceedingly important that even though the integrity of the feedback loop may be preserved, the sensitivity at each of the relay stations seen in early life often becomes blunted. Of paramount interest from the clinical standpoint is the need to evaluate tests of hormone function in the light of carefully selected age-matched controls.

GENERAL AND CELLULAR AGING

The passage of time after maturity is accompanied by physiologic decline measurable in virtually all systems.[131] In seeking root causes, a vast array of factors has been implicated, ranging from defective molecules within cells to neurohumoral feedback loops between organs. While the true source of these decrements is still unknown, two general concepts have emerged. First, aging may originate from a single focus or primary "pacemaker" which triggers senescence. Alternatively, aging may be an intrinsic property of all cells and, even though responsive to external signals, each cell may age autonomously. Whichever mechanism turns out to be primary must still be explicable in more fundamental molecular terms as the loss of genetic information (see below).

Several problems exist in identifying the origins of senescence, principally due to lack of agreement on its true nature. Age-dependent processes that are developmental are often not easily distinguished from those that are senescent. While embryogenesis and pubescence fit our notions of development, what about involu-

Table 151-1. Age-Dependent Changes in the Major Hormones of Normal Man

Hormone or Axis	Basal Output	Capacity to Augment Output	Concentration in Blood	Metabolic Turnover	Sensitivity of Target Organ(s)
Gonads					
Estrogen	↓	↓	↓	↓	↓ ?
Testosterone	↓	↓	↓	↓	↓ ?
FSH, LH	↑	↑	↑	?	↓
Thyroid					
T_4	⟷	⟷	⟷	↓	↑ ?
T_3	↓	↓	↓	↓	⟷ ?
TSH	⟷	↓ ♂ ⟷ ♀	⟷	?	⟷ ?
Adrenal cortex					
Cortisol	⟷	↓	⟷	↓	↓ ?
Androgens	↓	↓	↓	?	?
ACTH	⟷	⟷	⟷	?	⟷
Renin	↓	↓	↓	?	?
Angiotensin	↓	↓	↓	?	?
Aldosterone	↓	↓	↓	↓	?
GH	⟷	↓	⟷	?	↓ ?
PTH	↓	↓ ?	↓	?	↑
Epinephrine &	⟷*	↓	↑	?	↓
norepinephrine	↓†	?	?	?	?
Thymosin	↓	↓	↓	?	↓ ?
Insulin	⟷	↓	⟷	⟷	↓
Glucagon	⟷	⟷	⟷	?	?

Abbreviations: ↑, increase; ↓, decrease; ⟷, no change; ?, as yet uncertain.
*Medullary.
†Extramedullary.
Many hormones have been omitted because no information currently exists for them in human aging.

tion of the placenta during gestation, the thymus during childhood, and the ovary during menopause? Further confusion can arise in the failure to distinguish between primary molecular events and secondary macroscopic consequences, in short, the distinction between etiology and pathogenesis. For example, one must appreciate the difference between age-dependent decline of melanin production versus greying of hair, or increased cross-linking of collagen versus wrinkling of skin. Although both pairs of phenomena are interdependent and the molecular to macroscopic trend is evident, a precise etiologic basis is still lacking. In this sense, the temporal profile of the γ-chain of fetal hemoglobin may be regarded equally as development or aging at the molecular level, since its levels drop before birth and reach low values in the newborn period. Perhaps the major distinction that can be identified between development and aging is that during the latter no proteins, matrices, or organs with essentially new structures or functions arise. It is useful to define aging as a progressive, unfavorable loss of adaptation to a relatively constant external environment expressed as decreased viability and increased vulnerability to the normal forces of mortality during the passage of time.

QUANTITATIVE ASPECTS

Measurement of aging is complex because it is the summation of physiologic processes changing throughout life and it is responsive to environmental modifications.[132] An obvious corollary is that no single test can encompass the essence of organismic aging. Longitudinal studies are limited because of the long human life span and because repeated, invasive procedures are precluded on moral and ethical grounds. As a result, short-lived lower forms have usually been studied rather than man, and life span rather than the rate of aging, has served as a convenient but limited criterion. Therefore, relatively sparse information has hitherto been available for various indices of human aging apart from mortality. Primitive hunting and gathering populations fell prey to the vagaries of plague, famine, and predatory attack, and few survived beyond middle age. Over the centuries, the mean and median life span have been extended significantly (Fig. 151-6),[133] largely following the advent of agricultural and health technologies. In contrast, maximum life span has remained relatively fixed, with few individuals surviving beyond 100 years. This suggests the presence of a biologic barrier, even acknowledging that certain rare geographic isolates may live some decades beyond this time.[134]

Recently, a test battery has been proposed to shift the focus away from mortality.[135] It has been designed to measure the rate of human aging by combining 50 diverse anatomic, physiologic, biochemical, psychomotor, and pathologic parameters. In principle, such a scheme has merit because it could facilitate the short-term measurement of aging and also enable us to evaluate modification regimens, for example, nutrition and miscellaneous therapeutic agents. However, it calls for an expensive logistic enterprise, and a greater shortcoming from the etiologic standpoint is that several of the parameters may be more closely related to age-dependent disease rather than to the underlying aging process.

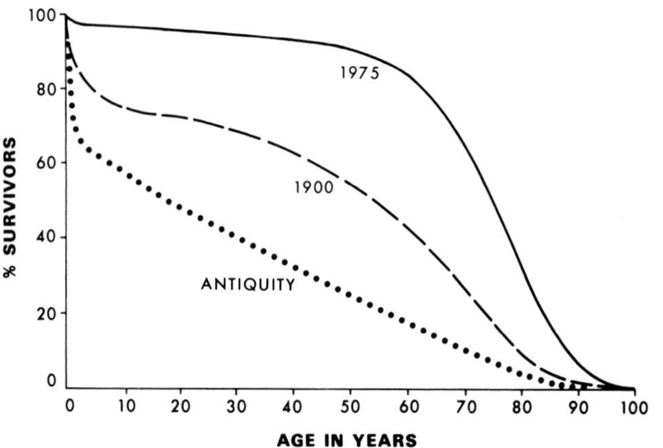

Fig. 151-6. Human survival trends from antiquity to the present. (Adapted from Strehler: Fed. Proc. *34:* 5, 1975.)

GENETICS

It seems clear that genetic factors contribute to aging for several reasons, particularly the fact that each species has a characteristic life span. Indeed, the modern survivorship curve for man (Fig. 151-6) can be applied equally well to any aging population of animals in protected captivity, substituting only the distinctive time scale for each species. Human longevity also appears to be heritable,[136,137] so that the life span of parents correlates positively with that of their offspring. Furthermore, monozygotic twins show mean intrapair differences in age at death that are smaller than those seen in dizygotic twins, which in turn, are smaller than those seen in other siblings. Indeed, the causes of death in monozygotic twins are similar more than twice as often as in dizygotic twins, even under diverse environmental conditions.[137]

Several human syndromes, often associated with a high incidence of glucose intolerance and insulin resistance (Table 151-2),[138] frequently show a decreased life span and the premature appearance of various forms of pathology normally regarded as age-dependent. Other features of these disorders are that most are hereditary and of unknown etiology, and often they are accompanied by stunting of growth. New syndromes will undoubtedly be added to the list as more testing is done, but even now it appears that a wide variety of genetic disorders, affecting many metabolic pathways, can simultaneously reduce glucose tolerance, abbreviate the life span, and impair somatic growth. In this context, notwithstanding the importance of adequate hormone balance, glucose tolerance may be no more specific an index than to reflect the state of health of the total cell mass at a given time.

Two syndromes of premature aging have become exceedingly important in our approach to the aging process and warrant further discussion.

Werner Syndrome

This disease is transmitted by autosomal recessive genes.[139] The full-blown clinical picture includes shortness of stature, early graying and loss of hair, juvenile cataracts, a tendency to insulin-resistant diabetes, atherosclerosis and calcification of the blood vessels, osteoporosis, and a high prevalence of cancer. Some doubt exists as to whether Werner syndrome constitutes a genuine model for the study of aging although various features are unquestionably common to both. Blood vessel involvement is qualitatively similar in character and distribution, but it occurs earlier and with greater severity in Werner syndrome than in natural aging. On the other hand, the very high frequency of cataracts, atrophy of the distal extremities, and mesenchymal neoplasia in Werner syndrome, in contradistinction to normal aging, militates against a simple relation between the two. Thus, Epstein et al.[139] have considered Werner syndrome to be a caricature of aging, reasoning that the various tissues of the human organism have only a limited number of reactions to degenerative processes. This argument may be academic at the present stage of limited knowledge and should

Table 151-2. Genetic Disorders Associated with Glucose Intolerance and/or Insulin Resistance, Many of Which also Have a Decreased Life Span

Familial
Alström syndrome
Ataxia telangiectasia
Cockayne syndrome
Cystic fibrosis
Fanconi anemia*
Friedreich ataxia
Glucose-6-phosphate dehydrogenase deficiency
Type 1 glycogen storage disease
Gout
Hemochromatosis
Huntington disease
Hutchinson-Gilford (progeria) syndrome
Hyperlipidemia, diabetes, hypogonadism and short stature syndrome
Hyperlipoproteinemias III, IV, and V
Isolated growth hormone deficiency
Laurence-Moon Biedl syndrome
Lipoatrophic diabetes
Muscular dystrophy
Myotonic dystrophy
Ocular hypertension induced by dexamethasone
Optic atrophy and diabetes
Optic atrophy, diabetes insipidus, and diabetes mellitus
Hereditary relapsing pancreatitis
Photomyoclonus, diabetes, deafness, nephropathy, and cerebral dysfunction
Pineal hyperplasia and diabetes
Acute intermittent porphyria
Pheochromocytoma
Prader-Willi syndrome
Retinitis pigmentosa, neuropathy, ataxia, and diabetes
Rothmund-Thomson syndrome
Schmidt syndrome
Werner syndrome
Nonfamilial (chromosomal)
Down syndrome†
Klinefelter syndrome
Turner syndrome

From Goldstein et al.: Fed. Proc. *34:* 56, 1975.
*From Swift et al.[250]
†A small percentage of cases, e.g., balanced translocation, is familial.

not deter investigation. Any disorder that produces a picture so reminiscent of aging, especially one determined by a single gene, merits intensive study.

Progeria

This condition has also been said to show autosomal recessive inheritance but the issue is still in doubt.[140] It begins much earlier in life than Werner syndrome and hence leads to severe stunting of growth. Endocrine function appears to be generally normal, although a marked resistance to exogenous insulin is a constant finding.[141] The most striking feature is generalized atherosclerosis involving all major vessels, including the aorta and coronaries, even in patients autopsied at 9 years of age. Recent postmortem studies have revealed severe focal myocardial fibrosis in the absence of coronary artery disease, which may reflect primary cell death independent of ischemia. Substantial deposits of the age pigment, lipofuscin, are also found within the cells of many organs. Progeria warrants intensive study for the same reasons that apply to Werner syndrome.

GENETIC PROGRAMMING OF CELLULAR PROLIFERATION DURING LIFE

The most cogent example of genetic programming is the complex sequence triggered by fertilization of the ovum. In precision of timing and efficiency of organogenesis, the 9 months of human gestation represent the highest order of program schedules. During fetal life, tissue expansion is accomplished by proliferation of enormously diverse cells with similar growth trajectories, but these peak just before birth (Fig. 151-7). Subsequently, during adolescence, growth of virtually all organs ceases as the somatic proportions of adulthood are achieved. Thereafter, tissue homeostasis is maintained with only a fraction of the mitotic activity seen during intrauterine life, except following cell injury or heightened physiologic demand. Tissues then respond with a variable blend of proliferation or increased cell size, depending on highly characteristic mitotic properties determined by differentiation. Parenchymal and supporting cells can be classified into three main types based on their mitotic capacity in adulthood, even though after this time the progressive trend in most tissues is from hyperplasia to hypertrophy.

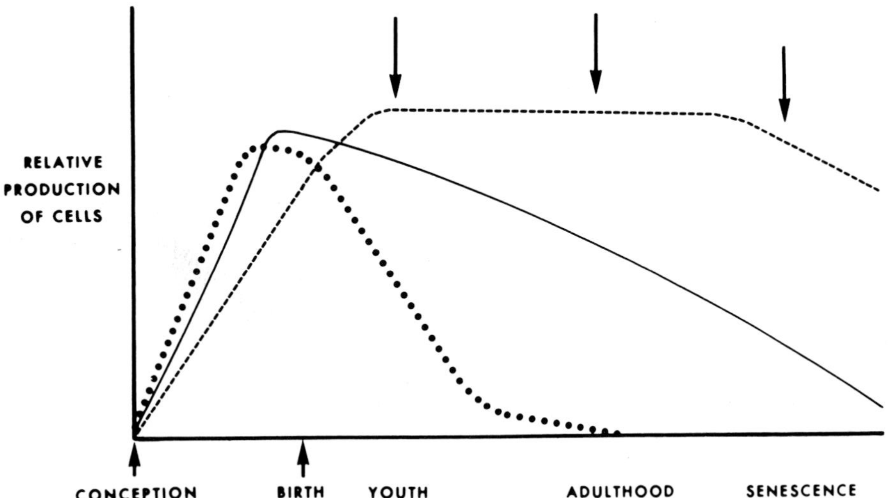

Fig. 151-7. Mitotic capacity of cells during life. Cells are classified according to their mitotic capacity after cessation of somatic growth. --/-, Continuous mitotics; ——, intermittent mitotics; . . . . , nonmitotics;↑, discrete events on a time scale that is otherwise a gradual and continuous sequence;↓, stimuli for cell division at various stages of life span. (Reprinted by permission from Goldstein: N. Engl. J. Med. *285:* 1120, 1971.)

Continuous Mitotics

Well-known examples of cells capable of dividing throughout life are those of the gastrointestinal, hematopoietic, epidermal, and spermatogenic systems. Blatant insufficiencies are rare in the elderly, although in all cases stem cell compartments gradually atrophy and surviving cells lose their replicative vigor.[142] Red marrow, the most widely distributed of these systems in early life, is gradually replaced by fat and is eventually found only in flat bones of the axial skeleton. It is generally asserted that marrow reserve does not diminish with aging, but it must be recognized that anemia and leukopenia are not unusual. Even after remediable causes such as inadequate nutrition, malabsorption, and intercurrent diseases are ruled out, over 50 percent of the anemic and leukopenic elderly still have an idiopathic hypoplastic marrow response, and this may be an underestimate.[143]. The term *myeloproliferative disorder,* while thought to be a primary nosologic entity, could in fact be secondary fibrotic replacement of a failing marrow.

Lymphocytes from elderly persons have a decreased proliferative response to plant mitogens and allogeneic lymphocytes compared to young persons.[144] This functional difference cannot be attributed to the plasma that bathes the lymphocytes, the number of stimulating cells, or the percentage of thymus-derived lymphocytes because each of these variables is identical in elderly and young subjects.

In aged mice, the number of immunocompetent splenic cells is reduced to one-tenth that found in young animals.[145] Additionally, an impairment in antigen processing appears since it is necessary to raise the immunizing dose of antigen 10-fold in old mice to achieve maximal stimulation. The plasma of old mice is also inhibitory, albeit to a far smaller degree than the defect intrinsic to cells. That the decline of the mouse immune system is related to a progressive inefficiency to proliferate and differentiate is borne out by studies on serial transplantation of an antibody-producing clone: secretion of a specific immunoglobulin eventually dies out as the growth capacity is exhausted.[146] A similar limit occurs in the transplanted hematopoietic cells whether they grow in the marrow or spleen of preirradiated recipients.[147] Only certain rare hematopoietic variants develop an unlimited proliferative capacity, but they lose the ability to differentiate and have other properties similar to neoplastic cells.

The recent demonstration that hematopoietic cells in certain mice can be serially transplanted for a calendar time well beyond the normal life span may be the exception that proves the rule. Even in this case, proliferative capacity measured by colony-forming units declines with successive transplantation.[148] This underscores the tissue-specific variation in mitotic potential and yet the inevitable occurrence of age-dependent decline.

Intermittent Mitotics

Cells in this group normally turn over slowly, but appropriate stimuli will trigger a proliferative response. In the liver, for example, partial hepatectomy or substantial necrosis brought about by toxic chemicals leads to a burst of regeneration in surviving cells. Although the regenerative rate decreases in senescent animals, the ability to completely replenish the original liver mass is not detectably impaired.[149] In other organs, the nature of regeneration undergoes a shift with age. Compensatory growth readily occurs in the remaining kidney after unilateral nephrectomy, but expansion of renal tubular mass is progressively hypertrophic with age rather than hyperplastic. In fact, after the neonatal period, no new glomeruli or nephrons are formed.[149] In bone, osteons are depleted with time, so that dead bone accumulates and prefractures appear.[150] Mammary tissue in inbred mice shows a progressive loss of division potential on serial transplantation, eventually resulting in complete loss of mitotic capacity.[151] Only certain kinds of breast tissue from strains of mice predisposed to mammary cancer are capable of indefinite proliferation.

Under normal steady-state conditions, connective tissue fibroblasts and nervous system glia divide infrequently to replace wear-and-tear losses, but they are capable of responding with a vigor that is proportional to the intensity of the stimulus. Although these cells maintain excellent proliferative capacity until advanced age, there is a noticeable decline seen in the healing of wounds in elderly animals, including man.[152] The proliferative life span of vascular cells also has definite limits that could become exhausted in meeting the repeated demands of low-grade injury, perhaps leading to the development of atherosclerosis.[153] In this regard, the smooth muscle cell of the medial layer seems particularly important.[154]

Nonmitotics

Neurons lose virtually all mitotic capability before adolescence, but once adult proportions are attained, brain weight does not normally change till much later in life. Glial cells ostensibly replace neurons to the extent that the proliferative reserve of this connective tissue cell ebbs as well. Cardiac and skeletal muscle also lose mitotic potential with advancing age, so that the response to injury and increased loading is effected via hypertrophy of preexisting cells.[155] Clinically, this correlates with the poor parenchymal healing and the gliosis and fibrosis that occur following stroke and myocardial infarction, respectively.

Miscellaneous Mitotics

Not all cell types are readily classified. Certain endocrine, cells such as the β cell of the pancreas, have a limited proliferative ability[156] perhaps intermediate to that of neurons and liver. Exhaustion of mitotic reserve in surviving β cells, whether following endogenous or exogenous insults, probably constitutes the basis of most forms of insulin-dependent diabetes. The transition in some individuals from mild adult-onset diabetes to the juvenile form may have a similar explanation but with an expanded time scale. Other cells, such as those of the anterior pituitary, appear to undergo relatively little depletion with age and, accordingly, the capacity for hormone production seems unimpaired.[157] However, the exact relationship between the proliferative and hormone-secreting capacities of endocrine cells is unknown. In the short run, demand for extra hormone should be met by augmentation of biosynthetic and secretory machinery within preexisting cells. Following extremely vigorous or prolonged stimulation, or even necrosis, signals should arise to increase cell mass, but this would be governed by the mitotic capacity, which in turn is a function of tissue-specific differentiation and cellular age.

AGING AS A LOSS OF GENETIC INFORMATION

Aging and the concept of a biologic barrier must somehow relate to impaired flow of information within the sequence from nuclear DNA to the final gene product (Fig. 151-8). Information could be lost in two ways: (1) via random deterioration related to the gradual accumulation of errors or other damage that reaches a threshold beyond which viability is impossible; or (2) via a genetic program emanating from differentiation and development that actively slows down biochemical processes—alternatively, the putative genetic program could become passively exhausted. No sound basis yet exists for choosing between the error and program con-

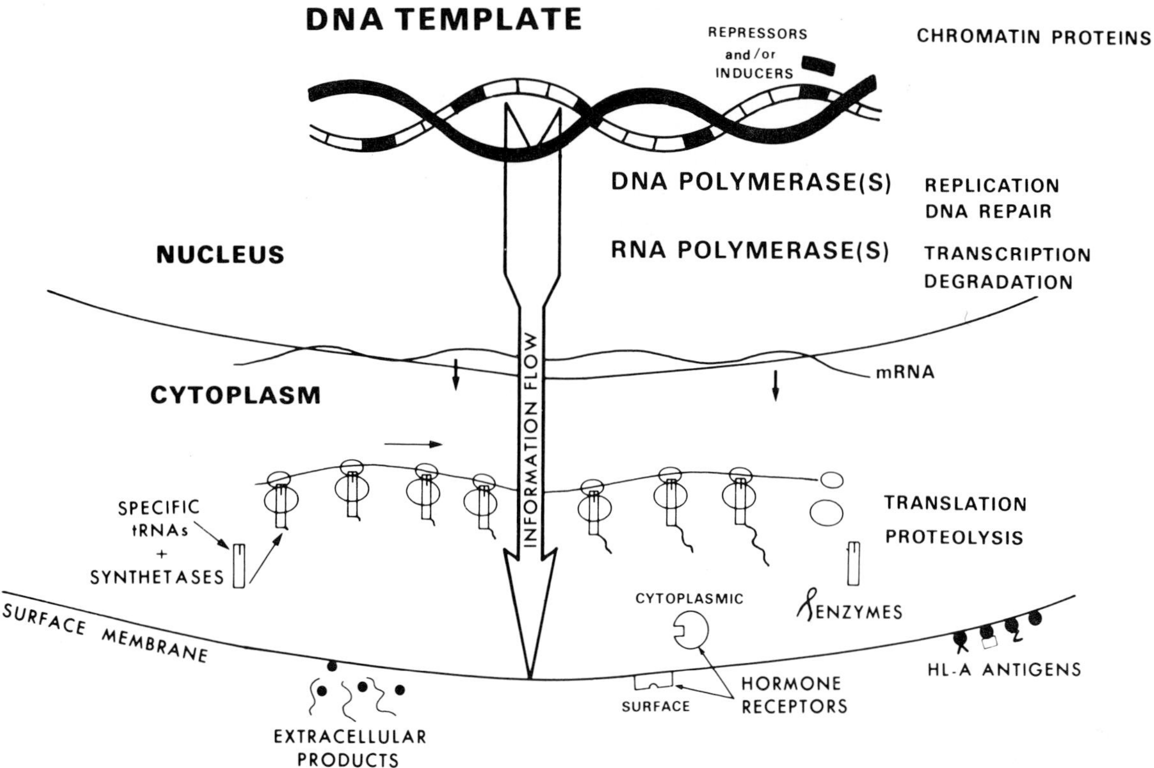

Fig. 151-8. Genetic information flow and potential sites for error production or programmed genetic changes during the aging process.

cepts. Indeed, both may be inextricably related, although overwhelming precedent and intuition favor the primacy of a program.

Molecular Error Theories

Defective Repair of Macromolecular Damage. It is now generally appreciated that cells from man phylogenetically on down to *Escherichia coli* normally possess sensitive mechanisms to recognize and eliminate abnormalities in the three major macromolecules by degradation and new synthesis. In the case of DNA, repair occurs either by replacing damaged segments following excision, or ligation of simple breaks in the base sequence. In contrast, aberrant molecules of RNA and protein, whether arising by faulty synthesis or from subsequent damage, are "repaired" by replacing whole molecules. Although there is no proof for causality in any mammalian species, aging of lower forms is clearly associated with the gradual accumulation of defective DNA and proteins, i.e., gene products, probably due to faltering of molecular surveillance mechanisms.[158–160]

Decreased Fidelity of Protein Synthesis. Information-handling proteins, such as aminoacyl synthetases, are particularly important since errors at the level of protein synthesis could jeopardize the functional integrity of a wide variety of proteins.[161] This could then lead to a vicious cycle that produces a cascade of defects and ultimately the demise of the cell. A major shortcoming of this theory as originally proposed is that it tends to ignore the surveillance function of proteolytic mechansims. Thus, before a defect in the synthetic limb could produce serious problems there would also have to be, a priori, a defect in proteolytic surveillance.[162]

Still another mechanism to safeguard that the synthesis of proteins proceeds correctly is known as *verification*. This process has so far only been documented for bacteria, in which it has the ability to intercept mischarged aminoacyl tRNAs before they reach the level of the ribosome.[163] If a given tRNA were charged with the wrong amino acid, then the verification mechansm could abort the synthesis of a faulty protein before it began. An obviously aberrant protein that breached this first line of defense would then meet the proteolytic mechanism, which could selectively degrade it after synthesis,[164] but the proteolytic sensitivity would be finite. It would depend on a threshold amount of configurational distortion consequent to insertion of the wrong amino acid in the primary sequence or some other posttranslational modification or denaturation. Some altered proteins would be too subtle for detection, but, by the same token, they should be near normal structurally and hence of little functional consequence.

Exhaustion of the Genetic Program

Codon-Restriction Theory This concept holds great appeal because it is comprehensive in scope and eminently testable in practice. Indeed, it has the potential to explain aging and link it to growth and development. It states that during life each differentiated cell synthesizes its own set of specific proteins based on a "language set" of code words taken from the genetic code, i.e., a group of tRNA molecules and their cognate synthetases.[165] Although gene sequences are composed of 61 usable triplets, there is abundant evidence in differentiating systems that only specific combinations are used in coding for any particular protein. In short, the group of codons needed is less than the 61 that are available. Furthermore, the choice of codons used is related to the types of aminoacyl tRNA species available as well as the cognate synthetases. Thus, the protein complement changes pari passu with the language set. As new proteins are evoked by the genetic program, old language sets are discarded or diluted out. Consequently, some proteins are no longer synthesized, or if they are, it is only in very small and increasingly limiting concentrations.

This concept fits nicely with the observations during early

differentiation when division of labor occurs within the body's community of cells. Tissue-specific proteins appear and others are jettisoned with the retention of a minimal complement of "housekeeping" proteins. These are needed, for example, to catalyze glycolytic reactions, maintain gradients, and serve as a structural components of membranes. As applied to aging, the concept predicts that various proteins will gradually ebb over the decades beyond human maturity. In fact, brains of aging dogs show a substantial reduction in the number of active genes coding for ribosomal RNA. Furthermore, this concept is consistent with the observation that there is a clear reduction in total body protein turnover during aging of man and lower forms.[166] Several reviews have concluded, at least with respect to the activity of several enzymes during life, that some decrease, some remain the same, and others actually increase.[167–169] It is noteworthy that the latter group (with increased activity) almost invariably comprises lysosomal enzymes involved in degradative functions, which suggests a general disturbance in macromolecular turnover.

Replication and Transcription Program. This concept is closely related to the previous one and presupposes that primary alterations occur within the nuclear chromatin, particularly in the acidic and basic (histone) proteins.[170,171] Regulation at this level could determine not only the types of tRNA and tRNA synthetases synthesized, but also the mRNA and subsequently the exact protein complement. Age changes in nuclear proteins could be the result of acetylation, phosphorylation, and methylation,[172] just as they are during development.[173] Another possible mechanism is the direct modification of DNA itself,[174] thereby altering its ability to unwind prior to replication and transcription or to bind specific repressors and inducers.

Gene Redundancy. This therapy promises to reconcile the rival camps of error versus program. It states that aging may relate to the amount of redundant information within the genome.[175] Long-lived species would have more genetic redundancy than short-lived species so that, as errors accumulated in functioning genes with time, reserve sequences with the same information would take over until the redundancy in the system was exhausted. In fact, using DNA–RNA hybridization techniques, it has recently been demonstrated that the transcription of DNA, that is, RNA synthesis, whether of unique or repeated sequences, undergoes a general decline in liver and brain of mice during aging.[176] These studies must first distinguish between shifts in parenchymal and connective tissue composition and then, of course, be extended to man.

IN VITRO STUDIES

Recent technical improvements have promoted our ability to grow a variety of cells in vitro. However, parenchymal cells, which in vivo show little or no mitotic potential, carry this property over to the in vitro situation.[177] The most comprehensive studies have been carried out in lower forms,[155,177] but the same patterns almost certainly apply to man.

Culture of Human Cells

The advantages of this system are so important as to justify repetition. Human cells can be studied directly rather than those of lower forms. Skin is usually used to initiate cultures because of easy access and minimal invasiveness of a brief, inocuous biopsy procedure. After this time, the subject's active participation ends, and, because all studies are then carried out in vitro, the moral and ethical constraints associated with human experimentation are no longer an issue. Cell culture also eliminates the troublesome in vivo variables of nervous, circulatory, and hormonal function. Perhaps the overriding advantage is a by-product of working with a dividing population in vitro: cells synthesize new machinery with building blocks provided by a relatively constant environment. Hence, we can analyze more "genotype" and less "phenotype" and compare metabolic variation between strains from known persons.

The ability to initiate growth from human skin tissue explants decreases with the advancing age of the donor.[178,179] Fewer fragments produce cellular growth, while an inverse correlation exists between the age of the donor and the latent period before the first emigrating fibroblasts appear.[178] Moreover, diabetics and prediabetics, compared to normal age-matched controls, show impairment of all of these parameters from the stage of explantation on through growth as secondary cultures.[179]

Development of Human Cell Strains

The term *cell strain* should be reserved for cultures obtained directly from normal somatic cells. Following adaptation and selection, the growing population rapidly loses the characteristics of the original parenchymal tissue. Virtually all differentiated cells, whatever their in vivo growth capacity, are soon overrun by connective tissue cells, predominantly of fibroblast morphology. Whether this "fibroblast" originates from its in vivo counterpart is uncertain. On the basis of histochemical and ultrastructural markers that identify cell-specific proteins, it has been asserted that the precursor cell may be vascular endothelium,[180,181] but other possibilities of fixed tissue histiocytes, smooth muscle cells, and circulating macrophages have not been ruled out. It is possible that all cells have some capacity to shift from one morphologic and functional class to the other. This fluidity, however, is clearly limited because anatomic site determines the metabolic and growth properties of cultured cells.[182,183] This may reflect subgroups of differentiation within connective tissue cells historically thought to be homogeneous. Perhaps critical in vivo cues that emanate from parenchymal tissues biochemically "fix" each fibroblast as tissue specific and site specific. Such evidence has recently been presented for neuron-specific fibroblasts within sympathetic ganglia.[184] In any case, the need to standardize the biopsy site in comparative studies is evident.

Thousands of human skin biopsies have now been developed into fibroblast cultures, and in all cases a three-phase phenomenon is observed (Fig. 151-9): Phase I begins at the time of tissue explantation and extends until formation of the first confluent cell sheet. Phase II begins with the first subculture and consists of a variable period of vigorous growth. Diploid cells divide until they fill the available surface, when they are arrested by a phenomenon known as *density-dependent inhibition of growth,*[185,186] Further subcultivation is then required to allow continued proliferation. Finally, phase III, the inevitable result of repeated subculture and proliferation, is heralded by progressive slowing of mitosis, cellular enlargement, increasing granularity, and finally cell death.

Development of Permanent Lines in Man and Lower Forms

Explantation of tumors often gives rise to cells that can be subcultured indefinitely and that retain certain biochemical properties of the original tumor. HeLa cells represent the best-known example of a permanent line, having been derived almost 40 years ago from a carcinoma of the cervix. Occasionally, even within originally diploid cultures derived from lower forms such as ro-

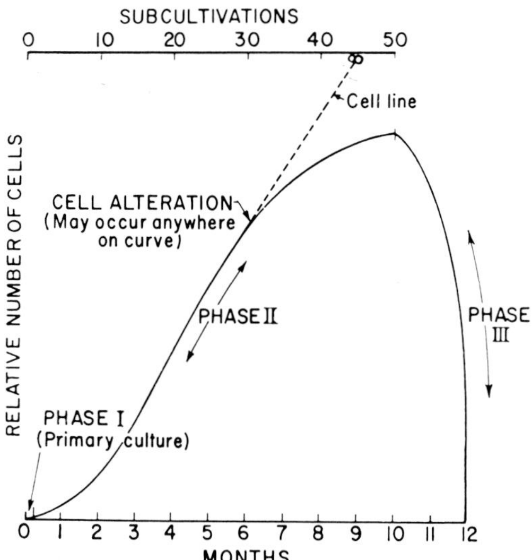

Fig. 151-9. In vitro history of cell strains and the phenomenon of cell alteration. (From Hayflick and Moorhead: Exp. Cell. Res. *25:* 585, 1961.)

dents, certain cells appear that seem better adapted to growth. They divide more frequently, often grow in suspension as well as in adherent culture, show a great tendency to develop aneuploidy, and, like HeLa cells, have an indefinite life span. This "transformation" may occur at any phase in the culture but it becomes more frequent with increasing levels of subculture.[185,187]

For obscure reasons, aging and the development of aneuploidy in vitro tend to occur concomitantly with the relaxation of repressive or differentiative controls of gene expression.[132] For example, cystathionase activity is present in permanent lines with chromosomal aberrations but not in diploid cells. Certain urea cycle enzymes are inducible in aneuploid lines, but not in the diploid fibroblast. The in vivo equivalent seems to be in endodermally derived gastrointestinal carcinomas, the reappearance of an antigen immunologically identical to that present in normal digestive tissues of the fetus.[188] This strongly suggests that aneuploidy and the acquisition of cellular "immortality" in vitro and in vivo are associated with derepression of certain genes. In any case, the properties of karyotypic and genetic instability, unlimited growth ability, and the propensity to form tumors when injected into suitable recipients make cellular transformation in vitro similar to the malignant state. Indeed, this phenomenon consitutes an excellent model for the study of carcinogenesis.[187]

Human Fibroblasts are Genetic Replicas of the Donor

In contradistinction to permanent lines, strains of human fibroblasts are stably diploid. However, toward the end of their finite replicative life span, there is an increasing frequency of aneuploidy and other chromosomal anomalies similar to those found with advancing age in vivo.[188a] Some prominent exceptions emphasize that human fibroblasts are genetic replicas of the donor, a fact amply borne out by the growing number of mutant genes now known to be expressed in culture.[189,190] For example, xeroderma pigmentosum is an autosomal recessive disorder associated with extreme sensitivity to sunlight, resulting in severe destruction and inflammation of skin and eventually multifocal cutaneous carcinomas. Cell strains derived from these individuals have a defect in DNA repair that specifically impairs their ability to excise pyrimidine dimers that are formed in DNA following exposure to ultraviolet and sunlight. When protected from ambient radiation, the phenotypes appear normal, but minimal exposure to ultraviolet light causes cell killing (Fig. 151-10)[191] and chromosomal breakage.[192] Fanconi anemia strains have a defect at a later stage of DNA repair and apparently show no sun or ultraviolet sensitivity, i.e., they show normal excision repair, although they suffer from severe chromosomal breakage in vitro and in vivo.

It is of great interest that cells from both these syndromes and others which supernumerary chromosomes, such as Down syndrome,[193] are more readily transformed to permanent lines by the oncogenic virus, simian virus 40 (SV40). Even senescent normal strains are more susceptible to viral transformation compared to early-passage adult fibroblasts or those from fetal tissues.[187] Although increased transformability by SV40 is not well understood, it is noteworthy that this phenomenon correlates with epidemiologic data that show an increasing incidence of malignancy in syndromes of chromosomal breakage and trisomy, and during natural aging.

Other examples of faithful genetic expression are cultures from individuals with galactosemia[194] and citrullinemia.[195] Not only do they maintain the specific enzyme defect in vitro, but they also exhibit auxotrophy. If these cultures are given galactose or citrulline rather than the regular nutrient factors (glucose and arginine, respectively) they fail to grow. In contrast, normal strains thrive because they possess the enzymes needed to convert the precursors to utilizable growth factors. In total, therefore, cultured human fibroblasts express the genotype of the donor with fidelity. The corollary is that any study that seeks to grow fibroblasts to explore a given parameter must take into account the genetic identity of the individual and his age (see below) since these factors set the limits for the successful adaptation of a cell to its environment, its vulnerability, and hence its potential longevity.

Physiologic (Rather than Chronologic) Age In Vivo as the Prime Determinant of Cellular Life Span In Vitro

In a population at large, the chronologic age of the donor in vivo appears to be the prime determinant of the replicative life span in vitro.[183,186,196] Several studies have revealed an inverse correlation between the age of the donor and the mean number of times that normal fibroblasts can divide—"mean population doublings" (Fig. 151-11). Considerable scatter has been observed even though all manipulations are rigidly controlled. However, it is now increasingly evident that physiologic rather than chronologic age is of paramount importance because fibroblasts from the premature aging syndromes of progeria and Werner syndrome have reduced growth capacity in comparison to age-matched controls.[183,197–200]

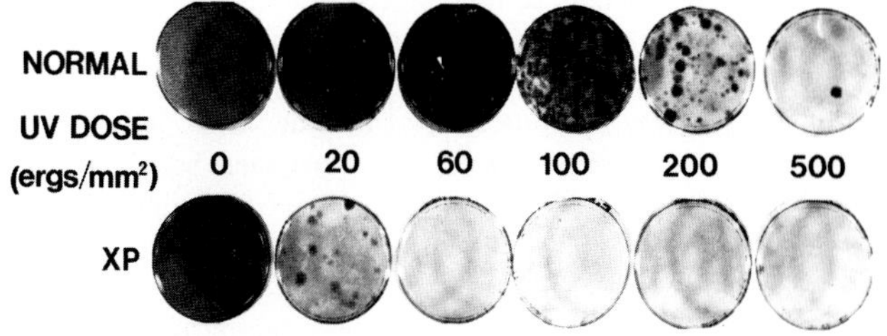

Fig. 151-10. Survival of cultured fibroblasts from a normal individual and a patient with xeroderma pigmentosum (XP); 300,000 cells were irradiated at the doses shown, inoculated into Petri dishes, and allowed to grow. After 14 days, cells were fixed and stained. Note that when the deleterious environmental factor, i.e., ultraviolet radiation, is zero, normal and XP cells have virtually identical growth vigor. At the lowest dose (20 ergs), most of the XP cells are killed, while there is no visible effect on normal cells until about 60 ergs, with progressive killing thereafter. (Adapted from Goldstein: Can. Med. Assoc. J. *105:* 738, 1971.)

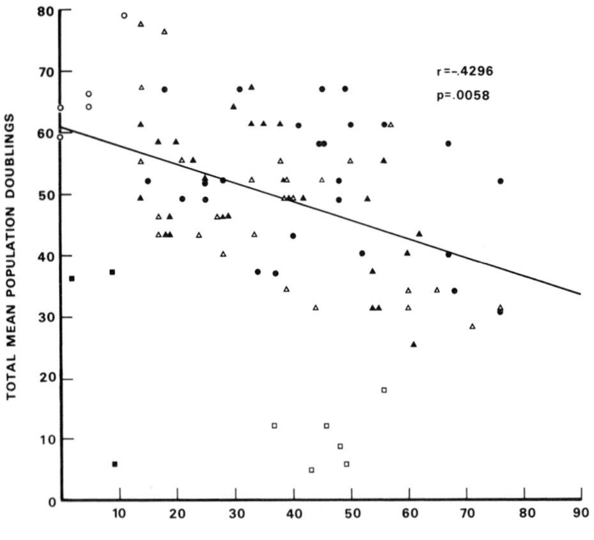

Fig. 151-11. Relationship between age of donor and the replicative life span of cultured skin fibroblasts. Most symbols represent a single comparative study of 3 groups of subjects: ●, 25 normal controls; ▲, 30 genetically prediabetic individuals; Δ, 25 overt diabetics. Additional symbols represent other cell strains interpolated to show the effect of accelerated physiologic aging on the cellular life span in vitro: ■, progeria; □, Werner's syndrome; ○, normal newborns and young controls. (Data from Goldstein et al.[197,198,200,256] and Martin et al.[183,199] and reproduced from ref. 257, courtesy of Plenum.)

The diabetic genotype also plays a critical role in the growth performance of cultured fibroblasts.[179,196] In fact, when the combined performances shown in Figure 151-11 are segregated into normals, overt diabetics, and prediabetics who are genetically predisposed but not yet glucose intolerant (the offspring of conjugal diabetics or an identical twin of a diabetic), only the two latter groups show an inverse proportion between age in vivo and the mitotic potential in vitro (Fig. 151-12). Normal controls are chosen on the basis of rather stringent criteria: subjects must have no family history of diabetes, no clinical evidence of metabolic, degenerative, or malignant disease, and repeatedly normal tests of glucose tolerance. Indeed, cultures derived from these fastidiously selected normals do not show the inverse proportionality; strikingly, many at middle and older age show fibroblast performances that, in fact, are as good as those of younger normals. This finding is not totally unexpected because the in vivo performances, particularly of older normals, clearly establish these subjects as physiologically elite. Hence, it is reasonable to expect their replicative totals to skew away from the inverse correlation.

Similarly, we might predict that geographic isolates of vigorously longevitous individuals[134] should also produce cultures capable of out-performing persons several decades their junior. This would be consistent with the concept that darwinian selection in no small part determines experimental selection. At the opposite end of the spectrum, individuals who have severely limited life spans, with or without manifest diabetes, do not survive to enter any of the three groups in such a series. In this context, even elderly individuals with overt diabetes are superior physiologic specimens.

Analysis of the limited life span of fibroblasts is at an early stage. It seems clear that many genetic determinants (including diabetes), other intercurrent pathologic states, and prior exposure to environmental factors will play a role. However, the frequent association between reduced fibroblast growth, the diabetic state, and accelerated aging suggests the existence of a common denominator in this triad.

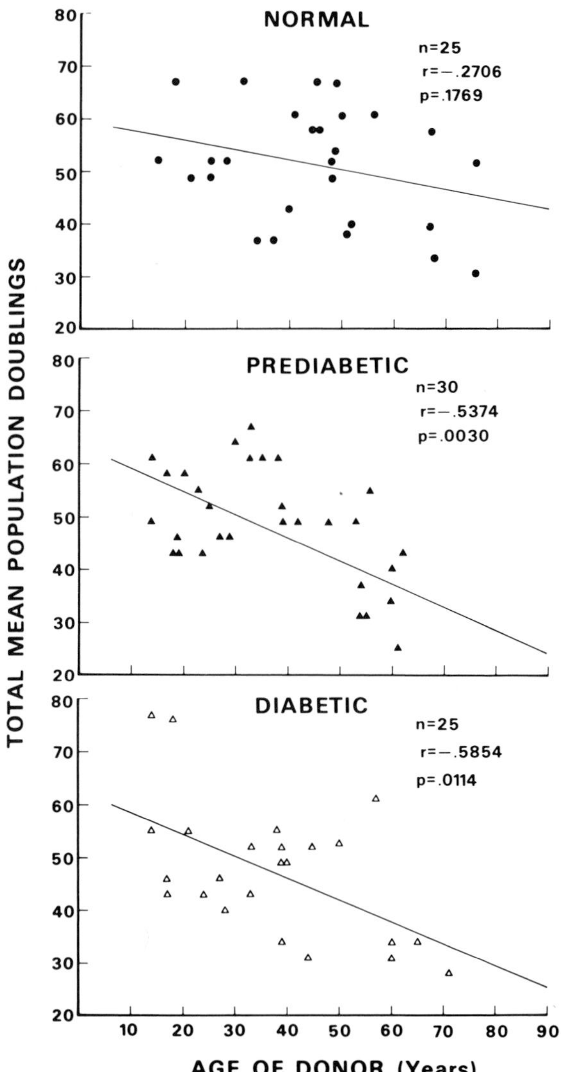

Fig. 151-12. Combined plot of normals, prediabetics, and diabetics shown in Figure 151-11 segregated into three groups, showing individual regression analyses. Note that in normal subjects the correlation between fibroblast life span and age is not significant, and the slope of the regression line is flatter than in prediabetics and diabetics, indicating a general trend toward greater fibroblast longevity in middle age and beyond. (Data from Goldstein et al.[179,256] and reproduced from ref. 257, courtesy of Plenum.)

Comparative Senescence of Cultured Cells from Various Animal Species

Studies are incomplete in this important area, but a pattern is now becoming apparent: the potential longevity of a species may determine the replicative life span in vitro (Table 151-3). It must be appreciated in evaluating these studies that intraspecies differences exist, each subgroup having its own longevity. Additionally, careful scrutiny must ensure that normal tissue has been explanted and that subtle genetic–chromosomal rearrangements have not occurred.[205] The exact culture medium and methods also influence the results, and, again, the age of the donor must be taken into account. Despite these reservations, a growing body of data now supports the direct relationship between in vivo and in vitro life spans. The polar extremes are defined by mouse embryo fibroblasts and the Galapagos tortoise. In fact, cultures from prehatchling tortoises would be expected to perform even better, but ethical constraints in this endangered species precluded the use of such material in the only studies so far reported.[201]

Table 151-3. Relationship Between the Maximum Life Span of an Animal Species and the Maximum Replicative Potential of Cultured Fibroblasts

Species	Maximum Life Span (yr)	Maximum No. of Mean Population Doublings	Reference No.
Galapagos tortoise	200	141	201
Man	110	90	202
Subhuman primates	40	70	203
Cow	40	68	187
Chicken	30	35	204
Mouse	3.5	28	204

Extracellular Possibilities for the Limited Replicative Capacity

Trivial explanations have been meticulously sought for the finite life span. Potential artifacts such as omission of nutrients from the culture medium, contamination by various microorganisms, and the presence of toxic materials have been ruled out. Some have suggested that cumulative damage from repeated environmental insults and stresses over the years, first delivered to the intact organism and then to the cultured cell, may cause cellular aging.[206,207] Often inculpated are the cumulative effects of repeated exposure to low levels of ionizing radiation. It is also possible that extracellular ground substances accumulate with age and mechanically restrict the migration of cells. Cells could have also incurred damage in vivo consequent to restricted access of nutrients or egress of toxic metabolites. One would predict, therefore, that cells with the poorest growth potential, such as adult neurons, would be surrounded by the densest connective tissue, but this is patently not so.[177]

Although these ideas of cumulative environmental damage and restriction by increasingly rigid connective tissue are consistent with several features, including the correlation between donor age and in vitro life span, it is unlikely that all individuals with disorders of accelerated aging have encountered more "environment" or metabolic restriction. Rather more reasonable is the premise that cells from these individuals are innately more vulnerable to a given set of environmental conditions. The same logic applies to cells from species with diverse life spans (Table 151-3). Hayflick and Moorhead were first to propose that the finite life span of human fibroblasts is a result of properties intrinsic to the cell and, therefore, intimately related to in vivo senescence.[185,186] Even if essential growth factors were found to be deficient, thus limiting the long-term growth of cells, the same lack would have to apply to the dwindling proliferative mass in vivo. Moreover, we would still have to explain why the physiologically aged fibroblast is more vulnerable. Indeed, if unlimited cell division occurs, either in vivo or in vitro, it should be considered quasi-neoplastic and hence abnormal.

Mitotic Versus Nonmitotic Cells

Whichever mechanism is ultimately responsible for limiting the life span must account for aging in both proliferating and nonproliferating cells. Cultured cells appear to have a clock that "counts" the number of mitotic events in preference to the total time of active metabolism.[208,209] This is remarkably like a taxi meter that charges more for distance traveled than for time. At the extreme, cells that are suitably frozen and stored in liquid nitrogen remain immortal. When reconstituted they demonstrate "memory" for the number of mitoses consumed (or that remain) prior to senescence, when compared to a continuously passaged cohort. Cells incubated under regular conditions but not allowed to divide, either by depriving them of serum[208] or by holding them up in stationary phase for several weeks in complete medium,[209] can resume their replicative activity when the regular serum content is restored or when additional growth surface is provided.

The exact nature of this counting apparatus is unknown, but it could reside in a mechanism that, for example, methylates DNA bases. In this scheme, each round of replication would be accompanied by the addition of one methyl group to DNA up to a given threshold number, which then terminates the program and/or commences an error cascade.[174] What about a nonmitotic cell, such as a neuron? Perhaps it contains a clock that counts, for example, the number of transcriptions of messenger RNA involved in the production of a specific neurotransmitter. Although such possibilities are at present only of theoretical interest, we must recognize that mechanisms of aging could be relatively unique in each cell.

Biochemical Changes in Aging Human Fibroblasts

Altered Enzymes. Recent studies are elucidating the nature of age-related biochemical changes. Simultaneously, they strengthen the view that this model represents aging of the intact organism. As normal fibroblasts traverse the in vitro life span they accumulate an increased fraction of heat-labile enzymes.[160,200,210,211] Such changes occur in late-passage cells from donors of all ages, but no differences have yet been reported between strains from fetuses, infants, young adults, and the elderly. Of the few enzymes studied, glucose-6-phosphate dehydrogenase and hypoxanthine–guanine phosphoribosyltransferase are particularly useful because they are X linked, and hence single-gene determined. Therefore, these gene products are composed of identical subunits that guarantee that allelic forms, and new isozymes will not be synthesized during the aging process.[212,213] As a result, any changes arising during the replicative life span must be ascribed to errors or programmed modifications.

Cells from individuals with Werner syndrome contain the highest fraction of heat-labile enzymes[197,214,215] (Fig. 151-13). Fibroblasts from progeric subjects appear to be intermediate between normal and Werner strains, but strikingly, progeric cells show their abnormalities early in the replicative life span, when

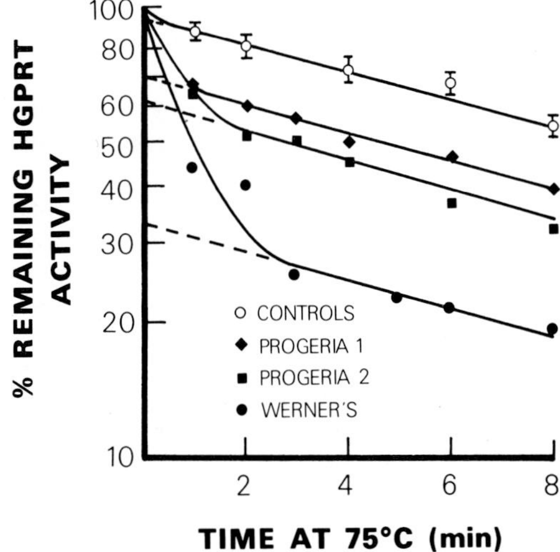

Fig. 151-13. Heat lability of hypoxanthine-guanine phosphoribosyltransferase in crude extracts of fibroblasts from normals (mean ± SEM). ◆, Progeria, age 2; ■, progeria, age 9; ●, Werner syndrome, age 56. (From Goldstein and Moerman; Nature *255:* 159, 1975; N. Engl. J. Med. *292:* 1305, 1975.)

their growth capacity is as vigorous as normal strains.[200] This is an important distinction because slowing of cell growth may in itself lead to altered proteins.

HLA Antigens. Normal fibroblasts, like all nucleated cells in vivo, contain histocompatibility (HLA) antigens on their surface membranes. These antigens undergo little or no change in expression during aging in vitro.[216] The fact that HLA phenotypes are first determined on circulating lymphocytes from each subject indicates that antigen expression is stable in cultured fibroblasts. However, a fraction of subclonal populations within the parental mass culture show altered antigen expression.[138] The most likely explanation is that clonal diversification develops within the parental mass culture during aging,[199,217] perhaps beginning in vivo and progressing in vitro.

Compared to these relatively subtle events in normal strains, there is a more severe disturbance in expression of HLA antigens in progeria and Werner cells that is concomitant with their increased enzyme heat lability. Parenthetically, the HLA phenotypes in these two syndromes are readily determined on peripheral lymphocytes and are not unusual inasmuch as they are frequently seen in normal populations. Because of the limited number of cases available for study, it is not yet possible to ascertain whether specific HLA antigens are preponderant in these disorders, as they are in certain disease states. In any event, still another form of gene product, a surface antigen that is apparently nonenzymatic, is altered configurationally or is in some way masked. It must be recognized that the composition of HLA antigens is not exclusively protein, but also includes carbohydrate components determined by glycosyl transferases, in themselves gene products. However, this does not affect the interpretation because the disturbance in antigen expression is more severe and uniform in progeria and Werner fibroblasts when compared to normal cells.

Hormone Receptors and cAMP. Hormonal responsiveness is now well documented in human fibroblasts, mainly via the cAMP system. Some of the hormones already tested are catecholamines, prostaglandins, glucagon, and insulin. Not unexpectedly, factors related to cell density and cell growth are critical in hormonal responsiveness and show specificity for each hormone.[218–220] Direct studies have confirmed the presence of an insulin receptor,[221–223] but the effects of cell aging have not yet been reported. Recent studies on progeric fibroblasts show a significant change in insulin binding, apparently due to altered receptor affinity.[224] This exciting finding may provide the explanation for the insulin resistance seen in vivo.[140,141]

More circumstantial evidence suggests that receptors for other hormones become altered during aging of normal cells in vitro.[219] Prostaglandin E_1 stimulates an enormous rise in cAMP concentration of young normal fibroblasts, up to 500-fold over basal; in senescent fibroblasts these levels increase only half as much, perhaps due to leakiness of aged cells.[225] Paradoxically, while epinephrine increases cAMP levels 8–10-fold in young cells, levels rise to 25-fold in old cells. Apparently, senescent cells change the expression of specific genes that regulate the concentration of each hormone receptor independently. It is noteworthy that basal cAMP concentration is not significantly different in young compared to old fibroblasts at any stage of growth or cell density. It seems unlikely, therefore, that cAMP has a significant role to play in fibroblast aging, although cGMP and its ratio to cAMP could still turn out to be important.

Clotting Factors. Circulating clotting elements interact extensively with fixed tissues such as endothelial and connective tissue cells,[226] thus linking the dual processes of hemostasis and wound healing. Recent studies indicate that polymerizing fibrin also interacts with cultured fibroblasts and that this process becomes impaired during normal aging in vitro.[227] Thus, less fibrin is bound by old cells and subsequently incorporated into the mature gelatinous clot. This effect may involve the loss of a membrane-associated receptor for fibrin or for the closely related activating enzyme, thrombin.[138]

Still another clotting defect occurs during aging in vitro. Normally, vigorous retraction of the fibrin clot occurs in young normal cells, so that it soon occupies less than half of the original volume. This retraction is significantly reduced in aging normal cultures and those from progeria and Werner syndrome.[128]

Human fibroblasts also contain a "tissue factor" with potent thromboplastic activity.[228] In effect, it short circuits the intrinsic clotting mechanism via the extrinsic system.[229] Activity of this factor increases in aging normal cells and is particularly high at all stages in strains from progeria and Werner syndrome.[230] Studies with a specific antiserum prepared against normal tissue factor suggest that, rather than being altered qualitatively, this material is more abundant in aging cells.

Molecular Basis for Altered Proteins. A primary basis has not yet been defined for aging in vitro nor for the diversity of altered proteins, but the familiar possibilities of error and program still apply. Preliminary results show that proteolysis is reduced in aging cultures despite the presence of an increasing fraction of defective proteins.[225] This would account for an enzyme complement that is more abundant but of a lower functional quality. These observations are compatible with most of the molecular theories of aging, although it is likely that a primary defect at one site will in time lead to diverse repercussions at many sites.

It must be appreciated that the slowdown of cell growth per se associated with aging may contribute to the findings. Thus, as the production of daughter cells containing newly synthesized complements of cell proteins diminishes, the turnover time of each cell protein is correspondingly prolonged. This in itself may lead to posttranslational modification and denaturation, which is entirely consistent with the picture during aging in vitro. However, progeria strains are clearly unique because they contain a relatively high percentage of defective proteins while they grow with normal vigor. In their case, therefore, a more primary defect in protein synthesis or degradation is the most likely possibility, although a disturbance at a higher level, such as multiple somatic mutations, cannot be dismissed. In fact, progeria cells may have a decreased capacity for DNA repair which appears earlier and with greater severity than in normal aging cultures.[231] This mechanism could provide a single common denominator to explain the diversity of altered proteins in early-passage progeria cells. It is also possible, however, that enzymes for DNA repair are only passively involved in a more generalized, fundamental disturbance of protein metabolism.

Other possibilities also exist. The ability of aging cells to maintain requisite concentrations of substrates and cofactors may deteriorate. It is known that these factors often stabilize the proteins that act upon them, and in fact old cells become leaky for amino acids.[225]

Other early results, which fit the program notion best, have recently been presented in fetal fibroblasts. Chromatin template activity for RNA synthesis, whether directed by endogenous or exogenous RNA polymerase, is decreased in aging cells.[232] Additionally, old cells contain an increased amount of a specific DNA-binding protein that binds preferentially to single-stranded DNA.[233] Perhaps the rise in DNA polymerase activity seen after continuous subculture of normal strains represents a feedback loop at the molecular level attempting to overcome a DNA template of diminished quality.[234]

PRACTICAL IMPLICATIONS OF AGING IN VITRO

Pathologic

There is clearly a large hiatus between cultured fibroblasts and in vivo realities, but some exciting patterns are already apparent. Although the general blunting of regenerative responses in vivo can be principally ascribed to the diminished mitotic capacity of cells, it would be naive to interpret every age-dependent decrement on this basis. In fact, lethal diseases intervene long before we have exhausted the mitotic capacities of all stem cells. Accordingly, impaired wound healing may not only be a result of impaired mitotic potential but could also reflect the diminished ability of cells to interact with circulating hemostatic factors such as fibrin. The recalcitrant ulcers of Werner syndrome are a particularly cogent example, although it may be argued that peripheral vascular occlusion is primarily responsible. However, growing evidence now links the vascular disease of diabetics and aging normal populations.[235–238] Thus, byproducts arising from repeated cell death could impair blood flow in the microvasculature by encroaching on the lumen. A similar mechanism could contribute to the rising prevalence of hypertension in aging populations, especially diabetics, and could also play a role in the macrovascular atherogenic process.[153,154] The augmented predisposition of patients with progeria. Werner syndrome and diabetes to atherothrombotic diseases may also relate to defective interaction of circulating elements, such as platelets and fibrin, with "fixed" cells in the blood vessel wall[154] whose proliferative ability, clot retraction, and production of coagulation factors is clearly abnormal.[138,230]

Insights from studies of HLA antigen expression are also potentially informative. Very early in the life of normal individuals cells would have a uniform growth capacity. Eventually, dominant clones would arise with a high growth capacity and stable HLA expression. Thus, during normal wear and tear, these clones would serve to repopulate a given microscopic patch of tissue. When the dominant clones begin to age, destabilization of HLA antigens (and other antigenic systems) would occur. The fate of lesser clones throughout this time is unknown, but perhaps each aging clone forms a nidus for the rising number of discrete pathologic foci seen during normal biologic aging.[239] There is abundant evidence that several age-related diseases in normal individuals are clonal in origin, including atherosclerosis,[240] solid tumors, myelomas, and leukemias,[241] as well as autoimmune and degenerative processes.[242] The rising incidence of these disorders during normal aging and their frequently precocious appearance in syndromes of accelerated aging (Table 151-2) could relate not only to impaired immune surveillance consequent to altered expression of crucial surface antigens, but also to defective enzyme proteins involved in regulating cellular metabolism.

Altered enzymes and hormone receptors may provide a basis for the explanation of such diverse but frequent observations as insulin resistance of diabetes and peculiar drug responses of the elderly. Defects similar to but of a smaller magnitude than familial hypercholesterolemia may also occur during aging of the cultured cell so that a lesion could develop in a membrane receptor for a low-density lipoprotein.[243] As a result, several contingent events would fail to occur, resulting in the build up of cholesterol in arterial cells and the development of atheromatous foci.

Therapeutic and Preventative

Rational approaches to therapy are almost always facilitated by understanding the problem in molecular terms. The best example is sickle cell disease, the first molecular defect to be elucidated. After it was found that hydrophobic valine substitutes for hydrophilic glutamic acid in the β chain of hemoglobin, we learned that hydrophobic bonds were responsible for the aggregation of hemoglobin molecules and the sickling phenomenon. This led to the use of urea (which disrupts hydrophobic bonds) and, currently, the more efficacious sodium cyanate.[244]

The present state of aging research suggests that many proteins are defective, perhaps for diverse reasons, so that intervention may be difficult at this level. Indeed, it may turn out that the primary defect is impaired information flow from RNA or DNA. However, influencing events at these levels may be unduly heroic and even harmful despite currently popular notions of gene therapy. Thus, it may be easier and preferable to carry out environmental rather than genetic engineering. For example, some enzyme defects respond nicely to increasing the cofactor concentration by megavitamin intake. In other cases, a harmful enzymopathy can be circumvented simply by proscribing the intake of a potentially harmful nutrient, e.g., galactose in galactosemia.

Other more empirical forms of treatment may also suffice. It seems clear that minimizing cell turnover, particularly in the vascular tree and in epithelial surfaces, may delay the appearance of certain age-related diseases. For example, good nutrition and maintenance of ideal, lean body weight may optimize hormone–fuel balance and, in particular, suppress the levels of insulin, a known mitogen. Reducing hypertension may retard atherogenesis, and shielding the skin from excessive exposure to the sun (especially in xeroderma pigmentosum), and the bronchi from cigarette smoke and pollution, may delay or prevent carcinoma. Recent evidence indicates that vitamin E added to the culture fluid of human fibroblasts not only prolongs their calendar life span, but also allows a significant number of additional, vigorous cell divisions prior to senescence.[207] Simultaneously, the appearance of the age pigment, lipofuscin, is delayed.[245] If vitamin E works as a general antioxidant that minimizes damage from free radical attack on vital cellular components, then perhaps vitamin C will also be of value. Additionally, cortisol has been shown to prolong the life span of cultured fibroblasts, perhaps by stabilizing the lysosome.[246] In any case, whether empirical or specifically tailored to discrete molecular lesions, intervention in the aging process should be enhanced by tissue culture research. It must be stated emphatically, however, that the aims of treatment and prevention are no different from those of standard medical practice: to extend the vigorous years of life with dignity.

CONCLUSIONS

Many gaps still exist in our understanding of the aging process. A primary pacemaker, perhaps hormonal and in the thymus, the hypothalamus, or at a higher level of function within the central nervous system, could still be discovered, although it is difficult to imagine that an identical primary pacemaker is at fault in each person. The multiplicity of aberrant genes that cause the diverse syndromes of premature aging (Table 151-2) makes this seem unlikely. Rather more plausible is the idea that the fundamental process is inherent in all or at least a majority of cells.

Meanwhile, it is reasonable to suggest that biologic aging is a physiologic process, an epilogue of development originating within the genome and the adaptive norm of the species. Errors undoubtedly arise at low frequency during normal genetic expression and, although most are rectified, subtle changes must escape detection even in the presence of fully functional surveillance mechanisms. Indeed, the correction of all deviations from the norm would have imperiled evolution itself. Senescence would still be consistent with high biologic fitness, since this concept implies only the capability to reproduce.

The inherited load sets the limits for the basic genetic program. At the polar extreme, homozygous lethal mutations, by definition, abort all programs soon after conception. Along a spectrum of severity are other homozygous recessive or even dominant mutations that allow gestation to proceed and a viable organism to be born; but such mutations may be expressed later in life as a wide variety of disease states, often incompatible with vigorous health or even attainment of maturity. However, most persons are probably heterozygous for a considerable number of "silent" recessive lethal and detrimental mutations that act between conception and postmaturity.

Moreover, it is probable that each member of the species is a unique chemical entity, in part due to subtle variants at several genetic loci, making many of us not homozygous but heterozygous at multiple alleles. In fact, several variant or polymorphic genes probably act in concert to determine the rate of aging as a multifactorial or continuously distributed trait. Some gene combinations may even confer a survival advantage in a given environment and at an early stage at the expense of premature aging in another environment or at a later stage. The example of sickle cell hemoglobin again comes to the fore. The heterozygous condition of sickle cell trait confers a survival advantage in areas where malaria is endemic, but it becomes disadvantageous in temperate climates. It has also been proposed that diabetes represents a multifactorial state, conferring a survival advantage under conditions of privation while being harmful during times of plenty.[247,248]

The salient point is that the functional genotype is dynamic. Although the genome of all cells is presumably identical, each differentiated cell performs a unique but changing function throughout life. Therefore, the viability of each cell is not only a function of the individual genotype and state of differentiation, but also of the elapsed time and cumulative environmental exposure. It follows that aging proceeds along a very uneven front, occurring sooner in some cells and later in others, even within clones of a given cell type. Indeed, as techniques allow, it may become possible to demonstrate that each cell ages uniquely.

To reintegrate and summarize, during the aging process the relationships between cells, tissues, and organs, organized as multitiered feedback loops that orchestrate bodily function into an efficient bodily whole, begin to break down. In the language of communications, the "signal-to-noise" ratio decreases.[249] Compensatory increases in signal output only aggravate the noise production and lead finally to systems failure. Senescence, then, is a normal physiologic process. It is the price we pay to maintain decorum in the bodily community of cells during the inexorable decline that culminates in the destruction of each individual organism but maximizes the adaptive fitness of future generations.

Addendum

Several articles on aging have appeared since concluding the original literature search, but only a selected few can be cited.

Following a review of the available data, Finch has espoused the idea of a neuroendocrine pacemaker of biologic aging rather than a process intrinsic to each cell.[251]

The previous claim[207] that vitamin E prolongs the replicative life span of cultured fibroblasts could not be substantiated;[252] in more recent experiments, fibroblast growth in media containing different lots of serum augmented with exogenous vitamin E at 10, 50, and 100 μg/ml failed to show any extension of life span due to the vitamin. Linn et al.[253] have shown, in contrast to others,[234] that DNA polymerase activity falls in late-passage fibroblasts. Of greater significance, "old" DNA polymerase had a substantial increase in error frequency in catalyzing the replication of artificial DNA templates. The implications of this synthetic infidelity for in vivo aging would be a generalized increase in the mutation frequency with ominous consequences for cell viability and the development of pathology. However, Schneider and Mitsui, while confirming that donor age is a prime determinant of replicative life span, have cautioned that aging in vitro, as related to passage level, may only have limited applications to biologic aging in vivo.[254]

Rowe et al. have demonstrated that growth is impaired in cultured skin fibroblasts from both juvenile- and adult-onset diabetics.[255] This strengthens the idea of Goldstein et al., based on earlier work[196] and a recent larger series,[256] that the diabetic genotype has a detrimental effect on fibroblast growth. The studies of Rowe et al. have also indicated that hydrocortisone stimulation of total protein synthesis and collagen synthesis is increased in adult-onset diabetics but decreased in the juvenile form or normal controls. Thus, hydrocortisone may unmask differences in protein synthesis that distinguish the two forms of diabetes.

REFERENCES

1. Norris, A. H., Lundy, T., Shock, N. W., Trends in selected indices of body composition in men between the ages 30 and 80 years. *Ann NY Acad Sci 110:* 623, 1963.
2. Wurtman, R. J., Cardinali, D. P., The pineal organ. In Williams, R. H. (ed): *Textbook of Endocrinology,* 5th ed. Philadelphia, Saunders, 1974, pp 832–840.
3. Frohman, L. A., Clinical neuropharmacology of hypothalamic releasing factors. *N Engl J Med 286:* 1391, 1972.
4. Schally, A. V., Arimura, A., Kasten, A. J., Hypothalamic regulatory hormones. *Science 179:* 341, 1973.
5. Bellamy, D, Hormonal effects in relation to aging in mammals. In Woolhouse, H. W. (ed): *Aspects of the Biology of Aging, Symposia of the Society for Experimental Biology,* No XXI. Cambridge, University Press, 1967, pp 427–453.
6. Gusseck, D. J., Endocrine mechanisms and aging. *Adv Gerontol Res 4:* 105, 1972.
7. Gregerman, R. I., Bierman, E. L., Aging and hormones. In Williams, R. H. (ed): *Textbook of Endocrinology,* 5th ed. Philadelphia, Saunders, 1974, pp 1059–1070.
8. Pincus, G., Romanoff, L. P., Carlo, J., The excretion of urinary steroids by men and women of various ages. *J Gerontol 9:* 113–131, 1954.
9. Pincus, G., Steroid hormones and aging in man. In Zarrow, M. X. (ed): *Growth in Living Systems.* New York, Basic Books, 1961.
10. Longcope, C., Metabolic clearance and blood production rates of estrogens in postmenopausal women. *Am J Obstet Gynecol 111:* 778, 1971.
11. Judd, H. L., Judd, G. E., Lucas, W. E., et al., Endocrine function of the postmenopausal ovary: concentration of androgens and estro-

gens in ovarian and peripheral vein blood. *J Clin Endocrinol Metab 39:* 1020, 1974.

12. Gherondache, C. N., Romanoff, L. P., Pincus, G., Steroid hormones in aging men. In Gitman, L. (ed): *Endocrines and Aging.* Springfield, Ill, Thomas, 1967, pp 76–101.
13. Hemsell, D. L., Grodin, J. M., Brenner, P. F., et al, Plasma precursors of estrogen: correlation of the extent of conversion of plasma androstenedione to estrone with age. *J Clin Endocrinol Metab 38:* 476, 1974.
14. Albert, A., Randall, R. V., Smith, R. A., et al, Urinary excretion of gonadotropin as a function of age. In Engle, E. R., Pincus, G. (eds): *Hormones and the Aging Process.* New York, Academic, 1956, pp 49–62.
15. Taymor, M. L., Toshihiro, A., Pheteplace, C., Serum levels of FSH and LH by radioimmunoassay. In Rosemberg (ed): *Gonadotropins 1968, Proceedings of the Workshop Conference, Vista Hermosa, Mor, Mexico.* Los Angeles, California, Geron-X, 1968, pp. 349–365.
16. Sherman, B. M., Korenman, S. G., Hormonal characteristics of the human menstrual cycle throughout reproductive life. *J Clin Invest 55:* 699, 1975.
17. Reyes, F. I., Winter, J. S. D., Faiman, C., Transition in pituitary–ovarian relationships preceding the menopause. *Clin Res 22:* 733A, 1974.
18. Seyler, E. L., Jr., Reichlin, S., Luteinizing hormone–releasing factor (LRF) in Plasma of Postmenopausal Women. *J Clin Endocrinol Metab 37:* 197, 1973.
19. Migeon, C. J., Keiler, A. R., Lawrence, B., et al, Dehydroepiandrosterone and androsterone levels in human plasma. *J Clin Endocrinol 17:* 1051, 1957.
20. Hollander, N., Hollander, V. P., The microdetermination of testosterone in human spermatic vein blood. *J Clin Endocrinol 18:* 966, 1958.
21. Rubens, R., Dhont, M., Vermeulen, A., Further studies on Leydig cell function in old age. *J Clin Endocrinol Metab 39:* 40, 1974.
22. Stearns, E. L., MacDonnell, J. A., Kaufman, B. J., et al, Declining testicular function with age. *Am J Med 57:* 761, 1974.
23. Vermeulen, A., Rubens, R., Verdonck, L., Testosterone secretion and metabolism in male senescence. *J Clin Endocrinol 34:* 730, 1972.
24. Kley, H. K., Nieschlag, E., Bidlingmaier, F., et al, Possible age-dependent influence of estrogens on the binding of testosterone in plasma of adult men. *Horm Metab Res 6:* 213, 1974.
25. Debeljuk, L., Arimura, A., Schally, A. V., Pituitary responsiveness to LH-releasing hormone in intact female rats of different ages. *Endocrinology 90:* 1499, 1972.
26. Spona, J., Luger, O., In vitro stimulation of LH release by LH-RH in female rat pituitaries of different ages. *FEBS Lett 32:* 52, 1973..
27. Snyder, P. J., Utiger, R. D., Response to thyrotropin releasing hormone (TRH) in normal man. *J Clin Endocrinol 34:* 380, 1972.
28. Snyder, P. J., Utiger, R. D., Thyrotropin response to thyrotropin releasing hormone in normal females over 40. *J Clin Endocrinol 34:* 1096, 1972.
29. Rubenstein, H. A., Bulter, V. P., Jr., Werner, S. C., Progressive decrease in serum triiodothyronine concentrations with human aging: radioimmunoassay following extraction of serum. *J Clin Endocrinol Metab 37:* 247, 1973.
30. Azizi, F., Vagenakis, A. G., Portnay, G. I., et al, Pituitary–thyroid responsiveness to intramuscular thyrotropin-releasing hormone based on analysis of serum thyroxine, tri-iodothyronine and thyrotropin concentrations. *N Engl J Med 292:* 273, 1975.
31. Gregerman, R. I., Effects on thyroid hormone economy: intrinsic physiological variables and nonthyroidal illness; environmental effects. In Werner, S. C., Sidney, H. I. (ed): *The Thyroid: A Fundamental and Clinical Test,* 3rd ed. New York, Harper & Row, 1971, pp 137–152.
32. Andrew, W., The anatomy of aging in man and animals. New York, Grune & Stratton, 1971.
33. Lutz, J. H., Gregerman, R. I., Spaulding, S. W. et al, Thyroxine binding proteins, free thyroxine and thyroxine turnover interrelationships during acute infectious illness in man. *J Clin Endocrinol Metab 35:* 230, 1972.
34. Jefferys, P. M., Hoffenberg, R., Farran, H. E. A. et al, Thyroid-function tests in the elderly. *Lancet 1:* 924, 1972.
35. Mayberry, W. E., Gharib, H., Bilstad, J. M. et al, Radioimmunoassay for human thyrotropin: clinical value in patients with normal and abnormal thyroid function. *Ann Intern Med 74:* 471, 1971.
36. Verzár, F., Anterior pituitary function in age. In Harris, G. W., Donovan, B. T. (eds): *The Pituitary Gland, vol. 2.* Berkeley, University of California Press, 1966, pp 444–459.
37. Gregerman, R. I., The age-related alteration of thyroid function and thyroid hormone metabolism in man. In Gitman, L. (ed): *Endocrines and Aging.* Springfield, Ill, Thomas, 1967, pp 161–173.
38. Keys, A., Taylor, H. L., Grande, F., Basal metabolism and age of adult man. *Metabolism 22:* 579, 1973.
39. O'Malley, B. W., Means, A. R., Female steroid hormones and target cell nuclei. *Science 183:* 610, 1974.
40. Surks, M. I., Koerner, D. H., Oppenheimer, J. H., In vitro binding of L-triiodothyronine to receptors in rat liver nuclei. *J Clin Invest 55:* 50, 1975.
41. Grad, B., The metabolic responsiveness of young and old female rats to thyroxine. *J Gerontol 24:* 5, 1969.
42. Geffner, D. L., Azukizawa, M., Hershman, J. M., Propylthiouracil blocks extrathyroidal conversion of thyroxine to triiodothyronine and augments thyrotropin secretion in man. *J Clin Invest 55:* 224, 1975.
43. Romanoff, L. P., Morris, G. W., Welch, P. et al, The metabolism of cortisol-4-C^{14} in young and elderly men. I. Secretion rate of cortisol and daily secretion of tetrahydrocortisol, allotetrahydrocortisol, tetrahydrocortisone and cortilone. *J Clin Endocrinol 21:* 1413, 1961.
44. West, C. D., Brown, H., Simons, E. L. et al, Adrenocortical function and cortisol metabolism in old age. *J Clin Endocrinol 21:* 1197, 1961.
45. Samuels, L. T., Effect of aging on the steroid metabolism as reflected in plasma levels. In Engle, E. T., Pincus, G. (eds): *Hormones and the Aging Process.* New York, Academic, 1956, pp 21–38.
46. Blichert-Toft, M., Assessment of serum corticotrophin concentration and its nyctohemeral rhythm in the aging. *Gerontol Clin 13:* 215, 1971.
47. Moncloa, F., Gomez, R., Pretell, E., Response to corticotrophin and correlation between excretion of creatinine and urinary steroids and between the clearance of creatinine and urinary steroids in aging. *Steroids 1:* 437, 1963.
48. Yamaji, T., Ibayashi, H., Plasma dehydroepiandrosterone sulfate in normal and pathological conditions. *J Clin Endocrinol 29:* 273, 1969.
49. Robertson, O. H., Wexler, B. C., Histological changes in the organs and tissues of migrating and spawning Pacific salmon (genus Oncohynchus). In Robertson, O. H. (ed): *Endocrines and Aging.* New York, MSS Information, 1972, pp 10–27.
50. Riegle, G. D., Nellor, J. E., Changes in adrenocortical function during aging in cattle. *J Gerontol 22:* 83, 1967.
51. Riegle, G. D., Przekop, F., Nellor, J. E., Changes in adrenocortical responsiveness to ACTH infusion in aging goats. In Robertson, O. H. et al. (eds): *Endocrines and Aging.* New York, MSS Information, 1972, pp 33–36.
52. Breznock, E. M., McQueen, R. D., Adrenocortical function during aging in the dog. In Robertson, O. H. et al. (eds): *Endocrines and Aging.* New York, MSS Information, 1972, pp 28–32.
53. Hess, G. D., Riegle, G. D., Effects of chronic ACTH stimulation on adrenocortical function in young and aged rats. *Am J Physiol 222:* 1458, 1972.
54. Oparil, S., Haber, E., The renin–angiotensin system. *N Engl J Med 291:* 389, 446, 1974.
55. Flood, C., Gherondache, C., Pincus, G. et al, The metabolism and secretion of aldosterone in elderly subjects. *J Clin Invest 46:* 960, 1967.
56. Tuck, M. L., Williams, G. H., Cain, J. P. et al, Relation of age, diastolic pressure and known duration of hypertension to presence of low renin essential hypertension. *Am J Cardiol 32:* 637, 1973.
57. Rapp, J. P., Age-related pathologic changes, hypertension, and 18-hydroxydeoxycorticosterone in rats selectively bred for high or low juxtaglomerular granularity. *Lab Invest 28:* 343, 1973.
58. Stewart, J., Genetic studies on the mechanism of action of aldosterone in mice. *Endocrinology 96:* 711, 1975.
59. Dunihue, F. W., Reduced juxtaglomerular cell granularity, pituitary neurosecretory material and width of the zona glomerulosa in aging rats. In Robertson, O. H. et al (eds): *Endocrines and Aging.* New York, MSS Information, 1972, pp 37–40.

60. Laragh, J. H., Sealey, J. E., Buhler, F. R. et al, The renin axis and vasoconstriction volume analysis for understanding and treating renovascular and renal hypertension. *Am J Med 58:* 4, 1975.
61. Hollenberg, N. K., Adams, D. F., Solomon, H. S. et al, Senescence and the renal vasculature in normal man. *Circ Res 34:* 309, 1974.
62. Laron, Z., Doron, M., Amikam, B., Plasma growth hormone in men and women over 70 years of age. In Brunner, D., Jokl, E. (eds): *Medicine and Sport, vol 4.* White Plains, N. Y., Phiebig, 1969, pp 126–131.
63. Dudl, R. J., Ensinck, J. W., Palmer, H. E. et al, Effect of age on growth hormone secretion in man. *J Clin Endocrinol Metab 37:* 11, 1973.
64. Cartlidge, N. E. F., Black, M. M., Hall, M. R. P. et al, Pituitary function in the elderly. *Gerontol Clin 12:* 65, 1970.
65. Sachar, E. J., Finklestein, J., Hellman, L., Growth hormone responses in depressive illnesses. I. Response to insulin tolerance test. *Arch Gen Psychiatry 25:* 263, 1971.
66. Carlson, H. E., Gillin, J. C., Gorden, P. et al, Absence of sleep-related growth hormone peaks in aged normal subjects and in acromegaly. *J Clin Endocrinol Metab 34:* 1102, 1972.
67. Aitken, J. M., Gallagher, M. J. D., Hart, D. M. et al, Plasma growth hormone and serum phosphorus concentrations in relation to the menopause and to oestrogen therapy. *J Endocrinol 59:* 593, 1973.
68. Root, A. W., Oski, F. A., Effects of human growth hormone in elderly males. *J Gerontol 24:* 97, 1969.
69. Pecile, A., Muller, E., Falconi, G. et al, Growth hormone–releasing activity of hypothalamic extracts at different ages. *Endocrinology 77:* 241, 1965.
70. Shire, J. G., Growth hormone and premature aging. *Nature 245:* 215, 1973.
71. Denckla, W. D., A time to die. *Life Sci 16:* 31, 1975.
72. Fujita, T., Orimo, H., Okano, K. et al, Radioimmunoassay of serum parathyroid hormone in postmenopausal osteoporosis. *Endocrinology 19:* 571, 1972.
73. Orimo, H., Fujita, T., Yoshikawa, M., Increased sensitivity of bone to parathyroid hormone in ovariectomized rats. *Endocrinology 90:* 760, 1972.
74. Davis, M. E., Lanzl, L. H., Strandjord, N. M., Estrogens and the aging process. The detection, prevention, and retardation of osteoporosis. *JAMA 196:* 219, 1966.
75. Hirsch, P. F., Munson, P. L., Thyrocalcitonin. *Physiol Rev 49:* 548, 1969.
76. Riggs, B. L., Jowsey, J., Kelly, P. J. et al, Treatment for postmenopausal and senile osteoporosis. *Med Clin North Am 56:* 989, 1972.
77. Kärki, N. T., The urinary excretion of noradrenaline and adrenaline in different age groups, its diurnal variation and the effect of muscular work on it. *Acta Physiol Scand 39*[*Suppl 132*]: 1, 1956.
78. Cohen, S. I., Shmavonian, B. M., Catecholamines, vasomotor conditioning and aging. In Gitman, L. (ed): *Endocrines and Aging.* Springfield, Ill, Thomas, 1967, pp 102–141.
79. Dilman, V. M., Age-associated elevation of hypothalamic threshold to feedback control, and its role in development, aging, and disease. *Lancet 1:* 1211, 1971.
80. Frolkis, V. V., Bezrukov, V. V., Duplenko, Y. K. et al, The hypothalamus in aging. *Exp Gerontol 7:* 169, 1972.
81. Christensen, N. J., Plasma noradrenaline and adrenaline in patients with thyrotoxicosis and myxoedema. *Clin Sci Mol Med 45:* 162, 1973.
82. Robinson, D. S., Changes in monamine oxidase and monamines with human development and aging. *Fed Proc 34:* 103, 1975.
83. Vernadakis, A., Neuronal–glial interactions during development and aging. *Fed Proc 34:* 89, 1975.
84. Finch, C. E., Catecholamine metabolism in the brains of aging male mice. *Brain Res 52:* 261, 1973.
85. Goldstein, A. L., Hooper, J. A., Schulof, R. S. et al, Thymosin and the immunopathology of aging. *Fed Proc 33:* 2053, 1974.
86. Goldstein, G., Scheid, M., Hammerling, U. et al, Isolation of a polypeptide that has lymphocyte-differentiating properties and is probably represented universally in living cells. *Proc Natl Acad Sci USA 72:* 11, 1975.
87. Marx, J. L., Inducers of T cell maturation. *Science 187:* 1183, 1217, 1975.
88. Tapp, E., Huxley, M., The histological appearance of the human pineal gland from puberty to old age. *J Pathol 108:* 137, 1972.
89. Friedman, S. M., Friedman, C. L., Nakashima, M., Adrenal–neurohypophyseal regulation of electrolytes and work performance age-related changes in the rat. In Gitman, L. (ed): *Endocrines and Aging.* Springfield, Ill, Thomas, 1967, pp 142–160.
90. Lindeman, R. D., Lee, T. D. Jr., Yiengst, M. J. et al, Influence of age, renal disease, hypertension, diuretics and calcium on the antidiuretic responses to suboptimal infusions of vasopressin. *J Lab Clin Med 68:* 206, 1966.
91. Weissman, P. N., Shenkman, L., Gregerman, R. I., Chlorpropamide hyponatremia: drug-induced inappropriate antidiuretic-hormone activity. *N Engl J Med 284:* 65, 1971.
92. Andres, R., Aging and diabetes. *Med Clin North Am 55:* 835, 1971.
93. Duckworth, W. C., Kitabchi, A. E., Direct measurement of plasma proinsulin in normal and diabetic subjects. *Am J Med 53:* 418, 1972.
94. Volk, B. W., Lazarus, S. S., Pathology of the pancreas and liver in diabetes mellitus. In Ellenberg, M., Rifkin, H (eds): *Diabetes Mellitus: Theory and Practice.* New York, McGraw-Hill, 1970, pp 150–177.
95. Gepts, W., Pathology of islet tissue in human diabetes. In Greep, R. O. et al, (eds): *Handbook of Physiology, section 7: Endocrinology, vol 1.* Washington, DC, American Physiological Society, 1972, pp 289–303.
96. Madsbad, S., Faber, O. K., Binder, M. D., et al, Prevalence of residual beta-cell function in insulin-dependent diabetics in relation to age at onset and duration of diabetes. *Diabetes* (Suppl 1): 262, 1978.
97. Boyns, D. R., Crossley, J. N., Abrams, M. E. et al, Oral glucose tolerance and related factors in a normal population sample. I. Blood sugar plasma insulin, glyceride, and cholesterol measurements and the effects of age and sex. *Br Med J 1:*595, 1969.
98. Sherwin, R. S., Insel, P. A., Tobin, J. D. et al, Computer modeling: an aid to understanding insulin action. *Diabetes 21* [*Suppl 1*]*:* 347, 1972.
99. Chlouverakis, C., Jarrett, R. J., Keen, H., Glucose tolerance, age, and circulating insulin. *Lancet 1:* 806, 1967.
100. Johansen, K., A new principle for the comparison of insulin secretory responses. 1. The effect of age on insulin secretion. *Acta Endocrinol 74:* 511, 1973.
101. Johansen, K., Mild diabetes in young subjects. Clinical aspects and plasma insulin response pattern. *Acta Med Scand 193:* 23, 1973.
102. Ginsberg, H., Kimmerling, G., Olefsky, J. M. et al, Demonstration of insulin resistance in untreated adult onset diabetic subjects with fasting hyperglycemia. *J Clin Invest 55:* 454, 1975.
103. Woods, S. C., Porte, D. Jr., Neural control of the endocrine pancreas. *Physiol Rev 54:* 596, 1974.
104. Adelman, R. C., Impaired hormonal regulation of enzyme activity during aging. *Fed Proc 34:* 179, 1975.
105. Olefsky, J. M., Reaven, G. M., Decreased insulin binding to lymphocytes from diabetic subjects. *J Clin Invest 54:* 1323, 1974.
106. Schwartz, R. H., Bianco, A. R., Handwerger, B. S. et al, Demonstration that monocytes rather than lymphocytes are the insulin-binding cells in preparation of human peripheral blood mononuclear leukocytes: implications for studies of insulin-resistant states in man. *Proc Natl Acad Sci USA 72:* 474, 1975.
107. Archer, J. A., Gorden, P., Roth, J., Defect in insulin binding to receptors in obese man. *J Clin Invest 55:* 166, 1975.
108. Amatruda, J. M., Livingston, J. N., Lockwood, D. H., Insulin receptor: role in the resistance of human obesity to insulin. *Science 188:* 264, 1975.
109. Dudl, R. J., Ensinck, J. W., The role of insulin, glucagon, and growth hormone in carbohydrate homeostasis during aging. *Diabetes 21:* 357, 1972.
110. Sakurai, H., Dobbs, R., Unger, R. H., Somatostatin-induced changes in insulin and glucagon secretion in normal and diabetic dogs. *J Clin Invest 54:* 1395, 1974.
111. Gerich, J. E., Lorenzi, M., Hane, S. et al, Evidence for a physiologic role of pancreatic glucagon in human glucose homeostasis: studies with somatostatin. *Metabolism 24:* 175, 1975.
112. Samorajski, T., Rolsten, C., Age and regional differences in the chemical composition of brains of mice, monkeys and humans. *Prog Brain Res 40:* 253, 1973.
113. Cicero, T. J., Ferrendelli, J. A., Suntzeff, V., Regional changes in CNS levels of the S-100 and 14-3-2 proteins during development and aging of the mouse. *J Neurochem 19:* 2119, 1972.
114. Kanungo, M. S., Patnaik, S. K., Koul, O., Decrease in 17β-oestradiol receptor in brain of aging rats. *Nature 253:* 366, 1975.

115. Walker, J. B., Walker, J. P., Properties of adenylate cyclase from senescent rat brain. *Brain Res 54:* 391, 1973.
116. Massa, P., Stupnicka, E., Kniewald, Z. et al, The transformation of testosterone into dihydrotestosterone by the brain and the anterior pituitary. *J Steroid Biochem 3:* 385, 1972.
117. Leathem, J. H., Albrecht, E. D., Effect of age on testis delta5-3beta-hydroxysteroid dehydrogenase in the rat. *Proc Soc Exp Biol Med 145:* 1212, 1974.
118. Weddington, S. C., McLean, W. S., Nayfeh, et al, Androgen binding protein (ABP) in rabbit testis and epididymis. *Steroids 24:* 123, 1974.
119. Clemens, J. A., Meites, J., Neuroendocrine status of old constant-estrous rats. *Neuroendocrinology 7:* 249, 1971.
120. Smithline, F., Sherman, L., Kolodny, H. D., Prolactin and breast carcinoma. *N Engl J Med 292:* 784, 1975.
121. Roth, G. S., Age-related changes in specific glucocorticoid binding by steroid-responsive tissues of rats. *Endocrinology 94:* 82, 1974.
122. Manganiello, V., Vaughan, M., Selective loss of adipose cell responsiveness to glucagon with growth in the rat. *J Lipid Res 13:* 12, 1972.
123. Forn, J., Schonhofer, P. S., Skidmore, I. F. et al, The effect of aging on adenyl cyclase and phosphodiesterase activity of isolated fat cells of the rat. *Biochem Biophys Acta 208:* 304, 1970.
124. Livingston, J. N., Cuatrecasas, P., Lockwood, D. H., Studies of glucagon resistance in large rat adipocytes: 1-labeled glucagon binding and lipolytic capacity. *J Lipid Res 15:* 26, 1974.
125. Bjorntorp, P., Effects of age, sex, and clinical conditions on adipose tissue cellularity in man. *Metabolism 23:* 1091, 1974.
126. Bitensky, M. W., Russell, V., Blanco, M., Independent variation of glucagon and epinephrine responsive components of hepatic adenyl cyclase as a function of age, sex and steroid hormones. *Endocrinology 86:* 154, 1970.
127. Cohen, M. L., Berkowitz, B. A., Age-related changes in vascular responsiveness to cyclic nucleotides and contractile agonists. *J Pharmacol Exp Ther 191:* 147, 1974.
128. Denckla, W. D., Role of the pituitary and thyroid glands in the decline of minimal O_2 consumption with age. *J Clin Invest 53:* 572, 1974.
129. Lefkowitz, R. J., Isolated hormone receptors—physiologic and clinical implications. *N Engl J Med 288:* 1061, 1973.
130. Williams, R. H., Thompson, W. J., Effect of age upon guanyl cyclase, adenyl cyclase, cyclic nucleotide phosphodiesterases in rats. *Proc Soc Biol Med 143:* 382, 1973.
131. Norris, A. H., Shock, N. W., Aging and variability. *Ann NY Acad Sci 134:* 591, 1966.
132. Goldstein, S., The biology of aging. *N Engl J Med 285:* 1120, 1971.
133. Strehler, B. L., Implications of aging research for society. *Fed Proc 34:* 5, 1975.
134. Leaf, A., Unusual longevity: the common denominators. *Hosp Practice 8:* 75, 1973.
135. Comfort, A., Measuring the human ageing rate. *Mech Ageing and Dev 1:* 101, 1972.
136. Lansing, A. I., General biology of senescence. In Birren, J. E. (ed): *Handbook of Aging and the Individual: Psychological and Biological Aspects.* Chicago, University of Chicago Press, 1959, pp 119–135.
137. Kallmann, Q. J., Jarvik, L. F., Individual differences in constitution and genetic background. In Birren, J. E. (ed): *Handbook of Aging and the Individual: Psychological and Biological Aspects.* Chicago, University of Chicago Press, 1959, pp 216–263.
138. Goldstein, S., Niewiarowski, S., Singal, D. P., Pathological implications of cell aging in vitro. *Fed Proc 34:* 56, 1975.
139. Epstein, C. J., Martin, G. M., Schultz, A. L. et al, Werner's syndrome: a review of its symptomatology, natural history, pathologic features, genetics and relationship to the natural aging process. *Medicine (Baltimore) 45:* 177, 1966.
140. DeBusk, F. L., The Hutchinson-Gilford progeria syndrome. *J Pediatr 80:* 697, 1972.
141. Villee, D. B., Nichols, G. Jr., Talbot, N. B., Metabolic studies in two boys with classical progeria. *Pediatrics 43:* 207, 1969.
142. Andrew, W., *The Anatomy of Aging in Man and Animals.* New York, Grune & Stratton, 1971.
143. Thomas, J. H., Powell, D. E. B., *Blood Disorders in the Elderly.* Bristol, Wright, 1971.
144. Weksler, M. E., Hutteroth, T. H., Impaired lymphocyte function in aged humans. *J Clin Invest 53:* 99, 1974.
145. Makinodan, T., Adler, W. H., Effects of aging on the differentiation and proliferation potentials of cells of the immune system. *Fed Proc 34:* 153, 1975.
146. Williamson, A. R., Askonas, B. A., Senescence of an antibody-forming cell clone. *Nature 238:* 337, 1972.
147. Till, J. E., McCulloch, E. A., Siminovitch, L., Isolation of variant cell lines during serial transplantation of hematopoietic cells derived from fetal liver. *J Natl Cancer Inst 33:* 707, 1964.
148. Harrison, D. E., Normal production of erythrocytes by mouse marrow continuous for 73 months. *Proc Natl Acad Sci USA 70:* 3184, 1973.
149. Bucher, N. L. R., Malt, R. A., *Regeneration of Liver and Kidney.* Boston, Little, Brown, 1971.
150. Urist, M. R., Accelerated aging and premature death of bone cells in osteoporosis. In Pearson, O. H., Joplin, G. F. (eds): *Dynamic Studies of Metabolic Bone Disease.* Oxford, Blackwell, 1964, pp 127–160.
151. Daniel, C. W., Aidells, B. D., Medina, D. et al, Unlimited division potential of precancerous mouse mammary cells after spontaneous or carcinogen-induced transformation. *Fed Proc 34:* 64, 1975.
152. Sussman, M. D., Aging of connective tissue: physical properties of healing wounds in young and old rats. *Am J Physiol 224:* 1167, 1973.
153. Martin, G. M., Sprague, C. A., Symposium on in vitro studies related to atherogenesis: life histories of hyperplastoid cell lines from aorta and skin. *Exp Mol Pathol 18:* 125, 1973.
154. Ross, R., Glomset, J., Kariya, B. et al, A platelet-dependent serum factor that stimulates the proliferation of arterial smooth muscle cells in vitro. *Proc Natl Acad Sci USA 71:* 1207, 1974.
155. Post, J., Hoffman, J., Cell renewal patterns. *N Engl J Med 279:* 248, 1968.
156. Logothetopoulos, J., Islet cell regeneration and neogenesis. In Greep, R. O. et al (eds): *Handbook of Physiology, Section 7: Endocrinology, vol 1, Endocrine Pancreas.* Washington, DC, American Physiological Society, 1972, pp 67–76.
157. Verzár, F., Anterior pituitary function in age. In Donovan, B. T., Harris, G. W. (eds): *The Pituitary Gland, vol 2.* Berkeley, University of California Press, 1966.
158. Price, G. B., Modak, S. P., Makinodan, T., Age-associated changes in the DNA of mouse tissue. *Science 171:* 917, 1971.
159. Chetsanga, C. J., Boyd, V., Peterson, L. et al, Single-stranded regions in DNA of old mice. *Nature 253:* 130, 1975.
160. Goldstein, S., Moerman, E. J., Defective proteins in normal and abnormal human fibroblasts during aging in vitro. *Interdiscipl Topics Geront 10:* 24, 1976.
161. Orgel, L. E., Ageing of clones of mammalian cells. *Nature 243:* 441, 1973.
162. Goldberg, A. L., Dice, J. F., Intracellular protein degradation in mammalian and bacteria cells. *Ann Rev Biochem 43:* 835, 1974.
163. Yarus, M., Corrective processes in replication, transcription and translation. *Gerontologia (in press).*
164. Capecchi, M. R., Capecchi, N. E., Hughes, S. H. et al, Selective degradation of abnormal proteins in mammalian tissue culture cells. *Proc Natl Acad Sci USA 71:* 4732, 1974.
165. Strehler, B., Hirsch, G., Gusseck, D. et al, Codon-restriction theory of aging and development. *J Theor Biol 33:* 429, 1971.
166. Young, V. R., Steffee, W. P., Pencharz, P. B. et al, Total human body protein synthesis in relation to protein requirements at various ages. *Nature 253:* 192, 1975.
167. Cristofalo, V. J., Animal cell cultures as a model system for the study of aging. *Adv Gerontol Res 4:* 45, 1972.
168. Finch, C. E., Enzyme activities, gene function and ageing in mammals. *Exp Gerontol 7:* 53, 1972 (review).
169. Wilson, P. D., Enzyme changes in ageing mammals. *Gerontologia 19:* 79, 1973.
170. VonHahn, H. P., The regulation of protein synthesis in the ageing cell. *Exp Gerontol 5:* 323, 1970.
171. Stein, G. S., Stein, J. S., Kleinsmith, L. J., Chromosomal proteins and gene regulation. *Sci Am 232:* 47, 1975.
172. Ryan, J. M., Cristofalo, V. J., Histone acetylation during aging of human cells in culture. *Biochem Biophys Res Commun 48:* 735, 1972.
173. Liew, C. C., Gornall, A. G., Covalent modification of nuclear proteins during aging. *Fed Proc 34:* 186, 1975.
174. Holliday, R., Pugh, J. E., DNA modification mechanisms and gene activity during development. *Science 187:* 226, 1975.

175. Medvedev, Z. A., Repetition of molecular-genetic information as a possible factor in evolutionary changes of life span. *Exp Gerontol 7:* 227, 1972.
176. Cutler, R. G., Redundancy of information content in the genome of mammalian species as a protective mechanism determining aging rate. *Mech Ageing Dev 2:* 381, 1973–74.
177. Soukupová, M., Holečková, E., Hněvkovský, P., Changes of the latent period of explanted tissues during ontogenesis. In Holečková, E., Cristofalo, V. J. (eds): *Aging in Cell and Tissue Culture.* New York, Plenum, 1970, pp 41–56.
178. Waters, H., Walford, R. L., Latent period for outgrowth of human skin explants as a function of age. *J Gerontol 25:* 381, 1970.
179. Goldstein, S., Moerman, E. J., Soeldner, J. S. et al, Diabetes mellitus and prediabetes: decreased replicative capacity of cultured fibroblasts. *J Clin Invest 53:* 27a, 1974.
180. Papayannopoulou, T. G., Martin, G. M., Albaline phosphatase "constitutive" clones: evidence for de-novo heterogeniety of established human skin fibroblast strains. *Exp Cell Res 45:* 72, 1966.
181. Franks, L. M., Cooper, T. W., The origin of human embryo lung cells in culture: a comment on cell differentiation, in vitro growth and neoplasia. *Int J Cancer 9:* 19, 1972.
182. Castor, C. W., Prince, R. K., Dorstewitz, E. L., Characteristics of human fibroblasts cultivated in vitro from different anatomical sites. *Lab Invest 11:* 703, 1962.
183. Martin, G. M., Sprague, C. A., Epstein, C. J., Replicative life-span of cultivated human cells. *Lab Invest 23:* 86, 1970.
184. O'Lague, P. H., Obata, K., Claude, P. et al, Evidence for cholinergic synapses between dissociated rat sympathetic neurons in cell culture. *Proc Natl Acad Sci USA 71:* 3602, 1974.
185. Hayflick, L., Moorhead, P. S., The serial cultivation of human diploid cell strains. *Exp Cell Res 25:* 585, 1961.
186. Hayflick, L., The limited in vitro lifetime of human diploid cell strains. *Exp Cell Res 37:* 614, 1965.
187. Pontén. J., Spontaneous and virus induced transformation in cell culture. In Gard, S., Hallauer, C., Meyer, K. F. (eds). New York, Springer, 1971.
188. Gold, P., Antigenic reversion in human cancer. *Ann Rev Med 22:* 85, 1971.
188a. Court Brown, W. M., *Human Population Cytogenetics.* Amsterdam, North-Holland, 1967.
189. Raivio, K. O., Seegmiller, J. E., Genetic diseases of metabolism. *Ann Rev Biochem 41:* 543, 1972.
190. Martin, G. M., Hoehn, H., Genetics and human disease. *Hum Pathol 5:* 387, 1974.
191. Goldstein, S., Somatic cell genetics. *Can Med Assoc J 105:* 738, 1971.
192. German, J., Genes which increase chromosomal instability in somatic cells and predispose to cancer. *Prog Med Genet 8:* 61, 1972.
193. Miller, R. W., Todaro, G. J., Viral transformation of cells from persons at high risk of cancer. *Lancet 1:* 81, 1969.
194. Nadler, H. L., Chacko, C. M., Rachmeler, M., Interallelic complementation in hybrid cells derived from human diploid strains deficient in galactose-1-phosphate uridyl transferase activity. *Proc Natl Acad Sci USA 67:* 976, 1970.
195. Tedesco, T. A., Mellman, W. J., Argininosuccinate synthetase activity and citrulline metabolism in cells cultured from a citrullinemic subject. *Proc Natl Acad Sci USA 57:* 829, 1967.
196. Goldstein, S., Littlefield, J. W., Soeldner, J. S., Diabetes mellitus and aging: diminished plating efficiency of cultured human fibroblasts. *Proc Natl Acad Sci USA 64:* 155, 1969.
197. Goldstein, S., Moerman, E. J., Heat-labile enzymes in Werner's syndrome fibroblasts. *Nature 255:* 159, 1975.
198. Goldstein, S., Lifespan of cultured cells in progeria. *Lancet 1:* 424, 1969.
199. Martin, G. M., Sprague, C. A., Norwood, T. H. et al, Clonal selection, attenuation and differentiation in an in vitro model of hyperplasia. *Am J Pathol 74:* 137, 1974.
200. Goldstein, S., Moerman, E. J., Heat-labile enzymes in skin fibroblasts from subjects with progeria. *N Engl J Med 292:* 1305, 1975.
201. Goldstein, S., Aging in vitro: growth of cultured cells from the Galapagos tortoise. *Exp Cell Res 83:* 297, 1974.
202. Goldstein, S., The role of DNA repair in aging of cultured fibroblasts from xeroderma pigmentosum and normals. *Proc Soc Exp Biol Med 137:* 730, 1971.
203. Hsu, T. C., Cooper, J. E. K., On diploid cell lines. *J Natl Cancer Inst 53:* 1431, 1974.
204. Hayflick, L., The longevity of cultured human cells. *J Am Geriatr Soc 22:* 1, 1974.
205. Stanley, J. F., Pye, D., MacGregor, A., Comparison of doubling numbers attained by cultured animal cells with life span of species. *Nature 255:* 158, 1975.
206. Szilard, L., On the nature of the aging process. *Proc Natl Acad Sci USA 45:* 30, 1959.
207. Packer, L., Smith, J. R., Extension of the lifespan of cultured normal human diploid cells by vitamin E. *Proc Natl Acad Sci USA 71:* 4763, 1974.
208. Dell'Orco, R. T., Mertens, J. G., Kruse, Jr. P. F., Doubling potential, calendar time, and senescence of human diploid cells in culture. *Exp Cell Res 77:* 356, 1973.
209. Goldstein, S., Singal, D. P., Senescence of cultured human fibroblasts: mitotic versus metabolic time. *Exp Cell Res 88:* 359, 1974.
210. Holliday, R., Tarrant, G. M., Altered enzymes in ageing human fibroblasts. *Nature 238:* 26, 1972.
211. Lewis, C. M., Tarrant, G. M., Error theory and ageing in human diploid fibroblasts. *Nature 239:* 316, 1972.
212. Beutler, E., Glucose-6-phosphate dehydrogenase deficiency. In Stanbury, J. B., Wyngaarden, J. B., Fredrickson, D. S. (eds): *The Metabolic Basis of Inherited Disease,* 3rd ed. New York, McGraw-Hill, 1972, pp 1358–1388.
213. Kelley, W. N., Meade, J. C., Studies on hypoxanthine-guanine phosphoribosyltransferase in fibroblasts from patients with the Lesch-Nyhan syndrome. *J Biol Chem 246:* 2953, 1971.
214. Holliday, R., Porterfield, J. S., Gibbs, D. D., Premature ageing and occurrence of altered enzyme in Werner's syndrome fibroblasts. *Nature 248:* 762, 1974.
215. Goldstein, S., Singal, D. P., Alteration of fibroblast gene products in vitro from a subject with Werner's syndrome. *Nature 251:* 719, 1974.
216. Brautbar, C., Pellegrino, M. A., Ferrone, S. et al, Fate of HLA antigens in aging cultured human diploid cell strains. II. Quantitative absorption studies. *Exp Cell Res 78:* 367, 1973.
217. Smith, J. R., Hayflick, L., Variation in the life-span of clones derived from human diploid cell strains. *J Cell Biol 62:* 48, 1974.
218. Kelley, L. A., Butcher, R. W., The effects of epinephrine and prostaglandin E_1 on cyclic adenosine 3′:5′-monophosphate levels in W1–38 fibroblasts. *J Biol Chem 249:* 3098, 1974.
219. Haslam, R., Goldstein, S., Adenosine 3′:5′-cyclic monophosphate in young and senescent human fibroblasts during growth and stationary phase in vitro. Effects of prostaglandin E_1 and of adrenaline. *Biochem J 144:* 253, 1974.
220. Rosenthal, J., Goldstein, S., The effect of insulin on basal and hormone-induced elevations of cyclic AMP content in cultured human fibroblasts. *J Cell Physiol 85:* 235, 1975.
221. Gavin, J. R. III, Roth, J., Jen, P. et al, Insulin receptors in human circulating cells and fibroblasts. *Proc Natl Acad Sci USA 69:* 747, 1972.
222. Hollenberg, M. D., Cuatrecasas, P., Insulin and epidermal growth factor: human fibroblast receptors related to deoxyribonucleic acid synthesis and amino acid uptake. *J Biol Chem 250:* 3845, 1975.
223. Rosenbloom, A. L., Goldstein, S., Rosenbloom, E. K. et al, The insulin receptor (InR) of cultured human fibroblasts (HF). *Clin Res 23:* 329A, 1975.
224. Rosenbloom, A. L., Goldstein, S., Yip, C. C., Insulin binding to cultured human fibroblasts increases with normal and precocious aging. *Science 193:* 412, 1976.
225. Goldstein, S., Cordeiro, R. A. J., Decreased proteolysis and increased amino acid efflux in aging human fibroblasts. *Mech Aging and Develop 5:* 221, 1976.
226. Niewiarowski, S., Markiewicz, M., Nath, N., Inhibition of the platelet-dependent fibrin retraction by the fibrin stabilizing factor (FSF, factor XIII). *J Lab Clin Med 81:* 641, 1973.
227. Niewiarowski, S., Goldstein, S., Interaction of cultured human fibroblasts with fibrin: modification by drugs and aging in vitro. *J Lab Clin Med 82:* 605, 1973.
228. Zacharski, L. R., McIntyre, O. R., Membrane-mediated synthesis of tissue factor (thromboplastin) in cultured fibroblasts. *Blood 41:* 679, 1973.
229. Maynard, J. R., Heckman, C. A., Pitlick, F. A. et al, Association of Tissue Factor Activity with the Surface of Cultured Cells. *J Clin Invest 55:* 814, 1975.
230. Goldstein, S., Niewiarowski, S., Increased procoagulant activity in cultured fibroblasts from progeria and Werner's syndromes of premature aging. *Nature 260:* 711, 1976.

231. Epstein, J., Williams, J. R., Little, J. B., Rate of DNA repair in progeric and normal human fibroblasts. *Biochem Biophys Res Commun 59*: 850, 1974.
232. Ryan, J. M., Cristofalo, V. J., Chromatin template activity during aging in W138 cells. *Exp Cell Res 90:* 456, 1975.
233. Stein, G. H., DNA-binding proteins in young and senescent normal human fibroblasts. *Exp Cell Res 90:* 237, 1975.
234. Giblak, R. E., McCoy, E. E., Studies on deoxyribonucleic acid polymerase from normal and Down's syndrome skin fibroblasts in vitro. *In Vitro 10:* 167, 1974.
235. Kilo, C., Vogler, N., Williamson, J. R., Muscle capillary basement membrane changes related to aging and to diabetes mellitus. *Diabetes 21:* 881, 1972.
236. Siperstein, M. D., Raskin, P., Burns, H., Electron microscopic quantification of diabetic microangiopathy. *Diabetes 22:* 514, 1973.
237. Vracko, R., Benditt, E. P., Manifestations of diabetes mellitus: their possible relationships to an underlying cell defect. *Am J Pathol 75:* 204, 1974.
238. Vracko, R., Benditt, E. P., Restricted replicative life-span of diabetic fibroblasts in vitro: its relation to microangiopathy. *Fed Proc 34:* 68, 1975.
239. Howell, T. H., Multiple pathology in a septuagenarian. *J Am Geriatr Soc 16:* 760, 1968.
240. Benditt, E. P., Benditt, J. M., Evidence for a monoclonal origin of human atherosclerotic plaques. *Proc Natl Acad Sci USA 70:* 1753, 1973.
241. Fialkow, P. J., Use of genetic markers to study cellular origin and development of tumors in human females. *Adv Cancer Res 15:* 191, 1972.
242. Walford, R. L., Immunologic theory of aging: current status. *Fed Proc 33:* 2020, 1974.
243. Brown, M. S., Faust, J. R., Goldstein, J. L., Role of the low density lipoprotein receptor in regulating the content of free and esterified cholesterol in human fibroblasts. *J Clin Invest 55:* 783, 1975.
244. Cerami, A., Peterson, C. M., Cyanate and sickle-cell disease. *Sci Am 232:* 45, 1975.
245. Deamer, D. W., Gonzales, J., Autofluourescent structures in cultured W1-38 cells. *Arch Biochem Biophys 165:* 421, 1974.
246. Christofalo, V. J., Metabolic aspects of aging in diploid human cells. In Holeckova, E, Cristofalo, V. J. (eds): *Aging in Cell and Tissue Culture*. New York, Plenum, 1970, pp 83–119.
247. Neel, J. V., The genetics of diabetes mellitus. In Camerini-Dávalos, R., Cole, H. S. (eds): *Early Diabetes, Advances in Metabolic Disorders, Suppl 1.* New York, Academic, 1970, pp 3–10.
248. Goldstein, S., On the pathogenesis of diabetes mellitus and its relationship to biological aging. *Humangenetik 12:* 83, 1971.
249. Goldstein, S., Commentary: biological aging—an essentially normal process. *JAMA 230:* 1651, 1974.
250. Swift, M., Sholman, L., Gilmour, D., Diabetes mellitus and the gene for Fanconi's anemia. *Science 178:* 308, 1972.
251. Finch, C. E., The regulation of physiological changes during mammalian aging. *Q. Rev Biol 51:* 49, 1976.
252. Packer, L., Smith, J. R., Extension of the lifespan of cultured normal human diploid cells by vitamin E: a reevaluation. *Proc Natl Acad Sci USA 74:* 1640, 1977.
253. Linn, S., Kairis, M., Holliday, R., Decreased fidelity of DNA polymerase activity isolated from aging human fibroblasts. *Proc Natl Acad Sci USA 73:* 2818, 1976.
254. Schneider, E. L., Mitsui, Y., The relationship between in vitro cellular aging and in vivo human age. *Proc Natl Acad Sci USA 73:* 3584, 1976.
255. Rowe, D. W., Starman, B. J., Fujimoto, W. Y., Williams, R. H., Abnormalities in proliferation and protein synthesis in skin fibroblast cultured from patients with diabetes mellitus. *Diabetes 26:* 284, 1977.
256. Goldstein, S., Moerman, E. J., Soeldner, J. S., Gleason, R. E., Barnett, D. M., Diabetes mellitus and genetic prediabetes: decreased replicative capacity of cultured skin fibroblasts. *Diabetes 27* (Suppl 2): 459, 1978.
257. Goldstein, S., Human genetic disorders that feature premature onset and accelerated progression of biological aging. In Schneider, E. L. (ed): The Genetics of Aging. New York, Plenum Press, 1978, pp. 171–224.

General Principles of Endocrine Pathophysiology

152

Quantitation of the Production, Distribution, and Interconversion of Hormones

Jack H. Oppenheimer
Erlio Gurpide

INTRODUCTION

The clinical effects of a hormone depend on a variety of kinetic factors not directly reflected by the amounts of the hormone, or its precursors and products, present in biologic fluids. Thus, if the average plasma concentration of a given hormone in a population is Z and a patient has a concentration of $3Z$, the clinician may anticipate evidence of *excessive* hormonal effects. In other words, a positive correlation between the concentration of that hormone and the hormone effect at a tissue level is assumed. Although such "common sense" assumptions are helpful in the transaction of everyday affairs, they are not universally reliable. For instance, elevation of serum thyroxine in a patient receiving estrogens does not necessarily connote increased hormonal activity since such elevation may result from increased plasma binding without changes in the free hormone plasma or total tissue concentrations.[1] A similar example is found with the glucocorticoids during pregnancy. In pregnancy or during estrogen treatment, the higher plasma concentration of the hormone is due to a slower fractional metabolism rather than to an elevated rate of secretion of the hormone.[2,3] Regarding the measurement of urinary metabolites, for example, the rate of excretion of testosterone glucuronoside in women does not reflect the amount of testosterone to which the patient is exposed, since the metabolite may be formed in the liver from precursors, such as dehydroisoandrosterone sulfate, without actual liberation of testosterone into circulation.[4] In these examples, any assumed positive correlation between hormone concentration and effect would be "counterintuitive."

In this chapter, we shall survey some of the principles involved in formal kinetic analysis of problems in tracer methodology. We shall address ourselves primarily to the general endocrinologist who looks to kinetic analysis as a tool to solve a set of specific problems. We shall try to provide a working definition of the basic concepts and to outline the general approaches that are commonly used to quantitate the production, distribution, and interconversion of hormones. Limitations in the applicability of these models will be emphasized. Special attention will also be directed to plasma-binding proteins because of their importance as factors in determining the concentration of steroid and thyroid hormones in plasma, their body distribution, and their clearance from plasma. For a more comprehensive treatment of the subject, the reader is referred to other publications.[5–8]

SINGLE-COMPARTMENT SYSTEM

A didactic introduction to tracer kinetics is provided by the consideration of a single-compartment system. Such a system would be adequate to describe a situation in which the intravenously injected tracer is rapidly mixed throughout the body with the endogenous hormone before being excreted or metabolized, and in which the hormone does not participate in reversible metabolic conversions.

The volume of the compartment (V) is defined as the ratio of the total mass of hormone in the compartment to the concentration of hormone in plasma (c), and is thus expressed in units of plasma volume equivalents. If the labeled hormone is concentrated in interstitial and cellular spaces, the volume of distribution may exceed both the plasma and interstitial body water. The significance of the concept of distribution volume lies in that it allows estimation of the total mass of hormone in the system. If the distribution volume of a substance per kilogram of body weight were reasonably constant for a species, one could estimate the mass of hormone simply by determining the plasma concentration and the weight of the animal.

An important kinetic parameter is the fractional removal rate (λ), which refers to the fraction of the total body mass or pool of hormone (P) removed per unit time under steady-state conditions,

Supported by National Institute's of Health Grant AM 19812 and National Cancer Institute Grant CA 15648.

i.e., when the rate of production of hormone equals the rate of total removal. Irreversible removal includes both metabolic and excretory processes. Thus, in a single-compartment system, the turnover rate equals λP.

The metabolic clearance rate (MCR) is another useful concept, which denotes the volume of plasma irreversibly cleared of hormone per unit time. By definition,

$$\text{MCR} = \frac{\text{Rate of removal}}{\text{Concentration in peripheral plasma}} = \frac{\lambda P}{c} = \frac{\lambda V c}{c} = \lambda V.$$

The concept of MCR is useful because, in general, it represents a relatively constant biologic characteristic of a given hormone in a given species within a physiologic range of concentrations. Once the MCR is known, it is possible to provide an estimate of the turnover rate of the hormone simply from its plasma concentration, and vice versa.

These parameters are estimated from isotopic studies in which the tracer is administered intravenously either as a single injection or as a constant infusion. Calculations are based on the following considerations.

PULSE INJECTION

The rate of removal of a tracer is proportional to the amount of tracer present in the compartment. In a single-compartment system, at any time *(t)* following injection,

$$\frac{dc^*}{dt} = -\lambda c^* \qquad (1)$$

where c^* is the concentration of labeled hormone (* indicates the isotopic label). This equation can be solved to yield

$$c^* = c_0^* e^{-\lambda t} \qquad (2)$$

where c_0^* is the labeled hormone concentration at $t = 0$. From equation 2, it follows that

$$\ln\left(\frac{c^*}{c_0^*}\right) = -\lambda t \qquad (3)$$

and

$$\ln c^* = -\lambda t + \ln c_0^*. \qquad (4)$$

This equation then predicts that for a single compartment the logarithm of the radioactive hormone concentration declines as a linear function of time, justifying the use of plots on semilogarithmic paper (Fig. 152-1). The slope of this decay line is λ, the fractional removal rate. It follows from equation 3 that when $c = \frac{1}{2} c_0^*$, $\ln \frac{1}{2} = -\lambda t_{1/2}$ or $\ln 2 = \lambda t_{1/2}$. Therefore,

$$\lambda = \frac{0.693}{t_{1/2}} \qquad (5)$$

where $t_{1/2}$ is the time when $c^* = \frac{1}{2} c_0^*$.

The $t_{1/2}$ of a substance in a single compartmental system is thus inversely related to the fractional removal rate. The initial concentration, c_0^*, can be determined from the ordinate intercept. From c_0^* and the injected dose (D^*), the volume of distribution can be conveniently calculated from the relationship $V = D^*/c_0^*$.

The average length of time that the tracer remains within the compartment is the mean residence time $(\bar{t})$. By definition, $1/\bar{t}$ of the total pool will be removed per unit time. Then $P/\bar{t} = \lambda P$ and

$$\bar{t} = \frac{1}{\lambda} \qquad (6)$$

From equation 5, it follows that $\bar{t} = 1.44\, t_{1/2}$.

CONSTANT INFUSION

A common technique for the administration of hormone is the continuous infusion of tracer at a constant rate. Following the start of the infusion there is a progressive increase in the concentration

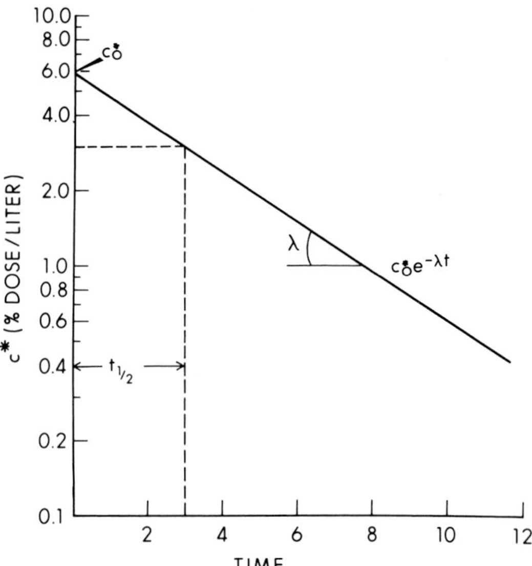

Fig. 152-1. Plasma decay of labeled hormone in an ideal single-compartmental system after pulse injection. c*, concentration of radioactively labeled hormone; λ, fractional rate of removal; $t_{1/2} = 0.693/\lambda$. The decay is represented by a straight line when plotted on semilogarithmic axes.

of radioactively labeled hormone (Fig. 152-2). Eventually, a steady-state relationship will supervene when the rate of infusion of hormone is equal to the rate of disposal. At that point, the concentration of the labeled hormone (c_{ss}^*) will be constant:

$$I^* = \lambda V c_{ss}^* = \text{MCR} \times c_{ss}^* \qquad (7)$$

where I^* is rate of infusion, or

$$\text{MCR} = \frac{I^*}{c_{ss}^*} \qquad (8)$$

In other words, the MCR can be simply calculated from the known rate of infusion of the labeled hormone, I^*, and the steady-state value of labeled hormone in plasma, c_{ss}^*. Equation 8 is not restricted to the single-compartment state, but is valid for any system regardless of compartmental complexity.

Also of interest is the curve describing the increase in labeled hormone from the start of infusion and the curve describing the fall off in the plasma concentration of labeled hormone following cessation of infusion. In a single-compartment system, at any time *(t)* during infusion of the tracer,

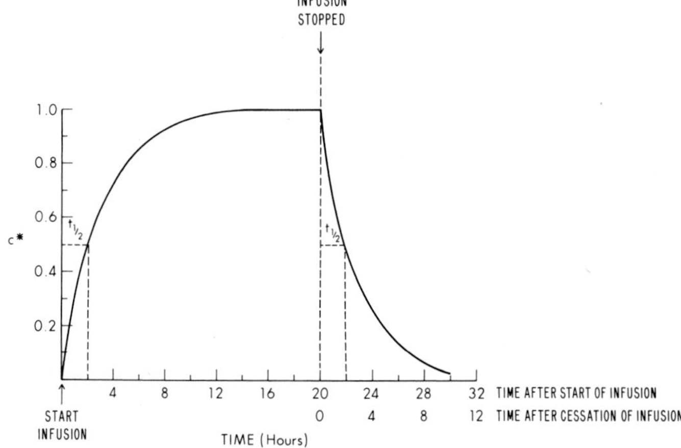

Fig. 152-2. Increase of plasma radioactivity (c^*) following start of constant infusion and decrement in plasma concentration after cessation of infusion in an ideal single-compartment system.

$$\frac{d\,(Vc^*)}{dt} = I^* - \lambda\,(Vc^*)$$

that is, the total body pool of labeled hormone ($P^* = Vc^*$) changes at a rate equal to the difference between the instantaneous rate of infusion and removal from the compartment. Solving this differential equation, we obtain

$$c^* = \frac{I^*}{\lambda V}(1 - e^{-\lambda t}). \tag{9}$$

Thus, when $t \to \infty$, $c^*_{ss} = I^*/\lambda V$, as already shown by equation 7. Similarly, if the infusion is discontinued at time t_s once the steady state is reached, it follows from equation 2 that

$$c^* = c^*_{ss}\; e^{-\lambda(t-t_s)} \tag{10}$$

It is thus apparent that λ can be obtained both from the rate of increase and from the decrease in radioactivity following the start and cessation of infusion. Since the MCR can be estimated from the steady-state value of the tracer concentration, it is possible to calculate the distribution volume from the relationship V = MCR/λ.

MEASUREMENT OF EXCRETED RADIOACTIVITY

The accumulation of radioactivity in urine and feces is sometimes used to calculate the metabolic parameters discussed above. This method is particularly useful in the study of iodothyronine metabolism.[9] For the purposes of simplicity of presentation, we shall consider the combined excretion by all pathways following a pulse injection of labeled hormone into a single compartmental system. Excreted radioactivity (U^*) may represent either the administered isotope or a metabolic derivative. If we assume no significant delay in excretion or accumulation of metabolites in the body, the rate of accumulation of radioactivity in the excretory compartment is the negative of the rate of decrease within the body, i.e.,

$$\frac{dU^*}{dt} = \frac{-dP^*}{dt} = +\lambda P^* = \lambda V\, c_0^* e^{-\lambda t} = \lambda D^* e^{-\lambda t}. \tag{11}$$

Solution of equation 11 yields

$$U^* = D^*\,(1-e^{-\lambda t}). \tag{12}$$

Equation 12 therefore represents the cumulative excretion of isotope following the pulse injection of labeled hormone under the idealized conditions specified above. The relationship in equation 12 is also readily apparent from equation 2 since

$$\begin{aligned} U^* &= D^* - \text{radioactivity remaining in body} \\ &= D^* - D^* e^{-\lambda t} = D^*\,(1-e^{-\lambda t}). \end{aligned}$$

or

$$\ln \frac{D^* - U^*}{D^*} = -\lambda t.$$

At the steady state during infusion of the tracer at a constant rate, $dU^*/dt = \lambda V c^*_{ss}$, or

$$\frac{dU^*/dt}{c^*_{ss}} = \lambda V = \text{MCR}. \tag{13}$$

The MCR could therefore be estimated at the steady state from the ratio of the total excretory rate and the plasma concentration.

MULTICOMPARTMENT SYSTEMS

Under most circumstances, the distribution and metabolism of a hormone cannot be accurately described by a single-compartment model. This situation becomes evident when the semilogarithmic plot of the plasma concentrations of the tracer versus time after an intravenous injection of the labeled hormone does not yield a straight line. Delayed reentry of the tracer into circulation after distribution in other spaces, or after reversible conversions to other compounds, is responsible for the deviation from a single exponential decay curve. The resulting curve can usually be described by a function consisting of 2–4 exponential terms. The values of the coefficients and exponents corresponding to the best fitting curve can be estimated using computer or graphic methods. The computer-implemented numerical methods yield a function that minimizes the deviations between the analytical curve and the data, within the limitations imposed by the estimated measurement errors. The basis for the graphic technique of "curve-stripping" is apparent in Figure 152-3 which represents a curve of disappearance of the tracer from plasma approximated by a function with 2 exponential terms:

$$c^* = Ae^{-\lambda_1 t} + Be^{-\lambda_2 t}. \tag{14}$$

The constant λ_2 characterizes the slope of the terminal plasma disappearance curve when plotted semilogarithmically. The intercept of the extrapolated terminal portion of the curve ($Be^{-\lambda_2 t}$) with the ordinate axis is B (Fig. 152-3). Moreover, subtraction of $Be^{-\lambda_2 t}$ from c^* yields $Ae^{-\lambda_1 t}$. This term will clearly be represented as a straight line when plotted as a function of t in the same graph, and therefore λ_1 and A can be evaluated graphically.

When the experimental points do not show a single exponential decline in the concentration of the tracer in plasma, hence preventing the application of a single-compartment analysis, two general approaches are usually followed: analysis of the data on the basis of multicompartment models or application of formulas derived from noncompartmental analysis.

In the multicompartmental approach, the number of compartments in the model used depends in part on the system under study and in part on the detail in which certain types of information are sought. For a complete description of the thyroid hormone system, Berman has proposed the use of 14 compartments.[8] Some problems in steroid dynamics have been analyzed on the basis of a restricted 2-compartment system,[10,11] partially justified by a satisfactory description of the experimental data (disappearance of labeled aldosterone or cortisol from plasma) by double exponential functions. However, most of the currently used parameters of hormone dynamics are obtained following a noncompartmental approach.

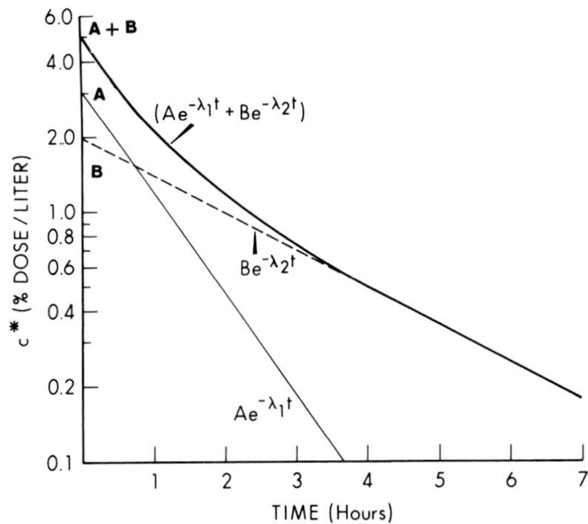

Fig. 152-3. The function $c^* = Ae^{-\lambda_1 t} + Be^{-\lambda_2 t}$ represents the decay in plasma radioactivity in a two-compartment model. This function is obtained from experimental data by the technique of "curve-stripping." See text for details.

NONCOMPARTMENTAL APPROACH

Whereas maximal information from the plasma disappearance curve is obtained when the number and the relationships of the compartments can be explicitly defined, the necessary data for such compartmental formulation are often not available. It is therefore desirable to employ noncompartmental techniques in which information can be obtained without the necessity of making specific assumptions about the number and relationships of the compartments in the system under study.

The analysis to follow is applicable to the interpretation of isotopic data obtained by using the two techniques for the intravenous administration of the tracer that have already been discussed.

CONSTANT INFUSION

We have previously described the process of infusing labeled hormone at a constant rate into the plasma compartment. Regardless of the number of compartments in the system, a constant plasma concentration of labeled hormone is attained when the system is at the steady state, i.e., when the rate of infusion of radioactive hormone is equal to the rate of irreversible removal of the tracer.

Since, by definition,

$$MCR = \frac{\text{Rate of irreversible removal from plasma}}{\text{Concentration in plasma}} \qquad (15)$$

and the infused and endogenous hormones entering the circulation have the same fate, then MCR $= I^*/c^*_{ss}$, where I^* is the rate of infusion and c^*_{ss} is the tracer concentration at the steady state. If all hormone produced in the body is secreted into circulation, it follows that MCR $\times\ c$ = PR, where c is the concentration of endogenous hormone and PR, the turnover rate, is the "plasma production rate." In order to shorten the time at which equilibrium is attained, a priming dose is frequently injected during the initial phase of the infusion. It is always necessary to be certain that an isotopic steady state has been attained by documenting the achievement of a constant plasma concentration of the labeled hormone. If the period of observation is not sufficiently long, a small but significant increase in concentration can easily be overlooked and false results may be obtained.[12]

PULSE INJECTION

The rate of irreversible removal of the labeled hormone from plasma is given, by definition, by the expression dm^*/dt = MCR $\times\ c^*$, or dm^* = MCR $\times\ c^*dt$. Integrating from $t = 0$ to $t = \infty$, we obtain

$$MCR = \frac{D^*}{\int_0^\infty c^*\,dt} \qquad (16)$$

where D^* is the dose injected. Since $\int_0^\infty c^*\,dt$ is the area under the plasma disappearance curve from $t = 0$ to $t = \infty$, metabolic clearance rate can be calculated simply by dividing the dose injected by this area. Formally, the calculation of the total area can be obtained by integration of the function fitting the experimental points derived by the computer or the "curve-stripping" method. Thus, if the function is that shown in equation 14, then

$$\int_0^\infty c^*\,dt = \int_0^\infty (Ae^{-\lambda_1 t} + Be^{-\lambda_2 t})\,dt = \frac{A}{\lambda_1} + \frac{B}{\lambda_2}$$

and

$$MCR = \frac{D^*\lambda_1\lambda_2}{A\lambda_2 + B\lambda_1}.$$

It should be noted, however, that in extrapolating from $t = 0$ and $t = \infty$, assumptions must be made about the nature of the disappearance curve beyond the limits of the sampling period.

A graphic procedure can be used to carry out the integration to $t = \infty$. In the semilogarithmic plot of the disappearance of the tracer from plasma, an arbitrary point, c^*_m, corresponding to t_m in the region where the fractional rate of disappearance becomes constant (terminal straight line), is chosen. It is then possible to evaluate the integral $\int_0^\infty c^*\,dt$ by breaking it into two components:

$$\int_0^\infty c^*\,dt = \int_0^{t_m} c^*\,dt + \int_{t_m}^\infty c^*\,dt.$$

The integral $\int_0^{t_m} c^*\,dt$ is evaluated graphically by measuring the area under the curve and the second integral

$$\int_{t_m}^\infty c^*\,dt = \int_{t_m}^\infty c^*_m\,e^{-\lambda(t-t_m)}\,dt = \frac{c^*_m}{\lambda} = \frac{c^*_m}{0.693}(t_{1/2})_{\text{terminal}}$$

is evaluated directly. The terminal slope of disappearance should be determined with precision since the second component may be a significant proportion of the total integral. A judicious distribution of sampling times is important in order to obtain a maximally reliable curve.

Whether to estimate the MCR by constant infusion or a single-dose injection should be determined primarily by the practical aspects of the problem. When equilibrium is rapidly attained, an infusion may be the simplest approach. When many days are required to attain equilibrium, constant infusion is no longer practical and a single-dose injection should be considered.

The product of the MCR and plasma concentration of the hormone is designated as its "plasma production rate," which represents a minimal estimate of total rate of production of the hormone. The reason for a potential discrepancy in the value of these parameters is easy to appreciate. Assume, for instance, that the hormone being traced is also produced outside of the initial distribution compartment as a result of conversion from a precursor. Assume at the same time that the hormone produced by conversion does not exchange with plasma hormone. It is readily apparent that the hormone resulting from conversion would not be adequately traced by an intravenous injection of label. Under many circumstances, however, exchange with the hormone formed outside of the initial distribution compartment is nearly complete. Under these circumstances, the plasma production rate will approximate the total turnover rate of the hormone. This appears to be the case for thyroxine (T_4) and triiodothyronine (T_3).

The volume of initial distribution of a hormone is usually estimated from isotopic data obtained following an intravenous injection of the tracer. As already discussed when a single compartment was considered, $V = D^*/c^*_0$, where c^*_0 represents the extrapolation to $t = 0$ of the curve of disappearance of the tracer from circulation. When this curve is multiexponential; c^*_0 can be evaluated from the sum of the coefficients of each term. For instance, in the case described by equation 14, $V = 100/(A + B)$, where c^* is expressed as 90 percent of the injected dose per unit volume plasma.

The volume of initial distribution is frequently desired in studies of rapidly metabolized steroid hormones, in which samples are obtained at short intervals after injection of the tracer. In contrast, studies of slowly metabolized T_4 or cholesterol have placed less emphasis on early sampling and showed more concern with the total volume of distribution of the compound in the whole body. An approximation to this total volume is provided by a parameter that can be estimated from tracer experiments—the "recirculation volume" (V_R), previously designated as the volume of the "exchangeable pool."[13] This volume stands in contrast to the volume containing hormone not returning to plasma, the "volume of nonrecirculation (V_N)" (Fig. 152-4). The total volume of distribution V_T is then the sum of V_R and V_N.

In order to derive a formula to calculate V_R from plasma concentrations of the labeled hormone, we shall consider the average length of time spent by a molecule in the recirculation volume (Fig. 152-4) before it disappears irreversibly from plasma. This average time is given by the expression

$$\bar{t} = \frac{\int_0^\infty tc^*\,dt}{\int_0^\infty c^*\,dt}. \tag{17}$$

When the hormone enters the system through the plasma compartment (Fig. 152-5), then the rate at which it is eliminated from the volume of recirculation $[(V_R \times c)/\bar{t}]$ equals MCR $\times\ c$. Therefore,

$$V_R = \text{MCR} \times \bar{t} \tag{18}$$

or, from equations 16 and 17,

$$V_R = D^* \frac{\int_0^\infty tc^*\,dt}{\left(\int_0^\infty c^*\,dt\right)^2}. \tag{19}$$

If an analytical function describing c^* as a function of time has been obtained by the computer or graphic methods already discussed, then V_R can be calculated directly. Thus, using the example in equation 14 and Figure 152-3, if $c^* = Ae^{-\lambda_1 t} + Be^{-\lambda_2 t}$, then

$$V_R = 100\,\frac{A\lambda_2^2 + B\lambda_1^2}{(A\lambda_2 + B\lambda_1)^2}.$$

The significance of the volume V_R is particularly evident when dealing with thyroid hormones and protein hormones, which are mainly subjected to irreversible metabolism. Some of the steroid hormones, however, are reversibly converted to other compounds, e.g., estrone to estrone sulfate. In these cases, the metabolic products are included in the calculated recirculation volume of the hormone.

A useful parameter to evaluate the extent of reentry of a hormone into systemic circulation is the fraction (ψ) of the material leaving the plasma pool that is irreversibly lost before returning to circulation. This parameter can be calculated from tracer data. For instance, if the disappearance of the tracer from plasma is biexponential, as described by equation 14, then [5,p56]

$$\psi = \frac{(A + B)^2\lambda_1\lambda_2}{(A\lambda_1 + B\lambda_2)(A\lambda_2 + B\lambda_1)}.$$

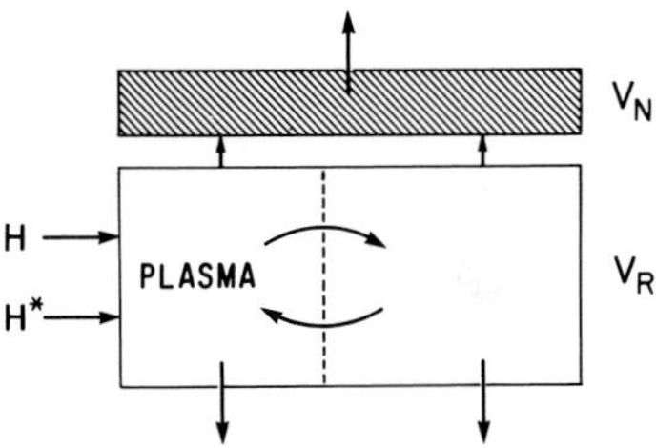

Figure 152-4. Representation of a noncompartmental model. Plasma is in equilibrium with one or many pools from which hormone returns before final irreversible exit. Some hormone, however, may leave directly without entering the recirculating volume (V_R). V_N, volume of hormone containing nonrecirculating hormone.

Application of this formula to experimental data for T_4, cortisol, and human chorionic gonadotropin gives values for ψ of 0.025, 0.23, and 0.64, respectively.

INTERCONVERSION OF CIRCULATING HORMONES

There are many examples of extraglandular formation of hormones from precursors secreted by endocrine glands. Of particular importance are the peripheral formation of estrogens from androstenedione, testosterone from other C_{19} steroids, estrogens from dehydroisoandrosterone sulfate during pregnancy, and T_3 from T_4. Therefore, the measurement of the fraction of a secreted precursor that is converted to another hormonally active circulating compound is of interest.

One procedure for estimating the extent of conversion involves the intravenous infusion of a mixture of tracers of the two compounds under study, each labeled with a different isotope, and the measurement of the isotopic ratios in compounds isolated from blood samples once an isotopic steady state is reached. It can be shown that if A and B are two such compounds and ^{3}H-A and ^{14}C-B are used as tracers, then

$$\text{Conversion factor of A to B} = \rho_{AB} = \frac{(^3\text{H}/^{14}\text{C})\text{ in B}}{(^3\text{H}/^{14}\text{C})\text{ infused}}$$

$$\text{Conversion factor of B to A} = \rho_{BA} = \frac{(^3\text{H}/^{14}\text{C})\text{ infused}}{(^3\text{H}/^{14}\text{C})\text{ in A}}.$$

It is intuitively evident that if the conversion of A to B were complete, all of the ^{3}H-A would go to B and the ^{3}H/^{14}C in B at the steady state would equal the infused ratio ($\rho_{AB} = 1$). If there were no conversion, there would be no ^{3}H in B ($\rho_{AB} = 0$). If 50 percent of A were converted to B, only half of the ^{3}H introduced with A would go to B and the ^{3}H/^{14}C in B would be half the infused ratio ($\rho_{AB} = 0.5$). The ^{3}H/^{14}C ratio in B is determined by the conversion of A to B and is not modified by further metabolism of this compound, including its possible conversion to A. These conversion factors include all pathways by which blood-borne A and B are interconverted, e.g., in various organs and through unspecified intermediates.

When the compounds are slowly metabolized and achievement of a steady state would require unacceptably long infusions, the mixture of tracers may be administered as a single injection and concentrations of the labeled compounds can be measured in blood samples drawn at various times following the injection. In this case,

$$\rho_{AB} = \frac{1}{(^3\text{H}/^{14}\text{C})\text{ injected}} \frac{\int_0^\infty c_B^{3H}\,dt}{\int_0^\infty c_B^{14C}\,dt}.$$

The integral values correspond to the areas under the corresponding concentration curves, extrapolated to $t = 0$ and $c^* = 0$, as already discussed.

The conversion factors can also be determined from experiments in which only one tracer (e.g., ^{3}H-A) is injected if the values for MCR_A and MCR_B are considered to be known. Thus, during infusion,

$$\rho_{AB} = \frac{\text{MCR}_B}{\text{MCR}_A}\left(\frac{c_B^{3H}}{c_A^{3H}}\right)$$

at the steady state, or, after a single injection of the mixture of tracers,

$$\rho_{AB} = \frac{MCR_B}{MCR_A}\frac{\int_0^\infty c_B^{3H}\,dt}{\int_0^\infty c_A^{3H}\,dt}.$$

Note that these formulas involve the value of MCR, whose determination had required the administration of labeled B.

Calculations of ρ and MCR involve only measurements of radioactivity, e.g., concentration of labeled compounds (cpm/ml). If data on concentrations of the endogenous compounds in plasma (pmole/ml) are also available, then production rates (PR = MCR × c) of the circulating compounds and rates of conversion can also be estimated. The rate of conversion of A in blood to B in blood (v_{AB} in pmole/h) by all paths can be calculated using values of PR_A, ρ_{AB}, and ρ_{BA}. Since v_{AB} is the sum of the rates at which material is transferred from A to B for the first time (ρ_{AB} PR_A), the second time (ρ_{AB} PR_A) ρ_{BA} ρ_{AB}, etc, then

$$v_{AB} = \rho_{AB}PR_A[1 + \rho_{AB}\rho_{BA} + (\rho_{AB}\rho_{BA})^2 + \cdots] = \frac{\rho_{AB}PR_A}{1-\rho_{AB}\rho_{BA}}.$$

Note that

$$\frac{1}{1-\rho_{AB}\,\rho_{BA}} = 1 + \rho_{AB}\,\rho_{BA} + (\rho_{AB}\,\rho_{BA})^2 + \cdots.$$

Similarly,

$$v_{BA} = \frac{\rho_{BA}\,PR_B}{1-\rho_{AB}\,\rho_{BA}}.$$

This type of measurements has been performed with a number of steroid hormone pairs[14] and also in the study of the conversion of T_4 to T_3.[15] In this case, $\nu_{T_4T_3} = \rho_{T_4T_3}PR_{T_4}$ since $\rho_{T_3T_4} = 0$.

SOURCES OF CIRCULATING HORMONES

The production rate of a hormone in blood describes the rate of its "de novo" appearance in circulation, either by secretion from one or more endocrine glands or by extraglandular formation from other precursors. For instance, circulating androstenedione (Δ) in an adult man derives from adrenal and testicular secretion and also from extraglandular conversion of testosterone (T) secreted by the testes. If the contribution of secreted T to Δ is estimated and subtracted from the production rate of Δ, a value that may represent the rate of secretion of Δ from the endocrine glands (Q_Δ) can be calculated as follows:[5]

$$Q_\Delta = \frac{PR_\Delta - \rho_{T\Delta}\,PR_T}{1-\rho_{T\Delta}\,\rho_{\Delta T}}.$$

Of course, discovery of other significant peripheral precursors of Δ would lead to a reevaluation of these estimates.

Infusion of ^{3}H-T and comparison of the steady-state specific activities (SA) of T and Δ isolated from blood at the steady state would also reveal the extent of contribution of T to circulating Δ, i.e.,

$$\text{Fraction of blood-borne } \Delta \text{ derived from T} = \frac{SA\ \Delta}{SA\ T}.$$

If all of Δ were derived from T, the two compounds would have the same specific activities. Formation of Δ from other sources will lower the specific activity of Δ and reduce the value of the ratio. If Δ were equally derived from T and from other sources, its specific activity would be one-half the specific activity of T and the fraction would equal 0.5.

NONSTEADY STATE

The rate of production of many hormones is not uniform and the plasma concentrations may show significant differences in samples taken 5 min apart. In addition to the observed circadian periodicity in the secretion of some hormones, and hormonal changes during the estrus cycle, truly intermittent secretion of adrenal hormones has been reported.[16,17] Similar rapid fluctuations in the secretion of gonadotropins have also been observed.[18]

When the production of hormones is variable, two situations must be clearly distinguished from each other. In one of them, the rate constants corresponding to the various metabolic and transfer processes involving the hormone remain constant during the period of observation. In this case, the MCR of the hormone will remain constant. It is worth noting that the concentrations (cpm/ml) of labeled compounds are solely determined by the values of the rate constants. Therefore, when the rate constants do not change, parameters such as MCR, which are estimated from isotopic data alone and do not involve values of concentration of the endogenous hormone, are not dependent on rates of production of the hormone. On the other hand, a situation in which rate constants, as well as rates, change with time is not rigorously manageable.

Examples of hormones whose MCRs are either not significantly affected or are dependent on their production can be listed. For instance, the MCRs of progesterone in men and in pregnant and nonpregnant women are very similar in spite of large differences in the rates of secretion of the hormone.[19] Similarily, the MCR of placental lactogen measured in men or nonpregnant women is not significantly different from the pregnancy value.[20] There are, however, clear examples of dependence of MCR upon the rate of production of the hormone. The MCR of testosterone, for instance, is affected by changes in its blood levels.[21] The MCR of cortisol measured in the morning differs from values obtained when the experiments are performed in the afternoon.[22] It should also be noted that considerable variations in MCR have been observed by changing the posture of the subject from the supine to the standing position, probably due to changes in the hepatic blood flow.[23]

If MCR is considered to be constant, the average rate of production of a circulating hormone can be estimated by taking proper mean values of the measured blood concentration of the hormone. The constant blood withdrawal technique, in which blood is collected at a constant rate after injection of the tracer, appears to be a feasible method for obtaining average values of rates of production.

ESTIMATION OF SECRETORY RATES OF HORMONES FROM URINARY METABOLITES

Rates of secretion of hormones were estimated from urinary data before more sensitive analytical methods were available for the measurement of hormones in blood. With the increasing awareness of the nonsteady-state situation of the endogenous hormones and of the difficulties in ascertaining an isotopic steady state of the hormones in blood during infusion of tracers or a proper extrapolation of experimental curves during single-dose injection of the labeled hormone, analysis of the specific activity of urinary metabolites may again be considered relevant.

The principle of the method can be easily shown in the case when there is one urinary metabolite derived from a single secreted hormone, e.g., tetrahydroaldosterone glucuronoside derived from adrenal aldosterone. If a dose of ^{3}H-aldosterone is injected into a peripheral vein, the tracer can be expected to be metabolized in the same manner as the secreted hormone since they immediately reach a common site, the right heart. If the MCR of aldosterone is not significantly altered during the day, the same fraction *(f)* of the tracer and of the endogenous hormone will be converted to the urinary metabolite. Therefore, the specific activity (SA) of the compound, isolated from pooled urine collected for about 2 days to ensure that all the radioactivity has been excreted, is

$$\text{SA of metabolite} = \frac{\text{Amount of radioactivity appearing in metabolite}}{\text{Amount of metabolite excreted}}$$

$$= \frac{\text{Dose injected} \times f}{\text{Secretion rate hormone} \times \text{Days of urine collection} \times f}$$

$$\text{Secretion rate (mg/day)} = \frac{\text{Dose injected (cpm)}}{\text{SA of metabolite (cpm/mg)} \times \text{Time of urine collection (days)}}.$$

A complication preventing the application of this single tracer method to the study of steroid hormones became evident in the early 1960s. The problem is that most steroid metabolites in urine derive from multiple precursors. For instance, urinary testosterone glucuronoside and the 17-ketosteroids derive from secreted testosterone, androstenedione, dehydroisoandrosterone, and dehydroisoandrosterone sulfate; estrone glucuronoside derives from secreted estradiol, estrone, and androsterone. This problem has been satisfactorily solved in cases when only two precursors contribute to a pair of urinary metabolites.[5] For instance, dehydroisoandrosterone glucuronoside and sulfate are two urinary metabolites that appear to be solely derived from dehydroisoandrosterone and dehydroisoandrosterone sulfate secreted by the adrenals. In this case, injection of a mixture of tracers of the two secreted compounds, labeled with ^{3}H and ^{14}C, respectively, produce doubly labeled metabolites that can be used to estimate the rates of secretion of the precursors.[24,25]

Application of competitive protein-binding techniques to the analysis of urine samples allows the measurement of minute amounts of the unconjugated hormones excreted. Measurement of the cumulative specific activities of these urinary compounds may be useful for the study of average production rates of the circulating hormone.

INFLUENCE OF PLASMA BINDING ON COMMON PARAMETERS OF HORMONE METABOLISM

It is generally recognized that a number of hormones are strongly bound to plasma proteins, including the thyroid hormones, estrogens, androgens, and glucocorticoids. In general, polypeptide hormones tend to be only weakly bound to plasma proteins if at all. The strength of plasma protein binding exerts a marked influence on the total concentration of hormone in plasma, the MCR, the net fractional removal of hormone, and the hormone distribution. By and large, however, plasma binding does not appear to affect the steady-state free hormone concentration nor to influence the hormonal state of the tissues.

Attention has been conventionally focused on plasma-binding proteins since the plasma proteins are more easily identified and quantitated than the cellular constituents. Nevertheless, the reversible binding of hormones to cellular components can account for a significant proportion of the total exchangeable hormone pool in the body. For instance, in man, approximately 80 percent of T_3 is bound to the cells, and only 20 percent to plasma proteins.[26] In the case of T_4, the intracellular pool is approximately equal to the extracellular protein-bound mass of hormone. The actual concentration of unbound thyroid hormone is extremely small, although the measurement of this small concentration may be important from a diagnostic point of view. Attention has been directed to an analysis of the exchange of iodothyronines between plasma proteins and cellular compartments. Similar processes have been demonstrated for bilirubin and BSP, and it appears highly probable that other plasma protein-bound hormones also exchange rapidly with cellular compartments.

If we can disregard the small proportion of total hormone present as free hormone, it follows that the volume of exchangeable T_4 can be considered to be the sum of the volume of distribution in the cellular compartment and the volume of distribution in the plasma protein compartment (including vascular and interstitial spaces). Thus,

$$V_R = V_p + V_c. \tag{20}$$

Moreover, one can define net cellular (B_c) and plasma binding (B_p) so that

$$\frac{V_c}{V_p} = \frac{B_c}{B_p} \quad \text{and} \quad B_c = \frac{V_c}{V_p} B_p. \tag{21}$$

In other words, net plasma and cellular binding is defined to be proportional to the pool (or equivalent plasma volumes) of hormone associated with the cellular compartment. The intensity of binding of protein (b_p) per unit volume of plasma can be determined experimentally by equilibrium dialysis from the relationship $b_p = (1 - \text{DF})/\text{DF}$, where DF is the dialyzable fraction[26] and appropriate correction is made for the dyalizing volume. It is also true that

$$b_p = \sum_1^n k_i(M_i - TP_i)$$

where k_i is the affinity constant of individual classes of binding proteins, TP_i, the concentration of hormone-bound to the ith class of binding protein, and M_i is the total concentration of individual classes binding proteins per liter.[26] The net binding to the plasma protein compartment can then be expressed as the product of the plasma protein volume (V_p) and the binding per liter (b_p). Since the distribution of serum albumin has been found to be characteristic of other plasma-binding proteins, the albumin distribution volume, determined isotopically, can be used as an index of V_p. Since $B_p = b_pV_p$, it follows from equation 21 that

$$\frac{V_c}{V_p} = \frac{B_c}{V_p b_p} \quad \text{and} \quad V_c = \frac{B_c}{b_p}. \tag{22}$$

Since $B_c = (V_R - V_p)b_p$, where V_R is the recirculating volume

$$V_R = \frac{B_c}{b_p} + V_p. \tag{23}$$

This equation indicates that, for a constant level of cellular binding, any decrease in plasma binding causes an increase in V_R, but this increase is not inversely related to b_p unless B_c is very much greater than V_p. Moreover, any change in B_c would also be reflected in a change in V_R but not in a proportional manner.

Moreover, let the fraction λ_c be the fraction of the cellular hormone pool that is irreversibly removed per unit time. This function has the virtue of being exclusively related to the cellular compartment and not primarily influenced by changes in plasma protein binding. It thus follows that, under steady-state conditions,

$$V_R\lambda_T = V_c\lambda_c = \frac{\lambda_c B_c}{b_p} \quad (24)$$

where λ_T is the total average fractional removal of hormone from the system. This equation shows that if the cellular attributes B_c and λ_c are held constant, the MCR of a given hormone is inversely proportional to the strength of plasma protein binding. Equation 24 indicates that a change in MCR can be due both to alterations in plasma protein binding and cellular determinants. If B_p can be evaluated before and after the physiologic perturbation, the effect of any stimulus on the cellular handling of the hormone ($\lambda_c B_c$) can be assessed. $\lambda_c B_c$ is numerically equal to the irreversible MCR of free hormone.

Similarily, the total fractional irreversible removal rate of a given hormone (λ_T) will depend both on plasma and cellular factors:

$$\lambda_T = \frac{\lambda_c B_c}{V_R b_p} = \frac{\lambda_c B_c}{\left(V_p + \frac{B_c}{b_p}\right) b_p} = \frac{\lambda_c B_c}{V_p b_p + B_c}. \quad (25)$$

Again, the larger b_p is, the smaller λ_T will be, but the relationship again is not inverse and depends upon the relative importance of cellular and plasma protein-binding components in the distribution equilibrium.

In vitro work involving superfusion of tissue slices with labeled steroid hormones has led to the definition and estimation of the intracellular clearance of a hormone;[5,27] This value denotes the ratio between the hormone's rate of "de novo" appearance per gram of tissue and its resulting steady-state intracellular concentration.

REFERENCES

1. Robbins, J., Rall, J. E.: Proteins associated with the thyroid hormones. *Physiol Rev 40:* 415, 1960.
2. Peterson, R. E., Nokes, G., Chen, P. S., et al: Estrogens and adrenocortical function in man. *J Clin Endocrinol Metab 20:* 495, 1960.
3. Migeon, C. J., Kenny, F. M., Taylor, F. H.: Cortisol production rate VIII. Pregnancy. *J Clin Endocrinol Metab 28:* 661, 1968.
4. Korenman, S. G., Lipsett, M. B.: Is testosterone glucuronoside uniquely derived from plasma testosterone? *J Clin Invest 43:* 2125, 1964.
5. Gurpide, E.: Tracer Methods in Hormone Research. New York, Springer, 1975.
6. DiStefano, J. J., III, Fisher, D. A.: Peripheral distribution and metabolism of the thyroid hormones: a primarily quantitative assessment. In Hershman, J. M., Bray, G. A., (eds): Pharmacology of the Thyroid Gland, International Encyclopedia of Pharmacology and Therapeutics. Oxford, Pergamon, 1975, ch 2 sect 1.
7. Tait, J. F., Burstein, S.: In vivo studies of steroid dynamics in man. In Pincus, G., Thimann, K. V., Astwood, E. G., (eds): The Hormones. New York, Academic, 1964.
8. Berman, M.: Iodine kinetics in the thyroid and biogenic amines. In Rall, J. E., et al (eds): Methods in Investigative and Diagnostic Endocrinology. Amsterdam, North Holland, 1972, ch 11, pp 172–203.
9. Ingbar, S. H., Freinkel, N.: Simultaneous estimation of rates of thyroxine degradation and thyroid hormone synthesis. *J Clin Invest 34:* 808, 1955.
10. Tait, J. F., Tait, S. A. S., Little, B., et al: The disappearance of 7-^{3}H-D-aldosterone in the plasma of normal subjects. *J Clin Invest 40:* 72, 1961.
11. Bradley, E. M., Waterhouse, C.: Effect of estrogen administration on extravascular cortisol. *J Clin Endocrinol 26:* 705, 1966.
12. Hembree, W. C., Bardin, C. W., Lipsett, M. B.: A study of estrogen metabolic clearance rates and transfer factors. *J Clin Invest 48:* 1809, 1969.
13. Oppenheimer, J. H., Schwartz, H. L., Surks, M. I.: Determination of common parameters of iodothyronine metabolism and distribution in man by noncompartmental analysis. *J Clin Endocrinol 41:* 319, 1975.
14. Baird, D., Horton, R., Longcope, C., et al: Steroid dynamics under steady state conditions. *Recent Prog Horm Res 25:* 611, 1969.
15. Surks, M. I., Schadlow, A. R., Stock, J. M., et al: Determination of iodothyronine absorption and conversion of L-thyroxine (T_4) to L-triiodothyronine (T_3) using turnover rate techniques. *J Clin Invest 52:* 805, 1973.
16. Hellman, L., Nakada, F., Curti, J., et al: Cortisol is secreted episodically by normal man. *J Clin Endocrinol 30:* 411, 1970.
17. Krieger, D.,. Allen, W., Rizzo, F., et al: Characterization of the normal temporal pattern of plasma corticocoid levels. *J Clin Endocrinol 32:* 266, 1971.
18. Midgley, A. R., Jaffe, R. B.: Regulation of human gonadotropins: X-episodic fluctuation of LH during the menstrual cycle. *J Clin Endocrinol 33:* 962, 1971.
19. Lin, T. J., Billiar, R. B., Little, B.: Metabolic clearance rate of progesterone in the menstrual cycle. *J Clin Endocrinol 35:* 879, 1972.
20. Kaplan, S., Gurpide, E., Sciarra, E., et al: Metabolic clearance rate and production rate of chorionic growth hormone–prolactin in late pregnancy. *J Clin Endocrinol 28:* 1450, 1968.
21. Southren, A. L., Gordon, G. C., Tochinoto, S.: Further study of factors affecting the metabolic clearance rate of testosterone in man. *J Clin Endocrinol 28:* 1105, 1968.
22. de Lacerda, L., Kowarski, A., Migeon, C.: Diurnal variation of the metabolic clearance rate of cortisol effect on measurement of cortisol production rate. *J Clin Endocrinol 36:* 1043, 1973.
23. Balikian, H. A., Brodie, A. H., Dale, S. L., et al: Effect of posture on the metabolic clearance rate, plasma concentration and blood production rate of aldosterone in man. *J Clin Endocrinol 28:* 1630, 1968.
24. MacDonald, P. C., Chapdelaine, A., Gonzalez, O., et al: Studies on the secretion and interconversion of the androgens. III. Results obtained after the injection of several radioactive C_{19} steroids, singly or as mixtures. *J Clin Endocrinol 25:* 1557, 1965.
25. Sandberg, E., Gurpide, E., Lieberman, S.: Quantitative studies on the metabolism of dehydroisoandrosterone sulfate. *Biochemistry 3:* 1256, 1964.
26. Oppenheimer, J. H., Surks, M. I.: Quantitative aspects of hormone production, distribution, metabolism, and activity. In Solomon, D. H., Greer, M. A., (eds): Handbook of Physiology, vol 3, Thyroid, section 7, Endocrinology. Washington, DC, American Physiological Society, 1974, ch 13 pp 197–214.
27. Tseng, L., Stolee, A., Gurpide, E.: Quantitative studies on the uptake and metabolism of estrogens and progesterone by human endometrium. *Endocrinology 90:* 390, 1972.

153

Receptors for Peptide Hormones

Jesse Roth

This chapter describes the role of peptide hormone receptors in disease states. It is not intended to be a comprehensive review of the subject. Instead, broad principles have been emphasized and selected examples chosen to illustrate the salient points. Sections of this chapter will (1) outline the role of receptors in hormone action, (2) characterize some of the physiological and experimental factors that modulate receptor concentration and affinity, and (3) describe endocrinological disorders in which changes in the receptor play a substantial role.

ROLE OF RECEPTORS

For a hormone to act, it must first bind to a specific receptor.[1–3] The receptor has two major functions. First, the receptor must recognize the specific hormone from all other materials to which the cell is being exposed; for example, in plasma the specific hormone is at $10^{-9} - 10^{-10}$M and thus represents only $1/10^6$ or $1/10^7$ molecules to which the target cell is exposed. The recognition process is carried out by binding of the hormone to the receptor. Second, the combination of hormone with receptor initiates the series of biochemical events by which the hormonal signal results in a specific action. The hormone molecule is totally dependent on the receptor to express its biological function. It is not clear whether the biological activity of the hormone-receptor complex resides in the hormone molecule, in the receptor molecule, or in a combination of the two. It is unclear also whether the receptor molecule exercises some biological activity even when hormone is not present. These points have been raised to emphasize that the hormone has no specific function in the absence of receptor and that the receptor is at least as important as the hormone in the production of the effects that we typically associate with the hormone.

CELLULAR LOCALIZATION OF HORMONE RECEPTORS

Hormones that are lipid-soluble, such as iodothyronines, steroids, and the vitamin D derivatives, which are sterols, readily traverse the plasma membrane of the cell; their receptors are intracellular, and the primary site of their action is at the nucleus. The peptide hormones, which constitute 75 to 80 percent of all hormones, and the catecholamines are hydrophilic and do not readily traverse the lipid bilayer of the plasma membrane of the cell. Their receptors are on the outer surface of the plasma membrane of the target cell.*[1–4]

HORMONE ACTION

The sequence of events for peptide hormones and catecholamines is illustrated in Fig. 153-1. Hormone released by the gland travels in the plasma to the target cell, where it binds rapidly and reversibly to a finite number of receptors on the outer surface of the plasma membrane of the target cell; the hormone itself is the extracellular messenger. The combination of hormone with receptor generates a transmembrane message. The nature of the transmembrane messenger(s) is not known, and it is not clear whether the hormone molecule and/or the receptor molecule act directly to

*Receptors for peptide hormones are also found on membranes of intracellular structures, including Golgi, rough and smooth endoplasmic reticulum, and nuclear membrane, which is an extension of the endoplasmic reticulum.[3,5–8] In the case of insulin receptors, the intracellular receptors are very similar to the plasma membrane receptors in their specificity and in most other characteristics but do differ from the plasma membrane receptors in several ways.[9] Whether the intracellular receptors are precursors for plasma membrane receptors or whether they have any role in hormone action is speculative at this time.

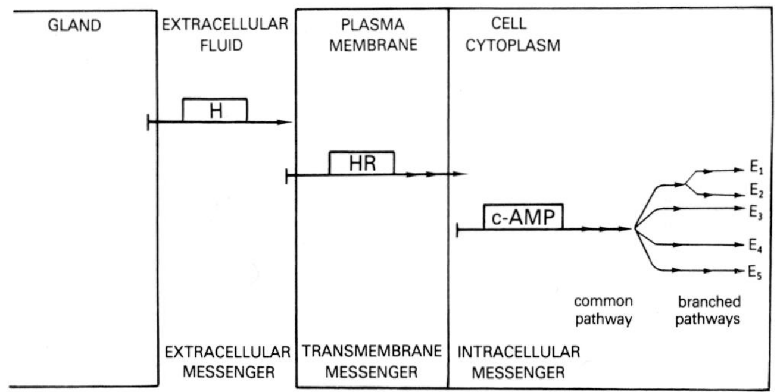

Fig. 153-1. Hormone action. This schematic representation of hormone action for peptide hormones and catecholamines is explained in the text (see section "Hormone Action"). There are an increasing number of examples in which a hormone that works through cyclic AMP has additional specific effects in the target tissue that appear to be independent of cyclic AMP. In these cases, *HR* generates some message(s) that stimulate cyclase (shown in figure) and some that bypass the adenylate cyclase system (not shown).

carry the message or act on the membrane to stimulate the production of other molecules that transmit the signal across the plasma membrane.* In Fig. 153-1, the next series of events is designated as the production of intracellular messenger(s) via some common intracellular pathway. For most of the peptide hormones and for the catecholamines that act through the β-adrenergic receptors, the common intracellular pathway includes activation of adenylate cyclase at the inner surface of the plasma membrane, elevation of the intracellular concentration of cyclic AMP, and activation of the cyclic AMP-dependent protein kinase.[16,17] The latter enzyme phosphorylates intracellular proteins and thereby activates or inactivates them. In the case of insulin, growth hormone, prolactin, α-adrenergic catecholamines, and other hormones that do not act through the adenylate cyclase–cAMP pathway, the nature of the common intracellular pathway for each of these hormones is unknown but has been assumed to be of similar design.† When a hormone acts on a cell, it typically produces multiple effects. Presumably beyond the common intracellular pathway there are numerous branches leading to the series of characteristic responses.

When a hormone fails to produce its characteristic response, or when the response of the cell to a given amount of hormone is abnormal, any one of the steps from the first to the last may be defective. Thus, abnormal responsiveness to a given concentration of hormone at the target cell can be observed owing to a change in receptor as well as a change in any of the steps beyond the binding of hormone to receptor.

*Initially the hormone-receptor interaction is fully reversible. Rapidly at 37° (and at lower temperatures more slowly or not at all), some of the hormone molecules become irreversibly bound or only slowly reversible; at about the same time, some hormone can be observed at sites that are not on the cell surface. Although some of the hormone radioactivity is detected in association with lysosomes, a substantial portion of these hormone molecules can be recovered intact.[10–15] The role of these transfers in hormone degradation, in receptor degradation and modulation, in initiation or termination of hormone action at the target cell, or in the production of a slowly releasable reservoir of intact hormone has not as yet been elucidated.

†Changes in cyclic AMP concentration, elevations of intracellular concentrations of cyclic GMP, and translocations of Ca^{2+} have been suggested but as yet are unestablished as representing an essential early intracellular event in the action of these hormones.[18,19]

QUANTITATIVE ASPECTS OF THE HORMONE-RECEPTOR INTERACTION

Free hormone in the medium (H) binds to receptors (R) on the cell surface reversibly to form hormone-receptor complexes (HR). The concentration of hormone-receptor complexes $[HR]$ determines the signal rate to the cell. The biological effect will be some function, f, of the concentration of hormone receptor complexes $[HR]$; $[HR]$ is determined by hormone concentration $[H]$, receptor concentration $[R]$, and the affinity of hormone for receptor, K. While it has always been clear that the signal rate can be increased by increasing the hormone concentration, it has only recently become clear that both the affinity and the concentration of receptors undergo rapid and substantial fluctuations.[8,20–31] All three (K, H, and R) are equal partners in determining the signal rate to the cell, and the signal generated by a given concentration of hormone will vary widely as receptor affinity and receptor concentration are varied (see Table 153-1).

ROLE OF EVENTS BEYOND THE RECEPTOR

Hormone-receptor complexes deliver a signal to the cell; the actual response to that signal depends on all the steps beyond the receptor. The steps distal to the receptor are also regulated quickly over a wide range, so that a given concentration of hormone receptor complexes will yield a particular response at a particular time that is determined by the current status of these distal steps. In summary, the target cell is not a fixed target but is by nature a highly regulated unit that responds to events both inside and outside the cell; a given concentration of hormone in the extracellular fluid will yield markedly different results, depending on the state of the receptor and of the steps distal to the receptor.

NATURE OF CELL SURFACE RECEPTORS

For hormones that bind at the cell surface, few receptors have been purified and none have been well characterized.[32–34] Molecular weights are grossly estimated to be in the range of 10^5 daltons. Receptors are proteins, since they are easily destroyed by the common proteolytic enzymes.[35–37] Because they cannot be removed from the membrane except by use of detergents, they are considered to be "integral" and presumed to have a region that is rich in lipid-soluble amino acids that reside in the membrane. Because receptors face the outer surface of the cell, they are thought to contain substantial complex carbohydrate moieties that keep some part of the receptor exposed to the extracellular fluid.[38]

Table 153-1. The Interaction of Hormone with Receptor*

1. The primary event:

$$H + R \rightleftarrows HR$$

2. The equilibrium constant (K_a) for this reaction:

$$K_a = \frac{[HR]}{[H][R]}$$

3. The biological effect (E) is some function (f) of the strength of the signal to the cell; the signal strength is directly related to $[HR]$.

$$E = f([HR]) = f(K[H][R]) = f\left(\frac{K[H][R_o]}{1 + K[H]}\right)$$

Thus the signal strength to the cell depends equally on K, H, and R (or R_o).

*H = free hormone, R = free receptor, HR = hormone-receptor complexes, R_o = total receptors (R + HR).

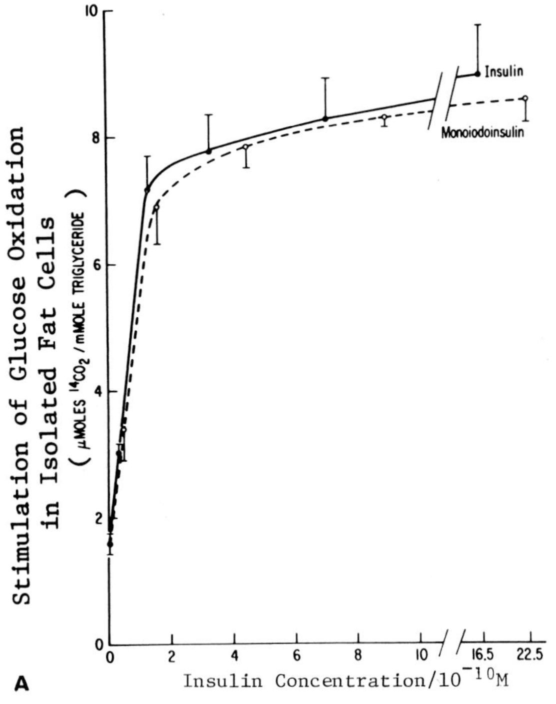

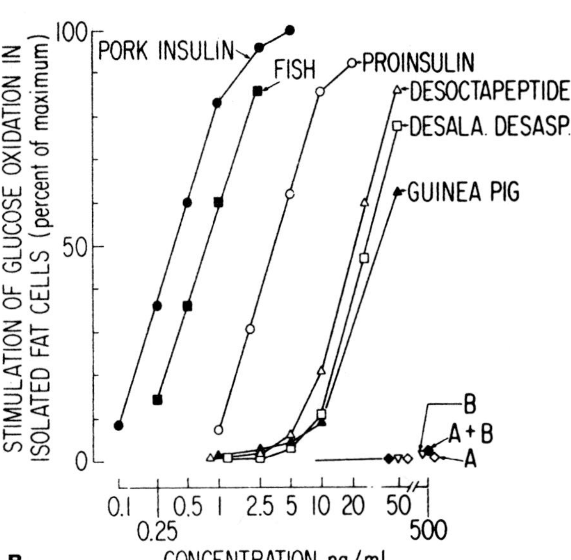

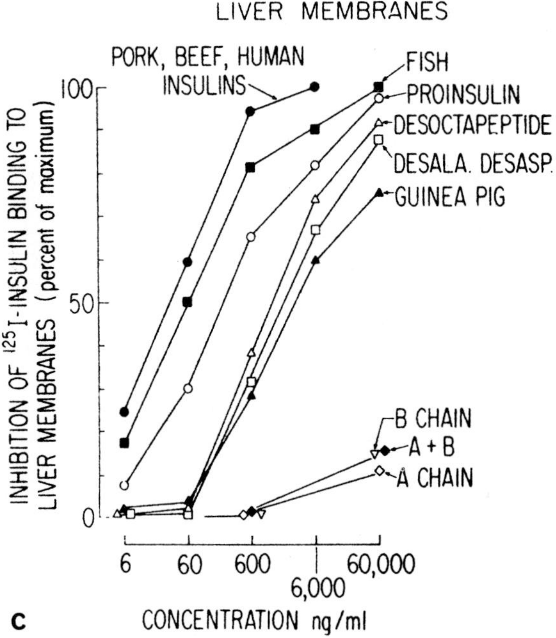

Fig. 153-2. Insulin receptor. (*a*) Monoiodoinsulin was compared with native insulin for its ability to stimulate glucose oxidation in isolated fat cells. It can be seen that the iodoinsulin has retained essentially the full biological potency of insulin. (*b*) Several species of insulin and insulin derivatives were compared for their biological potency in stimulating glucose oxidation in isolated rat adipocytes. (*c*) The same insulin preparations were compared for their ability to compete with ^{125}I-labeled pork insulin in binding to receptors on plasma membranes of rat liver. Notice that the rank order of potencies is the same for both stimulation of glucose oxidation and for binding to receptors. Thus the capacity of insulin to stimulate biological processes is predicted by its relative affinity for the insulin receptors. (From Freychet et al.[44,46])

It is not known whether receptor molecules span the plasma membrane or even extend into the interior of the cell, as has been described for several membrane proteins.[38] Commonly, a cell has on its surface 10^3 to 10^5 receptors for a given hormone, which represents, in most cases, less that 1 percent of the protein of the plasma membrane.[39]

METHODS OF MEASUREMENT

The hormone-receptor interaction is typically measured in vitro using receptor, radioactively labeled hormone, and unlabeled hormone in a fashion analogous to that used for radioimmunoassay or other competitive binding assays except that the cell's own receptor is used as the binding protein.[40,41] Typically, the radioactive hormone is labeled with ^{125}I under conditions such that the iodinated hormone retains most or all of the biological activity of the native hormone[40,42–45] (Fig. 153-2*a*). The receptors used for these studies are on whole cells, either freshly isolated or in culture, or membrane-rich fractions from broken cells, or highly purified preparations of plasma membrane. With some receptors, the receptor has been solubilized by treating cells or membranes with mild detergent, which allows the receptor to be freed of the membrane; the interaction of the hormone with the detergent-solubilized receptor can be studied in the continued presence of detergent.[31,40,47–50] (If the detergent is removed after solubilization, the receptor is usually denatured.) A fixed amount of labeled hormone in the absence and presence of various concentrations of unlabeled hormone is reacted with receptor. After an hour or two, the receptor-bound hormone is separated from the free hormone, and the binding of hormone to receptor is expressed as a function of the hormone concentration (Fig. 153-2). When the receptor is particulate, i.e., on cells or membranes, the bound and the free hormone are typically separated by centrifugation. When the receptor is soluble, the bound and the free hormone are usually separated by gel filtration or by precipitating the solubilized receptor with polyethylene glycol, which at appropriate concentrations will precipitate receptor-bound hormone and leave the free hormone in solution.*[51]

*New methods for direct measurement of the hormone-receptor interaction include: (1) the use in vitro of specific antireceptor antibodies labeled with radioactive iodine,[52] (2) the simultaneous injection of two individually labeled insulins, which differ in affinity for receptor, to measure hormone

BIOLOGICALLY RELEVANT FLUCTUATIONS IN RECEPTOR CONCENTRATIONS AND AFFINITY

Receptors, like most other cellular proteins, are being synthesized and degraded continuously, and under steady-state conditions, synthesis is equal to degradation.[57] The concentration and affinity of receptors at steady state vary widely under many biologically relevant conditions, as outlined in Table 153-2. Any major reprogramming of the cell can result in major changes in concentration of receptors. This can include changes in growth rate, differentiation, and culture conditions, or even differences in cell cycle. For example, fibroblasts that have stopped growing have many more insulin receptors than rapidly growing fibroblasts.[26] Similarly, transformed fibroblasts have fewer insulin receptors than nontransformed cells.[26] When cells become confluent and stop growing, cyclic AMP concentrations in the cells typically are elevated;[58] cyclic AMP itself in these cells is capable of increasing receptor concentrations twofold and may account for some of the increase in receptor concentrations in stationary confluent cells.[27] The effect of cell cycle on receptors is best illustrated with the receptor for alpha-MSH on Cloudman melanoma cells in culture. During one phase of the cell cycle (G_1), there are MSH receptors on the cell surface, and the adenylate cyclase is stimulated by MSH. At other times in the cell cycle, receptor concentrations are much lower, and the adenylate cyclase is no longer activated by alpha-MSH.[24]

Often, homologous hormone can regulate receptor concentration.[23,59,60] High hormone concentrations in a period of a few hours or even less can act on a cell to reduce the concentration of its own receptors. It should be emphasized that this is not simply occupancy of receptor by hormone but rather an active biological regulatory process. Typically, this regulation requires that biologically active hormone molecules bind to the receptor site. Biologically active hormones, but not specific antagonists, reduce receptor concentration, whereas both can bind to receptor. In addition to the binding of hormone to the receptor and the activation of the cell, in the case of the insulin receptor, this regulatory process appears to require an intact cell; disturbances in energy production, protein synthesis, or reduction of temperature block this effect of homologous hormone.[62] Regulation of receptor concentration by high concentrations of the ligand occurs not only with many peptide hormones and the catecholamines but also with many other ligand-receptor interactions.[63] Likewise, withdrawal of resting hormone concentrations in some cases can cause elevations of receptor concentrations.[60,64–66]

Homologous hormone can also regulate receptor affinity.[28,67] In the case of insulin and some other hormones, receptors are in the highest affinity state when all of them are unoccupied. Hormone bound to a small fraction of the receptors causes site–site interactions among receptors of the negatively cooperative type such that the average affinity of all the receptors is decreased. At some finite level of occupancy of receptors (with insulin, occupancy of 10 to 25 percent of the receptors), all the receptors are in the lowest affinity state. In the case of insulin, it has been shown that one portion of the hormone binds to one region of the receptor

binding to receptor in the whole animal in vivo,[53] and (3) the use in vitro of antireceptor antibody to precipitate detergent solubilized complexes of receptor with ^{125}I-hormone.[54] To localize the subcellular sites of hormone binding, investigators have used radioactively labeled hormones with electron-microscopic radioautography,[12] ferritin-labeled insulin with conventional electron microscopy,[55,56] and hormone labeled with fluorescent dyes for localization of fluorescence.[14]

Table 153-2. Biologically Relevant Changes in Receptor

	Total Concentration of Receptors (R_0)	Affinity of Hormone for Receptor (K)
1. Genetics, growth rate, cAMP, cell cycle, differentiation, transformation	√	?
2. Homologous hormone	√	√
3. Heterologous hormone	√	√
4. Antibodies to receptor	√	√
5. Ionic environment	?	√
6. Temperature	?	√

to generate the biological response, while another part of the hormone binds to another region of the receptor to generate the negatively cooperative interactions that regulate receptor affinity.[68] The effect of the hormone on the affinity of its own receptors, in contrast to its effect on receptor concentration, appears to be a simple physicochemical process that takes place readily in whole cells and purified plasma membranes, as well as in solubilized preparations of receptor.[2,3,28,50,69]

A hormone can have major effects on the biology of another hormone. One of the ways in which one hormone can affect another is by causing a change in either the concentration or affinity of the receptors of the other hormone. Thus, in the ovary, FSH binds to its own receptors to produce its own characteristic effect and in addition produces a marked elevation in concentration of LH receptors,[25] thereby heightening the responsiveness of the cell to LH. Other examples will be discussed later.

Autoantibodies directed against specific receptors have been reported for TSH,[29] insulin,[70] and acetylcholine,[71–75] and antibodies have been generated in response to injections of acetylcholine[76,77] and prolactin receptors.[78] The antibodies can act to change receptor concentration, affinity, or function. The clinical consequences are discussed later.

The affinity of a receptor is affected by the ionic environment, as might be expected for any protein-ligand interaction. The sensitivity of a hormone-receptor interaction to changes in the ionic environment varies quite markedly. The insulin receptor is extremely sensitive to pH[22,79] (Fig. 153-3*a*), and the change in pH from 7.4 to 6.8, as might occur with diabetic ketoacidosis, might well be associated with a major decrease in insulin binding as a result of an alteration in receptor affinity. The ACTH receptor from the adrenal is exquisitely sensitive to changes in Ca^{2+} concentration[31] (Fig. 153-3*b*). Fluctuations in calcium concentration in pathological situations in vivo might affect the ability of ACTH to stimulate the adrenal. Temperature has marked effect on hormone binding; with elevated temperatures, binding is more rapid, but the steady-state level of binding is lower than at lower temperatures.[80] This would be of trivial importance in mammals but might have substantial consequences in poikilotherms.

Since receptor concentrations and affinities have been shown to change rapidly in such a wide range of conditions, it is anticipated that other variables in the internal or external environment may have effects on receptors as well. For example, the insulin receptor is affected by dietary composition,[81] the timing of meals,[82] and other events such as increases in the concentration of ketone bodies.[83] Since the surface receptors are at the interface between the internal and external environment of the cell, retrospectively it is not surprising that it is so highly regulated by events both inside and outside the cell.

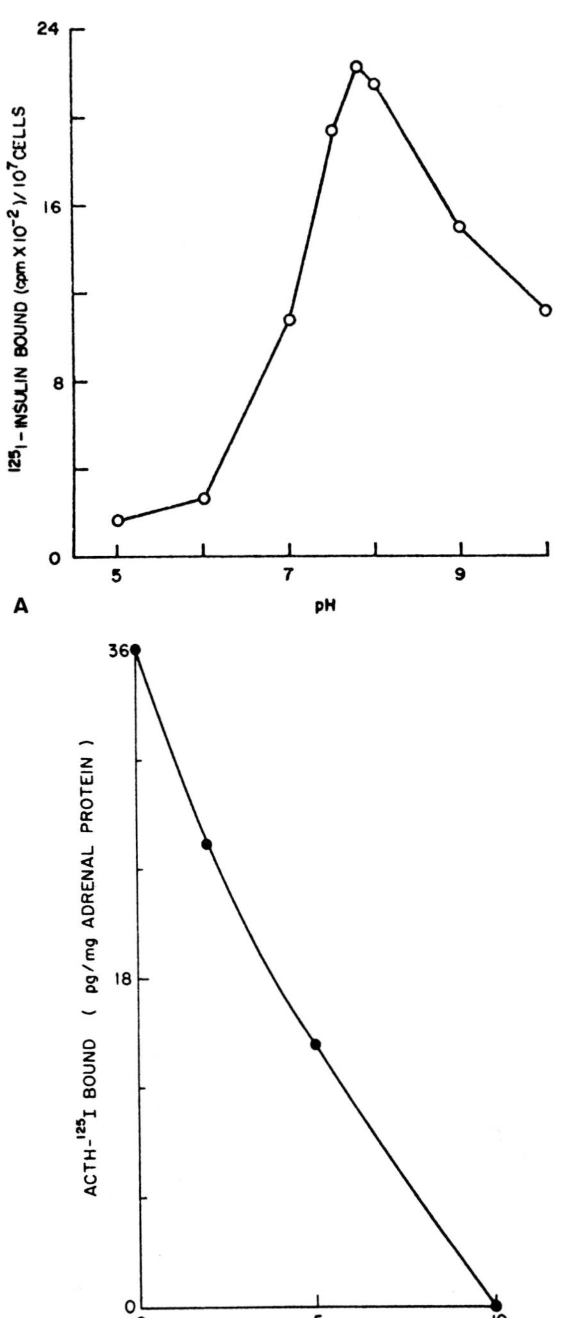

Fig. 153-3. Effect of ionic environment on hormone binding to receptor. (*a*) Specific binding of ^{125}I-insulin (10^{-11}M) to receptors on cultured human lymphocytes (IM-9 line) is plotted as a function of the pH of the medium. This sharp pH dependence of binding is characteristic of all insulin receptors. (From Gavin et al.[73]) (*b*) Specific binding of ^{125}I-ACTH to receptors derived from adrenal cells is plotted as a function of the [Ca^{2+}] in the medium. (From Lefkowitz et al.[31])

RECEPTOR DISEASES[2,84–87]

HUMAN OBESITY

The insulin resistance of obesity is the most common hormone-resistant state and is the first of the receptor diseases to be described[8,20] (see Table 153-3). Characteristically in obesity there is a high prevalence of glucose intolerance, but even more striking is the widespread occurrence of hyperinsulinemia.[88,89] The circulating insulin is qualitatively normal; the fraction of the immunoassayable insulin that is proinsulin is the same as in normal subjects,[90] and both the insulinlike and proinsulinlike components of plasma hormone have normal reactivity with receptors and are biologically intact.[91] In addition to resistance to endogenous insulin, there is resistance to exogenous insulin as well. In the typical obese patient, blood glucose will fall by less than 50 percent in response to 0.1 units of insulin per kilogram of body weight intravenously but will be reduced by 50 percent or more when the dose of insulin is increased to 0.3 units/kg.

Table 153-3. Outline of Receptor Diseases

1. "Down regulation"—receptor concentration inversely related to chronic level of circulating hormone
   Insulin—obesity, diabetes, uremia, acromegaly, insulinoma, type A extreme resistance insulin
   Other—catecholamine receptors reduced in asthmatics who are under treatment with adrenergic agents
2. Heterologous hormone—one hormone regulates receptor for another hormone
   Insulin—glucocorticoid excess and deficiency alter affinity of insulin receptor
   Other—thyroid hormone regulates concentration of β-adrenergic catecholamine receptors
3. Autoantibodies
   Insulin—type B extreme insulin resistance
   Other—Graves' disease, myasthenia gravis
4. Genetic
   Insulin—none known
   Other—receptors for low-density lipoproteins in familial hypercholesterolemia; steroid hormone resistance
5. Specificity spillover (see Table 153-7)
   Insulin—nonislet cell tumor hypoglycemia; macrosomia in babies of diabetics
   Other—many

The binding of ^{125}I-insulin to receptors is decreased[92] because the concentration of insulin receptors on cells of obese patients are decreased in number[93] (Fig. 153-4). The insulin receptors of circulating monocytes,[86,92–94] as well as adipocytes,[86,94,95] have been studied, and the results are comparable in both tissues[87,94] (Fig. 153-5). The residual receptors are normal by all criteria, including affinity of receptor for hormone.[93] The magnitude of the receptor deficiency is inversely related to the elevation of plasma insulin in the basal state (Fig. 153-4*b*). The severity of the receptor defect correlates with measurements of insulin resistance, both in vivo and in vitro[96] (Fig. 153-6). A minority of obese patients have normal binding of ^{125}I-insulin with normal receptor concentrations (e.g., patient A in Fig. 153-4*a*); these patients have basal insulin concentrations that are in or near the normal range (Fig. 153-4*b*) and show normal responsiveness to insulin.[86,93] With severe hyperinsulinemia, the receptor concentrations are reduced to about 25 percent of normal; we suspect that further increases in insulin concentration do not produce further decreases in receptor concentration.[86,87,93–96]

The receptor defect can be reversed. A low calorie intake for several weeks restores basal insulin concentrations to normal; simultaneously, glucose tolerance, insulin sensitivity and receptor concentrations are restored to normal (Fig. 153-4*c*). In markedly obese patients, the brief period of dietary restriction produces only a modest decrease in weight, so that adipose tissue is still massively in excess and yet the normal pattern of glucose and insulin metabolism is restored.[93] Total starvation for 1 to 2 weeks will also restore receptor concentrations as well.[97] Thus the overeating

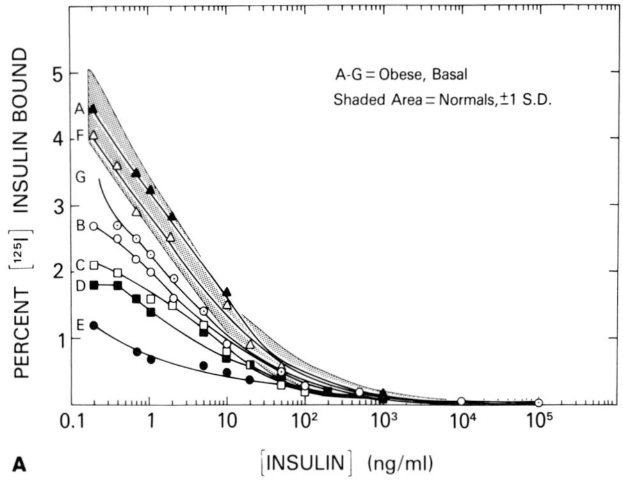

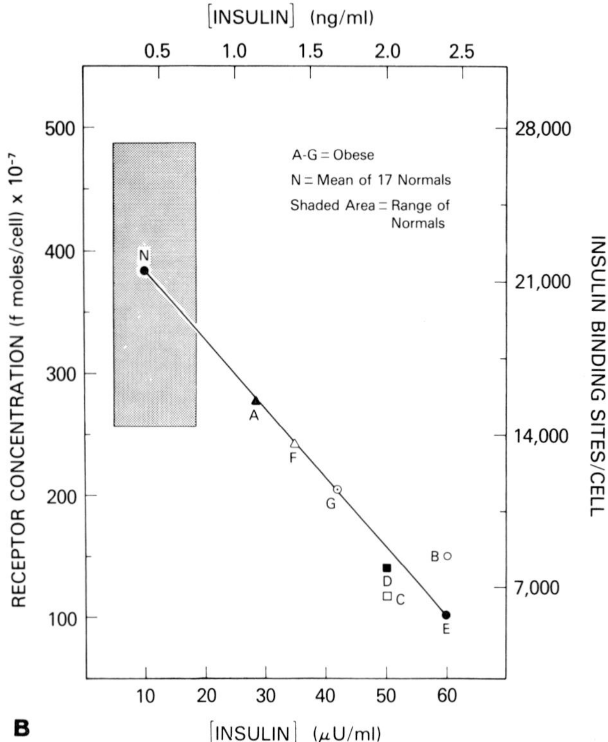

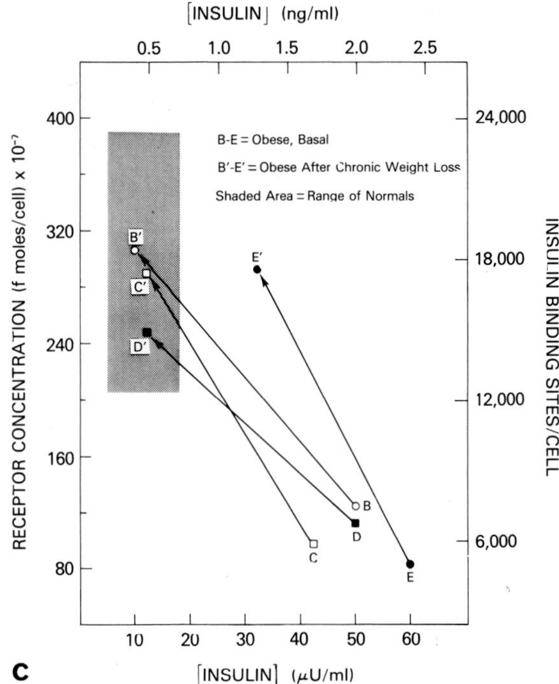

Fig. 153-4. Insulin binding to monocytes of obese patients. (*a*) Blood from a patient was centrifuged, and the plasma and red cells were returned to the patient. The buffy coat was applied to a Hypaque-Ficoll gradient and centrifuged, yielding a mononuclear cell fraction that is about 80 percent lymphocytes and 20 percent monocytes. ^{125}I-insulin is incubated with an aliquot of mononuclear cells in the absence or presence of unlabeled insulin. The binding of ^{125}I-insulin, expressed as a percentage of the total radioactivity, is plotted as a function of the insulin concentration in the assay. The shaded area represents results (mean ± 1 SD) from a large number of normal subjects. The results for individual obese patients (A-G) are also shown. It can be seen that two of the obese subjects (A and F) have insulin binding within the normal range, whereas most of the obese patients have depressed levels of insulin binding. The monocytes, although they constitute only about 20 percent of the cells, account for 85 percent or more of the insulin binding in the mononuclear cell preparations. Therefore, for greater precision, the binding of ^{125}I-insulin is expressed per 10^7 monocytes. The monocytes are identified by their ability to ingest latex beads or by a specific esterase stain. The data in part (*a*) can be plotted in another way as to yield values for the total receptor concentration per cell; the latter are presented in Part (*b*) for the same patients and plotted as a function of the fasting insulin concentration in vivo at the time that the cells were obtained. It can be seen that the receptor concentration per cell is inversely related to the circulating ambient insulin in vivo. To obtain the data in part (*c*), the 4 patients with the most severe degrees of hyperinsulinemia and insulin resistance were put on diets for several weeks. During this time the plasma insulin concentration fell, glucose intolerance improved, insulin resistance disappeared, and receptor concentrations were returned to normal. (From Bar *et al.*[93])

needed to maintain the obesity, rather than the mass of adipose tissue, appears to be the critical factor.

Acute starvation in obese people produces a unique response; the circulating plasma insulin falls markedly over the 24 to 72 hours of the fast, but receptor concentrations remain subnormal.[93] By 48 to 72 hours, there is a sharp increase in receptor affinity, but only at resting levels of plasma insulin (i.e., 0–20 microunits/ml). Under these conditions, insulin binding to its receptor is normal at low levels of insulin but subnormal at high concentrations of insulin (Fig. 153-7). Thin people who are fasted for 72 hours show no changes in their receptors.[93]

OBESITY IN RODENTS

The alterations in obese rodents are even of a more marked degree. In ob/ob mice, in whom obesity is inherited as a mendelian recessive, there is severe hyperinsulinemia, extreme resistance to insulin in vivo and in vitro, and a marked decrease in the concentration of insulin receptors. The magnitude of the receptor deficit is inversely related to the basal level of plasma insulin[60] (Fig. 153-8). The decrease in receptor concentrations has been demonstrated in multiple tissues including liver,[8,20,60] fat,[98] skeletal muscle,[99] heart muscle,[100] brain,[101] and thymus lymphocytes.[102] The defect is present when measured in whole cells, as well as in crude preparations of membranes and in highly purified plasma membranes.[8] The residual receptors are normal ones in all respects, including their affinity for hormone.[103] Restriction of food intake in the ob/ob mouse to the food intake of a normal littermate results in weight loss, reduction of plasma insulin concentrations, and a restoration or near restoration of receptor concentrations[60] (Fig. 153-8). Acute

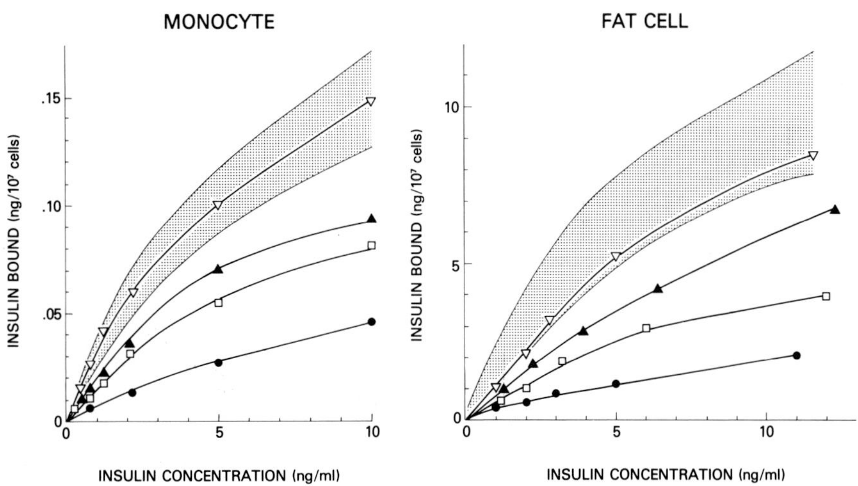

Fig. 153-5. Insulin binding to monocytes compared with adipocytes. Insulin binding was measured with circulating monocytes from obese patients and compared with similar studies of insulin binding to isolated adipocytes obtained from a separate group of obese subjects. The two series of obese subjects were studied in separate laboratories. Illustrated in each panel are the patient in each group with the most severe insulin binding defect, the patient with the mildest defect, and two that approximate median values. It can be seen that the mildly affected patient in each group falls within the normal range (shaded area) and that the most severely affected patient in each group has insulin binding that is reduced to a level of about 25 percent of normal. (The data are derived from experiments from Bar et al.[87,93] and Harrison et al.[95])

fasting of the obese animal for 24 hours results in a sharp fall in the circulating insulin concentration and a doubling of the receptor concentration. Thin littermates who are fasted for comparable periods also show an increase in receptor concentration of about 20 percent (in contrast to humans who are starved). When the ob/ob animals are fasted but their insulin concentrations maintained at high levels by injections of long-acting insulin, the receptor concentrations remain low. On the other hand, if the obese mice are fasted but insulin replacement is withheld until the last hour or two of the fast, receptor concentrations are raised to the level that were observed in animals that were fasted but not given insulin at all.[60,99]

The db/db mouse, another form of inherited obesity, shows similar degrees of hyperinsulinemia, insulin resistance, and receptor deficiencies[60] (Fig. 153-8). When normal mice are given gold thioglucose or other gold salts, neurons in the hypothalamus and related areas are destroyed, which results in a pattern of chronic overeating. As these animals overeat and gain weight, the plasma insulin concentrations in the basal state rise and receptor concentrations decrease. After these animals have become obese, if food intake is restricted, the process is reversed with a progressive fall in weight and fall in plasma insulin associated with restoration of receptor concentrations to normal (Fig. 153-8). As with the two forms of inherited obesity, the receptor concentration is predicted by the magnitude of the elevation of the plasma insulin (Fig. 153-8);

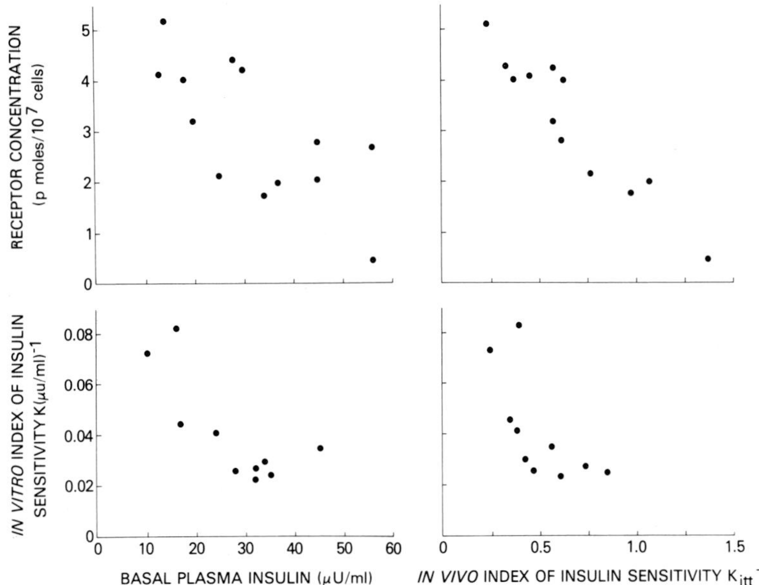

Fig. 153-6. Correlation of receptor defect with other features of insulin resistance in obese humans. A group of obese human adults were studied. Isolated fat cells were studied for their responsiveness to insulin in vitro, as well as the concentration of insulin receptors on the cell surface. This was compared to the level of insulin in the circulation under basal fasting conditions and to in vivo measurements of insulin sensitivity. It can be seen that the four variables correlate quite closely with one another. (From Harrison and King-Roach.[96])

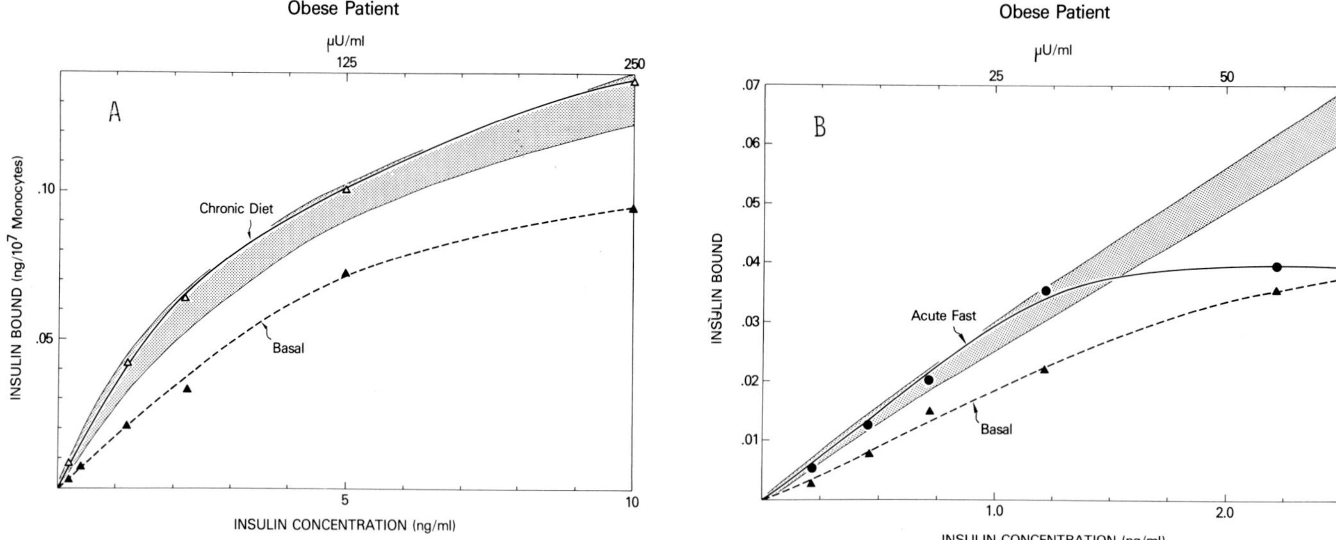

Fig. 153-7. Insulin receptor following chronic diet and acute fast in obese subjects. (*a*) The lower curve ("Basal"▲---▲) represents studies of insulin binding to specific receptors on monocytes from an insulin-resistant obese patient in the basal state. It can be seen that insulin binding is depressed in comparison with normal subjects (shaded area) over the entire range of insulin concentrations. Caloric restriction for several weeks ameliorates insulin resistance, improves glucose tolerance, and restores insulin binding to normal. In the curve labeled "Chronic Diet" Δ---Δ, it can be seen that insulin binding has been restored to normal over the entire range of insulin concentrations. This restoration has occurred despite the fact that the patient is still markedly overweight and has a multifold excess of body fat. Thus, overeating rather than excess fat tissue is probably the cause of the abnormalities. (*b*) Results of an insulin binding study in the same patient after an acute fast, i.e., less than 50 calories per day for 2 to 3 days. It can be seen that with an acute fast (●——●) insulin binding is restored to normal over the range of insulin concentrations that are characteristic of the basal or unstimulated state in vivo (i.e., less than or equal to 1 ng/ml). This results from an increase in the affinity of the unoccupied receptor ($\bar{K}_e$). At concentrations of insulin in excess of 1.2 ng/ml, insulin binding is depressed because concentration of insulin receptors remains depressed for the several days of the fast. (From Bar et al.[84,87])

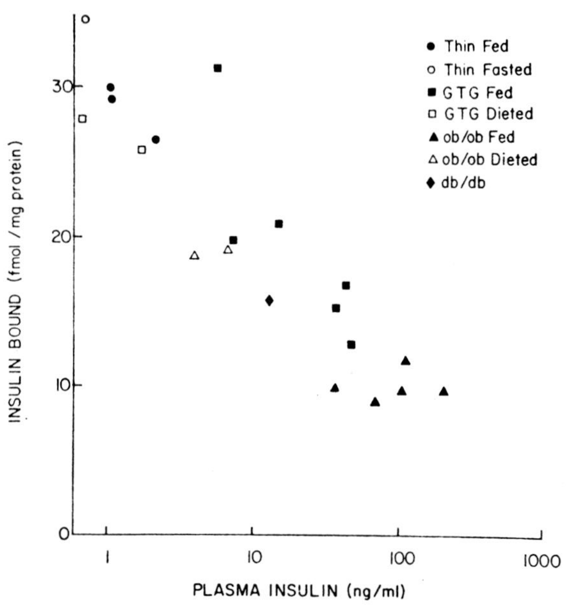

Fig. 153-8. Relationship of receptor concentration to basal plasma insulin concentration. This figure summarizes a large number of studies on mice with two forms of inherited obesity (ob/ob and db/db), as well as a group of normal mice who have become obese following treatment with gold thioglucose (GTG). The obese mice are compared to their thin littermates under a variety of experimental manipulations of feeding. Insulin receptor concentrations obtained from studies of ^{125}I-insulin binding to highly purified plasma membranes from liver are plotted as a function of the plasma insulin concentration in the basal state at the time of the experiment. It should be emphasized that this inverse correlation is related to the chronic level but not to the acute level of the ambient insulin. (From Soll et al.[60])

in all cases, the residual receptors are normal receptors and are only reduced in number. With severe degrees of hyperinsulinemia, 75 to 80 percent of the receptors are lost; further increases in plasma insulin concentration produce no further decreases in receptor concentration.[60,104,105]

EFFECT OF ELEVATED INSULIN CONCENTRATIONS IN VITRO

This relationship between receptor concentration and the chronic ambient insulin concentration has been reproduced in vitro with IM-9 lymphocytes, a continuous cell line of B-type lymphocytes.[23] These cells have insulin receptors that are indistinguishable from insulin receptors on all other tissues studied.[79,106] When these cells are grown in the absence of insulin, they have a full complement of receptors. If insulin is present in the growth medium, there is a rapid fall in receptor concentration, so that by 12 to 24 hours, the receptor concentration reaches a new steady state, and the steady-state concentration of receptors is inversely related to the concentration of insulin in the medium[23,62] (Fig. 153-9). At very high insulin concentrations, receptor concentrations are reduced to about 25 percent of normal. When insulins that differ in biological potency over a 100-fold range are used, the decrease in receptor concentration is proportional to the biological potency of the insulin, which is proportional to the ability of that insulin to bind to the insulin receptors. Insulin binding to the insulin receptor is a necessary but not sufficient condition for insulin-mediated loss of the insulin receptor. Thus, reduction in the temperature to 24°C or 20°C enhances insulin binding to its receptors but prevents insulin-mediated loss of receptors. Likewise interference with protein synthesis by cycloheximide or interference with energy production of the cells will also prevent the insulin-mediated loss of receptors.[62,107]

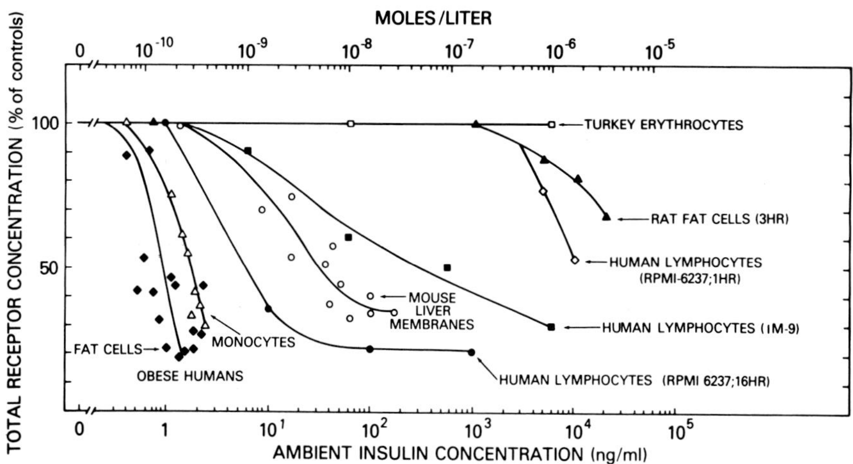

Fig. 153-9. Summary of relationship of receptor concentration to ambient insulin. The relationship of receptor concentration per cell as a function of the ambient insulin concentration is shown here for multiple systems. For obese humans, isolated fat cells and circulating monocytes were both studied. Insulin receptors on plasma membrane of liver from rats with hyperinsulinemia and hypoinsulinemia fit approximately the same relationship as in humans. With receptors in mice, there is a similar relationship, although over a different range of insulin concentrations (mice in vivo have higher insulin concentrations than humans). Human lymphocytes in cell culture have insulin receptors on their cell surface; the receptor concentration at steady state (16 to 18 hours) is predicted by the concentration of insulin in the medium. Cells that are incubated for shorter time periods show the same relationship but at higher insulin concentrations (rat fat cells incubated for 3 hours or human lymphocytes incubated for 1 hour). Turkey erythrocytes, incubated for up to 24 hours at 30° in the presence of insulin, showed no change in the concentration of their insulin receptors.

When IM-9 lymphocytes are maintained in the presence of insulin, they have a reduced concentration of receptors. Removal of the insulin results in a prompt increase in receptor concentrations; about half of the receptors are restored by 6 hours, and the full complement of receptors is restored by 18 to 24 hours. If the insulin is removed but protein synthesis is inhibited, restoration of receptors does not occur. While the concentration of receptors on these cells is sensitive to the chronic level of ambient insulin, they show little or no response to acute changes in ambient insulin.[23,62,107] In summary, it appears that insulin itself is capable of modulating the concentration of its own receptors. This process requires that biologically active insulin bind to the receptor, and the combination of hormone with receptor must act on an intact cell in order to produce receptor loss. Recovery of the lost receptors appears to require the synthesis of new receptor molecules. The fate of the lost receptor is unknown. They may be shed into the medium, destroyed at the cell surface, or internalized and destroyed intracellularly. The latter mechanism is the most likely, although as yet there are only scant studies of this process.*

POSTULATED SEQUENCE IN OBESITY

From these and related observations, we conclude that in obesity there is some defect in the regulation of food intake of unknown etiology. The excess intake of food, either of total calories or of carbohydrates, produces hyperinsulinemia in the basal state, probably mediated in part via hormones of the gastrointestinal tract. The hyperinsulinemia causes a reduction in receptor concentration and possibly also desensitization at steps beyond the receptor, both of which decrease sensitivity to insulin at the target cell. Resistance to the hormone leads to further hyperinsulinemia and its consequent receptor loss and desensitization, although to a reduced degree because of resistance to the hormone. A steady state is established in which we observe hyperinsulinemia, decrease in receptor concentration, and resistance at the target cell.

The brain has insulin receptors.[101] It is as yet unclear what role they play in appetite, satiety, and insulin resistance.

DIABETES WITHOUT OBESITY

The general pattern of relationships noted in obese patients also holds for thin diabetics.[108,109] Whereas most obese patients have elevations of the basal insulin, only a minority of thin diabetics have elevations of the plasma insulin in the basal state. The relationship of receptor concentration to the basal insulin is the same as that which has been observed in obese patients. Likewise, measurements of insulin resistance in vivo correlate well with the elevations of the basal insulin and reduction in receptor concentration.[108,109] (It should be emphasized that the majority of all diabetics are overweight.) In contrast with obesity, the sequence of events by which the thin diabetic patients reach the steady state of hyperinsulinemia, receptor deficiency, and resistance to insulin at the target cell is unknown.

ANIMAL MODELS OF INSULIN DEFICIENCY AND EXCESS

In other animal studies, hormone and receptor show a similar relationship. Chinese hamsters that are diabetic have hypoinsulinemia and elevated concentrations of insulin receptors.[65] Rodents made diabetic by the administration of alloxan have a fall in insulin associated with an elevation in receptor concentrations.[66,110] Insulin replacement causes restoration of receptor concentrations or may even produce a subnormal level of receptor concentrations.[66,110] Likewise, normal rats who were treated with insulin in gradually increasing daily doses had a progressive decrease in the concentration of their insulin receptors, with the magnitude of the loss being related to the ambient insulin concentration.[111]

*Regulation of the receptor concentration by homologous hormone is widespread.[95] However, the stringent conditions with the insulin system that the cell be intact and that protein synthesis be required for both receptor loss and receptor recovery are not matched in all systems. Thus, catecholamine receptors can be lost and recovered without new protein synthesis, and these alterations can be carried out in preparations of cell membrane.[43]

UREMIA

Uremia is frequently associated with glucose intolerance, hyperinsulinemia, and variable degrees of insulin resistance but the mechanisms are very complex and difficult to isolate. In uremic rodents, insulin receptors were decreased, and the magnitude of the receptor deficiency was predicted by the magnitude of the hyperinsulinemia.[112]

ACROMEGALY

Acromegaly is classically described as an insulin-resistant state associated with hyperinsulinemia. Receptor concentrations are decreased, and the magnitude of the decrease is related to the elevation of the basal insulin. In addition, there is an increase in the affinity of the insulin receptor, which is restricted to levels of insulin typically found in the resting state (0–20 microunits/ml); the receptor affinity is normal at insulin concentrations in the stimulated range (>20 microunits/ml). There were highly significant correlations between the magnitude of the elevation of the plasma growth hormone, the elevation of the basal insulin, the severity of insulin resistance, and the severity of the receptor defect.[113,114]

INSULINOMA

Patients with insulin-secreting tumors typically have inappropriate elevations of the plasma insulin in the basal state. Receptor concentrations in these patients are depressed and show the same relationship to the plasma insulin as have been observed in obese patients and in thin diabetics. As in obesity, the hyperinsulinemia precedes the receptor defect, but presumably the cause of the hormone excess is different in the two conditions. In some patients with insulinoma there are also some alterations in receptor affinity, and in these cases the speed of onset of the hypoglycemia following the cessation of eating seemed to correlate with these changes in receptor affinity.[115]

It is not clear whether patients with insulinomas are insulin resistant as a result of their receptor deficiency. While they do become hypoglycemic, indicating that they respond to insulin, they are clearly somewhat resistant to insulin; their resting insulin concentrations are elevated to levels that are rarely or only transiently achieved in normal individuals and carried for hours before producing hypoglycemia, and then only if food intake is omitted. Likewise they typically show glucose intolerance. In summary, the receptor concentration is inversely related to the chronic ambient insulin concentration, but we are unable to give these changes an unambiguous tie to "insulin resistance."

CAUTIONS IN INTERPRETATION

The triad at steady state of (1) elevated concentration of biologically active hormone, (2) resistance to the effect of hormone at the target cell, and (3) decrease in hormone binding to receptors can be reached by any of multiple routes. The primary defect or earliest defect in the cycle could be hormone excess, receptor deficiency, or distal defect in hormone action. Any one would yield the same triad at steady state, since excess hormone desensitizes the target cell (at the receptor and/or steps beyond receptor), and a resistant target cell (at the receptor or beyond) produces hypersecretion of hormone. Thus, elucidation of the sequence of events requires that the steady state be perturbed and that variables be dealt with individually when possible.

HETEROLOGOUS EFFECTS OF ONE HORMONE ON ANOTHER

As noted earlier, one hormone can affect the physiology of another hormone by a variety of mechanisms. At the receptor level, hormones frequently interact with one another.[3] For example, estrogens can have effects on oxytocin receptors,[116] growth hormones receptors,[117] their own receptors,[63] or progesterone receptors.[59] Likewise, FSH can cause a marked increase in LH receptors,[25] thereby sensitizing the ovary during maturation. The following two examples involve instances in which the effects of one hormone on the receptors of another appear to have major pathological consequences with possible applications in human disorders.

INSULIN RECEPTORS AND GLUCOCORTICOID STATUS[21,118–121]

Glucocorticoid deficiency is associated with supernormal sensitivity to the effects of insulin. Insulin receptors in rats that are glucocorticoid-deficient have an increase in affinity without any change in receptor concentration[121] (Fig. 153-10*A*). Conversely, glucocorticoid excess, which is associated with insulin resistance, is associated with a subnormal affinity of insulin for its receptors (Fig. 153-10*A*). In both cases, receptor concentrations show little or no change. This was a bit unexpected, since with glucocorticoid excess the severity of the hyperinsulinemia and insulin resistance is of the same magnitude as with acromegaly and obesity. Thus, in the case of steroid excess, the regulatory role of hyperinsulinemia in regulating the concentration of its own receptors appears to be nullified, and some mechanism other than hyperinsulinemia appears to be the primary regulator of the insulin receptor. The molecular mechanisms for this nullification and for the alteration in receptor affinity are as yet unknown.

HYPERTHYROIDISM AND CATECHOLAMINE RECEPTORS[122–124]

The hyperthyroid state in man and in experimental animals has many manifestations that appear to be an excessive effect of catecholamines, and many of these symptoms of thyrotoxicosis can be blocked by the administration of propranolol, a β-adrenergic antagonist. The mechanism for this heightened catecholamine state in hyperthyroidism has been speculated about for some time. Recent studies indicate that elevated levels of thyroid hormone increase the concentration of catecholamine receptors on the cell surface and may cause, at least in part, the magnified catecholamine effects (Fig. 153-10*B*).

RECEPTOR AUTOANTIBODIES

EXTREME INSULIN RESISTANCE ASSOCIATED WITH ACANTHOSIS NIGRICANS

There are a group of patients who have severe insulin resistance, extreme hyperinsulinemia, and severe defects in insulin binding to their own receptors, which were associated in most cases with the skin lesion of acanthosis nigricans.[125] The cases thus far have all been sporadic with no familial occurrence. The characteristic features of these patients are shown in Table 153-4.

Patients with the type A syndrome are female children or

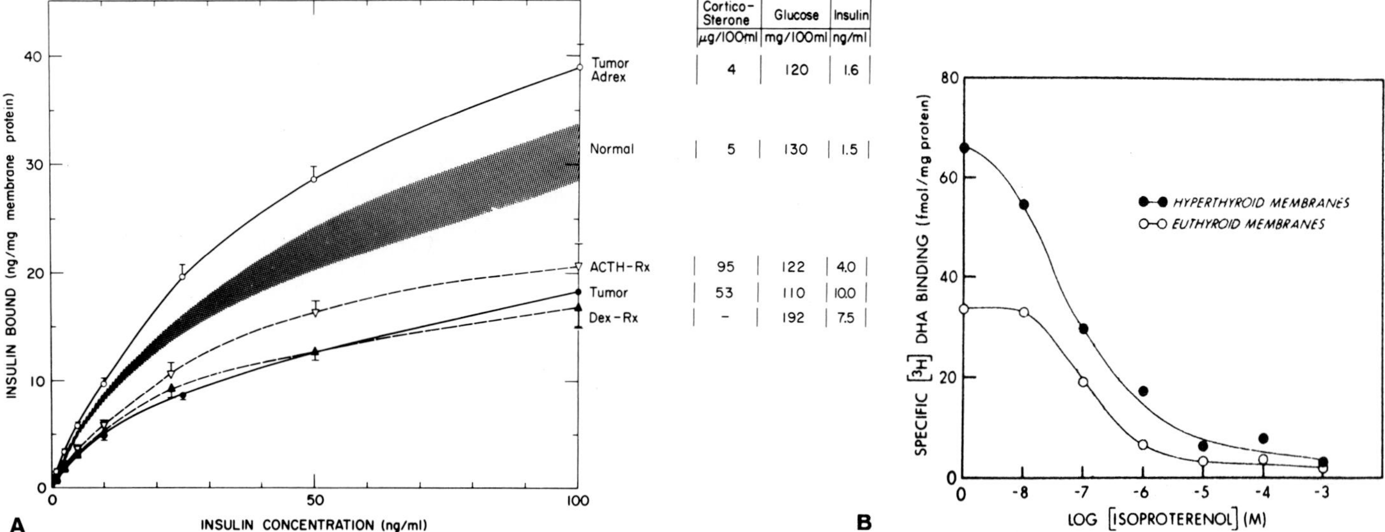

Fig. 153-10. Effects of glucocorticoid deficiency and excess on insulin binding. (*a*) Normal rats were treated with ACTH ("ACTH-Rx") or dexamethasone (Dex-Rx). The curve labeled "Tumor" represents rats bearing tumors that hypersecrete ACTH; the curve labeled "Tumor Adrex" represents the same animals following adrenalectomy. (Although these tumors also hypersecrete growth hormone and prolactin, the effect on the insulin receptor in these animals appears to reflect only the hyperadrenal and hypoadrenal states, with little or no effect from the other two hormones.) The depression of insulin binding resulting from glucocorticoid excess and the elevated level of insulin binding in adrenalectomized animals appears, on careful analysis, to be largely or entirely caused by changes in receptor affinity with little or no changes in receptor concentration. (*b*) Effect of thyroid hormone on β-adrenergic receptors. Rats were treated with thyroxine or triiodothyronine. β-adrenergic receptors on membrane preparations of cardiac muscle were measured by studying the binding of a leveled specific antagonist (dihydroalprenolol) as a function of the concentration of β-adrenergic agonist (isoproterenol). Analysis of the data indicate that in the hyperthyroid state there is an increase in receptor number, with little or no effect on receptor affinity. (From Williams et al.[122])

Table 153-4. Syndrome of Extreme Insulin Resistance with Acanthosis Nigricans

1. Extreme elevation of endogenous plasma insulin concentrations—basal and stimulated
2. Extreme resistance to exogenous insulin
3. Absence of other known causes of insulin resistance, including obesity and lipoatrophy
4. Glucose tolerance ranges from normal to severe hyperglycemia with moderate ketoacidosis
5. Marked impairment of insulin binding to its receptors on freshly obtained cells (monocytes)
6. No defect in insulin binding to cultured cells (fibroblasts)
7. Two or more clinical subtypes:

Type A—no immunological features
- Young females: children and adolescents
- Disordered sexual function: amenorrhea; hirsutism; enlargement of clitoris and/or labiae; polycystic ovaries
- Receptor concentration is decreased; receptor affinity is normal;
- Accelerated early growth; no autoimmune features; spontaneous remissions

Type B—autoimmune features
- Older; mostly females
- Immunological features: elevated erythrocyte sedimentation rate; leukopenia; alopecia; arthralgias; nephritis
- Antireceptor antibodies: bind to insulin receptor; block insulin binding and action, and also mimic insulin action
- Clinical course: insulin resistance may be replaced by hypoglycemia; nephritis and nephrotic syndrome associated with proliferation of cellular receptors with low affinity for insulin; remissions (spontaneous or drug-induced) and death in one case

Other types?

young adults who have no known cause of insulin resistance but do have problems with masculinization and hirsutism. On fasting, their plasma insulins fall substantially but are still somewhat elevated; over this interval, there is no change in receptor concentration or affinity. The mechanism for these defects is unknown, as is the sequence of events that leads to the receptor defect, hyperinsulinemia, and insulin resistance.

In another subgroup, designated type B, there are multiple features suggesting an autoimmune process, although few of the patients fit into the realm of previously defined autoimmune disorders. They have circulating immunoglobulins that have specificity for the insulin receptor. When these antibodies are bound to the insulin receptor, the binding of insulin to the receptor is impaired. The severity of the insulin resistance correlates well with the titer of antibodies. Both labeled insulin and labeled antibodies bind to the receptor, and the binding of both labeled ligands is competed for by biologically active insulins and by immunoglobulins from the same patient or from other patients with this disorder. When the disease remits, either spontaneously or as a result of the administration of agents that suppress immune functions, the circulating antibodies disappear along with the abnormality in insulin binding and hyperinsulinemia. Thus the presence and the titer of the antibodies correlates closely with the disease process.[52,125–130]

All the antibodies studied thus far, in binding to the receptor, not only block insulin binding but also display insulinomimetic properties, i.e., the antibodies are not pure antagonists but rather partial agonists.[131] Clinically, the insulin-blocking effect predominates most of the time, but in 3 of the patients, we have observed periods of hypoglycemia and in 2 patients it was quite severe. The factors that cause the insulin-blocking properties to predominate most of the time and the insulinlike properties to predominate at other times is as yet unclear.

GRAVES' DISEASE WITH ANTIBODIES TO THE TSH RECEPTOR

There are more than a dozen known causes of hyperthyroidism, but the major cause is diffuse hyperthyroidism associated with Graves' Disease. In addition to hyperthyroidism, these patients may manifest ophthalmopathy and, less commonly, pretibial myxedema. Plasma from these patients contains immunoglobulins with thyroid-stimulating bioactivity that can be demonstrated both in vivo and in vitro. Recent studies strongly suggest that these immunoglobulins have specificity for the TSH receptor of the human thyroid.[29,132] They bind to the thyroid and block TSH binding and, in addition, are capable of simulating TSH, i.e., the antibody-receptor complex mimics the TSH-receptor complex.[133–137] The role of these antibodies in causing the thyrotoxicosis is becoming increasingly accepted, but the role of these antibodies or of another antibody population in the ophthalmopathy or in pretibial myxedema is as yet unclear.

MYASTHENIA GRAVIS[71–77]

Patients with myasthenia gravis have circulating antibodies directed against the acetylcholine receptor located on motor endplates of skeletal muscles. This disease can be simulated in experimental animals by immunization with acetylcholine receptors from the electric organ of marine animals, and the disease can be passively transferred by immunoglobulins from immunized animals. The disease picture in animals is complicated by the coexistence of cellular immune components that cause substantial destruction of the motor endplates in addition to the interference by humoral factors.

Autoantibodies against the acetylcholine receptor, in contrast to those directed against the TSH receptor or insulin receptor, do not interfere with the binding of labeled ligand to the receptor but do appear to impair the capacity of the acetylcholine-receptor complex to generate its signal at the cell. In summary, specific antibodies directed against some region of the hormone (or neurotransmitter) receptor are capable of disrupting the system by blocking the binding of normal stimulating agents to its receptor (TSH and insulin), by interfering with the transmission of the message that would normally be generated by the ligand-receptor complex (insulin and acetylcholine), or by simulating the specific hormone signal (TSH and insulin).

SPECIFICITY SPILLOVER

DISEASE MANIFESTATIONS RESULTING FROM DEGENERACIES OF HORMONE RECEPTOR SPECIFICITY

As a first approximation, all cells in the body are exposed to the same concentration of all hormones. For a system to have specificity, the target cell must have a set of specific receptors that recognize the particular hormone. Ideally, each hormone is unique and has its own unique receptor (Table 153-5). In fact, each recognition unit is not unique. Among the peptide hormones there are families of hormones within which members have structural similarities, presumably because they evolved from a common ancestor. Likewise, overlaps exist with receptors. As shown in Table 153-5, the hormone has high affinity for its own receptors but also retains some finite affinity for the receptors of a structurally related hormone.

Table 153-5.

	Hormone (H)	Binds to Specific Receptor (R)	To Produce Characteristic Effects (E)
Ideal	H_A ⟶	R_A ⟶ ⟶	E_A
	H_B ⟶	R_B ⟶ ⟶	E_B
Within a Family of Hormones	H_A ⟶ (also ⤡ to R_B)	R_A ⟶ ⟶	E_A
	H_B ⟶ (also ⤢ to R_A)	R_B ⟶ ⟶	E_B

Note: Potential for spillover is present if hormone A (H_A) has any reactivity (i.e., has a finite, albeit low, affinity) for receptor of class B (R_B). Since the cross-reacting hormones typically have intrinsic activities that are normal or nearly normal, the signal strength of an H_AR_B complex should be the same as that of an H_BR_B complex. Since $[HR] = [H] \times K \times [R]$, spillover occurs when concentration of H_A is so high that $[H_A] \times K_{AB} \times [R_B]$ is equivalent to physiological range, i.e., $[H_B] \times K_{BB} \times [R_B]$.

Under normal circumstances, the spillover of one hormone on to the receptors of another is so slight that the fluctuations of the hormone concentration within the physiological range cause no significant biological effects via the receptor for other hormones. Under pathological circumstances, where the concentration of one hormone is elevated, disease manifestations can obviously result from excessive effect mediated through its own receptors. In addition, when the concentration of that hormone becomes sufficiently high, its weak affinity for another class of receptor now produces significant biological effects through that hormonal pathway (Table 153-6). Two examples from the insulin family will be presented and several other possible examples indicated (Table 153-7).

THE FAMILY OF INSULINLIKE PEPTIDES[84,138–149]

In addition to insulin and its precursors such as proinsulin, there exists in plasma or serum a series of closely related molecules designated somatomedins A and C, NSILA-s (IGF I and IGF II), and multiplication stimulating activity, which are insulinlike growth factors.* These peptides are similar to insulin and have molecular weights in the range of insulin and proinsulin but do not bind to anti-insulin antibodies and therefore do not react in the radioimmunoassay for insulin. They produce all the metabolic effects of insulin and at high concentrations are capable of maximally stimulating insulin-sensitive pathways. Biologically they are about 1 percent as potent as insulin on a molar basis, which is comparable to their reactivity for the insulin receptor, suggesting strongly that their insulinlike properties are exercised through the insulin receptor.[84,138–140]

These peptides are also growth-promoting agents; they stimulate cell division in numerous test systems. When they exercise their growth-promoting activities, they do so by binding to another set of receptors, which, in contrast to the insulin receptor, bind the insulinlike growth factors better than they bind insulin and proinsulin.

*Nonsuppressible insulinlike activity soluble in acid ethanol (NSILA-s) is composed of two closely related peptides, insulinlike growth factors (IGF) I and II.[141] Other related peptides that are not covered here include the insulinlike peptide that is found in the precipitate following acid ethanol treatment of plasma (NSILA-p or NSILP), which is of much higher molecular weight; somatomedin B, which has other biological characteristics; and nerve growth factor and relaxin, which, despite their extraordinary structural similarities to insulin and proinsulin, do not react significantly with the insulin receptor.

Table 153-6. Schematic Representation of Disorders with Specificity Spillover

Type I—Pure spillover

H_A excess ⟶ R_A: pathway blocked or absent
⟶ R_B ⟶ ⟶ ⟶ E_B excess only

Type II—Mixed: some excess effects through homologous receptor and some effects through spillover

H_A excess ⟶ R_A ⟶ ⟶ ⟶ E_A excess and
⟶ R_B ⟶ ⟶ ⟶ E_B excess

H = hormone; R = receptor; E = biological effect; A = homologous; B = spillover pathway.

Insulin and proinsulin also stimulate cell growth but are less potent on a molar basis than the insulinlike growth factors; the growth-promoting properties of insulin and proinsulin are probably not mediated via the insulin ("metabolic") receptor but rather through the receptors that prefer insulinlike factors ("growth" receptors). Thus, both insulin and insulinlike growth factors interact with their own receptors but, in addition, have weak yet significant reactivities for one or more closely related classes of receptors (Fig. 153-11). At low concentrations, each produces its own characteristic effects, whereas at very high concentrations, in addition to producing its own effects, each can produce effects mediated through the other receptors. It should be emphasized that these receptors are all highly specific. They discriminate totally between insulins and all noninsulin peptides, binding only insulin and insulinlike peptides; among the insulins, each receptor class has a different order of affinities.

HYPOGLYCEMIA ASSOCIATED WITH NONISLET CELL TUMORS

Islet cell tumors associated with hypoglycemia produce insulin and/or proinsulin inappropriately, and this can be detected by radioimmunoassay of plasma insulin. Nonislet cell tumors associated with hypoglycemia do not have inappropriate elevations of plasma insulin by radioimmunoassay; about 40 percent of those patients who have nonislet cell tumors with hypoglycemia have elevated levels of an insulinlike growth factor, NSILA-s, which is measured by radioreceptor assay that is highly sensitive to NSILA-s.[84,140,150,151] (The cause of the hypoglycemia in the other cases is as yet unknown.) Because under ordinary circumstances the concentration of NSILA-s is low relative to its affinity for the insulin receptor, NSILA-s has an insignificant role in glucose homeostasis and energy metabolism. When present at pathologically high levels, this growth factor interacts with the insulin receptor and produces hypoglycemia indistinguishable from that produced by insulin or proinsulin. From our studies, we estimate that the free NSILA-s in the plasma of these patients has as much insulinlike activity as does the insulin and proinsulin in a patient with an insulin-secreting tumor. Thus, an excess of a biologically active peptide in the circulation produces pathological effects, not by excessive stimulation through its own pathway, but by reacting with receptors of a closely related peptide.

INFANTS OF DIABETIC MOTHERS[152]

The offspring of diabetic mothers have chronically elevated levels of circulating insulin in utero, presumably owing to stimulation of the infant's β-cells by an excessive supply of glucose and/or amino acids from the mother. At term, the babies often have macrosomia and excessive deposition of stored substrates (fat, glycogen, and protein) and, in the first few postnatal days, hypoglycemia with inappropriate elevations in plasma insulin. The excess of stored substrates and the hypoglycemia are probably effects of insulin mediated through the insulin receptor, whereas the macrosomia, at least in part, may result from the effects of insulin mediated through one or more classes of receptors that have high reactivity for the insulinlike growth factors. Thus, excessive or inappropriately elevated levels of circulating hormone produce separate classes of pathological effects by reacting with its own receptors as well as with receptors of closely related peptides.

Table 153-7. Possible Examples of Specificity Spillover

Clinical Condition	Hormone in Excess	Reacts with Receptors for	To Produce
Nonislet cell tumors with hypoglycemia	NSILA-s*	Insulin	Hypoglycemia
Babies of diabetic mothers	Insulin	Insulinlike growth factor(s)	Macrosomia
Untreated Addison's disease; "Autonomous" overproduction of ACTH, pituitary or ectopic	ACTH	α-MSH	Skin darkening
Acromegaly	HGH	Prolactin	Syndrome of prolactin excess†
Choriocarcinoma	HCG	TSH	Hyperthyroidism
Primary hypothyroidism of childhood (Van Wyk-Grumbach)	TSH	LH, FSH	Precocious puberty
Glucocorticoid excess, especially of endogenous origin	Hydrocortisone	Aldosterone	Hypertension
Hypertension of pregnancy; Essential hypertension	? Oxytocin ? Other nonapeptide	Nonapeptide-specific pressor receptor	Hypertension

*NSILA-s is composed of two related peptides, IGF-I and IGF-II. The latter is likely to be the mediator of the hypoglycemia in these patients.

†Amenorrhea, galactorrhea, infertility, derangements in gonadotropic hormone secretion.

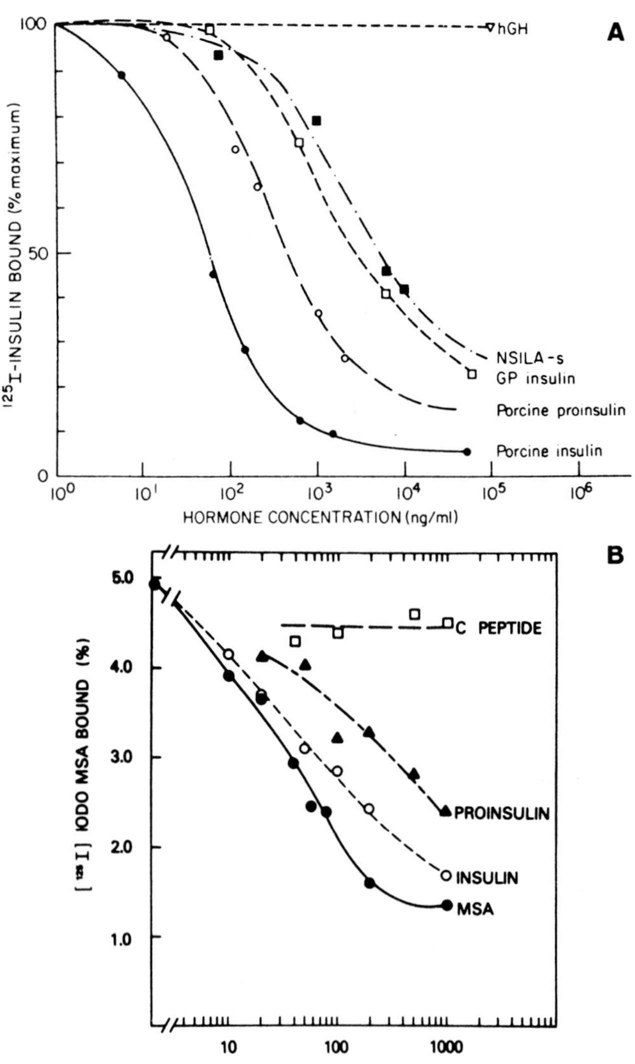

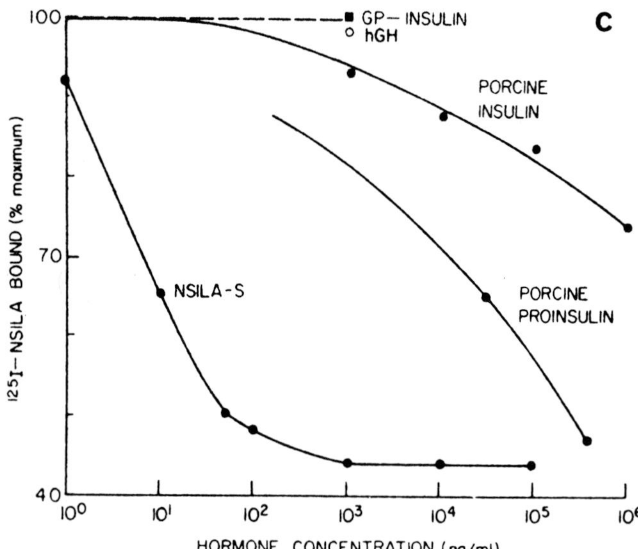

Fig. 153-11. Receptors for insulin and for insulinlike growth factors. (*a*) With the insulin receptor, which mediates the metabolic responses of insulin, it can be seen that insulin is about 10 times more potent than proinsulin, which in turn is many times more sensitive than NSILA-s or MSA, typical insulinlike growth factors. (*b*) A characteristic receptor for growth factors shows that the binding of growth factors is slightly higher in affinity than the binding of insulin, which in turn is slightly stronger than binding of proinsulin. (From Rechler et al.[146]) (*c*) The specific NSILA-s receptor, found on the plasma membrane of the rat liver, has an exceptionally high affinity for NSILA-s and MSA, with markedly less reactivity for proinsulin and insulin. (From Megyesi et al.[150]) It should be emphasized that all three sets of receptors are highly specific for insulin and insulinlike growth factors, but among the insulinlike materials the three receptors differ widely in their relative and absolute affinity for the hormones.

OTHER EXAMPLES: SKIN DARKENING WITH ACTH EXCESS

ACTH reacts strongly with its receptors in adrenal cortex (and mammalian fat) and has, in addition, a weak reactivity for MSH receptors; recall that N-terminal portion of ACTH contains a near-replica of the whole alpha-MSH molecule. With intact adrenal cortical tissue, excess levels of ACTH produce glucocorticoid excess through the ACTH receptor. In the presence or absence of a functioning adrenal, ACTH in excess can produce skin darkening, presumably acting through MSH receptors.

GALACTORRHEA WITH ACROMEGALY

In humans, prolactin, placental lactogen, and growth hormone are equally potent as lactogens and are all equally reactive with prolactin receptors.[153] In addition, human growth hormone reacts with receptors that are specific for growth hormone.[154,155] The effective prolactin concentration in vivo is the sum of the prolactin + HGH. Ordinarily HGH exerts no significant regulation of prolactin function because its circulating concentrations are too low. In cases of acromegaly where the HGH is substantially elevated, symptoms of prolactin excess (amenorrhea, galactorrhea, infertility, disordered gonadotropin secretion) may accompany the acromegaly, which may be in part or entirely due to the effect of the growth hormone interacting with the prolactin receptor.

CROSS-REACTIVITIES AMONG GLYCOPROTEIN HORMONES

In patients with choriocarcinoma, the extremely elevated levels of HCG typically produce little or no gonadotropic effect, probably because the extreme prolonged elevation of the hormone desensitizes the gonads, at the level of the LH-HCG receptor and/or at other steps beyond receptor. Because the four glycoprotein hormones (HCG,LH,TSH,FSH) are structurally so similar, it is not so surprising that HCG has a weak but finite reactivity with the TSH receptor,[156–158] which probably is the cause of the hyperthyroidism that occasionally develops in patients with choriocarcinoma. As expected, the hyperthyroidism responds dramatically to the successful treatment of the HCG excess. The weak reactivity of TSH for the gonadotropic receptors may possibly account in part for the precocious puberty that sometimes occurs with primary hypothyroidism in children and which can be halted by thyroid hormone replacement.[159]

HYPERTENSION

All naturally occurring glucocorticoids and mineralocorticoids, in addition to strong reactivities with their homologous receptors, have weaker but significant reactivities with receptors for the other.[160] With glucocorticoid excess, hypertension may be present,[161] which in some cases may result from interaction of the glucocorticoid hormone with the receptors for mineralocorticoids.

Another more speculative example relates to the nonapeptides of the neurohypophyseal family. All of these peptides react with all the classes of these receptors, but with widely differing affinities. It is remotely possible that in one or more subsets of patients with essential hypertension or hypertension during pregnancy, the etiologic agent will be excess levels of oxytocin or another related peptide that has high reactivity with receptors on smooth muscle of blood vessels to give pressor effects but relatively weak reactivity with receptors on tubular cells of the kidney that regulate water reabsorption.

SUMMARY

The first step in the action of peptide hormones and of catecholamines is binding to receptors on the cell surface. The receptors, which are at the junction of the intracellular and extracellular environments, are highly regulated, with major changes in both concentration and affinity in response to numerous influences. In multiple disorders in which the sensitivity of the target cell is altered, changes at the receptor have been demonstrated, mediated by the homologous hormone, heterologous hormone, or by autoantibodies to receptor. Disorders resulting from problems of specificity within a given family of hormones have been outlined.

REFERENCES

1. Roth, J.: Peptide hormone binding to receptors: A review of direct studies in vitro. *Metabolism 22:* 1059–1073, 1973.
2. Roth, J., Kahn, C. R., Lesniak, M. A., Gorden, P., De Meyts, P., Megyesi, K., Neville, D. M., Jr., Gavin, J. R., III, Soll, A. H., Freychet, P., Goldfine, I. D., Bar, R. S., and Archer, J. A.: Receptors for insulin, NSILA-s, and growth hormone: Applications to diseases states in man. *Rec. Prog. Horm. Res. 31:* 95–139, 1975.
3. Kahn, C. R.: Membrane receptors for hormones and neurotransmitters. *J. Cell. Biol. 70:* 261–286, 1976.
4. Pastan, I., Roth, J., Macchia, V.: Binding of hormone to tissue: The first step in polypeptide hormone action. *Proc. Natl. Acad. Sci., USA 56:* 1802–1809, 1966.
5. Bergeron, J. J. M., Evans, W. H., and Geschwind, I. I.: Insulin binding to rat liver golgi fraction. *J. Cell Biol. 59:* 771–776, 1973.
6. Posner, B. I., Josefsberg, Z., and Bergeron, J. J. M.: Intracellular (Golgi) insulin receptors in lean and obese rodents: Evidence for two distinct pools. *Diabetes 26* (suppl 1)*:* 368, 1977.
7. Goldfine, I. D., and Smith, G. J.: Binding of insulin to isolated nuclei. *Proc. Natl. Acad. Sci., USA 73:* 1427–1431, 1976.
8. Kahn, C. R., Neville, D. M., Jr., and Roth, J.: Insulin-receptor interaction in the obese-hyperglycemic mouse. *J. Biol. Chem. 248:* 244–250, 1973.
9. Goldfine, I. D., Vigneri, R., Cohen, D., Pliam, N. B., and Kahn, C. R.: Intracellular binding sites for insulin are immunologically distinct from those on the plasma membrane. *Nature 269:* 698–700, 1977.
10. Bradshaw, R. A., Jeng, I., Andres, R. Y., Pulliam, M. W., Silverman, R. E., Rubin, J., and Jacobs, J. W.: Structure and function of nerve growth factor. In: *Endocrinology, vol. 2,* Proceedings of the V International Congress of Endocrinology (James, V. H. T., ed.). Amsterdam, Excerpta Medica, 1977, pp. 206–212.
11. Carpenter, G., and Cohen, S.: ^{125}I-labeled human epidermal growth factor: Binding, internalization, and degradation in human fibroblasts. *J. Cell Biol. 71:* 159–171, 1976.
12. Gorden, P., Carpentier, J.-L., Freychet, P., Le Cam, A., and Orci, L.: Limited intracellular translocation of ^{125}I-insulin: Direct demonstration in isolated hepatocytes. *Science,* 1978 (in press).
13. Kahn, C. R., and Baird, K. L.: The fate of insulin bound to adipocytes: Evidence for compartmentalization and processing. *J. Biol. Chem.* 1978 (in press).
14. Schlessinger, J., Shechter, Y., Willingham, M. C., and Pastan, I.: Direct visualization of the binding, aggregation and internalization of insulin and epidermal growth factor on fibroblastic cells. Submitted.
15. Horvat, A., Li, E., and Katsoyannis, P. G.: Cellular binding sites for insulin in rat liver. *Biochim. Biophys. Acta 382:* 609–620, 1975.
16. Sutherland, E. W., Robison, G. A., and Butcher, R. W.: Some aspects of the biological role of adenosine 3′-5′-monophosphate (cyclic AMP). *Circulation 37:* 279–306, 1968.
17. Soderling, T. R., and Park, C. R.: Recent advances in glycogen metabolism. In: *Advances in Cyclic Nucleotide Research,* vol. 4 (Greengard, P., and Robison, G. A., eds.). New York, Raven Press, 1974, pp. 283–333.
18. Goldberg, N. D., and Haddox, M. K.: Cyclic GMP metabolism and involvement in biological regulation. *Ann. Rev. Biochem. 46:* 823–896, 1977.
19. Rasmussen, H.: Organization and control of endocrine systems. In: *The Textbook of Endocrinology,* 5th ed. (William, R. F., ed.). Philadelphia, W. B. Saunders, 1975, pp. 1–30.
20. Kahn, C. R., Neville, D. M., Jr., Gorden, P., Freychet, P., and Roth, J.: Insulin receptor defect in insulin resistance: Studies in the obese-hyperglycemic mouse. *Biochem. Biophys. Res. Commun. 48:* 135–142, 1972.
21. Kahn, C. R.: Membrane receptors for polypeptide hormones. In: *Methods in Membrane Biology,* vol. 3 (Korn, E. D., ed.). New York, Plenum, 1975, pp. 81–146.
22. Cuatrecasas, P.: Properties of the insulin receptor of isolated fat cells. *J. Biol. Chem. 23:* 7265–7274, 1971.
23. Gavin, J. R., III, Roth, J., Neville, D. M., Jr., De Meyts, P., and Buell, D. N.: Insulin-dependent regulation of insulin receptor concentrations: A direct demonstration in cell culture. *Proc. Natl. Acad. Sci., USA 71:* 84–88, 1974.
24. Varga, J. M., Dipasquale, A., Pawelek, J., McGuire, J. S., and Lerner, A. B.: Regulation of melanocyte stimulating hormone action at the receptor level: Discontinuous binding of hormone to synchronized mouse melanoma cells during the cell cycle. *Proc. Natl. Acad. Sci., USA 71:* 1590–1593, 1974.
25. Zeleznik, A. J., Midgley, A. R., Jr., and Reichert, L. E., Jr.: Granulosa cell maturation in the rat: Increased binding of human chorionic gonadotropin following treatment with follicle stimulating hormone in vivo. *Endocrinology 95:* 818-825, 1974.
26. Thomopoulos, P., Roth, J., Lovelace, E., and Pastan, I.: Insulin receptors in normal and transformed fibroblasts: Relationship to growth and transformation. *Cell 8:* 417–423, 1977.
27. Thomopoulos, P., Kosmakos, F. C., Pastan, I., and Lovelace, E.: Cyclic AMP increased the concentration of insulin receptors in cultured fibroblasts and lymphocytes. *Biochem. Biophys. Res. Commun. 75:* 246–252, 1977.
28. De Meyts, P., Roth, J., Neville, D. M., Jr., Gavin, J. R., III, and Lesniak, M. A.: Insulin interactions with its receptors: Experimental evidence for negative cooperativity. *Biochem. Biophys. Res. Commun. 55:* 154–161, 1973.
29. Mukhtar, E. D., Smith, B. R., Pyle, G. A., Hall, R., and Vice, P.: Relation of thyroid-stimulating immunoglobulins to thyroid function and effects of surgery, radio-iodine, and anti-thyroid drugs. *Lancet I:* 713–715, 1975.
30. Lefkowitz, R. J., Mukherjee, C., Limbird, L., Caron, M., Williams, L. T., Alexander, R. W., Mickey, J. V., and Tate, R.: Regulation of adenylate cyclase coupled β-adrenergic receptors. *Rec. Prog. Horm. Res.* (in press).
31. Lefkowitz, R. J., Roth, J., and Pastan, I.: Effects of calcium on ACTH stimulating of the adrenal: Separation of hormone binding from adenyl cyclase activation. *Nature* (London) *228:* 864–866, 1970.
32. Dufau, M. L., Ryan, D., Baukal, A., and Catt, K. J.: Gonadotropin receptors: Solubilization and purification by affinity chromatography. *J. Biol. Chem. 250:* 4822–4824, 1975.
33. Jacobs, S., Shechter, Y., Bissell, K., and Cuatrecasas, P.: Purification and properties of insulin receptors from rat liver membranes. *Biochem. Biophys. Res. Commun. 77:* 981–988, 1977.
34. Shiu, R. P. C., and Friesen, H. G.: Solubilization and purification of a prolactin receptor from the rabbit mammary gland. *J. Biol. Chem. 249:* 7902–7911, 1974.
35. Kono, T.: Destruction and restoration of the insulin effector system in isolated fat cells. *J. Biol. Chem. 244:* 5777–5784, 1969.
36. Kono, T., and Barham, F. W.: The relationship between the insulin-binding capacity of fat cells and the cellular response to insulin. Studies with intact and trypsin-treated fat cells. *J. Biol. Chem. 246:* 6210–6216, 1971.
37. Lefkowitz, R. J., Roth, J., and Pastan, I.: ACTH-receptor interaction in the adrenal: A model for the initial step in the action of hormones that stimulate adenyl cyclase. *Ann. N. Y. Acad. Sci. 185:* 195–209, 1971.
38. Singer, J.: Architecture and topography of biologic membranes. In: *Cell Membranes: Biochemistry, Cell Biology, and Pathology* (Weis-

mann, G., and Claiborne, R., eds.). New York, H. P. Publishing, 1975.

39. Ginsberg, B. H.: The insulin receptor: Properties and regulation. In: *Biochemical Actions of Hormones* (Litwack, G., ed.). New York, Academic Press, 1977, vol. 4, pp. 313–343.
40. Lefkowitz, R. J., Roth, J., Pricer, W., and Pastan, I.: ACTH-receptors in the adrenal: Specific binding of ACTH-^{125}I and its relation to adenyl cyclase. *Proc. Natl. Acad. Sci., USA 65:* 745–752, 1970.
41. Lin, S.-Y., and Goodfriend, T. L.: Angiotension receptors. *Am. J. Physiol. 218:* 1319–1328, 1970.
42. Lin, S.-Y., Ellis, H., Weisblum, B. A., and Goodfriend, T. L.: Preparation and properties of iodinated angiotensins. *Biochem. Pharmacol. 19:* 651–662, 1970.
43. Rodbell, M., Birnbaumer, L., Pohl, S. L., and Sundby, F.: The reaction of glucagon with its receptor: Evidence for discrete regions of activity and binding in the glucagon molecule. *Proc. Natl. Acad. Sci., USA 68:* 909–913, 1971.
44. Freychet, P., Roth, J., and Neville, D. M., Jr.: Mono-iodoinsulin: Demonstration of its biological activity and binding to fat cells and liver membranes. *Biochem. Biophys. Res. Commun. 43:* 400–408, 1971.
45. Thompson, E. E., Freychet, P., and Roth, J.: Monoiodo-oxytocin: Demonstration of its biological activity and specific binding to isolated fat cells. *Endocrinology 91:* 1199–1205, 1972.
46. Freychet, P., Roth, J., and Neville, D. M., Jr.: Insulin receptors in the liver: specific binding of ^{125}I-insulin to the plasma membrane and its relation to insulin bioactivity. *Proc. Natl. Acad. Sci., USA 68:* 1833–1837, 1971.
47. Pastan, I., Pricer, W., and Blanchette-Mackie, J.: Studies on an ACTH-activated adenyl cyclase from a mouse adrenal tumor. *Metabolism 19:* 809–817, 1970.
48. Cuatrecasas, P.: Affinity chromatography and purification of the insulin receptor of liver cell membranes. *Proc. Natl. Acad. Sci., USA 69:* 1277–1281, 1972.
49. Harrison, L. C., Billington, T., East, I. J., Nichols, R. J., and Clark, S.: The effect of solubilization on the properties of the insulin receptor of human placental membranes. *Endocrinology 102:* 1485–1495, 1978.
50. Ginsberg, B. H., Kahn, C. R., Roth, J., and De Meyts, P.: Insulin-induced dissociation of its receptor into subunits: Possible molecular concomitant of negative cooperativity. *Biochem. Biophys. Res. Commun. 73:* 1068–1074, 1976.
51. Desbuquois, B., and Aurbach, G. D.: Use of polyethylene glycol to separate free and antibody-bound peptide hormones in radioimmunoassay. *J. Clin. Endocrinol. Metab. 33:* 732–738, 1971.
52. Jarrett, D. B., Roth, J., Kahn, C. R., Flier, J. S.: A new direct method for detection and characterization of cell surface receptors for insulin using ^{125}I-anti-receptor autoantibodies. *Proc. Natl. Acad. Sci., USA 73:* 4115–4119, 1976.
53. Zeleznik, A. J., and Roth, J.: Demonstration of the insulin receptor *in vivo* in rabbits and its possible role as a reservoir for the plasma hormone. *J. Clin. Invest.* 1363–1364, 1978.
54. Harrison, L. C., Flier, J. S., Karlsson, F. A., Kahn, C. R., and Roth, J.: Immunoprecipitation of the insulin receptor: A sensitive assay for receptor antibodies and a specific technique for receptor purification. *J. Clin. Endocrinol. Metab.* (in press).
55. Orci, L., Rufener, C., Malaisse-Lagae, F., Blondel, B., Amherdt, M., Bataille, D., Freychet, P., and Perrelet, A.: A morphological approach to surface receptors in islet and liver cells. *Isr. J. Med. Sci. 11:* 639–655, 1975.
56. Jarett, L., and Smith, R. M.: The natural occurrence of insulin receptors in groups on adipocyte plasma membranes as demonstrated with monomeric ferritin-insulin. *J. Supramol. Struct. 6:* 45–59, 1977.
57. Schimke, R. T.: Turnover of membrane proteins in animal cells. In: *Methods in Membrane Biology,* vol. 3 (Korn, E. D., ed.). New York, Plenum, 1975, pp. 201–236.
58. Pastan, I., Johnson, G. S., and Anderson, W. B.: Role of cyclic nucleotide in growth control. *Annu. Rev. Biochem. 44:* 491–522, 1975.
59. Milgrom, E., Thi, L., Atger, M., and Baulieu, E.-E.: Mechanisms regulating the concentration and the conformation of progesterone receptor(s) in the uterus. *J. Biol. Chem. 248:* 6366–6374, 1973.
60. Soll, A. H., Kahn, C. R., Neville, D. M., Jr., and Roth, J.: Insulin receptor deficiency in genetic and acquired obesity. *J. Clin. Invest. 56:* 769–780, 1975.
61. Mukherjee, C., Caron, M. G., and Lefkowitz, R. J.: Catecholamine-induced subsensitivity of adenylate cyclase associated with loss of beta-adrenergic receptor binding sites. *Proc. Natl. Acad. Sci., USA 72:* 1945–1949, 1975.
62. Kosmakos, F. C., and Roth, J.: Cellular basis of insulin-induced loss of insulin receptors. *Endocrinology 98:* 69, 1976.
63. Lesniak, M. A., and Roth, J.: Regulation of receptor concentration by homologous hormone: Effect of human growth hormone on its receptor in IM-9 lymphocytes. *J. Biol. Chem. 251:* 3720–3729, 1976.
64. Olefsky, J. M.: Effect of fasting on insulin binding, glucose transport and glucose oxidation in isolated rat adipocytes. *J. Clin. Invest. 58:* 1450–1460, 1976.
65. Hepp, K. D., Langley, J., Von Funcke, H. J., Renner, R., and Kemmler, W.: Increased insulin binding capacity of liver membranes from diabetic Chinese hamsters. *Nature* (London) *258:* 154, 1975.
66. Davidson, M. B., and Kaplan, S. A.: Increased insulin binding by hepatic plasma membranes from diabetic rats. *J. Clin. Invest. 59:* 22–30, 1977.
67. De Meyts, P.: Cooperative properties of hormone receptors in cell membranes. *J. Supramol. Struct. 4:* 241–258, 1976.
68. De Meyts, P., Van Obberghen, E., Roth, J., Wollmer, A., and Brandenburg, D.: The receptor-binding region of insulin: Mapping of the residues responsible for the negative cooperativity. *Nature 273:* 504–509, 1978.
69. Ginsberg, B. H., Cohen, R. M., Kahn, C. R., and Roth, J.: The detergent solubilized insulin receptor: Properties and partial purification. *Biochem. Biophys. Acta 443:* 227–242, 1976.
70. Flier, J. S., Kahn, C. R., Roth, J., and Bar, R. S.: Antibodies that impair insulin receptor binding in an unusual diabetic syndrome with severe insulin resistance. *Science 190:* 63–65, 1975.
71. Almon, R. R., Andrew, C. G., and Appel, S. H.: Serum globulin in myasthenia gravis: Inhibition of α-bungarotoxin binding to acetylcholine receptors. *Science 186:* 55–57, 1974.
72. Bender, A. N., Ringle, S. P., Engel, W. K., Daniels, M. P., and Vogel, Z.: Myasthenia gravis: A serum factor blocking acetylcholine receptors of the human neuromuscular junction. *Lancet 1:* 607–608, 1975.
73. Aharonov, A., Abramsky, O., Tarrab-Hazdai, R., and Fuchs, S.: Humoral antibodies to acetylcholine receptor in patients with myasthenia gravis. *Lancet 2:* 340–342, 1975.
74. Lindstrom, J. M., Seybold, M. E., Lennon, V. A., Whittingham, S., and Duane, D. D.: Anti-acetylcholine receptor antibody in myasthenia gravis: Incidence, clinical correlates and usefulness as a diagnostic test. *Neurology 26:* 1054–1059, 1976.
75. Toyka, K. V., Drachman, D. B., Pestronk, A., and Kao, I.: Myasthenia gravis: Passive transfer from man to mouse. *Science 190:* 397–399, 1975.
76. Patrick, J., and Lindstrom, J.: Autoimmune response to acetylcholine receptor. *Science 180:* 871–872, 1973.
77. Tarrab-Hazdai, R., Aharonov, A., Silman, I., Fuchs, S., and Abramsky, O.: Experimental autoimmune myasthenia induced in monkeys by purified acetylcholine receptor. *Nature 256:* 128–130, 1975.
78. Shiu, R. P. C., and Friesen, H. G.: Blockade of prolactin action by an antiserum to its receptors. *Science 192:* 259–261, 1976.
79. Gavin, J. R., III, Gorden, P., Roth, J., Archer, J. A., and Buell, D. N.: Characteristics of the human lymphocyte insulin receptor. *J. Biol. Chem. 248:* 2202–2207, 1973.
80. Kahn, C. R., Freychet, P., Neville, D. M., Jr., and Roth, J.: Quantitative aspects of the insulin-receptor interaction in liver plasma membranes. *J. Biol. Chem. 249:* 2249–2257, 1974.
81. Sun, J. V., Tepperman, H. M., and Tepperman, J.: A comparison of insulin binding by liver plasma membranes of rats fed a high glucose diet or a high fat diet. *J. Lipid Res. 18:* 533–539, 1977.
82. Muggeo, M., Bar, R. S., and Roth, J.: Change in affinity of insulin receptors following oral glucose in normal adults. *J. Clin. Endocrinol. Metab. 44:* 1206–1209, 1977.
83. Merimee, T. J., Pulkkinen, A. J., and Lofton, S.: Increased insulin binding by lymphocyte receptors induced by β-OH butyrate. *J. Clin. Endocrinol. Metab. 43:* 1190–1192, 1976.
84. Kahn, C. R., Megyesi, K., Bar, R. S., Eastman, R. C., and Flier, J. S.: Receptors for peptide hormones: New insights into the pathophysiology of disease states in man. *Ann. Intern. Med. 86:* 205–219, 1977.
85. Bar, R. S., and Roth, J.: Insulin receptor status in disease states of man. *Arch. Intern. Med. 137:* 474, 1977.

86. Olefsky, J. M.: The insulin receptor: Its role in insulin resistance of obesity and diabetes. *Diabetes 25:* 1154–1162, 1976.
87. Bar, R. S., Harrison, L. C., Muggeo, M., Gorden, P., Kahn, C. R., and Roth, J.: Regulation of insulin receptors in normal and abnormal physiology in humans. In: *Adv. Intern. Med.* (in press).
88. Rabinowitz, D.: Some endocrine and metabolic aspects of obesity. *Annu. Rev. Med. 21:* 241–258, 1970.
89. Porte, D., Jr., and Bagdade, J. D.: Human insulin secretion: An integrated approach. *Annu. Rev. Med. 21:* 219–240, 1970.
90. Gorden, P., Sherman, B., and Roth, J.: Proinsulin-like component of circulating insulin in the basal state and in patients and hamsters with islet cell tumors. *J. Clin. Invest. 50:* 2113–2122, 1971.
91. Gavin, J. R., III, Kahn, C. R., Gorden, P., Roth, J., and Neville, D. M., Jr.: Radioreceptor assay of insulin: Comparison of plasma and pancreatic insulin and proinsulin. *J. Clin. Endocrinol. Metab. 41:* 438–445, 1975.
92. Archer, J. A., Gorden, P., and Roth, J.: Defect in insulin binding in receptors in obese man: Amelioration with caloric restriction. *J. Clin. Invest. 55:* 166–174, 1975.
93. Bar, R. S., Gorden, P., Roth, J., De Meyts, P., and Kahn, C. R.: Fluctuations in the affinity and concentration of insulin receptors on circulating monocytes of obese patients: Effects of starvation, refeeding and dieting. *J. Clin. Invest. 58:* 1123–1135, 1976.
94. Olefsky, J. M.: Insulin binding to adipocytes and circulating monocytes from obese subjects. *J. Clin. Invest. 57:* 1165–1172, 1972.
95. Harrison, L. C., Martin, F. I. R., and Melick, R. A.: Correlation between insulin receptor binding in isolated fat cells and insulin sensitivity in obese human subjects. *J. Clin. Invest. 58:* 1435–1441, 1976.
96. Harrison, L. C., and King-Roach, A. P.: Insulin sensitivity of adipose tissue in vitro and the response to exogenous insulin in obese human subjects. *Metabolism 25:* 1095–1101, 1976.
97. DeFronzo, R., Sherwin, R., Soman, V., et al: Dissociation of insulin binding to monocytes and insulin action in intact man during starvation and refeeding. *Clin. Res. 25:* 494A, 1977.
98. Freychet, P., Laudat, M. H., Laudat, P., Rosselin, G., Kahn, C. R., Gorden, P., and Roth, J.: Impairment of insulin binding to the fat cell membrane in the obese hyperglycemic mouse. *FEBS Lett 25:* 339–342, 1972.
99. Freychet, P.: Interactions of polypeptide hormones with cell membrane specific receptors: Studies with insulin and glucagon. *Diabetologia 12:* 83–100, 1976.
100. Forgue, M.-E., and Freychet, P.: Insulin receptors in the heart muscle. Demonstration of specific binding sites and impairment of insulin binding in the plasma membrane of the obese hyperglycemic mouse. *Diabetes 24:* 715–723, 1975.
101. Havrankova, J., Roth, J., and Brownstein, M.: Insulin receptors are widely distributed in the central nervous system of the rat. *Nature 272:* 827–829, 1978.
102. Soll, A. H., Goldfine, I. D., Roth, J., Kahn, C. R., and Neville, D. M., Jr.: Thymic lymphocytes in obese (ob/ob) mice: A mirror of the insulin receptor defect in liver and fat. *J. Biol. Chem. 249:* 4127–4131, 1974.
103. Soll, A. H., Kahn, C. R., and Neville, D. M., Jr.: Insulin binding to liver plasma membranes in the obese hyperglycemic (ob/ob) mouse: Demonstration of a decreased number of functionally normal receptors. *J. Biol. Chem. 250:* 7402–7407, 1975.
104. Le Marchand-Brustel, Y., Jeanrenaud, B., and Freychet, P.: Insulin binding and effects in the isolated soleus muscle of lean and obese mice. *Am. J. Physiol., 234:* E348–E358, 1978.
105. Le Marchand, Y., Freychet, P., and Jeanrenaud, B.: Longitudinal study in the establishment of insulin resistance in hypothalamic obese mice. *Endocrinology 102:* 74–85, 1978.
106. Gavin, J. R., III, Roth, J., Jen, P., and Freychet, P.: Insulin receptors in human circulating cells and fibroblasts. *Proc. Natl. Acad. Sci., USA 69:* 747–751, 1972.
107. Kosmakos, F. C., and Roth, J.: Insulin-induced loss of the insulin receptors in IM-9 lymphocytes: A biological process mediated through the insulin receptor (submitted).
108. Olefsky, J. M., and Reaven, G. M.: Decreased insulin binding to lymphocytes from diabetic subjects. *J. Clin. Invest. 54:* 1323–1328, 1974.
109. Olefsky, J. M., and Reaven, G. M.: Insulin binding to diabetes: Relationships with plasma insulin levels and insulin sensitivity. *Diabetes 26:* 680–688, 1977.
110. Vigneri, R., Pliam, N. B., Cohen, D. C., and Goldfine, I. D.: Regulation of intracellular binding sites for insulin by insulin. *Diabetes 26* (suppl 1)*:* 355, 1977.
111. Kobayashi, M., and Olefsky, J.: Effect of experimental hyperinsulinemia on insulin binding and glucose transport in isolated rat adipocytes. *Am. J. Physiol.,* 1978 (in press).
112. Soman, V., and Felig, P.: Glucagon and insulin binding to liver membranes in a partially nephrectomized uremic rat model. *J. Clin. Invest. 60:* 224–232, 1977.
113. Muggeo, M., Bar, R. S., Roth, J., and Kahn, C. R.: Two abnormalities in insulin binding to its receptor in the insulin resistance of acromegaly. *Clin. Res. 26:* 310A, 1978.
114. Muggeo, M., Bar, R. S., Roth, J., and Kahn, C. R.: Insulin resistance of acromegaly: Evidence for two alterations in the insulin receptor on circulating monocytes. *J. Clin. Endocrinol. Metab.* (in press).
115. Bar, R. S., Gorden, P., Roth, J., and Siebert, C. W.: Insulin receptors in patients with insulinomas. *J. Clin. Endocrinol. Metab. 44:* 1210–1212, 1977.
116. Soloff, M. S.: Uterine receptor for oxytocin: Effects of estrogen. *Biochem. Biophys. Res. Commun. 65:* 205–212, 1975.
117. Ranke, M. B., Parks, J. S., and Bongiovanni, A. M.: Modulation by estradiol of growth hormone binding to human lymphocytic cells. *Endocrinol. 94:* (suppl)*:* 73-A, 1974.
118. Olefsky, J. M.: Effect of dexamethasone on insulin binding, glucose transport, and glucose oxidation of isolated rat adipocytes. *J. Clin. Invest. 56:* 1499–1508, 1975.
119. Olefsky, J. M., Johnson, J., Liu, F., Jen, P., and Reaven, G. M.: The effects of acute and chronic dexamethasone administration on insulin binding to isolated rat hepatocytes and adipocytes. *Metabolism 24:* 517–527, 1975.
120. Bennett, V. G., and Cuatrecasas, P.: Insulin receptor of fat cells in insulin-resistant metabolic states. *Science 176:* 805–806, 1972.
121. Kahn, C. R., Goldfine, I. D., Neville, D. M., Jr., and De Meyts, P.: Alterations in insulin binding induced by changes *in vivo* in the levels of glucocorticoids and growth hormones. *Endocrinology* (in press).
122. Williams, L. T., Lefkowitz, R. J., Watanabe, A. M., Hathaway, D. R., and Besch, H. R., Jr.: Thyroid hormone regulation of β-adrenergic receptor number. *J. Biol. Chem. 252:* 2787–2789, 1977.
123. Banerjee, S. P., and Kung, L. S.: Beta adrenergic receptors in rat heart: Effects of thyroidectomy. *Eur. J. Pharmacol. 43:* 107–208, 1977.
124. Ciaraldi, T., and Marinetti, G. V.: Thyroxine and propylthiouracil effects in vivo on alpha and beta adrenergic receptors in rat heart. *Biochem. Biophys. Res. Commun. 74:* 984–991, 1977.
125. Kahn, C. R., Flier, J. S., Bar, R. S., Archer, J. A., Gorden, P., Martin, M. M., and Roth, J.: The syndromes of insulin resistance and acanthosis nigricans: Insulin-receptor disorders in man. *N. Engl. J. Med. 294:* 739–745, 1976.
126. Flier, J. S., Kahn, C. R., Roth, J., and Bar, R. S.: Antibodies that impair insulin receptor binding in an unusual diabetic syndrome with severe insulin resistance. *Science 190:* 63–65, 1975.
127. Flier, J. S., Kahn, C. R., Jarrett, D. B., and Roth, J.: Characterization of antibodies to the insulin receptor. A cause of insulin-resistant diabetes in man. *J. Clin. Invest. 58:* 1442–1449, 1976.
128. Flier, J. S., Kahn, C. R., Jarrett, D. B., and Roth, J.: Antibodies to the insulin receptor: Effect on the insulin-receptor interaction in lymphocytes. *J. Clin. Invest. 60:* 784–794, 1977.
129. Kawanishi, K., Kawamura, K., Nishina, Y., Goto, A., Okado, S., Ishida, T., Ofuji, T., Kahn, C. R., and Flier, J. S.: Successful immunosuppressive therapy in insulin resistant diabetes caused by anti-insulin receptor autoantibodies. *J. Clin. Endocrinol. Metab. 44:* 15–21, 1977.
130. Flier, J. S., Jarrett, D. B., Kahn, C. R., and Roth, J.: The immunology of the insulin receptor. *Immuno. Commun. 5:* 361–373, 1976.
131. Kahn, C. R., Baird, K. L., Flier, J. S., and Jarrett, D. B.: Effects of autoantibodies to the insulin receptor on isolated adipocytes: Studies of insulin binding and insulin action. *J. Clin. Invest. 60:* 1094–1106, 1977.
132. Smith, B. R., and Hall, R.: Thyroid stimulating immunoglobulins in Graves' disease. *Lancet II:* 427–430, 1974.
133. Levey, G. S., and Pastan, I.: Activation of thyroid adenyl cyclase by long-acting thyroid stimulator. *Life Sci. 9* (part 1)*:* 67–73, 1970.
134. Orgiazzi, J., Williams, D. E., Chopra, I. J., and Solomon, D.: Human thyroid adenyl cylase-stimulating activity of immunoglobulin G of patients wtih Graves' disease. *J. Clin. Endocrinol. Metab. 42:* 341–354, 1976.
135. Yamashita, K., and Field, J. B.: Effects of long acting thyroid

stimulator on thyrotropin stimulation of adenyl cyclase activity in thyroid plasma membranes. *J. Clin. Invest. 51:* 463–472, 1972.
136. McKenzie, J. M.: Does LATS cause hyperthyroidism in Graves' disease? (A review biased toward the affirmative). *Metab. Clin. Exp. 21:* 883–894, 1972.
137. O'Donnell, J., Silverberg, J., Row, V. V., and Volpe, R.: Thyrotropin-displacing activity (TDA) in serum immunoglobulins in Graves' disease. *Endocrinology 98:* (suppl 1) 367, 1976.
138. Van Wyk, J. J., Underwood, L. E., Hintz, R. L., Voina, S. J., and Weaver, R. P.: The somatomedins: A family of insulin-like hormones under growth hormone control. *Rec. Prog. Horm. Res. 30:* 259–295, 1974.
139. Daughaday, W. H., Hall, K., Raben, M. S., Salmon, W. D., Jr., Van den Brande, J. L., and Van Wyk, J. J.: Somatomedin: Proposed designation for sulfation factor. *Nature* (London) *235:* 107, 1972.
140. Megyesi, K., Kahn, C. R., Roth, J., and Gorden, P.: Pathophysiology of nonsuppressible insulin-like activity. In: *Endocrinology, vol. 2.* Proceedings of the V International Congress of Endocrinology, Excerpta Medica International Congress Series No. 403, (James, V. H. T., ed.), Amsterdam, Excerpta Medica, 1976, pp. 173–177.
141. Rinderknecht, E., and Humbel, R.: Polypeptides with nonsuppressible insulin-like and cell growth promoting activities in human serum: Isolation, chemical characterization, and some biological properties of forms I and II. *Proc. Natl. Acad. Sci., USA 73:* 2365–2369, 1976.
142. Dulak, N. C., and Temin, H. M.: A partially purified polypeptide fraction from rat liver cell conditioned medium with Multiplication Stimulating Activity for embryo fibroblasts. *J. Cell Physiol. 81:* 153–160, 1973.
143. Rechler, M. M., Fryklund, L., Nissley, S. P., Hall, K., Podskalny, J. M., Skottner, A., and Moses, A. C.: Purified human somatomedin A and rat Multiplication Stimulating Activity: Mitogens for cultured fibroblasts that cross-react with the same growth peptide receptors. *Eur. J. Biochem. 82:* 5–12, 1978.
144. Zapf, J., Mäder, M., Waldvogel, M., Schalch, D. S., and Froesch, E. R.: Specific binding of nonsuppressible insulin-like activity to chicken embryo fibroblasts and to solubilized receptors. *Arch. Biochem. Biophys. 168:* 630–637, 1975.
145. Rechler, M. M., Nissley, S. P., Podskalny, J. M., Moses, A. C., and Fryklund, L.: Identification of a receptor for somatomedin-like polypeptides in human fibroblasts. *J. Clin. Endocrinol. Metab. 44:* 820–831, 1977.
146. Rechler, M. M., Podskalny, J. M., and Nissley, S. P.: Characterization of the binding of Multiplication Stimulating Activity (MSA) to a receptor for growth polypeptides in chick embryo fibroblasts. *J. Biol. Chem. 252:* 3898–3910, 1977.
147. Rechler, M. M., Podskalny, J. M., and Nissley, S. P.: Interaction of Multiplication Stimulating Activity with chick embryo fibroblasts demonstrates a growth receptor. *Nature* (London) *259:* 134–136, 1976.
148. Baseman, J. B., and Hayes, N. S.: Differential effect of hormones on macromolecular synthesis and mitosis in chick embryo cells. *J. Cell Biol. 67:* 492–497, 1975.
149. Chochinov, R. H., and Daughaday, W. H.: Current concepts of somatomedin and other biologically related growth factors. *Diabetes 25:* 994–1007, 1976.
150. Megyesi, K., Kahn, C. R., Roth, J., and Gorden, P.: Hypoglycemia in association with extrapancreatic tumors: Demonstration by a new radioreceptor assay. *J. Clin. Endocrinol. Metab. 38:* 931–934, 1974.
151. Megyesi, K., Kahn, C. R., Roth, J., and Gorden, P.: Circulating NSILA-s in man: Preliminary studies of stimuli *in vivo* and of binding to plasma components. *J. Clin. Endocrinol. Metab. 41:* 475–484, 1975.
152. Cornblath, M., and Schwartz, R.: *Disorders of Carbohydrate Metabolism in Infancy,* 2nd ed. Philadelphia, W. B. Saunders, 1976.
153. Posner, B. I.: Growth hormone and prolactin receptors: Characterization and regulation. In: *Endocrinology, vol. 2.* Proceedings of the V International Congress of Endocrinology, Excerpta Medical International Congress Series No. 403, (James, V. H. T., ed.). Amsterdam, Excerpta Medica, 1976, pp. 178–185.
154. Lesniak, M. A., Gorden, P., Roth, J., and Gavin, J. R., III: Binding of ^{125}I-human growth hormone to specific receptors in human cultured lymphocytes. *J. Biol. Chem. 249:* 1661–1667, 1974.
155. Lesniak, M. A., Gorden, P., and Roth, J.: Reactivity of non-primate growth hormones and prolactins with human growth hormone receptors on cultured human lymphocytes. *J. Clin. Endocrinol. Metab. 44:* 838–849, 1977.
156. Nisula, B. C., and Ketelslegers, J.-M.: Thyroid-stimulating activity and chorionic gonadotropin. *J. Clin. Invest. 54:* 494–499, 1974.
157. Nisula, B. C., Morgan, F. J., and Canfield, R. E.: Evidence that chorionic gonadotropin has intrinsic thyrotropic activity. *Biochem. Biophys. Res. Commun. 59:* 86–91, 1974.
158. Taliadouros, G. S., Canfield, R. E., and Nisula, B. C.: Thyroid stimulating activity of chorionic gonadotropin and luteinizing hormone. *J. Clin. Endocrinol. Metab.* (in press).
159. Reichlin, S.: In: *The Textbook of Endocrinology,* 5th ed. (William, R. H., ed.). Philadelphia, W. B. Saunders, 1974, pp. 811.
160. Hayes, R. C., Jr., and Larner, J.: Adrenocorticotropic hormones: adrenocortical steroids and their synthetic analogs: inhibitors of adrenocortical steroid biosynthesis. In: *The Pharmacological Basis of Therapeutics* (Goodman, L. S., and Gilman, A., eds.). New York, Macmillan, 1975, pp. 1408.
161. Krakoff, L., Nicolis, G., and Anisel, B.: Pathogenesis of hypertension in Cushing's Syndrome. *Am. J. Med. 58:* 216–220, 1975.

154

Steroid Sex Hormone Receptors and Action

Elwood V. Jensen
Eugene R. DeSombre

The concept that drugs and hormones elicit response by interacting with cellular receptor sites has long been a tenet of pharmacology, but until relatively recently the receptor substances themselves were hypothetical entities. Recognition of specific receptors for steroid hormones dates from the late 1950s when the synthesis of estrogenic hormones labeled with carrier-free tritium made possible the determination of tissue distribution and intracellular localization of physiologic amounts of administered hormone. The striking ability of reproductive tissues to concentrate radioactive estrogen, without covalent binding or metabolic transformation of the steroid itself, indicated the presence in target tissues of active receptor systems. Within a few years, various types of steroid hormones labeled with tritium of high specific activity became commercially available, permitting studies of the disposition and chemical fate of these hormones in animal tissues. Investigations in many laboratories established that target tissues for all classes of steroid hormones contain high-affinity, low-capacity binding components and that the interaction with target cells takes place by the same general pathway first elucidated for estrogenic hormones in the immature rat uterus. In this process, often designated the two-step translocation mechanism, the steroid hormone enters the cell, apparently by passive diffusion, and associates with an extranuclear receptor protein, inducing its conversion to a biochemically functional form; this transformed or activated hormone-receptor complex is translocated to the nucleus where it binds in the chromatin and in some way alleviates restrictions on RNA synthesis that are characteristic of the hormone-dependent tissues.

This chapter describes the properties of receptor proteins for steroid sex hormones in reproductive tissues, summarizes the principal experimental evidence regarding the currently accepted translocation mechanism, mentions briefly the effects of hormone-receptor complexes on RNA synthesis, and discusses the relation of receptor content to hormone dependency in normal and neoplastic mammalian tissues. More detailed information, with specific references to the original literature, can be found in a number of comprehensive reviews and monographs.[1–15]

RECEPTOR PROTEINS IN TARGET TISSUES

RECEPTORS FOR ESTROGEN

The presence of a specific estrogen-binding component, now known as estrophilin, in organs of the female reproductive tract was first recognized by the striking ability of these tissues to take up and retain tritiated estradiol administered in vivo, without chemical change of the hormone itself. That this binding is involved in hormonal action was established by the ability of certain inhibitors of estrogen action, such as ethamoxytriphetol and nafoxidine, to prevent the specific uptake of labeled estradiol in target tissues and by the correlation of the reduction of hormone incorporation with the inhibition of uterine growth response when different amounts of nafoxidine are administered along with estradiol to the immature rat. In contrast, actinomycin-D and puromycin, which likewise block the uterotrophic response to estrogens, show no inhibition of estradiol incorporation, suggesting that the interaction of hormone with receptor is an early step in hormonal action, initiating a sequence of biochemical events that can be blocked at later stages by inhibitors of RNA and protein synthesis.

When excised uteri or other target tissues are exposed to dilute solutions of tritiated estradiol in vitro, there is specific uptake and binding of hormone by receptor that shows all the characteristics of the interaction in vivo. Both in vivo and at physiologic temperatures in vitro, most of the radioactive hormone (70 to 80 percent) becomes localized in the nucleus, as demonstrated by differential centrifugation of tissue homogenates and by autoradiography (Fig. 154-1), with a smaller portion appearing in the high-speed supernatant (cytosol) fraction of homogenates or in the extranuclear regions of autoradiograms. The radioactive estradiol is present in the cytosol in combination with a receptor protein, whereas the hormone bound in the nucleus can be extracted by 0.3 M or 0.4 M solutions of KCl or other salt as a macromolecular complex different from that found in the cytosol.

Most studies on the physical and chemical properties of estrophilin have been carried out with rat and calf uterus. However, specific binding of estrogens, both in vivo and in vitro, and the formation of cytosol and nuclear estrogen-receptor complexes have been observed with a large number of target tissues, including mammary gland, anterior pituitary, hypothalamus, and mammary, pituitary, and endometrial cancers. The technique of sucrose gradient ultracentrifugation, introduced by Toft and Gorski in 1966 for characterization of the estradiol-receptor complex of rat uterine cytosol, has provided a valuable means not only of detecting binding of steroid hormones to receptor proteins but also of distin-

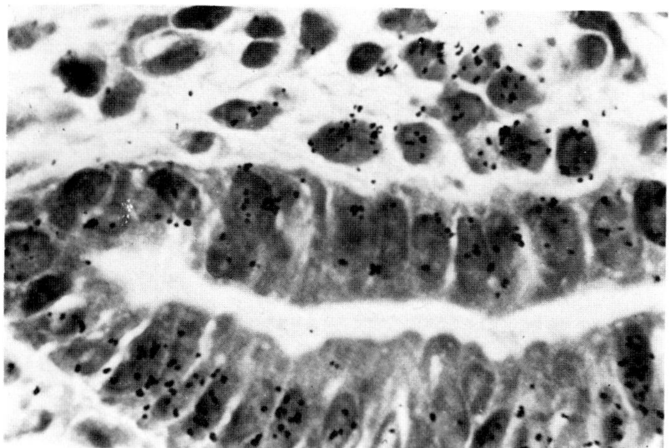

Fig. 154-1. Autoradiograph of frozen section of rat uterine endometrium excised 2 hours after subcutaneous injection of tritiated estradiol in saline. (Courtesy of Dr. W. E. Stumpf.)

guishing between different forms of the receptor, using the radioactivity of the bound hormone as a marker for the protein. In sucrose gradients of low ionic strength, the estrogen-receptor complex of uterine cytosol sediments at about 8S (Fig. 154-2), but is reversibly dissociated into a 3.8S estrogen-binding subunit in the presence of 0.3 M salt. In gradients of intermediate ionic strength (0.15 M), complexes sedimenting at about 6S have been reported, suggesting that the binding unit of estrophilin may undergo various degrees of association with as yet undefined components of uterine cytosol. The estradiol-receptor complex extracted from the uterine nucleus sediments at 5.2S in salt-containing sucrose gradients but aggregates to an 8–9S form in gradients of low ionic strength. In contrast to the 8S extranuclear complex or its 3.8S subunit, which can be generated simply by adding tritiated hormone to uterine cytosol in the cold, the 5.2S nuclear complex is not formed by direct treatment of uterine nuclei with estrogen in the absence of cytosol.

In addition to these two "physiological" forms of estrophilin, usually designated 4S and 5S for simplicity, certain nonaggregating modifications of both the cytosol and nuclear estrogen-receptor complexes have been observed. Uterine cytosol of immature rats and calves contains an enzymic factor which, when activated by the addition of calcium ions, converts the binding unit of the receptor to a form that sediments at 4.5S in either high-salt or low-salt sucrose gradients. The physiological significance of this "calcium-stabilized" modification of the cytosol receptor has not been established, although, as discussed later, this 4.5S receptor shows certain biochemical properties of the 5.2S nuclear form, even though the two are clearly different in physical properties. The uterus of the mature rat contains a proteolytic enzyme, apparently different from the calcium-sensitive factor of immature rat uterus, that during the course of homogenate preparation can change some or all of the cytosol receptor to a nonaggregating 4S form; adult human uterus behaves similarly, yielding a nonaggregating 3S form of the receptor. Conversion of the cytosol receptor to a nonaggregating entity, sedimenting at about 4S, also can be effected by limited proteolysis with trypsin or pronase. Recently it has been found that target tissues contain another proteolytic factor, inhibited by leupeptin, that degrades the cytosol receptor to the ultimate binding unit, a 2.8S entity that has been called the "mero" receptor.

On prolonged standing or during the course of purification the nuclear receptor is converted to a nonaggregating form that sediments at 4.8S and shows a marked difference from the 5.2S form on gel filtration. The 4.8S nonaggregating nuclear complex was once thought to be the same as the 4.5S calcium-stabilized cytosol complex, but the two can be distinguished by careful sedimentation as well as by acrylamide gel electrophoresis at pH 9, where the cytosol complex, with an isoelectric point of 6.4, migrates much faster than does the nuclear complex with an isoelectric point of about 5.8. The relations among some of these different forms of estrophilin are summarized in Figure 154-3.

Recently the 4.8S nonaggregating form of the nuclear estradiol-receptor complex of calf uterus has been isolated in highly purified form and used to immunize rabbits and goats. The antibodies thus obtained react not only with the different forms of cytosol and nuclear estrophilin of calf uterus but also with nuclear and

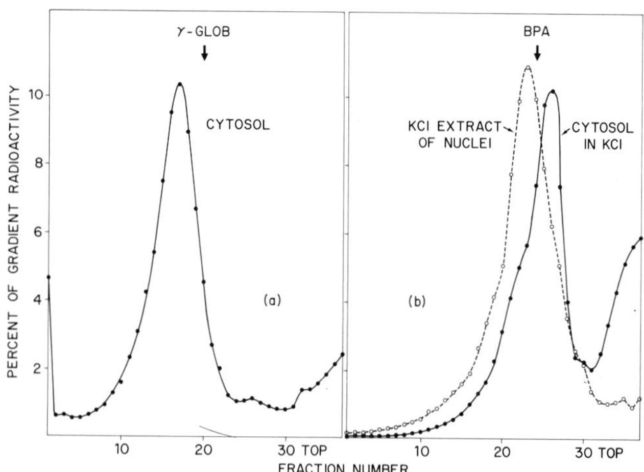

Fig. 154-2. Sedimentation patterns of radioactive estradiol-receptor complexes of cytosol and nuclear extract from uteri of immature rats excised 1 hour after the subcutaneous injection of 100 ng tritiated estradiol in saline. Gradients are: (a) 10 to 30 percent sucrose without added salt; (b) 5 to 20 percent sucrose containing 400 mM KCl. γ-GLOB and BPA indicate positions of bovine γ-globulin (7.0S) and bovine plasma albumin (4.6S) markers. (Reproduced from E. V. Jensen and E. R. DeSombre, Science 182:126–134, 1973.)

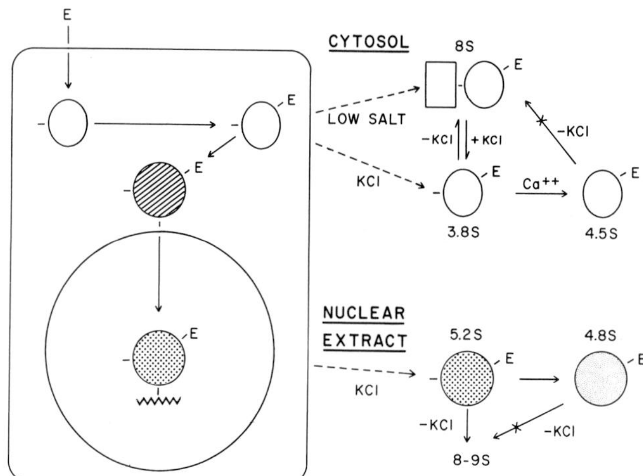

Fig. 154-3. Schematic representation of interaction pathway of estradiol in target cell. Diagram at left indicates estradiol combining with estrophilin to cause receptor activation followed by translocation of the transformed complex to bind to chromatin in the nucleus. Diagram at right indicates sedimentation properties of complexes extracted from cell after homogenization and the nonaggregating derivatives. (Reproduced from E. V. Jensen, S. Mohla, T. A. Gorell, and E. R. DeSombre, Vitamins and Hormones 32:89–127, 1974.)

cytosol estrogen-receptor complexes of normal and neoplastic target tissues of all mammalian species investigated. In contrast, these antibodies to estrophilin do not cross-react with progestin or androgen receptors. Thus, there appears to be immunochemical similarity among estrophilin from various sources, but not among receptors for different steroid hormones.

That estrophilin is predominantly protein in nature was first demonstrated by the ability of proteolytic enzymes, but not ribonuclease or deoxribonuclease, to liberate the hormone from the cytosol and nuclear complexes of rat uterus. Binding of the estrogen appears to depend on sulfhydryl groups in the receptor protein, inasmuch as sulfhydryl-blocking reagents not only prevent the association of hormone with receptor but also effect the release of bound steroid, in some instances accompanied by aggregation of the estrophilin. Recently it has been shown that the action of silver ions to eliminate estrogen binding can be reversed by the addition of a mercaptan such as dithiothreitol, a phenomenon that provides a simple means of exchanging receptor-bound endogenous estrogens for radioactive hormone at low temperatures.

The binding of estrogens by estrophilin, though noncovalent, is extremely strong. Dissociation constants ranging from 0.1 to 10 nM at 2°C have been reported for the cytosol estradiol-receptor complex. Because of the instability of estrophilin in crude tissue extracts and the fact that techniques used for estimating the concentrations of bound and free hormone disrupt the equilibrium, these procedures tend to underestimate the binding, which probably has a true dissociation constant of less than 0.1 nM in the cold. The strong binding apparently results from an extremely slow rate of dissociation; once bound, the hormone is not readily exchanged, even in the presence of a large excess of free estrogen. At temperatures of 25° to 40°C the affinity of estrophilin for estrogens is considerably reduced, especially in the case of estrone, and exchange of bound hormone in either cytosol or nuclear complexes can be effected, subject to the limitation that some of the receptor protein may be destroyed under these conditions. The bound hormone is readily removed from the receptor by organic solvents in the cold.

In addition to sucrose gradient ultracentrifugation, which has provided most of the detailed information concerning the interrelation of the different forms of estrogen-receptor complexes in target tissues, a number of other procedures have been used for demonstrating specific binding of steroid hormones to receptors and for estimating the receptor content in tissue specimens. All of these make use of radioactive hormone as a marker for the receptor protein and require the separation of the hormone bound to the receptor from unbound hormone often present in excess. Probably the most extensively employed method, especially for determining the estrophilin content of human breast cancers, has been that in which the excess unbound hormone is adsorbed on dextran-coated charcoal, leaving the receptor-bound estrogen in solution. The quantitative determination of total binding is best accomplished by making measurements at several estrogen concentrations and plotting the results according to the method of Scatchard in which the ratio of bound to free hormone as a function of that bound gives a straight line, the intercept of which represents the total binding at saturation and the slope of which represents the dissociation constant. Other methods of detecting and measuring binding of estrogens to receptors include separating bound from unbound hormone by agar gel electrophoresis, by gel filtration through Sephadex G-25, or by immobilized antibody to the steroid hormone, precipitation of the estrogen-receptor complex with protamine, and adsorption of the labeled complex on hydroxyapatite, powdered glass, or controlled pore glass beads. The recent preparation of specific antibodies to estrophilin afford, for the first time, a means of recognizing the receptor protein independent of its binding to estrogenic hormone and offers the possibility of estimating receptors by radioimmunoassay.

RECEPTORS FOR PROGESTINS

After it was recognized that the production of progesterone receptors in reproductive tissues depends on the action of estrogen, the administration of tritiated progesterone to estrogen-treated animals was shown to result in selective uptake and retention of labeled hormone in the mouse vagina; the guinea pig, rabbit, and hamster uterus; and the chick oviduct. The steroid incorporated is nearly all unchanged progesterone. Although the results of cell fractionation have not always been consistent, autoradiographic studies with guinea pig uterus clearly demonstrate selective nuclear concentration of radioactive hormone.

After exposure to hormone either in vivo or in vitro, the progesterone present in the cytosol and in the nuclei of target tissue cells is bound to receptor proteins (progestophilin) that can be characterized by sedimentation in sucrose gradients. These cytosol hormone-receptor complexes resemble those observed with estrophilin in that they sediment at about 4S in gradients of high ionic strength, but in low-salt gradients, they form larger aggregates, reported variously to sediment from 6.5S to 8S. Treatment with sulfhydryl-blocking reagents, as well as exposure to proteases but not nucleases, causes release of the bound hormone. Dissociation constants in the cold of 0.2, 0.5, and 0.8 nM have been reported for the cytosol progesterone-receptor complexes of rabbit and guinea pig uterus and chick oviduct, respectively.

The most extensive investigations of progesterone receptors have been carried out with the progestophilin of chick oviduct, where the cytosol complex is reported to sediment at 3.8S in salt-containing gradients and as a mixture of 5S and 8S entities in low-salt gradients. The progesterone-receptor complex extracted from the nucleus likewise sediments at about 4S in salt-containing gradients and has not been distinguished from the cytosol complex by ultracentrifugation. Oviduct cytosol contains a leupeptin-sensitive proteolytic enzyme which, in the presence of calcium or other divalent metal ions, degrades the receptor to a 2.6S subunit called the mero-receptor.

The cytosol progesterone-receptor complex of chick oviduct cytosol has been separated by ion exchange chromatography into two different components, each containing bound progesterone. Component A binds nonspecifically to DNA but not to chromatin, whereas component B does not bind to DNA but shows a specific affinity for chromatin from target tissues. Each unit has been purified to apparent homogeneity and its amino acid composition determined. Progestophilin A has a molecular weight of about 80,000 daltons and sediments at 3.8S, while progestophilin B has a molecular weight of 114,000 daltons and sediments at 4.2S. Both are acidic proteins, although there is some disagreement as to their actual isoelectric points. Under certain conditions, these two units combine to produce a 6S dimer.

RECEPTORS FOR ANDROGENS

The administration of tritiated testosterone to rats, mice, guinea pigs, and dogs results in the accumulation of radioactive steroid in the prostate, seminal vesicles, epididymis, and anterior pituitary. Except for the dog prostate, where microsomal binding is reported to predominate, the labeled hormone becomes localized chiefly in the nucleus, as demonstrated both by fractionation of tissue homogenates and by autoradiography. Specific uptake by the cellular receptors is prevented by simultaneous administration of such inhibitors of androgen action as cyproterone, cyproterone acetate, and flutamide.

Understanding of androgen-receptor interaction and the characterization of discrete hormone-receptor complexes was facilitated by the important discovery that 4,5α-dihydrotestosterone, formed by the reduction of the administered testosterone both in the liver and in the prostate itself, is the active form of the hormone in prostatic nuclei. When either tritiated testosterone or dihydrotestosterone is administered to castrate rats, the prostatic cytosol contains a dihydrotestosterone complex that sediments at 8S in low-salt sucrose gradients and is dissociated to a 3.8S subunit in the presence of salt. The same complex is formed on incubation of prostatic tissue with either substance in vitro or on direct addition of dihydrotestosterone to prostatic cytosol, whereas testosterone itself binds only weakly to the cytosol receptor. In contrast to the case of estrogen receptors in the uterus, where the nuclear complex sediments more rapidly than the salt-dissociated cytosol complex, or that of progesterone receptors, where the nuclear and cytosol complexes show similar sedimentation properties, the dihydrotestosterone-receptor complex extracted from prostatic nuclei of hormone-treated animals sediments at 3.0S, slower than the cytosol complex (Fig. 154-4). Like other steroid hormone receptors, the androphilic substances of rat prostate are proteins that appear to require intact sulfhydryl groups for their steroid-binding properties. Although larger values have been reported, there is good evidence that the dissociation constant for the dihydrotestosterone-receptor complex of prostatic cytosol is less than 0.1 nM.

While dihydrotestosterone appears to be the androgenic hormone showing the highest binding affinity and the greatest biological activity in the prostate, seminal vesicle, and epididymis, in certain other tissues, such as ovary, uterus, kidney, and adult testis, testosterone appears to be the active hormone that binds preferentially to the receptor. In the levator ani muscle, dihydrotestosterone binds more strongly to the receptor, but because little conversion of testosterone to dihydrotestosterone takes place in this tissue, testosterone itself appears to be responsible for biological action. In some species, testosterone but not dihydrotestosterone shows an effect on sexual behavior, an action that appears to result from its aromatization to produce estradiol in the brain cells involved.

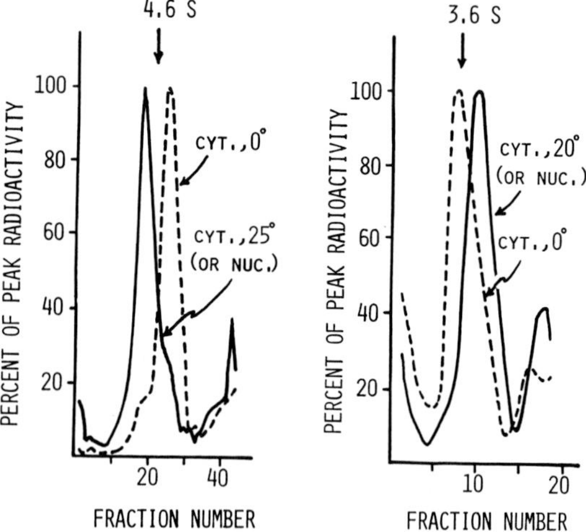

Fig. 154-4. Comparison of native (0°) and activated (25°) estradiol-receptor complex of calf uterine cytosol (left) with native (0°) and activated (20°) dihydrotestosterone-receptor complex of rat ventral prostate cytosol (right) on sedimentation in salt-containing sucrose gradients. Complex extracted from nuclei sediments in same position as activated cytosol complex. (Reproduced from S. Liao, International Review of Cytology 41:87–172, 1975.)

HORMONE-RECEPTOR INTERACTION

The elucidation of the relation between the cytosol and nuclear forms of the estrogen-receptor complex was an important advance, for the two-step pathway proposed for estradiol in uterine cells has provided a general model for the interaction of all types of steroid hormones in their respective target tissues. In this process, summarized in Figure 154-5, the hormone (E) enters the target cell and binds to the extranuclear receptor (R_C), inducing its conversion to an activated form (R_N) that is translocated to the nucleus where it binds in the chromatin and modulates RNA synthesis.

Although the foregoing reaction scheme is not proven unequivocally, it is supported by a wide variety of experimental evidence. A relation between cytosol and nuclear binding in immature rat uteri was first indicated by early in vivo studies in which varying doses of the antiestrogen, nafoxidine, were found to reduce nuclear and extranuclear binding proportionally, while an analysis of steroid uptake and retention when different amounts of estradiol are administered suggested that saturable retention of hormone in the nucleus is secondary to initial uptake by extranuclear receptor. The subsequent proposal that the nuclear estradiol-receptor complex is actually derived from the extranuclear complex by temperature-dependent, hormone-induced translocation was based on three experimental observations:

1. Excised uteri exposed to tritiated estradiol at 37°C in vitro show the same ability to concentrate labeled hormone in the nucleus as those exposed in vivo, whereas at 2°C the hormone taken up is mostly extranuclear, shifting to the nucleus if the tissues are then warmed to 37°C.
2. While the 8S estradiol-receptor complex or its 4S subunit can be readily formed by adding labeled hormone to uterine cytosol in the cold, direct treatment of uterine nuclei with estradiol does not yield any 5S complex unless uterine cytosol is also present, in which case incubation at 25°–37°C gives rise to extractible 5S complex, indistinguishable from that obtained in vivo.

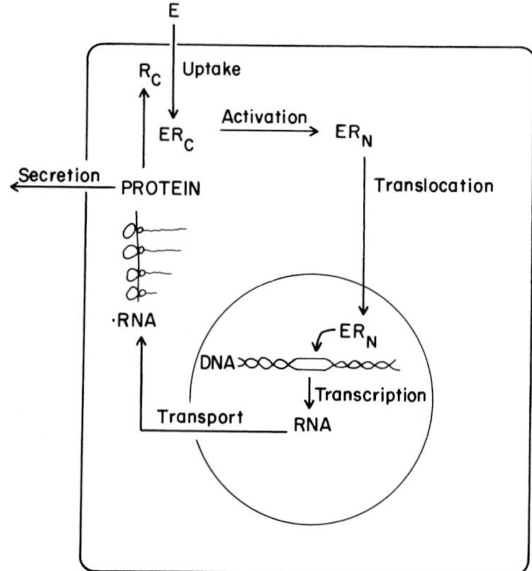

Fig. 154-5. General representation of hormone interaction pathway and biochemical responses in target cells.

3. Administration of estradiol in vivo causes a temporary depletion of the extranuclear receptor consistent with its migration to the nucleus; not only is there less estrophilin in uterine cytosol after a large dose of estradiol than after a smaller dose, but during the first 4 hours after the administration of a physiological amount of estradiol, there is a progressive fall in cytosol receptor level, after which the estrophilin is replenished, apparently by resynthesis.

Subsequent evidence has added further support to the two-step translocation hypothesis. Not only do antibodies to nuclear estrophilin cross-react with the cytosol receptor, indicating immunochemical similarity between the two forms, but transformation of the hormone-binding unit of estrophilin from the cytosol to the nuclear form can be effected in the absence of nuclei, simply by warming uterine cytosol to physiologic temperature in the presence but not the absence of estradiol or other estrogenic hormones. Under these conditions the 4S estrogen-receptor complex is converted to a 5S entity that resembles the complex extracted from uterine nuclei of estrogen-treated animals in two important characteristics not shown by the native 4S complex. These are the ability to bind strongly to isolated nuclei or chromatin preparations and, as discussed later, to enhance the RNA synthesizing capacity of isolated nuclei from hormone-dependent tissues and tumors. Because of these unique properties of the 5S complex, the transformation of estrophilin from the native (extranuclear) to the nuclear form has become known as receptor-activation.

In analogy with the foregoing observations with estrogen receptors, it was shown for progestin and androgen receptors that nuclear incorporation of labeled hormone in target tissues in vitro is markedly temperature-dependent, that exposure of isolated nuclei to hormone gives rise to nuclear complex only if cytosol receptor is also present, and that warming a mixture of cytosol and hormone endows the receptor with the ability to bind to nuclei or chromatin. Thus, hormone-induced, temperature-dependent conversion of the extranuclear receptor to an activated form that can bind in the nucleus appears to be a general characteristic of the interaction of all classes of steroid sex hormones in target cells.

The molecular basis of receptor activation is not well understood, but in the case of estrophilin the process represents more than simply a change in receptor conformation. On the basis of kinetic evidence for a second-order reaction and the elution properties on gel filtration of the 4S as compared to the 5S complex, it appears that activation of estrophilin involves an increase in molecular size, postulated to result from the dimerization of 4S units. In the case of progesterone receptor, a combination of progestophilin A and B units, sedimenting at 6S, has been obtained in vitro and is considered to be the biochemically active form of the progesterone receptor, although this heterodimer has not been demonstrated as yet in target cell nuclei in vivo. Because the cytosol and nuclear progesterone-receptor complexes show similar sedimentation properties and the nuclear dihydrotestosterone-receptor complex sediments more slowly than the cytosol complex (Fig. 154-4), the role of dimerization in the general phenomenon of receptor activation remains to be established. For all the sex hormones, precipitation of the cytosol receptor or its complex by ammonium sulfate in the cold yields a form of the receptor that can bind to chromatin; the relation of these "salt-activated" receptors, which in the case of estrophilin show an increased sedimentation rate (5.5S), to those produced by warming with the steroid hormone is not clear.

There is abundant evidence that, on translocation to the nucleus, the activated hormone-receptor complex binds in the chromatin. The exact nature of the nuclear "acceptor" sites and the biochemical mechanism by which the complex influences gene expression are poorly understood. In the case of the estrogens, the acceptor sites involved in hormonal action in vivo appear to be of limited capacity, inasmuch as physiologic amounts of radioactive estradiol are retained in the uterine cell nuclei for several hours, in contrast to hyperphysiologic doses of hormone, where the large amount of steroid taken up initially is rapidly lost from the nucleus. It has been difficult to identify specific acceptor sites in in vitro experiments because of the ability of activated estrogen-receptor complex to bind extensively to isolated chromatin of target and nontarget cells alike.

Physiologic doses of estradiol cause the disappearance, presumably to the nucleus, of about half the total number of cytosol receptors, estimated by different investigators to be between 20,000 and 40,000 per uterine cell, while nuclear exchange experiments indicate that about 6000 receptors appear in the nucleus of each cell. Whether all the receptor complexes entering the nucleus after a physiologic dose of hormone actually contribute equally to hormonal stimulation is not certain, but it would appear that the action of estrogen in the rat uterus probably involves the participation of several thousand hormone-receptor complexes per cell nucleus. This conclusion is consistent with observations that the uterotrophic action of estrogen requires the presence of the hormone-receptor complex in the nucleus for a prolonged period of time and is not simply the triggering of an initial step of a reaction sequence that then continues on its own.

The depletion of cytosol receptor, induced in uterine cells by interaction with the estrogenic hormone, appears to stimulate estrophilin synthesis, and replenishment of extranuclear receptor, evident after a few hours, is complete in 18 to 24 hours. Nafoxidine and similar antiestrogens, which compete with estrogenic steroids in binding to the cytosol receptor, also effect translocation of the receptor to the nucleus, but in this case, replenishment of extranuclear estrophilin does not take place. The prolonged depletion of receptor, depriving the nucleus of the continuing influx of estrogen-receptor complex needed for full uterotrophic response, is believed to be the basis of the antiestrogenic action of these antagonists, which themselves show weak estrogenic activity.

In contrast to the activated estrogen-receptor complex, which binds strongly to isolated nuclei or chromatin from many tissues, progestin- and androgen-receptor complexes show selective affinity for chromatin of target cell nuclei. In the case of progestin, extensive studies have been carried out on the nature of the acceptor site with which the transformed progesterone receptor complex associates in the chick oviduct nucleus. The enhanced binding of activated progesterone-receptor complex in oviduct nuclei appears to depend on the nonhistone (acidic) proteins of the oviduct chromatin. When chromatins from oviduct, heart, and erythrocyte nuclei are separated into DNA, histone, and acidic protein fractions and these components variously combined to produce reconstituted hybrid chromatins, only the chromatins containing the acidic protein fraction from oviduct show strong affinity for the progesterone-receptor complex. As mentioned earlier, the progesterone-receptor complex of oviduct cytosol has been separated into two components, progestophilin A, which binds nonspecifically to DNA, and progestophilin B, which shows specific binding to chromatin from target tissues. On the basis of these observations, it has been proposed (Fig. 154-6) that the active form of the progesterone-receptor complex is a dimer of A and B units, which can react with both the nonhistone protein and the DNA components of chromatin. The B unit of the receptor is

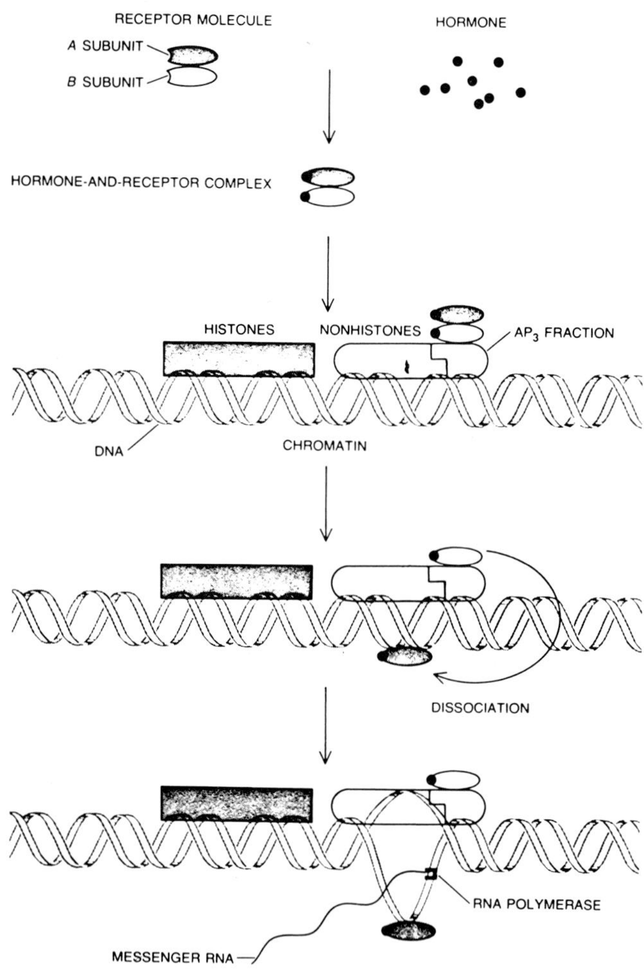

Fig. 154-6. Schematic representation of the mechanism of gene activation by interaction of dimeric progesterone-receptor complex with target cell chromatin. (Reproduced from B. W. O'Malley and W. T. Schrader, Scientific American 234:32–43, 1976.)

postulated to bind selectively to nonhistone proteins in oviduct chromatin, facilitating the reaction of the A unit with DNA at that location and resulting in an enhancement of template activity of the chromatin by making initiation sites available for the synthesis of mRNA for avidin and other oviduct proteins.

HORMONE-RECEPTOR COMPLEXES AND RNA SYNTHESIS

Studies by many investigators have established that enhancement of RNA synthesis is an important biochemical response to the action of steroid sex hormones in their target tissues. Soon after the administration of hormone, there is increased incorporation of labeled precursors into various types of RNA. In previously stimulated animals, the effect is most pronounced on the synthesis of mRNA for specific proteins, such as ovalbumin and avidin in chick oviduct and vitellogenin in frog liver, whereas in the primary stimulation of an undeveloped tissue, such as immature rat uterus or castrate rat prostate, the synthesis of preribosomal RNA, to provide for the translation of new messages, is also markedly enhanced. Extensive studies of the template activity of chick oviduct chromatin show that an increase in the number of initiation sites for the synthesis of ovalbumin mRNA is an important feature of estrogenic stimulation.

Administration of hormone also increases the capacity of nuclei isolated from target tissues to incorporate precursor nucleotides into RNA in vitro. In castrate rats receiving testosterone and in immature rats receiving estradiol, this RNA polymerase activity is increased in prostatic and uterine nuclei, respectively, whereas no effect is seen in the nuclei from nontarget tissues. Careful studies of the temporal sequence of this response have established that in uterine nuclei RNA polymerase-II activity, associated with mRNA production, shows a marked but transient increase 15 to 30 minutes after administration of estradiol, followed by a prolonged elevation after 2 hours, whereas RNA polymerase-I, the nucleolar enzyme associated with rRNA synthesis, becomes elevated about 1 hour after the hormone is given.

Enhancement of RNA synthesis, comparable to that observed after administration of hormone in vivo, can be effected in isolated target cell nuclei by direct treatment, not with hormone alone, but with hormone-receptor complex. In the case of prostatic nuclei, stimulation of both polymerase-I and, to a lesser extent, polymerase-II is observed after incubation with dihydrotestosterone and prostatic cytosol, whereas with rat or calf uterine nuclei, an effect of the estradiol-receptor complex has been observed only on polymerase-I. Enhancement of RNA synthesis in isolated uterine nuclei is effected by the 5S estradiol-receptor complex, either extracted from uterine nuclei or obtained by warming an estradiol-cytosol mixture, and by the 4.5S calcium-stabilized modification, but the native (4S) cytosol complex shows no stimulating activity. Sensitivity to stimulation by estradiol-receptor complex appears to be a characteristic of the RNA-synthesizing system in nuclei only from hormone-dependent tissues and tumors; it has been observed with nuclei from calf and rat uterus and hormone-dependent rat mammary tumor, but not from rat kidney, liver, diaphragm, or autonomous mammary tumor. These results offer support for the concept that the hormone interacts with an extranuclear receptor protein, inducing its conversion to a biochemically functional form that can bind in the nucleus and alleviate restrictions on RNA synthesis that are characteristic of hormone-dependent tissues.

RECEPTORS AND HORMONE DEPENDENCY

The fact that steroid hormones exert their principal biological actions in combination with receptor proteins carries the implication that hormone-dependent cells must contain sufficient quantities of receptor to permit the hormone to function. Although small amounts of hormone receptor appear to be present in most, if not all, animal tissues, a general property of target tissues is their relatively high content of receptor, at least in those cells in which the hormone acts. These considerations have had important clinical applications in the selection of therapy for patients with advanced breast cancer.

It has long been known that some human breast cancers retain the hormone-dependency of normal mammary cells in that, even when widely disseminated, they regress when deprived of hormonal support, either by ablation of the ovaries, adrenals, or pituitary gland or by the administration of large amounts of androgens, estrogens, or antiestrogens. For those patients who respond, endocrine therapy, especially ablation, affords the most effective treatment presently available. But since only 25 to 30 percent of patients with advanced breast cancer show objective remissions to endocrine therapy, some means has been needed to identify those women with hormone-dependent tumors and spare the majority of patients subjection to ineffective treatment. Determination of the estrophilin content of an excised specimen of the cancer provides considerable help in achieving this objective.

Since the first report in 1970 of a correlation between estrogen receptors and clinical response, studies by many investigators have established that patients whose breast cancers lack estrogen receptor have little or no chance of responding to any kind of endocrine therapy, with the possible exception, in a few instances, of the antiestrogen tamoxifen. Cancers that contain only small quantities of receptor likewise do not respond, in contrast to those with substantial levels of estrophilin, where most, but not all, patients show objective remissions to endocrine treatment. Thus, it has been helpful to classify breast cancers as receptor-rich and receptor-poor, rather than positive and negative, so that those patients whose tumors contain estrophilin but in small amount can be included in the nonresponding group.

Using an empirical definition of rich and poor based on clinical experience, it has been found that about 70 percent of human breast cancers may be classified as receptor-poor and that few if any of such patients respond to endocrine treatment. Of the patients with receptor-rich tumors, about two-thirds show objective remissions and a few others subjective remissions to some type of endocrine therapy. Thus the estrophilin content of a cancer specimen can aid in selecting the proper type of therapy for about 90 percent of the patients. It should be pointed out that some investigators still consider tumors with low but definite estrophilin content to be receptor-positive, and clinical data from such laboratories will list a larger percentage of patients as receptor-positive, with a correspondingly smaller fraction of the positive patients showing remissions to hormonal treatment.

The lack of response of some patients with receptor-rich breast cancers may result from different causes. In some cases the basis may be tumor heterogeneity. Most breast cancers probably are mixtures of hormone-dependent and autonomous cell populations, with the extent and duration of remission depending on the relative amounts of each population. If a patient from whom a receptor-rich metastasis is taken for assay possesses other metastases that are receptor-poor, she will fail to respond objectively to endocrine therapy.

In other instances, it appears that breast cancers may continue to produce estrophilin even though the tumor nuclei have escaped from the restrictions of hormone dependency and do not require stimulation by hormone-receptor complex. It has been proposed that such cancers containing nonessential estrophilin might be identified by measurement of their progesterone-receptor content, inasmuch as progestophilin synthesis in normal reproductive tissues is known to depend on stimulation by estrogen and thus on functioning estrophilin. Though the correlation of response with the presence in the tumor of both estrogen and progesterone receptors is somewhat better than with estrogen receptor alone, there are enough anomalies that the value of progesterone receptor measurements, especially from cost/benefit considerations, is not clearly established.

Although clinical correlations as yet are rather limited, preliminary data indicate that an estrophilin assay, carried out on the primary tumor at the time of mastectomy, can predict response to endocrine therapy at a later time if the cancer recurs in disseminated form. Because it is not always possible to obtain a suitable specimen of metastatic cancers, it is generally agreed that receptor assay should be performed on all primary breast tumors at the time of mastectomy, so that this information is available in the case of recurrence. It also has been found that if other parameters such as node involvement are comparable, receptor-poor primary breast cancers tend to recur more frequently and at an earlier time than do receptor-rich cancers.

REFERENCES

1. Raspé, G. (ed): Workshop on Steroid Hormone Receptors. *Advances in the Biosciences,* vol 7. Oxford, Pergamon-Vieweg, 1970.
2. Williams-Ashman, H. G., Reddi, A. H.: Action of vertebrate sex hormones. *Ann Rev Physiol 33:*31–82, 1971.
3. Jensen, E. V., DeSombre, E. R.: Mechanism of action of the female sex hormones. *Ann Rev Biochem 41:*203–230, 1972.
4. Jensen, E. V., DeSombre, E. R.: Estrogen-receptor interaction. *Science 182*:126–134, 1973.
5. O'Malley, B. W., Means, A. R.: Female steroid hormones and target cell nuclei. *Science 183:*610–620, 1974.
6. King, R. J. B., Mainwaring, W. I. P.: *Steroid-Cell Interaction.* Baltimore, University Park Press, 1974.
7. Liao, S.: Cellular receptors and mechanism of action of steroid hormones. *Int Rev Cytol 41:*87–172, 1975.
8. McGuire, W. L., Carbone, P. P., Vollmer, E. P. (eds): *Estrogen Receptors in Human Breast Cancer.* New York, Raven Press, 1975.
9. Gorski, J., Gannon, F.: Current models of steroid hormone action: A critique. *Annu Rev Physiol 38:*425–250, 1976.
10. Yamamoto, K. R., Alberts, B. M.: Steroid receptors: Elements for modulation of eukaryotic transcription. *Ann Rev Biochem 45:* 721–746, 1976.
11. O'Malley, B. W., Schrader, W. T.: The receptors of steroid hormones. *Sci Am 234:*32–43, 1976.
12. Jensen, E. V.: Receptor proteins: Past, present and future. *Research on Steroids 7:*1–36, 1977.
13. Liao, S.: Molecular actions of androgens, *in* Litwack, G. (ed): *Biochemical Actions of Hormones,* vol 4. New York, Academic Press, 1977, pp 351–406.
14. Jensen, E. V., DeSombre, E. R.: The diagnostic implications of steroid binding in malignant tissues. *Adv Clin Chem 19:*57–89, 1977.
15. O'Malley, B. W., Birnbaumer, L. (eds): *Receptors and Hormone Action,* vol 2. New York, Academic Press, 1978.

155

Endocrine Autoimmune Diseases

Aldo Pinchera
Gianfranco Fenzi

An essential function of the immune system is the discrimination of "self" from "nonself." A disturbance of this discriminatory recognition in an individual results in the development of immune responses directed against its own body constituents. Autoimmune reactions fall into a spectrum ranging from organ-specific to generalized forms, according to the distribution of the target antigen in the organism. Some of the best known organ-specific autoimmune disorders involve the endocrine system, as exemplified by Hashimoto's thyroiditis and idiopathic adrenocortical failure. The present review focuses on the immunologic aspects of endocrine diseases, all other aspects being considered elsewhere in this textbook. Immunology is a rapidly expanding branch of medical science, and knowledge in the field has greatly increased in the past few years. To facilitate further discussion, current concepts on autoimmunity and related problems are briefly outlined below. More detailed and comprehensive views on the subject may be found in several recent publications.[1–3]

GENERAL CONCEPTS ON AUTOIMMUNITY

The immune system consists of two major components: cellular immunity and humoral immunity. Lymphocytes are the principal mediators of immune responses and are composed of two independent but interrelated populations: T cells, which are derived from or depend on the thymus, and B cells, which are derived from the bursa of Fabricius in birds and probably from bone marrow in mammals. Both types of cells carry receptors on their surface that allow specific recognition of the antigen to which the cells are sensitized. Activation by antigen induces proliferation and differentiation of sensitized lymphocytes. T cells differentiate into effector cells, secreting soluble products (lymphokines) that mediate various functions of cellular immunity. B cells differentiate into antibody-forming cells (plasma cells) that are concerned with the functions of humoral immunity. Cooperation between T and B cells is required and is regulated by a series of complex interrelated processes in which secreted antibody itself may compete for antigen with cell receptors, while specialized subpopulations of T cells may either enhance (helper cells) or depress (suppressor cells) the intensity of the immune response. Accessory cells such as monocytes and tissue macrophages are also necessary for an immune reaction to occur.

Autoimmunity is characterized by an abnormal or excessive activity of the immune system, including autoantibody production by B lymphocytes and tissue infiltration by T lymphocytes and macrophages. This is said to reflect a loss of immunologic tolerance to self-antigens, but the mechanisms by which self-tolerance is normally maintained are not well defined. According to the "forbidden clone" theory, lymphocytes responding to autoantigens (and other antigens as well) during ontogeny would be eliminated before maturation. While the validity of this theory is supported by several data, recent evidence indicates that lymphocytes capable of reacting to self-antigens are normally present, suggesting that tolerance may be achieved through suppression or inactivation, rather than through elimination of sensitized cells as "forbidden clones." Mechanisms responsible for such suppression include blockade of lymphocyte receptor sites by soluble antigens or antigen-antibody complexes and inhibition of humoral and cell-mediated immunity by suppressor T lymphocytes. Whatever their relative importance, these mechanisms may be overcome or circumvented by a number of maneuvers. In general, injection of unmodified homologous or autologous antigens does not elicit an autoimmune response in the experimental animal unless an immunopotentiator such as Freund's complete adjuvant is used. Other means by which autoimmunity can be induced include an abnormal presentation or manipulation of autoantigens (alterations of the molecule, association with some new carrier), exposure to cross-reacting foreign antigens, binding of foreign haptens (such as drugs) to tissue components, nonspecific stimulation of helper T cells by infections or other agents, loss of suppressor T cell activity through disease, aging, or as a result of genetic factors. Viral infections are frequently implicated in human and animal autoimmune disorders. Viruses can act through several mechanisms: they may contain cross-reacting antigens, or produce carrier effects, or render autoimmunogenic the host antigens by alterating their molecule. In addition, viruses may interfere with the function of the immune system. It has also been postulated that self-antigens may become immunogenic because of genetic or environmentally induced abnormalities in their enzymatic degradation. There is now considerable evidence that autoimmunity is genetically controlled. It is well known that autoimmune phenomena are much more common in women that in men and that they frequently show familial aggregation. It appears that genes associated with the major histocompatibility locus in man (HL-A) are important in the pathogenesis of autoimmunity, since several autoimmune disorders have been found to be linked with certain HL-A haplotypes. The relationship between genetic factors and autoimmunity is best demonstrated by animal models, in which experimentally induced as well as spontaneously occurring autoimmune diseases, including thyroiditis, are clearly under genetic control.

Once established, an autoimmune reaction may affect tissues in several ways. Since in this respect there is no essential difference between immune responses to autoantigens and foreign antigens, the four basic types of pathogenetic mechanisms proposed by Coombs and Gell[4] may be considered (Fig. 155-1).

1. *Type I reactions (anaphylactic, reagin-dependent).* These are initiated by antigen reacting with antibody bound to basophils or mast cells through the Fc piece, leading to the release of pharmacologically active substances (vasoactive amines). The antibodies involved in these reactions are mostly IgEs and are termed homocytotropic or reaginic antibodies.
2. *Type II reactions (cytotoxic or cell-stimulating).* These involve the combination of IgG or IgM antibodies to either a tissue antigen or membrane-adsorbed antigen. Damage or death of the target cell may result from activation of the complement (complement-dependent antibody cytotoxicity), enhancement of phagocytosis through opsonization by antibody alone or antibody plus complement, or cytotoxicity by killer (K) cells acting in concert with antibody (antibody-dependent cell-mediated cytotoxicity). K cells are lymphocytes or monocytes with Fc receptors, by which they combine with antibody or antibody–antigen complexes. When the latter are attached to the surface of target cells, a lytic effect will be produced by K cells. Noncomplement-fixing antibodies reacting with cell surface antigens may stimulate rather than damage the target cell. An example are the thyroid-stimulating antibodies of Graves' disease.
3. *Type III reactions (immunocomplex-mediated).* These result from the formation of complexes between antigen and humoral antibody. The localization of these complexes in tissues leads to activation of complement followed by prominent inflammatory changes. Classical examples of these types of reactions are the Arthurs' phenomenon and serum sickness.
4. *Type IV reactions (cell-mediated, delayed hypersensitivity).* These are initiated by the reaction of actively sensitized T lymphocytes responding to specific antigen by the release of lymphokines, the development of direct cytotoxicity, or both. Antibody and complement are not involved. Lymphokines include cytotoxic factors (lymphotoxin) and other products that have the overall function to amplify the intial response by recruiting other lymphocytes (both B and T), by inducing mitogenesis of these cells (lymphocyte mitogenic factor), and by attracting and localizing macrophages and polymorphonuclear leukocytes at the site of the lesion (chemiotactic and migration inhibitory factors).

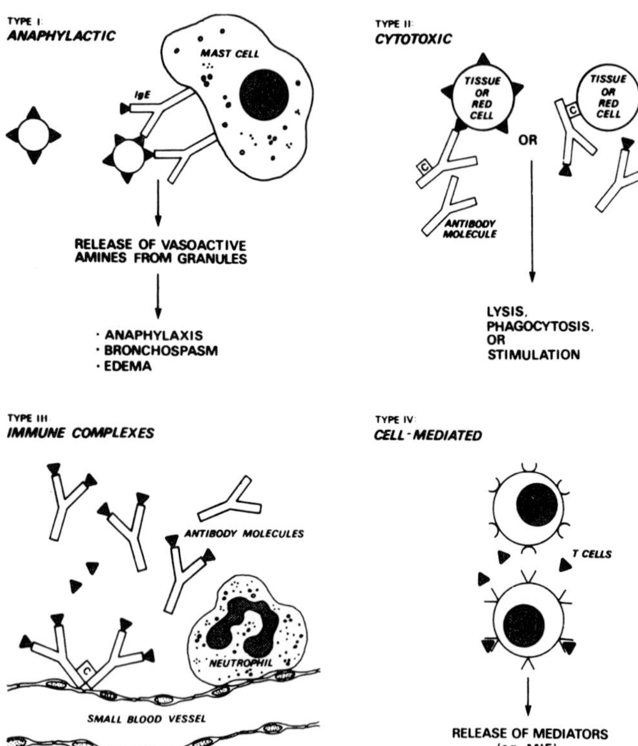

Fig. 155-1. The four types of immune reactions producing tissue damage. The diagrams are described in the text. C = complement, ▲ = antigen, U and V = cellular receptors for antigens. (From J. V. Wells, Immune Mechanisms in Tissue Damage, in H. H. Fudenberg, D. P. Stites, J. L. Caldwell and J. V. Wells, (Eds.), Basic and Clinical Immunology, Lange Medical Publ., Los Altos, 1976, p. 225, with kind permission of the author and the publishers.)

With the exception of type I reactions, all these mechanisms may participate in the pathogenesis of autoimmune disorders. It is worth emphasizing that autoimmune reactions are not necessarily harmful to the organism, and in fact, some may have a biological function by facilitating the disposal of cellular breakdown products. In principle, the term "autoimmune disease" should be restricted to those conditions in which the autoimmune process contributes to the pathogensis of the disease, rather than representing an apparently harmless reaction to tissue damage. Strict criteria for establishing the autoimmune origin of an organ-specific disease have been postulated by Milgrom and Witebsky.[5] These are listed in a modified version in Table 155-1. Admittedly, only

Table 155-1. Criteria for Organ-Specific Autoimmune Diseases

1. Lymphocytic infiltration of the target organ
2. Presence of circulating autoantibodies and/or cellular immunity against the target organ
3. Identification of the specific antigen(s)
4. Production of humoral and/or cellular autoimmune responses in animals sensitized by autologous antigen
5. Presence of organ-specific lesions in autosensitized animals
6. Close association with other autoimmune diseases

some of the endocrine disorders reported in Table 155-2 fulfill the above criteria, while others only partially do so. Nevertheless, they are also considered here because of their association with specific autoimmune phenomena.

THYROID AUTOIMMUNE DISEASES

Hashimoto's disease and idiopathic myxedema are commonly regarded as classic examples of organ-specific autoimmune disorders of the endocrine system. This concept was first formulated in 1956, when, independently, Roitt et al.[6] demonstrated thyroglobulin antibodies in the serum of patients with Hashimoto's disease, and Witebsky and Rose[7] produced thyroiditis lesions in the experimental animal by immunization with homologous thyroid antigens. The concept that Graves' disease should also be included in the group of thyroid autoimmune diseases stems from the discovery in 1956 by Adams and Purves[8] of the long-acting thyroid stimulator (LATS) and has gained support from the subsequent demonstration that this substance is one of the thyroid-stimulating antibodies that account for the hyperthyroidism of Graves' disease.

HISTOPATHOLOGIC CHANGES

In Hashimoto's disease the thyroid is usually moderately enlarged, and its histology shows variable but characteristic changes, with prominent inflammatory features. There is a diffuse

Table 155-2. Endocrine Diseases with Autoimmunity

Gland	Disease	Antigen	Detection of Antibodies
Thyroid	Hashimoto's disease or primary myxedema	Thyroglobulin	Precipitation Passive hemagglutination Immunofluorescence on fixed thyroid Competitive binding radioassay Coprecipitation with radioiodinated thyroglobulin
		Microsomes	Complement fixation Immunofluorescence on unfixed thyroid Competitive binding radioassay Passive hemagglutination
		Second colloid antigen (CA2)	Immunofluorescence on fixed thyroid
		Cell surface	Immunofluorescence on viable cells Mixed hemadsorption
	Graves' disease	TSH receptor-related antigen	LATS bioassay (stimulation of mouse thyroid in vivo) LATS-protector assay Colloid droplet formation in human thyroid slices Displacement of radiolabeled TSH from receptor Stimulation of human thyroid adenylate cyclase in vitro
Endocrine pancreas	Diabetes mellitus (insulin-dependent)	Cytoplasm of islet cells	Immunofluorescence on unfixed pancreas
		A cells	Double immunofluorescence
		D cells	Double immunofluorescence
		Cell-surface antigen of insulinoma cells	Immunofluorescence on viable insulinoma cells
	Diabetes with insulin resistance syndrome	Insulin receptor	Displacement of radioiodinated insulin from receptor
	Insulin autoimmune syndrome	Insulin (human)	Coprecipitation with radioiodinated insulin
Adrenals	Idiopathic Addison's disease	Adrenocortical cells (microsomes)	Complement fixation Immunofluorescence on unfixed adrenals
Ovary	Primary ovarian failure	Steroid-producing cells (ovary, testis, placenta, adrenals)	Immunofluorescence on unfixed sections
		Granulosa cells	C'-dependent cytotoxicity on cell cultures
Testis	Autoimmune testicular failure	Steroid-producing cells (testis, ovary, placenta, adrenals)	Immunofluorescence on unfixed sections
Parathyroid	Idiopathic hypoparathyroidism	Cytoplasm of parathyroid cells	Complement fixation Immunofluorescence on unfixed parathyroid
Pituitary	Stunted growth	GH-producing cells	Double immunofluorescence
	?	Cytoplasm of PRL-producing cells	Double immunofluorescence
	?	LH- and FSH-producing cells	Double immunofluorescence
—	Male infertility (autoimmunity to sperm in man)	Spermatozoa	Complement fixation Agglutination Immobilization Dye exclusion Immunofluorescence

mononuclear cell infiltration consisting mainly of lymphocytes. These may aggregate to form typical lymphoid follicles with germinal centers. Plasma cells are also present, and macrophages may be seen, especially within the colloid. The normal follicular architecture of the gland is disrupted, with partial degeneration and destruction of epithelial cells and fragmentation of the follicular basement membrane. The remaining follicular cells may be larger than normal and show oxyphilic changes in the cytoplasm (Askenazy or Hürthle cells). Fibrosis of some degree is demonstrable in most cases and is very pronounced in the fibrous variant, which is often associated with hypothyroidism.

In idiopathic myxedema the thyroid is reduced in size and shows marked atrophy of the follicular epithelium. There is extensive fibrosis associated with a more or less prominent lymphocytic infiltration, indicating that the basic histopathologic changes are similar to the thyroiditis of Hashimoto's disease.

In Graves' disease the thyroid is diffusely enlarged and vascular. The essential pathology is that of hypertrophy and hyperplasia of the parenchyma, but lymphocytic and plasma cell infiltration to a varying degree is a common finding, and lymphoid follicles with germinal centers may occur. Focal and occasionally diffuse lymphoid infiltration may also be encountered in other types of goiter and especially in papillary thyroid carcinoma. Lymphocytic infiltrates have been observed at autopsy even in subjects with no overt clinical manifestations of thyroid disease, notably in elderly women. The term "asymptomatic (or mild) atrophic thyroiditis" has been applied to this condition.[9,10]

THYROID ANTIBODIES AND RELATED ANTIGENS

Humoral antibodies specifically reacting with thyroid antigens are commonly detectable in patients with Hashimoto's disease, idiopathic myxedema, and Graves' disease, and less frequently in other thyroid disorders. Five antigen/antibody systems have been identified, involving different constituents of the thyroid gland: thyroglobulin, the microsomal antigen, the second antigen of the colloid, the cell surface antigen, and the antigen related to the thyrotropin (TSH) receptor (Table 155-2). The corresponding antibodies are mostly IgG, but some may be found in all other classes of immunoglobulins.[11]

Thyroglobulin Antibodies

Thyroglobulin is stored in the colloid and is enzymatically degraded within the thyroid follicular cells to release thyroid hormones, but some molecules escape proteolysis and eventually enter the bloodstream. Thyroglobulin is normally present in the serum, although in minute amounts, and its concentration rises under physiological or abnormal conditions leading to thyroid stimulation or thyroid damage.[12] This implies that thyroglobulin by itself does not evoke immune responses unless the normal tolerance to this protein is altered. Thyroglobulin antibodies are normally not complement-fixing and may produce precipitation reactions. On the basis of the antigen/antibody ratio at equivalence found in precipitin curves made with autoantibodies, it has been estimated that thyroglobulin contains two pairs of antigenic sites, compared to the over 40 antigenic sites found in heterologous systems. Thyroglobulin antibodies may be detected by a variety of techniques but are commonly determined by passive hemagglutination. By this technique, significant antibody titers are found in most patients with Hashimoto's disease and newly diagnosed idiopathic myxedema, in about one-third of those with Graves' disease, and in smaller percentages in thyroid carcinoma and other thyroid disorders. Measurements by the competitive binding radioassay[13] show a higher frequency of thyroglobulin antibodies in thyroid carcinoma and Graves' disease, but this may be due to the interference of elevated thyroglobulin levels which produce false-positive results in this system.[14]

Thyroid Microsomal Antibodies

The microsomal antigen has been localized in the apical cytoplasm of the thyroid epithelial cells. It is believed to be a lipoprotein in the membrane of exocytotic vesicles transporting newly synthetized thyroglobulin from the Golgi apparatus to the colloid.[15] Recent data indicate that active antigen may be solubilized from microsomes by the use of detergents and other agents.[16] Microsomal antigens are also involved in the humoral responses to gastric parietal cells, adrenocortical cells, and pancreatic islet cells. Thyroid microsomal antibodies are organ-specific and complement-fixing. The complement-dependent cytotoxicity observed in vitro with trypsinized thyroid cells has been ascribed to these antibodies. Microsomal antibodies may be detected by immunofluorescence, which is more sensitive than complement fixation but is not readily quantitated. Sensitive and quantitative methods are the competitive binding radioassay[13] and the hemagglutination technique.[17] which have been recently introduced. By these procedures, microsomal antibodies are found in virtually all the patients with Hashimoto's thyroiditis, most of those with primary myxedema or Graves' disease, and much less frequently in other thyroid disorders. Microsomal antibodies frequently occur in the absence of thyroglobulin antibodies, while only rarely can the reverse be observed.

Antibodies to the Second Colloid Antigen and the Thyroid Cell-Surface Antigen

The second colloid antigen consists of an noniodinated protein that is contained in the colloid and is unrelated to thyroglobulin. Antibodies to this antigen have been found by immunofluorescence on fixed thyroid sections in a few patients with Hashimoto's disease.[18]

Antibodies to cell-surface antigens(s) have been identified by immunofluorescence on viable suspensions of human thyroid cells and by a mixed hemadsorption technique using cell cultures.[19] They have been found in a large proportion of patients with Hashimoto's thyroiditis, primary myxedema, or Graves' disease. The antigens involved in this reaction are distinct from the microsomal antigen and appear to be unrelated to the TSH receptor.

THYROID-STIMULATING ANTIBODIES

An antigen closely related to the TSH receptor in the plasma membrane of the thyroid follicular cells is responsible for the production of the thyroid-stimulating antibodies (TSAb) that are present in the sera of patients with Graves' disease. All these antibodies react with the TSH receptor of human thyroid tissue, and some show cross-reactivity to a varying degree with receptors from mouse, guinea pig, sheep, and beef thyroid tissue.[20] This explains the low prevalence of LATS in hyperthyroidism, since the mouse bioassay measures only antibodies cross-reacting with murine thyroid. Human specific thyroid-stimulating antibodies are detected in human systems by methods based on their ability to (1) prevent binding of non-species-specific LATS to thyroid microsomes (LATS-protector assay);[21] (2) stimulate thyroid function in vitro as assessed by colloid droplet formation [human thyroid stimulator (HTS) assay][22,23] or adenylcyclase activity [human thyroid adenyl cyclase-stimulator (HTACS) assay];[24] and (3) displace TSH from thyroid plasma membrane [TSH-displacing immunoglobulin (TDI) assay].[25] By these methods, most of the sera from patients with Graves' disease are found to be positive, but TDIs have also been detected in Hashimoto's thyroiditis, with a frequency varying from 14 to 20 percent in two different series.[25,26] It appears that antibodies reacting with the TSH receptor do not necessarily produce thyroid stimulation, and some might even inhibit adenyl cyclase activity.[24]

CELL-MEDIATED IMMUNITY

Cell-mediated immunity in patients with thyroid disorders has been studied by leukocyte migration inhibition, lymphocyte transformation, and leukocyte-mediated cytotoxicity tests. By the former procedure, positive results are generally found in Hashimoto's disease, primary myxedema, and Graves' disease using thyroid microsomes,[27,28] whereas conflicting results have been obtained with thyroglobulin. Lymphocyte transformation in response to thyroglobulin has been observed in patients with Hashimoto's and Graves' disease.[29,30] Lymphocytes from patients with Hashimoto's thyroiditis, primary myxedema, and Graves' disease have been shown to release a "lymphotoxin" active on mouse fibrosarcoma cells when challenged with particulate thyroid antigens.[31] A direct cytotoxic effect of Hashimoto leukocytes on thyroid cells in monolayer cultures has been observed by some,[32] but not by others.[33] Cytotoxicity of Hashimoto's leukocytes on thyroglobulin coated target cells in the absence[34] or in the presence[35] of antibody has been reported.

ASSOCIATION OF THYROID AUTOIMMUNE DISORDERS WITH OTHER DISEASES

The occurrence of pernicious anemia in patients with Hashimoto's disease, primary myxedema, or Graves' disease is well documented.[36] Other associated disorders in which organ-specific autoimmunity is or seems implicated include idiopathic Addison's disease, insulin-dependent diabetes, lupoid hepatitis, and myasthenia gravis. Thyroiditis and hyperthyroidism are frequently found in patients with idiopathic hypoparathyroidism and in combination with other endocrine deficiencies as part of the rare polyendocrinopathies. Non-organ-specific autoimmune diseases such as rheumatoid arthritis, systemic lupus erythematosus, and Sjögren's syndrome are also said to occur in Hashimoto's and Graves' disease and in primary myxedema more often than expected. Other associations include idiopathic thrombocytopenic purpura, acquired hemolytic anemia, and vitiligo. Antibodies to gastric parietal cells, intrinsic factor, and adrenocortical cells may be found even in the absence of corresponding clinical manifestations in patients with serological or clinical evidence of thyroid autoimmunity. This also occurs in first-degree relatives of these patients.[9,37]

GENETIC ASPECTS

Hashimoto's disease, idiopathic myxedema, and Graves' disease frequently occur in the same family. Several cases of identical twins with either Hashimoto's or Graves' disease have been reported. Goiter or circulating thyroid antibodies are commonly found in the euthyroid twin of nonconcordant pairs. Interestingly, a similar frequency of hyperthyroidism has been found in the families of patients with proven colloid goiter or Hashimoto's thyroiditis, suggesting a dual heredity to autoimmunity and to thyroid diseases.[9] Thyroid antibodies are found in approximately 50 percent of first-degree relatives of patients with either Hashimoto's or Graves' disease.[38] Further evidence for a genetic control of Graves' disease has derived from recent studies on histocompatibility antigens. A strong association with HL-A-B8 and DW3 determinant has been documented in Caucasian hyperthyroid subjects,[39,40] while a highly significant increase in BW-35 antigen has been found in Japanese hyperthyroid patients.[41] So far, no significant association with histocompatibility antigens has been observed in patients with Hashimoto's thyroiditis or primary myxedema.

ANIMAL MODELS OF THYROID AUTOIMMUNITY

Experimental autoimmune thyroiditis following injection of homologous and autologous thyroid antigens plus Freund's adjuvant has been induced in several animal species, including rabbit, guinea pig, rat, mouse, dog, monkey, and chicken.[42] The thyroid lesions are strikingly similar to those of human lymphocytic thyroiditis, although oxyphilic changes are not observed in the experimental animal. Autoimmune thyroiditis may be induced by injection of soluble or particulate thyroid fractions, but the principal antigen is thyroglobulin.[43] Autologous thyroglobulin may be rendered immunogenic (without the need for adjuvants) by inserting foreign chemical determinants, such as arsanilic or sulfanilic groups, or by incomplete proteolytic digestion, indicating that minor modifications of the protein or exposure of unfamiliar sites of its molecule are sufficient to disrupt self-tolerance.[44] The appearance of circulating antibodies to thyroglobulin in immunized animals has been demonstrated by precipitation, passive hemagglutination, complement fixation, and immunofluorescence. At variance with human disease, antibodies to thyroid microsomal antigens are not detectable in most species, the monkey being a notable exception.[45] Delayed hypersensitivity to thyroglobulin is demonstrable by skin tests and has also been shown by leukocyte migration inhibition and lymphocyte transformation tests in some species. The precise role of humoral and cellular immune responses is still not determined. Experimental autoimmune thyroiditis is clearly under genetic control, since the responsiveness to a standard thyroglobulin challenge may vary considerably in different strains of the same animal species. In mice, one of the main genes controlling the response to thyroglobulin is linked to the major histocompatibility (H-2) complex.[46]

Spontaneous autoimmune thyroiditis has been described in chickens, rats, dogs, and monkeys.[47] This model is perhaps more relevant to human disease than the experimentally induced thyroiditis. There is a familial aggregation of the disease, and its hereditary transmission has been clearly demonstrated in certain strains of chickens, rats, and beagle dogs. Of particular interest is the obese strain (OS) of chickens, in which there is a severe lymphocytic infiltration of the thyroid associated with clinical and biochemical evidence of thyroid failure.

So far, no counterpart of Graves' disease has been found in the experimental animal. Thyroid-stimulating antibodies have been produced in rabbits by immunization with human thyroid homogenate,[48] microsomes,[49,50] or bovine thyroid plasma membranes,[51] but there was no evidence of hyperthyroidism in the immunized animals.

PATHOGENETIC AND ETIOLOGIC FACTORS IN THYROID AUTOIMMUNE DISEASES

Thyroiditis

From the clinical and experimental data described above it is apparent that Hashimoto's thyroiditis and its atrophic variant fulfill the common criteria for organ-specific autoimmune diseases. The precise mechanisms by which thyroid damage is produced are not yet well defined. It is unlikely that the lesions are primarily due to complement-dependent antibody cytotoxicity, since pretreatment of thyroid cells with trypsin is required for its demonstration in vitro, suggesting that the appropriate antigens are normally protected in vivo from the action of these antibodies. The question of whether placental transfer of maternal thyroid antibodies results in fetal thyroid injury is still debated. However, strong evidence for a pathogenetic role of humoral antibodies derives from studies on animal models. In the OS chickens, bursectomy at birth prevents the development of spontaneous autoimmune thyroiditis, whereas neonatal thymectomy in these animals and in rats results in an increased incidence and severity of the disease.[47] Experimentally induced thyroiditis has been transferred from immunized to normal animals by injecting antibody-containing serum.[52] Injected antibodies apparently interact with thyroglobulin emerging from the follicular cells, leading to thyroid lesions through the deposition of immune complexes along the follicular basement membrane.[53] With regard to human disease, electron-microscopic changes in this thyroid region closely resembling antigen–antibody deposits have been observed in Hashimoto's disease.[54] Soluble immune complexes have been demonstrated in the sera of subjects with thyroid autoimmune disorders,[55] and evidence has also been provided that these include thyroglobulin–antithyroglobulin antibody complexes.[56] Activation of K cells by these complexes is an additional mechanism by which an antibody-dependent cytotoxic effect could be produced.[57] On the other hand, a large body of data points to an involvement of cell-mediated immunity. Thyroid lesions of experimental autoimmune thyroiditis are in general better correlated with indices of delayed hypersensitivity than with antibody titers.[42] In some animal species, sensitized lymphoid cells are more effective than immune sera in passive transfer experiments.[58] Sensitized lymphocytes may destroy living target thyroid cells either by direct interaction or by releasing a soluble cytotoxic factor following stimulation by thyroid antigens, as suggested by recent in vitro studies in animal models.[59] The evidence for the occurrence of these cellular mechanisms in human disease has been discussed above.

The initiating event of thyroid autoimmunity is unknown. It was once postulated that any thyroid damage leading to the release of thyroglobulin could trigger an autoimmune response, on the assumption that tolerance to this protein could not be established because of its sequestration within the thyroid gland. This "hidden antigen" hypothesis has been disproven by the demonstration that thyroglobulin is a normal component of circulating plasma. Within the framework of the "forbidden clone" theory, it has been proposed that a self-reacting clone of lymphocytes escaping from elimination during ontogeny or arising through somatic mutation later in life could give rise to thyroid autoimmunity. This concept is difficult to reconcile with the finding that thyroid antibodies are of several immunoglobulin types and are frequently associated with other organ-specific antibodies, indicating that multiple clones of lymphocytes are involved. Perhaps the most telling argument against this hypothesis is the observation that lymphocytes capable of reacting with thyroglobulin are normally present in the serum,[60] implying that the potentiality for a thyroid autoimmune response exists in all individuals. Since these thyroglobulin-reacting lymphocytes are most probably of the B-cell type, it appears that normal tolerance to thyroglobulin affects only the T-cell compartment. Such selective unresponsiveness of T lymphocytes is in keeping with the "low-zone tolerance" produced by low levels of circulating antigens, such as those commonly found for thyroglobulin. Lack of cooperation of T cells could explain the inactivity of sensitized B cells under normal conditions. The need for such cooperation may be overcome in the experimental animal by an abnormal presentation or manipulation of thyroglobulin, obtained by maneuvers such as admixture with adjuvants, minor chemical modifications, or incomplete enzymatic digestion. It is theoretically conceivable that similar mechanisms might be implicated in human disease. For example, some defect in thyroid lysosomal enzymes or an unusual contact with tissue macrophages may result in an abnormal exposure of thyroglobulin antigenic determinants. Alternatively, structural abnormalities of thyroid antigens may occur, either because of a genetically determined defect or as a consequence of an acquired injury such as viral infection. At present, there is no evidence to substantiate any of these hypotheses. Inhibition by suppressor T cells may also explain the absence of activity of sensitized B cells in normal individuals. This is strongly supported by the observation that depletion of T lymphocytes by thymectomy and irradiation in rats leads to the spontaneous development of autoimmune thyroiditis.[61] However, there is no direct proof for a T-cell dysfunction in Hashimoto's disease. Whatever the nature of the primary abnormality, there is overwhelming evidence that it is genetically conditioned. The clinical and experimental data supporting this concept have been discussed previously. It is worth mentioning in this context, that genetic studies on the spontaneous autoimmune thyroiditis of the OS chicken have pointed to at least three different hereditary factors.[62] One of these is linked to the major histocompatibility locus and appears to be an "immune-response" gene that predisposes directly or indirectly to an enhanced response to thyroglobulin; the second consists of an abnormality in thymic suppression function; the third is an intrinsic defect in the thyroid gland itself. The relevance of these three defects to human disease remains to be proven.

Graves' Disease

Although in this disease the requirements for an autoimmune disorder have not all been met, available data clearly support the concept of an autoimmune pathogenesis of at least one of its cardinal features, namely hyperthyroidism. The demonstration that the levels of species-specific thyroid-stimulating antibodies are well correlated with the degree of thyroid hyperfunction[26] provides compelling evidence for a causative role of these antibodies. Additional evidence derives from neonatal thyrotoxicosis, which results from placental transfer of maternal thyroid-stimulating antibodies and subsides in coincidence with their disappearance from the bloodstream. Most probably, autoimmune mechanisms are also involved in the pathogenesis of infiltrative ophthalmopathy. Thyroglobulin–antithyroglobulin complexes deposited in the retro-orbital tissue[63] or antibodies reacting with receptors on fat, muscle, and fibrous cells in the orbit[64] may be implicated in this condition. Pretibial myxedema, which is an uncommon but characteristic manifestation of Graves' disease, might be related to autoimmune phenomena, but so far no direct evidence for this hypothesis has been obtained. With regard to the primary cause, essentially similar considerations to those made for Hashimoto's thyroiditis may be applied to Graves' disease. In this case the problem is rendered even more difficult by the lack of a suitable animal model.

DIABETES MELLITUS

Idiopathic diabetes is usually subdivided according to severity into an insulin-dependent and an insulin-independent type, the former accounting for most juvenile and some adult diabetics. The concept that these two types of diabetes are etiologically and pathogenetically distinct has gained increasing support over the last several years. There is now considerable evidence that insulin-dependent diabetes is frequently associated with autoimmune phenomena and that these may play a pathogenetic role at least in some cases.

HISTOPATHOLOGIC CHANGES

In insulin-dependent diabetes, the number of pancreatic islet cells is markedly reduced, and most of the remaining cells are inactive. Lymphocytic infiltration of the islet of Langerhans in the pancreas of young diabetics was first described by Schmidt[65] in 1902 and was later termed "insulitis."[66] Only recently, however, has it been recognized that this is a common finding in patients with juvenile diabetes dying shortly after the onset of the disease.[67] Insulitis is apparently a transient lesion, since it has never been seen in young diabetics who died more than a year after initial symptoms. Lymphocytic infiltration does not occur in insulin-independent diabetes but may be found in elderly diabetics requiring insulin therapy.[68] The inflammatory characteristics of insulitis are similar to the adrenalitis of idiopathic Addison's disease and the thyroiditis of Hashimoto's disease, suggesting an autoimmune origin. This hypothesis has received support from animal experiments in which lymphocytic infiltration and/or fibrosis of the islet have been induced by injection of homologous insulin in cattle[69] and sheep[70] or homologous endocrine pancreas in rodents.[71,72] The histological changes were frequently accompanied by a transient impairment of glucose tolerance[69,71] and by humoral[69] or cell-mediated[71] immune responses.

HUMORAL IMMUNITY

Early reports of humoral antipancreatic autoantibodies in diabetics could not be confirmed and were discarded as artifacts. In 1974, convincing evidence by immunofluorescence of antibodies to pancreatic islet cells in selected diabetics was provided by Bottazzo et al.[73] and MacCuish et al.[74] Islet-cell antibodies are mostly of IgG class, and some are complement-fixing. They react with all five cell types of the islet and are probably directed against the cytoplasmic organelles concerned in the synthesis or the delivery of the hormones (Fig. 155-2). More recently, antibodies specifically reacting with glucagon-secreting A cells or somatostatin-secreting D cells have been detected by a double immunofluorescence technique.[75] Antibodies reacting exclusively with insulin-secreting B cells have not yet been identified by this technique. Islet-cell antibodies were initially found in insulin-dependent diabetics with coexistent autoimmune disease.[73,74] Subsequent studies showed that these antibodies are very common in newly diagnosed juvenile diabetics,[76] their prevalence and titer declining with duration of the disease.[77,78] Islet-cell antibodies have been found to precede the onset of clinical diabetes in some instances and may therefore act as a marker of latent diabetes or prediabetes. They rarely occur in insulin-independent diabetics and, in these cases, may be indicative of subsequent insulin dependence. Two additional types of specific autoantibodies have been identified in the sera of diabetics: antibodies of IgM or IgG class reacting with a cell-surface antigen of viable human insulinoma cells, which have been detected by immunofluorescence in most juvenile diabetics of one series;[79] and antibodies to the insulin receptor, which are present only in patients with severe insulin resistance.[80,81] The latter antibodies are predominantly IgG and are polyclonal. They have been shown to affect receptor function in several ways and to prevent the binding of insulin to its receptors in a variety of tissue cells, thereby producing insulin resistance. This is distinct from the more common acquired insulin resistance, which is due to heterologous insulin-binding antibodies. In rare instances, insulin-binding antibodies of possible monoclonal origin have been demonstrated in patients who had never taken exogenous insulin and had spontaneous hypoglycemia.[82,83] The term "insulin autoimmune syndrome" has been applied to this rare condition.

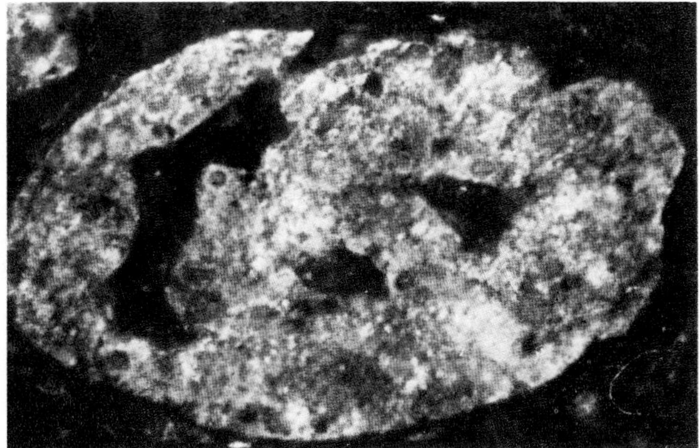

Fig. 155-2. Islet-cell antibody in insulin-dependent diabetes. Frozen section of human pancreas (blood group O) showing immunofluorescence with diabetes serum in all cell types of the islet. Exocrine pancreatic cells and vessel structures are unstained. (From G. F. Bottazzo, D. Doniach, and A. Pouplard, Humoral Autoimmunity in Diabetes Mellitus. Acta Endocrinol (Suppl. 205) *83:* 55, 1976, with kind permission of the authors and the editors.)

CELL-MEDIATED IMMUNITY

The occurrence of antipancreatic cell-mediated immunity in diabetes mellitus was first demonstrated by Nerup et al.[84] by means of the leukocyte migration inhibition test. By this technique, positive findings are found in about one-third of all diabetics, mainly in those with insulin-dependent diabetes of short duration. The antigen involved in this reaction is organ-specific but not species-specific and is different from insulin.[85] Cell-mediated immunity to a soluble antigen (insulin or insulin B-chain) is detectable by the lymphocyte transformation test in approximately 25 percent of insulin-taking diabetics, but it is also found in some young untreated and newly diagnosed patients.[86] Moreover, lymphocytes from insulin-dependent diabetics have been shown to produce cytotoxic effects on human insulinoma cells in vitro. This is apparently due to both antibody-independent and antibody-dependent lymphocyte-cytotoxic processes.[87]

ASSOCIATION OF INSULIN-DEPENDENT DIABETES WITH AUTOIMMUNE DISORDERS

The association of diabetes with diseases of established or putative autoimmune origin has been known for years. Pernicious anemia,[88] hyperthyroidism,[89] Hashimoto's thyroiditis,[90] primary hypothyroidism,[91] and idiopathic Addison's disease[92] are all encountered more commonly in diabetics than would be expected by chance. Diabetes may coexist with multiple autoimmune disorders, such as Schmidt's syndrome[93] and other rare polyendocrinopathies.[94] Antibodies to thyroid and gastric microsomal antigens,[88] intrinsic factor,[88] and adrenocortical cells[92] are more common in diabetic than in comparable nondiabetic control groups. Overt autoimmune disorders, as well as the high prevalence of organspecific autoantibodies, are mainly found in association with insulin-dependent diabetes, predominantly in female patients. A similar increase in antibody frequency is also observed in first-degree relatives of insulin-dependent diabetics.[95,96]

GENETIC ASPECTS

Studies on the prevalence of different antigens of the major histocompatibility system in man have shown a strong association between HL-A-B8 and BW15 and insulin-dependent diabetes.[97] It appears that the susceptibility to the disease conferred by B8 and BW15 involves two different mechanisms, since the risk of insulin-dependent diabetes is twice as high when both rather than either one of these antigens are present. An even stronger association has been demonstrated between insulin-dependent diabetes and HL-A-DW3 and DW4.[40] It is worth noticing that the frequency of HL-A-B8 and DW3 is also increased in idiopathic Addison's disease, Graves' disease, and premature ovarian failure. This provides further genetic evidence linking insulin-dependent diabetes with organ-specific autoimmune endocrinopathies.

POSSIBLE ETIOLOGIC FACTORS

Evidence that initiating factors of juvenile diabetes may be viral in nature has been reported. Mumps, rubella, infectious mononucleosis, as well as infections with the group B Coxsackie viruses, are known to produce pancreas damage in man.[98] Increased titers of antibody to Coxsackie virus B4 have been observed in recently diagnosed juvenile diabetics. In mice the M variant of the encephalomyocarditis virus[99] and Coxsackie virus B[100] produce a rapidly evolving insulitis leading to diabetes. The susceptibility to diabetogenic viruses in mice seems to be genetically determined, being observed only in certain strains.[101]

Available evidence indicates that autoimmunity, genetic constitution, and viral infections are all implicated in insulin-dependent diabetes. In an unifying hypothesis, it may be postulated that immune response genes associated with HL-A-B8 predispose the individuals carrying this HL-A type to develop diabetes mellitus when exposed to appropriate environmental factors such as pancreatotropic viruses, which in turn may lead to B-cell destruction either directly or by triggering autoimmune reactions. It has recently been proposed that there are at least two kinds of insulin-dependent diabetes, one of which is characterized by juvenile onset and a transient humoral response to islet-cell antigens, possibly as a consequence of viral infections. The second type is related to autoimmunity, occurs at any age and predominantly in women, and is associated with other organ-specific autoimmune disorders and with longer permanence of islet-cell antibodies.[102]

PRIMARY ADRENOCORTICAL INSUFFICIENCY

Primary adrenocortical insufficiency (Addison's disease) results from progressive destruction of the adrenal cortex, leading to deficiencies of cortisol, aldosterone, and adrenal androgen. In areas where active tuberculosis is well controlled, the most common cause of Addison's disease at present is idiopathic atrophy of the adrenal cortex. Unlike the tuberculosis form, idiopathic atrophy is seen more often in females than males, in a ratio of approximately 2:1 or 3:1. It may occur at any age, but its peak incidence is in the fourth and fifth decades.

HISTOPATHOLOGIC CHANGES

In idiopathic Addison's disease, both adrenal glands are in general greatly reduced in size. Histologically there is atrophy of the adrenal cortex, with complete disorganization of its normal three-layered structure. Some degree of diffuse mononuclear cell infiltration is invariably demonstrable. Infiltrating cells mainly consist of small lymphocytes, but plasma cells and macrophages are also present. The adrenal medulla is usually well preserved in idiopathic Addison's disease, whereas in the tuberculous form the whole gland is generally destroyed.[103] Focal lymphocytic adrenalitis has been rarely found in autopsy series of miscellaneous cases.[104] In this respect, the adrenals differ considerably from the thyroid gland, which is a common site of focal lymphocytic infiltration.

HUMORAL AND CELL-MEDIATED IMMUNITY

The presence of circulating adrenal autoantibodies in idiopathic Addison's disease was first demonstrated by Anderson et al. in 1957,[105] using a complement fixation test with saline extract of human adrenal. By indirect immunofluorescence on frozen sections of human or monkey adrenal tissue, adrenal antibodies have subsequently been detected in 65 to 74 percent of three large series of patients with idiopathic Addison's disease.[106–108] The overall incidence of these antibodies in tuberculous Addison's disease, as calculated from reported series, is approximately 8 percent, but it is even lower when only unequivocal cases of this type of adrenal insufficiency are considered.[107,108] Adrenal antibodies are undetectable in patients with adrenal insufficiency secondary to pituitary failure.[107] Antibody titers are unrelated to the duration of the disease and tend to persist for many years following adequate replacement therapy with adrenal steroids.

Evidence of cellular hypersensitivity to adrenal antigen as assessed by the leukocyte migration inhibition test has also been reported in patients with idiopathic Addison's disease with an incidence of 40 percent, while negative results were observed in tuberculous Addison's disease.[109]

The antigen has been found in normal, hyperplastic, or fetal human adrenal tissue but not in adrenocortical tumors. It is not strictly species-specific, since cross-reactions by immunofluorescence have been demonstrated with the adrenal of several species.[107,110] It may be found in all three layers of adrenal cortex, but some sera appear to react only with one or two layers, suggesting that multiple antigens are involved. These antigens are cytoplasmic components of cortical cells sedimenting mainly with the microsomal fraction[110] and appear to be constituted by a lipoprotein.[111] With regard to these aspects, the adrenal antigen is similar to the microsomal antigens involved in thyroid and gastric autoimmune disorders.

ASSOCIATION OF IDIOPATHIC ADDISON'S DISEASE WITH OTHER AUTOIMMUNE DISORDERS

The association of idiopathic Addison's disease with chronic lymphocytic thyroiditis has been known since 1926, when Schmidt[112] reported 2 patients with such condition. Since then it became apparent that the entire spectrum of thyroid autoimmune disorders (Graves' disease, Hashimoto's thyroiditis and idiopathic myxedema) is highly prevalent in patients with idiopathic Addison's disease but not in those with tuberculous adrenal insufficiency. Several other disorders believed to be autoimmune in nature, including pernicious anemia, idiopathic hypoparathyroidism, premature ovarian failure, and diabetes mellitus (predominantly the insulin-dependent type), have been reported in association with idiopathic adrenal atrophy.[108,113–115] The recognition of these diseases may precede, accompany, or follow the diagnosis of adrenal insufficiency. Antibodies to thyroglobulin, thyroid microsomal antigen, gastric parietal cells, intrinsic factor, parathyroid cells, and pancreatic islet cells are frequently detectable in patients with idiopathic Addison's disease, also in the absence of overt related disorders. The patients with premature ovarian failure have adrenal antibodies that are also reactive with steroid-producing cells of the ovary, the testis, and/or the placenta.[108]

EXPERIMENTAL AUTOIMMUNE ADRENALITIS

Adrenalitis and adrenal antibodies have been produced in the experimental animal by injection of adrenal homogenate emulsified with Freund's complete adjuvant, but variable results have been reported in different species. Guinea pigs have been shown to develop lymphocytic infiltration and necrosis of the adrenal cortex following immunization with homologous or autologous adrenal tissue.[116,117] In rabbits, adrenalitis after immunization with homologous or autologous adrenal gland was observed by some authors,[118] but not by others.[117] In both species the formation of adrenal-specific autoantibodies has been demonstrated, but no correlation was found between these autoantibodies and the development of histopathologic changes.[119] Inbred rats have been found to develop autoimmune adrenalitis following injection of syngeneic adrenal tissue with Freund's complete adjuvant and pertussis vaccine. Passive transfer of adrenalitis from actively immunized donors to normal recipients was obtained in these animals by means of living lymphocytic cells.[120] Autoradiographic studies suggest that the arrival in the adrenal of a few specifically sensitized lymphocytes migrating from the bloodstream is the initiating event of autoimmune adrenalitis in the rat.[121]

PATHOGENETIC AND ETIOLOGIC FACTORS IN IDIOPATHIC ADDISON'S DISEASE

The experimental and clinical data are consistent with an autoimmune pathogenesis of idiopathic Addison's disease. The fact that adrenal antibodies only rarely occur in tuberculous adrenal insufficiency indicates that the destruction of the adrenal gland by itself is not sufficient to stimulate the immune response. The remarkable difference in the incidence of associate autoimmune disorders between the two types of adrenal insufficiency suggest that the development of these conditions is unrelated to underactivity of the adrenal gland and that the patients with idiopathic adrenal atrophy have a peculiar susceptibility to organ-specific autoimmunity. The fundamental abnormality is unknown, but it is probably related to a disorder of immunologic tolerance. The possibility that this is genetically controlled is supported by recent studies indicating that HL-A-B8 and the DW3 determinant are strongly associated with idiopathic Addison's disease.[40] The mechanism by which adrenal damage is produced has not been elucidated. As in other organ-specific autoimmune disorders, there is probably a cooperation of circulating antibodies and cell-mediated immunity.

The detection of adrenal and other organ-specific antibodies in the presence of adrenocortical insufficiency is of diagnostic value insofar as it provides a clue to the etiology of the disease. The diagnosis of idiopathic adrenal atrophy implies that the patients should be observed and followed closely for the development of other autoimmune disorders. At present, immunosuppressive therapy of idiopathic adrenocortical insufficiency is unjustified in view of the effectiveness of replacement therapy with adrenal steroids and the lack of specificity of available immunosuppressive drugs.

PRIMARY OVARIAN FAILURE

Amenorrhea or oligomenorrhea with elevated serum and urinary pituitary gonadotropins is a frequent finding in women with idiopathic Addison's disease who are in the child-bearing period.[108,113] This cannot be explained by metabolic imbalance secondary to adrenal failure, since the menstrual disorders persist even after adequate steroid replacement. Histological findings in the ovary in this condition show either complete atrophy or lymphocytic infiltration predominantly in the vicinity of developing graafian follicles.[108] A high proportion of these patients have antibodies that are reactive with steroid-producing cells of the theca interna and the corpus luteum of the ovary, as well as interstitial cells of the testis, placental trophoblasts, and adrenocortical cells.[108,122] Immunofluorescence studies suggest that multiple antibodies reacting with different constituents of steroid-producing cells are involved, but most, if not all, of these antibodies can be absorbed out with extracts of adrenal cortex.[108] Some of the ovarian antibodies have a complement-dependent cytotoxic effect on human granulosa cells in culture.[123] Evidence of delayed hypersensitivity to ovarian as well as to thyroid and adrenal antigens, as assessed by the leukocyte migration inhibition test, has been reported in a patient with premature ovarian failure associated with autoimmune thyroiditis and adrenalitis.[134] Steroid-cell antibodies only rarely occur in patients with primary or secondary ovarian failure not associated with Addison's disease.[108,122] In patients with premature ovarian failure and idiopathic adrenocortical insufficiency, there is also a very high incidence of other organ-specific autoimmune disorders, especially idiopathic hypoparathyroidism and thyroid disease. Clinical manifestations of ovarian and adrenal failure occur at the same time, suggesting a causative role of autoimmune mechanisms involving antigens that are common to these two tissues.[108] Since hormonal replacement therapy is not expected to reinstate fertility in such cases, immunosuppressive therapy in selected patients might be considered.

AUTOIMMUNE TESTICULAR FAILURE

Impotence and loss of libido are commonly present in patients with Addison's disease, but these symptoms are usually reversed by adequate treatment of adrenal failure. Antibodies reacting with the interstitial cells of the testis, as well as with other steroid-producing cells, have been detected in male patients with idiopathic Addison's disease, but this occurred much less frequently than in female patients.[108,125] Moreover, most of these patients had no overt manifestations of gonadal insufficiency. Although there is little evidence that the hormonal function of the testis may be significantly affected by autoimmune processes, a considerable body of data indicate that sperm autoimmunity is implicated in several cases of infertility. This problem will be discussed in a later section.

IDIOPATHIC HYPOPARATHYROIDISM

Idiopathic hypoparathyroidism is a rare condition that is usually recognized in childhood or adolescence and is slightly more common in females than in males. Histologically it is characterized by lymphocytic infiltration and atrophy of the parathyroid glands. Autoimmune parathyroiditis with characteristic biochemical changes of hypoparathyroidism has been obtained in rats[125] and dogs[126] by injection of homologous parathyroid extracts plus Freund's adjuvant, but complement-fixing parathyroid antibodies were demonstrable in low titers only in the canine sera. Parathyroiditis with no apparent impairment of parathyroid function has been induced by rats by passive transfer of rabbit antiserum to rat parathyroid homogenate.[127]

Circulating antibodies specifically reacting with the cytoplasm of human parathyroid cells have been described in patients with hypoparathyroidism by Blizzard et al.,[128] using complement fixation and immunofluorescence techniques. By the latter method, these authors detected parathyroid antibodies in 38 percent of patients with hypoparathyroidism and in only 6 percent of control subjects. A relatively high incidence of these antibodies was also found in patients with idiopathic Addison's disease (26 percent) or Hashimoto's thyroiditis (12 percent), who had no clinical evidence of hypoparathyroidism. So far, only one laboratory[129] has been able to provide additional evidence for the occurrence of parathyroid antibodies by demonstrating antibodies reacting with both the oxyphil and the chief cells of the parathyroid in a patient with idiopathic hypoparathyroidism, idiopathic Addison's disease, and premature ovarian failure. The negative findings obtained by other authors have been attributed to the poor antigenicity of available specimens of human parathyroid.

In addition to idiopathic Addison's disease and primary ovarian failure, idiopathic hypoparathyroidism is often associated with other disorders of established or putative autoimmune nature, including Hashimoto's thyroiditis, idiopathic myxedema, pernicious anemia, and alopecia totalis. Antibodies to adrenal, thyroid, and gastric antigens are frequently detectable in patients with idiopathic hypoparathyroidism, even in the absence of overt associated disease.[108,128] A distinctive and unexplained feature of idiopathic hypoparathyroidism is its common association with refractory mucocutaneous moniliasis. There is familiar predisposition for the combination of moniliasis, hypoparathyroidism, and Addison's disease, which may also include one or more of the above disorders.[130] This condition is considered a separate entity[131] and is often referred to as moniliasis-polyendocrinopathy sydrome. Precipitating antibodies specifically reacting with a soluble adrenal antigen, distinct from the microsomal adrenal antigen commonly involved in idiopathic Addison's disease, have been described in patients with this syndrome.[132]

PITUITARY AUTOIMMUNITY

The occurrence of autoimmune hypophysitis resulting in hypopituitarism was first suggested by Goudie and Pinkerton,[133] when they found destructive lesions of the anterior pituitary with diffuse lymphoid infiltration at autopsy in a subject with associated thyroiditis and idiopathic Addison's disease. The presence of pituitary lymphoid infiltrates has also been described in other autopsy series.[134] Autoimmune hypothysitis has been produced in the experimental animal by injection of pituitary extracts in Freund's adjuvant.[135] Until recently, attempts to demonstrate circulating pituitary antibodies in patients with hypopituitarism have been unsuccessful. In 1975, Bottazzo and his co-workers[136] were able to detect complement-fixing autoantibodies to prolactin-secreting cells by a double immunofluorescence technique, using fresh pituitary gland obtained at hypophysectomy for breast cancer. The antigen involved in these reactions was not prolactin but appeared to be associated with cytoplasmic organelles involved in the synthesis or the delivery of the hormone. The clinical significance of these antibodies is unclear. Prolactin cell antibodies have mostly been detected in patients with autoimmune polyendocrinopathy and especially in those with idiopathic hypoparathyroidism, whereas neither this nor other types of pituitary antibodies have been found in cases of panhypopituitarism. So far, evidence for other pituitary antibodies has been obtained only in two subjects, including one girl with stunted growth and impaired growth hormone secretion in whom antibodies to growth hormone cells were found and one boy who had antibodies to either LH or FSH cells.[137] Antibodies to ACTH- or TSH-secreting cells have not yet been reported. Interestingly, ACTH-secreting cells have been shown to bind all human immunoglobulins by their Fc portions.[138] This is not an antigen–antibody reaction and is similar to the fixation of IgE and anaphylactic IgG on the mast cells, which also involves the Fc portion of the immunoglobulins and is known to be implicated in the release of histamine by these cells. The question of whether the affinity of the pituitary ACTH cells for human immunoglobulins has any physiological role remains to be established.

INFERTILITY

Male infertility, which accounts for more than 50 percent of childless couples, is usually unrelated to endocrine disorders. Although most of the infertile men have either azoospermia or profound oligospermia, a normal sperm count with spontaneous agglutination and early loss of motility of the otherwise normal spermatozoa is found in less than 10 percent of the cases. Evidence has been accumulated that the infertility of at least some of these subjects may result from autoantibodies that agglutinate and immobilize spermatozoa, preventing their penetration into the cervical mucus of the female partner. The question of whether nonobstructive azoospermia is related to autoimmune mechanisms remains to be proven. Isoimmunity to sperm has been recognized as a cause of unexplained infertility in women.

AUTOIMMUNITY TO SPERM IN MEN

The antigenicity of spermatozoa has been well established in several animal species by the demonstration of autoantibodies to spermatozoa following injection of homologous or autologous sperm. Spermatozoal antigens include intrinsic constituents of the spermatozoa and other substances that are acquired from the seminal fluid and are termed sperm-coating antigens. In humans, these antigens may derive from seminal vesicles, prostate, and epididymis and may include blood group substances A and B. Histocompatibility antigens have also been demonstrated. It appears that sperm autoimmunity of human males involves only intrinsic antigens, which are located in the head, tail, and tip of the tail according to agglutination patterns.[139]

The occurrence of agglutinating and immobilizing autoantibodies to spermatozoa in the sera of some infertile men was first described independently by Wilson[140] and Rümke[141] in 1954. Subsequent studies have shown that significant titers of serum agglutinating antibodies are present in 3 to 12 percent of infertile men with normal or low sperm counts, while negative or only low titers are found in control subjects. Spermagglutinins have been demonstrated in seminal fluid, occasionally in higher titers than in the serum, suggesting that these antibodies may also be produced locally.[142,143] Immobilizing antibodies are usually but not always present in sera with positive agglutination tests. These antibodies are generally complement-dependent and are probably identical to the cytotoxic antibodies detected by dye exclusion tests.[144] Antibodies that are demonstrable by immunofluorescence on fixed spermatozoa are probably directed against different antigens.[145] Serum antibody titers are correlated with the degree of spontaneous agglutination and loss of motility of spermatozoa in the ejaculates,[139] as well as with the inability of spermatozoa to invade cervical mucus in vitro.[146] Moreover, an inverse correlation between fertility and serum antibody titers has been found, although some subjects who had sperm agglutinins with normal sperm counts have subsequently fathered children.[147]

It has been postulated that formation of autoantibodies may be triggered by sperm extravasation into the interstitium of the epididymis, while removal of excess sperm by phagocytosis into the lumen of the epididymis occurring in physiological conditions would not induce an immunologic response. This explanation is strongly supported by the finding of sperm autoantibodies in more than 50 percent of vasectomized subjects.[148,149] Inflammation and trauma may also be important factors, since sperm antibodies are frequently found in patients with a history of inflammatory or traumatic disease.[150,151] Conflicting results have been obtained in therapeutical experiments with corticosteroids in immunosuppressive doses.

AUTOIMMUNE ASPERMATOGENESIS

Experimental autoimmune orchitis leading to aspermatogenesis has been induced in guinea pigs and several other species by immunization of male animals with homologous or autologous testis or sperm plus Freund's adjuvant.[139] Spermatozoal antigens are responsible for this reaction, and four different aspermatogenic antigens have been identified in the acrosome and proacrosomal structures of guinea pig spermatozoa.[152] Histological changes are limited to the germinal epithelium, which shows extensive degeneration with impaired maturation or complete aspermatogenesis, while Leydig cells are uninvolved. Focal lymphocytic and plasma cell infiltration with interstitial edema is demonstrable, but damage to the germinal cells has also been found in the absence of infiltrating cells.[153] Infiltration initiates and is most pronounced in the efferent ducts and rete testis,[154,155] possibly because in these regions there is a greater permeability of the peritubular barrier,[156] which normally provides an immunologic isolation of spermatozoa. Orchitis and aspermatogenesis have been transferred passively by means of humoral antibody, provided that the recipient animals had their tissue permeability increased by pretreatment with Freund's complete adjuvant.[157] Passive transfer by means of lymph node cells and macrophages was most effective when these materials were injected locally rather than systemically.[158,159] It would appear that the testicular damage results from an interplay of cellular and humoral immune mechanisms.

The relevance of these experimental data to human orchitis and aspermatogenesis remains to be established. Mumps orchitis rarely if ever occurs in children before spermatogenesis has begun, and its histological findings in the acute phase are not unlike that of experimental autoimmune orchitis. Interestingly, autoimmune orchitis has been produced in guinea pigs by immunization with the parotid gland,[160] but no further evidence has been provided that this mechanism is implicated in human disease. Volunteers with prostatic carcinoma have been submitted to immunization with autologous or homologous testicular homogenate, and 2 of the 4 cases studied developed testicular lesions in association with serum antibodies and delayed hypersensitivity to sperm antigen.[161] Agglutinating antibodies to sperm in infertile men are usually not associated with aspermatogenesis or histological changes of the testis, while cytotoxic antibodies have been found in several subjects with hypo- or aspermatogenesis and various testicular lesions.[162] Cell-mediated immunity to sperm antigens as assessed by blast-cell transformation has been reported in nonobstructive azoospermia,[163] but no correlation with the sperm count has been observed in a smaller series of infertile men.[164] At present the possibility that autoimmune orchitis with impaired spermatogenesis is a significant cause of male infertility remains an open question.

It has been reported that transient suppression of spermatogenesis with testosterone is followed in some infertile oligospermic subjects by an increase in total sperm counts over pretreatment values with restoration of fertility.[165] The effect might be attributed to a temporary depression of the immune response as a consequence of the diminished antigenic stimulus by spermatocytes. However, the overall experience with this treatment schedule has not been very encouraging. Similarly the beneficial effects of corticosteroids in immunosuppressive doses reported by some authors require further confirmation.

ISOIMMUNITY TO SPERM IN WOMEN

Early evidence for isoimmunity to sperm in women with unexplained infertility was provided in 1922 by Meaker,[166] who reported agglutination and immobilization of a husband's spermatozoa by the sera of two sterile women. Experimental support to this concept has derived from a number of studies indicating that immunization of female animals of various species with homologous sperm may result in a reduced fertility.[139] Sperm-agglutinating antibodies are frequently detectable in the serum of infertile women, but their incidence has varied considerably in different series. In a recent study of 150 infertile couples, positive results by a macroagglutination technique have been found in 23.1 percent of the female and 9.6 percent of the male partners, while only 2.7 percent of fertile women had detectable antibodies in low titers.[167] Complement-dependent immobilizing antibodies to sperm also occur much more frequently in the serum of women with unexplained infertility than in those with known causes of infertility or in fertile women,[168] whereas no clear difference between fertile and infertile women has been found by immunofluorescence tests.[145] Specific intrinsic antigens of spermatozoa are involved in these isoimmune reactions, but involvement of sperm-coating antigens has also been observed in some sera.[168,169] More relevant to infertility is probably the observation that cytotoxic[170] and agglutinating[171] antibodies to spermatozoa are also detectable in the cervical mucus of infertile women.

The formation of sperm isoantibodies is apparently related to sexual activity, since positive reactions have never been found in the sera of virgins. Evidence of immunization through the vaginal route has been obtained, but mating experiments in guinea pigs indicate that vaginal adsorption of homologous sperm is usually not sufficient to induce a primary immune response, while it may well act as a booster in animals with preexisting immunity induced parenterally.[172,173] Animal[174] and human[175] studies suggest that lesions in the epithelium of the genital tract may facilitate the induction of immune response. The concept that the sperm antibody production is sustained by resorption of sperm has led to the suggestion that the prolonged use of a condom by the male partner might result in a decreased immune response with restoration of fertility. Disappearance of sperm antibodies from infertile women during condom treatment[171] and the occurrence of pregnancy after resumption of normal intercourse[176] have been reported, but unsuccessful results with this therapeutic approach have also been described.[177]

REFERENCES

1. Roitt, I. M. Essential Immunology, ed. 2. Blackwell Scientific Publ., Oxford, 1974.
2. Gell, P. G. H., Coombs, R. R. A., and Lachmann, P. J. (Eds.). Clinical Aspects of Immunology, ed. 3, Blackwell Scientific Publ., Oxford, 1975.
3. Fudenberg, H. H., Stites, D. P., Caldwell, J. L., and Wells, J. V.

Basic and Clinical Immunology. Lange Medical Publ., Los Altos, 1976.

4. Coombs, R. R. A., and Gell, P. G. H. Classification of Allergic Reactions Responsible for Clinical Hypersensitivity and Disease, in Gell, P. G. H., Coombs, R. R. A., and Lachmann, P. J. (Eds.), Clinical Aspects of Immunology, ed. 3. Blackwell Scientific Publ., Oxford, 1975, p. 761.
5. Milgrom, F., and Witebski, E. Autoantibodies and Autoimmune Diseases. *JAMA 181:* 706, 1962.
6. Roitt, I. M., Doniach, D., Campbell, P. N., and Hudson, R. V. Auto-antibodies in Hashimoto's Disease (Lymphoadenoid Goiter). *Lancet 2:* 820, 1956.
7. Rose, N. R., and Witebsky, E. Studies on Organ Specificity. V. Changes in the Thyroid Glands of Rabbits Following Active Immunization with Rabbits Thyroid Extracts. *J Immunol 76:* 417, 1956.
8. Adams, D. D., and Purves, H. D. Abnormal Responses in the Assay of Thyrotropin. *Proc Univ Otago Med Sch 34:* 11, 1956.
9. Doniach, D., and Roitt, I. M., Thyroid Auto-Allergic Disease, in Gell, P. G. H., Coombs, R. R. A., and Lachmann, P. J. (Eds.), Clinical Aspects of Immunology, ed 3. Blackwell Scientific Publ., Oxford, 1975, p. 1355.
10. Neve, P., Ermans, A. M., and Bastenie, P. A. Struma Lymphomatosa (Hashimoto), in Bastenie, P. A., and Ermans, A. M. (Eds.), Thyroiditis and Thyroid Function. Pergamon Press, Oxford, 1972, p. 109.
11. Hay, F. C., and Torrigiani, G. The Distribution of Anti-Thyroglobulin Antibodies in the IgG Subclasses. *Clin Exp Immunol 16:* 517, 1974.
12. Torrigiani, G., Doniach, D., and Roitt, I. M. Serum Thyroglobulin Levels in Healthy Subjects and in Patients with Thyroid Disease. *J Clin Endocrinol Metab 29:* 305, 1969.
13. Mori, T., and Kriss, J. P. Measurement by Competitive Binding Radioassay of Serum Anti-Thyroglobulin and Anti-Microsomal Antibodies in Graves' Disease and Other Thyroid Disorders. *J Clin Endocrinol Metab 33:* 688, 1971.
14. Pinchera, A., Mariotti, S., Vitti, P., Tosi, M., Grasso, L., Pacini, F., et al. Interference of Serum Thyroglobulin in the Radioassay for Serum Anti-Thyroglobulin Antibodies. *J Clin Endocrinol Metab 45:* 1077, 1977.
15. Roitt, I. M., Ling, N. R., Doniach, D., and Couchman, K. G. The Cytoplasmic Autoantigen of the Human Thyroid. Immunological and Biochemical Characteristics. *Immunology 7:* 375, 1964.
16. Pinchera, A., Mariotti, S., Vitti, P., Fenzi, G. F., Grasso, L., Tosi, M., and Bindi, S. Studies on Thyroid Plasma Membrane Antigens, in Von Zur Muhlen, A., and Schleusener, H. (Eds.), Biochemical Basis of Thyroid Stimulation and Thyroid Hormone Action. George Thieme Publ., Stuttgart, 1976, p. 79.
17. Amino, N., Hagen, S. R., Refetoff, S., and Yamada, N. Measurement of Circulating Thyroid Microsomal Antibodies by the Tanned Red Cell Haemagglutination Technique: Its Usefulness in the Diagnosis of Autoimmune Thyroid Diseases. *Clin Endocrinol (Oxf) 5:* 115, 1976.
18. Balfour, B. M., Doniach, D., Roitt, I. M., and Couchman, K. G. Fluorescent Antibody Studies in Human Thyroiditis: Autoantibodies to an Antigen of the Thyroid Colloid Distinct from Thyroglobulin. *Br J Exp Pathol 42:* 307, 1961.
19. Fagraeus, A., and Jonsson, J. Distribution of Organ Antibodies Over the Surface of Thyroid Cells as Examined by Immunofluorescence Test. *Immunology 18:* 413, 1970.
20. McKenzie, J. M., and Zakarija, M. The Role of the Immune System in Graves' Disease, in James, V. H. T. (Ed), *Endocrinology,* Amsterdam, Excerpta Medica, 1977, p. 474.
21. Adams, D. D., and Kennedy, T. H. Occurrence in Thyrotoxicosis of a Gamma Globulin which Protects LATS from Neutralization by an Extract of Thyroid Gland. *J Clin Endocrinol Metab 27:* 173, 1967.
22. Onaya, T., Kotani, M., Yamada, T., and Ochi, Y. New in-vitro Tests to Detect the Thyroid Stimulator in Sera from Hyperthyroid Patients by Measuring Colloid Droplet Formation and Cyclic AMP in Human Thyroid Slices. *J Clin Endocrinol Metab 36:* 859, 1973.
23. Shishiba, Y., Shimizu, T., Yoshimura, S., and Shizume, K. Direct Evidence for Human Thyroid Stimulation by LATS-Protector. *J Clin Endocrinol Metab 36:* 517, 1973.
24. Orgiazzi, J., Williams, D. E., Chopra, I. J., and Solomon, D. H. Human Thyroid Adenylate Cyclase Stimulating Activity in Immunoglobulin G of Patients with Graves' Disease, *J Clin Endocrinol Metab 42:* 341, 1976.
25. Fenzi, G. F., Macchia, E., Bartalena, L., Mazzanti, F., Baschieri, L., and DeGroot, L. J. Radioreceptor Assay of TSH: Its Use to Detect Thyroid Stimulating Immunoglobulins. *J Endocrinol Invest 1:* 17, 1978.
26. Mukhtar, E. D., Smith, B. R., Pyle, G. A., Hall, R., and Vice, P. Relation of Thyroid Stimulating Immunoglobulins to Thyroid Function and Effect of Surgery, Radioiodine, and Antithyroid Drugs. *Lancet 1:* 713, 1975.
27. Calder, E. A., McLennan, D., Barnes, E. W., and Irvine, W. J. The Effect of Thyroid Antigens on the *in Vitro* Migration Inhibition of Leucocytes from Patients with Hashimoto's Thyroiditis. *Clin Exp Immunol 12:* 429, 1972.
28. Lamki, L., Row, V. V., and Volpé, R. Cell-Mediated Immunity in Graves' Disease and Hashimoto's Thyroiditis as Shown by the Demonstration of Migration Inhibition Factor (MIF). *J Clin Endocrinol Metab 36:* 358, 1973.
29. Ehrenfeld, E. N., Klein, E., and Benezra, D. Human Thyroglobulin and Thyroid Extracts as Specific Stimulators of Sensitized Lymphocytes. *J Clin Endocrinol Metab 32:* 115, 1971.
30. Delespesse, G., Duchateau, J., Collet, H., Govaerts, A., and Bastenie, P. A. Lymphocytes Transformation with Thyroglobulin in Thyroid Diseases. *Clin Exp Immunol 12:* 439, 1972.
31. Amino, N., Linn, E. S., Pyser, T. J., Moore, G. E., Mier, R., and DeGroot, L. J. Human Lymphotoxin Obtained from Established Lymphoid lines: Purification, Characterization and Inhibition by Anti-Immunoglobulin. *J Immunol 113:* 1334, 1974.
32. Laryea, E., Row, V. V., and Volpé, R. The Effect of Blood Leukocytes from Patients with Hashimoto's Disease on Human Thyroid Cells in Monolayer Culture. *Clin Endocrinol (Oxf) 2:* 23, 1973.
33. Ling, N. R., Acton, A. B., Roitt, I. M., and Doniach, D. Interaction of Lymphocytes from Immunized Hosts with Thyroid and Other Cells in Culture. *Br J Exp Pathol 46:* 348, 1965.
34. Podleski, W. K. Cytotoxic Lymphocytes in Hashimoto's Thyroiditis. *Clin Exp Immunol 11:* 543, 1972.
35. Calder, E. A., Penhale, W. J., McLennan, D., Barnes, E. W., and Irvine, W. J. Lymphocyte Dependent Antibody Mediated Cytotoxicity in Hashimoto Thyroiditis. *Clin Exp Immunol 14:* 153, 1973.
36. Irvine, W. J. The Association of Atrophic Gastritis with Autoimmune Thyroid Disease. *Clin Endocrinol Metabol 4:* 351, 1975.
37. DeGroot, L. J., and Stanbury, J. B. The Thyroid and Its Diseases, ed. 4. John Wiley & Sons, New York, 1975, p. 587.
38. Hall, R., Dingle, P. R., and Roberts, D. F. Thyroid Antibodies: A Study of First Degree Relatives. *Clin Genet 3:* 319, 1972.
39. Grumet, F. C., Rose, O. P., Konishi, J., and Kriss, J. P. HL-A Antigens as Markers for Disease Susceptibility and Autoimmunity in Graves' Disease. *J Clin Endocrinol Metab 39:* 1115, 1974.
40. Thomsen, M., Platz, P., Andersen, O. O., Cristy, M., Lyngsøe, J., Nerup, J., et al. MLC Typing in Juvenile Diabetes Mellitus and Isiopathic Addison's Disease. *Transplant Rev 22:* 125, 1975.
41. Grumet, F. C., Konishi, J., Rose, O. P., and Kriss, J. P. Association in Japanese of Graves' Disease with the HL-A Specificity W5, in Robbins, J., and Braverman, L. E. (Eds.). Thyroid Research. Excerpta Medica, Amsterdam, 1976, p. 376.
42. Rose, N. R., and Witebski, E. Experimental Thyroiditis, in Samter, M., Alexander, H. L., Talmage, D. W., Rose, B., Sherman, W. B., and Vaughan, J. H. (Eds.) Immunological Diseases. Little, Brown and Co., Boston, 1971, p. 1179.
43. Shulman, S. Thyroid Antigens and Autoimmunity. *Adv Immunol 14:* 85, 1971.
44. Weigle, W. O. Recent Observations and Concepts in Immunological Unresponsiveness and Autoimmunity. *Clin Exp Immunol 9:* 437, 1971.
45. Andrada, J. A., Rose, N. R., and Kite, J. H. Experimental Thyroiditis in the Rhesus Monkey: IV. The Role of Thyroglobulin and Cellular Antigens. *Clin Exp Immunol 3:* 133, 1968.
46. Tomazic, V., and Rose, N. R. Autoimmune Murine Thyroiditis. VIII. Role of Different Thyroid Antigens in the Induction of Experimental Autoimmune Thyroiditis. *Immunology 30:* 63, 1976.
47. Bigazzi, P. E., and Rose, N. R. Spontaneous Autoimmune Thyroiditis in Animals as a Model of Human Disease, *Prog Allergy 19:* 245, 1975.
48. Pinchera, A., Liberti, P., and Badalamenti, G. Attività Tireostimolante ad Azione Prolungata nel Siero di Conigli Immunizzati con Tiroide Umana. *Folia Endocrinol (Roma) 18:* 522, 1965.
49. Beall, G. N., and Solomon, D. H. Thyroid Stimulating Activity in

the Serum of Rabbits Immunized with Thyroid Microsomes. *J Clin Endocrinol Metab 28:* 503, 1968.
50. McKenzie, J. M., Experimental Production of Thyroid-Stimulating Anti-Thyroid Antibody. *J Clin Endocrinol Metab 28:* 596, 1968.
51. Ong, M., Malkin, D. G., Tays, K., and Malkin, A. Activation of Thyroid Adenyl Cyclase by Antisera to Thyroid Plasma Membrane Preparations. *Endocrinology 98:* 880, 1976.
52. Nakamura, R. M., and Weigle, W. O. Transfer of Experimental Autoimmune Thyroiditis by Sera from Thyroidectomized Donors. *J Exp Med 130:* 263, 1969.
53. Clagett, J. A., Wilson, C. B., and Weigle, W. O. Interstitial Immune Complex Thyroiditis in Mice. The Role of Autoantibody to Thyroglobulin. *J Exp Med 140:* 1439, 1974.
54. Kalderon, A. E., Bogaars, H. A., and Diamond, I. Ultrastructrual Alterations of the Follicular Basement Membrane in Hashiomoto's Thyroiditis. *Am J Med 55:* 485, 1973.
55. Calder, E. A., Penhale, W. J., Barnes, E. W., and Irvine, W. J. Evidence for Circulating Immune Complexes in Thyroid Disease. *Br Med J 2:* 30, 1974.
56. Takeda, Y., and Kriss, J. P. Radiometric Measurement of Thyroglobulin-Antithyroglobulin Immune Complexes in Human Serum. *J Clin Endocrinol Metab 44:* 46, 1977.
57. Calder, E. A., Irvine, W. J. Cell-Mediated Immunity and Immune Complexes in Thyroid Disease. *Clin Endocrinol Metabol 4:* 287, 1975.
58. McMaster, P. R. B., and Lerner, E. M. The Transfer of Allergic Thyroiditis in Hystocompatible Guinea Pigs by Lymphnode Cells. *J Immunol 99:* 208, 1967.
59. Lin, M. S., and Salvin, S. B. *In Vitro* and *in Vivo* Studies on the Mechanism of Experimental Autoimmune Thyroiditis in Guinea Pigs. *Cell Immunol 27:* 177, 1976.
60. Bankhurst, A. D., Torrigiani, G., and Allison, A. C. Lympocytes binding Human Thyroglobulin in Healthy People and Its Relevance to Tolerance for Autoantigens. *Lancet 1:* 226, 1973.
61. Penhale, W. J., Farmer, A., McKenna, R. P., and Irvine, W. J. Spontaneous Thyroiditis in Thymectomized and Irradiated Wistar Rats. *Clin Exp Immunol 15:* 225, 1973.
62. Rose, N. R., Becon, L. D., and Sundick, R. S. Genetic Determinants of Thyroiditis in the OS Chicken. *Transplant Rev 31:* 264, 1976.
63. Konishi, J., Herman, M. M., and Kriss, J. P. Binding of Thyroglobulin and Thyroglobulin-Anti-Thyroglobulin Immune Complex to Extraocular Muscle Membrane. *Endocrinology 95:* 434, 1974.
64. Etienne, J., Kohn, L. D., and Winand, R. J. Studies on the Mechanisms of Experimental Exophtalmos, in Robbins, J., and Braverman, L. E. (Eds.), Thyroid Research. Excerpta Medica, Amsterdam, 1976, p. 380.
65. Schmidt, M. B. Über die Beziehung der Langerhans'schen Inseln des Pankreas zum Diabetes Mellitus. *Munch Med Wochenschr 49:* 51, 1902.
66. Von Meyenburg, H. Über "Insulitis" bei Diabetes. *Schweiz Med Wochenschr 21:* 554, 1940.
67. Gepts, W. Pathologic Anatomy of the Pancreas in Juvenile Diabetes Mellitus. *Diabetes 14:* 619, 1965.
68. Le Compte, P. M., and Legg, M. A. Insulitis (Lymphocytic Infiltration of Pancreatic Islet) in Late Onset Diabetes. *Diabetes 21:* 762, 1972.
69. Renold, A. E., Soeldner, J. S., and Steinke, J. Immunological Studies with Homologous and Heterologous Pancreatic Insulin in the Cow, in Cameron, M. P., and O'Connor, M. (Eds.), The Aetiology of Diabetes Mellitus and Its Complications. Ciba Foundation Colloquia in Endocrinology, Churchill, London, 1964, vol. 15, p. 49.
70. Federlin, K., Renold, A. E., and Pfeiffer, E. F. Antigen Binding Lymphocytes in Patients and in Insulin-Sensitized Animals with Delayed Insulin Allergy, in Miescher, P. A., and Grabar, P. (Eds.), Immunopathology. Schwabe & Co, Basel, 1968, vol. 5, p. 107.
71. Nerup, J., Andersen, O. O., Bendixen, G., Egeberg, J., Poulsen, J. E., Vilien, M., and Westrup, M. Antipancreatic, Cellular Hypersensitivity in Diabetes Mellitus. III. Experimental Induction of Antipancreatic, Cellular Hypersensitivity and Associated Morphological B Cell Changes in the Rat. *Acta Allergol 28:* 231, 1973.
72. Heydinger, D. K., and Lacy, P. E. Islet Cell Changes in the Rat after Injection of Homogenized Islet. *Am J Surg 128:* 608, 1974.
73. Bottazzo, G. F., Florin-Christensen, A., and Doniach, D. Islet Cell Antibodies in Diabetes Mellitus with Autoimmune Polyendocrine Deficiencies. *Lancet 2:* 1279, 1974.
74. MacCuish, A. C., Barnes, E. W., Irvine, W. J., and Duncan, L. J. F. Antibodies to Pancreatic Islet-Cells in Insulin-Dependent Diabetics with Coexistent Autoimmune Disease. *Lancet 2:* 1529, 1974.
75. Bottazzo, G. F., and Lendrum, R. Separate Autoantibodies Reacting with Human Pancreatic Glucagon and Somatostatin Cells. *Lancet 2:* 873, 1976.
76. Lendrum, R., Walker, J. G., and Gamble, D. R. Islet Cell Antibodies in Juvenile Diabetes Mellitus of Recent Onset. *Lancet 1:* 880, 1975.
77. Lendrum, R., Walker, J. G., Cudworth, A. G., Theophanides, C., Pyke, D. A., Bloom, A., and Gamble, D. R. Islet Cell Antibodies in Diabetes Mellitus. *Lancet 2:* 1273, 1976.
78. Irvine, W. J., McCallum, C. J., Gray, R. S., Campbell, C. T., Duncan, L. P. J., Farquhar, J. W., et al. Pancreatic Islet Cell Antibodies in Diabetes Mellitus Correlated with the Duration and Type of Diabetes, Coexistent Autoimmune Disease, and HL-A Type. *Diabetes 26:* 138, 1977.
79. Mac Laren, N. K., Huang, S. W., and Fogh, J. Antibody to Cultured Human Insulinoma Cells in Insulin-Dependent Diabetes. *Lancet 1:* 997, 1975.
80. Flier, J. S., Kahn, C. R., Roth, J., and Bar, R. S. Antibodies That Impair Insulin Receptor Binding in an Unusual Diabetic Syndrome with Severe Insulin Resistance. *Science 190:* 63, 1975.
81. Flier, J. S., Kahn, C. R., Jarret, D. B., and Roth, J. Characterization of Antibodies to the Insulin Receptor. A Cause of Insulin-Resistent Diabetes in Man. *J Clin Invest 58:* 1442, 1976.
82. Hirata, Y., Nishimura, H., Tominaga, N., Arimichi, T., and Kogushi, T. An Insulin Autoimmune Syndrome. *Tonyobyo (Suppl) 15:* 179, 1972.
83. Folling, I., and Norman, N. Hyperglycaemia, Hypoglycaemic Attacks and Production of Anti-Insulin Antibodies without Previous Known Immunization. Immunological and Functional Studies in a Patient. *Diabetes 21:* 814, 1972.
84. Nerup, J., Andersen, O. O., Bendixen, G., Egeberg, J., and Poulsen, J. E. Antipancreatic Cellular Hypersensitivity in Diabetes Mellitus. *Diabetes 20:* 424, 1971.
85. Nerup, J., Andersen, O. O., Bendixen, G., Egeberg, J., and Poulsen, J. E. Antipancreatic, Cellular Hypersensitivity in Diabetes Mellitus. Antigenic Activity of Fetal Calf Pancreas and Correlation with Clinical Type of Diabetes. *Acta Allergol 28:* 223, 1973.
86. Mac Cuish, A. C., Jordan, J., Campbell, C. J., Duncan, L. J. P., and Irvine, W. J. Cell Mediated Immunity in Diabetes Mellitus: Lymphocyte Transformation by Insulin and Insulin Fragments in Insulin Treated and Newly-Diagnosed Diabetics. *Diabetes 24:* 36, 1975.
87. Huang, S. W., and Mac Laren, N. K. Insulin Dependent Diabetes: a Disease of Autoaggression. *Science 192:* 64, 1976.
88. Ungar, B., Stocks, A. E., Martin, F. I. R., Whittingham, S., and Mackay, I. R. Intrinsic Factor Antibody, Parietal Cell Antibody, and Latent Pernicious Anemia in Diabetes Mellitus. *Lancet 2:* 415, 1968.
89. Perlman, L. V. Familial Incidence of Diabetes in Hyperthyroidism. *Ann Intern Med 55:* 796, 1961.
90. Masi, A. T., Hartmann, W. H., Hahan, B. H., Abbey, H., and Shulman, L. E. Hashimoto's Disease: a Clinico-Pathological Study with Matched Controls. *Lancet 1:* 123, 1965.
91. Adreani, D. The Interrelation Between Primary Adult Mixedema and Diabetes, in Bastenie, P., and Gepts, W. (Eds.), Immunity and Autoimmunity in Diabetes Mellitus. Excerpta Medica, Amsterdam, 1974, p. 160.
92. Nerup, J. The Clinical and Immunological Association of Diabetes Mellitus and Addison's Disease, in Bastenie, P., and Gepts, W. (Eds.), Immunity and Autoimmunity in Diabetes Mellitus. Excerpta Medica, Amsterdam, 1974, p. 149.
93. Solomon, N., Carpenter, C. J. C., Bennett, I. L., and Harvey, A. M. Schmidt's Syndrome (Thyroid and Adrenal Insufficiency) and Coexistent Diabetes Mellitus. *Diabetes 14:* 300, 1965.
94. Blizzard, R. M., and Kyle, M. Studies of Adrenal Antigen and Antibodies in Addison's Disease. *J Clin Invest 42:* 1653, 1963.
95. Nissley, S. P., Drash, A. L., Blizzard, R. M., Sperling, M., and Childs, B. Comparison of Juvenile Diabetes with Positive and Negative Organ-Specific Antibody Titres. Evidence for Genetic Heterogeneity. *Diabetes 22:* 62, 1973.
96. Fialkow, P. J., Zavola, C., and Nielsen, R. Thyroid Autoimmunity: Increased Frequency in Relatives of Insulin-Dependent Diabetes Patients. *Ann Intern Med 83:* 170, 1975.
97. Nerup, J., Platz, P., Andersen, O. O., Christy, M., Lynsgoe, J., Poulsen, J. E., Ryder, L. P., Thomsen, M., Staub Nielsen, L., and

Svejgaard, A. HL-A Antigens and Diabetes Mellitus. *Lancet 2:* 864, 1974.
98. Steinke, J., and Taylor, K. W. Viruses and the Etiology of Diabetes. *Diabetes 23:* 631, 1974.
99. Craighead, J. E., and Mc Lane, M. F. Diabetes Mellitus: Induction in Mice by Encephalomyocarditis virus. *Science 172:* 913, 1968.
100. Coleman, T. M., Gamble, D. R., and Taylor, K. W. The Diabetogenic Effect of Coxsackie B Viruses. *Br Med J 3:* 25, 1973.
101. Craighead, J. E., and Higgins, D. A. Genetic Influence Affecting the Occurrance of a Diabetes Mellitus-Like Disease in Mice Infected with the Encephalomyocarditis Virus. *J Exp Med 139:* 414, 1974.
102. Bottazzo, G. F., and Doniach, D. Pancreatic Autoimmunity and HLA Antigens. *Lancet 2:* 800, 1976.
103. Nicols, J. Adrenal Cortex, in Bloodworth, J. M. B. (Ed.), Endocrine Pathology. Williams & Wilkins Co, Baltimore, 1968, p. 224.
104. Petri, M., and Nerup, J. Addison's Adrenalitis. *Acta Pathol Microbiol Scand Section A 79:* 381, 1971.
105. Anderson, J. R., Goudie, R. B., Gray, K. G., and Timbury, G. C. Auto-Antibodies in Addison's Disease. *Lancet 1:* 1123, 1957.
106. Blizzard, R. M., Chee, D., and Davis, W. The Incidence of Adrenal and Other Antibodies in the Sera of Patients with Idiopathic Adrenal Insufficiency (Addison's Disease). *Clin Exp Immunol 2:* 19, 1967.
107. Nerup, J., Addison's Disease—Serological Studies. *Acta Endocrinol 76:* 142, 1974.
108. Irvine, W. J., and Barnes, E. W. Addison's Disease, Ovarian Failure and Hypoparathyroidism. *Clin Endocrinol Metabol 4:* 379, 1975.
109. Nerup, J., and Bendixen, G. Anti-Adrenal Cellular Hypersensitivity in Addison's Disease: II. Correlation with Clinical and Serological Findings. *Clin Exp Immunol 5:* 341, 1969.
110. Blizzard, R. M., and Kyle, M. Studies of the Adrenal Antigens and Antibodies in Addison's Disease. *J Clin Invest 42:* 1653, 1963.
111. Goudie, R. B., Mc Donald, E., Anderson, J. R., and Gray, K. Immunological Features of Idiopathic Addison's Disease: Characterization of the Adrenocortical Antigens. *Clin Exp Immunol 3:* 119, 1968.
112. Schmidt, M. B. Eine Biglanduläre Erkrankung (Nebennieren und Schildrüse) bei Morbus Addinsonii. *Ver Dtsch Ges Pathol 21:* 212, 1926.
113. Turkington, R. W., and Lebowitz, H. E. Extra Adrenal Endocrine Deficiencies in Addison's Disease. *Am J Med 43:* 499, 1967.
114. Males, J. L., Spitler, A. L., and Gownsend, J. L. Addison's Disease. A Review of 32 Cases. *Oklahoma State Med J 64:* 298, 1971.
115. Nerup, J. Addison's Disease—Clinical Studies. A Report of 108 Cases. *Acta Endocrinol 76:* 127, 1974.
116. Colover, J., and Glynn, L. E. Experimental Iso-Immune Adrenalitis. *Immunology 1:* 172, 1958.
117. Barnett, E. V., Dumonde, D. C., and Glynn, L. E. Induction of Autoimmunity to Adrenal Gland. *Immunology 6:* 382, 1963.
118. Milcou, S. M., Pop, A., Lupulescu, A., and Taga, M. L'Autoimmunization Éxperimentale de la Surrénale chez les Lapin. *Ann Endocrinol (Paris) 20:* 799, 1959.
119. Witebski, E., and Milgrom, F. Immunological Studies on Adrenal Gland: II. Immunization with Adrenals of the Same Species. *Immunology 5:* 67, 1962.
120. Levine, R., and Wenk, E. J. The Production and Passive Transfer of Allergic Adrenalitis. *Am J Pathol 52:* 41, 1968.
121. Wederlin, O. The Origin, Nature and Specificity of Mononuclear Cells in Experimental Autoimmune Inflammation. *Acta Path Microbiol Scand Section A Suppl 232:* 3, 1972.
122. Ruehsen, M. de M., Blizzard, R. M., Garcia-Bunnuel, R., and Jones, G. S. Autoimmunity and Ovarian Failure. *Am J Obstet Gynecol 112:* 693, 1972.
123. McNatty, K. P., Short, R. V., Barnes, E. W., and Irvine, W. J. The Cytotoxic Effect of Serum from Patients with Addison's Disease and Autoimmune Ovarian Failure. *Clin Exp Immunol 22:* 378, 1975.
124. Edmonds, M., Lamki, L., Killinger, D. W., and Volpé, R. Autoimmune Thyroiditis, Adrenalitis and Oophoritis. *Am J Med 54:* 782, 1973.
125. Lupulescu, A., Pop, A., Merculiev, E., Neascu, C., and Heitmanek, C. Experimental Iso-Immune Hypoparathyroidism in Rats. *Nature 206:* 415, 1965.
126. Lupulescu, A., Potorac, E., Pop, A., Heitmanek, C., Merculiev, E., Chisiu, M., et al. Experimental Investigations on Immunology of the Parathyroid Gland. *Immunology 14:* 475, 1968.
127. Altenähr, E., and Jenke, W. Experimental Parathyroiditis in the Rat by Passive Immunization. *Virchows Arch [Pathol Anat] 363:* 333, 1974.
128. Blizzard, R. M., Chee, D., and Davis, W. The Incidence of Parathyroid and Other Antibodies in the Sera of Patients with Idiopathic Hypoparathyroidism. *Clin Exp Immunol 1:* 119, 1966.
129. Irvine, W. J., and Scarth, L. Antibody to the Oxiphil Cells of the Human Parathyroid in the Idiopatic Hypoparathyroidism. *Clin Exp Immunol 4:* 505, 1969.
130. Spinner, M. W., Blizzard, R. M., and Childs, B. Clinical and Genetic Heterogeneity in Idiopathic Addison's Disease and Hypoparathyroidism. *J Clin Endocrinol Metab 28:* 795, 1968.
131. Whitaker, J., Landing, B. H., Esselborn, V. M., and Williams, R. R. The Syndrome of Familial Juvenile Hypoparathyroidism, Hypoadrenocorticism and Superficial Moniliasis. *J Clin Endocrinol Metab 16:* 1374, 1956.
132. Krohn, K., Perheentupa, J., and Heinonen, E. Precipitating Anti-Adrenal Antibodies in Addison's Disease. *Clin Immunol Immunopathol 3:* 59, 1974.
133. Goudie, R. B., and Pinkerton, P. H. Anterior Hypophysitis and Hashimoto's Disease in Young Women. *J Pathol 83:* 584, 1962.
134. Zanchi, M., and Dova, E. Sugli Accumuli di Cellule Linfoidi nella Ipofisi Umana. *Folia Endocrinol (Roma) 3:* 3, 1950.
135. Levine, S. Allergic Adrenalitis and Adenohypophysitis: Further Observations on Production and Passive Tansfer. *Endocrinology 84:* 469, 1969.
136. Bottazzo, G. F., Pouplard, A., Florin-Christensen, A., and Doniach, D. Autoantibodies to Prolactin-Secreting Cells of Human Pituitary. *Lancet 2:* 97, 1975.
137. Bottazzo, G. F. Characterization of Specific Antibodies to Endocrine Pancreas and Pituitary, in International Symposium on Organ Specific Autoimmunity. Cremona, June 6–8, 1977, p. 6 (abstract).
138. Pouplard, A., Bottazzo, G. F., Doniach, D., and Roitt, I. M. Binding of Human Immunoglobulins to Pituitary ACTH Cells. *Nature 261:* 142, 1976.
139. Johnson, M. H., Hekman, A., and Rümke, P. The Male and Female Genital Tracts in Allergic Disease, in Gell, P. G. H., Coombs, R. R. A., and Lachman, P. J. (Eds.), Clinical Aspects of Immunology. Blackwell Scientific Publ., Oxford, 1975, p. 1509.
140. Wilson, L. Spermagglutinins in Human Semen and Blood. *Proc Soc Exp Biol Med 85:* 652, 1954.
141. Rümke, P. The Presence of Serum Antibodies in the Serum of Two Patients with Oligospermia. *Vox Sang 4:* 135, 1954.
142. Friberg, J. Clinical and Immunological Studies on Spermagglutinating Antibodies in Semen and Seminal Fluid. *Acta Obstet Gynecol Scand Suppl* 36, 1974.
143. Rümke, P. Autoantibodies Against Spermatozoa in Infertile Men: Some Unresolved Problems, in Centoro, A., and Cerretti, N. (Eds.), Proceedings of the First International Congress on Immunology in Obstetrics and Gynecology, Padua, 1973. Excerpta Medica, Amsterdam, 1974, p. 27.
144. Manarang-Pangan, S., and Behrman, S. J. Spermatotoxicity of Immune Sera in Human Infertility. *Fertil Steril 22:* 145, 1971.
145. Hjort, T., and Hansen, K. B. Immunofluorescent Studies on Human Spermatozoa, I. The Detection of Different Spermatozoal Antibodies and Their Occurrence in Normal and Infertile Women. *Clin Exp Immunol 8:* 9, 1971.
146. Fjällbrant, B. Interrelation Between High Levels of Sperm Antibodies, Reduced Mucus Penetration by Spermatozoa and Sterility in Man. *Acta Obstet Gynecol Scand 47:* 102, 1968.
147. Rümke, P. The Origin of Immunoglobulins in Semen. *Clin Exp Immunol 17:* 287, 1974.
148. Shulman, S., Zappi, E., Ahmed, V., and Davis, J. Immunologic Consequences of Vasectomy. *Contraception 5:* 269, 1972.
149. Ansbacher, R. Vasectomy: Sperm Antibodies. *Fertil Steril 24:* 788, 1973.
150. Fjällbrant, B. Spermagglutinins in Sterile and Fertile Man. *Acta Obstet Gynecol Scand 47:* 89, 1968.
151. Haensh, R. Fluorescenzimmunologische Spermienautantikörpen Befunde bei Männlichen Fertilitätsstörungen. *Arch Gynek 208:* 91, 1969.
152. Toullet, F., Voisin, G. A., and Nemirovsky, M. Localization Cytologique et Pouvoir Pathogène des Auto-Antigènes des Spermatozoides chez le Cobaye. *Ann Inst Pasteur 118:* 513, 1970.
153. Andrada, J. A., Andrada, E. C., and Witebski, E. Experimental Autoallergic Orchitis in Rhesus Monkey. *Proc Soc Exp Biol Med 130:* 1106, 1969.
154. Waksmann, B. H. A Histologic Study of the Autoallergic Testis Lesion in the Guinea Pig. *J Exp Med 109:* 311, 1959.
155. Brown, P. C., Glynn, L. E. The Early Lesion of Experimental

Allergic Orchitis in Guinea-Pigs: An Immunological Correlation. *J Pathol 98:* 277, 1969.

156. Johnson, M. H. Physiological Mechanisms for the Immunological Isolation of Spermatozoa. *Adv Reprod Physiol 6:* 279, 1973.

157. Pokorna, Z. Induction of Experimental Autoimmune Aspermatogenesis by Immune Serum Fractions. *Folia Biol (Praha) 16:* 320, 1970.

158. Tung, K. S. H., Unanue, E. R., and Dixon, F. J. Pathogenesis of Experimental Orchitis. I. Transfer with Immune Lympnode Cells. *J Immunol 106:* 1453, 1971.

159. Kantor, J. L., and Dixon, F. J. Transfer of Experimental Allergic Orchitis with Peritoneal Exudate Cells. *J Immunol 108:* 329, 1972.

160. Nagano, T., Okumura, K. Fine Structural Changes of Allergic Aspermatogenesis in Guinea Pigs. II. Induced by Homologous Parotid Gland as Antigen. *Virchows Arch [Zell Pathol] 14:* 237, 1973.

161. Mancini, R. E., Andrada, J. A., Saraceni, D., Bachmann, A. E., Lavieri, J. C., and Nemirovsky, M. Immunological and Testicular Response in Man Sensitized with Human Testicular Homogenate. *J Clin Endocrinol Metab 25:* 859, 1965.

162. Hamerlynck, J. V. T. H., and Rümke, P. Spermatotoxic Antibodies in Man, in Proc 6th World Congress on Fertility and Sterility. Israel Academy of Science and Humanities. 1970, p. 287.

163. El-Alfi, O. S., and Bassili, F. Immunological Aspermatogenesis in Man. I. Blastoid Transformation of Lymphocytes in Response to Seminal Antigen In Cases of Non-Obstructive Azoospermia. *J Reprod Fertil 21:* 23, 1970.

164. Gordon, L. H., Barsoles, P. B., Westerman, E. L., and Mumford, D. M. Microlymphocyte Transformation Studies with Seminal Antigen. II. Observations in Male Patients with Sperm Agglutinating Antibodies. *J Urol 105:* 858, 1971.

165. Rowley, M. J. M., and Heller, C. G. The Testosterone Rebound Phenomenon in the Treatment of Male Infertility. *Fertil Steril 23:* 498, 1972.

166. Meaker, S. R. Some Aspects of the Problem of Sterility. *Boston Med Surg J 187:* 535, 1922.

167. Shulman, S., Jackson, H., and Stone, M. L. Antibodies to Spermatozoa. VI. Comparative Studies of the Spermagglutination Activity in Groups of Infertile and Fertile Women. *Am J Obstet Gynecol 123:* 139, 1975.

168. Isojima, S., Tsuchiya, K., Koyama, K., Tanaka, C., Naka, O., and Adachi, H. Further Studies on Spermimmobilizing Antibodies Found in Sera of Unexplained Cases of Sterility in Women. *Am J Obstet Gynecol 112:* 199, 1972.

169. Hansen, K. B., and Hjort, T. Immunofluorescent Studies on Human Spermatozoa. II. Characterization of Spermatozoal Antigens and Their Occurrance in Spermatozoa from the Male Partners of Infertile Couples. *Clin Exp Immunol 9:* 21, 1971.

170. Parish, W. E., Carron-Brown, J. A., and Richards, C. P. The Detection of Antibodies to Spermatozoa and to Blood Group Antigens in Cervical Mucus. *J Reprod Fertil 7:* 163, 1967.

171. Shulman, S., and Friedman, M. R. Antibodies to Spermatozoa, V. Antibody Activity in Female Reproductive tissue. *Am J Reprod Fertil 122:* 101, 1975.

172. Isojima, S., and Ashitaka, Y. Absorption of Sperm Antigen from the Vagina in Guinea Pigs. *Am J Obstet Gynecol 88:* 433, 1964.

173. Behrman, S. J., and Nakayama, M. Antitestis Antibody: Its Inhibition of Pregnancy. *Fertil Steril 16:* 37, 1965.

174. Bratanov, K. Antibodies in the Reproductive Process in the Female, in Edwards, R. G. (Ed.), Immunology and Reproduction. International Parenthood Federation, London, 1969, p. 251.

175. El-Magoub, S. Antispermatozoal Antibodies in Infertile Women with Cervico-Vaginal Schistosomiasis. *Am J Obstet Gynecol 112:* 781, 1972.

176. Dukes, C. D. and Franklin, R. R. Spermagglutinins and Human Infertility; Female. *Fertil Steril 23:* 493, 1972.

177. Hanafiah, M. J., Epstein, J. A., and Sobrero, A. J. Sperm-Agglutinating Antibodies in 236 Infertile Couples. *Fertil Steril 23:* 493, 1972.

156

Endocrine and Other Biological Rhythms

Dorothy T. Krieger
Jurgen Aschoff

Although the constancy of the internal milieu is axiomatic, it is apparent that within this framework, rhythms in the levels of multitudinous bodily constituents and functions are pervasive throughout the evolutionary scale. The origin, interrelationships, and biological significance of such rhythms still are matters of speculation. It is evident, however, that disruption of a given bodily rhythm or of its relationship to other bodily rhythms may be associated with loss of well-being or symptoms of disease; in addition, new rhythms may appear in certain disease states. The susceptibility of an organism to toxic and therapeutic agents is also subject to rhythmic variation.

In the human, the most studied bodily constituents with regard to rhythmicity have been those of the endocrine system, making a chapter on biological rhythms most appropriate within the context of this book. Before considering endocrine and other rhythms in the human subject, however, it is important to analyze the properties that define any given rhythm and the factors that can modify such properties. To accumulate sufficient data to do so requires prolonged sequential observation of the organism and parameter in question. For this reason, many of the basic observations have been made on species and parameters (i.e., temperature, activity) that can be continuously monitored—the conclusions from such studies being applicable to the human, in whom such continuous monitoring is not ordinarily feasible.

The first two sections of this chapter therefore deal with the terminology and characterization of rhythms, based upon data obtained mostly from other than human species. Utilizing this as a background, hormonal and nonhormonal rhythms in health and disease in man will then be considered.

CLASSIFICATION, CAUSATION, AND TELEONOMY OF RHYTHMS

Biological rhythms cover a large range of frequencies, from about 1 cycle per millisecond up to 1 per several years. They can be observed in single cells, in networks of tissues and organs, in the whole organism, or only in populations. There are two possibilities with regard to the basis of such rhythms. If a rhythm can be proven to have its origin within the respective biological unit, it is called an endogenous rhythm. Alternatively, a rhythm is called exogenous if its manifestation depends on a rhythmic input from the environment. Of the four examples in Figure 156-1, two certainly belong to the class of endogenous rhythms: the heartbeat originates within the pacemaker of the heart, and the episodic secretion of luteinizing hormone (whatever its origin may be) does not depend on an environmental rhythm. In contrast to these two rhythms, the diurnal and seasonal rhythms depicted could also be endogenous or merely reflect responses to the periodic environment. Special experiments are necessary to determine whether these latter rhythms are endogenous periodic processes that are merely synchronized (see below) by the periodic environment or whether they are truly exogenous rhythms.

A different way of classifying rhythms is based on the theory of oscillation which distinguishes between autonomous systems, i.e., systems that are exposed to a constant (or nonperiodic) source of energy, and heteronomous systems, which are exposed to a periodic source of energy.[3] Im a simplified manner such as schematically drawn in Figure 156-2, autonomous systems can be divided into three groups according to their behavior after a single impulse: (a) systems that are not capable of (free) oscillations, (b) systems whose oscillations damp out as a result of the inevitable

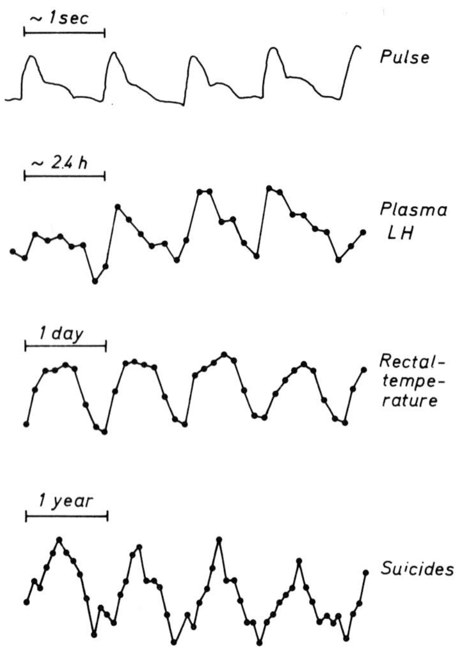

Fig. 156-1. Four examples of biological rhythms in man. LH (luteinizing hormone.[1,2] (Suicide data (in Austria) from Beitr. zur Osterr. Statistik, Heft 62, 1961.)

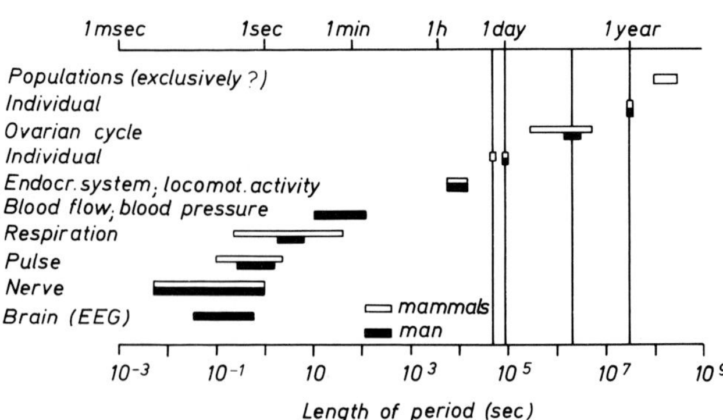

Fig. 156-3. Spectrum of biological rhythms. White bars (mammals) indicate interspecific variability; black bars (man) intraindividual variability. (Data from refs. 4 and 11.)

losses of energy (decaying or attenuated oscillations), and (c) systems that can make use of a constant source of energy to restore these losses and hence are capable of self-sustained oscillations (auto-oscillations). As heteronomous systems (d), i.e., when under the influence of a periodic source of energy, all three types show forced oscillations. The heartbeat represents a typical example of a self-sustained oscillation. Damped oscillations can be consequences of feedback loops with long time constants, as they partly are realized in the endocrine system.

To give an impression of the whole spectrum of rhythms, Figure 156-3 summarizes data from man (black bars) and from mammals (white bars). The higher frequencies at the left of the spectrum, which can be observed in the central nervous system, in the circulation, and in respiration, are often characterized by a large intraindividual variability. Contrary to this, some of the rhythms with lower frequencies, such as the ovarian cycle, show little intraindividual or intraspecific variability but differ among species. Finally, there are four rhythms (indicated in Fig. 156-3 by vertical lines) that, under natural conditions, are synchronized to cycles in the environment and hence normally do not vary in their frequency. These geophysical cycles are the tides, day and night, the phases of the moon, and the seasons. All four are reflected in tidal, diurnal, lunar, and seasonal rhythms of biological systems, and it has been shown for each of them, in at least a few organisms, that they can continue when shielded from the respective environmental cycle. Under these artificially constant conditions the period of the rhythm usually deviates slightly from that of the environment. For example, a rhythm that under ordinary environmental light-dark transition would have a period of 24 hours in all individuals exposed to such an environment may, under constant conditions, exhibit a period varying from 21 to 27 hours in different members of the group exposed to such constant conditions. The actual period length, however, will be constant in a given individual under such constant conditions. A rhythm that persists under such constant conditions is called "free running." v. i. If such a "free-running" rhythm can be shown to continue for many periods without attenuation, the conclusion is justified that the rhythm is (1) endogenous and (2) belongs to the class of systems capable of self-sustained oscillations (Fig. 156-2*c*). Since the period of the autonomous, free-running rhythm only approximates that of the cycle to which it is normally synchronized, the prefix "circa" has been introduced by Halberg[5] to characterize diurnal as "circadian" rhythms and was later on adopted for the three other rhythms (circa-tidal, circa-lunar, circannual rhythms).[6] The four "circa"-rhythms have some features in common that are characteristic of self-sustained oscillations. In the strict sense of the terminology as employed here, a rhythm whose manifestation depends on a periodic input from the environment is not a circa-rhythm.

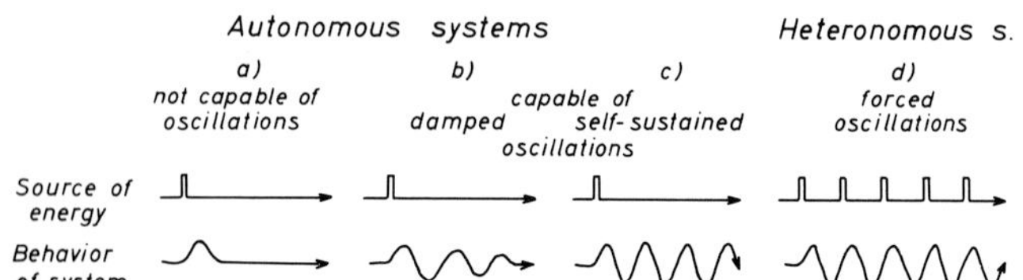

Fig. 156-2. Reactions of different systems to single and to periodic impulses.

Presumably, in view of their ubiquity and predominance in living systems, circadian rhythms have been used as a borderline to divide the spectrum into two parts: the ultradian rhythms (periods shorter than about 24 hours) and the infradian rhythms (periods longer than about 24 hours). Detailed descriptions of such classifications have been given by Halberg.[7–9]

Most rhythms of the spectrum probably have evolved under selective pressure to serve specific purposes, but some rhythms may also be mere by-products of other mechanisms, such as a noncritically damped feedback system. To illustrate teleonomic principles[10] by which rhythms may have originated during evolution, a few examples ought to suffice. Biological rhythms can be the necessary requirement for the fulfillment of a specific task such as the transfer of information within the central nervous system by varying spike frequencies or the transport of gases and liquids by rhythmic pumping. Rhythms further may be useful for the stabilization of a low-frequency rhythm by higher frequencies or for optimal synchronization of a variety of processes within the organism. (For a detailed discussion of these problems, see ref. 11.) The four circa-rhythms that have evolved as responses to geophysical cycles represent an adaptation to "niches in time" provided by the temporal structure of the environment.[12] In other words, during the process of evolution, the organism has acquired a periodic process whose period matches that of the environmental cycle. As a consequence, the periodicity of the environment, which ultimately provided the source of evolutionary selective pressure, no longer acts as the proximate cause for the biological rhythms but acts only as a synchronizing agent or "Zeitgeber" for an active, self-sustained oscillation within the organism. As a result of the acquisition of such internal temporal programs and their proper synchronization to the time structures of the environment, the organism at each time point is prepared in advance to cope with circumstances that ensue in the programmed environment.

Although all four circa-rhythms are of interest to a biologist, the circadian rhythms have attracted special attention in physiology and medicine. They are also better understood than the three other rhythms and hence are useful to outline the principles of self-sustained biological oscillations.

THE CIRCADIAN SYSTEM

INTRODUCTION TO SELF-SUSTAINED OSCILLATIONS

Since many of the properties of circadian rhythms correspond to properties of technical oscillators, it is justified and has been proven useful in describing rhythm parameters to apply the terminology used in oscillation theory. The analogy has been fruitful both in generating empirical research and in providing a theoretical framework.[13] Knowledge of definitions as well as of basic principles of oscillating systems facilitate the analysis of data and the correct interpretation of biological phenomena such as the synchronization of rhythms, their phase shifts, or their transitory states after a change of conditions. Some of the most common notions are explained in Figure 156-4. An oscillation is defined by its period, i.e., the time interval after which a distinct phase of the oscillation recurs; by its range of oscillation, i.e., the difference between the maximum and minimum value within one period; and by its mean value, i.e., the arithmetic mean of all instantaneous values of the oscillating variable within one period. (In sinusoidal oscillations, half the range of oscillation is called the amplitude.) Each instantaneous state of an oscillation represents a phase; it is defined by the value of the variable and all its time derivatives. The point on the abscissa that corresponds to a phase is called the phase angle θ; it is measured in fractions of the whole period from an arbitrary phase angle zero and expressed in units of time or in angular degrees (one period = 360°). If two oscillations are synchronized to each other by unidirectional coupling, i.e., one oscillation driving the other one, the two can either be in phase (which means that equal phases occur at the same time) or out of phase with each other. The phase relationship is described by the phase-angle difference ψ between corresponding phases in the two oscillations. The phase-angle difference has a positive sign if the driven rhythm leads in phase the driving rhythm; the sign becomes negative for lagging phases. Of the two oscillations shown in Figure 156-4, the driven one leads the driving one by 60° and therefore the phase-angle difference ψ is positive.

As mentioned earlier, the circa-rhythms are usually synchronized to periodic factor(s) in the environment, the Zeitgeber(s). A more specific term for the synchronization of self-sustained oscillations is entrainment; it implies that synchrony is achieved by phase control and that consequently a rigorously entrained oscillation maintains a distinct phase-angle difference to the entraining Zeitgeber. The sign and amount of the phase-angle difference depend on the ratio between the frequency of the driving and the (natural) frequency of the driven oscillation as measured before entrainment. If two oscillations with different natural frequencies (i.e., the frequency of the free-running oscillation) are entrained by the same Zeitgeber (Figure 156-5), the oscillation with a relative high frequency leads the Zeitgeber in phase (ψ positive), and the oscillation with a relative low frequency lags in phase (ψ negative). (Note that in the presence of the Zeitgeber the periods of the two oscillations now are identical with that of the Zeitgeber.)

Entrainment by a Zeitgeber means that the phase of the entrained oscillation is corrected at least once during each period. This correction is accomplished by either advancing (sign positive) or delaying phase shifts (sign negative), produced by stimuli from the Zeitgeber. Such phase shifts can be measured by applying single stimuli to a free-running oscillation, as illustrated in Figure 156-6. To achieve entrainment, the amount of phase shift resulting from a given stimulus must be (and the sign of the shift often is) a function of the phase of the oscillation to be entrained. A diagrammatic representation of this dependence of shifts on phase is called a phase-response curve.[14,15] Entrained oscillations can be shifted by advancing (Figure 156-6*B*) or delaying the phase of the entraining Zeitgeber once. After the shift of the Zeitgeber, it usually takes several periods (transients) until the oscillation again has reached its typical phase-angle difference.

Self-sustained oscillations can be entrained by Zeitgebers only to those frequencies that do not deviate too much from the natural frequency. Within this limited range of entrainment, the phase-angle difference changes systematically, large positive values coinciding with the low frequency end of the whole range (cf. Figure 156-11, right diagram) and large negative values with the higher frequency end. Second, smaller ranges of entrainment are possible around multiples and submultiples of the natural frequency. Outside one of the ranges of entrainment, the oscillation is no longer synchronized; it free-runs with its own frequency which, however, is often modulated by the still-present stimuli of the Zeitgeber. This phenomenon is called relative coordination (cf. Figure 156-11, left diagram). To determine rhythm parameters in biological time se-

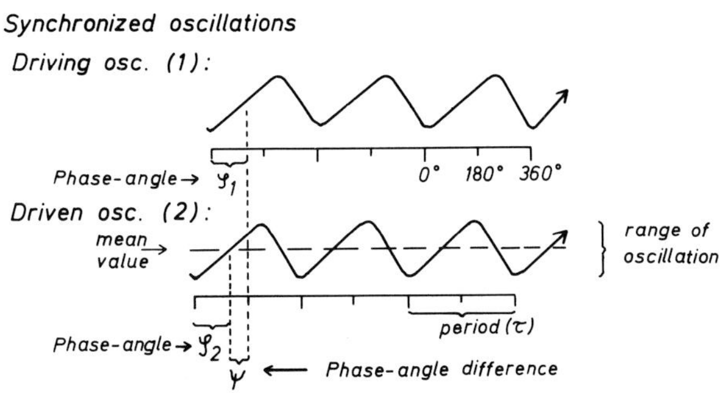

Fig. 156-4. Parameters of and phase relationship between two synchronized oscillations. (See text for definitions.)

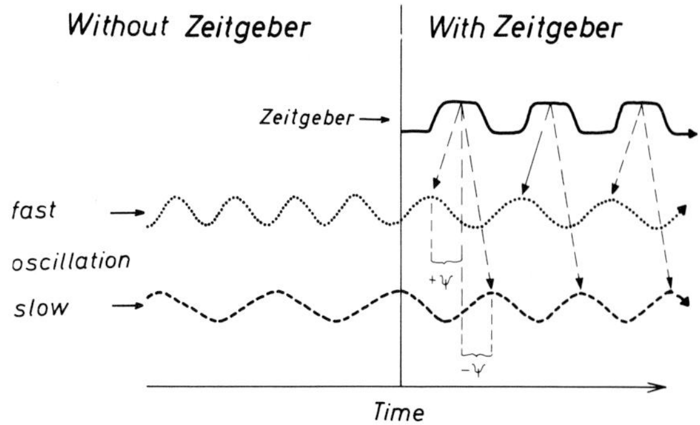

Fig. 156-5. Entrainment of two oscillations with different natural frequencies by the same Zeitgeber (See text for description.)

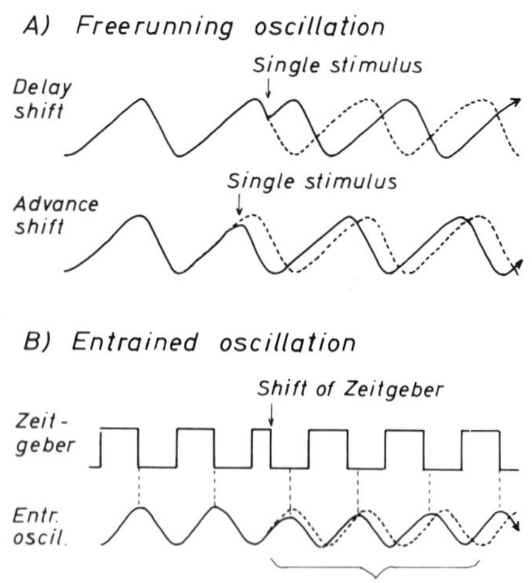

Fig. 156-6. *(A)* Delay and advance shift of a free-running oscillation resulting from a single stimulus (dotted line indicates period in absence of stimulus). *(B)* Advance shift of an entrained oscillation resulting from a shift of the Zeitgeber (dotted line indicates period of entrained oscillation as would be manifested without shift of Zeitgeber).

ries, laborious mathematical procedures are often unavoidable. Although biological rhythms rarely are sinusoidal, it is common usage to apply sine (or cosine) functions to the raw data either in the form of harmonic (Fourier) analysis or in determining the best-fitting curve by least-square techniques. Under the name of Cosinor, the latter approach has been especially adapted to the analysis of biological rhythms by Halberg.[7, 9, 16] Both of these approaches (Fourier and Cosinor) can give estimates for period, amplitude, and mean value of the rhythm. The acrophase, i.e., the crest of the fundamental period or of the best-fitting sine function, respectively, is often used as a reference phase instead of the maximum value of the raw data. A plot of computed amplitudes against the sequence of a variety of periods all applied to the same time series presents a least-square spectrum or a power spectrum, respectively, indicating with its highest value the period most prominent within the time series.

Several glossaries and vocabularies have been published that include explanations of terms and definitions of symbols and abbreviations.[17–19] Those used throughout this chapter are listed below.

L	Light (light-time)
D	Darkness (dark-time)
LD	Light–dark cycle
LL;DD	Continuous light; continuous darkness
τ	Circadian period
T	Zeitgeber period
Θ	Phase angle
ψ	Phase-angle difference
α	Activity time (wakefulness)
ρ	Rest time (sleep)
Acrophase	Maximal value of a sine function.
Circadian time, Zeitgeber time	A time scale covering one full circadian or Zeitgeber period, respectively; the zero point is defined arbitrarily.

PROPERTIES OF THE CIRCADIAN SYSTEM

Free-Running Circadian Rhythms

To demonstrate a free-running rhythm, an organism has to be kept in a soundproof chamber under conditions of constant illumination and temperature, with food and water available all the time. The results of such an experiment with a chaffinch are reproduced in Figure 156-7. After release from the Zeitgeber (LD, 12:12 hours) into constant conditions (LL), the rhythms of oxygen consumption and of locomotor activity persist, apart from an initial suppression of activity, nearly without change in the range of oscillation. The period, however, is now shorter than 24 hours, as can be seen from the drift of the minima of oxygen consumption and of the onsets of activity relative to the vertical lines drawn at midnight. This change in period becomes more conspicuous if the continuous records of activity from consecutive days are pasted beneath each other. In the record reproduced in Figure 156-8, each day the black bars representing activity of a dormouse move toward earlier hours (τ shorter than 24 hours) as long as the animal is kept in constant conditions with a very low level of illumination (0.006 lux); the bars move toward later hours each day (τ longer than 24 hours) after the intensity of illumination has been raised to 0.10 lux. In its last part (after day 55), the record indicates that, in the dormouse, there is also a dependence of the circadian period on ambient temperature.

In general, the effects of environmental conditions on the period of the free-running rhythm are slight and usually less so for temperature than for light. In fact, the often near-to-complete compensation of the circadian system against effects of temperature on frequency, especially well documented for the eclosion rhythm of *Drosophila*[20] and for the rhythm of luminescence in *Gonyaulax polyedra*,[21] has prompted the interpretation of the circadian system as a reliable biological clock;[20] its analysis is one of the puzzling problems in circadian rhythm research.

The data just mentioned from *Gonyaulax*, a unicellular organism, demonstrate that the manifestation of a circadian rhythm does not necessarily depend on a central nervous system. This is also indicated by the observation that circadian rhythms can persist in isolated tissues of higher vertebrates. Examples for such in vitro studies are rhythmic variations of heart rate in isolated hearts of the rat,[22] as well as circadian and ultradian rhythms of steroid production in isolated adrenals of the hamster.[23,24] A rhythm has been described in suspensions of rat liver cells in the activity of the enzyme tyrosine aminotransferase.[25]

A free-running circadian rhythm (period not calculated) in plasma corticosterone concentrations has been noted in blinded adult female rats[25] and in some instances where such animals were kept in constant light.[25]

As a last example of a free-running rhythm, Figure 156-9

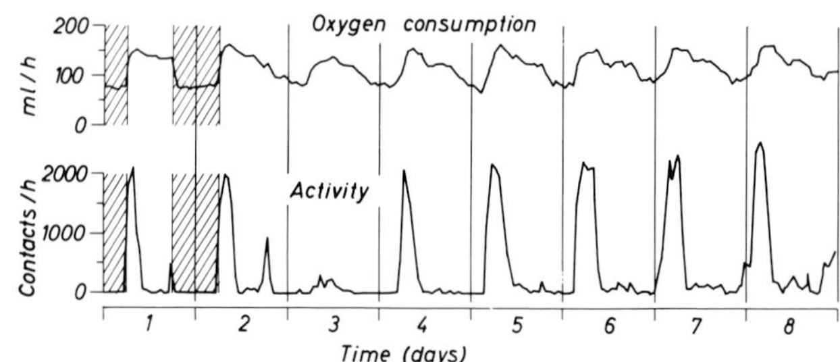

Fig. 156-7. Circadian rhythms of oxygen consumption and locomotor activity in a chaffinch (Fringilla coelebs) kept first in a light-dark cycle (shaded area) and, thereafter, in constant illumination. (See text for discussion.)

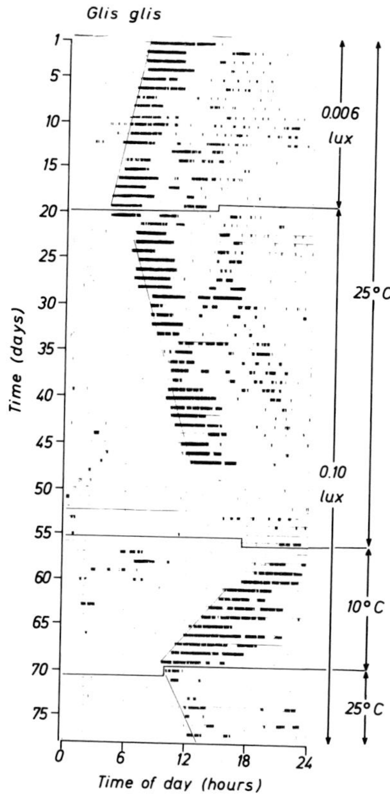

Fig. 156-8. Circadian rhythm of locomotor activity in a dormouse (Glis-glis) kept in constant conditions with two different intensities of illumination (0.006 and 0.10 lux) and at two levels of ambient temperature (10° and 25° C). (From H. Pohl, unpublished.)

presents data from a human subject who has lived in an underground isolation chamber for 22 days. During the first 7 days, the door of the chamber is open, and the subject knows the time of day. Therefore, his activity rhythm (wakefulness α, sleep ρ) as well as his rhythms of rectal temperature and of urinary cortisol excretion are entrained to 24 hours. Thereafter, when the door is closed and the subject is deprived of all time cues, all three rhythms start to free-run with a period slightly longer than 24 hours. The case is of especial interest, since the 27-year-old subject has been blind for the last 16 years. A closer inspection of the curves shown in Figure 156-9 reveals that the phase relationship between the three rhythms is different in the entrained and in the free-running system. To illustrate this in more detail, data from a similar experiment with a normal sighted subject are reproduced in Figure 156-10. During the first 7 days of entrainment, the rhythms of urinary steroid excretion reach their acrophase around the middle of the time of wakefulness. The acrophases slowly move toward earlier hours (relative to the rhythm of wakefulness and sleep) when the rhythms are free-running, eventually occurring just after the subject has woken up. During reentrainment to 24 hours, the acrophases again move back to their "normal" position. Implications of these findings are discussed in the section on multioscillator systems.

The period of circadian oscillations, whether under normal light–dark or under free-running conditions, remains remarkably stable. A recent report[25] is therefore of great interest, in which shortening of the free-running period of locomotor activity of blind hamsters occurred following continuous administration of estradiol benzoate by means of subcutaneously implanted capsules.

Entrainment by Zeitgebers

If a free-running rhythm becomes exposed to a Zeitgeber, it usually takes several periods until a stable phase relationship is reached. Specific models for the mechanism of entrainment, based on the principle of phase-response curves, have been developed by Pittendrigh.[29] One basic rule of coupled oscillations is that the rhythm with a short circadian period eventually keeps a positive phase-angle difference to the entraining Zeitgeber; a long circadian period becomes entrained with a slightly negative phase-angle difference.

For most animals, a light–dark cycle is the most powerful Zeitgeber, but entrainment is also possible by other periodic factors in the environment. A few points should be observed in experiments designed to test the effectiveness of a given Zeitgeber: (1) to avoid interference by other overlooked 24-hour Zeitgebers, the factor to be tested should preferably have a period that deviates slightly from 24 hours; (2) the experiment should include a phase shift; (3) before or after the test of the Zeitgeber, it should be demonstrated that the organism has a circadian rhythm that can free-run. Other cues[30] that can play the role of a Zeitgeber include periodic meal timing[31] or even cyclic variations of barometric pressure.[32] Of special interest are those factors that have social connotations. For birds, acoustical entrainment has been demonstrated by exposing isolated individuals periodically (via loudspeaker) to the song of their species,[33] and it is not unlikely that entrainment by smell can occur.

In analyzing data from entrainment experiments, one always should keep in mind that each Zeitgeber, besides its phase-controlling effects on the circadian oscillator, can have immediate direct (positive or negative) effects on the variable measured, i.e., on the overt rhythm that is coupled to the oscillator. Such "masking" effects[34] can obscure the phase-controlling effects and give rise to

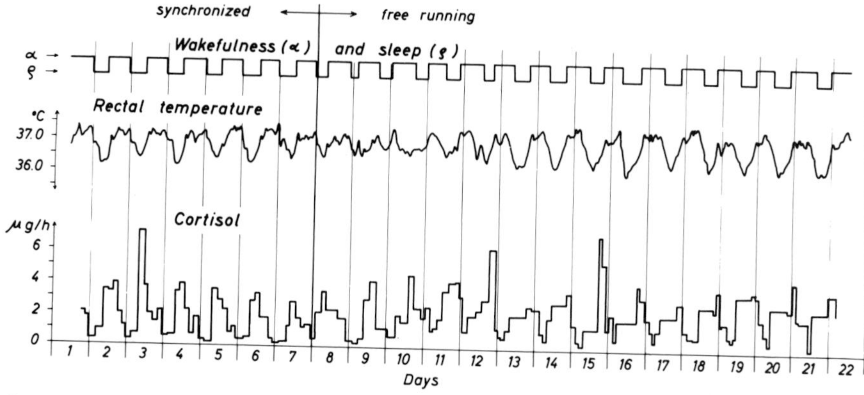

Fig. 156-9. Circadian rhythms of wakefulness (α) and sleep (ρ), of rectal temperature, and of urinary cortisol excretion in an isolated (blind) subject. (Data from ref. 26.)

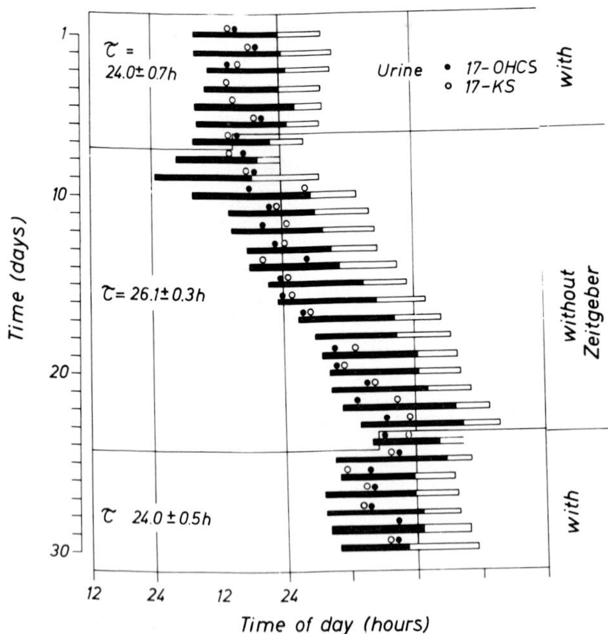

Fig. 156-10. Circadian rhythms in wakefulness (black bars) and sleep (white bars) and in urinary corticosteroid excretion (acrophases-maximal values indicated by circles) in an isolated subject. τ = circadian.

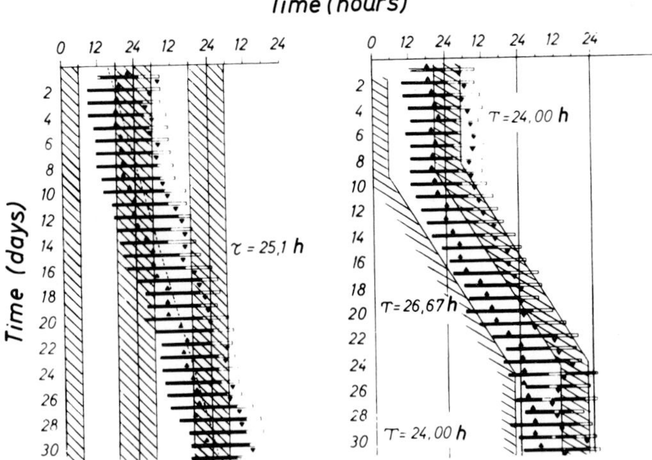

Fig. 156-11. Circadian rhythms of 2 human subjects exposed to artificial Zeitgebers in the isolation chamber. Black and white bars: wakefulness and sleep, respectively. Triangles: maxima (above bars) and minima (below bars) of rectal temperature. Shaded area: darkness including twilight. (Left) Light–dark cycle as the only Zeitgeber; small reading lamp available. (Note Zeitgeber period T = 24 hours, τ = mean circadian period of activity and temperature, Zeitgeber being LD cycle). (Right) Light–dark cycle supplemented by periodic acoustical signals. T = Zeitgeber (acoustical). Entrainmnent to the 26.67 as well as to the 24.00 T is shown in contrast to lack of entrainment to LD Zeitgeber alone in the left hand figure. See text for further discussion. (Data from ref. 35.)

misinterpretations of data from entrainment experiments, especially after a shift of the Zeitgeber.

For the entrainment of human circadian rhythms, social cues seem to be more important than a light–dark cycle. Apart from evidence that comes from observations of subjects during shift work and similar conditions, this conclusion is based on experiments in the isolation chamber. If a subject whose rhythm is free-running becomes exposed to an artificial 24-hour light–dark cycle, with the whole ceiling of the room brightly illuminated during light time, he often ignores the Zeitgeber as long as he can make use of a small reading lamp (Figure 156-11, left diagram). He continues to free-run despite the unpleasantness of being awake in a dimly illuminated room and sleeping in bright light while his rhythm is out of phase with the main light–dark cycle. A subject, however, becomes entrained if in addition to the main light–dark cycle, acoustical signals are applied in regular intervals that are a constant fraction of the Zeitgeber period (e.g., 3 hours in a 24-hour day). In contrast to the light–dark cycle, these signals are experienced by the subject as direct commands (e.g., for urine collection) given by the experimenter; they provide a kind of social contact and a time structure to which the subject can adhere. Exposed to such a "socially enriched" Zeitgeber, a subject can be entrained even to days deviating from 24 hours. The experimental results shown in the right diagram of Figure 156-11 demonstrate, in addition, the changes in phase relationship that are to be expected according to one of the rules of oscillation theory. The subject, who is a "late riser" in the 24-hour day, becomes (to his own surprise) an "early riser" in the unusual long day without being aware of the changed lighting schedule. Another important result of this experiment concerns the internal phase relationship between rhythms. As can be seen in Figure 156-11, the maxima and minima of rectal temperature (triangles) which occur in the second half of wakefulness and sleep, respectively, when the subject is entrained to 24 hours, both move toward earlier hours (relative to the activity cycle) during entrainment to the long day. These systematic changes in internal phase relationships, which are similar to those seen in free-running rhythms (cf. Figure 156-10), strongly contradict a simple cause-and-effect relationship between the activity rhythm and other rhythmic variables within the organism. In other words, the rhythm of rectal temperature is not simply a consequence of the alternation between wakefulness and sleep. The findings rather suggest that the circadian system consists of a multiplicity of (self-sustained?) oscillators to which the overt rhythms are coupled and whose phase relationship can change according to conditions.

Multioscillator Systems

In many ways, the circadian system of an organism behaves like a self-sustained oscillator, and it often has been postulated that there should be *one* driving (master-)oscillator by which all overt rhythms are driven. There are four sets of data, however, that indicate that this may not be the case.

1. A circadian rhythmic variable can "split" into several distinct components. The split phenomenon was first seen by Pittendrigh[14] in the locomotor activity of a ground squirrel and later confirmed in activity records of hamsters.[36] In tree shrews kept in constant conditions, a split can be induced by changing the light intensity, as shown in Figure 156-12. The solid block of activity that characterizes the free-running rhythm in 11.0 lux dissociates into two components when the intensity of illumination is lowered to 1.0 lux; activity again fuses into one block when the intensity is raised to 117 lux. The two split components keep a phase relationship of 180°. Similar findings in a variety of species, together with the often described bimodality of activity patterns,[38] have given rise to the hypothesis that the activity rhythm is based on two separate oscillators which, under conditions of entrainment to a light–dark cycle, are coupled to dawn and dark respectively.[36]
2. Another set of data indicating a multiplicity of oscillators comes from experiments with human subjects under conditions of free-run. In complete isolation, although the

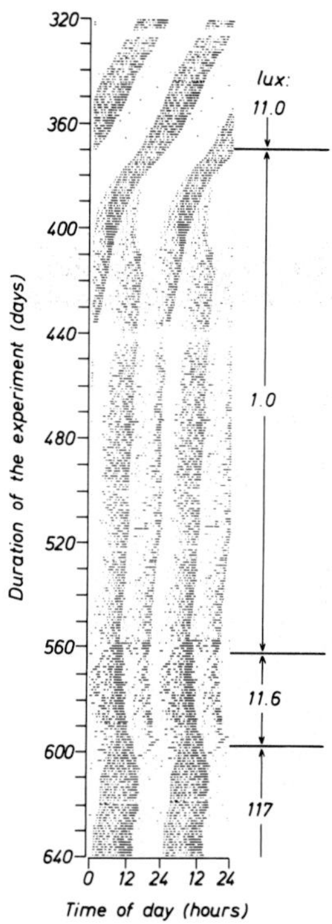

Fig. 156-12. Splitting of the free-running circadian rhythm of locomotor activity of a tree shrew *(Tupaia belangeri)* and refusion into one component, depending on the intensity of illumination. See text for discussion. (Data from ref. 37.)

free-running circadian system often remains internally synchronized, with all rhythms having the same period of about 25 to 26 hours (cf. Figures 156-9 and 156-10), in some instances the activity rhythm can lengthen or shorten to values far beyond this average circadian period. In these instances, other rhythmic variables such as rectal temperature desynchronize from the activity rhythm and continue to free-run with a period close to 25 hours. The records from two experiments reproduced in Figure 156-13 can both be separated into a section A, where the circadian system remains internally synchronized, and a section B, where it is desynchronized. The results can be interpreted as indicating a system with two (groups of) basic "driving" (self-sustained) oscillators which differ in their "degree of persistence"[3] and which both influence the two overt rhythms but to a different extent.[39,40]

3. Evidence of multiple oscillators can also be seen when the activity rhythm of a subject is entrained to artificial days that are outside the range of entrainment of other variables. The periodogram analysis shown in Figure 156-16 summarizes data from an experiment in which a subject had been entrained first to a 24-hour day and, thereafter, to a 28-hour day. For the first part of the experiment (*A* in Figure 156-14), the three measured rhythms (activity, temperature, cortisol excretion) all show a peak at 24 hours. In the data from the 28-hour day (*B*), only activity has its main peak at 28 hours, while rectal temperature and cortisol excretion have main peaks at 24.8 hours. This gives clear evidence that the rhythms of rectal temperature, as well as of cortisol excretion, can free-run *independently* from the rhythm of wakefulness and sleep.
4. In the cockroach, *Leucophaea maderae,* there are bilateral (optic lobe) pacemakers that control locomotor activity. Complete excision of either the left or right optic lobe or its surgical isolation from the central nervous system had no effect on the animal's ability to free-run in constant darkness, but such unilateral excision resulted in a significant increase in period. This suggests that the left and right pacemakers in the two optic lobes are mutually coupled and that the period of the compound pacemaker is shorter than that of either of its constituents.[40]

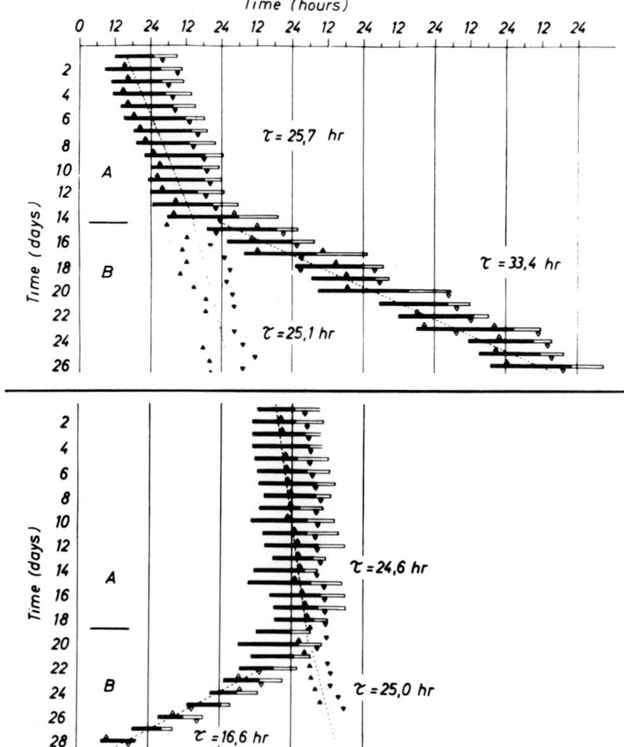

Fig. 156-13. Circadian rhythms of wakefulness and sleep (black and white bars) and of rectal temperature (triangles: maxima and minima) of two subjects, each living alone in the isolation chamber. *(A)* internal synchronization; *(B)* spontaneous internal desynchronization. τ :mean circadian period. In *A*, τ is similar for both temperature and wakefulness-sleep. In *B*, an 8.3 and 8.4 hour difference is present between T (temperature) and τ (wakefulness–sleep). (Data from ref. 30.)

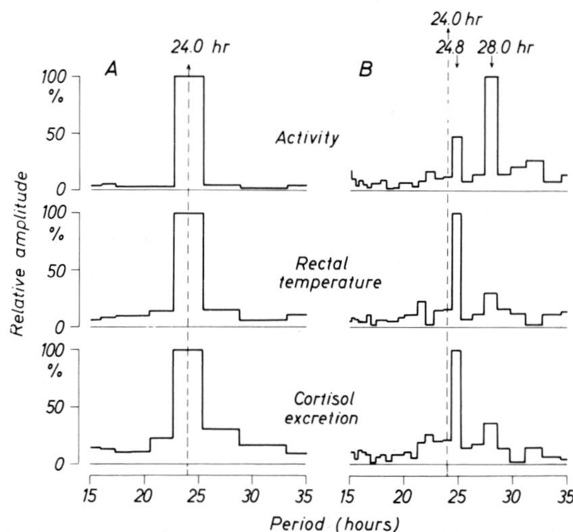

Fig. 156-14. Power spectra of the circadian rhythms of activity, rectal temperature and urinary cortisol excretion of a subject in the isolation chamber, entrained, first, to an artificial 24-hour day *(A)*, thereafter, to a 28-hour day *(B)*. (Data from ref. 39.)

THE ENTRAINED CIRCADIAN SYSTEM

Temporal Order

As stated in the introduction to this chapter, within the organism there is virtually no constituent nor function that does not manifest regular changes from day to night. These diverse rhythms keep distinct phase relationships to each other under normal conditions, representing a high degree of temporal order. In Figure 156-15, data are summarized from 6 subjects who have lived on a rigorous time schedule. Rectal temperature and urine constituents all show a rhythmic pattern, although the ranges of oscillation differ. Averaged from the 4 days, the mean curves can be drawn into one diagram constituting parts of a human "phase map." Patterns like those shown in Figure 156-15 are satisfactorily reproducible, not only when measurements are repeated with the same subjects[42] but also when results from different subjects and laboratories are compared.[43] Figure 156-16 summarizes data of plasma cortisol obtained by four groups of workers. There is good agreement with regard to the circadian maxima and minima, as well as to the two main episodes of cortisol secretion. (This coincidence is partly the result of the fact that middle of sleep is used as time zero on the abscissa; see below.) Numerous data show good agreement on time and level of maxima and minima of liver glycogen content and of plasma corticosterone concentrations in the rat and the mouse.[48–62]

Such temporal order is provided by passive dependence of some variables on other rhythms, by mutual coupling between circadian oscillators, and by the entraining effect of the Zeitgebers. In view of the latter factor it may be more meaningful when drawing phase maps to use as the abscissa, not time of day, but Zeitgeber time, with an arbitrary phase as time zero. When depicting rhythms of animals entrained to a light–dark cycle, the middle of light or dark time is a useful reference phase. In the human, it appears that the social environment may be a more important synchronizer than the light–dark cycle. Humans, however, display considerable interindividual differences in sleep time. Since it is felt that sleep may influence many physiological circadian variables, it has been suggested that in the case of human rhythms, the rhythmic variables may be related to sleep–wake rhythm, using the midpoint of sleep time as a reference phase.[63] The usefulness of this approach is illustrated in Figure 156-17 depicting the rhythms of plasma aldosterone from two groups of subjects who have slept at different times of day: there is better coincidence between the two curves when drawn with reference to sleep (lower diagram) than when drawn according to time of day (upper diagram). It

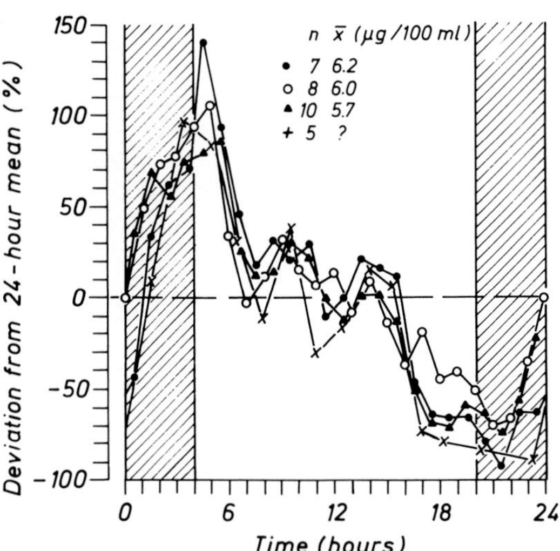

Fig. 156-16. Circadian rhythm of plasma cortisol concentration in man. Mean values from four groups of subjects. Shaded area: sleep. (Data from refs. 44–47.) Circadian rhythms of liver glycogen content and plasma corticosterone concentration. Shaded areas are: darkness. (Rat data from refs. 48–55. Mouse data from refs. 56–62.)

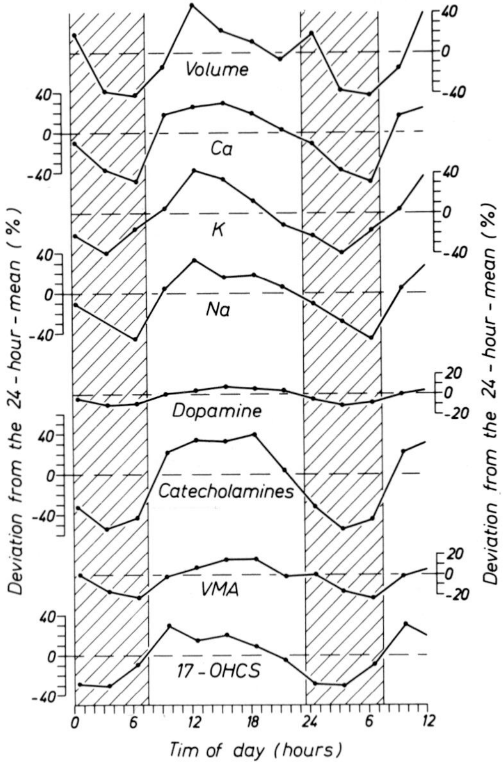

Fig. 156-15. Circadian rhythms of excretion of urinary constituents in man. Mean values from six subjects (average of observations on four consecutive 24-hour periods). Shaded area: sleep in darkness. (Data from ref. 41.)

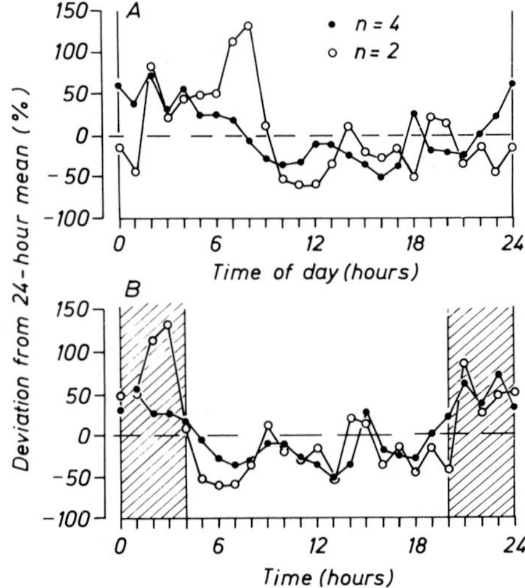

Fig. 156-17. Circadian rhythm of plasma aldosterone concentration in man. *(A)* Drawn with reference to clock time. *(B)* Drawn with reference to sleep time (shaded area). Zero time on abscissa = midsleep. Data from two groups of subjects with sleep from 23.00 to 7.00 (•) and from 2.00 to 8.00 (○). Shaded area: approximate sleep time. See text for discussion. (Data from ref. 64.)

should be noted that for many variables, it is not so much the sleep time on the day of experimentation but the habitual sleep schedule of the many days preceding the experiment that mainly determines the phase. Such phase-controlling effects of sleep which are suggested by a variety of observations, should not be interpreted as evidence for a direct dependence of a variable on sleep. Many of these rhythms probably represent separate oscillators differing in the strength by which they are coupled to the rhythm of wakefulness and sleep.

Circadian Rhythms in the Endocrine System

The temporal patterns of different hormones, as measured in an entrained organism, show a large variation in the range of oscillation. If it can be demonstrated that there is a statistically significant difference between a daily maximum and a minimum, and if it can be proven by experiments in constant conditions that this rhythm does not depend on an *exogenous* periodic factor, the rhythm can rightly be called circadian. It should be noted that the rhythms of many variables can be traced back to other variables that have been shown to be circadian in the strict sense; it is reasonable also to call the dependent variable "circadian," whether it is *passively driven* or whether it can be shown that it has the capacity for self-sustained oscillation and that it is hence entrained by the driving variable.

The pattern of plasma cortisol concentrations represents a paradigm of a circadian rhythm. It is also an example of a "driven" rhythm, as referred to above. Its phase follows that of the ACTH rhythm and ultimately that of the rhythm of hypothalamic CRF concentrations. The pattern of plasma cortisol concentrations manifests perhaps the largest range of oscillation of all the hormones and is less dependent on sleep than that of other hormones (see below), as shown by the length of time necessary for a phase shift following a shift of sleep time[66, 67] and by the persistence of the pattern during a prolonged 3-hour sleep–wake cycle.[68]

The rhythm of urinary corticosteroid excretion (whose relative independence from sleep has likewise been demonstrated in Figure 156-4) has only half the range of oscillation of the plasma cortisol rhythm (Figure 156-18). This may partly be due to the fact that urinary excretion is a value integrated over several hours, but it may also depend on the fact that different compounds are measured in plasma and in urine. The rhythm of corticosteroid excretion, furthermore, lags in phase to that of the plasma rhythm by several hours. A negative phase-angle difference may also be expected between the rhythm of a hormone in the plasma and the rhythm of its releasing factor in the hypothalamus. Data in accordance with this assumption have been obtained in the pigeon and in the rat (Figure 156-19). In both species the rhythm of hypothalamic CRF activity phase leads the plasma corticosterone rhythm. In the rat, this positive phase-angle difference amounts to about 2.0 hours in the male and to about 10.0 hours in the female. A similar large phase-angle difference has been observed in female mice between the rhythm of pituitary ACTH activity and the plasma corticosterone rhythm.[79,79a] Contrary to this, no major phase difference has been detected in animal studies between plasma ACTH and corticosterone rhythms. In man, similarly, it is possible by frequent sampling to demonstrate that in virtually all instances, a given ACTH peak precedes or is concordant with the plasma corticosteroid peak for a given time.[42, 80] There is recent evidence that plasma B-lipotropin levels also correlate with cortisol concentrations.[42a]

In contrast to the plasma cortisol rhythm, the secretory peaks of other hormones are said to be absolutely dependent on sleep.

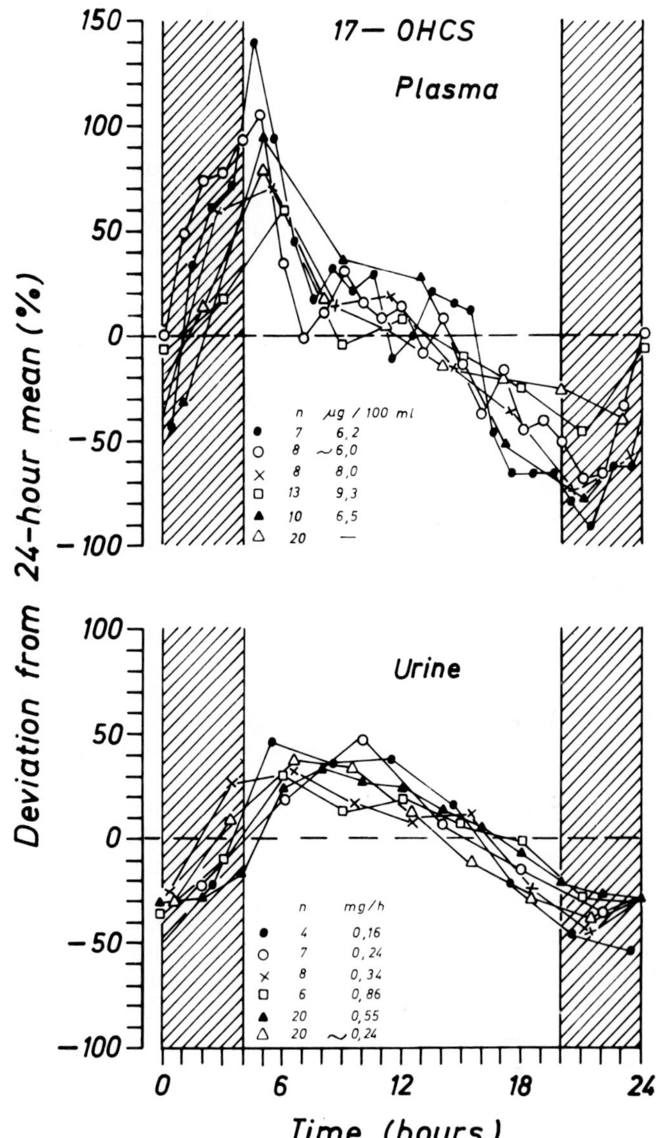

Fig. 156-18. Circadian rhythm of urinary and plasma corticosteroids in man. Shaded area: approximate sleep time. (Plasma data from refs. 45, 47, 69–72. Urine data from refs. 41, 69, 70, 73–75.)

The conclusion is usually based on experiments which show that the rhythm (e.g., of plasma growth hormone or prolactin) can immediately and completely be shifted by a shift of sleep time. Additional sleep-associated secretory peaks will also occur during the 24-hour period if the subject is awakened and then allowed to return to sleep again, thereby making the rhythm a noncircadian

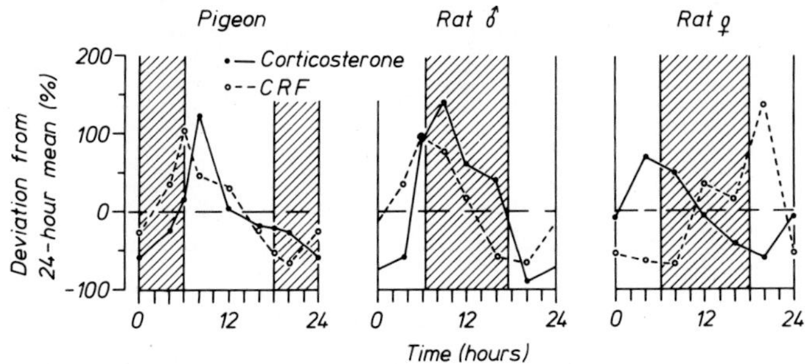

Fig. 156-19. Circadian rhythm of plasma corticosterone and of hypothalamic CRF in the pigeon and the rat. Shaded area: darkness. (Data sources: pigeon,[76] male rat,[77] female rat,[78].)

one. However, such a result is not necessarily in variance with the assumption that the rhythm may have a (weak) circadian component of its own. Two more types of experiments are needed to clarify the issue: one would have to test (1) whether hormone secretion occurs in circadian intervals during prolonged sleep deprivation, and (2) whether sleep introduced at different circadian times results in different amounts of hormone secretion. The second type of experiment, which searches for a rhythm in "sensitivity" to sleep, may also allow for a separation of phase-controlling effects from masking effects such as described for Zeitgebers.

Human plasma prolactin concentrations display a less pronounced 24-hour pattern than that of plasma cortisol (Figure 156-20). The phase of the pattern is immediately shifted following the time of sleep onset. In such shift experiments, no increase of the hormone has been observed at the time of day where it had occurred during normal sleep. Sassin and co-workers therefore conclude that the nocturnal rise depends on the occurrence of sleep and is "not based on an inherent rhythmic release . . . as is the case for ACTH."[84] However, neither of the experiments cited above have yet been performed with regard to prolactin secretion.

For growth hormone, the available data also suggest dependence of its rhythm on that of sleep. Although episodic growth hormone release has been observed in human subjects during the daytime, the results from many studies do not indicate any circadian trend apart from the major secretory peak in relation to the first hours of sleep. Some data, however, suggest a slight but steady increase in hormone level from late forenoon toward the evening.[84–88] It has recently been reported in children that the magnitude of the growth hormone peak following sleep onset (at unusual times of day) is dependent on the circadian phase during which such sleep occurs.[89]

Despite its relatively small range of oscillation, and despite a considerable interindividual variability, the circadian rhythm of plasma testosterone in the human male is well documented. Only 2 out of the 10 patterns reproduced in Figure 156-21 do not show a systematic trend from maximal values in the morning to minimal values in the late afternoon. In contrast with this clear picture, plasma FSH concentrations do not show any circadian rhythmicity (Figure 156-22*a*), there being only one contrary report.[99] The temporal pattern of plasma LH concentrations is a matter of controversy. For LH, all data available (from human adults only) are grouped in Figure 156-22 according to sex (*b*, female; *c* and *d*, male) as well as according to small (*c*) and large (*d*) variability. The

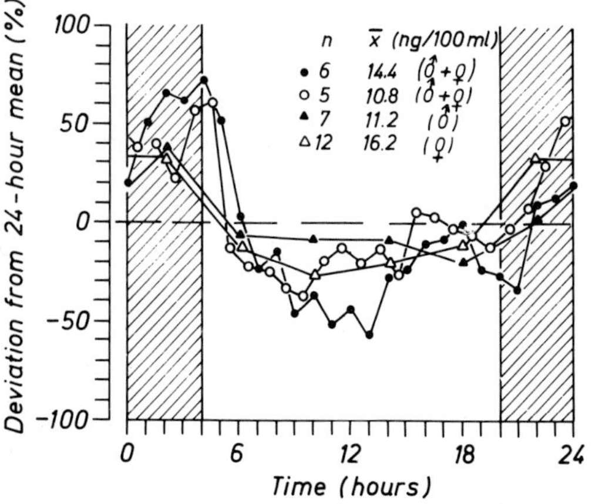

Fig. 156-20. Circadian rhythm of plasma prolactin in man. Shaded area: approximate sleep time. (Data sources: ▲, ref. 81; ○, ref. 82; ○, ref. 83. Circadian rhythm of plasma growth hormone in man. Shaded area: approximate sleep time. (Data sources: *A*, refs. 83, 85, 86: *B*, refs. 68, 80, 87, 88.)

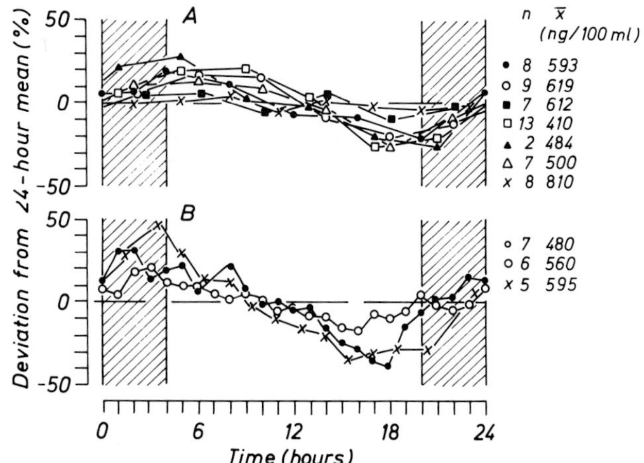

Fig. 156-21. Circadian rhythm of plasma testosterone in man. Shaded area: approximate sleep time. (Data sources: *A*, refs. 87, 90–95; *B*, refs. 46, 96, 97.)

number of female subjects is too small to warrant any conclusions. For male subjects, the two mean curves computed from diagrams *c* and *d* reveal a common pattern (Figure 156-22*e*): all but two of the mean values, which come from measurements during late sleep and during the forenoon, are above the 24-hour mean value, and all

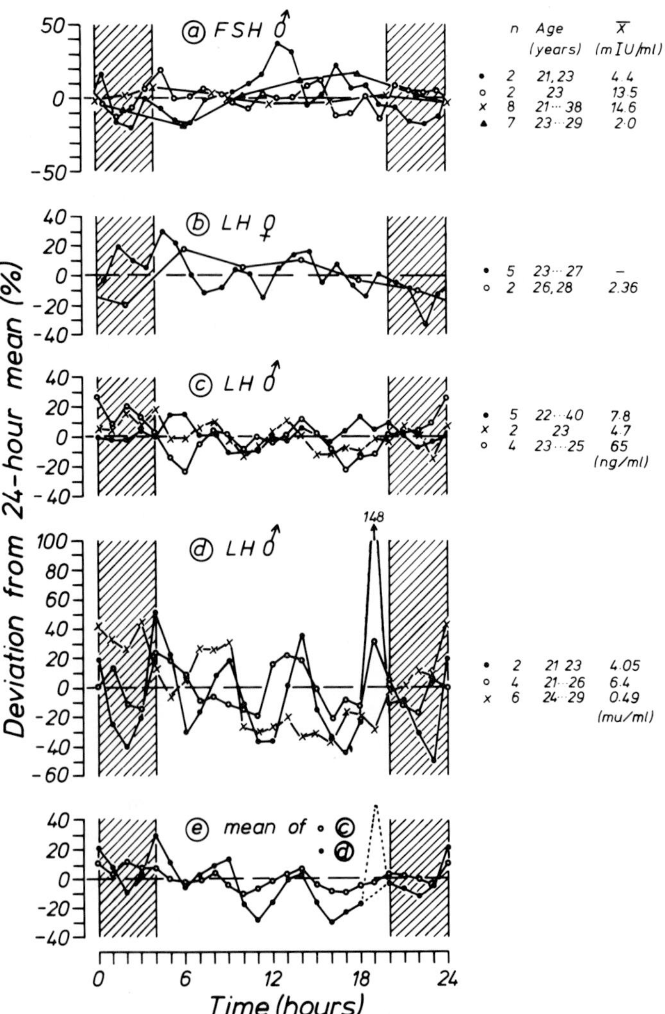

Fig. 156-22. Circadian variation of plasma FSH and LH in man. Shaded area: approximate sleep time. (Data sources: *a*, refs. 87, 90, 98; *b*, refs. 87, 100; *c*, refs. 1, 2, 101, 102; *d*, refs. 96, 98, 103.)

but two of the afternoon and early sleep values are below the mean value. Further search for a circadian component underlying the rhythm of plasma LH concentrations seems justified. For the gonadal and gonadotropic hormones, there is no available data with regard to effects of sleep deprivation or phase shifting.

The absence or near absence of a circadian rhythm in plasma LH concentrations has been used as an argument to reject the hypothesis that testosterone (which has a definite circadian rhythm) and LH are linked together in a feedback system.[90] Such a conclusion may not be justified. A rhythm of hormone secretion (e.g., in testosterone) can be generated on the basis of a more or less constant stimulus input (e.g., LH) provided that the target organ has a circadian rhythm of responsiveness. Furthermore, one has to keep in mind that "so far all of these investigations are based on total testosterone concentrations in plasma, neglecting the measurement of the biologically active free testosterone fraction, and that concentrations in peripheral plasma do not necessarily reflect those on cellular level."[104] In the rat there is a circadian variation of plasma TSH concentrations[104a] and of hypothalamic and amygdalar TRH concentrations,[104b] the zenith of both occurring at 1200. The periodicity of plasma TSH concentrations is not altered by adrenalectomy. Human subjects likewise exhibit a periodicity of plasma TSH concentrations,[104c] peak levels occurring just prior to or after sleep onset. Acute sleep–wake reversal does not appear to alter this periodicity but may modulate its amplitude.

There is insufficient data concerning the circadian variation of plasma vasopressin in man. Although a nocturnal increase has been described,[104d] with evidence of episodic secretion,[104e] complete reproducibility of pattern from day to day has not yet been obtained.

A survey of 24-hour patterns of the six hormones is shown in Figure 156-23. Figure 156-24 depicts patterns of three additional hormones: renin, TSH, and insulin. Patterns of plasma aldosterone, cortisol, and renin are correlated on a regular sodium diet and in recumbency.[104f,104g]

It remains to be seen whether endocrine rhythms fall into two

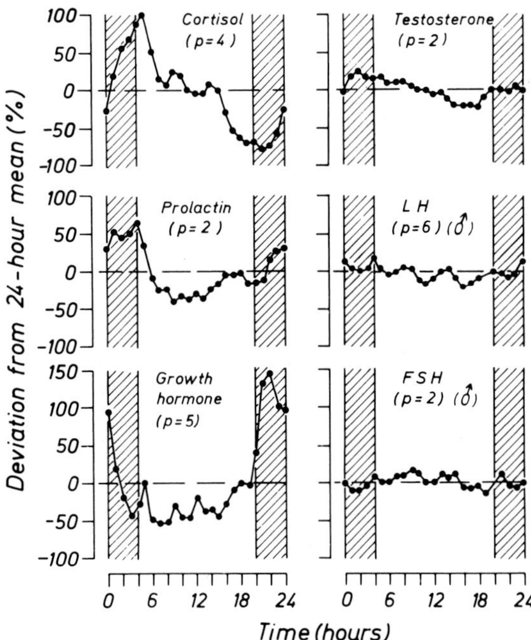

Fig. 156-23. Temporal pattern of several hormones in the plasma of man. Mean values from a number of studies *(p)* with sampling occurring for at least hourly intervals. Shaded area: approximate sleep time. (Data sources: see Figs. 156-19, 156-26 to 156-29.)

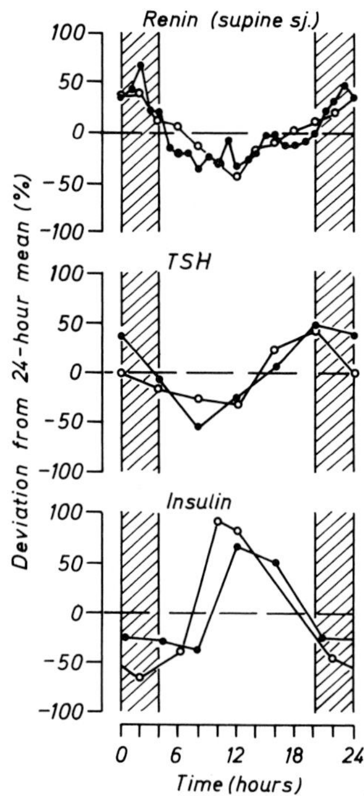

Fig. 156-24. Circadian rhythms of three hormones in the plasma of man. Mean values from several subjects each. Shaded area: Approximate sleep time. (Data sources: renin: • ref. 64, ○ ref. 105; thyroid-stimulating hormone: • ref. 71, ○ ref. 87; insulin: • ref. 80, ○ ref. 106.)

separate classes—those that are circadian and those that are exclusively sleep-dependent—or whether there is a continuum of rhythms with a trend from maximal to minimal range of circadian oscillation and from minimal to maximal dependence on sleep (either for phase control or with regard to the magnitude of "masking" effects).

In view of the basic structure of the circadian organization and its adaptive significance for proper adjustment to the environment's periodicity, it would be expected that representatives of related species or of species with similar temporal patterns of behavior (e.g., diurnal as opposed to nocturnal species) should have similarly phased rhythms. This assumption is supported by a comparison of plasma corticosteroid rhythms in diurnal birds and mammals.[76,107–109] There is a striking correspondence between the patterns in man and monkey, which both phase-lead the similarly corresponding bird patterns by about 2 hours. Such agreement, however, may not always occur, depending on the specific variable and on the species compared. An especially strange phase difference is indicated for at least one hormone in the circadian organization of man and rats. To facilitate a direct comparison, the patterns of the (nocturnal) rat have to be shifted with respect to the human patterns by 180°. This is done in Figure 156-25, in which zero at the abscissa represents the middle of sleep time for man and the middle of the entraining light–dark cycle for the rat. The patterns of rectal temperature and of plasma corticosteroid concentrations are in perfect agreement; that of plasma growth hormone also shows some similarity in the two organisms. The rhythm of prolactin, however, seems to reach maximal values in the rat at a circadian time when the values are minimal in man. So far, no explanation has been offered for this discrepancy.

Rhythms in Responsiveness

In view of the fact that the organism is in a different physicochemical state at each circadian phase, it is not surprising that the quantitative (and sometimes qualitative) responsiveness of the

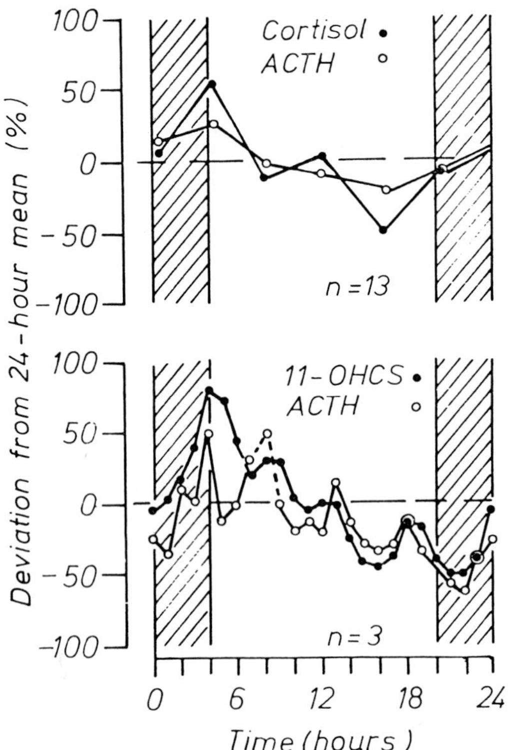

Fig. 156-25. Circadian rhythms in man (solid lines) as compared to those in the rat (dashed lines). Mean values from several sources (p = number of publications). Zero at the abscissa: middle of dark time for the rat and approximate middle of sleep time for man. (Data from: *a:* ○, ref. 110; •, refs. 111–114; *b:* ○, refs. 42, 65, 71, 115, 116; •, refs. 114, 172; *x*, refs. 117–119; Δ, refs. 50, 55, 120a; *c:* O, refs. 68, 83, 85, 86, 88; •, refs. 120, 121; *d:* O, refs. 81–83; •, ref. 118; *x*, ref. 123.)

organism to given stimuli differs according to the phase at which the stimulus is applied. Halberg and his co-workers first noted such differences with respect to the toxic effects of *E. coli* endotoxin[124] and of ethanol[125] in mice. As shown in Figure 156-26, there are circadian variations in mortality, with highest rates at the end of the light period and lowest rates in the middle or toward the end of the dark period. Further data that demonstrate rhythms in sensitivity to drugs, to noise, and to ACTH are summarized in Figure 156-27.

The duration of narcosis is 25 percent above the 24-hour mean when Nembutal is given in the middle of the light period and 25 percent below the mean when given in the dark period.[127] Mirror-like to this pattern are the patterns describing the percentage of

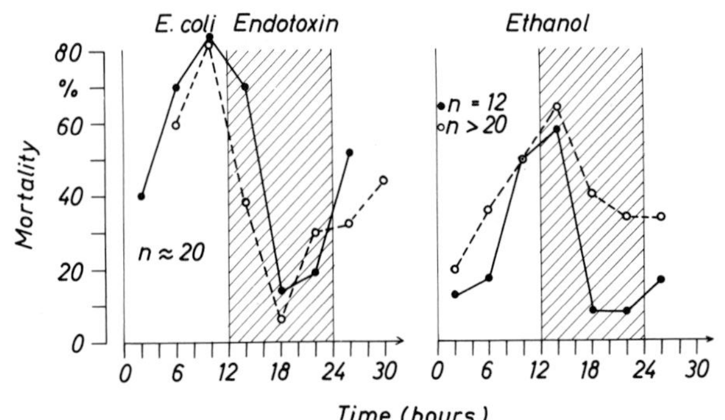

Fig. 156-26. Circadian rhythm of sensitivity to *E. coli* endotoxin and to ethanol in mice; two sets of experiments each. Shaded area: Darkness. (Data from: left, ref. 126; right ref. 125.)

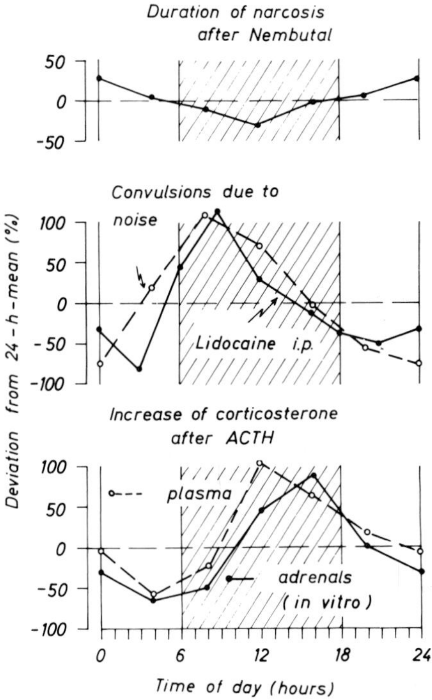

Fig. 156-27. Temporal pattern of sensitivity to Nembutal, to noise, and to lidocaine hydrochloride and of the adrenals to ACTH in mice. Shaded area: darkness. [Data from: top figure, ref. 127; middle figure, ref. 128 (noise) and ref. 129 (lidocaine); lower figure, ref. 130 (plasma) and ref. 131 (adrenals).]

convulsions elicited by a 1-minute noise (104 dc)[128] or by lidocaine (65 mg/kg ip).[129] The lowermost diagram in Figure 156-27 demonstrates that in mice the phase dependence of the response of adrenals to ACTH is not lost when the glands are taken out at different circadian phases and the hormone added in vitro.[130,131] This dependence may be explained by lack of prior adrenal priming by ACTH in the nonresponsive phase. In human subjects the decreased adrenal response observed following a 2300 as compared to an 0800 injection of ACTH becomes normal if the subject is given a prior submaximal injection of ACTH so as to have pre-ACTH 2300 corticosteroid levels similar to 0800 ones.[116] In addition, if a constant low infusion of small amounts of ACTH is administered to human subjects over a 24-hour period, plasma corticosteroid concentrations also remain constant, indicating no inherent periodicity in adrenal responsiveness to ACTH.[132]

Of theoretical as well as of practical interest are possible rhythms in responsiveness to stress situations. Scheving and co-workers[119,122] had reported a circadian variation in the response of plasma corticosterone and brain serotonin levels in rats to either brief exposure to ether–vapor immobilization (3 min supine, 12 min in holding cage), or novelty stress (putting the animals for 15 min in a strange situation). A lesser increment in plasma corticosteroid concentrations was noted when stresses were administered at the time of the circadian peak. Brain serotonin concentrations decreased following stress administered at the time of highest brain serotonin level and increased when animals were stressed at the time of the nadir of brain serotonin levels. More recent studies[132a] in which plasma ACTH as well as corticosterone were measured demonstrate that morning responses to stress may be greater, less than, or the same as the responses to the same stimuli applied to rats in the evening. It has been suggested that this represents an interaction between the potency of the stimulus, the magnitude and rate of increase of the corticosterone response, and the duration and magnitude of the ACTH response (i.e., when the corticosterone response is rapid and large, it will curtail subsequent ACTH secretion and further corticosterone responsiveness).

Zimmerman et al.[133] were unable to demonstrate such circadian periodicity in the corticosteroid response to stress. Furthermore, Allen and co-workers[134] found no absolute or incremental change in plasma ACTH concentrations following morning or afternoon tourniquet stress. (It is still possible that the same amount of ACTH could be put out at the trough and peak of the circadian cycle but that the adrenal would be differentially responsive at these times for the reasons cited above. It is also possible that at the peak of the circadian cycle, the increment seen following stress represents the maximal secretory capacity of the adrenal, so that a ceiling is reached independent of any alteration in sensitivity to ACTH.) The findings with regard to opposite changes in brain serotonin response dependent upon the magnitude of the baseline concentrations illustrate another general principle with regard to circadian responses—namely that the same perturbation of an organism may result in qualitatively different responses dependent upon the phase of the circadian cycle in which such a perturbation is introduced. For example, norepinephrine injected into the lateral hypothalamus of the rat increases fluid intake when applied during the light period but decreases intake (as compared to controls) when injected during the dark period.[135] Although rhythms of responsiveness are less well documented in man than in animals, the theoretical and practical significance of such alteration in responsiveness is evident.[136] A few examples are given in Figure 156-28. Increases of plasma 17-OHCS following an evening intravenous injection of pyrogen or of a corticotropic factor (CRA 4) are more than 100 percent above the 24-hour mean of all responses and are far below the mean when the drugs are given in the morning. Similarly, allergic reactions of the skin to histamine or to house dust, as measured by the size of the resulting erythema, are greater after an evening than after a morning injection.

The steadily increasing number of studies on rhythms of sensitivity in animals, either in vivo[130] or in vitro,[141] have opened the new area of chronopharmacology.[142–144] In the human, endocrine chronotherapy has been practiced with regard to the time of administration of corticosteroids.[145] First steps toward the use of chronotherapy in other fields are also being made.

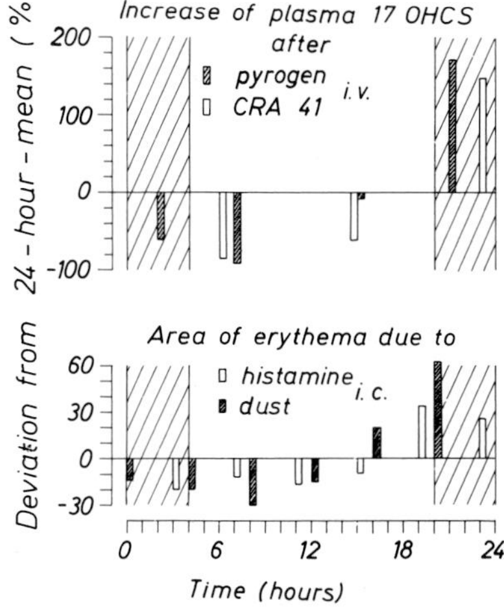

Fig. 156-28. Human sensitivity to drugs or allergens depending on circadian time (zero = approximate middle of sleep time). Plasma 17-OHCS after iv injection of pyrogen[137] or of the corticotropic factor CRA 41.[138] Size of skin erythema after i.c. injection of histamine[139] or of house dust.[140] Shaded area: approximate sleep time.

DEVELOPMENT OF CIRCADIAN PERIODICITY

In the human newborn, a circadian rhythm of rectal temperature is not detectable until the second or third week of life, and the normal range of oscillation is not attained until 1 year of age (Figure 156-29). In the lower diagram of Figure 156-30, the range of the temperature oscillation is drawn as a function of age (on a logarithmic scale), together with data on urinary water excretion. The upper graph shows the development of the evening-to-morning difference in plasma 17-OHCS levels, (morning value = 100 percent, right ordinate), together with the percentage of children awake at 3.00 A.M. (left ordinate). It seems that the age at which a rhythm first appears and the speed with which it develops differ with different functions and that, hence, different rhythms reach their full range of oscillation at different ages. The rhythm of wakefulness and sleep is more or less established at a time when the rhythms of urinary volume excretion and of plasma 17-OHCS concentration still have only half the normal range of oscillation. Of special interest are continuous records of the sleep–wake pattern such as first published by Kleitman and Engelman.[149] The example reproduced in Figure 156-31 indicates an initial development of an ultradian rhythm out of which the circadian rhythm emerges by "condensation" of ultradian periods, so that the circadian rhythm is at first free-running with a period longer than 24 hours and eventually (after 15 weeks of life) is entrained to 24 hours. These and similar findings support the hypothesis that the development of the rhythmic pattern of sleep (and that of other rhythms) is innately programmed, that development of rhythm depends on a maturational process, and that entrainment of the spontaneously emerging circadian rhythm occurs when the sense organs and the central nervous system allow for a coupling to the Zeitgebers in the environment.

Animal experiments also provide strong evidence for the innateness of circadian rhythmicity. Lizards or chickens raised in constant conditions from the day of hatching develop a free-running rhythm of locomotor activity;[154,155] in lizards, the period of this rhythm is about the same as that seen in animals whose eggs

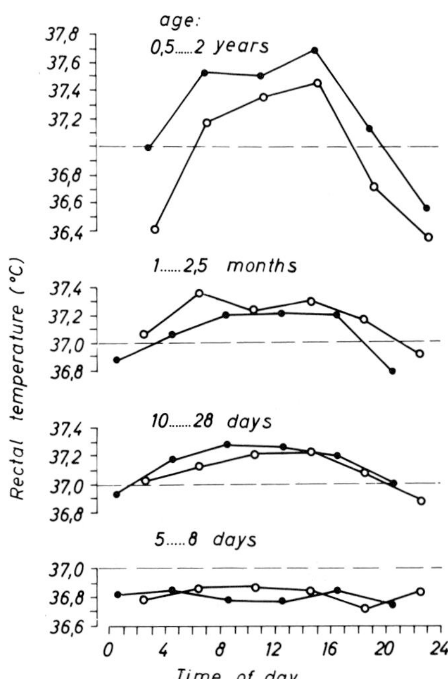

Fig. 156-29. Development of the circadian rhythm of rectal temperature in children. Mean values from two groups each (n = 5 to 17). (Data from ref. 147.)

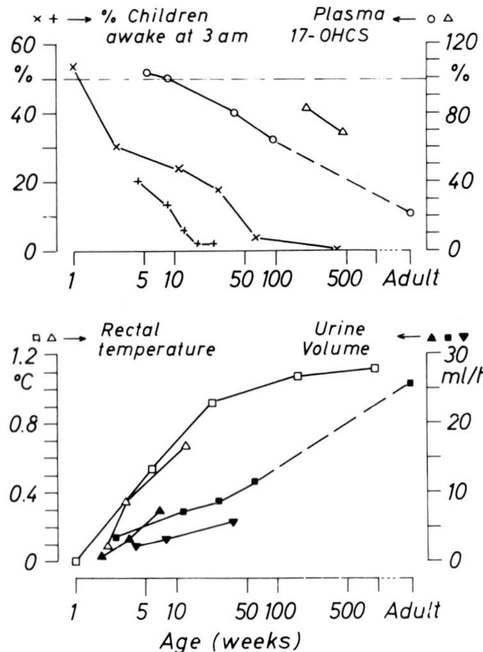

Fig. 156-30. Development of circadian rhythms in man. (Above) Percentage of children awake at 0300 (left ordinate) and evening value of plasma 17-OHCS as percent of the morning value (right ordinate). (Data from: *x*, ref. 148; +, ref. 149; ○, ref. 150; Δ, ref. 151.) (Below) Range of oscillation of rectal temperature (left ordinate) and of urinary water excretion (right ordinate). (Data from: ○, ref. 147; Δ, ref. 148; □, ref. 148; ∇, ref. 152; ▲, ref. 153.)

had been kept in a variety of artificial days (temperature and light cycle) deviating from 24 hours.[156] Under conditions of normal entrainment, the gradual development of the activity rhythm has been demonstrated for several mammalian species. Newborn monkeys (*Macaca mulatta*) are equally active during light and dark time; they start to be more active during daytime at an age of about 20 days, and they become fully day-active about 50 days later.[157] Nocturnal activity emerges at the 17th day in the hamster[158] and takes about 50 days to reach clear preponderance in the rat.[159] For several other variables that have been studied in the rat, no rhythm can be observed until about the 20th day of life.[159a]

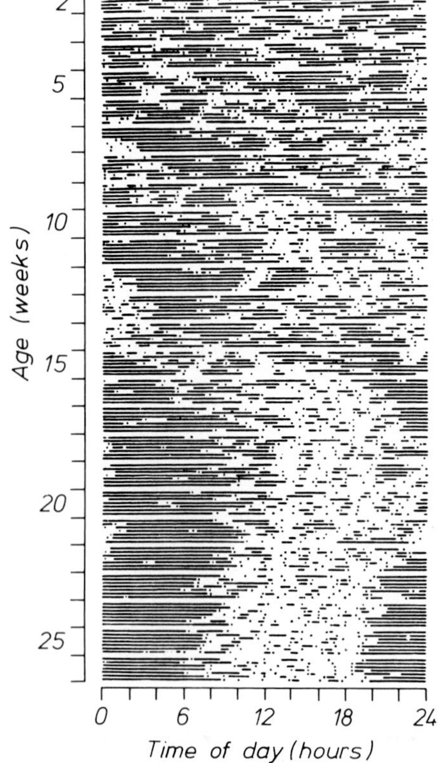

Fig. 156-31. Development of the rhythmic pattern of wakefulness and sleep in an infant. Bars: sleep. Dots: meals (From ref. 149.)

There is a suggestion that maternal factors may influence the rhythmicity of plasma corticosterone concentrations. Blind litters reared by blind mothers do not show a daily periodicity in plasma corticosterone levels at the expected time of appearance of such periodicity, whereas blind litters reared by normal mothers do display such periodicity. However, normally sighted litters (whether reared by normal or by blind mothers) have normal periodicity.[159b]

In animals, similar to what has been described for man, rhythms of different parameters develop at chronologically different rates.[160–165] The rhythm of hypothalamic CRF activity seems to appear earlier than the rhythm of plasma corticosterone; the rhythm of pineal N-acetyltransferase appears earlier than that of plasma tyrosine transaminase. The data further raise the question of whether there might be an inverse phase relationship to the light–dark cycle during the first days of life as suggested by sporadic observations on the development of the activity rhythm in several species.[166] Preliminary data on enzyme rhythms[167] and on the rhythms of serotonin and norepinephrine in the brain of the rat[168] seem to support such a hypothesis. The rhythm of plasma corticosterone is reported to appear on the 17th day in male and on the 25th day in female rats,[169] therefore raising the possibility of a sex difference in the rate of maturation. Neonatal administration of hydrocortisone is associated with absence of any circadian periodicity of plasma corticosteroid concentrations in 30-day-old animals, but such periodicity is evident when such animals are studied at 80 days of age.[170]* It should be noted that if hydrocortisone administration is delayed until animals are 12 days of age, normal periodicity is seen in the 30-day-old animals. This would imply that there is a "critical period" during which corticosteroids act on the presumed neural pathways involved in the regulation of such circadian periodicity, in some ways similar to the "critical period" described for the effects of neonatal androgenization on estrus cyclicity. Other studies[172] have shown that animals reared under constant conditions from birth until past the normal age of appearance of circadian periodicity of plasma corticosteroid levels have no periodicity under these conditions but that such periodicity develops subsequently when the animals are returned to normal environmental lighting. Conversely, adult animals with normal periodicity when placed under constant conditions do not appear to maintain such periodicity under the sampling conditions employed. This would indicate that there is no "critical age" for the appearance of nor an "imprinting" of the circadian periodicity of plasma corticosteroid levels.

Neonatal thyroxine treatment of rats has been reported[170a] to accelerate the time of appearance of the circadian periodicity of plasma corticosterone concentrations.

PHASE-SHIFT EXPERIMENTS

Experiments in which the phase of the Zeitgeber is abruptly shifted are often performed in order to test the effectiveness of an entraining agent or to study properties of the circadian system in a

*A recent study reports a sex difference in the time of restoration of normal periodicity in such neonatally treated animals, with female animals showing a normal rhythm at 55 days of age and males having a diminished rhythm on day 95 but normal on day 130.[171]

transitory state. From a survey of the results of many animal experiments, several rules can be derived.[35] As already shown in Figure 156-12, after the shift of the Zeitgeber it can take many periods until a circadian rhythm regains its normal phase relationship to the Zeitgeber. The time necessary for reentrainment depends on the species, on the properties of the Zeitgeber, and on the type of shift done. Two of the factors that are important in determining the number of transient cycles (i.e., time for reentrainment) are (1) the amount by which the Zeitgeber is shifted (reentrainment after a 12-hour shift usually takes longer than after a 6-hour shift) and (2) the strength of the Zeitgeber, which is related to its range of oscillation. With regard to the second point, it is reasonable to assume that reentrainment takes longer after the shift of a weak Zeitgeber (with a small range of oscillation) than after the shift of a strong Zeitgeber (with a large range).

Another important rule states that the time necessary for reentrainment depends on the direction of the shift. Reentrainment of a chaffinch's activity rhythm is accomplished within about four periods after a 6-hour delay shift of the entraining light–dark cycle but is present within two periods after a 6-hour advance shift. A similar "asymmetry effect," but with opposite signs, has been found in rodents: the transients last longer after an advance than after a delay shift. The natural circadian period seems to play a major role among the several factors that may contribute to the difference in the asymmetry effect between species (e.g., day-active versus night-active species, birds versus mammals).[173,174] Those species whose circadian period (as measured under constant conditions) has a tendency to be, on the average, longer than 24 hours, are usually reentrained faster after a delay shift of the Zeitgeber than after an advance shift; the opposite holds for species whose natural period tends to be mainly shorter than 24 hours.

In view of the fact that the circadian system has to be considered as a multiplicity of coupled oscillators and that these oscillators can become uncoupled from each other depending on various experimental conditions, one might expect differences in shift rate between different rhythmic variables. Some data from experiments with 12-hour shifts of the Zeitgeber support this idea. There seems to be a faster shift for the rhythm in rectal temperature than for the rhythm in plasma corticosterone in mice[175] and a faster shift for the rhythm in food intake than for the rhythm of the liver enzyme hydroxymethylglutaryl-CoA-reductase in rats.[176] In other words, the transitory state of reentrainment after a shift of the Zeitgeber is characterized by internal dissociation, i.e., by a temporary disturbance of the normal temporal order. The possibility of harmful consequences of such disorder, as occasioned by repeated phase shifting, cannot be excluded.

In contrast to most animal species which are effectively entrained by a light–dark cycle and which cannot help but follow a shifted Zeitgeber, man's circadian system is entrained by a variety of less well defined factors and is also less bound to follow such factors when they are shifted. Man can change the phase relationship of his sleep–wake cycle to Zeitgebers in the environment at will, and he often lives in unusual conditions where artificial and natural Zeitgebers provide contradictory cues. This is the situation of nightwork. Most shift workers live under the influence of conflicting Zeitgebers: the schedule of their working hours with all their concurrent signals tends to shift the circadian system, while the continuing relationship to the day-active society tends to keep the circadian system in its normal phase. As a consequence, circadian rhythms such as body temperature are "deformed" and flattened but remain basically unshifted (Figure 156-32).

Attempts to shift human circadian rhythms in the hospital or in the laboratory have failed as long as the subjects only shifted their sleep time and were not sufficiently shielded from unshifted

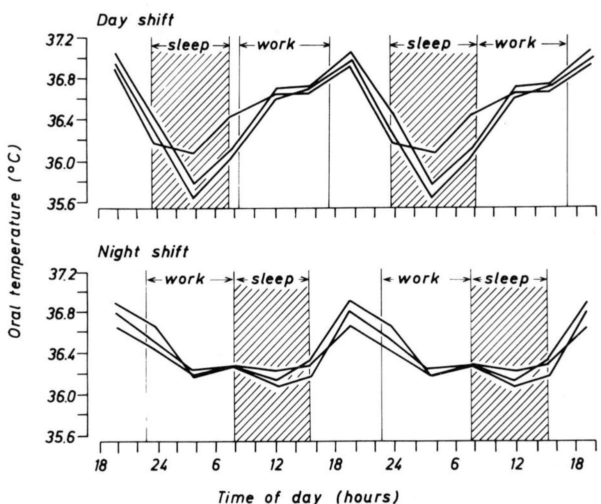

Fig. 156-32. Rhythm of oral temperature in 3 young male subjects before and after 12 weeks of night work (weekends off duty). (Data from ref. 177.)

(social) Zeitgebers. In a soundproof room, a shift of sleep time, together with a shift of the light–dark cycle and of other possible Zeitgebers, results in a gradual and eventually complete shift of the circadian system, as first demonstrated by Yorke and Blacklock[178] for the rhythm of microfilaria in the blood (Figure 156-33). Several later studies have shown, similar to animal studies, that different variables are shifted at a different rate and that 14 days may be necessary for a complete shift of some variables.[66,67,116] After 6 days of an inverse sleep–wake schedule, the rhythms of plasma cortisol and plasma magnesium may develop a bimodal pattern (masking?) but cannot be said to be really shifted.[179]

While only a limited number of subjects can be studied in the laboratory, thousands of tourists experience the problem of phase shift as a result of the speed of modern air transportation. The circadian system of a subject who has crossed several times zones by jet is out of phase with local time and has to be reentrained in the course of several days. As can be seen, the shift rate differs among variables. The two curves drawn in Figure 156-34 show the acrophases of the rhythms of oral temperature and of urinary 17-

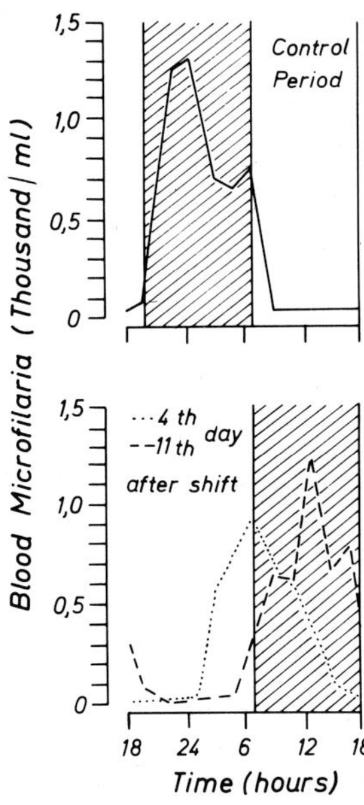

Fig. 156-33. Circadian rhythm of *Microfilaria nocturna* in the peripheral blood of a patient kept in isolation in a hospital room. Shaded area: Sleep in darkness. (Data from ref. 178.)

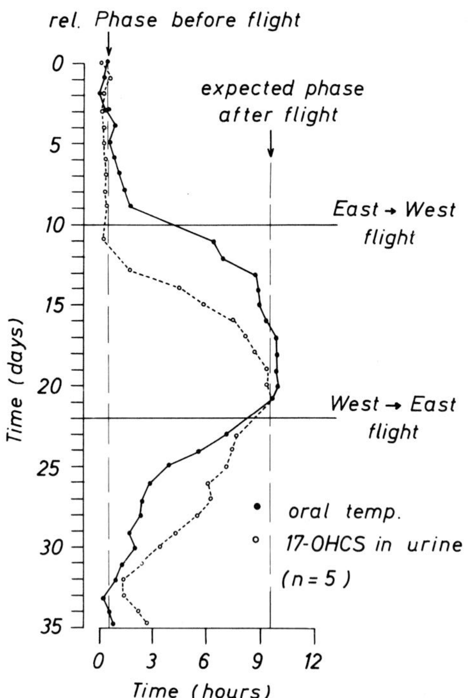

Fig. 156-34. Shift of acrophases of circadian rhythms in oral temperature and urinary 17-OHCS excretion after a westward and an eastward flight. Mean values from 5 subjects. Acrophases before first flight normalized to time zero at the abscissa. (Adapted from refs. 180 and 174.)

OHCS excretion before and after a flight over nine time zones, first in a westbound and thereafter in an eastbound flight. In both directions the rhythm of oral temperature has adjusted faster than that of the urinary excretion rhythm. Consequently, there is internal dissociation of the circadian system after both transmeridian flights. To what extent this temporal disorder contributes to the loss in efficiency and in well-being, often observed in such flights, is a still unanswered question.[35]

From Figure 156-34 it may also be seen that reentrainment takes somewhat longer after an eastbound flight than after a westbound flight. Although opposite directional effects have occasionally been observed, the majority of studies done so far agree with the data shown in Figure 156-34. When averaged from 10 publications and from a variety of rhythmic variables,[35] the mean shift rate comes out to be 92 min/day after a westbound flight and 57 min/day after an eastbound flight. Such mean shift-ratio values may vary considerably with regard to different parameters, and they also may vary according to conditions prevailing during flight and to those prevailing after the flight. For example, if it is correct that social Zeitgebers play an important role in the entrainment of human circadian rhythms, shift rates after a flight should depend on the nature of the passenger's activity, i.e., on the degree of social contact made possible by these activities. Experiments to test this hypothesis have been carried out by Klein and his coworkers.[181] Passengers who remain more or less isolated in their hotel room after a flight are not reentrained as quickly as when they are allowed to leave their rooms for outdoor activities every second day.[181]

NEURAL FACTORS INVOLVED IN THE REGULATION OF CIRCADIAN PERIODICITY

Evidence for Periodicity of Neural Function

Although the preceding discussion has provided ample evidence of periodic function on a cellular level, it has also suggested a hierarchy of rhythms (with either mutual or unidirectional coupling): cell–organ–organism.[36] It has also demonstrated the relationship of environmental influences—Zeitgebers—in the entrainment of the phase of many of the rhythms studied, with the implicit suggestion that in higher organisms such entrainment is mediated via the central nervous system (CNS) through thus far unknown anatomical and biochemical pathways.

Study of the sea hare, *Aplysia Californica,* has yielded important information with regard to the existence of circadian neuronal oscillators.[182] This organism has a circadian periodicity of locomotion that is abolished by blinding. The isolated eye of this organism has a circadian periodicity of optic nerve potential, although the site of the oscillator is undetermined. This oscillator can be phase-shifted by cell membrane depolarization in vitro (i.e., high K^+) or by incubation with inhibitors of RNA synthesis. A circadian periodicity in the parietovisceral ganglion of *Aplysia* has also been described. Such periodicity is resident in one identifiable neuron in this ganglion (R 15); periodicity in this neuron can persist even when impulse activity in the ganglion is abolished. It has also been shown that such pacemaker cells produce proteins of different molecular weight than those produced by nonpacemaker cells. The physiological and behavioral effects of the neurosecretion produced by such cells is not known.

Further evidence with regard to periodicity of neural function may be seen in reports of a circadian cycle in the group mean electrical output of the brain as measured by frequency analysis of the electroencephalogram.[183] A circadian rhythmicity in the activity of lateral hypothalamic neurons of the rat in response to glucose or hypotonic saline injected into the hepatic portal vein has also been reported.[184] In animals maintained under ad lib feeding conditions, circadian (reciprocal) changes in the frequency of firing of neurons in the ventromedial nuclei and in the lateral hypothalamic area have been described,[184a] associated with circadian changes in the responses of such neurons to stimulation of afferents. A circadian periodicity in morphological appearance of hypothalamic neurons has also been described.[184b]

A circadian rhythm of responsiveness in sensory (visual) and mechanoreceptors has been demonstrated in the crayfish.[185] Neuronal cells may be like all other body cells in that they manifest an inherent circadian periodicity. By virtue of their inherent hierarchical role, however, they are qualified to subserve an even more fundamental oscillatory function.

Role of the Pineal in Circadian Periodicity

Evidence for the neural (beta-adrenergic) regulation of the circadian periodicity of N-acetyltransferase concentrations (and consequently of serotonin, N-acetylserotonin, and melatonin) in the pineal gland has been exquisitely summarized by Axelrod.[186] The relationship of such changes to those of other bodily rhythms is far from clear. Although melatonin has been reported to block LH release if administered prior to the critical period on the day of proestrus[187] and pinealectomy to restore cyclicity in animals made constantly estrus by suprachiasmatic lesions,[188] there is no evidence that estrous cyclicity is destroyed in normal animals who are pinealectomized.[189] Similarly, although pinealectomy has been reported to be associated with an increase in adrenal corticosteroid levels and melatonin administration with a decrease in such levels,[190] superior cervical ganglionectomy (which denervates the pineal with regard to its response to light) causes no change in the circadian periodicity of plasma corticosteroid concentrations.[191] Pinealectomized sparrows become arrhythmic with regard to locomotor activity under constant dark conditions but show normal locomotor rhythms in normal light–dark conditions.[192] In contrast, pinealectomized rats maintain a circadian rhythm of locomotor activity in constant dim light,[193] and display normal circadian periodicity of plasma corticosteroid concentrations under light–

dark conditions, and shift periodicity with shifting of food presentation.[193a]

The evidence that the pinealectomized bird is arrhythmic in free-running conditions but can be entrained and the observations that surgical and chemical interference with pineal neural connections does not abolish the free-running rhythm, that pineal transplantation to the anterior chamber of the eye restores rhythmicity to pinealectomized birds,[193b] and that administration of melatonin, a pineal indoleamine, alters the period of free-running activity in pinealectomized birds[193c] all suggest that the pineal is hormonally, not neurally, coupled with other components of the circadian system.

The pineal may therefore act as a neuroendocrine transducer,[186] responding to a photic input by secretion of a family of hormones which may then act on other centers that mediate and synchronize other biological rhythms. The pineal, therefore, may not be involved in the genesis of the rhythm but may regulate it by virtue of the pineal's effect on other parts of the central nervous system,[194] thereby regulating the phase of such rhythms.

Central Nervous System Regulation of Nonendocrine Rhythms

Disruption of cerebral function in mice by electric shock is not associated with disruption of body temperature and eosinophile rhythms.[195] Lesions of the suprachiasmatic nucleus in the rat, abolish circadian rhythms of running and drinking activity[196] and of sleep–wakefulness.[196a] Lesions in this area have also been associated with loss of circadian periodicity of plasma corticosteroid concentrations.[197] In the hamster, suprachiasmatic nuclear lesions in female animals result in loss of estrous cyclicity and the occurrence of persistent estrus.[197a]

It has been demonstrated that, in addition to (1) the primary optic tract (which subserves visual function and projects to the lateral geniculate nuclei, pretectal area and tectum) and (2) the inferior accessory optic tract (projecting eventually to the pineal gland as well as to the hypothalamus), there is (3) a retinohypothalamic tract that projects ipsilaterally and contralaterally to the suprachiasmatic nuclei.[211] Such a projection has been identified in a number of mammalian species, including prosimian and anthropoid primates. Whether this area represents a primary oscillator to which other oscillators may be coupled remains a subject for further study. It is of interest that the age of appearance of the retinohypothalamic, pathway in the rat immediately precedes the age at which circadian periodicity of plasma corticosteroid levels is first evident.[198]

In the human there is also circumstantial evidence to link the central nervous system with circadian parameters. Central nervous system disease (diffuse or localized to the hypothalamic-limbic system area) is associated with disturbances in the circadian sleep–wake rhythm, temperature rhythm, and in the rhythm of plasma corticosteroid concentrations. Absence of a normal circadian temperature rhythm has been reported in patients with third ventricular neoplasms but only when ventricular obstruction with consequent increased intracranial pressure was present. When the ventricular obstruction was corrected, normal circadian periodicity of temperature returned.[199] Circadian rhythms of body temperature, sleep, urine flow, and plasma corticosteroid concentration are not present in the infancy of many species (including the human) and apparently require a certain degree of maturation of the organism (presumably of the central nervous system) before they appear (cf. section on development of circadian periodicity).

Central Nervous System Regulation of Endocrine Rhythms

The greatest degree of evidence of central nervous system control of a circadian endocrine rhythm is that with regard to the pituitary-adrenal system.[200] In this system, (1) neurotransmitter regulation of ACTH release has been established, (2) disruption of the circadian periodicity of plasma ACTH concentrations can be accomplished by either specific central nervous system lesions or by administration of agents that presumably alter central nervous system neurotransmitter content, (3) the central nervous system neurotransmitters, which have been implicated in the regulation of ACTH secretion, undergo circadian changes in concentration, and (4) the time of appearance of circadian periodicity of such neurotransmitter concentration is roughly correlated with the time of appearance of pituitary-adrenal periodicity.

Central nervous system control of estrous cycle rhythmicity has also been demonstrated. The initial observations were the classic ones of Everett and Sawyer[201] indicating a neurogenic timing factor in the control of the ovulatory discharge of LH in the cyclic rat. Atropine, ether, barbiturate, chlorpromazine, or reserpine administration several hours before the "critical period" for LH release on the day of proestrus will prevent ovulation. (The term "critical period" refers to two specific hours during which such LH release occurs.) Such ovulation will then occur during the "critical period" on the subsequent day if no further blocking agents are administered. The suggestion of a daily signal to gonadotropin-releasing hormone release is further supported by the findings of Fitzgerald and Zucker.[201A] They demonstrated that under constant conditions the estrous cycle free-ran with a period that was consistently a quadruple multiple of the period of the free-running circadian activity period. These studies indicated a 24-hour periodicity[202] in a signal for LH release, with the 4-day cyclicity of ovulation in the rat being a resultant of the interaction of appropriate hormonal concentration with this signal.

Sleep-Associated Hormone Release

The circadian nature of the sleep–wake cycle has been postulated to be regulated by variations in central neurotransmitter content or activity.[203] It has been suggested that serotoninergic mechanisms are involved in sleep induction and priming of paradoxical (REM) sleep, and catecholaminergic and possibly cholinergic mechanisms in waking and paradoxical sleep. A circadian variation in norepinephrine,[204] serotonin,[205] and acetylcholine[206] content of the central nervous system have been reported. Twenty-four-hour secretory patterns for growth hormone,[207] prolactin,[83] and pubertal LH release[208] have been found to be sleep-associated, with maximum levels noted for each of these hormones at specific intervals following sleep onset. Shifting the time of sleep onset immediately shifts the time when peak concentrations of growth hormone and prolactin are noted, the peak of each still maintaining the specific phase angle following sleep onset (Figure 156-35). In addition to the sleep-associated peak, there is suggestive evidence of a minor circadian component in the periodicity of plasma growth hormone levels.

In view of the considerable evidence implicating central neurotransmitter regulation of these hormones, it is tempting to interrelate variations in central nervous system neurotransmitter content, sleep state, and hormone concentration. Evidence suggests, however, that these may not be directly causally related. For example, although it has been stated that in the human, peak nocturnal growth hormone secretion occurs in association with slow-wave sleep,[27] there is human[209] and animal[210] evidence indicating the dissociation of these two parameters. If the secretion of a hormone such as growth hormone were exclusively triggered by sleep, one should expect secretion at any time sleep occurs. That this is not necessarily the case was demonstrated by Weitzman[68] in his study on the effects of a prolonged 3-hour sleep–wake cycle. The results summarized in Figure 156-36 show that after 10 days of such a schedule, the major secretory peak characterizing the first

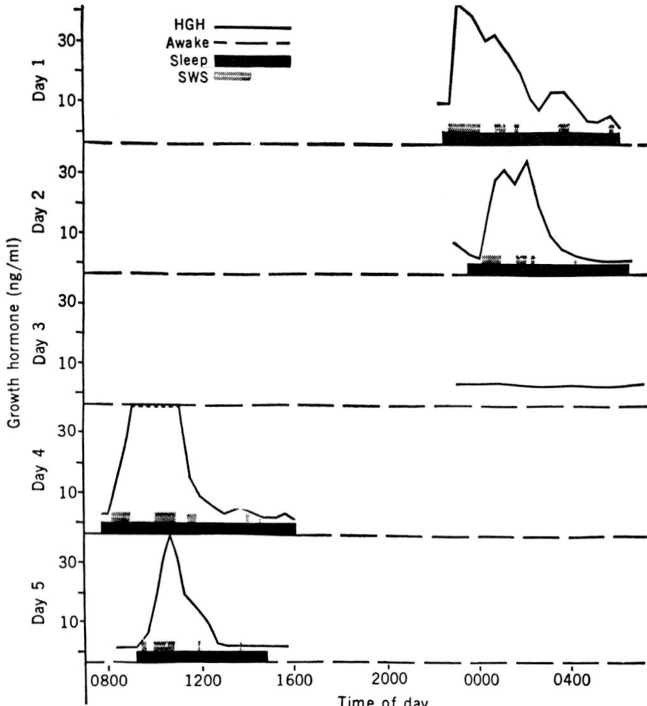

Fig. 156-35. Plots of nocturnal growth hormone patterns on 5 successive days of study of the reversal of the sleep–waking cycle. Note absence of growth hormone (HGH) secretion on third night, when subject was kept awake, and resumption of secretion on the fourth and fifth mornings when subject was asleep. SWS, slow-wave sleep. (From, ref. 212.)

few hours of normal sleep has disappeared, although in the 3-hour cycle the peak occurring just before the time of the "normal" sleep onset and the following peak are larger than any of the other observed peaks, that there are also five minor secretory episodes

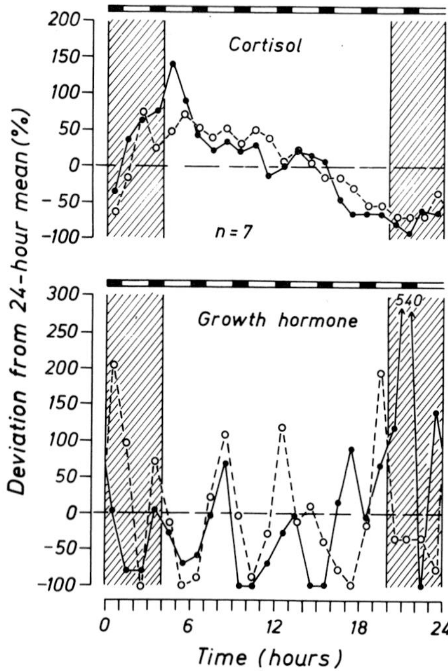

Fig. 156-36. Temporal pattern of plasma cortisol and growth hormone during (*a*) a normal sleep–wake schedule with 8 hours sleep (shaded area) and (*b*) after 10 days of a 3-hour sleep–wake cycle as indicated on top of both diagrams. (Black bars: sleep in darkness). Solid lines and closed circles for the normal schedule, dashed lines and open circles for the 3-hour cycle. (Data from ref. 68.)

that are present under both conditions, and that these episodes do not coincide with sleep during the 3-hour sleep–wake schedule.

All of the above observations are consistent with the theory that the periodic hormone secretion seen in association with sleep is mediated via the central nervous system. It may be, however, that different neural mechanisms are involved in the genesis of the sleep stages and in the periodicity of the nocturnal hormone rise.

Although, as cited above, there is evidence for central nervous system regulation of ACTH periodicity, such regulation does not appear to be via the same mechanisms as involved in growth hormone, prolactin, and LH periodicity. The early morning circadian rise in plasma ACTH concentrations does not appear to be a sleep-associated one, in that (1) there is a considerable lag (up to approximately 9 days) in the phase shifting of ACTH periodicity when the time of sleep onset is shifted, and (2) the circadian periodicity of plasma ACTH concentrations persists for at least a 2-day period of sleeplessness (the longest time period studied). In the case of the other hormones, no apparent periodicity has been seen in the sleep deprivation studies thus far. Therefore, although the phase of the periodicity of plasma ACTH concentrations is presumably entrained by the sleep–wake cycle, the factor or factors involved in the genesis of this periodicity may differ from those involved in the maintenance of the sleep–wake state. As noted previously (p. 2086), it may well be that periodicity of pituitary hormone release represents a continuum from those that are generated by mechanisms that have no direct relationship to the sleep–wake cycle (i.e., ACTH), through those that have a large sleep-dependent component (i.e., growth hormone, prolactin, possibly LH), to those with no demonstrated sleep or circadian component (i.e., FSH).

RHYTHMS IN HUMANS

IN NORMAL SUBJECTS

Ultradian Rhythms

Periodicity in vital signs and neuronal functions has already been cited (Figure 156-1). It has been recognized for the past 15 years that there is an approximately 90-minute cycle in the REM (rapid eye movement) EEG stage of sleep and that these cyclically recurring periods are accompanied by a similar periodicity of dreaming, penile erections, cardiac irregularity, and breathing. Kleitman[213] had suggested that this ultradian rhythm during sleep was a reflection of a "basic rest–activity cycle" which occurred during waking periods as well. There appears to be some confirmation of this in that an apparently similar periodicity in performance indices, telemetered gross motor activity and oral activity (i.e., observed episodes of food or water intake, smoking, or oral contact, as with a finger or pencil) has been reported by several observers during waking hours.[214–216]

The repetition of such episodes in hormonal secretion has also been referred to as a biological ultradian rhythm. So far, no rigorous proof has been provided that such pulsatile secretion represents a periodicity in its strict sense, and the possibility of a mainly random distribution of episodes cannot be excluded with certainty. A rhythmic process, however, underlying these patterns is suggested by the observed regularity of secretion, seen especially in the case of LH. The records from 3 subjects reproduced in Figure 156-37 all show 11 to 13 major peaks per 24 hours. Mean intervals between episodes of about 2.3 hours have been reported for males,[120] and 2.5 hours for females,[217] with such intervals varying from 1 to 4 hours, depending on the phase of the menstrual cycle.[218]

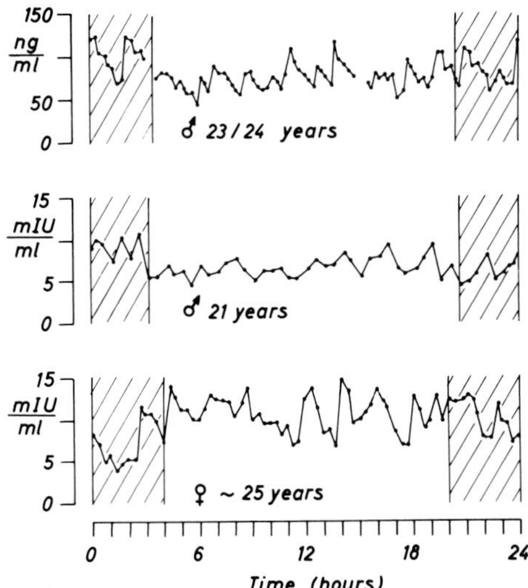

Fig. 156-37. Episodic secretion of luteinizing hormone in 2 male and 1 female subject. Upper curve measured in two half-day sessions, one year apart. Shaded area: approximate sleep time. (Data from: upper figure, refs. 1, 2; middle figure, ref. 98; lower figure, ref. 100.)

Episodic corticosteroid secretion has also been reported. In many of the 24-hour records based on frequent or integrated continuous sampling, three major peaks appear with superimposed minor fluctuations. The data from 6 subjects depicted in Figure 156-38 could be interpreted as indicating a close correlation between the major peaks and the three daily meals. The same study describes a shift of the noon peak following a shift of lunch time.[219] Other studies, however, do not confirm such a correlation.[44,168] The minor episodic fluctuations of cortisol secretion seem to be less regular and less frequent than those of LH secretion. All 5 subjects studied by Krieger et al.[42] showed six to nine episodes per 24 hours, a frequency similar to that noted in other studies.[44,47,220]

Although episodic secretion appears to occur with many hormones, no general principle for the generation of such episodes is applicable. It appears that with a decrease in the frequency of episodic secretion, the range of oscillation increases. When drawn on the same relative scale, the impressive episodes of LH secretion seen in Figure 156-37 become minor fluctuations when compared to those of ACTH and plasma corticosteroids, and these latter are less than those seen with prolactin and growth hormone secretion.

The physiological basis and significance of such periodicity are largely unknown. There have been no studies relating such secretory episodes to any of the nonhormonal parameters noted above, although there appears to be no correspondence between that of cortisol and REM rhythms. The role played by the central nervous system is still a matter of controversy. Yen[221] has described the LH secretory episodes as "reflecting an inherent ultradian rhythm of CNS-pituitary-gonadotropin regulation." In humans, immunoassayable plasma LRF concentrations have been demonstrated to undergo rapid fluctuations, but while increased numbers of LRF secretory spikes were associated with higher mean LH levels, episodic fluctuations in LRF concentrations were not correlated with subsequent episodic fluctuations in LH.[222] In 3 of 5 ovariectomized monkeys that were acutely stalk sectioned, and in whom a constant infusion of LRF was administered via the portal vein, evidence of pulsatile LH secretion was observed.[223] These same workers, however, have reported pulsatile release of LRF in studies in which stalk blood was collected over a 9-hour period.[224] Additionally, pulsatile LH release can be blocked by adrenergic blocking agents,[225] further suggesting a higher neuronal periodicity, if one accepts the assumption that such agents are acting at a central nervous system, not a pituitary level.

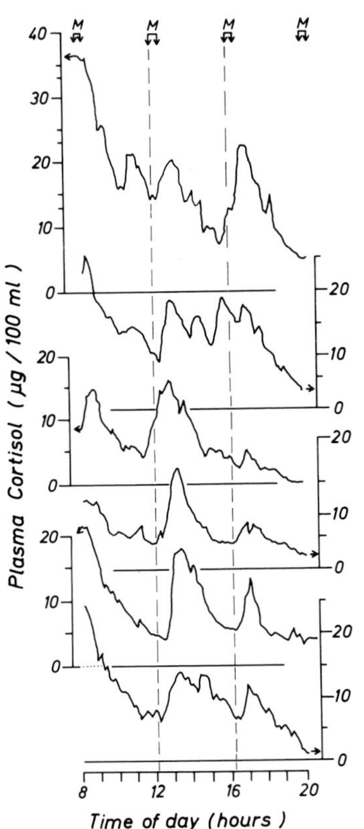

Fig. 156-38. Episodic secretion of cortisol in six subjects. M: meals. (Data from ref. 219.)

Circadian Rhythms

It is apparent that all bodily functions undergo rhythmic variations. Although detailed analysis of their exogenous or endogenous nature and the means by which they are entrained is lacking, many of these rhythms have been demonstrated to be endogenous. Circadian rhythms of hormones have been considered previously (p. 2087). A circadian variation in temperature, pulse, blood pressure, cardiac output, venous pressure, circulating blood volume, urinary volume, and intraocular pressure are well-recognized clinical phenomena. Obstetricians can testify to the circadian periodicity in the incidence of birth (with maximum frequency occurring in the early morning), and there is a similar peak incidence of deaths at this time.

A circadian variation in the concentration of various blood constituents has also been demonstrated (i.e., white blood cells, electrolytes, phosphorous, amino acids, etc.[226]). The periodicity of many of these parameters has been shown to be independent of sleep, posture, or feeding. A diurnal variation in plasma and urine glucose levels in diabetic subjects, maintained on constant feedings of equal glucose value at frequent intervals over the 24-hour period, was noted in a study performed in 1949. Highest levels were attained at 0600.[227] This did not appear to be related to variations in muscular activity; it should be noted that highest levels occurred at the time of the plasma cortisol peak. Such variation was not noted in normal subjects in a study that also confirmed the presence of such variation in diabetic subjects.[228] A diurnal variation in glucose tolerance test (all tests performed after a similar duration of fasting and a similar caloric meal prior to initiation of fast) has been well documented.[229] This is associated with a delayed insulin response to the glucose load. There is also evidence that a given dose of insulin produces a smaller hypoglycemic effect in the afternoon.[230] Such resistance is not explicable by any associated changes in plasma growth hormone or cortisol concentrations; it may be correlated with significantly higher afternoon levels of nonesterified fatty acids.

Another interesting aspect of circadian periodicity has to do with the phase of optimal performance (i.e., of learning, work speed, judgment, reaction time, computation, pattern recognition, sensorimotor coordination).[231] Most investigations agree that "peak" performance occurs in the late afternoon and that the "low" point occurs about 0400, this low point occurring whether subjects are awakened from sleep at this time or remain awake beforehand. Whether or not such periodicity is correlated with that of body temperature or is secondary to an inherent organizational pattern of the brain is a subject of controversy. Within this context, however, considerable intersubject variability occurs in both the amplitude and phasing of the performance rhythms that are found to exist. Speculation exists whether there are "day" people and "night" people, and differences in phase of physiological (i.e., temperature) and performance parameters have been found between subjects so categorized. It has also been suggested that there are measurable differences in personality characteristics of such subjects.[232] No studies have been performed to date with regard to the nature of hormonal or neurotransmitter periodicity in such "day" and "night" people.

A circadian variation in taste detection thresholds for sodium chloride is present in normal individuals but not in those with adrenal insufficiency.[233] It is of interest that normal detection threshold and periodicity occurs in the latter group when on replacement therapy, even though such therapy is administered in a pattern that does not approximate normal adrenal steroid periodicity. This would imply that the steroids play a permissive role in the expression of such periodicity but that the neural periodicity is not secondary to the adrenal periodicity.

Menstrual Periodicity

The most notable infradian periodicity is that of the human menstrual cycle. Such periodicity has been ascribed by some to be entrained to a lunar cycle. Inspection of Figure 156-39 shows this not to be the case. If there were entrainment to a lunar cycle, one would not expect a shift in cycle length with increasing age.

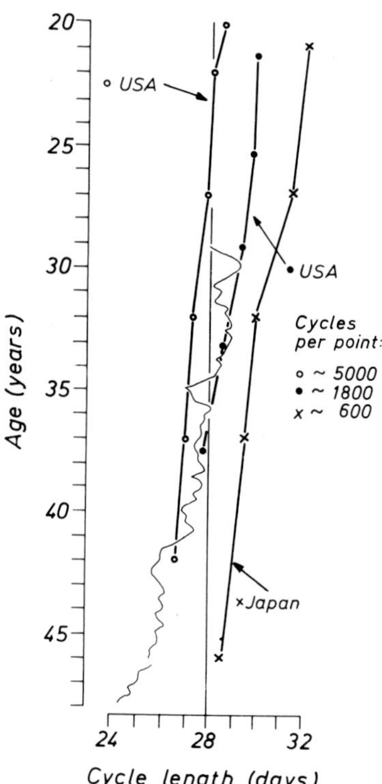

Fig. 156-39. Menstrual cycle length as a function of age. Thin line: record of one individual (data from ref. 232). Thick lines: mean values from many records. (Data from: ○, ref. 234; ∘, ref. 235; *x*, ref. 236.)

Discussion of the endocrine factors underlying this periodicity have been considered in Chapters 108 to 109. As noted above, superimposed on this <30 day rhythm is an ultradian pattern of gonadotropin release. In addition to the periodicity of these hormonal changes, there is a similar periodicity of various parameters of nervous system, cardiovascular, and respiratory function, as well as of many blood constituents. Figures 156-40 and 156-41 summarize some of the reported findings in this field.[19] It should be realized that in some of the studies, sampling was less than optimal in that the extent of circadian variation of the parameter was not considered, so that if a given parameter had a large amplitude of circadian variation and sampling was performed at random times

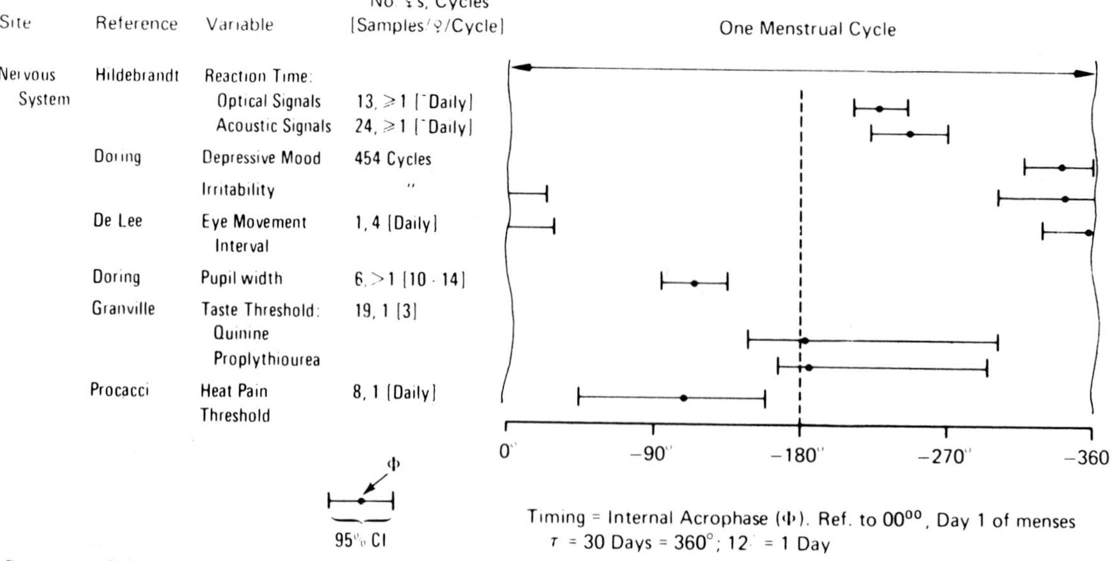

Fig. 156-40. Summary of the acrophase (the temporal peak of the 30-day cosine curve approximating time series data) and the 95 percent confidence interval for various menstrual rhythms of the nervous system.[237]

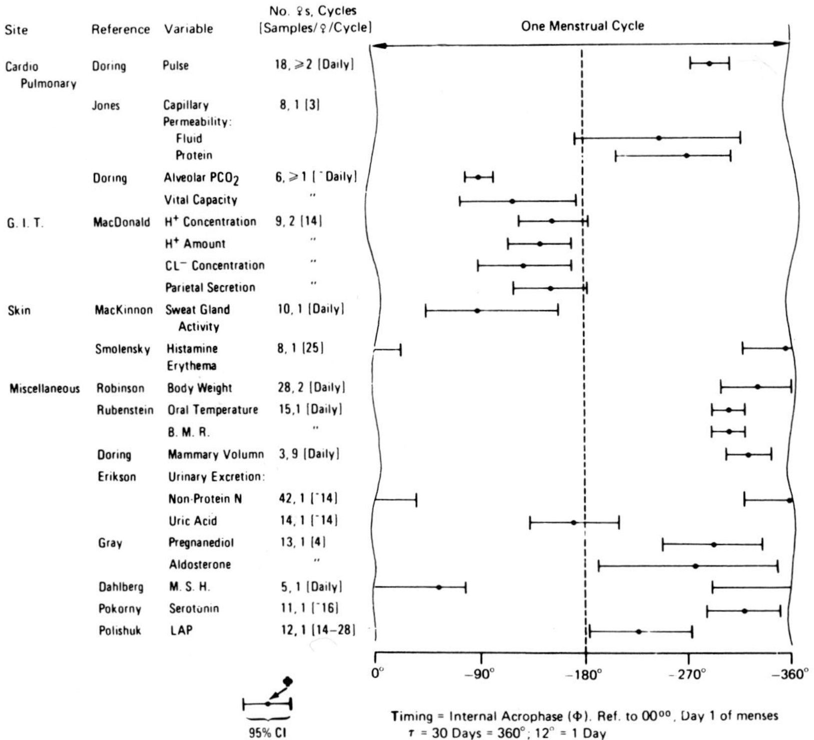

Site
Reference
Variable
No. ♀s, Cycles (Samples/♀/Cycle)
One Menstrual Cycle
Cardio Pulmonary
Doring
Pulse
18, ≥2 (Daily)
Jones
Capillary Permeability:
Fluid
Protein
8, 1 (3)
Doring
Alveolar PCO2
Vital Capacity
6, ≥1 (~Daily)
G. I. T.
MacDonald
H+ Concentration
H+ Amount
CL− Concentration
Parietal Secretion
9, 2 (14)
Skin
MacKinnon
Sweat Gland Activity
10, 1 (Daily)
Smolensky
Histamine Erythema
8, 1 (25)
Miscellaneous
Robinson
Body Weight
28, 2 (Daily)
Rubenstein
Oral Temperature
B. M. R.
15,1 (Daily)
Doring
Mammary Volumn
3, 9 (Daily)
Erikson
Urinary Excretion:
Non-Protein N
Uric Acid
42, 1 (~14)
14, 1 (~14)
Gray
Pregnanediol
Aldosterone
13, 1 (4)
Dahlberg
M. S. H.
5, 1 (Daily)
Pokorny
Serotonin
11, 1 (~16)
Polishuk
LAP
12, 1 (14–28)
0°
−90°
−180°
−270°
−360°
95% CI
Timing = Internal Acrophase (Φ). Ref. to 00⁰⁰, Day 1 of menses
τ = 30 Days = 360°; 12° = 1 Day

Fig. 156-41. Summary of the acrophase (the temporal peak of the 30-day cosine curve approximating time series data) for a number of menstrual rhythms including those of the cardiovascular, respiratory, and gastrointestinal systems.[237]

of a given 24-hour period during the monthly cycle, an approximately 30-day periodicity would be obscured. It should be noted that the circadian rhythm of a given parameter continues throughout the menstrual cycle, although with changing mean value (Figure 156-42). From this it is apparent that the circadian rhythm of oxygen uptake and of rectal temperature is similar in the follicular and luteal phases of the cycle but that the mean value for both is increased in the luteal phase.

There is an increased sensory detection acuity in the follicular phase of the cycle.[239] The relationship of these sensory changes to specific hormonal ones is inferred—there are, however, no studies of these parameters in women with spontaneous anovulatory cycles, menopausal women, patients with hypogonadism, or those on contraceptive pills. In another study on pain threshold,[240] a 30-day period was noted, the peak occurring in the follicular phase of 15- to 39-year-old women with spontaneous menses, but no periodicity was present in women taking contraceptive pills. Of interest was the presence of a 30-day period in pregnant and postmenopausal women, although the acrophase in these conditions occurred at a different point of time in the 30-day cycle than in the case of women with spontaneous menses.

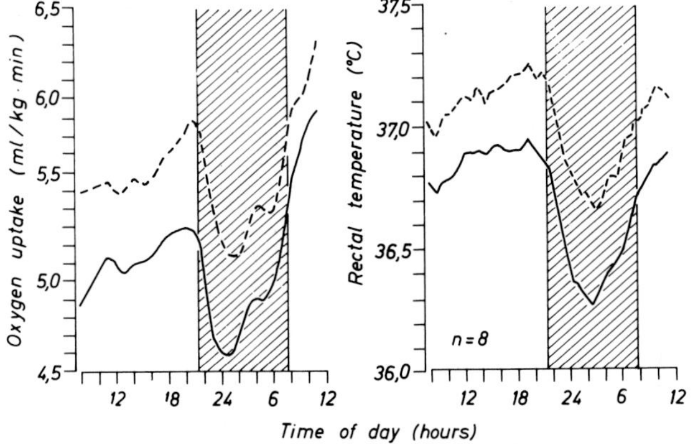

Fig. 156-42. Circadian rhythm of oxygen uptake and rectal temperature before (solid lines) and after ovulation (dashed lines). Mean values from 8 subjects, resting in a climatic chamber at 28° C. No meals, but 100 ml water every second hour. Shaded area: Sleep in darkness. (Data from ref. 238.)

When behavioral patterns were studied, there appeared to be three phases during the 30-day cycle in which deviations from chance expectancy were noted. There was increased occurrence of abnormalities 4 days premenstrually and 4 days postmenstrually and decreased occurrence in the postovulatory period. A pilot study of 3 healthy females who did not manifest any overtly abnormal behavioral patterns revealed a similar time variation of behavioral patterns, whereas the 1 anovulatory female studied did not manifest any relationship between mood–behavior changes and period phase.[241]

The human female has been described by some investigators as having fluctuating levels of sexual receptivity. These claims have not been mutually confirmatory with regard to phase of menstrual cycle associated with maximum receptivity. There are other studies that report no such fluctuations. It should also be noted that the cyclic differences noted are of an extremely lower order of magnitude than that noted for other species.

Seasonal Rhythms

With the exception of some tropical species, profound seasonal changes characterize the behavior, the physiology, and the morphology not only of the cold-blooded animals but also of most homoiothermic animals.[242] These seasonal rhythms have attracted new interest since it was shown that, similar to circadian rhythms, they can be based on endogenous, self-sustained oscillations. A first demonstration of a free-running "circannual" rhythm in hibernating mammals[243] was soon followed by observations on circannual rhythms of moult and migratory restlessness in birds.[244] Several recent articles review the literature on "circannual clocks."[245,246]

For man, seasonal rhythms are less well documented, and it is still an open question whether or not they represent circannual systems in a strict sense. Seasonal rhythms in birth rate were first documented at the beginning of the last century,[247] and several of the early statistics indicate a peak incidence of conceptions in spring and summer, a time of year at which conceptions still prevail in several European countries. However, the example presented in Figure 156-43 indicates that there is a tendency for a shift of this peak during consecutive decades. Similar, but more drastic phase shifts have been observed in Puerto Rico, where the peak of conceptions drifted within 15 years from August (in 1941–1945) to December (in 1956–1961), the typical peak month for the population of the United States.[249] Another parameter to be taken into account is geographical latitudes. According to an analysis made by Batchelet and co-workers,[250] the peak of conception occurs later in the year with increasing northern as well as southern latitude. It is highly probable that many of these phase shifts are culturally determined, but more data are necessary to allow for a detailed analysis of the contributing factors. Such studies would be of special interest in view of the hypothesis that changes in the hormonal state of the organism may underlie the rhythm of conception and also influence other season-dependent phenomena such as crimes and suicides (cf. Figure 156-1). In this regard, it should be noted that a seasonal rhythm of plasma testosterone levels has been reported in studies on 5 young Parisian males in whom blood samples were obtained at bimonthly intervals, with maximal values occurring in October[251] and correlating with a similar seasonal peak in reported sexual activity. A more extensive study (15 subjects, sampled at 3 monthly intervals) confirmed that October plasma testosterone levels were approximately 10 percent higher than those seen at other times of the year.[251a]

Seasonal rhythms in mortality have been even more extensively studied over the past 150 years. For many diseases, peak values for mortality occur in winter, with slight phase differences between the northern and the southern hemisphere. According to

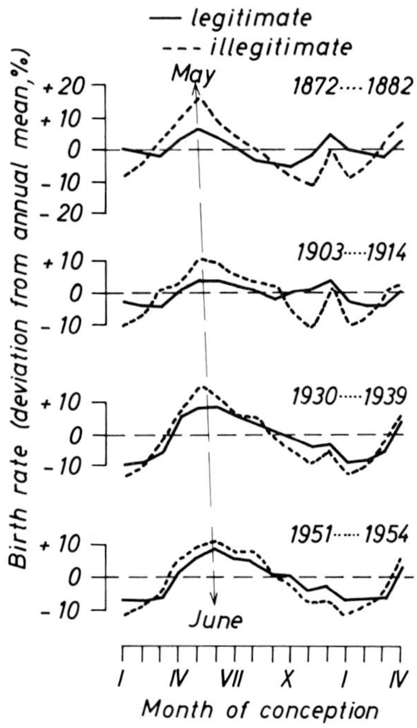

Fig. 156-43. Seasonal rhythm of birth rate, drawn according to month of conception, in Germany. (Data from ref. 248.)

Table 156-1. Reported Periodic Disease[a]

Intermittent hydrarthrosis or joint pain
Cyclic neutropenia, agranulocytosis (ulcers), thrombocytopenia (bleeding), reticulocytopenia (anemia)
Cyclic lymphocytosis, monocytosis, fever, Hodgkin's disease
Cyclic peptic ulcers, vomiting, diarrhea, fever
Benign paroxysmal peritonitis, pain, fever
Cyclic excessive sweating
Cyclic hematuria, oliguria, polyuria, fever
Familial periodic paralysis
Cyclic iritis, polyserositis
Cyclic purpura, urticaria, angio-neurotic edema, erythema, fever
Cyclic epilepsy, hypo- and hyperthermia, insomnia, hypersomnia, headache, migraine
Cyclic emotional disturbance (mania, depression, paranoia, stupor)

[a]Adapted from C. P. Richter, *Biological Clocks in Medicine and Psychiatry*, Springfield, Ill., Charles C. Thomas, 1965.

data summarized by Smolensky and co-workers,[252] the range of oscillation is more than twice as large for respiratory deaths as for cardiovascular deaths. In some countries, the range of oscillation has become smaller in the course of this century; this "deseasonalization" has again been attributed to changes in the mode of living, especially to changes in the system of room heating.[253]

There is little available data concerning seasonal rhythms in human physiology. There are reports on seasonal variations of concentrations of serum lipids,[254] choline,[255] hemoglobin and protein,[256] as well as in plasma vitamin D[257] and in the sensitivity of the skin to ultraviolet irradiation.[258] A seasonal rhythm of urinary 17-ketosteroid excretion has been described.[7] Earlier data suggesting a seasonal rhythm in catecholamine excretion[259,260] have not been confirmed.[261] Rather than citing additional examples (for an extensive review, see the monograph of De Rudder [262]), one further example may suffice. Figure 156-44 depicts the monthly weight gain of Swedish children, illustrating a seasonal rhythm with the pattern in part apparently depending on the latitude.[263]

Many natural environmental factors as well as cultural habits probably contribute to all these phenomena, but it is also likely that they may act on a residual endogenous rhythm. If the examples cited above can be considered as circannual rhythms, the question arises as to by what Zeitgebers such rhythms are synchronized. Again, social Zeitgebers may play a role, but other factors such as

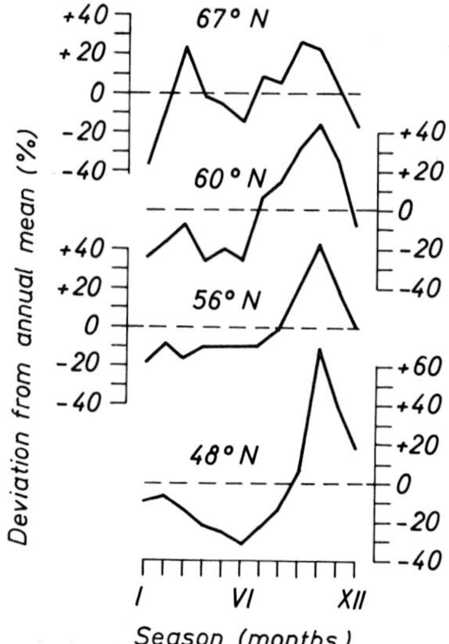

Fig. 156-44. Seasonal rhythm of gain in body weight in Swedish boys and girls, 6 to 14 years old. (Data from ref. 263.)

the changing photoperiod—one of the main Zeitgebers for circannual rhythms in animals—cannot be excluded. There is ample evidence for profound seasonal effects of light on man, as already claimed by Lindhard on the basis of his observations in the high Arctic.[264]

IN DISEASE

A disease state can be associated with malfunction of a normal "clock" or with the appearance of new periodic phenomena. These latter presumably arise from foci that have been removed from inhibition or have acquired de novo an innate periodicity. Previous discussions of periodic disease[265,266] have been concerned with the appearance of new periodic phenomena; it has only been recently that the first possibility, i.e., malfunction of a "normal" clock, has been considered as being etiological of disease.

Possible Malfunction of Normal Rhythms

Functional.

Cushing's Disease. One of the hallmarks of this disease is the absence of the normal circadian periodicity of plasma ACTH and cortisol concentrations. Morning levels may be normal or elevated and remain at this level throughout the 24-hour period. The observation of the lack of the normal nocturnal rise of plasma growth hormone[209] and prolactin[267] concentrations and absence of EEG slow-wave sleep[209] in patients with this disease, both when clinically active and in remission, has led to the suggestion that an abnormality in central nervous system function, perhaps in neurotransmitter action or content leading to loss of normal inhibitory mechanisms for CRF release, is the etiologic factor in this disease. It is of interest in this regard that patients with hypothalamic-limbic system disease also manifest abnormal periodicity of plasma ACTH and corticosteroid concentrations[268] (Fig. 156-45).

In addition to such postulated malfunction, there have been instances where the manifestations of Cushing's disease have appeared in a cyclic manner with evidence of interim clinical and laboratory remission between episodes. The most striking of these is presented in a case report wherein there was association of periodic fever, nausea and vomiting, hypertension, weight change, and increased urinary corticosteroid and epinephrine excretion.[269] It has long been known, however, that in the more classical form of Cushing's disease, continued studies will reveal alternating periods of normal and increased corticosteroid secretion.[270]

The phenomenon of intermittency of secretion is by no means limited to Cushing's disease. There is abundant clinical evidence of intermittency of secretion in patients with insulinomas, parathyroid adenomata, and pheochromytomas, although the reason for such intermittency is completely unknown.

Acromegaly. A similar suggestion of a functional central nervous system abnormality has been put forth with regard to acromegaly, even in those cases associated with evidence of a pituitary tumor. The lack of nonautonomy of some of these tumors in response to agents that provoke or inhibit growth hormone release, together with evidence of random episodes of growth hormone secretion unaccompanied by normal nocturnal rise, suggests that a loss of the rhythmic regulation of such growth hormone secretion may be etiologic in the pathogenesis of the disease.[271]

Stein-Leventhal Syndrome. This syndrome, which is characterized by uninterrupted estrogen production, anovulation, and moderately persistently elevated LH levels (without evidence of the

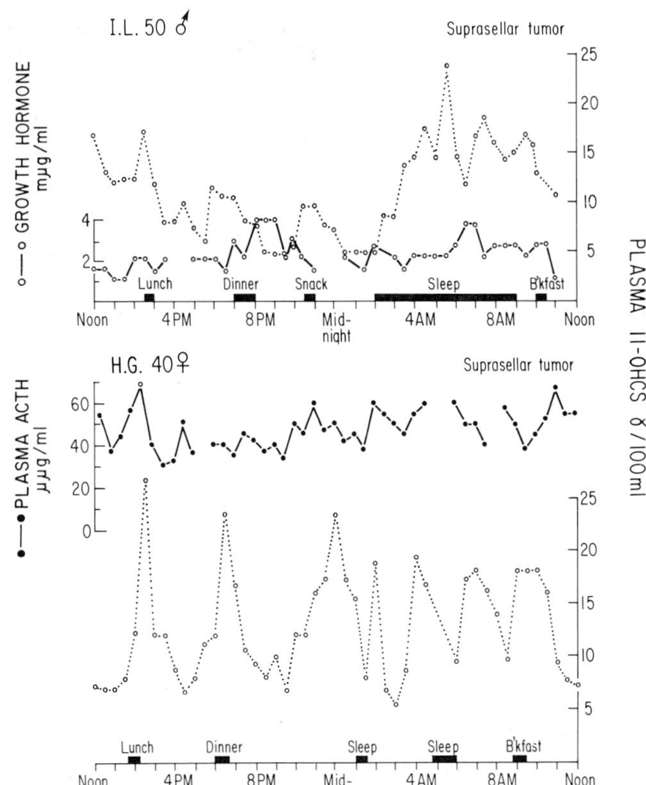

Fig. 156-45. Circadian periodicity of plasma cortisol and ACTH or growth hormone levels in two endocrinologically normal, nonobese patients with radiographically demonstrated hypothalamic tumors (normal sella turcica).

midluteal peak), bears a striking resemblance to the animal model of the neonatally androgenized female rat. In this latter model, it is assumed that there is a "masculinized" hypothalamus, with resultant constant, rather than cyclic, secretion of LH.

Organic Central Nervous System Disease. Several types of evidence may be cited in this regard. Abnormal periodicity of plasma cortisol concentrations[268] and of urinary electrolyte concentrations[272] has been reported in patients with disease involving the hypothalamic-limbic area in the absence of overt clinical endocrine symptomatology. Reiman has reported several cases of periodic nonendocrine disorders associated with lesions in the thalamus or hypothalamus.[273] There is a circadian periodicity in the time of occurrence of epileptic seizures, with the greatest number of such seizures occurring after the time of awakening.

In Blind Subjects. In view of the postulated (and somewhat controversial) role of the light–dark cycle as a Zeitgeber for circadian rhythms, the nature of hormonal periodicity in blind subjects is a matter of considerable interest. From a survey of 13 publications[26,66,274–284] which report measurements of a variety of rhythmic phenomena in a total of 190 patients without light perception (congenital or acquired) living under normal social conditions in normal environmental lighting, the following conclusions emerge: virtually no rhythms are seen in 16.0 percent of such patients, more or less normal rhythms in 30.5 percent, and rhythms with a reduced range of oscillation and with abnormal phase relations to Zeitgebers (light–dark or sleep–wake) in 53.5 percent. In discussing these figures, one has to keep in mind Lund's study[26] on 7 totally blind subjects, all of whom showed clear free-running circadian rhythms when living without time cues in the isolation chamber (see Fig. 156-9). These two observations, i.e., "abnormal'' periodicity in blind subjects living under natural conditions and free-running of periodicity under conditions of isolation, raise the question of whether the abnormality in blind subjects is one of less precise entrainment of an endogenous rhythm rather than an abnormality of the rhythm per se. The possibility that the various rhythms are free-running in blind subjects has been suggested in several studies[26,276,282] and recently confirmed for the plasma corticosteroid rhythm by Orth (unpublished observations).

Other Periodic Illness

Richter[265] has listed the major manifestations occurring in various categories of clinical periodic disease (Table 156-1). These diseases manifest different periodicities (though amazingly constant in a given patient), varying from every 12 hours to every 4 to 5 months, although longer periodicities of up to 2 years have been described (Fig. 156-46). The frequencies of longer duration are seen mostly in instances of psychiatric disease, where the time intervals may not exactly be duplicated in a given patient.[285]

The relationship of mania and depression to decreased and elevated levels respectively of urinary corticosteroid excretion has been commented upon by several investigators[268] (Fig. 156-47). "Disrupted" circadian patterns of plasma corticosteroid concentrations have also been reported in patients with depression; it appears that the abnormality is not one of period but rather one of an increased number and amplitude of secretory episodes.[287]

There is suggestive (unpublished) evidence that patients with

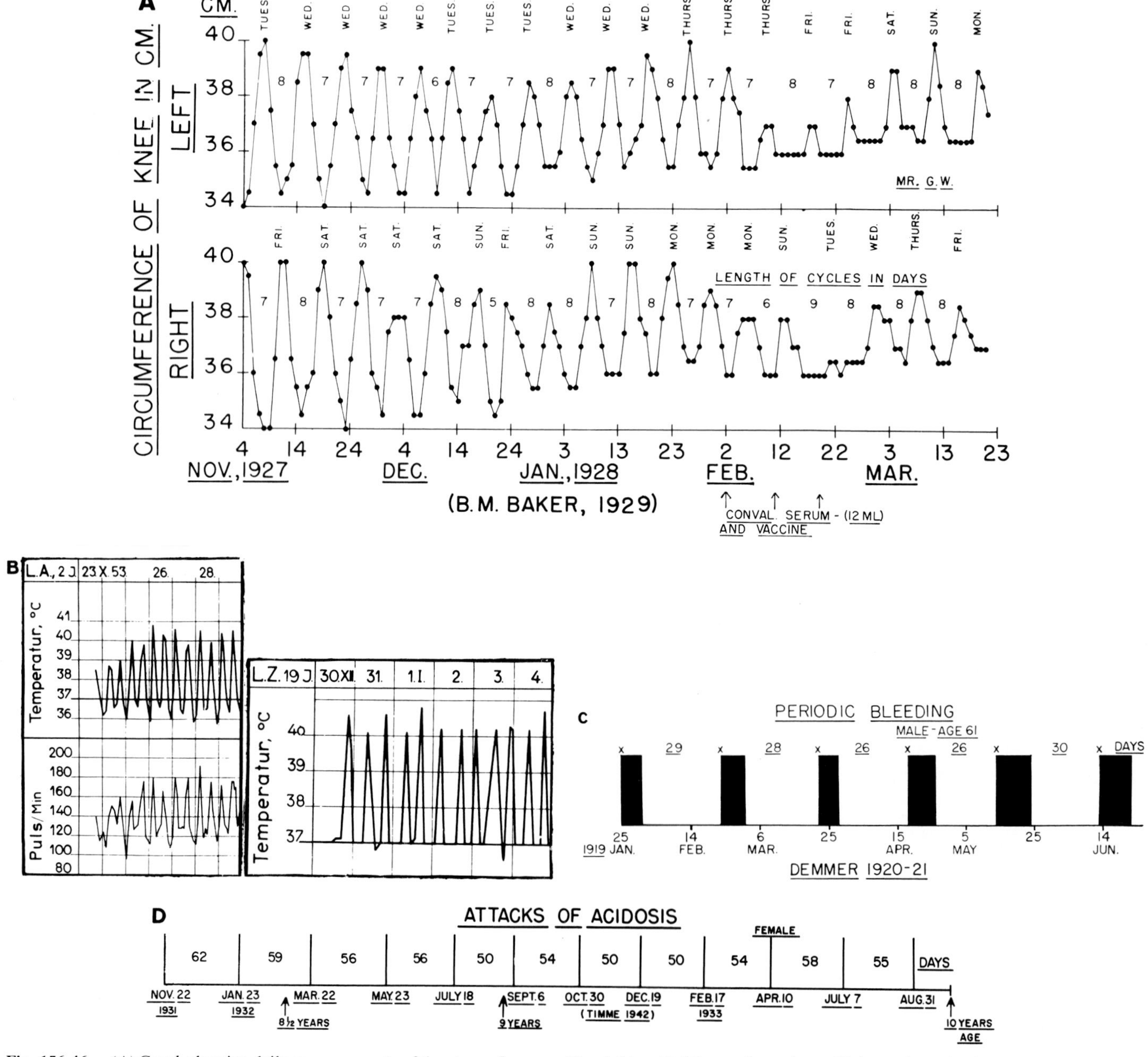

Fig. 156-46. *(A)* Graph showing daily measurements of the circumference of the right and left knee of a patient with intermittent hydrarthrosis. *(B)* Graph showing 12-hour peaks of body temperature and pulse rate of a 2-year-old girl (L.A.) and of the body temperature of her mother (L.Z.) at age of 19. *(C)* Record showing attacks of periodic bleeding in a 61-year-old man. *(D)* Record showing recurring attacks of acidosis in 8-year-old girl.

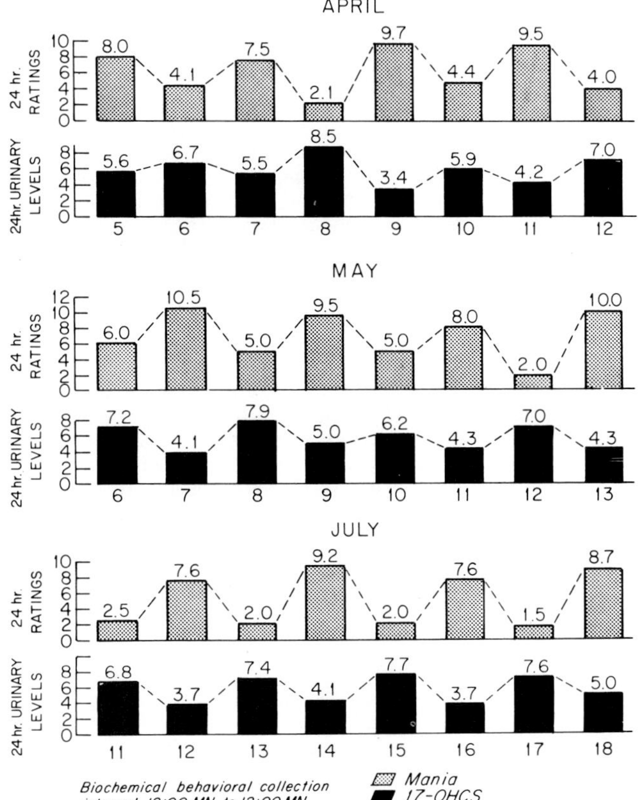

Fig. 156-47. Concordance of decreased urinary corticosteroid levels with increased rating of mania. (Data from ref. 286.)

manic-depressive psychosis may suffer from internal desynchronization of several body rhythms; i.e., such rhythms may not exhibit the phase relationship to each other seen in normal individuals. The observed desynchronization appears to be secondary to a shortening of the periodicity of some parameters. This is of interest in view of the reported efficacy of lithium treatment in such conditions, since it has also been observed that in plants, exposure to lithium results in an increase in period length.[288]

Chronotherapy

Apart from periodic phenomena in the genesis of disease, it is also becoming increasingly evident that periodic phenomena are involved in the therapy of a disease. The emerging field of chronopharmacology is based on the observations that at different points of the circadian cycle there are marked differences in the LD_{50} of a given drug and its therapeutic efficiency in terms of increased survival with a given dosage schedule (perhaps most dramatically shown in the treatment of mouse leukemia with adriamycin).[146] The basis for such circadian variation in drug efficacy remains to be fully explored—some possible factors that may be involved are the circadian periodicity of cell or bacterial division and function and the circadian periodicity of drug-metabolizing enzymes.

Endocrine "chronotherapy" has been practiced for several years, taking advantage of the observation that the pituitary-adrenal axis is much more sensitive to suppression by exogenous corticosteroid administration given prior to the time of the circadian rise in plasma ACTH and corticosteroid concentrations than when corticosteroids are administered after the circadian rise.

Such "chronotherapy" can and has been used in approximating the normal periodicity of hormonal secretion when replacement therapy is required, e.g., in Addison's disease, where patients report greater well-being on such a regimen than when replacement medication is given in equally spaced doses—which does not simulate normal adrenal circadian periodicity. It has also formed the basis for the alternate-morning method of steroid treatment for nonendocrine diseases requiring such treatment, whereby such a regimen lessens the likelihood of prolonged CNS-pituitary-adrenal suppression by allowing for the normal circadian rise on the "off" day of such a treatment schedule. Such morning steroid treatment may be of special importance in growing children in that the nocturnal rise of plasma growth hormone levels will not be suppressed (which may be the case in long-term around-the-clock steroid treatment). Conversely, when maximal pituitary-adrenal suppression is required, as in the case of the treatment of congenital adrenal hyperplasia, greater suppression with a given dose of corticosteroid is obtained when this is given at approximately midnight, so that the subsequent circadian rise is completely abolished.

There is suggestive evidence already that the time of thiazide administration may be associated with variation in diuretic response. From the discussion above with regard to circadian variation in insulin sensitivity, chronotherapy may be efficacious in the treatment of insulin-dependent diabetics. It is to be anticipated that in the near future, many new applications of this mode of therapy will be seen.

REFERENCES

1. Nankin, H. R., Troen P.: Repetitive luteinizing hormone elevations in serum of normal men. *J Clin Endocrinol Metab 33:* 558–560, 1971.
2. Nankin, H. R., Troen, P.: Overnight patterns of serum luteinizing hormone in normal men. *J Clin Endocrinol Metab 35:* 705–710, 1972.
3. Klotter, K.: General properties of oscillating systems. *Cold Spring Harbor Symp Quant Biol 25:* 185–187, 1960.
4. Hildebrandt, G.: Grundlagen einer angewandten medizinischen Rhythmusforschung. *Heilkunst 71:* 117–136, 1958.
5. Halberg, F.: Physiologic 24-hour periodicity; general and procedural considerations with reference to the adrenal cycle. *Z Vitam, Horm Fermentfsch 10:* 225–296, 1959.
6. Aschoff, J.: Adaptive Cycles: Their significance for defining environmental hazards. *Int J Biometeor 11:* 255-278, 1967.
7. Halberg, F., Engeli, M., Hamburger, C. H. et al: Spectral resolution of low-frequency, small-amplitude rhythms in excreted 17-ketosteroids; probable androgen-induced circaseptan desynchronization. *Acta Endocrinol 50:* 5–54, 1965.
8. Halberg, F., Reinberg, A.: Rythmes circadiens et rythmes de basses frequences en physiologie humaine. *J Physiol 59:* 117–200, 1967.
9. Halberg, F., Tong, Y. C., Johnson, E. A.: Circadian system phase—an aspect of temporal morphology; procedures and illustrative examples, in Mayersbach, H von (ed): The Cellular Aspects of Biorhythms. New York, Springer, 1965, p 20.
10. Pittendrigh, C. S.: Adaptation, natural selection and behavior, in Roe, A. and Simpson, G. G. (eds): Behavior and Evolution. New Haven, Yale University Press, 1961, p 390.
11. Aschoff, J., Wever, R.: Biologische Rhythmen and Regelung, in Bad Oeynhausener Gespraeche V, Probleme der zentralnervoesen Regulation. Berlin, Springer, 1961, p 1.
12. Aschoff, J.: Survival value of diurnal rhythms. *Symp Zool Soc Lond, 13:* 79–98, 1964.
13. Rusak, B., Zucker, I.: Biological rhythms and animal behavior. *Annu Rev Psychol 26:* 137–171, 1975.
14. Pittendrigh, C. S.: Circadian rhythms and the circadian organization of living systems. *Cold Spring Harbor Symp Quant Biol 25:* 159–184, 1960.
15. Aschoff, J.: Response curves in circadian periodicity, in Aschoff, J. (ed): Circadian Clocks, Proceedings of the Feldafing Summer School. Amsterdam, North-Holland, 1965, p 95.
16. Halberg, F., Johnson, E. A., Nelson, W., et al: Autorhythmome-

try-procedures for physiologic self-measurements and their analysis. *Physiol Teacher 1:* 1–11, 1972.

17. Aschoff, J., Klotter, K., Wever, R.: Circadian vocabulary, in Aschoff, J. (ed): Circadian Clocks, Proceedings of the Feldafing Summer School. Amsterdam, North-Holland, 1965, p XI.
18. Halberg, F., Katinas, G. S.: Chronobiologic glossary. *Int J Chronobiol 1:* 31–63, 1973.
19. Halberg, F., Lee J-K: Glossary of selected chronobiologic terms, in Scheving, L. E., Halberg, F., Pauly, J. E. (eds): Chronobiology. Stuttgart, Georg Thieme, 1974, p. XXXVII.
20. Pittendrigh, C. S.: On temperature independence in the clock system controlling emergence time in *Drosophila. Proc Natl Acad Sci 40:* 1018–1029, 1954.
21. Hastings, J. W., Sweeny, B. M.: On the mechanism of temperature independence in a biological clock. *Proc Natl Acad Sci 43:* 804–811, 1957.
22. Tharp, G. D., Folk, G. E.: Rhythmic changes in rate of the mammalian heart and heart cells during prolonged isolation. *Comp Biochem Physiol 14:* 225–273, 1965.
23. Andrews, R. V.: Temporal secretory responses of cultured hamster adrenals. *Comp Biochem Physiol 26:* 179–193, 1968.
24. Shiotsuka, R., Jovonovich, J., Jovonovich, J. A.: In vitro data on drug sensitivity: Circadian and ultradian corticosterone rhythms in adrenal organ cultures, in Chronobiological Aspects of Endocrinology. *Symposia Medica Hoechst 9.* Stuttgart, Schattauer, 1974, p 255–267.
25. Hardeland, R.: Circadian rhythmicity in cultured liver cells. I. Rhythms in tyrosine aminotransferase activity and inducibility and in (H) leucine incorporation. *Int J Biochem 4:* 581–590, 1973.
25a. Wilson, M. M., Rice, R. W., Critchlow, V.: Evidence for a free-running circadian rhythm in pituitary-adrenal function in blinded adult female rats. *Neuroendocrinology 20:* 289–295, 1976.
25b. Wilson, M. M., Greer, M. A.: Evidence for a free-running pituitary-adrenal circadian rhythm in constant light-treated adult rats. *Proc Soc Exp Biol Med 154:* 69–71, 1977.
25c. Morin, L. P., Fitzgerald, K. M., Zucker, I.: Estradiol shortens the period of hamster circadian rhythms. *Science 196:* 305–307, 1977.
26. Lund, R.: Circadiane Periodik physiologischer und psychologischer Variablen bei 7 blinden Versuchspersonen mit und ohne Zeitgeber. *Med Thesis,* 1974.
27. Kriebel, J.: Changes in internal phase relationships during isolation, in Scheving, L. E., Halberg, F., Pauly, J. E. (eds): Chronobiology. Stuttgart, Georg Thieme, 1974, p 451.
28. Aschoff, J., Wever, R.: Circadian period and phase-angle difference in chaffinches (Fringilla coelebs L.). *Comp Biochem Physiol 18:* 397–404, 1966.
29. Pittendrigh, C. S.: On the mechanism of the entrainment of a circadian rhythm by light cycles, in Aschoff, J. (ed): Circadian Clocks, Proceedings of the Feldafing Summer School. Amsterdam, North-Holland, 1965, p 277.
30. Hoffmann, K.: Zum einfluss der Zeitgeberstaerke auf die Phasenlage Periodik synchronisierten circadianen Periodik. *Z Vergl Physiol 62:* 93–110. 1969.
31. Stupfel, M., Halberg, E., Halberg, F.: L'accés alimentaire périodique des rats groupés surmonte l'alternance lumieŕe-obscurité comme synchroniseur du rhythme circadien d'emission de gaz carbonique. *CR Acad Sci Paris 277:* 873–876, 1973.
32. Hayden, P., Lindberg, R. G.: Circadian rhythm in mammalian body temperature entrained by cyclic pressure changes. *Science 164:* 1288–1289, 1969.
33. Gwinner, E.: Entrainment of a circadian rhythm in birds by species-specific song cycles (Aves, Fringillidae: Carduelis spinus, Serinus serinus). *Experientia 22:* 765, 1966.
34. Aschoff, J.: Exogenous and endogenous components in circadian rhythms. *Cold Spring Harbor Symp Quant Biol 25:* 11–28, 1960.
35. Aschoff, J., Hoffman, K., Pohl, H., et al: Re-entrainment of circadian rhythms after phase shifts of the Zeitgeber. *Chronobiologia 2:* 23–78, 1975.
36. Pittendrigh, C. S.: Circadian oscillations in cells and the circadian organization of multicellular systems, in Schmitt, F. O., Worden, F. G. (eds): The Neurosciences, Third Study Program. Cambridge, Mass., MIT Press, 1974, p 437.
37. Hoffman, K.: Circadiane Periodik bei Tupaias (Tupaia glis) in konstanten Bedingungen. *Zool Anz Suppl 33:* 171–177, 1970.
38. Aschoff, J.: Circadian activity pattern with two peaks. *Ecology 47:* 657–662, 1966.
39. Aschoff, J., Wever, R.: Human circadian rhythms: A multi-oscillator system. *Fed Proc 35:* 2326–2332, 1976.
40. Wever, R.: The circadian multi-oscillator system of man. *Int J Chronobiol 3:* 19–55, 1975.
40a. Page, T. L., Caldarola, P. C., Pittendrigh, C. S.: Mutual entrainment of bilaterally distributed circadian pacemakers. *Proc Nat Acad Sci 74:* 1277–1281, 1977.
41. Wisser, H., Doerr, P., Stamm, D., et al: Tagesperiodik der Ausscheidung von Elektrolyten, Katecholaminmetaboliten und 17-Hydroxycorticosteroiden im Harn. *Klin Wschr 51:* 242–246, 1973.
42. Krieger, D. T., Allen, W., Rizzo, F., et al: Characterization of the normal temporal pattern of plasma corticosteroid levels. *J Clin Endocrinol 32:* 266–284, 1971.
42a. Tanaka, K., Orth, D. N.: Diurnal rhythm in plasma β-lipotropin (β-LPH) in man. *Clin Res 25:* 15A, 1977.
43. Halberg, F., Reinhardt, J., Bartter, F. C., et al: Agreement in endpoints from circadian rhythmometry on healthy human beings living on different continents. *Experientia 25:* 107–112, 1969.
44. Lacerda, L. de, Kowarski, A., Migeon, C. J.: Integrated concentration and diurnal variation of plasma cortisol. *J Clin Endocrinol Metab 36:* 227–238, 1973.
45. Orth, D. N., Island, D. P., Liddle, G. W.: Experimental alteration of the circadian rhythm in plasma cortisol (17-OHCS) concentration in man. *J Clin Endocrinol 27:* 549–555, 1967.
46. Rose, R. M., Kreuz, L. E., Holaday, J. W. et al: Diurnal variation of plasma testosterone and cortisol. *J. Endocrinol 54:* 177–178, 1972.
47. Weitzman, E. D., Fukushima, D., Nogeire, C., et al: Twenty-four hour pattern of the episodic secretion of cortisol in normal subjects. *J Clin Endocrinol 33:* 14–22, 1971.
48. Fuller, R., Diller, E. R.: Diurnal variation of liver glycogen and plasma free fatty acids in rats fed ad libitum or single daily meal. *Metabolism 19:* 226–229, 1970.
49. Holmgren, H. J., Swensson, A.: Der Einfluss des Lichtes auf den 24- Stundenrhythmus der Aktivitat, des Leberglykogens und der Koerpertemperatur. *Acta Med Scand 278:* 71–76, 1953.
50. Peret, J., Macaire, I., Chanez, M.: Schedule of protein ingestion, nitrogen and energy utilization and circadian rhythm of hepatic glycogen, plasma corticosterone and insulin in rats. *J Nutr 103:* 866–874, 1973.
51. Seckel, H. P. G., Kato, K.: Development of the diurnal cycle of liver function in nursing rats. *Arch Pathol 25:* 247–360, 1938.
52. Critchlow, V., Liebelt, R. A., Bar-Sela, M., et al: Sex difference in resting pituitary-adrenal function in the rat. *Am J Physiol 205:* 807–815, 1963.
53. Krieger, D. T.: Circadian corticosteroid periodicity: critical period for abolition by neonatal injection of corticosteroid. *Science 178:* 1205–1207, 1972.
54. Moberg, G. P., Scapagnini, U., Groot de J., et al: Effect of sectioning the fornix on diurnal fluctuation in plasma corticosterone levels in the rat. *Neuroendocrinology 7:* 11–15, 1971.
55. Szafarczyk, A., Boisson, J., Assenmacher, I.: Effets du niveau d'éclairement sure le rythme circadien de la corticostéronemie chez la ratte. *CR Acad Sci Paris 273:* 2583–2586, 1971.
56. Haus, E., Halberg, F.: Persisting circadian rhythm in hepatic glycogen of mice during inanition and dehydration. *Experientia 22:* 113–114, 1966.
57. Haus, E., Lakatua, D., Halberg, F.: The internal timing of several circadian rhythms in the blinded mouse. *Exp Med Surg 25:* 7–45, 1967.
58. Mayersbach H. von: Seasonal influences on biological rhythms of standardized laboratory animals. In Mayersbach, H. von (ed): The Cellular Aspects of Biorhythms, Berlin, Springer, 1967, p 87–99.
59. Vilchez, C. A., Saffe de Vilchez, I. E.: Circadian rhythm in mouse liver phosphorylase activity. *J Interdiscipl Cycle Res 2:* 55–62, 1971.
60. Haus, E., Halberg, F.: Circannual rhythm in level and timing of serum corticosterone in standardized inbred mature c-mice. *Environ Res 3:* 81–106, 1970.
61. Halberg, F., Albrecht, P. G., Bittner, J. J.: Corticosterone rhythm of mouse adrenal in relation to serum corticosterone and sampling. *Am J Physiol 197:* 1083–1085, 1959.
62. Nelson, W.: Aspects of circadian periodic changes in phosphorus metabolism in mice. *Am J Physiol 206:* 589–598, 1964.
63. Halberg, F., Simpson, H.: Circadian acrophases of human 17-

hydroxycorticosteroid excretion referred to midsleep rather than midnight. *Hum Biol 39:* 405–413, 1967.

64. Breuer, H., Kaulhausen, H., Muhlbauer, W., et al: Circadian rhythm of the renin-angiotensin-aldosterone system, in Chronobiological Aspects of Endocrinology, Symposia Medica Hoechst 9. Stuttgart, Schattauer, 1974, p 101.
65. Grim, C., Winnacker, J., Peters, T., et al: Low renin, "normal" aldosterone and hypertension: Circadian rhythm of renin, aldosterone, cortisol, and growth hormone. *J Clin Endocrinol Metab 39:* 247–256, 1974.
66. Krieger, D. T., Kreuzer, J., Rizzo, F. A.: Constant light: Effect on circadian pattern and phase reversal of steroid and electrolyte levels in man. *J Clin Endocrinol Metab 29:* 1634–1638, 1969.
67. Weitzman, E. D., Goldmacher, D., Kripke, D., et al: Reversal of sleep-waking cycle: Effect on sleep stage pattern and certain neuroendocrine rhythms. *Trans Am Neurol Assoc 93:* 153–157, 1968.
68. Weitzman, E. D., Nogeire, C., Perlow, M., et al: Effects of a prolonged 3-hour sleep-wake cycle on sleep stages, plasma cortisol, growth hormone and body temperature in man. *J Clin Endocrinol Metab 38:* 1018–1030, 1974.
69. Doe, R. P., Vennes, I. A., Flink, E. D.: Diurnal variation of 17-hydroxycorticosteroids, sodium, potassium, magnesium and creatinine in normal subjects and in cases of treated adrenal insufficiency and Cushing's syndrome. *J Clin Endocrinol Metab 20:* 253–265, 1960.
70. Fullerton, D. T., Wenzel, F. J., Lohrenz, F. N. et al: Circadian rhythm of adrenal cortical activity in depression. II. A comparison of types in depression. *Arch Gen Psychiatr 19:* 682–688, 1968.
71. Nicoloff, J. T., Fisher, D. A., Appleman, M. D. Jr.: The role of glucocorticoids in the regulation of thyroid function in man. *J Clin Invest 49:* 1922–1929, 1970.
72. Sholiton, L. J., Werk, E. E., Marnell, R. T.: Diurnal variation of adrenocortical function in non-endocrine disease states. *Metabolism 10:* 632–646, 1959.
73. Doe, R. P., Flink, E. D., Goodsell, M.: Relationship of diurnal variation in 17-hydroxycorticosteroid levels in blood and urine to eosinophils and electrolyte excretion. *J Clin Endocrinol Metab 16:* 192–206, 1956.
74. Reinberg, A., Ghata, J., Halberg, F., et al: Distribution temporelle du traitement de l'insuffisance corticosurrenalienne. Essai de chronotherapeutique. *Ann Endocrinol 32:* 566–573, 1971.
75. Simpson, H. W., Lobban, M. C.: Effect of a 21-hour day on the human circadian excretory rhythms of 17-hydroxycorticosteroids and electrolytes. *Aerospace Med 38:* 1205–1213, 1967.
76. Sato, T., George, J. C.: Diurnal rhythm of corticotropin-releasing factor activity in the pigeon hypothalamus. *Can J Physiol Pharmacol 51:* 743–747, 1973.
77. Hiroshige, T., Sakakura, M., Itoh, S.: Diurnal variation of corticotropin-releasing activity in the rat hypothalamus. *Endocrinol Jpn 16:* 465–469, 1969.
78. Hiroshige, T., Abe, K., Wada, S., et al: Sex difference in circadian periodicity of CRF activity in the rat hypothalamus. *Neuroendocrinology 11:* 306–320, 1973.
79. Halberg, F., Galicich, J. H., Ungar, F. et al: Circadian rhythmic pituitary adrenocorticotropic activity, rectal temperature and pinnal mitosis of starving, dehydrated C mice. *Proc Soc Exp Biol Med 118:* 414–419, 1965.
79a. Ungar, F., Halberg, F.: In vitro exploration of a circadian rhythm in adrenocorticotropic activity of C mouse hypophysis. *Experientia 19:* 158, 1963.
80. Lakatua, D. J., Haus, E., Gold, E. M., et al: Circadian rhythm of ACTH and growth hormone in human blood; time relations to adrenocortical (blood and urinary) rhythms, in Scheving, L. E., Halberg, F., Pauly, J. E. (eds): Chronobiology. *Stuttgart, Georg Thieme,* 1974, p 123–129.
81. Nokin, J., Vekemans, M., L'Hermite, M., et al: Circadian periodicity of serum prolactin concentration in man. *Br Med J 3:* 561–562, 1972.
82. Parker, D. C., Rossman, L. G., VanderLaan, E. F.: Sleep related, nyctohemeral and briefly episodic variation in human plasma prolactin concentrations. *J Clin Endocrinol Metab 36:* 1119–1124, 1973.
83. Sassin, J. F., Frantz, A. G., Weitzman, E. D., et al: Human prolactin: 24-hour pattern with increased release during sleep. *Science 177:* 1205–1207, 1972.
84. Sassin, J. F., Frantz, A. G., Kapen, S., et al: The nocturnal rise of human prolactin is dependent on sleep. *J Clin Endocrinol Metab 37:* 436–440, 1973.
85. Perlow, M., Sassin, J., Boyar, R., et al: Reduction of growth hormone secretion following clomiphene administration. *Metabolism 22:* 1269–1275, 1973.
86. Quabbe, H. J., Schilling, E., Helge, H.: Pattern of growth hormone secretion during a 24-hour fast in normal adults. *J Clin Endocrinol Metab 26:* 1173–1177, 1966.
87. Alford, F. P., Baker, H. W. G., Patel, Y. C., et al: Temporal patterns of circulating hormones as assessed by continuous blood sampling. *J Clin Endocrinol Metab 36:* 108–116, 1973.
88. Goldsmith, S. J., Glick, S. M.: Rhythmicity of human growth hormone secretion. *Mt Sinai J Med NY 27:* 501–508, 1970.
89. Morris, H. G.: Circadian pattern of plasma growth hormone concentration. *Chronobiologia 2 (Suppl 1):* 49, 1975.
90. Faiman, C., Winter, J. S.: Diurnal cycles in plasma FSH, testosterone and cortisol in men. *J Clin Endocrinol 33:* 186–193, 1971.
91. Gordon, R. D., Spinks, J., Dulmanis, A., et al: Amplitude and phase relations of several circadian rhythms in human plasma and urine: Demonstration of rhythm for tetrahydrocortisol and tetrahydrocorticosterone. *Clin Sci 35:* 307–324, 1968.
92. Nieschlag, E., Ismail, A. A.: Diurnal variations of plasma testosterone in normal and pathological conditions as measured by the technique of competitive protein binding. *J Endocrinol 46:* 3–4, 1970.
93. Saxena, B. B., Leyendecker, G., Chen, W., et al: Radioimmunoassay of follicle-stimulating (FSH) and luteinizing (LH) hormones by chromatoelectrophoreses. *Acta Endocrinol Suppl 142:* 185–206, 1969.
94. Smals, A. G. H., Kloppenberg, P. W. C., Benraad, T. J.: Diurnal plasma testosterone rhythm and the effect of short-term ACTH administration on plasma testosterone in man. *J Clin Endocrinol Metab 38:* 606–611, 1974.
95. Southren, A., Gordon, G. G., Tochimoto, G. et al: Mean plasma concentration, metabolic clearance and basal plasma production rates of testosterone in normal young men and women using a constant infusion procedure: Effect of time of day and plasma concentration on the metabolic clearance rate of testosterone. *J Clin Endocrinol Metab 27:* 686–694, 1967.
96. Lacerda, L.de, Kowarski, A., Johanson, A. J., et al: Integrated concentration and circadian variation of plasma testosterone in normal men. *J Clin Endocrinol Metab 37:* 366–371, 1973.
97. Lincoln, G. A., Rowe, P. H., Racey, R. A.: The circadian rhythm in plasma testosterone concentration in man, in Chronobiological Aspects of Endocrinology. *Symposia Medica Hoechst*. Stuttgart, Schattauer, 1974, p 101–109.
98. Krieger, D. T., Ossowski, R., Fogel, M., et al: Lack of circadian periodicity of human serum FSH and LH levels. *J Clin Endocrinol Metab 35:* 619–623, 1972.
99. Faiman, C., Ryan, R. J.: Diurnal cycle in serum concentrations of follicle-stimulating hormone in men. *Nature 215:* 857, 1967.
100. Kapen, S. H., Boyar, R., Perlow, M., et al: Luteinizing hormone: changes in secretory pattern during sleep in adult women. *Life Sci 13:* 693–701, 1973.
101. Boyar, R., Perlow, M., Hellman, L., et al: Twenty-four hour pattern of Luteinizing hormone secretion in normal men with sleep stage recordings. *J Clin Endocrinol Metab 35:* 73–81, 1972.
102. Peterson, N. T. Jr., Midgley, A. R. Jr., Jaffe, R. B.: Regulation of human gonadotropins. III. Luteinizing hormone and follicle-stimulating in sera from adult males. *J Clin Endocrinol Metab 28:* 1473–1478, 1968.
103. Rowe, P. H., Racey, P. A., Lincoln, G. A., et al: The temporal relationship between the secretion of luteinizing hormone and testosterone in man. *J Endocrinol 64:* 17–26, 1975.
104. Nieschlag, E.: Circadian rhythm of plasma testosterone, in Chronobiological Aspects of Endocrinology. *Symposia Medica Hoechst 9*. Stuttgart, Schattauer, 1974.
104a. Fukuda, H., Greer, M. A., Roberts, L., Allen, C. F., Critchlow, V., Wilson, M.: Nyctohemeral and sex-related variations in plasma thyrotropin, thyroxine and triiodothyronine. *Endocrinology 97:* 1424–1431, 1975.
104b. Collu, R., Du Ruisseau, P., Tache, Y., Ducharme, J. R.: Thyrotropin-releasing hormone in rat brain: Nyctohemeral variations. *Endocrinology 100:* 1391–1393, 1977.
104c. Parker, D. C., Pekary, A. E., Hershman, J. M.: Effect of normal and reversed sleep-wake cycles upon nyctohemeral rhythmicity of

plasma thyrotropin: Evidence suggestive of an inhibitory influence in sleep. *J Clin Endocrinol Metab 43:* 318–329, 1976.

104d. Georg, C. P. L., Messerli, F. H., Genest, J., Nowaczynski, W., Boucher, R., Kuchel, O., Ortega, R. O.: Diurnal variation of plasma vasopressin in man. *J Clin Endocrinol Metab 41:* 332–338, 1975.

104e. Rubin, R. T., Poland, R. E., Ravessoud, F., Gouin, P. R., Tower, B. B.: Antidiuretic hormone: Episodic nocturnal secretion in adult men. *Endocrinol Res Comm 2:* 461–469, 1975.

104f. Gomez-Sanchez, C., Holland, O. B., Higgins, J. R., Kem, D. C., Kaplan, N. M.: Circadian rhythms of serum renin activity and serum corticosterone, prolactin, and aldosterone concentrations in the male rat on normal and low sodium diets. *Endocrinology 99:* 567–572, 1976.

105. Gordon, R. D., Wolfe, K., Island, D. P. et al: A diurnal rhythm in plasma renin activity in man. *J Clin Invest 45:* 1587–1592, 1966.

106. Deschamps, I., Heilbronner, J., Canivet, J., et al: Les variations spontanées de l'insuline au cours des vingt-quatre heures chez des sujets normaux. *La Presse Médicale 77:* 1815–1817, 1969.

107. Boissin, J., Assenmacher, I.: Entrainment of the adrenal cortical rhythm and of the locomotor activity rhythm by ahemeral photoperiods in the quail. *J Interdiscipl Cycle Res 2:* 437–443, 1971.

108. El-Halawani, M. E., Waibel, P. E., Appel, J. R., et al: Effects of temperature stress on catecholamines and corticosterone of male turkeys. *Am J Physiol 224:* 384–388, 1973.

109. Jacoby, J. H., Sassin, J. F., Greenstein, M., et al: Patterns of spontaneous cortisol and growth hormone secretion in rhesus monkeys during the sleep-waking cycle. *Neuroendocrinology 14:* 165–173, 1974.

110. Aschoff, J., Fatranska, M., Giedke, H., et al: Human circadian rhythms in continuous darkness: Entrainment by social cues. *Science 171:* 213–215,1971.

111. Fioretti, M. C., Riccardi, C., Menconi, E., et al: Control of the circadian rhythm of the body temperature in the rat. *Life Sci 14:* 2111–2119, 1974.

112. Friedman, A. H., Walker, Ch. A.: Circadian rhythms in rat midbrain and caudate nucleus biogenic amine levels. *J Physiol 197:* 77–85, 1968.

113. Kayser, C. H.: Recherches sur le rythme circadien de la consommation d'oxygene du rat blanc. *Arch Sci Physiol 24:* 439–456, 1970.

114. Krieger, D. T.: Food and water restriction shifts corticosterone, temperature, activity and brain amine periodicity. *Endocrinology 95:* 1195–1201, 1974.

115. Knapp, M. S., Keane, P. M., Wright, J. G.: Circadian rhythm of plasma 11-hydroxycorticosteroids in depressive illness, congestive heart failure and Cushing's syndrome. *Br Med J 2:* 27–30, 1967.

116. Perkoff, G. T., Eik-Nes, K., Nugent, C. A., et al: Studies of the diurnal variation of plasma 17-hydroxycorticosteroids in man. *J Clin Endocrinol Metab 19:* 432–443, 1959.

117. David-Nelson, M. A., Brodish, A.: Evidence for a diurnal rhythm of corticotrophin releasing factor (CRF) in the hypothalamus. *Endocrinology 85:* 861–866, 1969.

118. Dunn, J. D., Arimura, A., Scheving, L. E.: Effect of stress on circadian periodicity in serum LH and prolactin concentration. *Endocrinology 90:* 29–33, 1972.

119. Dunn, J., Scheving, L., Millet, P.: Circadian variation in stress-evoked increases in plasma corticosterone. *Am J Physiol 223:* 402–406, 1972.

120. Collu, R., Jequier, J. C., Letarte, J., et al: Diurnal variations of plasma growth hormone and brain monoamines in adult male rats. *Can J Physiol Pharmacol 51:* 890–892, 1973.

120a. Scheving, L. E., Pauly, J. E.: Effect of light on corticosterone levels in plasma of rats. *Am J Physiol 210:* 1112–1117, 1966.

121. Dunn, J. D., Schindler, W. J., Hutchins, M. D., et al: Daily variation in rat growth hormone concentration and the effect of stress on periodicity. *Neuroendocrinology 13:* 69–78, 1973–1974.

122. Scheving, L., Dunn, J. D., Pauly, J. E. et al: Circadian variation in rat serum 5-hydroxytryptamine and effects of stimuli on the rhythm. *Am J Physiol 222:* 252–255, 1972.

123. Kizer, J. S., Zivin, J. A., Jacobowitz, D. M. et al: The nyctohemeral rhythm of plasma prolactin: Effects of ganglionectomy, pinealectomy, constant light, constant darkness or 6-OH-dopamine administration. *Endocrinology 96:* 1230–1240, 1975.

124. Halberg, F., Stephens, A.: Twenty-four-hours periodicity in mortality of C mice from e. coli lipopolysacherida. *Fed Proc 17:* 439, 1958.

125. Haus, E., Halberg, F.: 24-hour rhythm in susceptibility of C mice to a toxic dose of ethanol. *J Appl Physiol 14:* 878–880, 1959.

126. Halberg, F., Johnson, E. A., Brown, B. W., et al: Susceptibility rhythm to *E. coli* endotoxin and bioassay. *Proc Soc Exp Biol Med 103:* 142–144, 1960.

127. Davis, W. M.: Day-night periodicity in pentobarbitol response of mice and the influence of socio-psychological conditions. *Experientia 18:* 235, 1962.

128. Halberg, F., Bittner, J. J., Gully, R., et al: 24-hour periodicity and audiogenic convulsions in I mice of various ages. *Proc Soc Exp Biol Med 88:* 169–173, 1955.

129. Lutsch, E. F., Morris, R. W.: Circadian periodicity in susceptibility to lidocaine hydrochloride. *Science 156:* 100–102, 1967.

130. Haus, E.: Periodicity in response and susceptibility to environmental stimuli. *Ann NY Acad Sci 117:* 292–319, 1964.

131. Ungar, F., Halberg, F.: Circadian rhythm in the in vitro response of mouse adrenal to adrenocorticotropic hormone. *Science 137:* 1058–1060, 1962.

132. Nugent, C. A., Eik-Nes, K., Kent, H. S. et al: A possible explanation for cushing's syndrome associated with adrenal hyperplasia. *J Clin Endocrinol 20:* 1259–1268, 1960.

132a. Engeland, W. C., Shinsako, J., Winget, C. M., Vernikos-Danellis, J., Dallman, M. F.: Circadian patterns of stress-induced ACTH secretion are modified by corticosterone responses. *Endocrinology 100:* 138–147, 1977.

133. Zimmermann, E., Critchlow, V.: Effects of diurnal variation in plasma corticosterone levels on adrenocortical response to stress. *Proc Soc Exp Biol Med 125:* 658–663, 1967.

134. Allen, C. F., Allen, J. P., Greer, M. A.: Absence of nyctohemeral variation in stress-induced ACTH secretion in the rat. *Aviation, Space Environ Med 46:* 296–299, 1975.

135. Margules, D. L., Lewis, M. J., Dragovich, J. A. et al: Hypothalamic norepinephrine: Circadian rhythms and the control of feeding behavior. *Science 178:* 640–643, 1972.

136. Reinberg, A.: The hours of changing responsiveness or susceptibility. *Perspect Biol Med 11:* 111–128, 1967.

137. Takebe, K., Setaishi, C., Hirama, M.: Effects of a bacterial pyrogen on the pituitary-adrenal axis at various times in the 24 hours. *J Clin Endocrinol 26:* 437–442, 1966.

138. Clayton, G. W., Librik, L., Gardner, R. L., et al: Studies on the circadian rhythm of pituitary adrenocorticotropic release in man. *J Clin Endocrinol 23:* 975–980, 1963.

139. Reinberg, A.: Hours of changing responsiveness in relation to allergy and the circadian adrenal cycle, in Aschoff, J. (ed): Circadian Clocks, Proceedings of the Feldafing Summer School. Amsterdam, North-Holland, 1965, p 214–218.

140. Reinberg, A., Zagula-Mally, Z., Ghata, J.: Circadian reactivity rhythm of human skin to house dust, penicillin and histamine. *J Allergy 44:* 292–306, 1969.

141. Ungar, F.: "In vitro" studies of circadian rhythms in hypothalamic-pituitary-adrenal systems. *Rass Neur Veg 21:* 57–70, 1967.

142. Haus, E., Halberg, F., Kuhl, J. F., et al: Chronopharmacology in animals, in Chronobiological Aspects of Endocrinology. *Symposia Medica Hoechst 9.* Stuttgart, Schattauer, 1974, p 269–304.

143. Reinberg, A., Halberg, F.: Circadian Chronopharmacology. *Annu Rev Pharmacol 11:* 455–492, 1971.

144. Scheving, L. E. Mayersbach, H. V., Pauly, J. E.: An overview of chronopharmacology. *J Europ Toxicol 7:* 203–227, 1974.

145. Aschoff, J., Ceresa, F., Halberg, F.: Chronobiological aspects of endocrinology. *Chronobiologia 1 (Suppl 1):* 1–509, 1974.

146. Halberg, F., Haus, E., Cardoso, S. S. et al: Toward a chronotherapy of neoplasia: Tolerance of treatment depends upon host rhythms. *Experientia 29:* 909–1044, 1973.

147. Jundell I: Uber die nykttremeralen Temperaturschwankungen im ersten Lebensjahr des Menschen. *Jahrb Kinderhlkd 59:* 521–619, 1904.

148. Hellbrugge, T. H., Lange, J., Rutenfranz, J., et al: Uber das Entstehen einer 24-Stunden-Periodik physiologischer Funktionen im Saeuglingsalter. *Fortschr Med 81:* 19–26, 1963.

149. Kleitman, N., Engelmann, T.: Sleep characteristics of infants. *J Appl Physiol 6:* 269–282, 1953.

150. Franks, R. C.: Diurnal variation of plasma 17-hydroxycorticosteroids in children. *J Clin Endocrinol Metab 27:* 75–78, 1967.

151. Genova, R., Olivi, O., Benatti, C., et al: Ricerche sul bioritmo fisiologico dei 17, 21-diidrossi-20 corticosteroidi liberi plasmatici nel

bambino normale della seconda e terza infanzia. *Folia Endocrinol 16:* 455–466, 1963.
152. Beyer, P., Kayser, C. H.: Etablissement du rythme nycthéméral de la sécrétion urinaire chez le nourisson. *CR Soc Biol 143:* 1231–1233, 1949.
153. Martin-Du-Pan, R., Vollenweider, L.: L'apparition du rythme circadien des 17-hydroxystéroides chez le nourrisson. Sa modification sous l'effet de la consommation de corticostéroides. *Praxis 4:* 138–144, 1967.
154. Aschoff, J., Meyer-Lohmann, J.: Angeborene 24-Stunden-Periodik beim Kuecken. *Pfluegers Arch 260:* 170–176, 1954.
155. Hoffmann, K.: Angeborene Tagesperiodik bei Eidechsen. *Naturwiss 44:* 359–360, 1957.
156. Hoffmann, K.: Die Aktivitatsperiodik von im 18- und 36-Stunden-Tag erbrueteten Eidechsen. *Z Vergl Physiol 47:* 422–432, 1959.
157. Tscherkowitschn, G. M.: Ontogenese der Tagesperiodik bei Affen, in Bykow, K. M. (ed): Studies on the Regulation of Physiological Functions Under Natural Living Conditions vol 2, (Russian). Moscow 1953, p 199–216.
158. Morin, J., Constant, P.: Contribution à l'étude de l'ontogenèse du rythme nycthéméral d'activité chez le hamster doré (Mesocricetus auratus). *CR Acad Sci Paris 265:* 1071–1074, 1967.
159. Richter, C.: A behavioristic study of the activity of the rat. *Comp Psychol Monogr 1 (No. 2):* 1922–1923.
159a. Ader, R.: Early experiences accelerate maturation of the 24-hour adrenocortical rhythm. *Science 163:* 1225–1226, 1969.
159b. Levin, R., Fitzpatrick, K. M., Levine, S.: Maternal influences on the ontogeny of basal levels of plasma corticosterone in the rat. *Horm Behav 7:* 41–48, 1976.
160. Allen, C., Kendall, J. W.: Maturation of the circadian rhythm of plasma corticosterone in the rat. *Endocrinology 80:* 926–930, 1967.
161. Hiroshige, T., Sato, T.: Postnatal development of circadian rhythm of corticotropin releasing activity in the rat hypothalamus. *Endocrinol Jpn 17:* 1–6, 1970.
162. Okada, F.: The maturation of the circadian rhythm of brain serotonin in the rat. *Life Sci 10:* 77–86, 1971.
163. Ellison, N., Weller, J. L., Klein, D. C.: Development of a circadian rhythm in the activity of pineal serotonin N-acetyltransferase. *J Neurochem 19:* 1335–1341, 1972.
164. Ulrich, R. S., Yuwiler, A.: Adrenocortical influences on the development of the diurnal rhythm in hepatic tyrosine transaminase. *Endocrinology 89:* 936–941, 1971.
165. Honova, E., Miller, S. A., Ehrenkranz, R. A., et al: Tyrosine transaminase: development of daily rhythm in liver of neonatal rat. *Science 162:* 999–1001, 1968.
166. Aschoff, K. J.: Spontane lolomotorische Aktivitaet, in Helmcke, J. G., Stark, D. V. (ed): *Handbuch der Zoologie,* vol 8. Berlin, Walter de Gruyter, 1962, p. 1–76.
167. Orr, E. L., Quay, W. B.: Hypothalamic circadian rhythms in histamine and evidence for a peripubertal phase shift. *Physiologist 17:* 385, 1974.
168. Asano, Y.: The maturation of the circadian rhythm of brain norepinephrine. *Life Sci 10:* 883–894, 1971.
169. Carter, D. B., Vernadakis, A.: Sexual differences in the development of the adrenocortical diurnal rhythm in rats. *Fed Proc 31:* 327, 1972.
170. Krieger, D. T.: Effect of neonatal hydrocortisone on corticosteroid circadian periodicity, responsiveness to ACTH and stress in prepuberal and adult rats. *Neuroendocrinology 16:* 355–363, 1974.
170a. Lengvari, I., Branch, B. J., Zimmerman, E., Taylor, A. N.: Accelerated development of the diurnal pituitary-adrenal rhythm by perinatal thyroxin treatment. *Neurosci Abstr 2:* 675, 1976.
171. Miyabo, S., Hisada, T.: Sex difference in ontogenesis of circadian adrenocortical rhythm in cortisone-primed rats. *Nature 256:* 590–592, 1975.
172. Krieger, D. T.: Effect of ocular enucleation and altered lighting regimens at various ages on the circadian periodicity of plasma corticosteroid levels in the rat. *Endocrinology 93:* 1077–1091, 1973.
173. Aschoff, J., Wever, R.: Resynchronisation der Tagesperiodik von Vogeln nach Phasensprung des Zeitgebers. *Z Vergl Physiol 46:* 321–335, 1963.
174. Halberg, F., Nelson, W., Runge, W. F., et al: Plans for orbital study of rat biorhythms results of interest beyond the biosatellite program. *Space Life Sci 2:* 437–471, 1971.
175. Haus, E., Halberg, F.: Phase-shifting of circadian rhythms in rectal temperature, serum corticosterone and liver glycogen of the male C mouse. *Rass Neur Veg XXIII:* 83–171, 1969.
176. Huber, J., Hamprecht, B.: Tageszeitlicher Rhythmus der Hydroxymethylglutaryl-CoA-reduktase in der Rattenleber. *Hoppe Seyler's Z Physiol Chem 353:* 307–312, 1972.
177. Loon van, J. H.: Diurnal body temperature curves in shift workers. *Ergonomics 6:* 267–273, 1963.
178. Yorke, W., Blacklock, B.: Observations on the periodicity of micro-filaria nocturna. *Ann Trop Med Parasit 11:* 127–148, 1917–18.
179. Lanuza, D. M., Marotta, S. F.: Circadian and basal interrelationships of plasma cortisol and cations in women. *Aerospace Med 45 (8):* 864–868, 1974.
180. Halberg, F., Halberg, E., Montalbetti, N.: Premesse e sviluppi della cronofarmacologia. *Quad Med Quant 8:* 7–54, 1970.
181. Klein, K. E., Wegmann, H. M.: The resynchronization of human circadian rhythms after transmeridian flights as a result of flight direction and mode of activity, in Scheving, L. E., Halberg, F., Pauly, J. E. (eds): Chronobiology. Tokyo, Igaku, 1974, p 504–570.
182. Strumwasser, F.: Neuronal principles organizing periodic behaviors, in Schmitt, F., Worden, F. G. (eds): The Neurosciences, 3rd Study Program. Cambridge, Mass., MIT Press, 1974, p 437–458.
183. Frank, G. S.: Circadian aspects of the normal human electroencephalogram, in Circadian Systems, Report of the 39th Ross Conference on Pediatric Research. Columbus Ohio, Ross Laboratories, 1961, p 48–50.
184. Schmitt, M.: Circadian rhythmicity in reponses of cells in the lateral hypothalamus. *Am J Physiol 225:* 1096–1101, 1973.
184a. Koizumi, K., Nishino, H.: Circadian and other rhythmic activity of neurones in the ventromedial nuclei and lateral hypothalamic area. *J Physiol 263:* 331–356, 1976.
184b. Armstrong, W. E., Hatton, G. I.: Morphological changes in hypothalamic neurosecretory neurons during the diurnal cycle. *Neurosci Abstr 2:* 2, 1976.
185. Arechiga, H.: Circadian rhythm of sensory input in the crayfish, in Schmitt, F., Worden, F. G. (eds): The Neurosciences, 3rd Study Program. Cambridge, Mass, MIT Press, 1974, p 517–523.
186. Axelrod, J.: The pineal gland: A neurochemical transducer. *Science 184:* 1341–1348, 1974.
187. Moszkowska, A., Kordon, C., Ebels, I.: Biochemical fractions and mechanisms involved in the pineal modulation of pituitary gonadotropin release, in The Pineal Gland, Ciba Foundation Symposium, Edinburgh and London, Churchill Livingstone, 1971 p 241–255.
188. Mess, B., Heizer, A., Toth, A. M., Time, L.: Luteinization induced by pinealectomy in the polyfollicular ovaries of rats bearing anterior hypothalamic lesions, in The Pineal Gland, Ciba Foundation Symposium. Edinburgh and London, Churchill Livingstone, 1971, p 229–240.
189. Alleva, J. J., Waleski, M. V., Alleva, F. R.: The Zeitgeber for ovulation in rats: non-participation of the pineal gland. *Life Sci 9:* 241–246, 1970.
190. Motta, M., Schiaffini, O., Pava, F., et al: Pineal principles and the control of andrenocorticotropin secretion, in The Pineal Gland, Ciba Foundation Symposium. Edinburgh and London, Churchill Livingstone, 1971, p 279–291.
191. Fiske, V.: Discussion, in The Pineal Gland, Ciba Foundation Symposium. Edinburgh and London, Churchill Livingstone, 1971, p 292.
192. Gaston, S., Menaker, M.: Pineal function: The biological clock in the sparrow. *Science 160:* 1125–1127, 1968.
193. Quay, W. B.: Pineal homeostatic regulation of shifts in the circadian activity rhythm during maturation and aging. *Trans NY Acad Sci 34:* 239–253, 1972.
193a. Morimoto, Y.: Relationship between the shift of circadian rhythm of plasma corticosteroid and that of food intake under various lighting conditions in normal and pinealectomized rats. *V Int Congr Endocrinol* 1976, p 154 (abstr).
193b. Zimmerman, N. H., Menaker, M.: Neural connections of sparrow pineal: Role in circadian control of activity. *Science 190:* 477–479, 1975.
193c. Turek, F. W., McMillan, J. P., Menaker, M.: Melatonin: Effects on the circadian locomotor rhythm of sparrows. *Science 194:* 1441–1443, 1976.
194. Anton-Tay, F.: Pineal brain relationships, in The Pineal Gland, Ciba Foundation Symposium. Edinburgh and London, Churchill Livingstone, 1971, p 213–220.
195. Halberg, F., Halberg, E., Barnum, C. P. et al: Physiologic 24-hour

periodicity in human beings and mice, the lighting regimen and daily routine, in Photoperiodism and Related Phenomena in Plants and Animals, vol. 5. Washington D.C., *Am Assoc Adv Sci Publ,* 1969, p 804–878.

196. Stephan, F. K., Zucker, I.: Circadian rhythms in drinking behavior and locomotor activity of rats are eliminated by hypothalamic lesions. *Proc Natl Acad Sci 69:* 1583–1586, 1972.

196a. Ibuka, N., Inouye, S. T., Kawamura, H.: Analysis of sleep-wakefulness rhythms in male rats after suprachiasmatic nucleus lesions and ocular enucleation. *Brain Res 122:* 33–47, 1977.

197. Moore, R. Y., Eichler, V. B.: Loss of a circadian adrenal corticosterone rhythm following suprachiasmatic lesions in the rat. *Brain Res 42:* 201–206, 1972.

197a. Stetson, M. H., Watson-Whitmyre, M.: Nucleus suprachiasmaticus: The biological clock in the hamster? *Science 191:* 197–199, 1976.

198. Campbell, C. B. G., Ramaley, J. A.: Retino-hypothalamic projections: Correlations with onset of the adrenal rhythm in infant rats. *Endocrinology 94:* 1201–1204, 1974.

199. Page, R. B., Galichich, J. H., Grunt, J. A.: Alteration of circadian temperature rhythm with third ventricular obstruction. *J Neurosurg 38:* 309–319, 1973.

200. Krieger, D. T.: Factors influencing the circadian periodicity of plasma corticosteroid levels. *Chronobiologia 1:* 195–216, 1974.

201. Everett, J. W., and Sawyer, C. H.: A 24-hour periodicity in the "LH-release apparatus" of female rats, disclosed by barbiturate sedation. *Endocrinology 47:* 198–218, 1950.

201a. Fitzgerald, K. M., Zucker, I.: Circadian organization of the estrous cycle of the golden hamster. *Proc Natl Acad Sci 73:* 2923–2927, 1976.

202. Everett, J. D., Sawyer, C. H., Markee, J. E.: A neurogenic timing factor in control of the ovulatory discharge of luteinizing hormone in the cyclic rat. *Endocrinology 44:* 234–250, 1949.

203. Jouvet, M.: Monoaminergic regulation of the sleep-waking cycle in the cat, in Schmitt, F., Worden, F. G. (eds): The Neurosciences, 3rd Study Program, Cambridge, Mass, MIT Press, 1974, p 499–508.

204. Reis, D. J., Weinbren, M., Corvelli, A.: A circadian rhythm of norepinephrine regionally in cat brain; its relationship to environmental lighting and to regional diurnal variations in brain serotonin. *J Pharm Exp Ther 164:* 135–145, 1968.

205. Reis, D. J., Corvelli, A., Conners, J.: Circadian and ultradian rhythms of serotonin regionally in cat brain. *J Pharm Exp Ther 167:* 328–333, 1969.

206. Hanin, I., Massarelli, R., Costa, E.: Acetylcholine concentrations in rat brain: Diurnal oscillation. *Science 170:* 341–342, 1970.

207. Takahashi, Y., Kipnis, D. M., Daughaday, W. H.: Growth hormone secretion during sleep. *J Clin Invest 47:* 2079–2090, 1968.

208. Boyar, R., Finkelstein, J., Roffwarg, H., et al: Synchronization of augmented luteinizing hormone secretion with sleep during puberty. *N Engl J Med 287:* 582–586, 1972.

209. Krieger, D. T., Glick, S. M.: Sleep EEG stages and plasma growth hormone concentration in states of endogenous and exogenous hypercortisolemia or ACTH elevation. *J Clin Endocrinol Metab 39:* 986–1000, 1974.

210. Willoughby, J. O., Martin, J. B., Renaud, L. P. et al: Pulsatile growth hormone and prolactin secretion: Absent correlation with sleep stages. *Endocrinology* (in press).

211. Moore, R. Y., Heller, A., Bhatnager, R. K., et al: Central control of the pineal gland: Visual pathways. *Arch Neurol 18:* 208–218, 1968.

212. Sassin, J. F., Parker, D. C., Mace, J. W., et al: Human growth hormone release: relation to slow-wave sleep and sleep waking cycles. *Science 165:* 513–515, 1969.

213. Kleitman, N.: Basic rest-activity cycle in relation to sleep and wakefulness, in Kales, A. (ed): Sleep: Physiology and Pathology. Philadelphia, Lippincott, 1969.

214. Orr, W. C., Hoffman, H. J., Hegge, F. W.: Ultradian rhythms in extended performance. *Aerospace Med 45:* 995–1000, 1974.

215. Globus, G. G., Phoebus, E. C., Humphries, J., et al: Ultradian rhythms in human telemetered gross motor activity. *Aerospace Med 44:* 882–887, 1973.

216. Friedman, S., Fisher, C.: On the presence of a rhythmic diurnal, oral instinctual drive cycle in man: A preliminary report. *J Am Psychoan Assoc 15:* 317–343, 1967.

217. Midgley, A. R., Jaffe, R. B.: Regulation of human gonadotropins: X. episodic fluctuation of LH during the menstrual cycle. *J Clin Endocrinol 33:* 962–969, 1971.

218. Yen, S. S. C., Tsai, C. C., Naftolin, F., et al: Pulsatile patterns of gonadotropin release in subjects with and without ovarian function. *J Clin Endocrinol Metab 34:* 671–675, 1972.

219. Brandenberger, G., Follenius, M.: Variations dirunes de la cortisolémie, de la glycémie et du cortisol libre urinaire chez l'homme au repos. *J Physiol Paris 66:* 271–282, 1973.

220. Sachar, E. J., Hellman, L., Roffwarg, H. P., et al: Disrupted 24-hour patterns of cortisol secretion in psychotic depression. *Arch Gen Psychiatr 28:* 19–24, 1974.

221. Yen, S. S. C., Vandenberg, G., Tsai, C. C., et al: Ultradian fluctuations of gonadotropins, in Ferin, M., Halberg, F., Richart, R. M., et al (eds): Biorhythms and Human Reproduction. New York, John Wiley, 1974, p 203–218.

222. Seyler, L. E., Reichlin, S.: Episodic secretion of luteinizing hormone-releasing factor (LRF) in the human. *J Clin Endocrinol Metab 39:* 471–478, 1974.

223. VandeWiele, R. L., Ferin, M.: The control of pulsatile gonadotrophin secretion, in Chronobiological Aspects of Endocrinology. *Symposia Medica Hoechst 9.* Stuttgart, Schattauer, 1974, p 203–211.

224. Carmel, P. C., Araki, S., Ferin, M.: Prolonged stalk portal blood collection in rhesus monkeys: Pulsatile release of gonadotropin-releasing hormone (Gn-Rh), Proceedings of the Endocrine Society, 1975 meeting, Abstract 107, p 104.

225. Bhattacharya, A. N., Dierschke, D. J., Yamaj, I. T., et al: The pharmacological blockade of circhoral mode of LH secretion in the anesthetized rhesus monkey. *Endocrinology 90:* 778–786, 1972.

226. Mills, J. N.: Human circadian rhythms. *Physiol Rev 46:* 128–171, 1966.

227. Izzo, J. L.: Diurnal rhythm in diabetes and mellitus. *Proc Am Diab Assoc 9:* 247–372, 1949.

228. Faiman, C., Moorhouse, J. A.: Diurnal variation in the levels of glucose and related substances in healthy and diabetic subjects during starvation. *Clin Sci 32:* 111–126, 1967.

229. Zimmet, P. Z., Wall, J. R., Rome, R., et al: Diurnal variations in glucose tolerance, Associated changes in plasma insulin, growth hormone and non-esterified fatty acids. *Br Med J 16* March 1974, pp. 485–488.

230. Gibson, T., Jarrett, R. J.: Diurnal variation in insulin sensitivity. *Lancet 2:* 947, 1972.

231. Colquhoun, W. P.: Circadian variations in mental efficiency, in Colquhoun, W. P. (ed): Biological Rhythms and Human Performance. New York, Academic Press, 1971, p 38–107.

232. Blake, M. J. F.: Temperature and time of day, in Colquhoun, W. P. (ed): Biological Rhythms and Human Performance. New York, Academic Press, 1971, p 109–148.

232a. Hosemann, H.: Bestehen solare und lunare Einflusse auf die Nativitat und den Menstrualcyclus? *Z Geburtsch Gynekol 133:* 263–285, 1950.

233. Henkin, R. I.: A study of circadian variation in taste in normal man and patients with adrenal cortical insufficiency: The role of adrenal cortical steroids, in Ferin, M., Halberg, F., Richart, R. M., et al (eds): Biorhythms and Human Reproduction. New York, John Wiley, 1974 p 397–408.

234. Chiazze, L., Brayer, F. T., Macisco, J. J., et al: The length and variability of the human menstrual cycle. *JAMA 203:* 377–380, 1968.

235. Treloar, A. E., Boynton, R. E., Behn, B. G., et al: Variation of the human menstrual cycle through reproductive life. *Int J Fertil 12:* 77–126, 1967.

236. Matsumoto, S., Nogami, Y., Ohkuri, S.: Statistical studies on menstruation: a criticism on the definition of normal menstruation. *Gunma J Med Sci 11:* 294–318, 1962.

237. Reinberg, A., Smolensky, M. J.: Circatrigintan secondary rhythms related to hormonal changes in the menstrual cycle, in Ferin, M., Halberg, F., Richart, R. M., VandeWiele (eds): Rhythms and Human Reproduction, New York, Academic Press, 1971, p 241–258.

238. Schmidt, Th. H.: Thermoregulatorische Groessen in Abhaengigkeit von Tageszeit und Menstruationszyklus. *Med Diss Munchen,* 1972.

239. Henkin, R. I.: Sensory changes during the menstrual cycle, in Colquhoun, W. P. (ed): Biological Rhythms and Human Performance. New York, Academic Press, 1971, p 277–285.

240. Procacci, P., Buzzelli, R., Passeri, I., et al: Studies on the cutaneous pricking pain threshold in man, circadian and circatrigintan changes. *Res. Clin Stud Headache 3:* 260–276, 1972.

241. O'Connor, J. F.: Secondary rhythms related to the menstrual cycle,

in Colquhoun, W. P. (ed): Biological Rhythms and Human Performance. New York, Academic Press, 1971, p 309–324.
242. Aschoff, J.: Jahresperiodik der Fortpflanzung bei Warmblutern. *Studium Generale 8:* 742–776, 1955.
243. Pengelley, E. T., Fisher, K. C.: The effect of temperature and photoperiod on the yearly hibernating behavior of captive golden-mantled ground squirrels (Citellus lateralis). *Can J Zool 41:* 1103–1120, 1963.
244. Gwinner, E.: Circannuale Periodik der Mauser und der Zugunruhe bei einem Vogel. *Naturwissenschaften 54:* 447, 1967.
245. Gwinner, E.: Circadian and circannual rhythms in birds, in Farner, D. S., King, J. R., Perkes, K. C. (eds): Avian Biology, vol V. New York, Academic Press, 1975, p 221–285.
246. Pengelley, E. T. (ed): Circannual Clocks. New York, Academic Press, 1974.
247. Quetelet, L. A. J.: Mémoire sur les lois des naissances et de la mortalite à Bruxelles. *Nouv Mém Acad R Sci Belles-Lettres Bruxelles 3:* 493–512, 1826.
248. Otto, W.: Jahreszeit und Geburtsfrequenz. *Z Hygiene Grenzgeb 5:* 106–113, 1959.
249. Cowgill, U. M.: The season of birth in man. *Man 1:* 232–240, 1966.
250. Batschelet, E., Hillman, D., Smolensky, M., et al: Angular-linear correlation coefficient for rhythmometry and circannually changing human birth rates at different geographic latitudes. *Int J Chronobiol 1:* 183–205, 1973.
251. Reinberg, A., Lagoguey, M., Chauffournier, J. M., et al: Rythmes annuels et circadiens de la testosterone plasmatique. *Ann Endocrinol (Paris) 36:* 44–45, 1975.
251a. Smals, A. G. H., Kloppenborg, P. W. C., Benraad, T. J.: Circannual cycle in plasma testosterone levels in man. *J Clin Endocrinol Metab 42:* 979–982, 1976.
252. Smolensky, M., Halberg, F., Sargent, II, F.: Chronobiology of the life sequence, in Ito, S., Ogata, K., Yoshimura, H. (eds): Advances in Climatic Physiology. Tokyo, Igaku Shoin, 1972, 281–318.
253. Momiyama, M., Katayama, K.: Deseasonalization of mortality in the world. *Int J Biometeor 16:* 329–342, 1972.
254. Paloheimo, J.: Seasonal variations of serum lipids in healthy men. *Ann Med Exp Biol fenn 39 (Suppl 7):* 24–88, 1961.
255. Schlegel, J. U.: Seasonal variations in the choline content of human serum. *Proc Soc Exp Biol Med 70:* 695–697, 1949.
256. Depner, M.: Ergebnisse der Haemoglobin-und Serumeiweiss-Bestimmung im Rahmen der Reihenuntersuchung in Hessen. *Klin Wschr 28:* 441–444, 1950.
257. Stamp, T. C. B., Round, J. M.: Seasonal changes in human plasma levels of 25-hydroxyvitamin D. *Nature 247:* 563–565, 1974.
258. Ellinger, F.: Die Lichtempfindlichkeit der menschlichen Haut, ihre bestimmung und Bedeutung fuer die lichtbiologische Konstitutionsforschung. *Strahlentherapie 44:* 1–82, 1932.
259. Hale, H. B., Ellis, J. P., Williams, E. W.: Seasonal changes among endocrine-metabolic indices of men residing in a subtropical climate. USAF School of Aerospace Medicine Brooks SAM-TR-66-114, 1–14, 1966.
260. Johansson, G., Frankenhaeuser, M., Lambert, W. W.: Note on seasonal variations in catecholamine output. *Percept Mot Skills 28:* 677–678, 1969.
261. Johansson, G., Post, B.: Catecholamine output of males and females over a one-year period. *Acta Physiol Scand 92:* 557–565, 1974.
262. De Rudder, B.: Grundriss einer Meteorbiologie des Menschen. Berlin-Goettingen-Heidelberg, Springer, 1952.
263. Nylin, G.: Periodical variations in growth, standard metabolism and oxygen capacity of the blood in children. *Acta Med Scand Suppl 31:* 1–207, 1929.
264. Lindhard, J.: Contribution to the physiology of respiration under the arctic climate. *Meddelelser om Grønland 44:* 77–175, 1917.
265. Richter, C. P.: Biological Clocks in Medicine and Psychiatry. Springfield, Ill, Charles C. Thomas, 1965, p 96.
266. Reiman, H. A.: Periodic Disease. Philadelphia, F. A. Davis, 1963, pp 1–189.
267. Krieger, D. T.: Lack of circadian periodicity of plasma prolactin concentrations in Cushing's disease. *J Clin Endocrinol Metab* (in press).
268. Krieger, D. T., Krieger, H. P.: Circadian variation of plasma 17-hydroxycorticosteroids in central nervous system disease. *J Clin Endocrinol 26:* 929–940, 1966.
269. Wolff, S. M., Adler, R. C., Buskirk, E. R., et al: A syndrome of periodic hypothalamic discharge. *Am J Med 36:* 956–967, 1964.
270. Birke, G., Plantin, L. O., Diczfalusy, E.: Fluctuation in the excretion of adrenocortical steroids in a case of Cushing's Syndrome. *J Clin Endocrinol. 16:* 286–289, 1956.
271. Cryer, P. E., Daughaday, W. H.: Regulation of growth hormone secretion in acromegaly. *J Clin Endocrinol 29:* 380–393, 1969.
272. Krieger, D. T., Krieger, H. P.: Circadian patterns of urinary electrolyte excretion in central nervous system disease. *Metabolism 16:* 815–823, 1967.
273. Reimann, H. A.: Hypothalamic-hypophyseal-neural influence in periodic disease. *Ann NY Acad Sci 117:* 589–594, 1964.
274. Appel, W., Hansen, K. J.: Lichteinwirkung, Tagesrhythmik der eosinophilen Leukozythen und Hypophysen-Nebennierenrindensystem. *Dtsch Arch Klin Med 199:* 530–537, 1952.
275. Bodenheimer, S., et al: Diurnal rhythms of serum gonadotropins, testosterone, estradiol and cortisol in blind man. *J Endocrinol Metab 37:* 472, 1973.
276. D'Allesandro, B., et al: Circadian rhythm of cortisol secretion in elderly and blind subjects. *Br Med J 2:* 274, 1974.
277. Fatranska, M.: Circadian rhythms of the urinary 17-OHCS and VMA in continuous light, during sound and light deprivation. *J Interdiscipl Cycle Res 2:* 247–254, 1971.
278. Hollwich, F., Dieckhues, B.: Circadian rhythm in the blind. *J Interdiscipl Cycle Res 2:* 291–302, 1971.
279. Krieger, D. T., Glick, S.: Absent sleep peaks of growth hormone release in blind subjects: Correlation with sleep EEG stages. *J Clin Endocrinol Metab 33:* 847–850, 1971.
280. Lobban, M. C., Tredre, B.: Perception of light and the maintenance of human renal diurnal rhythms. *J Physiol 189:* 32–33, 1966.
281. Migeon, C. J. et al: The diurnal variation of plasma levels and urinary excretion of 17-OHCS in normal subjects, night workers and blind subjects. *J Clin Endocrinol 16:* 622–633, 1956.
282. Orth, D. N., Island, D. P.: Light synchronization of the circadian rhythm in plasma cortisol (17-OHCS) concentration in man. *J Clin Endocrinol 29:* 479–486, 1969.
283. Remler, O.: Untersuchungen an Blinden uber die 24-Std-Rhythmik. *Klin Mbl Augenheilkd 113:* 116–140, 1948.
284. Weitzman, E. D., Perlow, M., Sassin, J. F. et al: Persistence of the twenty-four hour pattern of episodic cortisol secretion and growth hormone release in blind subjects. *Trans Am Neurol Assoc 97,* 1973.
285. Gjessing, R.: Beitrage zur Kenntnis der Pathophysiologie der katatonen Errregung. III. Mitteilung. Uber periodisch rezidierende katatone Errregung, mit kritischem Beginn und Abschluss. *Arch Psychiatr Nervenkr 104:* 355–416, 1935.
286. Bunney, W. E., Hartman, E. L., Mason, J. W.: Study of a patient with 48-hour manic depressive cycles. *Arch Gen Psychiatr 12:* 619–625, 1965.
287. Sachar, E. J., Hellman, L., Roffwarg, H. et al: Disrupted 24-hour patterns of cortisol secretion in psychotic depression. *Arch Gen Psychiatr 28:* 19–24, 1973.
288. Engelmann, W.: Lithium slows down the kalanchoe clock. *Z Naturforsch 27b:* 477, 1972.

157

Endocrine Management of Malignancies of the Prostate, Breast, Endometrium, Kidney, and Ovary

Richard L. Landau

INTRODUCTION

". . . It became apparent that cancer is an escape from homeostasis and the loi de balancement and that it may be important to discover not so much why cancer cells grow relentlessly, but rather how the growth of the normal cells is so wonderfully restrained."[1]

At the present time the endocrine management of these cancers, principally of the male and female reproductive systems, is confined to the treatment of advanced or disseminated disease. At this late stage the cancer cannot be irradicated by local excision or destroyed by ionizing radiation, although such approaches may be indicated for palliative purposes. The patient with metastatic cancer has a systemic disease; the clinical manifestations support this position. Accordingly, the rational therapeutic approach aimed at arrest or cure must reach all tissues in the body, exert an adverse or destructive influence on malignant cells, and have little or no effect on all others. The several forms of endocrine manipulation that have a place in the treatment of breast, prostatic, and endometrial malignancies approach this ideal more closely than all other therapeutic modalities.

The first evidence of endocrine-induced regression of a malignancy was Beatson's discovery in 1896[2] that bilateral oophorectomy resulted in substantial improvement in two patients with breast cancer. Many years later Huggins and his associates[3,4] reported the ameliorative influence of castration in some patients with advanced prostatic cancer; when cortisone became available for replacement therapy, Huggins and Bergenstal demonstrated the beneficial effects of adrenalectomy in prostatic and breast cancer.[5] With these discoveries the concept of hormonally dependent cancer was developed. The idea has flourished. It was natural to assume that, since the normal breast and prostate require estrogen and androgen, respectively, for full development, some derivative cancers would preserve a similar dependent state.

Although the discovery that some cancers regressed after the removal of endocrine glands is of unquestionable importance, the concept of hormonal dependency, while attractive and persuasive, may be a misleading partial truth. Thayer[6] has said: "Man is gifted above all at self-deception. To know a thing he must name it. To name it, he must distinguish it from other things. In distinguishing it from other things he makes it something it is not." Is it possible that the term *hormonal dependency* has made the hormonal regulation of malignancies something it is not? The analogy between the responses of normal hormonally dependent glands and hormonally responsive tumors leaves something to be desired.

The forms of endocrine therapy have multiplied. It is now possible to induce remissions by administering an excess of the very hormone upon which it is assumed that a dependency relationship may exist. Moreover, a hormonal dependency appears to be the hypothetical basis for the newest attempts to develop predictive tests for the responses to endocrine therapy. Knowledge that specific hormonal "receptors" exist in normal accessory sex tissues and the belief that this hormonal binding initiates accelerated synthetic activity and growth[7] is the basis for the search for similar receptors in malignant tissue as predictive tests. Even if such tests become useful, however, there is no proof at this time that the presence of a specific receptor indicates hormonal dependency of the tumor.

It is now possible to add months and sometimes years in reasonable health to the lives of many patients through hormonal therapy. Unfortunately, cures are almost never achieved, but the induction of spectacular remission or effective arrest of the progress of disease is now an old story. There is, furthermore, a tendency for cancers that respond to one form of endocrine therapy and then recur or relapse to then respond to another quite different hormonal approach. Without in any way depreciating the progress that has been made, it must be pointed out that both the therapeutic and investigative approaches to the management of these forms of cancer have become stereotyped. Can one ascribe the minimal progress of the past two decades to thinking of the hormonal responsiveness of cancer "as something it is not?"

In this spirit it seems appropriate to ask several questions: (1) If metastatic cancer is, as suggested, a systemic disease, should not the disease be regarded as systemic and controlled or limited from the moment the primary growth begins? (2) What are the local factors that encourage or permit metastatic proliferation in some tissues, and what is it that inhibits growth of metastases in others? (3) Do immunologic mechanisms play a role in tumor regression when endocrine therapy is effective? (4) Is the atrophy of tumors following gonadectomy, adrenalectomy, and hypophysectomy much the same process that occurs in normal hormone dependent tissues after the withdrawal of specific endocrine support? (5) After gonadectomy and adrenalectomy, virtually no steroid hormone is produced. Are we sure that the benefits that accrue can be ascribed to the absence of estrogen in breast cancer and testosterone in prostatic cancer? (6) Is the favorable response to the administration of hormone excess (estrogen, androgen, glucocorticoid, progestin) a demonstration of hormonal dependency? (7) Which hormone is breast cancer in the male dependent upon?

These and other questions are doubtlessly being asked by today's cancer researchers. Endocrine approaches to the management of malignancies are far too promising to abandon. No other form of treatment offers so much at so little cost to the host.

PROSTATIC CANCER

HISTORY

In his Nobel address Charles B. Huggins[8] tells the story of what appeared to be an easy and natural shift in research interest from his splendid studies on the endocrine physiology of the male genital tract to the investigation of the endocrine control of prostatic cancer. The dogs that were utilized in the study of the regulation of prostatic secretory activity frequently developed spontaneous tumors of the prostate. Castration carried out for other purposes resulted in the shrinkage of these tumors along with the rest of the gland.

In 1939 Abe Johnson developed symptoms of prostatic obstruction of the urine flow. He also experienced severe pelvic bone pain due to lytic metastatic lesions. Walking was almost impossible. Palpation of the prostate revealed symmetrical hypertrophy as well as nodular tumors. Abe Johnson arrived as Huggins' urology patient at about the same time as the idea to extend the dog experience to man, and he was accordingly the first patient to be castrated for prostatic cancer. He agreed that he had nothing to lose. Within 1 week of the operation his pain had diminished remarkably. Later he walked out of the hospital. The lytic bone lesions almost disappeared over a period of months. He went on to live quite comfortably for another 12 years.

Other patients who followed Abe Johnson experienced similar orchiectomy-induced remissions. The treatment, although cruelly mutilating in the psychologic sense, was almost trivial in the physical hazard imposed. Thus, in terms of the clinical pharmacologists' risk/benefit ratio, this therapeutic approach for a lingering, debilitating, often painful, and ultimately fatal disease of older men passed, almost at once, with a high grade. The era of hormonal control of advanced prostatic cancer had begun.

Huggins also proposed that the measurement of plasma acid and alkaline phosphatase concentrations would provide chemical indicators of the growth activity of the tumor. It had been previously shown that a phosphatase with maximum activity at an acid pH was often elevated in the serum of patients with a prostatic malignancy, and that a plasma phosphatase with maximal activity at an alkaline pH was increased with growing osteoblastic metastases in bone. Reactivity of both phosphatases dropped when orchiectomy resulted in shrinkage of the cancer and healing of the bone metastases. The administration of testosterone seemed to enhance tumor growth and the phosphatase concentrations rose promptly. Unfortunately, these phosphatase measurements could not be used as an unqualified test for the presence or absence of prostatic cancer, for not all such tumors release an excess of acid phosphatase, and the bone alkaline phosphatase may be elevated in any number of diseases besides prostatic cancer metastases to bone. However, in appropriate patients the tests have provided important objective indicators of the progress of the disease and its response to therapy.

If the growth of the malignancy was dependent upon the presence of circulating androgen, it was reasoned that estrogen therapy could serve as an effective substitute for castration. A very large amount should, it was anticipated, effectively block testosterone secretion by the testicular interstitial cells by suppressing pituitary gonadotropin secretion. Diethylstilbestrol, 5mg/day, at least 10 times the replacement dosage in a normal woman, became a usual dosage, and regression of the prostatic cancers was induced with approximately the same frequency as had been noted following orchiectomy.

It thus appeared that even the morbidity of minor surgery could be eliminated. At the time it was thought that the estrogen therapy would have no special side effects except for gynecomastia. Accordingly, urologists desiring to spare the patients the chagrin and embarrassment of castration adopted stilbestrol or equivalent activity in other compounds as a commonplace therapy for men with advanced prostatic cancer.

EFFECTS OF CASTRATION AND ESTROGEN

The inexorable, but usually slow, unfavorable progress of the disease was so well established by the experience of innumerable physicians, that no control cases were required to confirm Huggins' observations of remissions induced by castration or estrogen treatment. The general impression gained was certainly that not only was useful life often restored by these modes of therapy, but that the duration of life was extended. Accordingly, it became a widespread habit of urologists to initiate one of these courses of therapy when the diagnosis of carcinoma was made. One could easily rationalize that if far-advanced disease remitted, the results in earlier cases would be at least as remarkable. However, not until quite recently was the life-extending capacity of these treatments actually quantitated with appropriate staging and controls (see below). In all probability the disease is never eradicated by these procedures.

Results from many centers indicate that 45–70 percent of patients respond favorably to either estrogen or castration.[9,10] The criteria for response include symptomatic improvement, diminution of tumor size when visible or palpable. improvement in x-ray demonstrated bone metastases, and decreases in the plasma acid and alkaline phosphatase concentrations. There is no evidence that the response rate in castration is superior to the results of estrogen in a dosage roughly equivalent to 5 mg of diethylstilbestrol daily. There are also no studies that indicate that simultaneous treatment by castration and estrogen provides results superior to either one alone. It is true that when relapses recur following one of these courses, introduction of the other may sometimes be followed by clinical improvement.

VETERANS ADMINISTRATION UROLOGIC RESEARCH GROUP STUDY

This cooperative investigation of the efficacy of therapy is a model of the type of investigation that must ultimately be carried out to evaluate long-term treatment of all chronic diseases such as carcinoma of the prostate.[11,12] When this program was started in 1960, the endocrine management of the disease tended to be impressionistic, guided to a great extent by the prejudices and feelings of physicians. There was no basis for agreement on when to employ castration, when to treat with estrogen, or whether there was anything to be gained by combining the two therapies. There was general agreement on the dosage of estrogen, but that was because dose–response studies had not been carried out.

The patients (a total of 2314 entered the study) were classified in accordance with a rather widely accepted scheme (Fig. 157-1). Stages I and II were defined as early disease; stage I, being discovered by transurethral prostatectomy or needle biopsy, can be regarded as symptomatic, while patients in stage II were asymptomatic. The men in these two groups were randomized and treated *immediately* with either 5 mg stilbestrol/day or a placebo. The results obtained were astonishing to the profession (Fig. 157-2). Employing survival as the criterion of success, there was obviously no benefit from estrogen treatment. Detailed investigation of the causes of death did reveal a significant lowering of the death rate from prostatic cancer, but there was a compensating increase in deaths from cardiovascular diseases, especially pulmonary emboli. The patients with preexisting cardiovascular disease when treatment started were particularly liable to succumb to such complications.

The stage III and stage IV patients were randomized into four groups: orchiectomy plus placebo, orchiectomy plus 5 mg stilbestrol, 5 mg stilbestrol, and placebo alone. In these groups, too, there was little or no significant difference in survival over the 9 years. However, as in stages I and II, cardiovascular and pulmonary embolic deaths were definitely more numerous in those cases receiving estrogen. The combination of estrogen and orchiectomy offered no survival advantage.

The increase in cardiovascular deaths in all categories of patients treated with large doses of estrogen has been confirmed by an entirely independent carefully executed prospective investigation of the possible benefits of equine estrogens for patients with

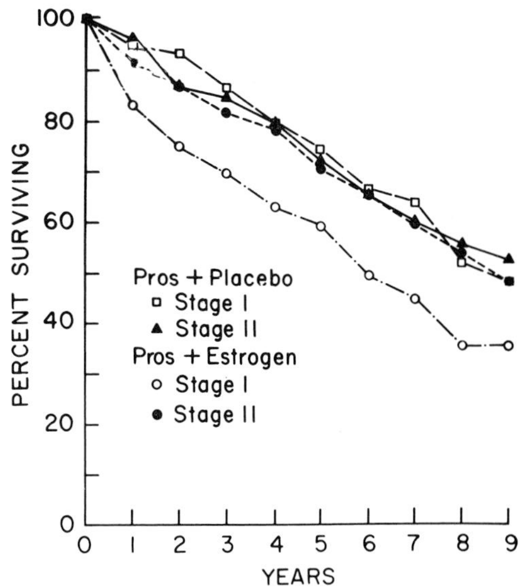

Figure 157-2. Survival curves by assigned treatment for stage I and stage II carcinomas of the prostate cases (From Byar: *Bull. N.Y. Acad. Med. 48:* 751, 1972.)

coronary atherosclerotic disease.[13] Furthermore, the slight increase in thromboembolic disease in young women taking estrogen-containing contraceptive pills is an observation that is quite consistent with these studies in older men.

In a second program the Veterans Administration Group has attempted to compare the results of placebo and 0.2, 1.0, and 5.0 mg stilbestrol/day given immediately to men in stages III and IV. After only 3 years the results of this study indicated that in stage III cardiovascular deaths were highest in the group receiving 5 mg stilbesterol; there was no significant difference in cardiovascular survival rates in the other three categories. In stage IV patients the overall survival rate was lowest in the placebo group. It must be emphasized, while pointing to the hazards of estrogen administration, that the results of this study clearly substantiate previous reports on the effectiveness of estrogen in rendering significant clinical benefit and in lessening the death rate from prostatic cancer (Fig. 157–3).

The awareness of the cardiovascular morbidity from high estrogen dosage led quite naturally to attempts to treat with smaller quantities. Because it was widely assumed (see below) that the estrogenic influence on the cancer was the result of suppression of

STAGE	RECTAL EXAMINATION	PROSTATIC ACID PHOSPHATASE		X-RAY OR BIOPSY EVIDENCE OF METASTASES
I	NO INDURATION	≤1.0 K.A.U.		0
II	LOCALIZED NODULE	≤1.0 K.A.U		0
III	EXTRA-PROSTATIC EXTENSION	≤1.0 K.A.U.		0
IV	EQUIVOCAL FINDINGS	>1.0 K.A.U.	OR	+

Fig. 157-1. Staging system employed by the Veteran's Administration Cooperative Urological Research Group. (From Byar: Bull. N.Y. Acad. Med. *48:* 751, 1972.)

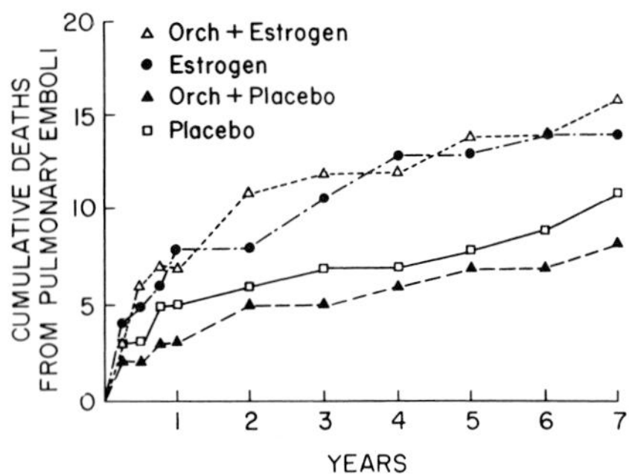

Fig. 157-3. Deaths due to pulmonary emboli by assigned treatment programs. (From Byar: *Bull. N.Y. Acad. Med. 48:* 751, 1972.)

testosterone secretion via gonadotropin suppression, a few studies have been carried out comparing the effect of several quantities of estrogen on plasma testosterone concentration. Stilbestrol, at a dosage of 5 mg/day, suppresses the plasma testosterone concentration to the female level; 1.0 mg three times a day is just about as effective; 1.0 mg/day lowers the level moderately; and 0.2 mg has virtually no influence.[12,14,15] In more or less comparable doses other estrogens also suppress plasma testosterone, with the notable exception of chlorotrianisene (Tace) in a therapeutically effective dose of 12 mg twice a day. Preliminary studies (2–3 years) suggest that therapeutic efficacy may be obtained with just 1 mg/day of stilbestrol, a dose that thus far appears safe from the cardiovascular viewpoint.

OTHER ENDOCRINE APPROACHES

Additional endocrine manipulations that have elicited at least occasional success fall into three categories: (1) the removal of other hormonally active materials that may support or stimulate tumor growth; (2) the administration of products that possess endocrine activity; or (3) the administration of endocrine products as a potential adjunct to other forms of anticancer treatment. Generally speaking, all of these approaches have most often been reserved for those patients who have failed to respond to castration or estrogen or have relapsed after an induced remission. Objective responses can be, indeed have been, noted and must be believed. However, careful quantitation of their effectiveness using controls as the Veterans Administration group did for castration and estrogen are badly needed. Without such studies these approaches must remain secondary and/or preterminal measures.

Adrenalectomy after castration, to remove the last vestige of testosterone, will, as previously mentioned, induce some dramatic remissions. However, they are almost always short lived,[16,17] and accordingly this major and hazardous surgical measure rarely seems justified. Hypophysectomy employing the transphenoidal approach, radioactive implants, or freezing is a substantially less morbid procedure and offers the theoretical and potential advantage of removing all androgen sources plus possibly important direct-acting pituitary principles by one maneuver. Clinically significant responses (complete remissions or partial relief of symptoms) and probable extension of life has been observed in 50–70 percent of cases. Interestingly, it seems to matter little whether there had been a prior response to orchiectomy or estrogen.[18–20] Hypophyseal removal, as indicated by plasma growth hormone measurements, need not be complete for therapeutic responses to occur, but a complete removal should be the aim of the operator. With improvements in the operative techniques, hypophysectomy would seem to be warranted for a trial as the primary endocrine therapy when symptoms and signs of dissemination are noted.

The synthetic progestin, cyproterone acetate, was developed as an androgen antagonist. It was only natural that it be tried in prostatic cancer. In the main it has been used in patients with previous castration or estrogen therapy and has been found to induce remissions in about one-half of the patients. It was recently shown to be effective as the primary therapy in one-half of 55 patients. It should be pointed out, however, that in addition to blocking the male hormone influence peripherally, it also results in a lowered circulating testosterone level.[21,22]

Attempts to utilize the growth-promoting effect of testosterone to enhance the uptake of radioactive phosphate by prostate cancer metastases in bone led to some successful results, but it was not established that the androgen therapy was required. However, the attempt did result in the wholly unexpected discovery that occasional patients in relapse respond favorably to testosterone alone.[23] This inexplicable result has occasionally been confirmed.[24]

A Swedish attempt to combine endocrine and nonspecific chemotherapy shows considerable promise. Estracyt is a chemical combination of long-acting estradiol-17-phosphate and nitrogen mustard that can be administered for some time with remarkably little toxicity. Benefit has been noted (1) in patients who had failed to improve when treated with estrogen alone, (2) in patients in relapse, and (3) in patients with advanced disease when used as the first systemic therapy. The histopathology of treated tissue indicates more than just an estrogen effect. This novel approach warrants further exploration.[25,26]

MECHANISMS OF ACTION

Much has been learned in the past decade about the mechanism of androgen action in accessory sex tissues, particularly in the rat ventral prostate. The unbound or free circulating male hormone, testosterone, enters prostate cells apparently without requiring an active transport process. Within the cytoplasm it is converted to dihydrotestosterone by the activity of Δ^4-3-keto-5α-oxidoreductase. At least for prostatic tissue, dihydrotestosterone is the active androgen.[27] Its specificity appears to be dependent primarily on the steric characterization of the molecule, which is relatively flat by comparison with testosterone. There are probably several cytosol proteins that bind this androgen. However, one highly specific receptor protein actually appears to envelop dihydrotestosterone; once bound to this receptor, the steroid cannot be freed by a potent specific antibody, as it can be from other binding proteins. After enveloping this androgen the receptor protein is able to penetrate the cell's nuclear membrane. Within the nucleus the receptor–dihydrotestosterone complex apparently initiates hormone action by combining with specific acceptors—deoxyribonucleoproteins and/or riboneucleoproteins. Within the nucleus the first detectable action of the androgen is an increase in the RNA polymerase activity. This is followed by an increase in ribosomal RNA. It is not known whether increased polymerase activity is the result of a negative action (i.e., the blocking of a genetic depressor) or a positive influence (i.e., a direct stimulation of polymerase activity in a specific region of the DNA template).

These concepts, based upon a series of detailed biochemical studies, are attractive indeed; but their translation into an explanation of the role of androgen in prostatic cellular and tissue activities remains to be accomplished. The action of androgen in other androgen-responsive tissues has not been analyzed in so detailed a fashion. As Liao says, "There is no compelling reason to believe these effects are carried out by a unique molecular process common to all (tissues)."[27] It seems obvious that the same precaution must be taken with any hypothesis that assumes that this mechanism holds true in malignant prostate tumors.

Moreover, it is essential to keep in mind the fact that almost the sole process with which the clinician is concerned in prostatic cancer is uncontrolled cell multiplication. When the tumor responds favorably to castration, cell division is at least temporarily arrested; cell necrosis occurs with the shrinkage and virtual disappearance of some tumors. The working assumption that all this is the result of the lack of androgen is appropriate enough. However, at this time it cannot be said that the androgen action that supports malignant prostate cell replication and maintains the life of the cell involves the biochemical processes that have been described above.

It is also premature to assume that testosterone or its active derivative, dihydrotestosterone, are the only hormones that directly affect cell division and growth of prostatic cancer. Huggins et al. pointed out initially that, in addition to suppressing testosterone secretion via the pituitary–hypothalamic system, estrogen might well act directly in suppressing the multiplication of prostate cells.[28] Such activity could be explained on the basis of an estrogen-induced inhibition of the conversion of testosterone to dihydrotestosterone in prostatic cells in vitro,[18] but other explanations are, of course, possible. It would seem to be of considerable importance to establish, if possible, a direct effect of estrogen on prostatic cancer cells. The existence of such targeted, effective, and safe chemotherapy should provide an important pharmacologic lead. To date, the most convincing evidence of direct cytotoxic action of estrogen in prostatic cancer is the previously mentioned report that the synthetic estrogen chlorotrianisene (Tace) is effective therapeutically without lowering the plasma testosterone concentration.[15] There is, in addition, an indication that the reticuloendothelial system may be stimulated by stilbestrol and other administered estrogens,[19] and it has been suggested that this may be a factor contributing to therapeutic effectiveness.

It was initially assumed that the beneficial influences of adrenalectomy, hypophysectomy, and the antiandrogen cyproterone acetate are due to the effective withdrawal of testosterone from dependent prostatic cancer cells, but in each case some doubts have arisen concerning this interpretation. Adrenalectomy in a castrated man reduces the circulating testosterone level from a value approximating that of the normal woman to virtually nil. One should question whether testosterone circulating at the normal female level is sufficient to support the growth of dependent cancer cells. Could it be the withdrawal of a much more plentiful adrenal product such as dehydroepiandrosterone that is responsible for the remissions? A complete hypophysectomy will, of course, eliminate virtually all testosterone; but the possibility that some pituitary principles may directly support some cancers must be considered. The prostates of hypophysectomized rats have a diminished affinity for testosterone,[20] and prolactin has been shown to augment the action of testosterone in hypophysectomized rats.[21] There are no reported studies bearing directly on prolactin and somatotropin and prostatic cancer, except that it must be pointed out that estrogen administration raises the circulating levels of both. Cyproterone acetate was assumed to be effective because it blocked the effect of testosterone in cancer cells. However, it also lowers the plasma testosterone concentration,[22] and one must also consider the possibility that, like estrogens, this compound may be directly cytotoxic via some mechanism not involving its antiandrogenic potential.

RECOMMENDED THERAPEUTIC APPROACH

The obvious must be said. When possible, prostatic cancer should be removed surgically by the appropriate procedure. A histologic diagnosis is highly desirable. The rare cancer of the uterus masculinus may simulate prostatic cancer clinically;[22] it is possible that estrogen treatment of this endometrial vestige would stimulate growth. When the cancer cannot be eliminated by prostatectomy, a variety of therapeutic modalities must be considered. Here we will concern ourselves only with the endocrine approaches. Three facts about the disease must dominate the plan in any particular case:

1. If the cancer has not been eliminated by prostatectomy, has extended locally, or has become widely disseminated, the disease cannot be cured by any presently available treatment program.
2. Prostatic cancer may be a slowly progressive disease permitting patients to survive for months or even years in reasonable comfort without local or systemic therapy.
3. A cancer may persist and advance despite all efforts to control its progress by endocrine means.

There is no conclusive evidence that early endocrine treatment offers more complete remissions, more enduring responses, or any other advantages over deferring such treatment until symptoms or physical signs require intervention. When the disease process is manifest, systemic therapy is indicated. At this time castration is probably the appropriate first treatment. Estrogen or antiandrogen should be reserved for those patients who refuse castration at this stage. When given, the dose of estrogen should *not* be in the range of the 5 mg/day of stilbestrol formerly employed with such great frequency. Satisfactory responses have been induced by one-fifth this dosage, an amount of estrogen less likely to result in cardiovascular morbidity. In the patients who fail to respond to castration or relapse following an induced remission any other endocrine approach should be attempted. No guide is suggested except to proceed from the courses with the least morbidity to the ones with greater hazard. It is often wise to delay a new course of treatment for several weeks following a relapse, because discontinuance of a previously effective treatment has been followed by another remission. There are no valid predictive tests. A cancer may respond to one endocrine approach after failing to be influenced by another. Even the administration of androgen may rarely result in improvement. Chemotherapy employing facilitating endocrine products such as the combination of estradiol and nitrogen mustard (Estracyt) has shown surprising promise in preliminary reports.

A carefully controlled comparison between the results of castration and hypophysectomy via the low-morbidity transphenoidal approach seems warranted. Theoretically, pituitary removal seems more advantageous. Until such a careful study has been completed, hypophysectomy by any route should be reserved for late in the course of the disease.

BREAST CANCER (FEMALE)

HISTORY

It is probably true that no endocrine-dependent tissue requires as many endocrine products for normal structural development and the regulation of function as do the mammary glands. Estrogen and progesterone stimulate parenchymal growth to maturity, and prolactin initiates milk formation and secretion. However, glucocorticoids, insulin, growth hormone, thyroid, and vasopressin are involved at one point or another for optimum function of the glands (see Chapter 131). It is conceivable that any or all of these hormones could influence the viability and growth of tumor tissue derived from mammary glands. However, only estrogen, progesterone, and prolactin have been implicated in the maintenance of malignant breast growth and have been demonstrated to be influential in regulating the disease process.

The early demonstration that mammary cancers that occur with high frequency in certain mice strains fail to develop in prepubertally ovariectomized animals[34] appears to fit logically with Beatson's discovery that cancer regressed after ovariectomy in premenopausal women. Application of the same logic to the fact that breast cancer flourished in the absence of ovarian function after the menopause led to the view that these cancers might be dependent upon residual ovarian function plus estrogen derived from the adrenal cortex. The dramatic response to adrenalectomy in many women with advanced breast cancer[5] has thus been interpreted as the result of the removal of the major source of residual estrogen. Treatment of the advanced disease by hypophysectomy was a reasonable extension.[35] Ovarian and adrenocortical atrophy were induced by one maneuver. Perhaps as important, the source of prolactin was also removed. Despite the technical difficulties of performing a complete hypophysectomy, the results of the procedure were at least as good statistically as adrenalectomy.

The results of endocrine product administration have been every bit as dramatic as those of endocrine removal, although the rationales do not flow so smoothly from physiology and pharmacology. The success of high-dose estrogen therapy in older women was unanticipated.[36] Androgen therapy probably had the initial retionale of nullifying the peripheral effect of estrogen.[37] Progestins were added to the high-estrogen therapy program only because the combination was unexpectedly effective in carcinogen-induced mammary cancer of rats.[38] High-dose glucocorticoid was initially thought to be effective by virtue of its suppressing adrenocortical secretory activity.

OVARIECTOMY IN PREMENOPAUSAL WOMEN

In premenopausal women the removal of ovarian sources of estrogen is unquestionably beneficial in some cases of advanced breast cancer. Remissions may also be induced in women at the menopause and perhaps 1 or 2 years beyond it. Ovariectomy is probably the approach to be favored since the procedure can now be carried out with minimal hazard, and one can be certain of a prompt loss of all ovarian estrogen. X-ray therapy administered in 4–6 days is also quite effective, but the decline in circulating estrogen is more gradual. In young women the complete eradication of ovarian function by x-ray is a bit less certain than in women over the age of 40. The results from several centers show response rates of 24.5–38 percent following surgical ovariectomy and 15–32 percent after radiation castration.[40 pp23–35] Remissions last on the average 8–20 months, depending on the series being reported. This considerable difference is difficult to explain but could be due to the fact that there may well have been significant variations from study to study in the extent of the disease process when the ovarian function was abolished.

Those patients with the longer interval between mastectomy and recurrence are most likely to respond. There are indications that the response rate with bone metastases is higher than in tumor located in soft tissue. However, neither the location of metastases nor the interval between mastectomy and tumor reappearances should alter the decision to abolish ovarian estrogen secretion as a therapeutic measure. In a field in which differing opinions and prejudices concerning treatment appear to be omnipresent, it is refreshing to note the universal agreement that ovariectomy (surgical or x-ray) is the first treatment for premenopausal women with advanced disease.

Since breast cancer is a particularly poignant and vicious disease in younger women, it seemed entirely rational to abolish ovarian function in young women at the time of mastectomy, particularly if lymph node metastases were evident. This has sometimes been termed a prophylactic ovariectomy. Unfortunately, the documented results of this approach have not lived up to the rational promise. There is no evidence that the proportion of cures is increased in these stage I and stage II cancers.[41] The time between mastectomy and recurrence is apparently prolonged by this approach—from 24 to 38 months. However, the total survival period following mastectomy is the same whether ovariectomy was done prophylactically or therapeutically. Thus the most that can be said is that a longer symptom-free period can be induced by the prophylactic removal of ovarian function. Clearly this limited benefit would have to be weighed against the disadvantages of early castration in any particular case.

ADRENALECTOMY AND HYPOPHYSECTOMY

As the major ablative techniques for the treatment of advanced breast cancer these two procedures will be considered in the same section. From the pragmatic viewpoint the clinician may well be faced with the decision of deciding between these two procedures for any particular patient. Thus a comparison of their efficacy, morbidity, endocrine pathophysiology, and theoretical assets is necessary.

Bilateral adrenalectomy, which should only be performed with simultaneous ovariectomy or in sequence with the elimination of ovarian secretory activity, results in significant objective remissions in approximately 35 percent of cases. Reported series range from 28 to 51 percent.[40 pp88–97] There are indications that the percentage of remissions is highest in older women and quite low about the time of the menopause and before the age of 30. The Joint Committee of the American Medical Association[42] provided a 31 percent estimate from pools of patients from several sources. Although some experiences suggest that metastases in one body area or another may be especially well treated by the procedure, there is not uniform agreement on this, and it seems wiser to accept the view that this is systemic therapy that may affect tumor tissue in any locale.

The rationale for the procedure has been to remove the last vestige of estrogen. The normal adrenal cortex does indeed secrete minute quantities of estrogen and estrogen precursors that are converted in peripheral tissues to minimal quantities of circulating estradiol. Except in rare instances in which accessory adrenal or ovarian tissues may remain and function, adrenalectomy and ovariectomy remove the source of all steroid hormones from a woman.

Thus far no evidence has been adduced to indicate that an early adrenalectomy and ovariectomy could cure the disease. However, palliation, when it occurs, is prompt and often dramatic, and life is prolonged. Because of the seriousness of the surgery, the procedure is usually deferred until the disease is moderately advanced—but usually not until the patient is in a preterminal state. In the hands of a competent surgeon and with optimum postoperative care, the morbidity and mortality of the procedure can be held to a sufficiently low point to justify the procedure.

Remissions following hypophysectomy occur with approximately the same frequency as those induced by adrenalectomy. In individual studies the remission rates range from 28 to 46 percent[40 pp88–97] and the Joint Committee of the American Medical Association pooled reports indicated a remission rate of 31–32 percent.[42] Despite the equality of published results a rather convincing argument can be made to support the superiority of hypophyseal removal or destruction.

The morbidity and mortality of the drastic transcranial approach has been lessened by modified approaches and techniques:[43] the implantation of radioactive isotopes such as yttrium and strontium, proton-beam irradiation, stalk section, freezing, and an improved transsphenoidal surgical approach. The incidence of complications such as diabetes insipidus and cranial nerve injuries has decreased. Replacement therapy with thyroid and glucocorticoids is not difficult. Although the incidence of induced remissions is not significantly greater than that from adrenalectomy, reports of remission from hypophysectomy following an adrenalectomy indicate a more broadly effective procedure.[44]

The argument that the removal of circulating prolactin and perhaps somatotropin in addition to the secondary loss of adrenocortical and ovarian estrogen provides additional benefit has acquired considerable support. The strongest evidence that prolactin supports mammary gland malignancy is derived from the study of carcinogen-induced mammary cancers in Sprague-Dawley rats. These model mammary cancers exhibit a number of similarities to the human disease. They regress after ovariectomy and are restimulated by estradiol administration.[45] The tumors also melt away after hypophysectomy, but in this circumstance estradiol fails to restore growth. However, prolactin administration promptly reactivates the tumor growth in the hypophysectomized rats.[46,47] Since these responsive tumors contain specific estrogen receptors, it appears that estradiol is a direct stimulus of tumor growth that reacts synergistically with prolactin. There is little doubt, however, that in these special cancers endogenous prolactin has a pronounced tumor-stimulating effect even in the absence of estrogen.[48] The blockade of prolactin secretion by the administration of ergocornine and other ergot drugs inhibits tumor growth.[49] Thus, prolactin removal has a favorable influence in this experimental cancer.

In humans the cancer-supporting influence of prolactin is comparatively slight. Indeed, the tumor regression induced by estrogen treatment and pituitary stalk section, both of which result in enhanced prolactin secretion,[50–52] point in the opposite direction. There is also no convincing evidence that the plasma prolactin concentrations are higher in women with advanced breast cancer than in matched noncancerous controls.[53,54] In such a series, however, it must be appreciated that an occasional case in which an elevated prolactin level may be stimulating cancer growth could be lost in the statistical analysis. Nonetheless, the suppression of plasma prolactin levels with a very potent ergot alkaloid failed to suppress the cancer growth in 19 patients with advanced disease.[55] The most convincing evidence of the importance of pituitary principles remains the occasional response of cancers in previously adrenalectomized women when the pituitary gland is removed.[44]

EFFECTS OF HORMONE ADMINISTRATION

Estrogen

The administration of supra-maintenance quantities of estrogen is the most effective single endocrine product treatment of advanced breast cancer. As originally reported by Haddow and his associates,[56] its major application is in postmenopausal women, but responses may occur at the time of the menopause and rarely even premenopausally.[56] The American Medical Association compilation indicated a regression rate of 38 percent, and this figure is very close to that adduced by individual investigators.[40,53,57] Of course, the average survival rate in all series was prolonged in comparison with that of untreated patients. There are indications that soft tissue metastases have a higher remission rate than those in bone. As in most endocrine manipulations, those patients with longer intervals between mastectomy and recurrence have the higher response rate, and old women are more likely to respond than those close to menopausal age.

It seems to matter little if at all whether synthetic estrogen, such as diethylstilbestrol, natural estrogens, or synthetic modifications of natural estrogens, such as ethinyl estradiol, are given. Doses have not been carefully worked out, but most quantities employed are at least 10 times the replacement range. The influence of such estrogen dosages on the cardiovascular system has been discussed (see Prostatic Cancer). This toxic influence is probably less important in breast cancer because the disease is characteristically much more rapidly progressive than prostatic cancer, even when spectacular remissions occur.

Exacerbation of the cancer by estrogen is frequent in premenopausal women and may occur rarely in older patients. Hypercalcemia may be an early sign of increased activity, especially in patients with bone lesions. It is important, however, to keep in mind that a mild acceleration of the disease process may occur prior to an induced remission, and such initial prompt exacerbations are often a favorable sign. This has been termed a *biphasic response*.[40 p54]

Remissions are not usually as prompt in developing as they are after extirpative therapy, and 6–8 weeks should be allowed before abandoning hope for improvement. If remissions are noted, therapy should be continued until toxic effect or relapse occurs. It is usually unwise to shift immediately to another treatment when a relapse is evident, because occasionally a second remission may follow the discontinuation of estrogen.

Androgens

The use of androgen stems from a report of its effect in mammary cancer of mice.[37] Since high androgen dosage is required for a favorable response, testosterone propionate was the product employed until about 15 years ago, when more potent long-acting and less virilizing androgens were developed and found to be effective. The American Medical Association compilation of results and the Cooperative Breast Cancer Group recorded objective regressions in 21.9 and 21.5 percent, respectively, of postmenopausal women.[40 p36,58,59] In premenopausal and menopausal women the response rate is somewhat lower (10–20 percent). As with estrogen, those patients with induced remissions lived about twice as long (19.1 months) as those in whom no benefits were documented. Data indicate that bone metastases respond more frequently that do tumors in soft tissues. Androgens are appropriate following a trial with estrogen or after an estrogen-induced remission. The response rate is somewhat better in those patients in whom estrogen was effective. As in the case of estrogens, a second response may occur during the 2 months following discontinuance.

There is, accordingly, considerable qualitative similarity between estrogen- and androgen-induced responses. However, in addition to the lower rate of effectiveness, the androgens (e.g., testosterone and fluoxymesterone) have the immense disadvantage of inducing disfiguring virilization and sometimes an insatiable stimulation of libido. Newer androgen derivatives that have little or nor virilizing potential retain the anticancer activity of testosterone. Two that are notable are testalolactone, with no androgenicity, and calusterone, which is a very weak androgen. Results with the latter compound indicate an effectiveness rate about the same as that of potent androgen.[59]

Antiestrogens

When compounds with antiestrogenic activity became available for clinical use, it was natural that they be tried in women with breast cancer. The fact that these compounds competitively bind with a specific intracellular protein in mammary tumors as well as in some normal estrogen-dependent tissues was supportive (see Prediction of Endocrine Response, below). It was hoped that at least the estrogen-dependent tumors would regress under the influence of such drugs. Reported results tend to be favorable, but the scattered short series of cases with objective improvement of 13–33 percent has not excited a great deal of interest.[60] It must be kept in mind that the antiestrogenic compounds possess slight intrinsic estrogenic activity, especially when given in large doses. Perhaps this is sufficient to undercut the estrogen antagonism in sensitive "dependent" tumors.

Glucocorticoids

Following the demonstration that adrenalectomy induced remissions in advanced breast cancer, it was proposed that suppression of adrenocortical function by large doses of glucocorticoids would have a similar effect by inducing a so-called "medical adrenalectomy." Remissions are induced by such therapy, but the results are not as effective as adrenalectomy.[39,40,p74] and a short intensive course of glucocorticoid cannot be employed as a test for the efficacy of adrenalectomy because some patients have been reported to have responded to removal of the adrenals after having failed to improve while receiving glucocorticoid.[61] Although some observers have reported an improvement rate as high as that of adrenalectomy, this has not been the usual experience. An improved state of well-being often accompanies this treatment, but in some cases this is certainly one of the toxic effects of hyperadrenocorticism and is not due to a favorable influence on the disease itself.

One of the problems with this therapeutic approach is that adrenocortical function cannot be obliterated by glucocorticoid excess—at least not in the time allowable. An atrophic gland persists that is probably able to secrete aldosterone for some time and may also liberate estrogen and other steroids that could stimulate growth of the cancers. Some of the benefits resulting from glucocorticoid therapy might well be ascribable to other actions of the steroid, such as nonspecific antiinflammatory action. It is also possible that the profound catabolic influence of glucocorticoid excess is exerted on cancer tissue, perhaps sometimes even in a relatively selective fashion to induce some tumor regression. The dramatic influence of induced hypercorticism on the hypercalcemia that occurs so frequently in preterminal breast cancer is a therapeutic tool that all physicians treating this disease must keep in mind. However, the explanation for this serum calcium-lowering action is obscure and does not appear to be the expression of a growth-inhibiting action of glucocorticoid on the malignant tumors.

Progestins

The earliest attempts to treat breast cancer with progesterone met with scant success. However, the development of very potent analogues permitting the easy administration of high progestin activity revived interest. The success of the combination of estrogen–progesterone and the clear demonstration that the results obtained could not be ascribed to the estrogen alone (see below) were undoubtedly encouraging. A number of trials with synthetic progestins have now been reported. All of the progestins have the clear advantage of being virtually free of significant side effects except for the rare hepatotoxicity of 17 alkylated steroids. Progesterone and the caproate ester of 17-hydroxyprogesterone must be given by injection. Medroxyprogesterone acetate is very effective both orally and by injection and is becoming the most widely employed steroid for progestational purposes. Reports indicate that favorable responses to large doses of progestins alone may be seen in 25–30 percent of the patients.[40 p68]

Estrogen–Progestin Combinations

Following Huggins' demonstration that the carcinogen (7,12-dimethylbenzanthracine, DMBA) induced mammary cancer of Sprague-Dawley rats responded most effectively to a combination of estradiol and progesterone, approximately the same relative doses on a weight basis were tried in patients with metastatic breast cancer.[62] In the first cases studied the patients had relapsed from or failed to respond adequately to adrenalectomy or hypophysectomy. One of the responding patients was a man whose tumors had previously regressed after castration and again after adrenalectomy. In one patient visible skin cancers continued to grow when estrogen alone was administered but promptly regressed when progesterone was added and remained under control for 8 years. Crowley and Mac Donald[63] confirmed these observations and noted 6 patients who responded to the combination after being unresponsive to estrogen alone. They then extrapolated from general experience with estrogen to reach the conclusion that more than 50 percent of postmenopausal women should experience remissions when subjected to estrogen–progestin therapy. This extrapolation may well be a bit optimistic.[40 p68,64] The combination of synthetic estrogens and progestins has also been found effective coupled with 0.1 and 0.05 mg dexamethasone/day in premenopausal as well as postmenopausal women.[65] The rationale of the slight excess of glucocorticoid was the suppression of ACTH secretion—a point of doubtful importance in evaluating the therapeutic efficacy of the combination.

Endocrine–Cytotoxic Combination

Estramustine phosphate (Estracyt), which is an ingenious clinical combination of estradiol and nitrogen mustard, has been given to women with breast cancer without notable benefit.[66] This is rather surprising, since results of prostatic cancer have been quite encouraging.

PREDICTION OF ENDOCRINE RESPONSE

Uncertainty that the cancer in any particular patient would respond to endocrine manipulation has led, quite naturally, to efforts to discover some factors in the tumor or the host that would correlate with endocrine-induced tumor regression. It was at first thought that histologic differentiation of the tumor was important—i.e., that those cancers most closely resembling healthy parenchyma would be hormonally dependent. However, such correlations were poor at best and attempts to make significant predictions on the basis of histology were soon abandoned.

The efforts of Bulbrook and his associates to employ the measurement of urinary corticoids and androgens in a ratio for predictive purposes has resulted in a good number of reports. These attempts to evaluate selective aspects of the endocrine milieu as being affected by or as influencing tumor responsiveness to adrenalectomy or hypophysectomy have been carried out in many patients. However, the predictive value of the procedure in the hands of its proponents has never led to sufficient precision to justify its application in a practical manner.[67] The procedure has not been taken up by others perhaps in large measure because it failed to shed light on the biology of the disease despite suggestively interesting results.

The estrogen dependency hypothesis, however, has spawned a promising predictive procedure. Tumors that demonstrated a capacity to take up more radioactively labeled estrogen in vivo than others tended to be the ones that regressed after adrenalectomy.[68] Jensen et al.[7] have pioneered in the development of an in vitro procedure based upon these hopeful observations. The test involves the demonstration that estrogen-responsive tissues such as the uterus contain a receptor protein that specifically binds to estradiol and thus induces its translocation to the cell nucleus. It has been shown that some experimental rodent mammary cancers contain such a protein, and this has also been demonstrated in some human breast cancers. This receptor protein, termed *estrophyllin,* was at first assayed on small tissue slices of about 0.5 g. However, the sensitivity of the assay has been enhanced by using cytosol purified by ultracentrifugation in a sucrose gradient. It can now be carried out on much smaller tissue fragments and more precisely quantitated. In their carefully evaluated series, approximately one-half of the patients with receptor-positive tumors responded to endocrine therapy, which in the overwhelming majority of these cases was hypophysectomy, adrenalectomy, and/or ovariectomy. Only occasional patients with no receptor protein responded favorably. These findings have been confirmed by others. It thus appears that those patients whose tumor contains no estrophyllin have little chance of responding to endocrine therapy.

The data apply better to extirpative endocrine treatments than to the array of hormone-treatment regimens. It is difficult to appreciate how an estrogen receptor could facilitate a favorable response to androgen, progestins, or glucocorticoid therapy. Perhaps the favorable correlations thus far are more a recognition of the fact that tumors that respond to one endocrine maneuver tend to respond to another rather than an indication that the presence of specific estrogen receptor facilitates any endocrine therapy.

MECHANISM OF HORMONAL EFFECTS

The regression of tumors that follows ovariectomy, adrenalectomy, or hypophysectomy can only be explained at this time on the basis of the withdrawal of growth-supporting endocrine products. The analogy between the need for estrogen of normal mammary gland development on the one hand, and the tumor-stimulating effect of estrogen (in some cases) and the clinical benefit of estrogen withdrawal on the other is almost totally persuasive. It is probably too glib to ascribe all of the effects of endocrine extirpation to the resulting decline or elimination of available estrogen. As noted elsewhere, prolactin withdrawal may be an important factor in some cases, and other pituitary principles could also be involved. The adrenal cortex probably secretes a small amount of estrogen; larger quantities are derived from the peripheral metabolism of adrenal products such as dehydroepiandrosterone and androstenedione.

It seems appropriate to question whether the very low levels of estrogen directly and indirectly derived from the adrenals is sufficient to promote dependent tumor growth. In ovariectomized women other sensitive indicators of estrogen's presence, such as the suppression of postmenopausal pituitary gonadotropin levels and full vaginal cornification, are not manifestations of these low estrogen levels. It is possible that some breast cancers may derive support from dehydroepiandrosterone, which is liberated from the functioning adrenal and circulates in the free form or as the sulfate in considerable concentrations. Dehydroepiandrosterone seems to be a biologically inert by-product of glucocorticoid synthesis, but it is conceivable that it could support the growth of some malignant cells, perhaps even indirectly via a metabolite developed in the cancer cells themselves.

The presence of specific estrogen receptors in most breast cancers that respond to endocrine gland removal (see Prediction of Endocrine Response) has been adduced as further support for the dependency theory. Since the presence of receptors in a tumor without estrogen dependency occurs with some frequency, the demonstration of the receptor alone cannot be accepted as proof of a dependent state. Thus, specific binding of estrogen may be unrelated to the processes of cell multiplication and tumor growth.

As in the case of testosterone, the binding of estradiol to a specific cytoplasmic protein is the essential first step to hormone action after the steroid enters the cell. The similarity to the mechanism of testosterone action continues, except that no metabolic modification of the estradiol occurs. The highly specific cytoplasmic estradiol-binding protein of uteri possesses a sedimentation coefficient of about 8 S. This protein probably contains the only specific binding site in estrogen-responsive tissues. Several rapid assays for the protein have been developed, and it has been found in uteri from a number of species including man. The estradiol, when bound to the 8 S protein, enters the cell nucleus; in the nucleus the estradiol-binding protein has a sedimentation coefficient of 4 S, which probably represents the disaggregated 8 S protein. It is apparently an identical receptor protein that has been measured in mammary cancer cells.[69,70]

Estradiol promptly stimulates several metabolic pathways within the responsive cells. Among them is increased protein synthesis, which appears to be closely related to an increase in RNA synthesis. These two effects are probably more closely involved with the aspects of estrogen action most important in relation to the control of breast cancer. Processes such as RNA and protein synthesis are generally thought to be hormonal actions resulting from gene expression. However, much more detailed investigation will be required to prove that the hormonal action of estradiol that leads to uncontrolled replication of mammary cancer cells is a direct outgrowth of this genetic action.

The possibility of prolactin dependency is less clear. In vitro receptors for prolactin have been described in some tumors,[71] but the relationship of this finding to tumor growth dependency has not yet been worked out. The growth of carcinogen-induced mammary tumors in rats may be stimulated by administered prolactin.[72] These results suggest that the favorable response to hypophysectomy in these rats, and similarly in some patients, may be due in part to prolactin withdrawal. If there is indeed prolactin dependency of tumor growth in these animals, it is not clear whether this hormone is acting alone or whether any growth-stimulating influence it possesses requires estrogen "permissively."

Several dilemmas face the enthusiast who believes prolactin has a substantial responsibility for encouraging breast cancer growth in women. The fact that estrogen is a most effective stimulus for prolactin secretion, inducing several-fold elevations in the plasma prolactin concentration, is not the least of them. It must be remembered that 30–50 percent of these patients respond favorably to the larger dose of estrogen or estrogen and progestin, despite this induction of hyperprolactinemia. The determinations of plasma prolactin have not been convincingly elevated in untreated patients with progressive breast cancer.

The most that can be said at this time is that prolactin may play a supporting role in the growth of some cancers. For these an elevated circulating concentration may not be required.

The interpretations of the influence of endocrine product administration range from uncertainty to confusion. Stoll has thoroughly reviewed the many studies that might have a bearing on the mechanisms by which estrogen administration favorably influences the course of the disease.[73] He then makes a heroic effort to weave the often contradictory facts into cohesive theories to explain the actions, but it just cannot be brought off.

Physiologically there is no parallel to the growth inhibition and cell-necrotizing influence of estrogen in mammary cancers. The fact that most of the cancers that respond appear to have specific estrogen receptors is intriguing, but it will be recalled that a substantial minority of cancers with receptors fail to respond. Thus the most that can be stated at this time is that the specific receptor may provide the vehicle for estrogen to reach the critically vulnerable cell function and/or structure within the cell. It is possible that some of those tumors that fail to respond to estradiol might respond if an intracellular vehicle in lieu of the cytoplasmic receptor protein could be provided.

The mechanisms of progestin, androgen, and glucocorticoid action are even more difficult to fathom. Estraphyllin is certainly not invoked since none of these steroids are bound by the estrogen receptor protein. Other specific receptors may be involved in some manner, but such possibilities have not been discovered. It is of at least passing interest that progesterone in large amounts does induce normal endometrial atrophy, and glucocorticoids are generally protein catabolic agents, but the relevance of these actions to their effect on mammary cancer is tenuous indeed. On the other hand, the androgens are somatically anabolic. In this instance it is attractive to consider the androgens as antiestrogens of sorts. It would seem more profitable, at the moment, to regard the anticancer influence of all these hormonal substances as remarkably discriminating chemotherapeutic agents and attempt to search for a more precise mechanism in that light.

What might be called the biology of the tumor cells seems to be important, for those tumors that respond to one endocrine manipulation are more likely to respond to another than those that are initially unresponsive. Cancers in older patients respond more frequently and more enduringly than those in younger women.

The key clinical feature of malignancies is their uncontrolled cell replication; the tumors grow in a manner suggesting that they are no longer the cells of the host. If the tumor is thus regarded as a foreign cell invasion, the immune resistance of the host becomes an important factor in the control of the disease. It thus seems important to look for the possibility that remissions induced by hormonal treatment could be due in part to a lowered resistance of the tumor to the host immune system or to enhancement of the resistance of the host tissues to the invading tumor. The latter possibility has been suggested as a factor in the response of tumors to large doses of estrogen.[30,74]

One of the more intriguing mysteries clinical investigators are considering is the fact that no matter how dramatic a remission has been induced, the disease almost inevitably recurs. Every cell with the capacity for uncontrolled mitotic activity cannot be eliminated. One possible explanation is that the recurring disease might be derived from a different genetic clone of cells, one that had not been previously multiplying. It is obvious that hormone "dependency" is not absolute, or that the endocrine chemotherapy and/or immunologic antagonism is incapable of abolishing the multiplying potential of every cell. Perhaps the disease is always too far advanced when endocrine treatment is initiated.

The importance of having an experimental model to explore the mechanism of hormone action and to develop new therapeutic approaches cannot be underestimated. Huggins' suggestion that the carcinogen (DMBA)-induced mammary cancer of Sprague-Dawley rats could be used for this purpose has already lead to some important developments. The model is not perfect. The rat mammary cancers do not metastasize and they differ in other ways that have been noted from the disease in man, but a number of the similarities are striking. One potentially important hint from Huggins' rat experiments has not been exploited in man. Only by very early treatment, when the cancers were microscopic, could Huggins et al. extinguish most of the tumors by the most effective treatment discovered, the combination of estradiol and progesterone in large quantities.[38] This finding has been confirmed by a "prophylactic" influence of the hormone in the same model.[75] Apparently, even the prophylactic ovariectomy in premenopausal women is too late.

SUGGESTIONS FOR THERAPY

Readers of the preceding sections describing the results of the several endocrine therapies must be left with practical uncertainties. There are good reasons for this.

Although the number of approaches to the management of this disease and the number of hormonal agents employed has multiplied, we find ourselves only slightly closer to the solution of this tantalizing problem than we were a quarter century ago. The tabulation of results indicates that with each therapeutic approach roughly the same percentage of effective responses can be anticipated (20–50 percent). The superiority of some methods has been indicated, but the differences are not great and individual circumstances must govern therapy. Controlled comparisons on randomized patients have rarely been made. It must also be pointed out that some of the percentages have been obtained from relatively small series of patients that could not possibly provide representation of all the diverse expressions of breast cancer. Most studies report objective remission rates, but to the responsible physician the induction of stability in the disease process is also an important gain.

There are also deficiencies in the pharmacologic details. These are inexcusible and yet are quite understandable. Dose–response data are sadly lacking. If patients responded to one dose, that dose was usually continued and replicated in other cases. This is the sort of problem that is almost inevitable in a serious chronic disease that, while relatively frequent, does not occur in epidemic proportions. A careful comparison of doses and responses with the several endocrine products that induce favorable effects would require years of careful observation—the sort of studies that seem to fail to excite and involve any researchers.

In devising a proposed treatment protocol several basic principles have been kept in mind: 1. Present information dictates that no protocol that is rigidly adhered to will serve all patients well. The wise physician will deviate intuitively to take advantage of unanticipated developments or special circumstances. 2. Radiation therapy for specific lesions may be indicated despite a favorable general response; for example, to forestall a pathologic fracture. 3. Six to twelve weeks may be required for a remission to be detected with certainty. 4. It is usually inadvisable to discontinue a course of treatment while the disease is in remission. 5. When the disease relapses after a remission induced by the administration of a hormonal product(s), treatment should be discontinued. Other systemic measures should be withheld for about 2 months to take advantage of a possible remission induced by endocrine withdrawal. 6. Predictive procedures such as the determination of the presence of specific estrogen receptors should be performed if readily available. At the present time their applied value lies in guiding the therapist away from relatively high morbidity approaches such as adrenalectomy. 7. Nonendocrine systemic chemotherapy for advanced cancer should not be employed prior to endocrine treatment programs. This relatively noxious therapy seems to lessen the response rate to endocrine approaches. 8. A response to one endocrine modality increases the likelihood of response to another. However, there are so many exceptions to this rule that it would be unwise to withhold a second endocrine approach because the first was a failure. 9. By starting with the simpler and more benign therapies and reserving the more traumatizing and hazardous efforts for later, maximum health and the capacity for a full life can be preserved for a longer period. 10. An exacerbation of signs and symptoms during the first week or two of treatment with endocrine products may indicate a subsequent favorable response.

In premenopausal women (and postmenopausal women up to 2 years after the last menstrual period) with estrogen receptor–positive tumors, bilateral ovariectomy or x-ray destruction of the secretory capacity of the ovaries is clearly the first therapeutic approach when metastases or local recurrence of the cancer is noted (Fig. 157-4). There appears to be little to be gained by removing the ovaries earlier, for example, immediately after mastectomy when lymph node involvement has been discovered. If removal of ovaries fails or when relapse occurs after a remission, medical management with estrogen and progestin or an androgen such as calusterone should be initiated. Following trials with one or both of these courses endocrine gland removal can be attempted. A transsphenoidal hypophysectomy is preferred to adrenalectomy because it is a less morbid procedure and offers the potential advantage of removing more endocrine secretions that might be stimulating some cancer cells. Systemic chemotherapy should probably be given to all patients without estrogen receptors in the cancer, but it should be reserved for the last and most heroic therapeutic attempt in those with receptor-positive tumors.

The management of advanced disease in postmenopausal women with estrogen receptors in the cancer can follow a very similar pattern (Fig. 157-5). Occasional patients without receptor-positive tumors have also responded favorably to endocrine measures, but some therapists would prefer to omit such attempts in these patients and proceed at once to systemic chemotherapy. The estrogen–progestin combination is preferred as the first endocrine approach, but newer androgens such as calusterone or one of the antiestrogens should be tried in selected cases. Adrenalectomy and ovariectomy or hypophysectomy may well be effective after the responses to endocrine product administration have ended, especially if estrogen receptors are present. The decision between these two surgical procedures is best made on the basis of availability of the appropriate surgical skill, but the transsphenoidal hypophysectomy is preferred. Systemic chemotherapy should probably be given to all patients without estrogen receptors in the cancer, but it should be reserved for the last and most heroic therapeutic attempt in those with receptor-positive tumors.

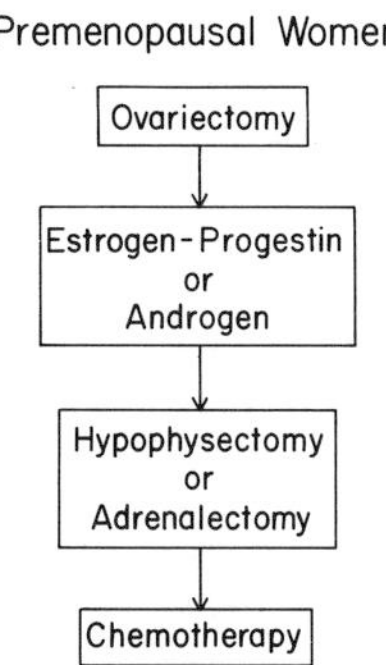

Fig. 157-4. Suggested protocol for managing premenopausal women with estrogen receptor–positive advanced breast cancer. An effective dose of estrogen–progestin is 40 mg estradiol valerate and 500 mg 17-hydroxyprogesterone caproate, both given intramuscularly once a week, or comparable daily oral doses of synthetics such as ethinyl estradiol and medroxyprogesterone acetate. The androgen suggested is calusterone in a dosage of 200 mg/day.

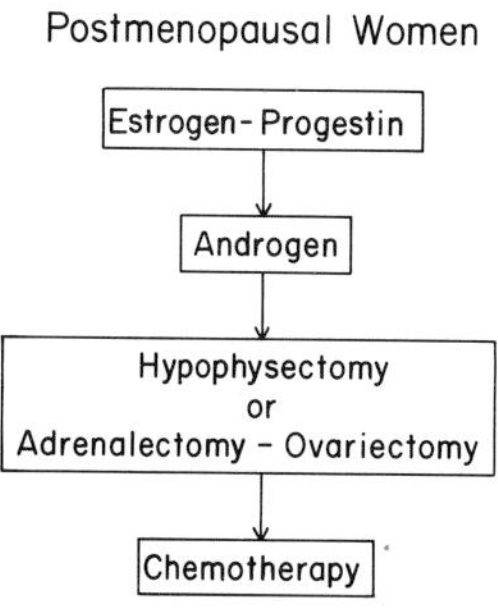

Fig. 157-5. Suggested protocol for managing postmenopausal women with advanced breast cancer (estrogen receptor–positive). Such exhaustive endocrine trials are probably not justified in patients with estrogen receptor–negative cancer. An effective dose of estrogen–progestin is 40 mg estradiol valerate and 500 mg 17-hydroxyprogesterone caproate, both given intramuscularly once a week, or comparable daily oral doses of synthetics such as ethinyl estradiol and medroxyprogesterone acetate. The androgen suggested is calusterone in a dosage of 200 mg/day.

MALE BREAST CANCER

There is a considerable body of evidence indicating that growth of mammary gland parenchyma under the influence of estrogen is a usual prerequisite for the development of mammary cancer in females. One can only speculate on the manner in which this applies to the development of the much rarer breast cancer in men. Mammary glands remain rudimentary in men as a result of the action of the male hormone. Exposure of the fetal mammary glands to small amounts of androgen is probably the most important factor:[76] in addition, during puberty and adult life, when the plasma estrogen concentrations of males overlap the normal concentrations of women, the high titers of androgen are probably inhibitory. The development of full breasts in the feminizing testis syndrome, in which the male hormone is genetically inoperative,[77] suggests that the concentration of estrogen derived from normal testicular activity is adequate to stimulate breast growth to feminine proportions when there is no virilizing androgen. On the other hand, the mild physiologic gynecomastia of puberty, gynecomastia induced by testosterone administration, and the suggestion that impressive gynecomastia might result from nonsuppressible hyperLeydigism[78] raise the possibility that growth of parenchymal tissue in the male mammary gland may be stimulated by androgen as well as by estrogen.

Entirely similar ambivalence prevails in the control of breast cancer in men. Castration in advanced cancer is more frequently effective than ovariectomy in women.[79] About two-thirds of men with metastases respond and life is significantly prolonged. Responses have also been reported following adrenalectomy, hypophysectomy, estrogen treatment, and estrogen–progestin therapy.[40 p127,80] The disease is exacerbated when androgen is administered after a castration-induced remission. The preponderance of reported results thus indicates that breast cancer in men may be dependent upon androgen. Just as in prostatic cancer, the withdrawal of androgen sources is followed by favorable responses. Because normal breast tissue is more responsive to estrogen, one may ask whether these responses might be in part due to estrogen withdrawal, since some estrogen is derived from the peripheral metabolism of testosterone as well as being secreted by normal adrenal cortices and testicular Leydig cells; but the answer is not forthcoming. No studies on the presence or absence of specific estrogen or androgen receptors in male breast cancer have been reported.

A relatively high response rate to endocrine manipulation is quite encouraging. The first therapeutic attempt when metastases are evident should be castration. Following this estrogen–progestin combinations should be given. Hypophysectomy and adrenalectomy are available as a last endocrine resource. As in women, those individuals who respond to one endocrine approach tend to respond to another.

ENDOMETRIAL CANCER

It is somewhat surprising that endometrial cancers were not shown to be hormonally responsive until 20 years after the first reports that prostatic cancer responded to castration. Histologic changes through the menstrual cycle are probably the most dramatic illustration of physiologic shifts in structure and function induced by modifications in the hormonal milieu. The proliferative growth under estrogen, the conversion of proliferative endometrium to a secretory phase with added progesterone, the slough of secretory endometrium after progesterone withdrawal, and the eventual atrophy of the epithelium and conversion of the stroma to a decidual reaction if progesterone secretion continues at a high level had been known for some years. The continuous administration of estrogen without the presentation of progesterone was known to produce endometrial hyperplasia, which may be a precancerous lesion. After the discovery by Kelley and Baker[81] how easy it is to see that progesterone should have been considered for the prevention and treatment of endometrial cancer much earlier.

A number of observations strongly suggest that endocrinologic and metabolic factors are important in the pathogenesis of endometrial malignancy. Women in whom the disease develops are usually postmenopausal and tend to be obese, mildly diabetic, nulliparous, and infertile. The continuous exposure of the endometrium to estrogen is a key factor in the pathogenesis of the disease, especially in younger women.[82] A history of dysfunctional uterine bleeding is not unusual. Women with functional ovarian tumors, granulosa, or thecal cell tumors that secrete estrogen have been shown to have associated endometrial cancers in 3–25 percent of the cases. Twenty-five percent of all cases of endometrial cancer that develop in women under the age of 30 are seen in patients with Stein-Leventhal syndrome, which is characterized by persistent estrogen secretion, polycystic ovaries, failure to ovulate, infertility, and intermittent bleeding or amenorrhea. Endometrial malignancy has also been reported in 5 cases of Turner's syndrome treated with rather large continuous doses of stilbestrol and no progestin.[83] In 1959 Kistner[84] reported that the unopposed action of estrogen, in its administration for up to 100 days in normal menstruating women, could induce varying degrees of endometrial hyperplasia and anaplasia. It was suggested that changes such as these, including carcinoma in situ occurring in postmenopausal women, could be successfully treated with large amounts of progestin by conversion of the endometrium to atrophic decidual-like states. This was the first hint that endometrial malignancies might be treatable by a progestin.

The first reported treatment of advanced metastatic endometrial cancer indicated excellent therapeutic responses in about 30 percent of the patients treated with large amounts of 17-hydroxyprogesterone caproate. Subsequent observations suggested that pulmonary metastases were more likely to be favorably influenced than tumors in other sites, but after the treatment of many cases, it became apparent that the site of the metastases was relatively unimportant. The dose of the synthetic progestins employed has varied greatly from one center to another, i.e., from a minimum of 500 mg 17-hydroxyprogesterone caproate/week to 1000 mg/day. Dose–response observations have not been made. A course of 1000 mg/week is suggested. Several other progestins, notably medroxyprogesterone acetate and megestrol, have also been employed with equal success. The most optimistic reports indicate that tumor regression, or at least an arrest of the tumor's growth, can be induced in up to 70 percent of all patients treated. Cures were actually suggested in about 20 percent of the patients in one series.[85] Some investigators have had the courage to discontinue progestin in favorable cases for a number of months without such discontinuance being followed by regrowth of the tumor. Most investigators have employed progestins alone. In one case, however, there was a favorable response to progestin and a relapse, at which point the addition of estrogen in large quantities was followed by a second tumor regression.[86] This observation is reminiscent of the fact that progesterone has no influence on the endometrium unless it has been previously prepared by estrogen. Perhaps the effectiveness of progestin would be enhanced in other cases if estrogen were administered simultaneously.

The antitumor effects of progestins have been assumed to be a direct influence of the steroid on cellular activity. Luteinizing hormone (LH) and follicle-stimulating hormone (FSH) are suppressed by these large doses of progestin, but it is difficult to see how this could contribute to the remissions induced. When large doses of progestin are presented to normal endometrial epithelial cells, they begin to atrophy, become cuboidal, and then flattened and very atrophic; finally mitoses cease. In endometrial cancer the same changes have been observed, followed in many cases by cell necrosis. The progestins actually appear to act as cytotoxic agents for the responsive tumor cells alone. The absence of toxic side effects with the huge doses of synthetic progestin administered in these cases is remarkable indeed.

OVARIAN CARCINOMA

Ovarian malignancies are the most recently reported to be responsive to endocrine therapy—in this case large doses of synthetic progestin. Publications are scattered, but some reports are quite convincing. Adenocarcinomas ranging from anaplastic to well differentiated in their histologic appearance have responded. Although the objective response rate ranges from about 10 percent to 30 percent, the duration of resulting benefit has usually been remarkably short lived and often was confined principally to the reduction of ascites.

Abdominal tumors were sometimes reported to be diminished in size. The infrequency of such reports for such a relatively common malignancy permits one to reach the conclusion that results are very seldom impressive.[87]

RENAL CANCER

It has long been appreciated that the growth-promoting influence of sex hormones is not restricted to the accessory sex apparatus in the two sexes.[88] The somatotrophic or growth-promoting influence of androgen is prominent and extends to some viscera, especially the kidneys. The general anabolic influence of estrogen is demonstrable but distinctly less effective and probably does not affect muscle. Progesterone is uniquely catabolic in man and has an appetite-stimulating effect in rats.[89] None of these effects prepare one for the known influence of the sex hormones in renal cancer.

The model that led to the studies in man was adenocarcinoma of the kidney of the golden hamster, which was induced by long-term estrogen treatment.[90] Surprisingly, this tumor has been shown to respond favorably to testosterone, progesterone, medroxyprogesterone acetate, cortisone, and orchiectomy. Castration-induced regression was overcome by estrogen therapy. This surprising array of responses to endocrine manipulations by Bloom and his associates[91] was the basis for the first trials of endocrine therapy for renal cancer in man. The successful results obtained cannot be explained on the basis of hormonal dependency or the blockade of a dependent state—at least so far as one can tell from available data.

Bloom's series[92] of 80 patients treated between 1959 and 1969 is the longest reported. Of 80 patients with advanced incurable disease treated with potent synthetic progestins (usually medroxyprogesterone acetate) in very large doses, subjective improvement was noted in 44 patients (55 percent) and 23 patients (29 percent) experienced demonstrable tumor regression of some degree; 16 percent were strikingly improved. As with other endocrine-responsive cancers, 6 weeks was sometimes required before improvement was demonstrable. Unfortunately, in only a few patients was there a clear indication that life was prolonged. In most the responses were limited and of short duration; occasionally tumor growth stimulation was actively suspected. Occasional patients also responded favorably to testosterone. Most of the responding renal cancers were in men, but it must be noted that a predominance of these malignancies occur in males.

Bloom's work has been confirmed by others, but it should be pointed out that Swiss investigators[93] failed to observe any remissions with androgen or progestin in 58 cases. The explanation for this discrepancy is not obvious, but this negative report does indicate that profound benefit, like that observed in breast and prostatic cancer, is relatively rare.

REFERENCES

1. Haddow, A. Sir Ernest Lawrence Kennaway FRS 1881–1958: chemical causation of cancer then and today. *Perspect Biol Med 17:* 543, 1974.
2. Beatson, G. T. On the treatment of inoperable cases of carcinoma of the mamma: suggestions for a new method of treatment, with illustrative cases. *Lancet 2:* 104, 1896.
3. Huggins, C. B., Hodges, C. V. Studies on prostate cancer I: the effect of castration, of estrogen and androgen injection on serum phosphatase in metastatic carcinoma of the prostate. *Cancer Res 1:* 293, 1941.
4. Huggins, C. B., Stevens, R. E. Jr., Hodges, C. V. Studies on prostatic cancer II. The effects of castration on advanced carcinoma of the prostate gland. *Arch Surg 43:* 209, 1941.
5. Huggins, C. B., Bergenstal, D. M. Inhibition of human mammary and prostatic cancers by adrenalectomy. *Cancer Res 12:* 134, 1952.
6. Thayer, L. On the functions of incompetence. *Prespect Biol Med 18:* 332, 1975.
7. Jensen, E. V., Polley, T. Z., Smith, S., et al. Prediction of hormone dependency in human breast cancer. In McGuire, W. L., Carbone, P. O., Vollmer, E. P. (eds.): Estrogen Receptors in Human Breast Cancer. New York, Raven, 1975, p 37.
8. Huggins, C. B. Endocrine-induced regression of cancers. *Science 156:* 1050, 1967.
9. Emmett, J. L., Greene, L. F., Papantoniou, A. Endocrine therapy in carcinoma of the prostate gland: ten year survival studies. *J Urol 83:* 471, 1960.
10. Brendler, H. Therapy with orchiectomy or estrogens or both. *JAMA 210:* 1074, 1969.
11. Veterans Administration Cooperative Urological Research Group. Carcinoma of the prostate treatment comparison by the Veterans Administration Cooperative Urologic Group. *J Urol 98:* 516, 1967.
12. Byar, D. P. Treatment of prostatic cancer. Studies by the Veterans Administration Cooperative Urological Research Group. *Bull N Y Acad Med 48:* 751, 1972.
13. Coronary Drug Project Research Group. Initial findings leading to modifications of its research protocol. *JAMA 214:* 1303, 1970.
14. Robinson, M. R., Thomas, B. S. Effect of hormonal therapy on plasma testosterone levels. *Br Med J 4:* 391, 1971.
15. Shearer, R. J., Hendry, W. F., Sommerville, T. F., et al. Plasma testosterone, an accurate monitor of hormone treatment in prostatic cancer. *Br J Urol 45:* 668, 1973.
16. Grayhack, J. T. Adrenalectomy and hypophysectomy for carcinoma of the prostate. *JAMA 210:* 1075, 1969.
17. Schoonees, R., Schalch, D. S., Reynoso, G. et al. Bilateral adrenalectomy for advanced prostatic carcinoma. *J Urol 108:* 123, 1972.
18. Fergusson, J. D., Hendry, W. F. Pituitary irradiation in advanced carcinoma of the prostate: analysis of 100 cases. *Br J Urol 43:* 514, 1971.
19. Schoonees, R., Bourke, R. S., Reynoso, G., et al. Hypophysectomy for reactivated disseminated prostatic carcinoma. *S Afr Med J 41:* 1278, 1972.
20. West, C. R., Murphy, G. P. Pituitary ablation and disseminated prostatic carcinoma. *JAMA 225:* 253, 1973.
21. Smith, R. B., Walsh, P. C., Goodwin, W. E. Cyproterone acetate in the treatment of advanced carcinoma of the prostate. *J Urol 110:* 106, 1973.
22. Wein, A. J., Murphy, J. J. Experience in the treatment of prostatic carcinoma with cyproterone acetate. *J Urol 109:* 68, 1973.
23. Corwin, S. H., Malament, M., Small, M., et al. Experiences with P-32 in advanced carcinoma of the prostate. *J Urol 104:* 745, 1970.
24. Prout, G. R. Jr., Brewer, W. R. Response of men with advanced prostatic carcinoma to exogenous administration of testosterone. *Cancer 20:* 1871, 1967.
25. Nilsson, T., Muntzing, J. Histochemical and biochemical investigation of advanced prostatic carcinoma treated with estramustine phosphate, Estracyt. *Scand J Urol Nephrol 7:* 18, 1973.
26. Lindberg, B. Treatment of rapidly progressing prostatic carcinoma with Estracyt. *J Urol 108:* 303, 1972.
27. Liao, S. Cellular receptors and mechanisms of action of steroid hormones. *Int Rev Cytol 41:* 87, 1975.
28. Huggins, C. B., Clarke, P. J. Quantitative studies of prostatic secretion II. The effect of castration and of estrogen injection on the normal and on the hyperplastic prostate glands of dogs. *J Exp Med 72:* 747, 1940.
29. Farnsworth, W. E. A direct effect of estrogens on prostatic metabolism of testosterone. *J Invest Urol 6:* 423, 1969.
30. Margarby, C. J., Baum, M. Estrogen and reticuloendothelial stimulant in patients with cancer. *Br Med J 2:* 367, 1971.
31. Lawrence, A. M., Landau, R. L. Impaired ventral prostate affinity for testosterone in hypophysectomized rats. *Endocrinology 77:* 1119, 1965.
32. Grayhack, J. T., Lebowitz, J. M. The effect of prolactin on citric acid of lateral lobe prostate of Sprague-Dawley rats. *Invest Urol 5:* 87, 1967.
33. Melicow, M. M., Tannenbaum, M. Endometrial carcinoma of uterus masculinus (prostatic utricle). Report of 6 cases. *J Urol 106:* 892, 1971.
34. Lacassagne, A. Hormonal pathogenesis of adenocarcinoma of the breast. *Am J Cancer 27:* 217, 1936.
35. Luft, R., Olivecrona, H., Sjogren, B. J. Hypophysectomie pa mannika. *Nord Med 47:* 351, 1952.
36. Haddow, A., Watkinson, J. M., Paterson, E., et al. Influence of synthetic oestrogens upon advanced malignant disease. *Br Med J 2:* 393, 1944.
37. Lacassagne, A. Attempts to modify by progesterone or testosterone the development in mice of mammary adenocarcinoma induced by oestrone. *C R Soc Biol (Paris) 126:* 385, 1936.
38. Huggins, C. B., Moon, R., Morie, S. Extinction of experimental mammary cancer I. Estradiol-17B and progesterone. *Proc Natl Acad Sci USA 48:* 379, 1962.
39. Nissen-Meyer, R., Vogt, J. H. Cortisone treatment of metastatic breast cancer. *Acta Unio Int Contra Cancer 15:* 1140, 1959.

40. Stoll, B. A. Hormonal Management in Breast Cancer. Philadelphia, Lippincott, 1969, pp 23–35.
41. Kennedy, B. J., Mielke, P. W., Fortuny, I. E. Therapeutic castration versus prophylactic castration in breast cancer. *Surg Gynecol Obstet 118:* 524, 1964.
42. Joint Committee on Ablative Procedures in Disseminated Mammary Carcinoma. *JAMA 175:* 137, 1961.
43. Juret, P., Hayem, M. Pituitary ablation in the treatment of breastcancer. In Stoll, B. A. (ed.): Mammary Cancer and Neuroendocrine Therapy. London, Butterworth, 1974, p 283.
44. Pearson, O. H., Ray, B. S. Hypophysectomy in the treatment of metastatic mammary cancer. *Am J Surg 97:* 544, 1960.
45. Huggins, C. B., Briziarelli, G., Sutton, H. Jr. Rapid induction of mammary carcinoma in the rat and the influence of hormones on the tumors. *J Exp Med 109:* 25, 1959.
46. Pearson, O. H., Llerena, O., Llerena, L., et al. Prolactin dependent rat mammary cancer: a model for man? *Trans Assoc Am Physicians 82:* 225, 1969.
47. Pearson, O. H. Biological problems regarding hormonal surgery. In Dargent, M., Romieu, C. (eds.): Major Endocrine Surgery for the Treatment of Cancer of the Breast in Advanced Stages, Colloque Internation de Lyon, 1967, p 215.
48. Nagasawa, H., Yanai, R. Effects of prolactin or growth hormone on growth of carcinogen-induced mammary tumors of adreno-ovariectomized rats. *Int J Cancer 6:* 488, 1970.
49. Herisen, J. C., Waelbroech-Van Gaves, C., Legros, N. Growth inhibition of rat mammary carcinoma and endocrine changes produced by 2-Br-a-ergocryptine, a suppressor of lactation and nidation. *Eur J Cancer 6:* 353, 1970.
50. Ehni, G., Eckles, N. E. Interruption of the pituitary stalk in the patient with mammary cancer. *J Neurosurg 16:* 628, 1959.
51. Turkington, R. W., Underwood, L. E., Van Wyk, J. J. Elevated serum prolactin levels after pituitary stalk section in man. *N Engl J Med 285:* 707, 1971.
52. Wilson, R. G., Buchan, R., Roberts, M. M., et al. Plasma prolactin and breast cancer. *Cancer 33:* 1325, 1974.
53. Boyns, A. R., Cole, E. N., Griffiths, K., et al. Plasma prolactin in breast cancer. *Eur J Cancer 9:* 99, 1972.
54. Kwa, H. G., DeJong-Bakker, Englesman, E., et al. Plasma prolactin in human breast cancer. *Lancet 1:* 433, 1974.
55. European Breast Cancer Group. Clinical trial of 2-Br-a-ergocryptine (CB154) in advanced breast cancer. *Eur J Cancer 8:* 387, 1972.
56. Nathanson, I. T. Clinical investigative experience with steroid hormones in breast cancer. *Cancer 5:* 754, 1952.
57. American Medical Association Committee on Research. Androgens and estrogens in the treatment of disseminated mammary carcinoma. *JAMA 172:* 1271, 1960.
58. Cooperative Breast Cancer Group. Testosterone propionate therapy in breast cancer. *JAMA 188:* 106, 1964.
59. Gordan, G. S., Halden, A., Horn, Y., et al. Calusterone (7B, 17a dimethyl testosterone) as primary and secondary therapy of advanced breast cancer. *Oncology 28:* 138, 1973.
60. Terenius, L Anti-estrogens and their role in mammary cancer. In Stoll, B. A. (ed.): Mammary Cancer and Neuroendocrine Therapy, London, Butterworth, 1974, p 82.
61. Dao, T. L. Y, Brooks, U. A comparative evaluation of adrenalectomy and cortisone in the treatment of advanced mammary carcinoma. *Cancer 14:* 1259, 1961.
62. Landau, R. L., Ehrlich, E. N., Huggins, C. B. Estradiol benzoate and progesterone in advanced human breast cancer. *JAMA 182:* 632, 1962.
63. Crowley, L. G., McDonald, I. Delalutin and estrogens for the treatment of advanced mammary carcinoma in the postmenopausal women. *Cancer 18:* 346, 1965.
64. Landau, R. L. Can endocrine therapy be expected to replace the surgical treatment of advanced breast cancer? In Dargent, M., Romieu, C. (eds.): Major Endocrine Surgery for the Treatment of Cancer of the Breast in Advanced Stages, Colloque International de Lyon, 1966, p 263.
65. Chemama, R., Jayle, M. F., Ennuyer, A. Progestin–oestrogen–corticosteroid combinations. In Stoll, B. A. (ed.): Mammary Cancer and Neuroendocrine Therapy. London, Butterworth, 1974, p 265.
66. EORTC Breast Cancer Group. Essai clinique du phenol bis (2-chloroethyl) conbamate diestradiol dans le cancer mammaire en phase avancie. *Eur J Cancer 5:* 1, 1969.
67. Atkins, H., Bulbrook, R. D., Falconer, M. A., et al. Ten years experience of steroid assays in the management of breast cancer. *Lancet 2:* 1255, 1968.
68. Folca, P. J., Glascock, R. F., Irvine, W. T. Studies with tritium labelled hexoestrol in advanced breast cancer. *Lancet 2:* 796, 1961.
69. Jensen, E. V., Jacobson, H. I. Basic guides to the mechanism of estrogen action. *Recent Prog Horm Res 18:* 387, 1962.
70. Gorski, J. Estrogen binding and control of gene expression in the uterus. In Handbook of Physiology, section 7, vol 2, part I, Endocrinology. Washington, DC, American Physiological Society, 1973, p 525.
71. Costlow, M. E., Buschow, R. A., McGuire, W. L. Prolactin receptors in an estrogen receptor deficient mammary carcinoma. *Science 184:* 85, 1974.
72. Meites, J., Cassell, E., Clark, J. Estrogen inhibition of mammary tumor growth in rats, counteraction by prolactin. *Proc Soc Exp Biol Med 137:* 1225, 1971.
73. Stoll, B. A. Mammary Cancer and Neuroendocrine Therapy. London, Butterworth, 1974, p 60.
74. George, W. D., Partridge, W., Blum, J. I. Macrophage activity and hormonal responsiveness in mammary cancers. *Br J Surg 60:* 317, 1973.
75. Kledzik, G. S., Bradley, C. J., Meites, J. Reduction of carcinogen induced mammary cancer incidence in rats by early treatment with hormones. *Cancer Res 34:* 2953, 1974.
76. Goldman, A. S., Neumann, F. Differentiation of the mammary gland in experimental congenital adrenal hyperplasia due to inhibition of Δ^5,3B-hydroxysteroid dehydrogenase in rats. *Proc Soc Exp Biol Med 132:* 237, 1969.
77. French, F. S., Van Wyk, J. J., Baggett, B., et al. Further evidence of a target organ defect in the syndrome of testicular feminization. *J Clin Endocrinol 26:* 493, 1966.
78. Goldfine, I., Rosenfield, R. L., Landau, R. L. Hyperleydigism: a cause of severe pubertal gynecomastia. *J Clin Endocrinol Metab 32:* 751, 1971.
79. Farrow, J. H., Adair, F. E. Effect of orchidectomy on skeletal metastases from cancer of male breast. *Science 95:* 654, 1942.
80. Trerres, N. The treatment of cancer, especially inoperable cancer of the male breast by ablative surgery (orchidectomy, adrenalectomy and hypophysectomy) and hormone therapy (estrogen and corticosteroids). *Cancer 12:* 820, 1959.
81. Kelley, R. M., Baker, W. H. Progestational agents in the treatment of carcinoma of the endometrium *N Engl J Med 264:* 216, 1961.
82. Gasberg, S. B. Hormone dependence of endometrial cancer. *Obstet Gynecol 30:* 287, 1967.
83. Wilkenson, E. J., Friedrich, E. G. Jr., Mattingly, R. F., et al. Turner's syndrome with endometrial adenocarcinoma and stilbestrol therapy. *Obstet Gynecol 42:* 193, 1973.
84. Kistner, R. W. Histologic effects of progesterone on hyperplasia and carcinoma in situ of endometrium. *Cancer 12:* 1106, 1959.
85. Sherman, A. I. Progesterone caproate in the treatment of endometrial cancer. *Obstet Gynecol 28:* 309, 1966.
86. Collins, J. Combined hormone therapy for recurrent adenocarcinoma of the endometrium. *Am J Obstet Gynecol 113:* 842, 1972.
87. Ward, H. W. L. Progesterone therapy for ovarian carcinoma. *J Obstet Gynecol 79:* 555, 1972.
88. Landau, R. L. The metabolic effects of anabolic steroids in man. In Kochakian, C. D. (ed.): Handbook of Experimental Pharmacology: Anabolic–Androgenic Steroids. Berlin, Springer, 1976, p 45.
89. Landau, R. L. The metabolic influence of progesterone. In Handbook of Physiology, section 7, vol 2, part 1, Endocrinology. Washington, DC, American Physiological Society, 1973, p 573.
90. Mathews, V. S., Kirkman, H., Baron, R. L. Kidney damage in the golden hamster following chronic administration of diethylstilbestrol and sesame oil. *Proc Soc Exp Biol Med 66:* 195, 1947.
91. Bloom, H. J. G., Baker, W. H., Dukes, C. E., et al. Hormone-dependent tumours of the kidney. II Effect of endocrine ablation procedures on the transplanted oestrogen-induced renal tumour of the Syrian hamster. *Br J Cancer 17:* 646, 1963.
92. Bloom, H. J. G. Medroxyprogesterone acetate (Provera) treatment of metastatic renal cancer. *Br J Cancer 25:* 250, 1971.
93. Aberto, P., Senn, H. J. Hormonal therapy of renal carcinoma alone and in association with cytostatic drugs. *Cancer 33:* 1226, 1974.

158

Radiologic Techniques in Tumor Localization

Harvey Eisenberg

Radiologists today have at their disposal a great variety of sophisticated imaging techniques for the morphologic evaluation of the endocrine glands. These include noninvasive scanning modalities such as computed axial tomography, gray-scale ultrasound, and nuclear imaging.

These scanning procedures have proven to be of considerable value in detecting tumors of 2–3 cm or above in size but are currently limited in spatial resolution capabilities below this level. Additional diagnostic information may be obtained by using these studies to guide percutaneous needle aspiration biopsies. Cytologic examinations have shown approximately 75 percent accuracy in differentiating benign from malignant tumors.[1]

Catheterization procedures continue to play an important role in endocrine diagnosis, while pneumatography has all but disappeared. Arteriography and venography are capable of detecting lesions as small as a few millimeters in size, particularly when magnification and selective techniques are employed.[2]

Equally, if not more important to the detection of endocrine abnormalities has been the use of selective venous sampling for the selective functional assessment of several endocrine glands, including the adrenals, the pancreas, the parathyroid, and the gonadals.

In addition to diagnostic studies, recent developments in the field of therapeutic angiography have offered, in selected circumstances, the transcatheter destruction of endocrine glands or tumors as an alternative to surgical resection. After a brief description of current radiologic techniques, their utilization will be illustrated in the discussions of several endocrine disorders.

RADIOLOGIC IMAGING MODALITIES

CONVENTIONAL RADIOGRAPHY

Plain film diagnosis in endocrine disease has generally been related to the detection of soft tissue mass, abnormal calcifications, or skeletal abnormalities. The development of microfocus x-ray sources for magnification radiography has improved detection of skeletal abnormalities such as subperiostal resorption, osteoporosis, and osteomalacia.[3] The more widespread application of tomography has improved the evaluation and detection of soft tissue masses and calcification.

The presence and definition of soft tissue calcifications are occasionally helpful in endocrine tumors. Psammomatas calcifications are generally thought specific for papillary tumors, and granular or coarse calcifications are always suggestive of a malignant process. Calcified phleboliths may be seen in hypervascular tumors, again suggesting malignancy, and curvilinear calcifications usually denote the presence of a benign process, such as a cyst.[4]

Barium studies are primarily useful for the differentiation of other tumors in the abdomen and are occasionally invaluable for demonstrating the effects of gastrin or glucagon-secreting tumors or malabsorption syndrome of the small bowel. Intravenous pyelography (IVP) with nephrotomography remains useful for demonstration of adrenal masses and will demonstrate the presence of such lesions in at least 70 percent of the cases.[5]

NUCLEAR MEDICINE TECHNIQUES

Radionuclides continue to offer the promise of labeling specific pathologic processes by selective uptake of specific radionuclides. These efforts, however, have met with only limited success and have been significantly limited by the relatively poor resolution of nuclear scanning equipment. ^{131}I-labeled steroids have recently been shown to be accurate in detecting adrenocortical masses and metastases[6] (Chap. 95), and ^{131}I-19-iodocholesterol scintigraphy has been of some use in detecting Conn's tumors[7] (Chapt. 98), although the incidence of false positives is relatively significant in this application. The greatest use of nuclide scanning has been in the diagnosis, detection, and treatment of thyroid abnormalities, as reviewed in Chapter 30. Parathyroid evaluation with selenomethionine have proved to be of little use because of the lack of specificity of this agent.

Multiple-array detectors for nuclear medicine application are currently under development, and these appear to increase resolution capabilities to the range of approximately 1.5–2.0 cm.

ULTRASOUND

Ultrasound offers the capability of defining the body's soft tissues without the use of ionizing radiation. Currently, resolution capabilities of 0.5–1.0 cm are possible with gray-scale equipment in both storage and real-time display. These techniques have proven highly accurate in differentiating solid from cystic structures (90 to 95 percent) and are particularly useful in evaluations of suspected masses in the pelvis,[8] thyroid,[9] and retroperitoneum,[10] and in the detection of liver metastases (Fig. 158-1).[11] Real-time ultrasonography is particularly valuable as a guide for percutaneous aspiration of cysts[12] and cytologic biopsy. It appears, however, that these techniques will always be limited in areas of overlying bone and gas, such as the chest and left adrenal. The technology of ultrasonic equipment is rapidly evolving. Current research with high-energy ultrasonic units has shown significant potential in improving both resolution and tissue differentiation, although with limited depth. These may be of considerable use in evaluations of the parathyroid and thyroid glands and the testes.[13]

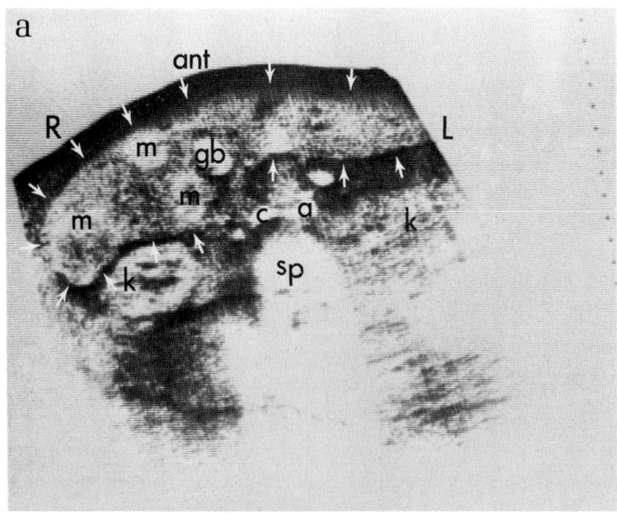

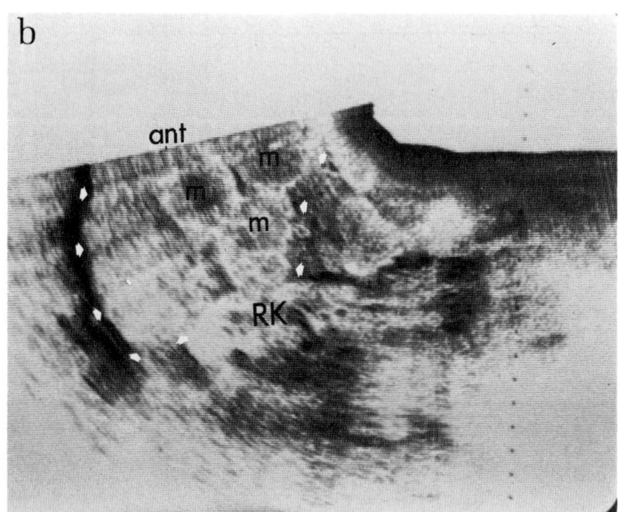

Fig. 158-1. (A) Transverse and (B) sagittal ultrasound scans over the liver showing liver metastases. The size of the masses (m) and their location relative to the body surface are noted and used to guide percutaneous needle aspiration biopsy for cytology. gb = gallbladder, K = kidney, Sp = spine, A = aorta, C = vena cava. (Courtesy M. Grossman, University of California, Irvine.)

COMPUTED AXIAL TOMOGRAPHY SCANNING

The most important recent advance in the use of ionizing radiation has been the development of computed axial tomography (CAT). This technique provides great sensitivity to differences in tissue contrast (1 to 2 percent) as compared to conventional radiography (25 to 75 percent), allowing one to visualize and quantify with absorption coefficients the soft tissues of the body. In addition, the technique presents an unobstructed view of axial tomographic slices throughout the body. Resolution has generally been limited to the detection of tumors above 2–3 cm in size, although high-density material such as calcium may be detected in very small quantities. Computed tomography can achieve higher resolution capabilities; however, this can only be accomplished by the use of high doses of radiation, which may only be acceptable in selected circumstances. This technique is proving particularly useful in the evaluation of adrenal and pararenal masses,[14] the pancreas,[15] abdominal lymph nodes,[16] tumor extensions, mediastinal tumors,[17] liver[18] and lung metastases,[19] pituitary masses and their extensions[20,21] (Fig. 158-2). This technique may also be used as a guide for needle aspiration, although it is appears to be less practical than real-time ultrasound.[22]

ARTERIOGRAPHY AND VENOGRAPHY

Advances in both catheter technology and x-ray imaging equipment have improved the technical success, quality, and safety of arteriography and venography. The great majority of endocrine tumors and their extensions are hypervascular and are well demonstrated by arteriography. In most circumstances, optimal demonstration necessitates the use of selective arterial injections rather than simple aortography. Differentiation between benign and malignant processes is often difficult, except by demonstration of large size, inflation metastases, or vascular invasion. Arteriography, with its higher resolution capabilities (70 μm to 300μm), remains the most sensitive test for detecting the usually hypervascular extensions or metastases of endocrine malignancy (Fig. 158-3). Selective magnification venography, particularly in

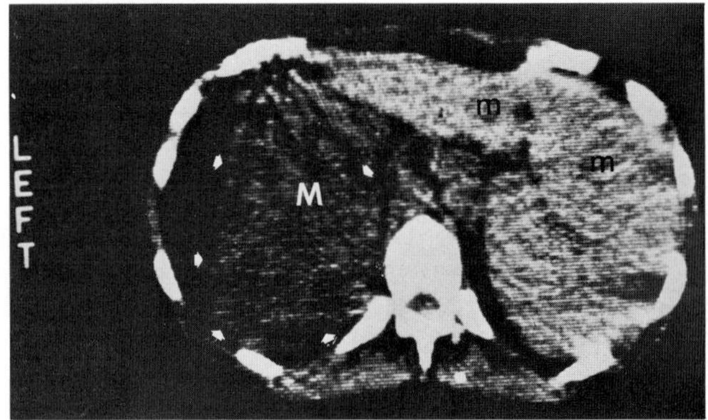

Fig. 158-2. (A) CT scan of the abdomen at the T-12 level shows a large (12 cm) mass (M) in the left suprarenal area representing adrenal cell carcinoma. (B) CT scan through the liver shows multiple round tissue density lesions from metastases (m). (Courtesy B. Carter, New England Medical Center, Tufts University.)

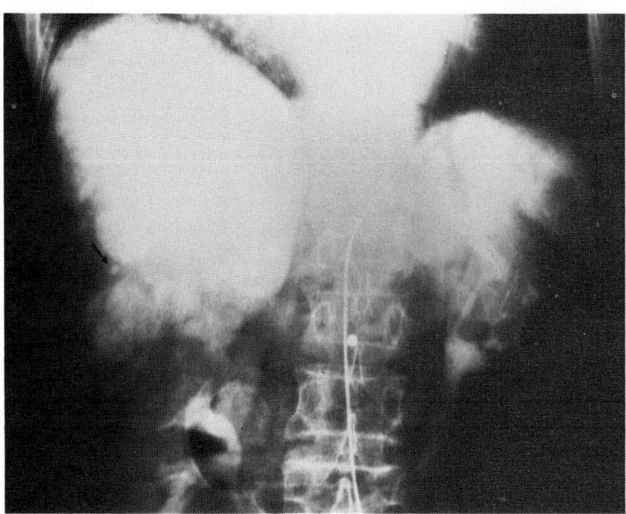

Fig. 158-3. Numerous liver metastases from adrenal cell carcinoma seen in the capillary (parenchymal) phase of a celiac trunk arteriogram. Even small lesions measuring down to a few millimeters in size (arrow) are well seen.

the adrenal, has, in our experience, proved to be a sensitive tool for detecting small tumors, as well as the hypervascularity usually associated with endocrine gland tumors and hyperplasia.[2,23] Venography has been extremely useful in demonstrating the presence of venous invasion, which carries a high specificity for defining a malignant process. Both arteriography and venography have proven very helpful in determining operability in malignant tumors. As these procedure are potentially hazardous, they should be carried out in experienced hands. Venography carries with it a 1 to 5 percent risk of extravasation of dye from veins, which may set up transient inflammatory reactions in areas such as the adrenal in patients with hyperaldosteronism or Cushing's syndrome. Although this produces a significant morbidity, the incidence of adrenal insufficiency is extremely low.[23]

VENOUS HORMONE ASSAY

Venous catheters may have their greatest value in the selective sampling of blood from the various endocrine organs, and in many circumstances, venography may not be necessary other than for test injections to confirm catheter positioning. In our experience[24–27] and that of others,[28–30] these techniques have detected significant functional endocrine abnormalities before those changes were even apparent on conventional histopathologic examination, let alone on morphologic evaluations provided by the techniques mentioned above or by the surgical assessment of gross pathology. Furthermore, we have frequently seen instances in which the gross morphology of endocrine glands (size, nodularity, vascularity) does not correlate with the functional status of these glands. Since the treatment of endocrine disease relates in most cases to functional rather than morphologic pathology, selective functional assessment may often be a better guide to therapy than peripheral functional evaluation or the morphologic conclusions reached by the radiologist, surgeon, or histopathologist.

Furthermore, if one considers the pathophysiology of endocrine disease and the unanswered questions relating to the relationship of hyperplastic and adenomatous disease, selective physiologic studies may in the future offer an understanding of the evolution and interrelationships of some of these endocrine disorders.

RATIONALE

In the rapidly evolving technology of radiologic localization techniques and the increasing awareness of the cost-effective approach to patient care, the radiologist must play an essential role in determining which procedures may be most applicable to diagnosing a particular endocrine problem. The choice of the specific modality will vary according to the disease process, the individual patient, and the availability of the various imaging modalities and technical expertise for the individual procedure. The optimal choice of diagnostic procedures should be based primarily on those considerations that will most affect subsequent patient therapy and the probability of success of such therapy. While noninvasive studies offer advantages for patient safety and comfort, often the more invasive procedures provide a more significant guide to therapy and thus play a more significant role in reducing overall patient morbidity, complications, and cost. The ability of these latter techniques to consistently detect small tumors or early disease implies their ability to rule out the presence of such disease, which is frequently as important in therapy planning as the detection of tumor masses. Finally, as noted above, therapy may best be directed by the evaluation of functional pathology rather than morphology.

When properly performed, the radiologic techniques mentioned above may be used for the following evaluations:

1. Specific localization of a functional endocrine gland abnormality
2. Localization of an extra-endocrine gland origin of excess hormone production
3. Differentiation between the solitary origin and multiplicity of origin of excess hormone production (adenoma vs. hyperplasia)
4. Establishing the diagnosis of endocrine gland abnormality in cases where peripheral chemical determinations are inconclusive or confused by concomitant therapy or disease
5. Establishing an optimal therapeutic approach, i.e., medical vs. surgical vs. radiotherapy
6. Planning optimal surgical approaches, including possibly the amount of tissue resection
7. Planning the postoperative management of suppressed endocrine activity
8. Understanding the evolutionary pathophysiology of endocrine disease
9. Alternative therapy (therapeutic angiography) to surgery.

These principles will be illustrated in the following discussions of specific endocrine disorders.

ADRENAL CORTEX

ALDOSTERONOMA

Primary aldosteronism originates from unilateral adenoma(s) (60 to 80 percent), bilateral adenomas (10 percent) or hyperplasia (15 to 30 percent). Bilateral disease is therefore common (20 to 40 percent), particularly in children (75 percent).[31] Fortunately, the incidence of malignancy is rare and not generally a consideration in the diagnostic workup. Radiologic techniques are primarily needed for differentiation of unilateral from bilateral disease and for lateralization so that most patients can be approached by single flank incision rather than bilateral flank or anterior abdominal surgery.

Establishing a diagnosis of hyperplasia may allow for medical rather then surgical therapy. Occasionally, diagnostic techniques may be needed to differentiate primary from secondary aldosteronism in patients with concomitant renal disease or those on diuretic therapy. Increased cortisol production may be seen in conjunction with hyperaldosteronism and thus confuse the relationship of functional and morphologic abnormalities.

The great majority of aldosteronomas are less than 2 cm in size, and hyperplasia is usually microscopic or in the form of millimeter-sized micronodularity. The use of radionuclide scanning agents (^{131}I cholesterol)[7] and, more recently, CAT scans[14] has been suggested for localization in Conn's syndrome. The consideration still exists, however, that if these techniques show a unilateral mass, they are incapable of ruling out contralateral disease, particularly the very small lesions frequently encountered in primary hyperaldosteronism. These scanning modalities may be definitive in the event that they demonstrate bilateral adrenal masses. Even when nodules are identified bilaterally, however, they may not correlate with hyperfunction (Fig. 158-4). In fact, nodularity of the adrenal is a common autopsy finding in patients with no known functional disease. Conversely, in functional hyperplasia, micronodularity identical to that found in normal autopsies may be the only pathologic finding.

Since the pathology requiring therapy is that of functional overactivity, preoperative diagnostic studies are best directed toward identifying that activity and determining unilateral vs bilateral hypersecretion. Selective venous sampling is the optimal approach, and we have routinely performed this bilaterally and simultaneously in over 100 consecutive patients with a variety of primary and secondary adrenal lesions, as well as for determination of normal ranges. These results will be amplified in the following sections. The general experience with adrenal venous sampling for aldosterone secretions has been that it represents the most accurate test for directing proper therapy. Successful lateralization has been achieved in 85 to 100 percent of cases.[30,32,33]

When adrenal venous sampling cannot be obtained bilaterally, Scoggins has been somewhat successful in using caval and left adrenal samples to deduce functional information about unilateral vs. bilateral functional disease.[35]

Adrenal venography is generally performed following sampling. Our experience with over 300 magnification adrenal venograms has been that this is the most sensitive test for showing both adrenal masses and the hypervascularity of hyperplasia or the remnant hypervascularity of necrotic tumors. These studies have proven more sensitive than subselective magnification adrenal arteriography.

Unfortunately, patients with hyperaldosteronism are particularly susceptible to extravasation on venography, and these injections must be performed with utmost care. Blushing of the gland is unnecessary, and one only need see the major venules. With recent quality image intensifiers, venography can be accomplished under direct vision and recorded on 35-mm cine or 100-mm spot films. An argument could be made for confining the catheterization procedure to confirming catheter position and relying on venous sampling for diagnosis. With proper technique, this remains the procedure of choice for diagnosis and determination of optimal therapy of primary hyperaldosteronism.

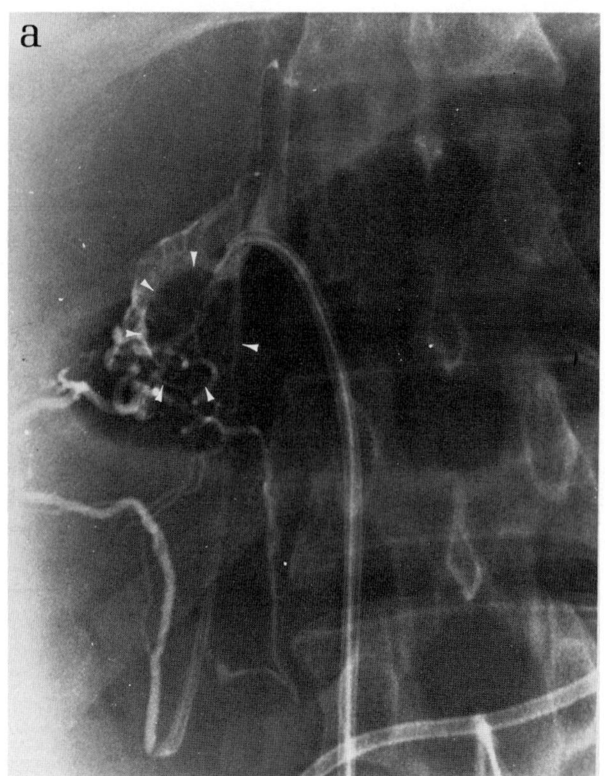

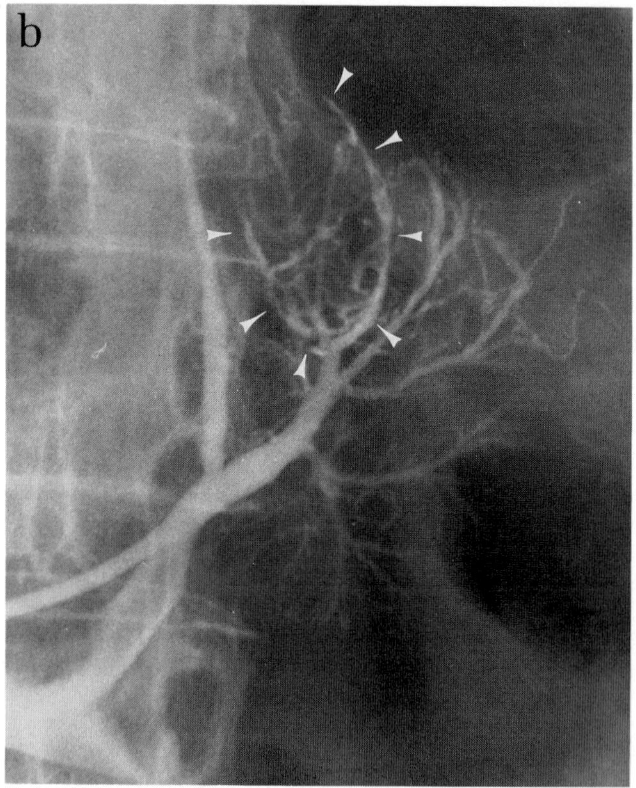

Fig. 158-4. Patient with primary aldosteronism showing nodules and enlargement of both the right (A) and left (B) adrenal glands. Adrenal vein aldosterone values were elevated only on the right (2000 ng/100 ml) and were low on the left (50 ng/100 ml). Unilateral adrenalectomy on the right resulted in restoration of normotension and normokalemia over a follow-up period of 5 years.

CUSHING'S SYNDROME

Cushing's syndrome may result from bilateral adrenal hyperplasia (approximately 70 percent), unilateral adenoma (approximately 12 percent), unilateral carcinoma (approximately 13 percent), bilateral adrenal tumors (approximately 3 percent), or ectopic ACTH production from tumor (oat cell, pancreas, etc.).[36] The pathologic entity of hyperplasia affecting the adrenal gland may be further divided into the diffuse variety, in which the glands may appear either histologically normal (10 percent), diffusely micronodular, or multinodular to the point that one or more macronodules may simulate a solitary adenoma. In multinodular hyperplastia (15 to 20 percent of hyperplasia in adults, 30 percent in children), the disease may be grossly asymmetric. The distinction between macronodular hyperplasia and a solitary adenoma is not always clear pathologically, as most patients with solitary adenoma have associated micronodules in the surgically resected gland, and when biopsies are available of the opposite gland, micronodules are found there as well.[36–39] The probability that solitary adenoma and macronodular hyperplasia represent a spectrum of disease, ending with one dominant nodule suppressing the others, has been suggested by several leading pathologists.[38,39] As noted previously, the pathology is further confused by the consideration that adrenal nodules, usually microscopic, are very commonly found at autopsy in patients with no functional adrenal disease.

It seems essential that in order to determine an optimal therapeutic approach in patients with Cushing's syndrome, one would need to determine exactly which pathologic entity is present or, more importantly, to specifically determine the presence of functional abnormality within the individual glands and to determine autonomy vs. pituitary-hypothalamic dependence. At present, most centers treat patients with suspected hyperplasia with bilateral adrenalectomies. This therapy may represent the most reliable way of obliterating abnormal cortisol production, but it exposes the patient to the perils of Addison's disease and lifelong exogenous therapy, as well as a 10 to 15 percent incidence of Nelson syndrome (pituitary tumor, often with local invasion, hyperpigmentation).[40]

If no functional autonomy exists in the adrenals, patients with hyperplasia may best be treated with proton-beam pituitary irradiation[41] or possibly with transsphenoidal pituitary microdissection surgery.[42] The latter approach is supported by the fact that 60 percent of patients with Cushing's syndrome have pituitary adenomas at autopsy,[43] and in limited series, the disease has been cured by pituitary adenonectomy.[44] In the case of unilateral autonomous adenoma, the optimal approach is a unilateral flank incision for adrenalectomy. In asymmetric nodular hyperplasia, autonomy may exist on one or both sides, and therapy may best be tailored to the individual functional abnormalities (Fig. 158-5). In the case of unilateral carcinoma the patients deserve an anterior abdominal approach more suitable for a wide resection and determination of metastasis. Preoperative studies must then provide accurate differentiation of these entities.

Traditionally, in the diagnosis of Cushing's syndrome, the determination of unilateral vs. bilateral disease and determination of autonomy is based upon the differential response to dynamic tests of adrenal function, including a low- and high-dose dexamethasone suppression test and response to stimulation with ACTH and metyrapone.[45]

A proper decision for therapy can often be reached by considering a lack of high-dose dexamethasone suppression as an indicator of autonomy from either adenoma or carcinoma and by differentiating these entities by preoperative determination of the size of a mass. Carcinoma generally presents as a mass greater than 5 cm, and adenomas generally present as masses in the range of 2–5 cm.[46] Masses of such size may usually be detected by noninvasive studies such as IVP, gray-scale ultrasound (Fig. 158-6), abdominal

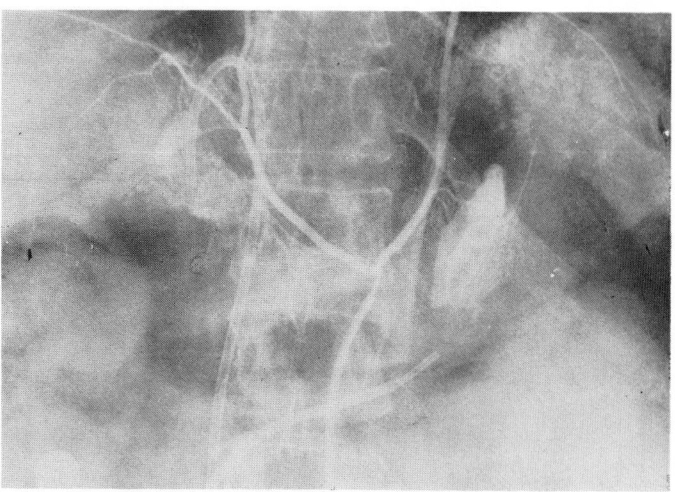

Fig. 158-5. A 52-year-old female with Cushing's syndrome and asymmetrical adrenal hyperplasia. Both adrenal glands appear slightly enlarged. Gross nodularity seems confined to the left. Selective venous sampling showed incomplete suppression on the left, suggesting some degree of autonomy without significant hyperfunction on the right. Patient underwent a left unilateral adrenalectomy and has remained well in a 6½ year follow-up.

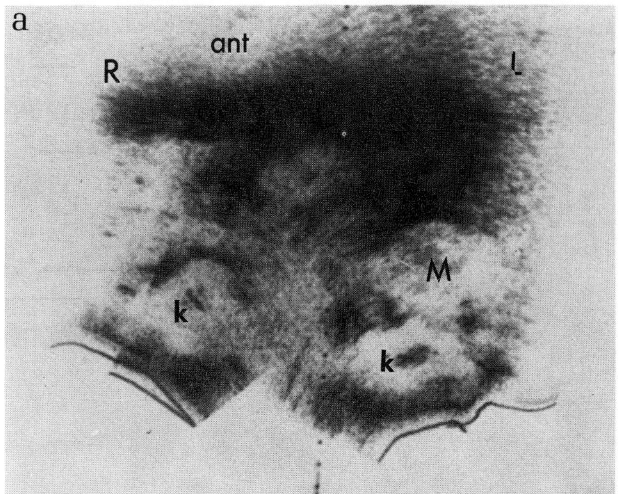

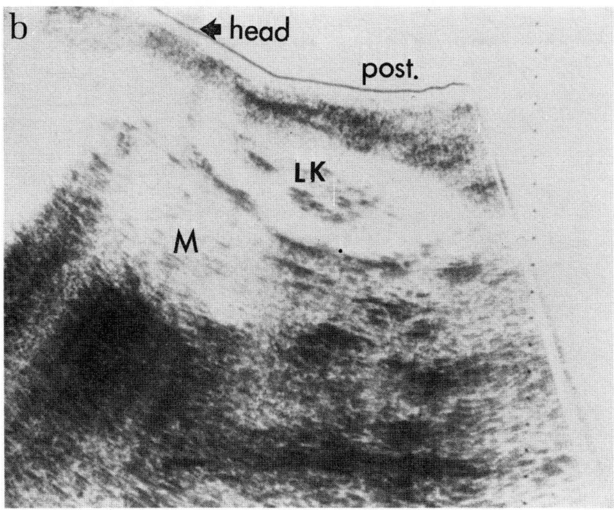

Fig. 158-6. (A) Transverse and (B) longitudinal gray-scale sonograms of a left upper quadrant suprarenal mass (M) shown surgically to be a mixed cystic, solid, and calcified pheochromocytoma. Mass was seen to be separate from the kidney (k).

CAT scanning (Fig. 158-2A), and recently, nuclear scanning with ^{131}I steroid. In the case of carcinoma, these latter modalities have also proven helpful in the determination of hepatic metastases (Fig. 158-3) and may be used as a guide for aspiration cytology. The consideration still exists, however, that in cases where these studies show a unilateral mass over 2–3 cm, they do not exclude the possibility of bilateral disease. This is particularly relevant with smaller masses, where unilateral adenoma may be confused with asymmetric nodular hyperplasia. They also may not differentiate benign from malignant disease in the absence of demonstrable metastases. Also, the absence of tumor demonstration does not necessarily imply hyperplasia.

In centers where selective arteriography and venous assays are available, there is much to be gained by the use of these techniques, particularly from simultaneous selective venous sampling for cortisol determination.[25,26]

The relatively higher sensitivity to cortisol dynamics of adrenal vein blood samples as compared to peripheral blood samples and the need for simultaneous sampling to eliminate variations seen with ACTH pulsing is illustrated in Figure 158-7. Hyperplasia was readily diagnosed by simultaneous sampling of the adrenals with assessment of cortisol dynamics after dexamethasone suppression and ACTH stimulation. Marked hypersecretion 5 minutes after ACTH administration was noted in hyperplasia, including those patients with normal-appearing glands (30 percent of hyperplasia) where the most sophisticated radiologic techniques, surgical evaluation, and even occasionally histopathologic evaluation would fail to detect any significant abnormality in the adrenal gland (Fig. 158-8). Magnification venography has provided the best demonstration of the hypervascularity seen in hyperplasia, including normal-sized glands (Fig. 158-9). Furthermore, these techniques are significantly more accurate than scanning in detecting or excluding adenomas and in assessing the opposite gland for size, mass, vascularity, and functional activity (Fig. 158-10). In addition, these studies are far more accurate than peripheral studies in assessing individual gland autonomy. Peripheral chemistry studies have, in our experience, often been misleading, both in suggesting adrenal autonomy in hyperplasia (40 percent) and in showing ACTH response with adenoma (50 percent) and carcinoma (10 percent).[47] In asymmetrical micronodular hyperplasia in particular, both the evaluation of autonomy from peripheral blood chemistries and surgical assessment may be erroneous, leading to a unilateral adrenalectomy when either bilateral excision or pituitary therapy without adrenal exploration would be the treatment of choice (Fig. 158-11). Conversely, in the case of the small solitary adenoma, undetected by preoperative morphologic studies or operative evaluation, a mistaken diagnosis of hyperplasia may ensue, and bilateral adrenalectomy may be performed or pituitary therapy given when unilateral adrenalectomy is indicated. Bilateral selective simultaneous venous sampling performed immediately after an abnormal overnight dexamethasone suppression test has provided a highly accurate and relatively inexpensive way of evaluating patients with Cushing's syndrome. These studies may allow one to: (1) proceed with pituitary irradiation or surgery with confidence in patients with hyperplasia, without exposing the patient to surgical evaluation of the adrenals; (2) identify the side for unilateral flank incision in patients with adenoma; (3) reliably rule out functional overactivity on the opposite side; (4) assess activity of suppressed glands for optimal postsurgical management; (5) individualize therapy in cases of asymmetric macronodular hyperplasia; and (6) rule out the diagnosis of Cushing's disease in patients in whom the diagnostic workup is inconclusive or confused by drug therapy (diphenylhydantoin), depression, etc. In addition, patients with carcinoma may be diagnosed by showing the almost constant finding of adrenal vein occlusion (Fig. 158-12) or invasion. Arteriography shows these hypervascular tumors well and provides a vascular road map for the surgeon. These are the most accurate

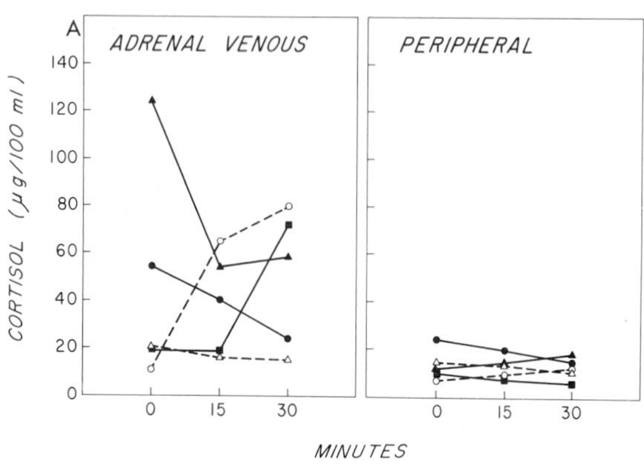

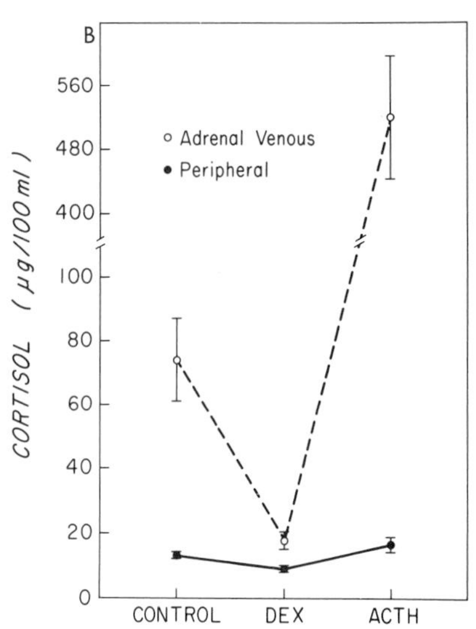

Fig. 158-7. (A) Adrenal venous and peripheral cortisol levels in normal patients. (B) Mean ± SEM adrenal venous and peripheral cortisols under baseline conditions, 30 minutes after peripheral intravenous dexamethasone injection (4.0 mg) and 5 minutes after injection of 250 μg of beta 1-24 ACTH. Note broken scale. (C) Comparison of simultaneous and nonsimultaneous adrenal vein sampling. Differences relate to pulsatile activity occurring within 50 to 30 minute time intervals. (Reproduced from R. Spark, Eisenberg, H., *J. Clin. Endocrinol. Metab. 39(2):* 305–310, 1974.)

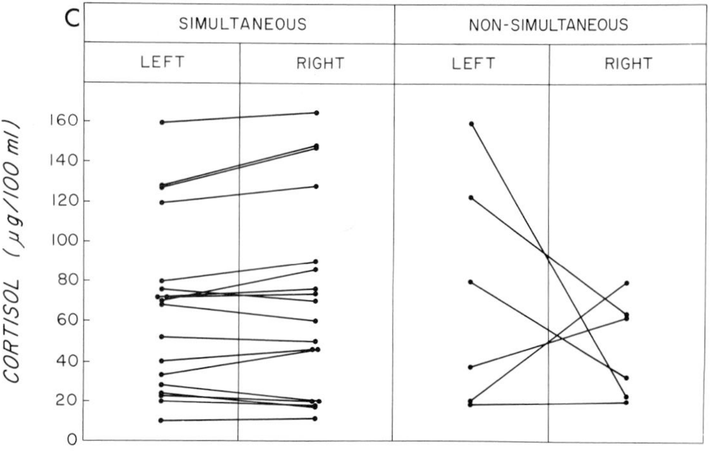

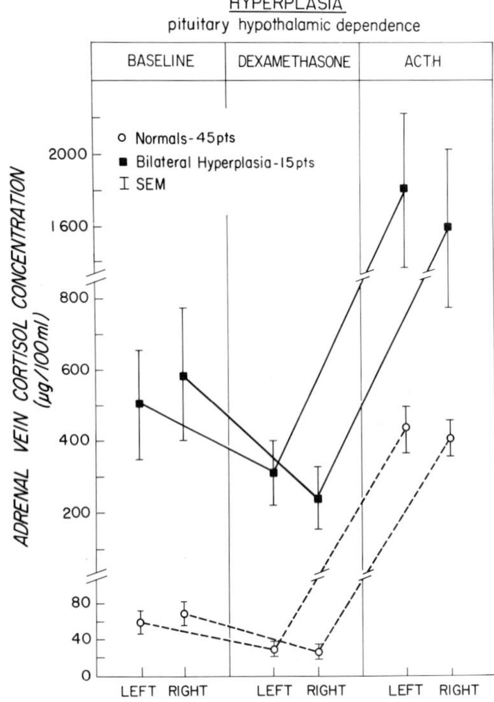

Fig. 158-8. Comparison of cortisol dynamics in hyperplasia (17 patients) with normal ranges (45 patients). No overlap between these groups was seen in the post-ACTH cortisol values. Forty percent of patients had peripheral studies of cortisol dynamics that suggested autonomy. All of these patients had nodular hyperplasia at surgery.

techniques for determining metastases or invasion of critical structures such as the vena cava. We have also used venous sampling to detect liver and bone metastases before other radiographic abnormalities could be discerned.

ADRENOGENITAL SYNDROMES

Here, the differentiation is between hyperplasia and adenoma and the occasional carcinoma. In the former two circumstances, one must differentiate between unilateral adenoma and bilateral hyperplasia. For the reasons previously proposed, it is thought that the optimal approach to these patients is adrenal venography and venous assay for androgen or estrogens. In addition, the ovarian veins should be catheterized. Several investigators have pointed out the value of combined ovarian and adrenal catheterization to assist in localization of the site of predominant androgen production.[23,48] Visualization of the ovaries may be obtained by a retrograde venography in the erect position following venous sampling. Gray-scale ultrasound has proven particularly valuable in this area, with positive identification of ovarian masses possible in over 90 percent of cases and should be the special exam (Fig. 158-13).

NONFUNCTIONING ADRENAL TUMORS

Not infrequently, patients present with a mass by palpation and IVP in the area of the adrenal without evidence of abnormal cortisol, aldosterone, or catecholamine secretions. Differential diagnosis may lie between a primary renal and adrenal tumor or a secondary adrenal tumor from direct extensions (renal, pancreas, liver), or metastases (lung, breast, thyroid, prostate). With left-sided masses, tumor of the pancreatic tail or retrogastric space (leiomyosarcoma, lymphosarcoma) must be excluded. With right-sided masses, one must differentiate tumors arising from the liver, the pancreatic head, or rarely, the duodenum.

These tumors are usually over 5 cm in size and may be detected by scanning. CAT is recommended for left-sided masses

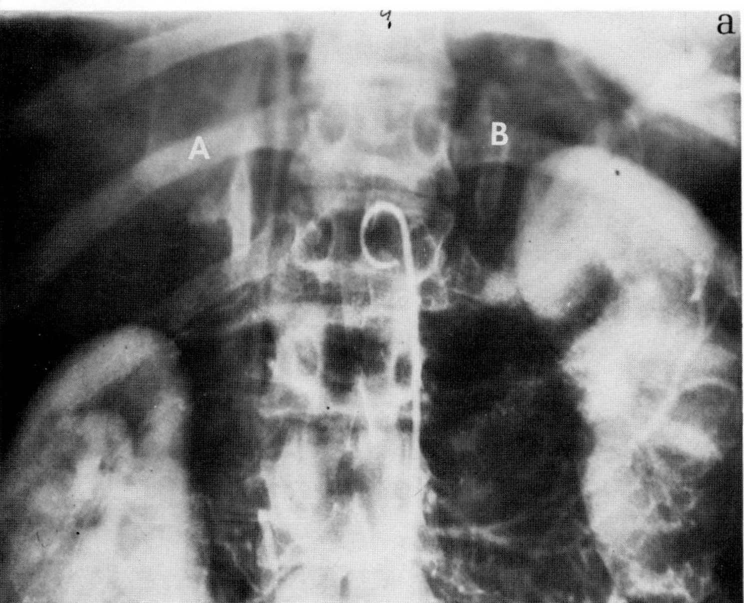

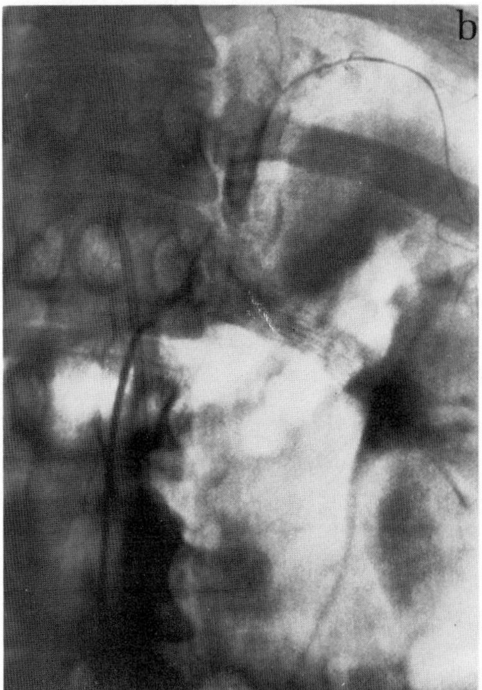

Fig. 158-9. A 23-year-old patient with florid Cushing's syndrome from adrenal hyperplasia. Outside selective arteriography suggested adrenal mass on right (A) and appeared normal on left (B). Bilateral adrenal venograms (C and D) show marked hypervascularity, disorganization, and slight enlargement bilaterally as compared to normal right (E) and left (F) venograms. Adrenal vein cortisols showed marked bilateral hypersecretion of cortisol and hypersensitivity to ACTH stimulation.

	Right Adrenal	Left adrenal
Baseline	560 (μg/100 ml)	630 (μg/100 ml)
Post-dexamethasone (30 min)	340 (μg/100 ml)	280 (μg/100 ml)
Post-ACTH (5 min)	1680 (μg/100 ml)	1830 (μg/100 ml)

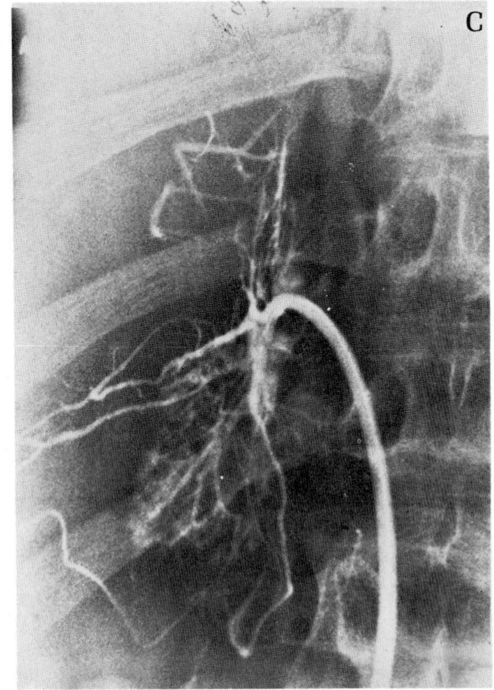

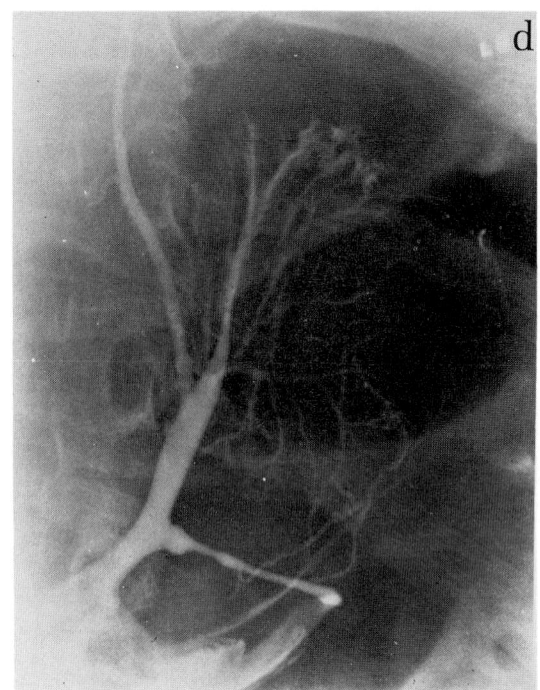

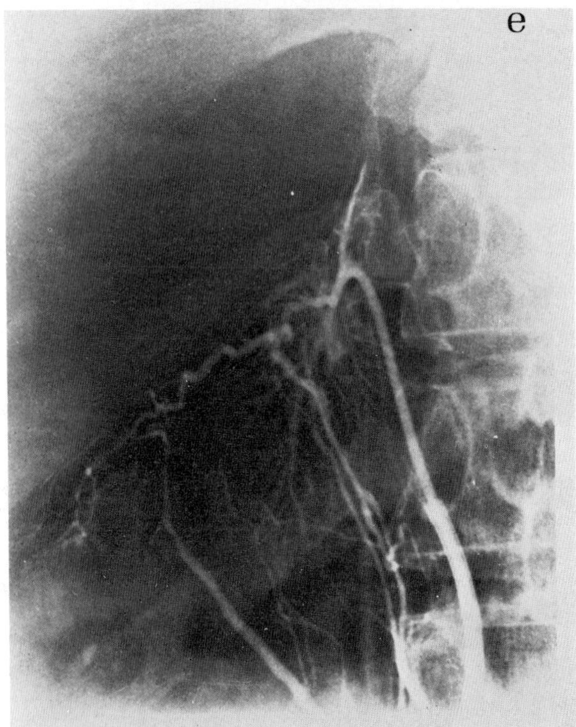

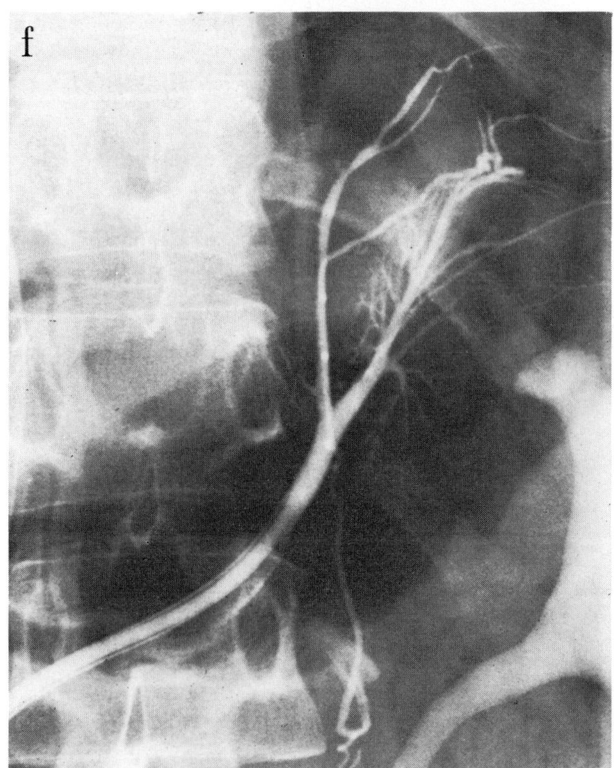

Fig. 158-9. (*Continued*)

and either CAT or ultrasound for right-sided lesions. These studies may be used to guide needle aspirations for cytologic examination of a solid mass or to identify and aspirate an adrenal cyst.

These large masses usually compress adjacent organs, and their site of origin may often be impossible to determine by scanning. Angiography is often performed to help assess operability (e.g., caval invasion). These studies will usually determine the site of origin by showing the origin of the major blood supply, which should be the adrenal arteries in a tumor growing from the adrenal. Hypervascular tumors (most adrenal, renal, and hepatic tumors) can parasitize blood supply, however, and this differentiation may at times be difficult.

Benign adrenal masses and some malignancies (neuroblastoma) are readily identified as primary adrenal tumors by adrenal venography. Most adrenal malignancies, both primary and metastatic, partially occlude the veins (Fig. 158-12). Venography is usually possible and will show splaying and expansion of the gland from intra-adrenal mass. We have used venous sampling and

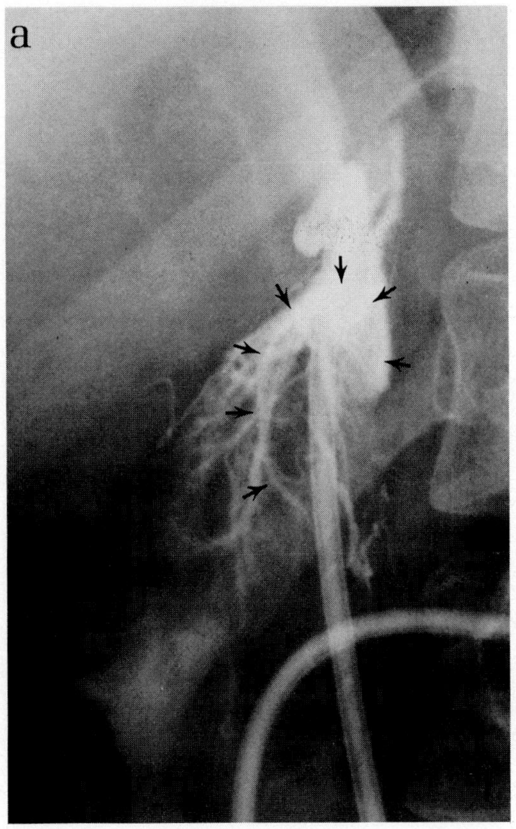

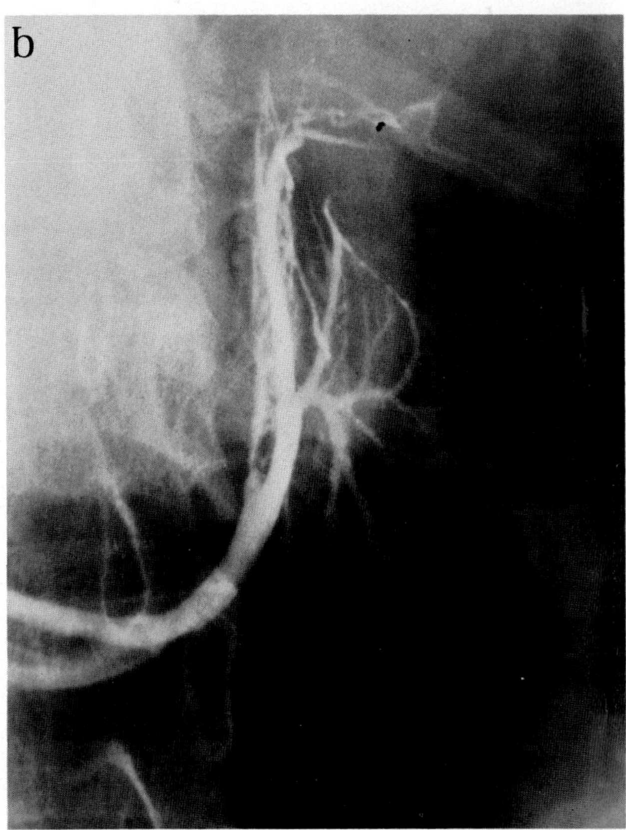

Fig. 158-10. A 27-year-old female with Cushing's syndrome. Venogram on right suggests adenoma; venogram is normal on left. Peripheral cortisol studies suggested autonomous cortisol production. Simultaneous adrenal vein sampling showed cortisol levels and dynamics typical of bilateral hyperplasia.

	Baseline	Post-dexamethasone	Post-ACTH
Right	1340	500	1460
Left	1020	555	1280

(Values are in micrograms per 100 ml.)

At surgery, the left gland was thought to be normal and only the right side was resected. Cushing's disease persisted, requiring subsequent resection on the left.

cortisol determinations to identify primary adrenal malignancy. Adrenal carcinoma, even when not functionally overactive, appears to produce some level of cortisol that is not responsive to dexamethasone or ACTH stimulation, as opposed to metastatic or invasive lesions, which either partially destroy the gland, leaving a reduced level of activity with normal cortisol dynamics, or completely destroy the adrenal and obliterate all function.

DISEASES OF THE ADRENAL MEDULLA

PHEOCHROMOCYTOMA

A diagnosis of pheochromocytoma is made from determination of excessive levels of catecholamines and their metabolites in the urine of hypertensive patients or patients suspected of having MEN syndrome. A significant percentage of pheochromocytomas is discovered incidently at autopsy in patients with and without hypertension. The problems of localization in pheochromocytoma reside with both the possibility of bilateral adrenal tumors (10 to 20 percent in sporadic cases and over 50 percent in MEN syndromes or associated disorders such as ganglioneuromas and neurofibromatosis) and the significant incidence of extra-adrenal location (10 to 15 percent). Uncommonly these tumors may appear both intra- and extra-adrenally (4 percent). Further, approximately 7 to 10 percent of pheochromocytomas are malignant, and these frequently metastasize to the liver and lungs. Only 2 percent of pheochromocytomas occur above the diaphragm, and these are often seen on chest x-rays or tomograms or palpated in the area of the carotid bifurcation.[49,50]

Therapy for pheochromocytoma is surgical removal. Traditionally, this has included an anterior abdominal approach with wide incision suited for exploration of the entire abdomen and pelvis. This approach has been largely determined by the uncertainty of preoperative information for precise localization and determination of single vs. multiple tumors, resulting in an underemphasized recurrence rate of 10 to 20 percent. In fact, 75 to 90 percent of pheochromocytomas occur sporadically, are unilateral and intra-adrenal, and are less than 10 cm in size. These would best be approached from a single flank incision if preoperative diagnosis could rule out mulitplicity, extra-adrenal site, and possible metastases.

The noninvasive techniques such as CAT scans and gray-scale ultrasound have the capability of detecting most pheochromocytomas and possible hepatic metastases.[51] Clear statistics as to the accuracy of these techniques are not yet available, but their

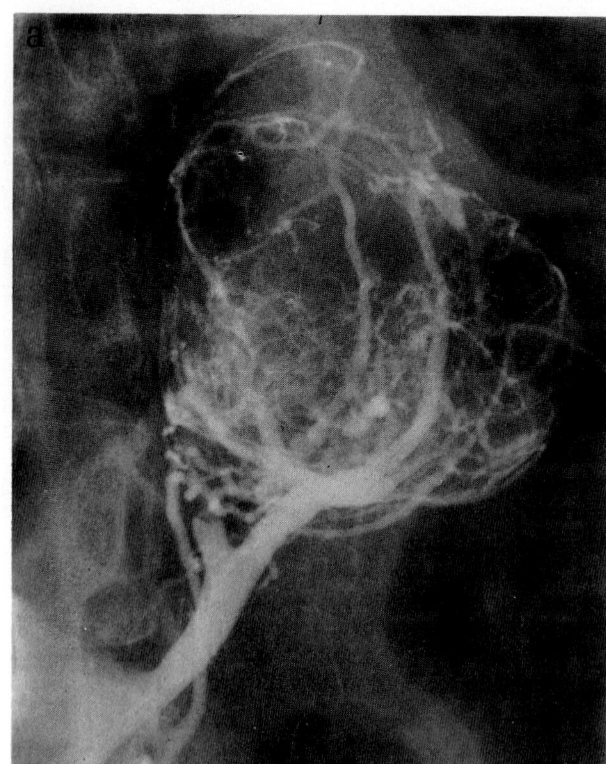

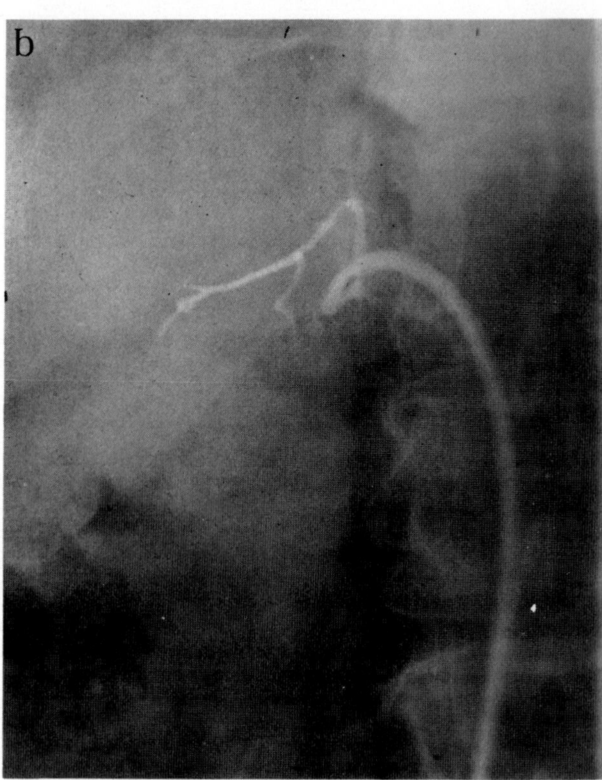

Fig. 158-11. Cushing's syndrome produced by an adrenal adenoma. Left adrenal venogram (A) shows 6-cm hypervascular mass. Right adrenal venogram shows an atrophic gland. (B) Cortisol dynamics indicated relative functional autonomy on the left with suppression on the right and are useful in predicting postoperative cortical function.

	Right	Left
Baseline	0	98
Post-dexamethasone (30 min)	0	89
Post-ACTH (5 min)	27.5	722

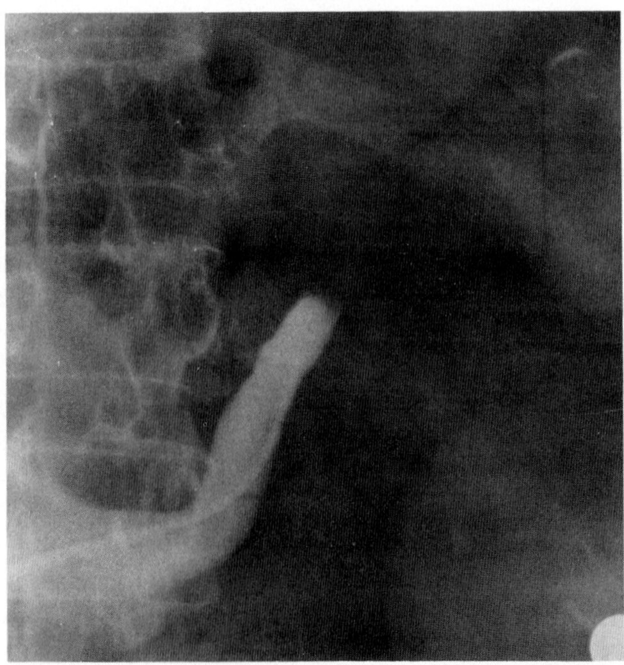

Fig. 158-12. Occlusion of the left adrenal vein by adrenal cell carcinoma.

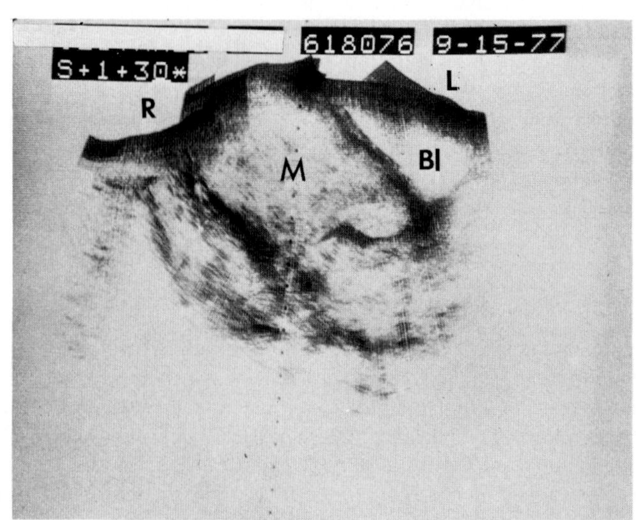

Fig. 158-13. Virilizing ovarian tumor. Transverse gray-scale ultrasound demonstration of an ovarian mass (M) with numerous reflected echos from within indicating solid structure. The bladder (Bl) is displaced to the left.

routine use seems justified. Again, their greatest value will lie in clear demonstration of bilateral adrenal tumors. If a unilateral mass is identified, these studies may not reliably rule out a smaller contralateral mass. The CAT scan may be additionally helpful in detecting a retroperitoneal, pararenal, or mediastinal extra-adrenal location but should be followed by arteriography for confirmation. Ultrasound may define bladder or perivesicular lesions.

Because exploring the entire abdomen, retroperitoneum, and pelvis involves considerable dissection, and because there is a high recurrence rate, most surgeons desire as much preoperative information as possible. Angiography is generally performed, as these tumors are hypervascular and show up readily on simple aortography in 80 percent of cases and on selective arteriography in over 90 percent.[23,52] In patients with hyperplastic syndromes, these lesions may be quite small and difficult to detect even on selective arteriography. In approximately 10 percent of cases, the tumors are hypovascular, which may be a feature of either very small lesions or of large tumors under tension within their capsule or undergoing partial necrosis (Fig. 158-14). In addition, the extra-adrenal lesions, even when hypervascular, may be very difficult to differentiate from superimposed blushes of other vascular structures. The overall accuracy of arteriography has been reported to vary from 75 to 90 percent.[34]

Plasma catecholamine assays on venous samples from multiple sites in the vena cava have been advocated for aiding in localization of missed extra-adrenal lesions and have occasionally been attempted for identifying adrenal lesions.[53] The use of such assays has been limited by the technical difficulty of obtaining a reliable plasma catecholamine assay and the unpredictability of catecholamine release. In our own laboratory, we have relied upon a selective adrenal venous approach as the primary study in patients with suspected sporadic pheochromocytoma. Bilateral simultaneous sampling is necessary because of the potentially large fluctuations in epinephrine release that may occur with anxiety state or catheter manipulation. Since these are centrally induced, false elevations will be present bilaterally. Unilateral elevations obtained with simultaneous bilateral sampling may be taken, based on our current data, as both diagnostic of intra- or para-adrenal ipsilateral tumor and exclusive of a contralateral adrenal pheochromocytoma. (Fig. 158-15). Selective simultaneous venous sampling combined with magnification venography has provided reliable detection of adrenal lesions as small as 2 mm (Fig. 158-16). In addition, venous sampling with minimally abnormal venograms has been successful in identifying and lateralizing tumors in several patients referred to us with adrenal lesions as large as 6 cm, which were missed on selective adrenal arteriography. In our opinion, the accuracy of such techniques in defining unilateral intra-adrenal disease should allow the single flank approach in the great majority of patients, with considerable reduction in overall patient morbidity and cost. When bilateral catecholamine elevations are encountered in the adrenal effluent, they must be correlated with masses seen on venography. In our total experience, we have not seen a false-negative adrenal venogram for masses over 4 mm.

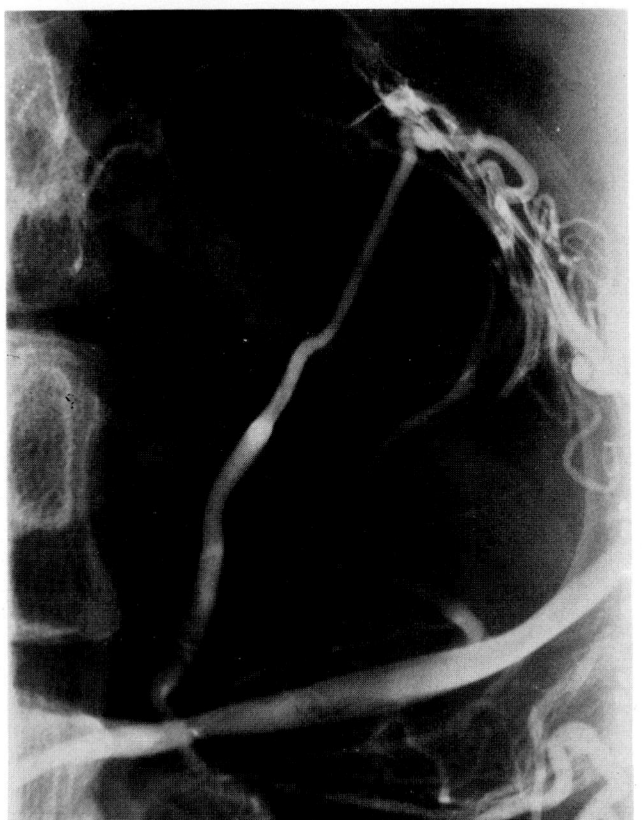

Fig. 158-14. Left adrenal venography shows marked expansion and draping from tumor. Catecholamine levels were elevated bilaterally (see Fig. 158-15, no. 3).

Bilateral elevations with normal venography should probably be considered as centrally induced excitation unless one is dealing with a suspected MEN patient, in whom microscopic medullary hyperplasia must be considered. If venograms are negative in patients with suspected sporadic tumor, then aortography may be performed. We have preferred to delay aortography and continue the venous study with multiple sampling from the jugular veins, the superior and inferior venae cavae and the renal and hypogastric veins. In this approach subsequent CAT scan or angiography may be performed with concentration on the area suggested by venous sampling.

If we are studying a patient suspected of having MEN syndrome and the venograms are negative, we generally proceed directly with selective arteriography to aid in the differential of small unilateral tumor vs. medullary hyperplasia.

It is impossible to differentiate arteriographically the bizarre vasculature of a benign pheochromocytoma from that of a malignant one. In fact, the pathologist relies upon the demonstration of venous invasion to make this diagnosis histologically. Venography has the capability of showing this venous invasion well. We have also used hepatic vein sampling for detecting liver metastases.

Hypertensive crises have been reported in approximately 2 percent of patients undergoing arterial studies. These patients should be treated with adrenergic receptor blocking agents (dibenzyline, 1 mg/kg/day) for several days before the procedure. In addition, regitine should be available for immediate injection during a procedure. Hypertensive crisis has also been noted on venous study. However, selective venography, when performed properly, should provide less stimulation to a tumor than selective adrenal arteriography. A large adrenal mass can easily be identified with a simple test injection into the mouth of the enlarged adrenal vein without the need for a full venogram in a patient who is particularly labile. In this case the diagnosis may be confirmed with the venous samples.

PANCREATIC ENDOCRINE TUMORS

The diagnosis of pancreatic endocrine disease is generally made by a biochemical determination of elevated insulin levels in association with hypoglycemia or elevated gastrin levels in patients

SIMULTANEOUS ADRENAL VEIN SAMPLING
FOR CATECHOLAMINES

	RT. ADRENAL		LT. ADRENAL			
	E	NE	E	NE		
1.	6.5	2.5	9.6	3.9		
2.	3.5	1.6	8.3	2.1		
3.	6.1	0	7.0	0		
4.	0.7	0.02	4.9	0.13		
5.	4.4	4.6	7.8	1.4		Typical
6.	2.7	0.4	2.1	0.3		Normals
7.	5.7	1.3	2.3	1.3		
8.	3.2	0.9	3.1	1.0		
9.	4.1	1.4	5.6	1.3		
Mean	±0.7	±0.5	±1.0	±0.5		
					Site	
1.*	352	288	4.5	1.8	L	
2.*	108	91	1.8	2.1	L	
3.*	42	3	21.0	6	Bilat.	Adrenal
4.	7.2	4.4	25.0	113	R	Pheds.
5.	2.2	1.3	26.4	143	R	
6.*	66	25	7.0	3.0	L	
7.	5.4	1.5	630	48	R	

*Missed on selective adrenal arteriography.

Fig. 158-15. Adrenal vein catecholamine levels in simultaneous samples taken from 9 normal patients and 7 patients with pheochromocytomas. In the pheochromocytoma group, all but 1 patient had a unilateral intra-adrenal tumor, ranging in size from 2 mm to 10 cm. Three patients were referred after negative selective adrenal arteriograms. (See also Figs. 158-16 and 158-22.)

with peptic ulcer disease. A high mortality rate is associated with these disorders, which relates primarily to their functional activity but also to a relatively high incidence of malignancy. Medical therapy has been generally unrewarding, and surgical intervention is usually indicated.

The optimal surgical approach to these disorders depends upon whether the functional abnormality is arising from a solitary lesion, from multiple individual lesions, or from diffuse disease, including microscopic hyperplasia. This assessment is often impossible to make in the operating room, as over 70 percent of the endocrine tumors of the pancreas tend to be small (1–3 cm) and difficult to palpate, even at autopsy.[54] Differentiation between benign and malignant tumors and the detection of the often small hepatic or lymph node metastases associated with malignancies are also difficult intraoperatively. Conventional radiologic examinations, CAT scanning, gray-scale ultrasound, and ERCP (endoscopic retrograde cholangiopancreatography) have been ineffective in pancreatic endocrine tumor diagnosis and localization. The resolution of the scanning modalities is inadequate to detect these generally small tumors, and ductography is unrewarding, as these lesions, unlike carcinomas, arise from the parenchyma rather than from the duct. Since most of these tumors are hypervascular, angiography has been used effectively in most series for localization of endocrine tumors and for defining metastases. Most recently, transhepatic cannulation of the portal vein and subsequent selective pancreatic venous sampling has been introduced for the diagnosis of pancreatic endocrine disease. Radioimmunoassays are available for the detection of gastrin, insulin, and the polypeptide of WDH syndrome.

INSULINOMA

The great majority of insulinomas are solitary lesions (90 percent), occurring with equal distribution throughout the pancreas. When multiple tumors occur, they tend to be localized and limited in number. Malignancy is encountered in approximately 10 percent of cases.[55] Specific tumor localization allows for local resection, most often in the form of a simple tumor enucleation, and will obviate the need for blind resections of the body and tail of the pancreas, which have been advocated in the surgical literature when pancreatic tumors cannot be identified intraoperatively. Blind resections are unsuccessful in 50 percent of cases and leave the subsequent surgeon with the difficult decison of performing a debilitating pancreatectomy.[56] Angiography has been effective in localization of insulinomas in from 50 to 90 percent of cases, with most angiographers averaging around 75 percent.[57–59]

Radiologic and catheter techniques play a large role in improving accuracy. The role of subselective pancreatic artery injection and magnification techniques are paramount to the success of these studies (Fig. 158-17). The most frequent angiographic finding is an increase in contrast accumulation in tumors with persistent staining, as is typical of most endocrine tumors. Histology will

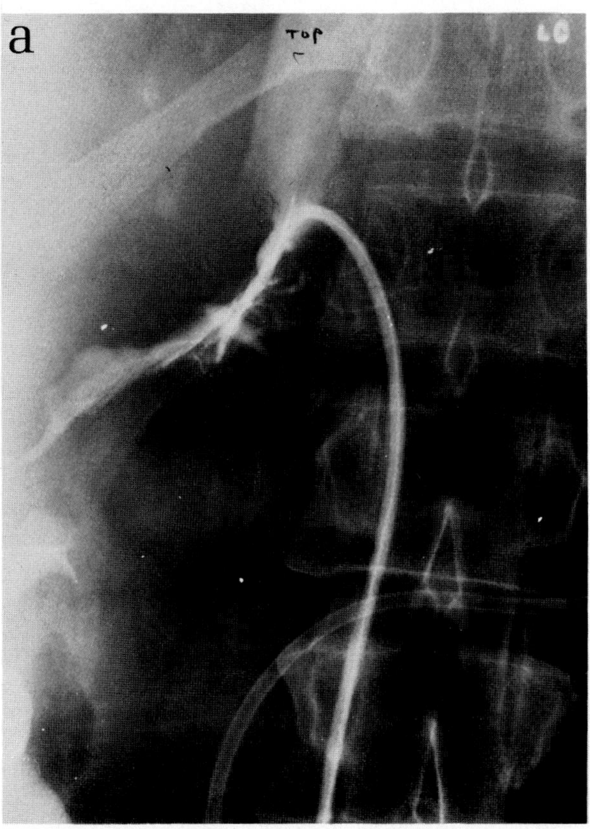

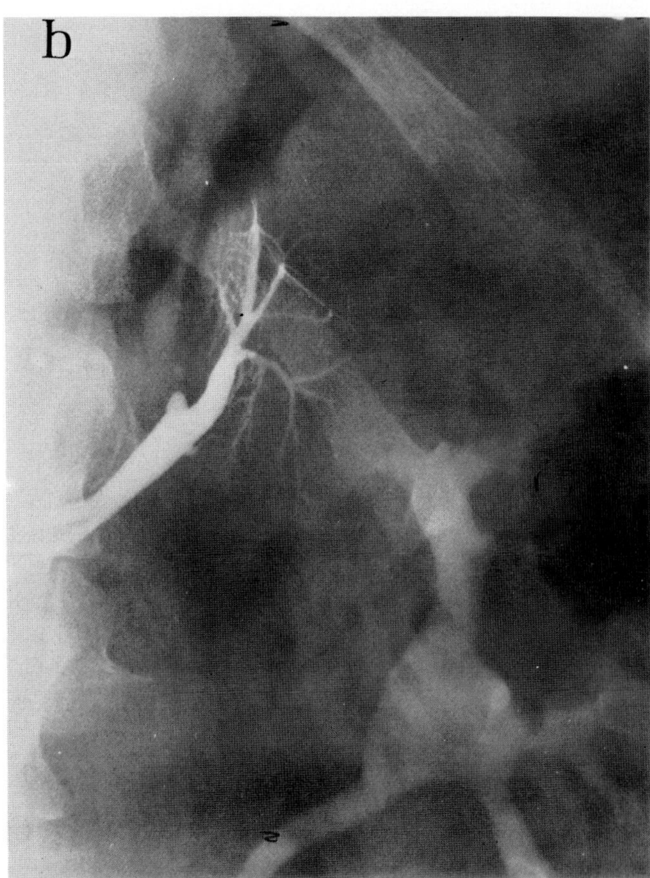

Fig. 158-16. A 47-year-old male with elevated urinary catecholamines. Abdominal aortography and selective adrenal arteriography were negative. Adrenal venography shows a bizarre pattern on the right (a) but no definite mass effect. There was also slight suspicion of an upper pole small nodule on the left venogram. (b) Selective simultaneous adrenal vein samples show a marked elevation on the right and normal levels on the left (see Fig. 15, No. 5). At surgery, a 3.5-cm right adrenal pheochromocytoma was removed with apparent "cure."

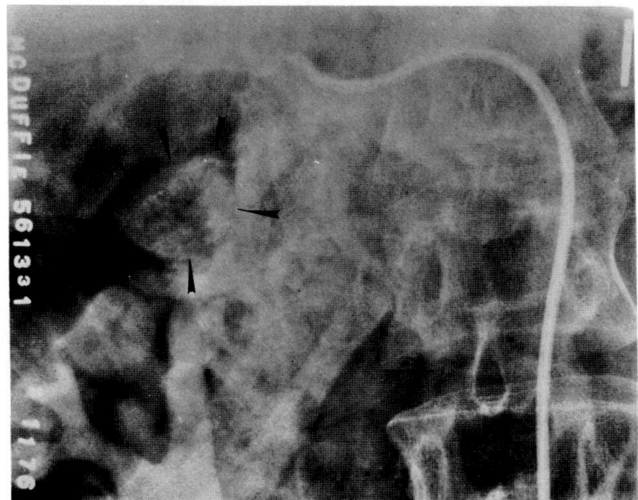

Fig. 158-17. A 24-year-old female with 1.5-cm insulinoma. Patient had the distal half of her pancreas resected at prior unsuccessful exploration and had two negative selective arteriograms prior to referral. Venous samples from posterosuperior pancreatic vein showed elevated insulin levels. At repeat angiography the lesion was only seen on a posterosuperior pancreatic injection following negative dorsal and anterosuperior pancreatic artery injections. An expert surgeon was unable to palpate the tumor at a repeat operation. Mobilization and careful dissection of the posterosuperior aspect of the pancreas uncovered the lesion, which was then shelled out.

confirm this hypervascularity when special elastic stains are used. The use of subselective high bolus injections to blush the pancreas will silhouette these tumors (Figs. 158-18 and 158-19) and may allow detection of tumors ranging in size from 1 to 2 mm, or 1 to 2 cm when vascularity is not increased. In a Mayo Clinic series using routine preoperative selective arteriography, successful localization was achieved in 123 out of 132 patients (93 percent) at first operation, as compared to the general success rate of 85 percent.[60] Most recently, Lunderquist introduced a technique of pancreatic vein sampling for insulin assay and has achieved successful localization in 5 consecutive patients, including 1 patient with multiple tumors.[61] Although experience with this technique is limited, there is precedence for its rationale in the successful use of the venous sampling techniques mentioned previously. Pancreatic vein catheterization does not appear to be a technically difficult procedure, and significant complication rates have not been reported from these studies or from similar catheter introductions in a large number of patients for study of portal hypertension.[62]

GASTRINOMAS

Approximately 20 percent of gastrinomas are solitary and benign, occurring with high frequency in the area of the head of the pancreas and in the wall of the duodenal loop. Hyperplasia is seen more frequently with gastrinomas than with islet cell tumors and occurs in approximately 5 percent of all cases and in 14 percent of patients with multiple endocrinopathies (MEA Type 1). Gastrino-

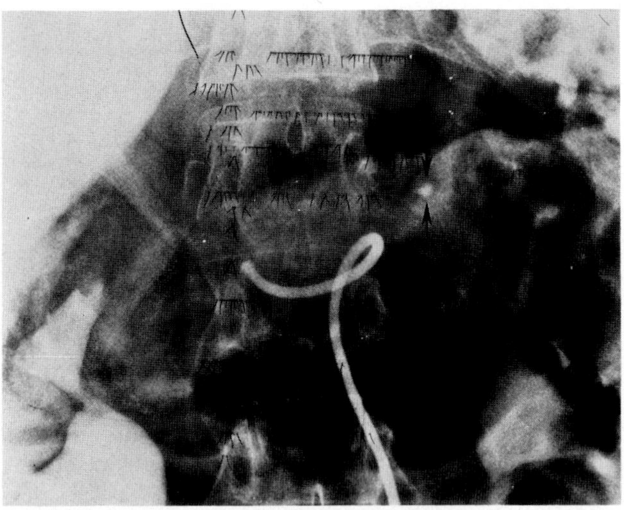

Fig. 158-18. A 2-mm nonpalpable insulinoma in the distal pancreatic body removed by blind wedge resection following angiographic localization. (Courtesy V. A. Millan, New England Medical Center.)

mas are most often malignant (60 percent), and 80 percent have associated metastases.[63] Patients most frequently die from their ulcer disease, rather than from extensions or metastases of the malignancies. Because of the multiplicity of the disease, and because of the difficulty in preoperative or intraoperative assessment of these tumors, the preferred surgical approach has been total gastrectomy.[64] Recent preliminary studies have shown Cimetadine to be an effective drug for control of the hyperacidity associated with these tumors,[65] and the current surgical approach may be redirected toward resection of the primary tumors. This will reemphasize the need for accurate preoperative localization studies. Arteriography has had a reported accuracy of 50 to 80 percent, and the findings are the same as with insulinomas.[66]

Experience with multiple direct pancreatic venous sampling for gastrin has been limited to the study of 5 patients with multicentric disease and 1 patient with a solitary lesion. These studies were successful in all patients.[67] As discussed previously, the sampling technique offers a significant potential advantage to preoperative localization and differentiating solitary from multifocal disease, even when microscopic.

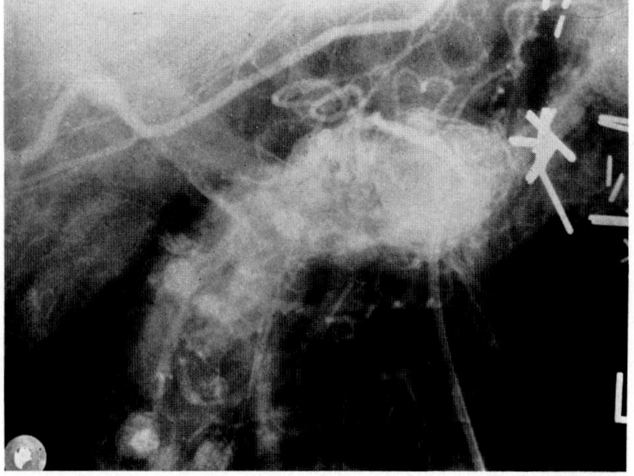

Fig. 158-19. Multiple hypervascular tumors throughout the pancreas typical of endocrine tumors. These range in size from 1 mm to several centimeters, and most are nonpalpable.

GLUCAGONOMAS

Angiographic studies in glucogenoma have been very limited, and findings have been similar to those in insulinoma. Two patients with glucogenomas have undergone venous sampling with successful localization of solitary lesions.[67] Although no experience has been obtained to date in WDH syndrome or in alpha cell tumors, one might predict similar success of these techniques in these disorders.

PARATHYROID

Parathyroid localization techniques have been discussed in Chapter 56. A need for localization studies is obvious in patients with prior unsuccessful explorations, which usually result from an unusual neck or mediastinal location or from difficulty in distinguishing single from multiple gland disease. Noninvasive modalities, to date, have proven of little value, while selective arteriography and venous assay provide high accuracy.

Arteriography is important for planning a specific surgical approach, but it may confuse thyroid pathology with parathyroid disease. Venous sampling is specific for parathyroid pathology, but drainage patterns must be carefully observed following surgical distortion of anatomy. There is also good reason to consider venous sampling in routine cases, since serious controversy exists as to the proper surgical approach. Some surgical groups routinely resect three and one-half glands at initial exploration because of the difficulty in distinguishing adenoma from hyperplasia on gross inspection or frozen section. Although there is a rough correlation between gland size and calcium level, histologically normal glands may hypersecrete, and large glands may be functionally inactive. An opposite surgical approach is for limited parathyroid exploration whenever possible. If rapid identification of an adenoma is achieved, additional exploration is limited to biopsy of a normal gland. Another important controversy is whether or not resection of three and one-half glands is always necessary in hyperplasia, as the disease process may be grossly asymmetric, morphologically and functionally. Venous catheterization studies may play a role in resolving these controversies and allowing more limited surgical approach. Recent developments suggest that high-energy ultrasound may have an important future role in parathyroid disease in the neck, and CAT scanning has been useful in identifying anterior mediastinal tumors.

CARCINOID TUMORS[68]

Hypervascular carcinoid tumors are found throughout the gut and bronchi, mostly occurring as small masses in the duodenum or distal ilium. These tumors are slow growing, even when malignant (40 percent), and survival may be prolonged.

Carcinoid syndrome occurs only in 1 in 40 patients with the tumor and is almost invariably associated with malignancy and liver metastases. Death results from the effects of the secretory products rather than from the tumor itself. Liver metastases are usually large enough to be demonstrated by scanning. The tumors are vascular and well demonstrated by angiography, which may be necessary for diagnosis of smaller tumors. The vascular pattern and histology are similar to endocrine tumors of the A.P.U.D. series. One sees an increased vascularity occurring in vessels below 100 μm in size, where it may only be perceived as well-circumscribed intensified vascular blush with persistent staining. These tumors may incite a serotonin-mediated fibroplastic reaction out of proportion to tumor size and appear as a predominantly avascular fibrous mass. Even in these cases, the metastases retain a hypervascular appearance.

PITUITARY DISEASE

Pituitary tumors are most likely to manifest themselves clinically by causing visual difficulties from supersellar extension and compression of the optic nerve or by inducing infertility and/or galactorrhea as endocrinopathies related to abnormal ACTH, TSH, ADH, or prolactin secretion. Occasionally, nonfunctioning tumors may present with headache, hypothyroidism, or hypogonadism. Biochemical or radioimmune assay will generally demonstrate abnormal hormone production and, along with metyrapone testing, will usually establish the diagnosis of a pituitary tumor. Therapy may involve conventional x-ray treatment, proton beam treatment, craniotomy with tumor resection, stereotaxic transnasal approach for cryosurgery or radio-frequency destruction, or transsphenoidal approach for removal with microdissection techniques.

Radiodiagnosis is directed toward determining: (1) the presence and size of the pituitary tumor; (2) the precise position of the tumor within the sella (central vs. lateral); (3) the presence and degree of suprasellar extension, as well as lateral extension and intrasphenoidal extension; (4) the degree of pneumatization and septation within the sphenoid sinus; (5) the relationship of the carotid artery to the pituitary tumor; (6) the presence of vascular invasion in pituitary malignancy suspected from transsphenoidal biopsy; (7) the presence or absence of a parasellar tumor (such as meningioma, aneurysm, or A-V malformation) or empty sella syndrome.

Details of the anatomy of the tumor, the sphenoid sinus, and local vasculature will be particularly important if the more sophisticated but blinder approach of transsphenoidal surgery is planned or if stereotaxic techniques are used. Decision for optimal therapy may be based upon the size and extensions of the tumor, which need to be carefully determined. Whenever possible, it would seem that microdissection techniques would be preferable for lower morbidity, for preservation of normal pituitary function, and for elimination of damage to the optic nerve, which may occur with either surgery or radiotherapy.[69] Surgery provides the advantage of lowering elevated hormonal levels instantly.

RADIOLOGIC APPROACH

Following plain skull films, tomography coned to the sellar region should be performed routinely. Large sellar or parasellar masses producing plain film abnormalities may be further characterized and localized by the presence and appearance of calcification as well as by the appearance of the bony erosions and remodeling that they produce. Most neuroradiologists do not rely upon volume measurements, but rather on the observations of localized erosions, ballooning, and cortical thinning. Microcalcifications may be seen in the sella in approximately 15 percent of chromophobe adenomas and are noted in and above the sella in approximately 50 to 70 percent of craniopharyngiomas. Calcifications are characteristically flecklike or conglomerate and must be differentiated from the ringlike calcification that may be seen in association with aneurysm and the dense flocculent calcifications seen in association with hyperostosis and meningiomas. Pluridirectional

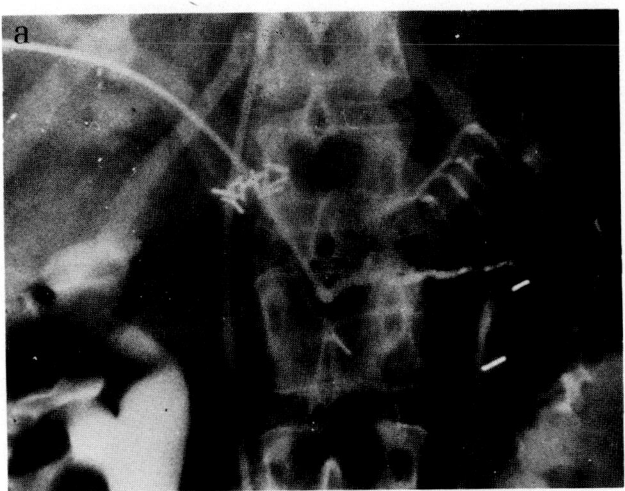

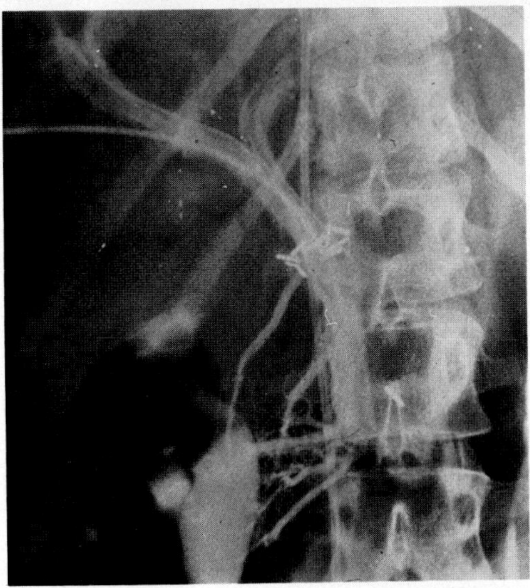

Fig. 158-20. Dorsal pancreatic (a) and superior pancreatic (b) venograms performed during venous sampling procedure which localized an adenoma missed at prior surgery and subselective angiography. (Courtesy of R. Coury.)

tomography is particularly helpful in patients with normal-appearing sellae on plain films and should especially be performed on patients with suspected microadenomas, as in prolactin-secreting, or basophilic tumors. Typically these produce a unilateral inferior bowing and erosion of the floor.

Computerized axial tomography should routinely follow tomography. This examination will provide most or all of the information needed for therapy.[20,21] It will generally define the size and abnormal tissue density of the pituitary mass, as well as the presence of even small amounts of calcification. Suprasellar extension may be defined by the deformity of the supersellar cistern or third ventricle. Intrasphenoidal extensions are also well seen, along with the degree of aeration and presence of septa within the sphenoid sinus. In the empty sella syndrome, there is decreased tissue density within the sella on CAT, but one must be careful to determine that the tissue density information is from the sella itself and not averaged information from the cisterns above the sella. Cystic pituitary adenoma must also be differentiated, as well as anterior herniation of a dilated third ventricle into the sella. Enhancement of the CAT with intravenous iodine injection is generally performed to improve visualization of the pituitary mass,

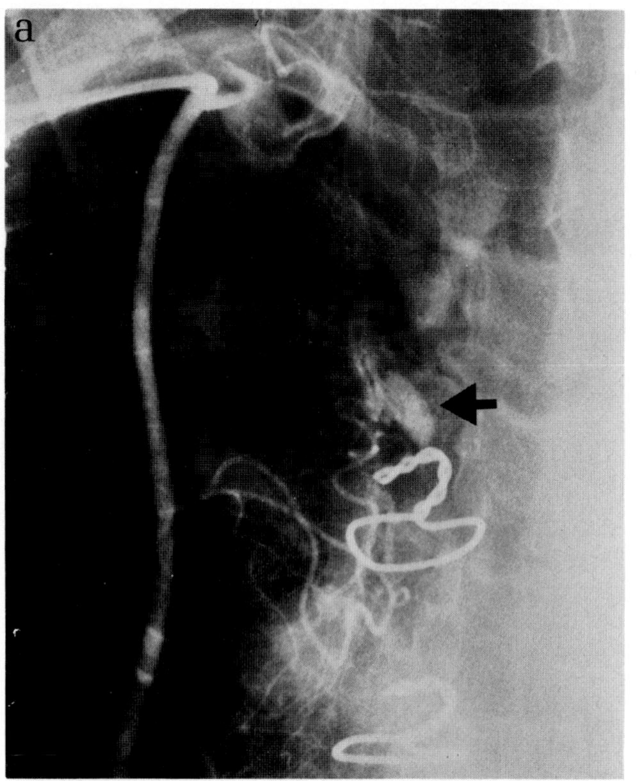

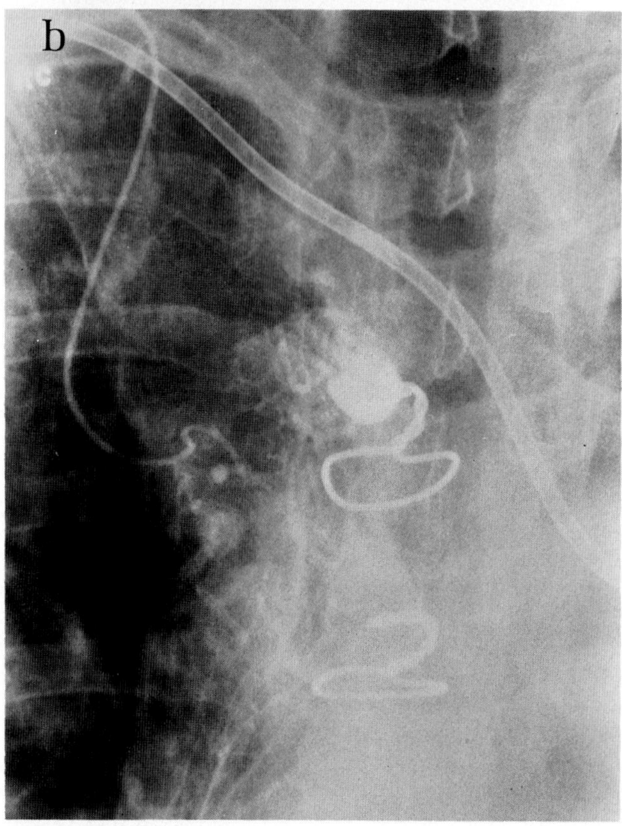

Fig. 158-21. Destruction of a parathyroid adenoma shown arising from the internal mammary artery (A) by intra-arterial embolization of short-ranged Y^{90} beta-radiation carbon microspheres directly into the feeding artery (B). Calculated tumor dose was 25,000 rads and produced no apparent radiation to normal tissues beyond 4 mm. This poor surgical risk patient, with Ca^{2+} ranging from 13.0 to 14.5, has remained normocalcemic in a 3-year follow-up post catheter destruction.

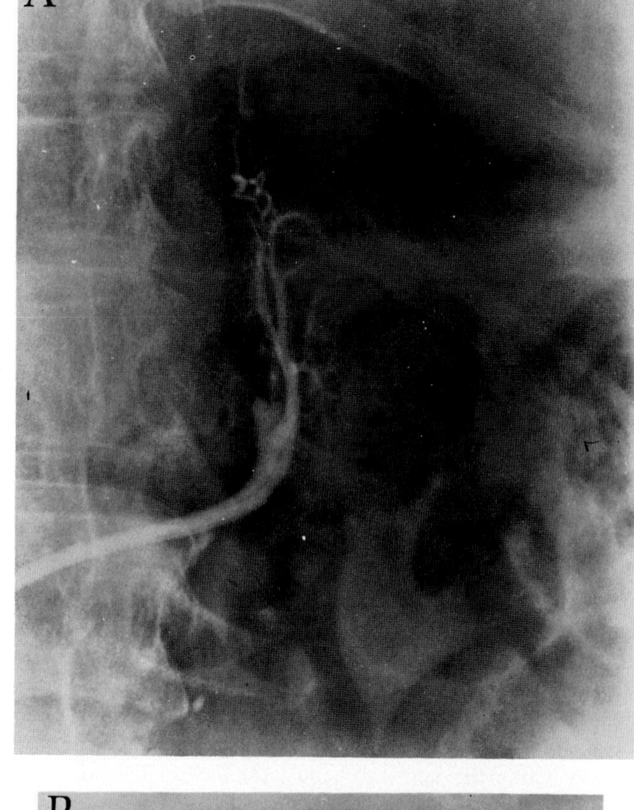

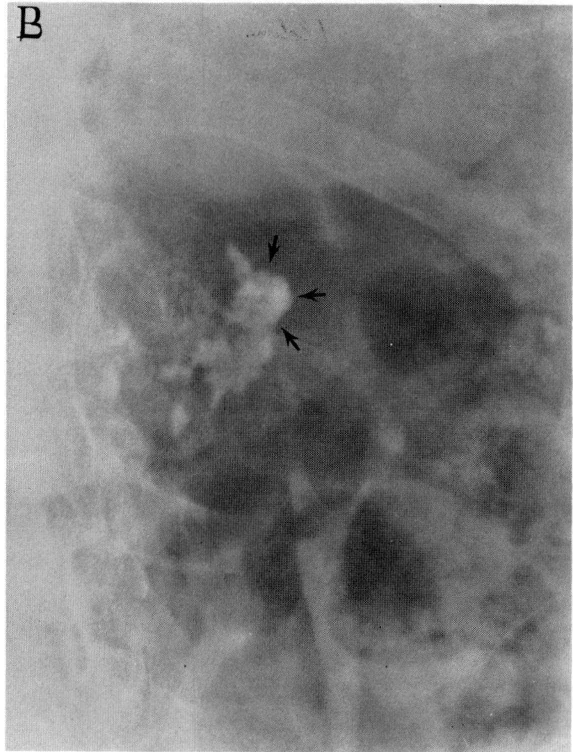

Fig. 158-22. A 32-year-old male with poorly controlled hypertension and a small left kidney on IVP, studied for suspected renal artery stenosis. Identification of suspicious blush above the left kidney on aortography prompted left adrenal venography following renin sampling. A nodule was noted on venography (A). Bilateral simultaneous adrenal vein samples confirmed the diagnosis of pheochromocytoma with marked elevation of catecholamines on the left and normal levels on the right. (See Fig. 15, No. 7). Accidental infarction of the tumor resulted from selective arteriography, and the patient has remained normotensive in a 5-year follow-up.

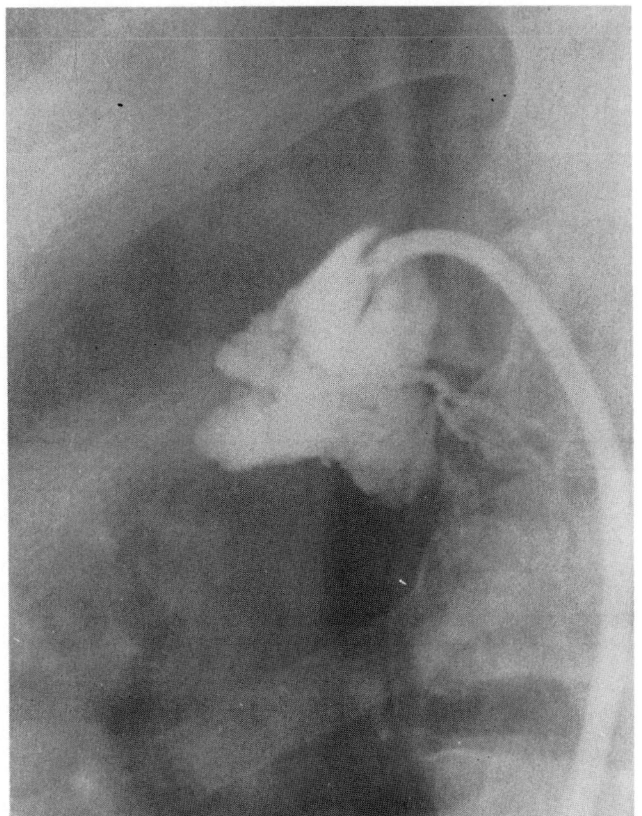

Fig. 158-23. Transvenous adrenal ablation. Intra-adrenal extravasation of a mixture of contrast material and nitrogen mustard (0.1 mg/kg).

which is usually moderately hypervascular, and also helps define cystic degeneration. Iodine enhancement will generally provide a clear diagnosis and visualization of parasellar meningiomas, which are typically highly vascular with prolonged retention of contrast. Parasellar aneurysm or vascular malformations are usually suspected but require further definition by arteriography. In approximately 5 to 7 percent of patients, the CAT scans will be falsely negative, particularly when dealing with microadenomas. Other examinations may then be performed if tomography and CAT scans are negative or if the supersellar space or parasellar spaces have not been adequately defined. At the present time, the most promising test appears to be CAT scanning, following intrathecal administration of water-soluble contrast (Metrizamide).[21] This examination is capable of showing even slight supersellar extensions, as well as providing better definition of size, shape, density, and site of origin of the pituitary mass (Fig. 158-24).

Several indications may exist for the use of internal carotid arteriography. This examination is best performed using magnification and subtraction and will provide the best possible resolution for pituitary adenomas, demonstrating tumor staining in most cases, along with visualization of capsular veins and meningohypohyseal blood supply.[70] Suprasellar and lateral extensions may be detected by displacements of the cavernous carotid artery, the anterior cerebral artery (M-1 segment), and the anterior choroidal arteries, along with the septal vein and veins of Rosenthal. Demonstration of the course of the cavernous carotid through the pituitary sella is important to avoid carotid cavernous fistula formation when a blind transsphenoidal surgical approach is used. Angiography will be diagnostic in determining the presence of aneurysm, vascular malformation, or meningioma and will show vascular encasement in the rare pituitary malignancies. Orbital venography will occasionally be helpful in defining the parasellar space.

Pneumoencephalography carries the greatest morbidity and should be reserved only to augment the previously mentioned studies. This examination will provide the best possible definition of the suprasellar space and may occasionally be required to demonstrate an empty sella. The examination is best performed with fluoroscopy and tomography to limit the amount of air.

THERAPUETIC ANGIOGRAPHY

Most recently, catheterization techniques have been developed for a number of therapeutic applications, including the control of hemorrhage[71,72] and the purposeful infarction of normal tissue[73] and tumors.[74] Catheter perfusion of tumor circulation with chemotherapeutic agents has been advocated for as long as selective catheterization procedures have been performed. However, the results of such therapy have been controversial. It should be

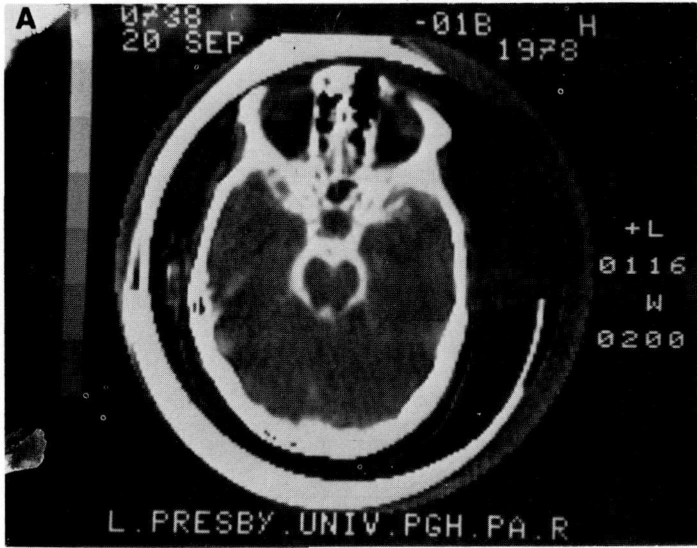

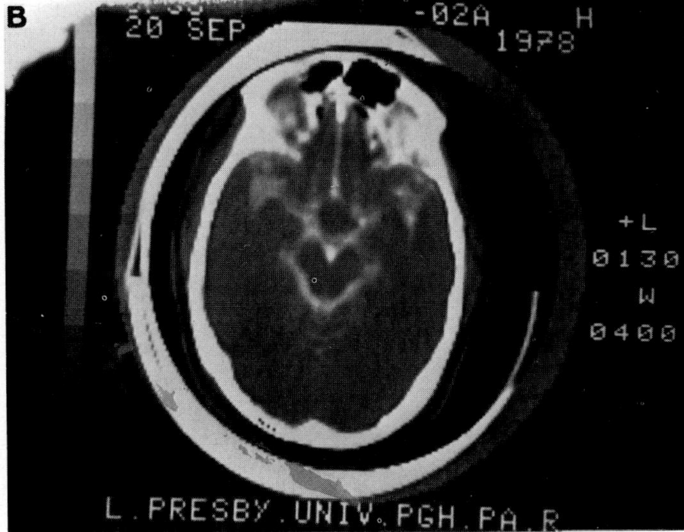

Fig. 158-24. (A) Filling defect within central portion of pentagonal-shaped suprasellar cistern. (B) Eccentricity of growth of suprasellar mass on slice obtained 13 mm. The plane of growth of this plane is more rightward, but it also encroaches on the interpeduncular cistern and interhemispheric fissure above previous figure. Note visualization of middle cerebral artery bilaterally within Sylvian vallecula.

pointed out that the circulation of most tumors in the body is relatively hypovascular, and even direct organ perfusion with such tumors would result in relatively little tumor uptake on a mechanical basis. Hypervascular tumors usually have considerable shunting, which again diminishes the mechanical advantages of direct organ perfusion. However, the circulation of most endocrine tumors consists of a fine plethoric vascular plexus, which tends to have a delayed circulation time with minimal or no shunting. This type of circulation appears to soak up and retain injected contrast media. Thus, direct perfusion of endocrine tumors and their extensions may provide a true mechanical advantage. Success has been reported in direct installation of streptozotocin into the dorsal pancreatic artery for destruction of malignant pancreatic islet cell tumors.[75] Microspheres loaded with short-range beta-radiation isotopes have been injected into the hepatic circulation with selective uptake and destruction of metastatic carcinoid tumors.[76] We have combined highly selective catheter placement with injection of vasoconstricting drugs to temporarily gain highly selective access to tumor circulation. During this brief period of tumor circulation control, we have embolized carbon microspheres with Y^{90} (pure beta emitter, range 4 mm) directly into tumors to achieve considerably higher radiation doses than are possible from external beam therapy. We have used such techniques for the destruction of parathyroid adenomas, as illustrated in Fig. 158-21. Damage to and possible destruction of endocrine tissue can also be achieved by mechanical blockage from embolic materials, such as Gelfoam,[77] or metallic microspheres, or from chemical toxicity (Fig. 158-22) achieved by high doses of contrast media. Improved survival curves have been obtained by mechanically blocking the circulation to more vascular shunting tumors such as hepatoma,[74] which have a circulation similar to that of adrenal carcinomas. It should be cautioned that if tumor destruction is attempted, particularly in benign disease, these techniques should be reasonably certain of producing total tumor destruction, since small nests of endocrine tumors are capable of growing back over long periods of time to produce excess hormone levels. If only partial tumor damage has been achieved, the subsequent surgical resection might be considerably more difficult because of the inflammatory reaction created by the initial transcatheter therapy. It is for this reason that we have favored use of beta radiation, which should have the advantage of being most destructive at the tumor level and which leaves the feeding vessels patent for subsequent therapy in the event of tumor regrowth. Selective tumor uptake of isotope in pulmonary and hepatic metastases may also be achieved through the bronchial and hepatic artery circulations.

We have also developed a technique for transcatheter adrenalectomy.[73] This involves the purposeful extravasation of nitrogen mustard into the adrenal glands and has been used as an alternative to surgical adrenalectomy for palliation of breast and prostatic cancer in patients who are relatively poor surgical risks. This procedure has a considerably lower morbidity than bilateral surgical adrenalectomy and produces an effective, although not total destruction of adrenal function (Fig. 158-23). Over the next several years, we will see a continuing effort and refinement of techniques for the transcatheter approach to destruction of both primary and metastic endocrine tumors.

REFERENCES

1. Holm, H. H., Pedersen, J. F., Kristensen, J. K., et al: Ultrasonically guided percutaneous puncture. *Radiol Clin North Am, 13 (3):* 493, 1975.
2. Eisenberg, H., Holland, W.: Magnification arteriography with grid biased focal spot x-ray tubes. *Laboratory and Clinical Analysis.* Stanford, Conn., Cathode Press, 1972.
3. Genant, H., Doi, K., Mall, J., et al: direct radiographic magnification for skeletal radiography: Assessment of image quality and clinical application. *Radiology 123:* 47, 1977.
4. Steinbach, H., Minagi, H.: The Endocrines. An Atlas of Tumor Radiology. Chicago, Year Book Medical Publishers, 1969.
5. Pickering, R., Hartman, G., Weeks, R., et al: Excretory urographic localization of adrenal cortical tumors and pheochromocytomas. *Radiology 114:* 345, 1975.
6. Watanabe, K., Kamoi, I., Nakayama, C., et al: Scintigraphic detection of hepatic metastases with 131-I-labeled steroid in recurrent adrenal carcinoma: A case report. *J Nucl Med 17:* 904–906, 1976.
7. Seabold, J., Cohen, E., Beierwaltes, W., et al: Adrenal imaging with ^{131}I-19-iodocholesterol in the diagnostic evaluation of patients with aldosteronism. *J Clin Endocrinol Metab 42:* 41–45, 1976.
8. Lawson, T., Albarelli, J.: Diagnosis of gynecologic pelvic masses by gray scale ultrasonography: Analysis of specificity and accuracy. *Am J Roentgenol 128:* 1003–1006, 1977.
9. Miskin, M., Rosen, I., Walfish, P.: Ultrasonography of the thyroid gland. *Radiol Clin North Am 13 (3):* 479, 1975.
10. Doust, B.: Ultrasonic examination of the pancreas. *Radiol Clin North Am 13 (3):* 467, 1975.
11. Green, B., Bree, R., Goldstein, H., Stanley, C.: Gray-scale ultrasound evaluation of hepatic neoplasms: Pattern and correlations. *Radiology, 124:* 203, 1977.
12. Scheible, W., Coel, M., Siemers, P., Siegel, H.: Percutaneous aspiration of adrenal cysts. *Am J Roentgenol 128:* 1013–1016, 1977.
13. Leopold, G.: Personal communication.
14. Sheedy, P., Hattery, R., Stephens, D., et al: CT scanning of the adrenal gland. Presented at the Third International Symposium and Course in Computed Tomography, Miami Beach, Fla., Apr. 3–8, 1977.
15. Haaga, J., Alfidi, R.: Computed tomographic scanning of the pancreas. *Radiol Clin North Am 25 (3):* 367, 1977.
16. Stephens, D., Williamson, B., Sheedy, P., et al: Computed tomography of the retroperitoneal space. *Radiol Clin North Am 25 (3):* 377, 1977.
17. Heitzman, E., Goldwin, R., Proto, A.: Radiologic analysis of the mediastinum utilizing computed tomography. *Radiol Clin North Am 25 (3):* 309, 1977.
18. Stanley, R., Sagel, S., Levitt, R.: Computed tomography of the liver. *Radiol Clin North Am 25 (3):* 331, 1977.
19. Kollins, S.: Computed tomography of the pulmonary parenchyma and chest wall. *Radiol Clin North Am 25 (3):* 297, 1977.
20. Leeds, N., Naidick, T.: Computerized tomography in the diagnosis of sellar and parasellar lesions. *Semin Roentgenol 12 (2):* 1977.
21. Drayer, B., Rosenbaum, A., Kennerdell, J., et al: Computed tomographic diagnosis of suprasellar masses by intrathecal enhancement. *Radiology 123:* 339, 1977.
22. Haaga, J., Reich, N., Havrilla, Q., Alfidi, R.: Interventional CT scanning. *Radiol Clin North Am 25 (3):* 449, 1977.
23. Lecky, J., Gartland, J.: Adrenal angiography. *In* Robbins, L. L. (ed): Selective Angiography, section 18. Golden's Diagnostic Radiology, Baltimore, Williams & Wilkins, 1972.
24. Eisenberg, H., Pallotta, J., Sherwood, L.: Selective arteriography, venography, and venous hormone assay in diagnosis and localization of parathyroid lesions, 3rd Keating symposium on hyperparathyroidism. *Am J Med 56:* 810–820, 1974.
25. Spark, R., Kettyle, W., Eisenberg, H.: Cortisol dynamics in the adrenal venous effluent. *J Clin Endocrinol Metab 39 (2):* 305–310, 1974.
26. Spark, R., Eisenberg, H.: Medical aspects of adrenal surgery. *Urol Clin North Am 3 (2):* 433–449, 1976.
27. Spark, R., Kettyle, W., Eisenberg, H.: Definitive diagnosis of Cushing's disease in 2 days. *Ann Intern Med.*
28. Doppman, J.: The venous sampler. *Invest Radiol 8:* 423, 1973.
29. Ingemansson, S., Lunderquist, A., Lundquist, I., et al: Portal and pancreatic vein catheterization with radioimmunological determination of insulin. *Surg Gynecol Obstet 141:* 705, 1975.
30. Kahn, P., Kelleher, M., Egdahl, R., Melby, J.: Adrenal arteriography and venography in primary aldosteronism. *Radiology 101:* 71, 1971.
31. Symington, T.: The adrenal cortex. *In:* The Functional Pathology of the Human Adrenal Gland. Baltimore, Williams and Wilkins, 1969, pp 3–216.
32. Horton, R., Finck, E.: Diagnosis and localization in primary aldosteronism. *Ann Intern Med 76:* 885–890, 1972.

33. Melby, J.: Identifying the adrenal lesion in primary aldosteronism. *Ann Intern Med 76 (6):* 1972, p 1039.
34. Davidson, J., Morley, P., Hurley, G., et al: Adrenal venography and ultrasound in the investigation of the adrenal gland: an analysis of 58 cases. *BR J Radiol 48:* 435–450, 1975.
35. Scoggins, B., Oddie, C., Hare, W., Coghlan, J.: Preoperative lateralisation of aldosterone-producing tumours in primary aldosteronism. *Ann Intern Med 76:* 891–897, 1972.
36. Neville, A.: The human adrenal cortex: Correlation of structure and function. *In:* The Functional Pathology of the Human Adrenal Gland. Baltimore, Williams and Wilkins, 1969, pp 219–324.
37. Cohen, R.: Observations on cortical nodules in human adrenal glands. Their relationship to neoplasia. *Cancer, 19 (4):* 552–556, 1966.
38. Dobbie, J.: Morphology of the human adrenal cortex. *In:* The Functional Pathology of the Human Adrenal Gland. Baltimore, Williams and Wilkins, 1969, pp 326–381.
39. Cohen, R., Chapman, W., Castleman, B.: Hyperadrenocorticism (Cushing's disease): A study of surgically resected adrenal glands. *Am J Pathol. 35 (3):* 537–561, 1959.
40. Orth, D., Liddle, G.: Results of treatment in 108 patients with Cushing's syndrome, *N Engl J Med 285:* 243, 1971.
41. Kjelberg, R.: Treatment of acromegaly by proton hypophysectomy. *In:* Zarco and Delaney (eds.) Controversy in Surgery. Philadelphia, Saunders, pp 392–405.
42. Hardy, J.: Transsphenoidal microsurgery for selective removal of functional pituitary microadenomas. *World J Surg 1(1):* 79, 1977.
43. Liddle, G.: The adrenal cortex. *In* Williams, R. H. (ed): Textbook of Endocrinology (eds). Philadelphia, Saunders, 1974, part I, chap 5.
44. Lagerquist, L.: Cushing's disease with cure by resection of a pituitary adenoma. Evidence against a primary hypothalamic defect. *Am J Med 57:* 826–830, 1974.
45. Tyler, F., West, C.: Laboratory evaluation of disorders of the adrenal cortex. *Am J Med 53:* 664, 1972.
46. Liddle, G.: The adrenals. *In* Williams, R. H. (ed): Textbook of Endocrinology. (ed 5). Philadelphia, Saunders, 1974, part I.
47. Weiss, E., et al: Evaluation of stimulation of suppression tests in the etiological diagnosis of Cushing's syndrome. *Ann Intern Med 71:* 941, 1969.
48. Kirschner, M., Jacobs, J.: Combined ovarian and adrenal vein catheterization to determine the site(s) of androgen overproduction in hirsute women. *J Clin Endocrinol Metab 33:* 199, 1971.
49. Levine, R., Landsberg, L.: Catecholamines and the adrenal medulla. *In* Bondy, P. K., Rosenberg, L. E. (eds): Duncan's Diseases of Metabolism (ed 7). Philadelphia, Saunders, 1974.
50. Harrison, T., Thompson, N.: Multiple endocrine adenomatosis—I and II. *Curr Prob Surg* August 1975, pp 2–52.
51. Morley, P.: Ultrasound in the investigation of the adrenal glands and the kidneys. *Neth J Med 19:* 74–84, 1976.
52. Kahn, P.: Adrenal arteriography. *In* Abrams, H. (ed): Angiography, vol II. Boston, Little, Brown, 1971.
53. Harrison, T., Freier, D.: Pitfalls in the technique and interpretation of regional venous sampling for localizing pheochromocytomas. *Surg Clin North Am 54 (2):* 339–348, 1974.
54. Edis, A., Ayala, L., Egdahl, R.: Manual of Endocrine Surgery. New York, Springer-Verlag, 1975.
55. Field, J.: Functioning islet cell tumors with hypoglycemia. *In* Astwood, E. B., Cassidy, C. E. (eds): *Clinical Endocrinology II.* New York, Grune and Stratton, 1968, p 390.
56. Warren, K., Hoffman, G.: Changing patterns in surgery of the pancreas. *Surg Clin North Am 56:* 3, 1976.
57. Fulton, R., Sheedy, P., et al: Preoperative angiographic localization of insulin-producing tumors of the pancreas. *Am J Roentgenol 123:* 367, 1975.
58. Schein, P.: Islet cell tumors: Current concepts and management *Ann Intern Med 79:* 239, 1973.
59. Clouse, M., Costello, P., Legg, M., et al: Subselective angiography in localizing insulinomas of the pancreas. *Am J Roentgenol 128:* 741–746, 1977.
60. Scholz, D., ReMine, W., Priestly, J.: Hyperinsulinism: Review of 95 cases of functioning pancreatic islet cell tumors. *Proc. Staff Meet. Mayo Clinic 35:* 545, 1960.
61. Lunderquist, A.: Personal communication.
62. Perieras, R., Viamonte, J., et al: New techniques for interruption of gastroesophageal venous blood flow. *Radiology 124:* 313, 1977.
63. Friesen, S.: Sollinger-Ellison syndrome. *In* Ravitch, M. (ed): Current Problems in Surgery. Chicago, Year Book Medical Publishers, 1972.
64. Fox, P., Hofman, J., et al: The influence of total gastrectomy on survival in malignant Zollinger-Ellison tumors. *Ann Surg 180:* 558–566, 1974.
65. Orchard, J. et al: Cimetidine therapy in Zollinger-Ellison syndrome. *JAMA 237 (20):* 2221, 1977.
66. Gray, R., Rosch, J., Grollman, J.: Arteriography in the diagnosis of islet-cell tumors. *Radiology 97:* 39, 1970.
67. Ingemansson, S., Lunderquist, A., Holst, J., et al: Selective catheterization of pancreatic vein for radioimmuneassay in glucagon-secreting carcinoma of the pancreas. *Radiology 119:* 555, 1976.
68. McDonald, R.: A study of 356 carcinoids of the gastrointestinal tract. *Am J Med 21:* 867–878, 1956.
69. Harris, J., Levene, M.: Visual complications following irradiation for pituitary adenomas and craniopharyngiomas. *Radiology 120:* 167–171, 1976.
70. Baker, H.: Significance of fine sellar, parasellar, and central cerebral arteries in diagnosis. *In* Hilal, S. (ed): Small Vessel Angiography. St. Louis, Mosby, 1973.
71. Athanasoulis, C., Waltman, A., Novelline, R., et al: Angiography: Its contribution to the emergency management of gastrointestinal hemorrhage. *Radiol Clin North Am 14(2):* August 1976.
72. Eisenberg, H., Steer, M.: The nonoperative treatment of massive pyloroduodenal hemorrhage by retracted autologous clot embolization (5-year experience). *Surgery 79(4):* 414–420, 1976.
73. Zimmerman, C., Eisenberg, H., Spark, R., Rosoff, C.: Transvenous adrenal destruction: Clinical trials in patients with metastatic malignancy. *Surgery 75(4):* 550–556, 1974.
74. Goldstein, H., Wallace, S., Anderson, J.: Transcatheter occlusion of abdominal tumors. *Radiology 120:* 539, 1976.
75. Stadil, F., et al: Treatment of Zollinger-Ellison syndrome with streptozotocin. *N Engl J Med 294(26):* 1440, 1976.
76. Simon, N., Warner, R., Baron, M., et al: Intra-arterial irradiation of carcinoid tumors of the liver. *Am J Roentgenol 102:* 552, 1968.
77. Doppman, J., Marx, S., Spiegel, A.: Treatment of hyperparathyroidism by percutaneous embolization of a mediastinal adenoma. *Radiology 115:* 37, 1975.

Index

B

C

D

E

I

J

K

L

P

T